7th INTERNATIONAL CONGRESS of ENDOCRINOLOGY

7th INTERNATIONAL CONGRESS of ENDOCRINOLOGY

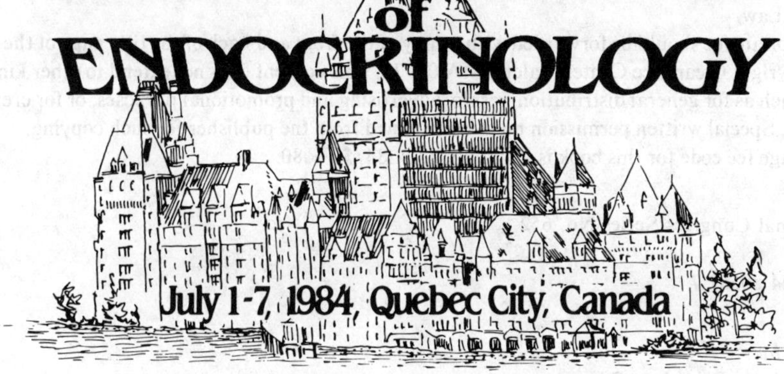

July 1-7, 1984, Quebec City, Canada

Under the sponsorship of

The International Society of Endocrinology
The Canadian Society of Endocrinology and Metabolism
Laval University

ABSTRACTS

1984

Excerpta Medica, Amsterdam-Oxford-Princeton

International Congress Series No. 652

ISBN 0 444 80587 7

Published by:
Elsevier Science Publishers B.V.
P.O Box 211
1000 AE Amsterdam
The Netherlands

Sole Distributors for the USA and Canada:
Elsevier Science Publishing Co. Inc.
52, Vanderbilt Avenue
New York, NY 10017
USA

Printed in The Netherlands

INTERNATIONAL SOCIETY OF ENDOCRINOLOGY

President:	Bryan Hudson, Australia
Secretary General:	Mortimer B. Lipsett, U.S.A.
Executive Committee:	Cesar Bergada, Argentina
	Raymond Hoffenberg, U.K.
	Hiroo Imura, Japan
	Ernst Knobil, U.S.A. (Chairman)
	Fernand Labrie, Canada
	Luciano Martini, Italy
	René Mornex, France
	Roger V. Short, Australia

OFFICERS OF THE CONGRESS

Honorary President:	Alfred Jost, France

ORGANIZING COMMITTEE:

Chairman:	Fernand Labrie, Canada
Secretary:	Georges Pelletier, Canada
Treasurer:	Alain Bélanger, Canada
Assistant-secretary:	Louise Proulx, Canada
Coordinator:	Jean-Denis Dubois, Canada
Members:	Pierre Borgeat, Canada
	Nicholas Barden, Canada
	André Dupont, Canada
	Jean Dussault, Canada
	Claude Fortier, Canada
	Claude Gagnon, Canada
	Maurice Normand, Canada
	Peter Walker, Canada

PROGRAM COMMITTEE:

Chairman:	Hiroo Imura, Japan
Members:	Daniel Cardinali, Argentina
	Pierre Corvol, France
	Jan A. Fischer, Switzerland
	Delbert A. Fisher, U.S.A.
	Henry G. Friesen, Canada
	Dorothy T. Krieger, U.S.A.
	Dennis W. Lincoln, U.K.
	Pierre De Meyts, Belgium
	Shigenobu Nagataki, Japan
	Jimmy D. Neil, U.S.A.
	Hugh D. Niall, Australia
	Miklos Palkovits, Hungary
	John G. Phillips, U.K.
	Henk J. van der Molen, Holland

Contents

Plenary Lectures

P.1 CONTROL OF TRANSCRIPTION BY STEROID HORMONES. Pierre Chambon, Laboratoire de Génétique Moléculaire des Eucaryotes du CNRS et Unité 184 de Biologie Moléculaire et de Génie Génétique de l'INSERM, Faculté de Médecine, Strasbourg - France.

Control of transcription at the level of RNA chain initiation plays a unique role in regulation of gene expression in eukaryotic organisms both during development and in terminally differentiated cells. We have dissected the organization of the promoter sequences which are involved in the control of initiation of transcription of genes coding for proteins. Several promoter elements, some of which having no counterparts in prokaryotic cells, have been identified. The interaction of steroid hormone-receptor complexes with some of these elements will be discussed and results demonstrating the role of oestrogens in the transcriptional induction of expression of a specific gene in some human breast cancers will be presented.

P.2 ADVANCES IN THE DIAGNOSIS AND TREATMENT OF PITUITARY DISEASE. Lesley H. Rees, Department of Chemical Endocrinology, St. Bartholomew's Hospital, London, EC1A 7BE, U.K.

High resolution CT scanning allows a clearer view of the pituitary/hypothalamic region and responses to treatment. In acromegaly the technique of radiotherapy may influence its efficacy; approximately 50% of tumours can be diminished in size by dopamine agonist therapy alone. Circulating GRF levels lay within the normal range (<10-60pg/ml) in 95% of 80 acromegalic subjects, four were elevated, three with obvious large pituitary tumours and one with the carcinoid syndrome and 'ectopic' GRF production. The optimal ablative therapy of prolactinomas is controversial. Thus, while dopamine agonist therapy is highly effective in the majority of patients, transsphenoidal hypophysectomy is the preferred treatment in some centres. Even in skilled hands, longterm surgical cure of hyperprolactinaemia only occurs in 40-80% of patients with a higher cure rate the smaller the tumour. An alternative approach is the use of supervoltage radiotherapy and recent data demonstrate that it results in eventual normalisation of levels after 2 to 10 years, dopamine agonists being used in the interim. Whilst surgery is the definitive treatment for large tumours it is often unsuccessful in normalising hormone levels and may cause hypopituitarism. Dopamine agonist therapy is effective in reducing tumour size in 66% of prolactinomas and a trial of therapy should be instituted prior to ablative manoeuvres since the tumour usually decreases in size and vision and pituitary function improves. In Cushing's disease, the obvious disadvantages of alternative treatments, have encouraged successful microdissection of small adenomas with little morbidity and mortality. Cushing's disease is not a single pathological entity and flexible management is mandatory and pituitary operations should be tailored to meet the requirements of individual patients. Identification in blood of fragments of pro-opiomelanocortin by some, usually large, tumours, in a manner reminiscent of ectopic ACTH secreting tumours, suggests the presence of an aggressive lesion demanding more radical pituitary surgery. In most cases pituitary surgery is now the treatment of choice for Cushing's disease. Diagnostically, differentiation between Cushing's disease and the ectopic ACTH syndrome still remains a problem as standard tests are often misleading. ACTH measurements in samples from the inferior petrosal sinus improve diagnostic accuracy. IR-CRF-41 was undetectable (<20pg/ml) in the plasma of 10 patients with Cushing's disease. However, elaboration of a GRP-like peptide by one medullary carcinoma of the thyroid caused Cushing's syndrome due to its potentiating effect on endogenous CRF activity. Use of LHRH, CRF-41 and the GRFs has produced interesting data concerning the site of the lesion both in patients with hypopituitarism due to pituitary tumours or isolated LHRH/ACTH or GH deficiencies, be they idiopathic or acquired. In most patients the lesion lies either in the hypothalamus itself or in the delivery of regulatory peptides to the pituitary. Use of LHRH continues to expand, and pulsatile administration via the mini-pump is successful in management of patients with LHRH deficiency and hypogonadism. In cases of "idiopathic GH deficiency" initial studies with GRF analogues are encouraging, as GH secretion can be promoted with rise in somatomedin-C.

P.3 HYBRIDIZATION HISTOCHEMISTRY : TISSUE LOCALIZATION OF GENE EXPRESSION. J. P. Coghlan*, H. D. Niall, J. Penschow and G. W. Tregear, Howard Florey Institute of Experimental Physiology and Medicine, University of Melbourne, Parkville, Victoria, 3052, Australia.

A procedure called Hybridization Histochemistry has been developed to locate in situ in specially prepared sections of tissues those cells which contain specific mRNA populations. This name was chosen to distinguish the technique from the widely used in situ cDNA mRNA hybridization procedures on solid supports and to emphasize the complementary nature of the technique to immunohistochemistry, and other histological localization procedures. The presence of specific mRNA populations indicates that a certain gene is "switched on" and that the production of a specific protein or peptide is highly probable.

The basis of the technique of hybridization histochemistry is the incubation of a labelled recombinant cDNA probe with a carefully prepared section of tissue. After appropriate washing and drying the tissue section, autoradiography is used to identify specific cell populations or tissue regions binding the labelled probe. ^{32}P labelled recombinant DNA probes were favoured initially because of the short time necessary for the autoradiographic detection of the binding sites, enabled the development of the procedure to proceed quickly. In the main we have continued to use ^{32}P labelled DNA probes complementary to several peptide hormones or enzymes of interest to us. The theoretical loss of resolution resulting from ^{32}P labelling can be minimized and is usually not disabling in the applications we have selected. The results indicate that the mRNA's of species we have examined are present in whole sections of tissue in a physical state which leaves them accessible to cDNA probes. The procedure has proven to be highly specific and reproducible.

Because the method allows a clear distinction to be made between those cells which manufacture a peptide or protein and those which have imported the material from elsewhere it will have special use in resolving many controversies over specific sites of origin of peptide and proteins, especially in tissues of the gut and CNS which are functionally complex and morphologically heterogeneous.

As more potential hormones are discovered by the molecular biological route hybridization histochemistry offers good initial access for physiological study. Recent significant advances in gene synthesis should allow synthetic DNA probes to be tailored to specific requirements in the near future.

P.4 PULSATILE GnRH - STUDIES OF PUBERTY AND THE MENSTRUAL CYCLE.

J. C. Marshall*, R. P. Kelch, S. Sauder, A. Barkan, N. Reame, and S. Khoury. Divisions of Endocrinology and Metabolism, Departments of Internal Medicine and Pediatrics, University of Michigan, Ann Arbor, MI 48109.

Puberty is associated with increased secretion of LH and FSH but the patterns of hormone secretion vary. In prepubertal girls, FSH secretion is initially predominant but declines with advancing maturation so that LH secretion exceeds that of FSH in adolesents. To determine whether the changing patterns of gonadotropin secretion result from increased pituitary stimulation by GnRH, we have studied the effects of pulsatile GnRH in prepubertal children and GnRH deficient adults (isolated GnRH deficiency, idiopathic panhypopituitarism, anorexia nervosa). GnRH was administered in a manner to mimic presumed physiological secretion, IV every 2 hrs at a dose of 25 ng/kg (which produced peak serum GnRH concentrations of approx. 200 pg/ml) for periods of 5 to 15 days. In GnRH deficient females, pulsatile GnRH resulted in a gradual increase in serum LH over 4 to 5 days. In contrast, FSH release was marked after the initial injections but after 1 to 2 days, FSH levels declined at the time that serum estradiol was rising. Pretreatment of GnRH deficient patients with estradiol abolished the FSH response indicating that estradiol exerts a selective inhibitory effect on FSH release by the pituitary. Thus, physiological administration of GnRH reproduces the patterns of gonadotropin secretion seen during pubertal maturation and the sequence of hormone changes, initial FSH predominance and subsequent increased LH, is very similar to that which occurs during the early follicular phase of the menstrual cycle. GnRH pulses for two weeks reproduced the gonadotropin and estradiol changes of the normal follicular phase but did not reliably induce a mid-cycle LH surge of normal magnitude in GnRH deficient woman, suggesting that increased amount or frequency of GnRH administration was required to produce a preovulatory LH surge. Analysis of serum gonadotropin concentrations (10 min. samples) in normal women during ovulatory cycles showed that LH pulse frequency, and by inference GnRH pulse frequency, increased by 30% between the early and late follicular phase. Pulse frequency declined during the luteal phase to 50% of late follicular values. Serum FSH was inversely correlated to estradiol being low or undetectable in the late follicular and luteal phases when estradiol was increased. These data show that the cyclical changes in pituitary and ovarian hormones seen during the normal menstrual cycle result from the varying stimulation of the pituitary by GnRH. After the mid-cycle LH surge, the rise in progesterone reduces GnRH pulse frequency which may impair LH synthesis. This together with intermittent release of LH will deplete pituitary LH stores while pituitary FSH content is maintained as estradiol inhibits FSH release in the luteal phase. With the decline of the corpus luteum, the fall in progesterone allows an increase in GnRH frequency which now stimulates FSH secretion as estradiol has also declined. The increase in serum FSH stimulates the next group of developing follicles and the subsequent rise in E_2 stimulates an increase in GnRH pulse frequency as well as pituitary sensitivity to GnRH resulting in the preovulatory LH surge. Thus, changes in frequency of GnRH secretion, and thus pituitary stimulation by GnRH may be critically important for the maintenance of normal menstrual cyclicity.

P.5 REGULATORY MECHANISMS COORDINATING RECEPTOR SIGNAL TRANSDUCTION,

Michael P. Czech, University of Massachusetts Medical Center, Worcester, MA, 01605

Although receptors for hormones, neurotransmitters, and other agonists have long been recognized as components that initiate cellular signalling pathways, it is also apparent that they serve as targets for regulatory mechanisms. We have investigated in detail types of receptor regulations whereby one receptor system is modulated by a signalling mechanism initiated by a second, distinct receptor system. We have studied in parallel three model systems of such regulation in order to gain insight to underlying mechanisms: I. Insulin action rapidly stimulates ^{125}I-IGF-II binding to intact adipocytes and H-35 hepatoma cells (1). In order to distinguish between an increase in IGF-II receptor number versus affinity, we raised potent anti-IGF-II receptor antiserum in a rabbit immunized with IGF-II receptor we purified (2). The anti-receptor Ig bound the receptor in the presence or absence of saturating concentrations of IGF-II. Insulin action increased ^{125}I-IGF-II binding as well as anti-receptor Ig binding to intact fat cells to the same extent, indicating an increase in receptor number. II. Tumor promoting phorbol diesters (PD) appear to decrease the number of high affinity EGF receptors on the surface of cultured cells. Because the PD receptor appears to be associated with C-kinase, we investigated PD action in ^{32}P-labeled A431 cells. Specific phosphorylation of the EGF receptor on serine residues localized to a unique peptide fragment of the EGF receptor upon tryptic hydrolysis was found in response to PD. III. β-adrenergic inhibition of ^{125}I-insulin binding to adipocytes appears to be mediated by cyclic AMP (3). Using anti-insulin receptor Ig, we find that the number of insulin receptors on the cell surface is not changed, but that a decrease in receptor affinity is responsible for the catecholamine-mediated ^{125}I-insulin binding inhibition. Furthermore, we find that the tyrosine kinase activity associated with insulin receptor purified from catecholamine-treated cells is markedly impaired in its ability to respond to saturating concentrations of insulin. Autophosphorylation of insulin receptor in response to insulin in intact cells is also inhibited by catecholamines. These studies demonstrate at least three modes of receptor modulation. In I, IGF-II receptors are expressed on the cell surface in response to insulin, while in II, EGF receptors appear to disappear from the cell surface in response to PD. In contrast, β-adrenergic action on the insulin receptor appears to involve no receptor number change, but rather structural alterations which lead to decreased affinity for ^{125}I-insulin and an impaired tyrosine kinase activation. These receptor regulatory mechanisms appear to be directly involved in modulating and coordinating receptor signalling.

1. Czech, M.P. (1982) Cell, 31, 8-10.
2. Oppenheimer, C.L., and Czech, M.P. (1983) J. Biol. Chem., 258, 8539-8542.
3. Pessin, J.E., Gitomer, W., Oka, Y., Oppenheimer, C.L., and Czech, M.P. (1983) J. Biol. Chem., 258, 7386-7394.

P.6 MEMBRANE PHOSPHOLIPIDS AND THE MECHANISM OF ACTION OF HORMONES. Yasutomi Nishizuka, Department of Biochemistry, Kobe University School of Medicine, Kobe 650, and Department of Cell Biology, National Institute for Basic Biology, Okazaki 444, Japan.

The Biochemical basis of signal transduction across the cell membrane has long been a subject of great interest. In recent years much attention has been turned to the role of inositol phospholipid turnover in membranes that is commonly observed immediately after the interaction of a wide variety of hormones, neurotransmitters, growth factors and many other biologically active substances with their specific cell surface receptors. In a manner as yet uncertain this membrane phospholipid turnover is normally associated with Ca^{2+} mobilization, which appears to mediate many of the subsequent physiological cellular responses. In our studies, a novel protein phosphorylation system of protein kinase C is shown to be firmly linked to the signal transduction by demonstrating that diacylglycerol, one of the earliest products of the signal-induced inositol phospholipid breakdown, greatly increases the affinity of protein kinase C for Ca^{2+}, thereby activating this enzyme without any increase in the intracellular Ca^{2+} concentration. The purpose of this talk is to summarize the evidence relating to the activation of protein kinase C and to the importance of this protein phosphorylation system for subsequent cellular responses. In the experiments to be described, protein kinase C is shown to be activated directly in intact cells by application of either tumour-promoting phorbol ester or synthetic diacylglycerol such as 1-oleoyl-2-acetyl-glycerol without any inositol phospholipid breakdown nor Ca^{2+} mobilization. It is worth noting that protein kinase C is a prime target of tumour-promoting phorbol esters. On the other hand, the intracellular Ca^{2+} concentration may be raised specifically by the addition of low concentrations of Ca^{2+} ionophore, A23187. Thus, the two routes, protein kinase C activation and Ca^{2+} mobilization by which information flows from the cell surface into the cell interior, are opened selectively and independently by the modification of cell membranes with the chemical substances mentioned above. Based on these procedures it is found that the activation of cellular responses by the route of protein kinase C is separate from and synergistic to those elecited by Ca^{2+} mobilization. Recent evidence will be presented that these two synergistic routes are of crucial importance in hormonal and neuronal control of many biological processes such as secretion and exocytosis, glycogenolysis as well as growth responses which are observed in a variety of cell types exposed to extracellular signals. (supported by the Ministry of Education, Science and Culture; the Ministry of Health and Welfare; and the Science and Technology Agency, Japan)

REFERENCES (review articles)

1. Nishizuka, Y., Phil. Trans. R. Soc. B., 302, 101-112 (1983).
2. Nishizuka, Y., Trends in Biochem. Sci., 8, 13-16 (1983).
3. Nishizuka, Y., Takai, Y., Kishimoto, A., Kikkawa, U. & Kaibuchi, K., Recent Progress in Hormone Research, 40 in press (1984).
4. Nishizuka, Y., Nature, in press (1984).

P.7 REGULATION OF PANCREATIC BETA CELL FUNCTION.

W.J. Malaisse*, Laboratory of Experimental Medicine, Brussels Free University, Brussels, B-1000, Belgium.

The functional organization of the pancreatic B-cell involves an array of sensor systems capable of identifying suitable insulinotropic agents. In the process of proinsulin biosynthesis and insulin release stimulated by nutrients, an increase in oxidative flux seems to provide the signal for activation of the B-cell. The knowledge that the B-cell behaves as a fuel-sensor organ raises questions regarding the nutrients utilized by the islet cells to cover their energy expenditure whether in the resting or active state. In isolated islets deprived of exogenous nutrient, the metabolism of endogenous fatty acids and amino acids accounts for the major fraction of basal respiration. In the presence of D-glucose, these endogenous nutrients are little spared. The regulation of glucose metabolism depends on a series of tightly interrelated reactions in which the hexose serves both as a substrate for glycolysis and as a precursor of activators of 6-phosphofructo 1-kinase. In the case of certain amino acids, including a nonmetabolized analog of L-leucine, the activation of glutamate dehydrogenase plays a critical role in the metabolic response of the islet cells. The coupling of metabolic to more distal events in the secretory sequence, could represent a multifactorial process involving changes in the generation rate and/or intracellular distribution of reducing equivalents, protons and high-energy phosphate intermediates. Such changes result in an extensive remodelling of ionic fluxes, with induction of bioelectrical activity. This culminates in the cytosolic accumulation of Ca^{2+} and the subsequent activation of motile events leading to the exocytosis of secretory granules. Current investigations aim at the identification of molecular systems participating in these ionic and mechanical responses. In this perspective, Ca-responsive targets include a protein kinase C susceptible to activation by diglycerides or tumor-promoting phorbol esters, quinine-sensitive K^+ channels, and the activation of enzyme (e.g. adenylate cyclase) by Ca-calmodulin. Changes in adenylate cyclase activity, such as inhibition by α_2-adrenergic agonists or stimulation by forskolin, indicate that cyclic AMP acts as an amplifier rather than initiator of insulin release. An increased turnover in the phosphatidylinositol cycle, as observed in islets exposed to nutrient or cholinergic secretagogues, may also participate in the stimulus-secretion coupling. The latter two phenomena illustrate mechanisms by which hormonal & neurohumoral agents may modulate the release of insulin evoked by circulating nutrients. The integrated control of insulin release by nutrients, hormones and neurotransmitter is well suited to adjust the output of this anabolic hormone to the metabolic requirements of extrapancreatic organs.

P.8 STRUCTURES, EXPRESSION AND PRODUCTS OF NEUROPEPTIDE AND RECEPTOR GENES.

Shosaku Numa, Department of Medical Chemistry, Kyoto University Faculty of Medicine, Kyoto 606, Japan.

A powerful tool for studying neural and hormonal peptides as well as neurotransmitter receptors has recently been provided by recombinant DNA technology. The primary structures of three opioid peptide precursors, i.e., the corticotropin-β-lipotropin precursor, preproenkephalin A and preproenkephalin B, have been elucidated by determining the nucleotide sequences of cloned DNAs complementary to their mRNAs. All of the endogenous opioid peptides thus far identified are derived from these three precursors. In addition, some novel neural and hormonal peptides have been discovered from the cDNA sequences. The three precursors each contain multiple repetitive units (melanotropin or enkephalin), thus representing multi-hormone precursors. The genes encoding the respective precursors have been isolated and characterized. The striking similarities found among the structural organizations of the three multi-hormone precursors as well as their genes suggest that these genes are evolutionarily related. Expression studies have identified the promoter region of the corticotropin-β-lipotropin precursor gene and the preproenkephalin A gene. The biological significance of the multi-hormone precursors is discussed. The structures of the corticotropin-releasing factor precursor and its gene are also presented.

The primary structures of all subunits of the Torpedo californica electroplax acetylcholine receptor (with a subunit structure of $\alpha_2\beta\gamma\delta$) have been deduced from the nucleotide sequences of cloned cDNAs encoding the respective subunit precursors. The four subunits exhibit marked amino acid sequence homology and are similar in hydrophilicity profile and predicted secondary structure, thus being most probably oriented in a pseudosymmetric fashion across the membrane. The transmembrane topology of the subunit polypeptides and the locations of functionally important regions, such as the acetylcholine binding site and the transmembrane segments which may be involved in the ionic channel, have been proposed. The amino acid sequence homology among the acetylcholine receptor subunits suggests that the genes encoding them have been generated from a single common ancestor by gene duplications. The primary structures of the α-subunits of the calf and human skeletal muscle acetylcholine receptors have also been deduced from the nucleotide sequence of cloned cDNA or genomic DNA. The mammalian acetylcholine receptor α-subunits exhibit conspicuous amino acid sequence homology with their fish counterpart. The protein-coding sequence of the human acetylcholine receptor α-subunit precursor gene is divided by eight introns into nine exons, which seem to correspond to different structural and functional domains of the subunit precursor molecule. The cloned cDNAs encoding the four subunit precursors of the Torpedo californica acetylcholine receptor, each carried by a simian virus 40 vector, direct the synthesis of the functional receptor of the nicotinic type in a combined expression system consisting of COS monkey cells and Xenopus oocytes. Studies on the effect of deletion of each subunit suggest that all four subunits are required to elicit a normal electrophysiological response to acetylcholine, whereas only the α-subunit is indispensable for α-bungarotoxin binding activity. This expression system will be useful for investigating the structure-function relationship as well as the antigenic determinants of the acetylcholine receptor by site-directed mutagenesis.

P.9 CHARACTERIZATION OF CORTICOTROPIN AND GROWTH HORMONE RELEASING FACTORS.

W. Vale*, C. Rivier, P. Plotsky, M. Brown, P. Sawchenko, T. Bruhn, H. Seifert, L. Bilezikjian, S. Pandol, M. Perrin, L. Swanson, L. Fisher, J. Spiess, M. Thorner and J. Rivier, The Salk Institute and UCSD VA Hospital, La Jolla, CA and University of Virginia, Charlottesville, Virginia USA.

Hypothalamic peptides reaching the anterior pituitary via portal vessels play a major role in the regulation of corticotropic and somatotropic cells. CRF initially identified in the sheep hypothalamus, has now been characterized in rat hypothalamus by peptide sequence analysis and in the human by deduction (Numa's group) from the DNA sequence of the CRF genome. Rat CRF and human CRF are identical to each other and differ from ovine by 7 out of 41 residues. Immunoneutralization studies with anti-CRF serum, results with recently developed CRF receptor antagonists, and observations of CRF dynamics in portal blood strongly support the key involvement of CRF in regulation of ACTH secretion under basal and stressful circumstances. Other weaker ACTH secretagogs, including catecholamines and neurohypophysial peptides enhance the response to CRF *in vitro* and *in vivo* and appear to modulate the action of CRF during stress. These functional interactions are particularly noteworthy in view of findings that the neurohypophysial peptides are co-expressed in the same paraventricular neurons under certain circumstances, and that pro-CRF and pro-vasopressin neurophysin are structurally related. Glucocorticoids can act at the pituitary level to non-competitively inhibit the response to CRF and also can act centrally to attenuate the stress-mediated secretion of CRF into the portal blood. The production of CRF by a human hepatic cell line is also inhibited by glucocorticoids. CRF-like immunoreactivity is widely distributed throughout the brain particularly in the limbic system and brainstem and exerts *in vitro* and *in vivo* actions on the brain including the modulation of hypophysiotropic peptide secretion and the stimulation of sympathetic and inhibition of parasympathetic activities. These results taken together with arousal-like behavioral effects of the peptide suggest that CRF may be involved in the integration of endocrine, autonomic and behavioral responses to stress.

The neuroregulation of GH secretion is mediated in part by a stimulatory GH-releasing factor (GRF) and an inhibitory peptide, somatostatin. Peptides with potent GH releasing activity have been characterized in two pancreatic tumors removed from acromegalic subjects in Charlottesville and Lyon. The most abundant human pancreatic (tumor) GRF (hpGRF) in both tumors, a 40 residue peptide (hpGRF-40), and the C-terminally extended, amidated peptide, hpGRF-44, found only in the Lyon tumor processed by Guillemin and co-workers, probably occur also in extracts of human infundibular fragments (courtesy of S. Reichlin). Rat hypothalamic (rh)GRF is a 43 residue peptide with a free C-terminus that differs from hpGRF by 33% and is more closely related to VIP, PHI and most other members of the glucagon family than is hpGRF. Accordingly certain VIP-like actions of rhGRF have been observed. GRF binds with high affinity and specificity to somatotrophs and leads to increases in rates of cyclic AMP production, GH gene transcription and GH biosynthesis and secretion. The action of GRF can be modulated by interactions between various factors including somatostatin thyroid hormones and glucocorticoids.

P.10 RECEPTORS AND ACTIONS OF HYPOTHALAMIC AND GONADOTROPIC HORMONES. Kevin J. Catt, Endocrinology and Reproduction Research Branch, National Institute of Child Health and Human Development, NIH, Bethesda, MD 20205, USA.

The integration of regulatory mechanisms within the hypothalamic-pituitary-gonadal axis is mediated by specific and high-affinity receptors for the peptides and glycoproteins concerned in signal transmission within this system. Whereas the hypothalamic peptides which elicit stimulation of gonadotropin and prolactin secretion (GnRH, TRH and angiotensin II) exert their pituitary actions via specific receptors coupled to calcium and phospholipid-dependent response mechanisms, the gonadotropins act primarily through cyclic AMP-dependent processes and prolactin through a plasma-membrane product that stimulates gene transcription. In serving as the major regulator of gonadotropin secretion, GnRH stimulates phospholipid turnover and calcium-dependent processes which act through both calcium-calmodulin and protein kinase C mechanisms to enhance the release of LH and FSH from pituitary gonadotrophs. Studies on the formation and actions of phospholipid metabolites in the gonadotroph suggest that arachidonic acid and its lipoxygenated derivatives are involved in the process of LH release. The prominent desensitizing action of GnRH agonist analogs on gonadotroph function is related to both receptor depletion and refractoriness of the plasma-membrane response mechanisms. The turnover and processing of GnRH receptors in vitro is increased during GnRH action, but not when the gonadotrophs are activated by depolarizing potassium concentrations. However, stimulation of LH release by phorbol esters and arachidonic acid is accompanied by GnRH receptor loss, implying that activation of the receptor-mediated secretion pathway at several levels causes an increase in GnRH receptor turnover. In contrast, potent GnRH antagonists that cause prolonged blockade of pituitary receptors are accompanied by a much slower rate of receptor turnover than that associated with GnRH receptor-agonist binding, and do not desensitize the gonadotroph. The dynamic changes in plasma-membrane receptors that accompany increased secretion or administration of the homologous hormone range from up- to down-regulation of sites but are not consistently associated with a corresponding change in target-cell sensitivity to the ligand. In most endocrine target cells the occupancy of a very small number of the total number of functionally active sites appears to be sufficient to elicit the maximum cellular response. Variations in receptor number may contribute to changes in sensitivity, but do not appear to be a determining factor in the pituitary-gonadal axis. The ability of GnRH to act as a neurohormone in fish and amphibia also applies to the mammalian brain, where specific binding of GnRH to central receptors is correlated with behavioural actions of the releasing peptide. The octapeptide angiotensin II also has receptors in several discrete brain regions, and acts as a neuroendocrine regulator in the hypothalamus and anterior pituitary gland by promoting the release of vasopressin, oxytocin, prolactin, and corticotropin. AII also influences gonadotropin release, and may modulate the secretion as well as the actions of CRF upon corticotropin release. The brain receptors and actions of regulatory neuropeptides including GnRH, AII and CRF emphasize the dual hypophysiotropic and neuromodulatory roles of these and other hypothalamic releasing hormones.

Symposia

S.1 IMMUNOHISTOCHEMISTRY OF HUMAN PITUITARY ADENOMAS. K. Kovacs*, Department of Pathology, St. Michael's Hospital, University of Toronto, Toronto, Ontario M5B 1W8, Canada.

Although clinical and biochemical findings often establish the underlying endocrine abnormality in patients with pituitary adenoma, the accurate identification of cells constituting the tumor can only be undertaken by morphologic techniques. Immunohistochemical methods are capable of detecting GH, PRL, ACTH, endorphins, TSH, FSH, LH and α-subunit in the cytoplasm of adenoma cells, providing evidence that all known adenohypophysial hormones can be produced by pituitary tumors. In addition, nonhormonal markers (keratin, neuron specific enolase, S-100 protein, GFA protein, factor 8, etc.) can be used to label certain cell types and separate pituitary adenomas from other neoplasms. The immunoperoxidase techniques have replaced previously applied immunofluorescence procedures in studies related to the pituitary. They are sensitive, reliable and reproducible; tissue fixed in formalin or embedded in paraffin and stored for a considerable length of time can be immunostained for adenohypophysial hormones. The original procedure was modified by several authors; currently we use the avidin-biotin-peroxidase complex method. Immunostainings can be performed at the light microscopic and ultrastructural levels. Immunoelectron microscopy localizes hormones at their subcellular sites. Immunohistochemical techniques are not quantitative; they demonstrate the presence of hormones, but fail to provide information on the amount of stored hormone, the rate of hormone synthesis and release. Rigorous control studies are necessary to avoid misleading conclusions. In many cases of pituitary adenoma, clinical and biochemical findings can be correlated with immunohistochemical results. The silent adenomas represent exceptions. These tumors are unassociated with clinical and biochemical evidence of hormone excess, but may contain various hormones, biologically inactive precursors or hormone fragments which may be detected by immunohistochemical methods. The immunohistochemical investigation plays a substantial role in the diagnosis of plurihormonal adenomas. These tumors, capable of producing two or more hormones different in chemical composition, immunoreactivity and biologic action, can be divided into monomorphous and plurimorphous adenomas. The former tumors consist of one cell type and two or more hormones are present in the cytoplasm of the same cell. The latter ones are composed of two or more cell types and each hormone is present in different cells. The most common variants of plurihormonal adenomas produce GH and PRL. Less frequently, unusual combinations occur, such as the production of GH and TSH; GH, PRL and TSH; GH, PRL and ACTH; GH, PRL and α-subunit, etc. In some plurihormonal adenomas, the hormones are discharged into the circulation leading to endocrine abnormality. In other tumors, one or more components are silent and hormone production can only be proven by the application of immunohistochemical techniques. Modern pituitary adenoma classifications are based on ultrastructural features, hormone content, cellular composition and origin. With more widespread availability of a growing number of antibodies, immunohistochemistry will not only play an important role in the diagnostic process, but it will have a profound impact on the better understanding of the endocrine function and cytogenesis of pituitary adenomas. This study was supported by the Medical Research Council of Canada.

S.2 PRODUCTION OF GROWTH HORMONE-RELEASING FACTOR BY TUMORS. L. A. Frohman*, Division of Endocrinology and Metabolism, University of Cincinnati College of Medicine, Cincinnati, Ohio 45267.

The association of extrapituitary tumors with acromegaly had been recognized for more than a decade before the possibility of ectopic growth hormone releasing factor (GRF) secretion was considered. Within a few years of the first demonstration of GRF in a bronchial carcinoid tumor associated with acromegaly (the "ectopic GRF syndrome"), the spectrum of tumors possessing GRF bioactivity had been defined and the sequence of human ectopic GRF determined from two pancreatic islet adenomas. Although the sequence of human hypothalamic GRF has not yet been identified, evidence points to a structure very similar, if not identical with that of ectopic GRF. Tumors most frequently found to contain GRF are carcinoid tumors (bronchial and intestinal), pancreatic islet adenomas, and small cell carcinomas of lung. The concentration of GRF in several of the tumors has been greater than that in human hypothalamus, and among those tumors with the greatest levels of GRF, a highly significant correlation exists between the concentrations of biological and immunological activity. Attempts to distinguish those patients with ectopic GRF production based on pituitary histology (hyperplasia vs adenoma) and GH responses to stimulatory or suppressive agents have not been successful, though measurement of plasma immunoreactive GRF levels appears more promising. Plasma immunoreactive GRF levels in normal subjects have uniformly been undetectable (<25 pg/ml) while in patients with proven or presumed ectopic GRF production, levels ranging from 2 to 6 ng/ml have been observed. In acromegalics without clinical evidence of an extrapituitary tumor, plasma GRF levels are either undetectable or near the lower level of assay sensitivity. On the basis of metabolic clearance studies of GRF(1-40) in normal subjects, the GRF secretory rate in patients with ectopic GRF production is in the range of 10 to 30 μg/day. Another form of ectopic GRF syndrome has recently been described in which intrapituitary gangliocytomas have been found in juxtaposition to somatotroph adenomas, and GRF-containing hypothalamic hamartomas have also been identified in patients with acromegaly. Thus, GRF production by neoplasms in both ectopic and eutopic sites may occur with the secreted GRF functoning in an endocrine, paracrine, or neuropeptidergic role in the pathogenesis of GH-secreting pituitary tumors.

S.3 PRODUCTION OF GASTRIN-RELEASING PEPTIDE (BOMBESIN) BY TUMORS.

K. Abe*, K. Yamaguchi and I. Adachi, Endocrinology Division, National Cancer Center Research Institute, Tokyo 104, Japan.

Gastrin-releasing peptide (GRP) is a peptide composed of 27 amino acids, and its C-terminal decapeptide sequence is bombesin itself except for the position 20 where His is replaced by Gln in bombesin. The tumor production of GRP and bombesin was examined by GRP and bombesin RIAs. The materials were 119 primary lung cancers (31 small cell carcinomas, 44 adenocarcinomas, 30 squamous cell carcinomas and 14 large cell carcinomas), 20 carcinoids, 63 pancreatic endocrine tumors, 19 pheochromocytomas, 33 neuroblastic tumors and 11 medullary carcinomas of the thyroid (MCT). Five fetal lung tissues were also examined. These tissues were extracted by the boiling water method with the recovery of over 85%. Some of these tissue extracts were subjected to Sephadex G-50 gel filtration. The presence of GRP and CT was also examined immunohistochemically in some tumors. Furthermore, the tumor production of calcitonin (CT), vasoactive intestinal peptide (VIP), somatostatin (SRIF) and pancreatic growth hormone-releasing factor (pGRF) were also examined by the respective RIAs. Our GRP RIA could not discriminate GRP from bombesin, but in the bombesin RIA, GRP cross-reacted only slightly (less than 0.03%). The tumor tissues were found to produce GRP in variable frequency associated often with the production of other hormones (Table), and the amounts ranged from 2.5 ng/g wet weight to 130 μg/g wet weight, but bombesin was detected only in a few cases with small amounts, which could be explained by the cross-reaction of GRP in the bombesin RIA. The gel filtration studies revealed 2 peaks which corresponded to GRP and its C-terminal fragment, but the ratio of these 2 peaks was different from tumor to tumor. GRP was detected in all 5 fetal lungs. In the cases of MCT, when the concentrations of GRP were compared with those of CT by use of their common logarithmic values, a significant correlation ($p < 0.02$) was found, although the amounts of GRP were 100-1,000 times less than those of CT. Immunohistochemically, some MCT tumor cells were found to contain both GRP and CT. These data indicate that GRP, not bombesin, is produced frequently by various types of tumors and that its production is often associated with the production of CT, VIP, SRIF and pGRF. There is some unknown but related mechanism between production of GRP and that of CT in MCT.

Frequency of hormone production in tumors (No.detected/No.examined)

Type of tumors	GRP	CT	VIP	SRIF	pGRF
Lung cancers					
small cell carcinoma	23/31	16/24	6/29	10/29	20/45
adenocarcinoma	9/44	4/39	5/39	18/39	7/47
squamous cell carcinoma	5/30	3/28	4/28	5/25	1/28
large cell carcinoma	1/14	1/14	1/14	4/14	2/13
Carcinoid	11/20	8/17	6/16	12/16	10/21
Pancreatic endocrine tumors	33/63	19/45	23/40	34/45	34/74
Pheochromocytoma	14/19	8/11	11/16	14/16	6/15
Neuroblastic tumors	13/33	5/26	21/28	23/28	9/21
Medullary ca. of the thyroid	10/11	16/16	8/14	11/13	5/ 7

S.4 FAMILIAL MEDULLARY CARCINOMA OF THE THYROID.

K. Melvin*, St. Vincent Hospital and Medical Center, Portland, Oregon, 97225, USA.

Familial medullary carcinoma of the thyroid (MCT) is unique amongst hormone secreting tumors, consistently secreting calcitonin, and frequently given also to the ectopic production of a variety of other peptides, and various bioactive molecules. The latter include ACTH, somatostatin, and katacalcin; prostaglandins, CEA, histaminase, dopa-decarboxylase, and serotonin. A C-cell tumor, of neural crest rather than of thyroid origin, MCT may occur either as familial or sporadic variants. The familial form is transmitted as a Mendelian dominant; is bilateral and often multifocal; is accompanied by diffuse C-cell hyperplasia; and is often associated to a varying degree with multiple endocrine neoplasia involving the parathyroids and adrenal medulla (M.E.N. II), and in some, with clinically evident neuroectodermal dysplasia. The sporadic form is unilateral and not accompanied by C-cell hyperplasia or other endocrine neoplasia. The distinction is of great clinical consequence for the relatives of affected individuals, amongst whom screening for hypercalcitoninemia permits early diagnosis of familial disease, even in its premalignant stage. Peak presentation is in the pediatric age group and most cases have declared by the age of 30. Screening of family members should commence at age 3 or 4, and continue annually until at least age 30, utilizing the intravenous administration of calcitonin secretagogues such as calcium or pentagastrin. Hyperparathyroidism and/or pheochromocytoma should be sought also. Hyperparathyroidism generally reflects parathyroid hyperplasia, although adenomata are not uncommon. When present, pheochromocytomas are usually bilateral, and often multiple and associated with adrenomedullary hyperplasia. A rarer variant of the familial disease is characterized by a distinctive phenotype with multiple mucosal neuromata. This form, often referred to as MEN IIb, may occur as a spontaneous mutation, without a family history to alert the clinician to the diagnosis. In such cases early diagnosis is imperative since the thyroid tumor tends to be more aggressive and may have already metastasized by the age of 3 years. When fully expressed, this phenotype can be recognized in infancy and will generally present with feeding difficulties. Mucosal neuromata and hypertrophied corneal nerves should be clinically evident within the first year or two. Screening for hypercalcitoninemia should be commenced as soon as the diagnosis is suspected. In MCT, hypercalcitoninemia is usually metabolically silent, but is probably the cause of the severe secretory diarrhea that may complicate disseminated disease. As a tumor-marker, serum calcitonin levels provide a means of assessing any response to treatment. The only effective treatment is surgical. Preliminary studies suggest the presence of chromosomal instability, or short arm deletion in chromosome 20p, in individuals carrying the gene predisposing to MCT. If confirmed this will have important epidemiologic implications for affected families.

S.5 PATHOGENESIS OF THE TYPE I DIABETES MELLITUS OF THE BB RAT. Errol B. Marliss,* McGill Nutrition and Food Science Centre, Royal Victoria Hospital, Montreal, H3A 1A1, Canada.

The spontaneous diabetic syndrome of the BB Wistar-derived rat shows multiple phenotypic similarities to that of the human, and it can provide insights into pathogenetic mechanisms potentially applicable in human studies. The syndrome shows a spectrum of severity, including classical insulin-dependent diabetes, impaired glucose tolerance and normal glucoregulation but with insulitis. These may represent different forms of the syndrome, or stages in the evolution to overt diabetes. Multiple lines of evidence implicate an immunologic disorder in lines bred for high incidence of diabetes. 1) A major histocompatibility complex association, with the $RT1^u$ type, occurs. 2) Morphological findings include the insulitis (mononuclear infiltration of the islets with beta cell loss), abnormal lymphoid tissue histology, frequent occurence of lymphocytic thyroiditis, a tendency to develop B cell lymphomas, and a possible index lesion termed "pancreatic lymphocytic infiltration". 3) A profound lymphopenia, antedating demonstrable beta-cytolysis, is a reliable association of the various forms. It is present within the first days of life. The T lymphocytes are most affected, and the helper subset shows the greatest quantitative deficit, though decreases in absolute number of suppressor T cells and B cells occur. 4) Lymphocyte function is abnormal. Though not inbred, BB rats show delayed allograft rejection. Lymphocytes generally show markedly decreased mitogenic responses to ConA, to mixed lymphocyte culture, and to Interleukin 2. 5) Islet cell surface antibodies (ICSA) are present, most often prior to onset of glycosuria, though with variable timing of peak values. Such ICSA identify a 64K beta cell membrane component. Diabetic sera inhibit insulin release and cause complement-dependent beta-cytolysis *in vitro*. Lymphocyte antibodies accompany the ICSA, and thyroid, gastric parietal cell and smooth muscle antibodies are frequently found. Islet cell cytoplasmic antibodies have not been shown. 6) Passive transfer of insulitis to nude mice and of insulitis and diabetes to other BB rats has been produced with diabetic rat lymphocytes but not with serum. 7) BB rats are highly susceptible to microbial infections, most often by mycoplasma. Diabetes occurs in animals kept in a gnotobiotic environment. 8) Diabetic rats, despite their immune deficiency, reject transplanted islets in an accelerated fashion. 9) The most dramatic findings have been the prevention and modification of diabetes by several immune interventions, including immunosuppression (thymectomy, antilymphocyte serum, irradiation, and Cyclosporin A) and reconstitution (neonatal bone marrow, circulating leucocytes). To the present, a unifying hypothesis which accounts for these disparate findings has not been proven. Attractive ones include a maturational defect in lymphocytes leading to subset imbalances, and a central role of the ICSA in the beta cell destruction. Though the human diabetic does not show lymphopenia, a helper T cell deficit, nor the T cell functional anomalies, further elucidation of the pathogenesis of the rat syndrome could point to possible mechamisms in the human. The BB rat has also served as an excellent "model" of the pathophysiology of the metabolic changes in diabetes as well as of neuropathy and gestational complications.

S.6 PATHOGENESIS OF TYPE I DIABETES MELLITUS. Å. Lernmark*, S. Bækkeskov, T. Dyrberg, G. Papadopoulos, B. Marner, H. Vissing, I. Gerling, A. Svenningsen, Hagedorn Research Laboratory, and C. Binder, J. Nerup and T.Mandrup-Poulsen, Steno Memorial Hospital, Gentofte, Denmark.

The clinical onset of insulin-dependent diabetes mellitus in man is associated with a number of immune related abnormalities. Islet cell antibodies reactive with either cell surface or intra-cellular determinants are present in many patients. Islet cell cytoplasmic antibodies represent primarily IgG and react with intra-cellular determinants in all endocrine islet cells. Islet cell surface antibodies in the serum of patients younger than 30 years of age at diagnosis are often β-cell specific. About 30-40 percent of new patients have islet cell surface antibodies which convey complement-mediated cytotoxicity against human and rodent islet cells as well as cloned rat islet tumor cells. Experiments with passive transfer or perifusion of rat islet cells with immunoglobulin prepared from the plasma of children with IDDM of short duration suggest that islet cell antibodies may interfere with the mechanism by which glucose stimulates insulin release. At the clinical onset the formation of islet cell antibodies seems to be an active process, since both islet cell cytoplasmic and complement-dependent cytotoxic antibodies reappeared in a rebound phenomenon following repeated plasmapheresis without immunesuppression.

Blood mononuclear cells from about 50% of newly diagnosed IDDM patients showed an increased ability spontaneously to produce immunoglobulin *in vitro*. This is taken as an indication of a polyclonal activation of B lymphocytes. Patients with increased numbers of spontaneous immunoglobulin producing cells tended to have higher titres of islet cell antibodies and fasting c-peptide. The presence of residual β-cell function may therefore determine the extent by which this polyclonal activation occurs. A prospective analysis of IDDM patients indicated that the decrease in the prevalence of islet cell cytoplasmic antibodies with increasing duration of IDDM was primarily due to a continuous decrease in antibody titres. Patients being islet cell antibody positive after 2 years of IDDM had significantly higher titres at diagnosis. Likewise, a high titre at diagnosis seemed to predict a lower fasting c-peptide after 3 years compared to islet cell antibody negative patients.

Immunoprecipitation of extracts of radioactively labelled human pancreatic islets with IDDM sera showed that many patients have antibodies against a M_r 64,000 protein. Antibodies against this islet cell component were present in about 80% of IDDM patients of short duration and was primarily detected in sera positive for β-cell specific islet cell surface antibodies. IDDM sera also detected the M_r 64,000 protein in radioactively labelled rodent islets. In one individual M_r 64,000 antibodies could be detected up to two years before the clinical onset of IDDM.

It is speculated that the loss of pancreatic β-cells is associated with an abnormal immune response, perhaps by non-specific effects on the immune system, but specifically reacting against certain β-cell antigens. The presence of this autoreactive process may result in a gradual diminution of insulin-producing cells, eventually leading to the onset of an insulin-dependency.

S.7 EFFECTS OF IMMUNOSUPPRESSION WITH CYCLOSPORIN IN TYPE I DIABETES MELLITUS.

J. Dupré, C.R. Stiller, M. Gent, M. Jenner, B. von Graffenried, M. Heinrichs, P.A. Keown, A. Laupacis, R. Martell, K. Mazabel, N.W. Rodger, B.M. Wolfe, London, Canada; C. Binder, T. Mandrup-Poulsen, B. Marner, J. Nerup, Gentofte, Denmark; A. Rabinovitch, Miami, Florida

In light of evidence for an autoimmune mechanism in beta-cell destruction in type I diabetes mellitus (TID) and given the morbidity of the disease under conventional treatment, the possible benefits of enhancement and/or preservation of residual function that might result from immunosuppression have prompted trials with various immunomodulatory agents in man, with inconclusive results to date. We have undertaken a pilot study with Cyclosporin (CyA) in recent-onset TID. CyA was administered as in management of organ transplantation, with adjustment of dosage in relation to blood levels of CyA and results of kidney and liver function tests. Among subjects entered <12 months after diagnosis, 23/58 (40%) developed non-insulin-requiring remission (NIR), with mean fasting plasma glucose 7.8 mmoles/litre after withdrawal of insulin for 12 weeks. Of these NIR subjects, 21 were found among 36 (58%) entered <6 weeks after diagnosis (recent onset group, 40). B-cell function was assessed by assay of plasma immunoreactive C-peptide (CP) and free immunoreactive insulin (FIRI) before and after IV glucagon, i.e. breakfast. In 20 subjects, stimulated CP levels (SCP) were subnormal and not significantly different in insulin-requiring (IR) and NIR sets at entry (IR .31±.04, NIR .40±.05 pm/ml), and rose within 30 days of CyA into the normal range in both groups (IR .83±.09, NIR .87±.05). Increments of FIRI after IV glucagon were similar in IR and NIR sets, and the CP/FIRI molar increment ratios were normal. With continued administration of CyA, mean plasma SCP levels were within normal range throughout the study in NIR subjects (n=8, mean 270±10 days) and all 23 subjects who became NIR exhibited SCP levels >0.6 pm/ml, but 8 of the 36 subjects with SCP>.6 remained IR. NIR subjects were glucose intolerant, with abnormal oral and IV glucose tolerance tests: FIRI and CP responses were present after oral but not IV glucose. Mean plasma levels of glycohemoglobin confirmed maintenance of target control of glycemia in NIR and IR groups. Of the 23 subjects who became NIR, 8 resumed insulin treatment because of loss of target control of glycemia. Transient relapses to IR occurred with intercurrent stress and no change in plasma CP, but there were 4 prolonged relapses. Of these, 2 were unexplained, with stable plasma CP, and 2 were associated with declining plasma CP levels, 1 during CyA, and 1 after discontinuation of CyA. Islet cell antibodies were detected at rates similar to those in historical controls (44%) and titres declined rapidly during CyA. Complement-dependent cytotoxic antibodies were present at rates similar to historical control (26%) and showed no change during the study. Phenotyping of lymphocytes showed declining proportions of peripheral OKT4+ and Ia+ cells during CyA. These studies have demonstrated apparently unprecedented enhancement and preservation of B-cell function for ≥1 year from diagnosis of TID during CyA. Recovery of insulin secretion into the normal range was essential for, but did not predict, development of NIR; this, and reduced erythrocyte insulin receptor affinity in IR subjects (30% tracer displaced with 1% more insulin) suggests the importance of insulin sensitivity as a factor in development of remission. The results indicate the need for a controlled trial to determine the magnitude and duration of the apparent effects of CyA on the remission phase of TID, and its clinical risks and benefits.

S.8 EFFECTS OF IMMUNOSUPPRESSION WITH CYCLOSPORIN IN TYPE I DIABETES MELLITUS.

J. Dupre*, C.R. Stiller, M. Gent, M. Behme, B. vGraffenreid, M. Jenner, P.A. Keown, A. Laupacis, R. Martell, R. Mazaheri, N.W. Rodger, B.M. Wolfe, London, Canada; C. Binder, T. Mandrup-Poulsen, B. Marner, J. Nerup, Gentofte, Denmark; A. Rabinovitch, Miami, Florida

In light of evidence for an autoimmune mechanism in beta cell destruction in Type I diabetes mellitus (TID), and given the morbidity of the disease under conventional treatment, the possible benefits of enhancement and/or preservation of residual function that might result from immunosuppression have prompted trials with various immunomodulatory agents in man, with inconclusive results to date. We have undertaken a pilot study with Cyclosporin (Cy) in recent-onset TID. Cy was administered as in management of organ transplantation, with adjustment of dosage in relation to blood levels of Cy and results of kidney and liver function tests. Among subjects entered <12 months after diagnosis, 23/48 (48%) developed non-insulin-requiring remission (NIR), with mean a.c. plasma glucose ≤ 7.8 mmoles/litre after withdrawal of insulin for >2 weeks: of these NIR subjects, 21 were found among 36 (58%) entered <6 weeks after diagnosis (recent onset group, RO). B-cell function was assessed by assay of plasma immunoreactive C-peptide (CP) and free immunoreactive insulin (FIRI) before and after IV glucagon, a.c.breakfast. In RO subjects, stimulated CP levels (SCP) were subnormal and not significantly different in insulin-requiring (IR) and NIR sets at entry (IR.44 $\pm$.04,NIR.46 $\pm$.05 pm/ml), and rose within 30 days of CyRx into the normal range in both groups (IR.88 $\pm$.06,NIR .87 $\pm$.05). Increments of FIRI after IV glucagon were similar in IR and NIR sets, and the CP/FIRI molar increment ratios were normal. With continued administration of Cy, mean plasma SCP levels were within normal range throughout the study in RO subjects (60-360,mean 270 $\pm$10 days). All 23 subjects who became NIR exhibited SCP levels >0.6 pm/ml, but 8 of the 36 subjects with SCP$>$.6 remained IR. NIR subjects were glucose intolerant, with abnormal oral and IV glucose tolerance tests; FIRI and CP responses were present after oral but not IV glucose. Mean plasma levels of glycohemoglobin confirmed maintenance of target control of glycemia in NIR and IR groups. Of the 23 subjects who became NIR, 8 resumed insulin treatment because of loss of target control of glycemia. Transient relapses to IR occured with intercurrent stress and no change in plasma CP, but there were 4 prolonged relapses. Of these, 2 were unexplained, with stable plasma CP; and 2 were associated with declining plasma CP levels, 1 during CyRx, and 1 after discontinuation of Cy. Islet cell antibodies were detected at rates similar to those in historical controls (44%) and titres declined rapidly during CyRx. Complement-dependent cytotoxic antibodies were present at rates similar to historical control (26%) and showed no change during the study. Phenotyping of lymphocytes showed declining proportions of peripheral $OKT4^+$ and Ia^+ cells during CyRx. These studies have demonstrated apparently unprecedented enhancement and preservation of B-cell function for ≤ 1 year from diagnosis of TID during CyRx. Recovery of insulin secretion into the normal range was essential for, but did not predict, development of NIR; this, and reduced erythrocyte-insulin receptor affinity in IR subjects (50% tracer displaced with 25% more insulin), suggests the importance of insulin sensitivity as a factor in development of remission. The results indicate the need for a controlled trial to determine the magnitude and duration of the apparent effects of CyRx in the remission phase of TID, and its clinical risks and benefits.

S.9 CHICKEN PROGESTERONE RECEPTOR: STRUCTURE AND FUNCTION. W.T. Schrader*, Department of Cell Biology, Baylor College of Medicine, Houston, Texas 77030, U.S.A.

The chicken progesterone receptor contains two hormone-binding subunits: A (Mr = 79K) and B (Mr = 108K). Both are phosphoproteins which have been purified to homogeneity. Monoclonal antibodies raised to these proteins have been used to identify forms of the subunits which lack hormone-binding activity. The antibodies have also been used to obtain cDNA clones of receptor mRNA from recombinant DNA expression libraries. Receptor B mRNA levels are acutely regulated by both estrogen and progesterone itself. Subunit A exists as a family of isoforms, each containing a DNA binding site. This protein binds to a specific DNA sequence of 150-200 base pairs upstream from the 5' end of the ovalbumin gene. Similar sequences flank some other hormone regulator genes. Subunit B lacks this DNA binding activity despite considerable structural similarity to subunit A.

S.10 ANDROGENIC REGULATION OF GENE EXPRESSION. M. Parker*, M. Needham and M. Page. Department of Molecular Endocrinology, Imperial Cancer Research Fund, Lincoln's Inn Fields, P.O. Box 123, London WC2A 3PX. England.

We are studying the mechanism whereby androgens regulate the expression of prostatic steroid binding protein. By applying gene transfer to introduce cloned genes into cells we are investigating the structural requirements for accurate and regulated gene expression.

Prostatic steroid binding protein is a tetramer consisting of C1, C2 and C3 polypeptides. We have selected two genes for C3, namely C3(1) and C3(2), to investigate in detail because, despite DNA sequence similarities, C3(1) is actively transcribed whereas C3(2) is inactive. When the intact C3 genes were introduced by transfection into heterologous S115 cells, an androgen responsive cell line, both genes were accurately expressed. Thus C3(2) is not a pseudogene and its lack of expression may be due to striking differences compared with the C3(1) gene in its state of DNA methylation. More importantly, gene expression was stimulated by up to 5-fold in approximately 1/3 of the clones which is appreciably less than occurs in vivo. Nevertheless we have attempted to investigate whether the hormone was acting directly on the promoter to stimulate transcription by constructing chaemeric genes. We have fused the C3(1) promoter to interferon DNA, as a marker gene, and analysed interferon expression both after transient expression and subsequently in stably transformed cell lines. Testosterone stimulated transient interferon expression only and supports the conclusion that androgens have a small effect directly on the promoter to stimulate transcription. However, in view of the magnitude of hormonal effects *in vivo* its clearly unsatisfactory to analyse gene expression in heterologous cells. Therefore we are attempting to culture rat prostate cells in order to transfer the genes into homologous cells.

S.11 STEROID HORMONE RECEPTOR-ACCEPTOR INTERACTIONS ON THE NUCLEAR MATRIX.

Evelyn R. Barrack,* Department of Urology, The Johns Hopkins University School of Medicine, Baltimore, Maryland 21205, U.S.A.

The importance of cellular structural proteins in the regulation of biological function is becoming increasingly apparent. Whereas the cytoskeleton provides structural and functional organization of cytoplasmic components, the nuclear matrix, a residual scaffolding of the nucleus, appears to play a fundamental role in the organization of the nuclear DNA and in many dynamic aspects of nuclear function, including DNA replication, heterogeneous nuclear RNA synthesis and processing, and steroid hormone receptor-acceptor interactions (reviewed by Barrack and Coffey, 1982, Recent Prog. Horm. Res. 38:133-195).

Using an *in vitro* exchange assay in which nuclear matrix fractions isolated from hormone-treated animals are incubated with radiolabeled steroid, we have identified and characterized specific androgen and estrogen receptors associated with the nuclear matrix of androgen and estrogen target tissues, respectively. The nuclear matrix-associated estrogen receptors in rat uterus and hen liver, and androgen receptors in rat and human prostate have all the properties of bona fide steroid hormone receptors, in that the binding of steroids to these sites is saturable, high affinity ($K_d \sim 1$ nM), and steroid specific. In addition, these receptors are tissue specific and increase or decrease appropriately, in response to the hormonal status of the animal. All these data are consistent with the conclusion that the specific binding of steroids to the nuclear matrix occurs via receptor proteins that had been translocated to the nucleus *in vivo* by endogenous hormone. A major proportion (50-90%) of the total nuclear receptor content is localized to the nuclear matrix, which contains only 10-15% of the total nuclear protein and 1-2% of the DNA.

The presence of significant receptor levels associated with the nuclear matrix suggests that the nuclear matrix contains the acceptor sites for these receptors. Direct evidence for the presence of acceptors on the nuclear matrix has been obtained using cell-free binding assays (Barrack, 1983, Endocrinology 113:430-432). In these experiments, androgen receptors in rat ventral prostate cytosol are charged with radiolabeled steroid (^{3}H-R1881) and increasing amounts of these labeled receptors are added to a constant amount of ventral prostate nuclear matrix isolated from castrated rats (to deplete the nuclei and matrix of endogenous androgen receptors). Under these conditions, we find that androgen receptors bind with high affinity ($K_d=10^{-10}$M) to a saturable number of sites (acceptors) on the prostate nuclear matrix. This binding is dependent on the presence of an activated androgen-receptor complex. In addition, the binding of receptors to nuclear matrix is tissue specific, since liver nuclear matrix contains only 15-20% as many acceptors for androgen receptors as the prostate nuclear matrix. The prostate nuclear matrix contains 75% of the acceptors of intact nuclei.

These studies will be discussed in relation to current concepts and models of the mechanisms of steroid hormone action. Our findings of receptor-acceptor interactions in association with the nuclear matrix may provide new insight into the mechanism of steroid hormone action and suggest mechanisms for the coordinated control of hormone-mediated nuclear events. (Supported by Grant AM 22000 from NIADDK, NIH).

S.12 GLUCOCORTICOID-REGULATED EXPRESSION OF MOUSE MAMMARY TUMOR VIRUS TRANSCRIPTION. B. Groner*[1], H. Ponta[2], P. Skroch[2], N. Kennedy[2], and H.E. Hynes[1]. Ludwig Institute for Cancer Research, Bern Branch, Inselspital, 3010 Bern, Switzerland [1], and Institute of Genetics, Kernforschungszentrum, D-7500 Karlsruhe, FRG [2].

Cloned proviral DNA of mouse mammary tumor virus, introduced into cultured cells, can be regulated in its expression by addition of glucocorticoid hormones to the culture medium. The DNA sequence responsible for hormonal regulation is contained within the long terminal repeat region (LTR) of the proviral DNA. This was shown by in vitro recombination of the LTR DNA with a thymidine kinase (tk) gene and transfection of the chimeric LTR-tk construct. RNA synthesis at the LTR and the tk gene initiation site is increased by dexamethasone. Deletions introduced from the 5' end into the LTR-tk gene showed that only 202 nucleotides of LTR DNA are necessary for full hormonal inducibility. Thus, 950 nucleotides from the 5' end of the LTR can be deleted without affecting hormone sensitivity. Deletions introduced from the 3' end of the LTR region showed that the proviral promoter (TATA box) and RNA initiation site are not part of the hormonal regulation sequence. Thus, 52 nucleotides upstream of the LTR cap site can be deleted without effect on the hormonal induction of the tk RNA initiation.

The hormone response sequence (HRS, -52 to -202) was recombined with the tk gene or with the α-globin gene in vitro and these constructs were transfected into cultured mouse fibroblasts. Both genes, the tk gene located 460 nucleotides 5' of the HRS and the α globin gene located 1100 nucleotides 5' of the HRS, are induced about 5-fold following hormone stimulation. The distance over which the regulation is functional is therefore flexible. The HRS-α globin genes transfected into mouse L cells only responded to dexamethasone with increased α globin transcription when the HRS was in the syn orientation (⟶ ⟶) and located 5' of the α globin gene. No or much weaker inducibility was observed in the anti orientation (⟵ ⟶) or in chimeras with the HRS at the 3' end of the α globin gene. These properties distinguish the HRS from enhancer elements.

The HRS sequence interacts preferentially in vitro with the glucocorticoid receptor. Two binding domains, at positions -72 to -124 and -163 to -192, have been identified. Functional glucocorticoid receptor has been found to be a prerequisite for hormonal induction in transfected cells. The receptor exerts its effect, in a process independent of protein synthesis, directly at the level of RNA initiation.

S.13 CELLULAR PRODUCTS RELATED TO ESTROGEN EFFECTS ON HYPOTHALAMIC NEURONS AND REPRODUCTIVE BEHAVIOR. R. Harlan*, D. Pfaff, B. Shivers, The Rockefeller University, New York, NY 10021 USA

Estrogen is concentrated by specific neurons in the basal forebrain, medial hypothalamus, amygdala and midbrain central gray (MCG). A subset of these estrogen-concentrating neurons, found in the mediobasal hypothalamus, is critical for the expression of female reproductive behavior, and is the main neural site at which estrogen acts to facilitate lordosis. Lordosis-facilitating neurons in the mediobasal hypothalamus send projections to the MCG. By analogy to other estrogen-responsive tissues, hypothalamic neurons are thought to respond to estrogen by production of specific cellular products. Moreover, hypothalamic protein synthesis is necessary for estrogenic facilitation of lordosis. Since estrogen-concentrating neurons communicate with other cells in the brain, one way in which estrogen may act is to augment synthesis of neuroactive peptides. Candidate lordosis-facilitating peptides should a) exist in cell bodies in the mediobasal hypothalamus with projections to the MCG, b) facilitate lordosis when applied to the MCG, and c) be regulated by estrogen. We have studied two candidates for lordosis-relevant, estrogen-modulated neuroactive peptides.

A lordosis-facilitating effect of luteinizing hormone releasing hormone (LHRH), especially when applied to the MCG, has been reported. A small number of fibers and, presumably, terminals containing LHRH can be found in the MCG. Immunocytochemical evidence suggests that estrogen increases the amount of LHRH released from terminals in the MCG (Neuroendocrinology 36: 1, 1983). Since few LHRH cells concentrate tritiated estradiol (Nature 304: 345, 1983), this effect of estrogen may be mediated by other neurons. Since the mediobasal hypothalamus contains few LHRH cell bodies, evidence so far does not suggest a major role for LHRH in the hypothalamus-to-midbrain, lordosis-facilitating circuitry.

Recently, we discovered that a prolactin-like substance is involved in estrogenic facilitation of lordosis (Science 219: 1451, 1983). Microinfusion of rat prolactin into the dorsal midbrain facilitated lordosis, while infusion of antiprolactin immune serum decreased lordotic responsiveness. The mediobasal hypothalamus contains 2-3000 cell bodies that can be stained immunocytochemically with antiprolactin immune serum (Abst. Soc. Neurosci. 9: 1018, 1983). These cells send a substantial fiber projection to the MCG. We now have evidence for the existence of prolactin mRNA in the rat hypothalamus (Schachter et al., this meeting), strongly suggesting that prolactin or a closely-related protein is synthesized in the brain. Studies are in progress to provide a physicochemical characterization of the prolactin-like substance and to determine whether it is regulated by steroids.

S.14 STRUCTURE OF THE COMMANDS FOR NEUROPEPTIDE-MEDIATED BEHAVIORS IN APLYSIA.
Felix Strumwasser* Dept. of Physiology, Boston University School of Medicine, Boston, MA. 02118.

From an evolutionary point of view, the nervous system is a conservative structure, since neurons utilize similar or identical mechanisms to carry out their functions in the simplest (coelenterates) and most complex forms (mammals). We can hope therefore to gain insights into neuroendocrine control of behavior from the study of model systems in simpler forms.

In the opisthobranch mollusc, Aplysia, there are two behaviors that are controlled by discrete and different neurosecretory structures in the nervous system. Egg-laying behavior (extrusion, attachment and winding of the egg-string) is controlled by the approximately 1000 peptidergic bag cell (BC) neurons in the abdominal ganglion, while circadian locomotor activity is controlled by a circadian oscillator in each of the two eyes.

The command for egg-laying is the peptide ELH (egg-laying hormone), synthesized and released by the BCs. ELH is a basic peptide (pI 9.1) containing 36 amino-acid residues with a calculated molecular weight of 4385 daltons. ELH acts directly on the ovotestis to release eggs into the reproductive tract and also acts back on targets in the nervous system to inhibit feeding (buccal ganglia) and locomotion (pedal ganglia). In the case of the buccal ganglion, one target of ELH is the motoneurons that cause retraction of the buccal mass. The command for ELH release is a 30 minute program of synchronized activity ("afterdischarge") in the BCs, the synchronization being mediated by electrical (gap-junction) coupling between BCs. The afterdischarge program is mediated by cyclic AMP-dependent protein phosphorylation changes. The evidence for this includes the demonstration that isolated BCs (in primary culture) contain the program for afterdischarge. Long-lasting afterdischarge, in such isolated BCs, can be released by priming with membrane permeant, phosphodiesterase-resistant, cyclic AMP analogs and directly firing a few calcium action potentials. The pre-command for egg-laying is partially worked out. Two peptides in the atrial gland, a part of the reproductive tract near the gonopore, cause egg-laying in a bag cell-dependent manner. These peptides are homologous with one another but share no significant sequences with ELH. Peptides A and B contain 34 amino-acid residues each, have molecular weights of 3924 and 4932 daltons, and pI of 8.0 and 9.1, respectively. These peptides induce bag cell afterdischarge, in vitro, and thus resemble releasing factors in their actions. However, the atrial gland has an exocrine structure and it remains to be seen whether peptides A and B have homologs in the CNS.

Circadian locomotion is controlled by a neuronal circadian oscillator in each eye. The isolated eye, in darkness, produces a pacemaker discharge, emitted in the optic nerve. The frequency of these action potentials varies smoothly over 24 hours, with peak activity near projected dawn and minimal activity near projected dusk. One of the output cells of this retina contains 100 nm dense core granules and, by autoradiographic criteria, is the most active protein synthesizing cell in the retina. Radioactive release experiments indicate that at least two peptides are released from the isolated eye with a circadian rhythm. It is likely that these peptides act in the cerebral ganglion, rather than the circulation, for animals with sectioned optic nerves are arhythmic in their activity.

S.15 EFFECTS OF SEX STEROIDS ON BEHAVIORAL AND BRAIN ORGANIZATION. R. Gorski*, Department of Anatomy and Laboratory of Neuroendocrinology of the Brain Research Institute, UCLA School of Medicine, Los Angeles, California, USA.

Sexual behavior is dependent upon the action of gonadal hormones on relevant brain regions. At the conceptual level it is convenient to describe two types of hormone action on the brain: activational or transient and organizational or permanent. In terms of feminine sexual behavior in the rat, two ovarian hormones (estrogen (E) and progesterone) interact in a complex way to facilitate lordosis, one index of sexual receptivity. Although the ventromedial hypothalamus may be one neural site critical for lordosis behavior, other areas such as the cerebral cortex and mesencephalic reticular formation are also probably involved. For masculine sexual behavior testosterone (T) is critical and one major site of its action is the medial preoptic area (MPOA). The response of the rat in terms of these behaviors is sexually dimorphic particularly in the case of lordosis; the male only rarely exhibits the lordosis reflex after priming with ovarian hormones following castration in adulthood. With respect to masculine behavior the sex dimorphism is less clear, particularly in terms of mounting behavior. A major research thrust has been to elucidate the basis of these sex differences in adult behavior. It is known that the organizational actions of steroids during development are responsible for sex differences in adult behavioral responsiveness to hormones. The rat brain is inherently female, or at least bipotential, and exposure to testicular hormones, or exogenous T or E, defeminizes and masculinizes the brain. Although it is possible that the organizational action of gonadal steroids is effected by neurochemical mechanisms we now recognize as activational, it is clear that there are also structural sex differences in the rat central nervous system, and that these differences are also under hormonal control, at least during development. We have focused on one such structural sex difference, the Sexually Dimorphic Nucleus of the Preoptic Area (SDN-POA), a morphological signature of the organizational action of gonadal steroids. Briefly, this nucleus is larger in volume and apparently comprised of more neurons in the male than it is in the female. The developing SDN-POA is sensitive to the hormonal environment, in fact, the SDN-POA of the female can be sex-reversed by prolonged administration of T or E perinatally. Our current understanding is that although neurogenesis and neuronal migration may be sensitive to hormones, steroid action on neuronal survival during a perinatal period of neuronal death may be the critical mechanism. To date, attempts to identify the function(s) of the neurons of the SDN-POA have been unsuccessful. Although hormonal implants in the region of the SDN-POA facilitate masculine sexual behavior, discrete lesions of the nucleus do not disrupt it. However, equally small lesions just dorsal to the SDN-POA are effective. Transplantation of the MPOA including the SDN-POA from the newborn male into the MPOA of littermate females facilitates masculine behavior of these females when adult, but lordosis behavior is also facilitated. Although it is logical to predict that the neurons of the SDN-POA form the neural substrate of some sexually dimorphic behavior or function, its identity remains unknown. Further study of the connectivity and neurochemical characteristics of the SDN-POA may lead to a better understanding of the role of this structure in neuroendocrine regulation. (HD-01182)

S.16 BEHAVIORAL EFFECTS OF NEUROHYPOPHYSEAL HORMONES.

Tj.B. van Wimersma Greidanus*, Rudolf Magnus Institute for Pharmacology, Medical Faculty, University of Utrecht, Vondellaan 6, 3521 GD Utrecht, The Netherlands.

Vasopressin and/or oxytocin induce a wide variety of behavioral effects which include extinction of a conditioned avoidance response, retention of a passive avoidance response, prevention and reversal of experimentally induced amnesia, learned helplesness, maze learning, development of tolerance to and physical dependence on opiates and alcohol, drug seeking behavior, maternal behavior etc. From these data it has been postulated that vasopressin and oxytocin affect memory processes and influence cognitive functions. In fact it has been hypothesized that vasopressin and oxytocin induce opposite effects on storage and retrieval processes in the brain.

Lesions of and microinjection into particular brain areas pointed to several limbic midbrain structures as the sites of action of neurohypophyseal hormones in this respect. The stimulatory effects of vasopressin on consolidation of memory processes seem to be related to its effects in the terminal regions of the coeruleo-telencephalic noradrenalin system, whereas it is likely that the effects of vasopressin on other transmitter systems (e.g. dopamine in the amygdala and serotonin in the hippocampus) correspond with the effect of this neuropeptide on retrieval processes.

Several experimental data point to a physiological role of the neurohypophyseal hormones in behavior, memory processes and/or cognitive functions: 1) the extrahypothalamic projections to various limbic regions; 2) the very small amounts resulting in behavioral effects following central administration; 3) changes in neuropeptide levels in cerebrospinal fluid of rats in relation to their behavioral performance; 4) the disturbed behavior of Brattleboro rats suffering from a lack of vasopressin and that of rats following central application of antisera to vasopressin or oxytocin.

The effects of vasopressin on memory processes are dissociated from its peripheral effects on blood pressure and water metabolism. Structure-activity relationship studies as well as investigations on the generation of fragments from vasopressin and oxytocin in brain synaptic membrane preparations *in vitro* revealed that these hormones may form higly potent and selective memory modulating neuropeptides. Therefore it is postulated that the neurohypophyseal hormones are precursor molecules of more potent and selective neuropeptides involved in the consolidation and/or retrieval processes of memory function.

References:

- Kovács, G.L. and G. Telegdy. Pharmac. Ther. 18, 375-395 (1982).
- De Wied, D. Prog. Brain. Res. 60, 155-167 (1983).
- Burbach, J.P.H., G.L. Kovács, D. De Wied, J.W. van Nispen and H.M. Greven. Science 211, 1310-1312 (1983).
- van Wimersma Greidanus, Tj.B., J.M. Van Ree and D. De Wied. Pharmac. Ther. 20, 437-458 (1983).

S.17 REGULATION OF MAMMALIAN PINEAL CIRCADIAN RHYTHMS. D. Klein;* Section on Neuroendocrinology, Laboatory of Developmental Neurobiology, NICHHD, National Institutes of Health, Bethesda, MD 20205

There is a 24-hour rhythm in melatonin in mammalian blood, CSF and urine, with high levels occurring at night; it is generated by the rhythmic production of melatonin in the pineal gland. Melatonin is synthesized from circulating tryptophan by a four enzyme pathway: tryptophan --→ hydroxytryptophan --→ serotonin --→ N-acetylserotonin --→ melatonin. The major pertubation in this pathway responsible for the daily melatonin rhythm is a 30- to 70-fold increase in N-acetylation at night. The enzyme responsible is a specific arylalkylamine N-acetyltransferase; arylamines are not substrates. It appears that two mechanisms are responsible for the increase in N-acetyltransferase activity. One is an inductive mechanism, dependent upon new gene expression. The second is stabilization or activation. Available evidence suggests that stabilization is required to prevent very rapid inactivation via protein thiol: disulfide exchange. The doubling time for the increase in enzyme activity is about 15 to 20 minutes. The decrease in enzyme activity which occurs at a dark --→ light transition at night has a halving time of about 3.5 minutes. This is the most rapid physiological inactivation of an enzyme known, and, as indicated above, appears to occur via protein thiol: disulfide exchange of thiol groups on the enzyme with a disulfide inactivator. The activity of N-acetyltransferase is regulated by cyclic AMP. It is not clear how cyclic AMP acts, but it seems that it acts in part to increase enzyme activity via a mechanism dependent upon membrane hyperpolarization. This might be related either to the inductive or stabilization processes necessary for the increase in activity. Cyclic AMP levels in the pineal gland are regulated by a mechanism involving both $alpha_1$- and $beta_1$-adrenoceptors. $Beta_1$ activation, which elevates cyclic AMP via actions on adenylate cyclase, is required; $alpha_1$ activation potentiates the effects of $beta_1$ activation. The mechanism of action of this is not clear; one possibility is that $alpha_1$-adrenoceptors control cyclic nucleotide phosphodiesterase activity. The neurotransmitter involved in the regulation of the pineal gland is norepinephrine. It is released from nerve terminals having their cell bodies in the superior cervical ganglia. These cells are regulated by a neural circuit originating in the suprachiasmatic nucleus (SCN) of the hypothalamus. The circuit from the SCN to the superior cervical ganglia passes through the paraventricular nucleus, medial forebrain bundle, reticular formation and intermediolateral cell column of the spinal cord; preganglionic cells there innervate the superior cervical ganglia. The SCN is a self-generating circadian oscillator, which continues to function in constant darkness. Light, which acts via a retinohypothalamic projection, has two effects on this system. First, it entrains the circadian clock to environmental lighting cues. Second, it gates suprachiasmiaic stimulation of the pineal gland. The available evidence indicates that the basic features of this system are seen in all mammals, including man.

PINEAL RHYTHMICITY AND SEASONAL REPRODUCTION. Fred J. Karsch* and Eric L. Bittman, Reproductive Endocrinology Program and Department of Physiology, The University of Michigan, Ann Arbor, Michigan, 48109, USA.

Experiments were conducted over the course of several years to evaluate the role of the pineal gland, and its nightly elevation of melatonin secretion, in mediating the reproductive response to photoperiod in the female sheep. The ewe is a seasonal breeder in which short days are inductive, and long days inhibitory to estrous cyclicity. The reproductive response to photoperiod is effected via the negative feedback system which controls the tonic mode of gonadotropin secretion. Long days inhibit estrous cycles by intensifying the negative feedback action of estradiol. Short days reverse this effect, causing estradiol feedback potency to diminish and estrous cycles to occur. Our initial experiments with the pineal revealed that this gland mediates the effect of **both** inductive and inhibitory photoperiods on estrous cyclicity as well as on the response to estradiol negative feedback in the ewe. Subsequent studies have indicated that this role of the pineal can be fully accounted for by its patterned secretion of melatonin. In the ewe, melatonin secretion is a circadian rhythm; it is elevated only at night; and the duration of this nighttime rise is directly proportional to the length of the night. In the pinealectomized ewe, restoration of a melatonin pattern typifying that which occurs in short days (by nightly iv infusion) leads to reproductive induction, whereas provision of a melatonin pattern characteristic of that in long days precipitates reproductive arrest. Furthermore, by mismatching the melatonin pattern with photoperiod in pinealectomized ewes (i.e., long-day melatonin pattern infused in short days or short-day melatonin pattern in long days), we have found that the reproductive response is invariably appropriate to the melatonin pattern, not the photoperiod. Our findings lead to the **conclusion** that the patterned secretion of melatonin determines the reproductive response to daylength in the short-day breeding ewe. In particular, the duration of nocturnal melatonin secretion is important in relaying photic information to the centers which govern tonic gonadotropin secretion, and in controlling the response of those centers to steroid negative feedback. By means of its rhythmic secretion of melatonin, therefore, the pineal gland participates in the measurement of daylength. (NIH-HD-11311, HD-05914 and the Michigan Society of Fellows).

S.19 BIOLOGICALLY ACTIVE COMPOUNDS IN PINEALS AND RETINAS OF ANIMALS EXPOSED TO DIFFERENT LIGHT CONDITIONS.

*I. Ebels[1] and G. Cremer-Bartels[2], [1]Department of Organic Chemistry, State University, 3522 AD Utrecht, The Netherlands, [2]Eye Hospital of the Westphalian Wilhelms University, 4400 Münster (Westf), Federal Republic of Germany.

Different pteridines have been isolated, purified and identified from ovine pineals in the last years. The pineal contains a very high amount of 6-L-erythrobiopterin, which compound in the reduced form is generally considered to be the natural cofactor of tryptophanhydroxylase, phenylalanine- and tyrosinehydroxylase. Therefore, 6-L-erythrotetrahydrobiopterin is very important for the biosynthesis of catecholamines, hydroxyindoles and for methoxyindole-biosynthesis. The results of experiments in which the influence of different pteridines and light of different wavelength on the activity of hydroxyindole-O-methyltransferase (HIOMT) were studied will be presented. HIOMT-preparations were isolated and purified from pineals and retinas by a flat-bed-gelelectrofocusing technique. Multiple forms of HIOMT-enzymes, which differ in the pH of the isoelectric point could be detected. The pattern of the concentrations of the enzymes differed in dependence on light adaptation. It was observed later on that partially purified ovine pineal gland- and retina-fractions can also suppress the activity of HIOMT, as some pteridines do. The mechanism of inhibition of HIOMT-activity is independent of the species and the organ from which the HIOMT-preparation was prepared; retinas or pineals from birds, cattle or sheep. The effects of (an) unknown natural suppressor(s) of HIOMT-activity is comparable to that of some antipsychotic drugs on HIOMT in _in vitro_ and _in vivo_ experiments. The results of the attempts to isolate, purify and identify the yet unknown ovine pineal inhibitor(s) of HIOMT will be presented and discussed.

S.20 REGULATION OF CIRCULATING MELATONIN AND N-ACETYLSEROTONIN.

G.M. Brown*, A.K. Ho, T.G. Burns, L. Harvey, L.J. Grota and J. Seggie, Department of Neurosciences, McMaster University, Hamilton, and Department of Psychiatry, University of Rochester, New York.

In all species studied serum melatonin (MT) and pineal N-acetyltransferase (NATase) show a distinct circadian rhythm with higher night than day levels. In the synthesis of MT, serotonin in the pineal is acetylated to N-acetylserotonin (NAS) by the enzyme NATase and NAS is further converted to MT by hydroxyindole-O-methyltransferase (HIOMT). NATase is particularly responsive to light and is thought to be the rate-limiting step in MT synthesis. It has been assumed that alteration in serum MT is produced by changes in pineal NATase activity. However serum rhythms of NAS and MT can be dissociated under certain lighting conditions and following stress. Moreover, MT and the enzyme HIOMT have been found in other tissues such as the retina which might conceivably give rise to serum MT hence influencing its rhythm.

The foregoing raises the following questions. Does pineal NATase reflect serum MT and does serum MT originate exclusively from the pineal? Male rats were studied under several light-dark (LD) cycles (LD 16:8 for 2 weeks, LD 12:12 for 2 weeks, LD 4:20 for 2 weeks and LD 4:20 for 4 weeks). Under all conditions a close parallelism of serum MT, pineal MT (measured by radioimmunoassay) and pineal NATase rhythms was established. Two separate studies of pinealectomy were also conducted. Undetectable serum MT was found throughout 24h in groups of rats sacrificed 3 and 7 weeks after pinealectomy. It can be concluded that immunoassayable MT in serum originates from the pineal where its synthesis is regulated by NATase.

Lack of dissociation of pineal NATase and serum MT rhythms raises the question of the source or sources of circulating NAS. NATase is found not only in pineal, retina and Harderian gland but also in the CNS and liver. Thus circulating NAS could originate from sources other than the pineal and hence be regulated independently of the pineal. The possibility that serum NAS may be related to the timing of their eating habit was investigated. After 4 weeks of different feeding schedules, the 24h pattern of circulating NAS and MT were examined by radioimmunoassay in male rats. A strong correlation of the NAS peak with feeding time was established while the MT rhythm remained in synchrony with the light-dark cycle. Thus the NAS but not the MT rhythm can be entrained by the time of food presentation. In male rats exposed to 4 different stressors (ether, cold, noise and novel environment) early in the light phase a clear serum MT rise occurred while NAS displayed a transient fall. Finally, in pinealectomized male rats there were no significant changes in the 24h serum NAS levels 3 and 7 weeks after pinealectomy. It can be concluded that the pineal is not the major source of serum NAS and that the serum NAS rhythm, unlike that of the MT, can be entrained by feeding rather than environmental lighting.

S.21 BIOCHEMICAL CHARACTERIZATION OF THE ADRENERGIC RECEPTORS: PURIFICATION, AFFINITY LABELLING AND RECONSTITUTION STUDIES. M.G. Caron*, R.A. Cerione, J.W. Regan, L.M.F. Leeb-Lundberg, J.L. Benovic, B. Strulovici, J. Codina, L. Birnbaumer and R.J. Lefkowitz. Howard Hughes Medical Institute, Duke Univ. Medical Center, Durham, N.C. 27710 U.S.A. and Baylor College of Medicine, Houston, Tex. 77030 U.S.A.

The specific α- and β-adrenergic receptors which mediate the various physiological actions of catecholamines appear to reside on distinct polypeptides. Identity of the polypeptides has been established by affinity chromatography purification and visualization by affinity and photoaffinity labelling as well as reconstitution studies. The β-adrenergic receptor (βAR) of mammalian lung has been purified to apparent homogeneity and its binding site resides on a single glycopeptide of M_r 62,000-65,000. The isolated peptide carries both functions of the βAR: 1) It binds catecholamines with a β-adrenergic specificity and 2) by reconstitution it confers β-adrenergic responsiveness to a previously unresponsive adenylate cyclase system. Moreover, coreconstitution of this purified βAR polypeptide with pure preparations of human erythrocyte nucleotide binding protein (N_s) results in the functional coupling of these proteins as assessed by the formation of a guanine nucleotide sensitive agonist high affinity state of the βAR and the establishment of a β-adrenergic sensitive GTPase activity. These results demonstrate that this single polypeptide does represent the physiological βAR and that no components other than pure βAR and N_s are necessary for these interactions.

Progress in the characterization of the αAR has also been accomplished. Using photoaffinity labelling with the prazosin analog [^{125}I]APDQ, the α_1AR binding peptide has been covalently labelled in several mammalian tissues including rat liver and cerebral cortex, rat, guinea pig and rabbit spleen and rabbit aorta vascular smooth muscle cells. Autoradiograms of membrane samples subjected to SDS-PAGE show that in the presence of protease inhibitors this photoaffinity probe incorporates with an α_1-adrenergic specificity into a peptide of M_r = 78,000-85,000. By peptide mapping this photoaffinity labelled polypeptide appears to be virtually identical within the various tissues of a species but slightly different from species to species. The α_2AR of human platelets has been partially purified (500-1,000 fold) by affinity chromatography on a benzazepine-Sepharose gel. In these partially purified preparations, the alkylating agent [^{3}H]phenoxybenzamine has been used to identify a peptide of M_r = 60,000 as the ligand binding site of this subtype of αAR. The availability of methods to purify and covalently label as well as functionally reconstitute receptors is proving to be useful in the elucidation of the biochemical properties of receptors for catecholamines and the mechanisms by which membrane signal transfer occurs.

S.22 ROLE OF N PROTEIN IN COUPLING OF ADRENERGIC RECEPTORS AND ADENYLATE CYCLASE.

Michio Ui*, Toshiaki Katada, Toshihiko Murayama and Hitoshi Kurose, Department of Physiological Chemistry, Faculty of Pharmaceutical Sciences, Hokkaido University, Sapporo 060, Japan.

Adrenergic receptors are classified into four subtypes; alpha-1, alpha-2, beta-1 and beta-2. Beta-1 and beta-2 adrenergic receptors are coupled to adenylate cyclase in such a manner as to activate the catalytic unit (C) of the cyclase. The activation is mediated by the N protein (Ns) which consists of an alpha-subunit (Mr=45,000) and a beta-subunit (Mr=35,000). The alpha-subunit of Ns possesses the binding sites for GTP (or GDP) and serves as a specific substrate of cholera toxin-catalyzed ADP-ribosylation. Ns communicates between beta-adrenergic receptors (R) and C by the following reaction sequence. Without stimulation of R, the three components of the receptor-adenylate cyclase system, R, Ns and C, are dissociated from each other in the plasma membrane. Under these conditions are the binding sites on Ns occupied by GDP. Upon stimulation of R by beta-adrenergic agonists (A), a ternary complex, A-R-Ns, is instantaneously formed with a high affinity for agonist binding. Then, GTP exchanges with GDP on Ns as the "turnon" reaction, since the GTP-bound Ns activates C. R detached from Ns is liable to discharge A due to a lower affinity for it, and GTP on Ns is finally hydrolyzed to GDP as the "turnoff" reaction; the initial unstimulated state of the system is then regained. The GTP-bound active form of Ns is irreversibly preserved, even without stimulation of coupled R, after it has been ADP-ribosylated by cholera toxin. Alpha-2 adrenergic receptors are coupled to adenylate cyclase contrarily in an inhibitory fashion. The N protein (Ni) involved in alpha-receptor-mediated inhibition of cyclase was identified as an entity distinct from Ns thanks to the discovery of an islet-activating protein (IAP), pertussis toxin, which ADP-ribosylates the membrane Mr=41,000 protein selectively. Ni purified as an IAP-specific substrate proved to be a dimer consisting of an alpha-subunit (Mr=41,000) with GTP-binding sites and a beta-subunit which is identical with that of Ns. The mechanism whereby Ni communicates between R and C is virtually the same as that for Ns, except for the fact that GTP-bound Ns activates, while GTP-bound Ni inhibits, C. Incubation of membranes from rat islets, rat or hamster adipocytes or NG108-15 cells with the active component of IAP and NAD resulted in ADP-ribosylation of the alpha-subunit of Ni in membranes. The addition of alpha-adrenergic agents to these IAP-treated membranes failed to reproduce their stimulatory effects on guanine nucleotide metabolism, such as GTP-GDP exchange or GTP hydrolysis, that should be observed with non-treated membranes. Thus, the communication between alpha-adrenergic receptors and Ni was blocked by IAP-catalyzed ADP-ribosylation. Moreover, GTP-induced inhibition of adenylate cyclase was totally reversed after the IAP treatment of membranes, indicating that Ni is not capable of interaction with C after being ADP-ribosylated. Thus, IAP-catalyzed ADP-ribosylation of the alpha-subunit of Ni results in a complete loss of the functions of Ni to communicate between alpha-adrenergic receptors and the adenylate cyclase catalytic component. This is because the ADP-ribosylated alpha-subunit of Ni is firmly associated with its beta-subunit, liberation of which is responsible for agonist-induced inhibition of adenylate cyclase.

S.23 THYROID HORMONE REGULATION OF ALPHA- AND BETA-ADRENERGIC RECEPTORS.

C.C. Malbon*, A. Cubero, M. Graziano, and C. Moxham, Department of Pharmacology, Health Sciences Center, The State University of New York at Stony Brook, Stony Brook, New York, 11794.

Thyroid hormones modulate the responsiveness of many tissues to the actions of catecholamines. β-Adrenergic catecholamine action in heart and adipose tissue, for example, is markedly potentiated by hyperthyroidism, while severely blunted by hypothyroidism. Research over the past 5 years has focused on elucidating the biochemical basis for the changes in catecholamine responsiveness observed in altered thyroid states. The hormone sensitive-adenylate cyclase system provides a useful model for these studies. The β-adrenergic catecholamine-sensitive adenylate cyclase system consists of at least three separable components: the β-adrenergic receptor (βAR), a guanine nucleotide-binding, stimulatory regulatory component (Ns), and a catalytic cyclase moiety (C). Ns plays a pivotal role in transducing agonist occupancy of the βAR into activation of C, a process dependent upon the presence of a guanine nucleotide triphosphate. Using a variety of new probes capable of detecting and quantitating βAR, Ns, and C activities, the biochemical basis of thyroid hormone effects on catecholamine action can be approached. The number of βARs in rat heart, liver, skeletal muscle, and submaxillary gland have been reported to be influenced by thyroid hormones. These changes in the number of βARs may explain, in part, the altered responses of these tissues.

We have focused our research on two model systems, the adipocyte and the hepatocyte of the hypothyroid rat. β-Catecholamine action is impaired in the former, while potentiated in the latter. In the adipocyte, the impaired response to β-catecholamine action does not involve changes in the affinity of βARs for antagonist ligands or in the amounts of βARs, Ns, or C, but appears to involve a loss of βAR function. Recently we have purified adipocyte β_1AR to apparent homogeneity. The adipocyte β_1-AR is a M_r=67,000 peptide, as determined by gel electrophoresis in sodium dodecyl sulfate under reducing conditions. The β_1AR of the hypothyroid rat has been purified also and is being analyzed in an effort to provide structural information that may explain the inability of this βAR to communicate with Ns. In the liver hypothyroidism potentiates rather than impairs β-catecholamine action. The basis for this potentiation appears to be a 3-fold increase in the number of βARs. We have also purified the βAR of liver. This β_2-AR is composed of M_r=60,000/67,000-peptides. Antibodies raised against these receptors should provide a new means with which to study the dynamics of βARs in both of these model systems. The effects of thyroid status on alpha-adrenergic responses are unclear. Thyroid hormone regulation of $alpha_1$- and $alpha_2$-adrenergic receptors will be discussed. (Supported by USPHS grants AM30111, AM25410, and K04-007886 from the National Institutes of Health).

S.24 BETA-AND ALPHA$_2$-ADRENOCEPTORS INTERPLAY AND THE REGULATION OF LIPOLYSIS IN HUMAN ADIPOSE TISSUE. M.Lafontan* and M.Berlan.

Institut de Physiologie,UPS,ERA412CNRS,Rue F.Magendie,31400 Toulouse,France.

It is well accepted that human fat cells are sensitive to the lipolytic action of norepinephrine(NEPI) and epinephrine(EPI);the lipolytic effect is mediated by the β-adrenoceptors.Biological studies and radioligand binding assays have also demonstrated the presence of α_2-adrenoceptors in human fat cell membranes;their stimulation promotes an inhibition of lipolysis.Our investigations were conducted to clear the status and delineate the advantages of this double signalling system in the regulation of lipolysis.

Alpha$_2$-and β-adrenoceptor binding studies,with antagonist radioligands, revealed the preponderance of α_2-over β-sites in human fat cell membranes; the β-adrenoceptor population being at least a third as numerous as the α_2-one.EPI and NEPI exhibit a higher affinity for the α_2- than for β-sites in "in vitro" biological studies and radioligand binding assays.Moreover,EPI as opposed to NEPI,is the major stimulant of α_2-adrenoceptors;EPI has a higher affinity than NEPI for α_2-sites while the two amines are equipotent at the β-sites(similar K_i:apparent dissociation constants).

Apparently,binding data do not correlate with receptor-mediated cellular response since,in standard conditions of lipolysis studies in human fat cell it is the beta-lipolytic action which appears to predominate.A better convergence between binding and biological assays would be expected if it is postulated that the efficiency of the amines is a function of affinity parameters and receptor number.A slight modification of the traditional incubation conditions,when adenosine is prevented from accumulating in the medium by inclusion of adenosine deaminase,EPI alone inhibited lipolysis at the lower concentrations(0.01 to 1μM),this effect was reversed at the higher doses corresponding to the commonly known lipolytic ones.NEPI is less potent in the initiation of the antilipolytic action.Thus, under these conditions, the α_2-adrenergic antilipolytic effect appears first, at the lower concentrations of EPI and it is followed by the β-effect which appears over the higher range of EPI concentrations.It is not exclusively the lowered adenosine level which explains the occurence of the biphasic effect of EPI since it also occurs when basal lipolysis has been increased by a small dose of β-adrenergic agonist....It is of interest to notice that the binding data now fits with receptor-mediated cellular responses in human fat cells.Alpha$_2$-adrenoceptors, with their higher number and higher affinity for physiological amines (mainly EPI) are the adrenoceptor population involved at the lowest concentration of the amines,the β-sites with a lower number and weaker affinity for EPI or NEPI are involved when higher concentrations of the amines reach the plasma membrane.

To conclude,the definition of the relationships between EPI,NEPI and β- and α_2-binding sites in human fat cells demonstrate that the adrenergic response of the adipocyte is really the resultant of β-and α_2-adrenoceptor stimulation.Alpha$_2$-receptors are of major interest in the control of lipolysis since they are the population first involved in the action of catecholamines although their stimulation is not able to counteract maximal lipolytic stimulations initiated by β-agonists or forskolin.Alpha$_2$-sites,with a higher affinity for EPI, seem to be a family of hormonal receptors mainly involved in the control of the state of activity of the human fat cell.

The investigations are supported by CNRS and INSERM(CRL and PRC)

S.25 LOCALIZATION OF PEPTIDES AND INTERACTIONS OF RF NEURONS IN THE CENTRAL NERVOUS SYSTEM. G. Pelletier*, MRC Group in Molecular Endocrinology, CHUL, Québec, G1V 4G2, Canada.

During the last decade, several neuropeptides involved in the regulation of anterior pituitary secretion have been isolated and characterized. The recent development of sensitive immunocytochemical techniques as well as the production of specific antibodies to these peptides have prompted neuroanatomists to search for the precise distribution of neuropeptides. The mapping of neuropeptides in the central nervous system was accomplished by immunocytochemistry at the light microscopic level whereas their subcellular distribution was performed by ultrastructural immunocytochemistry. It appeared soon that the peptides directly involved in the regulation of anterior pituitary function (regulatory factors, RF), namely TRH, LHRH, somatostatin, vasopressin, CRF and GRF, were located not only in the hypothalamus, but also in extra-hypothalamic areas. In the hypothalamus, these peptides were localized by immunoelectron microscopy in dense core vesicles in neuronal cell bodies and in free endings located in close proximity of the pituitary portal plexus, indicating that the peptides are probably released into the pituitary portal plexus to reach their target cells in the pituitary.

Other neuropeptides which are indirectly involved in the control of anterior pituitary secretion, such as enkephalins, endorphins, neurotensin and substance P, are also largely distributed throughout the central nervous system. At the ultrastructural level, these peptides are also mostly associated with dense core vesicles in neuronal cell bodies and axon profiles. In the dendrites, the immunostaining was more diffusively located without any association with specific organelles. These ultrastructural findings suggest that the neuropeptides could play a role as neurotransmitter or neuromodulator.

It is only very recently that the interactions between monoaminergic neurons and peptidergic neurons have been investigated with double staining techniques applied at the ultrastructural level. It has been demonstrated that LHRH neuronal cell bodies are contacted by other LHRH neurons. Similarly somatostatinergic neurons in the hypothalamus have been shown to be contacted by other somatostatinergic neurons. Finally, endorphinic neurons in the hypothalamic arcuate nucleus are receiving inputs from other endorphinic neurons as well as from serotoninergic neurons. These recent findings suggest an autoregulation of hypothalamic peptidergic systems.

S.26 REGULATION OF PITUITARY HORMONE SECRETION BY VIP AND RELATED PEPTIDES.

Y. Kato*, A. Shimatsu, N. Matsushita, H. Ohta, K. Tojo, Y. Kabayama, T. Inoue and H. Imura, Second Medical Clinic, Department of Medicine, Kyoto University Faculty of Medicine, Kyoto 606, Japan.

Vasoactive intestinal polypeptide (VIP), first discovered in the digestive tract, has been detected in the hypothalamus, suggesting a potential role in the hypothalamo-pituitary system. We first demonstrated that VIP stimulates prolactin (PRL) secretion in the rat in vivo (Endocrinology 103:554, 1978). Subsequent studies suggest that VIP is secreted into the hypophysial portal blood and can act directly at the pituitary level to evoke PRL release. VIP was effective to stimulate PRL release from superfused rat anterior pituitary cells and the stimulating action of VIP on rat PRL secretion was demonstrated even in the presence of dopamine and GABA which inhibit PRL release at the pituitary level. The concentration of VIP in rat hypophysial portal blood is sufficient to stimulate PRL release from pituitary cells in vitro. Serotonergic agents such as serotonin and 5-HTP, a precursor of serotonin, stimulated VIP release from the hypothalamus into the hypophysial portal vessel in vivo and from the hypothalamic fragments perifused in vitro. It is well known that serotonergic mechanisms stimulate PRL secretion. We found that PRL release induced by intraventricular injection of serotonin was blunted by anti-VIP rabbit serum which was injected into a lateral ventricle or infused into a single hypophysial portal vessel. It is concluded, therefore, that VIP may be a candidate for PRL releasing factor (PRF) and that PRL release induced by serotonergic mechanisms in the brain is mediated, at least in part, by endogenous VIP which is released from the hypothalamus into the hypophysial portal blood.
Intramuscular injection of VIP resulted in a significant increase in plasma PRL levels in normal women whereas plasma growth hormone (GH) and cortisol levels were not affected. VIP injection raised plasma PRL levels in most patients with prolactinoma and plasma GH levels were increased by VIP in some acromegalic patients. VIP stimulated PRL release in a dose-related manner from superfused pituitary adenoma cells which were obtained from patients with prolactinoma. VIP induced GH release from superfused pituitary adenoma cells in most patients with acromegaly. VIP concentrations in the cerebrospinal fluid (CSF) were increased in patients with hyperprolactinemia and a part of acromegalic patients. It is suggested, therefore, that VIP may play a role in regulating PRL secretion in man and may affect GH secretion from pituitary adenoma in acromegaly. It has been proposed that peptide histidine isoleucine (PHI) and VIP are derived from the same prohormone molecule. We found that plasma PHI-like immunoreactivity in rat hypophysial portal blood was 7 times higher than in the peripheral blood and was well correlated with VIP concentrations. PHI also stimulated PRL secretion in the rat in vivo and PRL release from superfused rat anterior pituitary cells. GH release from pituitary adenoma cells obtained from some acromegalic cases was also stimulated by PHI. These results may indicate that VIP and related peptides have a role in the regulation of pituitary function in man and rats.

(Supported in part by grants from the Ministry of Education and the Ministry of Health and Welfare, Japan.)

S.27 OPIOID PEPTIDES AND PITUITARY HORMONE SECRETION. A. Grossman*, Department of Endocrinology, St. Bartholomew's Hospital, London, UK.

The exponential growth in studies of opioid peptides has allowed us to gain considerable insight into the site and mode of action of these compounds in the control of pituitary hormone release. In the rat, early work demonstrating a stimulation of prolactin and GH release by opioid peptides and alkaloids has been repeatedly confirmed. Naloxone alone suppresses basal, stress-related, vasotocin- and suckling-induced release of prolactin, probably involving β-endorphin as the endogenous ligand. Although at least part of this activity of opioids is through a disinhibition of hypothalamic dopamine release, the additional involvement of serotonin-VIP mediation appears probable. The opioid control of GH release in the rat remains poorly characterised - many mediating neurotransmitters have been implicated. However, studies in our laboratory and elsewhere indicate that the predominant effect is via GH-releasing hormone rather than somatostatin; the site of action is different to that for prolactin. Opiate involvement in gonadotrophin release has been demonstrated to occur via changes in GnRH, probably through μ-receptors or ε-receptors, with β-endorphin as the endogenous ligand. There may be a separate pathway, of lesser importance, involving dynorphin modulation at K-receptors. Endogenous opioids may mediate the feedback effects of gonadal steroids in the hypothalamus. There is also persuasive evidence that during the process of pubertal maturation endogenous opioids modulate the activity of an incremental noradrenergic input. The opiate control of TSH is of relatively minor importance, and appears to involve the direct inhibition of TRH release ± a naloxone-independent direct pituitary component. ACTH release is complex, with evidence for both stimulatory and inhibitory modulation at both hypothalamic and pituitary levels. Similar considerations apply to AVP, but here the inhibitory control predominates, and may actually occur at the level of the pituicyte. Inhibitory modulation of oxytocin release may regulate interbirth intervals in the rat. CRF, AVP and oxytocin are all costored with opioid peptides, and part of the effects of opioids may be due to the corelease of dynorphin or met-enkephalin. In man, exogenous opioids stimulate prolactin, GH and (to a minor extent) TSH release. The receptors involved are probably ε-receptors for prolactin and μ-receptors for TSH. With the possible exception of prolactin and GH release induced by severe exercise in trained subjects, the opioid control of these hormones does not appear to be physiologically important. In contrast, the frequency of gonadotrophin release is constantly modulated by an endogenous opioid, probably β-endorphin, in males and females, with the effect contingent upon the steroid milieu. Unlike the rat, opioids do not appear to be involved in puberty, and do not operate via noradrenergic or dopaminergic neurotransmitters. However, there is good evidence that the hypothalamic gonadal dysfunction secondary to hyperprolactinaemia is due to opioid inhibition of GnRH release. Thus, certain amenorrhoeic states might respond to treatment with opiate antagonists. With regard to ACTH and AVP, there is evidence that both are inhibited by exogenous opioids; naloxone increases basal ACTH, probably via a noradrenergic mechanism. Naloxone-insensitive receptors of δ- or K-classes appear to be involved in these processes. The physiological significance of these observations is uncertain, but opiate agonists such as butorphanol or oxilorphan may be used to reduce AVP secretion in certain cases of the Schwartz-Bartter syndrome.

S.28 INTERACTIONS OF BRAIN PEPTIDES WITHIN THE HYPOTHALAMUS TO ALTER ANTERIOR PITUITARY HORMONE SECRETION.

S.M. McCann*, M.D. Lumpkin, N. Ono, O. Khorram, A. Ottlecz, J. Koenig, J. Bedran de Castro, L. Krulich and W.K. Samson. Department of Physiology, University of Texas Health Science Center at Dallas, Dallas, Texas 75235.

A host of peptides has been found to be resident within the hypothalamus. It now appears likely that ultra short-loop feedback actions of releasing and inhibiting hormones to alter their own release and that of other brain peptides are the rule rather than the exception. For example, somatostatin (panhibin) elevates rather than lowering GH release following its intraventricular injection, an action thought to be due either to inhibition of panhibin release within the hypothalamus and/or to stimulation of GH-releasing factor (GRF) release. Panhibin also inhibits release of TSH, FSH and LH suggesting that it reduces release of LHRH and TRH. GRF injected intraventricularly at doses too low to have a direct pituitary action lowers rather than elevating GH release, presumably by inhibiting its own release within the hypothalamus and/or stimulating panhibin release. Motilin, another peptide found in the hypothalamus, which can stimulate GH by direct action on the pituitary also inhibits GH release following its intraventricular injection, presumably due to reduction in output of GRF's. Corticotrophin releasing factor (CRF) injected intraventricularly in doses too low to act directly on the gland augments stress-induced ACTH release, presumably an example of positive ultra short-loop feedback of the peptide to augment its own release in stress. Under resting conditions, intraventricular CRF results in a decline in plasma GH and a decline in LH only at high doses in ovariectomized animals suggesting that it induces the stress pattern of release of LHRH and GRF. Oxytocin, which stimulates prolactin (Prl) release from male or lactating rat pituitary cells _in vitro_, inhibits Prl release following its intraventricular injection which is probably another example of ultra short-loop feedback. Various members of the secretin family of peptides such as VIP, secretin and PHI can directly stimulate the lactotrophs to release Prl and yet secretin has an inhibitory action on Prl release following its intraventricular injection. Another member of this family, gastric inhibitory polypeptide (GIP), directly stimulates pituitary FSH and LH secretion and yet when injected into the ventricle has a selective inhibitory action on FSH release, again reminisent of an ultra short-loop feedback mechanism. Similarly, angiotensin II which stimulates Prl release by direct action on the lactotrophs, inhibits Prl release when placed in the third ventricle. β-endorphin acts to stimulate Prl and GH at a hypothalamic level while inhibiting LH by actions on different opiate receptors within the hypothalamus. Hypothalamic α-MSH has a physiologically significant action to inhibit LH and Prl release via a dopaminergic mechanism. Thus, there are important hypothalamic peptide interactions which control the release of hypophysiotropic hormones. Supported by AM-10073 and HD-09988.

S.29 ALTERATION IN DISTRIBUTIONS OF PROLACTIN IN LACTOTROPHS UNDER VARIOUS PHYSIOLOGICAL CONDITIONS: IMMUNOELECTRON MICROSCOPIC INVESTIGATIONS. Paul K. Nakane*, Robert Y. Osamura, Departments of Cell Biology and Pathology, Tokai University School of Medicine, Isehara, Kanagawa, Japan.

The concept that a given physiological state reflects upon the morphology and visa versa has been well established at tissue and cell levels, however a little is documented at the subcellular levels. Because of its well defined effector and response to the effector, endocrine cells are best suited to study the subcellular morphological changes in response to environment. The lactotroph which may be stimulated to produce and secrete prolactin (PRL) by estrogen and may be suppressed by bromocriptine was investigated immunohistochemically using peroxidase-labeled antibody and the pre-embedding method. The pre-embedding method was used because it could define the intracellular sites of PRL in every cell organelles involved in protein synthesis. In the normal female rat with the serum PRL level of 0.3-0.4 μg/ml, the lactotrophs contained PRL in perinuclear space, cisternae of rough endoplasmic reticulum (RER), Golgi saccules and secretory granules. Four weeks after castration when the serum level of PRL was lowered to 0.1 μg/ml, the lactotrophs were hypotrophic and entered the storage phase. With these cells, cytoplasm was filled with PRL-positive condensed secretory granules. RER and Golgi saccules were reduced in size and contained little or no PRL. Four days after administration of estrogen to the castrated rats and the serum level of PRL was increased to 0.3-0.5 μg/ml, the lactotrophs were hypertrophic and entered the active secretory phase. With these cells, the cytoplasms were filled with lamellar or whorled RER with PRL. Golgi saccules and secretory granules were less in number and contained little PRL. At the periphery of the cytoplasm, PRL positive RER were found frequently in juxtaposition to the inner surface of plasma membrane. With estrogen-induced rat prolactinoma (serum PRL level of over 1 μg/ml) and with human prolactinoma (serum PRL level of 0.1-10 μg/ml), following treatment with bromocriptine (the serum PRL level was lowered to less than 0.1 μg/ml in rats and to 0.01-0.3 μg/ml in human), the sites of PRL was shifted from the cisternae of RER and Golgi saccules to condensed secretory granules as the number of secretory granules increased and RER and Golgi complexes atrophied. This phenomenon resembled the shift observed in the rat lactotrophs following castration and estrogen treatments and suggests that the bromocriptine treatment shifts the active PRL producing phase of the neoplastic cells to the inactive storage state. Depending upon the functional phase of lactotrophs, the size, shape and number of secretory granules and possibly the content of PRL in each secretory granule varied considerably and it was difficult to define the cell types without the aid of immunoelectron microscopy.

S.30 THE ROLE OF CALCIUM, ADENYLATE CYCLASE AND PHOSPHOLIPIDS IN THE CONTROL OF PROLACTIN SECRETION: RELATION TO DOPAMINERGIC INHIBITION.

R.M. MacLEOD,* Department of Internal Medicine, University of Virginia School of Medicine, Charlottesville, Virginia, U.S.A.

Prolactin release from the anterior pituitary may be mediated via several interacting biochemical systems whose activity may be modulated by TRH and dopamine. Calcium plays a major role in prolactin release since decreasing extracellular calcium or blockade of cellular calcium channels reduces basal prolactin release while, conversely, calcium ionophores or the calcium channel activator maitotoxin markedly increase Ca^{2+} influx and prolactin release. The intracellular effect of calcium may be partially mediated by calmodulin since basal and secretagogue-induced prolactin release is decreased by drugs that bind and inactivate calmodulin. TRH is well documented to increase cytoplasmic calcium, which may be an important step in TRH-induced prolactin secretion. Dopamine decreases the prolactin release induced by ionophore or maitotoxin and therefore exerts at least part of its action following calcium mobilization .

cAMP appears to increase prolactin release in primary pituitary cell cultures, while dopamine suppresses cellular cAMP content by reducing the activity of adenylate cyclase activity. It appears that the calcium and adenylate cyclase systems may interact because ionophore and maitotoxin cause an increase in prolactin secretion and cAMP content whereas dopamine inhibits both processes.

Phospholipid metabolism may likewise be associated with prolactin release because TRH increases while dopamine decreases pituitary phosphotylinositol turnover. These changes in phospholipid turnover may modify prolactin secretion directly or by altering the activity of phospholipid metabolites such as diacylglycerol or arachidonic acid. In support of the latter hypothesis, synthetic diacylglycerol has been demonstrated to stimulate prolactin secretion. This effect is markedly potentiated by low concentrations of either calcium ionophore or maitotoxin and may therefore be at least partially mediated by an activation of protein kinase C (phospholipid sensitive protein kinase). The finding that phorbol esters, which activate protein kinase C, stimulate prolactin secretion supports this hypothesis. Likewise arachidonate may be important in prolactin release because TRH increases pituitary arachidonate release within one minute, an effect attenuated by dopamine. Furthermore exogenous arachidonate stimulates prolactin release because pharmacological agents that alter arachidonate production modify basal and secretagogue-induced prolactin secretion.

In conclusion calcium, adenylate cyclase, and phospholipid metabolism may all have diverse and interrelated roles in regulating the release of prolactin.

S.31 STRUCTURE AND REGULATION OF THE HUMAN PROLACTIN (hPRL) GENE. J.A. Martial*, A.T. Truong, J.N. Laverrière, C. Duez, G.I. Bell[1] and A. Belayew, Laboratoire de Génie Génétique, Université de Liège, Belgium. [1] Present address: Chiron Corporation, Emeryville, California USA.

Prolactin, growth hormone (GH) and chorionic somatomammotropin (CS) form a group of related hormones which is thought to have evolved from a common ancestral protein. DNA copies (cDNA) of the messenger RNAs (mRNA) coding for PRL, GH and CS from several species have been cloned in bacteria. The cloned cDNAs have been used for several purposes. First, they have been sequenced leading to data from which the amino acid sequences of the proteins have been obtained or verified. Second, the cloned cDNAs have been used as probes to clone and characterize the genomic DNA coding for these hormones. In rat for example, GH and PRL are each encoded by a gene present only once per haploid genome. In human, by contrasts, 5 genes at least code for GH and CS. Recently, we screened the Maniatis human genomic DNA library in λ phage and isolated a single recombinant comprizing the whole human PRL gene. This gene was characterized by restriction endonuclease mapping and cDNA hybridization, by DNA heteroduplex analysis and by nucleotide sequencing. The hPRL gene is present as a single copy per haploid genome, is about 10 Kb long and contains 4 introns, 3 of which interrupt the coding sequence at the same locations as in the known GH and PRL genes. The origin of transcription was determined by S1 mapping using mRNA extracted from human prolactinoma : it corresponds to an A residue located 57 bp upstream of the initial ATG and 29 bp downstream of the TATA box. Several direct and inverted repeats, as well as dyad symmetries have been located in the 5' flanking region of the gene (about 1 Kb sequenced to date). No definite pattern however could be drawned since this region was very AT rich. We have also compared the hPRL gene with other members of the GH-CS-PRL gene family. Whereas the human GH and CS genes are very homologous, very little conservation remains between the hPRL and hGH genes. Interestingly a 15 bp sequence is present in the same position relative to the origin of transcription (-122 bp) in all the GH, CS and PRL genes sequenced to date. When the 5' flanking regions of the human and rat PRL genes were compared, five conserved DNA sequences were found (with 80-90% homology versus 73% in the coding regions) The largest one spans 136 bp and shows a 90% homology. In vitro studies of chromatin proteins and hormone receptors binding to the hPRL gene as well as in vivo assays are currently under way to find out the biological role, if any, of all these conserved sequences. Finally the cDNAs have been used to study the molecular mechanisms which control the in vivo expression of the GH and PRL genes. For example, TRH is known to inversely regulate GH and PRL synthesis by modulating the levels of their specific mRNAs. We have shown (work performed in collaboration with the team of A. Tixier-Vidal, Paris) that these changes in mRNA levels involve both transcriptional and post-transcriptional events. Indeed, on one hand, TRH increases in a rapid but transient manner the transcription of the PRL gene whereas, after a lag-time, it inhibits the GH gene transcription. On the other hand, our results show that without altering the processing or the transport of the mRNAs to the cytoplasm, TRH significantly increases the half-life of PRL mRNA while it decreases the half-life of GH mRNA.

S.32 IDENTIFICATION OF A PROLACTIN INTRACELLULAR MEDIATOR ACTING ON MILK PROTEIN GENES.
L.M. Houdebine*, J. Djiane, B. Teyssot, P.A. Kelly, E. Devinoy, I. Dusanter-Fourt, J.L. Servely and P. Martel, Laboratoire de Physiologie de la Lactation, CNRZ-INRA, 78350 Jouy-en-Josas, France and Laboratoire d'Endocrinologie Moléculaire, Université McGill, Montréal, Canada H3A 1A1

Prolactin is the major hormone controlling the expression of milk protein genes. Its effects are amplified by several hormones including insulin and glucocorticoids which are inactive alone and they are inhibited by progesterone. Prolactin induces casein synthesis in vivo and in cultured mammary explants. This induction is coincident with an accumulation of casein mRNAs and with a stimulation of casein gene transcription. Prolactin also favors casein mRNA stabilization and translation. Moreover, prolactin is responsible for the multiplication and the hypertrophy of the mammary cell. Hence, prolactin delivers multiple messages to the mammary cell. All these messages are transfered through specific receptors located in cell membranes. The prolactin receptor is down-regulated by the hormone through the internalization of the hormone-receptor complex but the hormonal stimulations are not abolished when this down-regulation is inhibited. The prolactin effects on casein mRNA accumulation and on DNA synthesis are mimicked by anti-prolactin receptor antibodies at low concentration of antibodies. Hence, prolactin is not required beyond its receptors and a relay must be formed at the membrane level. Mammary membranes incubated with prolactin release a soluble factor which directly stimulates casein gene transcription when added to isolated mammary nuclei. This factor is generated by other membranes containing prolactin receptor but not by those devoid of receptor. Only lactogenic hormones induce the generation of the factor and only mammary nuclei are sensitive to it. Bivalent (Fab'_2) but not monovalent (Fab) anti-prolactin receptor antibodies induce casein synthesis in explants and formation of the factor when added to isolated membranes. Several drugs (colchicine, phorbol esters sodium butyrate, amiloride) which inhibit prolactin actions in cultured mammary explants also prevent the generation of the factor when they are added to isolated membranes. The membrane supernatants containing the factor mimic prolactin action on casein mRNA accumulation when added to culture medium of isolated mammary cell. The factor stimulates specifically transcription of α_{s1}-, β-casein and α-lactalbumine genes. Its effect is totally abolished by various inhibitors of phosphatase but not by those acting on tyrosine phosphatase. Several inhibitors of RNA initiation prevent the action of the factor. As judged by the use of (γ-S)ATP, (γ-S)GTP and (α^{32}-P)UTP or of (β-^{35}S)ATP and (β-^{35}S)GTP followed by a chromatography on Hg-cellulose and an hybridization with the plasmid probes, the factor acts essentially on initiation of milk protein gene transcription and this effect is blocked by phosphatase inhibitors. This factor is a good candidate to be a prolactin intracellular mediator. It is thermostable and inactivated by proteases. It is eluted as a molecule of 5,000 - 6,000 molecular weight from A_cA_{202} gel and it is poorly retained on C-18 column in HPLC. Prolactin mediator stimulates several insulin sensitive enzymes in various cell-free systems whereas insulin mediator from liver and muscle stimulates casein gene transcription in mammary nuclei. These data incline to think that a new family of hormone mediators acting on enzymes or genes via an activation of phosphatase has been identified.

S.33 PHYSIOLOGICAL STUDIES OF A NEW ALDOSTERONE STIMULATING FACTOR. E. L. Bravo*, Research Division, Cleveland Clinic Foundation, Cleveland, Ohio, U.S.A.

We report the steroidogenic properties of an aldosterone-stimulating glycoprotein (MW = 26,000 daltons) isolated from urine of normal humans. When injected into normal rats, it produces sustained hypertension, hypervolemia, and increases in plasma aldosterone without alterations in plasma corticosterone. In *in vitro* studies utilizing the cat adrenocortical collagenase-dispersed cells, we have found that ASF produced dose-related increases in aldosterone and cortisol production following incubation at 37°C for 2 hours. However, its effect was not as potent as either angiotensin II or III. In addition, its steroidogenic effect was not associated with increases in cyclic AMP, could not be inhibited by specific competitive antagonist of angiotensin II and could be prevented by the absence of potassium in incubation media. These preliminary results suggest that the compound initiates steroidogenesis by mechanisms similar to that of angiotensin II; however, the inability to block its effect on steroidogenesis with a specific competitive antagonist of angiotensin II provides evidence of its action on a separate receptor site. In additional studies, it was also found that while a specific competitive antagonist of ACTH (Ile^9, $ACTH_{1-24}$) inhibited the response to both ACTH and beta-lipotropin, it had no effect on ASF-induced increases in aldosterone production. This strongly suggests that the new ASF interacts with receptor sites distinct from those of either ACTH or beta-lipotropin. In more recent studies, the requirements for its in vitro steroidogenic activity have been more clearly defined. Utilizing rabbit adrenocortical collagenase-dispersed cells, we have demonstrated that urinary ASF is less potent ($ED_{50} = 10^{-9}M$) than either angiotensin II ($ED_{50} = 8 \times 10^{-11}M$) or ACTH ($ED_{50} = 4 \times 10^{-11}M$). Increases in cyclic AMP accompanied the steroidogenic response to ACTH, but not to either urinary ASF or Ang II. Deprivation of potassium or calcium in incubation media or the addition of ouabain (1 mM) during incubation completely inhibited the steroidogenic response to either urinary ASF, ACTH, or Ang II. However, the aldosterone-stimulating activity of ASF did not appear to be as dependent on potassium concentration in media as that of angiotensin II. Whereas the aldosterone response to angiotensin II did not reach maximal until the potassium concentration was at least 4.0 mM, urinary ASF produced maximal responses with potassium concentrations of 2.0 mM. At potassium concentrations of 8.0 mM, the increase in aldosterone achieved was not different from that produced when combined with maximal doses of either Ang II, ACTH or urinary ASF. Thus the mechanisms by which urinary ASF stimulate aldosterone production are readily distinguishable from ACTH. In the first place, ASF-induced steroid responses are not associated with increased generation of cAMP, while those of ACTH are. Secondly, and more importantly, its ability to stimulate aldosterone production could not be inhibited by [Ile^9] ACTH, a specific competitive antagonist of ACTH. Although it shares some similarities with Ang II, the inability of a specific angiotensin II antagonist to inihibt its steroidogenic activity indicates that it acts at a separate receptor site. Finally, like Ang II and ACTH, urinary ASF is highly dependent on potassium for its steroidogenic action.

S.34 PHYSIOLOGICAL REGULATION OF ALDOSTERONE SECRETION IN THE RAT.

*G P Vinson, +B J Whitehouse, P W Raven and J P Hinson. Department of Biochemistry, St Bartholomew's Hospital Medical College, Charterhouse Square, LONDON EC1M 6BQ. +Department of Physiology, Queen Elizabeth College, LONDON W8 7AH

The study of aldosterone (aldo) production and the factors which stimulate it, has been carried out in a wide variety of in vivo and in vitro preparations, and in recent years much in vitro work has utilised the collagenase-treated dispersed cell preparation. Less attention has been paid to the way in which the nature of the preparation may affect the responses to stimulation, or the validity of extrapolating from the in vitro to the in vivo condition. In the rat adrenal the output of aldo greatly depends on the in vitro tissue preparation. Using intact capsules (to which the glomerulosa cells adhere) yields of aldo may be 50% of those of corticosterone (B) under basal conditions or when stimulated eg. by ACTH. Typical results are (aldo:B) basal 105 ± 8: 385 ± 14 ng/gland pair; ACTH-stimulated 405 ± 35: 855 ± 82 ng/gland pair. Much less aldo is produced both absolutely and relative to B in collagenase-dispersed capsule/glomerulosa cells, often only 5% of whole tissue yields. Typical results with ACTH stimulation are: aldo 39 ± 3; B 785 ± 34 ng/gland pair equivalent. These differences cannot be accounted for by changes in rates of aldo synthesis. Instead it seems likely that aldo is sequestered in intracellular pools. These are released by proteolytic mechanisms which are mimicked by trypsin. Incubation of whole capsule tissue with trypsin releases aldo (typical results are: basal 175 ± 26; trypsin (1mg/ml) 502 ± 41 ng/gland pair) but trypsin is ineffective in collagenase-dispersed cells. Thus differences in the output of aldosterone reflect a fundamental difference in the mechanism of secretion of aldo in intact tissue as compared with isolated cells. This has an important bearing on the interpretation of in vitro results. In studies on the role of α-MSH as a regulator of aldosterone secretion in the rat, stimulation of B production by dispersed glomerulosa cells was observed at 10^{-10} moles per l, whereas aldo was only stimulated at higher concentrations (10^{-7} moles per l). In the intact perfused gland, in contrast, aldo was preferentially stimulated. Typical results were: with 0.1μg α-MSH (bolus injection) aldo was increased 3.2 - fold, B was unaffected. With 1μg α-MSH stimulation ratios were 6.7 (aldo) and 1.78 (B). The results indicate that the function of the integrated glomerulosa tissue is to produce aldo, and not B: in this respect the perfused gland reflects in vivo results. In dispersed cells, the capacity to form aldo is greatly impaired, partly because of the loss of preformed aldo stores during preparation of cells. The nature of the response to stimulation is therefore greatly dependent on the tissue preparation used, with important implications for our understanding of the system. The results obtained with the in situ perfused gland suggest that α-MSH is potentially an important physiological regulator of aldo secretion in the rat.

S.35 INTERACTION OF POTASSIUM (K^+) AND THE RENIN-ANGIOTENSIN SYSTEM (RAS) ON ALDOSTERONE SECRETION IN NORMAL AND PATHOPHYSIOLOGIC STATES.

M. Schambelan* and A. Sebastian. University of California Medical Service, San Francisco General Hospital, San Francisco, CA 94110 USA.

Aldosterone secretion is known to be influenced by at least 5 factors: the RAS, ACTH, Na^+, K^+, and dopamine. Of these, the RAS and K^+ appear to be the predominant influences particularly in pathophysiologic states characterized by altered volume or electrolyte homeostasis. To determine the relative influences of renin (PRA, ng/ml/h) and plasma K^+ (mEq/L) on urinary aldosterone excretion ($U_{aldo}V$, μg/24h) we performed chronic metabolic balance studies in 21 normal subjects: during treatment with amiloride (AML), 30-40 mg/d for 10 days (N=5); after dietary NaCl restriction (LSD), 2-7 mEq/d for 14 days (N=4); while on a normal Na^+ and K^+ diet (NSD, N=17); and after 15 days of dietary K^+ restriction (LoK) with (N=4) and without (N=5) concomitant NaCl restriction. The mean ± SEM for these values and for the ratio $U_{aldo}V/K^+$ are:

Groups	PRA	Plasma K^+	$U_{aldo}V$	$U_{aldo}V/K^+$
AML	36.9±5.5	5.5±0.2	207.2±41.0	38.0±7.8
LSD	14.5±3.1	4.2±0.1	94.2±11.7	23.7±2.6
LSD LoK	9.1±2.4	2.9±0.1	9.9± 2.4	3.5±0.7
NSD	2.2±0.3	4.0±0.1	15.6± 1.4	3.9±0.4
NSD LoK	0.2±0.1	3.0±0.1	1.5± 0.2	0.4±0.1

PRA correlated with both $U_{aldo}V$ ($r=0.91$, $p < 0.001$, N=35) and $U_{aldo}V/K^+$ ($r=0.92$, $p < 0.001$); $U_{aldo}V$ also correlated with K^+ ($r=0.71$, $p < 0.001$). The interaction between PRA and K^+ was also examined in two well-known clinical disorders: Bartter's syndrome (N=12) in which $U_{aldo}V$ is "normal" (15.5±1.1 μg/24 h) despite hyperreninemia (12.7±1.6 ng/ml/h) as a consequence of profound hypokalemia (2.5±0.1 mEq/L); and isolated hypoaldosteronism (N=19) in which $U_{aldo}V$ is subnormal (3.2±0.4) despite hyperkalemia (5.3±0.1) as a consequence of hyporeninemia (0.3±0.1). $U_{aldo}V/K^+$ defines the presence of hyperaldosteronism (6.2±0.5) and hypoaldosteronism (0.6±0.2) in these two conditions. These data suggest a predominant role for the RAS in the control of aldosterone secretion that is modified by concomitant changes in K^+ in both physiologic and pathophysiologic states.

S.36 SIGNALLING TRANSMISSION PROCESS OF ANGIOTENSIN II AND POTASSIUM IN ADRENAL GLOMERULOSA PLASMA MEMBRANE. E.T. Marusic*, M.V. Lobo and R. Foster. Dept. Physiology and Biophysics, Sch. Medicine, Univ. of Chile, Santiago, Chile.

In the adrenal cortex, angiotensin II (A II) binds to specific receptor sites and exert direct stimulatory action upon adrenal glomerulosa cells. The mechanism of this effect is complex and poorly understood at the present time. Recent studies from this and other laboratories have shown that the activation of steroidogenesis in isolated glomerulosa cells by A II and potassium is mediated by calcium. Removal of extracellular Ca or addition of verapamil abolishes A II and potassium induced aldosterone release. Conversely the calcium ionophore (A 23187) can induce aldosterone secretion.- It has been postulated by several authors that A II and potassium exert their actions to stimulate steroidogenesis through a common pathway. However, although Ca is required for the steroidogenesic response of glomerulosa cells to A II and potassium, we will present evidence that membrane signalling transmission process for A II Action is different from that of potassium.

Previously we have demostrated that A II and potassium stimulate the uptake of ^{45}Ca into glomerulosa cells and that A II also increased significatly the efflux of Ca from preloaded cells. Furhher studies reveled that when Ca^{2+} was substituted by Sr^{2+}, there was a significant aldosterone response to A II, but no stimulus of potassium on steroidogenesis was observed in the presence of Sr^{2+}.- When membrane potential chnnges of adrenal cells were studied in the presence of both stimuli, the results revealed again a different pattern. Small changes in external potassium induced a calcium-dependent depolarization of glomerulosa cells concomitantly with the steroidogenic effect. The same concentration of potassium produced a minor depolarization in fasciculata cells.- On the other hand, A II induced a biphasic effect on membrane potential of glomerulosa cells; a short hyperpolarization, followed by membrane depolarization was observed.- To investigate the initial hyperpolarization induced by A II, we have measured Na, K - ATPase in the glomerulosa cells; enzyme activity was not modified by the polypeptide hormone. However, we were able to find a calcium-dependent potassium channel in the glomerulosa cells membranes that is activated by A II. The effect of A II in the potassium conductance was trasient. The relationship between this potassium channel and the steroidogenesis has to be established; nevertheles, quinine that blocks the effect of A II on calcium-dependent potassium conductance, also blocks its steroidogenic effect. The ionophore A 23187 has a stimulatory effect on both steroidogenesis and potassium permeability.

We suggest that multiple transduction mechanisms are likely involved in calcium mediated secretory events in adrenal glomerulosa cells.

S.37 ALLEVIATION OF SIDE EFFECTS PRODUCED BY GOSSYPOL USED AS MALE CONTRACEPTIVE. G.Z. Liu*, J. Cao and Kathy Ch'iu, Capital Hospital, Beijing, China and The Rockefeller Foundation, New York, U.S.A.

For over 10 years gossypol has been considered by Chinese workers an effective male antifertility agent. Recently progress has been made towards the goal of developing gossypol as a publicly available male oral contraceptive. However, despite its satisfactory antifertility effect and non-interference with sex hormones, gossypol is not without disadvantages which consist mainly of hypo-kalemia in a minority of cases. Supplementary potassium salts or potassium-sparing agents should be helpful in preventing hypo-kalemia. Our most recent study involves comparison of results in 4 groups of volunteers that take gossypol alone, gossypol plus potassium salt, gossypol plus triamterene and a 4th group taking nothing. It is anticipated that only the group taking gossypol alone will show tendency of serum potassium decline while the other 3 groups remain normo-kalemic.

S.38 GnRH ANALOGUES FOR FERTILITY CONTROL IN MAN. S.J. Nillius*, Section for Reproductive Endocrinology and Infertility, Department of Obstetrics and Gynecology, University Hospital, 751 85 Uppsala, Sweden.

The identification and synthesis of the hypothalamic gonadotropin-releasing hormone (GnRH) by Schally and his co-workers in 1971 provided the basis for a new class of contraceptives. It was anticipated that it might be possible to synthesize competitive inhibitors of GnRH which would exert contraceptive effects in the human. Antagonistic analogues of GnRH have been synthesized since then. During the last few years, their biological potency has steadily increased. However, no clinical contraceptive trials have been performed with GnRH antagonists as yet. Paradoxically, highly potent long-acting agonistic analogues of GnRH, which were synthesized for stimulation of fertility, proved on chronic administration to exert anti-fertility effects. The contraceptive potential of superagonists of GnRH has therefore been extensively explored during recent years.

In females, inhibition of ovulation can be acheived by prolonged intranasal GnRH agonist treatment. The daily superagonist administration results in pituitary desensitization with failure of estradiol to induce positive feedback on luteinizing hormone secretion. The induced anovulation causes acceptable bleeding disturbances, oligo-amenorrhea, but chronic GnRH agonist treatment has not resulted in any other serious adverse effects. Long-term studies of this new method of birth control have shown that continous intranasal GnRH agonist therapy can provide safe, effective and rapidly reversible contraception in women.

Luteolysis can be induced in women by mid-luteal phase administration of GnRH agonists. The timing of the superagonist administration is critical for its effectiveness. Furthermore, exogenous human chorionic gonadotropin prevents the luteolytic effect. Attempts to induce early abortion by high doses of superactive GnRH agonists have been unsuccessful. Results of clinical trials with early follicular phase GnRH agonist administration to produce defective luteal function have not been convincing. The contraceptive effectiveness of the luteolytic approaches remains to be established.

In males, spermatogenesis can be reversibly suppressed by long-term high dose GnRH agonist administration. The prolonged superagonist treatment results in pituitary desensitization with inhibition of gonadotropin secretion associated with a decline of testicular steroidogenesis. The result is highly undesirable side-effects of decreased libido and impotence. Thus, GnRH agonists alone can not be used as male contraceptive agents. Androgen replacement with testosterone injections is necessary to prevent the negative effects on libido and potency. Testosterone not only obviates these adverse effects but also has additive or synergistic inhibitory effects on the pituitary gonadotropin secretion. Combined therapy with superactive GnRH agonists and androgens is therefore at present being tested for male contraception.

Thus, to date inhibition of ovulation by daily intranasal GnRH agonist administration seems to be the most promising approach to peptide contraception in man.

S.39 THE IMMUNOLOGICAL DISRUPTION OF FERTILIZATION.

R.J. Aitken*
MRC Unit of Reproductive Biology, 37 Chalmers Street, Edinburgh EH3 9EW Scotland, U.K.

In our search for an immunological solution to the problem of contraception, the process of fertilization represents a logical point of attack. This process involves a complex series of specific interactions between the male and female gametes, many of which are thought to be mediated by glycoproteins and therefore susceptible to immunological interference.

One of the most promising targets for an anti-fertility vaccine is the zona pellucida, an acellular glycoprotein shell which is deposited around the oocyte during folliculogenesis and continues to protect the developing embryo upto the moment of implantation. In addition to the physical protection it affords, the zona pellucida contains species specific receptor sites which bind spermatozoa during the early stages of fertilization and then lose their binding affinity during the subsequent block to polyspermy. Antibodies directed against the zona pellucida block fertilization *in vitro* by inducing the formation of an immunoprecipitate on the outer surface of this structure and occluding the sperm binding sites by steric hindrance. Active immunization models employing heterologous zona antigens have been used to investigate whether anti-zona antibodies are also capable of blocking fertilization *in vivo*. Studies involving actively immunized laboratory rodents and primates have demonstrated that the induction of immunity against the zona pellucida *in vivo*, results in the generation of infertility without any overt adverse side effects. The duration of infertility is related to anti-zona antibody titre and is fully reversed when antibody titres decline. The feasibility of this approach to contraception has been strengthened by clinical data correlating idiopathic infertility with the presence of circulating auto-antibodies against the zona pellucida.

The production of auto- or iso-antibodies against sperm antigens has also been associated with human infertility, suggesting that the spermatozoon might be a suitable target for the development of a contraceptive vaccine. The mechanism of action of such antibodies is thought to involve the disruption of sperm migration through the endocervical canal, the inhibition of fertilization and the induction of abortion. Monoclonal antibodies are currently being used to identify unique sperm surface antigens which are critical to the process of fertilization and which might be used as the basis of a safe, effective antifertility vaccine.

S.40 THE ANTIPROGESTERONE STEROID RU-486 : A 'CONTRAGESTIVE' AGENT IN THE HUMAN.

E. Sakiz*, C. Euvrard and E.E. Baulieu, Roussel Uclaf and Inserm U33, Paris, France.

RU-486 (17β -hydroxy-11β(4-dimethylaminophenyl 1)-17α (prop-1-ynyl)-estra-4, 9-dien-3-one), is a new 19-norsteroid displaying antiprogesterone activity with no agonistic effect in the animal system so far studied. It shows very high affinity for the progesterone receptor and the binding is reversible. In animals, RU-486 antagonizes the effects of endogenous and exogenous progesterone in the genital tract and the pituitary. These remarkable antiprogesterone pharmacological properties led us to investigate the RU-486 efficacy in women during the menstrual cycle and for the interruption of early pregnancy. This was done after systematic verification of the absence of any toxic effect, as well as of the good tolerance of the molecule. Studies of the effects of RU-486 on the menstrual cycle were carried out through administration of the product on various days of the luteal phase, at various doses (50, 100 or 200 mg/day) and for various lengths of time (up to 4 days). In all cases, bleeding occurred within 3 days after the first intake. RU-486 was also administered to volunteers for the medical interruption of early pregnancy (4 to 10 weeks). This was performed by giving 50, 100 or 200 mg/day (divided in morning and evening administration) for 4 days. The results obtained until now show : a) the occurrence of bleeding in all cases between the 2nd and 4th day after treatment began ; b) the remarkable efficiency (over 80 %) for interrupting very early pregnancy (up to 7 weeks) ; further studies are in progress to improve the yield of interruptions in 8-10 week old pregnancies ; c) RU-486 was equally effective at all doses which have been used ; d) return to normal physiology was observed by the next cycle. RU-486 was always extremely well tolerated and no clinical or biological side-effects were observed. However, since the compound also demonstrates antiglucocorticosteroid properties, its effects on the pituitary-adrenal axis were examined in detail. No change in cortisol, ACTH and β -endorphin were observed after 50 mg/day ; after 200 mg/day, a significant rise in the three hormones was observed, ceasing when administration was stopped. No periphereal sign of adrenal insufficiency was ever recorded. These preliminary results confirm the antiprogesterone activity of RU-486 in women and the potential usefulness of this type of molecule for a new 'contragestive' approach of fertility control in human. Three protocols may be envisaged : 1. for medical interruption of early pregnancy ; 2. in case of delayed menstruation, as a 'menses inducer' ; 3. monthly, at the end of the cycle. In all cases, such a product has the advantage of maintaining the menstrual cycle and its hormonal balance until it is needed, and this should help towards its wide use in fertility control. Data reported here have been obtained with Pr. W. Herrmann, Dr. R. Wyss, Dr. A. Riondel and Dr. R. Gaillard (Geneva) ; Dr. L. Kovacs (Szeged) and Pr. M. Bygdeman (Stockholm), within the frame of WHO's Special Programme of Research in Human Reproduction ; with Dr. W. Bardin and Dr. I. Spitz (New York), in a Population Council programme ; Dr. G. Hodgen and Dr. D. Healy (Bethesda), thanks to The National Institute of Child Health and Human Development ; with Pr. A. Haspels (Utrecht) ; Dr. D. Elia (Paris), Pr. G. Schaison (Bicêtre) and our own colleagues.

S.41 ANALYSIS OF INSULIN GENE POLYMORPHISM IN NON-INSULIN DEPENDENT DIABETICS (NIDD).

Permutt, M.A.,* Andreone, T.A., Chirgwin, J., Elbein, S. and Rotwein, P. Washington University School of Medicine, St. Louis, MO

Monozygotic twins have a high concordance rate for NIDD indicating a strong genetic component, yet the nature of the gene defect is unknown. To evaluate the possiblity differences exist in either structural or regulatory regions of insulin genes in NIDD, blot hybridization analysis of leukocyte DNA was performed. Following digestion, the resulting DNA fragments were electrophoresed, blotted onto filters, and hybridized with radiolabeled cloned human insulin gene probes derived from various portions of the gene. A high degree of length polymorphism approximately 500 base pairs 5' (upstream) of the transcription inititation site was noted. This region has been shown by G. Belle, et.al. to be composed of a series of tandem oligonuceotide repeats of approximately 14 base pairs. The length polymorphism in individuals has been presumed to be due to the presence of variable numbers of repeats, although only two alleles have been sequenced to date.

We initially noted an association of a particular polymorphic insulin gene with NIDD. Observations have now been extended to approximately 500 non-related individuals of Caucasian, American Indian (Pima, in collaboration with M. Knowler and D. Pettit, NIH, Phoenix, Ariz.), and American Black racial groups. The frequency of polymorphic alleles differed in the three racial groups. There was no association of any particular insulin gene with NIDD in Caucasians or Pima Indians. In Blacks there appeared to be a significant increase in occurence of a particular polymorphic allele with NIDD in the homozygous state. Current investigation is focusing on extending the population sample size in Blacks and determining the nature of the polymorphic alleles and their effect on insulin secretion in the various groups.

S.42 RECEPTOR BINDING AND SIGNAL TRANSDUCTION IN DIABETIC SYNDROMES IN MAN.

C.R. Kahn*, F. Grigorescu, J. Flier, and O.P. Ganda, Joslin Diabetes Center, Boston, Massachusetts 02215 U.S.A.

The insulin receptor consists of two different subunits, the α subunit (M_r = 135,000) which contains the insulin binding site, and the β subunit (M_r = 95,000) which is an insulin-sensitive protein kinase and is believed to be important in receptor signal transmission. Previous studies have implicated alterations in both insulin binding and post-binding steps in insulin action in the pathogenesis of diabetes. The role of the kinase activity in signal transduction in diabetes is uncertain, as is the question of whether either of these abnormalities is a primary vs. secondary defect. We have attempted to answer these questions by studying insulin receptor binding and kinase activity in two different diabetic syndromes in man.

The syndrome of insulin resistance and acanthosis nigricans Type A is characterized by severe insulin resistance due to a primary defect in insulin action at the cellular level. The receptor defect in Type A patients is heterogenous. In some patients, the primary defect consists of a major decrease in insulin binding which is observed in several different cellular systems derived from the patients including erythrocytes, monocytes, and fibroblasts. This defect is also retained in the solubilized form of the receptor. In these cases, the kinase activity of the receptor is also markedly decreased, as evidenced by a decrease in insulin-stimulated receptor phosphorylation over the entire insulin dose-response curve. Interestingly, in one case, a significant reduction in kinase activity was observed in the presence of unaltered insulin binding. Thus, in this patient, the "post-binding" defect in insulin action seems to be located at the level of the receptor kinase activity.

We have also studied insulin binding and kinase activity in monozygotic twin pairs discordant for Type II diabetes, since in this setting it should be possible to distinguish genetic from acquired factors. Three twin pairs were studied in which the twins had been discordant for diabetes for 10-20 years. Two of the twin pairs were of normal body weight, while in the third pair, only the diabetic twin was obese. In all three pairs, insulin binding to circulating erythrocytes and monocytes was lower in the diabetic patient than in the non-affected twin mate. The average decrease in insulin binding was small, and thus in most cases, data on both twins actually fell within the normal range. Quantitative analysis of the binding data revealed that this decrease in binding was due to a decrease in receptor affinity rather than a decrease in receptor number. Insulin receptor autophosphorylation was studied using receptors extracted from the erythrocytes of one pair of twins. Although autophosphorylation was similar at maximal insulin concentrations, the dose-response curve for the diabetic twin was shifted to the right, consistent with the lower receptor affinity.

In summary, in both Type II diabetes and the Type A syndrome, there may be defects in insulin binding, receptor kinase activation, or in the coupling of binding to kinase activation. In Type II diabetes, these appear to be acquired defects, since they are observed only in the diabetic member of discordant twin pairs.

S.43 PATHOGENESIS OF TYPE II DIABETES. J.M. Olefsky*, University of California, La Jolla, California, 92093.

Insulin resistance is a characteristic feature of non-insulin dependent, or Type II diabetes mellitus. This insulin resistant state is characterized by multiple defects. Receptor and post-receptor defects contribute to the resistance to insulin's action to promote overall glucose disposal. In patients with mild fasting hyperglycemia, both receptor and post-receptor defects contribute to this abnormality. However, as the degree of diabetes and fasting hyperglycemia worsens, the overall insulin resistant state increases and the post-receptor defect becomes the predominant lesion. This post-receptor or post-binding defect is at least partially localized to an intrinsic defect in a glucose transport system. Abnormalities of hepatic glucose production also exist in NIDDM. Thus, accelerated hepatic glucose output is commonly seen in these subjects, and the degree of fasting hyperglycemia is well correlated to the magnitude of increase in hepatic glucose production. It would appear that increased hepatic glucose production as well as defects in overall glucose disposal contribute predominantly to the insulin resistance and hyperglycemia in NIDDM. In addition to these defects in insulin action, multiple abnormalities of insulin secretory dynamics have been described. Since all of these abnormalities co-exist, it is difficult to discern which defect is primary and which is secondary. Various forms of therapy such as insulin, oral sulfonylureas, and diet all lead to partial reversal of these abnormalities.

S.44 DETERMINANTS AND PATHOGENESIS OF NON-INSULIN DEPENDENT DIABETES IN THE PIMA INDIANS.

Peter H. Bennett*, C. Bogardus, J. Foley, W.C. Knowler and D.J. Pettitt, National Institute of Arthritis, Diabetes, and Digestive and Kidney Diseases, Phoenix, Arizona, U.S.A.

Extensive longitudinal studies in the Pima Indian population of Arizona have led to knowledge of some of the determinants and pathogenesis of non-insulin dependent diabetes (NIDDM). The Pima have the highest recognized incidence of NIDDM, which is associated with the development of the same characteristic specific vascular complications of diabetes seen in other populations.

Obesity, preexisting evidence of glucose intolerance and the occurrence of diabetes in at least one parent have each been shown to be strong predictors of the disease, but they also interact with each other.

Bimodality of the glucose tolerance distributions suggests that susceptibility to NIDDM in the Pima may be mainly due to the expression of a single major gene, the identity of which remains obscure, but environmental determinants and the genetic background almost certainly determine if and when the disease becomes manifest. In susceptible subjects, the risk of developing the disease is proportional to the degree of obesity, but in some this risk is also influenced by other factors, such as exposure to a diabetic intrauterine environment.

Hyperinsulinemia is a characteristic of the Pima Indians who are developing NIDDM. Among diabetics mean fasting insulin and C-peptide levels are high, but do not vary appreciably with increasing hyperglycemia although insulin responses to a glucose load diminish. In those with normal and impaired glucose tolerance, the fasting insulin and C-peptide levels rise proportionately with the degree of glucose intolerance, and are higher in the obese than in the non-obese. As no structural abnormality of insulin has been detected among the Pima, it appears that insulin resistance may be an important component in the pathogenesis of the disease.

Recent studies of in vivo insulin action, using glucose clamp techniques, have shown that insulin-mediated glucose disposal rates fall progressively with increasing glucose intolerance among those with normal and impaired glucose tolerance, whereas among the diabetics a uniformly high degree of insulin resistance is seen.

Failure of normal insulin action on glucose disposal, therefore, appears to precede decompensation to diabetes in the Pima, whereas in the established diabetic the degree of hyperglycemia is not directly related to the degree of impairment of insulin-mediated glucose disposal, but rather to hepatic glucose output.

The cellular basis of reduced insulin-mediated glucose disposal may be diminished sensitivity of insulin-stimulated glucose transport, which has been shown in vitro and which perhaps results from a post-binding defect in the coupling of insulin binding and glucose transport. In addition, in the diabetic, a diminished maximal capacity for insulin-stimulated glucose transport, possibly due to diminished transporter synthesis, occurs, but appears to be reversible.

Whether or not the diminished sensitivity of insulin-stimulated glucose transport is directly related to the primary inherited abnormality of NIDDM remains to be elucidated.

S.45 STRUCTURE AND EXPRESSION OF THE HUMAN PARTHYROID HORMONE GENE. H.M. Kronenberg*, J. Hellerman, T. Igarashi, M. Freeman, L. Ivashkiv, A. Rapoport, J.T. Potts, Jr., and R. Mulligan, Endocrine Unit, Massachusetts General Hospital and Harvard Medical School, Boston, Massachusetts 02114, and Department of Biology, Massachusetts Institute of Technology, Cambridge, Massachusetts 02139 USA.

We have isolated the gene encoding human parthyroid hormone (PTH), the major regulator of the level of calcium in blood. The gene was isolated from a lambda phage library, using both blot-hybridization with a cDNA probe, and also using the πVX vector of Seed. The gene contains two intervening sequences--one large one (3.4 kilobases) near the end of the 5'-noncoding sequence, and one small one (103 base pairs) separating the DNA encoding the signal sequence from the DNA encoding the mature hormone. Messenger RNA synthesis starts from two distinct clusters of bases separated from each other by about 30 base pairs. Each transcription start site is located about 30 base pairs downstream from a TATA-type sequence. The PTH gene is represented once in the haploid human genome. The restriction enzyme PstI can be used to detect a gene polymorphism located 2000 base pairs downstream from the gene; this polymorphism is present in about 30% of human chromosomes and therefore is useful for family studies. Classic linkage analysis, as well as the use of the mouse-human hybrid cell lines, have been used to show that the human PTH gene is linked to the β-globin and insulin genes on the short arm of chromosome 11.

Parathyroid hormone is synthesized as a larger precursor, preproparathyroid hormone. The "pre" or signal sequence is likely to direct the hormone across the endoplasmic reticulum and hence along the secretory pathway. During protein synthesis, the signal sequence binds to a signal recognition particle, which carries the polysome to the endoplasmic reticulum. How the protein crosses the membrane and the precise role of the "prepro" sequence in this process are unknown. To analyze the functions of different parts of the precursor sequence, we have used a retroviral vector to express PTH cDNA in cultured cells. Recombinant retrovirus encoding human preproPTH was generated using the psi-2 packaging cell line. This helper-free recombinant retrovirus was used to infect GH4 cells, a prolactin-secreting rat pituitary cell line. Clonal lines of the infected cells produce no infectious virus, synthesize and process preproPTH appropriately, and secrete PTH in response to a hormonal stimulus, thyrotropin-releasing hormone.

Several preproPTH genes encoding mutant proteins have been constructed and expressed in GH4 cells. A mutant missing the first 6 amino acids of the signal sequence functions as well as the normal gene. In contrast, mutants missing the first 10 or 13 amino acids are degraded rapidly without conversion to proPTH or secretiion of PTH from the cells. Another mutant which contains the hydrophobic portion of the signal, but is missing the residues bordering the signal cleavage site, accumulates in the cell without being secreted. A small fraction of the protein is cleavaged, and the cleavage product is efficiently secreted from the cell. Further analysis of these and other mutants will lead to a definition of the steps involved in protein secretion and the multiple roles that precursor sequences play in these steps.

S.46 EXPRESSION OF METALLOTHIONEIN-GROWTH HORMONE FUSION GENES IN TRANSGENIC MICE.

R. E. Hammer[1*], R. D. Palmiter[2] and R. L. Brinster[1]. Lab. of Reprod Phys., Sch. of Vet. Med., Univ. of Pennsylvania, Philadelphia, PA 19104. [2]Dept. Biochemistry, Howard Hughes Med. Inst., Univ. of Washington, Seattle, WA 98195.

Transgenic mice carrying a gene composed of the regulator/promoter region of the mouse metallothionein I-gene (MT-I) fused to the herpes virus thymidine kinase (TK) gene exhibit metal regulation of viral TK. This expression raised the possibility of using the MT-I promoter to regulate the transcriptional activity of a growth hormone (GH) gene and thereby control GH synthesis and growth. For this purpose we fused the MT-I promoter to the rat (r) and human (h) GH genes and microinjected linear DNA fragments containing these genes into the male pronuclei of fertilized mouse eggs. The resulting 122 animals that developed from these eggs were analyzed for the presence of the foreign gene by DNA dot hybridization. Forty mice contained the fusion genes and the majority (29) grew significantly larger than their littermates. Animals exhibiting this accelerated growth rate contained large quantities of MT-GH mRNA transcripts primarily in their livers and to a lesser degree intestine and heart. MT-GH transcriptional activity was induced by metal treatment and in some of the largest mice, about 1000 rat or human GH mRNA molecules per cell was detectable. High GH mRNA levels correlated with the presence of large quantities of either rGH or hGH. Although serum levels of GH could be augmented by chronic zinc treatment growth rates were not increased. Apparently the constitutive level of GH present from the MT-GH genes (~100ng) is sufficient to accelerate growth maximally. Transmission analysis revealed that the foreign gene was stably integrated into the host chromosome and the phenotype was heritable. The fusion gene has been passed into the fifth generation with continued expression of the foreign gene in every transgenic offspring. Growth rates remain accelerated with the average increase in adult size being about 2 fold. As a result of this success we sought to restore growth of the GH deficient dwarf mutant <u>lit/lit</u> mouse by gene transfer. While the rat and human GH genes were not expressed adequately in transgenic mice to affect growth, the MT-rGH fusion gene increases growth in transgenic mutants. Mutant mice that express the MT-rGH gene grew to about 3 times the size of these mutant siblings and approximately 1.5 times the size of heterozygous animals. In addition, the fusion gene was stably integrated into the host chromosome and was transmitted into the 3rd generation with continued expression. These results demonstrate that the mouse MT-I promoter when fused to the GH gene from two different species regulates GH mRNA production which in turn controls GH synthesis which alters the animals growth pattern. In addition we have demonstrated that the effects of a gene defect can be partially overcome by the introduction of a foreign replacement gene into the mutant germ line. These studies were supported by grants from NIH and NSF.

S.47 ORGANIZATION AND EXPRESSION OF LUTROPIN (LH) SUBUNIT GENES. W.W. Chin*
and J.F. Habener, Laboratory of Molecular Endocrinology, Massachusetts General Hospital and Howard Hughes Medical Institute Laboratories, Harvard Medical School, Boston, MA 02114

Lutropin (LH) consists of two different subunits, α and LHβ, which are encoded by separate genes. We are studying the structure and organization of these genes, and the mechanisms involved in the regulation of their expression by gonadal steroids and other factors. We have recently isolated and characterized cloned cDNAs encoding the precursors of the α and LHβ subunits from a cDNA library prepared from the poly(A) RNA of pituitary glands of ovariectomized rats. Using these cDNAs, we have further isolated and characterized the chromosomal genes that encode these subunits. There is a single gene in the rat genome which encodes the LHβ subunit. The transcriptional unit of this gene is ~1 kb in size, and consists of three exons and two introns in positions analogous to those reported for the human chorionic gonadotropin and LHβ genes. In addition, we have determined the site of transcriptional initiation of the LHβ gene by S1 nuclease and primer-extension techniques. We are now studying the regulation of expression of this gene introduced into foreign cells by DNA transfection. Next, in collaboration with Naylor et. al., we have demonstrated the localization of the two subunit genes to different chromosomes in mouse (α--4, LHβ--7) and man (α--6, LHβ--19). These studies were performed using subunit specific cDNAs in blot hybridization analyses of DNAs from well-characterized human-mouse and mouse-Chinese hamster somatic cell hybrids. Thus, the two subunits of LH are represented by separate genes on different chromosomes. Finally, we have determined the effects of gonadal steroids on the expression of the subunits genes as assessed by the steady-state levels of mRNAs encoding the subunits of LH in the rat pituitary gland using blot hybridization techniques. Ovariectomy produced gradual and parallel increases in RIA LH and subunit mRNA levels over 1--2 weeks. In contrast, replacement of ovariectomized rats with estradiol benzoate resulted in rapid declines of both RIA LH and subunit mRNA levels within 1 day. Thus, the expression of the LH subunit genes is regulated by gonadal steroids at the transcriptional and/or mRNA stability levels. Further studies concerning the effects of these hormones on the rates of transcription of the subunit genes and subunit mRNA turnover are in progress.

S.48 GROWTH HORMONE AND PLACENTAL LACTOGEN GENES. J. Parks,* Division of Pediatric Endocrinology, Emory University School of Medicine, Atlanta, GA 30322.

The growth hormone family of genes consists of five structural genes located over a distance of 55 kilobases (kb) on the long arm of human chromosome 17. These genes are oriented in the same 5' to 3' direction in the order 5' GH-N, CS-L, CS-A, GH-V, CS-B 3'. Each gene contains five coding sequences or exons interrupted by four intervening sequences or introns which are located at identical positions relative to amino acid codons. There is greater than 90% base sequence homology among the genes in their 5' flanking, 5' non-translated, coding, intervening and 3' non-translated regions. GH and CS genes begin to show class differences approximately 100 base pairs beyond the polyadenylation sites. The GH-N gene codes for normal, pituitary 22K human growth hormone (hGH). Through alternative splicing of premessenger RNA, it also codes for 20K hGH. Approximately 10% of GH-N gene transcripts undergo splicing between codons 31 and 47 of hGH. Codons for residues 32 to 46 are regarded as part of the second intron and the result is an mRNA for a shorter, 176 amino acid peptide with biological activities which differ from those of normal hGH. The GH-V gene codes for a variant peptide which differs from hGH at 13 of 191 residues. When GH-V is expressed in a transgenomic system, the peptide cross-reacts weakly with antibodies to hGH, but shows considerable activity in radioreceptor assays for hGH. The GH-V gene is not known to be expressed *in vivo*. The CS-A and CS-B genes each code for placental lactogen or human chorionic somatomammotropin (hCS). They specify the same mature hormone, but show one amino acid difference in the signal peptide and several silent base differences. The two genes are expressed at roughly equivalent levels in term placenta. The CS-L gene appears to be an unexpressed pseudogene. A single base substitution at the beginning of the second intron precludes normal mRNA splicing. Several studies have addressed the structural basis of tissue-specific expression of hGH and hCS through examination of cytosine methylation, DNase and restriction endonuclease sensitivity in preparations made from pituitary, placental and reference tissues. Some rare hGH and hCS deficiency states have been traced to deletions within the hGH gene cluster. Several different 5' deletions have shown that the GH-N gene is solely responsible for immunoreactive hGH and that the GH-V gene does not support normal growth when the GH-N gene is absent. Three different 3' deletions have shwon the neither hCS nor a GH-V gene product is required for normal fetal or postnatal development. There are no published examples of CS-L gene deletion. The next objective in relating GH gene structure to disease is to detect more subtle gene abnormalities which are responsible for deficiency or biological inactivity of hGH. Restriction fragment length polymorphisms have been used to trace hGH clusters through families and demonstrate that most mutations responsible for recessive deficiency of growth hormone are not linked to GH genes. Heterogeneity among children with the phenotype of "bioinactive hGH" implies that detection of a primary gene alteration will require cloning and sequencing of an abnormal GH-N gene.

S.49 INHERITANCE OF DEFICIENT RECEPTOR-CYCLASE COUPLING ACTIVITY IN PSEUDOHYPOPARATHYROIDISM. Henry R. Bourne* and Cornelis Van Dop, Departments of Pharmacology and Medicine and the Cardiovascular Research Institute, University of California, San Francisco, CA 94143, USA

Type I-pseudohypoparathyroidism (PHP-I) is an inherited syndrome of resistance to parathyroid hormone (PTH) and other hormones that act by stimulating the synthesis of cAMP. Many PHP-I patients exhibit hypocalcemia, associated with elevated serum PTH and resistance to metabolic effects of PTH. They also can suffer from mild hypothyroidism, associated with resistance to thyrotropin. Most of these patients also exhibit a typical body habitus called Albright's hereditary osteodystrophy (AHO). This laboratory and others (A.M. Spiegel et al., Am. J. Physiol. 243:E37, 1982) have reported that plasma membranes of the cells of many PHP-I patients show partial deficiency of the GTP-binding coupling protein, N, that couples hormone receptors to stimulation of adenylate cyclase. This laboratory quantitated N protein activity either by assessing the ability of membrane extracts to complement the biochemical defect of membranes from a genetically N-deficient tissue culture cell or by measuring incorporation of radioactive ADP-ribose from NAD into the N protein's α subunit, a reaction catalyzed by cholera toxin. These assays show that N activity is reduced by about 50% in erythrocytes, platelets, cultured fibroblasts, and virus-transformed lymphoblasts obtained from PHP-I patients. The observation of N deficiency in fibroblasts and lymphoblasts rules out the possibility that the defect results from a chemical or endocrine abnormality in the intact patient; instead, it indicates that the PHP-I defect is coded directly in the genome of individual cells of the patients. Downs et al. (J. Clin. Invest. 71:231, 1983) recently reported decreased N activity in an important PTH target organ -- the kidney -- of a PHP-I patient. It is reasonable to conclude that the N deficiency of PHP-I involves not only erythrocytes, platelets, fibroblasts, and lymphoblasts, but also endocrine target cells in the organs that exhibit resistance to PTH and other hormones. We have found both dominant and recessive inheritance of N deficiency and the PHP-I phenotype in different kindreds. This genetic heterogeneity indicates that more than one kind of molecular defect can cause N deficiency. The dominant disorder probably results from mutational loss of one of two normal alleles of a gene that encodes a polypeptide subunit of the N protein. This would be consistent with a 50% loss of N activity. In collaboration with R.M. Neer, we have recently studied a family in which N deficiency was inherited from father to son; this observation rules out X-linkage of the gene that encodes the mutant protein in PHP-I. In contrast, a recessive pattern of inheritance does not result simply from functional loss of the polypeptide encoded by a gene inherited from one parent; the molecular defect of recessively inherited N deficiency is not known. Finally, patients in some families with PHP-I do not show detectable N deficiency. In these "normal N" families, PHP-I is often not associated with AHO or endocrine disorders such as hypothyroidism. The molecular basis of this variant of PHP-I is unknown. Isolation of the genes that encode polypeptide subunits of the N protein and other components of the adenylate cyclase system will eventually contribute to understanding the molecular pathophysiology of the various subtypes of PHP-I.

S.50 BIOACTIVITY OF PTH IN PSEUDOHYPOPARATHYROIDISM. C. Nagant De Deuxchaisnes, Rheumatology Dept, Louvain University in Brussels, St-Luc University Hospital, 1200 Brussels, Belgium.

In untreated pseudohypoparathyroidism type 1 (PSP-I), there is a dissociation between circulating immunoreactive parathyroid hormone levels (iPTH) and bioactive PTH (BioPTH), as determined in vitro by a cytochemical bioassay at the level of the distal kidney tubule of the guinea-pig. The iPTH levels are invariably elevated in PSP-I, whereas the Bio-PTH values are low, normal or slightly elevated. More striking is the inhibitory property of PSP plasma on the activity of exogenously added PTH in the bioassay system. Whereas the recovery of PTH activity is of 69 ± 4% (49-90%) in normal, hyperparathyroid and hypoparathyroid patients, it falls to 7 ± 2% (< 1 to 23%) in patients with PSP-I (N = 15), I.E. There is no overlap between PSP values and those found in the other groups studied. In the parents (one father and 6 mothers) and other relatives (one sister, and one son) of the PSP patients, however, intermediate values of recovery are found: 44 ± 15% (< 1% to 130%). The recovery values in the patients with PSP-I are significantly lower than in their relatives ($p < 0.025$). One explanation is that there exists a factor in the circulation of PSP-I patients which partially blocks the receptors of PTH and interferes with the biological response of the hormone. That this factor originates in the parathyroid glands is shown by the following evidence. First, in a patient with PSP-I whose parathyroid glands had been removed in 1965, no inhibitory action of the plasma on the activity of exogenously added PTH could be demonstrated (recovery: 84%). Second, in two patients with PSP-I, this inhibitory action was suppressed during prolonged calcium infusions. In conclusion, a factor originating in the parathyroid glands (an inhibitor or an abnormal PTH) partially interferes with normal PTH responsiveness at the target organ level.

S.51 VITAMIN D RESISTANCE. U.A. Liberman*, C. Eil and S.J. Marx, Metabolic Diseases, Beilinson Medical Center, Petah Tiqva and the Tel Aviv University Sackler School of Medicine, Israel and Endocrinology Branch, National Naval Medical Center, Methesda, Md., and Metabolic Diseases Branch, NIADDK, NIH, Bethesda, Md., U.S.A.

We define resistance to vitamin D calciferol as a state where normal levels of the vitamin are associated with subnormal bioeffects; the bioeffects relevant to this discussion are the calcemic effect and the prevention of rickets and osteomalacia. Thus, vitamin D resistance can be associated with hypocalcemia, defects in bone matrix mineralization, or both. Resistance to vitamin D is a broad term that encompasses deficiencies in sensitivity and/or responsiveness. Deficient sensitivity is defined as a state where the level of vitamin D required to obtain a half maximal bioeffect is increased. Deficient responsiveness is defined as a state where the maximal bioeffect attainable in normals is not attainable with any level of the vitamin. Vitamin D can be considered a prohormone, that in order to become biologically active, it must undergo two distinct processes: a) a series of hydroxylations to active forms, the most potent natural metabolite being 1,25-dihydroxy-vitamin D ($1,25(OH)_2D$) that may be considered as a true hormone, and b) signalling by active metabolites in target tissues through a steroidal type receptor mechanism. Based on this scheme and the availability of assays for measurements of serum levels of calciferol and its metabolites, vitamin D resistant states can be divided into three groups: Type I - vitamin D resistance with low or inappropriately low circulating levels of $1,25(OH)_2D$, reflecting defects in the biosynthetic transformation of calciferol. Type II - vitamin D resistance with increased circulating levels of $1,25(OH)_2D$, reflecting defects in target tissue response to the hormone and an intact biosynthetic pathway of calciferol. Type III - vitamin D resistance with normal circulating levels of $1,25(OH)_2D$ and normal mineral metabolism, reflecting a primary disturbance in bone matrix mineralization not correlated to vitamin D or mineral fluxes. Vitamin D resistance types I and II can be subdivided into hereditary and acquired states, and the different entities in each can be defined according to the primary disturbance as hypocalcemic or hypophosphatemic. The classification presented is based on the pathogenesis of the different forms of vitamin D resistance, according to current knowledge. It puts the various syndromes into one scheme and may direct the choice of an appropriate therapy.

S.52 HORMONAL AND GENETIC REGULATION OF TYPE I COLLAGEN. D. Rowe*, B. Kream and J. Shapiro, Departments of Pediatrics and Medicine, University of Connecticut Health Center, Farmington, CT and Pratt Diagnostic Clinic, Tufts University Medical Center, Boston, MA. USA

Hormonal or genetic mechanisms that alter bone (type I) collagen production may result in osteopenic syndromes. Understanding these processes may explain why certain osteopenic disorders are limited to bone while others are associated with generalized connective tissue (CT) dysfunction. Type I collagen is synthesized at a low rate in a constitutive fashion by many mesenchymal cells; however the osteoblast produces it at a high rate and in a highly regulated manner. Three useful experimental models for studying the regulation of bone collagen production are available: the osteoblast-rich (central bone) portion of the rat calvaria, primary cultures of rat osteoblasts and an osteoblast-like cell line of a osteosarcoma (ROS 17/2). Fully differentiated osteoblasts in the calvaria produce 20-30% collagen which is all type I while the least differentiated ROS cell makes 5% collagen of which 90% is type I. Despite the degree of differentiation the hormonal modulations are identical. For example all these cell types reduce type I collagen synthesis over similar dose response curves of 1,25 dihydroxyvitamin D and PTH. The effect is mediated by a coordinated reduction in the α 1(I) and α 2(I) collagen mRNA as measured by cell-free translation and by dot hybridization using rat specific cDNA probes to collagen mRNA. Physiological levels of insulin enhance collagen synthesis and increase collagen mRNA. None of these hormones exert a similar effect on collgen synthesis in fibroblast-like periosteal cell. Thus, disorders involving these hormones manifest their clinical effect in bone. In contrast, prolonged exposure of tissues to glucocortocoids is inhibitory to collagen production in all cell types. This may account for the generalized CT abnormalities that occur in GC-treated patients. Type I collagen rather than type III collagen is preferentially reduced by GC due to a diminished content of type I collagen mRNA. However, the data are difficult to interpret since changes in cell growth, cell maturation and collagenase production may also be modified by GC.

Genetic disorders of type I collagen, such as found in Osteogenesis Imperfecta (OI), may also result in osteopenic syndromes associated with generalized CT abnormalities. This permits defining the abnormalities of bone collagen by studying collagen produced by dermal fibroblasts. In many cases either a regulatory or structural abnormality of type I collagen can be demonstrated. Type I OI is associated with low type I collagen production (high type III/type I ratio, low total collagen synthesis) and half-normal level of α 1(I) collagen mRNA. More severe forms of OI appear to result from structural mutations within the helical region of either collagen chain. Deletions of 30-100 amino acids from the α 1 or α 2 chain have been demonstrated in type II and type IV OI. A number of new techniques of protein chemistry and molecular biology are capable of detecting increasingly more subtle defects that compromise the stability of the collagen helix. Examples will be given that lead us to believe that application of these techniques to certain patients with osteopenic syndromes not readily identified as OI may reveal subtle abnormalities of type I collagen. This study was supported by the NIH, March of Dimes and Osteogenesis Imperfecta Foundation.

S.53 INTERACTION OF ADRENAL STEROIDS WITH MONO-AMINE SYSTEMS. E.R. de Kloet*
Rudolf Magnus Institute for Pharmacology, Medical Faculty, University of Utrecht, Vondellaan 6, 3521 GD Utrecht, The Netherlands.

Receptor systems for adrenal steroids in rat brain are heterogenous. Glucocorticoid receptors seem located in glial cells. These receptors resemble glucocorticoid receptors in the corticotrophs of the anterior pituitary. Synthetic glucocorticoids such as dexamethasone have highest affinity and are the most potent inducers of certain glial enzymes. The glucocorticoid receptors can be selectively occupied by RU 26988, a "pure" glucocorticoid. Inclusion of RU 26988 in brain cytosol leaves receptor sites available, that display high affinity to corticosterone, desoxycorticosterone and also aldosterone. Whether these receptor sites are mineralocorticoid sites and/or "corticosterone preferring" sites is not clear. Their principal localization is in neurons of the rat limbic brain, in particular of the hippocampus. A transcortin-like binding system shown to be present immunocytochemically in cells of the anterior pituitary, was not found in the neurons.

The function of these receptor systems in brain biochemistry, and behavior was studied after removal of the adrenals and subsequent replacement of adrenalectomized (ADX) rats with adrenal hormones (steroids, amines). Deficits in extinction of certain learned behaviors of ADX rats are restored with corticosterone replacement. Other stress-motivated behaviors are restored with adrenaline. The neural mechanism underlying the normalizing effect of adrenaline on behavior is, however, desensitized one thousand fold to the amine, if the ADX rats were also replaced with corticosterone.

Corticosterone stimulates in ADX rats the synthesis of serotonin in neurons that project from the midbrain raphe nucleus to the hippocampus. Replacement of ADX rats with aldosterone or dexamethasone did not restore reduced serotonin synthesis and deficient behavior. The specificity of the corticosterone effect on hippocampal associated serotonin and behavior supports the evidence from binding studies for the presence of "corticosterone preferring" receptors in hippocampal neurons.

The number of corticosterone receptor sites in the hippocampus is altered by changes in the serotonin input. In addition, the corticosterone receptor capacity is reduced at stress, at senescence and in certain endocrine diseases. Reduced receptor levels can be normalized by ACTH and vasopressin-related peptides. A compensatory increase in receptor sites is noted when part of the receptor containing neurons is removed surgically or with a neurotoxic lesion. Thus, it seems that the number of corticosterone receptors is adjusted to environmental need, which is expressed via neural and endocrine factors.

In conclusion, data were shown of the interaction of corticosterone with central and peripheral amine systems. Corticosterone action on stress-motivated behaviors and on central serotonin synthesis displays the specificity prescribed by "corticosterone-preferring" receptors in hippocampal neurons. Corticosterone desensitizes neural mechanisms against high peripheral catecholamine levels and corticosterone facilitates extinction of no more relevant behavior. The central serotonin response to corticosterone feeds back on hippocampal neurons, where serotonin affects the number of corticosterone receptors.

S.54 METABOLISM OF ANDROGENS IN THE BRAIN. F. Celotti* and L. Martini, Department of Endocrinology, University of Milan, Via A. del Sarto, 21, 20129 Milano, Italy.

The brain is a target structure for the action of various hormonal steroids and in particular of androgens. The brain possesses all the molecular mechanisms necessary to bind and metabolize testosterone. Two orders of metabolites are formed from testosterone: estrogens and 5alpha-reduced androgens {e.g.: 5alpha-androstane-17beta-ol-3-one (dihydrotestosterone, DHT); 5alpha-androstane-3alpha,17beta-diol (3alpha-diol); 5alpha-androstane-3beta, 17beta-diol (3beta-diol)}. It is generally believed that estrogens formed from testosterone play a relevant role in the control of perinatal differentiation of the brain towards male patterns and of male sexual behavior. On the contrary, the 5alpha-reduced metabolites of testosterone are involved in the feedback regulation of gonadotropin secretion. Among the brain structures, the hypothalamus possesses the highest levels of the enzymes (5alpha-reductase; 3alpha- and 3beta-hydroxysteroid dehydrogenases) which metabolize testosterone into the 5alpha-reduced metabolites. These enzymatic activities of the hypothalamus are rather insensitive to the effects of endogenous and exogenous sex steroids. This fact underlines a major difference between the mechanisms controlling these enzymatic activities in the brain and in the anterior pituitary; in the gland, sex steroids have been shown to play an important role in controlling the 5alpha-reductase - 3-hydroxysteroid dehydrogenase system. Some recent data suggest that the 5alpha-reductase activity of the hypothalamus might be regulated by nervous inputs. Data will be presented on the effects exerted on the hypothalamic 5alpha-reductase activity by different types of "hypothalamic deafferentations", and by the administration of drugs known to interfere with the synthesis, the release and the receptorial effects of various central neurotransmitters (e.g.: 5-hydroxytryptamine, catecholamines, acetylcholine, opioid peptides, etc.). The 5alpha-reduced metabolites of testosterone have been suggested to participate in the regulation of gonadotropin secretion, and especially of LH. DHT and 3alpha-diol are more active than testosterone in suppressing the high levels of LH induced by castration; 3beta-diol is less active than DHT and 3alpha-diol. This compound can be further hydroxylated in position 6 and 7. The effects of 3beta,6alpha,17beta-hydroxy-androstane (6alpha-triol), 3beta, 7alpha-17beta-hydroxy-5alpha-androstane (7alpha-triol), 3beta,6beta,17beta-hydroxy-5alpha-androstane (6beta-triol) and 3beta,7beta,17beta-hydroxy-5alpha-androstane (7beta-triol) have been evaluated on the secretion of LH, FSH and prolactin in castrated male rats. Only 7beta-triol possesses some inhibiting effect on LH secretion. Its action appears 2 hours after injection and disappears 24 hours later. No effect of the triols on FSH or prolactin secretion was noticed. (Supported by the Consiglio Nazionale delle Ricerche through the Project "Preventive and Rehabilitative Medicine").

S.55 NEURO-STEROIDS : 3β-HYDROXY-Δ5-DERIVATIVES IN THE RAT BRAIN. E.E. Baulieu*, P. Robel, C. Corpéchot, C. Clarke, A. Groyer and M. Synguelakis. Lab Hormones, 94270 Bicêtre, France.

Dehydroepiandrosterone (D), Pregnenolone (P) and their sulfate esters (DS and PS) have been characterized and measured in the brain of adult male rats. Their formation and/or accumulation depend on in situ mechanisms unrelated to the peripheral endocrine gland system (C. Corpéchot, P. Robel, M. Axelson, J. Sjövall, E.E. Baulieu, Proc. Natl. Acad. Sci. USA 78:1704, 1981 and C. Corpéchot, M. Synguelakis, S. Tahla, M. Axelson, J. Sjövall, R. Vihko, E.E. Baulieu, P. Robel, Brain Res. 270:119, 1983).

Brain P concentrations vary according to physiological or behavioral conditions : (i) In the newborn rats of both sexes, brain P is high at delivery and decreases steadily to reach adult levels at about the 6th hour of life. Brain corticosterone (B) is also high at delivery and decreases to very low levels between d 1 and d 10, a period of adrenal inactivity (in coll. with J. Roffi). (ii) In adult male rats, brain P undergoes a circadian rhythm with an abrupt rise between 9 and 12 am, high concentrations between 12 and 24 pm, and a fall between 0 and 6 am (lights on from 8 am, to 8 pm). (iii) Adult males were exposed for 1 week to the scent of either males (M/M) or females (M/F). P decreased in the olfactory bulb (OB) while increasing mostly in the amygdala (AMY) and to a lesser degree in the hypothalamus (HT). D content also decreased in the OB, but increased in the AMY and even more in the HT (in coll. with P. Brazeau).

P and D are metabolized in the brain. They yield their 3-oxo-Δ_4-counterparts (P → progesterone, D → androstenedione), and are converted into lipoidal derivatives (fatty acid esters) in certain parts of the brain (OB, AMY, HT), but not in others (cerebral cortex, cerebellum). The glioma C6 cell line also makes these metabolites, whereas the fibroblast like L 929 cell line does not.

DS, D and PS induce defined changes in the firing rate of single preoptic-septal neurons after direct application by iontophoresis or pressure (in coll. with P. Poulain and B. Carette). D inhibits the aggressive behavior of castrated male mice towards lactating female intruders. Whether this effect is direct or mediated by conversion into testosterone and/or estradiol is under current investigation. P is less active than D (in coll. with M. Haug and M.L. Schlegel).

In summary, 3β-hydroxy-Δ5-steroids are found in the brain of all mammalian species investigated so far. They undergo changes in relationship to central nervous system activity and may be active molecules in the brain. It is however premature to give a comprehensive account of their function.

S.56 HYPOTHALAMIC mRNA AND ITS ROLE IN SEXUAL DIFFERENTIATION. H.F. Stanley* and G. Fink, MRC Brain Metabolism Unit, Dept. of Pharmacology, 1 George Sq., Edinburgh, Scotland, U.K.

The adult patterns of gonadotropin secretion and sexual behaviour in the rat are dependent upon the endocrine status of the animal during a 'critical period' of development which ends at approximately postnatal day 10. Testosterone, largely through its central conversion to estradiol, has a permanent organising effect on neurons in and around the hypothalamus-preoptic-area (H-POA) resulting in a number of sexually dimorphic anatomical features. The precise mechanism of action of testosterone is not known although the fact that inhibitors of DNA, RNA and protein synthesis have been reported to block or partially protect against the masculinising actions of testosterone in the neonatal rat suggests that hormonal regulation of gene expression is an important factor in the differentiation process. In order to investigate whether sex differences in specific proteins occur during or as a result of sexual differentiation, an electrophoretic analysis of proteins from the H-POA of male, female and androgenised female (4 day female injected with 1.25mg testosterone propionate) rats at different stages of development was carried out. In one study mRNA was isolated from the H-POA and translated in vitro and in a second study proteins associated with various subcellular fractions of the H-POA were stained with Coomassie Brilliant Blue. Translation of mRNA showed that 4 and 12 day androgenised female and male rat H-POA had the capacity to synthesise greater amounts of a 55,000 - 58,000 molecular weight protein(s) than the respective control female H-POA. In addition, the H-POA content of a soluble protein of similar molecular weight was found to be approximately 30% higher in the male than the female at birth (day 0). The 55,000-58,000 molecular weight protein was found to migrate with the same R_f value as a standard preparation of tubulin. Two dimensional gel analysis of translation products showed that administration of testosterone to 4 day females for 6 hours inhibited the synthesis of an unidentified 20,000 molecular weight protein compared with the control female and that synthesis of this protein was further reduced in the 4 day male. These studies indicate that the synthesis of specific H-POA proteins appears to be influenced by androgen at the mRNA level in the neonatal rat. Of particular interest is the suggestion of a sex difference in a protein with the electrophoretic characteristics of tubulin. This finding could have important implications in that such a change may reflect structural alterations occuring in the developing H-POA, possibly involving enhanced neuritic outgrowth in the male. This study was supported by the MRC.

S.57 PROSTAGLANDINS AND OVULATION. K. Satoh*, University of Tokyo, Department of Obst. & Gynecol., Hongo, Tokyo, Japan 113

Prostaglandins (PGs) are biosynthesized by cyclooxygenase in the microsome from archidonic acid to PGs E_2, $F_{2\alpha}$, I_2 and thromboxane (TX) A_2 via PGs H_2 and G_2. Non-steroidal anti-inflammatory agents such as aspirin and indomethacin block PG biosynthesis. PGs E_2 and $F_{2\alpha}$ are applied clinically for induction and augmentation of labor. PGI_2, which is non-enzymatically converted to 6-keto $PGF_{1\alpha}$, has a strong effect to inhibit platelet aggregation. TXA_2 is a platelet aggregating factor.

Ovulation is a phenomenon in which oocyte is expelled out by luteinizing hormone (LH) from Graafian follicle matured by follicle stimulating hormone (FSH), followed by formation of corpus luteum. How is PG involved in the chain reaction to cause ovulation? No changes in PG levels were observed in the peripheral blood and urine in the rat, gilt and human in ovulation, whereas the preovulatory increases of PGs E, $F_{2\alpha}$ and 6-keto $PGF_{1\alpha}$ in the follicular fluid and ovarian vein blood were detected at regular intervals after LH stimulation. An increase of PG production in the follicular cells results from induction of cyclooxygenase by LH through the protein biosynthesis mechanism, since PG increases by LH stimulation were inhibited by actinomycin D and puromycin in follicle organ cultures. Immunohistochemical study revealed staining of the antiserum to cyclooxygenase intracellularly localized was observed by light microscopy in some of the granulosa cells. Cyclooxygenase inhibitors such as indomethacin and mefenamic acid and the antiserum to cylooxygenase block ovulation. But inhibition of superovulation in immature rats through suppression of PG production by indomethacin is recovered by the administration of PGs E_2, $F_{2\alpha}$ and I_2. Inhibition of ovulation by indomethacin does not affect luteinization and steroidogenesis, indicating the action of PGs in ovulation is independent of that of steroid hormones. This pathological state is designated "the luteinized unruptured follicle". Ovulation is usually followed by luteinization of the follicular cells, formation of corpus luteum. Therefore, ovulation and production of progesterone have been considered two sides of the same coin. But the present study suggests that it is possible to isolate the process of steroidogenesis and ovulation and offers a methodological direction for investigating pathogenesis of the luteinized unruptured follicle syndrome. The receptors for PGs E_1 and E_2 are indicated to be present in the ovarian follicle cells. A marked increase in specific binding of PGE occurs around the time of ovulation. Fibrinolytic system is activated by PGs correspondingly to the time of ovulation. PGs are involved in increases of plasminogen and plasminogen activator in the follicles.

In conclusions, the effect of LH on the follicle matured by FSH results in increasing PG production through the induction of cyclooxygenase in the follicle. The increased PGs act on the receptor for PGs, especially PGE and activate proteolytic enzymes such as plasmin to rupture the apex of the follicle and discharge oocyte.

S.58 PROSTAGLANDINS IN BONE CELL BIOLOGY. T.J. Martin*, N.C. Partridge and S.A. Livesey, Department of Medicine, University of Melbourne,Repatriation General Hospital, Heidelberg, Australia.

Prostaglandins are able to stimulate bone resorption in a manner similar to parathyroid hormone, with an increase in the number and activity of osteoclasts. Of all the arachidonic acid metabolites, the most potent bone resorber is PGE_2, and the major circulating metabolite of this compound, 13,14-H_2-diketo PGE_2, has virtually no bone resorbing activity. Prostacyclin (PGI_2) a very labile prostanoid is capable of promoting resorption but is appreciably less potent than PGE_2.

Although the net effect of PG's on bone is to increase osteoclastic activity, if endogenous PG production in bone is prevented by, e.g., glucocorticoid treatment, PGE_2 can be shown to stimulate collagen synthesis. Thus the possibility exists that PG's might have dual effects on bone, affecting both formation and resorption. Such effects could be brought about by pG's having different actions upon sub-populations of bone cells.

Osteoblasts produce PGE_2 and PGI_2, and each of these prostanoids acts upon the osteoblast to activate adenylate cyclase and cyclic AMP dependent protein kinase. As is the case with parathyroid hormone, full PGE_2 activation of cyclic AMP-dependent protein kinase requires only a small proportion of the total cyclic AMP generated by the cell. In osteoblasts PGE_2 and parathyroid hormone exhibit different patterns of selective activation of isoenzymes of cyclic AMP-dependent protein kinase, implying that there might be some differences in the physiological effects of the two agents. Indeed there is evidence for this.

The facts that cyclic AMP is thought to mediate the bone resorbing actions of PGE_2 and parathyroid hormone, and furthermore that both of those agents clearly act upon the osteoblast, have led to the view that the osteoblast might mediate the action of bone resorbing hormones, perhaps being responsible for production of factors which recruit and activate osteoclasts.

Although some animal cancers associated with humoral hypercalcemia may produce large amounts of PG's as the humoral agent, this seems to apply rarely, if ever, in human cancers. The role of PG's in malignant hypercalcemia remains to be established, but may be related to the mechanisms by which tumour cells begin to invade bone by resorbing from the marrow cavity.

Prostaglandins probably have an important role to play in normal bone physiology and pathological states. As is the case with PG's in other tissues, they probably function as locally active factors, perhaps in some circumstances mediating the effects of humoral agents.

S.59 PROSTAGLANDINS AND KIDNEY FUNCTION D. Schlondorff*, Dept. of Medicine, Albert Einstein College of Medicine, 1300 Morris Park Avenue, Bronx, New York 10461.

In the kidney, prostaglandins (PG) can influence such diverse parameters as blood flow and glomerular filtration as well as solute and water excretion by the tubules. PG are produced locally and affect cell function at the site of their synthesis. Hence, it is not surprising that PG synthesis is compartmentalized within specific segments of the nephron subserving specific functions.

Within the renal cortex PG are predominantly produced by arterioles and glomeruli where they modify the constrictor effects of e.g., angtiotensin II and platelet activating factor, a lipid mediator. Isolated glomeruli contract in response to these agents. This is mediated by glomerular mesangial cells which have characteristics of smooth muscle cells. In isolated glomeruli and cultured mesangial cells, the contraction induced by angiotensin II and platelet activating factor also causes increased synthesis of vasodilator PGs i.e., PGE_2 and PGI_2. This is mediated via stimulation of both phospholipases C and A_2, resulting in the release of arachidonic acid, the precursor for PGs. The increase in PGE_2 and PGI_2 synthesis in turn attenuates the constrictor effects of vasoactive agents closing a feed-back loop. Thus glomerular-mesangial PG production tends to preserve glomerular function in the presence of vasoconstrictors.

In the renal medulla PGE_2 inhibits the hydroosmotic effect of antidiuretic hormone (ADH). Isolated mammalian collecting tubules and their analogue, the toad urinary bladder, produce predominantly PGE_2. In these structures the hydroosmotic action of ADH is mediated by cAMP. Concomitantly to stimulating cAMP production, ADH also enhances PGE_2 synthesis in a cAMP independent fashion by activating phospholipase. The PGE_2 generated decreases cAMP production, via a mechanism that has not yet been determined. Thus a negative feed-back loop exists whereby ADH stimulates PGE_2 synthesis which in turn inhibits ADH's action.

On the other hand cAMP produced in response to ADH may inhibit phospholipase activation. This will result in a failure to release arachidonic acid and hence a fall in PGE_2 synthesis. Thus a double reciprocal feed-back mechanism may exist whereby ADH stimulates PG production in a cAMP-independent fashion but also inhibits PG-synthesis in a cAMP-dependent manner. Such an interlocked system would prevent an overshoot of both the ADH and PGE_2 response in either direction.

As a unifying hypothesis the role of PGs in different nephron segments can be visualized as that of local modulators for specific hormonal responses with the goal of maintaining local rather than total body homeostasis.

S.60 SEMINAL PROSTAGLANDINS AND SPERM FUNCTION. R.W. Kelly* & R.J. Aitken, MRC Reproductive Biology Unit, University of Edinburgh Centre for Reproductive Biology, 37 Chalmers Street, Edinburgh, EH3 9EW, UK.

Primate spermatozoa, at the time of ejaculation, are presented with the highest concentration of prostaglandin so far recorded. In humans the concentrations of PGE_1 and PGE_2 are seven orders of magnitude higher than those found in peripheral plasma and there are even higher concentrations of 19-OH PGE present. Although it has been suggested that these high PG levels are present to act on the female reproductive tract, possibly to enhance passive migration of spermatozoa, evidence for this hypothesis is still not forthcoming. The obvious possibility that PGs may act on the spermatozoa has been tested in several experiments to investigate the effect of PGs on sperm motility but the conditions of sperm incubation have not always been adequate and the results have generally been inconclusive. However, several observations in the last few years suggest an association between spermatozoa and PGs which might be elucidated by studying PGE function in other cells. In human polymorphonuclear leukocytes high E concentrations have the effect of inhibiting the release of lysosomal hydrolases both in response to phagocytotic and non-phagocytotic events. In macrophages PGE inhibits enzyme secretion and the metabolic burst as well as many other functions of the cell. PGE_2 has a biphasic effect on platelet aggregation and high PGE_2 concentrations inhibit aggregation secondary to other stimuli. All of the above effects involve the inhibition of cellular activation and enzyme release by high levels of PGE and are associated with an increase in cAMP concentration within the cell. The obvious inference is that seminal PGE inhibits leukocyte infiltration or macrophage function within the vagina which might indeed increase the fertility of the semen, but this overlooks the role of the spermatozoon as a secretory cell. The spermatozoal acrosome reaction, which is an essential process in the acquisition of fertilizing ability, is accompanied by enzyme release from the acrosome, an organelle of spermatozoa which is both developmentally and functionally a modified lysosome. PGE might therefore play a role in mediating capacitation and/or the acrosome reaction. We have tested this possibility by observing the effect of PGs on the in vitro fertilisation of zona-free hamster eggs. Paradoxically, PGE_2 stimulated ($p < 0.005$) oocyte penetration in this test at all dose levels studied (4.2 to 270 µg/ml). Increasing concentrations of PGE_1 gave a typical bell-shaped dose-response curve with highly significant stimulation at lower doses but at 270 µg/ml no stimulation was observed. 19-OH PGEs isolated from semen stimulated oocyte penetration but the effect was weaker than that of PGE. PGF_2 was without effect at all doses studied. In these experiments analysis of variance demonstrated that the effects of prostaglandins was to stimulate motility although the effect was moderate and did not account for the increased capacity for fertilization. These results do not yet explain the presence of seminal PGs since capacitation in semen is inappropriate but they provide additional evidence that prostaglandins interact with spermatozoa.

S.61 BIOSYNTHESIS AND STRUCTURE OF INSULIN RECEPTORS. M. Kasuga*[1,2,3], J. A. Hedo[1] and C. R. Kahn[1,2], Diabetes Branch[1], NIDDK, National Institutes of Health, Bethesda, Maryland 20205 U.S.A., Joslin Diabetes Center[2], Boston, Massachusetts 02215 U.S.A. and The Third Department of the Internal Medicine[3], School of Medicine, University of Tokyo, 7-3-1 Hongo, Tokyo, Japan 113.

The structure of the insulin receptor were identified in cultured human lymphocytes (IM-9 line) by means of metabolic and cell surface labeling, immunoprecipitation with anti-receptor autoantibodies and analysis on SDS-polyacrylamide gel electrophoresis and autoradiography under reducing conditions. With this approach, we have found there are two major, Mr = 135,000 (α), Mr = 95,000 (β) and one minor, Mr = 210,000 (γ) subunit. Tryptic fingerprints of ^{125}I-labeled these subunits suggested that the major peptides of the α and β subunits are different and the γ subunit contains peptides of both the α and β subunits. In nonreduced gels, free insulin receptor subunits are observed, as well as two higher molecular weight bands of Mr = 520,000 and 350,000. On reduction, the 520,000 band was composed primarily of Mr = 210,000 and 95,000 subunits, whereas the 350,000 band was composed primarily of Mr = 135,000 and 95,000 subunits. The biosynthesis and carbohydrate processing of the insulin receptor of the same cultured lymphocytes was also studied with similar approach. In addition to three subunits mentioned above, another subunit of Mr = 190,000 was detected. The α, β and γ subunits were labeled by [^{3}H]mannose, [^{3}H]glucosamine, [^{3}H]galactose and [^{3}H]fucose, and were bound by immobilized lentil, wheat germ, and ricin I lectins. On the other hand, the Mr = 190,000 band was labeled only by [^{3}H]mannose and [^{3}H]glucosamine and was bound only by lentil lectin. All four components could be labeled with [^{35}S] methionine; however, in contrast with the other three polypeptides, the Mr = 190,000 band was not labeled by cell surface iodination with lactoperoxidase, suggesting that it is not exposed at the outer surface of the plasma membrane. Pulse-chase studies with [^{3}H]mannose showed that the Mr = 190,000 was the earliest labeled component of the receptor and had a very rapid half-life ($t\frac{1}{2}$ = 2.5h). Radioactivity in this band reached a maximum 1 h after the pulse-chase. The other three subunits reached a maximum 6 h after pulse-chase. Monensin, an ionophore which interferes with maturation of some proteins, blocked both the disappearance of the Mr = 190,000 protein and the appearance of the α and β subunits. The mannose incorporated in the Mr = 190,000 component was fully sensitive to treatment with endoglycosidase H while that in the other three subunits was only partially sensitive. Considering the results of triptic fingerprints mentioned above, these data suggested that the Mr = 190,000 could be the high mannose precursor form of the insulin receptor that undergoes carbohydrate processing and proteolytic cleavage to generate the α and β subunits. In addition, the γ subunit is probably the fully glycosylated form of the precursor that escapes cleavage and is expressed in the plasma membrane.

S.62 INSULIN RECEPTOR: A PROTEIN KINASE FOR TRANSMEMBRANE HORMONE SIGNALLING.

E. Van Obberghen*, H. Gazzano, M. Fehlmann and A. Kowalski, INSERM U 145, Faculté de Médecine, 06034 Nice Cédex, France.

The insulin receptor is a high molecular weight integral membrane glycoprotein consisting of two major subunits with Mr 130,000 (α-subunit), and Mr 95,000 (β-subunit). The two subunits have distinct functions. Indeed, the α-subunit contains the insulin binding site, whereas the β-subunit is an insulin-activatable tyrosine-specific protein kinase, which is capable of self-phosphorylation and of catalyzing the phosphorylation of exogenous protein substrates. It is an appealing idea to envision that the insulin receptor-kinase complex functions as an integrated system for transferring hormonal information across the cell membrane. In this model the binding of insulin to its receptor at the cell surface stimulates the protein kinase activity of the receptor itself leading to autophosphorylation. The activated receptor protein kinase would then provoke the phosphorylation of cellular proteins, and through a cascade of phosphorylation-dephosphorylation reactions this would eventuate in the cellular responses to insulin. Major challenges for the relevance of this concept are the identification of native substrates of the insulin receptor kinase and the demonstration that receptor phosphorylation is a sufficient requisite for insulin to act.

S.63 MORPHOLOGICAL ASPECTS AND PHYSIOLOGICAL RELEVANCE OF INSULIN RECEPTOR INTERNALIZATION AND RECYCLING. J.-L. Carpentier*, M. Fehlmann, E. Van Obberghen, P. Gorden and L. Orci, Institute of Histology and Embryology, Geneva, Switzerland, INSERM U 145, Nice, France and Diabetes Branch NIADDK, NIH, Bethesda, Md., USA.

Using a ^{125}I-photoreactive insulin analogue that can be covalently coupled to its receptor we recently demonstrate that in rat hepatocytes (freshly isolated or in primary culture) the insulin receptor is concomitantly internalized with the labeled hormone and that the internalization of the ^{125}I-photoreactive insulin receptor complex is followed by a progressive recycling of the receptor back to the cell surface. By quantitative EM autoradiography we have tracked the intracellular pathway followed by the ^{125}I-photoreactive insulin receptor complex. Cells were preincubated for 2-3 h at 15^{0}C in the presence of ^{125}I-photoreactive insulin, exposed to UV for 3 min, washed and incubated for up to 6 h at 37^{0}C in the absence of labeled ligand. 15-20% of the cell associated radioactivity was cross-linked by UV and the hormone receptor complex remained apparently undegraded until the end of the 37^{0}C incubation. As determined by the hypothetical grain method, two intracellular compartments were preferentially labeled : electronlucent vesicles and lysosome-like structures. At 37^{0}C labeling of small vesicles decreased until 30 to 60 min of incubation and then slightly increased in a manner parallel to the reappearance of ^{125}I-photoreactive insulin receptor complexes on the cell surface. An inverse labeling pattern was observed for lysosome-like structures. NH_4Cl (2 x 10^{-2}M) and monensin (10^{-6}M) blocked insulin receptor recycling and induced an accumulation of labeled material within lysosome-like structures (mostly multivesicular bodies). These results provide evidence for the involvement of a vesicular compartment in the shuttling of the insulin receptor between the plasma membrane and lysosome-like structure.

On the basis of these morphological data we proposed that the loss of cell surface insulin receptors upon prolonged exposure of cells to the hormone (down-regulation) results from an internalization of the hormone receptor complexes occurring at a greater rate than recycling and synthesis of receptors. In order to test the role of recycling in the metabolism of insulin receptors we have tested the influence of an inhibitor of receptor recycling (monensin 10^{-6}M to 10^{-7}M) on insulin receptor down regulation. In U-937 monocyte-like cell that internalizes insulin receptor readily, monensin markedly enhanced insulin-induced down regulation. By contrast IM-9 lymphocytes, a slow internalizer, was less sensitive to monensin exposure. In both cell types monensin alone did not affect insulin binding and had little influence on ligand internalization as demonstrated by quantitative EM autoradiography. These data suggest that cells with a rapid internalization rate have an associated active recycling process while cells with a slow internalization rate poorly recycle their insulin receptors and demonstrate the key role played by insulin receptor recycling in the down regulation process.

S.64 USE OF THE HEAVY ISOTOPE DENSITY-SHIFT METHOD TO INVESTIGATE INSULIN RECEPTOR METABOLISM.

M. D. Lane*, Dept. of Physiological Chemistry, The Johns Hopkins Univ. School of Med., Baltimore, MD 21205, USA.

The responsiveness of a target cell to insulin depends upon the number of functional insulin receptors on its plasma membrane. Recent evidence shows that cells have the ability to modulate the level of cell-surface receptor in response to changes in physiological state. The total number of receptors a cell possesses depends upon the relative rates of receptor synthesis and degradation. We have employed the heavy isotope density-shift method to assess the rates of functional receptor synthesis, turnover and translocation in cells in different states. After shifting cells to medium containing heavy (>95% ^{15}N, ^{13}C and ^{2}H) amino acids, newly-synthesized receptors become "heavy." Following the shift, heavy and "light" receptors are isopycnically separated on CsCl density gradients and quantitated allowing calculation of the rates of synthesis of new heavy and the decay of old light functional (capable of binding insulin) receptors. During differentiation of 3T3-L1 preadipocytes into adipocytes insulin receptor number increases from 8,500 to 170,000 per cell. The heavy isotope density-shift approach reveals that this rise in receptor level is due entirely to an increased synthetic rate, from 800 to 15,400 receptors/-cell/h. The degradative rate constant is not altered by differentiation. In contrast, a different mechanism is used by cells for insulin-induced down-regulation of receptor level. Exposure of 3T3-L1 adipocytes or 3T3-C2 fibroblasts to insulin results in a 50-60% decrease in cell-surface and total cellular receptor level ($t_{1/2}$ = 2-3 h). Heavy isotope density-shift experiments show that in the down-regulated steady-state the rate of insulin receptor inactivation is increased 2-fold while the synthetic rate is not altered. The heavy isotope density-shift method was combined with covalent cross-linking of ^{125}I-insulin to surface receptors to study the transit of receptor to the plasma membrane. It was determined that 1.5 h are required for newly-synthesized receptors to acquire insulin binding capacity and an additional 1.5 h (3 h total) are needed for the receptor to reach the plasma membrane. Down-regulation does not alter the transit time to the surface, but causes a 2-fold increase in the inactivation rate of surface receptors. The heavy isotope density-shift method was used to study receptor decay in 3T3-C2 cells during the transition to the down-regulated state. A precipitous increase in receptor decay is preceded by a rapid translocation ($t_{1/2}$ < 10 min) of surface receptor to an intracellular compartment. Upon exposure to ligand, receptor rapidly redistributes from a cell-surface/intracellular ratio of 85/15 to a ratio of 40/60, without net loss of cellular receptors. Removal of insulin rapidly ($t_{1/2}$ < 20 min) reverses the process. Insulin-induced translocation of the receptor is followed by a slower inactivation/degradation of receptor in the intracellular compartment. Internalization of insulin receptor and its bound ligand are rapidly (< 10 min) blocked by phenylarsine oxide preventing their inactivation/degradation. Thus, upon exposure to ligand, insulin receptors are translocated from the cell-surface to an intracellular site resulting in accelerated receptor degradation and ultimately in a lower, i.e. down-regulated, steady-state receptor level.

S.65 A HIGH MOLECULAR WEIGHT PRECURSOR TO LUTEINIZING HORMONE RELEASING HORMONE (LHRH) FOUND IN HUMAN, RAT AND MOUSE HYPOTHALAMI IS ABSENT FROM THE HYPOTHALAMUS OF THE HYPOGONADAL (hpg) MOUSE. A. Curtis*, V. Lyons and G. Fink, MRC Brain Metabolism Unit, University Department of Pharmacology, 1 George Square, Edinburgh, EH8 9JZ, Scotland.

Many small peptide hormones and neurotransmitters are synthesised via a ribosome-dependent system into large polypeptide precursors of which the biologically active peptide represents less than 10% of the total sequence. We have demonstrated that the translation of hypothalamic mRNA produces a primary translation product with an apparent molecular weight of 28,000 containing an amino acid sequence immunologically similar to that of the biologically active decapeptide LHRH. Poly A^+ enriched fractions of total RNA extracted from rat, mouse and human hypothalami were translated in a mRNA dependent cell free system from rabbit reticulocyte lysate supplemented with tritiated amino acids. The translation products were immunoprecipitated using a specific anti-serum to LHRH (HC6). Following denaturing polyacrylamide gel electrophoresis and autoradiography of the immunoprecipitates, a single immunoreactive polypeptide was detected with a molecular weight of 28,000. The antiserum which recognised this polypeptide did not cross react with various analogues of LHRH or with several pituitary hormones though the free acid form of LHRH did compete for the anti-serum against the labelled polypeptide. The polypeptide was not detected amongst the translation products of the hypothalamic mRNAs when an excess of cold LHRH was added before immunoprecipitation, showing that the decapeptide is able to compete for the antiserum blocking its binding with the precursor completely. The 28,000 M_r band was also not detected by the identical immunoprecipitation of a translation mix to which no exogenous mRNA was added or in which normal rabbit serum replaced the anti-LHRH serum. In a second immunoprecipitation procedure, applied to the rat hypothalamic translation products, Staphyloccal Protein A replaced the anti-rabbit γ-globulin used as a second antibody in the precipitation of antigen-antibody complexes. A 28,000 M_r protein was immunoprecipitated using this technique thus confirming the previous results. When the translation products of the hypothalamic mRNA of hpg mouse, an animal which does not synthesise an immunoreactive or biologically active form of the LHRH decapeptide, were treated with the anti-LHRH serum in an identical procedure, no immunoprecipitated polypeptides were detected following electrophoresis and autoradiography. Specifically, the 28,000 M_r LHRH precursor was not present. Though the precise mechanism of the inherited hpg defect is unknown, these results suggest that it is unrelated to the processing mechanism of a large precursor molecule.which appears to be completely absent, or present in a mutated form not recognised by the anti-LHRH serum. The polypeptide is unlikely to be present at levels below our detection limits since the genetics of the hpg condition show that the primary defect represents an 'all or none' situtation. The identification of a large 28000 molecular weight LHRH immunoreactive polypeptide within the hypothalami of three different mammalian species, and the demonstration of its complete absence from the hpg mouse hypothalamus shows that LHRH is initially synthesized by way of a precursor molecule which is twenty times larger than the active peptide.

S.66 THE RELATIONSHIPS BETWEEN GnRH AND LH SECRETION. Iain J. Clarke*, Medical Research Centre, Prince Henry's Hospital, Melbourne, Australia.

Pituitary LH secretion is controlled primarily by gonadotropin releasing hormone (GnRH) from the hypothalamus. We have developed 2 animal models to study the interrelationships between GnRH and LH secretion. In the first model, GnRH secretion is monitored by sampling hypophyseal portal blood in conscious sheep (Clarke & Cummins, 1982). In ovariectomized (OVX) ewes, each pulsatile secretory episode ('pulse') of LH was coincident with a pulse of a GnRH. To examine the effects of estrogen, OVX ewes were injected (i.m.) with 50 μg estradiol benzoate (EB) and sampled for GnRH and LH; this treatment causes a biphasic LH response (decrease followed by increase). During the negative feedback phase there was a reduction in the frequency of LH pulses and plasma LH levels fell, but GnRH pulse frequency was not significantly reduced [mean ± SEM interpulse interval 46.2 ± 6.3 min (n=4) compared to 54.4 ± 8.4 min in untreated OVX ewes (n=7)]. At the onset of the positive feedback phase the GnRH pulse frequency was significantly ($P < 0.025$) increased [mean ± SEM interpulse interval 29.5 ± 4.1 min (n=7)]. The increased GnRH pulse frequency led to an elevation in the GnRH baseline. It is concluded that 1) the negative feedback effect of estrogen is a pituitary effect, 2) the positive feedback event is associated with an increase in the frequency of GnRH pulses and is therefore, at least in part, a hypothalamic event. In the second model we have surgically isolated the pituitary gland from the hypothalamus using a surgical method (Clarke et al., 1983). Restoration of gonadotropin secretion can be achieved by administering GnRH pulses. Using a constant dose per pulse, the amplitude of the LH pulses was seen to be dependent upon GnRH pulse frequency; increasing pulse frequency led to increases in baseline plasma LH levels and reductions in pulse amplitude and vice versa for reduced pulse frequency. In these situations the amplitudes of the LH pulses were directly related to the readily releasable pools of LH in the pituitary gland. To determine the pituitary effects of estrogen we used OVX ewes with isolated pituitaries and maintained gonadotropin output with hourly GnRH pulses. Injection (i.m.) of 50 μg EB to these ewes caused biphasic changes in the pattern of LH secretion qualitatively similar to those seen in hypothalamo-pituitary intact ewes, although the magnitude of the LH surge was reduced. These results are concordant with those obtained by measuring GnRH secretion and again show that the negative feedback effect of estrogen is due to a pituitary effect. Sensitization of the pituitary gland to GnRH during the positive feedback event also indicated a pituitary effect of estrogen but this alone does not account for the magnitude of the rise in plasma LH at this time. Thus, we conclude that the positive feedback action of estrogen is due to a hypothalamic effect to increase GnRH pulse frequency and a pituitary effect to sensitize the gland to GnRH.

References

Clarke I.J. and Cummins, J.T. (1982) Endocrinology 111, 1737.
Clarke, I.J., Cummins, J.T. and de Kretser, D.M. (1983) Neuroendocrinology 36, 376.

S.67 REGULATION OF PITUITARY GnRH RECEPTOR IN VIVO AND IN VITRO. R.N. Clayton,* S.I. Naik, A.Detta, H.M. Charlton*, L.S. Young, Dept. of Medicine, University of Birmingham, and *Dept. of Anatomy, University of Oxford, U.K.

Early studies in rats have shown a positive correlation between serum gonadotrophin levels and pituitary GnRH receptors (GnRH-R), suggesting an important role for GnRH-R in modulation of pituitary responsiveness to GnRH. Thus, GnRH-R are always elevated following gonadectomy (GDX) of rats, and endogenous GnRH is essential for this response. Indeed, neutralisation of GnRH reduces GnRH-R to below intact control values in rats. Exogenous GnRH or its agonist analogues are able to increase GnRH-R in vivo. Collectively, this evidence supports the concept of homologous ligand regulation of GnRH-R in vivo, and that GnRH-R measurement provides an index of prior pituitary exposure to endogenous GnRH. This concept seemed to extend to other species since the pituitary of the hpg mouse, which has isolated GnRH deficiency, has only 30% of the normal GnRH-R content. In mice with congenital GnRH deficiency (hpg) pulsatile GnRH restores GnRH-R within 3 days, an event followed 4 days later by normalisation of serum and pituitary FSH values. Prolonged (>40D) exposure of the hpg mouse pituitary to GnRH, by way of hypothalamic transplantation from normal donors, not only restores GnRH-R and pituitary gonadotrophin levels but also matures the gonads. Also, a single injection of GnRH (60 ng s.c.) to hpg male mice is followed by 2-3-fold increases in GnRH-R after 6-12 hrs, whereas the same treatment of normal male mice has no effect on GnRH-R. This GnRH effect is still evident in GDX hpg mice, and can be prevented by prior treatment with cycloheximide. The hpg mouse studies indicate that GnRH-R autoinduction is a prerequisite for 'normalisation' of pituitary gonadotroph function, a genuine trophic effect of the neuropeptide. Physiological studies in normal mice have shown that GnRH-R, serum LH, and FSH fall in lactating mice, as in lactating rats. However, GDX of male and female mice is accompanied by a sustained (up to 3 mths) 40-60% reduction in GnRH-R in the presence of 10-20-fold increases in serum LH and FSH, indicating that high levels of gonadotrophins can be maintained with a subnormal GnRH-R content. Thus, post-GDX GnRH-R changes in mice are the opposite to those in rats. The post-GDX decline of GnRH-R in mice is rapid (12-24 hrs) and cannot be prevented by GnRH injections or GnRH antiserum (GnRH-AS) treatment, implying that the GnRH receptor fall is unrelated to the homologous ligand. E_2 and progesterone (P) largely prevent the post-GDX GnRH-R fall, and restore the depleted GnRH-R content in pituitaries of female mice treated with GnRH-AS. E_2 + P also elevate GnRH-R in GnRH deficient hpg female mice, and exogenous GnRH increases GnRH-R in normal intact, but not GDX, female mice. These data suggest an essential role for gonadal steroids, acting directly on the pituitary, for maintenance of GnRH-R in female mice. Homologous ligand induction of GnRH-R in cultured pituitary cells follows a similar time-course as that shown in the hpg mouse pituitaries in vivo, and depends upon protein synthesis and extracellular Ca^{2+}. A possible role for cyclic nucleotides in gonadotroph function is suggested by the ability of DbcAMP to increase GnRH-R in vitro; this also being dependent on Ca^{2+} and protein synthesis. The induction of GnRH-R by DbcAMP is blocked by a GnRH antagonist, and cyclic nucleotides at mM concentrations appear to bind to pituitary GnRH-R. The results from the various experimental approaches presented indicate that GnRH-R changes play a significant, though not always critical, part in modulation of gonadotroph function.

S.68 THE ROLE OF ENDOGENOUS OPIOID PEPTIDES IN THE CONTROL OF GONADOTROPIN SECRETION IN THE PRIMATE. Michel Ferin*, Department of Physiology and Obstetrics and Gynecology, Columbia University, College of Physicians and Surgeons. New York, N.Y. 10032.

In this presentation, we will consider the physiological role that endogenous opioid peptides, and more specifically B-endorphin, play in the control of gonadotropin secretion and how they may affect the menstrual cycle in the rhesus monkey. The evidence in support for a role of endogenous opiates includes: 1) B-endorphin neuronal cell bodies are preferentially concentrated in the arcuate region, an area also rich in GnRH, allowing for interaction between the two peptides; 2) Opiate administration inhibits gonadotropin release; 3) naloxone, a competitive inhibitor of opiates, enhances gonadotropin secretion, indicating that there is an interaction between the endogenous opioid peptides and LH release. The action of naloxone, however, is restricted to specific phases of the menstrual cycle, suggesting that this regulatory mechanism is a complex one which involves gonadal hormones as well; 4) B-endorphin secretion by the hypothalamus, as measured by changes in concentration in hypophyseal portal blood, varies strikingly throughout the menstrual cycle, with maximal activity observed during the luteal phase and minimal activity seen at menstruation. Naloxone's effectiveness in modifying LH release during the menstrual cycle parallels hypothalamic B-endorphin immunoactivity. These results provide supportive evidence that endogenous opioid peptides control gonadotropin release at specific times of the menstrual cycle. Since prolonged naloxone infusion during the luteal phase increases LH pulse frequency, our present hypothesis is that endogenous opioid peptides participate in the decrease in GnRH and LH pulse frequency observed during the luteal phase. The rapid increase in pulse frequency observed at menstruation would then be related to the abrupt decrease in hypothalamic opioid activity observed at the end of the menstrual cycle. We postulate that the alternation of high and low B-endorphin hypothalamic activity, which we have shown to occur during the menstrual cycle, is an important causal phenomenon in cyclicity and that, in certain cases, amenorrhea may reflect abnormal hypothalamic B-endorphin activity. Supported by NIH grants HD 05077 and 10873.

S.69 COTRANSLATIONAL EVENTS IN PEPTIDE SECRETION

D.I. Meyer, Cell Biology Program, European Molecular Biology Laboratory, D6900 Heidelberg (Federal Republic of Germany)

The mechanism whereby nascent membrane and secretory proteins are selected for incorporation into or transport through the endoplasmic reticulum (ER) has been recently characterized. Briefly, the *signal recognition particle* (SRP), a cytoplasmic ribonucleoprotein complex, arrests translation of nascent secretory and membrane proteins at a point when the signal sequence has emerged from the ribosome (1). The arrest is maintained until the m-RNA-ribosome-SRP-nascent chain complex has contacted the correct membrane, the rough ER. At this point the complex "docks" with the membrane, the translation block is released and translocation commences. An ER specific component, the *docking protein*, mediates the interaction with the membrane by serving as a receptor for SRP and releases the SRP-induced translation arrest (2). The docking protein is an integral membrane protein, has a MW of 72,000 daltons, with a functional cytoplasmically-disposed domain of 60,000 Kd (3,4).

After the signal sequence has crossed the membrane of the ER, an endoprotease, the signal or leader peptidase, removes this portion of the nascent chain. What is still a complete mystery is the way in which the protein crosses the lipid bilayer and whether proteins other than SRP, Docking protein, leader peptidase and possibly a ribosome-binding component (5) are involved. We have begun to accumulate evidence that other, as yet undefined, proteins play a role.

The simplest approach to answering the question regarding the need for other proteins in the translocation process is to reconstitute the known components into a system including an artificial lipid bilayer. Initial results indicate that translocation cannot occur through a lipid bilayer which contains only purified docking protein.

Other experiments support this conclusion. By removing the 60 Kd cytoplasmic domain of the docking protein with mild proteolysis and high salt treatment an inactive microsomal vesicle is obtained. Under the appropriate conditions this proteolytic fragment can be added back to the inactive membranes to reconstitute function (6). When the inactive microsomes generated in this way are further proteolyzed the ability to recombine with the docking protein fragment is lost. This provides additional support for the existence of other ER proteins that are involved in translocation.

1. Walter, P. and Blobel, G. (1981) J. Cell Biol. 91, 545.
2. Meyer, D.I. et al. (1982) Nature 297, 647.
3. Meyer, D.I. and Dobberstein, B. (1980) 87, 503.
4. Meyer, D.I. et al. (1982) J. Cell Biol. 92, 579.
5. Kreibich, G. et al. (1978) J. Cell Biol. 77, 464.
6. Meyer, D.I. and Dobberstein, B. (1980) J. Cell Biol. 87, 498.

S.70 Abstract not received.

S.71 PROTEOLYTIC PROCESSING OF POLYPEPTIDE HORMONE PRECURSORS. K. Docherty, J. Hutton, B. SanSegundo, S.J. Chan, R.J. Carroll, and D.F. Steiner*, Department of Biochemistry, University of Chicago, 920 E. 58th Street, Chicago, Illinois 60637.

Proteolytic processing of hormone precursors occurs at several stages during their intracellular transport and storage. The processing enzymes are topographically organized along the secretory pathway and this discrete localization poses challenging problems in their identification and isolation. Two major levels of processing have been distinguished on the basis of timing, subcellular localization and cleavage mechanisms (Docherty, K. and Steiner, D.F. Ann. Rev. Physiol. 44, 625, 1981). The first is the signal cleavage mechanism which operates very rapidly, probably mainly cotranslationally, at the level of the R.E.R. (rough endoplasmic reticulum) membrane. Although a single endoprotease (signal or leader peptidase) located on the luminal side of the R.E.R. can accomplish this, evidence suggests that additional proteases associated with the R.E.R. may rapidly degrade the signal peptide after its removal. The signal peptide is thus not a normal secretory product.

The second major site of limited intracellular proteolysis can be broadly localized within the Golgi/granule system. Studies on the formation and processing of many proproteins including proinsulin, POMC and proparathyroid hormone have shown that processing of these forms begins only after their arrival in the Golgi apparatus and continues for many hours subsequently, as these products are stored in maturing cytosolic granules. In the case of some neuropeptides, maturation may occur as secretory vesicles move along nerve processes. Processing is almost always at pairs of basic residues by proteases having cleavage specificity similar but not identical to that of trypsin and carboxypeptidase B. Workers in several laboratories have described broken-cell systems which process precursors such as proinsulin or POMC *in vitro*. The endoprotease appears to be trypsin-like in specificity but with a thiol rather than serine in the active site and a lower, slightly acidic, pH optimum. Its inhibitory profile most closely resembles that of lysosomal cathepsin B. However, cathepsin B has too broad a cleavage specificity, as well as significant dipeptidyl carboxypeptidase activity against peptides such as glucagon, resulting in degradation or inappropriate cleavage. We have recently identified 31.5K and 39K cathepsin B-related proteases in islet granule fractions labeled with ^{125}I-Tyr-ALACK (Ala-Lys-Arg-chlormethyl ketone), an active site titrant of both trypsin-like and cathepsin B-like enzymes. These forms are precipitable with antibodies to cathepsin B (kindly provided by H. Kirschke) and the 39K form can be converted with pepsin to the approximate size of the smaller form. Further studies are in progress to determine the substrate specificity, mechanism of activation, and cleavage activity of the 39K protease against various prohormonal peptides. Biosynthetic studies indicate that cathepsin B is derived from a 44K precursor. Our results, taken together with those of others, clearly implicate cathepsin B-like enzymes, or their precursors in the endoproteolytic processing of prohormones. Secretory granule carboxypeptidase B-like enzymes from several tissues also exhibit properties more characteristic of catheptic enzymes, i.e. a more acid pH optimum, but with other features which tend to distinguish them from the lysosomal or pancreatic carboxypeptidases, including molecular size and stimulation by cobalt ions. It is of interest that while signal peptidase activity is distributed extremely widely in life forms, not all cells (e.g. Xenopus oocytes, monkey kidney cells, bacteria) appear to be able to process proproteins. Nonetheless, this form of processing appears to be of ancient phylogenetic origin, occuring in primitive vertebrates as well as molluscs and yeast cells (supported by USPHS AM 13914 and AM 20595).

S.72 PROTEOLYTIC PROCESSING OF PITUITARY PROHORMONES BY UNIQUE LYS-ARG SPECIFIC CONVERTING ENZYMES.

Y. Pen Loh* and D. Parish, Section on Cellular Neurobiology, Laboratory of Neurochemistry and Neuroimmunology, National Institute of Child Health and Human Development, National Institutes of Health, Bethesda, MD 20205, U.S.A.

It is well established from numerous studies that peptide hormones are synthesized from larger prohormones. The primary sequence of the prohormones reveal that the peptide hormones to be cleaved are flanked by paired basic amino acid residues, the most common being Lys-Arg pairs. Hence, it has been proposed that processing of prohormones involved specific proteolytic cleavages at these paired basic residues. Until recently, little was known about such prohormone converting enzymes.

We have been studying the proteolytic converting enzymes involved in the processing of pro-opiomelanocortin (POMC), a prohormone synthesized by the intermediate and anterior lobes of the pituitary. In both these lobes, POMC is cleaved at Lys-Arg residues to yield ACTH, β-LPH and β-endorphin. In the intermediate lobe, ACTH is further cleaved at Lys-Lys-Arg-Arg residues to form α-MSH. An enzyme activity which cleaves mouse POMC specifically at Lys-Arg pairs has been partially purified from bovine intermediate lobe secretory vesicles. This POMC converting enzyme (PCE) activity cleaved the prohormone to yield ACTH, β-LPH and β-endorphin, but did not form any α-MSH-like peptides. Further evidence for the cleavage of POMC by PCE at Lys-Arg pairs came from the ability to release stochiometrically appropriate amounts of free Lys from the cleavage products with carboxypeptidase B treatment. Characterization of the PCE activity revealed that it is a glycoprotein and has a pH optimum of 4.0, consistent with the acidic internal pH of these secretory vesicles. The PCE activity was not blocked by TLCK, PMSF and EDTA, agents which inhibit trypsin, and lysosomal cathepsin B; but was inhibited by PCMB (a thiol blocker) and pepstatin A. Thus, the PCE activity appears to be due to a unique enzyme.

A similar activity has also been found in neural lobe secretory vesicles which cleaves the Lys-Arg pair of pro-vasopressin and pro-oxytocin. Thus there exists, in both the intermediate and neural lobes, closely related paired basic residue specific enzymes which are capable of processing their endogenous prohormones. Further studies will determine if there is a universal or a family of enzymes involved in prohormone cleavage at paired basic residues.

S.73 INTRACELLULAR FUNCTION OF RENIN. T. Inagami*, K. Pandey, K. Naruse and M. Nakamaru, Department of Biochemistry and Hypertension Center, Vanderbilt University School of Medicine, Nashville, TN 37232, U.S.A..

While renin had been considered as a plasma enzyme with a highly specialized function to initiate angiotensin II formation from its prohormone angiotensinogen, renin-like activity has been reported in many types of tissues and cells. These include the brain, vascular bed, heart, liver, spleen, digestive tract and various endocrine glands such as the pituitary gland and adrenals. It was later found that some of the activities were artifacts due to non-specific action of cathepsins, the ubiquitous lysosomal proteases. However, we were able to demonstrate the presence of true renin in some of these tissues by chromatographic separation of cathepsin and renin and by the specific inhibition of renin by antibody to renin. Furthermore, we have detected the presence of mRNA for renin in the adrenal cortex, pituitary, testis, vascular endothelial and smooth muscle cell, and spleen. The role of local renin was not clear. We have asked whether local renin functions by an intracellular mechanism by studies using immunohistochemical methods and by using cultured cells. Several lines of cultured neuroblastoma cells were found to contain renin, angiotensin I, angiotensin I converting enzyme and angiotensin II. These cell lines were shown to synthesize angiotensinogen. Similar findings are have been made with pheochromocytoma cells, adrenal cortical cells, cloned juxtaglomerular cells, testicular Leydig cells, aortic smooth muscle cells and endothelial cells. By immunohistochemical studies using antibodies to renin, angiotensin I and angiotensin II, we found coexistence of these components of the renin-angiotensin system in rat and human juxtaglomerular cells, in the luteinizing hormone producing cells in rat anterior pituitary, and in testicular Leydig cells, indicating the intracellular production of angiotensin II by local renin. The physiological role of the intracellular renin-angiotensin system is not yet clarified. However, some interesting findings are being made. Except for juxtaglomerular cells and placental cholionic cells, renin does not seem to be secreted. It is angiotensin II which is secreted. Secretion of peptide hormone but not the peptide hormone forming enzyme is in agreement with other endocrine systems. Angiotensin II generated locally stimulates the secretory function of the same cells in the autocrine manner. For example, LH-gonadotrophs in culture secretes LH by angiotensin II stimulation, and zona glomerulosa cells in adrenal capsules are stimulated to synthesize and secrete aldosterone.

S.74 ACTIONS OF ANGIOTENSIN II ON THE BRAIN. Ian A. Reid,* Department of Physiology, University of California, San Francisco, CA 94143, USA.

Angiotensin II acts on the brain to produce a wide variety of cardiovascular, endocrine, renal and behavioral effects. These include elevation of arterial pressure, increased secretion of several pituitary hormones including vasopressin, oxytocin, ACTH and LH, inhibition of renin release by the kidneys, natriuresis, and stimulation of drinking and sodium appetite. The renin-angiotensin system is therefore in a position to exert important effects on cardiovascular regulation, fluid and electrolyte balance and even reproductive function.

During recent years, a considerable amount of information concerning the site and mechanism of the different central actions of angiotensin has been obtained. It has been established that the receptors for many of the actions are contained within the circumventricular organs, specialized areas of the brain which lack a blood brain barrier. The circumventricular organs which have received the most attention include the area postrema, subfornical organ, organum vasculosum of the lamina terminalis and the median eminence, and it is clear that many of the central cardiovascular, endocrine and behavioral effects of angiotensin are mediated via receptors in these structures. Many of the central effects of angiotensin II can be produced by centrally-administered angiotensin or by circulating, blood-borne angiotensin: these may act at common receptor sites in the circumventricular organs. Whether the different central effects of angiotensin II are normally produced by blood-borne angiotensin formed by the renal renin-angiotensin system, by angiotensin formed centrally by a brain renin-angiotensin system, or by both, remains to be determined.

The physiological significance of the central actions of angiotensin II is beginning to be understood. Dose-response studies have provided evidence that some of the actions, including elevation of arterial pressure, increased drinking and stimulation of ACTH secretion, can be produced by physiological levels of angiotensin II. Studies involving pharmacological blockade of the renin-angiotensin system or lesioning of receptor sites for angiotensin II have provided further evidence that the central actions of angiotensin II are physiologically important. Nevertheless, much additional research will be required before the significance of these actions will be completely understood.

S.75 NEW CLINICAL ASPECTS OF THE RENIN SYSTEM IN HYPERTENSION. A.F. Lever*, MRC Blood Pressure Unit, Western Infirmary, Glasgow G11 6NT, Scotland.

Angiotensin II is involved in the regulation of arterial pressure and it may be involved in the pathogenesis of hypertension. There are several ways in which the peptide could raise blood pressure: by a direct action where a 5-, 20-fold increase of plasma angiotensin II concentration is needed to produce a small rise of blood pressure by direct vasoconstriction. Blood-borne angiotensin II may also raise blood pressure gradually by a slow-developing action probably involving the nervous system. The rise of plasma angiotensin II concentration needed here is less, but the ultimate increase of blood pressure is much greater. The third possibility is that angiotensin II is generated locally within blood vessels; a fourth that it is generated and acts locally within the brain. In renin-secreting tumour increased plasma angiotensin II concentration is presumed to be the whole cause of the hypertension and yet the rise of blood pressure is greater than can be explained by the direct action alone. Renal artery stenosis in man and renal artery constriction in animals is a cause of hypertension where increased angiotensin II is almost certain to be responsible for the early stages of hypertension, but where some other mechanisms, possibly another action of angiotensin II, is responsible later. Essential hypertension is a state in which renin and angiotensin II are not likely to be involved in pathogenesis. This poses an interesting question: why is it that in all these different states relatively specific inhibitors of the renin-angiotensin mechanism are so successful in reducing blood pressure?

S.76 PHARMACOLOGIC INHIBITION OF RENIN AND ANGIOTENSIN CONVERTING ENZYME: RATIONAL BASIS AND COMPARISON OF RESULTS. VICTOR J. DZAU*Brigham and Women's Hospital, Harvard Medical School, Boston, MA

The renin angiotensin system plays a central role in blood pressure regulation. Specific inhibition of this system is likely to play a significant role in the therapy of hypertension. Since renin and angiotensin converting enzyme (ACE) are key enzymes in the generation of Angiotensin II, pharmacologic inhibition of these enzymes has become the major strategy in the development of antihypertensive drugs. ACE inhibitors have been synthesized based on a hypothetical model of the active site of ACE. Captopril, and enalapril are proline derivatives and are orally active. Several other ACE inhibitors are also under study. ACE inhibition is particularly effective in lowering blood pressure in sodium depleted subjects. The magnitude of acute depressor response appear to correlate with the pretreatment plasma renin activity. However, patients with normal or low renin essential hypertension also exhibit depressor responses of lesser magnitude. When combined with a diuretic, captopril controlled the blood pressure in over 90% of patients with essential hypertension. Part of depressor effect maybe mediated by increased bradykinin, vasodilator prostaglandins or decreased basoreceptor sensitivity. Preliminary evidence suggests that the prostaglandin accumulation may not occur with enalapril.

Chemical renin inhibitors include two major classes of compounds: general peptide inhibitors of acid proteases or angiotensinogen analogs. Pepstatin inhibits many acid proteases. Its application have been limited by its relative insolubility and nonselectivity. The addition of charged amino acids at the carboxyterminus have rendered it more useful. Analogs of angiotensinogen (minimal octapeptide substrate) have yielded highly selective competitive inhibitors. These analogs are highly species selective probably because of differing substrate specificity. Recent potent inhibitors are derived from a combined approach using substrate analogs with statine substitutions and/or reduced peptide bond at the cleavage site. These inhibitors have K_i of up to 10^{-11}M and increased stability when administered in vivo. All these compounds are limited by relatively short half life and susceptibility to digestive enzymes. In vivo studies with various peptide inhibitors have yielded overall results that appear somewhat different from those of ACE inhibitors. Substrate analog (RIP) administered to supine or upright man resulted in significant drop in blood pressure. More recently, the statine containing inhibitor SCRIP yielded no depressor response with increasing doses of the agent until the PRA was completely inhibited. Following this, blood pressure declined which was related to dose of drug infused. Taken together, both renin inhibitors and angiotensin converting enzyme inhibitors appear to be effective agents but produce somewhat different cardiovascular responses. The basis for this discrepancy is unclear. The differences in specificity, volume and tissues of distribution and effects on central nervous system may be responsible. Further investigations will be necessary to identify the advantages and disadvantage of these two approaches.

S.77 DIET-INDUCED THERMOGENESIS AND BROWN FAT. N.J.Rothwell* and M.J.Stock.
Department of Physiology, St.George's Hospital Medical School, Cranmer Terrace, London SW17 ORE, U.K.

Most mammals maintain a relatively constant body weight and energy content throughout most of their adult life, and although this can be partly ascribed to control of energy intake, the regulation of energy balance is also dependent on variations in energy expenditure. Extensive studies, performed largely on laboratory rodents, have demonstrated that voluntary hyperphagia is usually accompanied by compensatory increases in energy expenditure, referred to as diet-induced thermogenesis (DIT). This regulatory form of heat production, like most physiological parameters, is variable and dependent on a number of physiological and environmental factors, such as age, sex, genetic background, diet, season, temperature and housing conditions. Thus, some animals have a high capacity for DIT and maintain energy balance over a very wide range of energy intakes (e.g. young wild animals), while others develop obesity when consuming only slightly more food than normal.

The mechanisms of DIT are very similar to those responsible for the non-shivering thermogenesis (NST) seen in cold-adapted or hibernating animals. Both forms of heat production are activated by the sympathetic nervous system, and quantitative estimates of in vivo tissue oxygen consumption have shown that both result largely from heat production in brown adipose tissue, via an uncoupling of oxidative phosphorylation.

Brown fat activity, and hence diet-induced and non-shivering thermogenesis are controlled primarily by neural release of noradrenaline, but can be modified by other neural and hormonal systems. For example, there is some evidence that dopamine may activate brown fat and that noradrenaline stimulation of thermogenesis in the tissue may also involve histamine release. Conversely, the parasympathetic nervous system appears to inhibit DIT, since atropine treatment enhances the thermogenic responses to food.

Thyroid hormones, which exert potent effects on metabolic rate, seem to have only a permissive role in DIT, but may be involved in the trophic changes in brown fat during chronic hyperphagia. Adrenal steroids have important influences in DIT, and removal of the adrenal glands totally prevents the development of genetic and dietary obesity, largely due to stimulation of brown fat activity and DIT. These changes can be totally prevented by treatment of adrenalectomised rats with corticosterone.

The afferent signals relating the ingestion of food to activation of brown fat and metabolic rate are largely unknown, but it seems that insulin, possibly acting via the ventromedial hypothalamus, may mediate the thermogenic response to carbohydrate. DIT resulting from fat ingestion is not dependent on insulin release but could involve another gut hormone.

S.78 BROWN ADIPOSE TISSUE THERMOGENESIS AND OBESITY IN ANIMALS.

P. Trayhurn*
Dunn Nutrition Laboratory, Medical Research Council and University of Cambridge, Milton Road, Cambridge CB4 1XJ, U.K.

The mechanisms responsible for the increase in body fat that leads to obesity have been the subject of considerable debate over a number of years. The 'pathological' rise in fat stores in obesity must, of course, be differentiated from the 'physiologically programmed' increases in fat occurring at specific periods in an animal's life (e.g. during pregnancy and pre-hibernation), where the energy deposition relates to a subsequent energy demand. The problem of obesity is in essence one of energy balance - either food intake is higher than normal, or one or more components of energy expenditure is abnormally low. Animal models have been extensively used in the study of obesity, and a wide range of such models is available. These include animals where obesity is genetically determined - such as the obese (ob/ob) mouse, the diabetic-obese (db/db) mouse and the fatty (fa/fa) rat - and animals where the condition is experimentally induced. Examples of methods by which obesity can be induced experimentally include the administration of insulin, corticosteroids or gold thioglucose, lesioning of the ventromedial hypothalamus, and the provision of a high fat diet. In several types of animal obesity, notably the genetically inherited forms, it is clear that the condition can develop on a normal energy intake, with the subsequent development of hyperphagia exacerbating the disorder. This has led to interest in the routes by which energy expenditure can be reduced, with a particular emphasis on the activity of brown adipose tissue - the major site of thermoregulatory non-shivering thermogenesis in rodents. There is now considerable evidence from several experimental approaches, including blood flow measurements and various indices of the activity of the mitochondrial proton conductance pathway, that the thermogenic activity of brown adipose tissue is decreased in young ob/ob and db/db mice and that this is the principal reason for their ability to deposit excessive amounts of fat while receiving a normal energy intake. The price paid for this change appears to be a low body temperature. When hyperphagia develops secondarily in these mutants, and in the fa/fa rat, the increased energy intake does not lead to the same stimulation of brown adipose tissue thermogenesis as in normal animals i.e. the capacity for diet-induced thermogenesis is impaired. The effects of adrenalectomy in both fa/fa rats and ob/ob mice indicate that glucocorticoids inhibit brown adipose tissue thermogenesis in these mutants, adrenalectomy leading to a rapid increase both in mitochondrial mass and in the activity of the proton conductance pathway. This is consistent with results showing a suppression of thermogenesis in brown adipose tissue in mice treated chronically with corticosterone. Studies on noradrenaline turnover suggest that the activity of the sympathetic innervation to brown adipose tissue is reduced in obese mutants, and this is likely to be a key factor in determining thermogenesis in the tissue and thus the overall metabolic efficiency of the animal.

S.79 DIET-INDUCED CHANGES IN SYMPATHOADRENAL ACTIVITY: IMPLICATIONS FOR THERMOGENESIS. L. Landsberg*, J.B. Young, Beth Israel Hospital and Harvard Medical School. Boston, MA 02215, USA.

Utilizing a variety of of techniques including the measurement of norepinephrine (NE) turnover in the tissues of experimental animals, the measurement of urinary catecholamine excretion in human subjects and animals, and the measurement of plasma catecholamines in humans, the effect of dietary intake on the functional state of the sympathoadrenal system has been studied. Fasting suppresses sympathetic nervous system (SNS) activity in experimental animals as demonstrated by markedly diminished rates of NE turnover in a variety of organs including heart, liver, pancreas, and interscapular brown adipose tissue (IBAT). In human subjects fasting diminishes NE excretion while increasing urinary epinephrine, consistent with a suppressive effect on the SNS and modest stimulation of the adrenal medulla. In contrast, overfeeding markedly stimulates the SNS. NE turnover in heart and IBAT is increased 50-100% in rats fed a mixed "cafeteria" diet that substantially increases caloric intake. Fat and sucrose, moreover, when added to the diet increase NE turnover in these organs even when total caloric intake is not increased. Stimulation of the SNS by fat or sucrose requires intestinal absorbtion since the effect of fat is blocked by cholestyramine (a bile-acid binding resin) and the effect of sucrose is blocked by acarbose (a sucrase inhibitor). Addition of protein to the diet, in the form of casein, is, in contrast, without effect. Since hypoglycemia, induced by fasting in pregnant or phlorizin treated rats, and 2-deoxyglucose administration or streptozotocin diabetes (in freely feeding animals) are all associated with diminished NE turnover in rats, and since euglycemic hyperinsulinemia, induced by insulin infusions in normal human subjects increases plasma NE level, insulin-mediated glucose metabolism may be one signal in the relationship between dietary intake and sympathoadrenal activity. Experiments in the gold-thioglucose treated mouse indicate that insulin-glucose sensitive neurons in the ventromedial hypothalamus are involved in the integration of this signal since mice treated with gold thioglucose fail to suppress sympathetic activity with fasting. In conclusion: 1) Fasting supresses the SNS and stimulates the adrenal medulla; this pattern of sympathoadrenal response fosters substrate mobilization at a lower net energy cost. SNS supression during therapeutic dieting may, therefore, diminish energy output and reduce the efficiency of low energy diets. 2) Overfeeding a mixed diet stimulates the SNS, an effect attributable to carbohydrate and fat, since protein does not affect the SNS. The differential effects of various nutrients might permit an organism consuming a low protein diet to maintain energy balance while satisfying nitrogen requirements. The possibility that altered SNS responses to diet may contibute to obesity in some individuals by diminishing dietary thermogenesis warrants study. 3) The SNS may contribute to the cardiovacular changes that accompany alterations in dietary intake. The hypotensive effect of caloric restriction, on the one hand, and the association of obesity and hypertension on the other, may involve diet-induced changes in SNS activity. 4) Insulin-mediated glucose metabolism within the ventromedial hypothalamus is one (of many) signals in the coupling of ditary intake and sympathetic activity.

S.80 **THE MECHANISM OF CHANGES IN ENERGY EXPENDITURE IN RELATION TO CHANGES IN ENERGY INTAKE IN RATS.** G. R. Hervey* and G. Tobin,
Department of Physiology, University of Leeds, Leeds LS2 9JT, U.K.

'Thermogenesis' is an unsatisfactory term. All living processes produce heat, and no consensus exists as to which it refers to. After some uncertainty 'diet-induced thermogenesis' is now described as a regulatory mechanism, evoked by overfeeding, which dissipates up to 100 % of excess energy intake, and is distinct from the inevitable energy costs of increased feeding (Stock & Rothwell, J. Roy. Soc. Med. **76**, 71-73, 1983). This equates it with 'Luxuskonsumption', the existence of which has been controversial for many years.

Almost all claims that Luxuskonsumption exists have been based on estimates of energy intake and storage, and depend on the assumption that missing energy represents increased expenditure. We (Clin. Sci. **64**, 7-18, 1983) have reviewed these claims: evaluation requires careful, critical study of the experimental evidence. We consider the methods used inadequate to infer expenditure, or to show whether increases exceeded inevitable costs. There has been no evidence that the amplitude and time relationships of increased energy expenditure after overfeeding are consistent with a regulatory mechanism.

Our own studies have centred on measuring with the highest attainable accuracy energy intake, energy storage (by carcass analysis) and energy expenditure (by calorimetry). Energy balances over periods of up to 65 days show errors, mainly systematic, of not more than 3 %. The increase in energy expenditure with overfeeding by tube has been in the range 20 - 45 kJ / 100 kJ excess intake, and with overfeeding by 'cafeteria' diet 20 - 40 kJ / 100 kJ. Origin, strain and age of rats have no discernible influence.

There are at least three non-regulatory causes of increases in energy expenditure after overfeeding: increased activity of gut and liver; synthesis of fat; and the consequences of being heavier. We (Armitage et al., J. Physiol. **342**, 229-251, 1983) have reviewed published estimates, and our results support these. Metabolism is elevated over the 7 h after a meal by approx. 8 kJ /100 kJ intake on a mixed diet. We find the cost of synthesis of fat to be approx. 12 kJ / 100 kJ excess intake, when fat is added to a tube-fed maintenance diet supplying 84 % of energy as carbohydrate and 16 % as protein; and approx. 18 kJ / 100 kJ when carbohydrate is added. The cost of being heavier is approx. 0.1 kJ / g weight gain: usually a minor factor, but it accounts for the total exceeding 40 kJ / 100 kJ when gross obesity was produced by tube-feeding.

The total of the three components accounts for the measured increase in metabolism within attainable precision. It is impossible to show that there is no contribution from any other factor. The maximum possible unaccounted energy expenditure, however, is about 10 kJ / 100 kJ excess intake; this must be compared with the 90 or even 100 kJ / 100 kJ postulated for Luxuskonsumption. There may be further, modest, non-regulatory factors, for example increased locomotor activity. In any case the existence of discrepancies between estimates of energy intake and storage, which could be due to error, is not adequate evidence for a new or controversial mechanism. We believe there is no sound evidence for the existence of Luxuskonsumption.

When energy intake is reduced to 1.0 - 0.7 times normal intake, expenditure is reduced in the same proportion. There is thus overall a two-part relationship between intake and expenditure. The reduction of expenditure with reduced intake does appear to regulatory. Its mechanism is unknown.

S.81 MECHANISMS OF ESTROGENIC REGULATION OF HUMAN BREAST CANCER. M. Lippman*, R. Dickson, D. Bronzert and K. Huff, Medical Breast Cancer Section, Medicine Branch, National Cancer Institute, Bethesda, Maryland 20205.

In previous work we have shown that clonal lines of human breast cancer cells are responsive to estrogens and antiestrogens. At physiologic concentrations, estrogen can stimulate cell proliferation by stimulation of major de novo and scavenger pathways of DNA synthesis. We have measured activities of numerous enzymes involved in DNA synthesis (thymidine kinase, thymidylate synthetase, aspartate transcarbamylase, dihydrofolate reductase and DNA polymerase). All are increased by estrogens and decreased by antiestrogens. We have used a cloned cDNA for thymidine kinase and shown that regulation of mRNA for thymidine kinase in hormone responsive human breast cancer cells accounts for estrogen stimulation and antiestrogen inhibition of thymidine kinase activity. Alterations in thymidine kinase activity induced by estrogens and antiestrogens are not accompanied by apparent changes in gene methylation. In an effort to define critical steps required for growth regulation by estrogens, we considered the possibility that hormones might act by inducing the secretion of specific mammary growth factors which might stimulate growth. Using the conditioned medium from hormone responsive breast cancer cells it is possible to show potent growth stimulatory activity using other breast cancer cells as a target. The growth stimulatory activity present in conditioned medium is under estrogen control and can totally replace estrogen as a mitogen. Several fractions of growth activity have been partially purified using a system in which human breast cancer cells are grown in defined medium supplemented with transferrin and fibronectin. Estradiol, transferrin and fibronectin are sequentially removed from concentrated medium containing protease inhibitors followed by Sephacryl G200 chromatography and HPLC analysis. Several discrete growth stimulatory activities all of which are estrogen regulated have been identified. One of these activities cross reacts in a radioimmunoassay with IGF-1. We are currently preparing monoclonal antibodies to these growth factors and further exploring their biologic relevance. Finally, in an attempt to better understand the steps involved in the conversion from the hormone dependent to the hormone independent state we have prepared a series of variant cell lines using several selection procedures involving toxic concentrations of several antiestrogens or chronic exposure to ^{125}I estradiol. A variety of phenotypes have been obtained including cells able to show growth stimulation by estrogens but no induction of progesterone receptor. These cells are completely and stably uninhibited by antiestrogens. Since growth factor production is hormonally regulated we asked whether transfection of breast cancer cells with an oncgene capable of transforming 3T3 cells (V-ras) would result in a hormone independent phenotype. We have used co-transfection with a plasmid containing bacterial XGPRT'ase followed by incubation in selective medium. Such cells show stable integration of V-ras sequences and express high levels of mRNA derived from these V-ras sequences. V-ras RNA expression is not hormonally regulated. Implications of these experiments in understanding mechanisms by which hormones can regulate human breast cancer cell growth will be discussed.

S.82 AN ESTROGEN* REGULATED SECRETORY PROTEIN IN HUMAN MAMMARY CANCER.

H. Rochefort*, F. Capony, M. Garcia, O. Massot, F. May, F. Veith, F. Vignon and B. Westley, Unité d'Endocrinologie Cellulaire et Moléculaire (U 148) INSERM, 60 rue de Navacelles, 34100 Montpellier, France.

We have studied the proteins regulated by estrogens in metastatic breast cancer cells in culture in an attempt to find a better marker of hormone dependency and to analyse the mechanism by which estradiol stimulates the growth of breast cancer. In cell lines containing estrogen receptor, estrogens stimulate the total production of proteins in the medium and cell growth. In MCF7- and ZR75-1- cells, estrogens specifically increase the production of a 52,000 dalton (52 K) glycoprotein which is released into the culture medium (Cell 20, 352-362, 1980). The antiestrogens, Tamoxifen and Progestins, do not themselves induce the 52 K protein, but inhibit its induction by estrogens.

Several high affinity monoclonal antibodies to the purified secretory 52 K protein have been produced (in collaboration with Clin-Midy Laboratories). By immuno precipitation and western blot experiments the secreted and cellular 52 K protein have been quantified in various cell lines, and in primary cultures of several metastic breast cancers. By peroxidase-antiperoxidase staining, the 52 K protein has been detected in frozen sections of primary breast cancer but not in other estrogen responsive tissues.

The nature and function of the 52 K protein are unknown, but it is not a plasminogen activator or any other known E_2 regulated protein. Several indirect lines of evidence suggest that estrogens might stimulate the growth of breast cancer cells by inducing them to produce growth factors which would then auto-stimulate their proliferation (Autocrine mechanism). We have found that non dialysable, protease sensitive, estrogen induced factors from conditioned media promote the growth of E_2 deprived MCF7 cells. These factors are retained on Con A sepharose suggesting that they are glycoproteins. Monoclonal antibodies to the 52 K protein are currently being used to determine whether the 52 K protein or other estrogen regulated glycoproteins released by MCF7 cells are responsible for this mitogenic activity.

Antiestrogens decrease the production in the medium of the 52 K protein and cell growth in wild type MCF7 cells. However in two antiestrogen resistant cell lines, tamoxifen increases the production of the 52 K protein but not that of a specific estrogen regulated mRNA (pS2) (in collaboration with P. Chambon) suggesting that antiestrogen resistance might be due to production of growth factors by cancer cells.

The 52 K secretory protein may help to understand the mechanism by which estrogens and antiestrogens regulate protein synthesis and cell proliferation. Its assay in plasma and/or tissue might also be useful in clinical practice.

S.83 EPIDEMIOLOGY OF STEROID DEPENDENT CANCER. R.D. Bulbrook*, Imperial Cancer Research Fund, London, GB, WC213PX.

Evidence from epidemiological work indicates that endocrine function is intimately related to the incidence of breast and endometrial cancer. Age at menarche, first child, menopause are established determinants of risk: early oophorectomy markedly reduces incidence. Nulliparity, overweight and administration of oestrogens increase risk.

Attempts to replace inferences about endocrine mechanisms by actual measurements of hormonal status have generally been unsuccessful and this has led to a number of hypotheses such as oestriol as a protective agent; altered oestrogen metabolism; tissue sensitivity; a major role for prolactins or the androgens; and above all, to the luteal phase dysfunction thesis in which a controlling modulating effect of progesterone is postulated.

The recent appreciation that assays of total blood oestrogens might not be the appropriate measurement has led to some interesting new findings. In both endometrial and breast cancer, the fraction of oestradiol in blood thought to be biologically available (i.e. not bound to SHBG) is raised in patients compared with controls. Normal Japanese women have considerably less available oestradiol in their blood than British women and it is suggested that this finding may explain the differences in incidence in the two races. Japanese women with breast cancer have higher levels of available oestradiol than controls. The most persuasive evidence comes from a 22-year prospective study in Guerusey. Women who subsequently developed breast cancer had available oestradiol levels above the 80th percentile for the normal population.

The most important question is what controls the availability of oestradiol. While SHBG capacity declines with increasing weight, preliminary results indicate that other factors are more important and that diet may be involved.

S.84 DRAMATIC RESPONSE TO A NEW ANTIHORMONAL TREATMENT FOR PROSTATE CANCER.

F. Labrie, A. Dupont, A. Bélanger and members of the Laval University Prostate Cancer Program, Depts of Medicine and Molecular Endocrinology, CHUL, Quebec G1V 4G2, Canada.

During the last 40 years, a large number of large-scale studies have analyzed the benefits of endocrine therapy for the treatment of prostate cancer. Following surgical castration and estrogen administration, 60 to 70% of patients with advanced prostatic cancer experience subjective and/or objective improvement for a limited period of time. However, the results obtained are somewhat variable and left many physicians undecided about the real advantages of hormonal therapy. Since orchiectomy presents psychological limitations while estrogens have serious cardiovascular complications which often offset their benefits on the cancer, there was the need for a more acceptable means of neutralizing testicular androgens. It is now well established (Andrology 1, 209, 1980) that chronic treatment of adult men with LHRH agonists easily achieves medical castration with no secondary effects other than those related to low circulating levels of androgens. The mechanism of action of LHRH agonists in the human is blockade of gonadotropin secretion at the pituitary level, thus resulting in a medical hypophysectomy selective to gonadotrophs. Treatment with LHRH agonists alone, however, causes a transient increase in serum androgen levels lasting for 5 to 15 days before castration levels of androgens are reached after 2 to 4 weeks. In addition, 30-40% of total intraprostatic active androgens are locally synthesized from precursor adrenal androgens. In order to prevent the unacceptable risks of the transient rise in serum androgens at the start of LHRH agonist treatment and to neutralize adrenal androgens, we have administered simultaneously the LHRH agonist Buserelin in combination with a pure antiandrogen (Anandron or Flutamide) to 47 and 37 patients having stages D2 and C prostate cancer, respectively. A positive objective response assessed according to the criteria of the US National Prostatic Cancer Project (NPCP) was observed in all stage D2 patients as compared to 60 to 70% in previous studies. Moreover, after one year of treatment, remission is at 90% as compared to 50 to 60% in previous studies. After 1½ year of combined treatment, death has occurred in only 1 out of 30 patients (3.3%) as compared to 24 to 37.7% in all the large scale studies performed since 1950, thus representing a 8-to 11-fold improvement in survival. All 37 stage C patients showed a positive response and only one patient has shown progression to stage D2. A most important conclusion of this study is that previously untreated patients with prostatic cancer, even at the late metastatic stage, are exquisitively sensitive to androgens. In fact, when complete androgen blockade is achieved in previously untreated stage D2 or C patients, a positive objective response has been observed in all patients treated so far. Another most important conclusion is that a large proportion of the prostatic cancer cells which continue to grow under the influence of androgens of adrenal origin become insensitive to androgens in this androgen-poor milieu. The present data based on well-demonstrated endocrine principles clearly indicate that orchiectomy, estrogens and LHRH agonists alone should not be further used for the treatment of prostate cancer in the absence of a pure antiandrogen and that, instead, complete androgen blockade should be achieved at the start of treatment, at least at stages C and D of the disease.

S.85 HLA-DR EXPRESSION AS A FACTOR IN ENDOCRINE AUTOIMMUNE DISORDERS.

F. Bottazzo*, Immunology Department, The Middlesex Hospital Medical School, London, W1P 9PG, UK.

Organ-specific autoimmunity has been demonstrated in all the major endocrine organs, in hypothalamic nuclei and in paracrine cells of the gastrointestinal tract. The major question remains of how endocrine cells are able to provoke an efficient immune response to their own antigens. HLA-DR-positive cells such as macrophages, dendritic, interdigitating, and vascular endothelial cells usually initiate the immune responses to exogenous antigens by stimulating T-helper cells to divide. The same mechanism has been postulated for an efficient presentation of endocrine autoantigens. However we have shown that normal thyroid epithelial cells can be stimulated with mitogens to express DR in culture. Furthermore in thyrotoxicosis and in Hashimoto's disease, thyrocytes were found to express these molecules spontaneously. Gamma-interferon (IFN) is the best known inducer of HLA-DR expression in competent immune cells. Preliminary evidence suggests that interferon may induce the synthesis of these cell surface glycoproteins on normal thyrocytes when added to the cultures and it appears to act preferentially on glands removed from HLA-DR3 individuals. In the pathogenesis of autoimmune endocrine disorders we envisage the following sequence: local viral infection which would cause IFN production, or any other local environmental factor which would induce DR antigen expression, presentation of autoantigens, and subsequent autoimmune T cell induction. These T cells would activate effector B and T cells. Whether the initial induction of autoimmune T cells leads to autoimmune disease would depend on a variety of other factors such as abnormalities of the suppressor T cell pathway, reported to coexist with autoimmunity and necessary to induce autoimmune diseases in mice. This mechanism of autoimmune disease induction explains vague associations with viral infections, long latency periods before disease becomes manifest and provides a link for the well documented HLA-DR association with autoimmunity in man.

S.86 MECHANISM OF POSTPARTUM THYROID DISEASE

Nobuyuki Amino*

Department of Laboratory Medicine, Osaka University Medical School, Osaka 553, Japan

Pregnancy markedly influences the clinical course of Hashimoto's disease and Graves' disease. Both diseases are ameliorated during pregnancy. However diseases are aggravated after delivery and transient thyrotoxicosis and/or hypothyroidism are frequently observed. Subclinical autoimmune thyroiditis is also aggravated after delivery and thyroid dysfunction was found in 5.5 per cent of postpartum women in general population. The prevalence of persistent primary hypothyroidism was 0.2 per cent, which is 100 times higher than that for postpartum pituitary hypothyroidism. In Hashimoto's disease titers of antithyroid microsomal antibody and complement dependent cytotoxic antibody, and peripheral counts of total and K lymphocytes decreased during pregnancy but increased after delivery. Furthermore peripheral B lymphocytes and large granular lymphocytes, which have both natural killer and ADCC activities, increased after delivery, although there was no significant change of helper T/suppressor T cell ratio. Development of postpartum hypothyroidism could be predicted by MCHA titers and previous history, and could be prevented by short-term steroid therapy which was started immediately after delivery. In Graves' disease spontaneous changes of immune reactions as well as thyroid function were examined in the patients who were considered to be in a state of remission or near remission. About one-fourth of the patients relapsed Graves' thyrotoxicosis after delivery. At the time of postpartum relapse, activities of TSH-binding inhibitory immunoglobulins (TBII) were not detectable even by sensitive radioreceptor assay, although significant increase of peripheral B lymphocytes and decrease of $T\gamma$ lymphocytes were observed. However significant increase of TBII activity was observed 1-2 months later in all patients who relapsed Graves' thyrotoxicosis. Data suggest that cellular immunity may be more important than humoral immunity in the initiation of Graves' thyrotoxicosis, or that local immune reactions may be different from immunological abnormalities detected in peripheral blood. Postpartum relapse of Graves' thyrotoxicosis could be predicted by increase of free T_4 index at both 10-15 and 30-32 weeks of pregnancy. Short-term steroid therapy delayed the recurrence of thyrotoxicosis. It may be possible to prevent completely by more suitable steroid therapy. Other autoimmune diseases often ameliorate during pregnancy and are aggravated more frequently after delivery. "Immune rebound hypothesis" is proposed as the mechanism of postpartum development of thyroid dysfunction.

S.87 MODULATION OF LYMPHOCYTE FUNCTION IN AUTOIMMUNE THYROID DISEASE.

A.M. McGregor*, A.P. Weetman, R. Hassman, D.P. Rennie, M.E. Ludgate, C.Gunn and R. Hall, Department of Medicine, Welsh National School of Medicine, Heath Park, Cardiff CF4 4XN, Wales

Autoimmune thyroid disease (AITD) arises in genetically predisposed individuals and though the aetiology remains uncertain the pathogenetic mechanisms inducing the disease are increasingly well understood. Since AITD is due to immune-mediated events, the most effective means of controlling the disease will ultimately depend on modulating the aberrant autoimmune response. For this to be feasible a clear understanding of the immune response made to an autoantigen is necessary. Studies in vivo and in vitro in man and in rat models of AITD have begun to clarify the humoral and cell-mediated autoimmune responses and the influence of a wide variety of pharmacological and environmental factors such as lithium and iodide. The sites in the immune system where thyroid autoantibodies are synthesised has significance for successful modulation of AITD and within the immune response itself the role of the macrophage or antigen-presenting cell (APC) in regulating the autoimmune process by its uptake, handling and presentation of autoantigen is critical. Demonstration of the central role of the APC in the antigen-driven autoantibody response has permitted investigation of its susceptibility to modulation by the antithyroid agent methimazole (MMI) which inhibits autoantibody synthesis in vivo and in vitro. This may well result from an influence on APC which take the drug up and in which MMI can be shown to interfere with oxygen radical generation; a necessary step in APC activation. Similarly perchlorate can be shown to modulate the immune process and one might expect this agent to act in a similar way to MMI. In considering the conventional antithyroid agents therefore it is clear that a significant factor in their success in controlling AITD is their ability to influence the immune process itself. The conventional immunosuppressant cyclosporin A also ameliorates experimental AITD and we have recently obtained encouraging results in Graves' ophthalmopathy with this agent which in turn suggests a major role for T cells in the immunopathogenesis of the condition. Direct attack on the autoimmune process has traditionally relied on relatively non-specific immunosuppressive therapy such as this. In attempting to improve the specificity and selectivity of the agents used, "immunotoxins" consisting of the A-chain of the toxin ricin have been coupled to autoantigens and used in vitro to kill B cells recognising the antigen. Understanding the autoimmune process is permitting investigation of its therapeutic modulation. These studies are still in their infancy but ultimately AITD will be controlled by regulating the aberrant immune response.

S.88 MEMBRANE ANTIGENS IN THYROID AUTOIMMUNE DISEASES. A. Pinchera*, G.F. Fenzi, S. Mariotti, E. Macchia, L. Chiovato, P. Vitti, C. Marcocci. Cattedre di Endocrinologia and Patologia Medica 2, University of Pisa, Pisa, Italy.

The sera of patients with thyroid autoimmune disorders contain antibodies to various thyroid membrane antigens including microsomal, cell surface and TSH receptor components. Thyroglobulin (Tg) is the main colloid antigen, but antigenic determinants of this protein are also detectable in membrane structures as assessed: a) by binding of radioiodinated Tg antibodies to the surface of cultured human thyrocytes and to particulate or solubilized microsomal and plasma membrane preparations; b) by Tg antibody immunoprecipitation of solubilized radiolabelled thyroid plasma membrane. The question of whether colloid and membrane-associated Tg are antigenically heterogeneous remains to be elucidated and is currently under investigation using a panel of monoclonal Tg antibodies. The microsomal antigen is believed to be a lipoprotein membrane component of exocytotic vescicles transporting newly synthesized Tg from the Golgi apparatus to the colloid. Thyroid subcellular fractionation failed to separate antibodies reacting with microsomes and plasma membrane. Binding and absorption studies using cultured human thyroid cells clearly showed that the microsomal antigen is expressed on the surface of thyroid epithelial cells. These and other data are in keeping with the notion that exocytotic vescicles contribute to the membrane material of the apical cell surface. Antibodies to the TSH receptor are characterized by stimulation of thyroid adenylate cyclase and by inhibition of TSH binding. There is no correlation between these two activities suggesting that different pathways are involved. To study this problem monoclonal antibodies have been prepared fusing murine myeloma cells with peripheral lymphocytes of patients with Graves' disease. Two classes of monoclonal antibodies were obtained: one characterized by inhibition of binding and action of TSH and the other by partial hormone agonism. These and other data support the concept that TSH receptor antibodies may be directed to at least two different receptor components. Attempts have been made to separate the microsomal and the TSH receptor-related antigens. Immunoprecipitation studies with solubilized radiolabelled human thyroid plasma membrane showed that the TSH receptor cannot be readily separated from the microsomal-related cell surface antigen. Furthermore, microsomal antigenic determinants have been clearly detected by immunofluorescence on the surface of cultured $FRTL_5$ cells, a rat thyroid cell line which requires TSH for growth and expresses the TSH receptor on the surface. At contrary, negative results were obtained with FRT cells, a rat thyroid cell strain which does not require TSH for growing and does not express the TSH receptor. In addition, the microsomal antigen has also been identified in human thyroid coated vescicles. The significance of this finding is unclear but it is worth noting that these structures contain a high density of plasma membrane hormone receptors. These data raise the question of whether and to what extent the functional activity of the thyroid cell influences the expression of thyroid membrane antigen on the cell surface.

In conclusion, the present data indicate that several membrane antigens are involved in thyroid autoimmune disorders and suggest that their expression on the thyroid cell surface may be influenced by the functional state of the cell. This may account for the different clinical features of thyroid autoimmune disorders.

S.89 INSULIN-LIKE GROWTH FACTORS: IN VITRO AND IN VIVO EFFECTS

E.R. Froesch*, Chr. Schmid, U. Widmer, and J. Zapf
Metabolic Unit, Dept. of Medicine, University of Zurich, CH-8091 Zurich, Switzerland

IGF I and IGF II are the best characterized polypeptides of the somatomedin family. Somatomedin C is identical to IGF I. The IGFs are close relatives of insulin. In the A- and B-domain the amino acid sequence is homologous to that of the A- and B-chain of insulin. The C-region in the IGFs is much shorter (12 and 8 amino acids, recpectively) than the C-peptide of proinsulin. The homology is greatest in the biologically active centers of these hormones. - Most cells have receptors for insulin, IGF I and IGF II and all 3 respective molecules crossreact to some extent with these respective receptors. IGFs are present in human serum in large concentrations because they are bound to specific carrier proteins. - In contrast to most polypeptide hormones IGFs are synthesized and readily secreted by the liver without storage in granula. There is no measurable free IGF in serum. The IGFs exert insulin-like effects on the target tissues of insulin, such as adipose tissue, skeletal muscle, heart muscle etc. It is likely that IGFs act on adipose tissue via the insulin receptor and on heart muscle via the IGF receptor. IGF is 5 and 100 times less efficient in stimulating glucose uptake in the rat heart and rat adipose tissue, respectively, than insulin. The binding proteins appear to hinder IGF in reacting with the insulin receptor. - IGFs stimulate growth parameters and replication of mesenchymal cells in vitro. In this respect they are 100 - 200 times more potent than insulin. IGFs are not only potent growth factors but they also tend to stimulate the differentiation of mesenchymal precursor cells. This has been shown in the case of erythroid cells in fetal and adult mice, myoblasts in primary cultures of chick cells and osteoblasts in cultures of rat calvaria cells. - When IGFs are administered as a bolus in vivo together with anti-insulin serum in order to block insulin effects, adipose tissue and muscle are stimulated as if insulin had been injected, and acute hypoglycemia occurs. When IGFs are administered subcutaneously to hypophysectomized rats by means of Alza pumps, growth indices are stimulated, and the rats grow. IGF I is more potent than IGF II. These results prove that the hypothesis of Daughaday according to which the somatomedins mediate growth effects of growth hormone is valid. We have observed that the pattern of the IGF binding proteins is different in hypox animals treated with growth hormone and in those treated with IGF. Growth hormone appears to modulate the effects of IGF by changing their accessibility in the periphery.

S.90 INSULIN-LIKE GROWTH FACTORS/SOMATOMEDINS: PHYSIOLOGY AND GH DEPENDENCY.

L.E. UNDERWOOD*, J.J. VAN WYK, A.J. D'ERCOLE, D.R. CLEMMONS, & M.E. SVOBODA. University of North Carolina, Chapel Hill, NC 27514 USA

This presentation will focus on the factors which regulate immunoreactive somatomedin-C (Sm-C)/insulin-like growth factor I (IGF-I). Although it was originally believed that the liver was the principal site of synthesis, recent evidence suggests that somatomedins are produced by many tissues. A variety of organ explants from fetal mice, as well as cultured human fibroblasts, produce Sm-like peptides in vitro. We have developed methods for extracting Sm-C/IGF-I from tissues and have shown that most tissues from hypophysectomized rats contain far less activity than tissues from normal animals. Furthermore, after administration of oGH, tissue Sm-C/IGF-I concentrations rise earlier than serum values. In tissues peak values are reached 8-12 hours after GH, 6-10 hours before maximal serum concentrations are attained. The production of Sm-C/IGF-I by multiple tissues suggests that this peptide could act at or near its sites of production, through autocrine and/or paracrine mechanisms. Such mechanisms do not preclude actions by endocrine mechanisms.

Evidence for a close relationship between GH and Sm-C/IGF-I is strengthened by recent observations of the negative feedback relationship of Sm-C/IGF-I on GH secretion. In vitro, Sm-C/IGF-I stimulates somatostatin production by hypothalamic explants, and inhibits basal GH release and GRF stimulated GH release by primary cultures of pituitary cells. In unanesthetized, freely moving rats, intracerebroventricular injection of 500 ng Sm-C/IGF-I abolishes spontaneous GH release for up to 4 hours.

While the importance of GH as a regulator of plasma concentrations of Sm-C/IGF-I is accepted, recent studies provide convincing evidence that nutrient status is as important as GH, if not more so. When moderately obese young adults are fasted for 10 days, their plasma Sm-C/IGF-I concentrations decline into the hypopituitary range (mean prefast = 0.83 U/ml, mean postfast = 0.21 U/ml). A prompt increase occurs with refeeding. Additional fast-refeed studies done on normal weight adults indicate that both the energy and protein content of the refeeding diet are important in the restoration of Sm-C/IGF-I to normal. When either is reduced by as little as 30% of optimal intake, normalization of Sm-C/IGF-I after fasting is impeded. Furthermore, refeeding a protein-restricted diet supplemented with essential amino acids accelerates the rate of increase of Sm-C/IGF-I.

Studies in patients with disorders of nutrition indicate that dramatic increments in Sm-C/IGF-I occur within days of the institution of adequate nutrient intake. In preliminary studies on 6 such patients it appears that the change in Sm-C/IGF-I is a better indicator of nutrient repletion than albumin, prealbumin, transferrin or retinol binding protein. Studies directed at defining the relationship between nutrients and Sm-C/IGF-I appear to be crucial to understanding the mechanisms regulating this growth factor. They also suggest that measurement of Sm-C/IGF-I may be useful in defining changes in nutritional status in patients with malnutrition from malabsorption and other chronic illnesses.

S.91 IGF RECEPTORS. Helen A. Jonas* and Len C. Harrison, Endocrine Laboratory, University of Melbourne Department of Medicine, Royal Melbourne Hospital, 3050, Victoria, Australia.

Insulin-like growth factors (human IGF-I and IGF-II) share with insulin a high degree of amino acid sequence homology and biological effects ranging from acute stimulation of metabolism to nucleic acid and protein synthesis and mitogenesis. Competitive binding studies have defined distinct binding sites for IGF-I, IGF-II and insulin in a number of tissues. The insulin receptor has a low affinity for both IGF-I and IGF-II; the IGF-I receptor has a higher affinity for IGF-I than IGF-II and a low affinity for insulin; and the IGF-II receptor has a higher affinity for IGF-II than IGF-I and no affinity for insulin.

The homology between IGF-I and insulin receptors is further evidenced by the fact that IGF-I receptors can be down-regulated by either IGFs or insulin, are recognised by antibodies to the insulin receptor, and consist of similarly sized oligomers (M_r >300 K) composed of disulfide-linked ≃ 130 K and ≃ 90 K subunits. The 130 K subunits contain the hormone binding sites, while the 90 K subunits have tyrosine kinase activities which are stimulated by hormone binding. The identification of similarly sized biosynthetic precursors (M_r ≃ 180 K) and concordant receptor defects in some patients with severe insulin resistance suggest that both receptors are encoded by the same or at least very closely related genes.

IGF-II receptors, on the other hand, are antigenically distinct, consist of a single polypeptide (M_r ≃ 260 K) and do not possess intrinsic kinase activity. They are not subject to down-regulation, but can be up-regulated in adipocytes via their insulin-stimulated translocation from an intracellular compartment.

In most tissues IGFs promote growth more readily than does insulin, and in tissues containing no IGF-I receptors (e.g. adipocytes), ≃ 100 fold higher concentrations of IGFs are required to elicit insulin's metabolic actions. Therefore, it has generally been considered that insulin and IGF receptors mediate, respectively, the metabolic and mitogenic functions of these hormones. On the other hand, in some cells and tissues containing IGF-I receptors (e.g. soleus/cardiac muscle, BC_3H-I mouse myocytes and human skin fibroblasts) low concentrations of IGFs can stimulate glucose and amino acid transport, indicating that these acute metabolic responses can also be directly mediated by IGF binding to its receptor. Whether IGF-I exerts its metabolic and mitogenic actions via the same or different binding sites on IGF-I (or IGF-II) receptors is unknown. Recently, we showed that human placenta contains two species of IGF-I receptors with different binding affinities and susceptibilities to reducing agents, which can be delineated on the basis of their reactivity with auto-antibodies to the insulin receptor. This finding raises the possibility that cell or tissue-specific isotypes of the IGF-I receptor could mediate the different biological actions of IGF-I.

S.92 **SYMPOSIUM** IGF AND RELATED GROWTH FACTORS: MECHANISM OF ACTION OF CARTILAGE-DERIVED FACTOR (CDF) AND MULTIPLICATION-STIMULATING ACTIVITY (MSA).
F. Suzuki*, Y. Hiraki, H. Inoue and Y. Kato, Department of Biochemistry, Faculty of Dentistry, Osaka University, 1-8, Yamadaoka, Suita, Osaka 565, JAPAN.

We found that fetal bovine cartilage contains polypeptides that stimulate DNA synthesis, RNA synthesis, cell division and proteoglycan synthesis, a characteristic cartilage phenotype, in rabbit costal chondrocytes in culture. The role of this peptide, named the cartilage-derived factor (CDF), on skeletal growth was evaluated by comparing their effects on cultured chondrocytes with those of multiplication-stimulating activity (MSA), a somatomedin purified from conditioned medium of Buffalo rat liver cells, and other non-somatomedin growth factors. In cultures of rabbit costal chondrocytes exposed to medium containing CDF began to increase [^{3}H]thymidine incorporation into DNA after 14-16 h, reached a maximum at 24-28 h, after CDF addition, and then decreased. The time-course of MSA-induced DNA synthesis was similar to that of CDF-induced DNA synthesis. The incorporation of [^{3}H]uridine into RNA was also increased within 1-2 h in the cells incubated with the peptides. These stimulations of nucleic acid syntheses were followed by cell division in serum-free medium. On the other hand, CDF and MSA enhanced the synthesis of sulfated proteoglycans, as measured in terms of increased incorporation of [^{35}S]sulfate, [^{3}H]glucosamine or [^{3}H]serine into material precipitated with cetylpyridinium chloride, was consistently higher than the extent of CDF and MSA stimulation of total protein synthesis.

Epidermal growth factor (EGF) and fibroblast growth factor (FGF) also stimulated DNA synthesis, RNA synthesis and cell division of rabbit costal chodnrocytes in culture, but did not stimulate nor inhibit proteoglycan synthesis. MSA and EGF or FGF had synergistic effects on the growth of rabbit chondrocytes. CDF mimicked these effects of MSA: CDF and MSA had similar stimulatory effects on DNA synthesis in rabbit chondrocytes even in the presence of EGF, FGF or both. On the contrary, EGF and FGF had additive effects on DNA synthesis and cell division of chondrocytes. These findings suggest that somatomedin-like factors and non-somatomedin mitogens have complementary effects in chondrocytes.

DNA synthesis in cells treated with CDF or MSA for only the initial 5 h also increased 23 h after removal of CDF or MSA. Therefore, initial 5 h exposure of chondrocytes to CDF or MSA is sufficient for full stimulation of DNA synthesis. On the contrary, EGF or FGF, non-somatomedin family, must be continuously present in medium for more than 10 h for stimulation of DNA synthesis. Moreover, an early removal (5 h) of CDF or MSA from the medium did not affect the interaction of CDF or MSA with EGF or FGF for their synergistic stimulation of DNA synthesis in chondrocytes. Thus, a transient exposure to CDF or MSA with EGF or FGF followed by a continuous exposure to EGF or FGF resulted in $G_1 \rightarrow S$ transition. These findings suggest that somatomedin-related factors affect an early distinct state in G_1 phase in the cell cycle in chondrocytes and trigger some signals for entry into the DNA synthetic phase.

S.93 PARACRINE INTERACTION IN ANTERIOR PITUITARY. C. Denef* Dept. of Pharmacology, University of Leuven, School of Medicine, Campus Gasthuisberg, B-3000 Leuven, Belgium.

We recently presented evidence for the existence of a specific intercellular communication between gonadotrophs and lactotrophs (Denef and Andries, Endocrinology 112, 813, 1983) in anterior pituitary reaggregate cell cultures. In superfused co-cultures of enriched lactotroph and gonadotroph populations (obtained by unit gravity sedimentation), LHRH (10^{-11}-10^{-8} M) was capable of stimulating basal as well as dopamine inhibited PRL release but TRH did not affect LH release. Medium conditioned by purified gonadotrophs also stimulated PRL release, suggesting that gonadotrophs might activate the secretory activity of the lactotrophs by the release of a paracrine factor. Although the nature of this factor remains unknown, it was shown not to be LHRH itself, LH, FSH or PRL. The factor was ultrafiltrable and its M.W. was estimated to be smaller than 10,000. We now report our progress in this area.

In reaggregates containing gonadotrophs, lactotrophs, thyrotrophs and somatotrophs in about equal proportions (obtained from 14-day-old male rat pituitary), physiological concentrations of LHRH only stimulated PRL release. At 10^{-8} M there was no effect on TSH release but there was some stimulation of GH release. Corticotrophin-releasing factor (CRF) failed to influence PRL, GH, LH and TSH release. Human pancreatic growth hormone releasing factor [hpGHRF(1-40)] stimulated GH release but not LH, TSH or PRL release. Vasoactive intestinal peptide and angiotensin II (AII) stimulated PRL release but not TSH or LH release. These data further support the specificity of our pituitary reaggregate cell culture system as well as the relative selectivity of the gonadotroph-lactotroph interaction.

When gonadotrophs were co-cultured with somatotrophs, the GH response to hpGHRF and epinephrine (E) was strongly attenuated whereas gonadotrophs potentiated the PRL response to AII when co-cultured with lactotrophs. These data suggest that gonadotrophs not only seem to contain stimulatory factors but also agent(s) capable of inhibiting the response of other cell types to their specific secretagogues.

The secretory response of somatotrophs was also affected by β-endorphin and CRF β-endorphin did not affect basal GH or PRL release but potentiated the stimulation of GH by E and the stimulation of PRL release by AII. However, CRF attenuated the GH response to hpGHRF. These data suggest that the opio-melano-corticotrophs are capable of engaging in both stimulatory and inhibitory interactions with somatotrophs and lactotrophs.

Various steroid hormones and T_3 interfere with these cellular interactions, some being completely abolished, others being stimulated. The present data show that multiple and complex interactions may occur between different anterior pituitary cell types and that these interactions are not random. As far as studied, the underlying mechanism may be the release of paracrine factors.

S.94 MULTIPLE HORMONES IN A SINGLE CELL. Gwen Childs*, Dept. Anatomy, Univ. of Texas Med. Br. Galveston, Texas

The development of immunoperoxidase techniques in the late 1960's challenged the "one cell, one hormone" theory that had long been postulated for the pituitary. Early studies showed that corticotropes store both ACTH and MSH and gonadotropes store both LH and FSH. These data were obtained by matching serially sectioned fields (Phifer et al, 1972) or by the use of double stains applied to the same section (Nakane, 1970). During the next 10 years, various combinations of pituitary and non-pituitary hormones were found in pituitary cells. Some of the more unusual combinations were difficult to explain. Are the "non-pituitary" hormones stored in target cells following internalization? Do all the cells of a given type synthesize the same combination of hormones? What are the methodological pitfalls that must be considered when interpreting the data? Our studies of this phenomenon began when we localized ACTH and FSH in a subpopulation (<10%) of corticotropes and LH and FSH in a subpopulation of gonadotropes with the use of stains applied to ultrathin serial sections (Moriarty and Garner, 1976, 1977). Because of the sampling error associated with ultrathin sections, we added studies with thicker (1-2 μm) serial sections, and developed dual pre-embedding stains applied to whole pituitary cells. We also tested the effect of 4 fixation protocols (freeze-fixation, glutaraldehyde, picric acid formaldehyde and 4% p-formaldehyde) and 3 embedding protocols (water-soluble glycol methacrylate, Epoxy plastic, and paraplast) on hormone antigenicity. Stained gonadotropes or corticotropes were collected systematically following each of the above protocols and the data obtained thus far yield the following information: 1) In adult male rats, 70% of the gonadotropes are multihormonal (LH-FSH); diestrous female rats have 45-50% - LH-FSH cells. The rest contain only LH or FSH (monohormonal). These percentages do not vary with the fixation or embedding protocol. However, the relative percentages of LH-FSH cells are higher after GnRH stimulation, castration, or ovariectomy, and lower in estrous rats. 2) Small and medium sized (7-10 μm) gonadotropes are mostly monohormonal. This fact emphasizes the need to use serial thin sections or double stains for their detection. The use of 4-7 μm serial sections skew the data in favor of the larger (12-14 μm) multihormonal gonadotropes. 3) Multihormonal corticotropes that also contain LH and/or FSH are most abundant during neonatal development. Their percentages are unaffected by the fixation protocols tested. However, in 20% of the normal adult rat population, multihormonal corticotropes are increased to 7% - 12% of the pituitary cells. Ongoing studies relate this increase to environmental stresses. 4) Dual stains for biotinylated gonadotropin releasing hormone and biotinylated corticotropin releasing hormone show that both analogs bind specifically to their respective target cells. This is followed by rapid internalization (3-5 min). In summary, our studies show that hormone storage patterns in gonadotropes or corticotropes vary with the physiological state of the animal. Monohormonal cells may be reserve cells that are, in fact, multipotential. Multihormonal cells may point to a common stem cell of origin present during development. Finally, non-pituitary hormones inside target cells may reflect their internalization and intracellular processing. (NIH RO1 HD 15472, and RCDA HD 00306).

S.95 MONOAMINE-PEPTIDE INTERACTIONS IN THE REGULATION OF PITUITARY CELL FUNCTION.
A. Negro-Vilar*, Reproductive Neuroendocrinology Section, Lab. Reprod. Devel. Tox., NIEHS, NIH, Research Triangle Park, North Carolina 27709.

The release of ACTH and β-endorphin (β-end) from the anterior pituitary is under multiple control by neural peptides and aminergic neurotransmitters. In addition to the prominent role played by corticotropin releasing factor (CRF), other peptides such as arginine vasopressin (AVP), oxytocin (OXY), and angiotensin II (AII) are also active secretagogues of ACTH and β-end. On the aminergic side, catecholamines, particularly epinephrine and norepinephrine, as well as serotonin, can also enhance secretion of these hormones. Recent studies from our laboratory have been directed to evaluate the role of these modulatory agents, particularly in relation to the mechanism(s) and site(s) of action and also to determine possible peptide-peptide and peptide-amine interactions at the hypothalamic and pituitary levels. When tested in vitro for ACTH releasing activity, the above substances enhanced hormone release with the following minimal effective doses: CRF (10^{-11} M), AVP (10^{-10} M), OXY (10^{-9} M), AII (10^{-8} M), EPI (10^{-9} M), and 5-HT (10^{-8} M). In recent studies, we have characterized specific binding sites for AVP in dispersed anterior pituitary cells. Binding affinity for AVP is closely correlated with the ability of the peptide to elicit ACTH release, and the K_D for the receptor (1.6 nM) is consistent with the dose of peptide required to elicit a physiological response. Similarly, specific AII receptors in anterior pituitary cell membranes have a K_D (0.5 nM) in agreement with the dose of peptide required to stimulate hormone release. Since specific CRF receptors have also been demonstrated, it is evident that each peptide enhances ACTH/β-end release by interacting with a specific receptor. Peptide-peptide interactions are manifested by potentiating or additive effects between CRF, AVP, and AII at the anterior pituitary level, and by direct stimulatory effects of AII on AVP and CRF release at the hypothalamic level. The primary in vivo effect of AII on ACTH and β-end release seems to be centrally-mediated, since it is absent in centrally-blocked rats, and it may primarily involve release of CRF, as suggested by experiments in vasopressin-deficient Brattleboro rats. Both EPI and 5-HT can directly stimulate ACTH release in vitro, and these effects can be nullified by specific receptor blockers. We have recently shown that high concentrations of EPI from a central source are present in hypophyseal portal plasma, so central EPI may be physiologically involved in regulation of anterior pituitary cell functions. Our studies with 5-HT indicate that, in addition to a direct stimulatory effect of 5-HT on ACTH release from the rat pituitary, serotonin potentiates the in vitro effects of AVP on ACTH release. This intriguing peptide-amine interaction at the pituitary level is specific (it can be nullified by 5-HT receptor blockers) and selective (it does not occur with CRF or AII). Blockade of 5-HT receptors in anterior pituitary cells in vitro consistently blunted the release of ACTH elicited by ME extracts from normal rats but not from AVP-deficient Brattleboro animals, indicating that this peptide-amine interaction may be physiologically relevant. Taken together, these observations indicate that complex regulatory mechanisms involving peptidergic and aminergic systems interact at different control levels to effectively modulate ACTH and β-end release.

S.96 DISSIMILARITY IN THE CONCENTRATIONS OF DOPAMINE IN BLOOD OF THE VARIOUS HYPOPHYSIAL PORTAL VESSELS: CONSIDERATION OF THE CAUSES AND CONSEQUENCES.

John C. Porter*, Cecil H. and Ida Green Ctr for Reprod Biol Sci, Depts of Obstet and Gynecol and Physiol, Univ of Texas Hlth Sci Ctr at Dallas, Dallas, Texas, U.S.A.

When the concentration of dopamine, norepinephrine, or epinephrine in hypophysial portal blood is compared to that of the same hormone in arterial blood, it is found that the concentration of dopamine, but not norepinephrine or epinephrine, in portal blood is greater than that in arterial blood. Such evidence is supportive of the view that dopamine, but not norepinephrine or epinephrine, is released into portal blood by neurons of the hypothalamus. With respect to norepinephrine, the absence of such a finding is unexpected since there is an appreciable amount of norepinephrine in the median eminence. When the concentrations of dopamine in blood from the various portal vessels are considered, it is found that the concentration of dopamine in plasma from a portal vessel on the medial aspect of the pituitary stalk is two times that of dopamine in plasma from a portal vessel on the lateral aspect of the pituitary stalk. Thus, it appears that the concentrations of dopamine in portal blood of the various portal vessels are not the same. Inasmuch as a given portal vessel supplies blood to a discrete portion of the pars distalis, it is interesting to speculate that, as a result of different concentrations, the effect that dopamine on cells in some regions of the anterior pituitary gland is different from that in other regions. This lack of homogeneity in the concentration of dopamine in blood of the various portal vessels is believed to be due to different rates of entry of dopamine into the capillaries supplying blood to each portal vessel. Indeed, the rate of secretion of dopamine into a medial portal vessel is 2.5 times that into a lateral portal vessel. Although the basis for the difference in the rate of release of dopamine into the various portal vessels is unknown, it could be that dopaminergic neurons innervating the lateral median eminence secrete dopamine at a slower rate than do dopaminergic neurons innervating the medial median eminence. However, there is indirect evidence to suggest that this may not be the case. Selmanoff (Endocrinology 108:1716, 1981) was unable to demonstrate a significant difference in turnover of dopamine in the lateral and medial regions of the median eminence. In addition, the rates of biosynthesis of DOPA—the precursor of dopamine—in the lateral and medial median eminence are the same (Reymond et al., Endocrinology 112:1958, 1983). The slower release of dopamine into a lateral portal vessel than into a medial portal vessel may be due to the ease with which dopamine diffuses into the capillaries of the portal vessels. Although the consequence of the differences in the concentration of dopamine in blood of the various portal vessels is not established, it is worth noting that in general the lateral portal vessels supply blood to the lateral regions of the anterior lobe, whereas the medial portal vessels supply blood to the medial region of the gland. It is concluded that the release of dopamine into portal blood by dopaminergic neurons does not occur to an equal extent by all of the neurons, resulting in different concentrations of dopamine in blood of the various portal vessels. This disparity may be of significance in the regulation of normal as well as abnormal function of the anterior pituitary gland.

S.97 RELAXIN : STRUCTURE FUNCTION RELATIONS. Geoffrey W. Tregear,* Howard Florey Institute of Experimental Physiology & Medicine, University of Melbourne, Parkville, Victoria, Australia 3052.

The ovarian peptide relaxin is characterized by its action in remodelling the reproductive tract before parturition, thus facilitating the birth process. Although predominantly a hormone of pregnancy, relaxin has also been detected in the non-pregnant female as well as in the male.

The amino acid sequence of relaxin from pig, rat, mouse, tiger shark, dogfish shark and human have now been established. The hormone consists of two peptide chains (A & B) joined by disulfide bonds with an intrachain disulfide loop in the A-chain in a manner exactly analogous to that of insulin. The marked structural similarity between insulin, relaxin and IGF peptides strongly suggests that they were all originally derived from a common ancestral gene. A surprising difference between relaxin and most other peptide hormones is the considerable structural differences between species. For example, pig and rat relaxins differ in over 50% of amino acid positions whereas pig and rat insulins differ in only 8%. The shark and human relaxin sequences differ to a similar degree from one another and from the pig and rat structures. These differences explain the poor immunological cross-reactivity between relaxins of different species and also a number of the observed differences in their specific biological activity.

The application of recombinant DNA technology has led to the isolation and characterization of the genes coding for pig, rat, mouse and human relaxins. Analysis of the nucleotide sequence from cDNA and genomic clones and a comparison of the deduced amino acid sequences reveals a common structural organization for the relaxin precursor protein. There is a signal peptide of 25 residues followed by a B-chain of about 30 amino acids, a C-peptide of about 105 amino acids and an A-chain of 22 to 24 amino acids. In the human, pig and rat genomic clones , an intron interrupts the coding region of the C-peptide. The physiological role of the C-peptide,which is considerably longer than the related insulin peptides,and the nature of the enzymes responsible for its removal from the ends of the A and B chain are important unresolved issues. In the case of human relaxin two separate gene sequences have been characterized. Only one of these genes is expressed in the ovary during pregnancy and it is unclear whether the other gene is expressed at another tissue site or whether it represents a pseudogene.

The chemical synthesis of relaxin has been particularly difficult; however, preliminary studies have provided valuable information regarding the structural features important for biological activity. The full length of the A and B chains is not required for biological activity, and up to 6 amino acids may be removed from the C-terminus of the B-chain without affecting activity. Similarly, up to 3 amino acids may be removed from the N-terminus of the A-chain before activity is lost. There is evidence that one of the two inter-chain disulfide bonds may not be essential for biological activity, and many of the individual amino acids may be substituted with only minor activity changes. These studies and those provided by expression of chemically synthesized genes for relaxin in bacterial or yeast systems should provide sufficient human relaxin to permit detailed physiological studies of the hormone and will aid in the design of structural analogues for possible therapeutic use.

S.98 EXTRALUTEAL SECRETION OF RELAXIN. M. Bigazzi*, Poggiosecco Hospital, INRCA, Florence, Italy.

Relaxin (RLX) has been measured in blood only during pregnancy, its secretory granules have been identified in cells of the gestational corpus luteum and its extraction and purification was obtained from ovaries of pregnant pig, rat and shark. Therefore RLX has been considered an hormone exclusively of the pregnant female and solely secreted from the ovary. More recent studies demonstrated its presence in other tissues of pregnant or cycling female and also in male, and gave evidence that the major source of circulating RLX may vary in different species, as the ovary is not always the richest organ in RLX.

It is proved that RLX in blood during pregnancy is secreted by corpus luteum and, in some species, by placenta, while it has not been documented the endocrine secretion of RLX from the remaining tissues. Moreover their low content of RLX raised doubts whether the hormone is produced or simply stored in such tissues. The low sensitivity and the high species specificity of the bio- and radio-immunoassays in use, make difficult to clarify this problem through dynamic secretory studies, especially in man.

Anyway the extraluteal secretion of RLX is supported by these findings:

- RLX is contained in tissues and fluids, in physiological and pathological conditions, independently from pregnancy and also in the male.
- In such tissues immunofluorescence and immunoperoxidase methods can identify RLX and pre-proRLX in the cytoplasm of cells.
- Neo synthesis of RLX can be documented by aminoacids in corporation during in vitro cultures.

It is probable that in man the extraluteal sources of RLX do not secrete the hormone, or very little, in the circulating blood, but are rather used for local needs, in analogy with the extrapituitary secretion of PRL in decidua. The distinction between "systemic" and "local" RLX (Bryant-Greenwood, 1982), brings to a possible involvement of this hormone in many steps of reproduction other than the well recognized effects on the widening of the symphis pubic and the inhibition of uterine contractions. There is some existing evidence that could authorize to believe that RLX as "local hormone" can participate of the rupture of the follicular membrane and ovulation, of the embryo implantation and uterine quiescence, of the rupture of amniotic membrane and secondation and of sperm motility.

S.99 RELAXIN: A MULTIPURPOSE HORMONE. D.G. Porter* Pre-Clinical Veterinary Studies, Department of Anatomy, The Medical School, Bristol, U.K.

Relaxin has recently benefitted from a resurgence of interest. It had long been regarded as a hormone of pregnancy because of three classic actions of separating the interpelvic symphysis, of softening the cervix and of inhibiting myometrial activity. However even in the earlier literature there were glimpses of possible actions of relaxin over a wider spectrum. Thus its presence in birds, in an elasmobranch, in male animals and its actions on milk secretion suggested that it was unlikely that its responsibilities could be confined to the pre-partum period, a view which has been considerably strengthened in the last ten years. The demonstration of relaxin in a protozoan, its identification and sequencing in a shark and the confirmation of its presence in males points to functions on a broad scale. In mammals our concept of relaxin has been expanded. The demonstration of relaxin in the ovarian follicle begs the proposition that relaxin is involved in folliculogenesis or ovulation or both. Because of its classical actions on collagenous tissues relaxin may facilitate the expansion of the follicle within the connective tissue framework of the ovary, while its actions on uterine muscle point to a possible influence on smooth muscle of the follicle at ovulation. Whether or not it is also a hormone of lactation is uncertain, although earlier work had shown that relaxin affects the mammary gland. We have shown that relaxin reduces the sensitivity of the myoepithelium of the lactating rat to oxytocin, and also appears to inhibit the release of oxytocin centrally. The physiological significance of this for lactation is uncertain but it raises the exciting possibility that in the pre-partum animal relaxin may restrain myometrial activity by inhibiting spontaneous uterine contractions while at the same time preventing the premature secretion of oxytocin from the neurohypophysis. It is thus an appropriate hormone for the 'fine tuning' of the time of parturition. The action of relaxin on the myometrium contrasts with that of progesterone: it inhibits simultaneously spontaneous activity while enhancing co-ordination. Thus relaxin induced quiescence can be overcome by stimulatory agents such as oxytocin or $PGF_{2\alpha}$. These findings taken with reports of binding of relaxin to skin fibroblasts, actions of the hormone on fat cells, and its undisputed presence in the ejaculate and prostate gland present a picture of a hormone implicated in a wide range of reproductive and possibly non-reproductive processes. At present there is an irony in that there is no certainty that relaxin is essential for any of the processes in which it is involved.

S.100 CLINICAL STUDIES ON RELAXIN. G. Weiss* , Department of Obstetrics and Gynecology, New York University School of Medicine, New York, N.Y. 10016, U.S.A.

Relaxin is detectable in human serum throughout pregnancy from the time of the missed menses. The corpus luteum synthesizes immuno-and bioactive relaxin. Luteectomy results in a prompt fall in circulating relaxin levels. Relaxin levels are higher in the first than in either succeeding trimester of pregnancy. There is no detectable prelabor relaxin surge. Serum relaxin concentrations are lower in women during premature labor than in nonlabored women at the same stage of pregnancy. Relaxin secretion can be induced by hCG given on day 8-10 of the luteal phase. This treatment produces an abrupt rise in progesterone but relaxin does not become detectable for 2 to 6 days. The timing of the hCG is critical. When hCG injections are given on day 2 or 3 of the luteal phase, no relaxin was detectable. Human relaxin can inhibit spontaneous contractions of human myometrium <u>in-vitro</u> . Progesterone synergizes with relaxin in this effect. That relaxin is detectable from early pregnancy and inhibits human myometrium suggests a role for relaxin, in conjunction with luteal progesterone, in early pregnancy maintenance. Relaxin is detectable in human decidua and placenta at term in concentrations several orders of magnitude below that of luteal tissue. Relaxin is detectable in decidua of baboons months after luteectomy when peripheral levels are undetectable, suggesting local production as well as luteal production. Relaxin may be involved in the maintenance of uterine quiescence in late pregnancy. Relaxin is present in human seminal plasma. The presence of relaxin in the ejaculate of men with congenital absence of the vas deferens suggests a prostatic source. Washed human sperm are rendered immobile when treated with anti-relaxin antiserum. Pretreatment of this relaxin antiserum with relaxin abolishes its effect. Relaxin treatment inhibits the natural loss of motility of washed sperm. The addition of physiological concentrations of relaxin to washed human sperm increases the ability of the sperm to penetrate cervical mucus <u>in-vitro</u> . Improvement of penetration can be equally affected by addition of either whole seminal plasma or relaxin in buffer to washed sperm. Relaxin secretion in seminal plasma by the male represents a novel biological mechanism for hormone delivery. This exocrine male secretion is delivered to the female during coitus where it seems to subserve an endocrine function, the facilitation of sperm penetration through the female reproductive system.

S.101 PROBES FOR STEROID RECEPTORS. J.P. Raynaud*, Roussel-UCLAF, Paris 75007, France

By demonstrating in 1959 selective accumulation of tritium-labeled hexestrol in the reproductive organs of immature female goats and sheep, Glascock and Hoekstra initiated research into the mechanism of action of steroid hormones by the use of radiaoctive probes. These experiments were followed by those of Jensen who measured the radioactive uptake of tritium-labeled estradiol and estrone in estrogen target organs (uterus and vagina) of the rat. The ability to measure bound radioactivity in the high-speed supernatant (cytosol) from target organ homogenates led to rapid progress in the development of synthetic steroids for the detection and assay of steroid receptors. The first steroid probes were selected on the basis of their high biological potency since a ligand may be an excellent binder but trap the receptor in a non-functional state. 3H-dexamethasone was used to label the glucocorticoid receptor (GR). The highly labile progesterone receptor (PR) remained elusive for some time but the problem was solved by the introduction of 3H-promegestone (R 5020). In the case of the androgen receptor (AR), metabolism of dihydrotestosterone and plasma protein binding of testosterone were overcomed by the use of 3H-methyltrienolone (R 1881) with added triamcinolone acetonide to improve specificity. 3H-moxestrol (R 2858) fulfils all the criteria of an ideal ligand for the estrogen receptor (ER): high specific activity, high affinity, no binding to contaminating plasma proteins, no degradation in the assay medium. Thus, because of their long-standing experience in steroid synthesis, Roussel-UCLAF was able to develop several tags which have now become standard laboratory reagents for the detection and assay of steroid hormone receptors in animal and human tissues (E.G. in malignant breast, prostate and brain tumors). Over a thousand steroids have been tested at Roussel-UCLAF in a routine screening system to find improved ligands, potentially active drugs, and to construct images of the binding sites characteristic of each hormone class. Steroids can be labeled not only with tritium and studies are now in progress on labeling with iodine for imaging (but the affinity is often decreased), with metals such as boron for detection by spectometric methods, and with fluorescent markers for fluocytometry (but quantification is difficult). Attempts have also been made to exploit the natural fluorescence of synthetic high-affinity ligands with conjugated double bonds. These molecules can be used for affinity labeling or can be detected directly by observation with high-performance photomultipliers. Other teams have tried a different approach. For them the ideal ligand is the receptor antibody. In this case, the difficulty resides in the availability of a sufficiently pure receptor protein to raise antibodies and in species differences. The final aim in all these studies is quantification and visualisation of receptor in the absence and presence of ligand. The new techniques will have to relate the kinetics and subcellular distribution of the ligand with the momentary availability (or non-availability) of the receptor. In this respect, only techniques compatible with developments in, for example, scanning electron microscopy might be envisaged.

S.102 **ANTIESTROGEN BINDING PROTEINS.** B.S.Katzenellenbogen*, M.A.Miller, A.Mullick, and Y.Y.Sheen, Department of Physiology and Biophysics, University of Illinois and College of Medicine, Urbana, IL 61801.

Antiestrogens are non-steroidal compounds that are capable of antagonizing many of the actions of estrogens. They bind with high affinity to the estrogen receptor present in target cells and, in addition, they bind to an antiestrogen binding site (AEBS) that is estrogen-noncompetable. In contrast to the restriction of estrogen receptors to estrogen target cells, the AEBS is present in a wide variety of estrogen target and non-target tissues and in estrogen receptor - positive and - negative human breast cancer cell lines (MCF-7, T47D, MDA-MB-231) that differ markedly in their sensitivity to antiestrogens. The AEBS has a subcellular distribution and ligand binding specificity very different from that of the estrogen receptor. The order of affinities of different antiestrogens and related compounds for the AEBS (cis-tamoxifen = trans-tamoxifen > CI628 > trans-hydroxytamoxifen > CI628M > H1285 = LY117018 = tamoxifen aziridine) does not parallel their affinity for the estrogen receptor nor the potency of these compounds as antiestrogens. Affinity for estrogen receptor most closely correlates with the potency of these compounds as antiestrogens.

Studies with dense amino acid labeling of the estrogen receptor and with the covalently attaching antiestrogen, tamoxifen aziridine, reveal that antiestrogen-occupied receptor in MCF-7 cells is degraded at a rate ($t1/2$ = 4h) similar to that of the control unoccupied receptor, and only slightly slower than that of the estradiol-occupied receptor ($t1/2$ = 3h). In addition, while tamoxifen aziridine binds covalently to the estrogen receptor, it binds reversibly to the AEBS.

Studies with high affinity radiolabeled antiestrogens (CI628M, H1285, trans-hydroxytamoxifen) in MCF-7 and in ZR-75 human breast cancer cells indicate that these antiestrogens all favor maintenance of a 5.5S form (Mr ca. 130,000) of the nuclear estrogen receptor complex that may be an important aspect of the nuclear interaction of these compounds in these breast cancer cells.

Our findings raise questions about the role of the AEBS in mediating directly the estrogen antagonism of antiestrogens, and suggest that interaction with the estrogen receptor is most likely the mechanism underlying the growth-inhibitory effects of antiestrogens. However, the AEBS might influence the distribution of antiestrogens and, hence, their accessability to estrogen receptor in estrogen receptor-positive cells, or they might mediate actions of antiestrogens that are unrelated to estrogen antagonism. Supported by NIH Grants CA18119 and CA31870.

S.103 MONOCLONAL ANTIBODIES AS PROBES FOR ESTROGEN RECEPTOR. G.L. Greene*, W.J. King and M.F. Press. The Ben May Laboratory for Cancer Research and Department of Pathology, The University of Chicago, Chicago, Illinois 60637 U.S.A.

Monoclonal rat antibodies to MCF-7 human breast cancer estrogen receptor have been used to develop quantitative and qualitative assays for estrogen receptor (estrophilin) that do not depend on the binding of hormone to its receptor. Two monoclonal antibodies (D547, D75) were used to devise a simple enzyme immunoassay (immunocolorimetric [ICMA] or immunoradiometric [IRMA]) for estrophilin in extracts of reproductive tissues and tumors. When tested on 82 breast tumor cytosols, a linear correlation (m=0.94, r=0.98) of IRMA and ICMA results with sucrose gradient data (using 3[H]estradiol) was obtained. The sensitivity of the assay is about 17 fmol of receptor per milliliter of cytosol (1.7 fmol/mg protein). A newer version of this assay (with D547 and H222) has a sensitivity of a 2 fmol of receptor per milliliter of cytosol (0.2 fmol/mg protein). Several monoclonal antibodies (D547, D58, D75, H222, H226) have been used to develop an immunocytochemical assay (ER-ICA) for localizing estrogen receptor in reproductive tissues and in human breast cancers and tumor cell lines. Specific immunoperoxidase staining for receptor in fixed, frozen sections was confined to the nucleus of selected cell populations within each tissue or monolayer culture examined. In a study of 117 human breast cancers by the ER-ICA method, the presence or absence of nuclear staining was significantly associated with the concentration of cytosolic estrogen receptor determined by steroid-binding assay. When ER-ICA-positive tumors were further assessed for staining intensity, epithelial cellularity, and the proportion of tumor cells stained, epithelial cellularity showed the highest degree of correlation with the results of the steroid-binding assay. In view of the exclusively nuclear localization of specific immunoperoxidase staining for receptor in all estrogen-sensitive tissues and cells examined thus far, it appears that both cytosol and nuclear forms of the receptor may reside in the nuclear compartment in the presence and absence of steroid. We have seen little or no increase in nuclear staining intensity in MCF-7 cells and in uteri from immature or ovariectomized rabbits following short-term treatment of cells or animals with estradiol. These observations are consistent with the hypothesis that unoccupied estrophilin recovered in the low salt cytsol fraction of a tissue homogenate represents receptor that is loosely associated with nuclear components and that the binding of estradiol to its receptor leads to a tighter association, a phenomenon previously interpreted as indicating translocation of the receptor from the cytoplasm to the nucleus. These studies were supported by Abbott Laboratories, the American Cancer Society (BC-86), the NCI (CA-02897) and by the Women's Board of the University of Chicago Cancer Research Foundation. Antibodies H222 and H226 were prepared by Dr. Larry Miller at Abbott Laboratories.

S.104 GLUCOCORTICOID RECEPTORS AND THE PHYSIOLOGICAL ROLES OF GLUCOCORTICOID HORMONES. J. Funder*, Medical Research Centre, Prince Henry's Hospital, Melbourne, Australia 3004.

For over 40 years glucocorticoid hormones have been a physiological enigma, involved in an array of 'pleiotypic' and/or 'permissive' effects, and in an ill-defined 'stress' response. The term glucocorticoid derives from a classic bioassay, that of mouse liver glycogen deposition. Glucocorticoids are secreted upon demand from the adrenal cortex, under the immediate control of pituitary ACTH, and probably of other products of POMC in the longer term. ACTH has two patterns of secretion - circadian, with a major peak around waking, minor meal-related peaks and troughs of very low levels; and episodic, in response to stress (e.g. fever, hypoglycemia, trauma). In most species, including man, cortisol (hydrocortisone, compound F) is the predominant glucocorticoid; in the rat and mouse it is corticosterone (compound B). These glucocorticoids circulate >90% protein bound, largely to a high affinity globulin (corticosteroid binding globulin - CBG). Their specificity is not absolute; high therapeutic doses of hydrocortisone, for example, overlap into the mineralocorticoid (aldosterone) domain, and result in fluid and electrolyte retention. Recent studies have shown quite clearly that there exist two classes of glucocorticoid receptors. Classical glucocorticoid (Type II) receptors have been described over the past 15 years using ^{3}H-dexamethasone (^{3}HDM) as a probe, since it binds minimally to CBG, which may contaminate cytosol preparations. The affinity of steroids for these receptors parallels their anti-inflammatory potency; it is moderate for DM (K_d 3-10nM), and even lower for the natural glucocorticoids (B, F). Very recently, receptors with very high affinity for corticosterone (K_d ∿0.3nM), and much lower affinity for DM (∿10nM), have been found in some (hippocampus, kidney, mammary gland, epididymis) but not all (thymus) rat tissues. These (Type I) sites have equivalent affinity for corticosterone and aldosterone; in certain areas, e.g. renal inner medulla/papilla, there are mechanisms favoring receptor occupancy by aldosterone rather than corticosterone, suggesting a mineralocorticoid receptor role for such sites. However, in the hippocampus for example, such sites are occupied (at the peak of diurnal secretion) or unoccupied (at the troughs) by the glucocorticoid corticosterone; thus in these tissues such sites are best defined as glucocorticoid receptors. Glucocorticoids would therefore appear to operate in two modes. High-affinity receptors, filled and empty over the diurnal range of glucocorticoid levels, are ideally placed to mediate glucocorticoid effects on mood, appetite and sleep/wake patterns (hippocampus), or permissive effects on production of milk proteins (mammary gland). Type II glucocorticoid receptors have much lower affinity for natural glucocorticoids (but not, it should be noted, for dexamethasone); these sites are only substantially occupied by endogenous glucocorticoid in response to stressed levels of ACTH. Glucocorticoids, then, may play two overall physiological roles. The first is in a time dimension, serving as a zeitgeber for various neural and secretory processes; and the other as perhaps the endocrine equivalent of the sympathetic nervous system, serving to integrate cellular and organ adaptations to stress, probably primordially in response to substrate and/or temperature changes. Supported by the N.H. & M.R.C. of Australia.

S.105 NONTHYROID TSH RECEPTORS IN THE STUDY OF THE PATHOGENESIS OF GRAVES' DISEASE.

S.H. Ingbar*, Beth Israel Hospital and Harvard Medical School, Boston, MA, USA.

Abbreviations: IgG fractions from the serum of normals or patients with Graves' disease or Hashimoto's disease, N-IgG, G-IgG, H-IgG, respectively; factors in G-IgG specific to patients with Graves' disease (probably in the main TSH receptor antibodies) Graves'-related IgG or GR-IgG; guinea pig fat cell membranes, FCM; TSH-binding inhibition; TBI; *Yersinia enterocolitica*, YE.

Biologic materials other than thyroid tissue have proven useful in studies of the pathogenesis of Graves' disease. FCM contain a TSH receptor and bind GR-IgG, but not other antithyroid antibodies. Receptor-purification of GR-IgG using FCM yielded preparations highly and comparably enriched in TBI and adenylate cyclase activity and devoid of antimicrosomal antibodies. ^{125}I-labeled receptor-purified GR-IgG bound saturably to human thyroid membranes. Binding was disease-specific (inhibited by G-IgG but not H-IgG) and was at partly inhibited by TSH. Further, inhibition of labeled GR-IgG binding by various preparations of G-IgG correlated closely with their own TBI activity.

FCM were also used to explore cell-mediated immune responses in Graves' and Hashimoto's lymphocytes. We examined the mitogenic response of lymphocytes from patients with Graves' disease or Hashimoto's disease, and from controls, to membrane antigens from human thyroid, FCM, and kidney. As judged from ^{3}H-uridine incorporation, significant stimulatory responses to thyroid antigens were observed in both Graves' and Hashimoto's disease, but only in Graves' disease were significant responses to FCM seen. None responded to kidney. TSH blocked responses of Graves' lymphocytes to thyroid and FCM, but did not affect ^{3}H-uridine incorporation in other mixtures. These findings indicate that a TSH receptor is both the cell-sensitizing antigen and the antigen against which circulating GR-IgG are directed in Graves' disease.

Antibodies against the gram-negative enteric pathogen YE are found with inordinate frequency in the blood of patients with autoimmune thyroid disease, and immunofluorescent antithyroid antibodies appear transiently in a high proportion of patients recovering from YE infections. These findings, which suggest antigenic cross-reactivity between components of YE and those of the thyroid, led us to seek evidence of functional cross-reactivity. Saturable binding of bTSH to YE extracts, particularly the inner bacterial membrane, was demonstrated. bTSH binding sites in YE extracts shared many properties with the thyroid TSH receptor, including inhibition by GR-IgG. A similar site was identified in E. coli. Receptor-purification of G-IgG, but not N-IgG, yielded IgG with an enhanced concentration of antibodies against E. coli in an ELISA assay, and this interaction was blocked by TSH. These data demonstrate antigenic and functional cross-reactivity between the TSH receptors in thyroid and FCM with components of certain bacteria, and raise the possibility that an immune response to infection with such bacteria, in susceptible individuals, may give rise to persistent, self-directed anti-TSH antibodies. Efforts to create an animal model of Graves' disease by immunization are currently underway.

S.106 MONOCLONAL ANTIBODIES TO THE TSH RECEPTOR: A MULTIDETERMINANT STRUCTURE WITH COMPLEX RELATIONSHIPS TO GRAVFS' AUTOANTIBODIFS. L.D. KOHN*and E.F. Grollman, NIH, NIADDK, Bethesda, Maryland, U.S.A.

Monoclonal antibodies to the TSH receptor have been derived from fusions of spleen cells from mice immunized with solubilized bovine and human thyroid membrane preparations. Monoclonal antibodies also have been obtained from fusions using the peripheral B lymphocytes of patients with active Graves' disease in order to evaluate the relationship of Graves' autoantibodies to TSH receptor structure. TSH receptor monoclonals are defined by their ability to specifically and competitively inhibit TSH binding to membranes and cells or be themselves competitively inhibited in this respect by pure TSH. They must also act as competitive antagonists or, alternatively, be mimickers and competitive agonists of TSH function, i.e., stimulation of adenylate cyclase activity, iodide uptake, thyroid hormone secretion, and growth. Studies with >20 monoclonals derived and characterized as above allow the following conclusions.

The TSH receptor appears to be a functional complex of both a membrane glycoprotein and ganglioside; the complex is in equilibrium with its separated free components in the lipid bilayer; these components may have common antigenic determinants; the equilibrium state can account for the *in vitro* ability of cholera, tetanus, interferon, and other ligands to perturb TSH binding and function. Graves' autoantibodies which inhibit TSH binding and function, i.e., those positive in binding inhibition assays interact with the glycoprotein component; in contrast, thyroid stimulating antibodies (TSAbs) interact with the ganglioside component. Inhibitor antibodies of the first class can coexist in a patient with a TSAb; they do not inhibit TSAb activity, i.e., the phenotypic expression of the patient will always be hyperthyroidism. The glycoprotein component of the TSH receptor is a subunit structure, which in membrane preparations has a 20-25K and 45-55K component and can exist, apparently as both a 1:1 complex and its dimer. The antigen determinents of this high affinity TSH binding component do not appear to exibit significant species specificity. The TSH receptor ganglioside is a minor component (<0.1 to 1%) of the total ganglioside pool; appears to be thyroid specific; and may structurally account for the species specificity phenomenon exhibited by TSAbs.

The same TSH receptor complex is related to thyroid cell growth autoantibodies in Graves' patients. The growth message system is however, more complex than that for iodide uptake; antibodies to different determinants of the TSH receptor may thus effect thyroid cell growth by different pertubations of these systems. TSH receptor monoclonal antibodies isolated from spleen cell fusions and from the lymphocytes of patients with connective tissue complications of Graves', exophthalmos and pretibial myxedema, include a unique set also able to stimulate growth and/or collagen biosynthesis in human fibroblasts; TSH itself and most TSAbs are inactive in this respect. The TSH receptor already identified in binding studies in connective tissue and fat cells is thus structurally related to the thyroidal TSH receptor and may be pathologically expressed in the presence of certain specific TSH receptor autoantibodies.

S.107 TSH RECEPTOR BLOCKING ANTIBODY.

J. Konishi*, Y. Iida, K. Kasagi, K. Endo, T. Misaki, and K. Torizuka, Department of Nuclear Medicine, Kyoto University School of Medicine, Kyoto 606, Japan

It is now accepted that the serum of the patients with Graves' disease contains immunoglobulins which inhibit the binding of TSH to its receptor and elicit the thyroid stimulating activity. However, the correlation between these two activities is generally poor, and TSH-binding inhibitor immunoglobulins (TBII) have also been detected in about 15 % of patients with Hashimoto's thyroiditis who have no evidence of thyrotoxicosis. The most striking finding which indicated the presence of heterogeneity in TSH receptor antibodies with respect to TSH receptor binding and intrinsic thyroid stimulating activity was the detection of TBII in hypothyroid patients. Since the first case reported in 1978, we have found 11 myxedema patients who have remarkably potent TBII (>50 % inhibition of ^{125}I-TSH binding). All these patients were nongoitrous and rapidly developed hypothyroidism at ages ranging from 15 to 49. They had markedly elevated serum TSH levels and very low thyroid uptake.

IgG from these patients showed no thyroid-stimulating activity, inhibited human thyroid adenylate cyclase stimulation by TSH or Graves' IgG and caused significant inhibition of ^{131}I release induced by TSH or Graves' IgG in a McKenzie bioassay. Titers of TSH-binding inhibitory activity in these IgGs correlated well with their thyroid stimulation blocking activity. Analysis of TSH-binding under the presence of these IgGs by double reciprocal plots indicated the competitive nature of the inhibition of TSH-binding by these IgGs. Papain digestion of one IgG preparation resulted in the complete preservation of both activities in Fab fragment. The most potent TBII among these reacted only with anti-K antibody and the reaction resulted in loss of adenylate cyclase inhibiting activity as well as loss of TBII. The direct binding of the TBII to human thyroid membranes was observed after purification of the ^{125}I-labeled IgG by receptor adsorption using guinea pig fat cell membranes. The binding was significantly inhibited by TSH as well as the unlabeled TBII. In 4 families, transmission via the placenta of TBII to five babies was associated with temporary neonatal hypothyroidism. These data strongly suggest that TBII in these patients are blocking antibodies directed against TSH receptors. Both the biologic nature of the TBII and the familial setting of the transient hypothyroidism emphasize the importance of this type of antibodies as a cause of hypothyroidism.

Incidence of TBII in 43 consecutive patients with primary myxedema was 21 %. In contrast to the quantitatively close association of thyroid stimulation blocking activity with TBII in these cases as described above, many samples without detectable TBII were also inhibitory against TSH-induced cAMP increase in cultured human thyroid cells. The data suggest the presence of other types of antibodies in primary myxedema which block adenylate cyclase stimulation by TSH. Recently evidence has accumulated that TSH receptor blocking antibodies are also present in some patients with Graves' disease. These studies revealed heterogeneity in antibodies directed toward the TSH receptor-adenylate cyclase system in autoimmune thyroid diseases.

S.108 IMMUNOGENETICS OF GRAVES' AND HASHIMOTO'S DISEASE. H. Tamai*, H. Uno, Y. Hirota, S. Matsubayashi, K. Kuma, H. Matsumoto, T. Sasazuki, and S. Nagataki, Department of Psychosomatic Medicine, Faculty of Medicine, Kyushu University (H.T. Y.H. S.M.), Fukuoka; Department of Human Genetics, Medical Research Institute, Tokyo Medical and Dental University (H.U. T.S.), Tokyo; Kuma Hospital (K.K.), Kobe; Department of Legal Medicine, Osaka Medical School (H.M.), Takatsuki; and First Department of Internal Medicine, School of Medicine, Nagasaki University (S.N.), Nagasaki, Japan.

It has been reported from many laboratories that the susceptibility to autoimmune thyroid diseases is linked to certain immunogenetic factors. An increased frequency of certain HLA antigens has been found in patients with Graves' disease and those with Hashimoto's disease. Graves' disease and Hashimoto's disease are closely related to one another, both clinically and in familial incidence, and are considered by some to be variants of the same disorders. The present study was undertaken to investigate immunogenetic factors in Graves' and Hashimoto's diseases and elucidate the relation if any of genetic determinants in Graves' and Hashimoto's diseases. Haplotypes of the human major histocompatibility complex (HLA) and the immunoglobulin allotype (Gm) were analysed in all 243 members of 37 families in which more than two first degree relatives were affected with Graves' disease. In 27 families with 173 members, 70 (40%) had Graves' disease, and none was affected with Hashimoto's disease. In the other 10 families consisting of 70 members where more than one first degree relative was affected with Hashimoto's disease, 26 (37%) had Graves' disease and 14 (20%) had Hashimoto's disease. The disease-associated haplotypes of HLA and Gm for each family were identified by determining the haplotypes shared by the two members with Graves' disease. Among 96 members with Graves' disease in 37 families, 74 were used for the determination of disease-associated haplotypes, and among the remaining 22 members with Graves' disease, 21 had both disease-associated haplotypes in their families. In 10 families with Graves' and Hashimoto's diseases, all 14 members with Hashimoto's disease shared disease-associated haplotypes of both HLA and Gm with members with Graves' disease, in each family. Fifty subjects of 133 clinically and biochemically euthyroid relatives were followed for 3 to 6 yrs to observe changes in their thyroid function. Two subjects became clinically and biochemically thyrotoxic 3.5 and 4 yrs after their initial visits. These 2 subjects shared disease-associated haplotypes of both HLA and Gm with probands of Graves' disease. Our findings in these families suggest that 1) in Graves' disease as in Hashimoto's disease, two genes linked to HLA and Gm, respectively, control the susceptibility to the disease, 2) the same immunogenetic factors are involved in the pathogenesis of Graves' and Hashimoto's disease, and 3) those who do not have immunogenetic factors are very unlikely to develop Graves' or Hashimoto's disease.

S.109 EGF-RECEPTOR IS STRUCTURALLY RELATED TO TRANSFORMING PROTEIN ENCODED BY AN ONCOGENE. J. Schlessinger,* Department of Chemical Immunology, The Weizmann Institute of Science, Rehovot 76100, Israel.

Monoclonal antibodies were generated against the membrane receptor for EGF. One type of monoclonal antibody binds to EGF receptor of human, rat and mouse cells and induces various "EGF like" effects. Hence, it was concluded that the EGF-receptor is the active moiety and that the role of the growth factor is to induce the appropriate change in the receptor molecule leading to DNA synthesis. Studies, using the monoclonal anti-receptor antibodies have established two important points. First, receptor aggregation plays an important role in the initiation of the mitogenic signal. Second, tyrosine phosphorylation provides a necessary but insuffficent signal for DNA synthesis.

An immunological approach was used to compare the antigenic properties of transforming protein belonging to the src gene family (src, fes) and the EGF-receptor kinase. Antibodies were generated against various synthetic peptides from specific domains on $PP60^{src}$ and fes. It was found that an antibody generated against the major phosphorylation site of $PP60^{src}$ interacts specifically with the EGF-receptor and immunoprecipitates a functional EGF-receptor kinase. A similar result was obtained with an antibody directed against a synthetic peptide from fes. Another antibody which binds close to a region on the src molecule which is required for its kinase activity also binds to EGF receptor and prevents the autophosphorylation of the receptor molecule. Neither antibodies bind to intact cells but they do bind to various forms of the solubilized receptor. It was concluded that part of the cytoplasmic portion of EGF receptor is structurally related to the carboxy terminal region of the src gene family.

Using immunoaffinity chromatography with monoclonal antibodies against EGF receptor, large quantities of EGF receptor from human cells were purified and used for structural studies. Tryptic and cyanogen bromide cleaved peptides of the receptor molecule were generated and subsequently purified by HPLC. 16 peptides which were derived from the human EGF-receptor were sequenced (in collaboration with Dr. M. Waterfield). Comparison of the amino acid sequences with an oncogene sequence data base revealed striking similarity with an oncogene (1). Six peptides derived from the human EGF receptor very closely matched a part of the deduced sequence of the V-erb-B transforming protein of avian erythroblastosis virus (AEV) (1).

The V-erb-B is a member of the src gene family. These results support the view that the transforming protein encoded by V-erb-B acquired the cellular gene sequence of a truncated EGF-receptor lacking the external-binding domain but retaining the transmembranal domain and a domain involv involved in stimulating cell proliferation (1).

REFERENCES

1) Downward, J., Yarden, Y., Mayes, E., Scrace, G., Totty, N., Stockwell, P., Ullrich, A., Schlessinger, J. and Waterfield, M. Close similarity of epidermal growth factor receptor and V-erb-B oncogene protein sequences. Nature, February 9, 1984.

S.110 IN-VIVO CARDIOVASCULAR, RENAL AND ENDOCRINE EFFECTS OF EPIDERMAL GROWTH FACTOR IN SHEEP.

Bruce A. Scoggins*, Aldonna Butkus, John P. Coghlan, David T.W. Fei, John G. McDougall, Hugh D. Niall and Xaio-Ming Wang, Howard Florey Institute of Experimental Physiology and Medicine, Parkville, 3052, Australia.

Since the first demonstration of an 'epidermal growth factors' in extracts of mouse submaxillary glands by Cohen in 1962 and its subsequent characterisation as a 53 amino acid polypeptide there have been many studies on the biochemistry of its mechanism of action. There have however been few reports of the physiological effects of either mouse epidermal growth factor (mEGF) or urogastrone, a hormone isolated from human urine, in conscious animals. This report reviews the physiological effects of mEGF in conscious sheep and describes its cardiovascular, renal and effects of ACTH release for the first time. EGF was prepared from mouse submaxillary glands by homegenisation and extraction followed by gel permeation and ion exchange chromatography. EGF was infused intravenously into adult sheep (35-40kg). Although mEGF has been reported to stimulate cortisol production in-vitro (Singh-Asa & Waters 1983) it had no effect in-vivo on the cortisol, or aldosterone secretion rate when infused directly into the adrenal arterial blood supply, of Na replete or Na deplete sheep with an autotransplanted adrenal gland, for 30 min at 0.8 to 80 μg/hr. Systemic infusion of mEGF increased blood [cortisol] by stimulating ACTH release. The threshold dose for ACTH release was 37.5 μg/hr. The increase in plasma [ACTH] was observed after 30 min. At 125 μg/hr plasma [ACTH] rose from 41 ± 16 to 910 ± 163 pg/ml after 120 min. This response was greater than that seen with CRF or other stimuli to ACTH release. The ACTH response to mEGF infusion was not sustained beyond 6-12 hr. EGF (125 μg/hr) produces a fall in plasma [glucose] and [K]. Plasma [Na] did not change. Within 60 min of mEGF infusion cardiac output was increased from 5.4 ± 0.1 to 6.0 ± 0.1 L/min and to 8.3 ± 0.2 L/min at 4 hr due primarily to an increase in heart rate. There was a small fall in blood pressure after 3 hr. A fall in total peripheral resistance occurred within 60 min. There was an increase in the activity of the renin-angiotensin system and this plays an important role in the maintenance of blood pressure. Adrenalectomised sheep, on basal replacement steroid infusion, failed to maintain their blood pressure after 60 min during EGF infusion. EGF (125 μg/hr) produced a 3 fold increase in urinary Na and K excretion over the first 60 min associated with little change in GFR. After 2 hr GFR was reduced slightly. There were only small changes in ERPF. Urine volume was increased 5 fold within 30 min and remained elevated for the 5 hr of infusion. The rate of mEGF infusion (125 μg/hr) to produce these effects is similar to that known to produce fibre sheeding, a reduction in food intake and other endocrine changes such as a fall in plasma [insulin], [T3] and [T4], and an increase in [growth hormone], [TSH], [RT3], [progesterone] and [FSH] in sheep (Waters 1983). These studies establish that EGF has a number of cardiovascular, endocrine and renal effects. Further experiments will be required to determine the physiological significance of these effects.

S.111 HUMAN PLATELET DERIVED GROWTH FACTOR (PDGF): A PRODUCT OF THE HUMAN PROTO-ONCOGENE C-SIS WHICH INTERACTS WITH CELLS THROUGH A PDGF RECEPTOR/PROTEIN TYROSINE KINASE. T.F. Deuel*, S.S. Huang and J.S. Huang, Jewish Hospital at Washington University Medical Center, St. Louis, MO 63110.

PDGF is a potent mitogen for cells of mesenchymal origin. It is also a potent chemotactic factor for fibroblasts, smooth muscle cells, monocytes and neutrophils. The amino acid sequence of human PDGF has near identity to that predicted for $p28^{sis}$, the transforming protein of the simian sarcoma virus (SSV) which is encoded by the SSV oncogene v-sis. The A chain of PDGF appears to be the physiological gene product of the human cellular proto-oncogene c-sis. The growth promoting activity and immunological reactivity of $p28^{sis}$ in SSV-transformed cells has been shown to be effectively identical to PDGF. A growth promoting activity antigenically recognized by anti-PDGF antisera also has been demonstrated in the human tumor cell lines A172 (glioblastoma) and HOS (osteosarcoma). These results suggest that a PDGF-like growth factor activity is required to initiate and maintain the transformed state in SSV-transformed cells and perhaps in other human tumors as well. PDGF stimulates cell growth through specific cell surface receptors ($K_d \sim 1$ nM, for smooth muscle cells, fibroblasts, glial cells). The PDGF receptor protein from 3T3 cells has been purified to near-homogeneity. It is a glycoprotein of 180 KD with protein tyrosine kinase activity. PDGF stimulates the autophosphorylation of the purified protein kinase/PDGF receptor protein at tyrosine residues.

S.112 TUMOR GROWTH FACTORS; BIOLOGICAL AND BIOCHEMICAL CHARACTERIZATION

George J. Todaro; Oncogen, Seattle, Washington

Biologically active tumor growth factor (TGF) has been found to be produced by various solid tumors, including human lung, breast and colon cancers and is not produced by normal cells. It is also produced by various retrovirus-transformed cells, but not by DNA virus transformed cells. TGF has been purified and sequenced. It has 50 amino acids and three di-sulphide bonds; also, TGF has been chemically synthesized and this material has all of the activity of the biologically produced material. It stimulates cell division of resting mouse and human diploid cells, induces anchorage dependent cells to grow in semisolid medium, binds to the epidermal growth factor (EGF) receptors and activates a receptor associated tyrosine specific kinase. The underlying assumption is that this growth factor is not only a potential cancer "marker" but actually plays a key role in maintaining the growth of the various anchorage dependent cell types. It is released by the tumor cells and binds to external cell membrane receptors, where it stimulates the growth of the tumor cells, as well as surrounding normal cells (M. Sporn and G. Todaro, New Engl. J. Med. 303: 878, 1980).

We have synthesized a 17-residues peptide (TGF_{17}) which corresponds to the carboxy terminus of transforming growth factor (TGF). This peptide does not compete with epidermal growth factor (EGF) for binding to EGF membrane receptors and does not stimulate anchorage independent cell growth and, therefore, does not mimic TGF activity. The TGF peptide does, however, elicit a potent humoral response when administered into rabbits. A high titered polyclonal antisera (IgG fraction) can be recovered from immunized animals with specificity for native TGF as well as denatured TGF. Antibodies to TGF are also being tested for their ability to inhibit the growth of human tumors both in cell culture and in animal models.

S.113 A SYNTHETIC INHIBITOR OF PARATHYROID HORMONE (PTH) ACTION EFFECTIVE IN VIVO: DESIGN AND BIOLOGICAL EVALUATION. M. Rosenblatt*, S. Doppelt, N. Horiuchi, G.A. Tyler, R.M. Neer, J.T. Potts, Jr. Endocrine Unit, Massachusetts General Hospital and Department of Medicine, Harvard Medical School, Boston, Mass. 02114, USA.

Over the last decade, extensive studies of the structure and activity of PTH have delineated within the hormone molecule separable domains responsible for receptor binding and activation. There is an address core, or domain, responsible for receptor binding (that is, the 3--34 sequence) and a small but critical message region (positions 1 and 2) necessary for hormone action. These studies led to the design and synthesis of bovine parathyroid hormone (bPTH) analogs that are potent antagonists in multiple assay systems in vitro. An analog of the 3--34 sequence, with norleucine (Nle) and tryosine (Tyr) as substitutions, [Nle^{8},Nle^{18},Tyr^{34}]bPTH - (3--34)NH_2, proved to be the most potent in vitro antagonist of PTH yet designed. In vivo, however, [Nle^{8},Nle^{18},Tyr^{34}]bPTH-(3--34)NH_2 failed to display inhibitory properties; rather, the analog demonstrated weak, but definite, PTH-like agonist properties. To generate an in vivo inhibitor, we used two approaches: 1) We extended N-terminal truncation to position 7 to eliminate "agonism" without completely losing receptor avidity. 2) Theoretical considerations prompted development of new bioassays; rapid hormonal effects were explored. The analogue [Tyr-34]bPTH-(7--34) amide was synthesized and evaluated biologically. When infused I.V. (200 fold higher dose-rate than PTH), the analog caused complete inhibition of PTH-mediated phosphaturia and urinary cAMP excretion effects. No agonist properties were observed. In a newly developed in vivo calcemic assay which reflects predominantly PTH action on bone, the analogue inhibited completely PTH-mediated elevation of serum calcium when administered (in repeated doses) in a molar dose ratio of 30:1 of analogue:PTH. These studies establish this analogue as an effective inhibitor of several major parameters of PTH action in vivo, including elevation of blood calcium, phosphaturia, and urinary cAMP excretion. This analog should facilitate studies of PTH action, its role in normal physiology, and may ultimately prove useful in treating clinical disorders of calcium metabolism.

S.114 THE EFFECT OF PARATHYROID HORMONE ON BONE CELLS. G.A. Rodan, Department of Oral Biology, University of Connecticut Health Center, Farmington, CT 06032.

Bone resorption is one of the major physiological and pathological actions of parathyroid hormone (PTH). The target cells responsible for this effect and the mechanism of action of the hormone are major topics of current investigation. Osteoclasts are the recognized bone resorbing cells, however, current evidence, which is limited, suggests that they are not direct target cells for PTH. On the other hand, there is a vast amount of data convincingly showing that cells belonging to the osteoblastic lineage are PTH target cells. This led to the hypothesis that the increase in osteoclastic activity produced by PTH may be mediated by other cells. In addition to osteoblast-related cells, lymphocytes, which are also PTH target cells, were implicated in this process. It was proposed that the hormone either stimulates the release of osteoclast-activating mediators, blocks the release of inhibitors, or changes the shape of lining cells to increase matrix accessibility to osteoclasts. These effects are not mutually exclusive. Study of the interaction of PTH with osteoblastic cells, either from embryonic calvaria or osteosarcoma clonal lines, revealed the following. PTH binds to specific high affinity (K_d around 5 nM) receptors in the cell membranes and activates the membrane associated adenylate cyclase to produce a surge in cellular cyclic AMP, which peaks around 2 minutes. This event is followed by immediate desensitization (reduction in hormone responsiveness) and on a longer time scale, a decrease in the number of receptors accessible for binding. PTH stimulation of adenylate cyclase is subject to the GTP and Mg dependence observed for other hormones. Glucocorticoid treatment potentiates PTH activation of adenylate cyclase. The next step is activation of cyclic AMP dependent protein kinase (PK), which is detectable at lower concentrations than adenylate cyclase activation and peaks when only a fraction of the receptors are occupied. Recent data show unequal activation of PK-I and PK-II suggesting cellular compartmentalization. The dose response curve for PK activation corresponds to that observed for biological effects of the hormone. One of the earliest effects is a change in the cytoskeleton. One to 2 minutes after exposure to PTH, calvaria derived osteoblastic cells show a concentration dependent decrease in actin and myosin polymerization. Long term effects (24-72 hours) include inhibition of alkaline phosphatase and collagen synthesis, related to _de novo_ synthesis of these proteins. The effect on alkaline phosphatase and collagen synthesis is probably mediated by cyclic AMP and is potentiated by glucocorticoid treatment. PTH was also shown to stimulate bone cell proliferation and to promote bone formation _in vivo_, at concentrations which did not increase resorption. There is indication for PTH effects on calcium fluxes in bone cells, which may also be associated with the mechanism of action of the hormone. The effects of PTH on bone cells are probably pleiotropic (multiple) and at least some of them may involve regulation at the level of the genome.

S.115 OSTEOCLAST ACTIVATING FACTOR. G.R. Mundy*, Department of Medicine, Division of Endocrinology and Metabolism, University of Texas Health Science Center, 7703 Floyd Curl Drive, San Antonio, Texas, 78284.

Osteoclast activating factor (OAF) is the name given to the bone resorbing activity which is present in the supernatant media of leukocytes which have been activated by an antigen to which they have been previously exposed or a mitogen such as phytohemagglutinin. The effects of OAF on bone are inhibited by calcitonin, cortisol and phosphate. Production of OAF by lymphocytes is dependent on monocyte prostaglandin synthesis. The cell of origin is a lymphocyte which has been activated by a mitogen or antigen. OAF has been implicated as the mediator of bone resorption and hypercalcemia in myeloma and Burkitt's lymphoma.

Recently, it has become apparent that OAF represents a family of biologically active peptides with the same biological effect, namely stimulation of bone resorption in vitro. OAF(s) may represent different peptides produced by B lymphocytes, T lymphocytes and monocytes. Bone resorbing activity has been found in supernatant media bathing continuous cell lines with the surface characteristics of B lymphocytes and has been found in the supernatant media harvested from enriched unstimulated peripheral blood B lymphocyte cultures. This factor may be responsible for the bone resorption associated with hypercalcemia seen in patients with B cell malignancies. Recently, media harvested from activated mature T cell lines has been found to contain bone resorbing activity. These T cells are of the mature helper inducer type. This factor may be responsible for the bone resorption and hypercalcemia seen in a subset of T cell lymphomas which are associated with a Type C retrovirus known as Human T Cell Leukemia Virus (HTLV). Peripheral blood monocytes also produce bone resorbing activity. Monocytes produce prostaglandins of the E series, which stimulate bone resorption in vitro. In addition, they release a macromolecular bone resorbing factor which is present in partially purified preparations of interleukin 1, a monocyte product which stimulates T lymphocyte replication.

At the present time, the relationship of these various OAFs to each other is unknown. However, they may play important roles in formation of the normal bone marrow cavity and local bone remodeling and bone loss associated with chronic inflammatory diseases and in bone destruction associated with hematologic malignancies involving T cells, B cells, or cells of the monocyte-macrophage system.

These studies are supported by grant RR1346,AM21584 and CA-23957 from the National Institutes of Health.

S.116 MALIGNANCY-ASSOCIATED HYPERCALCEMIA (MAHC).
A.E. Broadus*, K.L. Insogna, E.C. Weir, A.M.C. Vignery, W.J. Burtis, J.W. Godsall, and A.F. Stewart, Department of Internal Medicine, Yale University, New Haven, CT 06510, U.S.A.

Two general mechanisms appear to be responsible for MAHC: a) local osteolytic hypercalcemia, which results from bone resorption mediated by malignant cells occurring primarily in or metastatic to bone (e.g., myeloma and breast carcinoma) and b) humoral hypercalcemia of malignancy (HHM), which results from bone resorption mediated by a circulating factor(s) produced by neoplasms remote from bone (e.g., squamous cell and renal carcinomas). The biochemical marker for HHM *in vivo* is an increase in nephrogenous cyclic AMP (NcAMP) excretion, and this abnormality has been observed in 100 of 125 patients with MAHC studied to date. In contrast to patients with primary hyperparathyroidism (1°HPT), the prototype of humoral hypercalcemia, patients with HHM display: 1) a marked increase in fractional calcium excretion, 2) a profound reduction in circulating 1,25-$(OH)_2$D, 3) normal or reduced serum iPTH in a variety of region-specific assays, 4) circulating cytochemical bioactivity which elutes ahead of PTH on gel filtration and which is largely uninhibited by preincubation with anti-PTH antisera, and 5) intense osteoclastic bone resorption and near-complete uncoupling of bone turnover on histomorphometric analysis. These findings portray HHM as a syndrome of purely resorptive hypercalcemia, with the mediator being "PTH-like" in only a very limited sense.

Our strategy for purifying the factor(s) in question was to assume that it would display *in vitro* the same actions it displays *in vivo*. Correspondingly, our detection systems include PTH-sensitive adenylate cyclase assays in canine renal membranes and cultured rat osteosarcoma cells, a bone resorption assay, and the cytochemical bioassay (courtesy D. Goltzman). The sources of material have included human tumors, the Leydig cell model in the rat, a novel carcinogen-induced squamous cell model in the mouse, and cultured cells from several of these systems. Cyclase-stimulating (ACSA) and cytochemical (CBA) activities have been regularly demonstrable in tumors from patients with HHM but are absent from control tumors. Both activities are completely inhibited by [Nle^{8}, Nle^{18}, Tyr^{34}]bPTH(3-34)NH_2($bPTH_{3-34}$), but the ACSA is untouched by preincubation with a variety of PTH antisera (courtesy G. Segre). A combination of solvent-precipitation, gel filtration, and reverse-phase HPLC has generated material which is 30,000-fold purified and which maintains maximal ACSA and bone-resorbing activities. The protein appears to be quite basic and has an estimated molecular weight of approximately 25,000 daltons. Material in conditioned medium from the cultured rat Leydig cell model has been similarly purified. In collaboration with H. Kronenberg, A. Webb, and D. Goltzman, mRNA prepared from human and animal model tumors has been microinjected in Xenopus oocytes and the medium shown to have dose-related activity in the CBA, inhibitable with the $bPTH_{3-34}$ analog.

HHM is a common syndrome which results from tumor secretion of a factor which is clearly not native PTH. The factor is a basic protein of about 25,000 daltons and is presently available in highly purified form in preparative scale.

S.117 Abstract not received.

S.118 THE ROLE OF PEPTIDE HORMONES IN THE CONTROL OF FOOD INTAKE AND ADIPOSITY BY THE BRAIN. Stephen C. Woods*, Department of Psychology, NI-25, University of Washington, Seattle, WA 98195, USA.

Considerable evidence implicates a number of endogenous peptide hormones in the normal control of meal size and adiposity. The term, 'satiety factors' has been applied to those hormones (and possibly other compounds) which are secreted during a meal and which help determine when the meal will terminate; i.e., when satiety will be manifest. Most of these peptides are important in the process of digestion, and they additionally provide information to the central nervous system (CNS), either directly or indirectly via peripheral nerves, that determines when eating will end. The peptides cholecystokinin (CCK), glucagon, bombesin (BBS), and somatostatin (SS) (among others) have been extensively investigated, and all have been found to reduce meal size in several species (including humans) and under many experimental conditions. Control experiments have ruled out the possibility that the reduction of meal size following the administration of any of these compounds is secondary to malaise or illness. Other peptides, especially several endogenous opioids, appear to increase meal size once feeding has begun. The oral presentation will cover what is known of the mechanism of action of these satiety peptides, how they interact with one another, and their potential as therapeutic agents. Insulin is a peptide hormone which also influences meal size, but which acts over a longer time interval and which is thought to help in the normal maintenance and defense of body adiposity. Insulin secretion from the pancreas is directly proportional to adiposity; the peptide gains access to critical CNS areas both directly from the blood and via the cerebrospinal fluid (CSF); there are specific insulin binding sites in the CNS; and the administration of insulin locally into the CSF or specific brain areas reduces food intake and adiposity in several species. The oral presentation will include discussion of animal models in which the brain-insulin system appears to be abnormal, and how this long-term adiposity regulatory system interacts with the within-meal satiety system. Research cited was supported by grant AM-17844 from the NIH.

S.119 CENTRAL NERVOUS SYSTEM PEPTIDES AND BLOOD PRESSURE CONTROL. D. Ganten*, R.E. Lang and Th. Unger, German Institute for High Blood Pressure Research and Dept. of Pharmacology, University of Heidelberg, FRG.

Evidence favouring a role of angiotensin, opioid peptides, substance P, vasopressin, kinins, corticotropin releasing factor, and other peptides such as bombesin and somatostatin in central blood pressure regulation arises from neuroanatomical observations as well as from pharmacological and biochemical studies (1,2): Peptides have been localized in brain areas known to be important in cardiovascular control. Specific peptide receptors with high affinity have been discovered in the brain. Upon central administration, a number of peptides produce blood pressure effects which can be prevented by competitive antagonists; they interact with other blood pressure-controlling neuroregulators, e.g. catecholamines or GABA. Central inhibition of endogenous brain peptide synthesis or interaction with brain peptide receptors results in marked cardiovascular effects. Peptide levels and the activity of synthesizing enzymes can be altered in hypertensive states (3), and finally, there is a supersensitivity to the pressor action of some brain peptides in certain experimental models of hypertension.

In addition to their occurrence in the brain, peptides also occur in peripheral afferent and efferent nerves innervating the target organs of blood pressure control, i.e. the peripheral resistance vessels, the heart and the kidney. The opioid peptides and peptides of the pancreatic polypeptide family are present in noradrenergic nerve endings where they appear to be related to and released with the catecholamines. They either modulate the release of noradrenaline by a presynaptic site of action or exert their effects at the postsynaptic level. Direct effects of neuropeptide Y on the sympathetically innervated blood vessels have also been described.

The observation that the peptides are confined to some selected areas suggests a suborganization of the sympathetic nervous system with respect to the colocalization of classical transmitters with neuropeptides. In the future the knowledge of this peptidergic organization of the autonomic nervous system may help to better understand cardiovascular disease processes and allow the development of new drugs influencing the sympathetic nervous system in a more selective manner.

1) Rettig R, Lang RE, Rascher W, Unger Th, Ganten D (1982) Clin Sci 63:269s-283s.
2) Holaday JW (1983) Ann Rev Pharmacol Toxicol 23:541-594.
3) Ganten D, Hermann K, Bayer C, Unger Th, Lang RE (1983) Science 221:869-871.

S.120 LOCALIZATION AND ACTIONS OF AII AND CRF RECEPTORS IN SPECIFIC REGIONS OF THE CENTRAL NERVOUS SYSTEM.

G. Aguilera*, P. C. Wynn, R. L. Hauger, M. C. holmes, M. A. Millan, F.A.O Mendelsohn, and K. J. Catt. ERRB, NICHD, NIH, Bethesda, MD 20205 USA.

Angiotensin II (AII) and corticotropin releasing factor (CRF) exert well-defined actions upon pituitary and adrenal function. Also, both peptides are present in the central nervous system and their injection into the brain causes responses unrelated to their recognized peripheral effects. Since the actions of hormones and neurotransmitters are initiated by interactions with plasma membrane receptors, we sought to identify and characterize receptors for AII and CRF in the brain, and to determine whether their anatomical distributions were correlated with the central actions of these peptides. Binding of ^{125}I-[Sar^{1}]AII to brain membranes showed similar properties to those found for adrenal and smooth muscle receptors. Autoradiographic analysis of AII binding to frozen brain sections revealed high concentrations of receptors in the subfornical organ (SFO), organum vasculosum of the lamina terminals (OVLT), medial preoptic area (MPA) and median preoptic nucleus (MPN), areas involved in the drinking response to AII. After 48 hrs water deprivation, AII receptors were increased in the SFO, but were unchanged in other circumventricular organs as shown by binding studies with particulate fractions of microdissected brain areas and autoradiographic analysis in brain sections. AII receptors were also concentrated in the nucleus of the tractus solitarius, locus coeruleus and area postrema, areas involved in the control of the symphathetic system and probably related to the action of AII in the central regulation of blood pressure. Other sites containing very high concentration of AII receptors were the paraventricular (PVN) and periventricular nuclei, and the median eminence, regions related to effects of AII in releasing vasopressin and probably CRF and other hypothalamic hormones. Supporting this possibility is the ability of central converting enzyme inhibition to reduce the ACTH responses to ether and hemarrhagic stress. AII receptors were also found in the suprachiasmatic, subthalamic, and inferior olivary nuclei, superior colliculus, nucleus of the spinal trigeminal tract, and subicular complex, areas of interest for future investigation of the actions of AII in the CNS. Central injection of CRF has been shown to increase sympathetic, activity and decrease parasympathetic outflow, and to induce behavioral responses associated with stress. Autoradiographic studies with ^{125}I-Tyr-CRF revealed abundant binding sites throughout the neocortex and cerebellar cortex, subiculum, lateral septum, olfactory tract, bed nucleus of the stria terminalis, amygdala complex, laterodorsal thalamic nucleus, interpeduncular nucleus and superior colliculus. Moderate to low binding was found in the hippocampus, nucleus accumbens, claustrum, nucleus periventricularis thalamus, mamillary bodies, subthalamic nucleus, periaqueductal gray, locus coerulus and nucleus of the spinal trigeminal tract. The location of CRF receptors in areas which are related to the limbic system, and involved in the control of hypothalamic and autonomic nervous functions, support the view that CRF has a key role in the integrated response to stress. The presence of specific receptors for AII and CRF in discrete, physiologically relevant areas of the brain provides an anatomical basis for elucidation of the multiple roles of these hormones as neuropeptides in the CNS.

S.121 REGULATION OF SERTOLI CELL FUNCTION *IN VITRO*. J.P. Mather*, G.L. Gunsalus, N.A. Musto, C.W. Bardin, Y. Salomon and V. Perez-Infante, The Population Council, 1230 York Avenue, New York, New York 10021 USA

The Sertoli cell is thought to play a critical role in supporting spermatogenesis in the testis. In order to ascertain which factors are capable of regulating Sertoli cell function we used Sertoli-enriched primary cultures prepared from 10-20 day old rats. Cells were cultured in a serum-free defined medium supplemented with hormones, vitamins, and growth factors. Cell survival, the secretion of two glycoproteins, transferrin (rTF) and androgen binding protein (rABP), and adenylate cyclase activity were studied as markers of Sertoli cell function.

Insulin (Ins), human transferrin (hTF), and epidermal growth factor (EGF) were used as additives (3F) for basal conditions. Ins was shown to increase cell survival and rABP and rTF secretion. EGF also increased all 3 parameters, although to a lesser extent than Ins. hTF increased survival and rABP secretion under conditions where rTF secretion was low (e.g., cultures from 10 day animals and low density cultures), but had no effect on rTF secretion.

Both rTF and rABP secretion were markedly affected by cell density with increased secretion per cell at increasing densities. The secretion of both rTF and rABP was a function of both animal age at the time of culture and duration of culture. rABP showed increasing rates of synthesis *in vitro* for the first 20 days (animal and culture) while rTF showed decreasing rates of synthesis. Cultures from animals older than 20 days had decreasing rates of rABP and increasing rates of rTF secretion.

Hormones which increase cAMP formation in Sertoli cell cultures include FSH, isoproterenol, prostaglandin E_1, and α-MSH. All of these factors increase rABP secretion to an extent proportional to their effect on cAMP formation. None of these factors increased rTF secretion over 3F control levels.

In the presence of 3F, testosterone, progesterone, hydrocortisone, and estradiol all increased rABP secretion. Of these steroids only testosterone increased rTF secretion.

The major stimulator of rTF secretion *in vitro* is retinoic acid (RA). RA had little or no effect on rABP secretion in the presence of 3F. RA pretreatment of cells diminished their response to FSH as measured by cAMP production or FSH-stimulated rABP secretion.

Cultures grown on extracellular matrix produced by a rat testicular cell line (TR-M) showed an increase in basal (3F, 2-fold) and FSH-stimulated (4.5-fold) rABP secretion as compared to cells grown on plastic or plastic coated with collagen, laminin or fibronectin. rTF secretion was affected to only a small (145% of control) extent by substrate.

It is concluded that a number of factors including peptides (Ins, FSH, MSH, EGF) prostaglandin E_1, steroids, and vitamins regulate Sertoli cell function *in vitro*. The secretion of rABP and rTF are regulated by different factors *in vitro* and seemingly *in vivo*.

(This work was supported by NIH P50 grant HD-13541.)

S.122 STRUCTURE, FUNCTION AND SYNTHESIS OF GLYCOPROTEINS SECRETED BY SERTOLI CELLS. Michael D. Griswold,* Jodi Huggenvik, Steven Sylvester, and Michael Skinner, Biochemistry/Biophysics Program, Washington State University, Pullman, WA 99164-4660, USA.

Sertoli cells secrete glycoproteins in response to stimulation by hormones. These glycoproteins presumably interact with germinal cells and may play important roles in the spermatogenic process. Our objective has been to identify, isolate and characterize the polypeptides synthesized and secreted by cultured Sertoli cells from 20 day old rats. Our studies have focused on 3 glycoproteins or glycoprotein complexes which together comrise nearly 90% of the mass of the total polypeptides secreted by the Sertoli cells. We have identified 2 of these glycoproteins as testicular transferrin and testicular ceruloplasmin. The third is a large glycoprotein complex consisting of 2 small subunits of 29,000 daltons and 41,000 daltons joined by disulfide bonds and a larger 70,000 dalton glycoprotein which associates non-covalently with the two small subunits. We have designated these glycoproteins as the dimeric acidic glycoproteins or DAG-protein complex. On a per cell basis, Sertoli cells secrete nearly as much transferrin as do hepatic cells. The testicular transferrin has the same polypeptide structure as does sero-transferrin but the 2 proteins differ in the composition of their oligosaccharide chains. The function of the testicular transferrin is apparently to deliver Fe^{+3} to specific stages of developing germinal cells. The sero-transferrin is excluded from the luminal portion of the tubule by tight junctional complexes between adjacent Sertoli cells. In the testis, immunofluorescence studies have shown that the testicular transferrin becomes associated with developing spermatids. The hormonal regulation of testicular transferrin synthesis in cultured Sertoli cells has been examined by a radioimmunoassay for transferrin. Sertoli cells secreted a maximum amount of transferrin when they were cultured in the presence of FSH, insulin, testosterone and retinol. A cloned cDNA probe for transferrin was used to quantitate the steady state level of transferrin mRNA. Again, FSH, insulin, testosterone and retinol were required for maximal amounts of detectable transferrin mRNA. Because of the development of the radioimmunoassay and the cDNA hybridization probe, the quantitation of the synthesis of transferrin provides a sensitive and reliable marker for Sertoli cell function. The DAG-protein complex is the major Sertoli cell secretion product, comprising about 50% of the total mass of the secreted proteins. Immunofluorescence studies have shown that the DAG-protein complex is associated with spermatozoa after spermiation and is still detectable on ejaculated spermatozoa. The complex binds to some extent to the entire sperm but is concentrated in the anterior acrosome and the distal tail. Using an antiserum to the DAG-protein complex, we have also shown that the complex is synthesized by the caput epididymis. All of the glycoprotein secretion products from cultured Sertoli cells can be purified and characterized by high performance liquid chromatography (HPLC) on reverse phase columns. This technique has been used to examine the rate of synthesis and secretion of all of the major secretion products from cells cultured in the presence of various hormones and vitamins. Supported by HD 10808 from the National Institute of Child Health and Human Development.

S.123 SERTOLI CELL-GERM CELL INTERACTIONS AND THE HORMONAL CONTROL OF SPERMATOGENESIS. J.A. Grootegoed*, R.B. Oonk, R. Jansen and H.J. van der Molen, Department of Biochemistry (Division of Chemical Endocrinology), Medical Faculty, Erasmus University Rotterdam, The Netherlands.

Spermatogenesis in mammals is under the control of testosterone and follitropin (FSH). There is ample evidence that Sertoli cells, but not germ cells, are target cells for testosterone and FSH. Hence, interactions between Sertoli cells and developing germ cells appear to play an essential role in spermatogenesis. Some important biochemical aspects of the Sertoli cell-germ cell interaction could involve simple mechanisms, such as the intercellular transport of compounds from Sertoli cells, which cannot be produced at a sufficiently high rate by germ cells. The reality of this possible mechanism was illustrated by the observation, that isolated pachytene spermatocytes and round spermatids require exogenous lactate, rather than glucose, for ATP production. Glucose was an effective energy substrate, however, if the germ cells were incubated in the presence of Sertoli cells. This can be explained, because Sertoli cells *in vitro* metabolize glucose via glycolysis at a high rate, which results in a high rate of net lactate production. In addition, it was found that Sertoli cells, but not germ cells, contain branched-chain amino acid aminotransferase activity and produce branched-chain α-ketoacids from branched-chain amino acids. When germ cells were kept in contact with Sertoli cells *in vitro*, the α-ketoacids were reduced to α-hydroxyacids. This reduction is catalyzed most likely by the lactate dehydrogenase isoenzyme LDH-C_4 (composed of male germ cell-specific C subunits). There is as yet no evidence, that the α-ketoacids play an essential role. However, this observation provides evidence that Sertoli cell products can be transported into germ cells and can be further metabolized by germ cells. With respect to a possible predominant role of lactate, the effect of hormones on net lactate production by Sertoli cells has been studied. It was found that FSH, dibutyryl cAMP and insulin, but not testosterone, stimulate the rate of glycolysis *in vitro*. After 3 days of incubation of Sertoli cells in the absence of hormones, the cAMP content of the cells was increased within 10 min after addition of FSH, whereas insulin had no effect on cAMP production. There was a 3-4 fold increase of the rates of glycolysis and net lactate production within several hours after addition of either of these two hormones, and a greater response (5-6 fold stimulation) was caused by the combination of FSH and insulin. The responses were not inhibited by inhibition of protein synthesis. Observations on lactate metabolism and ATP production by isolated spermatocytes and spermatids indicate that a high concentration of exogenous lactate (3-6 mM) may be essential to support the developing germ cells. In the spermatogenic epithelium *in vivo*, such high concentrations of lactate could result from a high rate of net lactate production by Sertoli cells in the presence of FSH and insulin.

S.124 HORMONAL REGULATION OF SPERMATOGENESIS IN PRIMATES.

E. Nieschlag* and G.R. Marshall, Max Planck Clinical Research Unit for Reproductive Medicine, Steinfurter Str. 107, D-4400 Münster, F.R. Germany

Hormonal regulation of spermatogenesis of primates has not been as well studied as that of rodents. We have done the following studies to investigate the regulatory roles of the various hormones on spermatogenesis in nonhuman primates. 1. When the pituitary gland was removed or the hypothalamo-hypophyseal portal circulation was permanently disrupted in macaques, the testes decreased to 30 % of presurgical volume 5 weeks after surgery and the seminiferous epithelia regressed, comprising Ad and Ap spermatogonia and Sertoli cells only. Testosterone, administered immediately after surgery and continuing for 13 weeks, elevated serum testosterone levels to 10 times normal adult concentrations. These concentrations were able to maintain spermatogenesis but at a reduced level, as shown by decreased numbers of all germ cells more advanced than Ad and Ap spermatogonia, as well as testes having only 60% of the presurgical volumes. 2. In both hypophysectomized and pituitary stalk-sectioned monkeys, testosterone at 10 to 25 fold higher than normal serum levels could also re-establish spermatogenesis. The testes increased to 60 % of presurgical volumes and complete spermatogenesis was restored. 3. On the other hand, immunization of monkeys against FSH also decreased testicular volume and reduced the seminiferous epithelium. These studies suggest a role for FSH in regulating normal spermatogenesis. 4. Administration of GnRH to out-ofseason monkeys, which have quiescent testes, resulted in stimulation of fully normal spermatogenesis. 5. In adult monkeys, having the pituitary stalk sectioned, pulsatile GnRH administration resulted in a complete restoration of testicular volume and spermatogenesis. These data together clearly lead to the conclusion that both FSH and LH are necessary for fully normal spermatogenesis in the adult primate. 6. This, however, leaves open the question of how the onset of spermatogenesis is stimulated in immature primates. Experiments in rats have indicated that androgens, although initiating the process, do not lead it to completion, i.e. spermatozoa were not produced. In prepubertal boys bearing testosterone secreting testicular tumors, complete spermatogenesis, however, occurred. We, therefore, treated prepubertal monkeys which have only spermatogonia and Sertoli cells, with testosterone and elevated serum levels 10 fold over normal adult levels. Although complete spermatogenesis was stimulated, fewer sperm than usual were produced. This suggests that the onset of spermatogenesis in primates can occur with testosterone alone, but the fully normal process probably requires both gonadotropins.

S.125 ENDORPHIN AND ENDOPSYCHOSIN: MU AND SIGMA OPIATE LIGANDS OF THE PITUITARY GLAND AND BRAIN. Thomas L. O'Donohue*, Experimental Therapeutics Branch, National Institute of Neurological and Communicative Disorders and Stroke, National Institutes of Health, Bethesda, MD 20205

At least three neuronal systems which contain opiate peptides have been identified. These systems are best characterized by the prohormones from which the opiates are derived: pro-opiomelanocortin (POMC), pro-enkephalin and pro-dynorphin. These three neuronal systems give rise to peptides which bind to the mu, delta and kappa opiate receptors.

All of the opiate prohormones give rise to multiple peptides. Unlike the other prohormones which contain only multiple opiate peptides, the POMC system contains ACTH and α-MSH in addition to β-endorphin (βE). The major secretary products of POMC in brain and the intermediate lobe of the pituitary gland are N-acetyl and des-acetyl forms of α-MSH, βE 1-31, βE 1-27 and βE 1-26.

A key to understanding the physiology of the POMC multiple hormone or multiple neurotransmitter system will be to determine the presynaptic and postsynaptic relationships of the different forms of α-MSH and βE. Recent results indicate that there are dynamic relationships of the different peptides secreted from the POMC cells and neurons. The ratios of α-MSH to βE in the pituitary and brain should be 1:1 based on the fact that equimolar amounts of the peptides are present in POMC. The data indicated, however, that different nuclei of the brain have different α-MSH: βE ratios. Furthermore, ratios of peptides derived from POMC in the intermediate lobe of the rat pituitary could be altered by increasing POMC synthesis and peptide secretion with chronic haloperidol treatment. This treatment also induced the enzyme, opiomelanotropin acetyltransferase which N-acetylates α-MSH and β-endorphin.

The postsynaptic actions of the POMC neurons can vary depending on which peptides are secreted. N-acetylation of the peptides resulted in a marked increase in the biological and behavioral potency of α-MSH and a marked decrease in the opioid potency of βE. βE and MSH also had post-synaptic or target cell interactions. For example, we have shown that βE 1-31 modulates the behavioral actions of α-MSH. Processing of the βE 1-31 to βE 1-27 or βE 1-26 completely eliminated the modulatory potential of β-endorphin. Similarly, Carter, et al. (Nature 279:74, 1979) have shown that β-endorphin 1-31 can modulate α-MSH actions on melanocytes and that the modulatory activity resides in the βE 28-31 fragment. It therefore appears that presynaptic processing in POMC neurons and cells can have functional significance on postsynaptic or target cells.

A fourth type of opiate receptor, the sigma receptor, was originally characterized by Martin and colleagues (J. Pharmacol. Exp. Ther. 197:517, 1976). This receptor mediates the psychotomimetic and delerium inducing effects of opiates. Phencyclidine (PCP or angel dust) induces its psycho-tomimetic actions via interaction with this receptor. An endogenous peptide ligand for the sigma opiate receptor has been isolated from porcine brain by its ability to inhibit ^{3}H-PCP binding. The peptide is in highest concentrations in the cortex and hippocampus and has a molecular weight of approximately 3500 daltons. The peptide, which has been named α-endo-psychosin, has behavioral and electrophysiological actions similar to PCP.

S.126 NEO-ENDORPHINS AND DYNORPHINS

Hisayuki Matsuo, Department of Biochemistry, Miyazaki Medical College, Kiyotake, Miyazaki 889-16, Japan

Since 1975 when the enkephalins were first identified in mammals, a number of endogenous opioid peptides have been isolated, which contain an enkephalin unit at N-terminus. It has been clarified that all the peptides are processed from either of three distinct precursors; pro-opiomelanocortin, proenkephalin A and proenkephalin B, whose precise structures have been determined by using recombinant DNA techniques. By focusing on neo-endorphins and dynorphins processed out of proenkephalin B, their distribution and biosynthetic feature will be discussed based on our recent results.

Successive discoveries of α-neo-endorphin and dynorphin A in 1980 lead us to a new field related to Leu-enkephalin, which had remained unclear at the time. Since α-neo-endorphin and dynorphin A both contain in common an N-terminal Leu-enkephalin, followed by paired basic residues, such as -Arg-Lys- or -Arg-Arg-, the peptides were thought to be the putative intermediates to Leu-enkephalin. Furthermore, a series of identifications of β-neo-endorphin, PH-8P(dynorphin[1-8]) and rimorphin(dynorphin B) followed. All the "big" Leu-enkephalins elicit an opioid activity much more potent than Leu-enkephalin itself and are distributed in their own fashion. These facts indicate a possibility that they may not only serve as biosynthetic intermediate of Leu-enkephalin, but also play a physiological function of their own, even though there still remain many questions to be answered.

The sequence of proenkephalin B, the common precursor for a series of "big" Leu-enkephalins mentioned above affords suggestive information about a still unsettled feature of opioid biosynthesis, which will be discussed by comparing proenkephalin B with proenkephalin A. In the molecule of proenkephalin B, the sequences of β-neo-endorphin and dynorphin A are bracketted by -Ly-Arg-, which is thought to be a typical processing signal. However, the fact that the sequence of Arg-Lys or Arg-Arg remains uncleaved in the molecules of "big" Leu-enkephalins, implies that Arg-Arg or Arg-Lys may not be an obligatory signal or more resistant to primary processing compared with Lys-Arg or Lys-Lys. Furthermore, natural occurrence of PH-8P and dynorphin B, whose C-terminal residues are not followed by a basic pair, indicates that another type of processing can take place at the site before -Arg-Pro- or special Arg residue. It has been evidenced that a similar processing of proenkephalin A results in the formation of adrenorphin (methorphamide), which is the first C-terminally amidated opioid peptide identified in mammals. Adrenorphin should be processed out of proenkephalin A by cleaving before the linkage of -Arg-Pro-, followed by C-terminal amidation. Another unique processing is observed in the case of α-neo-endorphin, which is likely formed by cleaving between Lys-Arg preceded by Pro residue.

In addition, our study on the enkephalin-converting enzyme will be presented.

S.127 CONTROL OF RELEASE AND BIOLOGICAL INACTIVATION OF OPIOID PEPTIDES

J-C. Schwartz*, B. Giros, C. Llorens, B. Malfroy, C. Rose, K. Zuzel, P. Chaillet, J. Costentin. Unité de Neurobiologie (U 109), Centre Paul Broca I.N.S.E.R.M., 75014 PARIS, France ; Laboratoire de Pharmacodynamie, U.E.R. de Médecine et de Pharmacie, 76800 St Etienne-du-Rouvray, France.

One possible way to analyse the biological roles of messenger peptides in brain could consist in inhibiting peptidases involved in their physiological inactivation and thereby reinforcing the messages they transmit.
However this approach requires that the relevant "inactivating neuropeptidases" should be identified, selective inhibitors developed and their possible effect on metabolism of various neuropeptidases assessed.
This task is not always easy since peptidases generally display limited specificity (a number of neuropeptides are potential substrates) and each neuropeptide can be substrate for several peptidases.
In the case of the enkephalins two metallo-peptidase activities identified in cerebral membranes (but also found in other tissues) seem involved in their synaptic inactivation : "enkephalinase" (EC 3.4.24.11) cleaving their Gly3-Phe4 amide bond and inhibited by thiorphan and aminopeptidase(s) inhibited by thiorphan and bestatin.
The role of these two enzymes as "inactivating neuropeptidase" is namely suggested by the effects observed following their selective inhibition.
In vitro, inhibition allows almost complete recovery of endogenous enkephalins released from depolarised brain slices which, otherwise, are hydrolysed to the extent of 80 %. Meanwhile, when their inactivation is prevented, the opioid peptides seem to inhibit their own release from the same preparation via a feedback mechanism that we have recently evidenced. In vivo inhibition of these peptidases is followed by a marked increase in enkephalin levels in brain and by various biochemical or behavioral effects similar to those induced by exogenous opiates like changes in monoamine turnover rate, antinociceptive and motor effects, all being prevented by naloxone. Interestingly, however, thiorphan does not produced in rodents signs of respiratory depression (acute administration) or withdrawal symptoms (chronic administration).
It is not yet established whether the same peptidases are also involved in the in vivo physiological inactivation of other neuropeptides, they are able to hydrolyse in vitro. However, as an example, while cholecystokinin (CCK-8) is an excellent substrate for "enkephalinase", inhibition of this enzyme does not significantly prevent the extensive hydrolysis of endogenous CCK-8 otherwise occuring when it is released from brain slices. Hence the localisation of the putative "neuropeptidases" is probably essential in determining which endogenous neuropeptide they inactivate. This localisation is being determined histochemically using monoclonal or conventional antibodies now available against the purified enzymes.
In conclusion, selective peptidase inhibitors can be powerful pharmacological tools to delineate the functional role of neuropeptides and show promise as possibly useful therapeutic agents.

S.128 REGULATION OF ENKEPHALIN BIOSYNTHESIS AND RECEPTOR INTERACTIONS. K.M. Braas* and S.H. Snyder, Departments of Neuroscience, Pharmacology and Experimental Therapeutics, and Psychiatry and Behavioral Sciences, The Johns Hopkins University School of Medicine, Baltimore, Maryland 21205, U.S.A.

Many peptidergic hormones and neurotransmitters have been shown to be synthesized from large MW precursors. The derived peptides require enzymatic processing for release in their biologically active forms. The opioid peptidergic families are synthesized from the precursor molecules proenkephalin A, proenkephalin B and proopiomelanocortin. The active opioid peptides are flanked by pairs of basic amino acids, a structural organization observed with many precursor proteins. Cleavage by trypsin-like enzymes yields peptide with basic amino acid carboxyl terminal extensions which are cleaved by carboxypeptidase B-like enzymes to the active opioid peptides. Recently, enkephalin convertase (EC), a carboxypeptidase-B-like enzyme with apparent specificity in the biosynthesis of the enkephalins from their extended precursor molecules, has been purified from brain, pituitary and adrenal gland (Fricker and Snyder, PNAS, 79: 3886, 1982; Fricker and Snyder, JBC, 258: 10950, 1983). EC has selective affinity for enkephalin containing peptides exhibiting micromolar affinities for the arginyl- and lysyl-hexapeptide of the enkephalins. The enzyme is stimulated by cobalt, specifically inhibited by analogues of arginine and lysine, and, in adrenal medullary cells, is localized to the chromaffin granules where enkephalin is stored with catecholamines. Carboxypeptidase-B, in contrast, is a lysosomal enzyme, possessed a much lower affinity for the extended enkephalin precursors, and is not stimulated by cobalt or inhibited by the basic amino acid analogues. Radioreceptor and autoradiographic methods have demonstrated regional opioid receptor distributions throughout the nervous system that are similar to those observed for the endogenous opioid peptides. Regional distribution of EC activity appears to parallel generally these receptor and peptide localizations, while carboxypeptidase-B is distributed homogeneously throughout the brain. We have employed immunocytochemical techniques to complement the distribution studies of EC activity, and investigate its cellular and subcellular localizations, specific polyclonal rabbit antisera and monoclonal mouse antisera have been produced against purified EC. These antisera have been utilized with the PAP complex and avidinbiotin complex immunocytochemical methods to demonstrate the localizations of EC in rat brain sections. Preliminary results indicate that EC immunoreactivity is localized to specific brain areas known to contain enkephalin. Serial sections stained using specific antisera to the enkephalins are being examined to compare the sites of enzyme with the neurotransmitter. In addition to those brain studies, neuroblastoma cell lines have been useful model systems for studies involving differentiated functions of mature neurons. Several cell lines possess both opiate receptors and their peptidergic ligands which we have utilized to examine regulation of enkephalin biosynthesis. EC activity and immunocytochemical staining patterns parallel the content and localization of the enkephalin in these cells. EC therefore, appears to be a specific enzyme selectively associated with the biosynthesis of enkephalins in both intact brain and neuronal cell lines.

S.129 PROCESSING OF PROSOMATOSTATIN EXPRESSED BY A METALLOTHIONEIN-SOMATOSTATIN FUSION GENE IN TRANSGENIC MICE AND CULTURED FIBROBLASTS.

J.F. Habener,* M.J. Low, R. Palmiter, R.E. Hammer, R. Brinster & R.H. Goodman, Laboratory of Molecular Endocrinology and Howard Hughes Medical Institute, Massachusetts General Hospital; Department of Medicine, New England Medical Center, Boston, Massachusetts; Department of Biochemistry, University of Washington, Seattle, Washington; School of Veterinary Medicine, University of Pennsylvania, Philadelphia, Pennsylvania.

Somatostatin is a ubiquitous neuropeptide of 14 (SS-14) or 28 (SS-28) amino acids that is expressed in multiple tissues and that regulates secretory activities. Both SS-14 and SS-28 arise by post-translational cleavages from prosomatostatin, a precursor of the somatostatins. To investigate the cellular mechanisms involved in the processing of prosomatostatin we have analyzed the products of the expression of a metallothionein-somatostatin fusion gene after introduction into fibroblasts and into the germ line of mice. We ligated a DNA fragment containing the entire coding sequence for rat pre-prosomatostatin into a plasmid containing the metallothionein promoter and the 3' end of the human growth hormone gene. To test the integrity of this recombinant DNA we introduced it by endocytosis into a hamster kidney fibroblast cell line. The fibroblasts synthesised and exported nanogram amounts of immunoreactive somatostatin and zinc induced ten-fold increases in the amounts of somatostatin synthesised indicating that the metallothionein promoter was active. We next introduced the recombinant DNA into the germ line of mice by micro-injection into fertilized mouse zygotes and transplantation of the zygotes into pseudopregnant mice. Eleven offspring born from these surrogate mothers contained rat somatostatin DNA sequences determined by DNA tail blots. Blood levels of immunoreactive somatostatin in four of the animals were 50 to 100 times above normal. The growth characteristics, however, of the transgenic mice expressing the rat somatostatin gene were no different from those of the control siblings without fusion genes. Extracts of 15 different organs of the transgenic mice contained elevated levels of somatostatin. 31 of 45 second generation mice resulting from transgenic probands contained fusion genes indicating multiple insertional loci of the genes which segregated independently. By gel filtration immunoreactive somatostatin in extracts of the cultured fibroblasts and in livers and kidneys of transgenic mice co-chromotographed in positions corresponding to prosomatostatin, SS-28, SS-14, and a 7K intermediate form of prosomatostatin. The successful introduction of an actively expressed somatostatin gene into the germ line of mice and into a stable cell line will facillitate further studies by site-specific mutagenesis of the structural elements in pre-prosomatostatin that are involved in the post-translational processing to SS-14 and SS-28. In addition analyses of the organ specific expression of the somatostatin gene in the transgenic mice may provide insights into specific organs that are, or are not, effective in specifically processing a prohormone to its bioactive products.

S.130 PRECURSORS AND PRODUCTS IN THE FORMATION OF NEUROHYPOPHYSIAL HORMONES.

B.T. Pickering* Department of Anatomy, University of Bristol, Bristol BS8 1TD, England.

The recent determination, by way of cDNA, of the amino acid sequences for the precursors of oxytocin and vasopressin [Land et al: Nature 295, 299 (1982); 302, 342 (1983)] has completed the first chapter in the biosynthesis of the hormones. It is now clear that oxytocin is derived from a precursor consisting of the hormone and its associated neurophysin, while the vasopressin precursor is similar but has an additional 39 residue glycopeptide at the carboxyterminus.

In the hypothalamo-neurohypophysial system the precursors are processed inside the secretory granules as they move along the axon towards the neurophysins. Movement through the axon, however, is not required for processing because normal products are formed inside granules whose transport has been arrested by treating the animal with colchicine.

When animals are treated with tunicamycin, a non-glycosylated form of the vasopressin precursor is formed. However, this is not packaged into secretory granules but builds up in the RER. Such a finding is compatible with a suggestion that the glycopeptide plays a rôle in the intracellular trafficking of the precursor but it is difficult to rationalise this with an oxytocin precursor which is apparently never glycosylated!

In our hands the rat appears to make two vasopressin precursors which do not have a precursor/product relationship. What is their significance?

There are some indications that the precursors may be processed differently in extrahypothalamic pathways in the brain. Gonadal oxytocin, however, is accompanied by a neurophysin-like protein, probably in equimolar amounts, and appears to arise from a precursor similar to that found in the hypothalamus.

S.131 BIOSYNTHESIS AND PROCESSING OF OPIOID PEPTIDE PRECURSORS.

D.L. Kilpatrick*, Roche Institute of Molecular Biology, Roche Research Center, Nutley, New Jersey 07110.

Over the past several years our laboratory has been involved in elucidating the biosynthetic pathway of the opioid peptides, [Met]enkephalin and [Leu]enkephalin. By using a combination of protein microsequencing and recombinant DNA techniques, it has been shown that in bovine adrenal medulla, these pentapeptides are derived from a multi-enkephalin precursor, proenkephalin. Proenkephalin not only gives rise to [Met]- and [Leu]enkephalin, but to a spectrum of different-sized enkephalin-containing (EC) peptides. While some of the larger EC peptides may only serve as precursors to enkephalins, others possess significant opioid activity and may themselves be important physiologically. Although the structure of proenkephalin and the EC peptides derived from it have been well characterized, little is known about the mechanisms involved in the biosynthesis and processing of this gene product. One model currently being examined is the rat adrenal medulla. The rat (as well as other rodents) differs from other mammalian species in having relatively low amounts of adrenal EC peptides (100-fold less). Of special interest is the fact that severing of the splanchnic nerve results in a marked increase in rat adrenal EC peptides. On re-investigating this phenomenon we observed a lag of about 10 hours before EC peptides started to increase. Maximal increases (10-15 times control values) were attained 48-72 hr after denervation. The initial increases occurred only in the high molecular weight EC peptides(s), mainly in what appears to be intact proenkephalin. Processing of the putative proenkephalin in rat adrenals occurs very slowly over a period of several days. The major processing product has been tentatively identified as peptide B, the 31 residue carboxyl terminal portion of the proenkephalin molecule.

The size distribution and time course for the increase in EC peptides following denervation is consistent with the stimulation of new proenkephalin synthesis. Using cDNA probes, it has now been demonstrated that denervation increases the steady state levels of proenkephalin mRNA several-fold. The earliest time point at which this increase can currently be detected is approximately 12 hr. This effect is not due to a non-selective increase in protein synthesis, since the tissue levels of poly A^+ mRNA actually decrease by as much as 50% after denervation. Furthermore, denervation did not increase the catecholamine content of the adrenal glands. Thus although catecholamines and EC peptides are stored within the same granules and are released together on exocytosis, regulation of their biosynthesis does not appear to be coordinated. This selective effect of denervation on proenkephalin biosynthesis together with the characteristically low EC peptide content in innervated rat adrenals suggests that rat adrenal proenkephalin gene expression is normally suppressed by splanchnic innervation at a pre-translational step. The physiological basis for this suppression is currently under investigation.

S.132 BIOSYNTHESIS AND PROCESSING OF HUMAN VIP/PHM-27 PRECURSOR.

H. Okamoto*, N. Yanaihara†, N. Itoh, K. Obata and Y. Hayakawa, Department of Biochemistry, Toyama Medical and Pharmaceutical University School of Medicine, Toyama 930-01, Japan, and †Laboratory of Bioorganic Chemistry, Shizuoka College of Pharmacy, Shizuoka 422, Japan.

Vasoactive intestinal polypeptide (VIP), a 28-amino acid peptide, is present not only in gastrointestinal tissues but also neural tissues possibly as a neurotransmitter, and exhibits a wide range of biological actions (e.g. relaxation of smooth muscle, stimulation of intestinal water and electrolyte secretion and release of insulin, glucagon and several anterior pituitary hormones). However, the biosynthetic mechanism of VIP remained to be elucidated. Recently, we have determined the primary structure of the VIP precursor and studied the regulatory mechanism of the precursor synthesis in human neuroblastoma cells in culture. We cloned the DNA sequence complementary to the mRNA coding for human VIP and analyzed the nucleotide sequence. The entire amino acid sequence deduced from the cDNA sequence indicated that the precursor protein consisted of 170 amino acid residues and that the sequence of human VIP was identical to that of porcine and bovine VIP and located near the carboxyl end of the precursor protein. The central region of the precursor contained a novel peptide of 27 amino acids. The peptide, designated PHM-27 (Peptide having an amino-ternimal Histidine and a carboxy-terminal Methionine amide and 27 amino acid residues), differed by only 2 amino acids from PHI-27, a peptide isolated from porcine intestine, and was also closely related in sequence to VIP. A glycine residue and a pair of basic amino acid residues, Lys-Arg, were adjacent to each carboxy-terminal residue of VIP and PHM-27. The glycine residue appears to serve as an amino donor to the carboxyl terminus of these peptides. VIP was preceded by a pair of basic amino acids (Lys-Arg) in the precursor protein, but PHM-27 was preceded by only one basic amino acid (Arg). This may reflect a differential tissue-specific post-translational processing pathway, yielding either VIP or PHM-27, or both. When neuroblastoma cells were grown for 48 h in the presence of 1 mM dibutyryl cAMP, the synthesis of the precursor, pro-VIP/PHM-27, was stimulated 11-fold. The amount of VIP/PHM-27 mRNA determined by hybridization with cloned VIP/PHM-27 cDNA was also increased 11-fold in the dibutyryl cAMP-induced cells. Transcription of VIP/PHM-27 mRNA in isolated nuclei was observed in the induced cells, but not in uninduced cells. These results indicate that the dibutyryl cAMP-induced pro-VIP/PHM-27 synthesis is achieved by enhancing the transcription rate of VIP/PHM-27 gene.

REFERENCES:

H. Okamoto, N. Itoh and K. Obata; Molecular cloning and sequence analysis of cDNA coding for human vasoactive intestinal polypeptide (VIP)/PHI-27 precursor. Regulatory Peptides 6, 320 (1983).

N. Itoh, K. Obata, N. Yanaihara and H. Okamoto; Human preprovasoactive intestinal polypeptide contains a novel PHI-27-like peptide, PHM-27. Nature (London) 304, 547-549 (1983).

Y. Hayakawa, K. Obata, N. Itoh, N. Yanaihara and H. Okamoto; Cyclic AMP regulation of pro-vasoactive intestinal polypeptide (VIP)/PHM-27 synthesis in human neuroblastoma cells. J. Biol. Chem. (1984) in press.

S.133 HORMONAL REGULATION OF GLOMERULAR ULTRAFILTRATION. K.L. Skorecki*, B. Ballermann, and B.M. Brenner. Brigham and Women's Hospital and Harvard Medical School, Boston, MA 02115, USA.

Studies employing micropuncture of surface glomeruli in Munich-Wistar rats have allowed precise definition of the hemodynamic determinants of glomerular filtration rate at the single nephron level. Among these the glomerular capillary ultrafiltration coefficient (K_f) varies through regulation of glomerular capillary patency by vasoactive hormones. Prominent among hormonal regulators of K_f is angiotensin II (AII). Infusion of subpressor doses of this peptide results in a fall in K_f. Furthermore, the fall in K_f which occurs in a number of experimental models of acute renal failure can be mitigated by angiotensin blockade. The fall in K_f associated with infusion of a variety of hormones which activate glomerular adenylate cyclase, as well as with the infusion of cAMP itself, can also be mitigated by angiotensin blockade. These hormones include prostaglandins E_1, E_2 and I_2 as well as parathyroid hormone. This suggests that these latter hormones may act through cAMP-mediated enhancement of renin release and local angiotensin production.

Using radioligand binding techniques applied to isolated glomeruli we and others have demonstrated the presence of a single class of high affinity AII receptors localized to the mesangial cells in the glomerulus. Occupancy of these receptors is associated with a mesangial contractile response, which is thought to regulate K_f through changes in glomerular capillary filtering surface area. The density of receptors (Ro) in isolated glomeruli is regulated by salt intake. With high salt intake and suppression of circulating AII levels there is a significant increase in Ro when compared to Ro in rats on a low salt intake with high circulating AII levels. There is no effect of salt intake on binding affinity. Administration of captopril to animals on a low salt intake also results in significant upregulation of Ro without a change in affinity. This indicates that the circulating level of AII per se, rather than any other effect of salt intake, regulates AII receptor density.

Reduced renal vascular sensitivity to AII and other vasoconstrictor hormones has been demonstrated in experimental diabetes mellitus. Accordingly, we determined the density and affinity of glomerular AII receptors in normal, untreated and insulin-treated streptozotocin diabetic rats 3 to 4 weeks following the induction of diabetes mellitus. With low, intermediate and high salt intakes, AII receptor density varied inversely with the plasma renin concentration in all three groups. However, despite lower plasma renin concentrations in untreated diabetic rats, AII receptor density was significantly reduced at all levels of salt intake. AII receptor affinity was not different among the groups studied. We postulate that reduced glomerular AII receptor density in the presence of a suppressed renin-angiotensin axis may contribute to the altered renal vascular responsiveness to AII in diabetes mellitus. Such hyporesponsiveness may contribute to the characteristic glomerular hemodynamic pattern observed in human and in experimental models of early diabetes, namely augmented single nephron glomerular capillary flow rates and glomerular hyperfiltration. These alterations in glomerular hemodynamics are thought to contribute to eventual development of diabetic glomerulopathy.

S.134 HORMONAL CONTROL OF TRANSEPITHELIAL SODIUM TRANSPORT AND Na^+,K^+ -ATPase IN EPITHELIAL CELLS.

B.C. Rossier*, Institut de Pharmacologie de l'Université de Lausanne, Bugnon 21, CH-1011-LAUSANNE, Switzerland

In amphibian epithelial cells (toad urinary bladder,TBM and A6 cell lines), the reabsorption of sodium is under the control of hormones such as aldosterone, oxytocin and T3 (1,2). The Na^+,K^+-ATPase is a plasma membrane protein which has been identified as the enzymatic expression of the sodium pump. In epithelial cells, this pump is the major driving force for the transcellular transport of salt and water. Na^+,K^+-ATPase is therefore a potential site of action for hormonal regulation. We have studied the effects of aldosterone on sodium transport and Na^+,K^+-ATPase, as well as the interaction with oxytocin (potentiation) and thyroid hormone (antagonism). Aldosterone (0.8-800nM) stimulated transepithelial sodium transport. At low hormone concentrations (0.8-8nM) the increase in sodium transport between 0.75 and 2.5 h was accompanied by a fall in transepithelial resistance (early response). Higher hormone concentrations (8-800nM) further increased sodium transport without changes in resistance (late response). Thyroid hormone (6nM) and sodium butyrate (3mM) selectively abolished the late mineralocorticoid response. Oxytocin (50mU/ml) induced a rapid (5-15min) increase in sodium transport but six hours after hormone addition a sustained response (2 fold over control) was recorded. Both types of response were dependent on cAMP generation but only the sustained response was sensitive to Actinomycin D. The effect of aldosterone and oxytocin were synergistic (potentiation). We further studied the effects of aldosterone, oxytocin, thyroid hormone and sodium butyrate on the relative rate of synthesis of the sodium pump subunits by measuring the incorporation of labeled aminoacids into the α and β subunit of Na^+,K^+-ATPase using published procedures(3). The results indicated that aldosterone and oxytocin were inducers of Na^+,K^+-ATPase during the late phase of their action. Both effects were additive. Thyroid hormone was totally inactive in these tissues of poikilotherm animals. Sodium butyrate specifically antagonized the effect of aldosterone on sodium transport and Na^+,K^+-ATPase. The induction of Na^+,K^+-ATPase by aldosterone was mineralocorticoid specific, mediated by Type I receptors and apparently at the transcriptional level. The induction by oxytocin was cAMP dependent but also sensitive to Actinomycin D, suggesting also a major action at the transcriptional level. Recently, we have also examined the affect of aldosterone on the expression of Na^+,K^+-ATPase at the cell surface. Using a ^{125}I-lactoperoxidase-glucose oxidase technique, an increased expression of the α and β subunits was observed upon addition of aldosterone. This could be secondary to the increased synthesis mentionned above (insertion of newly synthetized pumps) or it could be related to the action of an early regulatory aldosterone-induced protein (insertion of sodium pump from a preformed precursor pool).

1)B.C.Rossier,K.Geering, and J.P.Kraehenbühl, INSERM, Vol 85,pp185-194,1979
2)B.C.Rossier,A.Truscello and K.Geering INSERM Symp.21,pp 225,Elsevier,1982
3)B.C.Rossier in: Current Topics in Membrane and Transport,Vol 20, pp 125 - 144, 1984 (in the press)

S.135 RENAL MINERALOCORTICOID TARGET CELLS. Diana Marver* UTHSCD, Southwestern Medical School, Depts. Internal Medicine and Biochemistry, Dallas, Texas.

Aldosterone influences the renal handling of Na, K and H ions. Recent methodological advances have allowed investigators to delineate those mineralocorticoid target segments along the mammalian nephron which govern this aldosterone-sensitive fraction of ion transport. In general, four techniques have been used: in-vitro microperfusion of isolated tubule segments, autoradiography, individual tubule equilibrium steroid-binding assays, and biochemical studies using either NaK ATPase or citrate synthase activities as markers of steroid sensitivity. All of these techniques point to the cortical and medullary collecting duct as segments whose performance is altered by the presence of acute and/or chronic mineralocorticoids. However, acute addition of aldosterone to the bathing media surrounding cortical collecting tubules obtained from adrenalectomized rabbits results in an increase in the transepithelial transport of Na from lumen to bath, while addition of the same to the inner stripe of the medullary collecting duct increases the secretion of H ions, a process independent of luminal Na. These changes are manifest within some 3 hours after presentation of steroid to the tubules. Thus, while both segments contain mineralocorticoid receptors or binding proteins, it is clear that there is a functional heterogeneity along the collecting duct system as a consequence of binding to those receptors. Data obtained thusfar would also suggest that the enzyme citrate synthase is increased in both of these target segments following acute in-vivo hormone administration. Earlier studies in the toad bladder and rat kidney had suggested that this enzyme is one of the aldosterone-induced proteins. The physiological importance of an increase in the level of this Krebs cycle enzyme may be to enhance the cellular capacity to synthesize ATP, a substrate for both the active reabsorption of Na and secretion of H ions. More interestingly, acute administration of aldosterone enhanced the level of NaK ATPase activity in cortical collecting tubules of adrenalectomized rabbits. It did so within a time frame which was physiologically relevant (i.e. within 3 hours after hormone administration). The response was specific for aldosterone as opposed to dexamethasone and could be blocked by spirolactone. When amiloride was used to block luminal Na entry in this segment however, the rise in NaK ATPase following aldosterone, unlike the rise in citrate synthase, was abrogated, suggesting a Na-dependent step in the augmentation of NaK ATPase by steroid. In addition, chronic administration (10-15 days) of large doses of deoxycorticosterone (5 mg/kg body wt) results not only in a further rise in cortical collecting tubule NaK ATPase activity beyond that seen in normals, but is coincident with an increase in the basolateral membrane surface area. Finally a number of other possible target segments for aldosterone are currently under consideration. They include the thick ascending limb of Henle, the distal convoluted tubule (DCT) and the connecting segment, or that segment which joins the DCT and the collecting duct. It may well be that one or more of these segments may participate in aldosterone-mediated changes in K secretion.

S.136 THE HEART AS AN ENDOCRINE GLAND

M. CANTIN*, G. THIBAULT, R. GARCIA, J. GUTKOWSKA, N. SEIDAH, C. LAZURE, M. CHRETIEN, P. HAMET, M. ANAND-SRIVASTAVA, A. DE LEAN, E. SCHRIFFIN, and J. GENEST. MRC Group on Hypertension, Clinical Research Institute of Montreal.

Cell biology studies have shown that the atria of rats contain protein-rich secretory granules, a large Colgi complex and rough endoplasmic reticulum. The incorporation of 3H leucine and 3H fucose in atrial organelles and especialy in specific granules as revealed by ultrastructural radioautography is identical to that occuring in other peptide-secreting endocrine cells. Atrial extracts and isolated secretory granules produce a powerful diureris and natriuresis. By biochemical techniques, two peaks have been isolated from atrial homogenates. From the low molecular weight peak, a peptide of 33 amino acids has been isolated and sequenced. The synthetic 1-16 fragments is devoid of biological activity. The synthetic 8-33 fragment is as powerful as the native 3-33 fragment. From the high molecular weight peak, a peptide of 73 amino acids, 40 of which being an extension of the terminal portion of the 1-33 peptide , has been isolated and sequenced. This indicates that atrial cardiocytes contain only one peptide, a fraction of which is very active and the rest forming the propeptide. The native and synthetic peptide produce not only diuresis and natriuresis but have also vasorelaxant and vasodilatory effects. Antibodies against the 8-33 synthetic fragment have been used to localise the immunoreactive peptide in heart and salivary glands. In the heart only atrial cardiocytes are stained. The protein A -gold techniques revealed that the three types of atrial specific granules contain the immunoreactive peptide. In the rat, granularity is more extensive in the right atrium and measurement by radioimmunoassy has shown that the right atrium contains ~ 3 times more peptide that the left. The effect of the peptide on the kidney is accompanied by a marked rise in cGMP in the urine and vasorelaxation is alo accompanied by increased C-GMP in the arterial walls. In the aorta, mesenteric artery and in heart sarcolemma, the activity of adrenylate cyclase is greatly diminished following incubation with the 8-33 syntetic peptide. Administration to the rat of antiserum produced in the rabbit significantly diminishes the diuresis produced by blood expansion. During blood volume expansion the concentration of the peptide in the plasma as measured by RIA is increased severalfold. Exposure of cultured zona glomerulosa cells of the rat and beef to the peptide greatly diminish the aldosterone secretion induced by angiotensin or ACTH. Administration of a bolus injection of 1.0 ug of the 8-33 synthetic peptide significantly diminish blood pressure levelsin renal hypertensive and spontaneously hypertensive (SH) rats for relatively long ($\gg$ 30 min) periods of time. These results indicate that atrial cardiocytes may be probably considered as stretch-responsive endocrine cells which secrete a powerful diuretic, natriuretic and vasodilatory peptide which also inhibits aldosterone secretion.

(Supported by a group grant from the MRC).

S.137 ONTOGENESIS OF PITUITARY HORMONES. P.M. Dubois*[a], M. Begeot[a], M. Aubert[b], F. Hemming[a] and G. Morel[a]. a) CNRS-ERA 981, University of Lyon-Sud, Oullins, France ; b) Dept of Pediatrics, University of Geneva, Switzerland.

For fourty years, numerous reviews have shown the rapid increase in our knowledge of the ontogeny of pituitary hormones in man as well as in animals. However, little information exists concerning the initial differentiation of the cells secreting the pituitary hormones. Increased knowledge of factors which could act on the pituitary anlage between the first stage in the formation of Rathke pouch and the appearance of hormones offers possible insight into the differentiation of pituitary cells. To appreciate the nature and the origin of these factors, the methods used have included the study of congenital malformations in man or those induced either in experimental animals by ablation of fetal endocrine glands or by administration of drugs, grafts of pituitary primordia, and culture of pituitary anlage with enriched serum medium. It was then suggested that in early fetal life the pituitary cells have a capacity for self-differentiation and that the secretion of pituitary hormones is relatively autonomous and unrestrained. However, at present, culture of pituitary primordia in a synthetic medium, immunocytochemistry to detect the differentiated cells and radioimmunoassay to measure the quantities of secreted hormones seem to be more suitable methods for elucidating the nature, origin and time of action of the factors inducing the differentiation of pituitary cell types.

Using these methods in fetal rat, gonadoliberin (GnRH) has been shown to induce the differentiation of immunoreactive gonadotrophs (at 11 days of gestation) and immunoreactive lactotrophs (at 13 days of gestation) in synergy with insulin. GnRH may be of fetal origin since it has been detected by radioimmunoassay in the earliest brain tissues examined (12 days of gestation). Moreover, pituitary binding sites for GnRH have been detected as early as 12 days of gestation, and at 14 days GnRH can be localized inside the pituitary cells using immunocytochemistry, its concentration increasing from 16 days onwards. Estradiol, however, does not seem to be involved in the differentiation of lactotrophs. Growth hormone-Releasing Factor (GRF) does not seem to induce the differentiation of somatotrophs which is favoured by cortisol or corticosterone and by very low doses of insulin from 13 days of gestation only. Differentiation of corticotrophs is probably dependent on several factors whose nature and origin remain to be elucidated but whose influence could be felt even before 12 days. It is interesting that the time of appearance of the immunoreactive gonadotrophs and corticotrophs was the same in vitro as in vivo, independent of the day of explantation and of the time in culture. This suggests that the differentiated cells could be committed very early by the effective factors, programming the beginning of hormone synthesis. Thus, only some of the factors which regulate the secretion of pituitary hormones in the adult seem to be involved in the initial differentiation of these cell types. Whether or not the differentiation processes follow a common pattern in all the cells, there is evidence that the undifferentiated cells of the pituitary anlage are not capable of self-differentiation.

S.138 MATURATION OF NEUROENDOCRINE CONTROL OF PITUITARY HORMONE SECRETION - STUDIES IN THE OVINE FETUS. P. Gluckman*, Department of Paediatrics, University of Auckland, Private Bag, Auckland, New Zealand.

In the ovine fetus (term gestation 147 days), a neurally precocial species, circulating concentrations of growth hormone (GH) are markedly elevated compared to those after birth and fall rapidly from 2 days prior to birth. Multiple sampling shows that fetal GH secretion is characterised by a marked pulsatility (mean pulse amplitude 92 $\pm$ 89 (SD) ng/ml, n = 18) but the interpulse concentrations are also elevated (102 $\pm$ 65 ng/ml) compared to the postnatal lamb (pulse height, 23.7 $\pm$ 17.2 ng/ml; interpulse nadir, 5.8 $\pm$ 1.3 ng/ml, n = 7) or adult (height, 5.8 $\pm$ 2.2 ng/ml; nadir, 6.3 $\pm$ 1.2 ng/ml, n = 7). To examine the role of the fetal hypothalamus in the regulation of GH secretion, we studied fetuses 6 days after stereotaxic electrolytic destruction of the median eminence (n = 6) or arcuate-ventromedial region (n = 4) at 110 days and in 4 sham operated controls. In the lesioned fetuses, the pulsatility was abolished (mean pulse height; shams, 195 $\pm$ 91 ng/ml; median eminence 8.8 $\pm$ 9.1 ng/ml, arcuate 27 $\pm$ 17 ng/ml). The interpulse nadir was 64 $\pm$ 15 ng/ml in the shams and was less ($p < 0.05$) in the median eminence lesioned fetuses (17.5 $\pm$ 17.1 ng/ml). Exogenous synthetic GH releasing factor (hpGRF 1-44) given intravenously to the fetus and lamb (8 ug/kg) stimulates fetal GH release from 72 days. However the response decreases with advancing gestation ($r = -0.81$, $p < 0.001$, n = 12) whereas the pituitary content of GH is increasing. This suggests either changes in the responsiveness of the somatotrope or the progressive development of counteracting inhibitory mechanisms. We postulate that the high fetal GH concentrations reflect in part immaturity of the negative feedback loop controlling GH secretion. Neuropharmacological studies have failed to demonstrate a neurotransmitter tonically driving fetal GH release but demonstrate that differentiation of these systems occurs within the hypothalamus over a broad gestational range. Although somatostatin, isoprenaline, muscimol and apomorphine inhibit fetal GH release, none reduce fetal GH concentrations to levels seen after birth - further evidence for the immaturity of inhibitory control. Similarly multiple fetal sampling demonstrates marked pulsatility of TSH release in the sheep fetus from 90 days (mean pulse height 5.8 $\pm$ 5.4 uU/ml, n = 18) whereas in the lamb (n = 4) and ewe (n = 5) no such pulsatility is seen ($p < 0.01$, pulse height 0.4 $\pm$ 0.3 uU/ml). The amplitude and frequency of the TSH pulses decreases ($p \leq 0.1$) after 120 days and is reduced by lesions of the median eminence (shams, 10.2 $\pm$ 4.7 uU/ml; lesions, 2.0 $\pm$ 1.7 uU/ml). These pulses are not synchronous with GH pulses. Fetal hypothermia induced by circulating cool water through a coil in the amniotic cavity (n = 11, 106 - 135 days) stimulates a prompt increase ($p < 0.005$) in fetal TSH from 1.9 $\pm$ 0.5 uU/ml to 7.4 $\pm$ 1.9 uU/ml. While the neuroendocrine mechanisms for stimulating fetal TSH release are active by 100 days, the exagerated pulsatility is presumably a consequence of negative feedback. The marked pulsatility of fetal GH and TSH secretion has not been previously appreciated. Studies of both axes suggest that the hypothalamic stimulatory pathways are functional prior to the functional maturation of inhibitory control loops.

Supported by the Medical Research Council of N.Z.

S.139 PRENATAL DEVELOPMENT OF A FUNCTIONAL CIRCADIAN CLOCK.

S.M. Reppert* and W.J. Schwartz, Children's and Neurology Services, Massachusetts General Hospital and Harvard Medical School, Boston, MA, USA.

The suprachiasmatic nuclei (SCN) in the mammalian hypothalamus act as a circadian clock generating numerous hormonal and behavioral rhythms. This endogenous clock is entrained to the 24-hr period by environmental light acting via a monosynaptic retinohypothalamic pathway. Since circadian rhythms are not overtly expressed until well into the postnatal period, examination of the development of this system has been difficult. We have used the ^{14}C-deoxyglucose technique to study metabolic activity (glucose utilization) of the SCN itself at earlier developmental stages. Our studies have focused on investigation of SCN function during fetal life. Timed pregnant Sprague-Dawley rats were exposed to various environmental lighting regimens, outfitted with intra-atrial catheters on gestational day 10, and injected iv with 145 μCi ^{14}C-deoxyglucose at specified gestational ages and clock times. At 45 min after injection, the animals were sacrificed, fetal brains were removed and frozen, and serial 20 um coronal sections were cut and autoradiographed. First, dams were exposed to diurnal lighting (12 hrs light daily) until day 19 of gestation when they were placed and thereafter maintained in constant darkness until deoxyglucose injections on gestational day 21. Resultant metabolic activity of the SCN of both the maternal and fetal brains was high during the mother's subjective day (12-hr period when the lights would have been on) and low during her subjective night. Next, a 12-hr phase shift in the lighting cycle during pregnancy resulted in corresponding shifts in the rhythms of metabolic activity for both the mother and fetus. In a study using blind dams, we found that the timing of fetal SCN metabolic activity could not be directly influenced by environmental lighting, but could only be influenced through the mother's circadian system. A clear day-night oscillation of SCN metabolic activity was detectable in the fetus from the 19th through the 21st days of gestation. As the first step towards elucidating the mechanism of maternal coordination, we examined the effects of maternal SCN ablation on fetal timing. On gestational day 7, dams received either bilateral electrolytic SCN lesions or sham lesions. On gestational day 21, fetal autoradiographs from the sham-operated dams revealed that all the fetal SCN were metabolically active during the subjective day and inactive during subjective night. In contrast, after histologically confirmed complete SCN ablation in the dam, there was no significant day-night variation of SCN metabolic activity in the fetuses; activity was scattered over the inactive and active range within each of the three litters studied (8-10 fetuses/litter) at each of the two injection times. The results indicate that an entrainable circadian clock oscillates in the SCN during fetal life, and that the maternal SCN are an essential component of the mechanism by which the maternal circadian system coordinates the timing of the fetal clock to ambient lighting. Deoxyglucose studies with pregnant squirrel monkeys suggest that the SCN are also functional during late fetal life in the primate and that, as in the rat, the maternal circadian system coordinates the timing of the fetal primate SCN. The existence of this interesting form of maternal to fetal communication in such diverse species as the rat and monkey suggests that the phenomenon is generalized among mammals and may even be present in humans. Supported by PHS Grant HD 14427.

S.140 ONTOGENESIS OF FETAL CATECHOLAMINE BIOSYNTHESIS. G. Teitelman*, L. Iacovitti, T.H. Joh and D.J. Reis. Laboratory of Neurobiology, Cornell University Medical College, 1300 York Avenue, New York, NY 10021, U.S.A.

The autonomic neurons of the sympathetic and parasympathetic nervous systems, which in adults synthesize norepinephrine or acetylcholine, originate from undifferentiated precursors in the neural crest (NC). One of the critical issues in developmental neurobiology revolves around the question of whether the expression by neural crest cells of an overt neurotransmitter phenotype is predetermined or regulated by environmental cues. To analyze this issue, we sought to determine: 1) the ontongeny of appearance of a catecholaminergic (CA) phenotype in the developing sympathetic nervous system; 2) whether the appearance of CA properties is promoted by environmental signals; and 3) the stability of expression of CA traits. By tracking the biochemical differentiation of the sympathetic neuroblasts in developing rat embryo with immunohistochemical techniques, we determined that the cells express the CA biosynthetic enzymes tyrosine hydroxylase (TH) and dopamine B-hydroxylase (DBH) after they aggregate to form the sympathetic ganglia. This finding raised the possibility that environmental cues may promote the appearance of CA traits in neural crest cells or their progeny. To examine this possibility, we tested whether the neurons of the cholinergic ciliary ganglion, a neural crest derivative will express CA traits when maintained in vitro. It was found that ciliary neurons of chick embryo expressed TH and phenylethanolamine N-methyltransferase (PNMT) and that they probably contained dopa-decarboxylase (DDC) when maintained in culture. This observation indicates that the appearance of CA enzymes in NC cells is regulated by the environment. This signal may be instructive. However, the recent finding of cells containing TH in the ciliary ganglia (CG) from E6 and E14 of development in vivo suggests that all CG neurons may be intrinsically able to express a CA phenotype and that, in vivo, those traits are visualized in only a few cells. In vitro the expression of the CA enzymes is enhanced allowing their detection in most CG neurons.

The fact that tissue factors may promote the appearance of CA properties raises the question of whether the stability of such differentiation is also determined by the environment. Recent findings indicate that the initial expression of a CA phenotype is probably mutable. Thus, a population of cells containing TH has been found to populate the pancreas of mouse embryos from E11 to E14.5 of gestation. The fact that these cells disappear at later stages of development raised the possibility that this transient population of CA cells (TC cells) may be transformed into cells expressing other phenotypes in response to environmental cues. This possibility is supported by the finding that some of the TC cells of the mouse embryonic pancreas contain both TH and glucagon while others contain TH and insulin. The fact that TH is not detected in pancreatic cells after E15, while cells containing pancreatic polypeptides persist throughout life suggests that the glucagon and insulin cells arise from the transformation in situ of TC cells. Thus, the initial expression of a CA phenotype is labile and can be modified in response to environmental cues. In summary, our studies indicate that the appearance of an overt CA phenotype seems to be regulated by environmental signals which will also determine whether the cells retain this initial metabolic commitment or whether they interconvert and express other phenotypes.

S.141 CALCIUM AND STEROID RECEPTORS. G.G. Rousseau* and L. Hue,
International Institute of Cellular and Molecular Pathology, B-1200 Brussels, Belgium & J. Gannell and J.W. Funder, Medical Research Centre, Prince Henry's Hospital, 3004 Melbourne, Australia.

Steroid hormones regulate cell function by binding to and modifying the activity of specific proteins, called receptors, that interact with nuclear chromatin and control gene expression. We have found that the glucocorticoid hormone receptor is sensitive to calcium ions (van Bohemen et al., Molec. Physiol. 4: 95-110, 1983). In cytosol from rat (HTC) and human (IM-9) cell lines and from rat liver and kidney, calcium modulates the affinity of glucocorticoid agonists and antagonists for the receptor. Kinetic, thermodynamic, and physico-chemical studies suggest that calcium alters receptor conformation. This phenomenon can be demonstrated *in vitro* at free calcium ion concentrations (0.1-1 µM) known to occur within intact cells. A cell-free effect of calcium on the kinetics of steroid binding was also found with the mineralocorticoid receptor from rat kidney, but not with the androgen receptor from rat prostate, nor the estrogen or the progesterone receptor from rat uterus. This prompted us to study whether glucocorticoid binding and action could be modulated in intact cells by manipulating their calcium environment. Treatment with the calcium ionophore A23187 of calcium-loaded HTC cells exposed to radioactive dexamethasone, a semi-synthetic glucocorticoid, led to an increase in the ratio of nuclear-bound to cytoplasmic-bound steroid. Similarly, isolated rat hepatocytes in primary suspension culture accumulated in their nuclei more receptor-bound dexamethasone when the medium contained 2.5 mM $CaCl_2$ than when it contained 1 mM EGTA. The stimulation by dexamethasone of tyrosine aminotransferase activity in the hepatocytes was twice as much, after 8 h, in the calcium-containing than in the EGTA-containing medium. The data suggest that physiological variations in cellular calcium homeostasis can modulate the cell response to corticosteroid hormones via a steroid receptor-mediated effect. This study was supported in part by the F.R.S.M. (Belgium).

S.142 CALCIUM AND HORMONAL CONTROL OF MEIOSIS REINITIATION. M. Dorée*, A. Picard and J.G Demaille, Centre de Recherches de Biochimie Macromoléculaire, CNRS, B.P 5051, 34033 Montpellier Cedex, France.

In starfish, oocytes are released from prophase block by a hormone originating from follicle cells, which has been identified to 1-methyladenine (1-MeAde). The hormone reinitiates meiosis by interacting with stereospecific plasma membrane receptors, which triggers the release of Ca^{2+} and a transient increase of its intracellular concentration. Plasma membranes-rich fractions isolated from prophase-blocked but not from maturing oocytes exhibit a dose-dependent Ca^{2+} release when treated with 1-MeAde or with its biologically active structural analogs or mimetics. This led to propose that Ca^{2+} might act in starfish oocytes as a second messenger in meiosis reinitiation. Microinjection of EGTA into prophase-blocked oocytes does not however inhibit hormone-induced meiosis reinitiation, although it prevents oocyte activation by fertilization, by ionophore A 23187, or by subsequent microinjection of otherwise efficient Ca^{2+} buffers. In contrast microinjection of Ca^{2+} buffers inhibits 1-MeAde-induced meiosis reinitiation. Oocytes can be released from Ca^{2+} inhibition by raising hormone concentration or by the subsequent transfer of cytoplasm taken from maturing oocytes. Ca^{2+}-microinjected oocytes remain inhibited up to 1 h after microinjection although free Ca^{2+} concentration comes back to its resting value less than 30 sec after microinjection. Cyanide, which decreases ATP content and depresses Ca^{2+}-pumping activity, reversibly inhibits 1-MeAde-induced meiosis reinitiation. These results do not support the hypothesis that Ca^{2+} is the second messenger of the hormone in meiosis reinitiation, although they support the view that elimination of Ca^{2+} from some component of the oocyte cortex (perhaps the plasma membrane) might be a compulsory event from transduction of the hormonal message.

S.143 THE CALCIUM MESSENGER SYSTEM IN ENDOCRINE SYSTEMS. H. Rasmussen*, I. Kojima and W. Zawalich, Departments of Cell Biology and Internal Medicine, Yale University, New Haven, CT, USA, 06510.

It has now become clear in the past decade that Ca^{2+} is a major intracellular messenger in endocrine cells as well as in muscle and neural tissue. Recent experiments have provided data from which it is possible to construct a model of how the calcium messenger system operates to bring about sustained cellular responses. This model appears to be valid for both the glucose-dependent regulation of insulin secretion, and the angiotensin II-dependent regulation of aldosterone secretion. The basic observation explained by this model is that when a hormone or other extracellular messenger induces a sustained cellular response and employs the calcium messenger system to couple stimulus to response, the rise in cytosolic [Ca^{2+}] is transient even though cellular response is sustained. The model proposes that there are two branches in the calcium messenger system: the first, the calmodulin branch, which activated by the transient rise in cytosolic [Ca^{2+}], operates via amplitude modulation, and is responsible for the initial phase of cellular response; and the second, the C-kinase branch which is activated by a rise in the diacylglycerol content of the cell as a consequence of the hydrolysis of polyphosphatidylinositides, operates via sensitivity modulation, and is responsible for the sustained phase of cellular response. This model accounts for the known facts concerning both glucose-induced insulin secretion and angiotensin II-induced aldosterone secretion. In both cases, a rise in cellular [cAMP] leads to an enhancement of the response evoked by each branch of the calcium messenger system. It seems probable that cAMP acts by increasing the [Ca^{2+}] of the cytosol and/or increasing the sensitivity of components of each branch to activation by Ca^{2+}. This general model appears to be an equally valid description of how the calcium messenger system operates in a wide variety of cell types that display a sustained cellular response to the sustained presence of a particular extracellular messenger.

S.144 The Regulatory Action of Calmodulin. C.J. Pallen, R.K. Sharma, and J.H. Wang* Department of Medical Biochemistry, University of Calgary, Calgary, Alberta T2N 4N1

Many well characterized cascade regulatory systems are themselves regulated through the action of calmodulin (CaM). The mechanism of interaction of CaM with its target proteins is a multistep process involving the binding of Ca^{2+} to CaM followed by a series of conformational changes of CaM. The activated CaM can then associate with certain regulatory proteins to modulate their activities. Some of these regulatory proteins are protein kinases such as myosin light chain kinase and glycogen synthase kinase. In addition to mediating numerous phosphorylating enzymes, CaM may also regulate phosphatase activity, thus acting at both the initiating and terminating ends of a regulatory cascade. Recently a CaM-binding protein called calcineurin has been found to catalyze the dephosphorylation of phosphoproteins containing phosphoseryl and phosphothreonyl residues. Calcineurin phosphatase also acts on other phosphocompounds including p-nitrophenyl phosphate, phosphotyrosine, phosphoenol pyruvate, and phosphotyrosyl-containing peptides and proteins. Calcineurin appears to be a multifunctional phosphatase, implicating a role for CaM regulation of these various activities such as participation in a regulatory cascade involving phosphotyrosine protein phosphorylation/dephosphorylation.

The interaction between CaM and cyclic AMP regulatory systems is well established. One such specific interaction occurs between CaM and cyclic nucleotide phosphodiesterase (PDE) to stimulate the breakdown of the second messenger cAMP. Calcineurin was originally discovered as a competitive inhibitor of Ca^{2+}/CaM-stimulated PDE activity. Recent evidence suggests that the activation of calcineurin and cyclic nucleotide PDE by CaM have different metal ion requirements. For example, Ni^{2+} supports CaM activation of the phosphatase but not the PDE. The requirement for different metal-induced CaM conformations for the activation of different enzymes may be a manifestation of the stepwise conformational changes of CaM induced by Ca^{2+}.

S.145 THYROID HORMONE METABOLISM IN THE BRAIN. P.R. Larsen*, J.E. Silva, M.M. Kaplan, J.L. Leonard and T.J. Visser, Howard Hughes Medical Institute Laboratory and Thyroid Diagnostic Center, Brigham & Women's Hospital, Harvard Medical School, Boston, MA 02115.

It is now recognized that in the rat cerebral cortex approximately 80% of the T3 specifically bound to the thyroid hormone nuclear receptor derives from intracellular 5'-deiodination of T4. Only 20% of the T3 in this tissue can be accounted for by plasma T3 at ambient plasma T4 and T3 concentrations. The two enzymes identified in cerebral cortex which influence the concentration of T3 are the type-II 5'-iodothyronine deiodinase (5'-D-II) which has a low apparent Km for T4 and reverse-T3 (1-2nM), is insensitive to inhibition by propylthiouracil (PTU), and does not metabolize T3; and the 5-deiodinase (5-D-III) which metabolizes either T3 or T4. A type-I 5'-deiodinase (5-D'-I, PTU-sensitive) is also present in brain, but this enzyme dces not appear to deiodinate either T3 or T4.

The 5'-D-II produces all the local T3 in the brain, appears to be localized in plasma membrane fractions of whole cerebral cortex, increases severalfold over time in the neonatal rat, reaching peak levels between two and five weeks of age, and also increases when serum T4 concentrations fall. This increase in activity occurs within 24 hours of thyroidectomy and the 5'-D-II activity can be reduced to normal in a few hours by injection of T4, T3 or reverse-T3, of which T4 is the most effective. The mechanism for this effect is unknown but it does not require protein synthesis. The increase in 5'-D-II in the hypothyroid cortex appears to be a consequence of impaired degradation or inactivation of the enzyme rather than due to an increased synthetic rate. 5-D-III is elevated in newborn rats, decreasing to adult levels by four weeks of age. It is reduced in hypothyroid and increased in hyperthyroid rats. The apparent Km for T3 is 2-5 nM and this substrate is preferred over T4. The 5-D-III reaction is also PTU-insensitive but can be separated from 5'-D-II. All three enzyme activities have been identified in mixed cultures of embryonic rat neurons and glia, and results of these studies suggest that the 5'-D-II is present primarily in neurons. T3 is degraded rapidly by 5-D-III in such cultures and this may explain some of the difficulties in demonstrating T3-dependent effects in this system.

From a physiological viewpoint the increase in 5'-D-II and decrease in 5-D-III in hypothyroidism can maintain cerebrocortical T3-dependent enzyme activities at normal levels. In hypothyroid neonatal rats a significant increase in cerebrocortical T3 concentrations and a consequent increase in the T3-dependent enzyme aspartic transaminase can be induced by injection of 60 ng T4, but not by 50 μg of T3. This effect of T4 is abolished by iopanoic acid, i.e. by blocking conversion to T3. The same pattern of enzyme changes in the euthyroid neonatal rat might also act to ensure an adequate supply of T3 during a critical phase of central nervous system development. If similar protective phenomena occur in the human, it could explain why reduced serum T4 concentrations seen in endemic goiter regions and in incomplete forms of congenital hypothyroidism are not usually associated with the severe abnormalities in mental development seen in congenital athyreosis. It would also point to the importance of correcting the plasma T4 concentrations to provide adequate intracellular T3 concentrations in the treatment of congenital hypothyroidism.

S.146 BRAIN DEVELOPMENT IN THE IODINE DEFICIENT OVINE FETUS. B.S. Hetzel*, B.J. Potter, M. Mano, G. Belling, G. McIntosh and B. Cragg, CSIRO Division of Human Nutrition, Kintore Avenue, Adelaide, South Australia. 5000, and Department of Physiology, Monash University, Clayton, Victoria. 3168.

The causal relationship between severe iodine deficiency and endemic cretinism in man has been strongly suggested by epidemiological studies (Hetzel 1983). Final proof of the relation of iodine deficiency to brain development required the demonstration in an animal model which has now been achieved in the sheep. Merino ewes have been fed a specially developed iodine deficient diet (crushed maize and pelleted pea pollard) which provided only 5-8 μg iodine per day. Controls were fed the same diet with the addition of 1 mg of sodium iodide by subcutaneous injection twice weekly. Severe iodine deficiency caused reduction in fetal brain and body weights and in brain DNA and protein from 70 days gestation to parturition indicating a reduced number of cells, probably due to slower neuroblast multiplication, which normally occurs from 40-80 days in the sheep, and slowing of the development of neuroglia. In the cerebral hemispheres, an increased density of neurons was apparent histologically in the motor cortex and visual cortex and in the CA1 and CA4 areas of the hippocampus in comparison with controls. In the cerebellum, there was delayed migration of cells from external granular layer to the internal granular layer and increased density of Purkinje cells in the iodine deficient fetal brains. Evidence of fetal hypothyroidism was provided by low fetal thyroid iodine (29 μg versus 2.636 mg in controls) and low plasma T4 values (6 nmol/l versus 216 in controls) thyroid hyperplasia from 70 days gestation, significant reduction in body weight at the same time as the brain retardation, and absence of wool growth and delayed skeletal maturation near parturition.

Fetal thyroidectomy carried out at 60 and also at 98 days produced a similar but less severe retardation of fetal brain development. A combination of the effect of fetal thyroidectomy at 98 days with maternal thyroidectomy carried out 6 weeks before pregnancy resulted in similar but more severe changes. This was associated with more severe reduction in maternal and fetal T4 levels than in iodine deficiency.

Brain growth was considerably restored when pregnant iodine deficient ewes were given an iodised oil injection (400 mg iodine) at 100 days. Detailed histological studies revealed less complete recovery in cerebral cortex than in the cerebellum. Restoration of brain weight also occurred when thyroxine (T4) - 0.5 mg on alternate days - was given from 100 days; body weight however failed to increase in either case. Brain DNA and protein confirmed the restorative effect of iodine and T4 but the effect for T4 was less marked. Brain retardation was unaffected by the iodine free T4 analogue 3.5-dimethyl-3'-isopropyl-L-thyronine (DIMIT) - 2 mg on alternate days - injected from 100 days; failure to cross the placenta was suggested by lowered maternal but not fetal plasma thyroid stimulating hormone (TSH).

The findings indicate that the effects of iodine deficiency are mediated by a combination of maternal hypothyroidism (first half of gestation) and fetal hypothyroidism (second half). There is no evidence of a direct effect of iodine on fetal brain development in the sheep.

Hetzel, B.S., Lancet 2 : 1126-1129, 1983.

S.147 THYROID HORMONES AND MICROTUBULES DURING BRAIN DEVELOPMENT.

J. Nunez* CNRS-INSERM U 35, Hôpital Henri Mondor, 94010 Créteil, France.

The most dramatic effect of hypothyroidism which is seen during brain development is a hypoplastic neuropile; both *in vivo*, during the critical period of nerve cell differentiation (1,2) and *in vitro*, when added to primary cultures of embryonic nerve cells (3,4) thyroid hormones stimulate neurite outgrowth. Since neurite outgrowth requires massive microtubule assembly the assumption was made (5) that thyroid hormones stimulate nerve cell differentiation by changing the concentration or (and) activity of the different proteins (tubulin and "microtubule associated proteins", MAPs) which co-polymerize to form microtubules.

Preliminary informations were obtained by following the kinetics of microtubule assembly in crude brain supernatants. The data showed that 1) the rate of *in vitro* microtubule assembly increases with age during brain development; 2) hypothyroidism, when produced in the rat at late pregnancy, slowers this evolution; 3) early replacement therapy with thyroid hormones restore normal rates of assembly; 4) the addition of purified MAPs to normal young or 15 day old hypothyroid brain preparations restores normal rates of polymerisation. These and other data suggested that thyroid hormones regulate microtubule assembly by changing the composition or (and) concentration or (and) activity of one or more of the MAPs.

Further analysis (7) revealed that striking qualitative changes in MAPs composition occur during brain development. For instance the TAU fraction, a group of 4-5 proteins with a molecular weight of ∿ 60-68 K with is present in adult brain, is absent at early stages of post natal development: two other entities are present, TAU slow and TAU fast, with different molecular weights, lower activity and different peptide mapping. This latter observation suggests that different TAU genes are expressed during brain development a conclusion which has been confirmed by cell free translation of the m-RNas coding for these proteins (8). Analysis of the TAU fraction prepared from hypothyroid rat brains also revealed that a group of TAU proteins, "TAU_3", is almost missing, whereas thyroid hormone administration markedly increases its concentration. Two dimensional gel electrophoresis showed that the TAU fraction is composed with more than 15 entities with at least five of them being under thyroid hormone control (unpublished results).

The precise physiological significance of the heterogeneity of MAPs and of the changes in MAPs composition seen during development and in hypothyroid rat brain remains to be determined. Recent unpublished data suggest however that they might be of outmost importance to regulate the number and length of the microtubules as well as their stability.

1) Eayrs and Taylor, 1951. J. Anat. 83, 350.
2) Legrand, 1957. Arch. Anat. Microsc. Morph. Exp. 56, 205.
3) Puymerat *et al.*, 1982. Cold Spring Harbor Symp. 9, 1033.
4) Romijn *et al.*, 1982. Dev. Brain. Res. 2, 583.
5) Lennon *et al.*, 1980. J. Neurochem 35, 804.
6) Fellous *et al.*, 1979. Europ. J. Biochem. 101, 365.
7) Francon *et al.*, 1982. Europ. J. Biochem. 129, 465.
8) Ginzburg *et al.*, 1982. Proc. Natl. Acad. Sci. 79, 4892.

S.148 EFFECT OF EARLY THYROID TREATMENT ON BRAIN DEVELOPMENT. J.H. Dussault*, M.D., Thyroid Research Unit, Dept of Endocrinology and Metabolism, Centre Hospitalier de l'Université Laval, Ste-Foy, P.Q., Canada.

Thyroid hormones play an important role in the central nervous system. The most striking effects are observed during development where absence of thyroid hormones produces multiple morphological and biochemical alterations and in man finally leads to irreversible mental retardation. Since the brain is a very heterogenous organ, a first step to elucidate the mechanism of action of the thyroid hormone in this tissue is to identify the primary targets of the hormone, using the rat as a model for this purpose. The demonstration of local conversion of T_4 to T_3 in the brain with highly saturated T_3 receptor suggest that T_3 is particularly important in the brain. Saturation experiments reveals the presence of a single class of binding sites not evenly distributed in the cortex and concentrated in the neuronal population. Data on the morphological changes induced by hypothyroidism (de Escobar and coll.) shows that in the forebrain (maturation of pyramidal cells of the visual cortex) thyroidectomy (at 10 days of age) induce rapidly (20 days) a significant decrease in the number of spines/apical shaft of pyramidal cells which is restored with early treatment. In the cerebellum, arborization and ontogenesis of dendritic spines are markedly retarded in hypothyroidism with persistence of immature wiring pattern (Legrand). Biochemically, hypothyroidism induces a decrease of nucleic acid synthesis, of enzymes associated with synaptosomes (glutamate and succinate dehydrogenase). In the developing auditory system, perinatal hypothyroidism induce irreversible damage to the auditory function as determined by brainstem response audiometry (BSRA). This susceptibility to thyroid hormone deficiency occurs prior to 10 days postnatally and is prevented by early replacement therapy. Some recent data (Ruiz Marcos) suggest that the changes induced in auditory cortex pyramids are either very sensitive to a minor degree of hypothyroidism or have a shorter critical period during which treatment may reverse damage. " In vivo" the ornithine decarboxylase (ODC) activity in the immature rat cerebellum is regulated by thyroid hormones (decreased by hypothyroidism and restored by T_3) whereas " in vitro" , the activity of glutamyltransferase in immature astrocytes is also thyroid hormones dependent. In the same cell type, T_3 regulates specific soluble proteins phosphorylation: an increase of a 34 K protein and a decrease of a 20 and 21 K protein. As for neurotransmitters there is an increase in substance P and Dopamine in various anatomical regions of the brain in 60 days old rat rendered hypothyroid at birth. These data help to understand the mechanism of action and the importance of thyroid hormones on the developing brain as confirmed by the normal I.Q. attained by hypothyroid children at 5-6 year of age when detected and treated within 3 weeks of age.

S.149 MULTIPLE FORMS AND FRAGMENTS OF HUMAN GROWTH HORMONE. U.J. Lewis*, L.G. Frigeri, M.B. Sigel and W.P. VanderLaan, The Whittier Institute for Diabetes and Endocrinology, La Jolla, CA 92037 USA.

Two genes for variant forms of human growth hormone have been identified: one for the major form of the hormone (hGH) and the other for a variant with 13 amino acid substitutions (hGH-V, Seeburg). The substitutions are distributed throughout the amino acid sequence of hGH and are such that alteration in physico-chemical and biological properties are likely. There is no evidence that the hGH-V gene is expressed but there is no reason why this could not occur. One of the more interesting substitutions is the formation of the sequence Asn^{140}-Gln-Ser which makes glycosylation a possibility. The identification of an Asn-linked carbohydrate unit for ovine prolactin sets a precedent for glycosylation of the growth hormone-prolactin family of proteins. Essentially nothing is known regarding the biological activity of hGH-V.

Alternative processing of the mRNA transcript of the hGH gene is responsible for formation of the 20,000 dalton variant of hGH (hGH_{20K}). The coding sequences for amino acids 32-46 are treated as part of intron B and are thus eliminated during the splicing process of the precursor mRNA. The hGH-V gene could also produce a hGH-V_{20K} form. Deletion of the 15 amino acids from hGH alters the immuno and receptor binding activities as well as some of the biological properties of hGH. The hGH_{20K} lacks the early insulin-like properties (which may be insulin-potentiating activities) of hGH. The 32-46 sequence by itself has insulin-potentiating activity, an indication that this property resides in that region of the molecule. The mechanism for controlling the alternate splicing reaction is unknown but it must be influenced by the need for a noninsulin-potentiating form of the hormone. Noteworthy is that the 5,000 dalton peptide representing hGH (1-43) was isolated from pituitary extracts and has been found to be as potent an insulin potentiator as hGH in a number of test systems.

A peptide with a molecular weight of about 5,000 is thought to be the principal diabetogenic substance of the pituitary gland. Indirect evidence suggests it is a fragment of hGH.

Several posttranslational modifications of hGH have been identified: disulfide dimer, desamido forms, and a form with an acylated NH_2-terminus. Two alkaline forms of hGH have been identified in pituitary extracts but because their structures are unknown they are tentatively classified as posttranslational modifications.

Our hypothesis for the significance of these multiple forms is that their formation provides a mechanism for controlling proteolytic cleavage for production of specific, metabolically active fragments. Characteristic conformations of the forms could expose different yet specific regions, thus directing proteolytic cleavage.

S.150 HETEROGENEITY OF GROWTH HORMONE IN THE CIRCULATION. G. Baumann*, Department of Medicine, Northwestern University Medical School, Chicago, Illinois, USA.

Growth hormone (GH) in the human pituitary has recently been recognized as a family of related proteins. Growth hormone forms identified in pituitary extracts include the 22,000 dalton single-chain form (22K), the 20,000 dalton single-chain variant (20K), two deamidated forms, an acetylated form, 3 cleaved two-chain forms, and so-called slow-migrating forms. In addition, dimeric, trimeric and aggregated growth hormone are present in pituitary extracts. The biological significance of these various GH forms is unknown. Some of them could be generated during extraction from pituitary tissue. In order to gain a better understanding of the physiology of the various GH species, it is important to know which are secreted in vivo and what factors regulate the secretion of individual molecular forms. We therefore investigated the chemical nature of immunoreactive GH in human plasma under a variety of conditions. Blood was obtained from normal subjects after stimulation of GH secretion and during basal (unstimulated) conditions, as well as from patients with acromegaly. The stimuli for GH secretion were both endogenous (sleep, exercise, spontaneous release) and exogenous (L-DOPA, hpGRF, TRH, propranolol, estrogens). Plasma was subjected to gel filtration on Sephadex G-100, and GH was measured by RIA in collected fractions. Furthermore, GH was extracted and concentrated from whole plasma and from plasma prefractionated on Sephadex by immunoadsorbent chromatography, using an immobilized antibody which recognizes all GH forms in question. This procedure resulted in the recovery of GH and its various forms in high yield. The molecular nature of GH in the plasma extracts was then assessed by polyacrylamide gel electrophoresis (PAGE), SDS-PAGE with and without sulfhydryl reduction, and by isoelectric focusing. Gel filtration resulted in the separation of the previously recognized size isomers of GH (little, big and big-big GH). Analysis of little (monomeric) GH by the electrophoretic techniques showed that it consisted of at least 3 molecular forms, namely 22K (≈85%), 20K (≈10%) and one or more acidic forms (≈5%). The latter could represent deamidated, acetylated or cleaved GH; its small concentration precluded definitive identification. Analysis of big GH indicated that it represented a mixture of GH dimers, with the same monomeric GH species as building blocks. However, 20K was a particularly prevalent species in the big GH fraction. About 2/3 of big GH consisted of non-covalently linked monomers and 1/3 was composed of disulfide-linked monomers. Big-big GH was shown to be a series of GH oligomers up to pentameric GH, with the same monomeric components, again linked as simple oligomers (2/3) and disulfide oligomers (1/3). In addition, spurious GH immunoreactivity, not chemically related to GH, was present in the big-big fraction of some plasmas. All secretory stimuli, including those prevailing in acromegaly, resulted in a similar pattern of circulating GH forms. Plasma GH immunoreactivity under basal (non-stimulated) conditions was found to be quite heterogeneous, consisting of the known circulating GH forms in small amounts and several immunoreactive GH fragments. A 16,000 dalton fragment was a prominent component in several plasmas.

Conclusions: Circulating GH consists of several monomeric molecular forms (22K, 20K, acidic) and of several oligomeric moieties composed of these same monomers. The relative preponderance of the various GH species in the circulation reflects in part their proportions in the pituitary gland. Several immunoreactive GH fragments are also present in the circulation.

S.151 DISORDERS OF GROWTH HORMONE NEUROSECRETORY FUNCTION. B.B. Bercu*, Pregnancy Research Branch, NICHD, NIH, Bethesda, MD and University of South Florida College of Medicine, Tampa, FL, USA.

As a result of the commercial advancement of recombinant DNA technology, we are entering an era when the supply of human growth hormone (GH) will no longer be limited. This comes at a time when our understanding of GH physiology is expanding. Several investigators have identified children with short stature who are not GH deficient, but do benefit with accelerated linear growth after exogenous hGH therapy. The approach of several groups has been to explore the possibility of a biologically inactive GH molecule. We, however, have been interested in a different approach relating to the neuroregulation of GH secretion.

Based on several studies in nonhuman primates and children, we conclude that there is a subgroup of short-statured children with a disorder we have called growth hormone-neurosecretory dysfunction (GH-ND). These children are not GH deficient by classical definition and they also benefit from hGH treatment. In pathological states directly affecting the neurosecretion of GH (cranial radiation prophylactically in leukemic children and experimentally in monkeys), we have observed blunting of GH response after insulin induced hypoglycemia and a substantially decreased output of GH secretion during a 24 hour period (sampling interval of 20 minutes). In another study, we selected patients whom we defined as having GH-ND on the basis of the following criteria: height $<$ 1st percentile, growth velocity $\leqslant$ 4 cm/year, bone age $>$ 2 years behind chronological age, normal provocative tests (peak $>$ 10 ng/ml), low somatomedin-C concentration and abnormal 24 hour secretory GH when compared to age-matched and pubertal-stage matched control subjects and to GH deficient children. Several parameters of GH secretion including mean GH concentration, area under the curve, mean peak GH amplitude, and number of GH pulses were significantly reduced when compared to control children. These values were generally intermediate between those of the control and GH deficient subjects. These GH-ND children more than doubled their growth velocity when treated with a replacement dose of exogenous hGH. In this and another study using male monkeys, we established that there was no increase in GH secretion during pubertal development. Our studies also demonstrated that some GH deficient patients, who have markedly blunted GH responses ($<$ 5 ng/ml) after provocative stimuli, can still have normal nocturnal pulses (as high as 21 ng/ml) suggesting, at least in part, preservation of a physiologic neural stimulus of GH release.

As a result of these observations, we suggest that there is a spectrum of GH neurosecretory abnormalities from absolute deficiency to a problem in GH regulation not readily identified with provocative testing. We believe that this GH-ND subgroup of short children could represent a much larger group of children than GH deficient patients. We speculate that there may be many etiologies for GH neurosecretory malfunction ranging from an obvious defect, such as radiation damage and trauma, to more subtle defects in neurotransmittors and GH releasing or inhibiting hormones. Further studies are necessary to better define the parameters of growth hormone neurosecretory dysfunction and to determine whether these abnormalities are congenital or acquired in postnatal life.

S.152 DISORDERS OF GROWTH HORMONE AND IGF SECRETION IN MAN. T.J. Merimee*, Dept. of Medicine, University of Florida, Gainesville, FL 32610.

Several critical effects of growth hormone (GH) are mediated by secondary growth factors. Two such factors dependent upon pituitary GH have been described in man: insulin-like growth factor I (IGF I), which is identical in structure to somatomedin C, and insulin-like growth factor II (IGF II). Both are homologous to proinsulin; each is bound in serum by one or more proteins in what appears to be a complex carrier system. Pathological conditions may relate to primary disorders of GH, directly (A) (classical acromegaly and GH deficiency) or disorders primarily of IGF, with normal or only secondary defects in secretion of GH (B).

A. Primary Disorders of GH Secretion. As might be predicted decreased secretion of GH from a variety of causes is associated with lower values of IGF I and IGF II than in normal subjects. Measurement of IGF I or IGF II in preadolescent patients to document or confirm GH deficiency, however, is not exact since the overlap of values between normal and hypopituitary children is considerable. In states of excessive secretion of GH, serum concentrations of IGF I are increased but values do not correlate precisely with the serum concentrations of GH. Serum concentration of IGF II in acromegaly, is normal. This latter finding does not indicate a lack of dependence of IGF II on GH, as initially postulated, but rather a dose response difference of IGF I and II to GH. In Laron dwarfism with a deficiency of GH receptors, serum concentrations of IGF I and II are lower than recorded in any other state.

B. Primary Disorders of IGF. At least one type of dwarfism appears related to a primary disorder of IGF I secretion. This was initially described in pygmy subjects from Central Africa. Thirty-three pygmy subjects were shown to have low serum concentrations of IGF I but normal serum concentrations of IGF II. Mean serum concentration of IGF I in pygmy subjects was 57 ± 8.2 ng/ml (mean ± SE) which contrasted with the mean serum concentration of IGF I in normal subjects of 188 ± 16 ng/ml. GH given to pygmy subjects for 5 days (5 mg bid) failed to increase IGF I in the pygmies. This dose is effective for increasing IGF I concentrations in most patients with simple GH deficiency. This aberration in secretion of IGF I may occur sporadically in Caucasians. A similar defect has also been described in the animal model. Metabolic data from the treatment studies in subjects with an isolated IGF I deficiency have been important in clarifying which effects of GH depend upon IGF I.

Hypoglycemia associated with non-islet cell tumors is a condition that also may be related to IGF. In about 1/3 of the serum samples from patients with this condition, IGF II was shown to be high by one of several receptor assays. Another laboratory reported IGF II increased in 10 of 14 such samples, some of which have been assayed in the previous cited study. Yet another laboratory has reported, however, normal or low values of IGF II, especially by immunoassay. The possibility exists that non-immunoreactive IGF is secreted in such states.

S.153 NEWER PEPTIDES OF THE GASTROINTESTINAL TRACT. J.C. Brown,* C.H.S. McIntosh, S.C. Otte, R.A. Pederson, A. Buchan and S. Vincent, Department of Physiology, University of British Columbia, Vancouver, Canada.

A wide range of biologically active peptides have been isolated from the mucosa of the gastrointestinal tract and have been implicated in control mechanisms for gastrointestinal function. Methods of detection employed during the various stages of purification have undergone tremendous changes over the past few years, due to advances in technology. The classical approach was to study a defined physiological response, such as gastric or pancreatic secretion and to screen chromatographically purified fractions for their ability to mimic this response. In this way, gastrin was isolated from the mucosa of the gastric antrum and secretin, cholecystokinin, motilin, GIP, and VIP from duodenal mucosa. An approach using a chemical detection system based on fragmentation of peptides in tissue extracts and identification of the resulting C-terminal amide fragments has resulted in the isolation of peptide YY, neuropeptide Y and peptide HY. Generation of antibodies to existing gastrointestinal peptides with the subsequent development of radioimmunoassays has demonstrated that there are immunologically cross reacting peptides in brain tissue. Purification of these brain peptides has been achieved by employing radioimmunoassays to screen fractions. High performance liquid chromatography is a rapid and sensitive technique which has revolutionized small scale purification of peptides. This technique has allowed peptides from relatively small amounts of tissue to be purified and characterized based solely on retention times of peptides in a specific solvent system. As a result of this type of approach, biological data on these substances are usually not available. Hybridoma technology has been used to generate monoclonal antibodies to known gastrointestinal peptides. These antibodies have proven to be excellent tools for immunocytochemistry (somatostatin, VIP, GIP, motilin), radioimmunoassay (somatostatin) and affinity chromatography (GIP) when clones were screened using appropriate selection techniques. Affinity chromatography systems using monoclonal antibodies have been used to screen gastrointestinal extracts for immunoreactive species of GIP. To date, 2 immunoreactive GIP peptides have been isolated using this approach.

S.154 REGULATION OF SECRETION OF GASTROINTESTINAL HORMONES.

Y. Seino*, Second Division, Department of Medicine, Kyoto University Faculty of Medicine, Kyoto 606, Japan

Gastrointestinal (GI) hormone secretion is considered to be regulated by various factors such as intraluminal and hormonal secretagogues and neural activity. However, the details of the regulation of GI hormone secretion remain to be clarified. We have measured the effects of intraluminal, humoral, and neural factors on GI hormone secretion in man, dogs, and rats. In the fasting state some peptides, e.g., pancreatic polypeptide (PP) and motilin, were found to be fluctuating intermittently. Plasma motilin increased in accordance with the cyclical interdigestive contractions of the stomach. Nutrient ingestion produced an abrupt rise in the PP, somatostatin, gastrin, and gastric inhibitory polypeptide (GIP) secretions, but suppressed motilin release. Intravenous administration of some nutrients stimulated the gastrin, PP, and somatostatin secretion, but glucose and amino acids reduced motilin release. These GI peptides in turn influenced the secretion of other peptides. This interrelationship was observed in the secretion of gastrin, somatostatin, and PP. The GIP secretion, however, was not influenced by nutrients of GI hormones coming through the intravenous route except somatostatin, which suppressed it. Surgical modification of the food pathway also has been used to elucidate the mechanism of GI hormone secretion. The passage of nutrients through the duodenum plays an important role in the secretion of motilin and PP. In addition, the direct contact of food with GIP-producing cells seems to be a strong mechanical or chemical stimulus for GIP release. Neural regulation is also important. In order to elucidate the role of the vagus nerve in the regulation of gastric hormone secretion while excluding indirect effects via alterations of circulatory or metabolic states, we have established a new in vitro isolated perfused stomach method which leaves the vagus nerves attached. Using this procedure, the direct effect of vagal electrical stimulation on gastrin, gastric somatostatin, and gastrin releasing peptide (GRP) was studied. Vagal stimulation produced a significant rise in both GRP and gastrin, but a decreased somatostatin in the perfusate. Atropine sulfate, a muscarinic blocker, augmented the GRP release and reversed the decrease in somatostatin to a level above basal in response to vagal stimulation. However, the gastrin response to vagal stimulation was not affected by atropine. Hexamethonium bromide, a ganglionic blocker, suppressed both GRP and gastrin responses and completely blocked changes in somatostatin secretion induced by vagal stimulation. These findings suggest that intramural GRP neurons might play an important role in the regulation of gastrin as well as somatostatin secretion, and that somatostatin may be controlled not only by a cholinergic inhibitory neuron but also by a non-cholinergic, e.g., peptidergic, stimulatory neuron, both of which are under the control of preganglionic fibers via nicotinic receptors. These studies lead us to conclude that the secretion of most of the GI hormones is regulated by stimuli coming through both intraluminal and intravenous routes and, at least for some hormones, by neural activities. These seem to be factors organized in a complex system which regulates the secretion of GI hormones.

S.155 RECEPTORS OF SECRETIN, VIP (VASOACTIVE INTESTINAL PEPTIDE), GRF (GROWTH HORMONE RELEASING FACTOR) AND HELODERMIN IN THE RAT PANCREAS.

J. Christophe*, M. Waelbroeck, J.P. Dehaye, J. Winand and P. Robberecht, Department of Biochemistry, Medical School, Université Libre de Bruxelles, B-1000 Brussels, Belgium.

1/ Secretin and VIP responses of adenylate cyclase activity as well as ^{125}I-VIP binding are markedly reduced after 2-mercaptoethanol and dithiothreitol pretreatment in rat pancreatic plasma membranes, suggesting the participation of disulfide bridges in the organization of the corresponding secretin and VIP receptors (and especially so in the case of high affinity VIP receptors).

2/ Secretin-preferring receptors are discriminated from VIP receptors by the ability of secretin-(4-27), secretin-(5-27) and secretin-(7-27) to inhibit selectively the secretin-stimulated enzyme. In intact pancreatic acini the comparison of cyclic AMP elevations and concomitant amylase secretion suggests the presence of three classes of functional secretin receptors : high affinity receptors (EC50 0.3 nM) are probably related to centro-acinar cells as their occupancy does not lead to secretion, while the occupancy of intermediate (EC50 10 nM) and low affinity (EC50 100 nM) receptors is responsible for most of the exocrine secretion.

The action of helodermin, a newly isolated Mr = 5,900 peptide from the venom of Gila monster (Robberecht et al, FEBS Lett., 166: 277-281, 1984) is mediated through secretin receptors as : 1) helodermin activation of adenylate cyclase in plasma membranes is inhibited by secretin-(7-27), and 2) dose-effect curves of helodermin and secretin on cyclic AMP accumulation in dispersed acini are comparable.

3/ VIP-preferring receptors can be classified into two subtypes in plasma membranes with, respectively, high and low-affinity for VIP. These data when confronted with ^{125}I-VIP binding and dose-effect curves of amylase secretion from isolated acini, suggest that the first subtype only is involved in (modest) protein secretion. These results, as compared to those obtained with secretin, suggest that the efficiency of stimulus-secretion coupling via cyclic AMP depends on the type of receptors occupied and not on the total amount of cyclic AMP produced.

In plasma membranes where functional spareness of VIP receptors is observed, the key role of HIS^1 (with a free N-terminal amino group) is easily demonstrated by the decreasing order of efficacy and potency of the following VIP analogs : VIP > acetyl His^1-VIP > Phe^1-VIP = 3 Met His^1-VIP > D-His^1-VIP.

GRF(1-29)-NH_2 is a partial agonist of VIP acting on VIP receptors. GRF(1-29)-NH_2 analogs also display intrinsic activity (i.a) on adenylate cyclase activation through VIP receptors. This i.a is reduced when D-Phe^2, D-Arg^2, D-Asp^3, D-Ala^4, D-Phe^6, pCl.Phe^6 or D-Thr^7 replaces one of the corresponding natural amino acid residue. By contrast, D-Ala^2-GRF(1-29)-NH_2 and Phe^4-GRF(1-29)-NH_2 show high biological activity.

S.156 THE RELATIONSHIP BETWEEN GASTROINTESTINAL PEPTIDE PHYSIOLOGY AND CLINICAL SYNDROMES.

A. Shulkes,* Department of Surgery, University of Melbourne, Austin Hospital, Melbourne, Victoria, Australia.

With the development of recombinant DNA techniques, research on gut peptides is entering a new era - the genetic era. Research has passed through the classical secretory physiology era of Bayliss and Starling and the chemical era exemplified by Mutt and Gregory; currently we are in what Rehfeld has termed the immunological era. Despite this research, the clinical impact of gut peptides, termed regulatory peptides because of their ubiquitous distribution, has been disappointingly small. We still await a new era of physiology to assess the significance of these peptides in profusion.

The following physiological characteristics need to be addressed before pathophysiological roles for gut peptides can be established.

1. Mechanism of Action. Many of the gut peptides which are present in both nerves and endocrine cells do not act as endocrine hormones but probably act locally either as paracrine or neurocrine agents. The co-existence in nerve terminals of both gut peptides and classical transmitters is another possible control system and emphasizes the overlap of the endocrine system with the nervous system. A defect in one system can be compensated by the other systems.

2. Molecular Heterogeneity. Most gut peptides exist in multiple molecular forms with varying biological activities. The release of specific forms in various disease states is an important area for investigation. New families of peptides are being detected by both chemical and recombinant DNA techniques. The PP/NPY/PYY and the VIP/PHI/PHM families are examples which have immediate clinical significance. NPY normally found in adrenergic nerves is elevated in the tumour and the circulation of patients with phaeochromocytomas and may be of value in diagnosing these tumours. PHM is synthesized on the same gene as VIP and has similar effects on intestinal secretion. PHM may be the responsible agent in patients with secretory diarrhoea and normal VIP levels.

Other than gut peptide producing tumours, gut peptides have little clinical relevance at the present time. These endocrine tumours (e.g. VIPoma, gastrinoma, somatostatinoma) provide an in vivo system for studying the physiology and pharmacology of the gut peptides. Other diseases are characterised by disturbances of the peptidergic nervous system such as Hirschsprung's or Chagas' diseases. The involvement of regulatory peptides in brain diseases such as Alzheimer's disease and schizophrenia or in obesity are other possibilities. Many abnormalities of gut peptide secretion may be secondary to a gastrointestinal abnormality (e.g. coeliac disease). However, examination of the gut peptide profile can give information on the anatomical region of the disease and on the dynamic condition of the gut. Several therapeutic uses of gut peptides have been proposed including somatostatin for controlling gastrointestinal haemorrhage or for suppressing the secretions of endocrine tumours; VIP to produce bronchodilation in asthmatics or as a local vasodilator in patients suffering from penile erectile dysfunction. Progress in the future will depend on development of agents which can selectively inhibit a peptide or alter its secretion or metabolism. Several such agents are now available allowing individual peptide function to be assessed and therapeutic intervention to be contemplated.

S.157 SEASONAL CHANGES OF GONADOTROPIC AND GONADAL FUNCTIONS IN THE FEMALE JAPANESE MONKEY. M. Nozaki and K. Oshima*, Primate Research Institute, Kyoto University, Inuyama, Aichi 484, Japan.

Seasonal changes of menstrual cycles and of serum levels of LH, estrogen and progesterone have been studied in the mature female Japanese monkey (Macaca fuscata fuscata). Daily blood samples were collected throughout the year. Serum LH was measured by means of radioreceptor assay as described by Yoshida (Jap. J. Med. Sci. Biol. 36(4): 237, 1983), and LH value was expressed in terms of NIAMDD LER907. Sex steroid hormones were measured using radioimmunoassay. The first sign approaching to the breeding season was shown by the rise of the basal levels of serum LH from non-detectable level (to about 5 µg/ml from below 1 µg/ml) in late summer or early autumn, which was one to two months prior to the onset of the breeding season. Throughout this period serum levels of estrogen and progesterone maintained in the basal ranges (about 50 pg/ml and 0.5 ng/ml, respectively). The onset of breeding season was indicated by the rise of serum estrogen coinciding with preovulatory surge of LH followed by progesterone elevations and menstrual bleeding. During breeding season, autumn through winter, the menstrual bleeding was regularized at about one month intervals. Throughout this period, preovulatory surge of LH (about 20 µg/ml and 5-10 µg/ml for basal levels) was observed about 16 days prior to the onset of subsequent menstrual bleeding. Estrogen rises in late follicular phases (more than 300 pg/ml and about 100 pg/ml for luteal and early follicular phases) and progesterone elevations in luteal phases (more than 4 ng/ml and below 1 ng/ml for follicular phases) were also observed. During spring through early summer, the incidence of menstrual cycles varied in individuals: some showed regular cycles and others irregular. Accordingly, in most cases it was fairly difficult to know when the breeding season completely ceased only by the incidence of vaginal bleeding. However, the time course patterns of serum LH, estrogen, and progesterone were greatly different from those in the bleeding season, while conspicuous difference was not found between monkeys with apparently regular cycles and those with irregular cycles. The most remarkable hormonal fluctuations occurred in early spring, just after the cessation of breeding season: for example, serum LH levels decreased to non-detectable level for about 40 days, and after the mid-spring, subsequently serum LH levels increased and fluctuated in the range between the lowest level of the basal range in the breeding season and non-detectable level. In addition, throughout these periods including early spring through early summer, regardless of regularity of menstrual cycles serum progesterone levels maintained in the basal range (below 1 ng/ml), whereas serum estrogen levels were relatively high and fluctuated in the range between more than 300 pg/ml and 100 pg/ml, suggesting that several follicles have developed, but not ovulated. During mid-summer, menstrual bleeding was not observed in most animals and serum levels of estrogen and progesterone maintained in the basal ranges (about 50 pg/ml and 0.5 ng/ml, respectively). However, serum LH levels decreased again to non-detectable level for about 50 days. Thus, it was found that the marked changes in serum LH levels always preceded the initiation and cessation of the breeding season. Taking all findings mentioned above into considerations, it is concluded that seasonal change of reproductive functions in female Japanese monkey is controlled primarily by the brain-pituitary axis, but not by ovaries.

S.158 SEASONAL REPRODUCTION IN MARSUPIALS. M.B. Renfree* and R.V. Short, Depart-artments of Anatomy and Physiology, Monash University, Clayton, Victoria, 3168, Australia.

The majority of marsupials have a seasonal breeding pattern, with pouch emergence occuring at the most favourable time of the year. Photoperiod appears to be the primary cue in the regulation of this seasonal reproduction, although this has only been proven in three marsupial species. Investigations of the endocrine control of seasonal breeding have only been carried out in the tammar wallaby, Macropus eugenii. In the tammar, births usually occur about one month after the summer solstice, with pouch emergence the following spring. Females conceive within 24 hours of parturition, and the conceptus grows to about a 100 cell blastocyst before entering an 11 month period of embryonic diapause, when the corpus luteum is inactive. Removal of the sucking pouch young during lactational quiescence before the winter solstice causes luteal reactivation and a resumption of embryonic growth, but is without effect in seasonal quiescence after the solstice. During lactational quiescence, prolactin is thought to be the major inhibitor of the corpus luteum. However, during seasonal quiescence reactivation can be induced experimentally regardless of the prolactin levels. We have studied the role of the pineal gland in seasonal reproduction in the tammar. Bilateral removal of the superior cervical ganglion in female tammars denervated the pineal, and abolished the night time rise in blood melatonin concentrations. This was without effect on lactational diapause, but abolished seasonal diapause. Subcutaneous implants of melatonin to animals in seasonal quiescence caused a rapid resumption of embryonic growth and precocious births, whereas melatonin implants were without effect on lactational diapause. Since the melatonin implants failed to depress the prolactin levels, these findings once again suggest that hyperprolactinaemia cannot be the sole cause of seasonal diapause. Since hypophysectomy during seasonal diapause causes luteal reactivation and a resumption of embryonic development, the pituitary must be exerting some inhibitory effect on the ovaries at this time, one that can be overcome by either the removal or addition of melatonin.

S.159 THE SEASONAL REPRODUCTIVE CYCLE OF THE RAINBOW TROUT.

J.P.Sumpter*, Department of Applied Biology, Brunel University, Uxbridge, Middlesex, UB8 3PH, UK.

The rainbow trout is the major farmed fish in many temperate countries. It spawns once a year, but several times during its life. In both sexes gametogenesis takes at least a year to complete. Female trout have group - synchronous ovaries in which two distinct populations of oocytes can be distinguished - a population of primary oocytes and a population of synchronously developing secondary oocytes. One year prior to spawning the primary growth phase of the oocytes to be spawned a year hence is well advanced, and many have already entered the secondary growth phase. This comprises three separate processes, which are: endogenous vitellogenesis, characterized by the appearance of vesicles in the cytoplasm; uptake of lipid; exogenous vitellogenesis. The latter process, involving oestrogen - stimulated synthesis of vitellogenin by the liver, its secretion into the blood and sequestration by the developing oocytes, where it is processed and packaged as yolk, is responsible for the enormous growth of oocytes. During this process, which takes nine months, the gonadosomatic index increases from 0.1 to 15. This is made possible by the astonishingly high rate of vitellogenin production by the liver, with blood levels rising 10 000-fold as the female trout matures, to peak at 20mg/ml; the liver triples in weight to achieve this. The very large ovaries probably account for the high sex-steroid levels found in the blood: oestradiol levels rise steadily from 1ng/ml to peak at 50ng/ml two months before spawning, while testosterone levels, which can be very high in female trout, peak later, a week before spawning, when they are 300ng/ml. At this time there is a rapid switch from androgen production to progestagen production. The level of 17α - hydroxy - 20β - dihydroprogesterone, the principal progestagen, rises very rapidly to reach a peak (320ng/ml) 4 days before spawning, and plays an important role in final oocyte maturation and ovulation.

Male rainbow trout also show a pronounced annual gonadal cycle, with the testes comprising 10% of body weight when fully developed. During spermatogenesis there is a regular succession of germ cell stages. Testosterone and 11-ketotestosterone levels in the plasma increase steadily during the period when the testes are growing and spermatogenesis is most active, both peaking at levels around 150ng/ml. The levels start to fall when spermiation begins. It is not possible to correlate the level of either androgen with the volume, sperm number, or density of the milt. However, plasma levels of 17α - hydroxy, 20β - dihydroprogesterone do correlate closely with sperm production. Trout testes also have a high capacity to synthesize and secrete steroid glucuronides, the plasma levels rising and falling concomitantly with other androgens.

S.160 SEASONALITY OF REPRODUCTION IN INVERTEBRATES: THE CENTRAL ROLE OF A NEURO-ENDOCRINE SYSTEM IN THE REPRODUCTIVE STRATEGY OF THE SNAIL LYMNAEA STAGNALIS

J. Joosse*, Biological Laboratory, Vrije Universiteit, P.O. Box 7161, 1007 MC Amsterdam, The Netherlands.

Among the invertebrates knowledge of the effects of seasonal factors on reproductive activity is most detailed in insects and molluscs. Like in all animals integration of information about environmental factors occurs in the central nervous system and is transmitted to (neuro-)endocrine centres involved in control of reproductive activity. The neuroendocrine centres of some snails have great advantages for experimental studies: neurones have giant size, are located peripherally under the transparent perineurium and can be identified individually. Attention will be focussed on the reproductive strategy of the freshwater snail *Lymnaea stagnalis*. - Female reproductive activity of *Lymnaea* is controlled by two gonadotropic hormones. The Dorsal Body Hormone (DBH) is produced by endocrine Dorsal Bodies (DB) and stimulates the production of female components: vitellogenesis, and cellular differentiation, growth and synthetic activity of the female accessory sex organs, involved in egg and egg mass formation. The neurohormone CDCH is produced by about 100 Caudo-Dorsal Cells (CDC) and is released in considerable quantities only in relation to egg laying. CDCH induces ovulation, egg and egg mass formation and egg laying behaviour. - Environmental factors affecting the release of both hormones have been studied in detail: temperature, feeding conditions and photoperiod. - The central role of the CDC in the determination of the reproductive strategy is obvious from the following observations:

- A long day photoperiod accelerates sexual maturation and enhances egg laying frequency. The reactivity of snails in these conditions to injected CDCH is maximal and the CDC are more easily activated upon electrical stimulation. Under natural conditions egg laying is restricted to the LD period of the year.
- Isolated snails show a retarded sexual maturation. Once being mature the start of egg laying is also retarded. After only one insemination egg laying starts and continues. Apparently copulation decreases the threshold for CDC activation. This favours cross-fertilization.
- The developmental success of the eggs is highly dependent of the position of the egg mass in the heterogenous habitat. Fixation of the egg mass to a solid substrate in a region with clean water and a high oxygen content is important. These factors are identical to those which are able to activate the CDC: 5-10 minutes after a change of the snail to these conditions the CDC are firing and release CDCH. The snail stops locomotion, cleans the substrate and fixes the egg mass. Thus the CDC play a crucial role in selection of this microhabitat.
- At low temperature ($8^{o}C$) and during starvation egg laying stops in short day adapted snails but continues at a lower level in long day snails. In both conditions release of DBH is low which means that synthesis in the female structures decreases to prevent energy loss. This favours survival of the existing population. But the CDC of long day snails can still be activated. The small number of egg masses produced secures the development of a new generation. This dual strategy is expressed via the CDC and is advantagous for an annual species.

S.161 STUDIES ON THE SUPPRESSION OF OVARIAN ACTIVITY DURING LACTATION: IMPLICATIONS FOR THE CONTROL OF FOLLICULAR DEVELOPMENT.

A.S. McNeilly*, MRC Reproductive Biology Unit, University of Edinburgh, Centre for Reproductive Biology, 37 Chalmers Street, Edinburgh EH3 9EW, Scotland.

Epidemiological studies clearly show that breast feeding delays the resumption of fertility in women. However the precise mechaninsms whereby suckling suppresses follicular development and ovulation remain unclear. In a series of longitudinal studies on the resumption of ovarian activity in Edinburgh women we have shown that suppression of follicular development is dependent not only on the suckling frequency but also suckling duration. These parameters are equally important and both correlate with the basal levels of prolactin. Follicular development only resumes when suckling frequency and duration decline below 5 episodes and 65 min total duration per day, and while ovulation occurs it results in inadequate corpus luteum function in the majority of cases. Corpus luteum function in subsequent cycles improves towards normal and is associated with an increase in the amount of LH released during the preovulatory surge. Before ovulation resumes, follicle growth assessed by measurement of both urinary steroids and ultrasound is absent in 70% of women and is associated with normal plasma levels of FSH but reduced pulsatile LH secretion. In 30% of cases follicular development does occur and relates to the presence of apparently normal pulsatile LH secretion but ovulation does not occur suggesting a failure of positive feedback as shown previously by injection of oestrogen. Treatment of normal breast feeding women between 6 and 12 weeks post partum with pulsatile injection of GnRH at a dose and frequency which induces ovulation and normal corpus luteum function in hypogonadal women, induces normal follicular development in terms of oestrogen and ultrasound assessment of follicles, but development of an inadequate corpus luteum. This is associated with a reduced preovulatory LH surge. Studies in breast feeding women clearly show that the amount of suckling is of critical importance in the suppression of follicle growth and in the quality of the corpus luteum produced once ovulation resumes. While it remains unclear whether prolactin directly influences follicular development, studies in sheep suggest that hyperprolactinaemia can suppress oestradiol secretion when hormones are administered in physiological amounts, and only minor modifications in plasma levels of FSH can interrupt normal follicular development.

The present results suggest that suckling may suppress ovarian activity by a complex series of hormonal changes including hyperprolactinaemia, inadequate pulsatile secretion of LH, failure of positive feedback to oestrogen and, possibly, a failure to maintain normal FSH secretion during follicular development.

S.162 GRANULOSA CELL-THECAL CELL INTERACTIONS DURING FOLLICULAR DEVELOPMENT

J. Dorrington*, H. McKeracher, G. Garzo and M. Skinner, Banting and Best Dept. of Medical Research, University of Toronto, Toronto, M5G 1L6, Canada

The main objective of this study is to identify the intraovarian factors responsible for the development of the preovulatory follicle. In the sexually mature female the preovulatory follicle is the fastest orderly growing cell mass. We propose that the preovulatory follicle completes its developmental program as a result of the interaction between thecal cells of mesenchymal origin and granulosa cells of epithelial origin through the production of "inducer factors". The factors involved in both follicular development and also in atresia may be peptides, proteins, components of extracellular matrix or steroids. We have shown that steroids are important local regulators; testosterone synthesized in the thecal cells acts as a substrate for aromatization, and as a hormone to augment FSH-induced aromatase activity and cholesterol side-chain cleavage activity. Estrogen produced by the granulosa cells is an "autocrine" regulator of follicular development since it causes proliferation of granulosa cells and modulates FSH action.

The possibility that proteins synthesized by the follicle may also play a role in local regulation was suggested by the observation that insulin (and insulin-like growth factors) could augment the action of FSH on aromatase activity in human granulosa cells: Aromatase activity assessed by the release of tritiated water from [1β-^{3}H]testosterone was undetectable in granulosa cells from follicles with a diameter of less than 1.0 cm, thereafter, there was a direct correlation between aromatase activity and follicular diameter. FSH (200 ng FSH-15/ml) stimulated aromatase activity in cells isolated from all sizes of follicles from 0.4-1.5 cm. Insulin further augmented FSH-induced aromatase activity, as evidenced both by an increase in estradiol-17β production and by the release of tritiated water from [1β-^{3}H]testosterone. This study suggested that "insulin-like" factors may play a role in modifying FSH-dependent cellular differentiation. The concentration of insulin required however was higher than that found in human plasma suggesting that if these effects are important physiologically then "insulin-like" factors may be produced locally. This idea was supported by the finding that conditioned medium obtained from rat thecal cells will augment FSH-induced aromatase activity of rat granulosa cells.

Another approach was to examine electrophoretically the radiolabelled proteins secreted by cultured granulosa cells from immature rats. In control cultures a protein with a molecular weight of 220,000 dalton was the major protein secreted and comprised 20% of the total radiolabelled proteins. This was identified as fibronectin by immunoprecipitation and measured by ELISA assay. In the presence of FSH fibronectin secretion was less than 1% of the total radiolabelled protein. These studies indicate that as granulosa cells undergo cytodifferentiation in response to FSH, fibronectin synthesis is suppressed. Fibronectin is a component of extracellular matrix and promotes cell adhesion and cell proliferation. This may be a component of the substratum on which thecal cells and granulosa cells become organized during the early stages of folliculogenesis. In summary, thecal and granulosa cells communicate by the formation of steroids and proteins to establish an environment in which the oocyte can develop normally. (Supported by the MRC).

S.163 THE INTERACTION OF GONADOTROPHIN AND STEROIDS IN THE CONTROL OF OVARIAN CELL ACTIVITY.

A. Nimrod* and M. Pearlsman, Department of Hormone Research, The Weizmann Institute of Science, Rehovot, Israel.

The trophic effects of the pituitary glycoprotein hormones on gonadal cells are well recognized phenomena which have been studied in detail. The role of steroid hormones in the control of ovarian cell activity is less obvious, and the mechanisms involved are not fully known. We have chosen the system of cultured granulosa cells (GC) from hypophysectomized diethylstilbestrol-treated rats to study the synergistic action of androgen and FSH in the stimulation of progestin production. We have previously shown that androgen exerts its effect at a step in the biosynthetic pathway distal to cAMP. The mechanism of androgen action in GC was further investigated with respect to the conversion of cholesterol to progestins. Using intact cells and mitochondrial preparations from FSH and androgen-treated cells, it was found that both hormones increased cellular uptake of cholesterol in an additive fashion and had a synergistic effect on the mitochondrial side-chain cleavage enzyme, but had no effect on cholesterol ester hydrolysis and transport into the mitochondria.

In order to further examine the mechanism of androgen action, protein and RNA-synthesis inhibitors were used during critical periods of cutlure with FSH and androgen. It has been found that inhibition of the stimulatory effect of androgen on progestin production could be induced by protein synthesis inhibitors during the 4 hr of androgen addition, but not later on. Cordycepin, an inhibitor of RNA synthesis, failed to inhibit the androgen effect. A similar 4 hr-regimen of exposure to andorgen was used in combination with ^{35}S-methionine labelling, and cell lysates were then analysed by two-dimensional gel electrophoresis. FSH, but not androgen, had stimulated total ^{35}S-methionine incorporation and 3 specific proteins were enhanced by the glycoprotein hormone. No specific androgen-induced protein was detected.

S.164

LUTEAL PHASE DEFECTS

A.R.Genazzani,* G.D'Ambrogio, F.Facchinetti, F.Petraglia, and A.Volpe
Department of Obstetrics and Gynecology, University of Modena, ITALY.

Menstrual cycles associated to the luteal phase defects are normally present in two main periods of reproductive life: the postmenarchal and the premenopausal. When they are present in other periods of life they are considered as important risck factors for the development of neoplastic disease, dependent to the estrogen overstimulation. In fact the presence of repetitive ipaired luteal functions lead to the picture of unopposed estrogen stimulation in endometrial and mammary gland biopsies.

The luteal phase defects may be subdivided into three different groups according to the pattern and levels of circulating progesterone (P): aluteal, inadequate and short luteal phase. The aluteal cycle is charachterized by low estradiol levels in follicular phase suggestive for failure of follicular maturation, unable to induce adequate mid-cycle gonadotropin (Gn) rise and as consequence the formation of the corpus luteum. The inadequate luteal phase is charachterized by an impaired follicular maturation followed by a mid-cycle Gn rise leading to deficient luteal structures with P plasma levels lower than four/five ng/ml. The short luteal phase is charachterized by the presence of apparently normal follicular maturation with Gn mid-cycle peak and normal luteogenesis. The P levels reach values similar to those in the adequate luteal phase but the corpus luteum duration is shorter than normal and the total lenght of luteal fhase is less than 10 days.

In the pathogenesis of luteal phase defects three main mechanisms can be taken into account: central, peripheal and local factors. Central factors include: a) reduced FSH secretion in the early stage of follicular recruitment and the development of the dominant; b) premature activation of a mid-cycle LH/FSH secretion in presence of not completely developed pre-ovulatory follicle; c) increased baseline LH values leading to the policystic ovarian syndrome with associated excess of intraovarian androgens; d) hyperprolactinemia or pharmalogical hypoprolactinemia are also responsible for luteal phase defects due to the decreased pulsatility and to the lack of a specific trophic factor for luteal cells, respectively. The peripherial factors include all the situations where either the circulating steroid volume distribution or transport and clearance mechanism are impaired and all those conditions where excessive amounts of sex steroids from adrenal origin interfere with the hypotalamus-pituitary-ovarian axis. The local factors, besides the so-called hydiopatic or genetic alterations, mainly evoked to explain aluteal cycle, include those situations characterized by increased prostaglandin concentrations in the peritoneal fluid, which are know to originate the luteinized unruptured follicle syndrome.

The clinical pictures include oligo or polymenprrea, frequently associated with dysmenorrea, premenstrual syndrome, benign breast disease and frequently infertility. The treatment require a precise definition of the pathogenesis and the evaluation of the patients requirements, in relation to her infertility and age. As consequence the drugs which can be differently used variate from anti-estrogens, weack estrogens, direct or indirect dopamine-agonists, gestagens, FSH, HMG/HCG and recently Gn-RH.

Supported by C.N.R. "Gruppo endocrinologia".

S.165 GROWTH HORMONE-RELEASING FACTOR. AN UPDATE.

R. Guillemin*, N. Ling, F. Esch, P. Bohlen, P. Brazeau, W. Wehrenberg, A. Baird, B. Bloch, C. Mougin and F. Zeytin, Laboratories for Neuroendocrinology, The Salk Institute, La Jolla, Ca. 92037.

Growth hormone-releasing factor (GRF) was originally characterized as a 44 amino acid (aa) residue, COOH-terminal amidated polypeptide that was isolated along with several biologically active fragments (37 aa, 40 aa) from an islet cell tumor of the pancreas in an acromegalic patient with no pituitary adenoma (Science 218, 585, 1982). The 40 aa fragment was also recognized and characterized in another tumor recognized in similar circumstances (BBRC 109, 152, 1982; Nature 300, 276, 1982). We have now characterized hypothalamic GRF from several species (porcine, bovine, ovine). They are all 44 aa, COOH-terminal amidated peptides showing <5% aa substitutions from the sequence of the human material. Human hypothalamic GRF has recently been isolated; it also has 44 aa; we hope to have the aa sequence for the meeting. We have isolated, in the original tumor from which we obtained GRF, peptides corresponding to the fragments of pre-proGRF as postulated from the cDNA nucleotide sequence (PNAS 80, 4311, 1983). RIA's against such fragments show them also to be found in the hypothalamus. GRF appears to stimulate GH release by activating exocytosis of GH granules through a phosphorylation mechanism mediated by a granular receptor coupled with a cAMP-dependent protein kinase (PNAS 80, 6538, 1983). GRF does not affect the release of newly synthesized GH (<3 hrs after labelling) but only stimulates secretion of "old" GH (>12 hrs after labelling). Somatostatin, as well as somatomedin-C (IGF-1), are non-competitive antagonists of GRF on the release of GH. GRF stimulates the transcription of the GH gene 1-8 to 3.6 fold in rat pituitary cells in vitro. GRF also regulates pituitary GH transcription in vivo. There is a 1.8 and 2.5 fold increase in GH gene transcription at 10 and 20 min respectively, following the injection of GRF into anesthetized rats (Nature 306, 84, 1983). We have not observed any evidence of an effect of GRF on pituitary hormones other than GH, in vitro or in vivo. Continuous administration of GRF (24 hrs) in rats with an implanted cannula leads to decreasing responses to GRF in terms of GH release that can be correlated with massive depletion of pituitary GH content. Immunocytochemistry with several GRF antisera shows that most GRF neurons are located in the arcuate nucleus of the infundibulum, with only scattered GRF neurons in the n. ventromedialis (Nature 301, 607, 1983). The ontogeny of the GRF neurons in human fetuses does not correlate with previously published variations of fetal plasma GH throughout normal pregnancy. Clinical studies with synthetic GRF are proceeding in multiple clinical centers; they all show the high intrinsic activity of GRF in human subjects.

Research in our laboratories supported by NIH (HD-09690 and AM-18811) and the Robert J. Kleberg Jr. and Helen C. Kleberg Foundation.

S.166 DISTRIBUTION AND RELEASE OF GRF. A. Arimura*, I. Merchenthaler, K. Iwasaki, M. D. Culler, C. R. Thomas, and J. Kanda and M. Palkovits. Laboratories for Molecular Neuroendocrinology and Diabetes, Tulane University Hebert Research Center, Belle Chasse, La., 70037; Departments of Medicine and Anatomy, Tulane University School of Medicine, New Orleans, La.70112; and Laboratory of Clinical Sciences, NIMH, Bethesda, Md. 20205.

Growth hormone(GH) secretion from the pituitary gland is subject to dual control by GH releasing inhibiting (somatostatin,SS) and stimulating factor (GRF). Recent isolation and synthesis of human pancreatic tumor GRF (hpGRF) and rat hypothalamic GRF (rGRF) and the availability of these synthetic GRF preparations have prompted our investigation of GH secretory mechanisms. Studies on the distribution of SS containing structures in the central nervous system have revealed both intra- and extra-hypothalamic sites which suggests that this substance may have both neuroendocrine and neurotransmitter functions. To determine whether GRF and SS might be similar in distribution and have close functional relationships, we began a series of experiments. Before the isolation of GRF, we bioassayed extracts of various brain areas of the rat using superfusion of pituitary fragments. An increase in GH release was seen in extracts (stripped of SS by affinity chromatography) from the following areas; median eminence, arcuate N., paraventricular N., and suprachiasmatic N. These results were confirmed by ICC using both anti-hpGRF (SV97) and anti-rGRF (R565) sera with one exception, the suprachiasmatic region. One possible explanation for this may be the existence of two stimulators of GH release in the rat brain as is the case with the ovine brain (personal observation). Antiserum R565 stained perikarya in the hypothalamus in a similar fashion as that seen with antiserum SV97, and occasionally GRFpositive cellbodies were seen in the amygdala. GRF positive cell bodies were seen in the following areas of the colchicine treated rat brain: perifornical regions of the anterior and lateral hypothalamus, arcuate N., medial and lateral borders of the ventromedial N., paraventricular and dorsomedial N., and the lateral basal hypothalamus. In vivo studies to test the ability of anti-rGRF serum to suppress anti-SS induced GH release have provided strong evidence to support rGRF as a potent physiological stimulator of GH release. This in vivo model is now being used to test the effects of intraventricular injection of various neurotransmitters on GRF release. In addition, cultures of fetal rat hypothalami have been subjected to the addition of synthetic releasing hormones and neurotransmitters and then assayed for SS and GRF released in the incubation media by respective RIA and/or pituitary cell culture bioassay. Preliminary results demonstrate that three hypothalamic hormones, TRH, GRF, and CRF, significantly stimulate SS release from cultured neurons. This suggests that increased GRF release in neuronal tissues increases somatostatin release, possibly forming a short-circuit feedback in the central regulation of the GH secretion.

S.167 CLINICAL STUDIES WITH GROWTH-HORMONE-RELEASING FACTOR. M. O. Thorner*, W. S. Evans, M. L. Vance, J. L. C. Borges, R. M. Blizzard, A. D. Rogol, L. A. Frohman, R. L. Furlanetto, J. Rivier, and W. Vale. University of Virginia Medical Center, Charlottesville, VA 22908; University of Cincinnati Medical Center, Cincinnati, OH 45267; Children's Hospital of Philadelphia, Philadelphia, PA 19104; and Salk Institute, San Diego, CA 92138.

hpGRF-40 and hpGRF-44 are probably identical with the human hypothalamic growth hormone releasing hormone(s). In normal men hpGRF-40 (1 ug/kg iv bolus) stimulates GH release within five minutes but does not elevate serum prolactin, TSH, LH or ACTH (measured indirectly through plasma cortisol), or blood glucose or plasma levels of 8 enteropancreatic hormones. When graded doses hpGRF-40 (0.1 to 10 ug/kg) were given iv no differences were noted in the maximum levels of serum GH achieved. Doses of 1, 3.3, and 10 ug/kg hpGRF-40 elicited a prolonged and biphasic pattern of GH release. Twenty-four hours after hpGRF-40 administration serum somatomedin C increased in 66% of subjects tested. Side effects included a feeling of warmth and facial flushing in 66% (3.3 ug/kg) and 100% (10 ug/kg) of men given hpGRF-40. hpGRF-40 (3.3 ug/kg iv) selectively stimulates GH release and somatomedin C production in normal women, although no differences were found in GH responsivity during the menstrual cycle. hpGRF-40 given subcutaneously and intranasally to normal men requires approximately 10 and 100 fold higher doses than the iv route to achieve similar stimulation. The calculated metabolic clearance rate of hpGRF-40 is 194 $\pm$ 17.5 l/m^2/day; the disappearance rate occurs as two phases: an initial equilibration phase of 7.6 $\pm$ 1.2 minutes and a subsequent elimination phase of 51.8 $\pm$ 5.4 minutes. Seven adults with idiopathic GH deficiency (IGHD) were given hpGRF-40 0.33 ug/kg iv every three hours for five days and then were rechallenged with 10 ug/kg iv. The GH response to subsequent challenge was greater and serum somatomedin C (mean $\pm$ SE) increased significantly over the five-day period from 0.27 $\pm$ 0.14 to 0.89 $\pm$ 0.29 U/ml (normal 0.94 $\pm$ 0.3, mean $\pm$ 1 SD). Forty children with short stature were evaluated for GH reserve following pharmacological tests and after a single iv injection hpGRF-40 (3.3 ug/kg). The children were grouped into IGHD, organic hypopituitarism (OH), intrauterine growth retardation (IUGR), and constitutional delay of growth (CD) categories. In IGHD & OH patients' GH concentrations did not increase to more than 7 ng/ml following pharmacologic stimulation. However, the mean ($\pm$ SE) responses to hpGRF-40 were 3.4 $\pm$ 1.1 ng/ml and 8.2 $\pm$ 2.4 ng/ml in the OH and IGHD categories respectively. All children with IUGR, CD, and unclassified groups responded briskly to hpGRF-40 although there was wide variation of GH levels (5-25 ng/ml). Two GH deficient children were studied on constant diets and received hpGRF-40, 1 ug/kg q 3 h subcutaneously over 5 days. Both subjects demonstrated a reduction in nitrogen excretion and an increase in calcium excretion. Somatomedin C levels rose in both patients. Norleucine^{27} hpGRF(1-29)-NH_2 markedly stimulated GH secretion at 0.1 ug/kg in normal young men. Our studies suggest that GH deficiency in childhood often results from hypothalamic GHRH deficiency rather than pituitary disease. hpGRF-40 and its analogues may find therapeutic application of treatment of GH deficiency and in other disorders in which an increase or decrease in the secretion of GH would be beneficial.

S.168 SOMATOSTATIN: MECHANISMS OF RELEASE. J.B.Martin*, Neuroendocrine Laboratory, Department of Neurology, Massachusetts General Hospital and Harvard Medical School, Boston, Massachusetts, 02114.

Several experimental approaches have been used to determine the factors that regulate the release of somatostatin (SS) from the median eminence (ME) and to ascertain its function in the physiologic regulation of growth hormone (GH) secretion. This presentation will focus on four aspects of these studies; 1) the results of active and passive immunization inducing antibodies that bind endogenous SS; 2) the results of release of SS from *in vitro* studies of hypothalamic fragments or cultures; 3) release of SS into the pituitary portal blood and 4) attempts to assess physiologic SS release into the ME using push-pull perfusion techniques.

Passive immunization with somatostatin antibodies given to normal animals indicate that basal GH levels are suppressed by endogenous SS. Active immunization interrupts normal pulsatile GH secretion. *In vitro* studies show that several hypothalamic neurotransmitters can influence SS secretion. Similarly, measurement of SS in pituitary portal blood indicates that transmitters and hormones influence SS release. Of particular importance in this regard are dopamine (stimulates release) and GH, neurotensin and glucagon, which also stimulate release.

ME push-pull perfusion systems have been developed to sample directly the pituitary portal capillary bed, because of difficulties in measuring changes in pituitary portal concentrations in hypothalamic factors using techniques that require surgery and anesthesia. The push-pull system combined with chronic intra-atrial catheterization permits examination of the temporal patterns of neuropeptide release into the ME coincident with changes in plasma levels of anterior pituitary hormones. The push-pull system works on the following assumptions: 1) that there is continuous and consistent exchange between the perfusate and the extracellular fluid at the tip of the cannula, 2) that the perfusate or mechanical agitation by themselves do not alter the release of the substance being examined once perfusion is established and 3) that there is a sufficient number of undamaged neuronal elements present in the perfusion zone to permit physiologic interpretation of responses to a given stimulus in the area of the cannula tip. Measurable concentrations of SS in the ME are detected over 4-6 hr periods in rats, with a technically satisfactory placement of the cannula in the ME. SS is not detected with placements in the third ventricle or outside the ME in the adjacent hypothalamus. Gel chromatography of SS released from the perfusate suggests that SS is released in more than one molecular weight form. The bulk of the activity corresponded to SS-14 with other peaks that likely correspond to SS-28 and a higher molecular weight precursor form(s). Calculations of the amount of SS released higher molecular weight precursor form(s). The push-pull system permits assessment of the effects of feedback regulation by the introduction of a lateral ventricular cannula which permits administration centrally of agents thought to affect GH control. These experiments have shown that suppression of GH secretion after central administration of glucagon, HGH, and neurotensin is not accompanied by an increase in SS secretion in the ME, leading to the conclusion that GRF suppression may be more important than SS secretion in GH regulation.

S.169 RECEPTOR DEFECTS IN SYNDROMES OF EXTREME INSULIN RESISTANCE.
Simeon I. Taylor*, National Institutes of Health, Bethesda, MD.

The insulin receptor has two important functions: to bind insulin and to couple insulin binding to insulin action. Defects in either of these receptor functions may cause insulin resistance as has been demonstrated most clearly in syndromes associated with extreme insulin resistance and acanthosis nigricans. Several different types of molecular defects in receptor function have been identified in patients with these syndromes:

1. Quantitative defects in the insulin receptor.

a. Accelerated receptor degradation. Certain patients develop autoantibodies directed against the insulin receptor. Although the earliest effect of the anti-receptor antibodies in vitro is to mimic insulin action, prolonged exposure of the tissue to high concentrations of anti-receptor antibodies desensitizes target cells to the effect of insulin. This desensitization may result, at least in part, from the effect of anti-receptor antibodies to markedly accelerate receptor degradation, and thereby to decrease the number of insulin receptors at the cell surface.

b. Impaired receptor biosynthesis. In certain patients with genetic forms of extreme insulin resistance, insulin resistance results from a decrease in the number of insulin receptors at the cell surface. Using cultured lymphocyte cell lines derived from these patients, we have studied the biosynthesis of the receptor precursor (M_r = 190 kDa) by pulse-labelling with [2-^{3}H]mannose. The processing of the precursor to the mature receptor subunits (M_r = 135 and 95kDa) was followed during a subsequent chase period. Interestingly, these studies suggested the existence of at least two different biochemical defects in receptor biosynthesis among our patients with extreme insulin resistance: (i) a block in receptor biosynthesis at a step prior to the synthesis of the 190 kDa receptor precursor (2 patients); or (ii) the biosynthesis of an abnormal form of the receptor precursor with M_r = 148 kDa (1 patient).

2. Qualitative defects in the insulin receptor.

a. Abnormal binding affinity. We have studied a patient with leprechaunism whose receptors exhibit multiple qualitative defects in insulin binding including (i) abnormally high binding affinity and (ii) reduced sensitivity to alterations in pH and temperature. These abnormalities in insulin binding allowed for the detection of the defect in this patient's insulin receptor. Nevertheless, because the patient's receptors actually bind an abnormally large amount of insulin under conditions of physiological temperature and pH, it seems likely that insulin resistance results from a failure to couple insulin binding to insulin action.

b. Defective receptor phosphorylation. The 95 kDa subunit of the insulin receptor possesses a tyrosine-specific protein kinase activity which is stimulated by insulin and is capable of phosphorylating both the receptor itself as well as other proteins. It has been proposed that the receptor-associated protein kinase activity may play a key role in coupling insulin binding to insulin action. Using cultured lymphocytes derived from multiple patients with extreme insulin resistance, we have not identified any patients with selective defects in receptor phosphorylation. However, using solubilized insulin receptors from circulating monocytes and erythrocytes, other laboratories have identified insulin resistant patients whose receptors appear to have a selective defect in protein kinase activity.

S.170 THE SYNDROMES OF ANDROGEN RESISTANCE. J. D. Wilson*, Department of Internal Medicine, The University of Texas Health Science Center at Dallas, Dallas, TX, USA 75235.

Two secretions of the fetal testis, mullerian-inhibiting substance and testosterone, are responsible for male phenotypic differentiation during embryogenesis. Testosterone itself is responsible for the virilization of the wolffian duct system into the epididymis, vas deferens, and seminal vesicle, whereas dihydrotestosterone induces development of the prostate and male external genitalia. Analysis of the single gene defects that cause resistance to androgen action and impair male development and/or reproductive capacity have provided insight into the normal mechanisms by which male development occurs and into the pathological processes that impair normal development. 5α-reductase deficiency is an autosomal recessive disorder that impairs the conversion of testosterone to dihydrotestosterone and results in a characteristic phenotype in which the external genitalia are predominately female in character but the wolffian ducts virilize normally. In studies of subjects with 5α-reductase deficiency from 18 different families we have characterized two distinct types of enzyme abnormalities; most have a profound deficiency in the activity of the enzyme, and the remainder make qualitatively abnormal enzymes with distinct kinetic properties. No phenotypic difference is apparent between subjects carrying these two types of mutations. All subjects characterized to date have some residual 5α-reductase and measurable (but low) plasma dihydrotestosterone, and all virilize to a partial degree at the time of expected puberty. Studies performed by others suggest that the virilization at puberty is in fact mediated by the small amount of dihydrotestosterone formed by the residual enzyme activity and that raising the dihydrotestosterone to normal results in normal virilization. We interpret this evidence as indicating that virtually all androgenic actions at normal puberty are mediated by dihydrotestosterone. Mutations that impair the common receptor that mediates the action of testosterone and dihydrotestosterone are X-linked and result in a spectrum of phenotypic manifestations that vary from men with infertility to phenotypic women. We have studied the receptor from subjects from more than 40 families with endocrine, clinical, and phenotypic features of androgen resistance and have delineated several types of mutations: profound deficiency or absence of receptor function, qualitatively abnormal receptor, and a group (4 families) in which the defect is not yet identified. The group with qualitative abnormalities of the receptor have proved to be the most interesting; on the basis of cloning studies we believe that these mutations are allelic to those that cause deficiency of receptor function. These abnormal receptors have been characterized by different techniques in various laboratories. In our laboratory thermolability, failure of molybdate stabilization, and impairment of transformation of the hormone-receptor complexes to the DNA-binding state have been utilized as markers for characterizing the nature of impaired receptor function in these subjects. Analysis of the latter type of mutation has provided a new working model for the mechanism by which dihydrotestosterone formation amplifies the androgen signal.

S.171 GLUCOCORTICOID INSENSITIVITY. G.P. Chrousos*, M. Tomita, D. Brandon, D.L. Loriaux, and M.B. Lipsett, National Institute of Child Health and Human Development, National Institutes of Health, Bethesda, Maryland 20205.

Glucocorticoid insensitivity refers to the condition in which target tissues show decreased responsiveness to glucocorticoids (end-organ resistance). Since cortisol is essential for life in primates, complete glucocorticoid insensitivity would be incompatible with survival. Partial insensitivity, on the other hand, could be compensated for by elevation of circulating cortisol, a result of decreased negative feedback of glucocorticoids upon pituitary ACTH secretion. The syndrome of primary cortisol insensitivity in man is characterized by absence of signs and symptoms of Cushing's syndrome, elevated total and free plasma cortisol concentrations, high urinary free cortisol excretion, high plasma ACTH and in a severely affected case by hypertension and hypokalemic alkalosis. The latter is due to high plasma concentrations of deoxycorticosterone and corticosterone. In patients with this condition, dexamethasone, at the usual doses, fails to suppress the activity of the pituitary-adrenal axis. High dose dexamethasone therapy (3mg/d), however, corrected in our patient the hypertension and hypokalemic alkalosis, without causing signs of glucocorticoid excess. The glucocorticoid receptor in various tissues from these patients has a low affinity for glucocorticoids and is unstable, with excessive loss of specific bound ligand during thermal activation. Its molecular weight is similar to that of normal controls ($\sim$92,000) and the activation pattern per se appears normal. The amount of hormone-receptor complexes bound to nuclei is decreased. Patient B-lymphocyte transformation with the Epstein-Barr (EB)-virus leads to glucocorticoid receptor induction that is much less than that observed with cells obtained from normal controls. Thus, the glucocorticoid receptor in patients with glucocorticoid resistance is abnormal and its changes lead to the target tissue hyporesponsiveness.

New World primates also have glucocorticoid insensitivity, although no apparent pathology is present. These species have markedly elevated plasma cortisol - both total and free concentrations - increased urinary free cortisol excretion, and marked increases in plasma ACTH and β-endorphin. Similarly to the patients, the glucocorticoid receptors of these primates have a decreased affinity for glucocorticoids, are thermolabile, and fail to be induced by EB-virus transformation. Their molecular weight is indistinguishable from that of the normal human. Despite the high plasma cortisol levels there is no sodium retention and aldosterone levels are actually increased. The kidney aldosterone receptor in these animals crossreacts poorly with cortisol explaining the absence of sodium retention. In contrast to the patients with cortisol insensitivity, in whom the defect appears isolated to the glucocorticoid axis, the New World primates also have progesterone, estrogen, androgen, and vitamin D insensitivity, suggesting that their mutation(s) concerns some factor involved in more than one steroid hormone receptor system. It is of interest that the cortisol-binding globulin in the New World primates has a decreased affinity for cortisol, in addition to being present in lower concentrations. This finding, and the poor affinity of kidney aldosterone receptor for cortisol are probable examples of adaptive evolution in response to the mutation(s) affecting the glucocorticoid receptor.

S.172 INHIBITION OF FOLLICLE-STIMULATING HORMONE RECEPTOR BINDING BY CIRCULATING IMMUNOGLOBULINS.

E. H. Charreau,* Instituto de Biología y Medicina Experimental, Buenos Aires, Argentina.

An interesting new subset of receptor related diseases are those in which receptors seem to become the target of a disordered immune response and in which their function is altered by specific antireceptor antibodies.

We have characterized a circulating inhibitor of FSH receptor binding found in four patients with hypergonadotropic amenorrhea and myasthenia gravis which fulfill the criteria of the resistant ovary syndrome. Sera from twenty other patients with hypergonadotropic amenorrhea, including patients with chronic lymphocytic thyroiditis and systemic lupus erythematosus as well as patients with myasthenia gravis and normal menses failed to show inhibitory activity on FSH binding. The inhibitor behaves as an immunoglobulin according to several criteria, including precipitation by 30% ammonium sulfate, migration on DEAE-cellulose chromatography, specific binding to protein A-Sepharose, characterization as a 7S protein in sucrose density gradients, and immunoprecipitation with specific anti-human immunoglobulin G. In addition, activity is retained in the $F(ab')_2$ fraction of pepsin digested IgG.

When immunoglobulins from these patients were adsorbed on immature testicular tubule membranes, FSH inhibitory activity clearly diminished, however the exposure of the immunoglobulin fraction to interstitial tissue, prostatic tissue or acetylcholine receptors caused no change in FSH binding inhibitory activity, suggesting a tissue specificity for the interaction of this component.

Results of double reciprocal plot analysis obtained with different levels of immunoglobulins on the binding of ^{125}I-hFSH to membrane receptors, supported the view that they are tightly bound to the receptor itself or to a receptors related membrane domain with an apparent Ki of 2.94×10^{12} M^{-1}, a thousand times higher than the affinity constant for the FSH receptor interaction. The plasma level of this antibody was estimated as 10^{-10} M.

The "irreversible" nature of this inhibitory effect could also explain why the ovarian resistance could not be overcome by high FSH circulating levels in vivo. Further evidences of the biological implication of the serum inhibitor was given by the "in vitro" alteration in the production of the seminiferous tubules androgen binding protein secretion and cAMP production when this tissue is incubated in the presence of IgG fraction from patients with the resistant ovary syndrome.

An intrinsic failure in target cell machinery or a receptor down regulation phenomenum on the ovary due to the high circulating FSH levels can not be ruled out, nevertheless the presence of circulating antibodies to FSH receptors can explain the gonadotropin resistance in the patients.

S.173 SILENT THYROIDITIS. T. F. Nikolai*, Marshfield Clinic and Marshfield Medical Foundation, Marshfield, Wisconsin.

Within the past decade a new and unusual form of hyperthyroidism has been recognized with increasing frequency. It is usually manifested by a self-limited episode of hyperthyroidism. Early reports used different nomenclature to describe this syndrome such as silent thyroiditis, painless subacute thyroiditis, lymphocytic thyroiditis with spontaneously resolving hyperthyroidism, atypical subacute thyroiditis, hyperthyroiditis, and subacute non-suppurative thyroiditis. This syndrome was not recognized prior to 1970. Our studies found only 1-5 cases per 100,000 patients seen per year in the early 1970s. It gradually increased to a high of 20-25 cases per 100,000 patients seen per year in the late 1970s, but in the past 2-3 years a substantial decrease in the number of cases seen has occurred.

The clinical manifestations are those of a classic hyperthyroidism of a mild-to-moderate degree that runs its course in 2-5 months. Subsequently a period of transient hypothyroidism occurs in 20-35% of affected patients lasting 2-6 weeks. Occasionally the hypothyroidism is permanent. In about 50% of the cases a small residual goiter persists. Recurrent episodes of transient hyperthyroidism occur in 10-15% with up to 5 episodes being reported in a single patient 1-3 years apart.

The diagnosis of silent thyroiditis is usually first suspected when a suppressed radioactive iodine uptake is found in a patient who is initially felt to have hyperthyroidism of Graves' disease. As this disease runs a similar clinical course to that of subacute granulomatous thyroiditis, initial reports described this syndrome as a silent or painless form of subacute thyroiditis. Shortly thereafter multiple groups reported that biopsies of the thyroids in this syndrome showed only a focal or diffuse lymphocytic thyroiditis which could not be differentiated from chronic lymphocytic thyroiditis.

The frequent occurrence of silent thyroiditis and the confusion with making the differentiation from other forms of hyperthyroidism has resulted in a new classification of hyperthyroidism into that due to high (or normal) radioactive iodine uptake and that due to low radioactive iodine uptake. Silent thyroiditis is the commonest form of low radioactive iodine uptake hyperthyroidism.

Our studies show that about 10% of the cases are found in women within 6 months post partum. Several reports revealed a 5-10% incidence of silent thyroiditis in the postpartum period when groups of women were screened for thyroid disease. Actually a potpourri of thyroid disease including transient hyperthyroidism, transient hypothyroidism, and transient goiter with positive thyroid antibodies was found in these studies. The recurrence of the postpartum thyroiditis after subsequent pregnancies is common.

Long-term follow up of 5-10 years has shown that about 50% of patients retain normal thyroid size and function. The other 50% show a development of hypothyroidism in a few, gradually enlarging euthyroid goiters in others, and a loss of thyroid reserve as measured by the TRH test in the rest.

HL-A studies have shown an increase in DR-3 and DR-5 antigens in silent thyroiditis and the B-35 antigen in subacute thyroiditis indicating an autoimmune etiology for postpartum thyroiditis and a different etiology for subacute thyroiditis.

S.174 THYROID HORMONE RESISTANCE. B.D. Weintraub*, M.M. Menezes-Ferreira, P. Petrick and C. Eil, NIADDK, National Institutes of Health and Naval Hospital and Uniformed Services University of Health Sciences, Bethesda, MD, USA

Thyroid hormone resistance refers to a heterogeneous group of sporadic or familial syndromes in which patients demonstrate refractoriness to the action of endogenous or exogenous thyroid hormones. In the originally described syndrome, patients with generalized resistance display clinical and biochemical features of hypo- or euthyroidism as well as inappropriately elevated serum TSH despite elevated free T_4 and T_3. Subsequently patients were recognized with selective pituitary resistance who display elevated free thyroid hormones and TSH but peripheral hyperthyroidism. Recently a case of selective peripheral but not pituitary resistance was described. The molecular basis of these syndromes has not yet been elucidated, but we have found that certain patients with familial generalized resistance display decreased nuclear uptake of ^{125}I-T_3 in cultured fibroblasts. Such kinetic analysis appears more accurate than conventional equilibrium analysis in confirming the diagnosis in vitro.

Patients with thyroid hormone resistance must be distinguished from those with common forms of hyperthyroidism and from those with inappropriate TSH secretion resulting from a pituitary thyrotropic tumor. Certain euthyroid patients with generalized resistance may be well compensated and require no therapy, but children with delayed growth and development should be treated with thyroid hormone. Most patients with selective pituitary resistance should be treated with dopamine agonists or thyronine analogs that selectively suppress TSH; certain of these patients with apparent pituitary T_4 deiodinase deficiency may respond to T_3. Patients with selective peripheral resistance must be aggressively treated with thyroid hormone despite suppressed TSH. Since various peripheral tissues may differ in thyroid hormone sensitivity, therapy must be individualized using multiple indices of hormone action.

S.175 THERAPEUTIC DECISION MAKING IN ASYMPTOMATIC HYPERCALCEMIA AND PRIMARY HYPERPARATHYROIDISM.

H. Heath III*, Endocrine Research Unit, Mayo Clinic and Mayo Medical School, Rochester, Minnesota 55905.

Primary hyperparathyroidism was once considered an uncommon disease generally accompanied by symptomatic hypercalcemia, plus varying combinations of nephrolithiasis, renal failure, and skeletal disease. Since the early 1960s there has been growing recognition that primary hyperparathyroidism in western populations most commonly exists in a relatively mild form, with few symptoms or none at all. The principal mechanism of this discovery was the advent of automated multiphasic serum chemistry machines, which made inexpensive, accurate, routine determination of serum calcium possible. In western Europe and the United States, the average annual incidence rate for primary hyperparathyroidism is approximately 25/100,000 population. Approximately 50% of these patients will be "asymptomatic" or have no unequivocal hyperparathyroid complications. A distinction must be maintained between asymptomatic persons who have no detectable adverse effects of the disease, and those who are asymptomatic yet have medically detectable adverse effects of the disease. A clinical diagnosis of primary hyperparathyroidism is made with confidence by history, physical examination, and routine laboratory tests. Measurement of immunoreactive parathyroid hormone is of ancillary benefit. With care, the diagnosis can be made correctly without special studies in 90 to 95% of cases, and skilled surgeons achieve correspondingly high operative success rates. Since severe urolithiasis, renal failure, and hyperparathyroid bone disease are now uncommon, attention has turned recently to other possible adverse effects of the disease, such as arterial hypertension, psychological problems, and osteopenia. Recent studies, which will be reviewed, clearly document increased blood pressure and decreased bone mass even in patients with "asymptomatic" hyperparathyroidism. The pathogenetic mechanisms of these abnormalities are not yet known. Until the risks and benefits of surgical treatment versus medical followup are resolved, the clinical approach to these mildly hyperparathyroid patients must be based on probabilities, cost-benefit estimations, and common sense. A therapeutic strategy for decision making in suspected hyperparathyroidism will be presented and directions for new research suggested.

S.176 ANTIANDROGEN TREATMENT OF ACNE. F. Neumann* and U. Lachnit-Fixson, Schering AG Berlin/Bergkamen, Muellerstrasse 170-178, 1000 Berlin 65 (Germany West).

Of causal importance for the development of acne and seborrhoea is an increased sebaceous gland function. The skin surface lipid level in acne patients is significantly higher as compared with controls. There is a relationship between the sebum secretion rate and the severity of the disease. Because the sebaceous glands are under androgen control it was obvious to use antiandrogens for the treatment of this disease. The best known antiandrogen is cyproterone acetate (CPA). It has been shown in animal models that this antiandrogen inhibits sebocyte proliferation very effectively. Concerning the molecular mechanism of action, CPA competes with androgens for receptor sites in target organs for androgens and the sebaceous gland is a target organ. In most European and several other countries the therapy of acne with CPA containing preparations is well established. CPA is not only a potent antiandrogen but it has in addition progestational and antigonadotrophic properties. Based on this activity pattern it was possible to develop a contraceptive preparation containing 2 mg CPA in combination with 50 µg ethinyl estradiol (Diane[R]). Side effects and contraindications are more or less identical with other oral contraceptives. Pronounced improvement of acne and seborrhoea is seen after three to four treatment cycles. Improvement or healing in more than 90% of patients is seen after 9 to 12 months of therapy. In very severe cases of acne and severe hirsutism, this preparation has to be combined with a higher dose of CPA (10 to 100 mg) given in a reversed sequential schedule (21 days the low dose preparation, and during the first 10 days of the cycle in addition 10 to 100 mg CPA, depending on the severity of the disease).

S.177 EXPRESSION AND GENETIC DISORDER OF NEUROHYPOPHYSEAL HORMONES:

D. Richter*, H. Schmale, R. Ivell and M. Rehbein, Institut für Physiologische Chemie, Abteilung Zellbiochemie, Universität Hamburg, 2000 Hamburg 20, Martinistr. 52, Germany.

The hormones vasopressin and oxytocin are synthesized as composite precursors: pro-vasopressin consists of the hormone, its respective carrier protein called neurophysin and a glycoprotein; pro-oxytocin contains the hormone and another neurophysin carrier. Both precursors are produced by different populations of neurones in the supraoptic and paraventricular nuclei of the hypothalamus, packaged into neurosecretory granules and transported axonally to the posterior pituitary. During transportation the precursors are processed into their functional units.

The structural organization of the two precursors and their corresponding genes from calf and rat have been analyzed using recombinant DNA techniques (1-4).

Studies of the hereditary hypothalamic diabetes insipidus in mutant rats have shown that these animals lack the hormone vasopressin and its corresponding neurophysin carrier (5). To elucidate the molecular basis of this genetic defect the vasopressin gene from diabetes insipidus rats was isolated and sequenced. The results show that a single deletion in the gene leads to a new reading frame predicting a hormone precursor with a different carboxy terminus.

1. Land et al., Nature 295, 299 (1982).
2. Land et al., Nature 302, 342 (1983).
3. Schmale et al., EMBO J. 2, 763 (1983).
4. Ivell and Richter, PNAS in press.
5. Valtin et al. Handbook of Physiol. 7, 131 (1974).

S.178 ORGANIZATION OF THE PARAVENTRICULAR NUCLEUS.

M.Kawata* and Y.Sano, Department of Anatomy, Kyoto Prefectural University of Medicine, Kawaramachi-Hirokoji, Kamikyo-ku, Kyoto 602, Japan.

Recent studies have revealed that the projections of hypothalamic neurons which produce oxytocin, vasopressin and the related neurophysins are much more extensive and complex than had previously been assumed. In addition to the classical neurosecretory pathway extending from the supraoptic nucleus (SON) and the paraventricular nucleus (PVN) to systemic capillaries in the posterior lobe of the pituitary, a secondary pathway arising from the PVN has been discovered. It terminates at the median eminence and secretes vasopressin into the proximal capillary plexus of the hypophyseal portal system. This subsystem of the PVN could serve to regulate the secretion of ACTH from the corticotrophs in the anterior lobe of the pituitary. An increasing amount of evidence indicates that oxytocin- and vasopressin-containing nerve fibers are distributed in various regions of the central nervous system outside the hypothalamus. There have been a number of hypotheses concerning the physiological functions of these extrahypothalamic fiber networks. Oxytocinergic and vasopressinergic fibers distributed in the extrahypothalamic areas are believed to originate in the PVN. Since the physiological evidence suggests that the PVN is involved in various responses, it has been proposed that cytoarchitectonic subnuclei which consist of neurons of differing projections are present in the PVN. In addition to oxytocin, vasopressin and neurophysins, some neurons in the PVN produce peptides such as somatostatin, neurotensin, enkephalin, cholecystokinin, corticotropin-releasing factor and dynorphin. There appears to be a clear topographic segregation of these peptide-containing neurons. Moreover, the presence of peptides within the neurohypophyseal hormone-containing cells has been demonstrated. Noradrenergic fibers innervate the area of the PVN where vasopressinergic neurons predominate. In striking contrast to noradrenergic input, very few serotonergic fibers occur in this nucleus. Primarily noradrenergic neurons in the A1 (lateral reticular nucleus), A2 (solitary nucleus and dorsal motor nucleus of the vagus), and A6 (locus coeruleus) regions give rise to projections that terminate in the PVN. Like the SON, the PVN is extremely vascularized and a high density of capillaries occurs only in the magnocellular area.

These recent discoveries necessitate an investigation of the principal cellular organization of the PVN. We intend to focus on the morphological functions of this integrative nucleus, with the use of a combination of qualitative and quantitative morphological methods. These include silver impregnation, fluorescence histochemistry, immunohistochemistry, transmission electron microscopy, anterograde and retrograde tracer techniques and iontophoretic intracellular dye injection.

S.179 DESIGN OF MORE SPECIFIC ANTAGONISTIC ANALOGS OF THE NEUROHYPOPHYSIAL HORMONES. W. H. Sawyer* and M. Manning, Columbia University College of Physicians and Surgeons, New York, NY 10032 and the Medical College of Ohio, Toledo, OH 43699, USA.

Effective in vivo antagonists of some actions of the neurohypophysial hormones have only recently become available. These are potentially valuable pharmacological probes of the actions of endogenous neurohypophysial peptides and may have therapeutic applications. Antagonists of the vasopressor action of vasopressin have been widely exploited for assessing the contribution of endogenous vasopressin to vascular homeostasis under a variety of circumstances. Antagonists of oxytocic and antidiuretic actions have not yet proved as useful, partly because those available are neither as potent nor as specific as the vasopressor antagonists. Receptors mediating the well-known peripheral actions of neurohypophysial hormones have been characterized largely in studies using specific agonists. Oxytocin receptors in the uterus and mammary gland are similar but do differ somewhat in their pharmacological characteristics. Peripheral vasopressin receptors fall into two clearly distinct categories. Responses to V_1-receptors do not involve activation of adenylate cyclase. These include contraction of vascular smooth muscle and stimulation of glycogenolysis in isolated hepatocytes. Antidiuretic responses are mediated by V_2-receptors which are associated with activation of membrane-bound adenylate cyclase. Highly specific agonists are available that activate one or the other type of vasopressin receptor. This classification of vasopressin receptors, however, may only relate to those that mediate the familiar peripheral actions of the hormone. There are indications that other actions of vasopressin may involve receptors with differing properties. For example, V_1-antagonists can block the effects of vasopressin on delaying extinction of conditioned avoidance behavior in rats but some of the vasopressin analogs that are most potent in delaying extinction are devoid of V_1-agonistic activity. Improving and refining antagonists for specific receptor types appears to be a worthwhile goal. Even our most specific V_1-antagonists block behavioral responses that are not mediated by classical V_1-receptors. Presently available oxytocin antagonists are also potent V_1-antagonists. We have, however, made substantial recent progress toward improving the specificity of V_2-antagonists, although we have been unable to eliminate V_1-antagonism completely. Further efforts toward the design of antagonists that are more clearly selective for each receptor type should provide more incisive pharmacological tools and more sharply targeted agents for potential therapeutic uses. These studies were supported by NIH research grants AM-01940 and GM-25280.

S.180 A POSSIBLE ROLE FOR VASOPRESSIN AND OXYTOCIN IN NEUROTRANSMISSION.
M.Mühlethaler* and J.J.Dreifuss,Department of Physiology,University Medical Center,1211 Geneva 4,Switzerland.

Oxytocin(OT)and vasopressin(VP)are traditionally viewed as peptide hormones which are synthesized in hypothalamic perikarya and then carried by axoplasmic transport to the neurohypophysis where they are released into blood vessels.That both peptides act only as hormones affecting distal targets is today challenged on several grounds.1)It appears now that extrahypophysial fibres containing OT or VP are also present in other brain areas such as the limbic system,the brainstem and the spinal cord.Oxytocin fibres are believed to originate almost exclusively from the paraventricular nucleus of the hypothalamus.In contrast,most VP fibres are now thought to arise from newly described VP-containing cell bodies located outside the hypothalamus and which can only be visualized following colchicine pretreatment.2)Oxytocin and vasopressin-containing vesicles were demonstrated in presynaptic structures in the target fields of extrahypopysial pathways,and both peptides could be secreted in vitro from these areas upon depolarization by potassium or veratridine.The amounts present in and released from these territories were minute as compared to the neurohypophysis.However,since secretion was calcium-dependant,its mechanism in this regard is thus similar to that leading to the release of classical neurotransmitters. 3)Binding studies which were for a long time hampered by the lack of tritiated OT or VP of high specific activity have now succeded in showing high affinity vasopressin receptors on hippocampal synaptosomal membranes.4)In parallel with these biochemical and morphological studies,attention was also focused on the cellular actions of OT and VP in areas where extrahypophysial pathways were seen to terminate.Using hippocampal slices we found that both peptides directly excited a class of non-pyramidal neurones.In contrast,pyramidal cells were inhibited by these peptides through an indirect mechanism.Structure-activity studies using selective agonists of OT or VP allowed us to show that these effects were mediated by receptors for OT which were similar to those present in the uterus.A number of other in vivo and in vitro studies indicated that neurones sensitive to neurohypophysial peptides are also present in the supraoptic nucleus,locus coeruleus,brainstem and spinal cord.Taken together these data are clearly suggestive of a role of oxytocin and vasopressin within the central nervous system.However it is not clear yet what the link is,if any,between these studies and a number of hypothesis concerning the possible physiological role of these peptides with respect to memory consolidation,thermoregulation maternal behaviour or central regulation of certain autonomic fuctions.

S.181 AGING AND ADRENAL

H. IBAYASHI* and K. KATO, The Third Dept of Internal Medicine, Faculty of Medicine, Kyushu University, Fukuoka 812, Japan

In view of the hormonal regulation of homeostasis, considerable attention has been focused on the effect of aging on the adrenocortical function in man. The accumulation of lipofuscin pigment in zona reticularis of the adrenal gland is well known as the morphological characteristics in the aged.
Urinary excretion of 17-OHCS shows a slight decline with aging, however, urinary 11-deoxy-17KS demonstrates a markedly age-related and almost linear decrease in either sex.
Plasma cortisol(F) levels remain unchanged in advanced age, but the plasma levels of adrenal C_{19} androgens-DHEA sulfate (DHEA-S), DHEA and androstenedione(A-dione)-show significantly age-related and linear decline from 20 years of age. The age-dependent reduction in plasma aldosterone(Ald) concentration is due mainly to the decreasing renin production.
Plasma 19-OH-A-dione, one of the most active Ald amplifier, also exhibits a definite reduction in the aged.
Plasma pregnenolone(P_5) and P_5-S levels are significantly low in the aged, suggesting reduced production of steroid precursors in the adrenal gland in the aged compared with the young. Plasma F response to graded β^{1-24}ACTH infusions in the aged was not different significantly from that in the young, but the responses of plasma DHEA-S and DHEA demonstrated a significant decrease in the aged.
Despite no differences in the 24-hr secretion rate of F and Ald after ACTH-Z adminitsration between the young and the aged males, the secretion rates of DHEA-S and DHEA were significantly decreased in the aged, although that of 17α-OH progesterone was markedly increased. These results suggested the decrease in the activities of the enzymes for adrenal androgen biosynthesis, especially $C_{17,20}$lyase, in the aged adrenal glands. The basis for the decline in production of adrenal androgens in the aged was studied in connection with the prominent deposition of lipofuscin in the adrenocortical reticular cells of the aged. We determined the effect of lipoperoxidation on microsomal enzyme activity and the effect of microsomal vitamin E on malondialdehyde formation in the human adrenal gland in vitro. The in vitro lipoperoxidation of human adrenal microsomes caused a rapid and marked decrease in the activities of steroid-synthesizing enzymes, especially $C_{17,20}$lyase and 17α-hydroxylase in the microsomes. The microsomal vitamin E showed the protecting effect in a dose-dependent manner against the lipoperoxidation of adrenal microsomes and prevented the losses of enzyme activities resulting from lipoperoxidation.
This study was supported in part by a grant from the Ministry of Education, Japan.

S.182 ENDOCRINE PATHOGENESIS OF BENIGN PROSTATIC HYPERTROPHY. Jack Geller*, Mercy Hospital and Medical Center, San Diego, California 92103

Benign prostatic hypertrophy (BPH) is a common disease in aging males; eighty percent of males 70-80 years old will have histologic evidence of BPH; two-thirds of males over the age of 60 will have clinical symptoms related to BPH. The major established evidence for an endocrine role in the pathogenesis of BPH is as follows:

(1) Castration prevents BPH when performed in males prior to the age of 40.
(2) There is no development of the prostate whatsoever in androgen-resistant syndromes such as 5α-reductase deficiency or testicular feminization.
(3) Koch's postulates for an endocrinopathy have been satisfied in the dog which develops BPH when androstandiol with or without estrogen is administered to castrated animals.
(4) Increased tissue DHT with a decrease in the 3α-17β-androstandiols has been the universal finding in human BPH. Recently Walsh has challenged this data and indicated that the normal prostates which were compared with BPH were all obtained post mortem and that artifacts of DHT concentration may have been responsible for the low DHT in the normals. Nevertheless, DHT is the major intranuclear androgen in the prostate. DHT is increased in the nuclei of stromal cells in BPH compared to the nuclei of epithelial cells in the same tissue.
(5) Estrogen content of the nuclei of stromal cells is significantly higher than that of epithelial cells in the same human BPH tissue. Since estrogen receptors are found primarily in stroma, the predominant tissue in BPH, estrogen and stroma along with DHT may all have a significant role in the pathogenesis of the disease.

There is significant evidence from the work of several authors that 5α-reductase is indeed increased in patients with BPH compared to normal prostates; significant decreases have also been shown in the enzymes which remove DHT in BPH patients compared to controls. These combined effects would increase tissue DHT concentration.

No abnormalities in total androgen receptor have been noted between BPH and normal prostates with the best available receptor techniques. Nor is there evidence for a difference between plasma testosterone levels in BPH and normals.

We have recently found that tamoxifen, a competitor for the estrogen receptor, significantly decreases stromal protein synthesis as well as nuclear androgen receptor and cytosol progesterone receptor in the whole prostates of humans treated with tamoxifen for ten days as compared to controls. Tissue CPK concentrations were also decreased following tamoxifen administration. These findings support those of others who showed that increased estrogen levels in the stromal cells were associated with stromal proliferation in BPH. In view of the possibility that increased tissue DHT is not the sole or major factor in the pathogenesis of BPH the possility of the dominant role of the stroma and estrogen in the pathogenesis of this disease is now becoming more probable.

S.183 ANDROGENS, SEXUALITY AND THE AGEING MALE

John Bancroft, MRC Reproductive Biology Unit, Edinburgh, Scotland.

Evidence of a decline in both androgens and sexual behaviour in ageing men will be reviewed. As yet a causal relationship between the two trends has not been demonstrated and a variety of non-hormonal factors associated with ageing have to be taken into account. Recent evidence of the role of androgens in male sexuality will be presented. Androgens are necessary for maintaining normal sexual appetite and for ejaculation in men. Their role in erectile function is less clear. Nocturnal erections appear to be androgen dependent, whereas erection in response to erotic stimuli are not. Androgens may play a part in tactile sensitivity, as yet untested. So far, it is unclear whether there are threshold levels of testosterone above which additional hormone will have no behavioural effect. Evidence will be presented that sexual appetite can be enhanced by increasing testosterone levels initially within the normal male range. The implications of the finding for older men will be considered. Defining the role of relative androgen deficiency in the declining sexual interest of ageing men awaits the experimental evaluation of exogenous androgen administration in this age group. The methodological and clinical problems of doing so will be discussed.

S.184 EXPERIMENTAL ASPECTS OF AGE-RELATED CHANGES IN THE ENDOCRINE SYSTEM.

B.J. Merry* and A.M. Holehan, Wolfson Institute, University of Hull, Hull. HU6 7RX, England.

It is possible, through dietary intervention early in the post-weaning life of the female rat, to modify the timing of reproductive senescence to provide a model system for studying the endocrinology of reproductive decline. Chronic dietary restriction of Sprague-Dawley rats from weaning to maintain growth rate at 50% that of fully-fed control animals will result in both an increase in average (23 to 36 months) and maximum lifespan (36 to 47 months). Puberty is retarded to about 60 days and occurs over a wider age range in experimental animals after which greater than 70% of females exhibit normal five day oestrous cycles. At approximately 8-12 months control rats demonstrate irregular, lengthened oestrous cycles with the vaginal cytology characterised either by extended periods of oestrogen induced vaginal cornification or persistent dioestrus smears interrupted by 2-3 days of nucleated and cornified cells. In marked contrast age related irregularities of the oestrous cycle in restricted females are not observed until about 24 months. A rapid decline in fertility of control females is observed after 9 months and these animals are infertile by 16 months, the age of maximum fertility in the experimental females, with the age of the last litter prolonged to as late as 31 months. A decreased rate of atresia is observed in ovaries from dietary restricted females, the total number of follicles being greater when compared to aged-matched controls. It has been recognised that the incidence of abortions, stillbirths and congenital anomalies increase with maternal age, however, while the incidence of malformed young born to fully-fed females increases to about 1%, in over 1000 pups studied, no incidence of malformations in the offspring of restricted mothers has been observed. The hormonal profiles of rats on a restricted diet show no difference in the overall pattern of oestradiol-17β across the oestrous cycle but the total amount of this hormone released in dietary restricted females is 46% that of control animals. This is associated with elevated circulating FSH and an early release of the preovulatory LH peak in restricted females. Such an alteration in the hormonal profile has, as one result, a reduced exposure of the follicular ovum to high levels of oestradiol-17β. Therefore with increased age the oestrous cycle of dietary restricted female rats maintain a more precise synchrony between the priming of follicles by FSH, the increase in oestrogen and the release of LH to induce ovulation. These findings from the experimental manipulation of the rate of reproductive ageing will be reviewed in the context of recent experimental work from other groups on the hormonal manipulation of preovulatory ageing and reproductive senescence.

S.185 RNA PROCESSING OF CALCITONIN GENE EXPRESSION RESULTS IN THE PRODUCTION OF A NOVEL NEUROPEPTIDE. Michael G. Rosenfeld*, Susan G. Amara, Vivian Jonas, and Ronald M. Evans, UCSD and Salk Institute in La Jolla, California 92093 USA

Complex regulatory mechanisms restrict the expression in neural and endocrine tissues of genes encoding neuroendocrine peptides to precise groups of neurons or secretory cells. The calcitonin gene provides a model to study the molecular mechanisms which act during development to enable a tissue-specific differential expression of neuroendocrine genes. The calcitonin gene generates distinct mRNAs encoding either the calcium-regulatory hormone, calcitonin, or a novel neuropeptide, referred to as calcitonin gene related peptide (CGRP). The pattern of expression of the two mRNAs exhibits tissue-specificity; the thyroidal C-cell produces predominantly calcitonin mRNA, while CGRP mRNA is the product of calcitonin gene expression in the brain, spinal cord, and cranial nerve ganglia. The distribution of CGRP-producing cells and pathways in the brain and other tissues suggest potential functions in nociception, ingestive behavior, and modulation of the autonomic and endocrine systems. Effects of CGRP on blood pressure, catecholamine release, and gastric acid production have been documented. The presence of CGRP in thyroidal "C" cells implies co-secretion with calcitonin; hence, effects on hormonal metabolism are likely. CGRP is the peptide present in the islet baskets in the pancreas, as well as in exocrine pancreas, suggesting potential roles in digestive and metabolic regulation.

Because, as documented by analysis of calcitonin gene expression, RNA processing regulation is one strategy used in tissue-specific regulation of gene expression in the brain and endocrine organs, understanding the mechanisms of such decision-making is crucial for elucidation of the phenotypic development of these tissues. We have documented that these two RNAs use the same transcriptional initiation site but utilize distinct 3′ polyadenylation sites. Termination of transcription following the calcitonin exon does not dictate the production of calcitonin mRNA, implying that the selective use of polyadenylation sites dictates the pattern of mRNA production. Transfection of the calcitonin gene into a series of cell types establishes that this selection is adjudicated by a trans-acting factor(s). We have demonstrated that similar events operate both in the case of the human calcitonin gene, and for other genes of the neuroendocrine system.

S.186 THE CALCITONIN GENE PEPTIDE FAMILY AND THE CENTRAL NERVOUS SYSTEM.

H.R. Morris, M. Panico, T. Etienne, J. Tippins, S.I. Girgis and I. MacIntyre*

The calcitonin gene encodes a small family of peptides including calcitonin, katacalcin and a novel 37 amino acid peptide (hCGRP). Calcitonin is mainly concerned with calcium regulation and is co-secreted with katacalcin. The function of this last peptide still needs to be determined although it is likely that it is also involved with calcium regulation. hCGRP is present in the normal human central nervous system, including spinal cord, but is also present in C cells as well as in the adrenal medulla. It circulates in health and may well play a physiological role. All three peptides are present together in the central nervous system but the concentration of CGRP tends to be greater in nervous tissue than in the periphery. It is likely that all three peptides have a systemic role as well as a neurotransmitter or neuromodulator role in the central nervous system. Recent work on the physiology of these peptides (with special reference to the central nervous system) will be reviewed.

S.187 CALCITONIN BINDING SITES IN THE BRAIN. M. Koida*, H. Nakamuta and R. C. Orlowski, Department of Pharmacology, Faculty of Pharmaceutical Sciences, Nagasaki University, Nagasaki-852, Japan, Department of Pharmacology, Faculty of Pharmacy, Setsunan University, Hirakata 573-01, and Armour Pharmaceutical Co., Ill. 60901, U.S.A.

Salmon calcitonin (sCT) by intracerebroventricular (i.c.v.) injection induces a variety of behavioral effects in mammals. It is also a fact that the CT-specific binding sites occur in mammalian brains, exhibiting the properties expected of the "physiological receptor". On the basis of the available evidence, it is attempted to qualify the sites as the receptors.

a) In vitro binding studies: ^{125}I-sCT binds to the membrane fraction of the rat brain in the ways that are saturable, CT-specific, pH- and temperature-dependent, of the highest affinity to sCT and of low reversibility. The affinity decreased in the order of sCT > [Asu^{1,7}]-eel CT > porcine CT (pCT), sCT(11-32) > sCT(22-32) ≫ human CT (hCT) > sCT(1-11) = 0. The order of CTs is the same with that of the hypocalcemic activity assayed on rats. Scatchard plotting locates the sites of the lowest K and the highest B_{max} in the hypothalamus. The midbrain or brainstem follows in these parameters. In the subcellular fractions, the content decreased in the order of $P_3 > P_2 > P_1$, and among the subfractions of P_2 is highest in the synaptosomal one. The in vitro autoradiography results in a more detailed mapping of the sites. Most of the anterior hypothalamic nuclei exhibit the highest grain density which may mediate the anorectic effect. A series of other spots also heavily labeled such as brainstem, nucleus tractus spinalis nervi trigemini, some laminae of the spinal cord, etc., may be related to the antinociceptive action of sCT.
From a photoactive derivative of ^{125}I-sCT, the radioactive label is transferred by light to some macromolecules of the hypothalamus, including a distinct peak corresponding to BSA in size. sCT(11-32) of no anorectic activity depresses labeling of the peak to a large extent but not abolishes.
b) In vivo binding studies: After i.c.v. injection to rats, ^{125}I-sCT can survive in the brain for a long time as reflected in long-lasting anorexia. Of the radioactivity retained by the hypothalamus 3 hr after injection, more than one half can be recovered as ^{125}I-sCT on the HPLC.
c) In vitro effects: sCT ($\geqq$1 μM) stimulates the activity of adenylate cyclase in brain slices or in the homogenate, while the Ca-uptake by hypothalamic slices is inhibited by much lower concentrations (10 nM$\geqq$). The latter effect appears to be specific to sCT and also the brain region.
d) In vivo effects: Food-intake in rats is suppressed by an i.c.v. injection of 0.2-0.3 U of sCT or [Asu^{1,7}]-eel CT. pCT is a very weak suppressor and hCT is inert. Gastric acid secretion, intestinal motility and stress-induced feeding may be better measures of the sCT actions on the feeding-related phenomena since all respond well to 2 mM or less of sCT, but the actions of other CTs remain unknown. Antinociception can be a different measure. When estimated using the method of Randall & Selitto, sCT has no effect with 1 U/rat, while the ED_{min} of pCT is 0.04 or less.

It is concluded that some CTs given centrally interact with the receptors in the anterior hypothalamic nuclei, possibly affecting the Ca-flux, which then leads to inhibition of feeding behavior.

S.188 CALCITONIN: A CANDIDATE FOR A NEUROMODULATOR OF MULTIPLE PAIN INHIBITING SYSTEMS. A. Pecile*, F. Guidobono, V. Sibilia and C. Netti, Dept. of Pharmacology, Chemotherapy and Medical Toxicology, University of Milan, Milan, Italy.

Calcitonin (CT) administered in patients to counteract enhanced bone resorption in bone diseases induces analgesic effects. CT is now being proposed as analgesic for intolerable pain in terminal cancer patients. In several studies we have demonstrated that salmon calcitonin (sCT) administered directly into the brain induces analgesia which occurs without involvement of opiate receptors. Immunoreactive CT like material have been detected in various CNS areas. Binding sites for sCT were visualized by us and by others in areas anatomically involved in the transmission of nociceptive information. Thus calcitonin-like peptides were proposed as candidates for neural modulation of pain-inhibitory systems. A first hypothesis that we considered worthwhile to investigate for clarifying the suggested CT neuromodulation was that CT might exert its activity through the serotonergic (5-HT) or the catecholaminergic (CA) systems, or both, which are known to participate in central pain perception control. The integrity of 5-HT system was found not to be essential for sCT activity, but central (icv) administration of a selective neurotoxin for CA neurons (6-hydroxydopamine, 6-OHDA, 200 ug/rat) abolished the antinociceptive effect of sCT (2,5 ug/rat/icv) as measured by the hot-plate test. Treatment with an α-receptor blocker (phentolamine, 5 mg/kg/ip) did not counteract sCT-analgesia, but injection of a β-receptor blocker (propranolol, 10 mg/kg/ip) reduced the central analgesic effect of sCT. These results suggest that the CA system is involved in the analgesia of sCT, with β-receptors playing a predominant role. This conclusion is strengthened by the autoradiographic evidence that the treatment with 6-OHDA decreased the binding sites for sCT in CNS areas rich in the CA neurons involved in pain perception. Thus CT does appear to be a neuroactive peptide participating importantly in opioid-independent pain inhibitory system(s).

S.189 DITRIBUTION OF CRF IN THE BRAIN. S. Vigh* and I. Merchenthaler, Department of Anatomy, University Medical School, Pécs, 7643 Hungary.

Although the presence, in hypothalamic extracts, of a substance capable of stimulating corticotropin (ACTH) release and called "corticotropin - releasing factor (CRF)" was demonstrated more than 25 years ago (Saffran and Schally, 1955; Guillemin and Rosenberg, 1955), the chemical identification, and the localization of the CRF in the brain was delayed. Recent isolation, structural identification, and synthesis of ovine CRF (Vale et al. 1981) has made possible the generation of specific antibodies against this hypothalamic peptide. The distribution of CRF-containing perikarya, neuronal processes and terminals was examined in the central nervous system of normal and colchicine pretreated rats; in hypophysectomized or adrenalectomized animal models; and in animals with various brain lesions or microchirurgical cuts. CRF-immunoreactive neuronal elements were detected, using the peroxidase-antiperoxidase (PAP) immunocytochemistry combined with the recently developed silver-gold intensification method, in all major subdivisions of the brain. However, one well-described CRF system could be distinguished. The majority of the perikarya of this paraventriculo-infundibular (PV-IN) CRF system are located in the parvocellular division of the paraventricular nucleus of the hypothalamus (PVH). The CRF-positive fibers originating from the PVH form a medial, an intermediate and a lateral fiber pathway. The lateral and intermediate CRF tracts leave the dorsolateral part of the PVH and course laterally and medially of the fornix, respectively, ventrally toward the optic tract. Just dorsal to the optic tract they turn in caudal direction and run paralell with and very close to the basal surface of the hypothalamus. Individual fibers then turn medially to terminate in the external layer of the median eminence (ME). Only a few fibers originate from the medial-ventral part of the PVH (medial pathway). These fibers run in ventral direction along the walls of the 3rd ventricle and terminate in the ME. In comparison with untreated control rats, the adrenalectomy resulted in a dramatic increase in CRF-immunostaining of this system. In addition to the PV-IN system, cell bodies with CRF immunoreactivity were found in the following regions: olfactory bulb, olfactory tubercle, amygdala, septum, bed nuclei of the stria terminalis and anterior comissure, nucleus accumbens, supraoptic, medial preoptic and periventricular preoptic nuclei, cerebral cortex, hippocampus, periaqueductal gray of the mesencephalon and pons, raphe nuclei, lateral tegmental nucleus, parabrachial nucleus, cuneiform nuclei, locus ceruleus, medial vestibular nucleus, nucleus of the solitary tract, dorsal vagal complex, and most of the central sensory nuclei. CRF-immunopositive nerve processes were observed in all of the above areas as well as in the stria terminalis, thalamus, caudate-putamen, zona incerta, and the cerebellum. The widespread but selective distribution of CRF-immunoreactive neurons supports the neuroendocrine role of this peptide and reinforces the view that CRF, similarly to other neuropeptides, may also function as a neuromodulator througout the central nervous system.

S.190 HYPOTHALAMIC FACTORS REGULATING ACTH RELEASE: THE ROLES OF THE 41 AMINO ACID CRF AND VASOPRESSIN.
G.E.Gillies, E.A. Linton and P.J. Lowry*
Protein Hormone Unit, St. Bartholomew's Centre for Clinical Research, London EC1A 7BE.

Historically, the labile nature of CRF and the limitations and difficulties of bioassays for its detection have made it difficult to identify. Since the characterisation by Vale et al (Science 213: 1394, 1981), of a 41 amino acid peptide from ovine hypothalami, (o-CRF-41) with potent ACTH releasing activity, it has become apparent that this is not the sole hypothalamic factor controlling ACTH release, although abundant evidence has demonstrated that it plays a highly significant role in the stress response. The antidiuretic hormone, vasopressin, was an early CRF candidate but its role was soon discredited due to the high levels of vasopressin necessary to release ACTH. Using the superfused isolated rat anterior pituitary cell column coupled with an ACTH radioimmunoassay, as a CRF bioassay, three peaks of ACTH-releasing activity have been found after gel filtration of rat and porcine hypothalamic extracts. One peak co-elutes with ovine-CRF-41 immunoreactivity and another (the largest) with vasopressin. As yet there is no evidence for the identity of the third factor, although it elutes near oxytocin on both BioGel P2 and Sephadex G-50. An ACTH inhibitor may also exist. Typically, a dramatic loss of ACTH-releasing activity was observed after chromatography (>50%) which could be restored after re-combination of the peaks. We therefore have evidence that CRF is a multi-component system, two components of which appear to be CRF-41 and vasopressin,and they interact and synergise with each other to control ACTH release in a variety of stress situations. This conclusion has been supported both in vitro, using normal and the Brattleboro strain of rats, and in vivo. Synthetic o-CRF-41 and vasopressin act synergistically to produce supra-additive ACTH release. From radioimmunoassays of a rat stalk-median eminence extract the CRF-41 and vasopressin content can account for less than 10% and 30% respectively, of ACTH-releasing activity, and yet immunoneutralisation with either CRF-41 or AVP antisera, in vitro and in vivo, produces a 60% reduction of ACTH-releasing activity, and both antisera together cannot fully quench ACTH-releasing bioactivity. These results are indicative of a synergism of CRF-41 and AVP and the existence of other, as yet uncharacterised CRF's. In common with extracted ACTH-releasing activity, activity released from superfused rat hypothalami possessed an AVP and o-CRF-41-related component, as quenching with either antiserum produced a 50-60% reduction in CRF bioactivity. Interestingly, dilutions of hypothalamic superfusate which gave an ACTH-releasing activity equivalent to that of 1/40th SME extract contained only a tenth of the AVP immunoreactive content (35pg/ml) and undetectable o-CRF-41-like immunoreactivity. All in all these results suggest synergism between AVP, an ovine-CRF-41-like peptide and, as yet, unidentified factors. This work is supported by the Medical Research Council and the Joint Research Board of St. Bartholomew's Hospital.

S.191 THE EFFECT OF CORTICOTROPIN-RELEASING FACTOR (CRF) ON SOME ENDOCRINE FUNCTIONS. Catherine Rivier* and Wylie Vale, The Salk Institute, Peptide Biology Laboratory, La Jolla, CA 92037.

CRF was initially purified and isolated on the basis of its ability to stimulate the secretion of ACTH by the pituitary. Several laboratories, including our own, subsequently reported that the ACTH-releasing effect of CRF could be potentiated by a number of secretagogues, including catecholamines and vasopressin (VP). In an attempt to determine which class of VP receptors (V_1 = pressor like or V_2 = anti-diuretic-like) mediated the effect of VP, we have shown that the V_1 antagonist dPTyr(Me)AVP, but not the V_2 antagonist d(CH_2)$_5$DLeu ValAVP inhibited the ACTH-releasing as well as CRF potentiating effect of VP. This observation suggests that the action of VP on the corticotrophs is primarily mediated through pressor-like (V_1) receptors.

Glucocorticoids also regulate the action of CRF on the anterior pituitary through a well-documented negative feed-back. Acutely, both corticosterone and dexamethasone significantly inhibit CRF-induced ACTH release in intact rats. However, the long-term exposure of adult male rats to CRF results in significantly elevated plasma levels of both ACTH and corticosterone, suggesting that continuous stimulation of the pituitary can occur despite the presence of increased values of circulating corticosteroids.

Apart from controling ACTH release by a direct effect at the pituitary level, CRF has been found to act centrally to modulate the secretion of LH and GH. The ability of CRF to induce a dose-related inhibition of LH release in gonadectomized/adrenalectomized rats, indicates that this inhibition is not mediated through steroids of either adrenal or gonadal origin. Additionally, we have observed that neither the opiate receptor antagonist naltrexone nor the ganglionic blocker chlorisondamine would alter the CRF-induced decrease in plasma LH levels, thereby suggesting that CRF can exert delerious actions on reproductive functions which do not appear to directly involve opiate or peripheral catecholaminergic pathways.

Finally, we have observed that the intracerebroventricular administration of CRF caused a marked inhibition of GH secretion in freely-moving male rats, while the peripheral injection of the releasing factor was without effect. It is therefore possible that, either CRF acts centrally to inhibit growth-hormone-releasing factor production, or that, since CRF lowers the release of somatostatin (SS) by cultured brain cells, CRF-induced changes in brain levels of SS of intact rats modulate the ability of CRF to lower plasma GH levels *in vivo*. These results indicate that apart from its direct effect on the corticotrophs, CRF can act within the brain to modulate the secretion of LH and GH.

S.192 CLINICAL STUDIES WITH CRF.
D.N. Orth*, C.R. DeBold, G.S. DeCherney, R.V. Jackson, W.R. Sheldon, Jr., W.E. Nicholson, D.P. Island, A.N. Alexander, H. Uderman, W.S. Evans and M.O. Thorner, Departments of Medicine, Vanderbilt Medical Center, Nashville, TN, and University of Virginia Medical Center, Charlottesville, VA, USA.

Ovine corticotropin-releasing factor (oCRF) stimulates immunoreactive (IR)-ACTH and IR-β-endorphin (βEND) release from pituitaries of animals. Our studies were designed to elucidate the physiology and pharmacokinetics of oCRF in man. Synthetic oCRF, generously provided by Drs. J. Rivier and W. Vale, was administered iv to normal volunteers in late afternoon unless otherwise indicated. Subjects remained supine or semirecumbant. Blood was drawn at -15, 0, 2, 5, 10, 15, 30, 60, 90 and 120 min and at hourly intervals thereafter. The threshold dose appeared to be 0.01-0.03 µg/kg, half maximal dose 0.3-1 µg/kg and maximally-effective dose 3-10 µg/kg. Facial flushing, tachycardia and hypotension were observed with increasing frequency, severity and duration at doses of 3-30 µg/kg. Plasma IR-ACTH rose within 2 min after oCRF injection, and plasma IR-cortisol after 10 min or more. Other proopiolipomelanocortin peptides (lipotropins and βEND) were released concomitantly with ACTH. There was no effect on other anterior pituitary hormones. The oCRF response was biphasic and prolonged: IR-ACTH reached a peak at 15 min, fell until 1.5 h, then rose to a second major peak at 2-3 h. IR-cortisol reflected changes in IR-ACTH. After 30 µg/kg oCRF, IR-ACTH remained elevated for 8 h, IR-cortisol for 10 h. The prolonged effect of oCRF is due to its long half-life in blood. IR-oCRF had a triexponential plasma disappearance curve: an initial 6.1 ± 0.5 min distribution $t_{1/2}$ and metabolic $t_{1/2}$s of 55 ± 3.8 and 198 ± 54 min. After 90 min, the molecular size and bioactivity of IR-oCRF in plasma were identical to those of the injected peptide, indicating that it survives intact in blood for a long time. After doses of 3 and 30 µg/kg, the next morning's normal circadian rise in IR-ACTH and IR-cortisol was progressively diminished. This was due to the prolonged hypercortisolemia stimulated by oCRF, since Addisonian patients or normal subjects whose cortisol secretion was blocked with metyrapone had a normal circadian IR-ACTH rise the morning after oCRF. Their plasma IR-ACTH responses were also far greater, indicating that cortisol secreted as the early result of oCRF administration inhibits further ACTH release by oCRF still circulating in the blood. The responses of normal men and women to oCRF were not significantly different. The IR-ACTH increment was identical no matter what time of day oCRF was given, despite variations in basal plasma IR-ACTH, but the IR-cortisol increment was greater in the evening, when basal IR-cortisol was lower. Arginine vasopressin (AVP) 10 U im caused a 2.6x potentiation of the IR-ACTH response to oCRF 1 µg/kg when given 15 min earlier and a 4x potentiation when given simultaneously. The latter response was still somewhat less than the response to hypoglycemic stress. oCRF 1 or 10 µg/kg given at the time of hypoglycemia did not cause a further IR-ACTH increase, suggesting that the response to stress is maximal and probably involves CRF, AVP and possibly other ACTH secretagogues. Glucocorticoid inhibition of oCRF effect depended upon the dose of glucocorticoid and the interval between its administration and that of oCRF. The response of patients with untreated Cushing's disease to oCRF 1 µg/kg was very variable but, after successful transsphenoidal microadenomectomy, was markedly reduced. Thus, the microadenomas in these patients appear to respond to oCRF. However, because of the highly variable response, oCRF probably will not be particularly useful in the differential diagnosis of Cushing's syndrome. It will undoubtedly be useful in diagnosis of other hypothalamic-pituitary disorders. Administered together with GnRH, hpGRF and TRH as a combined anterior pituitary function test, individual anterior pituitary hormone responses were similar to those after injection of the individual peptides. Thus, CRF has both important investigative and potential clinical applications in man.

S.193 REGULATION OF GENE TRANSCRIPTION BY THYROID HORMONE IN CULTURED PITUITARY CELLS: ROLE OF THYROID HORMONE NUCLEAR RECEPTORS.

Barry M. Yaffe, Zebulun D. Horowitz, Juan Casanova and Herbert H. Samuels*, New York University Med. Ctr., N.Y., N.Y.

Using GH_1 cells we have shown that L-triiodothyronine (T3) increases growth hormone (GH) mRNA and also elicits a rapid reduction of receptor by decreasing receptor synthetic rates. In this study we utilized GC cells, a related cell line, to compare the abundance of T3-receptor complexes to the rate of GH mRNA synthesis and gene transcription stimulated by T3. Gene transcription was assessed by in vitro [α-^{32}P]UTP labeling of nuclei derived from cells incubated with hormone, while mRNA synthesis was determined in intact cells by [^{3}H]uridine labeling. Labeled GH mRNA and gene transcripts were quantitated by hybridization to immobilized plasmid containing GH cDNA. T3 decreased nuclear receptor levels in GC cells with kinetics similar to that in GH_1 cells. Within 3 h, T3 stimulated a 10-fold increase in GH mRNA synthesis which then decreased to 3- to 4-fold after 7 to 10 h in parallel with the T3 mediated reduction of receptor. No lag occurred between the kinetics of T3 binding to receptor and stimulation of GH gene transcription. At 30 min, T3-receptor complexes were 74% of the maximum 1 h level while T3 stimulation of transcription was 71% of the maximum 1 h rate. After 1 h, GH gene transcription decreased in parallel with T3-receptor levels. Using [^{3}H]uridine pulse-chase, GH mRNA was found to have a half-life of 50 h in agreement with the decay curve of GH production of deinduced cells. These studies indicate that stimulation of the GH response does not involve GH mRNA stabilization and that the thyroid hormone receptor acts directly to elicit positive control of GH gene transcription which is proportional to the concentration of thyroid hormone-receptor complexes. To study receptor structure we have utilized N-2-diazo-3,3,3-trifluoropropionyl-L-triiodothyronine (T3-PAL) which serves as an effective photoaffinity label probe of the thyroid hormone nuclear receptor in GH_1 cells. Irradiation at 254 nm covalently cross-links [^{125}I]T3-PAL to two nuclear receptor forms; an abundant (75%) 47,000 dalton (47K) component and a less abundant (25%) 57,000 dalton (57K) species. SDS-gel electrophoresis and autoradiography indicates that the 57K form is a doublet which differ in size by 1K to 2K. The various receptor forms are not an artifact of the [^{125}I]T3-PAL probe and identical forms can be labeled at 310 nm using underivatized [^{125}I]T3 with a 50-fold lower coupling efficiency. The 57K and 47K receptors are not identified in the extranuclear compartment. The 57K and 47K receptor forms are not generated by indiscriminate proteolysis, and irradiation at 310 nm indicates that the receptor forms do not result from UV peptide cleavage or zero-length protein-protein cross-linking. Micrococcal nuclease excises both the 57K and 47K forms and neither receptor is localized to the nuclear matrix. Both components show similar affinity for DNA as assessed by DNA-cellulose chromatography. By coupling dense amino acid and photoaffinity labeling of receptor we determined a half-life of 2.4 h for the 57K species and 5.6 h for the 47K form while both species have similar synthetic rates. One mM n-butyrate, which stimulates acetylation of chromatin, increases the 57K form by 25% and decreases the 47K form 50% by decreasing its half-life to 2.8 h. T3 stimulation of growth hormone synthesis and mRNA levels with n-butyrate parallels the abundance of the 57K species. These studies suggest that the 57K receptor form may mediate the action of T3 and may be a precursor of the abundant 47K species which could represent a biologically inactive form of the receptor.

S.194 TRANSPORT AND MOLECULAR ACTION OF TRIIODOTHYRONINE (T_3) AT THE NUCLEAR LEVEL.

J.H. Oppenheimer*, D.B. Jump, C.N. Mariash, H.L. Schwartz, S. Seelig and H.C. Towle, Departments of Medicine, Pediatrics, and Biochemistry, University of Minnesota, Minneapolis, MN 55455, U.S.A.

Nuclear receptors for T_3 play a central role in the initiation of thyroid hormone action. Recent isotopic studies in the intact rat have demonstrated a 40- to 80-fold gradient of free T_3 from cytoplasm to the nucleus in liver, kidney, brain and heart. Free hormone concentrations in the nuclei were estimated from the known fraction of T_3 sites occupied and the association constant of nuclear receptors determined by Scatchard analysis of isolated nuclei incubated at 37°C. These gradients and the preferential accumulation of the L enantiomer of T_3 point to a stereospecific energy-requiring system involved in uphill transport. Although little is known about the immediate events following occupation of nuclear receptors, recent studies involving endonuclease digestion of nuclei show that the receptor (M_r50,500, 3.5 S, Stokes radius 35Å) is a component of a larger discrete chromatin structure (M_r95,400, 5.5-6.0S, Stokes radius 42Å). The T_3 receptor-containing chromatin complex is found in all tissues studied which harbor T_3 receptors. In other studies we have identified specific hepatic mRNA sequences the activities of which are modified by T_3. Two-dimensional gel electrophoresis of *in vitro* translational products of hepatic RNA (mRNA activity profiles) indicate that approximately 8% of the mRNAs seen are influenced by T_3. Eleven sequences are stimulated, 7 inhibited, and 1 displays a biphasic response to T_3. Approximately 40% of the changes observed in hepatic mRNA activity profiles are mediated by L-T_3 induction of pituitary growth hormone. However, as demonstrated both in the intact rat and in primary cultures of adult rat hepatocytes, T_3 also exerts a direct effect on some 50% of the responding sequences. There is also an important interaction between T_3 and a carbohydrate-generated signal at the genomic level, analogous to the previously demonstrated multiplicative interaction of T_3 with carbohydrates in the induction of malic enzyme. The use of mRNA activity profiles allows analysis of sequential alterations of individual mRNA sequences in reponse to T_3. Such studies have identified a mRNA coding for Spot 14 ($mRNA_{S14}$) (pI 4.9, M_r17,500) which rapidly increases 20 mins. after T_3 administration and rises to a level 20-fold above the basal hypothyroid levels within 4 hrs. Administration of a high carbohydrate fat free lipogenic diet also results in a dramatic increase in hepatic $mRNA_{S14}$. The results of translational assays have been confirmed by hybridization studies with a specific cDNA probe to $mRNA_{S14}$. High levels of $mRNA_{S14}$ are found in liver and lactating breast with only small concentrations in heart, brain and spleen where there appears to be little regulation by T_3. A response of $mRNA_{S14}$ analogous to that observed in the liver of intact animals occurs in cultured rat hepatocytes. This finding indicates that the effects of T_3 and carbohydrate are not mediated by metabolic responses of other tissues. Moreover, the rapidity of the $mRNA_{S14}$ response in the liver strongly militates against the possibility that the T_3 effect on $mRNA_{S14}$ is mediated by the stimulation of an antecedent liver protein. Our results indicate that $mRNA_{S14}$ may be a useful model for elucidating T_3 action at the cellular level.

S.195 INFLUENCE OF THYROID HORMONE ON MESSENGER RNA LEVELS IN THE HEART.

W.H. Dillmann*, Department of Medicine, University of California, San Diego. San Diego, California 92103, U.S.A.

The heart is a major target organ for thyroid hormone action; however, influences of thyroid hormones on cardiac mRNA levels have been only incompletely characterized. It has recently been documented that rat ventricular myosin (M) contains three M isoenzymes (MI) (V_1, V_2, V_3) which are comprised of two isoenzymes of myosin heavy chain (MHC). MV_1 contains two MHC-α, MV_2 contains one MHC-α and one MHC-β, and MV_3 contains two MHC-β. In normal (N) rat hearts MV_1 predominates (70% of M), whereas in hypothyroid (Tx) hearts MV_3 predominates (90% of M). To determine if these changes in MI predominance were accompanied by changes in the levels of the mRNAs coding for the corresponding MHCs (N∼MHC-α, Tx∼MHC-β) RNA was isolated from the ventricles of N and Tx rats and translated in a modified rabbit reticulocyte lysate system. Purified in vitro formed MHC was partially digested with chymotrypsin and protease V8 and the generated peptides were separated by S.D.S. gel electrophoresis. The peptide maps of MHCs synthesized in vitro under the direction of N and Tx mRNA showed reproducible differences. These findings indicate therefore that thyroid status related changes in MI predominance are caused by alterations in the levels of the mRNA species coding for MHC-α and MHC-β. Similar thyroid hormone-induced changes in the levels of MHC-α and MHC-β mRNA have been documented in the rat and rabbit heart by other investigators using cDNA probes specific for MHC-α and MHC-β. To determine if thyroid hormones exert an influence on other mRNAs, the translational activity of specific cardiac mRNA was determined by in vitro translation of RNA isolated from the heart of N, Tx, and T_3-injected Tx rats. Proteins synthesized in vitro in the presence of [^{35}S]methionine were separated by two-dimensional gel electrophoresis and quantitated by digital matrix photometry. A total of 421 translational products were detected by fluorography and changes in the predominance of 12 of these were influenced by the thyroid state of the animals. The relative predominance of 8 species was increased in N animals, whereas 4 translational products were increased in Tx animals. The majority of these thyroid hormone-related alterations occurred in spot pairs of similar molecular weights (Mr), but slightly different isoelectric points (pI). In contrast, the relative predominance of mRNAs coding for several major contractile proteins, light chain 1, light chain 2, tropomyosin and actin was not altered by the thyroid status of the animals. In recent experiments Tx rats were injected with T_3 and mRNA levels were quantitated 3, 5 and 24 h after T_3 administration. Two mRNAs (spot 71-72, Mr 81,000, pI 5.54 and 5.50) which were markedly decreased in Tx rats were significantly increased 3 h after T_3 administration, while mRNAs coding for proteins increased in Tx rats were not affected at 3 h (spot 247: Mr 35,000, pI 6.02; spot 253: Mr 33,000, pI 6.24). However, 24 h after T_3 injection the two latter spots were decreased to levels found in N rats.

In vivo effects of thyroid hormone on cardiac RNA levels are complex. In addition to a general increase in total RNA and mRNA levels, increases or attenuations in the predominance of a small number of specific mRNA species including those coding for MHC-α and MHC-β are observed when normal and hypothyroid animals are compared. A subset of these mRNAs respond rapidly to T_3 administration.

S.196 ONTOGENESIS OF THYROID HORMONE RECEPTORS.

J. Bernal*, Departamento de Endocrinologia Experimental, C.S.I.C Facultad Autonoma de Medicina, Madrid-34. Spain.

According to present views on thyroid hormone action, the sensitivity of a given tissue to thyroid hormone is determined primarily by the concentration of nuclear T_3 receptors. The study of receptor appearance during ontogenesis is important since it would define what tissues are potential targets of thyroid hormone during fetal life. This is specially relevant in the case of the human brain. Thyroid hormone plays an essential role in brain development, but there are uncertainties as to whether intrauterine brain maturation is dependent on thyroid hormone. Nuclear receptors for T_3 have been found in fetal tissues from rabbit, rat and human, and in chick embryos In the rat, high concentrations of nuclear T_3 receptor have been found in the cerebrum 2 days before birth. According to the stage of brain development, this would correspond to the fourth month of intrauterine life in the case of the human fetus.

In the human brain, the T_3 receptor is present at 10 weeks of gestation at a low concentration, 46 fmol/mg DNA, a figure similar to that of cells considered to be little or non responsive to thyroid hormones, such as peripheral blood mononuclear cells. The concentration of receptor increases progressively at 12 and 16 weeks by factors of six and ten, respectively, without changes of affinity. During the same period, the brain experiences a rapid cell proliferation, as indicated by 80 times increases of the total brain DNA. The receptor in fetal brain and liver shows the following order of analog binding affinity: triac > L-T_3 > L-T_4 > rT_3, which is identical to the analog binding specificity displayed by the rat liver receptor.

Other human fetal organs also contain T_3 receptors, namely liver, heart and lung, at 16-18 weeks of gestation.

The only presence of receptor does not, by itself, ensures that these tissues are dependent on thyroid hormone. In particular, tissue concentrations of T_3 might be too low to account for a significant degree of receptor occupancy. Although the timing of receptor appearance in the brain seems to parallel the development of the thyroid gland, it is known that the main product of the fetal thyroid gland is T_4 , and that little, if any, T_3 is formed periferally from T_4 in fetal tissues. Plasma T_3 is undetectable before the 30th week of gestation, and its concentration is low until birth. To investigate this problem further, levels of T_4 and T_3 were measured in fetal tissues. In brain, both, T_4 and T_3 were present. However, in other organs, only T_4 could be detected. These results suggest that the development of thyroid hormone sensitivity is dependent, at least, on two factors. First the appearance of nuclear receptor, which in some organs (liver, lung and heart) has the significance of an anticipatory mechanism, preceeding the neonatal surge of T_3. Second, the development of tissue 5'-deiodinases, which would make possible the production of local T_3 from T_4. The coordination of these two mechanisms would account for a differential timing of appearance of tissue sensitivity to thyroid hormones during development. The signal triggering receptor appearance in fetal tissues is not known.

S.197 POSTRECEPTOR MECHANISMS AND THYROID HORMONE ACTION. L.J. DeGroot*, The University of Chicago, Chicago, IL USA

If thyroid hormone (T_3) works via nuclear receptors (R), it may do so by causing an alteration in the physical state or compartmentalization of the R, altering binding to chromatin, altering its function as a receptor for phosphorylation, or dissociation of inhibitor. T_3 might cause allosteric activation of an enzymatic function of R. Conceding primacy to the action of R via transcription, the sequence of events may start with "zero order" effects as direct effects on transcription followed by "first order" responses such as increased polymerase activity, "second order" responses such as increased transcriptional products, "third order" reactions such as increased translational products, and "fourth order" responses such as increased gross metabolic and clinical effects. Recent investigations on "third order" responses emphasize formation of Na+, K+ ATPase, liver phosphoenylpyruvate carboxykinase, and glucokinase, and increased GH, malic enzyme, and α-glycerophosphate dehydrogenase. Cardiac myosin isozyme distribution is altered. These responses are blocked by agents such as α-amanitin and cycloheximide. T_3 causes an increase in one nuclear globulin and may cause 67 of 500 identifiable liver protein subunits to be increased. Cytosolic and nuclear protein kinase (PK) is altered within a few hours of administration of thyroid hormone, and the pattern of protein phosphorylation is altered. The changes in phosphorylation of cytosolic protein appear to be dependent upon increased activity of casein kinase. Both phosphorylation and dephosphorylation are stimulated. Phosphorylation of pyruvate kinase and acetyl-co-A-carboxykinase are seen. These changes are inhibited by cycloheximide and are probably "third order". "Second order" responses include detection of new mRNA for GH, $\alpha\text{-}_{1}\mu$globulin, albumin, and malic enzyme occurring within 8 hours after T_3 administration to hypothyroid (H) animals. New mRNA synthesis occurs within 10 min of exposure of T_3 to an H rat; possibly this activity is inhibited by cycloheximide. Increased transcriptional products imply increased transcription, and liver and brain polymerase are possibly increased within 1-1/2 hours of administration of T_3. Increased liver nuclear polymerase activity occurs 3-8 hours after T_3, but this must be preceded by other polymerase activity as noted above. Template capacity is not increased at 12 hours by T_3, but is increased in normal animals as compared to H animals, apparently representing a more delayed effect of T_3. Nuclear PK activity with casein and protamine substrates is increased 1-1/2 hours after T_3, and increased phosphorylation of nuclear proteins has been reported. Increased DNA digestibility of chromatin is caused by T_3. Possibly all of these phenomena, including ADP ribosylation and nuclear protein phosphorylation, cause alterations in template availability or polymerase function. Polymerase subunits are substrates for PK, and their activities are altered by phosphorylation. Phosphorylation of histones may alter the ability of polymerase to read genes. While most attention is focused on a direct effect of T_3-R on transcription, it is possible that, concomitantly, there are T_3-R induced alterations in phosphorylation, acetylation, and ribosylation, which may also have direct effects on transcription and may be, in the classification scheme above, "zero order" actions of the hormone.

S.198 CENTRAL AMINES AND NEUROPEPTIDES THAT REGULATE SYMPTHOADRENAL NEURONS

R. Elde*, Department of Anatomy, University of Minnesota, Minneapolis, Min. 55455, U.S.A.

Preganglionic sympathetic neurons whose cell bodies and dendrites lie within the intermediolateral cell column of the thoracic spinal cord integrate input from a variety of brain areas and thereby regulate activity within sympathetic ganglia and the adrenal medulla. We have studied a discrete subpopulation of these preganglionic sympathetic neurons which project to and regulate the adrenal medulla. The fluorescent dye fast blue was injected into the adrenal medulla and was transported retrogradely to the cell bodies of origin. These sympathoadrenal neurons lie as clusters of cells among the general population of sympathetic preganglionic neurons. Major synaptic input to the sympathoadrenal neurons is derived from several supraspinal sites. The neurotransmitters contained within these input systems include substance P, serotonin, norepinephrine, the enkephalins, dynorphin, somatostatin and oxytocin. The region of the intermediolateral cell column contains high densities of binding sites for numerous neurotransmitters. However, alpha-2 adrenergic and serotonergic binding sites were autoradiographically localized in even higher concentrations over the fast blue-marked, sympathoadrenal neurons. Muscarinic cholinergic and μ opiate binding sites were not enriched over sympatoadrenal neurons. Thus, central serotonergic and noradrenergic systems are likely to be important regulators of sympathetic activity important to adrenomedullary regulation.

S.199 ENKEPHALINS IN THE ADRENAL MEDULLA: REGULATION OF SYNTHESIS AND PROCESSING BY CATECHOLAMINES AND cAMP IN CULTURED BOVINE CHROMAFFIN CELLS AND BY SPLANCHNIC INNERVATION IN THE RAT. C.D. Unsworth, S.P. Wilson and O.H. Viveros*, Dept. of Medicinal Biochemistry, The Wellcome Research Labs., Research Triangle Park, NC 27709 and Dept. of Pharmacology, Duke University Medical Center, Durham, NC 27710, U.S.A.

The mammalian adrenal medulla contains large amounts of opioid peptides (OP) derived from proenkephalin A. Total opioid peptides (TOP) can be measured by the displacement of radiolabeled [D-ala^2,D-leu^5]enkephalin from rat brain membrane receptors by tissue or cell extracts treated with trypsin and carboxypeptidase B. The native opioid peptide activity (NOP) in the untreated extracts is due mainly to met- and leu-enkephalin and the difference between TOP and NOP, or cryptic opioid peptides (COP), is an estimate of the amount of precursor present in the extracts. Addition of cAMP to bovine chromaffin cells in primary culture, activation of cell adenylate cyclase by forskolin or inhibition of cyclic nucleotide phosphodiesterase increased both NOP and COP in a dose and time dependent manner. These effects could be obtained in the absence of significant changes in protein or cellular catecholamine (CA) content. Depletion of total CA in the cultures by a variety of treatments that do not induce secretion of OP or of other chromaffin vesicle components (reserpine, tetrabenazine, inhibitors of CA synthesis enzymes) increased cellular NOP and TOP but not of COP. These effects were roughly proportional to the depletion of cellular CA but had no apparent relation to extracellular CA levels nor were OP affected by the addition of adrenergic receptor agonists or antagonists to the culture medium. Apparently these agents do not increase the cellular content of cAMP, nor did they decrease the spontaneous or the stimulated release of OP to the medium. These results suggest that both decreases in some intracellular CA pool and elevation of cellular cAMP may trigger increases in the synthesis and processing of OP in adrenomedullary cells. Several reports have shown an apparent increase in adrenomedullary OP in the rat after unilateral splanchnic denervation, thus suggesting a different mechanism for the regulation of adrenomedullary enkephalins in this species. After 3 hr of increased neurogenic stimulation by insulin hypoglycemia adrenomedullary NOP had decreased to 10% of original values (7.08 ± 1.20 and 1.04 ± 0.08 pmole/pair for control COP and NOP, respectively). Values were completely recovered 48 hr later, had increased to 2.5 times control at day 3 and were still doubled after 14 days. COP decreased initially to a lesser extent than NOP, then increased 3-fold compared to untreated controls by day 3. This increase in COP clearly preceded the rise in NOP. Unilateral adrenal denervation resulted in an immediate fall in OP of both glands as a result of the surgical stress. CA and NOP reached their lowest values at 24 hr, recovered in the left denervated gland by 48 hr but right adrenomedullary NOP recovered only between 7 and 14 days. COP in the right gland decreased by 24 hr and was normal by 14 days but never increased over initial values. Left adrenal COP had increased 5-fold 48 hr after surgery. The pattern of NOP and COP changes in the denervated gland was similar to that produced from the short reflex neurogenic stimulation induced by the 3 hr of insulin hypoglycemia. Since neurogenic stimulation produces both a decrease in adrenomedullary CA levels due to secretion and an increase in cAMP the same mechanisms shown to affect OP synthesis and processing in culture may regulate these processes *in vivo*.

S.200 VASOACTIVE INTESTINAL POLYPEPTIDE(VIP)-MUSCARINIC RECEPTOR INTERACTIONS.

Britta Hedlund*, Janis Abens, Anita Westlind and Tamas Bartfai, Department of Biochemistry, Arrhenius Laboratory, University of Stockholm, S-106 91 Stockholm, Sweden.

In nerve endings of the postganglionic nerve innervating the cat and rat submandibular salivary gland, it has been shown that acetylcholine coexists with VIP, vasoactive intestinal polypeptide.

In membranes from the rat salivary gland a number of mutual interactions take place between occupied muscarinic receptors and VIP-receptors. 1). VIP, in nanomolar concentrations, increases the time the muscarinic receptor is in a high affinity conformation. This receptor conformation is most likely the one coupled to the secretory response. Longer incubation times shifts the muscarinic receptor towards a conformation with lower affinity for agonists. 2) Occupancy of muscarinic receptors by either agonists or antagonists (!!) enhances the VIP-mediated stimulation of adenylate cyclase in a GTP-dependent manner. 3). VIP attenuates the muscarinic receptor mediated increase in cGMP levels. Atropine and oxotremorine affect the binding of ^{125}I-VIP to VIP-receptors. Atropine, in nanomolar concentrations, does most likely act as a noncompetitive inhibitor of ^{125}I-VIP binding. These effects are easiest studied in membranes from cerebral cortex.

Chronic treatment of rats with the muscarinic antagonist atropine, 20 mg/kg for 14 days s.c., results in a muscarinic supersensitivity, measured as an increased number of receptors, in all tissues tested. Furthermore, the tissue levels of VIP in the submandibular salivary gland are virtually depleted and the number of ^{125}I-VIP binding sites increased. The same treatment also induced an increase in the number of VIP-receptors in the cerebral cortex, where coexistence of VIP and acetylcholine has not yet been reported, but the presence of both VIP and acetylcholine is known.

The results indicate widespread interactions between VIP receptors and muscarinic receptors.

S.201 PEPTIDE AND AMINE INTERACTIONS IN CENTRAL NERVOUS SYSTEM (CNS) AND PITUITARY FUNCTIONS: FUNCTIONAL AND CLINICAL ASPECTS.

W.H. Rostène* and G. Charpentier
INSERM U.55, Hôpital Saint-Antoine, 75012 Paris, France

In spite of extensive research, current notions about peptide-amine interactions remain far from satisfactory and many discrepancies are due to the complex neural circuits which control physiological responses and to the various ways in which a peptide exhibits its effects on aminergic transmission. We will try to illustrate, by means of one particular neuropeptide, the Vasoactive Intestinal Peptide (VIP), how a peptide can influence the activity of aminergic systems (serotoninergic (5HT), cholinergic and dopaminergic (DA)) in CNS and anterior pituitary functions.

One possibility for a neurotransmitter/modulatory role of VIP is that the peptide may regulate aminergic neurotransmission through an action on specific enzymatic activities which lead to the synthesis of the neurotransmitter. For instance, VIP is able to stimulate the activity of 5HT-N-acetyltransferase in the pineal gland as well as tyrosine hydroxylase in the superior cervical ganglion and choline-acetyltransferase in the anterior hypothalamus and in the hippocampus. VIP may also modulate transmitter receptor sensitivity at the postsynaptic level. By means of isolated membrane preparations and/or <u>in vitro</u> binding of ^{3}H-5HT on brain sections coupled with visualization by quantitative autoradiography, we showed that VIP alters the binding of ^{3}H-5HT to $5HT_1$ receptors in the suprachiasmatic nucleus (SCN) and in the dorsal subiculum of the hippocampus. VIP may also increase the release of 5HT from the SCN, an other way of peptide-amine interactions. The importance of the endocrine environment for these modulatory effects of VIP will be discussed.

On the other hand, VIP release from the hypothalamus into the hypophyseal portal blood is stimulated by 5HT which may explain the stimulatory effect of both substances on prolactin (PRL) secretion. In the pituitary, DA is able to counteract VIP-stimulation of PRL release, an effect which probably takes place on the coupling of VIP receptors with adenylate cyclase (AC) activity. <u>In vivo</u> administration of VIP in normal women and in patients with prolactinoma suggests an impairment of the PRL response in prolactinomas. However, the stimulatory effect of VIP is restored when patients are treated with DA in order to lower PRL secretion. Moreover, VIP is only able to stimulate AC activity if AC levels are previously decreased by DA. Modulatory peptides can thus exhibit, under various endocrine conditions, multiple effects on aminergic transmission in both CNS and pituitary functions, which result in refined physiological responses.

S.202 CHARACTERIZATION OF NORADRENERGIC AFFERENTS TO HYPOTHALAMIC MAGNOCELLULAR NEURONS.

L.P. Renaud*, T.A. Day, J.C.R. Randle, C.W. Bourque and A.V. Ferguson, Neurosciences Unit, Montreal General Hospital and McGill University, Montreal, Quebec, H3G 1A4, Canada.

The hypothalamic supraoptic (SON) and paraventricular (PVN) magnocellular vasopressinergic and oxytocinergic neurosecretory neurons both receive a dense catecholamine innervation. Recent anatomical studies indicate that fibers to SON arise almost exclusively from the A1 noradrenergic neurons in the ventrolateral medulla, while those to PVN arise from A1, A2 and A6 noradrenergic neurons (Sawchenko & Swanson, Brain Res. Rev. 4, 275-325, 1982). In order to clarify noradrenaline's role in regulating the release of neurohypophyseal hormones, we have utilized electrophysiological methods to examine the effects of A1 and A2 noradrenergic afferents on the excitability of SON and PVN neurosecretory neurons and the influence of exogenously applied noradrenaline on the activity and membrane properties of SON neurons.

Extracellular recordings in pentobarbital anesthestized male Sprague-Dawley rats reveal that electrical stimulation in A1 exerts a selective activation of the majority (80%) of putative vasopressinergic neurons while most putative oxytocinergic cells are inhibited (15%) or unresponsive (85%). The effects of electrical stimulation in A1 can be mimicked by the direct application of low concentrations(100 µM) of noradrenaline to these cells. In contrast, A2 stimulation enhances the firing of 60% of PVN vasopressinergic neurons and 70% of PVN oxytocinergic cells. In each nucleus, neurosecretory neurons recorded 24 hrs after pretreatment with 6-hydroxydopamine, sufficient to abolish the endogenous catecholamine histofluorescence, display no response to stimulation in either A1 or A2 regions, but continue to respond to activation of peripheral baroreceptors.

Recordings from SON neurons maintained in-vitro in a perfused hypothalamic explant indicate that 85% of neurons are activated by bath or pressure application of noradrenaline and the α-adrenergic agonist methoxamine, but not the β-adrenergic agonist isoproterenol. At threshold concentrations (10 µM) insufficient to induce an increase in firing, SON neurons demonstrate increased bursting behaviour; higher concentrations (up to 100 µM) increase the overall firing rate with the appearance of both bursting and phasic activity. During intracellular recordings, the effects are associated with membrane depolarization but are not accompanied by any consistent change in membrane conductance, and can be blocked by the α-adrenergic antagonist prazosin (12 nM).

Although it is commonly held that noradrenaline decreases vasopressin release, these in-vivo and in-vitro data argue for a predominantly facilitatory action of noradrenaline on the excitability of neurosecretory neurons, mediated through an α-adrenoreceptor. In both the SON and PVN, the neural circuitry favors a selective A1 projection to vasopressinergic cells; in PVN, the A2 input appears to be distributed to both oxytocinergic and vasopressinergic neurons. This research was supported by the MRC, FRSQ and AHFMR.

S.203 PATTERNS OF ELECTRICAL ACTIVITY AND HORMONE RELEASE FROM NEUROSECRETORY CELLS. G. Leng* and R.J. Bicknell, AFRC Institute of Animal Physiology, Babraham, Cambridge, CB2 4AT, U.K.

The release of oxytocin and vasopressin from nerve terminals in the neurohypophysis is determined primarily by the electrical activity of the neurosecretory neurones in the supraoptic and paraventricular nuclei of the hypothalamus. The vasopressin and oxytocin cells in these nuclei evolve distinctive patterns of activity during physiological conditions associated with hormone release: we have sought to establish the significance of this patterning for stimulus-secretion coupling at the neurosecretory terminals.

The vasopressin cells are osmoreceptors, and dehydration, which demands a high and continuing release of vasopressin for antidiuresis, causes each vasopressin cell to discharge "phasically": periods of electrical discharge at 8-15Hz for 20-40s are separated by periods of electrical silence. This phasic activity does not lead to pulsatile hormone release into the circulation as the phasic discharge of neighbouring neurones is not synchronised. Instead, the purpose of the phasic activity appears to be to optimise the amount of hormone released by each action potential. From in vitro studies of secretion from the rat neurohypophysis we have shown that continued electrical stimulation of the terminals does not produce sustained high levels of secretion. During regular 13Hz electrical stimulation, the release of vasopressin is subject to a dramatic fatigue: more than 50% of the vasopressin released by 20 min of stimulation is released within the first 2 min, and analysis of the total hormone released by brief periods of stimulation suggests that the highest rates of release are only sustained for 20-40s. However brief silent periods (of 30s duration) enable the terminals to recover from this fatigue. Thus the pattern of activation of vasopressin neurones appear to be ideally matched to the demands of effective stimulus-secretion coupling at the terminals. Similar phasic patterning has been observed in other secretory cells, including pancreatic B cells: it remains to be seen whether the same explanation holds true for other phasic cells.

Whereas vasopressin secretion must be maintained at a high tonic level, oxytocin secretion is markedly pulsatile during suckling, to produce repeated, abrupt contractions of the mammary gland to effect milk let-down. The background electrical discharge of oxytocin cells is slow and asynchronous, but suckling-induced reflex milk-ejection is characterised by brief, synchronous discharge at a high frequency (40-80Hz for 2-4s), probably involving every oxytocin cell in the hypothalamo-neurohypophysial system. The different secretory requirements for oxytocin are reflected by the different electrophysiological characteristics, but again the patterns of nerve activation are optimally efficient for releasing oxytocin in a way that achieves effective contraction of the mammary gland. The neural mechanisms responsible for the bursting behaviour are not established, but lactation is accompanied by morphological changes within the hypothalamus which may modify direct or indirect communication between oxytocin cells to provide the basis for orchestrated activation.

S.204 CENTRAL ELECTROPHYSIOLOGIC CORRELATES OF PULSATILE LUTEINIZING HORMONE SECRETION IN THE RHESUS MONKEY. R.C. Wilson* and E. Knobil, University of Texas Medical School, Departments of Neurobiology and Anatomy and Physiology and Cell Biology, Houston, TX 77025, USA

In the rhesus monkey, as in other mammals, luteinizing hormone (LH) is secreted from the pituitary gland in discrete circhoral pulses as a consequence of the periodic secretion of hypothalamic luteinizing hormone releasing hormone (LHRH) into the pituitary portal circulation. LHRH release is governed, in turn, by a neuronal "pulse generator" resident in the medial basal hypothalamus (MBH). Our preliminary attempts to monitor the electrical activity of this LHRH pulse generator using single electrodes acutely placed into the MBH of ovariectomized rhesus monkeys occasionally yielded evidence of striking increases in hypothalamic multiple unit activity (MUA) synchronous with LH pulses in the peripheral circulation. Subsequent studies, using multiple electrodes chronically implanted in the MBH, have confirmed those initial observations and have permitted characterization of this unique and reproducible MUA pattern.

In 16 of 21 animals chronically implanted with multiple electrodes, dramatic and characteristic increases in hypothalamic MUA were recorded in conjunction with the initiation of LH pulses. Typically, in awake animals restrained in primate chairs, these periodic MUA volleys took the form of a square wave with an initial "overshoot" on the ascending limb. This overshoot ranged in magnitude from 50-500% of baseline and declined precipitously within 1-2 min to enter a plateau phase of still markedly increased activity lasting 5-15 min. Variations of this pattern were occasionally observed including the absence of a plateau phase with the initial overshoot returning directly to baseline and the appearance of additional spikes of activity during the plateau phase, most typically just prior to its termination. The onset of circhoral MUA volleys was invariably followed, within 2-5 min, by a rise in plasma LH concentration. Barbiturate anesthesia decreased the frequency of the MUA volleys to one every 2-3 h and prolonged the duration of the plateau phase to approximately 30 min. α-adrenergic blocking agents such as phenoxybenzamine and prazosin also slowed the frequency of the MUA volleys but did not increase the duration of the MUA rise. These pharmacologic treatments did not alter the exclusive association of LH pulses with the characteristic MUA volleys.

We conclude that the dramatic increase in neural traffic accompanying the initiation of each plasma LH pulse reflects the activation of a hypothalamic pulse generator which controls LHRH secretion. The neuronal origin of the pulse generator and the mechanisms which govern its rhythmic activation and deactivation remain to be investigated.

Supported by NIH grants HD03968 and HD08610 to E.K.

S.205 INTRACELLULAR RECORDINGS FROM NORMAL PITUITARY CELLS: REGULATION OF ELECTRICAL EVENTS LEADING TO HORMONE RELEASE BY HYPOPHYSIOTROPIC PEPTIDES.

W.T. Mason*, C.D. Ingram, R.J. Bicknell and D.W. Waring, ARC Institute of Animal Physiology, Babraham, Cambridge CB2 4AT UK

The secretion of hormones by cells of the anterior pituitary gland is controlled by hypothalamic peptides secreted into the portal blood. Electrophysiological study of the 'target' pituitary cells has not generally been possible because of tissue heterogeneiety. Most workers have used clonal pituitary tumour cell lines, and some of these generated action potentials. However, early work on normal pituitary cells suggested that most did not generate action potentials. The role of electrical events in stimulus-secretion coupling in normal pituitary cells has thus been an elusive topic. However, recent work has suggested that a small percentage of pituitary cells, putative mammotrophs and melanotrophs, may generate action potentials.

Recent work in this laboratory has centred on the electrophysiology *in vitro* of two purified pituitary cell types. Firstly, gonadotrophs containing luteinizing-(LH) and follicle stimulating-hormone (FSH) have been isolated from the ovine pars tuberalis which contains gonadotrophs as the exclusive hormone-secreting cell type. Secondly, we have prepared purified bovine somatotrophs by a Percoll density gradient procedure. Gonadotrophs isolated by enzymatic dispersion and maintained in culture secrete LH in response to the peptide gonadotrophin releasing hormone (GnRH) under conditions in which our electrophysiological recordings have been made.

Intracellular recordings made from both cell types indicate that injection of depolarising current activates a voltage-dependent Ca^{+2} conductance which causes a graded, non-regenerative, 3-5 msec depolarisation, but spontaneous activity in the form of all-or-none action potentials is never observed. Our work has therefore been directed at mechanisms whereby hormone might be released in the absence of action potentials.

GnRH applied to gonadotrophs does not elicit all-or-none action potentials, but induces membrane voltage fluctuations in 95% of tested cells. Power spectra of this 'noise' indicate that GnRH activates long duration (30-40 msec), Ca^{+2}-dependent ion channels. These spectra fit a single Lorentzian indicating that such channels are the main contribution to agonist-evoked membrane noise. Preliminary experiments with somatotrophs suggest they behave in a qualitatively similar fashion, in that GRF elicits 2 to 10 fold increases in the variance of voltage noise. GRF induces Ca^{+2}-dependent voltage fluctuations of varying amplitude and duration, up to 30 mV magnitude and 10-500 msec duration.

Our results suggest that hormone release by normal pituitary gonadotrophs and somatotrophs can occur in the absence of action potentials, and the hypophysiotrophic peptidergic agonists for release of LH, FSH and GH act to evoke discrete conductance fluctuations indicative of the opening of ionic channels. These agonist-induced channels may play a role in the initial stage of stimulus-secretion coupling leading to hormone release and could prove to be a general signal in the electrophysiological control of pituitary hormone secretion.

This work was supported in part by Burroughs Wellcome Foundation.

Meet-the-Professor Sessions

MP.1 INFERTILITY IN THE FEMALE. B. Lunenfeld*, D. Vardimon, B. Goldstein, World Health Organization Collaborating Center for Research on Fertility Promoting Agents, Institute of Endocrinology, Chaim Sheba Medical Center, Tel Hashomer, Israel.

The possibilities for classifying and treating the infertile couple are virtually unlimited. Thus the striking lack of uniformity in the process by which these couples are evaluated and treated. Because of the historical variability of the infertility workup, comparison of data from different investigations and treatment schemes has seldom been appropriate, and our ability to properly assess the relative merits of each has been poor. Coordinated multicentered research using standardized procedures helps to clarify many issues, as well as to improve diagnostic precision and the results of subsequent management in terms of effectiveness, cost and risk. In this session we will attempt: 1) Tc describe the components for a rational workup of the couple complaining of infertility. 2) Propose standardized definition of diagnostic categories. 3)Present algorithmic flow charts for arriving with optimal cost effectiveness of different therapeutically oriented diagnostic entities. 4)Suggest the treatment of choice as well as alternative treatments for specific diagnostic groups (see table). Note that the couple must be considered as a single unit since each partner contributes a share to the fertility potential of the other. Management of one partner only, may therefore in some instances delay the recognition and possible therapy of the fertility problem of the other partner and decrease the cost or time effectiveness of the management of the couple.

—ETIOLOGICAL DIAGNOSIS AND SUGGESTIONS FOR TREATMENT OF CHOICE OR ALTERNATIVE TREATMENT

ETIOLOGICAL DIAGNOSIS	TREATMENT OF CHOICE	ALTERNATIVE TREATMENT
Gonadotropic insufficiency due to pituitary or hypothalamic insufficiency	Menotropins (HMG) followed by HCG	LH–RH (pulsatile)
Impaired hypothalamic-pituitary responsiveness and/or function:		
Inappropriate sensitivity of the hypothalamic pituitary system to feedback signal.	Clomiphene Citrate (CC)	CC + HCG CC + Estrogens HMG/HCG
Impaired pituitary responsiveness secondary to excessive prolactin secretion	Ergoline derivatives (ED) (bromocriptine, lysuride, metergoline)	ED + CC ED + HMG/HCG HMG/HCG
Impaired hypothalamic/ pituitary responsiveness and/or function by inappropriate secretion of adrenal steroids	Corticosteroids (COR)	COR + CC COR + HMG/ HCG
Impaired hypothalamic-pituitary responsiveness and/or function induced by inappropriate secretion of ovarian steroids	Cyproterone acetate and estrogen for six months followed by CC or HMG/HCG, or FSH.	Wedge resection
Impaired hypothalamic-pituitary responsiveness and/or function due to primary hypothyroidism	Thyroid hormone or their analogues (TH)	TH + CC TH + HMG/HCG

MP.2 DISORDERS OF WATER METABOLISM - Meet the Professor Session. Alan G. Robinson, M.D.*, Division of Endocrinology and Metabolism, School of Medicine, University of Pittsburgh, Pittsburgh, PA, 15261, USA.

This session will be primarily for questions and answers regarding the role of vasopressin in disorders of water balance. Recent evidence has proven conclusively that vasopressin is synthesized as part of a prohormone consisting of vasopressin, vasopressin-neurophysin, and a glycopeptide. While the classical system of the neurohypophysis for secretion of vasopressin into the peripheral blood is still thought to consist of the supraoptic nucleus, the paraventricular nucleus, and the supraopticohypophyseal tract to the posterior pituitary, it is now clear that vasopressin is also released at the median eminence, into cerebrospinal fluid, and as a neurotransmitter in diffuse areas of the central nervous system. The predominant regulation of vasopressin release is through the osmoreceptors which are close to the magnocellular neurons which synthesize vasopressin, but which are separated by at least one synapse. Acetylcholine and angiotensin may work as independent neurotransmitters in osmoreceptor regulation of vasopressin secretion. The concept of volume receptors has been expanded in recent years to include all "non-osmotic" regulation of vasopressin release. While the diseases of the neurohypophysis are opposites (diabetes insipidus with hypernatremia and SIADH with hyponatremia), pathogenic mechanisms for the two are similar and include tumors, trauma, infiltrative lesions of the hypothalamus, vascular lesions, pulmonary disease, infectious diseases, metabolic disorders, and a variety of drugs. Diabetes insipidus can usually be diagnosed by standard indirect tests with dehydration and response to administered vasopressin - providing true hyperosmolality is achieved with the dehydration. Primary polydipsia may be difficult to distinguish from partial diabetes insipidus and in this situation measured vasopressin is useful. Measured vasopressin is especially helpful in the diagnosis of nephrogenic diabetes insipidus where the levels are diagnostic. Variants of diabetes insipidus which produce special clinical problems include diabetes insipidus with inadequate thirst, and absent osmoreceptor function with intact volume receptor function. DDAVP intranasally or parenterally is the treatment of choice for diabetes insipidus although other agents may be used where DDAVP cannot be obtained. Inappropriate secretion of antidiuretic hormone produces hyponatremia. Recent experimental models of SIADH have studied the relative contribution of expanded body water and of natriuresis as the cause of the hyponatremia. Fluid restriction is the primary therapy for SIADH but demeclocycline may be used in chronic situations and acute hypertonic NaCl with diuretics in acute situations. Some recent work has suggested the therapeutic effectiveness of orally administered urea. Abnormally elevated levels of vasopressin have recently been reported in other illnesses with abnormal retention of water including cirrhosis, congestive heart failure, adrenal insufficiency, and myxedema. New antagonists to the antidiuretic effect of vasopressin may help in the elucidation of the exact role which vasopressin plays in the pathophysiology of these disorders.

MP.3 NEW DEVELOPMENTS IN HORMONAL FEMALE CONTRACEPTION. C. Wayne Bardin, The Population Council, 1230 York Avenue, New York, New York 10021 USA

A large fraction of women are sufficiently dissatisfied with their present method of contraception that they would be willing to change to a new method were it available. The questions most frequently asked by these women are, "when will something new be available?" and "will it be safe?". It is the goal of this seminar to review new contraceptive technologies with regard to effectiveness, mechanism of action, availability to the public, and major and minor side effects compared to existing methods.

The most recently approved contraceptive technology is the Norplant[R] subdermal implant system. This five year method is based on the continuous release of levonorgestrel (30μg/day) from subcutaneously placed capsules. This is one of the most effective methods yet devised with cumulative pregnancy rates of 1% after 3 years and 2.7% after 5 years. No serious side effects have been detected in over 7,000 women that have used this method in 14 countries. Menstrual irregularities like those associated with all progestin only methods occur, but do not usually result in discontinuation when women are told what to expect prior to acceptance. These implants inhibit ovulation and thicken cervical mucous making sperm penetration difficult. When implants are removed there is return to fertility at the same rate as following discontinuation of barrier contraception.

Contraceptive vaginal rings have been developed by several organizations, and should be ready for introduction in 1-3 years. Some rings deliver continuous low dose progestin and may not block ovulation; others deliver estrogen and progestin in doses sufficient to block ovulation. The latter ring is removed monthly to allow for cyclic bleeding. Vaginal rings provide a level of efficacy and continuation rates comparable to the pill. Since the estrogen is not delivered via the splanchnic circulation, the pattern of major and minor side effects should differ from those of the pill.

The effectiveness of an IUD can be improved by the addition of a progestin to the device. The levonorgestrel IUD is now in extended trials. The cumulative pregnancy rate for 5 years is 0.3%. The common side effects associated with IUDs such as bleeding, pain, and infection appear to be reduced with the levonorgestrel device. It is anticipated that the levonorgestrel IUD could be available in 3-5 years.

Novel approaches to contraception for the future are offered by LHRH analogs for ovulation inihibition and antiprogestins for menses induction. Both of these approaches are currently in early clinical trials. Both appear to be free of the side effects associated with current methods.

Conclusion: New contraceptive methods which are safe and effective should be introduced in the next decade.

MP.4 ANOREXIA NERVOSA: A COMPULSIVE BEHAVIOUR DISEASE. Ivor H. Mills, Department of Medicine, University of Cambridge, Addenbrooke's Hospital, Cambridge, CB2 2QQ, England.

Anorexia nervosa is a condition which mainly occurs in young women between 15 and 25 years. It has increased greatly since the early 1960's when the slim image for women became fashionable. Many young females start dieting but only the perfectionists refuse to give in to hunger and develop anorexia. They are, therefore, self-selected for determination. Dieting then becomes compulsive and thoughts of food, weight, size and diet get fixed in their brains like a record-player stuck in a groove. They become incapable of differentiating between the thoughts associated with the compulsive mechanism in the brain and those arising from rational thinking. Compulsive thinking about food and size can only be excluded from the brain by intense concentration on something else. Excessive mental drive produces high arousal which predisposes to compulsive behaviour. About 75% of the young females start "crash dieting" when they are working for examinations: most of the other 25% are trying to cure insoluble social problems, such as broken families. They discover by accident that starvation excites the brain, makes it more active and more efficient (Benedict, 1915, Carnegie Inst., Washington). Later with weight loss the mental body image becomes enlarged and they diet even more strictly to slim down this mental image. When forced to eat they feel guilty to eat when "so fat": in hospital they then hide food or dispose of it or may start vomiting. In 20% they swing to compulsive eating and this is commonly the fore-runner of compulsive vomiting. On our compulsion questionnaire (Medlicott & Mills, 1984) the mean ($\pm$ S.E.) compulsion score for normal young women (controls: $n = 42$) was 13.1 ± 1.1 and for pure anorexics ($n = 34$) 32.1 ± 1.9: $P < 0.005$. In compulsive eating anorexics ($n = 28$) the compulsion score was 35.8 ± 1.9: $P < 0.005$. Treatment was successful in outpatients in 50% by the combination of tricyclic antidepressants and constantly reminding them that if they wish to be able to have a family in the future it is important to make themselves eat NOW. The success of this therapy makes it unlikely that the primary cause of anorexia is fear of the responsibility of sexual maturity. Fighting the compulsion to starve causes depression and they give up without antidepressants. In 30%, a single admission to hospital is sufficient to cure them: 10% leave the clinic because they cannot stand the pressure on them and 10% require repeated admissions. In the severe cases weight gain is greatly accelerated in hospital by continuous intravenous naloxone infusion for many weeks. Plasma non-esterified fatty acids and ß-hydroxybutyrate are reduced to very low levels by this treatment. Without it, excessive rate of weight gain stimulates metabolism (up to a BMR of +30%) and may cause the plasma tri-iodothyronine to rise to hyper-thyroid levels. The role of naloxone in extinguishing the compulsive thinking and learned behaviour is still being assessed. Training the young women to run their lives without the use of starvation to excite their brains is essential for long term cure. With achievement of normal weight, menstruation returns but in 20% ovulation does not occur until clomiphene is administered.

MP.5 OSTEOPOROSIS. R. Lindsay, M.B.Ch.B., Ph.D., M.R.C.P.*, Helen Hayes Hospital, West Haverstraw, New York, and Department of Medicine, Columbia Presbyterian Medical Center, New York City, New York.

Osteoporosis is being increasingly recognized as a major public health problem. Estimates of affected individuals range up to 5 million and above in the U.S.A., and the disorder contributes to at least 300,000 femoral neck fractures per year. In addition to an annual health care cost of $4 billion, these fractures are associated with almost a 10 per cent mortality. Recent evidence indicates that, at least in the U.S.A. and the United Kingdom, osteoporosis prevalence is increasing at a rate in excess of the increments in the at-risk population, for reasons which are currently obscure. The most common variety of osteoporosis, postmenopausal osteoporosis, affects white or caucasian women, generally of higher social class. A positive family history of the disorder is often evident as well as a history of early menopause (or oophorectomy), poor diet and life-style. In the pathogenesis of osteoporosis, dietary factors probably include reduced intake of calcium and excessive intakes of phosphorus and protein. Lifestyle factors include high caffeine intake, cigarette smoking, alcohol abuse, and lack of exercise. Obesity appears to be protective, probably by increasing conversion of adrenal androgens to estrogens in postmenopausal women. Since the introduction of non-invasive methods of measurement of bone mass, it has become evident that bone loss may begin sometime between the ages of 20 and 40 years, with an acceleration in the immediate postmenopausal years. The sexual dichotomy in the presentation of the disorder may result from the lower bone mass at maturity in women as well as this exaggeration of bone loss following ovarian failure. The rate of bone loss in such women depends on remaining sex hormone status and can be prevented by therapy with estrogens or certain progestogens. The mode of action of these sex hormones appears to be normally associated with calcium homeostasis, perhaps through stimulation of calcitonin production. However, a direct non genome dependent action of estrogen on bone cannot be ruled out. Other advice on prevention of bone loss includes increasing calcium intake and exercise. After fracture, treatment becomes more difficult. Standard techniques usually rely on a polypharmaceutical approach with calcium, estrogen, fluoride, vitamin D, and other agents. Newer approaches depend on manipulation of the bone remodeling cycle to obtain a large number of synchronous cycles in which subsequent behavior of osteoclasts can be reduced, allowing osteoblasts to lay down excessive bone with a resulting positive bone balance (so-called "ADFR" approach). The pathogenesis of other forms of osteoporosis, particularly steroid osteoporosis, is also poorly understood, and prevention and therapy are even more difficult to provide. Advances in measurement, developments in the understanding of the pathogenesis of the disease, and new developments in prevention and therapy may revolutionize our approach to this disorder in the coming years.

MP.6 Abstract not received.

MP.7 ENDOCRINE HYPERTENSION. E. G. Biglieri*. San Francisco General Hospital, San Francisco, CA

Excessive production of known and unknown hormones from the adrenal gland is the usual cause of endocrine hypertension. The mineralocorticoid hormones (MCH) aldosterone (A) and deoxycorticosterone (DOC) are both causative and contributory factors to steroid-induced hypertension. Primary aldosteronism due to adenoma (APA) is the index model of MCH excess, with hypertension, hypokalemia, and suppressed renin the hallmarks of the disorder. Primary aldosteronism is also characterized by: increased levels of precursor steroids in peripheral blood, plasma A levels that decrease with upright posture and do not suppress with saline. Computed tomography localizes the tumor in 80%. Extended spironolactone therapy, with normalization of blood pressure, hypokalemia, and renin fails to effect A production only in APA. These features of APA distinguish it from idiopathic hyperaldosteronism (hyperplasia) which is likely not a primary adrenal disorder. A new type of primary aldosteronism due to unilateral or bilateral primary hyperplasia is described with all the above findings of APA. Reduction of adrenal mass produces sustained cures. Glucocorticoid remediable hyperaldosteronism (hyperplasia) is a rare form that reveals a link between the pituitary and an adrenal aberration. DOC excess is the cause of hypertension in the non-virilizing 17α-hydroxylase deficiency syndrome and the virilizing 11β-hydroxylase deficiency. Heterozygotes for 17-hydroxylase deficiency can be identified by the ACTH stimulated divergence of the 18-hydroxycorticosterone:A ratio. DOC levels must be very high to produce hypertension in both. Glucocorticoid insensitivity leads to excess ACTH levels with subsequent stimulation of the zona fasciculata MCH pathway (DOC). In Cushing's disease the same pathway is activated. A still perplexing MCH excess state occurs in children with the biochemical marker being a deficiency of 11-hydroxysteroid dehydrogenase (metabolic conversion of cortisol to cortisone). No causative steroid is identified but dependency in ACTH and the corrective value of spironolactone, indicate a steroid of mixed functions may be present. Recognition and management of these disorders is possible. Unknown MCHs still await identification.

MP.8 Abstract not received.

MP.9 EUTHYROID HYPERTHYROXINEMIA

J.R. Stockigt
Ewen Downie Metabolic Unit, Alfred Hospital, Melbourne 3181, Australia.

The term euthyroid hyperthyroxinemia (EH) indicates that T_4, either total or free, is increased in a euthyroid subject - an imperfect definition in view of difficulty defining the euthyroid state. This difficulty arises because: (i) we still lack a precise, convenient index of thyroid hormone action, and (ii) a normal TSH with normal response to TRH does not always indicate euthyroidism (e.g. in hyperthyroidism due to selective pituitary resistance to T_4). Hence, the diagnosis of EH rests on a combination of clinical and laboratory findings.

EH may be persistent or transient, and may be associated with high, normal or low levels of T_3. In some instances, laboratory artifacts may result in apparent EH. Where possible, the precise reason for T_4 excess should be identified so as to minimize the risk of misdiagnosis in euthyroid individuals or kindreds with EH.

Classification of EH (*indicates that T_3 is usually also increased)
1. Abnormal binding: *excess thyroxine binding globulin; familial dysalbuminemic hyperthyroxinemia (FDH); prealbumin-associated hyperthyroxinemia (PAH); *autoantibody-associated hyperthyroxinemia (AAH).
2.*Generalized hormone-resistance syndromes.
3. Drug-related effects: amiodarone; cholecystographic contrast agents; propranolol; amphetamines.
4. Ingestion of thyroxine.
5. Transient hyperthyroxinemia of psychiatric or other nonthyroidal illness.
6. EH of unknown cause (? defect in cell uptake or deiodination of T_4).

Suggested diagnostic approach to anomalous or unexpected T_4 excess:
1. Clinical re-evaluation, including drug exposure and family history.
2. Assessment of T_3 level, with correction for variations in TBG.
3. Evaluation of the TSH response to TRH.
4. Authentic free T_4 estimate, avoiding methods known to give spurious results in EH.
5. Serial observation. Is the anomaly transient or persistent?
6. Laboratory assessment for unusual binding using appropriate buffer, tracer, serum dilution, added hormone load and separation method. Electrophoretic binding studies will be required to confirm new variants.
7. Family studies to identify others at risk of misdiagnosis.

Diagnostic methods for unusual binding abnormalities:
1. FDH: charcoal uptake of ^{125}I T_4; serum 1:100 + unlabeled T_4 $10^{-6}M$; phosphate buffer. (T_4 excess accentuates binding of a particular capacity).
2. PAH: ^{125}I T_4 immunoprecipitation by anti-prealbumin, or T_4 uptake test as for FDH, using $5x10^{-8}M$ unlabeled T_4 with serum 1:100.
3. AAB: precipitation of ^{125}I T_4 by 15% PEG 6000, or immunoprecipitation with anti-IgG.

Conclusions: The distinction between EH and true thyroid disease depends on clinical perception, valid estimates of free T_4, assessment of the TSH response to TRH and exclusion of known binding abnormalities. Some so-called free T_4 methods are invalid in conditions causing EH. Serial observation is preferable to therapeutic trial where diagnostic doubt persists.

MP.10 RECEPTORS IN BREAST CANCER. W. L. McGuire*, The University of Texas Health Science Center, Department of Medicine/Oncology, 7703 Floyd Curl Drive, San Antonio, Texas 78284, USA.

Site of metastasis is said to be of prognostic importance in recurrent breast carcinoma. Our analysis of estrogen receptors, sites of metastasis, and survival in 431 women with recurrent breast cancer suggests a more complex picture. Estrogen receptor-negative patients recur more frequently in brain and liver than estrogen receptor-positive patients. Regardless of site, estrogen receptor-positive patients survive longer than estrogen receptor-negative patients. Site of metastasis is an important prognostic factor in estrogen receptor-negative patients but is relatively unimportant in estrogen receptor-positive patients. The prognostic importance of ER, progesterone receptor (PgR), and other risk factors were examined in a randomized clinical trial of adjuvant therapy for Stage II breast cancer. Both ER and PgR were significant predictors of prolonged disease-free survival when analyzed separately, independent of the presence of an endocrine component in the adjuvant regimen. However, when ER and PgR were analyzed together in multivariate models, ER was not a significant predictor of recurrence. On the other hand, PgR and the number of positive nodes always remained significant prognostic factors. This implies that the additional knowledge of PgR status may help predict disease-free survival even if ER status is already known, while if PgR levels are available, then the ER status provides little additional prognostic information in this setting. Therefore, it is clear that PgR should be routinely measured and incorporated into future adjuvant therapy trials. A review of assay results from more than 5500 patients revealed 283 patients in whom multiple breast cancer specimens were analyzed for PgR. All assays were performed in a single laboratory between 1975 and 1982 using the sucrose gradient technique. We considered only the 8S fraction of PgR, defining PgR+ = greater than 10 fmol/mg cytosol protein, PgR- = less than 5 fmol/mg protein. Simultaneous assays in 109 patients yielded 14% discordance (one assay PgR+ and one assay PgR-). Among 161 sequential assays there was an overall discordance of 19%: 8% (9/106) when the initial assay was PgR-, but 44% (24/55) when the initial assay was PgR+. Among PgR+ patients initially assayed at the time of diagnosis, there was a tendency to greater receptor loss in patients with positive axillary lymph nodes (44% vs. 11%). The length of time between biopsies did not increase the discordance, but endocrine therapy within this interval did increase it (56% of initially PgR+ patients who received interim endocrine therapy were PgR- at second biopsy). To evaluate the significance of interval loss of PgR, we compared survival from first biopsy in initially PgR+ patients who subsequently lost their receptor, versus those whose receptor persisted. The latter group experienced a significantly longer survival ($p < .02$). In summary, we observed an ominous loss of PgR in sequential biopsies, particularly with intervening endocrine therapy, and those patients whose tumor cells lost PgR experienced poorer survival than patients retaining PgR. Therefore, patients with PgR+ primary tumors require repeat biopsy for PgR upon disease recurrence for optimal treatment planning.

MP.11 INFERTILITY IN THE MALE. E. Nieschlag*, U.A. Knuth, L. Belkien, H. Bents, Max Planck Clinical Research Unit for Reproductive Medicine, Steinfurter Str. 107, D-4400 Münster, F.R. Germany

Male infertility is an extremely frustrating, yet challenging field. First, male infertility is an ill-defined status in terms of diagnostic assessment. Comparison of those men attending an infertility clinic but finally impregnating their wives with such patients who fail to do so shows that there are no seminal or endocrine variables that clearly discriminate between fertile and infertile men (with the exception of azoospermia). Second, infertility is a problem of the couple and female infertility adds another dimension to the evaluation of male infertility. Third, the pathophysiological causes of male infertility are obscure in most cases and thus a rational basis for treatment is lacking. In this dilemma andrologists usually concentrate their therapeutic efforts on the improvement of seminal parameters. However, what does a small yet significant increase in sperm motility from 45 ± 20 to 52 ± 17 % as we could demonstrate in 160 men treated with kallikrein really mean? Similar marginal improvements can be achieved with hormonal treatment such as androgens, antiestrogens or gonadotrophins. As pregnancy rates and not seminal parameters should be the ultimate criterion for evaluating treatment diagnostic procedures to assess sperm function are required. For the first time *in vitro* fertilisation (ivF) makes it possible to assess the fertilizing capacity of sperm directly without the imponderabilities of other female factors. In our experience fertilisation of human ova does indeed correlate well with sperm motility so that it appears most important to obtain highly motile sperm for ivF. Motility may also be most important for the *in vivo* situation and attempts to improve motility may thus be well justified. The results of the heterologous ovum penetration test (HOP-test) using hamster ova shows quite good correlation with the fertilization of human ova so that this test may be used to predict fertility. The elaborate HOP-test can possibly be replaced by simpler techniques such as the "sperm swelling test". The evaluation of current or future forms of treatment should be conducted as controlled clinical trials (randomized and double blind) which require the patients' informed consent and are laborious. The importance of such design is emphasised by a trial we recently performed using high dose testosterone plus hCG in an attempt to overcome presumed androgen resistence: the best response was seen in the placebo group. In addition to rigorous evaluation of medications currently applied, male infertility research requires new impetus which may derive e.g. from ivF and genetics. Otherwise the cynic may prefer to turn to psychotherapy immediately which we now apply as a last resort and - as a pilot study in our clinic showed - with quite good results.

MP.12 NEUROENDOCRINE STRATEGIES IN THE ELUCIDATION OF THE PATHOPHYSIOLOGY OF NEUROPSYCHIATRIC DISORDERS.

Kenneth L. Davis,*[1] and Bonnie M. Davis,[2] [1]Psychiatry Service, VA Medical Center, Bronx, NY and Depts. of Psychiatry and Pharmacology, Mt. Sinai School of Medicine, New York, NY and [2]Medical Service, VA Medical Center, Bronx, NY and Depts. of Medicine and Psychiatry, Mt. Sinai School of Medicine, New York, NY

Attempts to understand the neurotransmitter basis of a series of neuropsychiatric diseases have utilized neuroendocrine parameters in the hope of elucidating the pathophysiology of these diseases. This approach has been used in patients with a diagnosis of depression, schizophrenia and Alzheimer's disease (AD). An overview of the general strategy that investigators have employed, and the kind of data gathered to date will be reviewed. The strengths and weaknesses of the approach will be elaborated. Particular emphasis will be given to the use of the dexamethasone suppression test (DST), neuroendocrine responses to dopaminergic probes and prolonged studies of the secretion of various pituitary hormones. The unique problems that occur when a neuroendocrine strategy is used in neuropsychiatric patients will be discussed.

MP.13 CLINICAL APPLICATIONS OF LHRH AND ITS ANALOGUES. W. Crowley*.
Reproductive Endocrine Unit, Departments of Medicine and Gynecology, Vincent Research Laboratories, Massachusetts General Hospital, Boston, MA 02114.

The pituitary response to LHRH and/or its long-acting agonistic analogues is critically dependent upon the dosage, frequency of administration, and duration of LHRH effect which can be lengthened by LHRH agonists. Pituitary responses can be divided into, a) a 'priming' response which is characterized by continued physiologic secretion of LH and FSH from the anterior pituitary and is evoked by pulsatile administration of the native sequence decapeptide, and b) a 'desensitization' response or a refractoriness of gonadotropin secretion from the pituitary which appears with continued administration of LHRH and/or long-acting LHRH agonists. The physiologic responses can be elicited in those circumstances in which pulsatile replacement of the hypothalamic peptide is undertaken such as induction of ovulation in females and induction of puberty in LHRH deficient males. LHRH agonist-induced desensitization is useful as a non-steroidal contraceptive, a chemical castration therapy of malignancies, a reversible pituitary suppression of gonadotropins in polycystic ovarian disease and endometriosis, and as the only effective therapy of central precocious puberty.

A. Physiologic effects of LHRH. Pulsatile LHRH therapy has been administered to 17 consecutive men with hypogonadotropic hypogonadism by portable Ferring infusion pumps at 2 hour intervals for periods varying from 3-30 months. By means of adjusting the dose of the subcutaneous LHRH it is possible to achieve normal adult testosterone levels in all subjects, a marked increase in their gonadal size, and mature spermatozoa in the ejaculate of 66% of the patients whose pituitary-gonadal has become normalized for greater than 6 months. During therapy it is possible to dissect several aspects of the pubertal process into its various components including pituitary and gonadal amplification and to chronicle these changes during long-term studies. In addition, pulsatile LHRH in a dose of 100 ng/kg used intravenously is capable of inducing ovulation in women with hypothalamic amenorrhea when administered in frequencies of 60-120 minute intervals. Altering the frequency of LHRH administration across the induced menstrual cycle of women with hypothalamic amenorrhea results in restoration of the normal sequence of physiologic events such as folliculogenesis, ovulation, formation of a corpus luteum, and luteolysis.

B. Antifertility effects. Long-term studies of LHRH analogue administration in precocious puberty have demonstrated a complete suppression of pulsatile gonadotropin release during both day and night, an ablation of pituitary responsiveness to exogenous LHRH testing, a restoration of prepubertal growth velocity, striking retardation of skeletal maturation, and improvements in predicted height. Such a reversible suppression of gonadarche also permit a more precise dissection of the normal sequence of pubertal events such as gonadal maturation, adrenarche, and the role of gonadal steroids in the pubertal growth spurt. Conclusions: LHRH and its analogues represent promising new modes of therapy which will impact widely in Reproductive Endocrinology and investigation.

MP.14 **CONGENITAL HYPOTHYROIDISM.** Harvey J. Guyda, Division of Endocrinology, Montreal Children's Hospital, Montreal, Canada.

Newborn screening has proven to be the only systematic approach by which early diagnosis and treatment of congenital hypothyroidism (**CH**) can be achieved. Mass screening for **CH** has been instituted in most developed countries, usually with a centralized laboratory for the reliable assay of hormone levels (T4 and/or TSH) in the biological specimen employed for screening. Over 50 million infants have been screened, with over 12,000 infants detected (2000 annually). Successful programs consist of seven components: (1) access to and screening of all liveborn infants, (2) reliable assays of T4 and/or TSH, (3) reliable interpretation of results, (4) rapid and complete follow up of infants with positive tests, (5) specific diagnosis of infants with abnormal test results, (6) appropriate institution of therapy, and (7) formalized evaluation of outcome variables. Cost-benefit analysis of newborn thyroid screening reveals a highly favorable ratio of benefits to cost. While the major stigmata of cretinism can be avoided by early diagnosis and treatment, some persistent sequelae of **CH** (mild abnormalities of perception and co-ordination) remain, particularly in severely affected infants.

The results of screening programs have indicated that the incidence of the sporadic form of **CH** is approximately 1/4000 live births worldwide. In certain endemic goitre areas this incidence is markedly increased. Only 3% of infants with documented **CH** have been suspected on clinical grounds in North America. The Quebec Program has systematized the clinical features into a Neonatal Hypothyroid Index (**NHI**) which shows a negative correlation with serum T4 and T3 levels and with bone maturation at diagnosis. The etiology of **CH** in most infants diagnosed in the Quebec Program is due to congenital absence or dysplasia of the thyroid gland (73%), with goitrous forms (11%) and secondary and tertiary forms (5%) being relatively uncommon. Transplacental passage of TSI or antithyroid drugs has uncommonly resulted in neonatal thyroid dysfunction. A new syndrome of transient hypothyroidism has been recognized as a result of universal screening. Its incidence is low in Quebec (11%) whereas in Europe it approaches 50% of that of sporadic **CH**, and may be as high as 10% in acutely ill premature infants in some areas. The pathogenesis is uncertain but immaturity of the newborn thyroid and /or altered iodine intake have been implicated. Although a higher set point for TSH suppression has been recognized in **CH**, prompt institution of adequate treatment with L-thyroxine (100 ug/M^2) will quickly normalize serum T4 and TSH levels. Frequent clinical and biochemical assessment is required to optimize therapy. The mean developmental indices of infants with **CH** treated before 1 month of age fall in the normal range. However, motor function may be developmentally delayed and the need for longitudinal assessment through school age has been stressed.

MP.15 INTENSIVE TREATMENT OF INSULIN DEPENDENT DIABETES: HOW AND WHY. W. Tamborlane*, Department of Pediatrics, Yale School of Medicine, New Haven, Ct., U.S.A.

Recent advances in management of insulin-dependent diabetes mellitus including more physiologic approaches in insulin delivery (using continous infusion devices or multiple injections) and more precise methods of assessing diabetic control with self blood glucose monitoring and glycosylated hemoglobin assays will be discussed. A practical approach to incorporate these technologies in a comprehensive, intensive treatment program will be outlined. These new treatment strategies have provided a means to achieve and maintain near normal glucose control of diabetes for extended periods and have provided new opportunities to examine the relationship between metabolic control and diabetic complications. Results of studies examining whether the reduction in blood glucose is accompanied by correction of other metabolic, hormonal or functional microvascular (e.g. capillary permeability) abnormalities which characterize poorly controlled diabetes will be reviewed. Potential risks and adverse effects of intensive therapies will be detailed. We will also discuss results of preliminary studies designed to ascertain whether intensive treatment provides the requisite degree of metabolic control to delay the progression of diabetic retinopathy or nephropathy.

MP.16A HYPERPROLACTINEMIA: COMBINED MEDICAL AND SURGICAL TREATMENT OF PROLACTINOMAS
Jules Hardy*, Division of Neurosurgery, Department of Surgery, University of Montreal, Canada.

Prolactinomas are the most frequent pituitary tumors and the major cause of hyperprolactinemia. The optimum treatment should encompass complete eradication of the tumor, normalization of prolactin secretion and preservation of the other pituitary functions.

Transsphenoidal microsurgery resulted in complete tumor removal and normalization of prolactin levels in 77% of patients with microadenoma. The cure rate was increased to 84% when preoperative levels of prolactin were below 250 ng/ml. In macroadenomas, despite satisfactory removal of tumor, hyperprolactinemia persisted and residual levels of prolactin increased progressively with the size of the remnant of the tumor. In those cases where the preoperative prolactin level was higher than 500 ng/ml, the success rate of surgery was 38%. We have recently reported a 45% relapse of hyperprolactinemia six years following surgery in a selective group of patients. The dopaminergic agonist Bromocriptin is successful in inhibiting prolactin secretion and reducing the size of the tumor in 40 to 60% of the cases. Complete disappearance of the tumor, however, was only incidental. Following the withdrawal of Bromocriptin, hyperprolactinemia resumed rapidly to pretreatment levels and the tumor reexpanded.

From a series of 364 cases of prolactinomas in female, 80 patients were previously treated with Bromocriptin. In the group of 188 patients with a microadenoma, normalization of prolactin occurred in 76% of cases after selective adenomectomy and there was no statistical significant difference between patients with or without previous Bromocriptin treatment. In a subgroup of patients previously treated with Bromocriptin, there was a higher cure rate (90%) in those treated for less than six months prior to the operation than in the group treated for more than six months (52%).

Fibrosis, as a consequence of long term treatment with Bromocriptin, was recently advocated as a possible cause of surgical difficulty in achieving normalization of prolactin levels. In our series, there is no significant difference in the incidence of fibrosis in patients not treated (47%) from those treated with Bromocriptin (45%) prior to surgery. In the group of non-cured patients previously treated with Bromocriptin, however, there was a higher incidence of fibrosis (62%) and even more so in the group of patients who were treated for more than six months.

Combined medical and surgical therapy is the optimal therapeutic approach for the treatment of prolactinomas. A preoperative attempt of Bromocriptin treatment to reduce the tumor may result, if effective, in a further improvement in success rate of complete removal provided surgery is not delayed over six months of Bromocriptin therapy.

MP.16B CLINICAL MANAGEMENT OF HYPERPROLACTINAEMIA. G.M. Besser*, Department of Endocrinology, St. Bartholomew's Hospital, London, EC1A 7BE, UK.

Hyperprolactinaemia is a common cause of gonadal dysfunction. In women it may cause amenorrhoea, usually secondary, oligomenorrhoea or infertility due to deficient progesterone secretion or anovulation. In men, impotence is a cardinal feature and secondary sexual characteristics may be entirely normal. Arrested or delayed puberty is less common but is being recognised more frequently as aetiologically related to hyperprolactinaemia. Drugs and pituitary tumours are the commonest cause of hyperprolactinaemia. Most tumours are microadenomas (<1cm, often only 2-3mm in diameter) but macroadenomas are not uncommon and occur disproportionately often in men. Hypothalamic disease, such as craniopharyngiomas or other tumours, also may present with hyperprolactinaemic syndromes. Response to dopamine agonist therapy does not distinguish between pituitary and hypothalamic causes necessarily. Galactorrhoea occurs only in a minority of patients, approximately 30%. Dopamine agonist drugs lower circulating prolactin levels and then, in most cases, normal gonadal function returns. In half the patients menses return within 2 months of dopamine agonist therapy, even though many years of amenorrhoea may have been present. After the occurrence of 3 regular ovulatory cycles, 50% of patients conceive within 2 months of attempted conception, even though they have had many years of infertility. In men, lowering of prolactin results in rapid return of gonadal function and normal potency. Only with massive pituitary tumours does hypopituitarism continue but even then this may return to normal if the pituitary tumour shrinks under dopamine agonist therapy. The widest experience has been obtained with bromocriptine. Doses of 7.5mg a day are usually sufficient, but up to 60mg a day may be required. A small number (perhaps 5%) of pituitary tumours may be resistant to bromocriptine and such patients may fail to achieve normal prolactin levels despite high doses of bromocriptine. Alternative medications are pergolide or mesulergin, but experience is limited with these agents. Macroadenomas respond as well as microadenomas. It is now clear that even massive macroadenomas frequently show shrinkage of the tumour right back into the pituitary fossa and with alleviation of the neighbourhood pressure effects and frequently complete resolution of hypopituitarism as the pressure on the portal capillary vessels of the pituitary stalk is relieved. Such dramatic responses occur in two thirds of the patients avoiding hypophysectomy. Radiotherapy, using a linear accelerator and administering 4,500 rads in fractions of less than 200 rads a day in 25 treatments over 36 days, has been shown to be safe and extremely effective in long term ablation of prolactinomas, but it may take up to 10 years to achieve normal prolactin levels; bromocriptine or alternative dopamine agonist therapy is indicated in the interim. Since gonadotrophin deficiency does not occur during the first 10 years after such therapy, the patient is assured of completing her family in this time. The radiotherapy not only produces long term control of prolactin hypersecretion, it also protects against the risk of rapid enlargement of such tumours during pregnancy. Should such an event occur during pregnancy, bromocriptine is the treatment of choice, as an emergency, since it will then rapidly shrink such oestrogen-stimulated tumours.

Wass, J.A.H. & Besser, G.M. The medical management of hormone secreting tumours of the pituitary. Ann Rev Med 34; 283-94, 1983.

MP.17 HIRSUTISM. - F. Kuttenn, Dept of Reproductive Endocrinology, Hôpital Necker, 75015 PARIS, France.

Hirsutism provides endocrinologists with an experimental model for the investigation of androgen secretion, metabolism and mechanism of action. Plasma androgen assay, free testosterone measurement, hepatic and extrahepatic androgen metabolic clearance and androgen metabolism in the skin are the different steps which were studied by many groups in the past 10 years and represent valuable parameters of the mechanisms of hirsutism.

Determination of the origin of androgen oversecretion has become easier by technical progress in differential effluent venous catheterism, which makes it possible to compare androgens in adrenal or ovarian effluent veins to their peripheral levels, and to determine the ovarian or adrenal source of the androgen oversecretion as well as the responsible side, essential in the case of tumors.

The study of androgen metabolism and the discovery of androgen receptors in the skin confirm the latter as an actual target cell for androgens. This target cell uses the circulating active androgen, i.e., testosterone and can also metabolize local inactive androgens into T and also DHT. The capacity of the skin to transform inactive androgens into active ones varies from one individual to another. That would support the concept of variable skin receptivity from one woman to another and from one ethnic group to another.

Concerning therapy, it may be easy to suppress an androgen oversecretion in the case of a virilizing tumor, but it is more difficult to inhibit androgen oversecretion of non tumoral ovarian or adrenal origin which in any case will be incomplete. Moreover, skin "overuse" of circulating androgens often remains unaltered, even if the oversecretion is corrected. The antiandrogens have opened a new therapeutic era. Cyproterone acetate is the most interesting due to both its antigonadotropic and peripheral antiandrogen effects. Its administration in moderate sequential doses (50 mg x 21 days per cycle) associated with percutaneous 17β-estradiol provides considerable efficiency without the classic side effects of higher doses and of synthetic estrogens orally administered. Its use in hirsutism has transformed the prognosis of this disease.

MP.18 CLINICAL USE OF VITAMIN D ASSAYS. R. BOUILLON*

Katholieke Universiteit Leuven, Rega Instituut, Minderbroedersstraat 10, B-3000 Leuven, Belgium.

Vitamin D_2 or D_3 are metabolized to a large number of metabolites by hydroxylation in either the side chain (positions 23,24,25 or 26) or in the A ring (1α position). Several assays are therefore necessary for a complete evaluation of the vitamin D metabolism.

The serum concentration of vitamin D_3 is relatively low (a few ng/ml) and increases for only a few days after exposure to ultraviolet light. The serum concentration of vitamin D_3 therefore reflects only the recent access to this compound.

25-Hydroxyvitamin D_3 is the metabolite with the highest serum concentration (10^{-8} à 10^{-7} M with seasonal variation), tightly bound to a plasma protein (DBP) and a prolonged half-life (2-3 weeks). It therefore represents the best parameter to assess the vitamin D stores of the organism. In vitamin D deficiency rickets or osteomalacia the serum concentration of 25-OHD is usually below 5 ng/ml. Similar values are frequently observed in other diseases or in infants, especially when born in winter or when they do not receive oral vitamin D supplements. The dark-skinned immigrant population in Western Europe, especially women and children, also have a high prevalence of low 25-OHD concentrations. The largest group of 25-OHD deficiency is certainly found in the elderly especially when their sun exposure is minimal. The disease states associated with vitamin D deficiency include nephrotic syndrome, biliary cirrhosis and several forms of malabsorption.

25-Hydroxyvitamin D concentrations well above 100 to 150 ng/ml represent an imminent risk for vitamin D toxicity. Such levels are not normally found even after prolonged exposure to sunshine or artificial ultraviolet light and thus are nearly also iatrogenic.

The serum concentration of the hormonally regulated $1,25-(OH)_2D_3$ metabolite ($\pm$ 0.1 nM) does not show a seasonal variation but usually predicts the physiological state of activation of the vitamin D status. The renal 25-OH-D-1α-hydroxylase activity is mainly stimulated by parathyroid hormone and low (serum) phosphorus concentration. Low circulating concentrations will therefore be observed in case of renal insufficiency and primary or secondary hypoparathyroidism. Several physiological or disease states with increased calcium demands are associated with high serum concentrations of $1,25-(OH)_2D$. As for other steroid hormones, the unbound (not DBP-bound) metabolite is probably a better indicator for its state of activity than the total concentration of $1,25-(OH)_2D$.

The serum concentration of $24,25-(OH)_2D$ and $25,26-(OH)_2D$ are usually present in a constant proportion to the circulating 25-OHD concentration. Unusually low concentration of $24,25-(OH)_2D$ have however been observed in kidney diseases, increased calcium need or diabetes mellitus. It is unclear whether this creates a separate and specific effect on target cells.

The 25-OHD-23,26-lactone is unusually high in case of vitamin D intoxication but its separate measurement is usually not necessary for this diagnosis.

The true diagnostic contribution for vitamin D measurements can be found in recognizing clinical and subclinical forms of vitamin D deficiency or excess and in the differential diagnosis of osteoporosis versus osteomalacia or in the unravelling of difficult cases of rickets or hypercalcemia.

MP.19 DIAGNOSIS AND TREATMENT OF THE SOLITARY THYROID NODULE.

Yoshihide Fujimoto*, Department of Endocrine Surgery, Tokyo Women's Medical College, Ichigaya-Kawada, Shinjuku, Tokyo, 162 Japan.

As an introduction to this session, the general principle on the diagnosis and treatment of the solitary thyroid nodule will be presented with particular emphasis on palpation, ultrasonography, neck x-rays and fine needle aspiration biopsy. Active participation of the attendants in the discussion on this problem using as many illustrative cases as possible will be highly appreciated.

Considerable controversy still remains in the diagnostic procedure of the solitary thyroid nodule and the selection of patients for surgery. For the evaluation of thyroid nodules, the knowledge of pathological classification, relative frequency and biological behavior of nodular lesions of the thyroid is required.

The frequency of solitary thyroid nodule in adults has been estimated to range from 1 to 5%. The incidence of thyroid carcinoma was estimated as 3.7 cases per 100,000 individuals in the United States. Population survey on the prevalence of thyroid carcinoma carried out in a non-endemic region, Japan, over 6 years revealed a rate of as high as 1 per 1,000 individuals.

In the evaluation of thyroid nodule, the most common diagnostic problem concerns whether it is malignant or not. A history of exposure to external irradiation, progressive enlargement of the nodule and recent onset of horseness, all these indicate increased possibility of thyroid malignancy. The careful physical examination of the neck remains a fundamental procedure. Patient's age, sex and race are also considered.

Useful employment of diagnostic measures will be discussed in details at the meeting. In our experience over 25 years, we have recently adopted considerably practical approach, in which physical examination of the neck, supplemented by ultrasound scanning and neck x-rays (lateral projection being taken by a soft tissue roentgenography technique) are all we need to make a diagnosis in the majority of thyroid nodules, other than follicular carcinoma. A fine needle aspiration biopsy is useful particularly in the diagnosis of papillary and anaplastic carcinomas. It meets the cost-effective policy, but it needs a highly trained cytologist. Thyroid scintigraphy has been overutilized. ^{131}I or ^{99m}Tc scan can detect a "hot" nodule, although its frequency ranges only 2 to 5% of all solitary nodules. Selection of patients for surgery, based on the finding of "cold" nodule on ^{99m}Tc scan and ^{201}Tl accumulation to the nodule, is simple, but the method cannot tell the underlying pathology of the nodule and is quite expensive. Diagnostic thyroid suppression therapy may be applied for the patients who have probable benign nodules.

If a patient is selected for surgery, lobectomy is the procedure of choice for the grossly solitary nodule, with preservation of the ipsilateral parathyroid glands,when possible. Any further surgical procedure will be determined by the macroscopic findings of cut sections of the specimen, occasionally along with frozen sections.

MP.20 ENDOCRINE MANIFESTATIONS OF PANCREATIC TUMOURS Bloom S.R*, Department of Medicine, Royal Postgraduate Medical School, Du Cane Road, London W12 OHS, UK.

The number of recognised pancreatic endocrine tumours (apudomas) is constantly increasing and now includes insulinomas, gastrinomas, glucagonomas, VIPomas-PHMomas, PPomas, neurotensinomas, somatostatinomas, CRFomas, GRFomas, carcinoids and NPYomas. Many of these tumours produce multiple hormones and may be best regarded histologically as islet cell tumours. They are usually slow growing and, with the marked exception of insulinomas, usually malignant. Attention is drawn to them by the main effect of the secreted peptide rather than tumour bulk as such. Successful resection is possible in more than half and results in excellent palliation but the majority will recur, usually within a few years. Therapy is then directed towards:

1) Blocking the effect of the hormone causing clinical symptoms.
2) Reducing tumour bulk.

A good example of the first possibility is the use in gastrinomas of the potassium ATPase inhibitor, omeprazole, which completely inhibits gastric acid. This allows the patient to return to normal health (without the burden of a gastrectomy) and the slow-growing tumour may allow a normal life for many years. Reduction of tumour bulk depends on surgical resection, reduction of metastases by hepatic arterial embolisation and cytotoxic therapy (streptozotocin). These tumours have provided useful information as to the long-term effects of their respective peptides and recently provided a source of messenger RNA for VIP, resulting in the discovery that the VIPoma syndrome also results from co-synthesis and co-secretion of a second active peptide PHM.

New Technical Development Sessions

NTD.1 METHODS FOR DETECTING GENE POLYMORPHISMS. G. I. Bell*, Chiron Corporation, Emeryville, California 94608.

Variations in the nucleotide sequence of a gene can be studied by cloning and sequencing its alleles. This strategy reveals all of the differences between alleles but is time consuming and not amenable to examining large numbers. In contrast, restriction endonuclease digestion in combination with the blotting technique developed by Southern (J. Mol. Biol. 98, 503 [1975]) is well suited to studies of variation in populations but detects only a subset of polymorphic sites, those associated with restriction endonuclease cleavage sites and polymorphic regions. In this procedure, the DNA fragments generated by an appropriate restriction endonuclease are separated by electrophoresis through an agarose gel and then denatured in situ. They are then immobilized directly by drying the gel or transferred to a nitrocellulose filter or nylon membrane. The DNA fragments of interest are identified by hybridization with a radioactively labeled or "immunologically tagged" cloned segment of the gene, its mRNA or a chemically synthesized DNA oligonucleotide. The hybridizing DNA fragments are visualized by autoradiography or immunological staining and the polymorphic fragments identified by their different size.

NTD.2 ANALYSIS OF LIPOXYGENASE PRODUCTS OF ARACHIDONIC ACID BY REVERSED PHASE (RP)-HPLC.

P. Borgeat* and S. Picard, Groupe de Recherche sur les Leucotriènes, Laboratoire d'Endocrinologie Moléculaire, Centre Hospitalier de l'Université Laval, Québec G1V 4G2, Canada.

Recent studies indicated that several metabolites of arachidonic acid derived from lipoxygenase pathways may be involved in endocrine functions; therefore, the availability of assay methods for some of these substances such as the hydroxyeicosatetraenoic acids (HETEs) and the leukotrienes (LTs), is essential for the assessment of the role of these compounds in hormone release and action. HPLC is particularly convenient for the analysis of lipoxygenase products since most of these substances carry an ultraviolet (UV) chromophore (conjugated dienes, λ max 230-235 nm and conjugated trienes, λ max 260-290 nm) which make their detection relatively easy and specific using sensitive photometers. The major advantage of HPLC over other methods of analysis available, lies in the possibility of profiling arachidonic acid metabolites, as opposed to the measurement of a single compound. The use of an internal standard in HPLC analysis also enables absolute quantitation. The main drawback of HPLC is the relatively high limit of detection (1-5 ng per compound using UV photometry). We have developed a RP-HPLC analysis method which enables fast and reliable separation and quantitation of ω-COOH-LTB_4, ω-OH-LTB_4, LTB_4, Δ^6-trans-LTB_4, Δ^6-trans-12-epi-LTB_4, 5S,12S-DiHETE, 5S,15S-DiHETE, HHT, 15-HETE, 12-HETE, 5-HETE, ω-OH-12-HETE, LTC_4, LTD_4, LTE_4 and LTF_4 using UV photometers; radiolabeled PGs and TXB_2, as well as other compounds lacking UV chromophores, could also be analyzed using an HPLC radioactivity detector. Briefly, biological samples (tissue or cell homogenates, tissue perfusates or incubation media) are denaturated with an equal volume of methanol:acetonitrile (1:1, V:V) and centrifuged at 600 g x 5 min to remove precipitated material. The supernates are acidified to pH 3 with H_3PO_4 and injected (injection volume up to 4 ml) onto a Radial Pak C18 cartridge (100 x 8 mm, 10 µm particles, Waters Scientific). The various compounds are eluted with water/organic solvent (methanol and acetonitrile) mixtures including pH gradients at a flow of 2.5 ml/min (see ref. 1 for exact solvent compositions and elution program). This new method features high sensitivity and selectivity for the analysis of LTC_4, LTD_4 and LTE_4, which are eluted separately following the previous elution of cyclooxygenase products and hydroxy acids (HETEs, LTB_4 and isomers). The procedure is fast and the analysis highly reliable since sample preparation only involves denaturation and centrifugation, without extraction, concentration or derivatization, thus minimizing the possibility of loss or deterioration of some components. The recovery of tritium labeled LTB_4 and LTC_4 was over 90% on 40 pg injected (carrier free). Profiles of arachidonic acid metabolites obtained from biological systems rich in lipoxygenase products will be shown to illustrate the procedure (see ref. 1 for chromatograms).

This study was supported by the MRC and the NCI (Canada).

1. Borgeat P, Fruteau de Laclos B, Rabinovitch H, Picard S, Braquet P, Hébert J, Laviolette M, 1984 Eosinophil-rich human polymorphonuclear leukocyte preparations characteristically release leukotriene C_4 upon ionophore A23187 challenge. J All Clin Immunol, in press.

NTD.3 DEVELOPMENTS IN AFFINITY CHROMATOGRAPHY OF STEROID HORMONE RECEPTORS

J. Mester*, G. Redeuilh, T. Buchou and J.M. Renoir, Lab. Hormones, 78 Rue du Général-Leclerc, 94270 Bicêtre, France.

1. Classical approach. Matrices containing immobilized steroid residues have been proposed for purification of most steroid hormone receptors. We have improved considerably the effectiveness of procedures based on the use of such matrices by including a step where the column with specifically retained receptor is washed with urea (2.5M to 3M according to case). Most non-specifically adsorbed proteins are removed by urea, and at biospecific elution approx. 25% to 40% purity can be obtained for the chicken oviduct progesterone receptor both in "activated" and "non-activated" forms.

2. Use of soluble affinity ligands. Molecules which bind to the receptor and possess also an additional feature permitting subsequent isolation of the complex have been developed. The first such compound we have used is a high $M_r$dextran-estradiol (E_2) conjugate which allows separation of the ER from other proteins by size-shift (Hubert et al, PNAS 75: 3143, 1978). Further advantages are offered by recently synthesized E_2-biotin adducts. The difficulty to surmount was the requirement for a long spacer chain so that the ligand can bind simultaneously to ER and to avidin. Purification of the calf uterus ER has been accomplished by this approach (Redeuilh et al., in preparation).

NTD.4 THE REVERSE HEMOLYTIC PLAQUE ASSAY FOR DETECTION OF HORMONE SECRETION BY INDIVIDUAL CELLS.

P. Smith*, Dept. of Physiology and Biophysics, University of Alabama in Birmingham, Alabama 35294 USA

Functional or morphological heterogeneity within each of the pituitary cell types has been described using cell separation techniques and immunocytochemistry. To understand how the secretion of a hormone is regulated requires knowledge of the extent of functional heterogeneity on a single cell level. A method for detecting secretion by single cells, the reverse hemolytic plaque assay (RHPA), has been adapted in our laboratory for detection of hormone secretion by dispersed anterior pituitary cells incubated as a monolayer with ovine erythrocytes. This assay, based on complement mediated lysis of protein A-coated ovine erythrocytes in the presence of an antiserum directed against a secretory protein, results in a zone of hemolysis, a plaque, surrounding each cell which has secreted that protein. Using antisera against ACTH, LH, Prl and GH we have been able to calculate the percentage of the total pituitary cell population that secretes each hormone, and generally these values agree with those obtained with immunocytochemistry (ICC) on cells from the same dispersion. Cells taken from rats at certain physiological states demonstrate a divergence between the number of hormone-containing and hormone-secreting cells. In the neonatal period there are a number of ACTH, LH and Prl containing cells that do not secrete that hormone in response to maximal doses of secretagogue. This is also true of LH containing cells in the adult male and diestrus I female rat. By plotting the amount of LH secreted per gonadotrope (determined by RIA) versus the mean plaque area per gonadotrope we generated a standard curve. The sensitivity of the RHPA for LH is $\sim$ 2-5 pg LH RP-1. Furthermore there is a >1000 fold difference in the amount of LH secreted by individual cells from the same pituitary gland. This heterogeneity in amount of hormone secreted by individual cells is also apparent with other cell types.

The plaque assay can be performed repeatedly on the same pituitary cells using different antibodies to look for cells capable of secreting more than one hormone. Using this "sequential RHPA" we have observed cells which can secrete both Prl and GH (Frawley and Neill, unpublished) as well as cells which secrete both ACTH and LH, each in response to the appropriate secretagogue.

Using the plaque assay in conjunction with pulse labeling of cells with ^{3}H-leucine followed by autoradiography we have demonstrated the presence of a subpopulation of lactotropes which preferentially secretes newly synthesized Prl. This technique relies on the fact that ^{3}H-labeled hormone released from a cell remains bound to antibody, and hence to the lysed erythrocytes. Comparison of the plaque area and the number of developed silver grains over that area gives an index of the specific activity of the bound hormone. We are at present performing electron microscopy on individual cells functionally defined by the RHPA to determine the morphological correlates of functionally distinct subpopulations of lactotropes and gonadotropes.

In summary the RHPA is useful to study the heterogeneity in secretory response of individual cells in a mixed population of cells and can probably be used to study cells secreting any hormone for which an antibody is available.

NTD.5 IN SITU cDNA:mRNA HYBRIDIZATION: A TECHNIQUE TO STUDY GENE EXPRESSION IN INDIVIDUAL CELLS. J.L. Roberts*, J.N.Wilcox and C.E.Gee, Center for Reproductive Sciences and Department of Biochemistry, Columbia University, New York, New York, 10032, U.S.A.

In situ cDNA:mRNA hybridization is a technique that has been developed for the visualization of specific mRNAs at the level of the individual cell. Briefly, fixed cryostat sectioned tissue is incubated with a radioactive cDNA probe favoring cDNA:mRNA hybrid formation. At the end of the hybridization step, the tissue is washed to remove unhybridized cDNA probe and processed for autoradiography. After a suitable exposure period the slides are developed and counterstained to visualize the cells. The distribution and density of silver grains then yields information regarding the presence or absence of mRNAs complementary to the cDNA probe used. We have used this technique to visualize and in some cases quantify GH, betaLH, and POMC mRNA in the rat pituitary. We have also used this technique to successfully identify POMC mRNA in scattered cells in the periarcuate region of the rat hypothalamus co-localized with POMC peptides. The *in situ* cDNA:mRNA hybridization technique has great potential in the understanding of the control of gene expression in complex systems such as the brain. The ultimate goal of our work is to use it as a semi-quantitative assay for mRNA levels in individual neurons. We have therefore been optimizing the *in situ* cDNA:mRNA hybridization technique for the demonstration of mRNAs in the brain using POMC as a model system. Previously, the use of this technique to localize specific brain mRNAs has met with limited success due to high backgrounds and variable results. We haverecently identified some of the parameters contributing to this limited success. Basic proteins such as myelin appear to have an affinity for the cDNA probes and preincubation of the tissue section with buffers containing low concentrations of nucleic acids appears to reduce non-specific binding of the probes to myelinated structures. Ribonuclease appears to be very active even after fixation of the tissue with paraformaldehyde and care must be taken in the isolation and preparation of neural tissue for *in situ* cDNA:mRNA hybridization to minimize ribonuclease degradation of the mRNA prior to hybridization.

NTD.6 MONOCLONAL ANTIBODIES AGAINST MEMBRANE RECEPTORS: LESSONS LEARNED FROM THE INSULIN RECEPTOR.

R.A. Roth*, M.L. Mesirow and D.J. Cassell, Mt. Zion Hospital and Medical Center, San Francisco, CA 94120

The development of the monoclonal technique by Kohler and Milstein in 1975 greatly facilitated the study of plasma membrane receptors for hormones, neurotransmitters and other ligands. This technique allowed the production of large quantities of homogeneous antibodies to limited amounts of antigens in impure preparations. However, the production of a particular monoclonal antibody can be an arduous task. Numerous immunization schemes abound, fusion protocols vary and the possible screening procedures are endless. Thus, the finding of a suitable monoclonal antibody may appear to be more an art than a science. To further aid anyone undertaking such a task, we will outline some of our experiences in the production of a monoclonal antibody to the insulin receptor. First, we found that immunization of mice with intact IM-9 cells, a human lymphocyte cell line with insulin receptors, readily produced antibodies to the insulin receptor. In fact, it was easier to obtain antibodies to the insulin receptor by this immunization protocol which contained only ~200 fmoles of receptor in a highly impure form than by the immunization of 20 pmoles of highly purified receptor. In addition, in vitro immunizations of mouse spleen cells with purified receptor also gave only poor yields of anti-receptor antibody. Thus, these results would suggest that the use of purified antigens need not necessarily simplify the task of producing a monoclonal antibody. Second, we found that the mice with the highest titer of antibody to the insulin receptor were the ones that were most likely to yield a hybridoma producing the desired antibody. All three hybridomas that produced antibodies to the receptor arose in fusions which utilized the spleen cells of the mice with the highest titer of antibody to the receptor. Thus, prescreening the antisera could decrease the number of hybridomas that need to be screened. Third, we found that the characteristics of the monoclonal antibody we obtained were similar to that of the antisera of the mice. For example, the antisera inhibited insulin binding to several human tissues but not to rat tissues. In addition, the antisera precipitated the insulin-receptor complex. The monoclonal antibody exhibited the same characteristics; it inhibited insulin binding to human but not rat tissues and could precipitate the insulin-receptor complex. Thus, by finding an immunization scheme that yields an antisera with a particular property, one may increase the likelihood of getting a monoclonal with the same characteristics. Finally, one must carefully consider the screening procedure to be utilized. Since we were interested in an antibody that inhibited insulin binding, we screened the hybridomas for the production of such an inhibiting antibody. The monoclonal antibody we isolated was very good at inhibiting binding. However, it was not very good in certain other assays. For example, it was poor at binding purified insulin receptors insolubilized on nitrocellulose paper. Thus, it is important to utilize a screening method which reflects the ultimate planned use of the monoclonal antibody. In summary, time spent in optimizing the immunization procedure and choosing the screening assay are very important in obtaining the desired monoclonal antibody. This study was supported by the Juvenile Diabetes Foundation and the National Institutes of Health.

NTD.7 NON-ISOTOPIC IMMUNOASSAYS. W.P. Collins*, Diagnostics Research Unit, King's College School of Medicine, Denmark Hill, London SE5 8RX, UK

Recent advances in biotechnology and microelectronics are changing the study and practice of diagnostic medicine. Novel immunochemical tests have been developed for use in the central or research laboratory, the outpatient clinic or ward, and in the home. Different assay systems (e.g. limited or excess reagent, separation or non-separation) using monoclonal or polyclonal antibodies (in solution or attached to a solid-phase) will be reviewed in the context of alternative labels, end-points and instrumentation (e.g. spectrophotometry, nephelometry, radioluminometry, chemiluminometry and fluorimetry). In particular, assay systems involving the use of enzymes, isoluminol derivatives, acridinium esters and rare earth chelates as labels will be compared for sensitivity, speed, ruggedness, clinical utility and cost. An assessment will be made of the extent to which the technological developments are fulfilling the requirements of the assayist for well-defined applications.

NTD.8 POLYPEPTIDE MICROSEQUENCE ANALYSIS WITH THE COMMERCIALLY AVAILABLE GAS-PHASE SEQUENCER. F.S. Esch, Laboratories for Neuroendocrinology, 10010 N. Torrey Pines Rd., La Jolla, California, USA, 92037.

An evaluation of the commercially available gas-phase sequencer with regard to its sensitivity, ease of operation and reliability is presented. Techniques for the preparation of ultra-pure reagents and solvents for this new technology are reviewed as is a highly sensitive reverse-phase liquid chromatography program for the identification and quantitation of phenylthiohydantoin amino acid residues from the new sequenator.

WTD.9 **PURIFICATION OF HUMAN INSULIN RECEPTOR WITH HIGH INSULIN-BINDING AND KINASE ACTIVITIES.**

Y. Fujita-Yamaguchi *, Beckman Research Institute of the City of Hope, Duarte, CA. 91010

Since the first purification of the receptor from rat liver by Jacobs *et al.* in 1977, purification of insulin receptor had been reported from different laboratories. However, their results were controversial because no one had purified insulin receptor with specific activity of 20μg of insulin bound per mg of protein, which would be expected if insulin receptor with Mr=300,000 binds one molecule of insulin. The low specific activities achieved by them could be due to contaminants in the preparation or to inactivation of the receptor.

While purification of the receptor had been unsuccessful, progress has been made in elucidating the subunit structure of the receptor by the use of affinity-labeling methods and immunoprecipitation techniques in the last 5 years. Insulin receptor appears to have multi-subunits with Mr=125,000-135,000 (α), Mr=90,000-95,000 (β), Mr=210,000 (possibly a precursor molecule of α and β), and Mr=40,000-50,000. The most popular structural model for insulin receptor with Mr=300,000 is $\alpha_2\beta_2$ that has been proposed by Czech *et al.* However, the information obtained by these affinity-labeling methods is inconclusive, because only specifically labeled proteins can be detected. Thus, it is necessary to completely purify fully active insulin receptor to determine the stoichiometry and amino acid sequence of the receptor subunits and to study the exact mechanism of insulin and the receptor interaction.

Among the methods originally proposed, we have realized that insulin-sepharose affinity chromatography is the most practical and efficient method to purify insulin receptor, since we take advantage of the high affinity and specificity of the receptor to insulin. This approach has been pioneered by Cuatrecasus and used by his colleagues and others but unfortunately resulted in purifying the receptor with poor insulin binding activity. We have reevaluated the synthesis of insulin-Sepharose and, systematically investigating different elution conditions, have developed a new elution method (pH5 with high salt) without using urea to purify insulin receptor with full insulin-binding activity. Insulin receptor was purified 2400-fold with a yield of 40% from human placental membranes by affinity chromatography on wheat germ agglutinin-Sepharose and insulin-Sepharose. Approximately 50 μg of purified receptor was obtained from 2 placentae. The receptor was eluted from insulin-Sepharose using mild conditions (50 mM acetate buffer, pH 5, containing 1M NaCl and 0.1% Triton X-100) so that it was stable and retained full insulin binding activity. Specific activity of the purified receptor determined by Scatchard analysis was 28 μg of insulin bound per mg of protein, whereas the receptor eluted by previously used conditions (pH6.0 with 4.5 M urea) resulted in only 6μg of insulin bound per mg of protein. This indicates that four to five-fold increases in specific activity can be obtained by using the new conditions.

SDS-gel electrophoresis of the purified receptor showed two major protein bands with Mr 125K (α) and 90K(β) and a minor band with Mr 50K under reducing conditions. All three components were immunoprecipitated by anti-insulin receptor sera. Peptide mapping of isolated subunits revealed that the α subunit is distinct from the β subunit and that the 50K subunit is a degradation product of the β subunit. Further analysis by two-dimentional SDS-gel electrophoresis provided conclusive evidence that a disulfide-linked complex (α_2,2β) is the basic structural unit of insulin receptor. The purified receptor showed a curvilinear Scatchard plot as well as autophosphorylation of β subunit, indicating that our receptor preparation retains basic functions of native insulin receptor. This biologically active insulin receptor has been proven to be useful in investigating the structure-function relationship of the receptor molecule itself and the mechanism of the signal transmission upon hormone binding. This study was supported by NIH Grant 29770.

NTD.10 RNA BLOT HYBRIDIZATION ANALYSIS. F. Carter Bancroft, Memorial Sloan-Kettering Cancer Center, and Molecular Biology and Virology Program, Sloan-Kettering Division, Cornell University, New York, NY 10021.

With the advent of recombinant DNA technology and the consequent availability of pure probes for the RNA products of specific genes, attention has been focused on the development of convenient and reliable methods for employing these probes to follow the concentrations of specific RNAs in animal cells or organs during induction by hormones, differentiation, etc. RNA blot techniques have been developed by a number of investigators for performing such measurements, in which the common theme is immobilization of RNA on nitrocellulose, followed by hybridization with a ^{32}P-labeled cloned probe. Examples of such techniques will be described, including gel electrophoresis of RNA followed by blotting of the RNA to nitrocellulose, dotting of samples of total RNA, and dotting of cellular fractions containing RNA plus other cellular macromolecules.

NTD.11 TISSUE CULTURE IN CHEMICALLY DEFINED MEDIA. G. Sato*, W. Alton Jomes Cell Science Center, Old Barn Road, Lake Placid, New York 12946, U.S.A.

The development of hormonally defined media for various functionally differentiated cell types reveals unsuspected complexities of hormonal interactions. These findings enable us to delineate a new sub-discipline: cellular endocrinology. An important area for future investigation in the extrapolation of culture studies is that cells in culture require high density for satisfactory growth indicating that animal cells produce many of the factors that are significant in their local environment. We are embarked on a systematic program to elucidate these secretory products and to relate them to animal physiology with the use of monoclonal antibodies to receptors and cDNA complementary to factor messengers.

NTD.12 HIGH PERFORMANCE/PRESSURE LIQUID CHROMATOGRAPHY (HPLC): AN IMPORTANT TOOL IN THE LIFE SCIENCES.

Jean Rivier*, R. McClintock, J. Vaughan and W. Vale. The Salk Institute, Peptide Biology Laboratory, La Jolla, CA 92037

In 1976, two antipodean laboratories independently described the use of reversed phase (RP) HPLC for the separation of unprotected peptides greater than a few amino acids long, and illustrated the extreme potential of this new technique [R. Burgus, J. Rivier, (1976) In Peptides 1976, J. Loffet, Ed., Editions de l'Universite de Bruxelles, pp. 85-94 and W.S. Hancock, C.A. Bishop and M.T.W. Hearn, (1976) FEBS Lett. 72:139]. Peptides could be separated on the basis of their composition and chirality. For the first time, a reliable and quantitative analytical system existed which could assess the purity of a synthetic peptide whether it had been synthesized using solution chemistry (classical approach) or Merrifield's solid phase strategy. HPLC was also recognized in our original paper as the method of choice for the purification of new peptides from natural sources as illustrated by the isolation of α-endorphin. Similarly, we used HPLC to separate peptide analogs semi-preparatively in order to assess their biological potencies. There seemed to be no limitations to the use of this new technique. Very quickly however we realized that recoveries of certain peptides (those with strong amphiphilic character) such as β-endorphin and corticotropin releasing factor, were poor. New solvent systems were described [Triethylammonium phosphate buffer (TEAP) by J. Rivier (1978) J. Liq. Chrom. 1:343- 367; and .1% TFA or HFBA by H.P.J. Bennet, H.M. Hudson, C.McMartin and G.E. Purdon (1977) Biochem. J. 168:9-13] and the use of columns packed with spherical, large pore size 300 Å end capped silicas were suggested in order to increase resolution and recoveries [J. Rivier, C. Rivier, J. Spiess and W. Vale (1982) Analy. Biochem. 127:258-266; J. Rivier, R. McClintock (1983) J. Chrom. 268:112-119]. This approach was illustrated by the isolation of both rat hypothalamic CRF and GRF [J. Rivier, R. McClintock and W. Vale (1984) J. Chrom. submitted] which took advantage of the selectivity brought about by the appropriate use of supports (C_{18}/C_4/Diphenyl) and buffer systems (TEAP/TFA/HFBA). Similarly, partial characterization of known biological or immunologically defined entities have been addressed by HPLC. Taking the above mentioned isolation and characterization projects as examples we will discuss some of the pitfalls and limitations presently associated with this technique.

Poster Presentations

Monday 2nd July	*(Abstracts 1-552)*
Tuesday 3rd July	*(Abstracts 553-1104)*
Wednesday 4th July	*(Abstracts 1105-1379)*
Thursday 5th July	*(Abstracts 1380-1929)*
Friday 6th July	*(Abstracts 1930-2470)*
Saturday 7th July	*(Abstracts 2471-2781)*

1 CORTICOSTERONE INFUSIONS IN CYANOKETONE-TREATED RATS LOWER ACTH LEVELS PROVIDING EVIDENCE FOR RESET IN THE ADRENOCORTICAL SYSTEM. S. F. Akana*, J. Shinsako and M. F. Dallman. Dept. of Physiology, University of California, San Francisco, CA 94143 USA.

We have reported that treatment of rats with the adrenal enzyme inhibitor cyanoketone (CK) results in a diurnal corticosterone (B) rhythm of normal amplitude and normal ACTH levels in the AM compared to vehicle-treated controls (DMSO) (Endo. 113:2232, 1983). When chronically cannulated rats were continuously sampled (65 ul/5 min) for 2 h periods during the day (12:12 h light cycle), mean 2 h B and ACTH values were normal in the AM (CK vs DMSO, n.s.); however mean B levels were lower and ACTH levels were higher in CK than in DMSO rats during 2 h before lights out (PM). (Both $p < 0.05$.) Thus CK resulted in a PM error signal in average plasma B that might explain the high PM ACTH levels. To test this possibility CK and DMSO rats were infused sc in the PM for 2 h with saline or with 8 ug B. Four days later, the other infusate was similarly administered so that each rat participated in 2 experiments. Plasma ACTH was decreased by B infusion in CK rats (saline: 620 ± 76 vs B: 294 ± 48 pg/ml, n = 5) but not in DMSO rats (saline: 105 ± 11 vs B: 107 ± 15 pg/ml, n = 5). Mean plasma B in CK rats was not altered by exogenous B (saline: 11.5 ± 0.5 vs B: 11.1 ± 0.4 ug/dl), and was decreased in DMSO rats (saline: 15.1 ± 0.6 vs B: 8.9 ± 0.5 ug/dl). We conclude that the small PM error signal in plasma B in CK rats is responsible for the elevated ACTH, and that diurnal reset of the feedback setpoint in the adrenocortical system controls the diurnal rhythm in ACTH. (Supported by AM06455 and AM28172.)

2 ELEVATED B- ENDORPHIN PLASMA LEVELS IN A GROUP OF WOMEN WITH POLYCYSTIC OVARIAN DISEASE. F. Aleem*, T. McIntosh, Dept. Obs/Gyn New York Medical College, N.Y., and Trauma Research Center, Boston University Medical School, Boston, Mass.

Recent studies demonstrated a concomitant increase of LH and FSH after the administration of Naloxone (a specific B-endorphin antagonist) to normal menstruating and amenorrheic women. Other recent studies in rodents suggest the possibility of an association between elevated B-endorphins and overeating and obesity. Our study measured plasma levels of B-endorphin in conjunction with plasma gonadotropins and androgens in a group of patients with polycystic ovarian disease (19) and a group of normal menstruating women (16). Using a specific RIA technique for B-Endorphin, B-Lipotrophin (B-L PH) was entirely removed from the sample by preincubation of the plasma with anti B-LPH sepharose complex. The incubated plasma was extracted using octadecyl silica (C-18) high performance liquid chromomatrography and B-EP was eluted with glacial acetic acid/95% ethanol, then RIA of B-EP. Of the study group 19/19 amenorrheic, 19/19 hirsute, 15/19 obese, 14/19 had ratio LH/FSH $>$ 2, 15/19 $\uparrow$ total testosterone levels, and 10/19 had abnormally high free testosterone. The mean level of B-EP in the study group was 185.30 ± 93.40/Pg/ml which was significantly higher ($P < 0.001$) than in the control group mean B-EP = 86.86 ± 27Pg/ml. These data suggest that central nervous system inhibitory opioid pathway may be involved in control of gonadotropin secretion in normal cycles and that the excessive production of B-EP may play a role in the pathophysiology of polycystic ovarian disease especially when amenorrhea, obesity and hyperandrogenism are common findings.

3 DIFFERENT EFFECTS OF TWO SYNTHETIC ACTHS ON STEROIDOGENESIS AND CYCLIC AMP IN ISOLATED LUTEAL CELLS FROM RAT OVARIES. R. Asakai*, A. Kumai, S. Sassa, and R. Okamoto, Dept. of Endocrinology, Med. Res. Inst., Tokyo Med. & Dent. Univ., Tokyo 113, Japan.

Effects of synthetic Acthormon ($ACTH^{1-18}$) and Cortrosyn ($ACTH^{1-24}$) on the synthesis of progesterone(PRG), 20α-OH-progesterone(20α-OH-PRG) and cyclic AMP(cAMP) in isolated luteal cells from PMS plus hCG primed immature rats were studied. Luteal cells were isolated using a sucrose density gradient after digestion with trypsin and collagenase. Hormones in the medium and intracellular cAMP were assayed following a 6 hr-incubation. Effect of 10-100 ug of $ACTH^{1-24}$: PRG increased in a dose dependent manner at an ED_{50} value of 6.4 ug, while 20α-OH-PRG decreased in a dose dependent manner at an ID_{50} value of 15 ug. cAMP also increased significantly. Effect of 10-100 ug of $ACTH^{1-18}$: No change in PRG level was noted and 20 -OH-PRG decreased in a dose dependent manner at an ID_{50} value of 10 ug. cAMP also decreased in dose dependent manner. The present data demonstrate that ACTH has direct effects on PRG and 20α-OH-PRG synthesis in luteal cells and suggest that the effect of ACTH is mediated by cAMP. Difference in the effects between two synthetic ACTHs is thought to be resulted from a difference in chemical structure.

4 THE ROLE OF OPIATES IN THE MECHANISM OF THE DISTURBED PITUITARY HORMONES SECRETION. B.Baranowska*, W.Jeske and M.Abdel-Fattah Endocrinology Clinic, Cegłowska 80, 01-809 Warsaw, Poland

It has been shown that opiate peptides are involved in the control of pituitary hormones secretion in men. The aim of the study was to evaluate the effect of naloxone upon ACTH, β-endorphine-like substance, growth hormone /GH/, prolactin /Prl/, LH and FSH in patients with Cushing's disease, prolactinomas, "functional" amenorrhoea-galactorrhoea syndrome and acromegaly. The above hormones were estimated by RiA methods at 30,45,60 min following opiate receptors blockade with Naloxone /Narcan-Whinthrop/. In 3 out of 7 patients with Cushing's disease naloxone caused diminution of the serum ACTH and β-endorphine-like substance concentrations. Naloxone administration failed to induce any changes in GH levels in 6 acromegalic patients and in Prl concentrations in 6 patients with prolactinomas. However, a significant increment of LH but not FSH in response to naloxone was observed both in patients with prolactinomas and with "functional" amenorrhoea-galactorrhoea syndrome. Moreover, naloxone restored or increased the frequency and the amplitude of LH pulsatility. Conclusions: 1.Increased opioid activity may lead to inhibition of LH secretion in hiperprolactinemic patients. 2.The paradoxical effects of naloxone in some patients with Cushing's disease may point to its important therapeutical role.

5 RATE SENSITIVITY OF THE PITUITARY-ADRENAL RESPONSE TO HEMORRHAGE IN THE CAT

D.A.BEREITER*, A.M. ZAID AND D.S.GANN. Brown Univ. R.I. Hospital Endocrine Lab, Providence, R.I. 02902 USA

The ACTH response to graded hemorrhage(H) of brief duration is proportional to the volume of blood removed. However, previous studies have frequently confounded magnitude with rate of H which initiates ACTH release. To assess the effect of rate of H, acutely prepared cats anesthetized with chloralose/urethane sustained moderate H(20% of measured blood volume) or large H(30%) at a slow removal rate(2%/min) or at a rapid rate(10%/min) and withheld until 20min. Peripheral plasma samples were collected every 2min for 20min after onset of H and assayed for ACTH, cortisol, catecholamines and glucose. Results include: a) no evidence for rate sensitivity in the ACTH response to 30%H, b)the rise in ACTH after 20%H was greatest with the slower rate of H, c)catecholamine release, by contrast, increased with increasing rate of H, d) mean arterial pressure(MAP) decreased steadily during 20% or 30%H withdrawn at 2%/min with only slight recovery towards baseline during the post-H period, e)MAP during 20% and 30%H withdrawn at 10%/min showed a large transient decrease during H with recovery towards baseline proportional to the magnitude of H and the magnitude of the early increase in catecholamines, and f)the steady state change in ACTH after H correlated($r=.65, P<.005$) with the post-H change in MAP, but not to the early change in MAP during H. These data indicate H-induced ACTH release is level-sensitive and not rate-sensitive over the range of blood withdrawal rates employed (2%/min and 10%/min). Catecholamine release by H is both rate-and level-sensitive and the early rise in catecholamines by rapid H indirectly attenuates ACTH release by markedly improving the recovery of MAP after a rapid 20%H. Funded by NIH Grants AM-26831 and GM-27946.

6 IMPORTANCE OF CATECHOLAMINES IN STRESS-INDUCED ACTIVATION OF THE PITUITARY-ADRENAL SYSTEM.

F. Berkenbosch+, F.J.H. Tilders, I. Vermes. Dept. Pharmacology, Free University, 1007 MC, Amsterdam, The Netherlands.

We investigated the effects of catecholamines on ACTH secretion from the anterior pituitary. Intravenous infusion of epinephrine in rats in physiological doses (30-1000 ng/kg.min.) caused a dose-dependent increase in plasma ACTH and corticosterone. This effect could be mimicked by the β-adrenoceptor agonist l-isoproterenol, blocked by peripheral administration of β-adrenoceptor antagonist l-propranolol (2.5 mg/kg i.p.) and was slightly potentiated by peripheral administration of the α-adrenoceptor antagonist phentolamine (2.5,10 mg/kg i.p.). Central administration of l-propranolol (30 /ug/5 /ul i.c.v.) inhibited the l-isoproterenol-induced pituitary -adrenal activity, without affecting the increase in heartrate and the stimulating effect on MSH secretion from the intermediate lobe. Passive immunisation with antibodies directed against CRF1-41 and hypothalamic deafferentation, which results in a disappearence of CRF-immunostaining in the median eminence, caused a nearly complete blockade of the epinephrine or isoproterenol-induced increase in plasma ACTH and corticosterone. Propranolol (2.5,10 mg/kg i.p.) or phentolamine (2.5,10 mg/kg i.p.) did not significantly change the increase in plasma ACTH 2-4 min. after exposure of rats to a variety of stress stimuli. These data indicate that although catecholamines can trigger ACTH release via a permissive β-adrenoceptor mechanism in the brain, they do not play an important role in the acute activation of the pituitary-adrenal system during stress.

7 EFFECT OF KETANSERIN,A NEW SPECIFIC 5-HT2 RECEPTOR ANTAGONIST,ON ACTH SECRETION:IN VITRO AND IN VIVO STUDIES. M.Boscaro*,A.Menegus,G.Merola,F.Mantero Istituto di Semeiotica Medica,Università di Padova,Padova,Italy.

Serotonin(5-HT) is considered to be involved in ACTH regulation.Antiserotoninergic drugs(e.g.cyproheptadine)may inhibit ACTH secretion both in normal subjects and in some cases of Cushing's disease(C.D.),and occasionally in cultures of pituitary adenoma cells. The availability of the new,more specific 5-HT2 receptor antagonist Ketanserin(Janssen) has prompted us to study its effect on ACTH secretion,both in vitro and in vivo in patients with various forms of ACTH hypersecretion:4 C.D.,1 ectopic ACTH production,1 Nelson's s. and 2 Addison's d. The in vitro studies were done in a continuous perfusion system of rat anterior pituitary cells or human pituitary ACTH secreting adenoma cells. The cell preparations were stimulated with 5-HT 10^{-6} M , Lysine-vasopressin (LVP) 10^{-7} M or Adrenalin (A) 10^{-6} M alone or during Ket. (10^{-5}-10^{-7} M) infusion. 5-HT failed to directly stimulate ACTH secretion. Ket. did not modify the basal and LVP- or A-stimulated ACTH secretion. In vivo: I.v. bolus of 10 mg of Ket.did not significantly inhibit basal or LVP-stimulated ACTH and cortisol secretion. These data do not support the hypothesis of a direct activity of 5-HT on ACTH secretion;furthermore they show a lack of acute effect of the very specific 5-HT2 antagonist Ket. in states of ACTH hypersecretion. A longer treatment period with this drug is probably needed before drawing any conclusion.

8 EXERCISE-ASSOCIATED DISTURBANCES IN THE RAT ESTRUS CYCLE CAN BE REVERSED BY NALTREXONE. C.A. Caldwell and J.M. Davis*, Dept. Phys. Ed., University of South Carolina, Columbia, S.C. 29208, U.S.A.

An animal model was developed in order to study the possible involvement of endogenous opioid peptides (EOP) in exercise-associated disturbances of the reproductive cycle. Female Sprague-Dawley rats (220-260 gm) with normal estrus cycles (4-5 days) were randomly assigned to 3 groups: Exercisers (EX;n = 7), Waders (W;n = 6) and Controls (C;n = 8). EX were subjected to 60 min. swim sessions twice daily with weights (3% of body wt.) attached to their back. W were placed in shallow water to control for the effect of immersion without exercise; the C group received no treatment. Body weight and vaginal smears were monitored daily. Following 4-weeks of training body weight was similar in all groups, however, 6 of the 7 EX animals displayed cycle irregularities (> 5 days in length; n = 3 ; or complete cessation of cycles; n = 3). Both W and C groups continued to cycle normally. Of the EX with irregular cycles, 4 were given naltrexone (EX-NALT; 10 mg/kg) and 2 received saline injections (EX-SAL) twice daily prior to exercise over a 10-day period. One EX-NALT animal immediately began to cycle normally, two were in estrus following a normal cycle by day 9, and the fourth began to cycle but failed to display the estrus phase. EX-SAL animals remained in diestrus. By one week following cessation of exercise and drug treatment all but one animal regained normal cycles. These results suggest that EOP play a role in disturbances of the rat estrous cycle associated with strenuous swimming exercise and moreover, they demonstrate the potential of the rat model for future studies of this nature. Supported by NIH Biomedical Research Support Grant #RR07160-08.

9 AN ACTION OF CORTICOSTERONE(B) ON BRAIN MAY PROTECT ADRENALECTOMIZED(ADX) RATS FROM STRESS-ASSOCIATED MORTALITY. Caren S. Cascio*, Nancy Levin and Mary F. Dallman. Dept. Physiology, Univ. of Ca., San Francisco, CA 94143

Bilaterally ADX rats are exceedingly sensitive to stress and succumb to insults that sham-operated control rats(SHAMS) weather well. Although given 0.5%NaCl to drink, ADX rats do not gain weight normally during the first 48h post-surgery (ΔBW ADX<SHAM, $p<0.05$). Replacement of B by supplying it in the drinking fluid(20μgB/ml) results in normal food intake and weight gain during the first 24h compared to SHAM(both $p>0.1$) and greater food intake and weight gain than after ADX-saline(both $p<0.05$). When subjected to the nutritional stress of restricted access to food(4h/day), ADX rats died within 5d whereas all ADX-B and SHAM rats lived. To test whether B infused into brain protects ADX rats from other stresses, rats(n=4/group) were ADX and provided with osmotic pumps that delivered either saline or B in saline into a lateral ventricle(ICV) at a rate of lul/h. Four-5d after ADX and pump placement or SHAM surgery, rats were given pentobarbital(45mg/kg) and prepared with femoral arterial and venous cannulae for subsequent measurements. Three of 4 ADX rats infused with saline ICV died before vascular cannulation was completed whereas all 4 ADX rats infused with B ICV survived the planned procedure. There was no difference in mean arterial blood pressure or plasma glucose levels between SHAM and ADX-B rats(n=4/gp). B levels in brains of ADX-saline rats were lower than those of ADX-B rats(0.8 vs 3.6ng/g, n=2/gp), whereas plasma B levels were similarly low in both groups (1.1 vs 0.5 ug/dl). We conclude that it may be a lack of B in the central nervous system that results in the well known vulnerability of ADX rats to stress. Supported in part by USPHS grant AM28172.

10 INTRAVENOUS INFUSION DEXAMETHASONE (DEX) SUPPRESSION TEST. A.B.Abou Samra, B.Estour, H.Dechaud, M.Pugeat, F.Claustrat, C.Baret, D.Chalendar and J.Tourniaire*. Laboratoire de la Clinique Endocrinologique and Laboratoire Central de Biochimie, Hôpital de l'Antiquaille, 69321 Lyon Cedex 05 France.

The Classical oral DEX suppression test is widely used for the diagnosis of Cushing's syndrome. However, variations in intestinal absorption of DEX modify its plasma level. To avoid these variations a pump was used to infuse DEX phosphate intravenously (iv) from 11.00 to 15.00 (1mg/hour). 9 normal subjects and 8 patients Cushing's syndrome were studied. Blood samples were withdrawn every 20 minutes between 09.00 and 15.00, then every 2 hours until midnight and at 08.00 the next day. Plasma cortisol (F) and β-lipotropin (β-LPH) concentrations were measured by specific methods. In the controls, 50% suppression of plasma β-LPH and F occured within 30-90 mn of DEX infusion. F and β-LPH levels were respectively lower than 3 μg/dl and 40 pg/ml at the end of the infusion and remained so till 08.00 the next day. In the 4 patients with Cushing's disease, 50% suppression occured within 120-180 mn of DEX infusion and a rapid escape from suppression occured between 16.00 - 24.00. All these patients recuperated more than 75% of plasma F and β-LPH at 08.00 the next day. In the 3 patients with adrenal tumor, β-LPH levels were low and F levels were not suppressed by DEX infusion. In the patient with ectopic ACTH secretion, β-LPH levels were high without any suppression by DEX infusion. In conclusion, this test is useful for the clinical investigation of Cushing's syndrome and for the evaluation of the sensitivity of the hypothalami-pituitary-adrenal axis to glucocorticoids.

11 ADRENAL SENSITIVITY TO ACTH IS DECREASED AFTER ADRENAL TRANSPLANTATION IN RATS. C. F. Allen-Rowlands* and W. C. Engeland, Brown Univ/RI Hospital, Providence 02902, USA

We have previously reported that transplantation(T) of the neonatal adrenal to the anterior chamber of the eye(NTE) of adrenalectomized(ADX) adult rats resulted in elevated plasma ACTH but normal diurnal rhythmicity of plasma corticosterone(B). To determine whether the age of the adrenal at T affects the pituitary-adrenocortical response to T, groups of rats were sacrificed in the AM and in the PM at 5wks after either NTE, ADX and unilateral neonatal(NTK) or adult(ATK) adrenal T to the kidney capsule, or unilateral ADX with sham T(STK). Plasma ACTH and B concentrations were determined by RIA. Normal diurnal rhythmicity in plasma B was seen within all groups ($p<0.01$). Plasma B was similar in the AM for all groups but plasma B in the PM was less in each T group vs STK($p<0.05$). Plasma ACTH was similiar in the AM for all groups but plasma ACTH in the PM was increased in each T group vs STK($p<0.05$). Adrenal sensitivity(AdS) to ACTH was tested in the PM in anesthetized, dexamethasone-blocked rats by measuring plasma B response to submaximal doses of ACTH. Serial samples were collected prior to and post iv ACTH(3 and 10ng). Results showed the plasma B response of each T group was less than that of STK($p<0.05$) and that the response of the neonatal group was less than that of adult T($p<0.05$). AdS was also assessed in vitro by measuring B response to graded [ACTH] of acutely dispersed adrenal cells obtained at 5wks post T. Comparison of the B response to ACTH showed that transplanted adrenal cells have an increased ED50 vs intact cells. These results demonstrate that adrenal T disrupts normal pituitary adrenal feedback relationships. In addition, the age of the adrenal at time of T is important as evidenced by greater impairment observed in the groups with transplanted neonatal adrenals. Finally, the data indicate that this impairment results in part from decreased AdS to ACTH. Supported by NIH AM26831 and RI Hosp grants 7653 & 7655.

12 ADRENOCORTICOTROPIN REGULATES ANGIOTENSIN II RECEPTORS IN ADRENAL CELLS IN VITRO. G. Andoka, J.M. Saez and A.M. Morera*. INSERM U. 162, Hôpital Debrousse, 69322 Lyon Cedex 05, France.

The role of ACTH-(1-24) on angiotensin II (A-II) receptors has been studied on bovine adrenal glomerulosa cells in primary culture. A-II receptors were measured in cells pretreated or not by ACTH-(1-24) on day 4 of culture. ACTH-(1-24) decreased A-II binding sites in a time- and dose-dependent manner. The maximal inhibitory effect was obtained after 24 hours of treatment with 10^{-8}M ACTH-(1-24). The minimal effective dose of ACTH-(1-24) was 10^{-11}M after 24 hours of treatment. Moreover ACTH-(1-24) (10^{-8}M) decreased significantly A-II receptors after 6 hours of treatment. Scatchard plot analysis showed that ACTH-(1-24) treatment did not modify the affinity of A-II receptors (Ka = $0.84 \times 10^{9}M^{-1}$ in the controls and $0.87 \times 10^{9}M^{-1}$ after ACTH treatment) but reduced the A-II sites number per cell from 25,190 to 13,600. Like ACTH-(1-24), 8-Bromo-cAMP (1 mM), Forskolin (5×10^{-5}M) and cholera toxin (10 µg/ml) decreased A-II receptors. Prolactin (10^{-5}M) had no effect. After removal of ACTH or 8-Bromo-cAMP the A-II receptors reappeared progressively during 48 hours. Cycloheximide (20 µg/ml) prevented this receptor reappearance. It has been suggested that the decrease of A-II receptors following an in vivo ACTH administration could be due to a decrease of plasma renin activity. Our studies in vitro demonstrate for the first time that ACTH decreases A-II receptors on glomerulosa cells by a direct mechanism. In addition they also suggest that this effect is mediated by cAMP.

13 THE EFFECT OF INDOMETHACIN ON THE ADRENAL RENIN RESPONSE TO NEPHRECTOMY IN THE RAT. K. Baba, Y. Izumi, F. Atarashi, R. Franco-Saenz* and P.J. Mulrow
Department of Medicine, Medical College of Ohio, C.S. 10008, Toledo, Ohio USA, 43699

The presence of active renin in adrenal glands has been reported by several investigators. Recently our laboratory showed that adrenal renin increases after low Na or high K diet and after nephrectomy (NEPEX). Hypophysectomy (HYPOX) abolishes the response to NEPEX and ACTH treatment restores the response to nephrectomy of HYPOX rats. Since prostaglandin (PG'S) appear to play a role in the release of renin by the kidney, in this study we investigate the effect of PG'S inhibition on the adrenal renin response to NEPEX. Male S.D. rats were nephrectomized and received indomethacin (INDO) 8 mg/kg by gastric lavage immediately after NEPEX and q 9 h therefore for a total of 3 doses. The rats were decapitated 20 h after NEPEX. The adrenals were removed and adrenal renin, aldosterone and PGE_2 were measured by previously described techniques. NEPEX increased adrenal renin from a control of 13.2 ± 1.37 ng Al mg/Prot to 166.5 ± 17.3 ng/mg/Prot. ($P<0.001$). INDO treatment significantly suppressed the adrenal renin response to NEPEX: NEPEX + INDO = 47.8 ± 5.22 ng Al/ng/Prot. Adrenal aldosterone was also suppressed by INDO: control 44.6 ± 2.07 ng/mg, NEPEX 75.1 ± 4.0 ng/ml NEPEX + INDO 64.0 ± 2.89 ng/ml ($p<0.05$). Adrenal PGE_2 increased after NEPEX from 1.49 ± 0.03 ng/mg/Prot to 1.96 ± 0.19 ng/ml/Prot and decreased after INDO to 0.90 ± 0.13 ng/ml/Prot. Plasma corticosterone did not change significantly after INDO suggesting no effect of INDO on ACTH release. In conclusion PG's appear to play a role in the adrenal renin response to nephrectomy. The mechanism by which PG'S influence adrenal renin is presently unknown.

14 STUDIES ON ^{32}P INCORPORATION INTO THE PHOSPHATIDYLINOSITOL (PI), PHOSPHATIDIC ACID (PA) AND PHOSPHATIDYLCHOLINE (PC) OF THE RAT ZONA GLOMERULOSA (ZG) AND FASCICULATA-RETICULARIS (ZFR) ADRENAL CELLS.
J. B. G. Bell, F. W. Chu, G. St. J. Whitley*, J. F. Tait and S. A. S. Tait. Middlesex Hospital Medical School. London W.1. England.

Angiotensins (AII, AIII), which slightly decrease cAMP output but markedly increase the ^{45}Ca efflux of capsular (95% ZG) cells, raised the ^{32}P incorporation into PI and PA, but not into PC. The rise in incorporation into PA, unlike that into PI, was well correlated with increases of steroid output. Serotonin and ACTH, which increased cAMP, had no effect on the ^{45}Ca efflux or on the incorporation of ^{32}P into PA, PI or PC. Under our incubation conditions, increases in K^+ concentration also raise cAMP output but do not affect ^{45}Ca efflux or ^{32}P incorporation into PA (although there is a small effect on incorporation into PI). The incorporation of ^{32}P into PA is the basis of a Ca messenger bioassay using adrenal capsular cells, satisfactory in specificity and also in sensitivity (threshold concentration $5x10^{-11}$ M AII) and precision (index of presision 0.23). ACTH, at certain concentrations, had a significant but small effect on the ^{32}P incorporation into the PI, PA and PC of ZFR cells. These results are in agreement with the data of Farese and coworkers. However, we also find that the angiotensins caused a marked increase in the ^{32}P incorporation into PI (and a smaller increase in incorporation into PA), although they had no effect on steroid output. Therefore, there seems to be a defect in the connection between changes in phospholipid metabolism and steroidogenesis in ZFR cells.

15 PERIODIC, STROBOSCOPIC AND REGRESSION ANALYSES OF CORTISOL (F) AND CORTICOSTERONE (B) SECRETION RATES IN CONSCIOUS, NORMAL DOGS.
L.A. Benton*, L.L. Loring and F.E. Yates, Crump Institute for Medical Engineering, UCLA, Los Angeles, CA 90024, U.S.A.

Both cortisol and corticosterone secretion rates (FSR, BSR) oscillate separately at 90 min. To look for correlations between BSR and FSR that are either monotonic or periodic, we collected over 1000 adrenal blood samples in 17 experiments in 7 dogs. We used linear regression, spectral analysis, and our new method of digital stroboscopy. Stroboscopy keeps waveshapes together instead of separating them into harmonic components. Results: By all 3 methods BSR and FSR were well correlated over experiments lasting 4-8 hr (r^2, 0.74-0.94 in 5/8 cases). In 6/8 cases BSR and FSR showed a joint 90 min oscillation at zero phase. In experiments of less than 30 min, however, BSR and FSR were uncorrelated (r^2, 0.0-0.5 in 8/9 cases). BSR was usually low compared to FSR; BSR/FSR typically was 0.2. (In one case, however, BSR showed a striking increase, opposite to FSR, and BSR/FSR was nearly 2.0.) After a 1 U i.v. bolus of ACTH peak FSR was approximately 40 ug/min, and peak BSR 20% of that value. In 5/6 cases BSR led FSR to peak by 7 min; but BSR lagged increases in adrenal blood flow by 11 min. Conclusions: These results are consistent with either a series (B as precursor to F) or parallel (B and F derived by separate paths from common precursor) relation between B and F in steroidogenesis. 90 min again appears to be a strong organizing rhythm in the normal dog, as we have now reported for BSR, FSR, adrenal blood flow, blood pressure, heart rate, glucose and insulin. (Supported by NIH Grant GM 23732.)

16 INTERFERENCE OF GONADOTROPIN BINDING AND ACTIVATION OF ADENYLYL CYCLASE BY SYNTHETIC ESTROGENS IN THE HUMAN TESTIS.
M.I. Berman* & M.R. Sairam. Reproduction Research Laboratory, Institut de Recherches Cliniques, 110 Ave des Pins O., Montréal H2W 1R7, Canada.

The synthetic estrogens diethyl stilbestrol (DES) and its water soluble derivative diethyl stilbestrol sodium phosphate (DES-NaP), directly inhibited ^{125}I-hFSH and ^{125}I-hCG binding to the human testicular FSH and LH receptors in a dose dependent manner. FSH binding to the receptor was affected to a greater degree than the LH-receptor interaction (60% vs 25% inhibition) suggesting a preferential inhibitory effect of the synthetic estrogens. The pattern of inhibition was similar using either compound, with DES-NaP being more effective. Two other estrogenic compounds, estradiol (E2) and estradiol-benzoate (E2B) had no influence at 400 μg/ml). The steroids testosterone (T), androstendione (A), and progesterone (P) were also without effect at a concentration of 400 μg/ml. Preincubation of the human FSH receptor with DES and DES-NaP, followed by washing, prevented subsequent binding of the labeled FSH, indicating a strong effect. Similar to effects on binding, only DES and DES-NaP affected adenylate cyclase activity. Both effectively inhibited basal and FSH stimulated adenylate cyclase activity in the human and rat systems. Thus, synthetic estrogens may directly inhibit human testicular function by binding to membrane components and inducing conformational changes resulting in decreased binding ability of the gonadotropin receptor and loss of adenylate cyclase activity.
(Supported by MRC of Canada).

17 ANTIGLUCOCORTICOID ACTION OF RU486 IN PATIENTS WITH CUSHING'S SYNDROME.

X.Bertagna, C.Bertagna, M.H.Laudat, J.M.Husson, F.Girard and J.P.Luton*, Centre de Recherches Endocrinologiques, Cochin, Paris 75014; INSERM U142, Trousseau, Paris 75012; Institut Roussel-Uclaf, Paris 75007; France.

The antiglucocorticoid action of RU486 was evaluated in patients with Cushing's syndrome. 400mg of RU were administered at 0800h to 3 patients with Cushing's disease; in contrast to normal subjects there was no significant change in plasma cortisol (F) over the next 10 hours: 0800h 220 ± 32 (ng/ml,mean ± SE),1000h 235 ± 21,1200h 207 ± 33, 1400h 251 ± 28, 1600h 202 ± 48,1800h 246 ± 30. Administration of RU 400mg daily for 3 days increased steroid secretion; variations from baseline (mean of 5 collections) to maximum levels were: 1) for urinary free cortisol (µg/day) 727 to 5720 (case 1), 126 to 586 (case 2), 321 to 990 (case 3); 2) for 0800h plasma F (ng/ml) 237 to 640, 144 to 261, 241 to 413. Plasma ACTH and LPH, (pg/ml), showed parallel although attenuated variations from 30 to 86 and 240 to 477 (case 1), from 10 to 23 and 180 to 220 (case 2). Hormone variations were apparent on day 2, maximum on day 3, and lasted 3 to 4 days after the drug was discontinued. Vital signs were stable; blood glucose, electrolytes, angiotensinogen, leukocytes, as peripheral markers of glucocorticoid action showed no appreciable change. Subjective manifestations of headache (case 2) or malaise (case 3) occurred at the end of treatment and were relieved within minutes by iv dexamethasone (4mg). A fourth patient with the ectopic ACTH syndrome had no steroid secretion rise with RU. In conclusion, RU induced a delayed and prolonged corticotropic response in Cushing's disease; further studies will evaluate whether the resulting F overproduction overcomes the peripheral effect of RU.

18 INTERNALIZATION PATHWAYS OF ^{125}I-AII IN THE ZONA GLOMERULOSA OF THE ADRENAL CORTEX.

C. Bianchi*, J. Gutkowska, A. De Léan, J. Genest, M. Cantin, Clinical Research Institute of Montreal, Quebec, Canada, H2W 1R7.

Female Sprague Dawley rats (40g) were injected with 10^8 CPM of ^{125}I-AII in 0.1 ml of 0.9% NaCl containing 0.1% BSA into the aorta. The animals were sacrificed by intracardiac perfusion first of Locke-Ringer fluid (30 sec) and then with 2% glutaraldehyde (10 min) buffered with cacodylate-HCl at 2, 5, 10 and 20 min after the injection. Controls were infused either with saralasin, the angiotensin III inhibitor or ACTH $^{1-39}$ (5 nmoles) during 30 min before injection of ^{125}I-AII. The adrenal radioactivity was estimated and then the cortex was processed for LM and EM radioautography according to the flat substrate technique. Saralasin almost completely inhibited radioactive uptake and binding, AIII inhibitor was less effective while ACTH had no such effect. In rats injected with ^{125}I-AII, silver grains were localized predominantly over zona glomerulosa cells (ZG) at 2 min and exclusively there at later time intervals. At the EM level most of the radioactivity was associated with the cell surface of ZG cells at 2 min after injection (half distance of 90 nm). At 5 min, clusters of grains were found in coated pits, in coated vesicles and at later time intervals in receptosomes, multivesicular bodies, Golgi complex and finally lysosomes. Concomitant studies of eluted material from the adrenals at 2, 5, 10 and 20 min by chromatography and binding to adrenal cortical beef membranes show that at least half the radioactive material corresponds to ^{125}I-AII. These studies indicate that AII follows the degradative pathway of several peptide hormones. (Supported by MRC group grant).

19 AN EFFORT TO CHARACTERIZE OSTEOPENIA AMONG ELDERLY HYPOPITUITARY FEMALES (SHEEHAN'S SYNDROME). F. Aguiló *& staff, Endocrine Division, University of Puerto Rico Sch Med, San Juan PR

In order to characterize the extent and possible mechanism of bone loss among elderly hypopituitary females, a metabolic, hormonal, radiologic and densitometric survey was done among 43 of our patients with Sheehan's syndrome. A subgroup (42%) with "active bone disease" as shown by their high thermolabile alkaline phosphatase was compared with those with "silent" disease: Twelve patient pairs matched for age and disease duration failed to show statistically significant differences as to: serum Ca, OHproline, Ca intake, sun exposure, Singh's index or % I.V. Ca retained (high vs. N alk. p'tase). Neither could we find differences among 5 patient pairs as to serum PTH, 25 OH vit D, 1,25 diOH vit D, ponderal index, mineral content at distal radii (0.62 vs 0.58 Gm/cm), age (60.9 vs. 61.2 yrs), nor disease duration (30.3 vs. 31.7 yrs). There was a significant inverse correlation between age (not duration), and bone mineral content, only for the group with increased alk. P'tase ($r = -0.67$, $p<0.01$). Thus, through non-invasive means we are unable to distinguish between osteoporosis and osteomalacia among these subjects, in keeping with findings by Miller (Clin. Res. 31:392A, 1983), who propose that only bone histology can distinguish them. This will be particularly relevant among these patients with ample sun exposure (lat 18°N) and prolonged estrogen deficiency as models for hormonal deficiency and aging.

20 AGE-RELATED REDUCTIONS IN THE CONCENTRATIONS OF LH, α AND LH-β, BUT NOT FSH OR FSH-β, IN SERUM OF HEALTHY OLDER COMPARED TO YOUNGER POSTMENOPAUSAL WOMEN. M. R. Blackman*. Dept. of Medicine, Baltimore City Hospitals, and Gerontology Research Center, NIA, NIH, Baltimore, MD 21224 USA.

Several investigators have reported there to be an age-related decline in serum levels of both LH and FSH in older vs younger postmenopausal women. We have measured basal serum concentrations of LH, FSH, α, LH-β, and FSH-β in unfractionated sera from 66 healthy, ambulatory, clinically euthyroid postmenopausal women, aged 36-88y (mean, 58y). Serum glycoprotein levels (ng/ml; mean±SE) in the entire group were as follows: LH, 14.9±1.1; FSH, 17.3±1.0; α, 5.0±0.3; LH-β, 2.8±0.1; and FSH-β, 5.5±0.2. There was a significant decrease in serum α-subunit levels with increasing age ($r=-0.477$; $p<0.001$), such that serum α levels ≥ 7.0 occurred in 8/37 (22%) women below the age of 60, but in only 1/29 (3%) women ≥ 60 years old. Similarly, there were significant decreases in serum levels of LH ($r=-0.304$; $p<0.05$) and LH-β ($r=-0.334$; $p<0.01$) with increasing age. Serum LH values ≥ 18.8 and LH-β values ≥ 4.0 occurred in 10/37 (27%) and 5/37 (13%), respectively, of women below age 60, but in 2/29 (7%) and 0/29 (0%), respectively, of women ≥ 60 years old. In contrast, there were no significant age-related alterations in serum levels of FSH ($r= -0.130$; $p > 0.1$) or FSH-β ($r= -0.061$; $p > 0.1$). These data reveal that, in healthy aging postmenopausal women, there are progressive declines, albeit to differing extents, in circulating levels of LH, α, and LH-β, but not FSH or FSH-β. Since the MCR of LH has been reported not to change significantly after the menopause, these data also suggest there to be a selective decrement in the production of LH, compared with that of FSH, in healthy older vs younger postmenopausal women.

21 MENARCHE AND MENOPAUSE IN HIGHLAND NEW GUINEA. K. Campbell* and J. Wood,
Dept. of Biology, U. of Massachusetts, Boston, MA 02125, and Reproductive Endocrinology Program, U. of Michigan, Ann Arbor, MI 48109.

The Gainj of highland New Guinea have one of the lowest total fertility rates ever recorded in a noncontracepting human population. As part of a series of studies of reproductive endocrinology in this population, we have developed a procedure for estimating age at menarche and menopause--and hence length of the reproductive span--from cross-sectional data on steroids and gonadotropins. Serum samples were drawn from 172 females aged 10 to 60 and assayed by RIA for progesterone (P_4), total estrogen (E) and LH/hCG. Detailed reproductive histories were also obtained. Subjects were classified as pregnant (LH/hCG>100 mIU, P_4>20 ng/ml, E>100 pg/ml), in the luteal phase of the ovarian cycle ($1<P_4<20$ ng/ml), lactating (based on self-assessment) or unclassifiable on hormonal grounds. A probability argument permits categorizing unclassified subjects as either acyclic or in the follicular phase of the cycle. Finally, a weighted maximum likelihood version of probit analysis is used to estimate median age at menarche and menopause from these data. We find that the median age at menarche is 20.9 ± 0.9 years. Although this figure appears extraordinary, it is consistent with morphological data collected among the Gainj, as well as evidence from neighboring populations. The estimated median age at menopause is 46.2 ± 1.1 years, not greatly different from what is observed in Western populations. We conclude that one reason for the low reproductive output of Gainj women is a reproductive lifetime that is truncated at younger ages. Supported by NSF, NIH and the Mellon Foundation.

22 DYNAMICS OF STEROID METABOLISM IN AGING MALE RATS. S.W.C. Chan* and A. M. Hasan. Dept. Biology, SUNY Brockport, NY USA.

There is a paucity of information on age-related changes in dynamics of steroid metabolism in rats. This study examined changes in metabolic clearance rates (M.C.R.) of testosterone (T) and estradiol (E_2) in aging Sprague-Dawley rats using the non-equilibrium method of single dose of ^{3}H-steroid injected via the cannulated jugular vein. ^{3}H-steroids were extracted, processed by LH-20 columns and results were analysed using the 'peel-off' method for a two-compartment model. M.C.R. of T for the 4m rats (66.94 l/d or 124.6 l/kg/d) were approximately 7 times higher than the 18m rats (9.32 l/d or 16.36 l/kg/d). Half-lives ($T_{1/2}$) also differed significantly for the two age-groups (4m vs 18m: α-7.63 vs 12.56 min; β-105.2 vs 241.8 min). Both the inner and outer metabolic pool sizes for the 4m are twice that of the 18m rats. Production rates of T in the young greatly exceded that of the aged rats (261 μg/d vs 8.67 μg/d). M.C.R. for E_2, however, remained unchanged; $T_{1/2}$ for the inner but not the outer compartment were similar in the two groups. Chronically castrated animals of both age groups showed significant decline in M.C.R. and increases in $T_{1/2}$ when compared with their respective intact controls. Interestingly, both M.C.R. and $T_{1/2}$ values of the young castrates now approximated those of the aged intact rats.These results testify to an interaction of age and androgen status to bring about senescent dysfunction of the testis in rats.

23 A COMPARISON OF THE EFFECTS OF CHRONIC CORTICOTROPHIN TREATMENT ON ALDOSTERONE SECRETION BY RAT ADRENAL TISSUE IN VITRO AND IN VIVO.
D.R.E.Abayasekara, B.J.Whitehouse*, H.Vazir, G.P.Vinson & M.E.McAuley, Department of Physiology, Queen Elizabeth College London W8 and Department of Biochemistry, St.Bartholomew's Medical College, London EC1, U.K.

The reported effects of chronic corticotrophin (ACTH) treatment on aldosterone secretion *in vitro* and *in vivo* are inconsistent and a systematic comparison has therefore been made. Sprague Dawley rats (250-300 gm body weight) were injected for 8 days with varying doses of ACTH (Synacthen Depot; 25, 50 or 100 µg/day) and maintained on normal or low sodium or high potassium diets. Aldosterone levels were measured by RIA, and corticosterone and 18-OH-DOC were measured by gas chromatography. Results are expressed as the ratio of experimental values to controls (R). In all experiments aldosterone production by capsular tissue from ACTH treated animals was suppressed (R=0.17 ± 0.02), whereas corticosterone and 18-OH DOC production was stimulated (R=6.2 ± 0.6 and R=4.9 ± 1.1 respectively). In contrast, peripheral plasma aldosterone levels were found to be significantly elevated in ACTH treated animals (R=1.5 ± 0.14). However, when adrenal vein blood was sampled aldosterone production was again found to be suppressed (R=0.06 ± 0.01). The results show therefore that chronic ACTH treatment does suppress aldosterone secretion both *in vivo* and *in vitro*, but that paradoxically peripheral plasma aldosterone levels appear to be increased. This phenomenon may be accounted for by changes in metabolism and clearance of aldosterone in ACTH treated animals.

24 ALTERED REGULATION OF ADRENAL SENSITIVITY TO ANGIOTENSIN II (AII) IN THE SPONTANEOUS HYPERTENSIVE RAT.
G. Aguilera*, W. Hausdorff and K. J. Catt. ERRB, NICHD, NIH, Bethesda, MD 20205, U.S.A.

The normal regulation of adrenal and vascular sensitivity to angiotensin II (AII) during changes in sodium intake has an important role in the maintenance of circulatory homeostasis. To determine whether adrenal regulation is altered in hypertension, we analyzed the effects of dietary sodium on plasma aldosterone (aldo), adrenal AII receptors and 18 hydroxylase activity in 10 week old spontaneous hypertensive rats (SHR) and Wistar Kyoto (WKY) controls. Basal plasma aldo levels were lower in SHR than in WKY rats (6.8±1.3 and 11.5±3.2 ng%, n=23), and the aldo responses to sodium intake were correspondingly lower in the SHR (63±8 and 5.8±1.3 ng%, low and high sodium diet) than in WKY rats (143±15 and <2 ng% respectively). On the other hand, the SHR showed an exaggerated aldo response to ether stress, with aldo levels of 98±5 compared to 57+5 in WKY. When adrenal AII receptors were compared during dietary sodium changes, their concentrations in WKY rats were 730±68 and 1842±183 fmol/mg with high and low sodium diet, respectively, whereas SHR showed little change (947±80 and 1152±45 fmol/mg). This blunted response in SHR rats was also reflected in the 18-hydroxylase activity, with aldo formation of 43 and 59 nmol/mg/min in adrenal mitochondria from sodium-loaded and restricted SHR, while responses were normal in the WKY (25 and 78 nmol/mg/min). The inability of SHR to adjust their adrenal responses to altered sodium intake reflects a defect in the mechanisms that modulate the responsiveness to AII, and may be an important factor in the pathogenesis of hypertension in these animals.

25 URINARY KALLIKREIN: SEX DIFFERENCE, MENSTRUAL VARIATION, SHORT AND LONG TERM RELATIONSHIP TO ALDOSTERONE. J.D.M. Albano, S. Campbell, A. Farrer, D. Kirk and J.G.B. Millar*, University of Southampton Department of Medicine, St. Mary's Hospital, Portsmouth PO3 6AD, United Kingdom.

A close relationship between urinary kallikrein (UK) and mineralocorticoid activity has been well documented, but other hormonal influences on UK are less clear. A comparison between healthy male subjects and healthy females with regular periods showed a range of 84 - 1262 units (U)/24 hrs (mean 350.6) in males and 239 - 1832 U/24 hrs (mean 929.9) in females, which is a significant difference ($p < 0.01$). Levels were constant in individual males, within subject variance accounting for only 1.6% of the total. In females a clear-cut variation was seen within the menstrual cycle, mid luteal levels for UK averaging more than double the mid-follicular levels, and paralleling the changes seen in plasma renin activity (PRA) and plasma aldosterone (PA). A close correlation ($r = 0.82$, $p < 0.001$) was found between UK and serum progesterone. This variation was abolished both by the administration of spironolactone during the luteal phase and by administration of a combined oestrogen-progestogen oral contraceptive. In contrast to PA there was no nyctohemeral variation in UK excretion; day/night rates of excretion correlated closely within subjects ($r = 0.98$, $m = 0.978$). Addisonian patients had very low levels of UK, which returned to normal on treatment while in primary hyperaldosteronism high levels were found, again returning to normal after treatment. We concluded that over periods of several days or weeks a close relationship between PA and UK can be seen, but short term changes in PA have no demonstrable effect on UK excretion.

26 EVIDENCE THAT CALCIUM IS A SECOND MESSENGER FOR RENIN RELEASE. I. Antonipillai* and R. Horton, Section of Endocrinology, Department of Medicine, LAC/USC Medical Center, Los Angeles, Ca.

To more directly study the role of calcium in renin release, independent of vascular tone or sodium flux, we used rat renal cortical slices. At physiologic temperature, osmolarity, Ca (10^{-3}M) and an energy source (KRBG buffer), 95% O_2 and 5% CO_2, our preparation was stable for periods >1 hr. (96+10%). Each slice acted as its own control using 15 min. periods. Renin release was measured by RIA of generated angiotensin I using homologous renin substrate from anephric animals. Isoproterenol 10^{-6}M induces a significant release of renin (160±10%, $p < 0.05$). Ca-free buffer does not alter this response (151±21%) supporting a primary role of cAMP as the 2nd messenger of this β adrenergic agonist. AII 10^{-6}M inhibits renin release as it does in vivo (69±7%, $p < 0.05$), but Ca-free buffer blocks this effect (100±6%). Nifedipine, a Ca channel inhibitor, 10^{-5}M induces a marked increase in renin release (182±37%). TMB-8 10^{-4}M, a specific intracellular inhibitor of Ca release causes a marked increase in renin release of 2 1/2-3 fold control values. Trifluoperazine (TFP), a calmodulin inactivator (10^{-4}M) induced a significant stimulation in renin release (154±15%), all studies $p < 0.01$. We conclude that 1) the adrenergic signal for renin release is independent of extracellular Ca. 2) Angiotensin II acts via Ca++ as it does on vessels and adrenal glomerulosa cells. 3) Inhibition of calcium entry, intracellular calcium action, or calmodulin activity increases renin release indicating that unlike its effect upon other systems, reduced Ca++ levels act as a renin secretogogue.

27 CLEARANCE OF ANGIOTENSINOGEN AND DES-ANGIOTENSIN I-ANGIOTENSINOGEN IN RATS IN DIFFERENT PHYSIOLOGIC STATES.
J.Bouhnik*, D.J.Campbell, P.Corvol and J.Ménard. INSERM U36, 17, rue du Fer-à-Moulin. 75005 Paris. France.

In order to define the role of renin in the clearance of plasma angiotensinogen (Aogen), we have investigated the clearance of both ^{125}I-labeled intact Aogen and ^{125}I-Des-AI-Aogen in 3 groups of rats: normal, binephrectomized and captopril-treated. The extent of hydrolysis of Aogen in vivo was determined from the change in the proportion of radioactivity released after incubation with an excess of renin. Thus, we are able to measure the plasma clearance of Aogen in rats with high plasma renin levels and demonstrable Aogen hydrolysis in vivo. Clearance data were fitted to a two-compartment model; compartment 1 representing the initial rapid phase and compartment 2, the second slower phase of clearance.

	Plasma half-life (min ± SEM)		
	Normal	Binephrectomized	Captopril
Des-AI-Angiotensinogen			
Compartment 1	57 ± 6	79 ± 9	77 ± 5
Compartment 2	362 ± 35	542 ± 43	296 ± 8
Angiotensinogen			
Compartment 1	87 ± 7	82 ± 6	83 ± 3
Compartment 2	290 ± 35	458 ± 28	215 ± 34

These results demonstrate 1. In binephrectomized rats, clearance of Des-AI-Aogen and intact Aogen is similar. 2. Binephrectomy prolongs the second phase of clearance of both Des-AI-Aogen and Aogen indicating a role for the kidney in the clearance. 3. High plasma renin levels in captopril-treated rats accelerate the second phase of clearance of Aogen but not Des-AI-Aogen.

28 APPARENT CORRELATION BETWEEN RATE OF PREKALLIKREIN ACTIVATION AND CRYO-ACTIVATION OF HUMAN PLASMA PRORENIN.
C.F. Brown* and D.H. Osmond, Dept. of Physiology, Univ. of Toronto, Toronto, Ontario, M5S 1A8, Canada.

Human plasma "prorenin" can be converted to renin in vitro by incubating plasma at -4°C. This "cryoactivation" (CA) of prorenin is protease-dependent, continues for several days at -4°C, and is markedly inhibited in plasmas deficient in either factor XII or plasminogen. Plasma prekallikrein has also been implicated in prorenin activation. During CA of 6 individual human plasmas for 6 days the rates of activation of prekallikrein (PK), plasminogen (PLG) and prorenin (as increased plasma renin activity, PRA) were determined. Subjects 1 and 2 had the highest prorenin, and subject 6 the lowest. Prekallikrein was almost completely activated in subjects 1 and 2 after 1 day of CA, and scarcely activated in subject 6, suggesting an apparent correlation between the rate of PK consumption and the rate of prorenin activation. Subjects 3 to 5 had intermediate degrees of activation of both prorenin and PK. Surprisingly, there was no evidence of plasminogen activation in any subject, despite the probable presence of kallikrein (from activated prekallikrein), a known PLG activator. Thus, our data suggest a possible role for prekallikrein-kallikrein in prorenin activation without further defining any likely cooperative actions of plasminogen and factor XII.

Supported by the Ontario Heart Foundation.

29 CHARACTERIZATION OF PRECURSOR AND SECRETED FORMS OF HUMAN ANGIOTENSINOGEN.

D.J.Campbell*, J.Bouhnik, E.Coezy, J.Ménard, P.Corvol, INSERM U 36, Paris, France.

We have investigated the basis of the heterogeneity of plasma angiotensinogen (Aogen) using two complementary approaches. ^{35}S-Methionine labeled Aogen precursor synthesized by rabbit reticulocyte lysate primed with human liver RNA was compared with ^{35}S-methionine labeled Aogen secreted by human hepatoma cells (Hep G2) using immunoprecipitation, sodium dodecyl sulfate polyacrylamide gel electrophoresis and autoradiography. Cell free translation of RNA revealed a single precursor (MW~50k) which was cleaved by renin resulting in nonglycosylated des-AI-Aogen (MW~45.6k). Cell free translation of RNA in the presence of microsomal membranes suggested two sites of N-glycosylation. Subsequent removal of oligosaccharides with endoglycosidase H revealed a proAogen of MW~46.7k which was of higher MW than nonglycosylated secreted Aogen suggesting that the precursor contains a prosequence of MW~0.6k. Whereas secreted glycosylated Aogen showed electrophoretic heterogeneity (MW 53-67k), tunicamycin treated cells secreted a major nonglycosylated form of MW~46.1k which, after cleavage by renin, had identical electrophoretic mobility to des-AI-Aogen synthesized by cell free translation. Despite complete inhibition of N-glycosylation, 10% of Aogen secreted by tunicamycin treated cells had a higher MW (46-50k) which, after cleavage by renin showed a reduction in MW of ~1k. These results demonstrate that the major contribution to heterogeneity of secreted Aogen is variation in N-glycosylation. However, there is also evidence for another post-translational modification of secreted Aogen. Pure human Aogen was the gift of Dr D.A.Tewksbury.

30 CYTOSOLIC FREE CA^{++} AND ALDOSTERONE PRODUCTION IN BOVINE ADRENAL GLOMERULOSA CELLS: EFFECTS OF ANGIOTENSIN II AND POTASSIUM.

A. Capponi*, D. Lew, L. Jornot and M. Vallotton, Divisions of Endocrinology and Infectious Diseases, University Hospital, CH-1211 Geneva, Switzerland.

Quantitative changes in cytosolic free calcium, ($[Ca^{++}]_i$), membrane potential and aldosterone production in response to angiotensin II and extracellular potassium were measured in intact bovine adrenal glomerulosa cells loaded with the fluorescent calcium indicator, quin 2. Angiotensin II (10^{-9} M) induced a rapid rise in $[Ca^{++}]_i$ from 124±26 nM to 204±63 nM (n=7), which was followed by aldosterone production, as measured in dynamic studies with superfused adrenal cells, and by slower changes in membrane potential, as assessed with the fluorescent probe, 3,3'-dipropylthiadicarbocyanine (diS-C_3-(5)). Both $[Ca^{++}]_i$ rises and functional response were blocked by the antagonist analogue, (Sar^1, Ala^8)-angiotensin II, in a dose-dependent manner. Potassium (3 - 10 mM) provoked dose-dependent increases in $[Ca^{++}]_i$, with ED_{50} of 6.5 mM, associated with rapid changes in membrane potential, a response superimposable to the dose-related aldosterone production induced by potassium in static incubations of quin 2-loaded glomerulosa cells (ED_{50} = 6.8 mM). Verapamil (20 µM) decreased resting $[Ca^{++}]_i$ and blocked entirely the rise in $[Ca^{++}]_i$ induced by potassium, but not that induced by angiotensin II. These findings indicate that two important physiological regulators of aldosterone secretion, extracellular potassium, by the opening of voltage-dependent calcium channels, and angiotensin II, by a receptor-mediated mechanism, induce rapid rises in cytosolic free calcium, which precede, and presumably trigger the biological response.

31 AGGRESSIVE BEHAVIOR AUGMENTS SERUM βNGF IN MOUSE - COMPARISON OF RADIOIMMUNOASSAY AND BIOASSAY. J. Alm*, J. Lakshmanan, U. Beri, H. Kim, T. Macaso and D.A. Fisher. Harbor-UCLA Medical Center, UCLA School of Medicine, Torrance, CA 90509

Using adult Swiss-Webster female and male mice we studied serum βNGF under basal conditions and changes due to aggressive behavior. The mice were housed 1, 2 or 5 per cage for 1 week before killed. Aggressive behavior was induced by grouping 6 previously isolated mice together in one cage during 20-40 minutes before killing. A new sensitive RIA was used with a sensitivity of 20 pg/tube. The RIA was validated by tests of parallelism, recovery studies, evaluation of crossreactivity and comparison with PC-12 bioassay (neurite outgrowth). Results: Serum NGF in ng/ml (means ± SD were:

Housing:	1 mouse/cage	2 mice/cage	5 mice/cage	Aggressive mice
Females	1.5±0.20	1.6±0.046	1.6±0.11	-
Males	1.7±0.093	1.7±0.13	2.7±1.7	115±90

Bioassay was performed on serum samples from the aggressive males and confirmed the RIA results. The increase of serum βNGF in male mice housed 5 per cage and in aggressive males was significant ($p<0.05$).
Conclusions: 1) The results confirm that stress associated housing conditions in male mice increase basal serum βNGF levels; 2) This phenomenon is further augmented by 2 orders of magnitude when aggressive behavior is induced by fighting; 3) The high serum βNGF levels in aggressive male mice provides a way to validate serum βNGF-RIA with bioassay systems.

32 BIOCHEMICAL CHARACTERIZATION OF A FSH SUPPRESSING FACTOR FROM HUMAN SEMINAL PLASMA. N.J. Arbatti*[1,2], A.R. Sheth[1] and M.R. Sairam[2]. Institute for Research in Reproduction, Parel, Bombay, India[1]. Reproduction Research Lab., Clinical Research Institute of Montreal, Qué. Canada[2].

Human seminal plasma appears to contain proteinaceous substance of differing molecular weights with the ability to suppress FSH release from the pituitary. Employing a three step purification scheme a protein with inhibin like activity was obtained from steroid free ethanolic powder of human seminal plasma. The isolation procedure consisted of gel filtration on Sephadex G-100, ion exchange chromatography on DEAE-Sephadex A 50 and rechromatography on Sephadex G-75. The protein with a molecular weight of about 15,000 daltons was acidic in nature as suggested by electrophoretic behavior at pH 8.9. Its homogeneity was established by FPLC on Mono Q column and reverse phase HPLC. The active fraction decreased the LH-RH response of mouse pituitaries incubated *in vitro*. FSH release was preferentially suppressed. The active fraction did not inhibit the basal release of FSH in cultured rat pituitary cells. However, the increase in serum FSH induced by castration in adult male rats was preferentially suppressed suggesting that this inhibin like factor acts when pituitaries are sensitized by LHRH or castration. Hexoses were not detectable but the protein contained about 0.1% of glucosamine and galactosamine. Approximately 140 amino acid residues were estimated to be present in the homogeneous protein which had serine at the NH_2-terminus and isoleucine at the COOH terminus. The homogeneous protein has no effect on the binding of labeled FSH or LH to their respective receptors.
(This work was supported by a Research Training Grant to NJA from W.H.O.).

33 OSTEOMALACIA IN PATIENTS WITH HIP FRACTURES - A FREQUENT PROBLEM, BUT A DIAGNOSTIC DILEMMA.

S.H. Doppelt*, X.W. Meng, G.V. Segre, M. Holick, H.J. Mankin and R.M. Neer, Massachusetts General Hospital, Boston, MA 02114

To evaluate the pathogenesis of their osteopenia, 187 patients with hip fractures admitted to the Massachusetts General Hospital had measurements of serum calcium, phosphorus, alkaline phosphatase, 25-Hydroxyvitamin D (25-OH-D), amino-terminal parathyroid hormone (PTH), 1,25-dihydroxyvitamin D (1,25-$(OH)_2$D), and quantitative histomorphometric analysis of randomly selected bicortical iliac crest biopsies.

21% had serum 25-OH-D levels below normal (normal = 8-55 ng/ml), and an additional 12% were in the very low normal range (8-10 ng/ml). 35% had an elevated PTH value ($>$25 pg/ml) and 22% had sub-normal 1,25$(OH)_2$D levels (normal = 26-65 pg/ml. 20% of patients biopsied had osteomalacia. The serum calcium, phosphorus and alkaline phosphatase were in general normal and showed no correlation with the other measurements. 57% had either an elevated PTH or a low or borderline low 25-OH-D; 39% had either an elevated PTH or a low 1,25-$(OH)_2$D, but PTH and D-metabolite levels were not correlated in 2-way or 3-way comparisons, nor were D-metabolite levels correlated with each other; no combination of hormone levels predicted bone histology. We conclude: there is a high incidence of osteomalacia and an even higher incidence of vitamin D deficiency among the elderly with hip fractures; serum 1,25-$(OH)_2$D levels cannot be used to exclude vitamin D deficiency or osteomalacia; unmeasured factors significantly affect bone histology and modify interactions of the calcium-regulation hormones in this disease, and therefore must be involved in its genesis.

34 IMMUNOREACTIVE VASOACTIVE INTESTINAL POLYPEPTIDE (VIP) IN HYPOPHYSIAL PORTAL VESSEL BLOOD: EFFECTS OF ANAESTHETICS AND GUT REMOVAL.

A.K. Brar*, W.H. Rostene+ and G. Fink, MRC Brain Metabolism Unit, 1 George Sq., Edinburgh, Scotland; +INSERM U55, Hopital St-Antoine, 75012, Paris, France.

There is growing evidence for a role of VIP as a PRL-releasing factor. Since the peripheral blood (PB) concentration of PRL varies during the rat oestrous cycle, we measured the release of VIP into PB and hypophysial portal vessel blood (HPVB) during the cycle. As anaesthetics modify the release of hypothalamic peptides, the effect of i.p. Althesin (A), Ketalar (K), Urethane (U) or Sagatal (S) on HPVB VIP levels was determined. The concentration of VIP in PB and HPVB was also measured after removal of the gut to determine the contribution of gut VIP secretion to VIP levels in PB and HPVB. PB was obtained from the jugular vein before cutting the pituitary stalk. HPVB was collected for two 30 min periods between 15:30-18:30 h daily during the oestrous cycle. In all groups of rats, VIP concentration in HPVB was significantly ($P < 0.01$) greater than in PB. The release of VIP into HPVB but not PB, on any particular day of the cycle varied with the anaesthetic used, e.g. on pro-oestrous (the day of PRL surge) rats given K but not A, U, or S had significantly ($P < 0.05$) higher VIP values in HPVB than on diestrus (192 $\pm$ 35 vs 70 $\pm$ 12 pg/ml). Removal of the gut (lower oesophagus to rectum) significantly ($P < 0.01$) decreased VIP concentration in PB. VIP released into HPVB was unaffected by removal of the gut. Conclusions: (1) Since K but not A suppresses oestrogen-induced surges in PRL in PB the increase in VIP in HPVB in rats given K may not be related to the pro-oestrous surge of PRL; (2) The main source of VIP in HPVB is the hypothalamus; (3) PB VIP is derived mainly from the gut.

35 STRESS HORMONE CHANGES IN BLOOD AND CEREBROSPINAL FLUID (CSF): EFFECT OF INTRACEREBROVENTRICULAR (I.C.V.) CAPTOPRIL. V. Cameron*, E. Espiner, G. Nicholls, R. Donald and M. MacFarlane, Department of Endocrinology, The Princess Margaret Hospital, Christchurch, New Zealand.

Acute moderate hemorrhage (15 ml/kg over 10 min) was used to study stress hormone changes in blood and CSF in conscious sheep with indwelling I.C.V. cannulae. Plasma hormone levels (mean ± SEM, n = 8), before and after hemorrhage (H), were: arginine vasopressin (AVP) pre 8 ± 5, peak (20 min) 1506 ± 475 pmol/L; ACTH pre 169 ± 27, peak (20 min) 2360 ± 836 ng/L; angiotensin II (AII) pre 16 ± 4, peak (10 min) 72 ± 23 pmol/L; cortisol pre 38 ± 7, peak (45 min) 125 ± 15 nmol/L; epinephrine (epi) pre 235 ± 48, peak (10 min) 621 ± 170 pg/ml. After H, CSF AVP increased to peak levels at 15 min whereas the rise in CSF ACTH, AII and cortisol was slower (peak at 90 min) and independent of levels observed in plasma. Despite signs of increased sympathetic activity and rise in plasma catecholamines, CSF epi fell after H. A possible role of the brain renin angiotensin system in mediating the hormone response to H was assessed in separate experiments using I.C.V. captopril. When captopril was infused into the lateral ventricle (2.8 ng/min) 1 hr pre and during H, the peak plasma ACTH and AVP response was markedly reduced in 3 of 4 sheep whereas the plasma AII response to H remained unimpaired. These results show that there is a selective increase in stress hormones in ventricular CSF after H and suggest that the brain renin angiotensin system may be involved in the plasma ACTH and AVP response to acute H in sheep.

36 TRYPSIN-SENSITIVE SITES ON 1,25-DIHYDROXYVITAMIN D_3 RECEPTORS ARE ASSOCIATED WITH HORMONE, DNA, AND MONOCLONAL ANTIBODY BINDING DOMAINS. E. A. Allegretto* and J. W. Pike, Department of Biochemistry, University of Arizona Health Sciences Center, Tucson, Arizona, USA.

Chick 1,25-dihydroxyvitamin D_3 (1,25$(OH)_2D_3$) receptors were subjected to limited tryptic digestion as a means of evaluating the interrelationship between its binding domains for hormone, DNA, and antibody. Hormone-labeled intestinal cytosol receptors exhibited enzyme concentration dependent changes which were characterized via DEAE ion exchange HPLC, gel filtration, and sedimentation analysis, as well as through binding to DNA-cellulose and antibody. The effects of trypsin were multiple, and suggest that the 1,25$(OH)_2D_3$ receptor contains at least two sites differentially sensitive to the enzyme. Action at site I (3 µg trypsin/A_{280}), caused dissociation of high-salt receptor aggregates, loss of DNA binding, and an apparent 10-fold reduction in affinity for monoclonal antibody. No evidence of hormone dissociation, or changes in charge, shape, or size were discernible. Activity at site II (100 µg trypsin/A_{280}), produced a major cleavage fragment which retained 1,25$(OH)_2D_3$, evidenced reduced charge, sedimented at 2.5S, M_r = 45,000, and was unreactive to antibody. Prolonged exposure resulted in unique polypeptides concomitant with loss of hormone binding. These observations suggest that the receptor's 1,25-$(OH)_2D_3$ binding region is separate from the domains associated with binding sites for both DNA and antibody, although the latter appear to be interrelated. This approach, utilizing enzymatic digestion, coupled with DNA, radioligand, and immunologic probes, should prove useful in deciphering the topology of the 1,25$(OH)_2D_3$ receptor. Supported by AM-32313.

37 HUMAN MEDULLARY THYROID CARCINOMA (MTC) IN CULTURE PROVIDES A MODEL RELATING GROWTH DYNAMICS, ENDOCRINE CELL DIFFERENTIATION, AND TUMOR PROGRESSION.

C.L.Berger*, A.deBustros, B.A.Roos, S.S.Leong, G.Mendelsohn, M.S.Gesell and S.B.Baylin, The Johns Hopkins Medical Inst., Balto., MD 21205, Case Western Reserve Univ., Cleveland, OH, Roswell Park Memorial Inst., Buffalo, NY.

Tumor tissues from patients with virulent MTC have an increased ratio of L-dopa decarboxylase activity (DDC) to calcitonin (CT) and a high degree of cellular heterogeneity for CT immunostaining (JCEM 54:233,1982). Using the TT culture line of human MTC, obtained from a patient who died of metastatic MTC, we studied relationships among DDC, CT and growth and differentiation. During exponential growth, DDC increased by 70%, CT decreased by 40%, and the resultant ratio of DDC to CT increased by 3-fold. In 54 clones derived from parent cells, intracellular CT levels varied more widely than DDC (15-fold vs. 4-fold). Growth curves performed on the highest and lowest CT producing clones exhibited the same dynamics between DDC and CT as the parent line. However, in the low CT producing clone, the DDC/CT ratios were 3-4 fold higher and in the range seen only in tumor tissue from patients dying from MTC. Cells from the parent line and the two clones were grown on embryonic chick skin. Cellular heterogeneity for CT immunostaining was greatest in the clone with the lowest CT levels. Heterogeneity increased dramatically in the parent line and in both clones during growth. We conclude that in human MTC: (1) the inverse relationships between DDC and CT are determined by the fraction of actively proliferating cells; and (2) the magnitude of the ratio is a function of the differentiation potential of individual cell clones. In patients with virulent MTC, a high fraction of rapidly growing cells and of immature clones would well explain the biochemistry previously observed.

38 1,25 DIHYDROXYVITAMIN D ($1,25(OH)_2D$) INCREASES CALMODULIN BINDING TO SPECIFIC DUODENAL BRUSH BORDER MEMBRANE PROTEINS.

D.D. Bikle*, S. Munson, Veterans Administration and University of California, San Francisco, and J. Chafouleas, Baylor College of Medicine, Houston, Texas.

The administration of 1,25 dihydroxyvitamin D ($1,25(OH)_2D$) to vitamin D deficient chicks increases the calmodulin (CaM) content of the subsequently isolated duodenal brush border membranes (BBM). This increase in CaM parallels the increased ability of the BBM to accumulate calcium; the increased ability of the BBM to accumulate calcium is blocked by specific CaM antagonists (trifluoperazine, W_7, W_{13}). To evaluate the mechanism by which $1,25(OH)_2D$ increases the CaM content of the BBM we separated the proteins of the BBM using SDS-PAGE and analyzed the ability of proteins so separated to bind to ^{125}I-CaM. We observed that 3 proteins with the molecular weights of 102K, 88K, and 78K bound CaM. Unlike the CaM binding proteins of the basolateral membrane, these CaM binding proteins did not require calcium for the binding of CaM to occur. However, binding was abolished by both 10^{-4}M trifluoperazine and excess nonradioactive CaM. The administration of $1,25(OH)_2D$ increased the extent of CaM binding to all 3 proteins with a time course of response that paralleled the increase in CaM content of and calcium uptake by the BBM. We conclude that $1,25(OH)_2D$ increases the ability of specific proteins in the BBM to bind CaM, and this increased CaM binding may mediate the ability of $1,25(OH)_2D$ to stimulate calcium flux across the BBM.

39 PARATHYROID HORMONE(PTH) AND INSULIN(IRI) RESPONSES TO THE DOPAMINERGIC AGONIST 2-AMINO-6,7-DIHYDROXY-1,2,3,4-TETRAHYDRONAPHTHALENE(ADTN). J.Blum* and J.Fischer, Inst.for Animal Prod., Swiss Fed.Inst.of Techn., 8092 Zurich, and Res.Lab.for Calcium Metab., Dept.of Orthoped.Surg.and Med., Univ.of Zurich, 8008 and 8091 Zurich, Switzerland.

The administration of dopamine(DA) is followed by increased blood plasma levels of norepinephrine(NE) and epinephrine(E), which interact with α- and β-adrenergic receptors. The DA-like agonist ADTN is not metabolized to NE and E. We have studied effects of ADTN on plasma PTH and IRI levels in cattle. During ADTN infusions (.2, 1 and 5 μg/kg/min for 7 min) plasma levels of ADTN, PTH and glucose increased within min in a dose-dependent manner, whereas IRI decreased and calcium remained unchanged. The administration of glucose and tolbutamide raised IRI in the absence but not in the presence of ADTN, whereas IRI responses to the β-adrenergic agonist isoproterenol were maintained during simultaneous ADTN infusions. PTH, IRI and glucose responses to ADTN were not modified by the β-adrenergic blocker propranolol, infused in amounts lowering basal IRI levels and earlier shown to suppress PTH responses to isoproterenol and E. During infusions with the α-adrenergic blocker phentolamine, IRI increased within min and PTH remained unchanged. Superimposed ADTN infusions caused PTH to increase, while IRI decreased and glucose responses were suppressed. In conclusion, although the increase of glucose was due to intrinsic α-adrenergic properties of ADTN, the DA-like agonist caused a direct stimulation of PTH secretion, not mediated by hypocalcemia or β-adrenergic receptors on parathyroid cells, and a direct inhibition of IRI secretion.

40 IMMUNOCYTOCHEMICAL EVIDENCE FOR ENDOGENOUS HORMONES IN OSTEOBLASTS OF NEONATAL MICE CALVARIA. G. Boivin*, G. Morel°, P.J. Meunier and P.M. Dubois°, INSERM unité 234, Faculté A. Carrel, 69008 Lyon, France; ° CNRS ERA 981 et Laboratoire d'Histologie et Embryologie, Faculté de Médecine Lyon-Sud, 69921 Oullins, France.

Immunoreactivity to endogenous calcitonin (CT), endogenous parathyroid hormone (PTH), endogenous estradiol (E_2) and estradiol receptors (E_2-receptors) were studied in osteoblasts from neonatal mouse calvaria by immunocytochemistry, using ultrathin sections obtained by cryoultramicrotomy. Tissues were fixed in glutaraldehyde, post-fixed in osmium tetroxide and frozen under liquid nitrogen. Ultrathin sections obtained at -140°C with an ultrotome III fitted with a cryokit, were incubated with the different antiserums. The antigen-antibody reactions were detected by peroxidase conjugated complex revealed by 4-chloro-1-naphthol. E_2 and E_2-receptors could not be detected in osteoblasts, whereas CT- and PTH-like immunoreactivities were observed in this cell-type. CT and PTH had similar subcellular localizations: at the plasma membrane level, in the cytoplasmic matrix — but not in organelles —, and in the nucleus (nuclear membrane; euchromatin in the vicinity of heterochromatin). These results provide immunocytological evidence for: 1) the internalization of CT and PTH in osteoblasts; 2) a direct participation of CT and PTH in osteoblastic function; 3) the absence of E_2-receptors and E_2 in osteoblasts. Other hormones as testosterone, growth hormone and 1,25 dihydroxyvitamin D_3 are under investigation.

41 CALCITONIN RECEPTORS IN RAT KIDNEY ; PURIFICATION AND CHARACTERIZATION.
Bouizar*, Z., Taboulet, J., Fouchereau-Peron+, M., Milhaud, G., and Moukhtar, M.S., U113 INSERM, 27 rue Chaligny, 75012 Paris, FRANCE.

+Laboratoire de Biologie Marine du Collège de France, 29110 Concarneau, FRANCE.

Specific receptors for calcitonin have been reported in kidney and bone, two physiological target organs of the hormone. We have characterized the binding parameters of renal receptors (Scatchard analysis revealed the presence of two sites : Site I, $ka_1 = 1.29 \times 10^9\ M^{-1}$, number of binding sites I = 9.9×10^6/ug protein and site II, $ka_2 = 4.2 \times 10^8\ M^{-1}$, number of binding sites II = 1.86×10^7/ug protein) and studied the effects of solubilization. A 4000 fold purification was achieved using molecular sieving and affinity chromatography (synthetic salmon calcitonin bound to sepharose 4B). Binding parameters were obtained for the purified fractions, and SDS polyacrylamide gel electrophoresis carried out. Synthetic salmon calcitonin was also bound to renal membranes using chemical or photoaffinity cross-linking. When solubilized membranes were subjected to S-200 chromatography, specific binding of sCT was observed in a fraction eluting in a volume consistent with an apparent M.W. of 447.000 daltons. Cross-linked receptors also eluted in the same volume. SDS polyacrylamide gel electrophoresis showed the presence of two protein bands specifically binding sCT, of molecular weight 68.000 and 38.900 respectively. The partial purification of calcitonin receptors will allow the development of antibodies specific for the hormone receptors a powerfull tool for further studies involving these receptors.

42 EVIDENCE THAT 1,25-DIHYDROXYVITAMIN D_3 ENHANCES OSTEOCLAST RECRUITMENT IN VITRO. I.P. Braidman*, C.M. Taylor and D.C. Anderson. Bone Research Unit and Department of Medicine (University of Manchester), Clinical Sciences Building, Hope Hospital, Eccles Old Road, Salford M6 8HD, U.K.

$1,25(OH)_2D_3$, which induces HL60 cells to differentiate into mature monocytes (Abe *et al*, 1981; PNAS 77 2936) might similarly promote bone resorption by enhancing recruitment of osteoclast precursors. We have examined this possibility in vitro with cells (Type C) which contain osteoclasts (Oc) and their precursors, obtained from 21 day foetal rat calvaria by enzyme digestion and Percoll gradient isopycnic centrifugation, as described previously (Braidman *et al*, 1983; J Endocr 99 387). Gross examination of the foetal rat calvaria stained with 0.1% neutral red reveals at least two populations of strongly neutral red-positive cells, namely multinucleated Oc on the inner surface and within perivascular channels, and small granular (NR-1) cells, mainly in the meninges and on the inner bone surface. In 18-19 day calvariae, NR-1 cells are plentiful, but Oc's scanty; after 24-40h culture numerous Oc's were found. Cultured Type C cells from 21-day calvariae probably contains both Oc's and NR-1 cells. Such cells were cultured with or without $1\text{-}2 \times 10^{-9}$M $1,25(OH)_2D_3$ on plastic discs, and these were removed at 16,24 and 48h, stained with acid haematoxylin and examined by light microscopy. After 24 ahd 48h the cell populations cultured with $1,25(OH)_2D_3$ contained significantly more multinuclear cells (a 50% increase over control after 48h). This appears to be the first direct evidence in vitro that $1,25(OH)_2D_3$ may induce differentiation and/or fusion of osteoclast precursors into osteoclasts.

43 LENGTH REQUIREMENT FOR PRECURSORS OF SECRETED PEPTIDES. S. Brand*, J. Hellerman, R. Tepper, J. Potts, Jr. and H. Kronenberg, Endocrine Genetics Unit and Department of Medicine, Massachusetts General Hospital, Boston, Massachusetts 02114 USA

All secreted peptides are synthesized as large precursors. Signal sequences that direct peptides to the endoplasmic reticulum account for only a small portion of a precursor's length; the remainder of the precursor's length may be required for the unknown mechanism used to transport proteins across the reticular membrane. To test this hypothesis and help define the mechanism of membrane transport, we have constructed mutant preproparathyroid hormone (preproPTH) genes encoding progressively shorter preproPTH-related peptides. PTH cDNA was cut with SstI endonuclease, digested with Bal 31 exonuclease, and then ligated to a synthetic oligonucleotide containing the TGA termination codon. DNA sequence analysis revealed which clones contained the termination codon in the correct translational reading frame. A mutant cDNA encoding the first 69 residues of preproPTH was ligated into a retroviral vector and stably integrated into rat pituitary GH4 cells. Further, we have used a linked transcription-translation system to transcribe the mutant cDNA into RNA and translate the RNA into protein. After translation using a reticulocyte lysate, [^{35}S]-methionine labeled proteins were immuno-precipitated and analyzed by gel electrophoresis and fluorography. The mutant DNA directed the synthesis of an immunoreactive protein smaller than PTH. Further analysis of the cell-free processing of this protein and the fate of this protein in the GH4 cells will define the length requirement for precursors of secreted peptides.

44 THE MECHANISM OF THE HYPOCALCEMIC EFFECT OF WR2721. M. Attie*, J. Wolf, and S. Goldfarb. University of Pennsylvania, Philadelphia, PA

WR2721 (S-2-(3-aminopropylaminoethyl) phosphorothioate) a drug undergoing trials as a chemo- and radioprotector, produces acute hypocalcemia in humans. We have shown that WR2721 lowers serum immunoreactive PTH and inhibits PTH release *in vitro* from bovine parathyroid cells (NEJM 309:1137, 1983). Hypocalcemia after WR2721 infusion occurs more rapidly than after acute parathyroidectomy suggesting that, acutely, it is mediated by mechanisms other than inhibiting PTH secretion. To determine whether WR2721 produces hypocalcemia independent of its effect on the parathyroid gland, 8 chronically parathyroidectomized rats on high Ca/low PO_4 diet were given WR2721 (30 mg/kg) i.v. WR2721 reduced serum Ca from 9.4$\pm$.6 to 7.7$\pm$.5 mg/dl(p<.01) at 3h, while in sham operated rats on the same diet, WR2721 calcium fell from 9.7$\pm$.7 to 8.0$\pm$.5(p<.01). To localize the site of action of WR2721, radiocalcium kinetic studies were performed. WR2721 (30 mg/kg) lowered fasting serum Ca (10.5 $\pm$.4 to 8.5$\pm$.5 and 8.5$\pm$.2 at 1.5 and 3h) but did not affect the rate of disappearance of ^{45}Ca (injected 3 hours previously) from serum compared to vehicle injected rats. However, serum ^{45}Ca specific activity was higher at 1.5h (p<.01) and 3h (p<.05) in rats given WR2721 than in rats given vehicle alone indicating that WR2721 inhibits dilution of isotopic calcium by cold calcium release, presumably from bone. When bone Ca was labelled by injecting ^{45}Ca 18 days before the experiment, WR2721 lowered both ^{45}Ca and total Ca in serum. These data indicate that WR2721 can produce hypocalcemia independent of its effect on PTH secretion. WR2721 causes hypocalcemia by decreasing flux of Ca into extracellular fluid, most likely as a result of decreased bone resorption.

45 MULTIPLE FORMS OF THE GLUCOCORTICOID RENAL RECEPTOR DURING EMBRYOGENESIS.

D. Bellabarba,* S. Bélisle, and J.G. Lehoux , Faculté de Médecine, Université de Sherbrooke, Québec, J1H 5N4, Canada.

In the present study, we have examined the variations of the components of the glucocorticoid renal receptor during chick embryo development. Cytosol prepared in a TTEG (Tes, Thioglycerol, EDTA, glycerol) buffer at ph 7.4 was labeled with a (^{3}H) triamcinolone acetonide and then chromatographed on Agarose A-1.5 M columns equilibrated in the same buffer plus 0.05 or 0.4 M KCl. Simultaneous filtration of "markers" was performed to determine the distribution coefficient (KD) and the approximate M.W. of the various receptor forms. In some experiments Sodium Molybdate (30 mM) was added to the homogenization and elution buffers. The cytosol of 12-day old embryos revealed, with low and high salt buffer, a single component with a KD:0.26 ± 0.06 and an estimated M.W.: 120,000. With Sodium Molybdate, the single component had a KD: 0.12 ± 0.01 and a M.W.: >200,000. In the cytosol of 15-day old embryo, with low salt buffer, there was a small component excluded from the column and a very large peak (KD: 0.22 ± 0.04; M.W.: 150,000). With high salt buffer only the larger component was evident. No difference from day 12 were observed with Sodium Molybdate. Before hatching (day 19), the elution profile with 0.05M KCl did not differ from day 15, but with 0.4M KCl we found the major component (KD: 0.26 ± 0.02) and another fraction of smaller M.W.(KD: 0.5 ± 0.03; M.W.: 45,000). The results with Sodium Molybdate were similar to those of days 12-15. These results indicate that the renal glucocorticoid receptor of chick embryo changes with maturation from a single to multiple components. Such changes are probably related to the transformation of the receptor since they occur in presence of 0.4M KCl and they are inhibited by Sodium Molybdate.

46 PROSTAGLANDIN E (PGE) BINDING AND MAMMARY TUMOR REGRESSION.

H. Abou-Issa*, J. P. Minton and C. Petrucelli, The Ohio State University College of Medicine, Columbus, Ohio 43210 U.S.A.

The in vivo relationship between Prostaglandin E (PGE) binding and tumor regression was studied in hormone dependent MTW9 rat mammary tumors following ovariectomy or dibutyryl cAMP (DBcAMP) treatment of the hosts. During growth arrest by DBcAMP there was a significant increase in the production of PGE_2 (threefold) and in PGE_1 or PGE_2 binding (twofold). cAMP binding activity was also increased in tumor cytosol (twofold) and nuclei (fourfold). Concomitant with the increase in PGE and cAMP binding activities were also increases in cAMP content and cAMP dependent protein kinase activity. The increases in PGE and cAMP binding activities were reversed when resumption of tumor growth was induced by cessation of DBcAMP treatment. Ovariectomy of rats bearing the MTW9 tumors, or DMBA-induced mammary tumors also caused an increase in PGE binding (twofold) and cAMP content (twofold) in regressing tumors compared to growing tumors in intact rats. On the other hand, autonomously growing hormone independent MTW9D mammary tumors showed no significant increase in PGE binding, and consequently no changes in the cAMP system, following either ovariectomy or DBcAMP treatment. These tumors failed to regress and continued to grow actively. The similarity of the increase in PGE binding that occurred upon induction of regression by two different treatments indicate that PGE binding may represent an important initial step in the regulation of mammary tumor regression.

47 PRODUCTION OF MULTIPLE HORMONES IN MEDULLARY CARCINOMA OF THE THYROID.
I. Adachi*, K. Yamaguchi, S. Kimura and K. Abe, Endocrinology Division, National Cancer Center, Tokyo, Japan.

Production of calcitonin (CT), gastrin-releasing peptide (GRP), somatostatin (SRIF), vasoactive intestinal peptide (VIP) and ACTH in medullary carcinomas of the thyroid (MCT) was examined. Methods: Three primary tumors were obtained from 3 patients with Sipple's syndrome, and 4 primary and 7 metastatic tumors from 11 sporadic cases. The tumor tissues were extracted with the boiling water method, and the hormone contents were examined by RIA of the respective hormone. In a sporadic case with the liver metastasis, calcium (4.5 mg/kg/10 min) and tetragastrin (1 μg/kg, bolus) were administered intravenously at a separate occasion, and plasma levels of CT and GRP were determined before and serially after injection. Results: Immunoreactive (IR-) CT and IR-GRP were detected in all of the MCT tissue extracts and IR-SRIF in 11 of the 13 tissue extracts examined. IR-VIP was detected in 7 of the 14 and IR-ACTH in 5 of the 12 MCT tissue extracts examined. When compared the amounts of IR-CT, those of IR-GRP and those of IR-SRIF with each other by use of their common logalithmic values, it was found that there was a significant correlation between each two of these hormones ($p < 0.02$), although the amounts of IR-GRP were 100-1,000 times and those of IR-SRIF were 1,000-10,000 times less than those of IR-CT. Plasma IR-CT and IR-GRP levels were increased concomitantly in response to both calcium and tetragastrin loads. Conclusion: MCT produces multiple hormones, and there is a significant correlation among the amounts of IR-CT, IR-GRP and IR-SRIF produced by the tumor.

48 QUANTITATIVE IMMUNOASSAY FOR 24K, A MAJOR ESTROGEN-REGULATED PROTEIN IN HUMAN BREAST CANCER.
D. Adams,* G. Chamness, D. Edwards and W. McGuire, Department of Medicine, University of Texas Health Science Center at San Antonio, San Antonio, Texas 78284, U.S.A.

Although about 60% of human breast tumors contain significant levels of estrogen receptor (ER), only half of these patients respond to endocrine therapy. To identify this responsive subset, markers of a functional pathway of estrogen action have been sought. Progesterone receptor (PgR) is one such marker that has proved to be an important clinical prognostic factor. Recently, our laboratory has identified another estrogen-regulated protein in human breast tumor cells, a 24,000 mol wt cytoplasmic glycoprotein (24K), that unlike PgR represents 1-2% of cytosol protein. We have developed monoclonal antibodies against 24K and have used these antibodies to purify the protein and to immunostain 24K in breast tumor biopsies. To quantitate 24K in cultured breast cancer cells and in breast tumor biopsies, we have now developed a competitive enzyme-linked immunoassay (ELISA) and find that: 1) estrogen stimulates release of 24K by the MCF-7 human breast cancer cell line, 2) human breast tumors contain significant amounts of 24K (as much as 10 ug/mg cytosol protein) that can be measured even after long-term storage of cytosols (at least 5 yr at -70°C), and 3) the presence of 24K correlates with that of steroid receptors, particularly ER. CONCLUSION: Preliminary results using a quantitative ELISA for 24K indicate that this major cytoplasmic glycoprotein is shed or secreted by ER positive breast tumor cells in vitro, suggesting that 24K may be a potential marker for differentiation in human breast cancer.

49 ESTRONE SULFATASE ACTIVITY IN BREAST CARCINOMA TISSUES AND ESTRONE-SULFATE PLASMA LEVELS IN POST-MENOPAUSAL WOMEN.

G.L. ADESSI*, O. PROST and M.O. TURREL, INSERM U 198, Route de Dole, 25000 BESANCON, FRANCE.

Estrone-sulfate (E_1-S) in blood provides a potentially high flux of free estrogens to mammary carcinoma due to the presence of a membrane bound estrone sulfatase. In 21 tested breast carcinoma (12 from post-menopausal women and 9 from non-menopausal women) estrone sulfatase was consistantly present. The mean values of Km and Vmax (6.8μM and 59.2 pmol of E_1/mg protein per min) were not statistically different for menopausal and non-menopausal women. The estrone sulfatase activities were not correlated to the estrogen or progesterone receptor status of the tumors. It may be concluded that estrone sulfatase activity is present in all breast tumors regardless of their hormonal status. E_1-S, the substrate of estrone sulfatase, was measured in plasma of post-menopausal women. The mean values (nmol/l) were higher in post-menopausal women with breast cancer (n=51) than in post-menopausal women without breast cancer (n=39). For the first class of age (48-55 years) the difference was not statistically significant : 1.91±1.06 vs 1.50±1.04 (mean$\pm t_{.95}\frac{s}{\sqrt{n}}$). For the two other classes of age (56-65 and 66-80) the differences were significant : 1.46±0.43 vs 0.77±0.21 ($P<0.02$) and 1.77±0.53 vs 0.81±0.22 ($P<0.01$). The mechanism implicated in the increase of circulating E_1-S in elderly post-menopausal women with breast carcinoma remains to be elucidated. Estrone sulfatase controls the transport of E_1-S from the plasma to the tumoral cells as free estrogens. In post-menopausal women with hormone sensitive breast carcinoma, circulating E_1-S, which represents the majority of the plasma estrogens, appears to be the main source of active estrogens.

50 CULTURED HUMAN CHORIOCARCINOMA JEG-3 CELLS: RETINOIC ACID (RA) BLOCKS THE EFFECT OF EPIDERMAL GROWTH FACTOR (EGF) ON CHORIOGONADOTROPIN (hCG) PRODUCTION.

Thomas Alderson, John Ilekis* and Robert Benveniste, Division of Reproductive Endocrinology, Dept. OBGYN, Michael Reese Hosp. Med. Cntr., University of Chicago, Chicago, IL 60616, USA.

The JEG-3 cell is an interesting model to study the mechanism of action of co-carcinogens since it has specific receptors for EGF and phorbol esters , the occupancy of which induces an increased hCG production (Ilekis & Benveniste, Trophoblast Research 1:289,1983). Herein, we used the JEG-3 cell to study the influence of RA (which in several In Vivo and In Vitro systems has an anti-tumor promoting activity) on the activity of EGF. Cell culture media (serum-free Dulbecco's modified Eagles medium, DMEM) were replaced by DMEM alone or DMEM with and without EGF (3.3 nM) or RA; media and cells were collected 24 hr later for hCG and cell protein measurement. Results (ng hCG/ mg cell protein; means ± SEM) were:

		DMEM + EGF	
DMEM	95 ± 3.2	+ RA (3.5 M)	115 ± 3.8
DMEM + RA (3.5 M)	97 ± 5.8	+ RA (350 nM)	130 ± 4.3
DMEM + EGF	216 ±12.7	+ RA (35 nM)	170 ± 9.3
		+ RA (3.5 nM)	192 ± 6.7

The RA inhibition on EGF stimulatory effect occured without significant effect on (i) cell number, (ii) EGF binding, and (iii) EGF internalization and degradation. Conclusion. In the JEG-3 cell, RA inhibits EGF activity. Our results suggest that the block induced by RA on EGF occurs at a post-receptor level.

51 COMBINED KETOCONAZOLE AND LHRH ANALOGUE:EFFECTIVE TREATMENT FOR PROSTATE CANCER:

J.M. Allen*, T. Yeo, D. J. Kerle, C. Smith, H. Ware, G. Williams, S.R. Bloom: Depts. of Medicine and Urology, Royal Postgraduate Medical School, London. W12 UK.

Prostate cancer is androgen dependent. Relapse is common and is considered due to loss of this dependency. Current endocrine therapy is based on suppression of testicular androgens and adrenal androgen synthesis is largely ignored. Ketoconazole blocks gonadal and adrenal 17 OH progesterone aldolase. 16 patients with progressive prostate cancer who had relapsed on treatment with a superactive LHRH analogue received in addition ketoconazole (400 mg tds). A prompt reduction in serum androstenedione was observed within eight hours (basal 9.6 ± 1.0 nM/l to 4.4 ± 0.8 nm/l) and concentrations remained suppressed over the next 30 days. Serum testosterone although at orchidectomy level before starting ketoconazole, showed further reduction in all patients. As ketoconazole has been shown to inhibit steroidogenesis in vitro, plasma ACTH was measured, and rose from 61± 18 ng/l to 252 ± 86 ng/l. Synacthen tests before and after two weeks of treatment were normal. The acid phosphatase fell by over 50% in 7 patients, and objective evidence by NMR of tumour shrinkage was recorded in 1 patient. Since suppression of androgen synthesis alone would result in a disadvantageous rise in gonadotrophins, combination of LHRH analogue with ketoconzole is required for maximum effect. The remarkable response of these patients indicates this combined therapy may have advantage in treatment of prostate cancer.

52 ANTIESTROGENS ARE PARTIAL ESTROGENIC AGONISTS FOR STIMULATION OF GH_4C_1 CELL GROWTH.

Jane F. Amara*and Priscilla S. Dannies, Department of Pharmacology, Yale University School of Medicine, New Haven, CT, USA.

To test whether the stimulation of GH_4C_1 cell growth by 17β-estradiol (E_2)is specifically dependent on serum, we grew cells for one week, with or without 3 x 10^{-11} M E_2 (which maximally stimulates growth), in medium containing various concentrations of serum. Serum concentrations up to 1% increased cell number in a concentration dependent manner; concentrations above 1% decreased cell number relative to the value at 1%. E_2 had no effect at serum concentrations below 2.5%, and increased cell number relative to controls between 2.5% and 15% serum. E_2's growth effect thus depends on interactions with serum factor(s). We therefore used medium containing 10% gelding serum to study further the estrogenic effect on growth. We compared the potency of estrogen agonists for stimulating prolactin production, increasing growth, and inhibiting ^3H-E_2 binding to GH_4C_1 cells. The orders of potency for the 3 effects were the same: ethynyl estradiol $\simeq$ E_2 $\simeq$ moxestrol > estriol $\simeq$ estrone > 17α-estradiol. All were full agonists, and all were about 10 fold more potent stimulators of cell growth than of prolactin production. The antiestrogens tamoxifen citrate and LY117018 increased cell number to 2 to 3 fold of control values, always less than the E_2 effect in the same experiment, which ranged from 3 to 7 fold. The antiestrogens' relative potency for growth stimulation correlated with their relative binding activities, when compared with the full agonists, consistent with the mediation of the growth stimulation caused by estrogens and antiestrogens through the same receptor.

53 TIGHTLY BOUND STEROID-PROTEIN COMPLEXES IN HUMAN BREAST TUMOURS.
Anderson, E.*, Vinson, G.P. and Gilmore, O.J.A.+ *Dept of Biochemistry, Medical College of St Bartholomew's Hospital, LONDON, U.K. +Breast Unit, St Bartholomew's Hospital, West Smithfield, LONDON, U.K.

Low speed supernatants (2000g) were prepared from human breast tumours and incubated (1h, 37°) in 5ml medium containing KH_2PO_4 (10mM), sucrose (0.25M), KCl (20mM), triethanolamine (15mM), $MgCl_2$ (5mM) and $CaCl_2$ (2mM) (pH7.4). This yielded an ethyl acetate extractable oestrogen measurable by a rat uterus radio receptor assay (RRA) and a non-specific total oestrogen radio-immunoassay (RIA) but not by a specific oestradiol-17β RIA. Oestrogen receptor (ER) content was measured routinely using a dextran-coated charcoal method and tumours containing 5 fmole/mg protein or less were regarded as being ER-ve. In ER+ve (but not ER-ve) tumours, the addition of excess trypsin (4mg/ml) to incubations of supernatants prepared in the presence of TAME (10mM), a low molecular weight competitive inhibitor of trypsin, caused an increase in extractable oestrogen measurable by RRA (305 ± 145 to 428 ± 183 pg/200mg tissue, n=14; $p<0.05$, paired t-test). Preparation of ER+ve tumour supernatants in the presence of soya bean trypsin inhibitor (1mg/ml), a high molecular weight inclusion inhibitor, caused a significant increase in extractable oestrogen, (305 ± 145 to 1103 ± 240 pg/100mg tissue, n=16; $p<0.01$ Students t-test). In these preparations trypsin caused a small decrease in extractable oestrogen (1103 ± 240 to 932 ± 225 pg/100mg tissue, $p<0.01$ paired t-test). Trypsin had variable effects on supernatants prepared without inhibitor. Inter alia the data suggest that there are tightly bound steroid protein complexes other than conventional steroid-receptor complexes present in human breast tumours.

54 THE INFLUENCE OF HORMONE ADDITIONS ON THE GROWTH OF N-NITROSOMETHYLUREA (NMU) INDUCED RAT MAMMARY TUMORS IN VITRO USING SERUM-FREE MEDIA IN SOFT AGAR. B. M. Arafah* and O. H. Pearson. Department of Medicine, Case Western Reserve University, Cleveland, Ohio 44106, U.S.A.

Hormone dependency of NMU rat mammary tumors has been established in vivo where estradiol (E_2) and prolactin (PRL) stimulate tumor growth (Arafah, et al., Endocrinology 111, 584, 1982). The clonogenic soft agar technique has provided a new approach to study the growth of various tumors in vitro. This technique has been widely used to study the chemosensitivity of tumors in vitro. We have adapted the technique to study the influence of hormones (PRL, E_2) on the growth of NMU-induced rat mammary tumors in vitro. We studied the influence of these hormones in media lacking serum but to which insulin was added. Cells from all 10 tumors studied formed colonies in vitro. The lack of serum from the media resulted in a significant decrease in the number of colonies formed in 6 of 10 tumors. In these 6 tumors, the reduction ranged between 25 and 65% with a mean of 50%. The addition of E_2 (10^{-8}M) in serum free media resulted in a significant increase in the number of colonies formed in 6 tumors. Similarly PRL addition (100 ng/ml) resulted in a significant increase in the number of colonies formed in 5 tumors. Neither E_2 nor PRL influenced colony formation in 3 tumors. The influence of adding both hormones was studied in 5 tumors. There, the effect of both hormones was additive in 2 tumors and similar to the effect of either hormone in the remaining 3 tumors. These data indicate that the growth of NMU-rat mammary tumors can be stimulated in vitro with E_2 and/or PRL. This is in agreement with the known hormone dependency of these tumors in vivo.

55 PARATHYROID HORMONE AS A TRANSFORMING GROWTH FACTOR IN ACUTE LEUKEMIA ?
M.J.Atkinson, H.Bodenstein and R.-D. Hesch *, Abteilung für Klinische Endokrinologie, Medizinische Hochschule Hannover, D3000 Hannover 61, West Germany.

Viral or carcinogen treatment of cultured cells has been associated with the production of specific transformation-inducing growth factors (TGF's). The TGF's are able to sustain cell growth in vitro in the absence of normally essential growth promoting substances. Production of TGF's, which are believed to be closely related to normal cell products, is thought to occur ectopically. We have recently demonstrated that human acute leukemia blast cells are able to ectopically produce Parathyroid hormone (PTH). As the PTH production was shown to coincide closely with the proliferative activity of the blast cell populations we have considered the possibility that PTH is itself closely involved in the modulation of blast cell proliferative activity. Indeed, investigations have shown that PTH is a potent stimulator of rat thymic lymphocyte mitosis in vivo and in vitro. Moreover, both normal and malignant human lymphoid cell populations have been shown to contain both PTH specific receptors and a PTH responsive system of secondary messengers.
Thus, we postulate that ectopically produced leukemic blast cell PTH is able to stimulate or sustain uncontrolled malignant cell growth, acting upon the PTH-producing blast cells in an autocrine loop. By acting in this fashion PTH may be considered as a transforming growth factor.

56 BIOCHEMICAL EFFECTS OF TRILOSTANE & DEXAMETHASONE IN POST-MENOPAUSAL WOMEN WITH BREAST CANCER.
C. G. Beardwell*, J. St.John, A. C. Hindley and P.M. Wilkinson. Christie Hospital & Holt Radium Institute,Manchester M20 9BX,UK.

Trilostane is an inhibitor of adrenal steroid biosynthesis thought to act by blocking 3β hydroxysteroid dehydrogenase. The combination of trilostane 960 mg daily & dexamethasone (D) 1 mg daily produces objective response in 32.3% (10/31) post-menopausal women with breast cancer and stabilisation of disease in a further 9.7% (3/31). We have studied the biochemical changes in these patients by measuring cortisol (F), dehydroepiandrosterone sulphate ($D\text{-}SO_4$), pregnenolone (Pe), progesterone (P) 17OH pregnenolone (17pe), 17OH progesterone (17P), androstenedione (A), testosterone (T), oestrone (E_1) and oestradiol (E_2). Samples were taken before treatment, after 3 days on trilostane 240 mg daily, 3 days on 480mg daily, 3 days on 960 mg daily & at intervals after addition of dexamethasone 1 mg daily. F levels showed no change on trilostane alone but were undetectable after adding D. Significant increases were seen in 17Pe,P, $D\text{-}SO_4$ and A in patients on trilostane alone with a return to baseline levels after D was added. A significant fall in E_1 levels was seen during trilostane therapy which was maintained after the addition of D (basal median 58 pmol/l; median after 45-94 days 28 pmol/l). The ratio A/E_1 increased from a median value of 0.03 before treatment to 0.208 on trilostane 960 mg daily, only to fall to 0.056 after 8-12 weeks' therapy. We conclude that, as well as inhibiting 3β hydroxysteroid dehydrogenase, long term treatment with trilostane also produces inhibition of aromatase

57 EFFECTS OF BROMOCRIPTINE ON SERUM GONADOTROPINS AND GONADAL SEX STEROIDS LEVELS AND THEIR PULSATILE PATTERNS IN NORMAL WOMEN AND MEN. K. Aisaka*, H. Mori, T. Ogawa and T. Kigawa, Dept. of Obstetrics & Gynecology, Oita Medical College, Oita, Japan.

To elucidate the sites of the actions of bromocriptine on hypothalamo-pituitary-ovarian axis in normoprolactinemia, 5mg of bromocriptine was administered to five normally cycling women (in menstrual, follicular, ovulatory and mid-luteal phases) and five men who were normal in their endocrinological states. Blood samplings had been done every 15 min. before two hours and after six hours of the administration, and serum levels of FSH, LH, estradiol and progesterone (in women), and testosterone (in men) were measured by RIA. The basal levels of serum FSH and LH were significantly decreased ($p<0.001$-$p<0.05$) from 4 to 6 hours after the administration both in women and men. In women, there was no significant change in serum estradiol level in every phase of the menstrual cycle, but in mid-luteal phase, serum level of progesterone was significantly decreased ($p<0.005$) from 4 to 6 hours after the administration. In men, serum level of testosterone decreased significantly ($p<0.01$) from 4 to 6 hours after the administration. The pulsatile patterns of serum FSH, LH, estradiol and progesterone, and testosterone did not show significant changes by the administration. From these facts mentioned above, it is suggested that bromocriptine affects not hypothalamus but pituitary and gonadal glands, which decreases serum levels of gonadotropins and sex steroids consequently.

58 TRANSIENT HYPERTHYROIDISM AFTER UNILATERAL ADRENALECTOMY IN TWO PATIENTS WITH CUSHING'S SYNDROME. F. Akasu*, K. Haraguchi, K. Hiramatsu[1] and T. Onaya, The Third Department of Internal Medicine, University of Yamanashi Medical School, Tamaho, Yamanashi-ken 409-38; Department of Medicine (K. H.[1]), Institute of Adaptation Medicine, Shinshu University School of Medicine, Matsumoto 390, Japan.

We found transient hyperthyroidism in two patients who had underwent unilateral adrenalectomy to resect cortisol-hypersecreting adenoma. A 38-yr-old woman showed clinical thyrotoxicosis 3 months after the surgery. Serum T_4, T_3 and TBG levels were 11.9 µg/dl, 310 ng/dl and 16.5 µg/ml, respectively. One month later, she eventually recovered to the euthyroid state. The other 34-yr-old man showed very mild clinical symptoms of hyperthyroidism 2 months after the surgery. Serum T_4, T_3 and TBG levels were 10.4 µg/dl, 240 ng/dl and 14.5 µg/ml, respectively. Two to three months after the onset of hyperthyroidism, he returned to the euthyroid state spontaneously. We carefully denied factitious thyrotoxicosis in both cases. These patients had neither neck pain nor fever. Both had low radioactive iodine uptake by the thyroid.

Murayama and his coworkers have recently reported a transient thyrotoxicosis which occurred after the cessation of steroid therapy in a patient with autoimmune thyroiditis and rheumatoid arthritis. It is of interest to note that there is much similarity between their case and ours. It seems proper to say that this type of transient thyrotoxicosis is one of the steroid withdrawal syndrome. The mechanism of this syndrome, however, remains to be investigated further.

59 THE INCIDENCE OF PARATHYROID ABNORMALITIES IN AN AUTOPSY MATERIAL

G. Åkerström*, C. Rudberg, L. Grimelius, H. Johansson, S. Ljunghall, J. Rastad, University Hospital, Uppsala, Sweden.

In an autopsy material of 503 individuals the parathyroid glands were examined with the aim to determine the incidence of histological abnormalities and to try to elucidate the development of parathyroid disease. Parathyroid adenomas were diagnosed in 2.7%, hyperplasia in 5%. One third of the cases with hyperplasia had a greatly asymmetric nodularity of their parathyroids, which mimiced adenoma formation. The finding of similar though smaller nodules in the associated glands constituted evidence of multiglandular disease. Serumcalcium was elevated in cases with adenomas or asymmetric nodular hyperplasia, but normal in those with diffuse hyperplasia although also their total parenchymal cellmass was elevated. In the individuals not fulfilling criteria for adenomatous or hyperplastic disease nodular formation was common in the older age groups. Similar findings were noted also in cases with long standing renal disease. The results suggest that an important incident in the development of parathyroid disease is the formation of nodules of various size. The occurrence of rather large nodules seemed to be mandatory for the development of hypercalcemia. That tumor growth may be initiated in glands exhibiting multiple nodular formation has been recognized in many endocrine glands but has not been adequately considered in parathyroid pathology. The high incidence of parathyroid abnormalities in the present material may indicate that stimulating factors exist.

60 PREVALENCE AND CLINICAL ASSOCIATIONS OF INTRAOCULAR PRESSURE (IOP) CHANGES IN GRAVES' DISEASE.

C.B. Allen*, D. Stetz, S.H. Roman, S. Podos and T.F. Davies, Departments of Medicine and Ophthalmology, Mount Sinai School of Medicine, New York, New York, Veterans Administration Hosp., Bronx, N.Y., U.S.A.

It has recently been reported that >75% of patients with Graves' disease exhibit a rise in IOP (ΔIOP) when measured in the upward gaze position. We have investigated an unselected series of 55 patients with treated/untreated Graves' disease and assessed their clinical and laboratory status in addition to ophthalmological evaluation with applanation tonometry. In contrast to earlier reports, we observed a significant ΔIOP (≥3mmHg) in only 22% of Graves' patients (mean ΔIOP=3.5±1.6mmHg). ΔIOP showed no correlation with age, sex, age at disease onset, duration of disease, mode of treatment or thyroid function testing at the time of examination. Hertel exophthalmometry measurements in patients with increased ΔIOP was 22.0±2.9mm compared to 18.4±3.7mm in those with ΔIOP<3mmHg ($p<0.027$ by rank sum). Although only 58% of these patients exhibited exophthalmos, CT scanning revealed significant proptosis and/or orbital muscle involvement in all patients with increased ΔIOP. Our data indicate that increased ΔIOP is not present in most patients with Graves' disease. ΔIOP findings do not support the concept of ophthalmic involvement as an intrinsic component of the Graves' thyroid diathesis.

61 PLASMA AMINOACID VALUES AND PANCREATIC B-CELL FUNCTION IN PHENYLKETONURIA (PKU). I. Antonozzi, S. Morano, L.Vestri , R. Dominici, M. Andreoli, F. Monaco* Child Neuropsychiatry Institute and IMS,CNR,c/o II Clinica Medica Policlinico Umberto I 00100 Rome, Italy.

Aim of the study was to correlate plasma glucose, insulin (IRI) and C-peptide (CP) values with plasma aminoacids (AA). In 16 PKU patients, aged 5.5-12.3 years, blood glucose, IRI and CP and plasma AA were measured in basal condition and under OGTT. A highly significant correlation was observed between B-cell function tests (e.g.basal blood gluc values vs basal CP:r=.650; p 0.01, blood gluc vs CP and IRI areas :r=.610;p 0.01 and r=.846; p 0.001 respectively). Basal blood gluc was in the low range (70.62± 10.24mg/dl) while basal IRI and CP values in the high range of normality, being respectively 5.?9+4.99 and 1.77±1.12uU/ml. PHE did not show, during OGTT, any significant variation, while val leu and tyr showed a highly significant decrease (p 0.01) from 30min.on. Plasma PHE, under different dietary regimens, varied from 3.47 to 169uM/dl and were correlated with basal blood gluc (r=.709,p 0.001), with IRI area (r=.559,p 0.02), with basal CP levels (r=.729,p 0.001),leu and valwere also correlated with gluc CP and IRI values under OGTT. Thus these data suggest that in PKU patients an inappropiate insulin secretion is related to the aminoacid imbalance.

62 FREE PLASMA TESTOSTERONE AND SEX-HORMONE-BINDING GLOBULIN IN THE EVALUATION OF HIRSUTE WOMEN. M. Asai*, M. Osawa, Y. Ichikawa, MC. Wu, N. Suganuma, T. Masahashi, O. Narita, Y. Tomoda, and N. Matsui, Department Obstetrics and Gynecology. The Research Institute of Environmental Medicine, Nagoya University School of Medicine, Nagoya, Japan.

To investigate the relation between plasma androgen levels and hirsutism, plasma total testosterone (T), free T, and sex-hormone-binding globulin (SHBG) were measured in 39 hirsute patients. These patients were divided into 3 groups according to degree of hirsutism. SHBG was determined as a DHT binding capacity, which was measured by a modification of the method used by Rosner. Free T concentrations were determined by an equilibrium dialysis. Plasma T and other androgens were determined by radioimmunoassay. Total T levels were significantly elevated in group 3, but not in group 1 and 2 when compared with normal women. In group 2 and 3 SHBG binding capacities were lower but free T concentrations were higher than normal women, significantly. In 13 of all patients, total T levels were within the normal range. Suppressed SHBG binding capacity and elevated free T concentrations were evident in these patients. These results suggested that SHBG and free T concentrations separated the hirsute population better than total testosterone.

63 HYPOGONADOTROPIC HYPOGONADISM IN MALES WITH 46XX/46XY MOSAICISM.
H. A. ASKARI, Institute of Endocrinology, Behjatabad, Tehran, 15, Iran.

Two phenotypically male individuals , aged 21 and 27, with abscence of puberty and 46xx/46xy sex chromosome mosaicism were studied, Plasma FSH and LH levels were in prepubertal range, and plasma testosterone concentrations were low, 0.10 and 0.35ng per ml. The response to a bolus injection of LHRH was absent in the first and markedly subnormal in the second. The plasma testosterone following administration of HCG, 1500units daily for ten days increased to 0.75 and 1.55 ng/mlrespectively, a markedly subnormal response.

Hypogonadism associated with sex chromosome anomalies is usually of gonadal origin and hypergonadotropic. Our findings in these patients suggests disorders of hypthalamo-pituitary function along with the abnormal testicular function, probably due to the developmental disorder of the hypothalamo- pituitary-testicular axis.

64 EFFECTS OF TESTOSTERONE TREATMENT IN PUBERTAL MALES WITH XXY KARYOTYPE.
J.D. Bailey*, D.A. Stewart, E. Park and C.T. Netley, Hospital for Sick Children, Toronto, Canada.

Eight randomly selected boys with XXY karyotype diagnosed at birth were started on I.M. long-acting testosterone cypionate 100 mg q4wk at age 13y. Assessments of physical growth, pubertal development and personality with measurements of serum gonadotropins and sex hormones were made at 6 monthly intervals. Results were compared with those from nine similar untreated boys with XXY karyotype. Although the control group was taller and heavier at 13y, the treated group on average grew faster (9.46 vs 6.27cm/y) and gained weight faster during the first year of the study. During this period, bone age mean of 12.4 y in both groups at age 13 y advanced to 13.7 y in the treated group vs 13.5 y in controls. Mean testicular volume was 3 ml at 13 y and 3.5 ml at 14 y in both groups. Pubic hair and penile length increased more rapidly in the treated group. Mean serum levels of FSH (14IU/L),LH(7IU/L),androstenedione and estradiol were similar at 13y. FSH rose by age 14 when 5 boys from each group showed levels above the normal upper adult male of 14 IU/L. Serum LH concentrations became elevated in one boy of each group at age 14 y. Four of the treated but only one of the untreated boys reached low normal adult male levels of testosterone by 14 y. Two-way analysis of variance on all 12 subtests of the Piers-Harris and Sentence Completion self-report personality tests showed no significant difference in the two groups before or after one year of treatment. Conclusion: Testosterone treatment of XXY pubertal males caused a slight advance in the rate of pubertal development but no significant changes in growth, personality or endocrine function.

65 IMPAIRED WATER EXCRETION IN PANHYPOPITUITARISM WITH ARGININE VASOPRESSIN (AVP) - DEFICIENCY. F. Bakiri*, M. Benmiloud and M.B. Vallotton. Services d'Endocrinologie, Centre Pierre et Marie Curie, Algiers, Algeria and Hopital Cantonal, Geneva, Switzerland.

Inappropriate secretion of AVP has been implicated as a cause of the delayed water excretion associated to adrenal insufficiency and hypothyroidism. To evaluate the import of this factor we have studied the response to a water load test in 20 post-partum panhypopituitary patients with confirmed AVP deficiency(1), before treatment(P), after cortisol(F) and cortisol + thyroid hormones (F+T) replacement, and in 12 normal females (C). Urinary AVP excretion was similarly suppressed in the four groups and remained so throughout the study. In P, urinary volume was 24 % and urinary osmolality 558 % that of C ($p < 0.001$); despite the well-hydrated status free water clearance was negative. Dilutional ability was improved in F ($p < 0.001$) and not modified further in F+T. In both groups it remained lower than in C ($p < 0.01$). Basal plasma osmolality, sodium and potassium were similar in P and C ; a significant ($p < 0.01$) increase was observed in F and a further increase in F+T ($p < 0.05$). Conclusion : The excess of AVP is not a prerequisite factor in delayed water excretion since the phenomenon is clearly observed in AVP deficient patients. The incomplete recovery in treated patients could be due to hypovolemia and / or basal aldosterone deficiency which occured after substitution with cortisol and thyroid hormones (2).

1. Bakiri et al : J Clin Endocrinol Metab 1984,58:in press
2. Bakiri et al : Acta Endocrinol 1983,103 (Suppl 256):180

66 LONG TERM DRUG THERAPY REGIME FOR GRAVES' DISEASE. A PROSPECTIVE FEASIBILITY STUDY. H. BANK*, I. BANK, Z. EISENSTEIN, M. WEISS, Thyroid Clinic, Sheba Med. Center, Sackler Med. School, Tel-Aviv University, Israel.

170 patients with Graves' Disease were followed from 3 to 24 years after commencement of treatment with once daily methimazole administration. Once euthyroidism was achieved a regime was instituted with gradual weekly dose reduction administered 5 to 2 times a week, the object being to maintain remission on minimal dosage. The average weekly dose was 95 mg at 5 yrs and 55 mg at 17 yrs. After the first year clinic visits were once or twice yearly. 50% of patients were receiving the drug 2 or 3 times weekly. 78 relapses were recorded; the maximal number in the early period (3-4 yrs) but also at very late periods. Calculated per patient population percentage relapses were 10% at 3 yrs, declining to 3% at 6 yrs and increasing to 12% at 15 yrs. Relapses were due to treatment stoppage or too rapid dose reduction and easily corrected. 35 patients remained euthyroid on cessation after varying lengths of time on treatment. Their prestoppage weekly dose was significantly lower than patients still on treatment (48.2 mg). TSH values are available for 95 patients. The difference in TSH average at 3-5 yrs (3.04 ± 1.30) and 15-18 yrs (6.35 ± 5.68) was marginally significant ($P<0.1$). 2 cases were overtly hypothyroid after 18 years. 14 patients had alternative treatment, 9 of these for undesirable high dose requirements. Long term therapy by this regime appeared feasible, economical and with good patient compliance. Relapse rates are minimized and compared to "so called" definitive therapies unattended by hypothyroidism or significant complications.

67 ENDOGENOUS OPIOID ACTIVITY IN POLYCYSTIC OVARY SYNDROME (PCO). R. Barnes,* D. Shoupe, and R. Lobo. Univ. So. Calif. Sch. of Med., L.A., Calif.

Peripheral plasma β-endorphin (βEP) has been found to be elevated in polycystic ovary syndrome(PCO). However, these measurements may not reflect brain opioid activity. Since the effect of βEP on hypothalamic GnRH secretion may be influenced by dopamine (DA), and because there is evidence to suggest a relative central deficiency of DA in PCO, we studied the effects of Naloxone (Nal) infusions before and again one week after daily L-Dopa (400mg) with carbidopa(C) 100mg in 5 patients with PCO and 5 ovulatory controls studied in the mid follicular phase. Patients with PCO had hirsutism, increased body weight, serum LH:FSH ratios >3, oligoamenorrhea, perimenarchial onset of symptoms and signs and LH levels averaging 28±1.7 mIU/ml. Serum LH was measured every 15 min before, during and after a 4 hr. infusion of Nal (2mg/hr.). Weight and E_2 levels were similar in patients and controls. After Nal, LH responses were similar in controls and PCO (18±2, 17±2% change). These elevations in LH were of borderline significance except for a marked increase in LH in one patient with PCO (36% change). After 1 wk. of L-Dopa-C in patients with PCO, baseline serum LH was unchanged (27.8±1.7 vs. 26±1.8 mIU/ml). However, LH responses after Nal were elevated (36±10% increase, $p<.005$) and on an individual basis, Nal responses were greater after L-Dopa-C compared to pretreatment in 4 of the 5 patients. These data suggest that endogenous opioid activity may be heightened in PCO.The dopaminergic status of patients with PCO may influence Nal-evoked responses. The elevated LH in PCO may be unrelated to increased endogenous opioid activity.

68 EVIDENCE FOR HYPOTHALAMIC DYSFUNCTION IN ENDURANCE ATHLETES SUFFERING FROM THE OVERTRAINING SYNDROME. J.L. Barron[+], T.D. Noakes and R.P. Millar, Department of Chemical Pathology and Metropolitan Sports Science Center, University of Cape Town Medical School, Observatory 7925, South Africa.

Some athletes exposed to heavy training loads for a prolonged period of time develop the overtraining syndrome. Hypothalamic-pituitary function was studied by the hormonal response to insulin hypoglycaemia in four overtrained athletes and in five asymptomatic marathon runners during a four month period in which they ran 42- , 56- and 92-km races. The response of the asymptomatic runners was not different when tested one month before and within 48h after the 42- and 92-km races. All four overtrained athletes presented with impaired training and racing times, apathy and a heavy-legged feeling and were tested when overtrained and again after four weeks rest. The plasma cortisol, ACTH and GH responses in the four overtrained athletes were significantly lower (p 0.05) compared to their levels after rest and to the asymptomatic runners. The integrated responses (mean ± SEM) were

		Overtrained(n=4)	Rested(n=4)	Asymptomatic(n=15)
Cortisol	umol min/ℓ	1.92±2.09	15.66±1.71	14.40±1.44
ACTH	ng min/ml	0.22±0.13	2.51±1.30	3.71±0.54
GH	ug min/ml	0.98±0.37	2.14±0.28	2.13±0.14

The impaired hormonal responses to insulin-induced hypoglycaemia and recovery after rest, indicate hypothalamic dysfunction and may be a diagnostic marker of the overtraining syndrome.

69 PRE-OPERATIVE MANAGEMENT OF NEONATAL NESIDIOBLASTOSIS WITH SOMATOSTATIN-28. F. Bonnici*, R.P. Millar and P. White, Departments of Paediatrics and Chemical Pathology, University of Cape Town, South Africa.

Persistent neonatal hypoglycaemia due to nesidioblastosis is a serious condition which should be recognised promptly. Urgent medical treatment is mandatory to prevent central nervous system damage and surgery is often required. Three newborn infants reported here developed unremitting non-ketotic hyperinsulinaemic hypoglycaemia within hours of birth. Medical therapy (high rate of glucose infusion, hydrocortisone, diazoxide, glucagon) was ineffective in maintaining normoglycaemia and urgent pancreatectomy was comtemplated in each case. The use of synthetic cyclic somatostatin-14 (SS-14) has been advocated in the preoperative control of hypoglycaemia in such infants. In order to restore blood glucose levels to normal, we successfully employed somatostatin-28 (SS-28), a higher molecular weight, 28 amino acid species of somatostatin, with 14 additional amino acids on the NH_2 terminus. The beta cells were extremely sensitive to infusions of SS-28 (4-12 μg/kg/hr IV) with a dose-dependent rise in blood glucose (pretreatment average of <1 mmol/ℓ rising to a range of 4-15 mmol/ℓ) and concomittant suppression of serum insulin levels. In one infant, SS-28 was more effective than SS-14 in maintaining normoglycaemia and suppressing hyperinsulinaemia, possibly by the preferential inhibition of insulin with a relatively lesser effect on the counter regulatory hormones glucagon and growth hormone. We conclude that SS-28 effectively suppresses abnormal insulin secretion in infants with nesidioblastosis and we define its therapeutic role in the pre-operative management of this condition.

70 THE INFLUENCE OF NIMODIPINE ON THE ENDOCRINE STRESS RESPONSE - ADH, HGH, ACTH, CORTISOL, INSULIN - IN PATIENTS UNDERGOING OPEN HEART SURGERY. B. v.Bormann*, J. Boldt, G. Sturm°, B. Weidler and G. Hempelmann, Dept. of Anesthesiology and Intensive Care, Univ. D 6300 Gießen, and Dept. Gynaecol. Obstetrics°,Univ. D 3550 Marburg, FRG.

Nimodipine (NMDP), a new calcium entry blocker, seems to influence the response to surgical stress presumably by interaction with drugs used for general anesthesia. We have observed that its use leads to a massive reduction of the need of the opiate fentanyl during open heart operation (OP). In order to elucidate whether this is due to the very strong cardiovascular activity of NMDP or to an analgesia attenuating the endocrine stress response, the plasma levels of some "stress hormones" in two groups (n=10) of patients have been determined during OP. Both groups had identical premedication and an anesthesia induction with 0.1 mg fentanyl. The group under investigation received further on only NMDP(60μg/kgbw x h), the control group as usual a mean dosage of 2.4 mg fentanyl/patient during OP. While in the control group ADH increased from basal levels of 2.8 ± 1.7 pg/ml before sternotomy to 34 - 42 pg/ml during extracorporal circulation (ECC), the NMDP-group showed a lowered increase. Cortisol levels in the NMDP-group remained unchanged during OP (50-90 ng/ml); the control group showed up to 4 fold elevated cortisol levels. ACTH levels in the NMDP-group started to increase from 30-100 pg/ml before to 600-900 pg/ml after the ECC; in the control group ACTH levels already short after OP begin. Similar results were obtained for hPRL, HGH and insuline plasma levels. At least concerning the studied endocrine stress response the NMDP-procedure seems to be superior to the usual anesthesia.

71 IMMUNOHISTOCHEMICAL LOCALIZATION OF NEUROPEPTIDES IN THE FOREBRAIN AND PITUITARY GLAND OF A TELEOST FISH. T.F.C. Batten*, M.L. Cambré, W.A. Verdonck, F. Ollevier and F. Vandesande. Dept. of Zoology, Univ. of Sheffield, S10 2TN, UK, and Zoological Institute, Naamsestraat 59/61, B-3000 Leuven, Belgium.

Using the PAP immunohistochemical method, the gonadotrophin releasing hormone system in the brain and pituitary of the green molly has been recently described (Batten and Goos, 1984, Gen.comp.Endocrinol. 53, in press). Now, by single and double staining PAP methods, and using antisera raised in our laboratories and tested for specificity, the location of the following neuropeptides has been investigated: somatostatin (SRIF), corticotrophin-releasing factor (CRF), vasotocin (AVT), cholecystokinin (CCK), thyrotrophin-releasing factor (TRH), growth hormone-releasing factor (GRF), substance P (SP) and enkephalin (ENK). In the parvocellular preoptic nucleus (NPO), cell bodies stained for SRIF, AVT,CCK (very few cells) and CRF (small, poorly defined cells): no two antisera were seen to stain the same cell. The magnocellular neurons of the NPO stained only for AVT. AVT-positive fibres formed distinct tracts towards the nucleus lateralis tuberis (NLT) and pituitary; anti-SRIF and anti-CRF stained fibres occurred difusely in the preoptic, tuberal and posterior hypothalamic regions, and SRIF-positive fibres were also seen in the dorsal telencephalon. Antisera to SRIF, CRF, ENK and AVT stained numerous fibres in the neurohypophysis. Anti-ENK also stained a few large cells of the lateral NLT. No specific staining was observed with antisera to TRH, GRF or SP.

72 CULTURE AND SUB-CULTURE OF EPITHELIAL CELLS FROM BOVINE AND RABBIT OVIDUCTS: PREPARATION AND CHARACTERIZATION. M.Boulanger*, M.A.Fortier, R.D.Lambert, M.A.Sirard and C.Bernard. Molecular Genetic (reproduction), CHUL,Quebec, G1V 4G2,Canada.

Epithelial cells from oviducts of estrous rabbits and heifers were obtained by digestion with trypsin. The cells were grown in RPMI 1640 supplemented with 10% fetal calf serum (FCS), whole or steroid depleted by treatment with dextran-saturated charcoal (DC). Two types of cells were obtained in both species: ciliated and secretory cells. Attachement of the cells to the culture plate was observed within 24 hours and confluency within 4 or 5 days. The growth rate of the cells was slighty diminished after culture in FCS-DC. In heifers, this effect was more pronounced after the cells had reached confluency. E_2 and P added in physiological concentrations to rabbit cells cultured in DC serum could not increase the growth rate to the level observed in whole serum. Also, their was no significant effect of increasing doses of E_2 and P (10^{-9} M to 10^{-6}M) on protein secretion of the primary cultured cells. However, E_2 from 10^{-8}M to 10^{-6}M, seemed to slightly inhibit secretion of rabbit cells while the opposite was observed with bovine cells. Bovine sub-cultured cells were more sensitive to P and produced a maximum quantity of secretion from 10^{-7}M to 10^{-6}M. Similarity of the function of the cultured cells with those *in vivo* was tested by *in vitro* capacitation of rabbit and bull spermatozoa. Futhermore, other aspects of gamete and embryo-interactions with the oviduct cells in culture are under current investigation.

73 ADRENAL HORMONES IN THE WHALE. A. Carballeira*, J. Brown, L. M. Fishman, D. Trujillo and D. Odell, V.A. Medical Center and Departments of Medicine and Marine Science, University of Miami, Miami, Florida 33125, U.S.A.

Adrenal hormonal content and steroid synthesis were studied in 3 pygmy sperm whales (*Kogia breviceps*) and 1 Gulfstream beaked whale (*Mesoplodon europaeus*) stranded on local beaches. Using HPLC, the following catecholamines (mg/g tissue) were found in the medulla: norepinephrine (1.4), epinephrine (0.4) and dopamine (0.08). Using RIA, corticosterone (B) was the predominant steroid in the cortex (7.1 μg/g tissue) and the only compound whose elaboration from endogenous sources increased during in vitro studies. Incubations of monolayer cell cultures and of cellular organelles with radioactive precursors were consistent with the following biosynthetic scheme: cholesterol → pregnenolone → progesterone → DOC → B. Only traces of aldosterone could be isolated from some incubates. Cholesterol cleavage enzymes (CCE) and 11β-hydroxylase (11βOH) were associated with mitochondria, 21-hydroxylase with microsomes and steroid dehydrogenase-isomerase with both fractions. Exogenous NADPH supported all steroid enzymes studied; CCE and 11βOH activities were lost (75-100%), however, when Krebs cycle intermediates (KCI, 10 mM each) were substituted. Metyrapone inhibited CCE and 11βOH maximally at 1.0 and 0.1 mM concentrations, respectively. B formation was stimulated in cell cultures by ACTH and cAMP. These studies thus demonstrate major similarities in adrenal biochemistry between the whale and B-producing terrestrial mammals such as the rat. Though changes resulting from agonal events cannot be excluded, difference in catecholamine ratios, in aldosterone production and in the apparent role of KCI may reflect biologic adaptation of this aquatic mammal to a marine environment.

74 IN VITRO EFFECT OF SOMATOSTATIN AND DOPAMINERGIC AGENTS ON CYCLIC NUCLEOTIDE PHOSPHODIESTERASE IN THE PITUITARY GLAND. T. Aono*, A. Nagasaka, H. Hidaka°, K. Iwase, H. Nakagawa, A. Nakai and T. Ohyama, Fujita-Gakuen Univ. and °Mie Univ. School of Med., Toyoake, Aichi 470-11, Japan.

Growth hormone secretion is affected by somatostatin and dopaminergic agents which may act directly to the anterior pituitary gland. The action of these hypothalamic hormones and dopaminergic agents to the pituitary gland is induced by the alteration of intracellular cyclic nucleotide levels. Therefore, we studied the effect of these compounds on cyclic nucleotide phosphodiesterase(PDE) partially purified by a DEAE cellulose column chromatography. Cyclic nucleotide PDE activities were measured by a modification of the procedure of Butcher and Sutherland. The effect of somatostatin(cyclized form) and dopaminergic agents was tested by adding into the reaction mixture. The elution profile from DEAE cellulose column chromatography revealed a dominant cyclic AMP-PDE activity as compared to cyclic GMP-PDE activity in the anterior lobe and vice versa in the posterior lobe. Somatostatin, L-DOPA, dopamine and CB-154(2-bromo- -ergocriptine) inhibited low Km enzyme of cyclic AMP-PDE in the anterior lobe. Kinetic studies of cyclic AMP-PDE inhibition by these compounds indicated that the inhibition was competitive with the substrate. Potent inhibition was observed with somatostatin and CB-154. These results suggest the possibility of the direct action of dopaminergic agents on the anterior pituitary gland, with more potent inhibition of cyclic AMP-PDE activity which is dominant in the anterior lobe.

75 RELATIONSHIPS BETWEEN THE GTP CONTENT AND THE TSH STIMULATED ADENYLATE-CYCLASE ACTIVITY OF CULTURED THYROID CELLS. J.L. Aublin, S. Champion* and C. Jacquemin, U.E.R. Sciences, 51062 Reims-cédex, FRANCE.

As previously reported, the acute TSH (25 mU/ml) stimulated adenylate-cyclase activity of a crude membrane fraction derived from cells cultured for 4 days in the presence of TSH (0.1 mU/ml) (TSH cells) is 5-8 times higher than that derived from control cells. It was suggested that changes in the intracellular content of GTP resulting from the presence of minute amounts of TSH in the culture medium, were responsible of the modified responsiveness of the cyclase. A method for GTP determination has been developped. The steady concentration of GTP in 4 days TSH cells is 2-3 times higher than in 4 days control cells (126 and 275 pmol/10^6 cells respectively). The increase in GTP content is dose dependent between 5 and 500 uU/ml TSH in the culture medium. It presents a maximum on day 4 of culture but remains elevated up to day 5. Nevertheless the GTP content it not the only factor controlling the cyclase activity, indeed the addition of 0.1 mM GTP to membranes from control cells does not increase the response to the level obtained with membranes from TSH cells. Cross-experiments were performed between 10000 g pellets and supernatants from control and TSH treated cells homogenate. If the supernatant from TSH cells is unable to increase the cyclase activity of a control cells derived pellet, the supernatant from control cells decreases the cyclase activity of a pellet from TSH cells. Chronic TSH treatment exerts the modulation of adenylate-cyclase activity through several effects : increase in the GTP content, increase of the enzyme activity, decrease of the activity of a soluble inhibitor.

76 **GENE DOSAGE EFFECT ON THE ACTIVATION OF ADIPOCYTE ADENYLATE CYCLASE BY AGONISTS AND GTP IN THE OB/OB MOUSE.** **Nicole Bégin-Heick*, Department of Biochemistry, University of Ottawa, Ottawa, K1H 8M5, Canada.**

GTP is known to produce both stimulatory and inhibitory effects on rat adipocyte adenylate cyclase (AC). The stimulatory effects have been ascribed to interactions of GTP with N_s and the inhibitory effects to interactions with N_i, respectively the stimulatory and inhibitory components of the guanine nucleotide regulatory complex (N) of AC. In the course of studies on the regulation of adipocyte AC in the ob/ob mouse, I discovered that in the tissue of obese mice, the response to GTP was different than the response found in the homozygous (+/+) and heterozygous (+/ob) lean mice. In the +/+, the response to GTP was similar to that expected from the data on rat adipocytes: a biphasic curve with stimulation by increasing GTP concentrations to a maximum at 0.3μM GTP, followed by an inhibitory phase. In the ob/ob mouse, the dose response curve was shifted to the right, with no visible inhibitory phase. Half maximal stimulation occurred at luM and maximal stimulation at 0.3mM. With adipocyte membranes from heterozygous mice (+/ob), a multiphasic GTP dose response curve was obtained which was close to the theoretical values predicted from the contribution of one + and one ob gene. These data indicate a gene related effect on the regulation of adenylate cyclase in the ob/ob mouse. Studies with bacterial toxins will allow to define the system further. **Supported by MRC.**

77 POLYCLONAL PANCREATIC TUMOR RESPONSIBLE FOR CUSHING SYNDROME AND ZOLLINGER - ELLISON SYNDROME. Genton P. *, Thomas J.L., Hartemann P., Leclere J., Kahn J.P., Boman F., Burlet A., Guedenet J.C., Boissel P., Berger G., Trouillas J., C.H.U. de NANCY, FRANCE; Faculté de Médecine A. Carrel, LYON, FRANCE.

In an endocrine tumor of the pancreas with Cushing syndrome, multiple gastric ulcerations and liver metastases we assessed high, non-suppressible plasma cortisol and ACTH levels as well as markedly elevated gastrin. The tumor and liver metastases were tested for immunoreactivity against ovine 41-CRF, ACTH (1-39, 1-24 and 17-39), β - LPH, MET- and LEU- enkephalin, α- and β-endorphin, MSH, hGH, hPRL, hLH, gastrin, glucagon, Somatostatin, pancreatic polypeptide and insulin. On light microscopic examination the tumor showed marked polymorphism. The pituitary was analysed when the 38 yr-old female patient, who responded poorly to streptozotocin, died 7 months after the first admission : no pituitary adenoma was found. In the tumor, insulin secreting cells were grouped in one single nodular area. ACTH- and βLPH- reactive cellular groups represented 5 % of the tumoral mass. 50 to 60 % of all cells reacted to antigastrin serum while in other vast compact tumoral masses 100 % cells were reactive. The peculiar distribution of endocrine activity correlated with microscopic polymorphism. Electron microscopy found one single type of secretion granule per cell. All findings favor the hypothesis of polyclonal development within this singular endocrine tumor of the pancreas.

78 CONTRIBUTION OF EPIDIDYMIS TO α-GLUCOSIDASE CONTENT OF RAM SEMINAL PLASMA. J. Besançon*, J.-L. Dacheux, R. Paquin and R.R. Tremblay. Endocrinology and Metabolism, CHUL, Québec, G1V 4G2, Canada.

We have recently shown that physiological (in lamb) or drug-induced immaturity of sperm (α-chlorohydrin in adult ram) was associated with low specific activity (SA) of ram seminal plasma (SP) acid α-glucosidase (α-G) like in vasectomised ram (less than 1 mU/mg prot.). To determine the origin of this enzyme in reproductive organs, the epididymis was initially selected. Acid α-G and L-carnitine (a well known epididymal marker) were measured in rete testis (RTF) and epididymal fluids (EF) collected respectively by selective catheterism or by micropuncture technique. Both parameters remained at a low and constant level in RTF and EF of caput and corpus. Then they increased parallely in epididymal cauda to levels greater than those in seminal plasma (5 mU/mg prot. and 10 mM respectively). A pH optimum study of α-G activity in these fluids showed two well separated peaks in RTF and caput EF around pH 4 and 7 respectively but a single one in cauda EF (pH 4) comparable to the one in SP. A sucrose density gradient analysis performed at pH 4 and 7 in presence or absence of SDS 1%, a selective inhibitor of acid α-G activity, allowed the demonstration of 2 enzyme forms in RTF sedimenting in the 7 and 4S regions of the gradients while the unique 4S form was encountered in cauda EF and SP. These results suggest that there is a major contribution of cauda epididymis to the α-G content of ram SP. Two (acid and neutral) forms of α-G would be secreted by testis but only the acid form would be accumulated (or secreted) in cauda epididymis. This study was supported by the MRC.

79 ENHANCED SUPPRESSION OF GONADAL FUNCTION BY CONSTANT INFUSION OF GnRH AGONIST IN THE HUMAN MALE: A POTENTIAL APPROACH TOWARDS MALE CONTRACEPTION. S. Bhasin*, M. Peterson, B.S. Steiner, R.S. Swerdloff, Harbor-UCLA Medical Center, Torrance, CA. 90509

Studies employing single daily injection of GnRH agonist (GnRH-A) alone or in combination with testosterone failed to induce azoospermia in man over 16 week treatment period. To determine if constant infusion of GnRH-A will result in greater suppression of gonadal function in the human male than single daily injections by providing constant and optimum blood levels, we administered 200 μg of $D(Nal_2)^6$GnRH to two groups of 5 normal males for 28 d either by single daily injection (Group I) or by constant subcutaneous infusion by an insulin pump (Group II). Serum LH, FSH and T were measured on days 0,1,4,7,9,10,14,18,22,26 and 28. On d 28, both basal (22±7 vs 85±47% of baseline) and 24 h integrated T (-10.2±4.5 vs 1.0±7.9 μg-h/dl) conc. were lower in group II vs. group I. Serum T fell to castrate range in 2 out of 5 in group II in contrast to none of 5 subjects in group I. LH and FSH were not significantly different in the two groups. Decline in serum T in both groups occurred in face of little or no change in serum LH. We conclude: 1) Constant infusion of GnRH-A leads to more consistent and greater suppression of gonadal function than its intermittent administration, 2) Antigonadal effects of intermediate term GnRH-A treatment in man cannot be fully explained on basis of downregulation of gonadotropin secretion alone. Studies currently underway to assess the effects of long term infusion of GnRH-A on spermatogenesis in man could provide feasibility data for development of biodegradable implants of GnRH-A and androgen for male contraception.

80 EFFECT OF hCG AND OTHER FACTORS ON GROWTH (THYMIDINE INCORPORATION) OF HUMAN FETAL ZONE ADRENAL CELLS IN MONOLAYER CULTURE. M. Abu-Hakima, C.L. Branchaud, C. Goodyer and B.E. Pearson Murphy*, Reproductive Physiology Unit, Montreal General Hospital, and Montreal Children's Hospital Research Unit, Montreal, Canada.

Evidence for the effects of hCG on growth and steroidogenesis in the human fetal adrenal gland (HFA) is conflicting. Relative adrenal weight varies during gestation, with a large peak at 15 weeks and a smaller peak at the time of birth; the fetal zone comprises about 80% of the total mass. HFA of anencephalics is normal up to 20 weeks gestation in the absence of a functional pituitary, suggesting that factor(s) other than ACTH are responsible for its development. To investigate growth, thymidine incorporation (TI) into fetal zone adrenal cells in monolayer cultures was assessed. DHAS levels were measured by RIA. Two preparations of hCG were used; one highly purified (NIH:CR-121) and one crude, obtained from human pregnancy urine (Sigma); also ACTH (Duracton or Cortrosyn), hLH (NIH:LER 960) and EGF (Collaborative Research) were added to the incubation medium (Ham's F-10 + fetal calf serum). TI was 2-10-fold higher in wells exposed to EGF or crude hCG compared to control. Pure hCG, LH and ACTH, alone or in combination, had no effect on TI. When ACTH was combined with EGF or crude hCG, TI was decreased. DHAS was stimulated by ACTH but not by LH, hCG or EGF. Both EGF and crude hCG had an antagonistic effect on DHAS production in the presence of ACTH. These results suggest that crude hCG contains a potent growth factor (which remains to be identified), but that pure hCG has no mitogenic or steroidogenic effect on the fetal zone of the human fetal adrenal gland.

81 IN VITRO INFLUENCE OF STEROIDS, OXYTOCIN, HISTAMINE, BRADYKININ AND ANGIOTENSINS I AND II ON SECRETION OF PROSTAGLANDIN E_2 (PG E_2) BY HUMAN FETAL MEMBRANES. G.Acker,* A.Pesty, A.Bianchi and E.Papiernik. INSERM U.187 32, rue des Carnets. 92140 - Clamart. France.

The precise mechanisms controlling the initiation of human parturition are still unknown. The fetal membranes are believed to play a central role in the metabolic events that lead to the initiation of woman parturition. There is also considerable evidence that PG E_2 produced in these tissues act directly to initiate labor. This study was undertaken to determine the factors that influence PG E_2 synthesis during delivery. Amnion and chorion in primary culture were used. These cultures were characterized by rapid cell multiplication : $2.3x10^5$ at day 4, $1.4x10^6$ at day 8, $3.0x10^6$cells at day 10 of culture. PG E_2 was measured by R.I.A. Cells were incubated 30 minutes with different drugs. Chorionic and amniotic cells react in different ways to stimuli. Steroids (progesterone, 17β estradiol,corticosterone) 10^{-9}M have no action on the synthesis of PG E_2 by amnion. The same steroids increased the PG E_2 secretion by chorion. The response to bradykinin (10^{-5}M) is a 5 fold increase in PG E_2 level, while histamine (10^{-5}M) produces a 13 fold increase and oxytocin (500µg/ml) is a 9 fold increase over controls in chorionic cells. In amniotic cells the stimulation is weak. Angiotensins I and II (10^{-9}M) stimule PG E_2 production by chorion but inhibe the secretion by amnion. We have shown in these *in vitro* studies that fetal membranes secrete PG E_2 . The chorion is a fetal membrane that reacts most dramatically to the stimuli. We conclude that the chorion playes a major role in human parturition.

82 SPECIES-SPECIFIC TRANSLATION PRODUCTS OF THE PRO-OPIOMELANOCORTIN GENE ARE PROCESSED TO SPECIES AND LOBE-SPECIFIC END PRODUCT HORMONES IN ADULT AND FETAL PITUITARY TISSUES. R. G. Allen*, J. Stack, J.W. Kendall, School of Medicine, Dept. of Medicine, and J.A. Resko, Dept. of Physiology, The Oregon Health Sciences University, Portland, OR, 97201.

The amino acid sequences of pro-opiomelanocortin (POMC) molecules produced in rat, human, cow, and monkey are different. We have investigated species-specific POMC processing. Acid extracts of pituitary lobes from rat and monkey were fractionated by sodium dodecyl sulfate/polyacryamide gel electrophoresis and analyzed by radioimmunoassay for five POMC domains. The major POMC-derived peptides present in monkey anterior pituitary tissue were 1-39 ACTH, β-lipotropin (β-LPH), smaller amounts of γ-LPH (1-58 β-LPH), and 3.5 K-size endorphins. No α-melanocyte stimulating hormone (α-MSH) or 2K-size β-MSH were detected. Approximately 20% of the 3.5K size endorphins were α-N-acetylated. The major POMC-derived peptides present in monkey intermediate pituitary were α-N-acetylated endorphins, α-MSH, and 2K-size β-MSH. These findings also predict that 1-37 γ-LPH, or a derivative, is produced in monkey intermediate pituitary. We have confirmed these lobe-specific processing differences using embryonic day 80 fetal monkey pituitary tissues. In contrast, the major forms of POMC-derived peptides present in rat intermediate pituitary are α-MSH, α-N-acetylated endorphins and relatively large amounts of "shortened" γ-LPH, no 2K-size β-MSH was detected. The production of a "shortened" γ-LPH in rat intermediate pituitary and the production of 2K-size β-MSH in monkey intermediate pituitary suggests that the differences in the amino acid sequences (e.g. a dibasic cleavage site in the monkey γ-LPH region) of the POMC molecule produced in each specie, may be the basis for different lobe-specific POMC processing in rat and monkey pituitary. By simultaneously comparing the POMC peptides in monkey and rat pituitary tissues, we have demonstrated species-specific POMC processing. POMC-derived peptides in the anterior pituitary are different from the intermediate pituitary POMC products in both species. Between species, the anterior POMC products are similar but the intermediate pituitary products are different. Further studies of species-specific POMC-derived end products in developing and differentiated monkey and rat pituitary tissues will be important to fully understanding the expression of the enzyme activities responsible for lobe-specific post-translational POMC processing.

83 STREPTOZOTOCIN INDUCES SEVERE DEPLETION OF PANCREATIC TRH IN NEONATAL RAT.
S. Aratan-Spire*, B. Wolf, B. Portha, and P. Czernichow. INSERM U.30, Hôpital des Enfants-Malades, 149, rue de Sèvres 75743 PARIS CEDEX 15, FRANCE.

Contrary to hypothalamic TRH, pancreatic TRH concentrations (P.TRH) are elevated at birth, reaching a peak on day 2-3 and decreasing thereafter. The selective β-cells destruction by Streptozotocin (STZ) injection at birth was used as a new approach to characterize the cellular location of TRH in the pancreas. Following blood glucose determination, P.TRH and P.insulin concentrations were measured by RIA between d1 and d35 and at 4 months in STZ injected and control animals. Results are expressed as percentage of controls. In order to gain more information about TRH turnover, pancreatic TRH-degrading activity (P.TRH-DA) was quantified in 4 months-old STZ and control rats: following incubation of constant amounts of pancreatic homogenates with tritiated TRH, chromatography of the degraded products and remaining TRH, ng of TRH degraded/min. was taken as an indice of P.TRH-DA. In STZ injected rats: (1)on d2, P.TRH decreases to 21.9±1.9% of control, as well as P.insulin : 9.0±0.9% of control (2)on d35, TRH concentrations remained severely diminished : 8.9±3.3% of control while the recovery of P.insulin was 42.5±5% of control, remaining at the same level up to 4 months ; (3)however the recovery of P.TRH reached 83.1±5.2% in 4 months-old STZ rats. (4) at the same time, P.TRH-DA in STZ rats was significantly higher to that of control 29.1±1.9 vs 16.1±2.3 $ng.min^{-1}$ TRHdegraded. In conclusion : TRH is mainly localized in STZ-sensitive cells. However, recovery pattern of TRH is different from that of insulin. Depletion of TRH stores may be related to increased turnover. This model in which neonatal P.TRH surge is abolished allows further studies on the role of this peptide in the pancreas.

84 ONTOGENY OF HYPOTHALAMIC GnRH AND PITUITARY GnRH RECEPTORS IN FETAL RATS.
M.L. Aubert*, M. Begeot, B.P. Winiger, G. Morel, P.C. Sizonenko and P.M. Dubois, Dept. of Pediatrics, Univ. of GENEVA, Switzerland, CNRS-ERA 981, Univ. of LYON, Oullins, France.

LH secretion starts at 17 days of gestation in the rat and GnRH is involved in this primitive surge. However a role for GnRH at an earlier stage has been postulated. We have shown that when pituitary primordia are removed at 13 days of gestation and maintained in culture, functional gonadotrophs appears spontaneously in absence of GnRH. When removed at 11 days, no such development occurs unless GnRH is present for 24 h in the culture medium (Begeot et al. Neuroendocr. 1984). To clarify the exact role of GnRH during gestation, the ontogenesis of GnRH and of pituitary GnRH receptors was evaluated in Wistar rats. GnRH was present in the earliest brain tissue examined (12 days), remained low until 17 days when it increased markedly as documented by RIA. There was no immunoreactive GnRH in placentae. Pituitary binding sites for GnRH were present as early as 12 days but remained low until 16 days ($K_A = 10^{10}$ M^{-1} at 17 days). Intracellular GnRH in gonadotrophs as seen by immunocytochemistry at the EM level was first detectable at 14 days. LH was first detectable in the pituitary gland by RIA at 17 days, FSH, at 21 days, and PRL at birth. In summary, 1) hypothalamic GnRH appears very early in fetal life and potentially can induce differentiation of the pituitary anlage, 2) the primitive pituitary gland displays binding sites for GnRH largely before LH biosynthesis has started, 3) rat placenta does not synthesize GnRH. It can be concluded that GnRH appears to be essential both for the differentiation of gonadotrophs and for the induction of the first LH secretion.

85 CORTICOSTEROIDS AND THYROID HORMONES PRODUCE SUPRA-ADDITIVE STIMULATION OF PHOSPHATIDYLCHOLINE (PC) SYNTHESIS IN CULTURED FETAL LUNG.

P.L. Ballard* and L.K. Gonzales, Department of Pediatrics and Cardiovascular Research Institute, University of California, San Francisco, CA

We investigated the interaction of T_3 and dexamethasone (dex) on surfactant production by characterizing effects on PC synthesis in organ cultures of fetal rabbit (23 d) and human (15-20 w) lung. Tissue was cultured in serum-free Waymouth's medium without hormones or with optimal concentrations of T_3 (2 nM) and/or dex (10 nM). PC synthesis was assessed by incorporation of choline (or glucose, glycerol, acetate); PC content correlated with rate of choline incorporation. Stimulation by T_3 + dex was additive or greater with each precursor (rabbit) and at all times of exposure (1-7 d). After 2-3 d culture, for example, the increase with T_3, dex, and T_3 + dex was 50 ± 6, 62 ± 7, and $161 \pm 11\%$, respectively, in rabbit tissue (n=22) and 12 ± 5, 37 ± 12, and $107 \pm 36\%$ (n=7) in human. The maximal response to T_3 + dex occurred by 2-3 d in rabbit and 4-6 d in human. Differences in the action of T_3 and dex were: increased saturation of PC by dex (26.4%) but not by T_3 (20.9%) vs control (19.9%) (human); increase in % of (^3H) acetate cpm into PC vs other phospholipids by dex but not T_3; effect of T_3 more sensitive to inhibition by actinomycin D and cycloheximide; prior exposure to dex enhanced response to T_3 but not vice versa (rabbit). We conclude that T_3 and dex synergistically stimulate pulmonary PC synthesis through action at different biochemical sites. Combined hormonal treatment may be more effective than glucocorticoid alone in stimulating surfactant production and preventing neonatal Respiratory Distress Syndrome.

86 DISTRIBUTION OF SERUM AND TISSUE ANDROGEN BINDING PROTEIN IN NEONATAL RATS.

Russell R. Becker* and Donna J. Iles, Department of Anatomy, Bowman Gray School of Medicine, Wake Forest University, Winston-Salem, North Carolina 27103. U.S.A.

While the presence of androgen binding protein (ABP) in adult serum and tissue compartments has been studied, little is known about its distribution during the neonatal period. We have examined the ABP distribution in male and female rats daily for the first 6 days after birth. Tests for independence show that there was no significant difference in serum ABP concentrations between litters at the same age. The serum concentration for males was 183 ± 27 ng/ml at birth and decreased very rapidly to 60 ng/ml at day 4. Similar levels were observed for females during this period. Neonate liver of both sexes and ovary showed no ABP concentrations of any import. From birth to day 6, total epididymal ABP increased from 1.26 to 3.59 ng. Total testicular ABP increased along a power exponential curve from 0.74 to 32.69 ng during the same period. At birth, only 37% of the tissue ABP pool was found in the testis; by day 6, this had risen to 90%. The observed dramatic increase in testicular ABP when compared to the modest increase in epididymal ABP and the rapid decrease in serum ABP suggests that ABP is retained in the seminiferous tubules and is not released to the blood or transported to the epididymis during the immediate postnatal period.

Supported in part by NIH-NIADDKD Training Grant #5T35 AM 07400 and a United Way/Bowman Gray Venture Grant.

87 DIFFERENTIATION OF IMMUNOREACTIVE LACTOTROPES IS INDUCED BY α-SUBUNIT OF LH. M. Begeot*, F.J. Hemming, Y. Combarnous, M.L. Aubert, M.P. Dubois and P.M. Dubois, CNRS-ERA 981, Univ. of LYON, Oullins, INRA, NOUZILLY, France, Dept. of Pediatrics, Univ. of GENEVA, Switzerland.

The differentiation of immunoreactive lactotropes in the rat occurs late in gestation but it can be induced in fetal hypophyses in vitro by GnRH as early as 13 days of gestation (Begeot et al. Endocrinology, 1983). Whether this action is direct or mediated by another cell type had to be investigated. Adenophypophysial primordia explanted from 13-day-old rat fetuses were maintained for 8 days in organ culture in synthetic Parker's 199 medium and then studied using immunocytochemical staining with anti-rat prolactin serum on paraffin and ultrathin sections and radioimmunoassay of prolactin in cultured tissue and culture medium. The use of synthetic medium alone was characterized by the absence of immunoreactive material in cultured tissue and in culture medium. The action of GnRH (10^{-9} M) added to the synthetic culture medium was abolished by simultaneous addition of anti-rLH but was not altered by the addition of anti-LHβ serum. The action of GnRH could therefore be mediated by the α-subunit of LH elaborated by gonadotropes. To verify this hypothesis, pure α-subunit of porcine LH was added (10^{-7} and 10^{-9} M) to the synthetic culture medium throughout the culture period. After 8 days of culture, lactotropes were observed by immunocytochemistry, and PRL was detected by RIA in both tissue and culture medium. Even at 10^{-7} M, β-subunit of porcine LH was ineffective. This study suggests that differentiation of lactotropes can be induced by LHα which may be the mediator involved in the action of GnRH.

88 HUMAN PLACENTAL 11β-HYDROXYSTEROID DEHYDROGENASE. A López Bernal*, P J R Phizackerley, G E Newman and A C Turnbull. Nuffield Department of Obstetrics & Gynaecology and Clinical Biochemistry, University of Oxford, UK

Placental tissue obtained at term was incubated with tritiated cortisol or cortisone and the metabolites were extracted and separated by thin layer chromatography. Placental slices in a buffered salt solution under 95% O_2, 5% CO_2 converted cortisol to cortisone at a rate (pmol/g dry weight per min) of 2460 ± 481 compared with 61 ± 25 for the reverse conversion and similar results were obtained in homogenates incubated with NADP or NADPH. In slices the apparent Km was 0.35 μM for cortisol and 0.21 μM for cortisone. Placental microsomes had apparent Kms of 0.07 μM for cortisol, 0.08 μM for cortisone, 0.21 μM for NADP and 264 μM for NADPH. Although many detergents used were inert or inhibitors, treatment with Tween 80 selectively increased microsomal conversion of cortisol to cortisone with little release of enzyme from the microsomal pellet. 11β-HSD activity in placental slices was not influenced by glucose, insulin, pyruvate, citrate, malate or glutamate; nor by malonate or 2,4 dinitrophenol. Potassium cyanide decreased activity by 35%. Furthermore, when slices were incubated under anoxic conditions (100% N_2 in the presence of yellow phosphorus) the oxidation of cortisol to cortisone remained linear for up to 60 min. These data indicate that 11β-HSD is a complex membrane-bound enzyme whose activity is largely independent of aerobic metabolism. The strong oxidative activity appears to be due to the high affinity of the enzyme for NADP relative to NADPH and the capacity of placental tissue to convert cofactors to their oxidized form. This work was supported by the Lalor Foundation.

89 NERVE GROWTH FACTOR (NGF) AND CORTICOSTERONE (CS) STIMULATION OF NEURAL ENZYMES IN DIFFERENTIATING RAT EMBRYOS IN VITRO DURING ORGANOGENESIS. W. Biggers, E.R. Barnea*, M. Sanyal and F. Naftolin, Dept. Ob/Gyn, Yale University School of Medicine, New Haven, CT 06510

Profiles of 3 adrenergic (tyrosine hydroxylase, TH; monoamine oxidase, MAO; catechol-o-methyl transferase, COMT) and 2 cholinergic (choline acetyl transferase, CAT; acetyl cholinestrase, AChE) neural enzyme activities indicate that these enzymes are first expressed in embryos at different time periods during organogenesis in vivo (pregnancy days 10 through 15). COMT activities were highest during pregnancy days 11-13, MAO during 13-14, AChE during 13-15, and TH and CAT activities elevated gradually from day 10, reaching a plateau by day 13 of pregnancy. To assess the possible role of hormonal factors in expression of these marker neural enzymes, pregnancy day 10 rat conceptuses (Witschi stage 13, neurula) were cultured for 45 hr in male rat serum in roller bottles to which NGF and CS were added at various concentrations. In control cultures under standard conditions, the embryos differentiated numerous primary organs, including closed neural tubes with brain segments and sensory organs during this period of culture. A dose response effect was observed in replicate experiments exhibiting anomalous embryogenesis at higher doses of NGF (1-5 μg/ml) and CS (10-100 μg/ml). However, in low concentrations of 100 ng NGF and 1 μg CS per ml serum medium, embryogenesis was normal, and TH, MAO and CAT activities in embryonic tissues were markedly stimulated. Thus, these in vitro studies indicate that these hormones may play a significant role in neural enzyme differentiation, even during early neural development. (Supported by NIH 5 R01 HD14587 and NIH Post-doctoral Fellowship 06324)

Quebec, Canada G1V 4G2

90 CO-RELEASE OF G34 N-TERMINAL FRAGMENT WITH G17 IN PERFUSED ISOLATED RAT STOMACH. H. Akai*[1,3], M. Kawamura[2], K. Iguchi[2], C. Yanaihara[2], T. Toyota[3], Y. Goto[3] and N. Yanaihara[1,2], [1]National Institute for Physiological Sciences, Okazaki 444, [2]Shizuoka College of Pharmacy, Shizuoka 422, and [3]Tohoku University School of Medicine, Sendai 980, Japan.

Big gastrin (G34) and its related peptides were measured by a G34 N-terminal specific RIA, which had been developed with use of synthetic human G34(1-15). The RIA was shown to recognize G34(1-5) sequence, especially the terminal pGlu residue and have no crossreactivity with G34 C-terminal little gastrin (G17) sequence at all. Throughout the rat gastrointestinal tract, G34 N-terminal immunoreactivity (IR-G34-N) was detected in the highest concentration (1108.8 ± 380.0, mean ± SD, pg/mg wet weight of tissue) in the antral mucosa. The IR-G34-N was attributed mostly to the G34 N-terminal pentadecapeptide-like component. Methacholine and synthetic porcine gastrin releasing peptide (GRP) 10^{-8} - 10^{-5}M produced a biphasic dose-dependent release of IR-G34-N from the vascularly perfused isolated rat stomach. The release was concomitant with that of IR-G17 during the methacholine or GRP stimulation. However, the integrated IR-G34-N released was not stoichiometric with that of IR-G17 and IR-G34-N was constantly lower. Gel filtration of the perfusate revealed the presence of the G34 N-terminal pentadecapeptide-like component as almost sole major component. The present results demonstrate that post-translational processing of the gastrin precursor in the rat antrum produces, but not necessarily, G34, which is further converted in the tissue to G17-related peptides and that the G34 N-terminal fragment formed in the G34 conversion is stored and released concomitantly with G17-related peptide(s).

91 AUTOANTIBODY AGAINST IODINATED GASTRIN. E. Aoki*, H. Adachi and K. Torizuka, Kyoto University School of Medicine, Kyoto, Japan.

Autoantibodies against hormones influence measured values of serum hormone levels by radioimmunoassay(RIA). In this study, we found autoantibody against iodinated gastrin. [Methods]: Gastrin was iodinated by chloramine-T method. Diiodinated gastrin(DIT-G) was separated from monoiodinated gastrin(MIT-G) by linear gradient elution of DEAE sephadex A-25. [Results]: Four sera, which showed lower serum gastrin levels than zero in gastrin RIA using charcoal dextran method for B/F separation, had an ability to bind DIT-G selectively. Immunoglobulin G fractions prepared by protein A affinity column chromatography and gel filtration with sephadex G-200 were fully responsible for the binding. The binding was displaced by non-radioactive DIT-G alone but not by non-radioactive MIT-G and synthetic human gastrin. All of these cases showed positive anti-thyroglobulin antibody. [Conclusion]: In sera of patients who had positive anti-thyroglobulin antibody, specific binding ability of DIT-G was found. The binding was due to immunoglobulin. Occurance of these autoantibodies against DIT-G is unknown but will have close co-relationship with the development of anti-thyroglobulin antibody. Clinically the existence of these autoantibody will have a significant effect on measured serum gastrin level by RIA. In RIA of gastrin, DIT-G is better to be removed from tracer gastrin.

92 RAPID GASTRIN ASSAY FOR LOCALIZING GASTRINOMA DURING SURGERY. I. Chen*, E. Barnes, C. Volle, M. Chen, H. Maxon, and S. Joffe, Depts. of Radiology and Surgery, Univ. of Cincinnati Medical Center, Cincinnati, Ohio 45267, USA.

Percutaneous transhepatic venous sampling for measurement of gastrin has been used to localize gastrinoma in the pancreas, duodenum, and liver, but difficulty in portal vein catheterizatin and uncertainity in the sites of venous sampling have been experienced. Such problems can be minimized by performing the selective venous sampling at the time of exploratory surgery. We developed a rapid gastrin assay for use in this intraoperative procedure by modifying assay conditions of a commercial gastrin kit (Becton Dickinson Immunodiagnostics). The modified procedure (parentheses are for the original procedure) involved incubating a mixture of 200 (200) μl of standard or sample, 100 (100) μl of radiolabeled gastrin, and 200 (100) μl of gastrin antiserum for 10 (120) minutes at 37° (25°) C. This was followed by addition of 1000 (1000) μl of precipitating antiserum, centrifugation at 3500 x g (1500 x g) for 2 (15) minutes, and counting for 1 minute in a 6-well γ-counter. By increasing the amount of antiserum and assay temperature, we could reduce the total assay time for 42 tubes (5 standards, 2 controls, and 12 samples in duplicate) from more than 4 hours to less than 40 minutes and thus were able to make gastrin values available during exploratory surgery. Coefficients of variation of the modified procedure were less than 7.6%. Gastrin values obtained by the two procedures correlated well (r = 0.935), but values obtained by the modified method tended to be higher. This was attributed at least partly to increased affinity at higher assay temperature of antibody to various molecular species of gastrin relative to the little gastrin (G-17) used as standard in the assay.

93 HLA-DR3 AND DRw6: POSSIBLE PROGNOSTIC FACTORS FOR THE INCIDENCE OF HYPOTHYROIDISM IN RADIOIODINE TREATED GRAVES'DISEASE.

B. Althaus*, J.J. Staub, T. Neri, A. Ryff, J. Müller, W. Berger. Div. of Endocrinology, Dept. of Medicine, University of CH - 4031 Basle

It was the aim of the present study to examine if different grades of hypothyroidism in radioiodine (RI) treated Graves'disease were immunologically heterogeneous according to HLA pattern and thyroid autoantibodies. Patients and Methods: 45 patients with Graves'disease after RI therapy were studied, 27 had preclinical hypothyroidism (pc hypo) and 18 overt hypothyroidism (ov hypo). Controls: 87 healthy blood donors. 56 alleles of the 4 HLA-loci A,B,C, and DR have been determined. Statistical analysis was made by Fisher's exact test.

Results and Conclusions:	%DR3	%DRw6	p value vs for DR3	controls for DRw6
whole group of pat. (N=45)	33 (N=15)	36 (N=16)	<0.05	<0.04
pc hypo (N=27)	37 (N=10)	26 (N= 7)	<0.05	n.s.
ov hypo (N=18)	28 (N= 5)	44 (N= 8)	n.s.	<0.04
controls (N=87)	16 (N=14)	17 (N=15)	-	-

Patients without thyroid antibodies had a marked elevation of DRw6 (p <0.01) and those with antibodies of DR3 (p<0.03). - DR3 represents a possible protective factor and DRw6 a risk factor for the development of overt hypothyroidism. Thus, the knowledge of DR3 and DRw6 could be of importance in the management of patients with Graves'disease.

94 DETECTION OF ENDOGENOUS RAT TESTES LH-RECEPTOR COMPLEXES USING A LABELED MONOCLONAL ANTIBODY WHICH BINDS hCG BETA SUBUNIT.

D.M.Anderson*, G.J.Macdonald, T.Guan, P.H. Ehrlich, and W.R.Moyle. UMDNJ-Rutgers Medical School, Piscataway, NJ 08854, USA.

Our topological map describing the orientation of hCG when it binds to rat testes LH receptors shows that some sites on the beta subunit project away from the receptor binding site and can be detected using ^{125}I-monoclonal antibodies (PNAS 79:2245,1982). For example, antibody B105 binds to hCG-receptor complexes formed when hCG is pre-incubated with rat testes homogenates. Since B105 also binds with high affinity to human LH and with lower affinity to ovine LH, we anticipated that ^{125}I-B105 might bind to rat LH-receptor complexes which had been formed in vivo. To test this idea we measured the binding of ^{125}I-B105 to testes homogenates in the absence and presence of 1 ug hCG or unlabeled B105/100 ul. Both the excess hCG and the B105 reduced binding of ^{125}I-B105 to the same extent indicating that B105 was binding to testes sites through its Fab but not its Fc components. By 5 hours after hypophysectomy (APX), the high affinity specific binding (K_a~10^8M^{-1}) was reduced 4-fold. It was barely detectable 11 days later. APX did not alter non-specific binding. Injection of 10 ug hCG into 60 day old APX rats increased the binding of ^{125}I-B105. To learn which fraction of the testes contained the specific binding sites for B105, we manually dispersed the testes by shaking them at the end of a glass rod in a 50 ml centrifuge tube filled with 0.9% NaCl solution and separated the interstitial cells from the tubules which rapidly settled to the bottom of the tube. We compared the ability of ^{125}I-hCG and ^{125}I-B105 to bind to each fraction and observed that the interstitial fraction contained most of the specific B105 binding sites. Collagenase treatment of the testes destroyed the B105 binding sites suggesting that they were localized on the cell surface. These observations support the notion that B105 is binding to endogenous rat LH-receptor complexes. This antibody probe should be useful in studies of LH physiology since it should enable us to measure occupied receptors. In principle, measurements of occupied receptors would give a better index of biological function than measurements of unoccupied receptors (i.e., those detected with ^{125}I-hCG). Supported by NIH grants HD14907 and HD15454.

95 EFFECT OF GONADOTROPIN SECRETION RATE ON THE SENSITIVITY OF THE GONADOTROPH TO IONIZING RADIATION. K.M. Barnes*, J. Winterer, A. Lichter, A.M. De Luca, D.L. Loriaux and G.B. Cutler,Jr., Developmental Endocrinology Branch, NICHHD, and Radiation Oncology Branch, NCI, NIH, Bethesda, MD, 20205, USA.

Radiotherapy to the hypothalamus and pituitary has the unwanted side-effect of damage to normal pituitary cells, including the gonadotroph. We explored the possibility that the functional state of the gonadotroph during or after irradiation might affect its susceptibility to radiation damage. We initially determined the dose-response relationship and time course for the effect of radiation on the LH & FSH response to castration. Male rats were given a single dose from a ^{60}Co source with shielding of the esophagus. Radiation doses from 3000-5000 rads significantly decreased plasma LH and FSH at 24 wk after irradiation: 5000 rads decreased LH to 18% and FSH to 16% compared to non-irradiated control levels ($p<.001$). To assess the influence of LH & FSH suppression at the time of irradiation, rats were castrated, implanted with either 4-cm testosterone (T) containing or empty silastic capsules, irradiated 2 wk after castration (after which the capsules were removed), and bled 8 wk after irradiation. The rats bearing T capsules had increased radiation damage at 8 wk:LH & FSH were 72% and 80% of the levels in the control rats bearing empty capsules ($p<.005$). In a third experiment, rats were castrated, irradiated 2 wk later, given T or empty capsules for 6 wk, and bled 2 wk after capsule removal. The rats bearing T capsules showed no significant difference compared to the control rats with empty capsules. We conclude that a single dose of 5000 rads impairs the gonadotropin response to castration, and that suppression of gonadotropins by testosterone before and during, but not after, irradiation augments the radiation-induced impairment of gonadotropin secretion.

96 CLONING AND EXPRESSION OF cDNAS CODING FOR HUMAN CHORIOGONADOTROPIN AND LUTEINIZING HORMONE. A. Beck*, V. Vellucci, E. Bernstine, N. Hsiung, V.B. Reddy and R. Pelham. Integrated Genetics, Inc., 31 New York Ave., Framingham MA 01701 and Serono Laboratories Inc., Randolph MA 02368, U.S.A.

Human choriogonadotropin (hCG) and luteinizing hormone (LH) are members of the glycoprotein hormone family. They are very similar both functionally and structurally but are expressed in different tissues. They consist of two dissimilar non-covalently linked alpha and beta subunits. The alpha subunit is common to all the glycoprotein hormones and the beta subunits are unique to each hormone and specify the biological activity. cDNA clones coding for the alpha and beta subunits of hCG have been isolated from a placental cDNA library using complimentary DNA probes. For the isolation of a beta LH CDNA clone, a ^{32}P labeled cDNA fragment of beta hCG was used to screen a cDNA library prepared from human pituitary mRNA. Sequence analysis of several positively hybridizing clones showed that they code for human LH. The homology between the beta chains of hCG and LH is 92% on the nucleotide level and 82% on the amino acid level. Several differences between the amino acid sequence derived from our cDNA sequence and the published protein sequencing data were found: There is an additional methionine at position 42, an additional valine at position 55 and the carboxy terminus is 7 amino acids longer than previously reported. The beta LH chain is thus 121 amino acids in length. The cDNAs were inserted into SV40 vectors as well as expression vectors based on Bovine Papilloma Virus (BPV) in which the expression of the cDNAs is under control of the mouse metallothionein promoter. hCG and LH were produced in both expression systems at high levels. Both hormones have been shown to bind receptors and to exhibit biological activity both in vitro and in vivo.

97 ROLE OF OPIOID PEPTIDES IN PULSATILE RELEASE OF GONADOTROPINS IN THE RAT. J.C. Bedran de Castro*, O. Khorram, S.L. Petrovic and S.M. McCann. Dept of Physiology, University of Texas Health Sci Center at Dallas, Dallas, TX 75235.

To further elucidate the role of opioid peptides in the release of gonadotropins, the opiate receptor blocker, naloxone, was injected i.v. (0.6 and 6.0 mg/kg) into ovariectomized, conscious rats. The lower dose increased plasma LH transiently at 10 and 20 min, while the higher dose produced an elevation of LH that was maintained for 60 min. The overall levels of FSH increased. The frequency of sampling was increased from every 10 to every 5 min and naloxone (3.0 mg/kg) was given i.v. twice at 30 min intervals. The overall mean levels of LH and FSH increased as did the LH pulse amplitude but pulse frequency decreased. To determine the opioid peptide involved, a highly specific anti-β endorphin antiserum (3 µl) was injected into the 3rd ventricle. Anti-β endorphin serum induced a biphasic effect on plasma LH, with a significant lowering at 10 min followed by an elevation at 20 min. The increase in LH levels at 20 min suggests that β endorphin is the LH release-inhibitory opioid peptide. The transitory lowering of plasma LH may be due to low initial levels of antiserum in the tissue which suppressed an ultrashort loop feedback leading to an increase in endorphin release. The experiments with naloxone suggest that opioids are involved in determining the frequency and magnitude of pulsatile LH discharge and overall levels of FSH secretion in ovariectomized rats. (Supported by FAPESP and PHS grant HD 09988).

98 EFFECTS OF MICROWAVES ON MATURATION OF GONADOTROPHIN FUNCTION IN THE MALE RAT NEONATALLY IRRADIATED. G. Beraud*, J.M. Renou and J. Maniey, Physiologie des Régulations, Université de Rennes, Campus de Beaulieu, 35042 Rennes-Cedex, France.

Endocrine effects of microwaves exposure of male rats were studied on the maturation of gonadotrophin function. Newborn rats (SHERMAN) were exposed, in an anechoic chamber, to pulsed microwaves (3GHz ; pulse frequency 500Hz ; level power density 6.1 mW/cm^2) from day 1 to day 15 of life. Animals were then housed in the laboratory until decapitation at 30, 45, 60 and 90 days of age. Plasma luteinizing hormone (LH), follicule stimulating hormone (FSH), testosterone and the pituitary content of gonadotrophins were assayed by radioimmunoassay. The irradiation increased the plasma LH at 30, 45 and 60 days and FSH at 45 days. The main increase was observed at 45 days (2.75 fold-increase for LH and 2.38 for FSH). Only a significant increase of the pituitary FSH **content** was seen at 30 days. There was a slight, but non-significant, increase at 45 and 60 days of plasma testosterone, and a decrease ($p < 0,05$) at 90 days, in spite of no modification of plasma LH and FSH at that age. These data demonstrate that neonatal irradiation affects significantly the control of gonadotrophin secretion in maturing rats. It is impossible to know if microwaves act directly on the pituitary and testis or through an alteration of hypothalamic functions. As they affect also the pituitary-thyroidal axis, it is hypothesized that, because the first days after birth are very critical in the development of brain functions in the Rat, they act probably at the hypothalamic level. This work was supported by D.R.E.T.

99 CONFORMATIONAL COMPARISON OF NATIVE AND DE-GLYCOSYLATED OVINE PITUITARY LUTROPIN. T. A. Bewley* and M. R. Sairam, Laboratory of Molecular Endocrinology, University of California, San Francisco, CA 94143, USA and Reproduction Research Laboratory, Clinical Research Laboratory of Montréal, Montréal, Québec, H2W 1R7, Canada.

Second-order (second derivative) spectra of both native and partially de-glycosylated ovine lutropin (pH 7.5) contain a maximum at 287.6 nm which can be assigned to the two tyrosyl residues, known from previous circular dichroism studies, to be buried within the interior of the non-covalent complex. In all other respects the conformation of the de-glycosylated protein also appears to be essentially equivalent to the native hormone as judged by second-order and circular dichroism spectra. Titration of either protein to pH 2.5 produces rapid dissociation of the complex, with complete loss of the 287.6 nm band. Back titration of the native protein to pH 7.5 is followed by recombination of the subunits and a slow repair of the conformation to its original state. At 0.5 mg/ml (25°C) this repair is 90% complete in 72 hrs. In sharp contrast, under the same experimental conditions, recombination and conformational repair of the de-glycosylated form is 95% complete in less than 3 hrs. These results suggest that during biosynthesis, non-covalent combination of the α and β subunits would be more efficient if carried out prior to completion of the glycosylation. This study was supported in part by NIH Grant AM-6097.

100 AN IMMUNOCHEMICAL METHOD TO ASSESS THE STRUCTURE OF THE CARBOHYDRATE AND PEPTIDE COMPONENTS OF THE β COOH-TERMINUS OF HCG AND APPLICATION TO STUDIES OF EXPRESSED HCG. S. Birken*, R. Canfield, A. Beck, E. Bernstine, E. Cole, C. Bryant and N. Hsuing. Department of Medicine, Columbia University College of Physicians and Surgeons, New York, NY 10032 and Integrated Genetics Inc., Framingham, MA. 01701.

A system for assessment of the state of the O-serine oligosaccharides as well as the peptide chain structure of the β COOH-terminal portion (βCTP)of human chorionic gonadotropin (hCG) has been developed. This immunochemical evaluation procedure is based on the use of three specific immunoassays. Total hCG and hCG βCTP content is measured by a general antiserum, R525 which recognizes the βCTP region composed of residues 123-145 independent of its carbohydrate content. Native hCG is measured by antiserum R561, which binds intact βCTP but reacts poorly with its desialylated form and fails to bind the synthetic peptide analogue. Desialylated βCTP is quantitated by antiserum R141, which requires the N-acetylgalactosamine and galactose portions of the O-serine oligosaccharides and is also specific for peptide residues between positions 123 to 141. This immunochemical method system was applied to assess the nature of the βCTP region of hCG and the free hCGβ subunit secreted by mammalian cells which contain expression vectors encoding the subunits of hCG. The expressed proteins were purified chromatographically from the cell growth media and compared on a molar basis with urinary hCG. It was found that the purified expressed hormone and β subunit were indistinguishable from the urinary products in their reactivities in this assay system.

101 EPISODIC GONADOTROPIN SECRETION IN AZOOSPERMIC MEN WITH SELECTIVE INCREASE IN PLASMA FSH. J.D. Booth*, G.R. Merriam, D.L. Loriaux, and R.J. Sherins. DEB, NICHD, NIH, Bethesda, MD 20205, U.S.A.

Testosterone (T) modulates the pulsatile secretion of gonadotropins in men. Hypogonadal subjects have an increased frequency of gonadotropin (Gn) pulses, which can be reduced by T supplementation. We have recently shown that azoospermic men with a selective increase in plasma FSH have low free T levels and diminished T production (3.5 ± 0.8 mg/day, mean ± SE) vs. controls (7.5 ± 0.8 mg/day, p<0.01), despite normal plasma LH and total T concentrations. To determine whether this degree of T deficiency changes Gn dynamics, which could in turn alter the LH:FSH ratio, we measured Gn's at 20 min. intervals in 13 such men (6 for 24h. and 7 for 8h. beginning at 0800h.), 15 normal men (24h.), and 6 hypogonadal men (24h.). LH pulses were analyzed using a modification of the method of Santen and Bardin (peaks defined as a rise of 4 assay CV's above preceding minimum).

	Mean T (ng/dl)	Mean LH (mIU/ml)	Mean FSH (mIU/ml)	LH Pulses/24 h.	LH Pulse amp (mIU/ml)
Normal Controls	580±49	8.4±0.6	7.2±1.6	9.7±0.5	9.0±1.6
Azoospermic Men	382±47*	14.8±1.3*	38.1±4.1*	11.3±0.9	10.5±1.2
Hypogonadal Men	98±33*†	51.4±7.3*†	108±15*†	16.3±1.0*†	13.4±2.0

Results: Means ± SE; * p<0.01 vs. normals; † p<0.01 vs. azoospermic men. Thus FSH levels appear to be a more sensitive index of reduced T production, since LH pulse frequency is maintained at normal values by T concentrations insufficient to reduce FSH to within normal limits.

102 THE NUMBER OF EPIDERMAL GROWTH FACTOR (EGF) RECEPTORS DIFFERS IN MALE AND FEMALE RAT LIVERS. R. Benveniste, Z. Steynbok and S. A. Carson*, Division Reproductive Endocrinology, Dept. OBGYN, Michael Reese Hosp. Med. Cntr., University of Chicago, Chicago, IL 60616, USA.

The understanding of EGF and EGF receptors' role in normal cell growth and differentiation, and during tumor promotion, is of much interest. Herein, we report a sex difference in the number of EGF receptors present in cell membrane preparations from adult male (n = 9) and female (n = 10) rat livers. Membrane preparations were used in a RRA to generate EGF competitive binding curves, and Scatchard plot of binding data at equilibrium provided the number of EGF receptors (N) per mg of liver preparation. To limit inter-assay variations, the same human term placental membrane preparation was assayed with each liver preparation, and its EGF receptor number (Nr) served as a reference; further procedural details have been published (Am. J. Obstet. Gynecol. 147: 932, 1983). Results (mean ± SEM) were:

	N ($x 10^{-8}$)	N/Nr (x 100)	
Female	1,116 ± 136	11.4 ± 1.49	p< .005
Male	2,946 ± 228	32.4 ± 3.33	

Conclusion. The number of EGF receptors in liver membrane preparations from age-matched adult female rats is about 65% lower than that found in males. Discussion. The decreased EGF receptor number appears not to result from a higher EGF content in female rat liver. Although reasons for decreased EGF receptors in the female need to be established (estrogen vs androgen milieu, neonatal imprinting, etc.) this observation leads to interesting speculation on cell differentiatiation and on tumor incidence in sex-hormone-responsive tissues.

103 RAT PLACENTA RECEPTORS FOR BASIC SOMATOMEDIN AND MULTIPLICATION STIMULATING ACTIVITY.

B. Bhaumick* and R.M. Bala, Dept. of Medicine, University of Saskatchewan, Saskatoon, Saskatchewan, S7N 0X0, Canada.

Basic somatomedin (B-SM), one of the Type I group of somatomedins (SM) binds preferentially and specifically to a Type I SM receptor (Mr ~140K in the presence of reductant or > 300K in the absence of reductant) in human placenta. However, the presence of Type I SM receptors in rat placenta has been controversial. As multiplication stimulating activity (MSA) binds specifically to Type II SM receptors, we have now compared the binding of [^{125}I]B-SM with that of [^{125}I]MSA in rat placenta from days 16 to 21 of gestation. Specific binding of [^{125}I]MSA was constant at ~20% while that of [^{125}I]B-SM was significantly lower in placentas from day 16 (13%) but in those from days 17 to 21 was similar (~18%) to that of MSA. [^{125}I)B-SM binding was inhibited by MSA (~1/3 the potency of B-SM) and weakly by insulin while binding of [^{125}I]MSA was inhibited by B-SM (1/10 the potency of MSA) but not by insulin. SDS-gel electrophoresis after affinity cross-linked binding of [^{125}I]B-SM revealed binding components of Mr ~ 140K in the presence of reductant and Mr >300K in the absence of reductant and in addition a component of Mr ~220K with or without reductant. [^{125}I]MSA bound only to a Mr ~220K component (Type II receptor). These studies confirm the presence of Type I receptors in rat placenta and suggest that B-SM binds to Type I and Type II receptors in the rat placenta while MSA binds only to a Type II receptor. Supported by M.R.C. MSA was the gift of Dr. S.P. Nissley.

104 RELAXIN INDUCES GROWTH OF MOUSE MAMMARY GLAND : A LIGTH AND ELECTRON MICROSCOPIC STUDY.

M.Bigazzi, G.Bani, R.Cecchi and F.Petrucci, Endocrine Unit, INRCA and Dpt of Animal Biology, Univ. of Florence, Florence, Italy.

A mammotropic effect of relaxin (RLX) can be expected from early studies and recent finding on RLX-receptors. Therefore we investigated the morphological changes at M.O. and M.E. of the mammary gland induces by porcine RLX standard (NIH) and human decidual RLX. Intact and ovariectomized virgin mice were treated with: a) estrogen (E_2), b) E_2+ RLX. E_2 x 7 days initiated deep changes in the mammary gland structure with stimulation of epithelial cells and connective tissue. Both RLX preparation induced in 18 hs a further enhancement of the growth of mammary tissue. We observed a strong increase in number and size of ducts, the active proliferation of epithelial cells with development of myoepithelial cells. The connective tissue was stimulated with loosening of the intercellular matrix and increase of periductal stroma and the fibroblasts and adipocytes. Blood vessels became more numerous and wide taking strict contact with the growing ducts. Ovariectomy did not changed the RLX effect. Our study shows that RLX is a growth factor for the mice mammary gland, synergistic with E_2. This hormone may play an important role in the physiological and pathological growth of the gland also in the human, since significant RLX-levels have been found in milk and cystic fluid of fibrocystic disease of women.

105 IGF STIMULATES THE PRODUCTION OF IGF BINDING PROTEIN (IGF BP) BY THE LIVER.
M. Binoux* and C. Lassarre, INSERM U 142, Hôpital Trousseau, 75012 Paris, France.

The results of our "in vivo" and "in vitro" studies suggest that the biosyntheses of IGFs and their BPs, though interdependent, are regulated by hormones in different ways : 1) compared with IGF, BP levels are increased to a lesser extent in acromegalics and depressed to a lesser extent in hypopituitary patients; 2) in contrast with IGF, BP levels do not change significantly after short-term administration of GH; 3) GH and insulin both stimulate IGF production by rat liver in organ culture but have no significant effect on BP. Cortisol inhibits the production of IGF but stimulates that of BP (Acta Endocrinol. 1982, 99, 422).

We have made the hypothesis that IGFs and BPs are involved in the control of each other biosynthesis. In order to evaluate the effect of IGF on BP production by rat liver explants, we have added to the culture medium increasing concentrations of a partially purified preparation of IGF, from 10 to 100 mU/ml (serum units). The BPs released into the media after 3 day's culture were separated from IGFs by gel filtration in acetic acid and titrated with the aid of $[^{125}I]$ IGF I (generous gift of R. Humbel, Zürich). Results of 5 experiments show a dose dependent stimulatory effect of IGF on BP production. Maximum stimulation was obtained with 25 or 50 mU/ml. For these doses, the BP concentrations in the media ranged from 2.5 to 15 times those of controls. These results support our hypothesis of a control of BP biosynthesis by IGFs and provide a new insight in understanding the regulation of IGFs and their BPs.

106 ISOLATION OF FOUR PEPTIDES OF THE SOMATOMEDIN FAMILY FROM HUMAN PLASMA.
W.F.P. Blum*, M.B. Ranke, J.R. Bierich, Children's Hospital, University of Tübingen, D 7400 Tübingen, Germany.

Our primary aim was to develop methods for small-scale purification of SmC/IGF-I and IGF-II from human plasma. For monitoring at various steps the following assays were used: stimulation of SO_4-incorporation into porcine cartilage, a heterologous insulin RRA, a competitive binding assay using crude IGF-binding protein, and SmC RIA (NIADDK antibody). Isolation involved the following steps: 1) diafiltration at pH 8.6 (MW cut-off 30 K), 2) diafiltration in 1 M HAc (MW cut-off 30 K), 3) gel filtration on Sephadex G 75 in 1 M HAc, 4) chromatofocusing (CF): a) pH 6.8 - 5.9; b) pH 9.0 - 7.9; c) pH 5.5 - 4.5; d) pH 9.4 - 8.6, 5) HPLC on a reverse phase C18 column using an acetonitrile gradient (29-40%), giving base-line resolution. The conditions of CF were optimized thus giving 10-fold higher resolution compared to conventional IEF. Peptides isolated in steps 4a) and 4b) showed chemical and biological characteristics described for IGF-I/SmC and IGF-II respectively. One liter of plasma gave a yield of approx. 10 µg of each peptide. In addition two other peptides were constantly co-purified. The basic one (step 4d, pI = 9.2 showed activity in all assay systems, while the acidic one (step 4c, pI = 5.0) was barely active in the SmC RIA. The structural and biological relation of these peptides to the known insulin-like growth factors will be studied in further detail.
Supported by DFG Bi 77/16-2.

107 ISOLATION FROM BOVINE PITUITARY AND PARTIAL MOLECULAR CHARACTERIZATION OF A GROWTH FACTOR FOR MESODERM-DERIVED CELLS. Peter Böhlen*, Andrew Baird, Fred Esch, Nicholas Ling, Roger Guillemin and Denis Gospodarowicz†. Laboratories for Neuroendocrinology, The Salk Institute for Biological Studies, La Jolla, CA 92037, †Cancer Research Institute, UCSF School of Medicine, San Francisco, CA 94143.

From a preparation of partially purified fibroblast growth factor (FGF) of pituitary origin (Gospodarowicz et al., J. Biol. Chem. 253 3736, 1978) a mitogenic protein was purified to homogeneity by cation-exchange HPLC and two reverse-phase HPLC steps. Isolation was monitored by testing column fractions for their ability to stimulate proliferation of cultured bovine aortic endothelial cells. Amino acid composition and N-terminal amino acid sequence of the protein (MW 15,800 by polyacrylamide gel electrophoresis) indicate that its structure is different from that of other known growth factors including brain FGF. The pituitary-derived growth factor is highly active in vitro in stimulating division ($ED_{50} \sim 1$ ng/ml) of vascular (aortic and umbilical vein) endothelial cells, smooth muscle cells, adrenal cortical cells, chondrocytes and granulosa cells but not basal epithelial cells and resembles in this respect the activity of partially purified FGF preparations from brain and pituitary. Antibodies were raised in rabbits against a synthetic decapeptide representing the amino terminal sequence of the pituitary-derived growth factor. The antisera recognize the synthetic peptide and the growth factor on an equimolar basis and are capable of inhibiting the mitogenic activity of the native protein in vitro.

108 GROWTH REQUIREMENTS OF HUMAN AND CANINE PROSTATIC FIBROBLASTS IN CULTURE. P. Boulanger*, S. Chevalier, G. Bleau, K.D. Roberts and A. Chapdelaine. Maisonneuve-Rosemont Res. Center and U. of Montreal, Quebec, Canada.

In human benign prostatic hyperplasia, both fibromuscular and epithelial elements contribute to the hyperplastic changes and the stroma can represent up to 90% of the tissue. Monolayer cultures of human prostatic fibroblasts were established from explants isolated from hyperplastic glands in order to define their growth requirements. When compared to serum-free cultures, cell proliferation was highly dependent upon added serum; after six days of culture in the presence of charcoal-treated human, fetal bovine and dog serum, increases in cell number were found to be 9, 7 and 3-fold, respectively. The proliferative responses of fibroblasts to human serum were dose (up to 50%) and time dependent. In presence of fetal bovine serum, their growth was also linear up to 20%; higher concentrations were toxic. Upon gel filtration of human serum, one peak of activity was found with a low molecular weight. The addition of $3\alpha,17\beta$-androstanediol, dihydrotestosterone or estrogens, at concentrations of 10^{-8} and 10^{-6}M, did not influence fibroblast division. When compared to the effect of human serum on cell division, EGF and FGF show no, or minimal, activity. Similar results were obtained with canine prostatic fibroblasts. Thus, as described for the epithelial cells of human and canine prostates, the growth of prostatic fibroblasts in vitro is also influenced by non-steroidal serum factor(s). Their role in the development of prostatic hyperplasia remains to be elucidated. (Supported by MRC, FRSQ and FCAC).

109 INCREASED SERUM LEVELS OF SOMATOMEDIN-C IN WOMEN WITH MILD HYPERANDROGENISM

A. Caufriez*, J. Golstein, D. Bosson, C. Robyn and G. Copinschi, St Pierre Hospital, University of Brussels, Belgium.

While it has recently been shown that the rise in somatomedin-C (Sm-C) concentrations during early puberty is partially related to the increasing testosterone levels, no data exist in the literature concerning Sm-C values in adult women with hyperandrogenism. In 31 menstruating women, aged 19-48 off contraceptive pills for at least 6 months, blood was drawn at random once during the menstrual cycle at 0900 h for hormonal determinations; 19 of them had progesterone values $\leqslant$ 0.80 ng/ml, averaging 0.32 $\pm$ 0.04 ng/ml (mean $\pm$ SE), and were considered for this study. Sm-C levels averaged 0.80 $\pm$ 0.07 U/ml. Sm-C presented significant positive correlations with testosterone (T) ($r = 0.66$, $P < 0.01$), LH ($r = 0.64$, $P < 0.01$) and LH/FSH ($r = 0.50$, $P < 0.05$). Within this group, T values were normal in 8 women ($\leqslant$ 0.45 ng/ml; mean 0.33 $\pm$ 0.02 ng/ml), elevated in 6 subjects ($\geqslant$ 0.60 ng/ml; mean 0.73 $\pm$ 0.06 ng/ml), borderline in 5 individuals (0.50-0.55 ng/ml). Sm-C was significantly higher ($P < 0.01$) in the hyperandrogenic (1.05 $\pm$ 0.13 U/ml) than in the normal women (0.64 $\pm$ 0.05 U/ml); intermediate values (0.77 $\pm$ 0.10 U/ml) were found in the borderline subgroup. These data suggest that in adult women as well as in early puberty, mild pathophysiological increases of androgens may induce Sm-C elevations.

110 BINDING OF GH TO IM-9 CELLS INVOLVES THE PORTION ASSOCIATED WITH ITS BIOACTIVITY.

S. Agarwal*, S. Chalew, S. Dhawan and A. Kowarski, Department of Pediatrics, University of Maryland School of Medicine, Baltimore, Maryland, USA.

The established GH radioreceptor assay requires fresh preparation of liver membrane and may not necessarily reflect GH bioactivity.

We have documented the presence of GH receptors on IM-9 cells (a lymphoid cell line growing in culture). Of 71 monoclonal antibodies (MAB) to GH which were raised in our lab, 3 inhibited GH binding to receptors on both IM-9 cells and rabbit liver membrane. Five MABs did not inhibit GH binding to the IM-9 cells or to the liver membrane. The 8 MABs reacted with 22K hGH but not with hPRL or hCS.

We previously reported the presence of structural variants of GH in plasma of patients, using one of our MAB which binds to regular 22K GH but not to GH of variant structure (GH Symposium 1983).

We compared the binding of each MAB to identical concentrations of 22K GH and GH from 5 patients with bioinactive GH syndrome. The fraction of patients' GH bound by the 3 inhibitory MABs was 53%$\pm$13%, while the GH fraction detected by the 5 noninhibitory MAB was 100%$\pm$5% ($P<0.001$).

We interpret our results as indicating that the inhibitory MABs block epitopes on 22K GH responsible for binding to receptors on IM-9 cells. These epitopes are not present on GH from patients with bioinactive GH syndrome. Consequently, we conclude that GH binding to IM-9 cells involves the portion of the GH molecule which is associated with its growth promoting activity.

111 SERUM IMMUNOREACTIVE PROCOLLAGEN LEVELS IN CHILDREN OF SHORT STATURE DURING GROWTH HORMONE TREATMENT. K Albertsson-Wikland*, G Lindstedt and P-A Lundberg, Depts of Pediatrics, Physiology and Clinical Chemistry, University of Goteborg, Sweden.

Radioimmunoassay of serum procollagen-III offers an alternative to the more laborious urinary hydroxyproline assay in the evaluation of growth hormone (GH) therapy. 25 children, with integrated GH concentration <400 mU/l per 24 h (72 intervals) were characterized according to GH response to provocative tests as well as to growth rate before and during GH treatment (Crescormone, KabiVitrum, 0,1 IU/kg s c once daily). Serum procollagen-III peptides were measured with reagents from Behring-Werke AG (Marburg; FRG), using a serum pool from thyrotoxic patients as secondary calibrator.

Group	n	Increase in growth*	Basal serum procollagen-III before treatm.	% increase during treatment day 2	day 5, 10	month 1, 3	month 6, 9, 12
IΔ	4	>twice	23 ± 3	14	92 ± 25	157 ± 46	127 ± 26
II°	12	twice	31 ± 2	13	34 ± 4	57 ± 5	55 ± 4
III°	7	<twice	36 ± 5	2	11 ± 5	16 ± 4	15 ± 4
IV°	2	none	19 ± 5	0	12 ± 7	9 ± 7	0 ± 0

*Growth velocity (cm/year) above the growth rate during the year before treatment. Δ No increase in GH after provocative tests. ° Increase in GH after provocative tests.

A significant increase was observed in group I-II from day 5 to month 12. Conclusion: Serum procollagen-III may be a useful biochemical marker of the growth response to growth hormone treatment in short children.

112 EVALUATION OF BASAL SOMATOMEDIN-C (SmC) LEVELS IN A NORMAL SPANISH POPULATION. C. Arraiza, J. Saavedra, R. Rodriguez, M. Goena, I. Cano, J. Salvador, J.J. Barberia and E. Moncada, Dept. of Endocrinol., Univ. Hosp. of Navarra and Faculty of Medicine, Univ. of Navarra, Pamplona, Spain.

In order to know the normal range of SmC levels and its relationship to sex, age, height and bone maturity a population of 799 spanish children (412 males and 387 females) has been studied. The subjects were aged between 4 and 17 years and they were divided in 28 groups according to sex and chronological age. There were 17 subjects at least in each group. In all cases height and weight were measured, bone maturity was evaluated by both Greulich-Pyle and TW2 methods and the basal levels of SmC estimated by RIA (Nichols Institute, California). Highest levels of SmC were observed at 15 years in males and at 13 years in females, when the menarche took place (12,4 ± 1 years). SmC values at postpuberal age were significantly greater than those obtained before puberty in males (1,83 ± 0,80 U/ml vs 0,88 ± 0,35 U/ml*) as well as in females (2,16 ± 0,84 U/ml vs 1,18 ± 0,42 U/ml*). A good correlation between bone age and SmC concentration was found in both sex groups (r=0,67** in males and r=0,59** in females). Likewise, height (r=0,69** in males and r=0,60** in females), weight (r=0,70** in males and r=0,56** in females), body surface (r=0,70** in males and r=0,58** in females) showed a positive correlation with SmC levels. It is concluded that the estimation of the basal level of SmC is an accurate parameter to indicate a normal development, showing a significant increase at the pubertal stage. Since there are obvious differences between our results and those observed in other countries, it is necessary to compare the individual levels to those found in a population with similar nutritional and developmental conditions. Results are mean ± SD. *p 0.001, **p 0.01.

113 TREATMENT OF ACROMEGALY WITH CU-32-085, A NEW DOPAMINE AGONIST. P.Aschner* C.Tafurt, W.Villamil and G.Cano, Hospital Militar Central, Bogotá -Colombia

Long-term treatment of acromegaly with bromocriptine is controversial. We have been treating 3 actively acromegalic patients with a new dopamine agonist, CU-32-085, an 8α-aminoergoline with an in vitro hypoprolactinemic potency 4Xgreater than bromocriptine. 2 patients (female and male) had no absolute indication for surgery and the third (male) underwent transsphenoidal hypophysectomy but relapsed 4 months later. Basal leveles of hGH and response to a glucose load (100 g orally) were determined before treatment. 1 patient showed also suppression with L-dopa. hGH was then measured at specific follow-up intervals in 2 basal samples within one hour. Initial CU dose of 0.3 mg/d was increased according to response. A significant and sustained hGH decrease was observed after reaching 1.2 mg/d. The hGH levels in the female patient fell from 42 ng/ml to normal range after 3.5 months and have kept normal for 2 months with 2.5 mg/d. In the males the hGH has fallen from a range of 226-318 ng/ml to a range of 60-115 ng/ml after 7 months treatment and with a present dose of 3.5 mg/d. No neuroradiological signs of further tumour growth have been noted. No haemathological or hepatic side effects have been observed and the drug has been well tolerated. These results suggest the feasibility of alternative therapy with CU-32-085 in selected acromegalic patients.

114 GROWTH HORMONE FAILS TO STIMULATE THE LIPOLYTIC ACTIVITY OF RABBIT ADIPOCYTES INCUBATED IN VITRO. B. BARENTON,* Y. COMBARNOUS, M.P. DUBOIS and V. BATIFOL, INRA, Station de Physiologie Animale, 34060, Montpellier, France.

The supernatant (S) and pellet (P) from the soluble fraction of pig hypophyseal homogenate were compared for lipolytic activity on rabbit adipocytes with ACTH (Synacthen), ovine placental lactogen (oPL) and GH of human (h), ovine (o), porcine (p) and rabbit (Rb) origin. All the GH preparations and oPL were equivalent in inhibiting the binding of ^{125}I-oGH to liver plasma membranes from pregnant rabbit (IC_{50} value of 3-4 ng/ml). In this binding system the activity of S and P were respectively 0.1% and 20% of that of oGH-NIH-S5. Immunohistochemical studies showed that S had a high $ACTH_{1-24}$ activity. Free fatty acid (FFA) production by isolated adipocytes ($5x10^5$ cells/dish) incubated for 3h was stimulated by ACTH (ED_{50} value of 8 ng/ml ; R max of 5.7 mEq/3h). When incubated with 200 mIU adenosine deaminase (AD) the ED_{50} of ACTH was reduced to 3 ng/ml but Rmax unchanged. The Ed_{50} of S and P were respectively 80 and 10,000 ng/ml in absence and 25 and 1500 ng/ml in presence of AD. The Rmax for S and P was similar to that for ACTH and did not change with AD. The addition of 100 µg of either pGH, oGH or oPL did not stimulate the FFA production even in presence of AD but the same doses of RbGH and hGH induced the release of 3 and 4.7 mEq/3h respectively. The ED_{50} value for hGH was reduced from 10 to 1 µg/ml when AD was added. Thus, GH and oPL have no effect on lipolysis at physiological dose. The lipolytic effect of pig pituitary extracts was lost during the purification of GH. The increased sensitivity of adipocytes incubated with AD suggests that lipolytic activity is mediated through the adenylate cyclase system.

115 IMMUNOLOGIC HETEROGENEITY OF CIRCULATING GH. S. Blethen*, F. Chasalow and K. Bieser, Dept. of Pediatrics, Washington Univ., St. Louis,MO, 63110,USA

We have screened a number of monoclonal antibodies (Ab) to GH and have found 3, each specific for a different epitope, which were sensitive enough for use in RIA's (B/Bo = 0.5 at GH added from 0.15-0.35 ng). With these Abs and affinity-purified [^{125}I]hGH, we measured the GH response to sleep or pharmacologic stimuli in 43 subjects (5 normal adults, 17 short children, 8 other children, 8 short children with normal GH in a polyclonal RIA and accelerated growth following treatment with exogenous GH and 5 similar short children who did not respond). For the monoclonal RIA's, each sample was diluted on the basis of its presumed GH concentration as determined in a polyclonal RIA and assayed at 3 concentrations with each Ab. Although not all samples had the same estimated GH content in each RIA (microheterogeneity), concordant results were observed in 28 of 30 individuals from whom multiple samples were available. In 6 of 8 short children who responded to exogenous GH, the 3 monoclonal RIA's and the polyclonal RIA gave similar estimates of the GH content. However, the GH secreted by one of the two others had NO cross-reactivity in one monoclonal RIA and a non-parallel dose-response curve (NPDRC) in a second. The second child had an NPDRC in one assay. No normal individuals had undectable GH or NPDRC with any of the monoclonal RIA's. Conclusions: We have found immunologic microheterogeneity in the circulating GH of both normal adults and children. Two children who responded to GH therapy appear to have immunologically distinct forms of GH in their circulation which are different from the microheterogeneity noted above. Supported by R01-AM05105-21 Monoclonal Abs obtained from Hybritech.

116 HUMAN PANCREATIC TUMOR GROWTH HORMONE RELEASING FACTOR (npGRF) STIMULATES NITROGEN (N) RETENTION IN TWO GROWTH HORMONE (GH) DEFICIENT CHILDREN. R. Blizzard,* J. Reschke, A.D. Rogol, S. Jackson, F. Beziriannidis, J. Chitwood, R. Furlanetto, J. Rivier, W. Vale, M. Thorner. University of Virginia, Charlottesville, VA; Children's Hospital of Philadelphia, PA; Salk Institute, San Diego, CA, USA.

The anabolic effects of GH include N retention in association with hypercalcuria. hpGRF stimulates GH release in some GH deficient children. To study the therapeutic potential of hpGRF, hpGRF (1 ug/kg) was administered s.c. by Pulsamat pump (courtesy Ferring Inc) for the last 6 days of a 16 day constant diet study period. Two short boys (8.3 & 9.6 yr), height ages (4.7 & 5.0 yr) and bone ages (5.5 & 3.5 yr) had low serum somatomedin C levels (0.13 & 0.05 U/ml) and subnormal peak GH responses to arginine/L-Dopa (5 & 1 ng/ml). Peak GH response to i.v. bolus npGRF (3.3 ug/kg) were 12 & 20 ng/ml. In response to 6 days hpGRF therapy N excretion (mean $\pm$ SE) fell in both children (24.6$\pm$0.2 to20.6$\pm$0.6 & 19.2$\pm$1.2 to 15.2$\pm$0.6 gm/gm creatinine; $p < 0.05$). Urinary calcium increased in both children (140$\pm$10 to 200$\pm$10 & 120$\pm$10 to 210$\pm$20; $p < 0.01$). Somatomedin C levels increased markedly in one child and slightly in other (0.13 to 0.56; & 0.02 to 0.08 U/ml). These children are currently receiving a 6 month course of hpGRF therapy. These results lead us to be optimistic about the therapeutic potential of hpGRF.

This work is supported by General Clinical Research Grants #RR-847 and #AM-32632.

117 NON-MAMMALIAN GROWTH HORMONES HAVE DIABETOGENIC AND INSULIN-LIKE ACTIVITIES

C.M. Cameron*,[1] J.L. Kostyo[1] and H. Papkoff,[2], Univ. of Mich. Med. Sch., Ann Arbor, MI[1], and Univ. of Calif., San Francisco, CA[2].

Pituitary growth hormones (GHs) from a number of non-mammalian species possess growth-promoting activity in the rat, although the degree of activity follows no phylogenetic pattern. Since mammalian GHs also have intrinsic diabetogenic and insulin-like activities, this study was undertaken to determine if the structural determinants for diabetogenic and insulin-like activities are also present in non-mammalian GHs (ostrich, sea turtle, snapping turtle, bullfrog and a teleost, Tilapia). Diabetogenic activity was determined by the ability of the GHs to increase fasting blood glucose and decrease glucose tolerance when given for 3 days to the ob/ob mouse. Insulin-like activity was assessed by the *in vitro* ability of the GHs to stimulate glucose oxidation to CO_2 by isolated epididymal fat from hypophysectomized rats. Human GH (A-type monomer) gave threshold responses in these assays when used at a dose of 10 μg/day and at a concentration of 2-5 nM, respectively. Ostrich and bullfrog GHs exhibited threshold diabetogenic activity at a dose of 100 μg/day, and sea turtle, snapping turtle, and Tilapia GHs at a dose of 200 μg/day. Thus these GHs possess ca. 5-10% the diabetogenic activity of human GH in the mouse. Ostrich GH and bullfrog GH gave threshold responses in the assay for insulin-like activity at concentrations of 250 and 50 nM, and thus possess ca. 5 and 10% the insulin-like activity of human GH, respectively. Therefore diabetogenic and insulin-like activities are also intrinsic properties of non-mammalian GHs, indicating that the structural determinants required for the expression of these activities in mammals appeared early in the evolution of the GH molecule.

118 QUANTITATIVELY DISHARMONIOUS TISSUE EFFECTS OF ANDROGENS: AN OBVIOUS BUT UNDISCUSSED ISSUE AND ITS NEUROENDOCRINOLOGICAL IMPLICATIONS.

A.G. Alias* St. Louis State Hospital Complex, St. Louis, Mo. 63139, U.S.A.

The three major and well known tissue effects of androgens in humans are promotion of body hair growth and of mesomorphism and deepening of voice. These physical parameters are rarely seen in equal proportions in a given individual, male or female, though more obvious in the male. For example, there are many men who have strikingly high pitched voice and/or are very low in mesomorphism but with liberal body hair and beard growth. Conversely, there are many men (of the same race) who have no more body hair or beard than that in slightly hirsute women, but have strikingly deep voice and/or are very high in mesomorphism. Further, racial and ethnic make up modulates these parameters, especially body hair growth; the latter is most in caucasians and least in east asians. Examples for these disharmonious tissue effects of androgens in different forms will be presented.

This conspicuous disharmony may be the result of (a) differential production rates of different androgens at the glandular level, and/or altered "peripheral" metabolic rates of these androgens and/or variable responses at the tissue level due to differential distribution of specfic androgen receptors as well as modulation by other steroids. There are no known methods to precisely determine the chemistry behind this disharmony.

It is, however, possible that a particular combination of these obvious "extraneuronal" tissue effects of androgens have an influence at the CNS level, determining or modulating the personality make-up or behavior -some interesting, though preliminary, observations in this regard will be presented.

119 PROLACTIN ADMINISTRATION ENHANCES THE SYNTHESIS AND RELEASE OF HYPOTHALAMIC GABA. J. Apud, G. Gudelsky*, C. Masotto, V. Locatelli, D. Cocchi, G. Racagni and E.E. Muller. Dept. of Pharmacology and Pharmacognosy, University of Milan, Italy and Dept. of Psychiatry, University of Chicago, Chicago, IL. USA

Increasingly, evidence has been obtained that is supportive of the view that GABA functions as an endogenous inhibitor of PRL secretion in the rat. The purpose of the present study was to address the issue of whether PRL can modulate via a feedback mechanism the synthesis and release of hypothalamic GABA. GABA was measured in the anterior pituitary gland and in hypophysial portal plasma of urethane-anesthetized male rats after the intraventricular injection of PRL (2 ug) or the solvent vehicle. Plasma PRL concentrations and the activity of the GABA synthesizing enzyme, glutamic acid decarboxylase (GAD), in the hypothalamus also were measured. The concentration of GABA in hypophysial portal plasma was increased 16 h but not 4 h after the administration of PRL. GABA concentrations in portal plasma of control and PRL-treated rats were 719 $\pm$ 106 and 1425 $\pm$ 266 pmol/ml, respectively. Associated with the PRL-induced increase in the portal plasma concentration of GABA was a 63% increase in the activity of GAD in the hypothalamus and a 135% increase in the concentration of GABA in the anterior pituitary gland. Neither GAD activity in the hypothalamus nor GABA concentrations in the anterior pituitary gland were significantly altered 4 h after PRL administration. Plasma PRL concentrations in control rats were 16 $\pm$ 6 ng/ml and were reduced to 2 $\pm$ 1 ng/ml 16 h after the injection of PRL. Thus, exogenous PRL exerts a delayed effect to increase the synthesis and release of hypothalamic GABA. The PRL-mediated feedback regulation of hypothalamic GABAergic neurons may be part of the mechanism by which PRL regulates its own secretion.

120 PURIFICATION, SEQUENCING AND SYNTHESIS OF AURICULIN, A VASOACTIVE AND NATRIURETIC PEPTIDE FROM RAT ATRIUM. S. Atlas*, H. Kleinert, M.J. Camargo, A. Januszewicz, J. Sealey, J. Laragh, T. Maack, J. Schilling, J. Lewicki and L. Johnson, Cornell University Medical College, New York NY, and California Biotechnology, Inc., Mountain View CA, USA.

Mammalian atria contain potent natriuretic factor(s) which also antagonize hormone and non-hormone induced contraction of the isolated rat kidney vasculature and isolated rabbit aorta. For purification, atria from 1400 rats were homogenized in 1N acetic acid with protease inhibitors; the neutralized and lyophilized supernatant, applied to a Sephadex G-50 column, gave two regions of natriuretic and vasorelaxant activity (MW >15,000 and <6000). The low MW peak was further purified by reverse phase HPLC (μBondapak C_{18} column, 15 to 55% acetonitrile in 0.1% trifluoroacetic acid). Of the two major peaks of coincident natriuretic and vasorelaxant activity, the more active was re-applied twice to the C_{18} column (20-36% and 22-29% gradients) and then to a μBondapak CN column (10-30% gradient). The homogeneous active peak obtained was, by automated microsequence analysis, the 24-residue peptide Arg-ser-ser-cys-phe-gly-gly-arg-ile-asp-arg-ile-gly-ala-gln-ser-gly-leu-gly-cys-asn-ser-phe-arg-OH. The peptide was produced by solid phase synthesis; after reduction, gel filtration and re-oxidation, the synthetic peptide, like purified native peptide, caused: increases in GFR, renal resistance and natriuresis of isolated kidneys (IK) perfused without vasoconstrictors; vasodilation of IK perfused with vasoconstrictors; and relaxation of angiotensin-, histamine- or K^+-contracted aortic rings. Since the physiological function of this substance is uncertain, we suggest the term "auriculin" to describe its tissue source. If secreted, it could represent a new class of natriuretic and vasoactive hormone.

121 DIFFERENCES BETWEEN FREE AND COMBINED α SUBUNITS OF HUMAN CHORIOGONADOTROPIN (hCG) IN PREGNANCY. D.L. Blithe* and B.C. Nisula.
DEB, NICHD, NIH, Bethesda, MD 20205, U.S.A.

HCG is a glycoprotein hormone with two subunits, α and β. This hormone and its α subunit are secreted by a variety of malignant cells, as well as by trophoblastic cells during pregnancy. Free α is incapable of combining with purified β subunit to form intact hormone, while α subunit dissociated from hCG can recombine. We have purified these two molecules from pregnancy urine by dissociation of α from hCG by urea, followed by affinity chromatography using anti-α antisera linked to Sepharose. SDS-PAGE of the two preparations showed that dissociated α consisted of a single component. Free α consisted of multiple components. The components of free α appeared homogeneous on Sephadex G-100 eluting earlier than dissociated α. Radioactive labeling of the sialic acid by limited periodate oxidation and $NaB[^3H]_4$ reduction resulted in more incorporation of ^3H into free α suggesting that free α contains more sialic acid per immunoreactive molecule. This was supported by DEAE chromatography in which free α eluted at higher ionic strength than dissociated α. The $[^3H]$-dissociated α but not the $[^3H]$-free α was able to combine with β subunit. Alkaline hydrolysis of the purified subunits released the radioactivity in the form of free oligosaccharides. Comparison of oligosaccharides from free α with those from dissociated α indicated distinct differences. Most of the material from dissociated α bound to Con A-Sepharose (73%) and could be eluted with α-methyl-mannoside. Significantly less material from free α (23-40%) was capable of binding to Con A. DEAE chromatography of the oligosaccharides revealed that a larger proportion of di- and tri-sialo oligosaccharides were contained on the free α compared with those which were present on α combined with β subunit.

122 Acute ACTH, α MSH, and cortisol response to CRF in Cushing's and Nelson's syndromes. M.Abalovich, A. Guitelman *, S. Belli, E.Emeric-Sauval, P. Mileikovsky, B. Espinola, and A. Negro-Vilar.
Endocrinology Unit, Hospital Alvarez. Buenos Aires, Argentina.

Corticotropin-releasing factor (CRF) has been previously shown to stimulate ACTH secretion in patients with Nelson's syndrome and Cushing's disease. The present study was undertaken to demostrate its action in a group of patients pre and post-surgery (Cx). A dose of 100 μg was administered intravenously to 3 groups of patients: I) Nelson's syndrome (n=1); II) Active Cushing's disease (n= 2) ; III) Pituitary (n=2) and adrenal (n=1) Cushing's syndromes with a prolonged remission post-Cx. Results. Group I: Pre-Cx CRF: ACTH hyperresponsiveness (B= 560 pg/ml, Δmax 640 pg/ml) and normal α MSH response (B= 34 pg/ml, Δmax 38 pg/ml); post-Cx CRF (2 months): deficient ACTH response. Group II: Pre-Cx CRF: 1 case with hyperresponsiveness of ACTH (B= 76 pg/ml, Δ max 384 pg/ml) and cortisol (B=280 μg/dl, Δ max 440 μg/dl); in the other case, no response was detected, but post-Cx CRF induced a normal ACTH response (B= 18 pg/ml, Δ max 42 pg/ml). Group III: normal ACTH and cortisol responses. Conclusions: a) CRF was capable of stimulating ACTH and α MSH release in Nelson's syndrome; b) A large variation in individual responses to CRF is observed in those cases with active Cushing's disease. After surgery, responses may be normal or suppressed, according to the resumption of the activity of normal corticotrophs; c) Pituitary or adrenal Cushing's syndromes evidencing a prolonged remission post-surgery, show a normal response to CRF, suggesting, in the first case, the pituitary etiology of the disease.

123 LHRH PULSATILITY AND POSITIVE FEEDBACK IN THE INDUCTION OF OVULATION.
N A Abdulwahid*, M Tucker, J Adams, P Mason and H S Jacobs, Cobbold Laboratories, The Middlesex Hospital, Mortimer Street, London W1.

Pulsatile LHRH infusion can produce follicular development and ovulation in patients with hypogonadotrophic hypogonadism, whereas intermittent bolus administration of high-dose LHRH is less effective. We therefore contrasted the effect of continuous intravenous LHRH infusion (250 mcg daily) with that of pulsatile infusion of the same dose in a 28 year old patient with primary amenorrhoea. Following initiation of continuous LHRH infusion, the serum LH levels rose from 8 to 24 U/l and the FSH levels from 6.8 to 12 U/l within 2 days. Ultrasonic examination of the ovaries showed development of multiple follicular structures (4 to 10 mm in size), and the serum oestradiol concentration rose from 130 to 940 pmol/l. A dominant follicle (25 mm) evolved on the eighth day of treatment, with an associated rise in E2 to 1240 pmol/l and suppression of the LH and FSH levels to 7.2 and 1.0 U/l respectively. Treatment was prolonged for a further 22 days, the follicle continued to grow, but ovulation did not occur. A second cycle of continuous LHRH therapy failed to produce dominance although follicular size increased to 10 mm by the 4th day. Treatment was then converted to pulsatile LHRH therapy. Within 7 days a dominant follicle had evolved and ovulation in association with an LH peak (32 U/l) occurred; successful conception resulted. These findings indicate that although follicular evolution can occur in the presence of constant exposure to LHRH, the oestrogen mediated LH surge does not occur. The latter phenomenon is dependant on exposure of the pituitary to pulsatile LHRH.

124 CORTICOTROPHIN-RELEASING ACTIVITY OF HUMAN FETAL HYPOTHALAMIC TISSUE.
Jacqueline Ackland*, Sally Ratter, G.L. Bourne and Lesley H. Rees, Departments of Chemical Endocrinology and Obstetrics and Gynaecology, St. Bartholomew's Hospital, London, EC1A 7BE, U.K.

Although human fetal pituitaries of at least 12 weeks gestation are known to contain and secrete ACTH little is known of the hypothalamic factors controlling this release. We have developed a RIA for ovine corticotrophin releasing factor (oCRF-41) and used it to measure CRF-like immunoreactivity (CRF-LI) in hypothalamic extracts from human fetuses of 12-26 weeks gestation. The concentration of CRF-LI ranged from 4.4-26.3pg/mg wet weight tissue and there was no significant correlation with gestation. The corticotrophin releasing bioactivity of these extracts was measured using dispersed rat anterior pituitary cells and showed a significant positive correlation with gestation ($r=0.80$, $p<0.02$) with adult hypothalamic extracts having even greater bioactivity. The bioactivity of fetal, but not adult, extracts was potentiated by up to 300% by the addition of arginine vasopressin (AVP). AVP levels measured by RIA in these extracts ranged from 4.5-82.0pg/mg wet weight tissue in the fetal hypothalami, 500-1150pg/mg in the adult and showed a significant correlation with gestation in the fetus ($r=0.82$, $p<0.05$). Pre-incubation of hypothalamic extracts with CRF and/or AVP antisera resulted in a reduction of bioactivity of up to 60% with anti-CRF, 80% with anti-AVP and 90% with both antisera together. These results are in agreement with others in proposing that AVP as well as CRF is required for full ACTH releasing activity and also suggest that the increase in bioactive CRF with gestation is due more to increasing AVP levels than CRF levels.

125 THE USE OF GROWTH HORMONE-RELEASING FACTOR (GHRF) TO DETECT THE SITE OF DAMAGE IN RADIATION-INDUCED GH DEFICIENCY. S.R. Ahmed*, S.M. Shalet and C.G. Beardwell. Department of Endocrinology, Christie Hospital, Manchester.

Pituitary hormonal deficits may be caused by external irradiation for intracranial and extracranial tumours. In patients with multiple hormonal deficiencies, either the pituitary or the hypothalamus may be the site of the radiation damage, however GH is always the first hormone to be affected by such damage. In order to determine if the hypothalamus is more radiosensitive than the pituitary we have studied GH secretion in 10 patients, aged 11-23 (mean 16) years, with abnormal GH responses to standard pharmacological stimuli but no other abnormality of anterior pituitary function. All 10 had received cranial irradiation during childhood for a brain tumour which had not directly involved the hypothalamic-pituitary axis. After a mean time of 8 (range 3-18) years following irradiation all 10 patients showed subnormal GH responses to insulin hypoglycaemia (mean peak 6.2 mU/l ; range 1-12 mU/l: normal $\geq$ 20 mU/l) and to arginine stimulation (range 1.6-15 mU/l; normal $\geq$ 20 mU/l). Subsequently the GH response after I.V. administration of a bolus of 100 µg GHRF (1-44) was monitored in each child. A significant rise in GH was seen in 6 patients (mean peak 27.8 mU/l ; range 14-57 mU/l). No GH response was seen in the remaining 4. Conclusion: An acute bolus GHRF test showed that in 6 out of 10 children, radiation -induced GH deficiency was due to hypothalamic damage. In the remaining 4 it was not possible to determine the site of damage. Pulsatile administration of GHRF may provide more information than a single bolus of GHRF. This may be of practical significance in determining which GH deficient children might benefit from GHRF therapy in the future.

126 CHARACTERIZATION OF THE ACUTE, BIPHASIC RESPONSE TO TRH IN GH_4C_1 RAT PITUITARY TUMOR CELLS. Toru Aizawa and Patricia M. Hinkle, Dept. of Pharmacology, Univ. of Rochester Medical Ctr., Rochester, N.Y. 14642 USA

TRH induced acute PRL and GH secretion in GH_4C_1 cells was studied in perifusion and in static culture systems. Acute PRL and GH secretory responses were identical. TRH elicited maximal secretion of PRL and GH in 5 sec. and 30 sec. in the static and perifusion systems without a detectable lag. The initial secretory rate remained high (250-1000% of basal) for 5-10 min. (1st phase), declined sharply despite continuous exposure to TRH, and plateaued at a lower rate (130-150% of basal, 2nd phase). The ED_{50}s for 1st and 2nd phase TRH responses were 3.0 and 0.5 nM, respectively. Experiments with cycloheximide and ^{35}S-Met incorporation indicated that the 1st phase consists of release of stored hormone and the 2nd phase includes the release of some newly synthesized hormone. Exposure to low Ca^{2+} medium for 15 sec. markedly depressed both phases of TRH-induced secretion. Continuous exposure to depolarizing concentrations of K^+ elicited only a single rapid burst of PRL and GH release. GH_4C_1 cells exhibited only partial (50%) desensitization to repeated pulses of TRH given every 5 min. In cells chronically exposed to TRH (48 h), TRH receptor concentrations are low due to downregulation, PRL synthesis is increased, and GH synthesis is decreased. When these cells were washed and challenged acutely with fresh TRH, there was a right shift of the dose-response curves for both the 1st and 2nd phases with increased PRL and decreased GH responsiveness. These data indicate that acute secretion in response to TRH is very rapid and biphasic. The absolute amount of PRL and GH secretion is determined by intracellular hormone stores, while the sensitivity to TRH is determined by receptor availability.

127 PATHWAYS OF TRH-INDUCED CHANGES IN CYTOSOLIC FREE [Ca^{++}] AND HORMONE SECRETION IN PITUITARY CELLS, Paul R. Albert* and Armen H. Tashjian, Jr., Dept of Pharmacology, Harvard Medical School and Lab of Toxicology, Harvard School of Public Health, Boston, MA 02]]5, U.S.A.

We have described the biphasic action of TRH on cytosolic free [Ca^{++}] ([Ca^{++}]$_i$) in GH-cells loaded with non-toxic concentrations of Quin 2 (Prog. of the Endocrine Soc. Meet., p. 37, Abs. 275, 1983). The TRH-induced spike in [Ca^{++}]$_i$ correlated with a burst (within 1 min) of PRL and GH secretion from GH-cells in suspension, and the plateau phase of [Ca^{++}]$_i$ was associated with prolonged enhancement of the rate of secretion of both hormones. The initial spike in [Ca^{++}]$_i$ after TRH was resistant (50-70% of control) to 5-min pretreatment with EGTA, and was not detectably affected by blockade of voltage-sensitive Ca^{++}-channels with verapamil (VML, 100 μM) or nifedipine (NIF, 2.5 μM). The plateau phase in [Ca^{++}]$_i$ after TRH was abolished by EGTA, and only partially blocked by VML and NIF to 63±12% (±S.D., n=5) and 34±3% of control, respectively. EGTA, VML, and NIF each decreased basal [Ca^{++}]$_i$ by 80±20%, 9±3%, and 27±6%, respectively. Both phases of TRH-stimulated PRL and GH secretion were blocked completely by EGTA, while VML attenuated (25-40% of control) both the initial burst and the plateau phase of TRH-enhanced PRL secretion. Ionomycin (100 nM), a Ca^{++}-ionophore, produced a TRH-like spike in [Ca^{++}]$_i$ which returned to basal [Ca^{++}]$_i$. Ionomycin prevented a subsequent TRH-induced spike in [Ca^{++}]$_i$, but allowed development of a normal plateau phase. We conclude that the TRH-induced spike in [Ca^{++}]$_i$ and PRL secretion are mediated primarily by a release of cellular Ca^{++} from an ionomycin-sensitive pool, while the plateau phase of [Ca^{++}]$_i$ and sustained PRL secretion are caused by influx of extracellular Ca^{++} through voltage-sensitive and VML/NIF-resistant Ca^{++}-channels.

128 A NEW LONG-ACTING SOMATOSTATIN ANALOGUE (SMS 201-995) - EFFECTS IN ACROMEGALIC PATIENTS. P.-H. Althoff*, B. Böttger, C. Rosak, M. Neufeld, H. Knigge, E. Jungmann, F. Lacey, K. Schöffling, Dept. of Endocrinology, Center of Internal Medicine, University of Frankfurt, Germany (FRG).

There are two problems with genuine somatostatin: its wide spectrum of effects and its very short duration in action. Now a new long-acting somatostatin analogue (SA = SMS 201-995, Sandoz AG, Basel) has become available. After a 1h base-line study, a constant infusion of 50 μg SA was administered over a period of 120 min. in 9 patients with active acromegaly. Blood samples were taken from -60 min. to +300 min. in order to measure blood glucose (BG), FFA, lactate, ß-hydroxybutyrate (BOHB), IRI, c-peptide, gastrin, cortisol, ACTH, aldosterone, prolactin and growth hormone (GH). During administration of SA there was a prompt and progressive decrease in GH-levels from 12,7 ± 7,8 ng/ml to 2,4 ± 1,2 ng/ml; ($\bar{x}$ + SE; p < 0,01) at the end of the infusion; mean maximal decrease was 83,5 %. The GH-suppression persisted for more than 3h after the end of the SA-infusion without rebound phenomenon. The mean IRI-level decreased during SA with a small increase but no rebound at the end of the test. BG-levels were not significantly changed. An increase of FFA-levels followed by a decline near to preinfusion-levels was paralleled by corresponding BOHB-level changes. Whereas there was a clear-cut inhibition of c-peptide, cortisol and gastrin, no changes in prolactin or aldosterone were seen. The tested somatostatin-analogue (SA) has a clearly more specific, enhanced and prolonged GH-inhibiting potency than genuine SA with much less pronounced inhibiting effects on IRI and the resulting changes of FFA and BOHB.

129 GROWTH HORMONE-RELEASING FACTOR (GRF) ON GROWTH HORMONE (GH) SECRETION AFTER HYPOPHYSIAL STALK TRANSECTION IN PIGS. L. L. Anderson*, J. J. Ford, J. Klindt, W. W. Vale and J. Rivier, Department of Animal Science, Iowa State University, Ames, IA 50011; USDA, ARS, Roman L. Hruska U.S. Meat Animal Research Center, Clay Center, NE 68933; and Peptide Biology Laboratory, The Salk Institute, San Diego, CA 92138.

Hypophysial stalk transection (HST) abolishes episodic release and elevates basal concentrations of porcine GH even though pituitary reserves of GH are reduced. The dose-response characteristics of human pancreatic GRF (hpGRF-1-40) on plasma GH concentrations were determined in 6 HST and 10 intact control prepuberal Yorkshire gilts averaging 55.4 kg BW. Blood was sampled via an indwelling juglar catheter at -45, -30, -15, 0, 7.5, 15, 30, 45, 60, 75, 90, 105 and 120 min, with injection of GRF or diluent at time 0. After diluent, circulating GH remained similar ($P>0.05$) in HST (4.5 ± 0.4 ng/ml; mean ± SE) and control (4.1 ± 0.6 ng/ml) gilts. Plasma GH peaked within 7.5 min after 0.1 μg GRF/kg BW in HST gilts (19.2 ± 5.3 ng/ml; ($P<0.025$) and controls (7.0 ± 1.9 ng/ml), and returned to basal levels within 60 min. After 0.5 μg GRF/kg BW, GH peaked within 15 min both in HST (37.8 ± 8.1 ng/ml; $P<0.005$) and control (15.1 ± 3.8 ng/ml; $P<0.025$) gilts. During first hour of 2 h constant infusion of somatostatin (SRIH; 500 μg/h) in intact gilts plasma GH remained low (2.8 ± 0.5 ng/ml). GRF (0.5 μg/kg BW) injected during SRIH infusion elicited greater ($P<0.05$) peak release of GH (32.3 ± 6.7 ng/ml) than controls (15.1 ± 3.8 ng/ml). These results indicate that GRF causes an immediate peak release of GH into peripheral blood in intact pigs, and this response is increased after HST. Furthermore, increased secretion of GH by GRF occurs during infusion of SRIH. Supported by USDA Cooperative Agreement 58-519B-M-1369.

130 CHARACTERIZATION OF A NOVEL TYPE OF VASOPRESSIN RECEPTOR IN RAT PITUITARY AND ITS DOWN-REGULATION UPON ADRENALECTOMY. F.A.Antoni*, M.C.Holmes[+] and J.Z. Kiss, Lab. Cell Biology,NIMH,NIH, [+]Endocrin.Reprod.Res.Branch,NICHD NIH, Bethesda,MD 20205, U.S.A.

Vasopressin appears to be an important mediator of the hypothalamic control of pituitary ACTH secretion.We have studied the binding of ^{3}H-AVP to rat pituitary membranes in order to characterize pituitary AVP receptors and examined their regulation under various conditions. Radiolabeled AVP interacted with a single class of high affinity ($K_d \approx 0.4$ nmol/l) and low capacity($B_{max} \approx 90$ fmol/mg pr) binding sites. The binding reaction required Mg^{2+} while Ca^{2+} had no effect. Displacement studies with various AVP analogs revealed that the specificity of pituitary binding is distinct from that in the liver (V_1 type) and from that in the kidney (V_2 type). Adrenalectomy (adrex) decreased the pituitary binding of AVP as early as 4h after operation, and only very low binding (≈10 % of control) remained 4 days later. Lesioning of the hypothalamic paraventricular nuclei attenuated the effect of adrex, however, it also decreased binding to appr. 70% of control. Adrex also reduced AVP binding in pituitaries of rats genetically lacking AVP (di/di Brattleboro rats). We conclude, that pituitary AVP binding sites represent a novel type of receptor and are affected by manipulations of the hypothalamo-pituitary-adrenal axis.

131 DIFFERENTIAL EFFECTS OF COLD AND PAIN STIMULI ON IN VIVO TRH AND SRIF RELEASES FROM THE MEDIAN EMINENCE IN UNANESTHETIZED RATS.

S. Arancibia, J. Epelbaum, L. Tapia-Arancibia, I. Assenmacher and H. Astier *, Neuroendocrinology Lab (CNRS, ERA 85) University of Montpellier II, France, and Neuroendocrinology Unit (INSERM, U 159), Paris, France.

Acute exposure to cold leads to a rapid rise in plasma TSH which seems closely correlated to a cold-induced TRH release, recently reported by us. Since passive immunization with somatostatin antisera enhances the TSH response to cold exposure, we tried to determine the possible relationships between the patterns of SRIF and TRH releases.In parallel,we checked if an other kind of acute stress such as pain,was able to induce changes in the release of these two neurohormones.In a first group of experiments,IR-TRH and SRIF releases from the ME,were directly estimated in conscious rats during 130 min of cold exposure(4°C),using a push-pull cannula stereotaxically implanted one week before.In a second group of experiments,both hormones were measured in rats kept at 24°C,during a pain stress("pinching tail"). Our data show that:(I) SRIF release from the ME decreased as soon as the rats were transferred to a 4°C perfusion room ; peak values of SRIF release (50 to 100 pg/15 min in amplitude) were blunted while basal values scarcely exceeded 2-3 pg/15 min along the experiment. It seems,thus,that a decrease in SRIF release could precede the peak of TRH release occurring 40 min after the begining of cold exposure.(2)the acute pain stress induced an abrupt SRIF release which was correlated with no changes in TRH release.Our results strengthen the successful use of the push-pull perfusion system in studying physiological neuroendocrine responses, and these results will be discussed.

132 IMMUNOHISTOCHEMICAL LOCALIZATION OF GROWTH HORMONE-RELEASING FACTOR IN HUMAN TISSUES.

S.L.Asa*, N.Ryan, K.Kovacs, D.A.Leong, M.O.Thorner, J.Rivier and W.Vale. Department of Pathology, St. Michael's Hospital, University of Toronto, Toronto, Ont., Canada; Department of Medicine, University of Virginia Medical Center, Charlottesville, VI, U.S.A., and Peptide Biology Laboratory, The Salk Institute, San Diego, CA, U.S.A.

Two growth hormone-releasing factors (hpGRF-40, hpGRF-44), isolated from pancreatic islet cell tumors, appear to play a role in the regulation of pituitary growth hormone (GH) secretion. In this immunohistochemical study, we examined formalin-fixed, paraffin-embedded human tissues for the presence of hpGRF-40 using the avidin-biotin-peroxidase complex technique. Immunopositivity was demonstrated in hypothalamus and in pancreatic islet cell tumors, bronchial and thymic carcinoids which were associated with acromegaly, GH excess and pituitary somatotroph hyperplasia or adenoma and/or were shown to contain GRF by radioimmunoassay or bioassay. Among 20 pancreatic islet cell tumors unaccompanied by clinical acromegaly, no hpGRF-40 was detected in 18 cases; slight positivity was noticeable in 2 cases. Several cases of small cell anaplastic carcinoma of lung seemed to contain hpGRF-40 and some medullary carcinomas of thyroid showed immunoreactivity. No conclusive immunopositivity was found in 11 intestinal carcinoids, 10 pheochromocytomas, in nontumorous adult and fetal pancreatic islet cells, exocrine pancreas, intestine or lung. It can be concluded that hpGRF-40 may be localized by immunohistochemistry in some tumors arising from and composed of peptide-hormone secreting endocrine cells. Further work is required to establish the prevalence and functional significance of GRF-containing tumors.

133 HYPOTHALAMIC GROWTH HORMONE RELEASING FACTOR IMMUNOREACTIVITY (GRF-LI IN HUMAN AND RAT TISSUE: QUANTITATION AND LOCALIZATION.

T. Audhya, N. Kanie, T. Nakane, M. Manzione, J. Passarelli, M. Russo and C.S. Hollander*. Endocrine Division, Dept of Medicine, NYU School of Medicine, New York, NY USA.

To evaluate the physiological role of the growth hormone releasing peptides recently isolated from human pancreatic tumors ($hpGRF_{1-44}$, $hpGRF_{1-40}$ as well as rat hypothalamus (rGRF), we have raised antibodies to synthetic rGRF and $hpGRF_{1-44}$ by injecting these weak immunogens, emulsified with complete Freund's adjuvant in the presence of activated charcoal, directly into the spleen. High titer antibodies, raised after subsequent booster injections by conventional routes, were employed in specific radioimmunoassays for rGRF and $hpGRF_{1-44}$. Utilizing antibodies with an apparent Ka of 10^{-12} (human) and 10^{-11} (rat) the sensitivity of these assays was 1 femtomole in both species. Serial dilutions of both human and rat hypothalamic extracts demonstrated parallelism with species-specific standard and ^{125}I labeled tracer. At antibody dilutions of 1:20,000, hypothalamic content in fm/mg wet weight tissue was 20±5.1 for the rat and 3.6±0.2 for the human. Immunocytochemical studies in the rat revealed cellular localization of rGRF-LI mostly in perikarya of the arcuate nucleus and, to a lesser extent, in the dorsomedial and ventromedial nuclei as well as in the amygdala. Levels of rGRF-LI in the amygdala were approximately 1/10th those in the hypothalamus but were readily detectable, and serial dilutions of extracts demonstrated parallelism with synthetic rGRF. In conclusion (1) femtomole quantities of species-specific GRF-like molecules are present in human and rat hypothalamus, with predominant localization in the arcuate nucleus and (2) immunoassay and immunocytochemical studies reveal the presence of detectable, albeit smaller amounts of GRF-LI in the amygdala of the rat.

134 THE EFFECTS OF TWO GROWTH HORMONE (GH) RELEASING PEPTIDES ON GH SECRETION IN PERIFUSED PITUITARY CELLS OF ADULT MALE RATS.

T.M. Badger, W.J. Millard*, G.F. McCormick, J.B. Martin & C.Y. Bowers, Departments of Gynecology & Neurology, Mass. Gen. Hosp., Vincent Res. Labs, Boston, MA, USA.

GRF-44 is a peptide containing 44 amino acids first isolated from a pancreatic tumor of a patient with acromegly and GHRP is a synthetic peptide (His-DTrp-Ala-Trp-DPhe-Lys-NH2). Both peptides stimulate GH secretion <u>in vitro</u> and <u>in vivo</u> in several species. The present study was conducted to determine the GH secretory activity of these two distinctively different peptides. Dispersed pituitary cell columns were prepared as described (Endo. 112: 793, 1983) and experiments were performed 24 h postdispersion. GRF-44 was 60 times more potent than GHRP and stimulated linear increases in GH secretion between 0.3 to 30ng ($y = 3109x + 2063$); whereas the GHRP dose range was 30 to 300ng ($y = 766x + 800$). Hourly pulses of GHRP (3 to 300ng) and GRF-44 (12 to 30ng) elicited consistent GH responses. However, a priming effect was observed at doses below 4 ng GRF-44. Continuous infusion of 30 ng/ml GHRP or 3 ng/ml GRF-44 resulted in desensitization. GH secretion during continuous GHRP infusion was monophasic; whereas biphasic GH secretion occurred during GRF-44 infusion. Cells desensitized by continuous GHRP infusion did not respond to subsequent GRF-44 stimulation, but cells desensitized with GRF-44 infusion responded to GHRP stimulation. These results suggest that; 1) GRF-44 and GHRP stimulate GH secretion by different mechanisms, and 2) structurally unique peptides such as GRF-44 and GHRP may prove to be valuable probes to identify mechanisms of GH secretion. Supported by HD15788 (TMB), AM26252 (JBM) & AM06164 (CYB) & the Vincent Research Fund.

135 IDENTIFICATION OF A NOVEL PEPTIDE DERIVED FROM THE PRECURSOR TO GROWTH HORMONE-RELEASING FACTOR. Andrew Baird, Peter Böhlen, Frederick Esch and Nicholas Ling*. Laboratories for Neuroendocrinology, The Salk Institute for Biological Studies, P.O. Box 85800, San Diego, CA 92138.

The structures of two mRNAs coding for two forms of the precursor for growth hormone releasing factor (proGRF) have been elucidated (Gubler et al, Proc Natl Acad Sci 80:4311, 1983). They differ by the presence of a serine codon in the carboxyl terminal portion of pro-GRF. Therefore, the possibility exists that processing of pro-GRF to GRF in vivo gives rise to two forms of a novel peptide representing the carboxyl-terminal portion of each of the precursors. Using antisera raised against synthetic peptides predicted from the pro-GRF mRNAs, we have developed an RIA specific for the carboxyl-terminal peptide sequence of pro-GRF (CTPG). The antibodies crossreact with CTPG and des-Ser CTPG on an equimolar basis. CTPG-like immunoreactivity (mol wt by gel filtration = 4000) has been detected in acid extracts of the human pancreas tumor from which GRF was originally isolated and in extracts of bovine, porcine and ovine hypothalami-stalk-median eminence. One form of immunoreactive CTPG has been isolated from the human pancreas tumor (4 nmol/g). Amino acid analysis indicates that the peptide is a specific cleavage product of pro-GRF processing. Complete structural characterization is in progress.

Research supported by grants from NIH (AM-18811 and HD-09690) and a grant from the Robert J and Helen C Kleberg Foundation.

136 ISOLATION & CHARACTERIZATION OF BOVINE CORTICOTROPIN-RELEASING FACTOR. Andrew Baird, Nicholas Ling, Peter Böhlen, Robert Benoit, Frederick Esch*. Laboratories for Neuroendocrinology, The Salk Institute for Biological Studies, P.O. Box 85800, San Diego, CA 92138.

A peptide with high intrinsic activity to release ACTH, β-endorphin and γ_3-melanotropin from bovine anterior pituitary cells in culture was isolated from side fractions of approximately 2,500 fragments of bovine median eminence used in the isolation of growth hormone-releasing factor (GRF). The unretained material in the eluate from an anti-GRF immunoaffinity column was used as the starting material. Corticotropin-releasing factor-like immunoreactivity (CRF) was monitored using a radioimmunoassay against ovine CRF developed with antisera raised against [Tyr^{21}]oCRF(21-41). The sample was pumped directly onto an anti-ovine CRF(21-41) immunoaffinity column prepared by coupling purified IgG to Affi-gel 10. Immunoreactive CRF was recovered in the acid eluate of the immunoaffinity column and purified to homogeneity by gel permeation chromatography and two steps of reverse phase HPLC (yield: 8nmoles). Amino acid analysis shows that the peptide contains 41 amino acids and is similar in composition but not identical to the known CRF's of other species. Complete structural characterization is in progress.

Research supported by grants from NIH (AM-18811 and HD-09690) and a grant from the Robert J and Helen C Kleberg Foundation.

137 LH RELEASE BY SUPERFUSED RAT PITUITARY CELLS IN RESPONSE TO THE SUPER-AGONIST (Des-gly^{10})-[D-trp^{6}, pro^{9}-ethylamide]-GnRH. C.J. Baird*and L. Tamarkin, DEB, NICHD, NIH, Bethesda, MD 20205, USA.

LH release stimulated by (Des-gly^{10})-[D-trp^{6}, pro^{9}-ethylamide]-GnRH agonist (GnRH-a) and by native GnRH (n-GnRH) was studied in dispersed, anterior pituitary cells from pubertal (30 day old), female rats. Cells were cultured on Cytodex I, loaded onto columns, and perfused (0.5 ml/min) at 37°C. LH release was dose-related for both GnRH's given as 6 min pulses. The linear response range was $10^{-10.5}$M - 10^{-9}M for GnRH-a and 10^{-10}M - 10^{-7}M for n-GnRH. Return to baseline after each LH peak was slower for GnRH-a than n-GnRH (30 vs 15 min). Desensitization of pituitary cells was induced by continuous exposure to 10^{-9}M GnRH-a and 10^{-8}M n-GnRH. Cells desensitized by n-GnRH rapidly responded to 6 min pulses of 10^{-6}M n-GnRH, but GnRH-a desensitized cells were unresponsive to 10^{-7}M GnRH-a. If cells desensitized by 10^{-9}M GnRH-a were given 10^{-6}M n-GnRH pulses, there was no response initially, but within 60 min, responsiveness returned. When pituitary cells were desensitized by lower GnRH-a doses (10^{-11}M or $10^{-10.5}$M), LH release was stimulated by high doses of GnRH-a, but only a single, initial LH response occurred despite repeated stimulation, whereas multiple pulses of n-GnRH resulted in multiple responses. These differences in LH release by superfused pituitary cells in response to GnRH-a and n-GnRH show that these GnRH's act on gonadotrophs differently. It is suggested that these differences may occur at the receptor level.

138 COPPER: A POTENT RELEASER OF LHRH FROM RAT MEDIAN EMINENCE (ME) EXPLANTS. A. Barnea*, M. Colombani-Vidal, Dept Ob/Gyn, Physiol, Green Cntr for Reprod Biol Sci, Univ of Tx Hlth Sci Cntr, Dallas, Tx 75235.

Copper, administered to female rabbits, is known to stimulate LHRH release into the hypophysial portal blood. We have shown that one site of action of copper is the LHRH secretory granule. Since copper is present in the circulation in a chelated form and since histidine (His) is known to facilitate copper uptake by tissues, we wished to ascertain if CuHis stimulates LHRH release from hypothalamic neurons. ME explants were incubated in a buffered medium (medium was changed every 15 min) and LHRH release into the medium was quantified by RIA. When ME were incubated with 50 μM CuHis for 15 min and then without CuHis for an additional period of 75 min, LHRH release was (pg/ME/15 min):

Time (min)	0	15	30	45	60	75	90
Control	3.0	2.4	2.4	2.2	2.8	2.6	2.8
CuHis	2.6	7.8	12.8	9.8	7.0	5.8	5.0

Thus, CuHis markedly stimulated the rate of LHRH release; maximal rate attained 30 min after initiation of the exposure to CuHis. When ME were exposed to a second 15-stimulus by CuHis (between 90 and 105 min), LHRH release was again stimulated and the temporal pattern of this release was similar to that noted after the first exposure to CuHis. In contrast to CuHis, $CuCl_2$ did not stimulate LHRH release. Thus, Cu, complexed by a putative circulating chelator, markedly stimulates LHRH release from LHRH neurons. The temporal pattern of the stimulated release is suggestive that Cu, taken up by the LHRH neuron, leads to the release of LHRH from a definite releasable pool of the peptide.

139 RATIONAL DRUG DESIGN OF LONG-ACTING SOMATOSTATIN ANALOGUES

W. Bauer, U. Briner, W. Doepfner, R. Haller, R. Huguenin, P. Marbach*, T.J. Petcher, and J. Pless, Sandoz Ltd., Pharmaceutical Division, Preclinical Research, Basle, Switzerland.

SMS 201-995, a potent octapeptide analogue of somatostatin, exhibits a markedly prolonged action in vivo after s.c. application. To further improve this favourable pharmacodynamic profile, N^{α}-acylated derivatives with the common structure R-DPhe-Cys-Phe-DTrp-Lys-Thr-Cys-Thr-ol have systematically been synthesised.' Their potency in inhibiting growth hormone (GH) secretion was determined 1 and 6 hours after s.c. application in rats. The ratio of ED50's at 6 and 1, hours respectively, taken as a measure of the duration of action, varied from 0.2 to 480 depending on the lipophilicity of R. The in vitro activity was also dependent on R. The decanoyl derivative of SMS 201-995, Code No. 203-306, had the best combination of potency and duration of action, having ED50's of 10, 16 and 28 μg/kg one, 6 and 18 h after s.c. application, respectively. When the drug was infused for one hour and GH measured after this time, ED50 was 14 μg/kg/h. These data suggest that 203-306 is slowly released into the circulation from a subcutaneous depot. Measurement of circulating plasma levels of the drug by means of RIA support this hypothesis - the concentration remained constant for at least 2h after s.c. application of 100 μg/kg.

It has been demonstrated that N^{α}-acylation of SMS 201-995 with lipophilic substituents can lead to analogues with dramatically prolonged duration of action.

140 SIMULTANEOUS IDENTIFICATION OF CATECHOLAMINE NEURON IN THE RAT HYPOTHALAMUS BY FLUORESCENCE AND IMMUNO-ELECTRON MICROSCOPY.

K.Ajika*, H.Seto, K.Arai and S.Okinaga, Department of Obstetrics and Gynecology, Teikyo University School of Medicine, Itabashi-ku, Tokyo, Japan.

Aqueous solution containing 4% paraformaldehyde and 1% glutaraldehyde was used to simultaneously localize catecholamine neuron by the formation of fluorescent products and to fix hypothalamic tissue for electron microscopy. Pregnant rats were subjected to cardiac perfusion of the above mentioned solution. Hypothalamic sections of about 15μm thickness which were cut with vibratome were maintained in the fixative and observed under fluorescence microscope. Many fluorescent cell bodies were observed in the arcuate nucleus region. If vibratome sections were rapidly dried with hair drier, the intensity of the fluorescence was enhanced and the sections could be permanently mounted. The same areas were rephotographed with white illumination to locate non-fluorescent structures close to the fluorescent cells. The same section was then washed in buffer, osmified and processed for electron microscopy. The chosen cell was positively identified by its shape and relation to other structures, such as blood vessels, myelinated axons and axon bundles. In the cytoplasma rough endoplasmic reticulum (rER) was well developed and a few small dopamine vesicles were observed. In the immuno-electron microscopical experiment, the tissue section which had been observed under fluorescence microscope was washed and processed for immunostaining of catecholamine synthesizing enzyme, tyrosine hydroxylase (TH), according to Sternberger's PAP method. The rER, dopamine vesicles and Golgi apparatus in the precisely the same neuron which had been regarded as fluorescent were specifically stained with TH antiserum.

141 RADIOAUTOGRAPHIC EVIDENCE FOR EXTRAHYPOTHALAMIC EFFERENCES FROM THE SUPRAOPTIC NUCLEI IN THE RAT. G. Alonso, A. Szafarczyk and I. Assenmacher*, Lab. Neuroendocrinology, ERA 85-CNRS, University of Montpellier II, France.

Whereas recent studies have traced a number of extrahypothalamic pathways originating in the paraventricular nuclei, the supraoptic nuclei (SON) -which at the present stage appear to include essentially vasopressinergic and oxytocinergic neurons- are generally considered to project mainly into the neurohypophysis. The present study was designed to explore systematically the efferences from the SON with a radioautographic tracing method after local stereotaxic injections of ^{3}H-Leu or ^{3}H-Pro (10 μCi in 15 nl saline). In addition to the classical dense axonal bundle projecting down to the posterior pituitary, six extrahypothalamic axonal pathways were found to project into various brain areas. Two of them are directed rostrally and project respectively to the olfactory bulb and to the cortex via the rostral divisions of the cingulum. The other axonal pathways are directed caudally and project to 1) the medial nucleus of the amygdala via the stria medullaris, 2) the lateral habenula, 3) the subcommissural organ via the stria medullaris, and 4) the mammillary bodies. These data suggest that at least some of the vasopressinergic and oxytocinergic fibers which were previously described within some of these specific extrahypothalamic regions may originate from the SON. The possible functional implications of these specific neuronal pathways are discussed.

142 INDUCTION OF MENSTRUAL BLEEDING IN EXPLANTS OF HUMAN ENDOMETRIUM TRANSPLANTED TO THE HAMSTER CHEEK POUCH. M.H. Abel*, C. Zhu and D.T. Baird, Department of Obstetrics, University of Edinburgh, Scotland, U.K.

Explants of follicular and luteal phase human endometrium have been maintained in the immunologically privileged site of the hamster cheek pouch for periods of 14 days. Female Syrian hamsters were ovariectomised two weeks before transplantation and given silastic implants of oestradiol-17β and progesterone to produce plasma levels comparable with those found during the luteal phase of the human menstrual cycle. The grafts were visualized through a perspex window inserted in the cheek wall and observed microscopically in the anaesthetised animal by transillumination via a fibre optic cable inserted through the mouth. Vascularization of the explants began 3-4 days after transplantation and a vascular network was present by day 5. Growth of the explants coincided with the appearance of a vascular network and was maximal on day 7. Withdrawal of progesterone and oestradiol-17β on day 11 induced bleeding within the endometrial explants in six out of six animals. Mean time to onset of bleeding = 60±8.9h. Withdrawal of progesterone alone resulted in bleeding in 9 out of 15 animals (60%), in 64.6±5.5h. Bleeding was not seen after withdrawal of oestradiol-17β alone and bleeding was never observed from the cheek pouch vessels. No change was seen within the explants during the first 24h after steroid withdrawal. Thereafter the explants became red in colour due to dilatation of vessels within the graft. Blood flow in these vessels was reduced and was followed by blurring of the vessel walls due to escape of red cells. As this increased distinct areas of bleeding could be identified. Thus this model allows direct observation of the vascular changes during menstruation.

143 SECRETORY PATTERNS OF RHESUS MONKEY PREGNANCY SPECIFIC BETA-1-GLYCOPROTEIN (rSP-1) THROUGHOUT PREGNANCY. G.D. Braunstein* and R.H. Asch, Departments of Medicine, Cedars-Sinai Medical Center, UCLA School of Medicine, Los Angeles, CA, 90048 and Department of Obstetrics and Gynecology, The University of Texas Health Science Center, San Antonio, TX, 78284, USA.

Although rSP-1 has been detected in maternal blood during pregnancy in the rhesus monkey, no information is available concerning the maternal serum concentrations of rSP-1 throughout pregnancy, its half-life ($T\frac{1}{2}$) or secretory patterns in individual monkeys. We studied these parameters in 16 pregnant monkeys. rSP-1 was measured by a heterologous RIA (sensitivity 20 ng/ml) using an antiserum against rSP-1 and purified human SP-1 as a standard and for iodination. No rSP-1 was detected in sera from 8 normal males, 8 castrates, or during the normal menstrual cycles in 10 female monkeys. rSP-1 was detected in the maternal serum 23 days after conception and the concentrations rose rapidly until day 70 followed by a more gradual increase until term (mean = 1654 mcg/ml), a pattern similar to that found in the human. Secretory peaks of rSP-1 occurred at approximately 60 minute intervals when animals (n=3) were sampled every 10-20 minutes for 8 hours. Serial blood samples obtained at 2-4 day intervals demonstrated marked day-to-day variation in maternal serum rSP-1 concentrations. The $T\frac{1}{2}$ of rSP-1 following delivery averaged 49 hours (n=5). These data indicate that (1) rSP-1 is undetectable (<20 ng/ml) in sera from nonpregnant rhesus monkeys; (2) the pattern of rSP-1 secretion throughout pregnancy is qualitatively similar to that found for human SP-1; and (3) rSP-1 is secreted approximately hourly throughout the day. rSP-1 measurements may provide a useful index of placental function during rhesus pregnancy.

144 TESTOSTERONE PRECURSORS IN SPERMATIC VEIN OF VARICOCELE PATIENTS: AN EVIDENCE OF IMPAIRED TESTOSTERONE BIOSYNTHESIS. S. Ando*, C. Giacchetto, E. Beraldi, M.L. Panno and M. Maggiolini, Department of Cell Biology, University of Calabria, Arcavacata di Rende (CS), Italy.

In the present study we determined progesterone (P), 17-OH-progesterone (17-OH-P), Δ_4-androstenedione (Δ_4), dehydroepiandrosterone (DHEA) and testosterone (T) in spermatic venous blood of 34 varicocele patients (V) and in 12 normal subjects (N). We also used DHEA/Δ_4 ratio as an index of Δ_5/Δ_4 pathway ratio in T biosynthesis. The mean of T and Δ_4 in the spermatic blood of V appeared to be significantly lower with respect to that of N (T: N=1708.7± 223.8 (SEM) nmol/l, n°10; V=1190± 101.1 (SEM) nmol/l, n°29. $P<0.03$. Δ_4: N=56.4±5.6 (SEM) nmol/l, n°12; V=38.1±4 (SEM) nmol/l n°27. $0.02>P>0.01$). A negative correlation was observed between the individual age of V and 17-OH-P (n°34, y=30.66x+1300, r=0.57, $P<0.01$) and Δ_4 values (n°27, y=-1.981x+96.52, r=-0.67, $P<0.01$). When was evaluated the ratio of T precursors, we observed a positive correlation between P/17-OH-P ratio and age of V (n°33, y =0.00652x-0.091, r=0.45, $P<0.05$). The 17-OH-P/Δ_4 ratio was greatly increased with respect to that of N (N=5.12±0.93 (SEM), n°12; V=10.77±1.31 (SEM), n°27. $P<0.01$). These data suggests that the reduced T levels in spermatic venous blood of V was due to the enzymatic deficiency of 17-20 lyase firstly and secondly to that of 17α-hydroxylase activity as the patients grow relatively older. A negative correlation between DHEA/Δ_4 ratio and Δ_4/T ratio was observed in N (n°10, y=-0.00432x+0.0542, r=-0.67. $P<0.03$) as well as in V (n°27, y=-0.00399x+ 0.0587, r=-0.48. $0.02>P>0.01$). This indicates that in the testis of V the T remains prevalently supplied by the Δ_5 pathway of biosynthesis. This is confirmed by the positive correlation between DHEA and T spermatic levels despite the absence of such a relationship between T and Δ_4 in such patients.

145 GESTRINONE IN TREATMENT OF ENDOMETRIOSIS : LIFE-TABLE ANALYSIS OF FERTILITY AND RECURRENCE

G. Azadian-Boulanger*, M. Hucher, J.M. Husson.
Institut Roussel-Uclaf, Paris 75007 France

Gestrinone (R 2323) is an anti-gonadotropic compound which has been proposed recently for the treatment of endometriosis. We report here the results on fertility and recurrence for 250 female patients with endometriosis, as demonstrated by laparoscopy, coming from three different centers. Patients received 2.5 mg of gestrinone two or three times a week. The mean duration of therapy was 6.5 months and the mean duration of follow-up after treatment was 10.5 months. Data were analyzed by life-table methods to take into account the variability in the duration of follow-up. In sterile patients, the actuarial fertility rate was 50.3 % at 12 months ; three patients characteristics were shown to influence significantly the fertility rate : age, duration of infertility and presence of a sterility factor other than endometriosis. The actuarial recurrence rate was 24.3 % at 12 months ; four factors were predictive of recurrence : age, duration of endometriosis, cure of macroscopic lesions, as assessed by a post-treatment laparoscopy, occurrence of a pregnancy. Three conclusions can be drawn from this study : 1) gestrinone compares favourably with the best existing therapies of endometriosis (surgery and danazol), 2) life-table analysis is needed to compare fertility and recurrence rates reported by different centers, 3) predictive factors must be taken into account in the evaluation of a therapy for infertility.

146 ADMINISTRATION OF "PURE FSH" TO INDUCE FOLLICULAR MATURATION IN WOMEN WITH POLYCYSTIC-OVARY-SYNDROME (PCO-S) AND LONG-STANDING INFERTILITY.

M.H. Birkhäuser and P. Huber*, Div. of Endocrinology, Universitäts-Frauenklinik, Kantonsspital, 4031 Basel, Switzerland.

10 patients with PCO-S and long-standing primary infertility characterized by elevated basal serum LH values (LH : FSH > 2), elevated serum androgens and amenorrhea or chronic anovulation had been selected for stimulation of follicular growth by "pure FSH" (Metrodin Serono). During the first 3 days of treatment, 225 - 300 IU FSH/d was administered. From day 4 until a mature follicle was evidenced by sonography and serum estradiol values the daily dose was decreased to 150 - 225 IU FSH. Ovulation was induced by administration of 10'000 IU HCG. 3 pregnancies occured during the first, 1 during the second treatment cycle. 9 other treatment cycles in various patients resulted in normal follicular maturation and luteal phase. In an additional cycle luteinization without ovulation was observed. Hyperstimulation of grade I or II occured in 3 out of 14 cycles following HCG administration. In 3 cycles treatment had to be interrupted before induction of ovulation because of threatening hyperstimulation or the appearance of a benign cyst. No serious complications were observed. In conclusion, treatment by "pure FSH" of long-standing infertility due to PCO-S seems to be a promising and low-risk alternative to classical stimulatory methods.

147 EFFECTS OF A TRANSPLANTABLE INSULINOMA ON HOST INSULIN GENE EXPRESSION.
M. Appel*, E. Kislauskis and L. Villa-Komaroff, University of Massachusetts Medical School, Worcester, MA 01605, U.S.A.

Transplantation of an insulinoma to inbred NEDH rats results in progressively severe hyperinsulinemia and hypoglycemia. Endogenous pancreatic B-cells of tumor bearing animals evidence atrophy, secretory degranulation and impaired insulin secretion and a transient 2-3 day interval of insulinopenia and hyperglycemia occur after tumor ablation. Electron microscopic, autoradiographic and morphometric studies were performed to characterize the suppressed pancreatic islets, B-cell replication and islet cell changes that follow tumor removal. In addition, the concentration of pancreatic proinsulin mRNA was measured to determine the effects of the tumor on insulin gene expression. With the tumor in-situ, suppressed islets contain reduced B-cell numbers (B-cells 33%, non-B-cells 67%, n=5) compared to controls (B-cells 74%, non-B-cells 26%, n=5) which fail to incorporate ^{3}H-thymidine and are functionally inactive. Autoradiographs obtained by filter hybridization to a cloned rat proinsulin I cDNA probe revealed undetectable proinsulin mRNA levels at this time. Profoundly increased proinsulin mRNA concentrations observed at 2 days following tumor resection preceded the initiation of B-cell replication and insulin biosynthesis. Restoration of B-cell number, morphology and function was achieved at 5 days. These data suggest that the tumor produces morphological and functional suppression of host pancreatic B-cells which is reversed by tumor removal. Since accumulation of proinsulin mRNA preceded the accumulation of insulin, it is likely that insulin synthesis is modulated by transcription of the insulin gene.

148 IS THE USE OF THE LOWEST POSSIBLE IMMUNOGENICITY INSULIN RATHER THAN PARTIALLY PURIFIED MORE IMMUNOGENIC INSULIN OF CLINICAL RELEVANCE IN CHILDREN WITH DIABETES? C.M. Asplin*, J.P. Palmer, P.K. Raghu, P. Clemons, K. Lyen, O. Tatti, and B.McKnight, Universities of Cinncinnati, Pennsylvania, Kansas, and Washington, U.S.A.

To determine if any clinical benefit accrues from the use of high purity insulin (HP1) (which is of the lowest possible immunogenicity) rather than partially purified (PP1) insulin (which is much more immunogenic) in childhood onset insulin dependent diabetics (IDDs). 112 children with newly diagnosed IDD were randomly assigned to insulin therapy. HP1, or PP1, twice daily, regular and isophane were used. Follow-up occurred at 1,2,4, 6,9, and 12 months. Insulin binding antibody (IBA) formation (specific % binding of tracer), fasting blood glucose, C-peptide, and glycosylated hemoglobin, insulin dose, skin reactions, nocturia, and growth of the IDDs were recorded. IBA formation which reached a plateau at 2 months, the mean % binding in the PP1 group being 38% nearly thrice that in the HP1 group (14%), the respective 12 month values being 36% and 15%. Skin reactions, (redness and/or irratation, hives and fat hypertrophy) were virtually all confined to the PP1 group. However, C-peptide insulin dosage, glycosylated hemoglobin, fasting blood glucose, growth, and nocturia were similar for HP1 and PP1 treated IDDs. Thus, the use of HP1 rather than PP1 is essential to minimize IBA formation and local skin reactions but no other clinical benefit such as diabetes regulation (as judged by growth, nocturia fasting glucose and glycosylated hemoglobin), insulin dosage or the preservation of endogenous insulin accrues from the use of HP1 rather than PP1 in the first year of treatment of the childhood IDD.

149 NEUROTENSIN STIMULATION OF INSULIN SECRETION IN GENETICALLY OBESE-DIABETIC MICE. C.J. Bailey*, P.R. Flatt, M.C. Sheppard and S.K. Swanston-Flatt. Department of Biological Sciences, University of Aston, Birmingham, UK, Division of Nutrition and Food Science, Department of Biochemistry, University of Surrey, Guildford, UK, and Department of Medicine, Queen Elizabeth Hospital, Birmingham, UK.

Neurotensin, a tridecapeptide found in brain, intestine, pancreas and plasma, has recently been ascribed a function in the control of the endocrine pancreas. To investigate possible abnormalities of neurotensin which might contribute to the hyperinsulinaemia of genetically obese-diabetic mice, we examined tissue and plasma immunoreactive neurotensin concentrations and insulin responses to exogenous neurotensin in Aston obese hyperglycaemic (ob/ob) mice and C57BL/KsJ diabetic (db/db) mice at 16-20 weeks of age. The obese-diabetic mutants showed normal concentrations of neurotensin in brain and plasma, but the amounts of intestinal neurotensin were doubled. Pancreatic neurotensin was also doubled in ob/ob mice which show very severe hyperinsulinaemia, but pancreatic neurotensin was normal in db/db mice which show only moderately raised insulin concentrations. Intraperitoneal injection of neurotensin (500 µg/kg) in 24h fasted ob/ob mice caused a rapid elevation of plasma insulin, approximately 2-fold after 5 min and 3-fold after 15 min, returning to pretest values by 60 min. Injection of neurotensin with glucose produced a smaller insulin response which only marginally exceeded the small insulin response to intraperitoneal glucose alone. The results demonstrate a marked but transient insulin response to neurotensin under conditions of basal hyperglycaemia which was suppressed at very high glucose concentrations in ob/ob mice.

150 EFFECTS OF STRICT GLYCEMIC CONTROL AND AUTONOMIC NERVE FUNCTION ON GLUCAGON RESPONSE TO INSULIN-INDUCED HYPOGLYCEMIA IN DIABETES MELLITUS. K.BANDO*, Y.GORIYA, M.KATSURA, R.KAWAMORI, M.SHICHIRI and H.ABE, First Department of Medicine, Osaka University Medical School, Osaka, Japan.

In order to elucidate the mechanism of A-cell dysfunction during hypoglycemia in diabetes mellitus, effects of strict glycemic control and autonomic nerve function were investigated. Subjects examined included 15 insulin-dependent diabetes mellitus (IDDM), 19 noninsulin-dependent diabetes mellitus (NIDDM), 1 Shy-Drager syndrome and 7 healthy controls. In diabetics, Actrapid insulin in amount of 0.1 U/kg was infused bolusly before and after 3-month strict glycemic control by continuous subcutaneous insulin infusion and multiple insulin injections. Autonomic nerve function was checked by measuring coefficient of variation (CV) of 100 R-R intervals on ECG. Although any significant glucagon responses were found in neither IDDM nor NIDDM before the strict glycemic control, glucagon responses improved significantly after the control in both IDDM and NIDDM who had intact autonomic nerve function. In the diabetics whose CVs were below 2.5 %, however, the rise in glucagon could not be recognized despite hypoglycemic stimulations identical to healthy subjects were obtained. A case of Shy-Drager syndrome who had marked autonomic nerve disturbance and normal glucose tolerance showed no remarkable glucagon response to hypoglycemia. From these observations, it was concluded that blunted glucagon response to hypoglycemia in diabetics is secondary to insulin lack and that autonomic nerve function is essential to raise glucagon in response to hypoglycemia.

151 SITE AND MECHANISM OF INSULIN DEGRADATION BY ERYTHROCYTES.
D.D. Bansal*, S. Kashyap and S. Sharma. Department of Biochemistry, Panjab University, Chandigarh - 160014, India.

The presence of highly specific insulin receptors on erythrocytes has been demonstrated earlier. However, erythrocyte hemolysates have been shown to degrade insulin. The present studies were carried out on normal and alloxan diabetic monkeys and normal, diabetic(NIDDM) human subjects to find out the site and mechanism of insulin degradation by erythrocytes. Blood was withdrawn after an overnight fast. Erythrocytes were separated, washed twice in 1 % NaCl in 30 mM tris HCl (pH 7.4). Hemolysates were prepared using a hypotonic buffer (10 mM tris HCl, pH 8.0). RBC ghosts were prepared by centrifugation at 12000 x g for 40 min. at 2-4° C. A portion of the supernatant (SI) was preserved. Three subsequent washings were given which resulted in the formation of ghosts. Insulin degradation was carried out using RBCs, hemolysates, RBC ghosts and SI. Both the normal and diabetic erythrocytes were found to bind insulin. Only hemolysates and SI degraded insulin. Insulin degradation by normal erythrocytes was significantly more than diabetic erythrocytes. N-ethylmaleimide inhibited the degradation of insulin significantly. Reduced glutathione content of normal erythrocytes was significantly more than diabetic erythrocytes. It is concluded that insulin is degraded by the erythrocyte cytosol fraction and SH groups play a role in this process.

152 ALTERATIONS IN THE DISTRIBUTION OF COLLAGEN TYPE IV IN GLOMERULAR BASAL LAMINAE OF STREPTOZOTOCIN-DIABETIC RATS AS REVEALED BY IMMUNOCYTOCHEMISTRY
M. Bendayan* and H. Stephens. Departement of Anatomy, Université de Montréal, Montréal, Québec Canada.

Collagen type IV antigenic sites were revealed in the basal laminae of renal structures in normal and streptozotocin-induced diabetic rats applying the protein A-gold immunocytochemical technique with specific antibodies. In normal rat kidney, the labeling by gold particles was found to be preferentially located over the central lamina densa of the basal laminae of the renal tubules and Bowman's capsule as well as over that of the glomeruli. Chronic hyperglycemia was induced in rats by intravenous injection of streptozotocin. The animals were studied at 10, 12 and 15 months after induction of the hyperglycemic state. Basal laminae, particularly that of Bowman's capsule and glomeruli were thickened. When collagen type IV was revealed, the labeling was found to be present over the entire thickened width of the epithelial basal laminae. However, in contrast to the normal distribution, the labeling present over the thickened glomerular basal laminae was preferentially located on the subendothelial side of the laminae. Thus, glomerular basal laminae deposits occurring in hyperglycemic states, seem to be antigenically different from collagen type IV and/or the distribution and proportions of this component are markedly altered. These results demonstrate that, in addition to the morphological, biochemical and functional alterations already established for the glomerular basal laminae in diabetic microangiopathy, modifications of the collagen type IV component occur during hyperglycemia.
This study was supported by the MRC and the Canadian Diabetes Association.

153 ANALYSIS OF ANTISULIN ANTIBODIES (A-I Ab) IN A CASE OF EXTREME INSULIN RESISTANCE. A.S. Brown,* G. Antony, S. Cooper, N. Gürtunca and A.W. Steinbeck, Department of Endocrinology & Department of Paediatrics, The Prince of Wales Hospital, Sydney, Australia.

In a 19 year old diabetic female, only centrally administered insulin provided adequate metabolic control. All other routes of administration resulted in high insulin requirements, low circulating free insulin and elevated blood glucose levels. Other known methods having failed, we used plasma exchange (PE) to treat the insulin resistance. This treatment restored metabolic control. Since A-I Ab were found in the plasma, we investigated them as a possible cause of the resistance. Between weekly PE, the insulin requirements rose. A-I Ab, which fell by 50% post PE, also rose between exchanges and correlated directly with insulin dose. A-I Ab were identified as immunoglobulin G (IgG). Electrophoretic studies of the patient's plasma after overnight incubation with ^{125}I-insulin, showed 80% of the bound radioactivity localised in the IgG region, the remainder was found in the $\alpha 2$ microglobulin band. Deinsulinised pre- and post- PE samples were compared by Scatchard analyses and produced curvilinear plots. The A-I Ab were predominantly low affinity (up to 10^5l/mole) and high capacity (approx. 10^6moles/ml). Post PE samples showed a 50% reduction in initial binding (Bo) but the affinity was unchanged in these samples compared to the pre PE samples. The decrease in Bo reflected a reduction in the total number of binding sites. We conclude that these A-I Ab, with such low affinity, cannot alone account for the extreme insulin resistance observed. We suspect a defect in insulin absorption may be contributory.

154 BRAINSTEM AUDITORY EVOKED RESPONSES (BAER) IN EXPERIMENTAL DIABETES MELLITUS. N. Buller*, Z. Shwahny, N. Laurian and L. Laurian, Endocrinological Department, Ichilov Medical Center, Tel Aviv University Medical School; Experimental Surgery Laboratory, B. Gattegno Research Institute, and Institute of Audiology, Hasharon Hospital, Petah-Tiqva, Israel.

Brainstem auditory evoked responses (BAER) examination is a sensitive and accurate method to detect any disturbances in the transmission of the auditive stimulus in the brainstem. The prolongation of latencies of BAER's waves is evidence of a central conduction delay at the corresponding level of the brainstem. We study the possibility to use BAER in the detection of central diabetic neuropathy. 80 adults albino rats turned diabetic by intravenous administration of alloxan monohydrate 40-50 mg/kg after 48 h of starvation were studied. BAER was performed before the injection, 3 days later and at weekly intervals afterward. Peak latencies of the 3 most important waves (I,III,V) were compared with the values obtained before alloxan administration. The average latencies of all waves were significantly altered in the diabetic rats. No alterations in brainstem response were seen in non-diabetic rats. The percentage of BAER disturbances was 48% for the rats with mild diabetes (Gl. 150-300 mg%) and 82% in those with severe diabetes (gl. 300-700 mg%). The duration of diabetic state showed no significant relation to BAER. On the other hand, the alterations of BAER were more frequent in the rats with unbalanced and severe hyperglycemia. From the above results it appears that BAER can be utilised for the detection of subclinical central diabetic neuropathy.

155 GASTRIC ACID OUTPUT AND PANCREATIC POLYPEPTIDE (PP) SECRETION IN RESPONSE TO SHAM FEEDING IN DIABETIC AUTONOMIC NEUROPATHY (AN).
M. Buysschaert*, J. Donckier, A. Dive, J.-M. Ketelslegers and A.E. Lambert, Unité de Diabète et Nutrition, University of Louvain, B-1200, Brussels, Belgium.

In order to assess the relationship between cardiac and extra-cardiac dysfunction in diabetic AN, the gastric acid output and PP secretion in response to sham feeding were evaluated in three groups of age matched subjects; group I: normal controls (n=7); II and III: diabetics without (n=7) and with (n=9) cardiac AN (CAN). All patients assigned to the group with CAN exhibited an impaired beat to beat heart rate variation during deep breathing. The basal gastric acid output was equivalent in the 3 groups (I: 3.0 ± 1.2; II: 2.8 ± 1.5; III: 1.3 ± 0.5 mmol/hr; mean ± SEM). In contrast, the gastric acid output stimulated by sham feeding (chewing a mixed meal without swallowing the food for 30 min. followed by a 30 min. rest) was significantly lower in patients with CAN than in controls ($P<0.05$) or in diabetics without CAN ($P<0.01$)(group I: 10.3 ± 2.0; II: 15.0 ± 3.5; III: 5.2 ± 1.3 mmol/hr). In contrast, the maximal gastric acid secretion capacity, determined after pentagastrin, was similar in all patients. Mean basal PP concentrations were not different in the 3 groups (I: 122 ± 21; II: 131 ± 29; III: 185 ± 53 pmol/ml). In the controls and diabetics without CAN a significant mean 60% increase of the PP levels above basal values was observed during sham feeding. In contrast, no significant PP response occurred in the group with CAN. These data suggest that diabetic CAN is associated with dysfunctions of the vagal pathways controlling the gastric acid output and the PP secretion.

156 HORMONAL FACTORS ASSOCIATED WITH RECOVERY OF SYRIAN HAMSTERS FROM CHEMICALLY-INDUCED DIABETES MELLITUS.
G.T. Campbell* and S. Clawson, Dept. Physiol. and Biophys., Univ. Neb. Coll. Med., Omaha, NE 68105, USA

We measured serum glucose, glucagon, and insulin levels and examined immunostained alpha (α) and beta (β) cells in male hamsters given streptozotocin (SZ:40mg/kg BW;IP) for 3 days. Glucosuria was used as an indicator of altered β cell function. Animals were killed 60 and 120 days after the injections. Values in vehicle-treated animals (n=5) at 60 days were: glucose (104±7mg/dl); insulin (39±2μU/ml) and at 120 days (n=5) were: glucose (100±5mg/dl); insulin (49±5μU/ml); glucagon (108±10pg/ml). In islets of control animals, α cells were located at the periphery and β cells in the center. All SZ-treated animals (n=20) displayed glucosuria for at least 45 days. Five animals killed 60 days after the SZ had persistent glucosuria, hyperglycemia (glucose 483±25mg/dl); insulinopenia (21±3μU/ml). Islets in these animals were disordered with only a few β cells; numerous α cells were scattered throughout the islets. Another 5 animals (with intermittent glucosuria between 45-60 days) killed at 60 days were normoglycemic and insulinopenic. Islet morphology appeared normal in these animals. Four animals (with persistent glucosuria) killed at 120 days had: glucose (458±31mg/dl); insulin (21±1μU/ml); glucagon (258±64pg/ml). Pancreatic β cells were scarce. Six animals (with intermittent glucosuria) killed at 120 days had normal circulating levels of glucose, insulin and glucagon and islet morphology. Thus, this model may be amenable for studying factors responsible for the "recovery" of hamsters from chemically-induced diabetes mellitus which is associated with return of β cell function. AM 19170

157 TOLAZAMIDE (T) AND GLYBURIDE (G) BUT NOT CIGLYTAZONE (C) ENHANCE INSULIN ACTION IN THE LIVER. J.F. Caro,* O. Ittoop and M.K. Sinha, Department of Medicine, Endocrinology and Metabolism, East Carolina University School of Medicine, Greenville, North Carolina 27834.

We have studied the effect(s) of T (first generation sulfonylurea), G (second generation sulfonylurea), and C (non-sulfonylurea antidiabetic agent) on insulin action in rat hepatocytes cultured in serum-free medium. The cells were incubated for 20 hrs in the presence and absence of the drugs (1-100μg/ml) and insulin ($1x10^{-9}$M-$1x10^{-7}$M) to study ^{14}C acetate or $^{3}H_2O$ incorporation into total lipids. T and G were more effective at the lowest concentration (1μg/ml). At this concentration T and G alone stimulated lipid synthesis 22% and 17%, respectively, above control. Maximal insulin responsiveness in the control was 40% above basal, but when the cells were incubated with T or G, the insulin responsiveness increased by 95% and 60% respectively without any change in ED_{50}. C did not significantly affect either basal or insulin stimulated lipid synthesis. However, since C has been shown to be effective only in insulin resistant animals, we induced an in vitro insulin resistant state by incubating the hepatocytes with 1/100 dilutions of uremic serum. Under these conditions C was also ineffective. None of the three drugs altered ^{125}I-insulin binding or receptor structure as determined by SDS-PAGE of ^{125}I-insulin receptor complex cross-linked with DSS. We conclude that T and G enhance insulin responsiveness in the liver at a post receptor level. C is ineffective in the liver. Thus it is likely that C's site of action is at other tissue sites.

158 CIRCULATING ANTIBODIES AGAINST PANCREATIC ISLET CELL IN BRAZILIAN DIABETIC PATIENTS. A.R.Chacra*,S.A.Dib, E.M.K.Russo and B.Dean. Escola Paulista de Medicina,Sao Paulo,Brazil and Middlesex Hospital Med.School, London, UK.

Pancreatic islet cell antibodies (ICA) were first detected in sera of patients with insulin-dependent diabetes mellitus (IDDM) associated with autoimmune polyendocrinopathies. Later,ICA were also detected in sera of diabetics without autoimmune disease. Most of these studies were performed in North American and European populations,with but a few reports in populations of South America. Studies in different geographyc areas and different ethnyc backgrounds may give insight into the pathogenesis of the disease. With this aim we determined the incidence and prevalence of ICA,antibodies to: thyroglobulin (Thg), thyroid microssomes (TMc), gastric parietal cytoplasma (GPC) and adrenal cortex (AC) in blood samples of 112 Brazilian diabetic patients (68 IDDM, 39 IIDM, 5 with diabetes secondary to chronic pancreatitis (PDM) and 19 non-diabetic controls (C). Sera were tested for ICA, GPC and AC by an indirect immunofluorescence technique and for Thg and TMc by haemaglutination. Results below are % of positivity :

	ICA	GPC	Thg	TMc	AC
IDDM	48.5	7.3	7.3	10.2	4.4
IIDM	17.0	12.8	2.0	0	0
PDM	0	0	0	0	0
C	10.0	0	0	0	0

According to the duration of IDDM the prevalence of ICA was: 70.8% within the first year of diagnosis, 44.7% after 1-3yr, 33.3%, after 3-12yr and 28.5% over 12yr after diagnosis. This higher prevalence of ICA in IDDM was similar to that obtained in North-American and European populations providing evidence that IDDM in Brazil may have the same ethiologic pattern.

159 EFFECTS OF ESTROGEN ON PROLIFERATION OF SYNCHRONIZED MCF-7 MAMMARY TUMOR CELLS ARE DEPENDENT ON NEW RNA SYNTHESIS. S.C. Aitken, M.E. Lippman and D.R. Schoenberg*, Dept of Pharmacology, Uniformed Services University and Medical Breast Cancer Section, NCI, Bethesda, MD, USA.

MCF-7 mammary carcinoma cells synchronized by isoleucine (ILE) deprivation respond to ILE replenishment with increased thymidine (TdR) incorporation at 24h. Administration of 5 nM estradiol (E_2) with ILE causes a shift in this time course such that TdR incorporation begins after 14h and reaches a level twice that of the control. The increased TdR incorporation is preceded 6-8h by increased uridine (UdR) incorporation in both the E_2-treated and control cultures. UdR incorporation in the E_2-treated cultures reached a level twice that of controls. To determine if the E_2-induced increase in TdR incorporation is dependent on new RNA and protein synthesis, synchronized cells were repleted with ILE ± E_2 in the presence of increasing concentrations of actinomycin D, α-amanitin and cycloheximide. At concentrations of actinomycin D that inhibit pre-ribosomal RNA synthesis there was no effect on the E_2 stimulated TdR incorporation. Greater levels inhibited this in a dose-dependent manner. Alpha-amanitin caused a 75% inhibition of TdR incortion at a concentration of 1 µg/ml. With both antibiotics the inhibition of TdR incorporation was reflected by a parallel inhibition of UdR incorporation. Thus the proliferative response to E_2 is dependent on mRNA, but not rRNA transcription. The inhibition of protein synthesis by cycloheximide blocked the stimulation of TdR incorporation. Experiments are underway to determine the effects of E_2 ± ILE reversal on the transcription of dihydrofolate reductase mRNA as a marker for the enzymes of DNA synthesis.

160 PROSTAGLANDIN-INDUCED LUTEOLYSIS LINKED TO INHIBITION OF CALCIUM PUMP ACTIVITY. P.J. Albert*, S.L. Preston and H.R. Behrman, Reproductive Biology Section, Departments of Ob/Gyn and Pharmacology, Yale University School of Medicine, New Haven, CT 06510.

We have previously shown that $PGF_{2\alpha}$-induced luteolysis occurs by an uncoupling of the LH receptor complex in intact luteal cells. This action of $PGF_{2\alpha}$ is mimicked by agents which increase Ca_{in} (eg. A23187). Ca, but not $PGF_{2\alpha}$, inhibits activation of adenylate cyclase by LH in membranes. The anti-LH action of $PGF_{2\alpha}$ is not dependent on Ca_{ex} and Ca channel blockers have no effect on the response of luteal cells to $PGF_{2\alpha}$. The objective of the present studies was to evaluate if $PGF_{2\alpha}$ may increase Ca_{in} by inhibition of calcium extrusion which is regulated by a high affinity Ca^{2+} pump. A high affinity Ca-ATPase was characterized in "heavy" and in "light" rat luteal plasma membranes with $K_{1/2}$ of about 0.8 nd 0.35 µM, respectively. A lower affinity calcium activated ATPase was also evident in the same fractions ($K_{1/2} = \sim 15 \mu M$). Treatment of rats (7 day old corpora lutea) with 400 µg $PGF_{2\alpha}$ (sc) resulted in an almost complete loss of high affinity Ca-ATPase activity after 1 and 2 hr of treatment. Low affinity Ca-ATPase was also reduced by about 50%. In membranes isolated from luteal cells incubated with $PGF_{2\alpha}$ (2 µM), high affinity Ca-ATPase activity was reduced by about 50% within 15 min of $PGF_{2\alpha}$ treatment; a similar level of inhibition was also evident after 30 and 120 min of treatment. We suggest that an acute response of the luteal cell to luteolytic hormones may be an increase in intracellular calcium which occurs by inhibition of a high affinity, membrane bound, calcium extrusion pump. (Supported by NIH grants HD 15403 and HD 10718).

161 BLOCKING OF ION TRANSPORT AND LYSOSOMAL FUNCTION PREVENTS RECEPTOR-MEDIATED ENDOCYTOSIS AND DEGRADATION OF hCG IN RAT GRANULOSA CELLS.
A. Amsterdam*, A. Azrad, D. Malkin, N. Becker and U. Zor, Department of Hormone Research, The Weizmann Institute of Science, Rehovot 76100, Israel.

It has been demonstrated (Amsterdam et al., 1979, Am.J.Physiol. 5, E129) that receptor bound ^{125}I-hCG is internalized and degraded within lysosomes $t_{1/2}$ = 6-8 h). In order to examine the role of ion transport and lysosomal function in this process we preincubated granulosa cell cultures with 25 μM monensin (MON), or 1 mg/ml leupeptin (LEU) for 1 h at 37°C and thereafter cultures were incubated with ^{125}I-hCG, washed (x3) with hormone free medium and then incubated with the appropriate drug for up to 10 h. Cells were tested for binding capacity of ^{125}I-hCG and localization of the radiolabeled hormone by high resolution autoradiography. The extent of hormone degradation was assessed by release of TCA soluble radioactive material from incubated cells. None of the drugs applied to the cultures changed the amount of initial binding of ^{125}I-hCG to cells. However, MON and LEU reduced the liberation of TCA soluble material from cells by 50-90% compared to drug free cultures. Autoradiography revealed that labeled hormone was mainly trapped in lysosomes in the presence of LEU, while after treatment with MON most of the hormone still remained on the plasma membrane even after the 10 h incubation. MON also induced formation of large smooth-membrane vesicles within cells, probably derived from Golgi cisternae. It is concluded that interference with lysosomal function by LEU leads to accumulation of internalized but non-degraded hormone molecules within lysosomes. MON interferes mainly with receptor mediated endocytosis and transport of hormone molecules to lysosomes.

162 EFFECTS OF AMINOGLUTETHIMIDE IN NORMAL AND DESENSITIZED LEYDIG CELLS: D.R. Aquilano*, C-H Tsai-Morris and M.L.Dufau. NICHD, NIH, Bethesda, MD 20205.

To obtain sustained inhibitory effects of aminoglutethimide (AG) on testicular steroidogenesis we have optimized the use of this inhibitor *in vitro* and *in vivo* for the study of hCG-induced early and late steroidogenic lesions. AG inhibited Leydig cell (LC) steroidogenesis *in vitro* at a dose of 100 μg/ml. The minimal serum concentration of AG necessary for maximal inhibition of testosterone (T) *in vivo* was also 100 μg/ml (1 h after the i.p. administration of 20 mg AG). However, T levels were normal 5 hr later, coincident with a marked fall in the serum AG levels. The $t_{1/2}$ of AG in serum was 5 ± 0.7 h on the 1st day of treatment but was reduced to 3.0 ± 0.4 and 2.25 ± 0.35 h at 2 and 3 days of treatment. At the dose eliciting maximal and sustained side-chain cleavage (SCC) and aromatase inhibition (60 mg/d) AG was able to prevent the E_2-dependent late steroidogenic lesion induced by 1 μg hCG, with no effect on the steroid-independent early lesion caused by 10 μg hCG. The *in vivo* accumulation of cholesterol (C) in the inner mitochondrial membrane (IMM) induced by AG (by 50%) caused the LC to increase T and pregnenolone (P) production when subsequently incubated *in vitro*. The C content of the IMM was also increased in desensitized LC (by 52%); however, the conversion of C to P was substantially blocked in animals with the early lesion. Our findings explain the requirement of increasing high levels of AG to inhibit C metabolism, and provide a dose-schedule suitable for studies on C availability and inhibition of aromatase in the rat. These results also support the hypothesis that the early lesion in desensitized LC is due to inhibition of SCC activity rather than to a decrease in the amount of metabolically available C.

163 LECTIN-STAINING OF RAT EPIDIDYMIS AFTER CASTRATION. M. Arya* and T. Vanha-Perttula, Department of Anatomy, University of Kuopio, Kuopio, Finland.

Androgens maintain the epididymal secretory function responsible for induction of progressive motility and fertilizing capacity of spermatozoa.Seven lectins (ConA, SBA, DBA, UEA, PNA, RCA, WGA) labeled with rhodamine were used to stain glycoproteins in distal caput (cp) and proximal cauda (cd) of the rat 0, 2, 4 and 7 days after castration. In the control rat the surface of cp epithelium was strongly stained with WGA, moderately with ConA, DBA, RCA and PNA but not with SBA and UEA. Similarly, the intraluminal sperm mass (sm) had an even staining with the respective lectins. The acrosomes, however, were stained with SBA, DBA and UEA. A weak/moderate staining of the apical part of the principal cells (PC) was found with ConA,DBA, RCA and WGA, while the clear cells (CC) gave a staining with PNA, RCA and WGA. In cd the surface staining was stronger and sm staining weaker than in cp. The acrosome staining was equal but the CC differed only slightly from PC in their staining. After castration the surface staining in cp and cd initially (2-4 d) intensified with simultaneous fading of sm staining. CC rapidly lost their staining, while the apical part of PC gradually showed a stronger staining with all lectins. After 4 d the acrosomal staining diminished with occasional swelling of cells. This was accompanied by migration of macrophages around the tubules with increasing staining by all lectins. It is concluded that glycoproteins with terminal sialic acid (WGA), D-gal (RCA), D-galNAc (DBA) and D-gal-(1-3)-D-galNAc (PNA) groups are secreted mainly by PC and/or CC of cp and mixed with sm. During passage to cd, part of this material is absorbed and phagocytosed by PC. After castration this process is markedly increased and the phagocytic activity is enhanced by migration of macrophages which accumulate degradable glycoproteins.

164 PLASMA 3αANDROSTANEDIOL (3αAd): A MARKER OF PERIPHERAL ANDROGEN METABOLISM. R. BALDUCCI *,V.TOSCANO°,S. CAIOLA°,M.V. ADAMO°,M. DONARELLI °and B.BOSCHERINI ,Istituto di Clinica Pediatrica and°Istituto di V Clinica Medica,University of Rome,00100 Rome Italy.

3αAd is undoubtedly correlated to the androgenization of the subject.In fact,plasma levels are higher in man than in women,in young men than in elderly men and in hirsute females than in normal women.However,the mechanism with which this androgen exerts its action is not very clear. In fact 3αAd is not bound to cytosolic or nuclear androgen receptors,at least in vitro conditions.The aim of the present investigation was to better clarify the role of this androgen in the androgenization of the subject.The 3αAd plasma pattern was studied in basal conditions and after hCG,3500 I.U./m^2 B. S., in 2 cases of male pseudoermaphroditism with normal 5αreductase activity.17 hirsute women with isolated increase in plasma 3αAd were also studied in basal conditions and after 50mg/day for 14 days of Cyproterone Acetate(CPA).Results show a lack of increase of 3αAd after hCG,even if DHT increased similarly to the controls.In the hirsute females CPA treatment induces a significant increase of DHT/3αAd ratio,due to an isolated decrease in 3αAd plasma levels.No modifications of T/DHT ratio were observed before and after treatment. The lack of the increase of 3αAd plasma levels after hCG in male pseudoermaphroditism due to receptors deficiency and the isolated decrease of 3αAd after CPA in the hirsute females may be obviously correlated.It may be hypothesized on the basis of these data that a complete availability of the cellular receptors is necessary for the transformation of DHT into 3αAd.

165 ELECTRICAL EFFECTS OF ACTH AND VASOPRESSIN ON CULTURED GLOMERULOSA CELLS.
M. Benabderrazik*, N. Gallo-Payet and M.D. Payet, Dép. Médecine et Biophysique (Spon: D. Bellabarba), CHUS, J1H 5N4, Sherbrooke. It has been demonstrated that ACTH and Vasopressin triggered the secretion of mineralocorticoids in isolated glomerulosa cells (Payet et al., J. Physiol. Paris, 78, 317, 1982). Electrical events possibly involved in the excitation-secretion coupling were assessed by recording membrane potential in control and under hormones perfusion conditions. The glomerulosa cells cultures were obtained according to Payet et al., J. Steroid Biochem. 20, 1 (1984). The resting potential was recorded with microelectrode (60-80 MΩ) and ranged, in control conditions, between -20 to -45 mV. Once a stable potential is obtained, the hormone is apply in the medium through another electrode (1-2 MΩ) positionned near the cell under recording. Positive pressure allowed repetitive applications of small quantities of hormone. With a 10^{-7} M ACTH filled pipette, the first application induced a transient depolarisation of 4 mV and the following of 9, 16 and 16 mV respectively; the resting level decreased from -46 mV to -36 mV. As a function of time, the ACTH induced depolarisation increased rapidly and after the maximum, showed an exponential decrease. Several responses may be summed until saturation is obtained. Vasopressin (10^{-8} M) application gave basically the same results. These results indicate that a depolarisation of the membrane is involved in the excitation-secretion coupling for both ACTH and Vasopressin. The induced hormone depolarisation may be produced by a potassium channels closure or the opening of channels allowing an influx of cations (possibly Ca^{2+}). In the case of Vasopressin, recordings of single channel current by patch clamp show that K^+ channels closure hypothesis is more probable.
Supported by MRC, N. Gallo-Payet is MRC Scholar and M.D. Payet CHF Scholar.

166 THE UNSATURATED NON ESTERIFIED FATTY ACIDS (NEFAs) HIGHLY POTENTIALIZE THE ESTRADIOL BINDING TO HUMAN TISSULAR PROTEINS : TRUE ESTROGEN BINDING RECEPTOR OR ESTRADIOL METABOLITES ? Benassayag, C., Hassid, J.,* Vallette, G., Raymond, J.P.*, Nunez, E.A. - U. 224, INSERM - ERA 881, CNRS - Faculté de Médecine Xavier Bichat - Laboratoire de Biochimie 16, rue Henri Huchard - 75018 PARIS - * Hôpital Bichat Service d'Endocrinologie - 75018 PARIS.

We have demonstrated that, in human, the estradiol binding by healthy, neoplasic or fibromatous cytosoluble uterine proteins appears to be 2-5 fold enhanced by the presence of physiological concentration of unsaturated NEFAs (80 nmoles/mg cytosoluble proteins). The same studies conducted on healthy or cancerous breast tissues or on melanoma tissues show also a similar 7-10 fold increase.
The apparent potentialization of the estradiol binding to cytosoluble uterine proteins in presence of unsaturated NEFAs is due, in part, to an increase of the organosoluble compounds (2 fold) and especially to a dramatical formation of hydrosoluble metabolites (10 fold) when compared to the incubations without fatty acids. These hydrosoluble compounds are in part TCA precipitable and seem to be estradiol derivatives covalently linked to proteins i.e. "estroproteins". The non precipitable TCA molecules might be $^{3}H_2O$ or/and the result of covalent binding between small peptides and estradiol metabolites. The biological role of these "estroproteins" in the target tissues has to be elucidated. Furthermore the existence of such hydrosoluble metabolites could be spuriously interpretated as a true binding of the specific hormone to the cytosoluble receptor when the dextran coated charcoal method is used.

167 INTERACTION BETWEEN ADENOSINE AND FSH IN REGULATING ATP CONTENT IN RAT GRANULOSA CELLS. Håkan Billig*, Sten Rosberg and Kurt Ahrén, Department of Physiology, University of Göteborg, Sweden

It has been shown that adenosine can serve as modulator of hormonal response as well as ATP content in ovarian cells (Behrman et al, J Steroid Biochem 19,789,1983). In the present study the ATP metabolism was studied in isolated preovulatory rat granulosa cells from PMSG-treated rats.

Freshly isolated cells were incubated in Eagle's MEM in presence and absence of FSH (NIH S-13) and adenosine. ATP content was determined by the luciferine-luciferase method. In the absence of adenosine the ATP content was constant at least up to 90 min of incubation. In the presence of adenosine the ATP content increased linearly with time up to 90 min. In the presence of FSH and adenosine the rate of increase was less than half of that in the presence of adenosine alone. Adenosine (50 uM) increased the ATP content from 1.2 to 2.6 ng/1000 cells at 45 min. FSH depressed the ATP content 30-60% in a dose-dependent way, with maximal effect at 100 ng/ml. The decrease by FSH was evident both in control and adenosine treated cells.

We conclude that adenosine increases ATP content in rat granulosa cells analogously to luteal cells (Brennan et al, Endocrinology 112,499, 1983). However, in contrast to LH which did not alter the ATP content in luteal cells, FSH caused a profound decrease in granulosa cell ATP content. It is possible that adenosine serves as a modulator of hormonal response in granulosa cells and/or as an important factor to reestablish functional metabolism in isolated granulosa cells.

168 LYMPHOCYTE CHOLESTEROL SYNTHESIS (LCS) IN NEWLY DIAGNOSED INSULIN-DEPENDENT DIABETICS (IDD) BEFORE AND AFTER INSULIN THERAPY. S. Arslanian*, V. Warty, D. Becker, A. Drash, A. Sanghvi, Univ. of Pgh., School of Med., Dept. of Pediatrics, Children's Hospital of Pittsburgh, Pittsburgh, PA 15213, USA

LCS from C^{14} acetate was studied in freshly isolated lymphocytes in 12 newly diagnosed IDD before (Day 0) and 5 days after insulin therapy, and in 5 controls (C) who were nondiabetic siblings of IDD. An index LDL_{50} was calculated for each subject. This is the concentration of LDL cholesterol (µg/ml) in the medium necessary to reduce cholesterol synthesis to 50% of that in lipoprotein deficient serum (LPDS). The patients (8 females and 4 males) had ketonuria or ketonemia. The mean age at diagnosis was 9.6 yrs. (4.6-14.8 yrs). On the basis of LCS in LPDS, the patients could be segregated into 2 distinct groups: GI (n=7) and GII (n=5). Results were as follows: DAY 0: GI had normal maximum LCS in LPDS compared to C. GII had significantly higher maximum LCS compared to C and to GI (1580.4±241.9 pmoles/hr/mg vs 440.4±45.7, P=0.0005 vs 469.4± 170.2, P<0.0005). LDL_{50} was above 100 µg/ml in all 3 groups. DAY 5: Following insulin therapy, maximum LCS in GI was no different from Day 0; however, in GII, maximum LCS dropped significantly from that of Day 0 (530.8±520.9 vs 1580.4±241.9, P= 0.006) and was similar to C and GI. LDL_{50} was the same in the 3 groups and no different from Day 0. At Day 0, GI had a significantly higher HDL and glucose levels and lower B-OH butyrate than GII. Triglycerides, LDL, VLDL, insulin, C-Peptide, glucagon, bicarbonate, and PH were no different. These results indicate that nondiabetic siblings of IDD may have abnormal LDL metabolism, i.e. the nonsuppressibility of endogenous cholesterol synthesis by LDL. Abnormalities in LDL degradation and cellular cholesterol metabolism are present in IDD and can be corrected partly with insulin.

169 ANALYSIS OF LIPOPROTEIN ABNORMALITIES IN VENTROMEDIAL HYPOTHALANIC OBESITY IN RATS. M. Asami*, S. Inoue, T. Sugimasa, M. Egawa, S. Satoh, Y. Takamura, T. Murase, M. Okazaki and I. Hara. 3rd Dept. Int. Med., Yokohama City Univ., Yokohama, 3rd Dept. Int. Med., Univ. of Tokyo, Tokyo and Lab. of chemistry, Tokyo Medical and Dental Univ., Ichikawa, Japan.

Ventromedial hypothalamic (VMH) obese rats have hyperlipidemia. No report has yet been appeared which has analized lipoprotein abrormalities in VMH obese rats. The present study investigated the hyperlipidemia in VMH obese rats by analizing serum lipoproteins using the method of high performance liquid chromatography developed by Hara, Okazaki and Ohno (J. Biochem. 87 : 1863, 1980, J. Chromatogr. 221 : 257, 1980) Female Sprague-Dawley rats weighing about 200 g. were divided into two groups (N=9) : VMH lesioned and sham operated rats. Twelve weeks after operations, various parameters were determined. VMH lesioned rats revealed 1) remarkable weight gain (463 ± 19 g. vs 294 ± 7 g, controls), 2) elevated serum cholesterol, triglucerides and phospholipids, 3) hyperinsulinemia, 4) increased postheparin lipoprotein lipase activity, 5) increased triglyceride secretion rate and 6) elevated very low density lipoprotein (VLDL) and high density lipoprotein (HDL) in cholesterol analysis, and elevated chylomicron and VLDL in triglyceride analysis.

It was suggested that lipoprotein abnormalities in VMH obese rats depend on mainly hepatic overproduction probably due to hyperinsulinemia and partly hyperphagia.

170 INFLUENCE OF THE ROUTE OF ADMINISTRATION ON THE PROTEINEMIC, LIPEMIC AND HORMONAL RESPONSES TO 17β ESTRADIOL. A. Basdevant*, B. De Lignières, J. Conard, P.N. Guyenne, B. Guy-Grand, CHU Broussais-Hôtel-Dieu. 75181 Paris Cedex 04 France.

Alterations of hepatic functions are responsible for most of the metabolic side effects of oral estrogen therapy : ie hyperlipidemia, alteration of clotting factors, increased hepatic synthesis of Renin Substrate (RS) and other proteins. In this study we compared the hormonal and metabolic effects or oral (OE) versus percutaneous (PE) administration of 17βEstradiol (E2) to determine whether parenteral route which initially by passes the portal circulation would result in less impairment of hepatocyte functions. OE (2 mg/24 h) and PE (3 mg/24 h) were given during 6 weeks in 40 post menopausal women. Both regimen reduced FSH and increased E2 significantly to the same levels. OE was predominantly converted to Estrone (E1) resulting in low (0.3) E2/E1 ratio whereas PE led to normal E2/E1 premenopausal levels. OE resulted in significant increase in triglycerides (TG) very low density lipoproteins (VLDL)-TG, RS levels and decreases in Antithrombine III activity (ATIII) and low density lipoprotein (LDL)-CT as observed with oral synthetic estrogens. By contrast PE resulted in a significant decrease of TG and VLDL-TG, and no change in LDL-CT, RS and ATIII. The increase in high density lipoprotein-CT observed in both groups was not significant. These data indicate that parenteral route (i.e. percutaneous) : 1) may be used to provide estrogen replacement ; 2) reproduce the premenopausal physiologic E2 and E1 status more closely than oral therapy ; 3) as judged from the lipemic and proteinemic response caused less stimulation of hepatic metabolism ; 4) there fore, should be, prefered to oral route.

171 NON-SPECIFIC RESULTS OBTAINED WITH A MONOCLONAL ANTIBODY IN AN RIA FOR HCG. D T Carrick, J P Foster, K C Tovey, A J Brockas, *K Mashiter, Clinical Reagents Development, Amersham International plc, Amersham, Bucks, England.

An anti-Human Chorionic Gonadotrophin (HCG) monoclonal antibody raised against whole HCG was evaluated for use in an RIA in which 100μl of sample was incubated with 100μl of ^{125}I-HCG followed by a solid phase second antibody separation step. The antibody had an exceptionally high affinity constant of 7 x 10^{11} lit/mole and attained equilibrium following incubation at 37°C for 30 min. Assay sensitivity was 1mIU/ml. Antibody specificity was evaluated using pure luteinising hormone (LH) and 42 normal male and 108 postmenopausal female sera. LH cross-reactivity was less than 5% - adequate for the clinical need. However 2 of the male sera and 4 of the postmenopausal female sera gave elevated HCG values close to, or above, the normal pregnancy cut-off value of 25mIU/ml (range 18-108mIU/ml). These elevated values were not associated with any known clinical condition nor to non-specific sera related effects. The sera gave the expected values within the normal range (<10mIU/ml) when assayed using the Amersham Amerlex β-HCG RIA kit. These results serve as an important reminder that the specificity of a monoclonal antibody is directed against a single epitope which may also be found in other serum constituents. Great care must therefore be taken in the evaluation of monoclonal antibodies for use in single antibody immunoassays.

172 PRODUCTION AND CHARACTERIZATION OF MONOCLONAL ANTIBODY DIRECTED TOWARD RAT LIVER GLUTATHIONE-INSULIN TRANSHYDROGENASE. D.B. Dawson* and P.T. Varandani, Fels Research Institute and Biomedical Sciences Program, Wright State University, Yellow Springs, Ohio 45387, U.S.A.

Glutathione-insulin transhydrogenase (GIT) is an ubiquitous enzyme which cleaves insulin's disulfide bonds resulting in the formation of separate A and B chains. Purified rat liver GIT was used to immunize BALB/cByJ mice for the subsequent production of monoclonal antibodies (McAb's). Spleen cells removed from the immunized mice were fused to an established myeloma cell line in the presence of polyethylene glycol (M_r 1450). Of the 300 original hybridoma cultures, 8 were determined to be positive for GIT specific antibody production by the use of an enzyme (peroxidase) linked immunosorbent assay (ELISA). Of the 8 positive cultures, 7 have been cryogenically preserved. On the eighth positive culture, a limiting dilution was performed from which 10 positive monoclonal cultures were utilized for the production of ascites fluid. The McAb obtained was characterized as IgG, γ_1 isotype, with κ light chains. The McAb has been used to screen GIT separated from various rat tissue extracts following SDS/Urea polyacrylamide gel electrophoresis and electrophoretic transfer to nitrocellulose. All tissues showed an immunoreactive protein band corresponding to the purified GIT. Using constant amounts of enzyme activity for each tissue, the degree of immunoreactivity was: Liver, Fat > Kidney > Heart, Spleen > Testis > Skeletal muscle. An additional immunoreactive band of lower molecular weight was noted in the spleen tissue extract. This phenomenon of the occurrence of GIT in multiple immunoreactive forms is under further investigation. This work was supported in part by NIH Grant AM 24057.

173 SUPPRESSION OF BASAL LUTEINIZING HORMONE (LH) CONCENTRATION BY MELATONIN IN POST-MENOPAUSAL WOMEN. F. Aleem*, U. Weinberg, E. Weitzman, Montefiore Medical Center, Dept. of Gynecology and Neurology, Albert Einstein College of Medicine, Bronx, N.Y., New York Medical College, N.Y.

The large volume of literature implicating melatonin in the regulation of the hypothalamic pituitary-gonadol axis prompted our study to establish the possible role of melatonin in the regulation of this axis in menopause. The effect of a continuous IV infusion of melatonin (5-methoxy N-acetyl tryptamine) on plasma concentrations of LH in three post-menopausal women was studied. Melatonin was infused IV (125 mg/hr) for 48 hours. Prior to the melatonin infusion, 24 hour basal LH pattern was determined in each subject as a control. Pharmacological concentrations of serum melatonin was maintained throughout the infusion. The melatonin infusion induced a dramatic suppression of serum LH concentrations below baseline levels in all three women (LH suppresion precentages are: 58.03%, 57.74%, 54.66% respectively). This data indicates a possible modulatory rate of melatonin on the hypthalamic pituitary axis in menopause.

174 CHRONIC PARTIAL DOPAMINERGIC BLOCKADE IN NORMAL WOMEN - EFFECT ON PITUITARY HORMONE SECRETION. A. Nyboe Andersen*, C.Hagen and H. Djursing. Department of Internal Medicine and Endocrinology, Herlev University Hospital, 273o Herlev, Denmark.

Eight normal women were given the dopamine (DA) receptor blocker metoclopramide (MTC) orally 2.5 mg three times daily for 4 weeks. Prior to and after 4 weeks of drug administration, serial measurements of basal prolactin (PRL) luteinizing hormone (LH), follicle stimulating hormone (FSH) thyroid stimulating hormone (TSH) and growth hormone (GH) and the acute responses to lo mg of MTC i.v., was assessed in the early follicular phase. Chronic MTC administration significantly increased serum PRL ($p < o.o2$) and reduced basal levels of LH ($p < o.o2$), whereas basal levels of FSH, TSH and GH were unchanged. Before chronic administration MTC i.v. evoked significant increments in serum PRL ($p < o.oo1$), TSH ($p < o.oo1$) and GH ($p < o.oo5$). The acute TSH response was significantly ($p < o.o2$) diminished after 4 weeks of treatment.

The altered LH and TSH secretion may be the result of a competitive effect of a stimulatory influence of DA receptor blockade, and an opposing inhibitory influence of an increased hypothalamic DA activity evoked by the hyperprolactinemia. With low doses of DA receptor blocking agents, the latter mechanism may be dominant.

The study was supported by the Danish Medical Research Counsil.

175 PHENOL SULFOTRANSFERASE (PST) IN RAT BRAIN: A POTENTIAL MODEL OF THE HUMAN THERMOSTABLE ENZYME. R. ANDERSON* and B. JACKSON, VA West Side and University of Illinois Medical Centers, Chicago, IL., USA, 60612.

PST catalyzes the sulfate conjugation of dopamine (DA) and of 6-OH-melatonin. In human tissue a thermolabile form (TL) of PST acts on DA and a thermostable form (TS) acts on micromolar concentrations of 6-OH-melatonin and p-nitrophenol (p-NP). Rat brain PST measured with DA is biochemically unlike human TL PST. To learn whether the rat brain enzyme might be useful as a model of human TS PST, we studied high speed supernatant preparations of the rat tissue with p-NP as the substrate. The pH optimum was 6.1. Apparent Km values for p-NP and for 3'-phospho-adenosine-5'-phosphosulfate were 1.01 and 0.06 μM, respectively. After preincubation at 41°C for 15 minutes, rat brain preparations assayed with p-NP, DA, and 3-methoxy-4-hydroxyphenylglycol (MHPG) retaind 56.7 ± 4.3, 63.5 ± 6.2 and 54.1 ± 0.8% of the PST activity, respectively (mean ± SEM, n=3). Activity with p-NP expressed per mg protein was significantly correlated with activity measured with MHPG (r=0.84, n=21, $p < 0.0000i$). Mean activities with p-NP expressed as units per mg protein and units per gm tissue were 1.54 ± 0.06 and 46.1 ± 1.64, respectively (mean ± SEM, n=21). The biochemical properties of the rat brain enzyme are similar to those of partially purified rat brain and human platelet PST. Correlation and thermal stability studies suggest that rat brain PST with DA is different from human TL PST. The results raise the possibility that rat brain PST may serve as a model of human tissue TS PST. Supported by the VA Medical Research Service.

176 CALCIUM AND CALMODULIN-DEPENDENT REGULATION OF ENDOGENOUS DOPAMINE RELEASE FROM TUBEROINFUNDIBULAR NEURONS

L.Annunziato*, S.Amoroso, M.Taglialatela and G.F.Di Renzo

Dept. Pharmacology, IInd School of Medicine, University of Naples, Via S.Pansini 5, 80131 Naples,Italy

The role played by extracellular calcium ions and calmodulin on endogenous dopamine (DA) release was investigated in a short-term organ culture of arcuate-periventricular nucleus-median eminence fragment containing cell bodies and nerve endings of tuberoinfundibular DA (TIDA) neurons.

Stimulus secretion-evoked release was completely Ca^{++}-dependent. Thus the removal of extracellular Ca ions in presence of the Ca^{++} chelator EGTA blocked both the basal and 35 mM K^{+}-stimulated release. In addition the blockade of Ca^{++} influx across the plasma membrane obtained with the Ca^{++} organic blocker verapamil (10 and 100 μM) prevented K^{+}-elicited endogenous DA release.

Once Ca is entered into the cells, calmodulin appears to be its major receptors. This interaction takes part in the mechanism of neurotransmitter release.

The possible role played by calmodulin in the stimulated DA release from TIDA neurons was studied by means of the selective calmodulin antagonist N-(6-aminohexyl)-5-chloro-1-naphtalene sulphonamide (W-7). This compound, in a dose-dependent manner (2, 20 and 200 μM), was capable to prevent the K^{+}-stimulated DA release. By contrast W-5, a chlorine deficient analog of W-7 provided of the same hydrophobicity but that interacts only weakly with calmodulin, failed to modify the stimulated DA release.

These results are indicative of the calcium and calmodulin involvment in the events leading to release of DA from the prejunctional site of TIDA neurons.

(This study was partially supported by Ministero Pubblica Istruzione, 40 and 60 per cent funds)

177 MU RECEPTORS IN SPECIFIC BRAIN NUCLEI MEDIATE THE OPIOID PEPTIDE STIMULATION OF CATECHOLAMINE SECRETION. N.M. Appel*, J.A. Kiritsy-Roy and G.R. Van Loon. Veterans Administration Medical Center and Department of Medicine, University of Kentucky, Lexington, Kentucky 40511 USA.

We have previously reported that intracisternal administration of synthetic human β-endorphin to rats stimulates central sympathetic outflow, thus increasing catecholamine secretion from adrenal medulla and sympathetic nerves. To further define the receptor mediation of this opioid peptide effect, we compared the plasma epinephrine, norepinephrine and dopamine responses to intracisternal β-endorphin with those to two specific mu agonists. Morphine was less potent and [D-Ala^2, $MePhe^4$, Gly^5-ol]enkephalin (DAGO) was more potent than β-endorphin in stimulating catecholamine secretion. Next, we defined the brain sites mediating this mu receptor stimulation of catecholamine secretion. DAGO (0.1 nmol) increased plasma catecholamine secretion when administered directly into either the paraventricular nucleus or the nucleus of the solitary tract, but not when administered into frontoparietal cortex. Thus, endogenous opioid peptides appear to increase central sympathetic outflow and catecholamine secretion by stimulating mu receptors in both the paraventricular nucleus and the nucleus of the solitary tract.

178 IMPLICATION OF THE CENTRAL NUCLEUS OF THE AMYGDALA AND BRAIN CATECHOLAMINES IN THE ACTH RESPONSE TO STRESS. S. Beaulieu*, T. Di Paolo and N. Barden, Dept. of Molecular Endocrinology, CHUL, Quebec G1V 4G2, Canada.

We have studied the role of the central nucleus of the amygdala (ACE), which contains high levels of corticotropin-releasing factor, in the modulation of the ACTH response to immobilization stress. Normal rats and rats bearing bilateral lesions of the stria terminalis and/or the ACE were submitted to a period of immobilization of one hour during which blood was sampled by a chronically implanted jugular cannula. Control animals (lesioned and normal) were maintained in a sound-proof room and submitted to the same procedure. Each control or stressed animal was decapitated at completion of its blood sampling. Brains were rapidly frozen and kept at -70°C until microdissected and assayed for norepinephrine (NE) and dopamine (DA) contents by HPLC with electrochemical detection. In response to stress, plasma levels of ACTH, measured by radioimmunoassay, are significantly lower in lesioned compared to normal rats. In normal rats, stress produces a rise in the concentration of DA in the cortical and central nuclei of the amygdala, the hypothalamic dorsomedian nucleus and the ventral tegmental area. DA concentration increases in the hypothalamic ventromedial nucleus of control lesioned rats compared to normal controls and no further enhancement is produced by stress. NE concentration is diminished in the anterior hypothalamic area and lateral hypothalamus of normal rats submitted to stress while such a response is abolished in lesioned animals. It is proposed that the ACE plays a role in the modulation of the secretion of ACTH in response to immobilization stress by the intermediary of NE and DA in specific hypothalamic areas. (Supported by the MRC)

179 THE ROLE OF PEROXIDASE IN LUTEAL HORMONE REGULATION IN RATS.
P. Agrawal*, M.J.K. Harper and M.M. Laloraya, Department of Life Sciences, Vigyan Bhawan, Khandwa Road, Devi Ahilya Vishwavidhyalaya, Indore-452001, India.

A study of the enzymes, Δ^5-3β-hydroxy steroid dehydrogenase (Δ^5-3β-HSD) and peroxidase, has been made in ovaries taken from rats treated with luteinizing hormone (LH) on different days of the estrous cycle. Peroxidase activity is increased within 3h in females injected with LH on the morning of diestrous day 1 (D1) at 0800 h, and is associated with a depletion of ascorbate which is maintained upto the afternoon of D1. Peroxidase and ascorbate then reverted towards basal values by the morning of D2; however, a second injection of LH at 0800 h on D2 produced effects similar to those seen after LH on D1. Females treated with LH did not display greater Δ^5-3β-HSD activity than did controls on D1 after one LH injection, but did on D2 after two LH injections. The peroxidase-ascorbate system appears to be involved in the mechanism responsible for the extended function of the corpus luteum during the estrous cycle. The importance of peroxidase in luteal steroidogenesis is indicated.

180 NOREPINEPHRINE (NE) SYNTHESIS BY THE NEONATAL OVARY AND BY ISOLATED FOLLICLES DURING THE ESTROUS CYCLE. L. Arbogast, T. Rhoades, D. Peleg and N. Ben-Jonathan*, Department of Physiology, Indiana University Medical School, Indianapolis, Indiana 46223, USA

The aims of the study were: 1. To compare catecholamine (CA) synthesis by the neonatal ovary during development with that by other organs, and relate it to plasma gonadotropin levels, and 2. to determine if cyclic changes occur in NE synthesis by the mature ovary, and identify the structures involved. Ovaries, spleen and posterior pituitary (PP) removed from 5-15 day old rats were incubated with ^{3}H tyrosine and labeled CA determined by HPLC. Whereas ovarian NE synthesis was 1750 dpm/ovary on day 5 and decreased 90% by day 15, splenic NE synthesis rose from non-detectable levels on day 10 to 515 dpm/tissue by day 15. Dopamine synthesis was 780 dpm/PP on day 5 and increased 7 fold by day 15. Plasma FSH was 780, 1400 and 1000 ng/ml on day 5, 10 and 15, respectively, whereas LH and PRL (10 ng/ml) were unchanged. Follicles and CL were dissected from adult ovaries at 1300h on each day of the cycle and NE synthesis determined as above. NE synthesis (dpm/10 follicles) was 250 on diestrus I and II, rose to 1200 on proestrus and reduced to 350 on estrus. In contrast, NE synthesis by the CL (150-300 dpm/10 CL) was unchanged during the cycle.

Conclusions: 1. The marked reduction in NE synthesis from days 5-15 of life is unique to the ovary and contrarious to other adrenergically innervated tissues. 2. Based on the temporal relationship with plasma FSH, we postulate that CA in the immature ovary are regulated by FSH. 3. The marked increase in NE synthesis by the preovulatory follicles on proestrus, may be related to the concomitant changes in ovarian steroid levels. Supported by NIH grants NS 13234, HD 14348 and RCDA NS 219.

181 LACTATIONAL AMENORRHEA WITH FAILURE OF PULSATILE GNRH TO INDUCE OVULATION: SYNERGISTIC ACTIONS OF LH AND PROLACTIN REJUVENATE THE CORPUS LUTEUM OF PREGNANCY. T. Aso and R.F. Williams*, Pregnancy Research Branch, NICHD, NIH, Bethesda, MD 20205, USA.

To test the hypothesis that the suckling stimulus induces lactational amenorrhea by diminishing GnRH secretion from the hypothalamus, 6 nursing (120 days postpartum) rhesus and cynomolgus monkeys were chronically administered GnRH (6-9ug, iv, Q 90 min). In 3 of 4 monkeys with secondary amenorrhea, this GnRH regimen induced ovulation within 21 to 35 days of treatment. In the current study, daily femoral blood samples were collected for the measurement of LH, FSH, estradiol, progesterone, and prolactin. Weekly laparoscopies were performed to assess ovarian status. In the course of two months, none of these 6 nursing monkeys demonstrated endocrine patterns indicative of ovulation, nor was follicular maturation culminating in ovulation observed by laparoscopy. In three of the six nursing monkeys, a burgeoning corpus luteum developed during the GnRH treatment. Its emergence was not preceeded by an ovulatory rise of LH and FSH, an antecedent estradiol rise, nor an identifiable dominant follicle. After the initiation of GnRH therapy, peripheral progesterone levels were up to 4 ng/ml. Unlike monkeys having secondary amenorrhea, the pituitary-ovarian axis in nursing monkeys does not respond to this GnRH regimen with follicular growth culminating in ovulation. We hypothesize that the recrudescent corpus luteum observed in these monkeys was rejuvenated from the latent CL of pregnancy. Presumably, prolactin secretion during lactation prevents total luteolysis of this corpus luteum; in turn, the rejuvenation of this CL was stimulated by LH secretion during the GnRH therapy.

182 LUTEOLYSIS IN THE RHESUS MONKEY: EVIDENCE FOR THE CORPUS LUTEUM AS THE SITE OF PROSTAGLANDIN $F_2\alpha(PGF_2\alpha)$ ACTION. F. J. Auletta*, D.K. Paradis, M. Wesley, and M. Gibson. University of Vermont College of Medicine, Depts of Ob/Gyn and Biochemistry, Burlington, Vermont 05405, U.S.A.

In our investigations to elucidate the mechanisms involved in primate luteolysis, we reported that $PGF_2\alpha$, infused directly into the corpus luteum (CL) via an Alzet osmotic pump-ovarian cannula system at a rate of 10 ng/µl/hr, caused premature functional luteolysis. Infusion of $PGF_2\alpha$ at the same rate to the stroma of the non-CL ovary or subcutaneously had no effect on luteal function, suggesting that the site of $PGF_2\alpha$ action was the CL. The purpose of this study was to determine the source of $PGF_2\alpha$ in luteolysis. Monkeys were chronically infused with $PGF_2\alpha$(10 ng/µl/hr, a dose consistent with the production rate by the primate ovary) or vehicle directly into the stroma of the CL-bearing ovary, beginning 5-7 days after the preovulatory estradiol surge. Peripheral blood was drawn daily until menses for the determination of estradiol and progesterone. An additional group of monkeys were similarly infused with a high dose of $PGF_2\alpha$(5 µg/µl/hr). Results show that low dose $PGF_2\alpha$ or vehicle did not impair luteal function, as seen by the normal secretory pattern of the steroids and normal luteal phase and menstrual cycle lengths. Conversely, the high dose infusions resulted in premature luteolysis. These data strongly suggest that luteolysis results from the action of $PGF_2\alpha$ on the CL and that the source of the luteolytic signal is the CL. Supported by NIH grant R01 HD-15444.

183 MODULATION OF CHOLESTEROL METABOLIZING ENZYMES IN RELATION TO GONADOTROPIN INDUCED DESENSITIZATION OF STEROIDOGENIC RESPONSE IN LUTEINIZED RAT OVARY. S. Azhar*, Y-D.I. Chen and G.M. Reaven, Dept. of Medicine, Stanford University and VA Medical Center, Palo Alto, CA 94304, U.S.A.

We have recently demonstrated profound changes in high density lipoprotein receptor concentration and cholesterol metabolism of luteinized ovary in association with gonadotropin induced desensitization of steroidogenic response. In the present study, we explored how the increased receptor number influences the activity of cholesterol metabolizing enzymes. The enzymes examined include HMG CoA reductase, acylCoA : cholesterol acyltransferase (ACAT) and cholesteryl esterase (CEstrase). Human chorionic gonadotropin (hCG) treatment caused a time and dose dependent increase in HMG CoA reductase activity from a low level of 183 ±37 to peak levels of 3757 ±491 pmol · min^{-1} · mg $protein^{-1}$. Maximal stimulation occurred at 24h with ~10 IU of hCG. The half maximal response (ED_{50}) was seen at 2.5 IU. The effect was specific for LH and hCG as other peptide hormones failed to modulate enzyme activity. Furthermore, hCG mediated increase in HMG CoA reductase activity was independent of cellular depletion of sterols. hCG treatment produced a biphasic effect on soluble and microsomal associated CEstrase activity: a marked increase in activity was observed at 1.5h followed by a significant reduction of 70-90% below the control value for up to 24h. In contrast, activity of acidic CEstrase (lysosomal) was unaffected by hCG treatment. Gonadotropin also produced a slight but significant decrease in microsomal ACAT activity at 24h. This decrease was noted both in the presence and absence of exogenous substrate (cholesterol) and loss in enzyme activity was not related to depletion of endogenous substrate. From these studies we conclude that gonadotropins exert a profound and specific effect on cholesterol metabolizing enzymes in luteinized ovary.

184 RELAXIN DEMONSTRATION IN THE WALL OF HUMAN CAVITARY FOLLICLES. G.C.Balboni[+], M. Bigazzi, G. Scarselli and G. Vannelli, Institute of Human Anatomy and Obstetrics and Gynecology Department, Univ. of Florence, Florence, Italy.

The presence of Rlx was observed in the follicular fluid (Noci et al., 1983). Its production by granulosa cells was demonstrated in vitro (Bryant-Greenwood et al., 1980). However, according to Evans et al. (1983) the principal source of Rlx in porcine preovulatory follicles is represented by theca cells. In previous research (Balboni et al., 1983) we have detected immunoreactive Rlx-like substances in both porcine and human isolated granulosa cells from cavitary follicles. These investigations concern the demonstration of Rlx in the cells of the wall of whole human cavitary follicles 7-9 mm in diameter, using the immunofluorescence and immunoperoxidase methods, as well as the electron microscopy. Our results have shown an evident positivity for the immunohistochemical methods in a number of granulosa cells. Only few theca cells exhibit a modest positivity. With the E.M. the presence has been detected in some granulosa and theca cells of dense granules 200-300 nm in diameter, very similar to the Rlx granules described in different sites by previous Authors.

185 HORMONAL REGULATION OF THE STEROIDOGENESIS IN CULTURED PORCINE GRANULOSA CELLS. J.L. Baranao* and J.M. Hammond, Dept. of Medicine, Division of Endocrinology, The Milton S. Hershey Medical Center, The Pennsylvania State University, Hershey, PA 17033

FSH, LH and estradiol (E_2) are known to modulate ovarian follicular differentiation. However, the cellular site of action and relative importance of the three hormones have remained uncertain. The recent development of a serum-free medium (SFM) for the culture of immature porcine granulosa cells has enabled us to reinvestigate this issue under hormonally defined conditions. Progesterone production in response to FSH (200 ng/ml) was higher in cells cultured in SFM (10-fold increase over basal) than in those grown in the presence of 10% fetal calf serum (10% FCS) (1.5-2 fold). Ovine LH alone (200 ng/ml) was also able to stimulate progesterone production in SFM (6-fold). This effect could not be accounted for by FSH contamination. The LH stimulation, however, was enhanced by FSH. E_2 (1 µg/ml) stimulated progesterone production *per se* (2-3 fold) and also enhanced both the FSH and LH actions. Maximal levels of progesterone after 6 days were observed when a combination of FSH, LH and E_2 were present from the onset of the culture (25-fold). Incubations carried out in the presence of 25-hydroxycholesterol indicated that the hormonal interactions take place, at least in part, at the level of the side-chain cleavage enzyme. Conclusions: FSH is the most important hormonal stimulus for progesterone synthesis in immature granulosa cells. However, E_2 and LH exert direct actions on the granulosa cell that may be required for the development of optimal steroidogenic potential.

186 INSULIN STIMULATES ANDROGEN ACCUMULATION IN INCUBATIONS OF HUMAN OVARIAN STROMA AND THECA. R.L.Barbieri*,A.Makris,K.J. Ryan, Laboratory of Human Reproduction and Reproductive Biology, Harvard Medical School, Boston, MA 02115.

Recent clinical observations suggest that a strong association exists between hyperinsulinemia and hyperandrogenism in women of reproductive age. To further characterize this relationship the effects of insulin on ovarian steroidogenesis *in vitro* were examined. Ovarian wedge biopsies were obtained from a woman with hyperandrogenism, severe insulin resistance and acanthosis nigricans(HAIR-AN), and from a normally cycling woman. The effects of insulin on ovarian steroidogenesis were examined in 4-day incubations of minced stroma and theca. Incubation media was changed daily and assayed for steroids using specific antibodies. In incubations of theca obtained from the patient with HAIR-AN, LH(25ng/ml) stimulated androstenedione(A)(+780%),testosterone(T)(+1170%),progesterone(P) (+310%) and estradiol(E)(810%). Insulin alone(500ng/ml), stimulated A(+432%),T(+700%) but not P or E in the thecal incubations. In the incubations of stroma obtained from the patient with HAIR-AN, LH alone stimulated A(+350%) and T(260%) but not DHT. Insulin stimulated A(+562%),T(+460%)and DHT (+560%) accumulation. FSH did not alter steroid accumulation in the theca or stoma. In incubations of stroma from the normally cycling woman, LH plus insulin acted synergistically to stimulate A(+510%) and T(+380%) accumulation compared to LH alone. Insulin may regulate human ovarian steroidogenesis.

187 ISOLATION AND STRUCTURE OF THE COMMON PRECURSOR TO MSEL-NEUROHYPOPHYSIN AND COPEPTIN (A GLYCOPEPTIDE) PRESENT IN GUINEA-PIG NEUROHYPOPHYSIS. R. Acher*, J. Chauvet, M. T. Chauvet, D. Sunde, A.N. Thorn, Laboratory of Biological Chemistry, University of Paris VI, 96 Bd Raspail, 75006 Paris (France) and Institute of Medical Physiology C, University of Copenhagen, DK 200 Copenhagen (Danemark).

From frozen guinea-pig posterior pituitaries, three polypeptides corresponding to the three putative fragments of the vasopressin precursor, namely vasopressin (9 residues), MSEL-neurophysin (93 residues) and a glycopeptide (39 residues) referred to as copeptin, have been isolated and characterized. On the other hand a 17 000-dalton protein precursor has been purified, by successive molecular sievings, until homogeneity as shown by SDS electrophoresis with reducing agent. This protein, performic acid-oxidized, was subjected to tryptic hydrolysis and resulting fragments separated by peptide mapping. 9 tryptic peptides corresponding to those of MSEL-neurophysin (6) and of copeptin (3), respectively, were obtained. However the C-terminal peptide of MSEL-neurophysin was replaced by a more basic peptide having the same sequence with an additional C-terminal arginine. It is concluded that MSEL-neurophysin and copeptin are hyphened by an arginine residue in a common 133-residue precursor. The processing of the three-domain vasopressin precursor seems to involve two steps: first the release of vasopressin from the N-terminal end, then the cleavage of the remaining fragment into neurophysin and copeptin.

188 PROTEIN REPLETION CORRECTS DDAVP-INDUCED HYPONATREMIA BY DECREASING NATRIURESIS. E.F. Baldwin*, J.G. Verbalis, P.R. Neish and A.G. Robinson, Department of Medicine, University of Pittsburgh, Pittsburgh, PA, USA.

In an animal model of SIADH, protein deprived rats became significantly more hyponatremic after chronic DDAVP infusions than rats fed a 20% protein diet. To further study this effect 22 adult rats were infused with DDAVP (10 ng/h) X 4d. On days 1 and 2 they received only D_5W causing hyponatremia, then on days 3 and 4 Group I (n=11) was refed a 20% protein diet while Group II (n=11) continued to be protein deprived (isocaloric 0% protein diet). By day 4 the protein repleted rats had a significantly increased p[Na+] despite no change in osmolar-free water clearance (C_{H_2O}). However, a significant decrease in sodium clearance (C_{Na}) and increase in sodium-free water clearance (C_{NaFW}) was observed:

	I & II, day 2	I, day 4	II, day 4	day 2 vs 4
p [Na+], mEq/L	119.6±1.7	130.4±2.4***	114.7±3.4##	*p<.05
BUN, mg/dl	8.0±0.7	12.5±0.9***	8.1±0.9##	***p<.001
Uosm, mosm/l	2028±117	2369±196	1897±270	day 4, I vs II
C_{H_2O}, µl/min	-24.1±1.4	-29.2±2.5	-21.2±2.6#	#p<.05
C_{Na}, µl/min	2.1±0.3	0.7±0.2*	1.8±0.4#	##p<.01
C_{NaFW}, µl/min	1.9±0.3	3.4±0.4***	2.0±0.6###	###p<.001

Renal inner medullary urea content and concentration were both significantly increased in the protein repleted rats (64% and 76% respectively). Thus, dietary protein corrects DDAVP-induced hyponatremia in rats by decreasing natriuresis, an effect probably mediated by the observed increases in renal inner medullary urea. The same mechanism likely accounts for the similar responses of patients with SIADH treated with urea.

189 SYNCHRONIZATION OF OXYTOCIN CELL FIRING IN THE FOUR MAGNO-CELLULAR NUCLEI: SIMULTANEOUS RESPONSES TO INTRAVENTRICULARLY INJECTED DRUGS. V. Belin, F. Moos and Ph. Richard *.
Laboratoire de Physiologie, ULP, LA 309 CNRS, 21, rue René Descartes 67084 STRASBOURG Cedex, France.

For the pulsatile release of oxytocin (OT) during suckling, the neurosecretory bursts which induce such a release must appear almost simultaneously on all or most cells in the para-ventricular (PV) and supraoptic (SO) nuclei. In suckled rats, simultaneous recording of two identified OT cells (15 times with PV and SO cells coupled and twice with left and right SO cells coupled) shows a possible time-lag between the beginning of two corresponding neurosecretory bursts. For a given couple of cells, this time-lag can vary one way or the other for successive bursts but never exceeds 100msec. Milk ejection reflex stimulants (OT, dopamine) or inhibitors (OT or dopamine antagonists) injected into the third ventricle act simultane-ously and similarly on PV and SO nuclei OT cells. Phasic vaso-pressin cell activity in PV and SO nuclei is never synchro-nized.

190 VASOPRESSIN FRAGMENTS ARE PRESENT IN THE BRAIN BUT NOT IN THE PITUITARY
J.P.H. Burbach[+], X-C. Wang, J.A. Ten Haaf and D. De Wied, Rudolf Magnus Institute for Pharmacology, Vondellaan 6, 3521 GD Utrecht, The Netherlands.

Findings of central activities of Arg-vasopressin (AVP-(1-9)) that are retained or modified by partial sequences of the peptide prompted biochemi-cal investigations on a role of AVP as precursor of centrally active oligo-peptides. Recently, these studies showed that brain synaptic membranes pro-cessed AVP-(1-9) by sequential aminopeptidase cleavage into C-terminal frag-ments[1]. One of them [$pGlu^4$,Cyt^6]AVP-(4-9) and its (4-8)-derivative were thou-sand times more potent than AVP in affecting avoidance behavior but had no peripheral activity[2]. Here these findings are further elaborated by experi-ments on the endogenous presence of AVP fragments in brain. Using an anti-serum that reactied with C-terminal AVP peptides as small as AVP-(5-9) immu-noreactivity was detected in rat brain extracts in addition to AVP-(1-9). Characterization by two HPLC systems showed similarity of immunoreactive components with [Cyt^6]AVP-(2-9), -(3-9), -(4-9), -(5-9) and likely reduced forms of them. Extraction of [^3H]AVP excluded artifactual generation of the peptides. Relatively highest amounts of AVP fragments were found in brain areas having terminals of AVP fibers; e.g. in the hippocampus they represen-ted 3-18% of the AVP-(1-9) content, while in the hypothalamus, having AVP cell bodies, only 1-3%. In contrast, the pituitary had virtually no AVP frag-ments (<0.1%). The data demonstrate the existence of C-terminal AVP fragments in the brain but not in the pituitary gland, pointing to a role of these peptides selectively in the brain. They may have a role as neuropeptides of the central vasopressinergic system.
[1]: J.Biol. Chem. (1983)258, 1487; [2]: Science (1983)221, 1310.

191 INCREASES IN PLASMA VASOPRESSIN-ASSOCIATED NEUROPHYSIN (VP-RNP) LEVELS BY ACUTE INFUSION OF HYPERTONIC SOLUTIONS THAT CAN NOT BE TOTALLY EXPLAINED BY OSMORECEPTORS AND SODIUM RECEPTORS.

S.W.T. Cheng* and W.G. North, Dept. of Physiology, Dartmouth Medical School, Hanover, NH 03756, U.S.A.

The effects of acute iv infusion of 18% NaCl, 25% D-mannitol and a combination of 15% D-mannitol and 1.35% NaCl on plasma concentrations of VP-RNP ([VP-RNP]) were studied using conscious, chronic catheterized Long-Evans rats. In each case infusion was performed at a rate of 10ul/100g b.w./min for 60 min using a Sage infusion pump. Plasma samples at 0,10,20, 40 and 60 min were evaluated for [VP-RNP], plasma osmolality (Posm) and plasma sodium concentration [Na+]. All three infusions produced similar rises in Posm and there was a significant drop in [Na+] in animals receiving 25% mannitol while those receiving the combination maintained approximately normal [Na+]. The slopes for the relationship between Δ[VP-RNP] and ΔPosm were almost identical for the 18% NaCl and 25% mannitol infusions (92 and 98 $pg \cdot ml^{-1} \cdot mosm^{-1}$ kg), but infusion of the combination of 15% mannitol and 1.35% NaCl produced much smaller rises in [VP-RNP] with changes of Psom (48 $pg \cdot ml^{-1} \cdot msom^{-1} \cdot kg$). These results suggest that: (1) Sodium receptors (if they exist) are not involved to a measurable extent in the release of neurohypophysial principles under the experimental conditions used. (2)There is a coincidence between Posm and the ability of hypertonic NaCl or mannitol to induce the release of VP-RNP, but that certain effects of the substances are not additive when NaCl and mannitol are used in combination. This study was supported by grants CA 19613, AM 08469, CA 00552 and the Albert J. Ryan Foundation.

192 DIFFERENTIAL RESPONSE OF UTERINE ESTROGEN RECEPTORS TO MELATONIN IN ADULT AND JUVENILE SYRIAN HAMSTERS.

O.F.X. Almeida* and L. Tamarkin, Developmental Endocrinology Branch, NICHHD, NIH, Bethesda, MD 20205, USA.

The reproductive effects of melatonin (MEL) may be due to its action upon steroid receptors in peripheral, pituitary or brain tissues. The concentration and affinity of uterine estrogen receptors (ER) was determined by a dextran-coated charcoal assay to compare the effects of MEL on ER in intact 20 d.o. juveniles and 45 d.o. adults (ovariectomised at 34 d.o.). The hamsters received either 25 ug MEL or saline (s.c.) at 1400h (lights on: 0100-1500h), 40 min. prior to sacrifice. ER affinity remained unchanged in both juveniles and adults following MEL (Kd = 10^{-10}-10^{-11} M/L). In agreement with our earlier data for juveniles, MEL caused a 62% increase in ER number (11 groups; n=6/group). In contrast, MEL caused a 26% decrease in ER number in the adults (14 groups; n=4/group). This latter finding is consistent with that obtained by others in adult rat brains (Science: 213, 1525). The above data were confirmed by measuring the specific uptake of 60 ng of ^3H-E_2 by the uteri of juvenile and adult hamsters injected with MEL or saline in the same way as above. Half the animals were injected with 60 µg diethylstilbestrol 40 min. before the ^3H-E_2 injection in order to determine specificity of uptake. The MEL treatment resulted in a 27% increase, and 36% decrease, in the specific uptake of ^3H-E_2 in the juveniles and adults respectively. We conclude that there are differential effects of MEL upon ER numbers in juveniles and adults; the biological significance of these differences remains to be determined.

193 SHORT PHOTOPERIOD-INDUCED INCREASE IN HYPOTHALAMIC DOPAMINE TURNOVER IN MALE HAMSTERS. B. Benson*, Univ. of Arizona, Tucson, AZ., U.S.A.

Transfer of male Syrian hamsters from long photoperiod (LP) to short photoperiod (SP) results in pineal-mediated reductions in pituitary and blood levels of prolactin (PRL), gonadotropins and gonadal weight, although hypothalamic mechanisms are not clear. Adult male Syrian hamsters were acclimated to LP (L/D=14/10 hrs) for three weeks, after which half were transferred to SP (L/D=10/14 hrs). Groups of 8-10 SP- and LP-treated hamsters were sacrificed two, four, eight and 12 weeks later. Testes and accessory organs were weighed and pituitary and serum levels of PRL, FSH and LH determined by radioimmunoassay. One hour after either saline or α-methyl-paratyrosine injection, hypothalamic norepinephrine (NE) and dopamine (DA) were determined by high pressure liquid chromatography with electrochemical detection. Significant reductions in pituitary and serum levels of PRL were noted as early as two weeks after transfer into SP; whereas FSH and LH levels were not significantly depressed until twelve weeks. No significant differences were noted in hypothalamic catecholamine content or NE turnover between LP- and SP-treated animals. On the other hand, DA turnover was significantly increased at eight and 12 weeks of SP-treatment, at which time serum and pituitary levels of PRL and gonadal/accessory organ weights were markedly depressed. This increased hypothalamic dopaminergic activity may be important to SP effects on the reproductive system in hamsters.

194 LOCALIZATION, CHARACTERIZATION AND BINDING OF A NOVEL RAT PITUITARY POLYPEPTIDE: ALPHA 2u GLOBULIN. Antakly, T.,* M.G. Zelechowska and S. Raguet-Horowitz, Dept. of Anatomy, McGill University, Montreal, Canada.

Recent reports have demonstrated the presence of a number of novel exogenous polypeptides in the pituitary such as substance P, Angiotensin II, EGF and IGF's. We have localized in the rat anterior pituitary (PNAS 80:4000,1983) a rat serum and urinary protein α 2u globulin, which is largely secreted by the hepatocytes essentially under pituitary hormone control (Am.J.Anat. 165:211,1982). The presence of α 2u globulin in the pituitary raises the possibility that a hepatic protein might modulate pituitary function. A double-labelling immunocytochemical technique was used to determine which of the pituitary cells contain α 2u globulin. Somatotrophs, gonadotrophs and prolactin cells reacted with anti-α 2u globulin antibodies. To further validate that the anti-α 2u globulin antibody is indeed detecting authentic α 2u globulin, we performed Western blot analysis on pituitary and liver S-100's as well as on HPLC purified α 2u globulin. Results showed essentially one protein band common to all 3 samples which reacts with the anti-α 2u globulin antibody (Mr≃19K). Alpha 2u globulin is not seemingly synthesized by pituitary cells since α 2u globulin mRNA could not be detected using Northern blot analysis. Our hypothesis is that exogenous α 2u is internalized by the pituitary cells via receptor-mediated endocytosis. Indeed, binding sites could be demonstrated as ^{125}I α 2u globulin (HPLC purified) specifically bound to pituitary cells in primary culture. Seventy percent of the labelled protein was displaced by the addition of unlabelled pure α 2u globulin (50 μg/ml). (Supported by the MRC, Canada and FRSQ, Quebec).

195 FOUR CASES OF ACTH-DEPENDENT CUSHING'S SYNDROME WITH CYCLICAL VARIATIONS IN CORTISOL PRODUCTION.

A.B.Atkinson*, B.Sheridan, D.J.Carson, D.R.Hadden, A.L.Kennedy and J.A.Weaver, Metabolic Unit, Royal Victoria Hospital, BELFAST BT12 6BA, N. Ireland.

Cushing's Syndrome is said to be a rare variant of hypercortisolism with only a few documented single case reports. In the last 18 months 4 cases of ACTH-dependent Cushing's syndrome have been proven by us to have cyclical patterns, with, in all patients, nadir values of cortisol production which were strictly normal. Each patient has been studied for at least 100 days continuously. In each case there was extreme variation in urinary free cortisol (UFC) excretion e.g. in patient 1, UFC values varied from a nadir of 136 nmol/24 hours (normal $<$ 450 nmol) to a peak of 15,400 nmol. Cycle length has varied between 4 and 64 days. In all 4 cases the serotonin antagonist cyproheptadine has proven ineffective in controlling the syndrome while in 2 of 3 cases the combination of cyproheptadine with the dopamine agonist bromocriptine has also been without effect. In the third case the combination treatment has been associated temporally with a decrease in the height of the cortisol peaks - cyclicity is still apparent. The precise incidence of cyclical Cushing's syndrome is unknown but these 4 cases suggest that it may be underestimated and the diagnostic pitfalls of these cases requires recognition. The neuroendocrine mechanism responsible for cyclicity remains unknown.

196 PITUITARY-DERIVED GROWTH FACTOR IS SECRETED BY THE BOVINE ADENOHYPOPHYSIS IN VITRO.

Andrew Baird* Peter Böhlen, Frederich Esch, Nicholas Ling, Roger Guillemin and D Gospodarowicz†. Laboratories for Neuroendocrinology, The Salk Institute for Biological Studies, La Jolla, CA 92037, †Cancer Research Institute, UCSF School of Medicine, San Francisco, CA 94143.

We have recently isolated and identified by partial sequence analysis a pituitary derived growth factor that has high intrinsic activity to stimulate proliferation in mesoderm-derived cells. Using this sequence information, we have raised antisera and developed a specific radioimmunoassay. Rabbits were immunized with a synthetic replicate of an N-terminal fragment of the growth factor after conjugation to BSA via a BDB linkage. Serum collected after the 4th boost (715B4, 716B4) had titers of 1:10,000 and 1:5,000 respectively as assessed by their ability to bind the iodinated synthetic antigen. Specificity for a free amino terminal was determined by the low crossreactivity of the N-acetylated fragment (<0.1%). The radioimmunoassay recognizes the native protein on an equimolar basis when quantitation is compared by RIA and amino acid analysis. Furthermore, the antiserum can neutralize mitogenic activity from samples containing the native growth factor. Using the RIA we have established that it is actively secreted by bovine anterior pituitary cells in culture. The secretion of this molecule can be stimulated by depolarization with KCl (50 mM) or by activation of adenylate cyclase with forskolin (10^{-4} M). Its release under basal and stimulated conditions is also highly dependent on cell density. The application of these antisera to the immunolocalization of the pituitary derived growth factor in various tissues and the regulation of its secretion in the adenohypophysis is in progress.

197 **IN VITRO EFFECT OF GNRH ON LH RELEASE, SYNTHESIS AND ISOELECTRIC FORMS AS RELATED TO THE HORMONAL STATE.** **D.M. Baldwin* and R.F. Highsmith, Dept. of Physiology, Univ. of Cincinnati College of Medicine, Cincinnati, OH 45267 USA**

Previous studies have suggested that the hormonal state may influence both the quality and the quantity of LH. The objective of this sutdy was to determine whether in vitro differences in GnRH-stimulated LH secretion for pituitaries from proestrous (P) vs 72h-ovariectomized (OVX) rats could be related to qualitative and/or quantitative changes in pituitary and secreted LH. Using an in vitro static incubation system, three paired hemipituitaries from P or OVX rats were incubated for 4h with or without 10 nM GnRH (n=4-5/grp). Media and pituitary extracts were analyzed quantitatively for LH by RIA and qualitatively by isoelectric focusing (IEF) in polyacrylamide gel, pH 3-10. GnRH-stimulated LH synthesis was estimated by comparing total LH content (med + tiss) in experimental (GnRH) vs its paired control (no GnRH). GnRH-stimulated LH release was significantly greater in P vs OVX (10.1 vs 4.5 μ g/mg/4h). Two isoelectric forms were evident in all treatment groups (i.e. P vs OVX, tiss vs med, ± GnRH): one in the alkaline (pH 8.1-8.6, alk LH) and one in the acidic range (pH 5.5-6.5) with the alk LH representing ∽ 67% and the acidic ∽ 32% of the total LH recovered from the gel. GnRH significantly stimulated total LH synthesis in P (62% ↑) and OVX (18% ↑) with the increase significantly greater in P vs OVX (6.2 vs 2.2 μ g/mg). Net synthesis of alk LH was similar to that for total LH, whereas net synthesis of acidic LH was only observed in the P group (69% ↑). We conclude that 1) the distribution of isoelectric forms of pituitary and secreted LH is similar in pituitaries from P and OVX rats and that these forms are not preferentially released, 2) GnRH-stimulated synthesis of acidic LH may be influenced by ovarian steroids, and 3) GnRH-stimulated LH release is closely associated with GnRH-stimulted LH synthesis. Supported by NIH 16994.

198 STANDARDS AND STANDARDIZATION IN ENDOCRINOLOGY. D.R. Bangham*, A.F. Bristow, R.E. Gaines Das, S. Poole, D. Schulster, P.L. Storring and J.M. Zanelli. National Institute for Biological Standards and Control, London NW3 6RB, UK.

The need for standards and standardization in endocrinology is more prevalent and evident than ever, despite the advances made in methods of analysis and synthesis. Standards - attested reference materials - serve to calibrate assays for hormones used clinically and in diagnosis, eg. kits, 'define' certain protein hormones, and evaluate specificity of assay systems. The poster outlines the background to International Standards for hormones; their characterization, preparation and evaluation in international collaborative studies; and describes the mechanism and implications of their establishment by the Expert Committee on Biological Standardization of the World Health Organization. The concept of the 'International Unit', its continuity and its application are discribed. The nature of the (international) unit derived from comparative assays requires an understanding of the differences between in vivo and in vitro bioassays, receptor- and other ligand assays , and the significance of the difference between standard and hormone analyte. Examples of recent problems of standardization (of gonadotrophins, hPRL, hGH, PTH and Insulin) are given.

199 A PLURIHORMONAL AND A SEPARATE NULL CELL ADENOMA REMOVED BY SURGERY FROM THE PITUITARY OF AN ACROMEGALIC MAN. T.A. Bayley*, E. Horvath, K. Kovacs, Depts. of Medicine, St. Joseph's Health Centre, and Pathology, St. Michael's Hosp., University of Toronto, Toronto, Ont. M5B 1W8, Canada.

Two simultaneously occurring pituitary adenomas differing in histologic characteristics, hormone content and ultrastructural features are very rarely recognized clinically. A 55-year-old man with typical clinical and biochemical features of active acromegaly accompanied by goiter and mild hypertension underwent transsphenoidal removal of a pituitary tumor which was believed to be single. However, morphologic investigation, including immunocytology and transmission electron microscopy, revealed two, structurally markedly different, sharply demarcated, separate pituitary adenomas in close approximation. One tumor was an acidophilic adenoma and the avidin-biotin-immunoperoxidase complex technique demonstrated GH, PRL and TSH in the cytoplasm of adenoma cells. The other tumor was a chromophobic adenoma containing no adenohypophysial hormones, as shown by immunocytologic methods. By electron microscopy, the first adenoma was monomorphous, the cells resembling densely granulated growth hormone cells of the nontumorous adenohypophysis. The second tumor possessed sparse, small secretory granules. This tumor was also composed of one cell type and was diagnosed as a null cell adenoma. It appears that neoplastic transformation occurred in two different cell types, resulting in two distinct adenomas.
(Supported in part by the St. Joseph's Health's Centre Research Foundation and the Medical Research Council of Canada)

200 THE INFLUENCE OF PITUITARY HORMONES ON ADJUVANT ARTHRITIS. I. Berczi*, E. Nagy, S.L. Asa, K. Kovacs. Dept. of Immunology, University of Manitoba, Winnipeg, Manitoba, and Dept. of Pathology, St. Michael's Hospital, Univ. of Toronto, Toronto, Ontario.

Adjuvant arthritis (AA) was induced in female Fischer and Wistar-Furth rats by injecting their right hind paw with 0.1 ml Freund's complete adjuvant. The development of AA was inhibited by hypophysectomy (Hypox) and by daily treatment of intact animals with the dopaminergic agent, bromocriptine (BRC). AA developed normally if Hypox or BRC-suppressed animals were treated with either prolactin or growth hormone. Additional treatment with adrenocorticotropic hormone inhibited this restoration. Treatment of Hypox rats with follicle-stimulating hormone, luteinizing hormone and thyroid-stimulating hormone had no effect. These results indicate that pituitary hormones have a regulatory influence on AA.
(This study was supported by the Arthritis Society of Canada).

201 GONADOTROPIN RELEASING HORMONE (GnRH) PULSATILE ADMINISTRATION RESTORES NORMAL TESTOSTERONE LEVELS IN MALE WITH HYPERPROLACTINEMIA.

P. Bouchard*, A. Reinberg and G. Schaison, Service d'endocrinologie et des maladies de la reproduction, Hopital Bicêtre, 94270 Le Kremlin-Bicêtre and CNRS 105 75490 Paris - France.

Hyperprolactinemia in men is frequently associated with hypogonadism. Normalization of Prolactin (PRL) levels is generally associated with an increase in serum Testosterone (T) to normal. In order to determine the level of the inhibitory effect of hyperprolactinemia on the hypothalamus-pituitary-gonadal axis, we studied the effect of intermittent circhoral GnRH administration on LH pulsatility and T levels in 4 patients with prolactinomas. All patients had high PRL values (80-3000 ng.ml, low LH (2.2 ± 0.1 $mIU.ml^{-1}$) and low T values (2.3 ± 0.3 $ng.ml^{-1}$), with no other apparent abnormality of pituitary function. GnRH was administered IV using a pump delivering a bolus of 10µg every 90 min for 15 days. Samples for T, LH, and PRL RIA were collected daily. All subjects had blood sampled every 15 minutes for 4 hours once before and during the pulsatile GnRH administration. No pulse of LH could be detected before treatment. GnRH pulsatile administration resulted in a significant increase in LH basal levels (6.7 ± 0.6 $mIU.ml^{-1}$) ($p < 0.001$), and restored LH pulsatility. In addition T levels increased significantly to normal values in all patients (7.8 ± 0.4 $ng.ml^{-1}$) ($p < 0.001$). T levels remained normal during pulsatile LHRH administration, although PRL levels remained elevated. In conclusion : in hyperprolactinemic males, GnRH pulsatile administration resulted in increased basal LH levels, restored LH pulsatility and increased serum T values to normal. These data therefore suggest that hyperprolactinemia produces hypogonadism primarily by interfering with GnRH pulsatile release.

202 ANTI-IDIOTYPES TO PRL ANTIBODY HAVE PRL-LIKE ACTIVITY AND BIND TO THE PRL RECEPTOR. T. Amit*, M. Gavish, R.J. Barkey and M.B.H. Youdim, Rappaport Institute for Research in Medical Sciences,Technion,POB 9697,Haifa, Israel.

Anti-idiotypic antibodies have been raised against antibodies to ovine prolactin (oPRL). Rats and rabbits were immunized with oPRL and the anti-serum chromatographed on an oPRL-Sepharose-4B affinity column. The specific antibodies against oPRL (1mg/ml) in Freund's complete adjuvant were injected into rabbits followed by boosters on alternate weeks for three months. IgG fractions from the anti-idiotypic antisera were isolated by affinity chromatography on a Sepharose-4B-Protein A column and further chromatographed on the oPRL affinity column to remove residual PRL antibodies. The IgG fraction (10µg/ml) of the anti-idiotypic antibodies inhibited the binding of ^{125}I-PRL to the immunizing anti-oPRL antibody (by 85%). A tenfold higher concentration of this anti-idiotypic IgG only partially inhibited PRL binding to its membrane-bound receptor (by up to 30%). ^{125}I-Protein A caused a dose-dependent precipitation of the anti-idiotype-receptor complex, which was competitively and specifically inhibited by the immunizing anti-oPRL antibody. Preliminary data showed that the anti-idiotypic antibody also exhibited PRL-like physiological activity in mammary gland explants in culture: anti-idiotypic IgG (300µg/ml) increased both basal as well as PRL-stimulated (1µg/ml) α-lactalbumin secretion (14.3 ± 1.0, 25.4 ± 2.6 ng/ml) compared with non immune IgG (300µg/ml) (4.8 ± 0.3, 12.4 ± 0.7 ng/ml). Anti-idiotypic antibodies will provide a further useful tool in elucidating the structure-function relationship of PRL with its receptor. Furthermore the development of a PRL-like antireceptor antibody through the anti-idiotypic pathway could explain changes reported in the receptor activity of circulating PRL in some pathological situations.

203 HEMOLYTIC PLAQUE ASSAY OF RAT PROLACTIN (PRL) ANTERIOR PITUITARY CELLS (AP): EFFECTS OF DOPAMINE (DA), FORSKOLIN AND MAITOTOXIN (MTX).

J. Anderson*, D. Keefer+, D. Yasumoto# and M. Cronin, Univ. Virginia, Charlottesville, VA., +Loyola of Baltimore, MD., USA, #Tohoku Univ., Sendai, Japan.

The reverse hemolytic plaque assay was applied to enzymatically dispersed, male AP (ENDOCRINOLOGY 112:1135, 1983). This allowed us to monitor the response of single mammotrophs to increased cAMP production via 3 uM forskolin, enhanced calcium flux with 5 ng/ml MTX, and DA receptor activation with 10 uM DA for 45 min. The % of total cells forming plaques (400-600 cells scored/slide) and the average plaque area (u^2: 35 plaques measured/slide) were determined in 3 independent studies as listed (Table).

	% Plaques	Area of Plaques[b]
control	27 ± 1	1,970 ± 70
DA	14 ± 1	1,130 ± 60
Forskolin	35 ± 1	3,560 ± 130
Forskolin + DA	27 ± 1[a]	2,590 ± 100
MTX	35 ± 1	4,910 ± 530
MTX + DA	29 ± 2[a]	2,790 ± 100

a = not different from control
b = all groups different from each other

The DA inhibition was blocked by 10 nM spiperone, a potent DA receptor antagonist. The responses to bromocriptine were similar to DA. We conclude that: 1) individual PRL cells respond to increased cAMP and calcium tonus by amplifying PRL release; 2) DA receptor activation ± secretagogues reduces the number and size of identifiable PRL plaques; 3) because alterations in the % of plaque-forming cells were observed after several treatments, subpopulations of mammotrophs must exist *in vitro*. (Supported by a DuPont Fellowship, RCDA 1K04NS500601, NS18409.)

204 PROLACTIN (PRL) SHORT-LOOP FEEDBACK IS OVERCOME BY INHIBITION OF DOPAMINE (DA) IN VIVO.

R.L.W. Averill*, Zoology Department, Victoria University of Wellington, New Zealand.

Intrahypothalamic grafts of anterior pituitary (AP) tissue prevented the luteotropic PRL surges following coitus. 81 fertile matings in 17 rats were followed by 76 normal cycles (4-6 days), 5 pseudopregnancies (7-12 days) and no pregnancies. α-Methyl-p-tyrosine (AMT) or Reserpine (RES) treatments (200 mg/kg i.p. and 1 mg/kg s.c. respectively) were given following matings by the same males to test whether the graft-induced failure of PRL surges was due to enhanced DA secretion. 80% of 15 normal unmated rats became pseudopregnant with a single dose of RES given on the day following oestrus compared with only 31% (4/13) graft-bearing mated rats. To permit pseudopregnancy (or pregnancy) in >60% of the graft-bearing rats required AMT or RES treatments for 2, 3 or 4 successive days, and despite RES treatment 31 out of 60 matings were followed in 3-5 days by prooestrous smears. Clearly graft PRL creates a considerable block to normal PRL while pharmacological blockade of DA permitted PRL release in most cases. It is concluded that short-loop feedback of PRL is due to elevated DA inhibition.

205 EFFECTS OF LONG TERM TREATMENT WITH 2-α-BROMOCRIPTINE IN FEMALE PATIENTS WITH THE HYPERPROLACTINEMIC SYNDROME.

D.Ayalon*, A. Eshel, S. Avidan and N. Eckstein, Timsit Institute of Reproductive Endocrinology, Ichilov Hospital, Tel Aviv Medical Center, Tel Aviv, 64239, Israel.

Seventeen hyperprolactinemic patients with or without radiological evidences of a pituitary adenoma, were submitted to a long term (7-36 months) suppressive treatment with bromocriptine. Nine patients conceived during the treatment. All of them had a normal pregnancy and delivered normal babies. In all patients (including those who underwent a pregnancy) the post treatment prolactin levels were significantly lower than the pretreatment values suggesting a long lasting suppressive effect of this dopamine agonist on the pituitary lactotrophs.All patients reported normal menstrual bleeding during the 3 months no-treatment interval.Three of them were followed throughout a whole menstrual cycle 3-10 months after cessation of therapy, and demonstrated clinical and endocrinological presumptive signs of ovulation in spite of relatively elevated immunoreactive prolactin concentrations.These data might suggest a permanent change in the biological activity of the hormone secreted by the pituitary lactotrophs following the prolonged treatment with the dopamine agonist drug. This hypothesis is currently under research by our group.

206 PROLACTIN AND THYROTROPIN-RELEASING HORMONE RESPONSES TO DOPAMINE RECEPTOR BLOCKADE IN HYPERPROLACTINEMIC STATES.

A.Barbarino*,L.De Marinis,A.Mancini,C.Anile,and G.Maira.Institutes of Internal Medicine,Division of Endocrinology,and Neurosurgery,Catholic University School of Medicine,L.A.Gemelli 8,00168 Rome,Italy.

Recent reports have indicated increased dopaminergic(DA)activity in patients with PRL-secreting pituitary microadenomas and have suggested that increased DA activity is induced by augmented PRL secretion from the adenomatous cells via a short loop feedback.We have studied the PRL and TSH responses to DA receptor blockade with metoclopramide(MCP,10 mg p.o.) in prolactinoma patients,both pre- and post-operatively,and patients with hypothalamic tumors(n.7),primary empty sella(n.7),lactating postpartum women(n.5)and normal female subjects(n.5).PRL responses to MCP were normal in postpartum women,normal or increased in the empty sella syndrome,absent in hypothalamic tumors and prolactinomas.A TSH response(greater than 0.5 μU/ml)was present in patients with microprolactinomas and absent in the other groups of patients.Postoperatively,in all prolactinoma patients with prolonged clinical remission and normal PRL dynamic tests TSH did not respond to MCP (n.11).In 7 patients with normal or borderline PRL levels in the immediate postoperative period,the TSH response to MCP disappeared,but became evident later together with progressive elevation of PRL levels.TSH increases after MCP occurred in all patients who had abnormal PRL levels after surgery. These results confirm the existence of increased DA activity in patients harbouring a microprolactinoma.The TSH test after MCP administration can readily detect after surgery increased DA activity in prolactinoma patients even when PRL levels remain normal or borderline,and thus predict persistence or recurrence of the disease.

207 HYPOTHALAMIC-PITUITARY FUNCTION IN HYPERPROLACTINEMIC MALE MICE.

A. Bartke*, W.W. Morgan, R. Clayton, T.A. Parkening and T.J. Collins, Depts. of Ob/Gyn and Anat., Univ. of Texas Health Sci. Center, San Antonio, TX 78284; Dept. Med., Univ. Birmingham, Birmingham B15 2TH, Great Britain; and Dept. Anat., Univ. Texas Medical Branch, Galveston, TX 77550.

In humans and in rats, hyperprolactinemia (hyperPRL) is associated with suppression of gonadotropin release. However, in mice with hyperPRL, plasma LH and FSH levels are elevated rather than suppressed. To identify mechanism(s) which may be responsible for these differences, we have examined the effects of two ectopic pituitary isografts on several indices of hypothalamic, pituitary and testicular function in adult DBA/2J male mice. Pituitary-grafted animals had elevated plasma PRL ($P<.01$), LH ($P<.025$) and FSH ($P<.005$) and enlarged seminal vesicles ($P<.01$). Testicular and pituitary weights and pituitary content of GnRH receptors were not altered. Turnover rates of dopamine (DA) and norepinephrine (NE) in the median eminance (ME) were estimated from DOPA accumulation after treatment with NSD-1015, an inhibitor of L-aromatic amino acid decarboxylase, and from depletion of NE after administration of U-14,624, an inhibitor of DA-β-hydroxylase. HyperPRL increased the turnover of DA ($P<.001$) and NE ($P<.001$). The increase in DA turnover fits well with the ability of PRL to stimulate tuberoinfundibular dopaminergic neurons, but the increase in NE turnover was opposite from the effects of hyperPRL in the rat. Thus, species differences in gonadotropin response to hyperPRL may be related to divergent effects of PRL on hypothalamic adrenergic neurons. In the mouse, increase in ME-NE turnover probably mediates stimulatory action of hyperPRL on LH and FSH release. (Supported by HD 12671.)

208 A SUCCESSFUL BROMOCRIPTINE TREATMENT IN HABITUAL ABORTION IN CASES OF PREOVULATORY TRANSIENT HYPERPROLACTINEMIA.

M. Ben-David and R. Bornstein, Department of Pharmacology and Obstet. & Gynec. Hebrew Univ. - Hadassah Medical School, Jerusalem, Israel.

Most cases of habitual abortion (HA) have chromosomal abnormalities, uterine defects or inadequate C.L. function. However, about 15% of HA cases are still of unexplained cause. The possible association between the idiopathic HA and the preovulatory transient hyperprolactinemia (TH) (J Clin Endocr & Metab, 57: 442, 1983) was studied in thirty patients who have had multiple (3-8) consecutive first trimester miscarriages. Serum E_2 and iso-prolactin-B (SPRL) levels were determined at mid-follicular phase, during the period around ovulation and at mid-luteal phase. Twenty five out of thirty (83%) of these patients exhibited an evident preovulatory E_2-provoked-TH detected during at least two cycles that randomly monitored prior to treatment. To prevent elevation of SPRL, individually adjusted doses of bromocriptine were given to all patients, and when pregnancy was confirmed in sixteen patients, treatment was not stopped and patients were kept under a low dose during the entire period of pregnancy. So far nine patients gave birth to healthy babies. Other five are presently in various stages of advanced pregnancy and only two patients (12.5%) aborted at the end of the fifth month. These results indicate that in certain patients with HA, the egg exposure to a high SPRL may have destructive effects on processes that take place in the decidua-chorio-aminon complex, the prevention of which, results in a successful pregnancy in the vast majority of cases.

209 Treatment of hyperprolactinaemia with a new dopamin agonist CU 32-085 (Mesulergin)

J. Beyer*, D. Oppermann, U. Schaffner, J. Happ, U. Krause, E. del Pozo, Department Internal Medicine, Endocrinology and Metabolism, University Mainz, FRG, and Department Experimental Therapeutics Sandoz Ltd., Basle, Switzerl.

CU 32-085 (Mesulergin) is an 8α-amino-ergoline with a 5 times higher prolactin((PRL)-inhibiting potency than bromocriptine and with low incidence of side effects. In this open study the efficacy and toleration of CU 32-085 was studied by the treatment of patients with prolactinomas. Furthermore, the influence of prolonged suppression on tumor development will be investigated.

22 patients with prolactinomas were treated for 8 to 14 months with daily doses of CU 32-085 ranging from 0.5 to 15 mg. To gain indentical suppressive effects we needed 3 to 10 times higher doses of bromocriptine than with Mesulergin. The toleration of Mesulergin was clearly better than that of bromocriptine. Most side effects disappeared under therapy with Mesulergin. Only in 2 patients the normal PRL-level was not reached, because of a history of servere complications under bromocriptine (bradycardia, circulatory collapse, apoplectic stroke).One of these 2 patients showed normal PRL-levels with 5 mg Mesulergin on some occasions. The basal PRL-levels from the other patients decreased to normal. No case of tumor progression occured. In single cases, however we found a dramatic normalisation of the PRL-values and a tumor regression.

210 STUDIES ON THE MODE OF ACTION OF MUSCARINIC AGONISTS ON PROLACTIN AND GROWTH HORMONE SECRETION. B.L. Brown*, R.J.H. Wojcikiewicz and P.R.M. Dobson. Dept of Human Metabolism & Clinical Biochemistry, University of Sheffield Medical School, Beech Hill Road, Sheffield S10 2RX, UK.

It is known that muscarinic cholinergic agonists stimulate growth hormone secretion and inhibit prolactin secretion from normal rat pituitary cells. In an attempt to elucidate the respective modes of action of these agents on mammotrophs and somatotrophs we have studied the possible role of the adenylate cyclase-cyclic AMP system. Normal and tumour (GH_3) anterior pituitary cells, cultured for three days in the presence or absence of dexamethasone and triiodothyrone (T_3), were incubated with or without cholinergic agonists. Prolactin and growth hormone in the medium and cyclic AMP in the cell layer were assayed by radioimmunoassay. Oxotremorine caused a decrease in cyclic AMP accumulation in normal as well as in tumour cells. Growth hormone release from normal cells was stimulated whereas the release of prolactin was inhibited. However, the release of both hormones from GH_3 cells was decreased. The effect on cyclic AMP was more pronounced in GH_3 cells (possibly reflecting the heterogeneity of normal pituitary tissue) and was blocked by atropine. This lowering of cyclic AMP was also abolished by pertussis toxin (which uncouples inhibition of adenylate cyclase). Pre-treatment of cells with dexamethasone/T_3 had little effect on the response to oxotremorine but did lower the EC_{50} of the stimulatory effect of GHRF on cyclic AMP accumulation. These results indicate that the inhibitory effects of muscarinic agonists on prolactin secretion are mediated by an inhibition of adenylate cyclase activity in both normal and tumour cells.

211 GALACTORRHEA IN NORMOPROLACTINEMIC AMENORRHEIC WOMEN.PROPOSED MECHANISMS FOR ITS APPEARANCE.

A.Hernández Bueno*,H.Porias,C.Salazar,(Spon:V.Cortés Gallegos)Reproductive Endocrinology.Hospital General de Mex.SSA,Mex Cty.(Durango 290-607,Mex 06700,DF)

Still there is no explanation for the appearance of galactorrhea in normoprolactinemic(NPRL)amenorrheic women.We have found some possibilities in the literature.1.-Isoprolactines 2.Stress(latent hyperprolactinemia(HPRL)3.Previous HPRL.4.Receptor disturbances.5.Local influences at the mammary gland.In order to clarify some pathophysiological aspects,we compared 2 groups of 5 patients.I NPRL and II HPRL.The general clinical aspects of both groups were amenorrhea,chronic anovulation,galactorrhea and no evidence of pituitary tumor.A minimum of 6 basal samples for each patient showed in I:PRL9.4$\pm$5.6ng/ml($\bar{x}\pm$SD)vs51.3$\pm$27in II. LH:47$\pm$37mIU/ml vs15.9$\pm$6.3for I&II respectively.E1&E2 levels did not reveal statistical differences in both groups with aE1/E2ratio greater than 1.A 10mgIV bolus of metoclopramide(MCP)elicited(Δ %)inI;LH72.7andPRL3654vsII;LH43&PRL189.One week later2.5mg bromocriptine was given orally with no significant changes for LH during 4hrs.and a depression of PRL occurred in both groups,without statistical differences.Dopamine(DA)is exerting a very important inhibitory role on the lactotroph in I in comparison with II.So far that this overrole of DA on the lactotroph could be an"escape"that modify the levels of PRL at the time of the study resulting in normoprolactinemia.Indeed we are not able to assume or discard the possible theories enunciated before.By the other hand,DA seems to inhibit the GnRH neurons in both groups according with the LH behaviour.

212 EFFECTS OF PROSTAGLANDIN D_2 ON SECRETIONS OF ANTERIOR PITUITARY HORMONES.

Masayoshi Arisawa*, Tsunehisa Makino, Toranoshin Ohno, Masaki Shiina, Shun-ichiro Izumi, Takashi Seki and Rihachi Iizuka, Department of Obstetrics and Gynecology, School of Medicine, Keio University, Tokyo, Japan

Prostaglandin D_2(PGD_2), which is highly concentrated in the rat hypothalamic-pituitary axis, was investigated for its effects on pituitary hormone secretions from the rat anterior pituitary in vitro and in vivo. More than 200 µg of PGD_2/ml induced a marked increase of cyclic adenocine 3', 5' monophosphate (cAMP) formation in the anterior pituitary and this effect was observed within 10 minutes after stimulation by PGD_2. The increase of cAMP continues for at least 30 minutes after stimulation. In contrast, PGD_2 did not affect pituitary cyclic cytidine 3',5' monophosphate (cCMP) formation at any dose. Significant increases in the release of luteinizing hormone and follicle-stimulating hormone were observed when the anterior pituitaries were incubated for 4 hours in vitro in the presence of 500 µg PGD_2 /ml. In contrast, more than 100 µg PGD_2/ml significantly suppressed the secretions of prolactin and growth hormone in vitro. In the second experiment, intravenously administered PGD_2 significantly suppressed the serum PRL levels but little affected the serum LH, FSH GH levels and hypothalamic contents of LHRH at the doses of 250 and 500 µg/animal. These results indicate that PGD_2 directly stimulates LH and FSH secretions and also directly suppresses PRL and GH secretions from rat anterior pituitary. The mechanism of these effects of PGD_2 could be mediated in part by cAMP formation, but not by cCMP formation.

213 ARACHIDONIC ACID (AA) METABOLISM INVOLVEMENT IN PRL AND LH RELEASE FROM THE PITUITARY GLAND: IN VITRO STUDIES. D. Conte°, P. Falaschi^, A. Proietti^, R. D'Urso^, F. Citarella, F.G. Conti, M. Motta^^, A. Isidori^, Cattedra di Andrologia and ^Clinica Medica V, University of Rome, ^^Cattedra di Fisiologia, Ist. di Endocrinologia, University of Milan, Italy.

AA metabolites seem to be involved in the control of pituitary hormone release. It is unclear if some metabolites, prostaglandins (PGs) and leukotrienes (LKT) in particular, play their role at hypothalamic or pituitary level, or both. The action of AA and of its derivatives directly at the pituitary level was studied in a system of male rat adenohypophyseal cells isolated and dispersed in perfusion. Both PGE_2 and $PGF_{2}\alpha$ in the eluate showed a dose-related rise after the addition to the perfusion medium of increasing AA doses (0.05, 0.16 and 0.3 mM). These data suggest that adenohypophyseal cells metabolize AA into its prostanoid derivatives. AA, added at the same doses, stimulates PRL secretion (from 5 to 15, 20 and 50 ng/ml respectively). AA exerts on LH secretion a stimulatory effect which is maximal (from 50 to 4000 ng/ml) at the lower dose of 0.05 mM (rPRL and rLH kits, NIAMDD, USA). Using the association of AA with 0.05 mM indomethacin (IND), inhibitor of PGs synthesis, the action on PRL release is highly potentiated (from 2.5 to 320 ng/ml). No significant modifications were observed using either AA with 0.05 mM nordihydroguaiaretic acid (NDGA), inhibitor of LKT synthesis, or with both inhibitors. IND and NDGA failed to modify PRL and LH levels. In presence of 0.05 mM IND the stimulatory action of AA on LH release is more evident (from 50 to 5000 ng/ml); AA + NDGA or AA + both inhibitors exert on LH release an effect similar to that observed on PRL. LKT could play a stimulatory role both on PRL and LH secretion at the pituitary level.

214 FAMILIAL MALE PSEUDOHERMAPHRODITISM (FMP) IN A TURKISH VILLAGE DUE TO 5α-REDUCTASE DEFICIENCY (5α-RD). S. AKGÜN*, N.H.ERTEL, J.IMPERATO-McGINLEY, B.S. ŞAYLI and C.SHACKLETON. VAMC, E.ORANGE, UMDNJ N.J., CORNELL MED COLL. N.Y.; ANKARA U., TURKEY; OAKLAND CHILDREN'S HOSPITAL, OAKLAND, CA.

FMP due to 5α-RD in the Dominican Republic was described in 1974 by Imperato-McGinley, et al. We identified another isolated community with FMP in southern Turkey and studied 8 of 13 affected males ages 5-56. Adults studied were raised as females; one was married to a man. After puberty they developed male gender identity and libido, deepening of the voice, and male musculature of varying degree. There was no temporal hairline recession and scanty facial and pubic hair. The phallus was 1.5-5 cm in 5 adults. They all had pseudovaginal perineoscrotal hypospadias. The testes, when descended, were of normal size and consistency. Buccal smear for chromatin bodies in subjects 4 and 5 was negative. Chromosome analysis in patient 2 was XY. Plasma T_4 and TSH were normal.

(*Brothers)		PLASMA					URINARY 5B/5α-METABS.	
	Age	LH	FSH	T	DHT	T/DHT	11BOH E/A	THE/alloTHF
(Nl values)		(0-9)	(2-10)	(300-950)	(30-70)	(8-17)	(0.1-0.6)	(0.8-1.5)
1	24	35	34	141	7	20	--	--
2*	34	41	18	1636	20	81	--	--
3	56	13	27	666	13	51	--	--
4*	36	13	6	632	15	42	1.6	12.5
5	44	30	34	220	8	28	3.3	14.3

The elevated T/DHT and urinary 5B/5α ratios and the clinical findings are compatible with FMP due to 5α-RD in a second community. The Dominican Republic disorder is autosomal recessive; the genetics of the Turkish pedigree may be different and is currently under investigation.

215 ACUTE SHBG RESPONSE TO TESTOSTERONE IN THE ANDROGEN INSENSITIVITY SYNDROME.
A.Belgorosky and M.A. Rivarola*, CEDIE,Hospital de Niños, B.A., Argentina.

Adequate distinction between an abnormality in androgen secretion or in target cell response is important in the diagnosis of male pseudohermaphroditism. We have studied the acute response of serum SHBG to exogenous testosterone (T) in a control group, in 6 patients with various abnormalities of gonadal function but normal male external genitalia, and in 8 patients with the androgen insensitivity syndrome (AIS). The diagnosis of AIS was made in 46 XY patients with 2 testicles and female external genitalia, who, after puberty, developed large breasts in the absence of clinical signs of virilization, despite of male serum T levels between 309 and 1228 ng/dl.Two mg/kg body weight of T enanthate was given im and blood was taken 1 week later for serum T and SHBG determination. Results are given as % of basal values. In 8 control subjects with serum T below 100 ng/dl, SHBG decreased to 64.4 ± 8.03 % ($\bar{X} \pm$ SD). In 6 subjects with male external genitalia and hypogonadism, SHBG dropped to 54.2 ± 20.2 %. In 4 patients with AIS and low serum T because of castration, SHBG ranged between 90 and 124 % of basal, while in another 4 patients with male adult levels of serum T, SHBG ranged between 100 and 131 % of basal after exogenous T. It is concluded that patients with AIS don't decrease their serum SHBG after exogenous T as normal subjects or patients with hypogonadism do. This different biological response could be used as a clinical test of androgen sensitivity.

216 REPRODUCTIVE HORMONES AND INITIATION OF PUBERTY IN THE FEMALE DOG.
P.K. Chakraborty*, A.P. Stewart, and D.R. Knab, Dept. of Obst. and Gyn., Uniformed Services University of the Health Sciences,Bethesda,MD 20814,USA

Hormonal regulation of initiation of puberty was studied in 12 purebred Labrador bitches between weaning (8 wks.) and the first behavioral estrus. Blood samples were collected 3 times weekly until proestrus and once daily thereafter until one week following cessation of estrus. Serum samples were analyzed for luteinizing hormone (LH), estradiol (E_2) and progesterone (P) concentrations by radioimmunoassay. Age of puberty and durations of proestrus and estrus were recorded. In addition to the examination of individual animals, all data were aligned to the day of first preovulatory LH surge (Day 0) and analyzed with respect to the first estrus. Episodic release of LH of varying magnitude (range 5-40 ng/ml) and duration was detected in all animals from weaning until 5 wks. prior to Day 0, occuring at decreasing frequency with the approach of puberty. Three significant elevations in mean E_2 were detected between 24 and 20, 16 and 12 and again beginning at 4 wks. prior to Day 0 (range 25-55 pg/ml). Post-weaning episodic release of greater than basal level of P (>1 ng/ml) was detected in all animals. A sustained rise in mean P was detected starting at 20 wks. before estrus which did not reach basal concentration until 4 wks. prior to Day 0 (range 2-9.5 ng/ml). The age at puberty ranged from 10 to 16 months and the mean durations of proestrus and estrus were 4.1 and 5.4 days, respectively. The data suggest that continued episodic release of LH can cause preovulatory lutenization; ovulation can occur without the expression of estrus; and sustained exposure to P is a prerequisite to the initiation of puberty in the female dog.

217 CYCLIC CHANGE IN ACTIVATION OF HUMAN ENDOMETRIAL PROGESTERONE RECEPTOR.

M. Asai*, Y. Sagara and Y. Takeda, Dept. of OB/GYN, Kochi Medical School, Kochi 781-51, M. Ito and H. Okada, Kyoto Prefectural University of Medicine, Japan.

Since activation is required for the effectve binding of progesterone receptor(PR) to chromatin, the evaluation of capability of PR to be activated seems to be important for predicting the response of target tissues to progesterone(P). We have investigated whether the capability of human endometrial PR to be activated shows cyclic change during menstrual cycle in cell-free system. Cytosolic PR from endometrium on various days in menstrual cycle was labeled with ^{3}H-P. Then, the labeled PR was processed for the activation at 0°C, low ionic strength and neutral pH, where it can be activated for chromatin binding more effectively than by heating at 25°C. The activated PR was estimated by its affinity for ATP on ATP-sepharose column chromatography. Because the activated PR showed markedly higher affinity for ATP than non-activated PR and the increased binding to ATP paraleled that to chromatin. Freshly prepared PR in human endometrium had little affinity for ATP through menstrual cycle. However, following the activation maniplation, the PR in the mid secretory phase showed markedly high affinity for ATP, whereas the PR in the proliferative phase did not.

Our data indicate that although unoccupied cytosolic PR determined by dextran-charcoal method was highest in the late proliferative phase, this PR has little capability to be activated. And it was suggested that the action of P may be regulated by not only quantitative but also qualitative change of cytosolic PR in human uteri through menstrual cycle.

218 COMPARISON OF UTERINE NUCLEAR ESTROGEN RECEPTORS (ER) BOUND TO [^{3}H] ESTRADIOL (E_2) OR [^{3}H] 4-HYDROXYTAMOXIFEN (OH TAM).

B. Attardi* and K. Happe, Dept Physiology, Univ Pittsburgh Sch Med, Pittsburgh, PA, U.S.A.

Our previous results demonstrating a difference in the sedimentation rate of nuclear ER labeled by in vitro exchange with [^{3}H] E_2 (predominantly 3 S) vs [^{3}H] antiestrogens (4 S) suggested that these complexes might exist in alternative conformations differentially susceptible to endogenous proteases. We have further characterized uterine nuclear ER labeled by exchange with [^{3}H] E_2 or [^{3}H] OH Tam. Both ligands bound with high affinity to nuclear ER (K_d's: 0.34 and 0.96 nM for [^{3}H] OH Tam and [^{3}H] E_2, respectively), and the number of binding sites was equivalent (473 and 501 fmol per uterus). Complexes between nuclear ER and [^{3}H] E_2 or [^{3}H] OH Tam dissociated with biphasic kinetics at 0° or 23°C in the presence of excess DES and had similar half-lives. The 3S and 4S forms of nuclear ER had mol wts of 33K and 54K and axial ratios (for prolate ellipsoids) of 2.5-3.0 and about 4.0, respectively. Neither in vitro labeled form bound appreciably to calf-thymus DNA-cellulose (~3%); in contrast, about 30-40% of the nuclear ER labeled in vivo with [^{3}H] E_2 or [^{3}H] OH Tam (4.5-5.0 S) was retained on DNA-cellulose columns, eluting with ~ 0.22M KCl. In conclusion, (1) the properties of the ligand-binding site on uterine nuclear ER are similar whether this site is occupied by E_2 or OH Tam; (2) nuclear ER labeled in vivo with [^{3}H] E_2 or OH Tam have comparable affinities for non-specific DNA; (3) processing of nuclear ER by nuclear extracts leads either to predominantly 33K (E_2) or 54K (OH Tam) species, both of which appear to have lost the DNA-binding site.

Supported by NIH grant 1 R01 HD12099.

219 IN THE PLASMA MEMBRANE OF XENOPUS LAEVIS OOCYTES, PROGESTERONE BINDS TO A 30kDa "RECEPTOR", AND SPECIFICALLY INHIBITS THE PHOSPHORYLATION OF A 48kDa PROTEIN.

J.P. Blondeau*, and E.E. Baulieu, INSERM U 33, Lab. Hormones, 94270 Bicêtre, France.

The meiotic maturation of Xenopus laevis oocytes is induced in vitro by progesterone (P), hormone released in vivo at the time of ovulation, and by many other steroids. Neither an intracellular receptor nor transcriptional events are implicated, and the steroid interaction occurs at the cell surface. Using ^{3}H-R 5020, a synthetic progestagen, we covalently photo-labeled proteins in vitellin envelopes, yolk platelets, melanosomes, microsomes, nuclei, cytosol and the 10^3-10^4 g pellet (p-10,000) fraction. Only in p-10,000 was P binding to a 30kDa peptide demonstrated, using competition studies and SDS-PAGE. The apparent Ki was ∿ 4 μM, compatible with the active hormone concentration inducing maturation. Binding specificity of steroids and analogues was highly correlated with their maturing activity, as expected for a true "receptor". In vitro p-10,000 phosphorylation by ^{32}P-ATP revealed, after SDS-PAGE, a 48kDa peptide, the phosphorylation of which was specifically inhibited by P, while protein phosphatase activity was unchanged. Half-maximum inhibition occured with ∿ 8 μM P. The potent agonists, testosterone and deoxycorticosterone inhibited 48kDa phosphorylation whereas the non-agonist cholesterol did not. Phosphorylation was not affected by cAMP, cGMP, polyamines, calmoduline and phospholipids + diolein. Ca^{2+} was inhibitory. These results, together with the previously reported inhibition of p-10,000 adenylate cyclase activity by P substentiate an alternative pathway of steroid action in plasma membrane of target cells.

220 ENHANCED END-ORGAN SENSITIVITY TO STEROID HORMONES IN VITAMIN B_6 DEFICIENCY

J F Bowden, D A Bender, W F Coulson* & E K Symes
The Courtauld Institute of Biochemistry, London W1P 5PR

There is enhanced tissue and nuclear uptake of [^{3}H]testosterone into the prostate of vitamin B_6 deficient rats and the circulating testosterone is lower in the deficient animals even though the circulating LH and the weight of the prostates are unchanged. This suggests an enhanced target organ sensitivity to steroid hormones in vitamin B_6 deficiency. We have now studied the uptake and retention of [^{3}H] oestradiol into the uterine cytosol and nuclear compartments in vitamin B_6 deficient and control rats at different phases of oestrus. Except in anaphase, there was a greatly enhanced nuclear uptake in the deficient animals in the first hour and in prooestrus and oestrus there was a very much greater retention at 8 hours. This supports the view that pyridoxal phosphate is involved in the recycling of the receptor from the nucleus. Also ovariectomised rats were treated with different doses of ethinyl oestradiol for 4 days, the uteri were removed, and the peroxidase activity determined. In both control and deficient animals there was a good correlation between administered dose of ethinyl oestradiol and peroxidase activity. The deficient animals showed greater sensitivity to uterine peroxidase induction, the activity being twice as high as in the controls on the highest dose. (3μg/kg body wt./day). Plasma LH was also more markedly depressed by low doses of ethinyl oestradiol (25 ng/kg body wt./day) in the deficient animals. These results confirm the enhanced oestogen sensitivity of target tissues in vitamin B_6 deficiency.

221 DISTRIBUTION OF ANDROGEN-BINDING SITES WITHIN THE OVINE OVARIAN FOLLICLE.

Stella Campo*, Ronald Carson and Jock Findlay, Medical Research Centre, Prince Henry's Hospital, Melbourne, Australia, 3004.

Interaction of androgens with target cells is thought to be mediated by extracellular androgen-binding proteins (ABP), cytoplasmic androgen receptors (AR) and possibly plasma membrane androgen-binding sites. We have studied the distribution of androgen-binding sites in the ovine follicle. Serum, follicular fluid and granulosa cytosol and particulate (membrane 27000xg pellet) fractions were pretreated with charcoal to remove endogenous steroids. Follicular fluid and serum exhibited similar affinity (5-20 x 10^{-9}M) and capacity (600 fmol/mg) for ^{3}H.T and ^{3}H.dHT but did not bind appreciable quantities of ^{3}H.R1881, a synthetic androgen. Granulosa particulate fractions bound ^{3}H.T and ^{3}H.dHT with comparable capacity but with 10-fold greater affinity than that of follicular fluid and serum, but did not bind ^{3}H.R1881. Granulosa cell cytosol bound ^{3}H.R1881 (Kd = 2.7 x 10^{-9}, 84 fmol/mg) in addition to ^{3}H.T and ^{3}H.dHT. Displacement times of 50% bound ^{3}H.T from serum (2 mins) and granulosa particulate fraction (30 mins) were different from that required for displacement of ^{3}H.R1881 from granulosa cytosol (>24h). Specificity of each fraction for each androgen was also different, follicular fluid T ≃ dHT > R1881, granulosa particulate dHT > T > R1881; granulosa cytosol R1881 > T ≃ dHT. Whereas androgen-binding sites in serum and follicular fluid are similar and most probably represent ABP, those of granulosa particulate fractions are distinct from both ABP and AR in granulosa cytosol. The effects of androgens on ovarian follicles might be modulated by the relative distribution of specific androgen-binding sites within the follicle.

222 ESTRADIOL-RECEPTOR TRANSLOCATION AND SATURATION OF RAT UTERINE ACCEPTOR SITES IN VITRO IN MATURE AND AGED ANIMALS.

R. C. Chuknyiska*, M. Hall, R. H. Foote, G. S. Roth, Endocrinology Section, Clinical Physiology Branch, NIA, NIH, Baltimore City Hospitals, Baltimore, MD 21224.

Binding of Estradiol-receptor complex (E_2R), purfied from rat uteri with CNBr activated agarose according to the Kon and Spelsberg procedure (Endrocinology 111 1925, 1982), to isolated nuclei is saturable and sensitive to circulating estrogen levels *in vivo*. Saturation was achieved at 3-4fmol E_2R/mg DNA. Mature (7-10 months) and old (24 months) Wistar rats were used in the experiments. E_2R translocation was performed during the incubation of 100 µl nuclei (50-100 µg DNA) and 200 µl purified cytosol (0.3-6.0 fmol E_2R) at room temperature (22°C) with intermittent vortexing. The saturation time for both age groups was about 90 min. Four different combinations of cytosol-nuclear mixtures were examined: mature cytosol-mature nuclei; old cytosol-old nuclei; mature cytosol-old nuclei; old cytosol-mature nuclei. No age differences in the binding affinity of E_2R for nuclei were found. Ka's for both mature and old rats were about 3.2-3.8x10^9 $M^{(-1)}$ and Kd's were found to be between 2.6-3.2x10^{-10}M. However, the number of nuclear acceptor sites, calculated from Scatchard plots was found to vary with the age both the E_2R and nuclei. Mature E_2R-mature nuclei mixture exhibited Bmax=2.0mol/mg DNA. For all other combinations in which old E_2R or old nuclei were present B max's were lower: 1.3±0.2 1.5±0.1x10^{-12} mol/mg DNA. The present data demonstrate that there is a decrease in the number of acceptor sites in old nuclei and some deficiency in the old E_2R which are not able to bind to all available acceptor sites in young nuclei.

223 THE EFFECTS OF TAMOXIFEN ON STEROID RECEPTORS IN THE HUMAN PROSTATE.
J. Albert*, J. Geller, J. Liu, P.-K. Ku Tai and L. Faber, Mercy Hospital and Medical Center, San Diego, California 92103 and Medical College of Ohio, Toledo, Ohio 43669.

Estrogen synergizes with androgen to produce benign prostatic hypertrophy (BPH) in the dog, and estrogen increases nuclear androgen receptor (AR), a potentially important event in the pathogenesis of BPH. Because of the potential relevance of these findings to human BPH, we have studied the putative role of estrogen in regulation of nuclear AR, as well as estrogen (ER) and progesterone receptors (PR) in patients administered an anti-estrogen, tamoxifen (Tm, 20 mg b.i.d.) for ten days prior to prostate resection. Using published methods, we measured steroid receptors, PR, ER, and AR in cytosol and nuclear preparations of these resected prostate tissues. Blood levels of Tm were 200-500 picomoles/ml at the time of surgery. Statistically significant decreases ($P < 0.05$) were found in cytosol PR (159 femtomoles/mg DNA in 12 Tm-patients vs. 308 in 10 control patients) and in nuclear AR (123 fmol/mg DNA in 16 Tm-patients vs. 273 in 15 controls). Cytosol AR was unchanged (257 fmol/mg DNA in 15 Tm-patients vs. 346 in 17 controls, $P > 0.6$), ruling out recycling of NAR. Nuclear PR was always undetectable, mitigating against translocation of CPR by Tm. ER (53 fmol/mg DNA in 6 of 15 patients, not detected in 9) may be decreased in prostate cytosol by Tm (not detected in 5 of 5 patients). These results indicate that estrogen has a role in the biological regulation of steroid receptors in the human prostate. This study was supported by NIH Grants Nos. CA 18003-08 and AG-02776.

224 PLASMA ANDROGEN ACTIVITY MEASURED BY RADIORECEPTORASSAY:METHOD AND CLINICAL APPLICATIONS:D.ARMANINI*#,I.KARBOWIAK,C.SCARONI,L.DE BESI,F.MANTERO, Istituto Semeiotica Medica,University of Padua,Italy.#Present address Medizinische Klinik Innenstadt,University Munich,West Germany.

Kidney cytosol from castrated mice was incubated with 2nM 3HRU1881 either with different amounts of cold RU1881 in stripped plasma or with the plasma of each patient.Incubations were 2h 4°C and separation by charcoal dextrane technique.Results are expressed as nM Eq RU1881.Evaluation of the method:RU1881 was used because its lack of binding to plasma proteins.The cross binding to glucocorticoid and progesterone receptors was negligeable in this assay model(no change of the Kd after addition 500fold excess triamcinolone).Intra and interassay variations were satisfactory.Results: normal subjects(n=10,mean$\pm$SD)male(M)1.7$\pm$0.6;female(F) 0.85$\pm$0.45.Single values in nMEq in human pathology:

		M	F
Cushing's	hyperpl.	2.2 1.4 1.3	7.1 3.9
syndrome	adenoma		4.2
21hydroxyl.	simple f.	8.0 4.6	5.0 2.9
deficiency	late onset		1.7 1.2 0.6 0.5
(21OHDS)	cryptic		3.5
11OHDS		5.1	
17OHDS		0.2	

Conclusions:this method can offer useful indications which are complementary with those obtained by RIA of androgens and by SSHBG determination,specially in cases with discrepancy between clinical and biochemical findings (e.g. "cryptic" 21OHDS, hirsutism, some forms of pseudohermaphroditism,etc).

225 HUMAN LIVER CONTAINS ANDROGEN AND ESTROGEN RECEPTORS. R.F. Aten*, A.J. Eisenfeld, Dept. of Ob/Gyn, Yale University School of Medicine, New Haven, CT 06510 and C.W. Beattie, Div. of Surgical Oncology, University of Illinois School of Medicine, Chicago, IL 60612, USA.

Sex steroids are known to influence the function of human liver. Human liver specimens, obtained during surgery from twenty one adult men and women, were examined for androgen, estrogen and progestin receptors. Some specimens were analysed shortly after surgery while others were frozen and studied later. All specimens were homogenized in a glycerol, sodium molybdate and monothioglycerol buffer. Specific binding was determined by incubating cytosols with ^{3}H-methyltrienolone (^{3}H-MT), ^{3}H-moxestrol (^{3}H-MOX), or ^{3}H-promegestone (^{3}H-PROM). All liver cytosols examined contained ^{3}H-MT (androgen) and ^{3}H-MOX (estrogen) binding. There was no sex difference in these binding levels. The ^{3}H-MT specific binding averaged 38 ± 3 femtomoles/mg protein with a K_d of 1.0 ± .1 nM. The specificity pattern was consistent with androgen receptor. Of note, some progestins (including norethindrone, norgestrel and medroxyprogesterone acetate) reduced the ^{3}H-MT binding. The ^{3}H-MOX specific binding averaged 2.3 ± .3 femtomoles/mg protein with a K_d of 1.8 ± .4 nM. The specificity pattern was consistent with estrogen receptor. In comparison to the high levels of ^{3}H-MT binding only low or negligible levels of ^{3}H-PROM specific binding were observed and the properties were not consistent with progestin receptor. In conclusion, human liver contains cytosol androgen and estrogen receptors. We suggest that progestins may act in the liver via the androgen receptor. The progestin and estrogen interactions with these liver receptors may be of particular importance in contributing to the side effects of oral contraceptives. (Supported by HD8280)

226 EFFECT OF DITHIOTHREITOL ON THE KINETICS OF INTERACTION OF DEXAMETHASONE WITH MAMMARY CYTOPLASMIC GLUCOCORTICOID RECEPTOR. R.H. Buell*, L.O. Wosu and G. Shyamala, Lady Davis Institute for Medical Research, Jewish General Hospital, Montreal, Quebec, Canada H3T 1E2.

Lactating mouse mammary gland cytosol requires sulfhydryl reducing agents such as dithiothreitol (DTT) to elicit maximal binding of ^{3}H-dexamethasone to the native glucocorticoid receptor. Little is known, however, about the possible effects of DTT on the kinetics of dexamethasone-receptor interaction. Therefore, we have examined these parameters for the untransformed complex formed with near saturating concentrations of ^{3}H-dexamethasone (50 nM) in the presence and absence of 20 mM DTT. There was little difference in the association rate constants: 3.1±0.07 $\times10^5$ $M^{-1}min^{-1}$ in the presence and 4.1±0.06$\times10^5$ $M^{-1}min^{-1}$ in the absence of DTT (mean±S.E.). When dissociation was initiated by removal of free steroid by charcoal stripping, there was little difference in the dissociation rates with a $t_{\frac{1}{2}}$ of 21.5±0.3 hours in the presence and 19.0±1.2 hours in the absence of DTT. When dissociation was initiated by the addition of excess unlabeled dexamethasone, however, a monophasic dissociation was seen in the presence of DTT with a $t_{\frac{1}{2}}$ of 5.2±0.1 hours while in the absence of DTT a biphasic curve was obtained. The first, relatively small component (11±3%) had a $t_{\frac{1}{2}}$ of 5.7±0.6 hours while the major component had a $t_{\frac{1}{2}}$ of 17±0.3 hours. Since the $t_{\frac{1}{2}}$ differed with the two methods used for dissociation, it suggests the binding of dexamethasone to the receptor may include site-site interactions, detectable with DTT.
(Supported by a grant from the Medical Research Council of Canada)

227 NUCLEAR BINDING AND BIOLOGICAL ACTIVITY OF DEXAMETHASONE MESYLATE IN HUMAN CELLS. J.A. Cidlowski, T.M. DeLorenzo, and R.E. Susek. Departments of Physiology and Biochemistry, Univ. of North Carolina, Chapel Hill, NC 27514

Nuclear glucocorticoid receptors from HeLa S_3 cells have been labeled *in situ* with the site specific affinity label [^{3}H]dexamethasone mesylate ([^{3}H]DM). Nonsaturable binding of [^{3}H]DM to non-receptor proteins was minimized by using low ($2x10^{-8}$M) ligand concentrations. The accumulation of saturable [^{3}H]DM receptor was temperature dependent. At 0°C ≈ 1000 [^{3}H]DM receptors were measured in nuclei and at 37°C ≈ 13,000 were found. Nuclear [^{3}H]DM receptor was effectively extracted (≈80%) with either 10mM pyridoxal phosphate or 0.4M KCl. Polyacrylamide gel analysis and western blotting revealed a single polypeptide having a molecular weight of ≈90,000 kDa. The isoelectric focusing pattern of nuclear [^{3}H]DM receptors differ substantially from that observed for cytoplasmic receptors. Cytoplasmic [^{3}H]DM receptors which are equal in mass exist in at least 4 forms displaying microheterogeneity in isoelectric points (pI 6.5-8.0). In contrast nuclear [^{3}H]DM receptors appear as a distinct more basic species having a pI of ≈ 8.1. Analysis of the biological activity of dexamethasone mesylate indicates that dexamethasone mesylate fails to alter basil alkaline phosphatase activity in HeLa S_3 and effectively inhibits the production of this enzyme by glucocorticoids. We conclude that: 1) the human nuclear glucocorticoid receptor can be effectively *in situ* affinity labeled with [^{3}H]DM, 2) the [^{3}H]DM receptor exists as a single polypeptide, 3) nuclear [^{3}H]DM receptors are equal in mass to cytoplasmic forms, but are more basic and less heterogeneous in charge, 4) dexamethasone mesylate behaves as a glucocorticoid agonist despite temperature dependent activation and nuclear accumulation. Supported by AM32440.

228 IMMUNOCHEMICAL PURIFICATION OF AFFINITY-LABELED GLUCOCORTICOID RECEPTOR. Laura P. Eisen[*+], Marsha E. Reichman[+], Bahiru Gametchu[§], Robert W. Harrison[§] and Howard J. Eisen[+], [+]LDP, NICHD, NIH, Bethesda, MD 20205 USA; [§]Vanderbilt University School of Medicine, Nashville, TN 37232.

We have used a monoclonal antibody to purify the glucocorticoid receptor from rat liver. Ammonium sulfate-precipitated rat liver cytosolic fractions were treated with [^{3}H]dexamethasone 21-mesylate to label covalently the glucocorticoid receptor. The fractions were treated with hybridoma (BuGR1) tissue culture supernatants containing the monoclonal antibody, and were "batch" adsorbed to protein A-Sepharose. The covalently labeled receptor was subsequently purified by preparative polyacrylamide gel electrophoresis (0.1% sodium dodecyl sulfate). The denatured, reduced M_r ≅ 98,000 receptor and the H and L chain of the antibody were the major proteins detected on Coomassie-blue stained gels. The receptor band was sliced from the gel and was electroeluted with a yield of ~50%. In order to isolate proteolytic fragments of the receptor, we treated unpurified cytosolic fractions with protease and then used immunoadsorption and polyacrylamide gel electrophoresis. V_8 protease digestion of crude preparations produced multiple covalently-labeled receptor fragments. Only those covalently-labeled fragments of M_r >45000 reacted with the monoclonal antibody. These methods are suitable for large-scale purification of the glucocorticoid receptor and proteolytic fragments that contain the immunoreactive region.

229 BOTH TYPE 1 AND TYPE 2 ALDOSTERONE RECEPTORS OF TOAD BLADDER ARE INVOLVED IN THE MINERALOCORTICOID RESPONSE.

M. Claire* , K. Geering , J.L. Steimer , M.E. Oblin and B.C. Rossier , INSERM U.36, 17 rue du fer-a-moulin, PARIS 75005, FRANCE.

The physiological response to aldosterone by the toad bladder is characterized by 1) an increase in the transepithelial Na^+ transport (NAT), 2) a fall in the transepithelial resistance (R) and 3) an increase in the biosynthesis rate of Na-K-ATPase (KNATPA). Initially we analysed by mathematical modeling the kinetics of cytoplasmic and nuclear aldosterone uptake in intact bladder at 25°C for various aldosterone concentrations. The model involved 2 types of cytoplasmic aldosterone receptors which were precursors of the chromatin bound nuclear aldosterone receptor-complexes. Nuclear translocation was assumed to obey first order kinetics. This model achieved a satisfactory fit to the experimental data. We have examined the relationship between the physiological responses (NAT, R and KNATPA) and the steady-state chromatin occupancy as a function of aldosterone concentration predicted from this model for each type of receptor-complexes. NAT was measured by the technique of short circuit current and KNATPA biosynthesis by using monospecific antibodies. A linear relationship was observed between R and KNATPA and both responses were closely related to chromatin occupancy by the high affinity type 1 receptors. In contrast, NAT was related to occupancy of both type 1 and type 2 sites contrary to accepted opinion that only the type 1 receptors mediates the mineralocorticoid response. Our results suggest that both types of aldosterone receptors are involved in the full mineralocorticoid response.

230 INSULIN-STIMULATED RECEPTOR CYCLING AND INSULIN ACTION IN RAT ADIPOCYTES.

G. Arsenis*, G. Hayes and J. Livingston. Univ. of Rochester, Rochester, N.Y.

Insulin (I) is known to cause internalization of its own receptor. It is not known however if I-receptors recycle back to the cell surface and are coupled to cell effector systems. Adipocytes incubated in the presence or absence of 0.1 μM I for 30 min at 37° were treated with pronase (0.5 mg/ml for 30 min at 12°) which destroys > 95% of cell surface I receptors. I-binding studies with Triton X-100 solubilized cells showed an increase in internal receptors from 10% of total receptor content (control) to 20% with I treatment. Warming pronase-treated cells to 37° (5 min with 0.1 mM cycloheximide) allowed reinsertion of receptors into the cell surface; control cells had 8% of original surface receptors whereas I-treated cells had 16%. Thus, receptors internalized after I-treatment are returned to the cell surface. Studies of I action were used to examine the functional integrity of the cell surface receptor after its reinsertion following pronase treatment. Control cells (8% of original receptors) had a marked rightward shift in the I-dose response curve for the stimulation of glucose incorporation into lipids (ED_{50}=1900 μU/ml) compared to normal cells not treated with pronase (ED_{50}=26 μU/ml); maximum I-response was depressed to 43% that of normal. In contrast, cells pretreated with 0.1 μM I before pronase had an ED_{50} value of 240 μU/ml with a maximum I-response of 77% that of normal cells. I-mediated antilipolysis was also studied and shown that I-pretreatment before pronase generated a more I-responsive cell in agreement with the studies of glucose metabolism. Conclusion: I-treatment rapidly drives I receptor into the cell interior. These receptors rapidly return to the surface and are coupled to cellular effector systems. The changes in I dose-responses are consistent with spare receptor theory.

231 INSULIN-BINDING TO ERYTHROCYTES IN NEWLY DIAGNOSED TYPE I DIABETES MELLITUS TREATED WITH CYCLOSPORINE. M.T. Behme*, J. Dupre, C.R. Stiller, M. Jenner, P. Keown, N.W. Rodger and B.M. Wolfe, University Hospital and University of Western Ontario, LONDON, Ontario N6A 5A5 Canada.

To investigate the effect of treatment with insulin and cyclosporine on insulin receptors, the binding of 125-I-insulin to erythrocytes was examined in newly diagnosed type I diabetics during immunosuppression; 18 patients developed non-insulin requiring remission and 21 continued to receive insulin, with maintained target control of glycemia in both groups. Blood samples from fasted subjects were treated with hypaque-ficoll gradient to isolate erythrocytes. For the patients in remission, total specific binding was 8.7 ± 1.66% and did not differ significantly from that for insulin-dependent patients (8.3 ± 2.47%); however, the concentration of unlabelled insulin required to decrease binding by 50% was 4.4 ± 1.07 ng/ml, significantly lower than that for insulin-dependent patients (6.0 ± 1.17 ng/ml, p 0.001). Blood levels of cyclosporine did not differ between the two groups. In previous studies, specific binding was 9.8 ± 1.4% in normal subjects and 8.9 ± 1.6% in long-term type I diabetics; 50% inhibition occurred at 4.1 ± 0.96 and 5.6 ± 2.64 ng/ml, respectively. These results suggest that exogenous insulin or other factors affect the affinity but not the number of insulin receptors in newly diagnosed diabetes mellitus during cyclosporine treatment.

232 MAJOR ROLE OF PLASMA MEMBRANE IN INSULIN DEGRADATION BY INTACT HEPATOCYTES. W. G. Blackard*, C. Ludeman and J. Stillman, Department of Medicine, Medical College of Virginia, Richmond, Virginia, U.S.A.

Bacitracin, a surface active antibiotic which inhibits insulin degradation by membrane proteases, was incorporated into either the association phase or the dissociation phase media, bathing cultured primary rat hepatocytes in monolayer. During the 90 min association phase the hepatocytes were exposed to ^{125}I-Insulin and degradation into TCA-soluble products was assessed during a 60 min dissociation period. Extra-cellular degradation was negligible. At 37°, bacitracin inhibited insulin degradation by 50% or more with a compensatory increase in release of TCA-precipitable hormone. At 15°, bacitracin inhibited insulin degradation by 80%, but without the compensatory increase in release of TCA-precipitable hormone. Bacitracin's effect on insulin degradation at 37° was observed only if bacitracin was present during the dissociation (phase when degradation assessed), whereas at 15° the antibiotic had a much more potent effect when present in association media. These findings suggest that at 37° bacitracin-inhibitable insulin degradation accounting for over 50% of degradation takes place on the membrane after either primary binding or diacytosis. At 15°, bacitracin-inhibitable degradation probably begins on the membrane but requires internalization for sequential degradation to TCA-soluble products. The fact that chloroquine as well as bacitracin inhibits degradation by 80% at this temperature suggests involvement of a chloroquine-sensitive pathway at 15° which is not required at 37°.

233 EVIDENCE FOR GASTRIC INHIBITORY PEPTIDE (GIP) RECEPTORS IN THE CULTURED HAMSTER INSULINOMA CELL LINE, IN 111. B. Amiranoff,* N. Vauclin-Jacques and M. Laburthe, INSERM U.55, CNRS ERA 494, Hôpital Saint-Antoine, 75012 Paris, FRANCE

The mechanism of GIP action on insulin release is unknown. In the present work, we demonstrate the presence of specific GIP receptors in a insulin-secreting pancreatic tumor cell line, In 111. The specific binding of ^{125}I-GIP is dependent on time, temperature and cells concentration. Under steady state conditions, i.e. at 10°C, for 2 hours and with 10^6 cells per assay, specific binding of the tracer is inhibited by native GIP in the concentration range between 10^{-10} - 10^{-6} M, half maximal inhibition being induced by 1 nM GIP. No other peptide of the gastrointestinal tract interacts with GIP binding sites. Scatchard analysis indicates the presence of two types of binding sites, a high affinity ($K_D = 4 \times 10^{-10}$ M)/ low capacity (10^3 sites/cell) site and a low affinity ($K_D = 10^{-7}$ M)/high capacity (10^4 sites/ cell) site.

GIP is able to stimulate cyclic AMP production in the In 111 cells. At 37°C, in the presence of IBMX, GIP is active in the 10^{-9} - 10^{-6} M range of concentration with a maximal 3 fold increase of basal level . Half maximal stimulation is observed in the presence of 5 nM GIP. In conclusion, those data provide the first evidence arguing for a direct physiological action of GIP on a insulin-secreting β cell. Furthermore, the evidence for a GIP receptor coupled to a cyclic AMP production system in the In 111 cell line provides a unique tool to further investigate the regulation by GIP of insulin secretion. This is currently under investigation. (We thank Dr. Uchida for his generous gift of In 111 cells).

234 INSULIN DOES AND HUMAN GROWTH HORMONE (hGH) DOES NOT STIMULATE PHOSPHORYLATION OF ITS RECEPTOR. K. Asakawa*, G. Grunberger, A. McElduff, and P. Gorden. Diabetes Branch, NIADDK, National Institutes of Health, Bethesda, Maryland 20205 U.S.A.

Insulin stimulates phosphorylation of a tyrosine specific artificial substrate, poly(GluNa,Tyr) 4:1, casein and histone H2b in the presence of partially purified plasma membranes of cultured human lymphocytes (IM-9). Since these cells also contain hGH receptor, we incubated hGH (5×10^{-11} to 5×10^{-6}M) with membranes derived from 2 - 8 x 10^9 IM-9 cells with the same exogenous substrates. Unlike insulin, hGH had no effect on phosphorylation. Similarly, hGH did not stimulate phosphorylation of poly(GluNa, Tyr) 4:1 by lectin purified rat liver membrane preparation, while insulin (10^{-7}M) increased phosphorylation four-fold. When the partially purified IM-9 plasma membrane preparation was preincubated with hGH, phosphorylated in the presence of Mn^{++}, and processed by SDS-polyacrylamide gel electrophoresis under reducing conditions, and autoradiographed, there was no effect of the hormone on any phosphorylated protein in the region of hGH receptor. Crosslinking experiments using disuccinimidyl suberate demonstrated the hGH receptor to migrate as an ∿140K protein. In contrast, insulin markedly stimulated phosphorylation of a 95K protein, known to correspond to the β-subunit of its receptor. Thus under these experimental conditions, hGH does not stimulate phosphorylation of either endogenous or exogenous substrates by the IM-9 plasma membrane preparation. While hGH and the growth promoting peptides (insulin, IGF, EGF, and PDGF) share several common features, i.e. receptor binding and internalization, receptor phosphorylation did not appear to be required for these early common steps.

235 MODULATION OF PITUITARY ANGIOTENSIN II RECEPTORS BY ESTRADIOL.
P.D. Carrière*, A. De Léan, J. Gutkowska, J. Genest and M. Cantin, MRC Hypertension Group, Institut de Recherches Cliniques de Montréal, Montréal, Québec, H2W 1R7, Canada.

Recently, angiotensin II has been shown to directly stimulate the secretion of prolactin. Since estrogens are known to be important modulators of pituitary cell function, we proposed to study the effect of estradiol treatment on the angiotensin II receptor in the anterior pituitary. We report here the use of a radiolabeled antagonist: $[^{125}I]$ (Sar^1, Ile^8) angiotensin II $[^{125}I]$ SARILE to measure angiotensin II (AII) receptors in target tissues of male and female rats under different hormonal states. Castrated male and female rats were injected daily with 25 μg of estradiol valerate for 1 and 2 weeks. AII receptors were measured in the homogenates of anterior and posterior pituitary. Specific AII binding was undetected in the posterior pituitary. Within 1-2 weeks, estradiol treatment had markedly reduced the density of AII receptors in the anterior pituitary of both male (60%) and female (80%) castrated groups with no significant change in the affinity for $[^{125}I]$ SARILE. Preliminary results suggest that the *in vivo* responsiveness of lactotrophs to AII stimulation is paradoxically enhanced by estradiol treatment. Furthermore, initial results indicate that following two weeks of estradiol treatment, AII receptors were reduced in the adrenal cortex of both male (35%) and female (45%) castrated rats. These data suggest an important modulatory role of estrogens on the effect of AII on anterior pituitary function. This study was supported by the MRC.

236 PHYSICOCHEMICAL PROPERTIES OF THE PITUITARY GnRH RECEPTOR. M. C. Carson*, K. Hirota, and M. Iwashita. ERRB, NICHD, NIH, Bethesda, MD 20205, U.S.A.

Pituitary GnRH receptors have been solubilized by extraction with 5 mM CHAPS and shown to retain the binding affinity ($6.7 \times 10^9\ M^{-1}$) and specificity of the original membrane sites. We also observed higher binding of the potent GnRH antagonist, ^{125}I-[Ac-D-p-Cl-Phe^{1,2},D-Trp^3,D-Lys^6,D-Ala^{10}] GnRH, than of radioiodinated GnRH agonists to solubilized receptors and relatively greater stability of the solubilized receptors. During gel filtration under non-denaturing conditions, both free and prelabeled receptors behaved as high molecular weight species with M_R of about 700,000. The CHAPS-solubilized receptor also behaved as a high molecular weight species on sucrose density gradient centrifugation, with a sedimentation coefficient of about 10S. To compare the holoreceptor with its binding subunits, and to compare the binding sites in different species, GnRH receptors in rat, mouse, and rabbit pituitaries were analyzed by photoaffinity labeling using ^{125}I-[N$^{\varepsilon}$-azidobenzoyl-D-Lys^6]-des-Gly^{10}-GnRH-N-ethylamide. After photolysis of the specifically bound photoaffinity label, SDS-PAGE on 5-15% polyacrylamide gels showed two major bands of $M_R \approx 60,000$ and 40,000 in rat and rabbit pituitary membranes, and major and minor bands of M_R 53,000 and 37,000, respectively, in the mouse pituitary. These results demonstrate that the subunit nature of the GnRH receptors, as well as their biochemical functions, are similar in the various species studied, and that at least two components with binding activity can be detected in the multimeric GnRH receptor.

237 GROWTH HORMONE INDUCES ITS OWN RECEPTORS IN BOTH MALE AND FEMALE RAT LIVER. Robert C. Baxter*, Zena Zaltsman and John R. Turtle, Department of Endocrinology, Royal Prince Alfred Hospital and Department of Medicine, University of Sydney, NSW, Australia.

We recently described hepatic GH receptor induction in intact female (F) rats by homologous GH (rGH) infusion, and in rats of both sexes bearing GH-secreting tumors. This contrasts with reports of down-regulation of GH receptors by rGH in male (M) rats. To resolve the question of sex differences we have measured GH receptors in normal (N) and hypophysectomized (H), M and F rats with or without rGH or rPRL replacement (NHPP, 200μg/day for 7 days). Liver microsomal membranes were desaturated with 3M $MgCl_2$ prior to binding studies using bovine GH tracer. The effect of hypophysectomy on specific bGH binding (% of total radioactivity) in rats not receiving infusions (n=10-12) was: 2.98±1.41 (N-F) vs 1.08±0.73 (H-F) [$p<0.001$] and 1.91±0.65 (N-M) vs 1.46±0.68 (H-M) [not signif.]. However without $MgCl_2$ stripping, there was an apparent 3-fold higher binding in H-M vs N-M ($p<0.001$). Infusion of rGH, which significantly ($p < 0.001$) increased immunoreactive somatomedin-C in H, but not intact, M and F rats, caused increases in binding in all 4 groups to 7.63±2.14 (N-F), 6.79±2.24 (H-F), 4.68±1.37 (N-M) and 5.37±2.50 (H-M) [all highly signif. vs no rGH], while rPRL infusion had no effect in N rats and a diminished effect in H rats. This study indicates that rGH is a potent inducer of GH receptors in M and F rats, that the effect is not mediated by somatomedin-C, and suggests that the reported apparent down-regulation by rGH in males may have been due to receptor occupancy. Supported by NH&MRC Australia.

238 ADRENAL INVOLVEMENT IN THE LOSS OF HEPATIC GH AND PRL RECEPTORS IN DIABETIC FEMALE RATS. J.M. Bryson* and R.C. Baxter. Department of Medicine, University of Sydney and Department of Endocrinology, Royal Prince Alfred Hospital, Sydney, N.S.W., Australia.

Both somatogenic (GH) and lactogenic (PRL) receptors are decreased in female rat livers following streptozotocin (strz) induction of diabetes, and are restored to normal levels by treatment with insulin. We have reported that the loss of receptors is accompanied by an increase in serum testosterone (T) which is also normalized by insulin therapy. Since adrenalectomy (adx) prevents the rise in T levels in diabetic (D) female rats, we have now investigated the effect of adx on the receptor loss in female Wistar Furth rats. Diabetes was induced by 100mg/Kg strz i.v. Bilateral adx was performed 3d after the induction of diabetes; control (C) rats were sham-operated. All rats were killed 3d after adx. Binding of bGH to microsomal membranes decreased by 66% (C:3.1±1.0%, D:1.0±0.4%, p 0.001) in diabetic animals and binding of oPRL by 56% (C:18.0±3.2%, D:9.9±2.8%, p 0.001) This was accompanied by a 2.5-fold increase in serum T levels (C:2.1±0.5nM, D:5.4±1.5nM). Adx had no effect on GH or PRL receptors or serum T levels in C animals but prevented the fall in oPRL binding in diabetic animals and partially prevented the fall in bGH binding (adx-D:2.0±0.6%, 33% below controls, p 0.01). Serum T returned to control levels. The fall in serum somatomedin-C (SM-C) levels seen in diabetes was also partially prevented by adx with a strong correlation seen between bGH binding and SM-C levels (r=0.759, p 0.001). It is concluded that changes in GH and PRL receptors in diabetes are mediated by the adrenals. Supported by NH&MRC and Kellion Diabetes Foundation.

239 CHARACTERIZATION OF 3,5,3'-TRIIODO-L-THYRONINE BINDING SITE ON PLASMA MEMBRANE FROM HUMAN PLACENTA. R. Alderson*, I. Pastan and S.-y. Cheng, Laboratory of Molecular Biology, National Cancer Institute, Bethesda, Maryland 20205.

The binding of 3,5,3'-[^{125}I]triiodo-L-thyronine ([^{125}I]T_3) to sites on human placenta plasma membranes was characterized and the binding site was solubilized following affinity labeling with N-bromoacetyl[^{125}I]T_3 (BrAc-[^{125}I]T_3). Two classes of T_3 binding sites were detected. One class has a high affinity (k_d = 2.0 nM) and a low capacity (321 fmol/mg protein); the other has a low affinity (k_d = 18.5 μM) and a high capacity (2.2 pmol/mg protein). The binding sites were found to be specific for T_3 in that other thyroid hormone analogues (D-T_3, reverse-T_3, D-thyroxine, L-thyroxine) were less effective in displacing the bound [^{125}I]T_3. BrAc[^{125}I]T_3 was found to specifically label a protein with an apparent molecular weight of 65,000 as determined by SDS-PAGE. The BrAc[^{125}I]T_3 labeled protein was solubilized with the detergent, 2 mM 3-[(3-cholamidopropyl)dimethylammonio]-1-propane sulfonate. The apparent molecular weight of the labeled, solubilized protein was found to be between 140,000 and 150,000 by Sephadex G-200 gel filtration. These data demonstrate that a high affinity binding site specific for T_3 is present on plasma membranes obtained from human placenta and that the binding site is a protein, most likely a dimer with a native molecular weight between 140,000 and 150,000. The physiological significance of the membrane T_3 binding sites is now under investigation.

*Supported by NIH research fellowship #1 F32 NS07002-01A1.

240 Peripheral Dopamine Receptors: Characterization of Dopamine Receptors In Renal Cortical Homogenates and Tubules, and Adrenal Glomerulosa and Myocardial Homogenates. F.W.J. Beck* and J.R. Sowers V.A. Medical Center and Medical College of Virginia, Richmond, VA 23249

There is increasing support for the existence of a peripheral dopaminergic system modulating cardiovascular function and sodium homeostasis. Accordingly, we have attempted to characterize dopamine receptors in rat kidney, adrenal glomerulosa and myocardial tissue using H^3-Spiroperidol bind. Specific binding was defined as total H^3-Spiroperidol binding minus nonspecific binding in the presence of 10^{-5}M butaclamol. The results are expressed as means ± SEM:

Tissue	K_d (nM)	Bmax (fmole/mg prot.)
Renal Homogenates	(1) 1.19±0.26	86±16
	(2) 5.41±0.79	253±34
Renal Tubules	1.55±0.48	68±8
Adrenal Glomerulosa	1.40±0.17	48±19
Myocardium	1.91±0.30	158±23

These studies indicate that there are high affinity dopamine receptor binding sites in rat renal cortical, adrenal glomerulosa, and myocardial tissue. The presence of two distinct binding affinities in renal cortical homogenate probably reflects binding at renal tubule as well as vascular binding sites. Thus, dopaminergic regulation of such physiological events as renal blood blow, natriuresis, inhibition of aldosterone secretion and myocardial contractility are probably affected through dopamine binding to high affinity binding sites in these tissues.

241 ESTROGENIC AND ANDROGENIC EFFECTS OF DEHYDROEPIANDOSTERONE (DHEA) IN MICE.

W. G. Beamer*, E. H. Leiter, and D. L. Coleman, The Jackson Laboratory, Bar Harbor, ME 04609, USA

Potent anti-hyperglycemic effects in genetically-diabetic mice are mediated by either 17β-estradiol (E2) administered in the diet or SC injection or by DHEA (effective in diet only). Dietary testosterone (T) or dihydrotestosterone were minimally effective. To determine whether the palliative effects of DHEA might be mediated via its conversion to E2 through T, we studied the effects of DHEA, E2, and T on sex steroid target tissues in normal and gonadectomized C57BL/6J and C57BL/Ks mice. In ovariectomized females, dietary or implanted E2 restored uterine wet weights and vaginal cytology to typical estrus conditions. Dietary or implanted T gave a proesterus-like effect on these parameters. Dietary DHEA (0.4%) resulted in a profuse vaginal cytologic pattern (leucocytes, nucleated and cornified epithelia) and a diestrus-like uterine weight. Thymic weights in normal females were twice that of males. Male castration eliminated this sex difference. DHEA feeding to gonadectomized mice yielded intermediate weights for both sexes. Serum T in ovariectomized females following DHEA feeding, but not implantation, was significantly increased. Preliminary data for serum E2 also indicated substantial increases. The threshold for the increased E2, but not T, levels was 0.2% DHEA. This was also the threshold for strong anti-hyperglycemic action. Since genetically diabetic female mice fed DHEA showed the same stimulation of the above-cited parameters, we conclude that DHEA administration by diet but not by implantation may exert its anti-hyperglycemic action via conversion to estrogen.

242 CARBON MONOXIDE INHIBITION OF ANDROSTENEDIONE AROMATIZATION BY PURIFIED RECONSTITUTED ESTROGEN SYNTHETASE (AROMATASE) FROM HUMAN TERM PLACENTAL MICROSOMES.

F.Bellino*and J.Lobo,Dept.Biol.Sci.,SUNY/Buffalo,NY 14260 USA

The inability to demonstrate carbon monoxide (CO) inhibition of androstenedione (A) aromatization in placental microsomes was attributed to either low steady-state levels of cytochrome P-450 (P-450) reduced heme iron-substrate complex (Thompson&Siiteri, J.Biol.Chem.,1974) or to reduced P-450 affinity for CO caused by A (Juchau et al.,BBRC,1975). The aromatase stimulation after mixing with purified NADPH-cytochrome c reductase(Bellino J.Ster.Biochem.,1982) suggests that reductase is rate-limiting in placental microsomes, thereby possibly limiting the entry of the first electron into the P-450 hydroxylation cycle. The dependence of the relative ratio of reductase/P-450 on the ability of CO to inhibit A aromatization was tested using reconstituted aromatase: purified NADPH-cytochrome c reductase(Bellino,see above) and partially purified P-450 (cholate solubilized,purified thru octyl Sepharose and DEAE-cellulose) from placental microsomes, and phosphatidylcholine. Neither protein fraction individually exhibited aromatase activity, but in combination gave an aromatase specific activity of about 500 pmol/min/mg prot. The reconstituted system was incubated at two different reductase/P-450 in the absence and presence of CO (CO/O_2=10) with constant % O_2. At low reductase (aromatase proportional to reductase) and saturating reductase, CO inhibited A aromatization by 12 and 26%,respectively. Microsomal aromatase was not inhibited under identical conditions. Therefore,the ability of CO to inhibit reconstituted aromatase appears to depend primarily on the reductase/P-450. However modifications of the P-450 due to solubilization and purification cannot be excluded. Supported by grant HD 16593 from U.S.D.H.H.S.-Nat. Inst. of Health

243 CORRELATION OF PEAK LUTEAL PHASE SALIVA PROGESTERONE (P_4) WITH OVARIAN FOLLICULAR VOLUMES. N. Besch*, W. Gibbons, I. Rossavik, and P. Besch, Reproductive Research Laboratory, St. Luke's Episcopal Hospital and Department of Ob/Gyn, Baylor College of Medicine, Houston, TX 77030, USA.

Ten women underwent serial ultrasound determinations of ovarian follicular size to determine the day of ovulation. Both natural and clomiphene-stimulated cycles were studied. Follicular volumes were determined on the day prior to ovulation (peak follicular volume) by taking the average of three diameters (one in each plane). The total follicular volume was the sum for all follicles greater than 1.0 cm in size. Saliva specimens were collected daily during the luteal phase starting on the day of ovulation. Saliva was kept frozen after collection, centrifuged after thawing to remove debris, and the supernatant assayed. Duplicate 0.5 ml aliquots were extracted twice with 3.0 ml of diethyl ether. Quantification was by RIA using a ^3H-P_4 label and charcoal separation. Peak saliva P_4 concentrations varied between 250 and 1400 pg/ml and were in the range of 300 pg/ml per follicle (averaging 318 $\pm$ 103 pg/ml) with no differences noted for stimulated (n = 6) versus natural (n = 4) cycles. The correlation coefficient for the relationship between peak luteal P_4 secretion in pg/ml and total follicular volume was 0.75 which was significant at the level of $p < 0.02$. In conclusion, there is a relationship between follicle size and luteal P_4 secretion. Saliva collections are non-invasive and can be done at home resulting in high patient acceptance for daily sampling. Since the concentration of P_4 in saliva can be correlated to ovarian function its determination may have practical clinical usefulness.

244 PROGESTINS BLOCK DNA SYNTHESIS IN UNSTIMULATED NEONATAL MOUSE UTERINE EPITHELIUM. R.M. Bigsby* and G.R. Cunha, Dept. of Anatomy, University of California, San Francisco, CA, USA, 94143.

It is known that the tissues of the neonatal mouse uterus proliferate rapidly and that the rate of DNA synthesis is not affected by ovariectomy plus adrenalectomy (Ogasawara, et al, Endocrinology 113:582, 1983). We have examined the effects of progesterone (P) and medroxyprogesterone acetate (MPA), injected as a suspension i.p., on DNA synthesis in 5 day old mouse uteri by 3H-thymidine (3H-TdR) autoradiography. Twenty-four hr after P administration (0.4-40 mg/kg) the thymidine labelling index (L.I., percent cells labelled 1 hr after 3H-TdR injection i.p.) of uterine epithelium is reduced in a dose dependent manner, stromal cell L.I. is not affected. Following P (40 mg/kg) injection, L.I. decreases progressively after an initial 1.5 hr lag, reaching nadir after 16 hr. This time course suggests that the cells are inhibited early in the G1 phase of the cell cycle, similar to the P effect observed in the estrogen-stimulated adult uterus. MPA maintains the block to epithelial L.I. but had no effect on stromal cell L.I. during a 72 hr experimental period. These results suggest that progestins have a direct effect on uterine epithelial DNA synthesis; therefore, inhibition of estrogen-stimulated adult epithelial proliferation may be a result of this direct effect rather than due to interference with the mechanism of estrogen action.

245 INHIBITION OF ESTROGEN METABOLISM IN MICROSOMAL AND HEPATOCYTE INCUBATIONS.
R.W. Brueggemeier*, J.G. Kimball and F. Kraft, College of Pharmacy and OSU Comprehensive Cancer Center, The Ohio State University, Columbus, Ohio 43210, USA.

The abilities of inhibitors and other agents to alter the metabolism of estradiol and the irreversible binding of estradiol to proteins were examined in microsomal and intact hepatocyte incubations. In studies with rat liver microsomal preparations containing estradiol and an NADPH-generating system, 2-bromoestradiol and 4-bromoestradiol were effective inhibitors of estrogen 2-hydroxylase, with K_i's of 2 μM, and also decreased the irreversible binding of radiolabeled steroid metabolite(s) to the microsomal proteins. In addition, these haloestrogens were effective inhibitors in intact hepatocyte cells, decreasing the amounts of organic metabolites, aqueous-soluble conjugates, and protein-bound materials. Ascorbic acid and cysteine, nonspecific modifiers of oxidative pathways of metabolism, also affected estradiol metabolism in microsomal and hepatocyte incubations. However, neither agent was able to decrease the irreversible binding of estrogen to proteins. Investigations of steroid metabolism in the isolated hepatocytes thus provide an effective in vitro technique for examining the overall oxidative, reductive, and conjugative pathways that are functional in the liver and enables one to investigate the abilities of inhibitors, regulators, and modifiers to affect the metabolic processes. Also, these hepatocyte studies demonstrate that the bromoestrogens, inhibitors of estrogen 2-hydroxylase, can enter and act in the intact cell. Consequently, these agents may be useful pharmacological probes for examining the functions of catechol estrogens in other tissues.

246 MODE OF MAINTENANCE WITH GONADOTROPIN INFLUENCES THE RESPONSE OF THE LEYDIG CELL TO ESTRADIOL IN THE HYPOPHYSECTOMIZED RAT.
D. B. Barr and D. K. Pomerantz*, MRC Group in Reproductive Biology, Univ. Western Ontario, London, N6A 5C1, Canada.

The physiologic role of estradiol (E) in controlling testosterone (T) production via intratesticular mechanisms is not understood. A common experimental model is the hypophysectomized (HX) rat whose Leydig cell integrity is maintained by gonadotropin treatment. The effect of E treatment of such animals on T secretion is controversial and may be due in part to different experimental designs. We have administered luteinizing hormone (LH, 10 μg NIAMDD-24) and follicle stimulating hormone (FSH, 5 μg NIAMDD-15) daily via osmotic mini-pumps to HX rats. Infusion sites were s.c. or i.v. The animals also received empty Silastic capsules or capsule programmed to cause plasma concentration of E of 350 pg/ml. After 5 days the gonads were removed and in vitro T secretion in response to a maximal dose of LH was determined. I.V. infusion of LH/FSH caused a higher rate of basal ($P < 0.01$), but a lower rate of LH stimulated T secretion ($P < 0.05$). E inhibited both basal and stimulated in vitro T secretion when LH/FSH had been infused s.c. ($P < 0.001$) but increased basal and stimulated in vitro T secretion 2-fold when LH/FSH had been infused i.v. The data show that the nature of the LH/FSH stimulus used to maintain Leydig cell function in HX rats influences the response of the testis to E.

247 DEMONSTRATION OF AROMATASE IN A LEYDIG CELL TUMOR. Mark Brandt*, Stephen Zimniski, Michael Melner, Douglas Covey and David Puett. Vanderbilt Univ., Nashville, TN 37232, REPSCEND, Univ. of Miami School of Medicine, Miami, FL 33101, and Washington Univ., St. Louis, MO 63110.

Aromatase, the enzyme that converts androgens to estrogens, is found in many tissues, including normal testicular Leydig cells. Leydig cells have relatively high levels of estrogen receptors; however, the function of estrogen is difficult to study since these cells synthesize this steroid. We have used the Leydig cell tumor to study the function of this enzyme in testicular tumors in which estrogens are known to have an effect. The objective of these experiments was to verify the presence of aromatase activity in the M5480A murine Leydig cell tumor and compare it to that of human placenta. M5480A Leydig cell tumors, maintained by serial transplantation in C57BL/6J mice, were homogenized and microsomes prepared. The crude microsomal preparation was assayed for aromatase activity by following the production of tritiated water from ($1\beta,2\beta\ ^3H$) testosterone by the method of Rabe et al., (J. Steroid Biochem., 17: 305, 1982). The resulting activity was about 1/2000 that of a placental microsome preparation when expressed per mg microsomal protein. In vitro experiments with specific aromatase inhibitors, e.g. 10-Propargylestr-4-ene-3,17-dione, showed that the measured enzymic activity was inhibited in both preparations, thus confirming that the activity can be attributed to aromatase. This is the first report of aromatase activity in this tumor. The role, if any, remains to be elucidated. (Supported by NIH: GMO7319, CA23582, HD07129 and AM33973.)

248 IMPAIRMENT OF TESTICULAR FUNCTION OF THE MALE RAT PROVOKED BY A SINGLE LOW DOSE OF γ-IRRADIATION PRIOR TO SEXUAL MATURITY. A. Canfi* and E. Bedrak[+], Department of Radiochemistry, NRCN, and [+]Department of Biology, Ben-Gurion University of the Negev, Beer-Sheva 84120, Israel.

The testicular function of mature rats, exposed to a single low dose of γ-irradiation (Ir-192) prior to sexual maturation, was investigated. The rats were allocated according to the exposure-dose (1 or 5 Rentgen, R) and age on day of irradiation (5,6,7,8,9,17,27 and 42 days). Fertility trials were conducted with control young multiparous females and hormone analysis was carried out in the serum and adenohypophysis along with histological examination of the testes. The results indicated that a single dose of 1 or 5 provoked: 1) a decline (approx. 40%) in the reproductive capacity irrespective of the animal's age on day of irradiation; 2) a decrease in the testicular weight; 3) hyperplasia and hypertrophy of the Leydig cells coupled with aberrations of the seminiferous tubules; 4) an increase in serum concentration of testosterone ($P < 0.05$), FSH ($P < 0.05$), LH ($P < 0.05$), and prolactin ($P < 0.05$); 5) a decline ($P < 0.005$) in the prolactin content of the adenohypophysis with little effect on the gonadotropins content of the pituitary. In general the high serum testosterone level was compatible with the histological changes observed in the testes. In conclusion, exposure of the sexually immature rat to small doses of γ-irradiation induces alteration in the hypophyseal-testicular axis which lead to malfunction of the exocrine and endocrine moities of the testes once the animal reaches sexual maturity.

249 ARGININE VASOTOCIN STIMULATES CHOLESTEROL SIDE CHAIN CLEAVAGE ACTIVITY OF CULTURED RAT TESTICULAR CELLS. E.Y. Adashi* and C.E. Resnick, Division of Reproductive Endocrinology, Department of Obstetrics and Gynecology, University of Maryland School of Medicine, Baltimore, MD 21201, USA.

The neurohypophysial hormones were recently shown to exert direct and varied effects on testicular function, including a direct stimulatory effect on testicular progestin biosynthesis(J Biol Chem 257:1301, 1982). To further study this "progestin-stimulatory" activity, we examined the effect of treatment with arginine vasotocin(AVT) on testicular cholesterol side chain cleavage (CSCC) activity as estimated by the rate of conversion of 25-hydroxycholesterol to pregnenolone during a 5h incubation. Treatment of testicular cells from adult hypophysectomized rats for 72h with increasing concentrations (10^{-11}-10^{-6}M) of AVT, led to dose-dependent increments in CSCC activity with minimal,median and maximal effective doses of 3.6±0.4x10^{-10}, 6.2±0.8x10^{-9} and 2.1±0.4x10^{-7}M, yielding a maximal response 3-fold greater than control. The CSCC-stimulatory effect of AVT was time-dependent becoming significant ($P<0.05$) by 24h of treatment and peaking 48h thereafter. Similar effects were observed with related, naturally occurring, pressor-dominant(arginine and lysine vasopressin) but not oxytocic-dominant (oxytocin, mesotocin and isotocin) neurohypophysial principles. Significantly, concomitant treatment with increasing concentrations (10^{-10}-10^{-6}M) of the pressor-selective antagonist d(CH_2)$_5$Tyr(Me)AVP, led to dose-dependent blockade of AVT(5x10^{-9}M)-stimulated CSCC activity. These findings suggest that AVT exerts a direct stimulatory effect on CSCC activity via putative pressor-selective testicular recognition sites and that this effect may account, in part, for the "progestin-stimulatory" property of the neurohypophysial hormones. Supp: Frank C. Bressler Research Fund.

250 MEMBRANE FLUIDITY AND POLARITY CHANGES IN MAMMALIAN SPERMS DURING MATURATION AND CAPACITATION BY SPIN LABEL PROBES. P. Agrawal* D.C. Wharton, and M.J.K. Harper, Department of Life Sciences, D.A. Vishwavidhyalaya, Indore-452001, India.

The stearic acid spin labels, 5NS and 16NS, have been used as probes of the hydrocarbon portion of the membrane bilayer of rat and rabbit spermatozoa recovered from various portions of the male and female genital tract. These spin labels enter membranes and become oriented with the -COOH groups near the water:lipid interfaces. EPR spectra obtained with these labels show that they are quite strongly immobilized and bound in more than one environment. The degree of immobilization is determined by an empirical motion parameter (R_i) and the polarity of the local environment by calculation of the nitrogen hyperfine coupling constant (A_N). R_i falls noticeably when these labels are bound to spermatozoa from the epididymis (caput and cauda) and the ejaculate compared to ones from the testes. A_N is lower for testicular than for other more mature sperm. Thus, fluidity of the sperm membrane increases and the polarity of the environment decreases as sperm move from the testis to the ejaculate. When sperm are in the genital tract of the female, R_i declines further, but A_N is unchanged as they move from the vagina to the oviduct. Studies were also done with the spin label, Malnet, which probes proteins with reactive sulfhydryl groups. The increased immobilization during epididymal transport may indicate changes in protein conformation. The increased fluidity of the sperm membrane might be one of the important changes associated with the process of maturation and this may be an essential prerequisite for fusion.

251 ONTOGENY OF RAT TESTICULAR ANDROGEN PRODUCTION IN RESPONSE TO LUTEINIZING HORMONE AND ISOPROTERENOL IN VITRO. O.O. Anakwe* and W.H. Moger, Depts. of Physiology & Biophysics and of Obstetrics & Gynecology, Dalhousie University, Halifax, Nova Scotia, Canada, B3H 4H7.

The in vitro effects of the β-adrenergic agonist L-isoproterenol (Isop) and luteinizing hormone (LH) on androgen production by testes from fetal and postnatal rats was studied. Isop (10^{-4}) significantly increased androgen production 1.2-3.3 fold (stimulated/basal) on 18.5, 19.5, 20.5 and 21.5 days of fetal life and on 1, 15, 20, 30, 40 and 60 days of postnatal life during the 3 h incubation in medium 199. No response to the β-agonist was observed on days 6 and 10 of postnatal life. For the ages studied, LH (100 ng/ml) induced large increases (2.8-120.4 fold) in androgen production. Isop was 0.4-18.9% as potent as LH. The least, half-maximum (EC_{50}) and maximum increase in androgen production by testes from 20.5 day fetuses was induced by 10^{-8}, $4x10^{-7}$ and 10^{-5}M respectively. A time-lag of 30 min was needed for Isop (10^{-5}M) to induce a significant ($p \leq 0.01$) increase in androgen production. The response to the β-agonist (10^{-5}M) was abolished by a β-adrenergic antagonist propranolol (10^{-5}) indicating that the agonist effect is mediated via β-adrenergic receptors. The response to the β-agonist was also stereo-specific, since the D-isomer of Isop did not stimulate androgen production. The results suggest that catecholamines may play some important role(s) in testicular development, especially at fetal ages.

Supported by the MRC of Canada and a Nigerian Government Scholarship.

252 DEVELOPMENTAL CHANGES IN THE SYNTHESIS AND ACTIVITY OF CHOLESTEROL SIDE CHAIN CLEAVAGE CYTOCHROME P-450 (P-450scc) IN THE FETAL RABBIT TESTIS. C.M. Anderson* and C.R. Mendelson, Depts. Biochemistry., Ob-Gyn, and The Cecil H. and Ida Green Ctr. for Reprod. Biol. Sci., Univ. Texas Southwestern Medical School, Dallas, Tx., U.S.A.

Synthesis of androgens by the fetal testis is mandatory for the development of a normal male phenotype. In the rabbit, testicular testosterone content reaches a detectable level between 17-18 d of gestation, rises sharply until 21-22 d, and then declines (Wilson et al., Biol. Reprod. [1980] 22:9). Since the conversion of cholesterol to pregnenolone by P-450scc is an important site of regulation of steroid synthesis, we investigated the changes in the synthesis and activity of this enzyme in the fetal rabbit testis during the critical period of sexual differentiation. The relative concentrations of gonadal P-450scc at several gestational ages were determined by immunoblotting. P-450scc content was low at 19 d; the concentration rose to a maximal level 3 times the 19 d value at 24 d, then declined to a level 1.8 times the 19 d content at 31 d. P-450scc activity at 19 d was 0.6 pmol pregnenolone produced/min/mg gonadal protein. Enzyme activity reached a maximum at 21 d of 5.2 pmol/min/mg protein, and then declined rapidly to 0.1 pmol/min/mg protein at 29 and 31 d. Both the concentration and activity of testicular P-450scc followed developmental patterns similar to that described previously for testosterone content. The decrease in enzyme activity at 29 d to a nearly undetectable level, while enzyme content declined only slightly, is suggestive that synthesis of P-450scc in an inactive form or lack of available cholesterol may be responsible for the decrease in testosterone synthesis by the fetal testis late in gestation.

253 EFFECTS OF SERTOLI CELLS AND FSH ON LEYDIG CELLS ACTIVITY. ORGANIZATION OF THE TWO CELL TYPES IN VITRO.

M. Benahmed+, J.Reventos, P.Leduque, E.Tabone, and J.M.SAEZ. INSERM-U.162. Hôpital Debrousse ; Centre Léon Bérard and Faculté de Médecine Lyon-Sud. 69322 Lyon Cedex 05. France.

In order to precise the role of Sertoli Cells (SC) on Leydig Cells (LC) function, purified LC and SC from immature porcine testes were cultured alone or together on extracellular matrix coated dishes in the presence or absence of FSH. The activity (hCG binding sites number and hCG stimulated Testosterone (T) secretion), ultrastructural aspect of LC as well as the cells organization were studied. LC were identified by immunocytochemical visualization of hCG receptors and 3β-hydroxydehydrogenase staining while SC were identified by visualization of FSH receptors. The results indicate that: a) FSH had not effect on purified LC cultured alone, b) Coculture of SC with LC increased T production; addition of FSH further increased T production and increased hCG binding sites number; c) FSH pretreatment of the Coculture produced a marked development of the smooth endoplasmic reticulum and Golgi complex in LC; d) after 3-4 days the Coculture in the absence or presence of FSH was organized into "tubules-like" structures containing mainly SC while the LC were located in the "interstitial " space. In summary, our results clearly show a positif effect of SC on LC activity; the action of FSH on LC activity is mediated by SC. In addition, these data show that in our experimental conditions, cocultured SC and LC organize into structures similar to that observed in vivo.

254 OPIATE RECEPTOR BINDING IN RAT TESTIS.

C. Boitani*, C. Shaha, C.W. Bardin and E.F. Hahn, Population Council and Rockefeller University, New York, NY 10021

Pro-opiomelanocortin (POMC)-derived peptides have been shown to be present and synthesized in a number of tissues, such as pituitary gland, central nervous system, placenta, gastrointestinal tract. Recent immunocytochemical evidence have demonstrated that these peptides are also present in the testis of several mammalian species, and that they are localized in the Leydig cells, but not in Sertoli, myoid, epithelial and germ cells. Recently the effects of opiate antagoinst administration on Sertoli and Leydig cell functions have been described, suggesting that POMC-derived peptides might play a role in the regulation of spermatogenesis. We therefore investigated whether specific opiate receptors are present in the testis and their localization in different cellular compartments of testes from adult males.Since several subclasses of opiate receptor have been reported with a range of affinities for various ligands, we have used an antagonist which binds to all types of opiate receptor. Specific saturable binding of tritiated naltrexone was observed in crude membrane preparations from adult testis and in the interstitial tissue obtained after collagenase treatment. No significant binding was detected in the tubular compartment. The binding in total testis preparations amounted to 10-15% of that from brain preparations. These findings demonstrate the existence of opiate receptors in rat testis. These receptors are on or near the cells which contain immunoreactive POMC-like material, supporting the hypothesis that POMC-derived peptides may have autocrine and/or paracrine effects on the testis.

255 EVALUATION OF THE HYPOTHALAMIC-PITUITARY-TESTICULAR AXIS (HPTA) IN MEN WITH GRAVE'S DISEASE. Abelin,N.*, Nicolau,W & Mattar, E., Endocrinology Unit, - Medical School, University São Paulo - CP 8091 - São Paulo, Brazil.

HPTA was evaluated in 8 men with Grave's disease. Mean (ng/dl±SE) - dihydrotestosterone and total testosterone (T) were significantly ($P \leq 0,05$) higher (227±122 and 1425±275) than in control (C) group (37±14 and 580±149) Four patients presented high basal levels (> 60 pg/ml) of 17 B estradiol - (E_2). The mean total sperm cells counts in 5 patients was significantly - lower than in controls. All the patients had normal testicular volume and- do not presented gynecomastia. There was an inverse correlation between - basal levels of E_2 and sperm cells count (r= .80). Basal LH were significantly higher than controls and hyperresponded to 100mcg LHRH administra - tion. The mean FSH basal levels and its response to LHRH was normal. On - fluoximesterone (40mg/day for 5 days) the relative decrease of serum FSH - and T levels was not significantly different from controls and the decrease of LH levels (-91%) was significantly higher than controls (-50%). The relative increment of LH, (62%), FSH (43%) and T (47%), on clomifene citrate (200mg/day during 10 days) were comparable to those obtained in controls. These results suggest: 1) The genesis of the alterations concerning LH - behaviour founded in hyperthyroidism was not due to an inability of the - hypothalamic-pituitary system to respond to the negative feed-back effect- of androgen. 2) integrity of hypothalamic mechanisms involving LH secre - tion and 3) integrity of LH endogenous action on the testis.

256 PERIPHERAL T-LYMPHOCYTE SUBSETS BEFORE AND DURING CARBIMAZOLE THERAPY IN GRAVES'S DISEASE(G D) Y. ABRAMOVICI*, M. SIMONNEAU, G. NGUYEN, E. TERRIER and J. BAILLET, Hôpital BROUSSAIS Université PARIS VI, PARIS, FRANCE.

Since a variety of abnormalities in peripheral T lymphocyte subsets has been reported in patients with G D and since Carbimazole has been shown to interfere with the autoimmune process in G D, the purpose of this work was to study the time course of blood T-cell populations in patients with G D and Carbimazole therapy. Lymphocytes were isolated from peripheral blood by Ficoll-Hypaque gradient centrifugation, stained with the monoclonal antibodies OKT3, OKT4 and OKT8 and counted using an epifluorescent microscope. 14 patients with untreated hyperthyroid G D were compared to 13 normal subjects. Collectively, the patient population showed an increase in the mean ratio of helper to suppressor cells (mean ± SD : 2,25 ± 0,82 vs 1,83 ± 0,25) although the difference was not statistically significant. Compared to controls, only 5 patients exhibited significant (>2 SD) decrease in the percentage of suppressor cells and increase in the ratio of helper to suppressor cells. No correlation was found between these abnormalities and thyroid size, degree of eye involvement, serum thyroid hormone levels, presence or titer of antithyroglobulin or antimicrosomal antibodies and HLA antigens. The same parameters were evaluated during antithyroid drug therapy, with a 3 months follow-up in 10 Carbimazole-treated patients. In 2 patients the initial abnormalities in lymphocyte subsets were no longer detectable, while they persisted in 3 other patients. In 2 patients, transient disturbances of T-cells supervened. Values remained normal throughout the follow-up period in the remaining 3 patients. In the 2 cases with both antithyroid antibodies and abnormal T lymphocyte populations before Carbimazole, the evolution of T-cell subgroups did not parallel the changes in circulating antibody titers. These preliminary results stress the need for redefining G D in view of the heterogeneity in clinical and immunological features in individual patients. This heterogeneity might reflect a spectrum of pathogenetic mechanisms in G D and/or different steps in the autoimmune conflict, and thus provide an explanation for the variable changes in T-cell subsets in our Carbimazole-treated patients.

257 ABNORMAL TSH-BINDING IMMUNOGLOBULINS IN 3 PATIENTS WITH GRAVES' DISEASE. T. Akamizu*, H. Ishii, T. Mori, T. Ishihara, K. Ikekubo and H. Imura, 2nd Division, Department of Medicine, Kyoto University Faculty of Medicine 54 Shogoin Kawaharacho, Sakyo-ku, Kyoto 606, Japan

Among 379 patients tested, 3 male patients with active Graves' disease were found to have TSH-binding immunoglobulins (Ig) of high affinity by the thyrotropin binding inhibitor Ig (TBII) assay. These Igs gave extremely high polyethyleneglycol (PEG) precipitable radioactivities (69, 83 and 69 %), higher than the maximal specific binding (33%) in TBII assay. Such findings were detected even in the absence of TSH receptors. The addition of bovine TSH (bTSH) or human TSH (hTSH) resulted in a dose-dependent reduction of PEG precipitable radioactivity, though the latter was much less effective. Scatchard analysis using b-TSH revealed that Ig of one patient had the dissociation constant of 4.0×10^{-11} M and the maximum specific binding of 1.6×10^{-14}M/mg Ig. Gel filtration chromatography of patient sera followed by incubation with ^{125}I-bTSH showed that the 7S fraction was a major binding component. Immunoelectrophoresis and subsequent autoradiography using ^{125}I-bTSH revealed the TSH binding material as being the IgG with k-chain in patients studied. These patients were concluded to have anti-TSH antibody. Anti-TSH antibody with such a high affinity in Graves' patients seems to be a useful tool for studying the anti-idiotype antibody for TSH.

258 INCREASE OF T8 CELLS DURING TREATMENT COURSE AND IN REMISSION IN A PROSPECTIVE STUDY OF MEDICAL TREATMENT FOR GRAVES'DISEASE. H. Allannic*, N.Genetet Y. Lorcy, A.M. Lequerrier, B. Genetet, Unit of Endocrinology, GURIFA, RENNES, FRANCE.

In a prospective study of patients with hyperthyroïd Graves'disease treated for 18 months with progressively reduced doses of carbimazole without hormone substitution and followed up for an additional 2 years period, peripheral total T lymphocyte counts (HTLA+ and E.ROS+) and OKT4, OKT8 subsets were compared using t test between patients at various times during treatment course and follow up as well as with age and sex matched controls. Compared to controls, patients showed decreased OKT8 counts at diagnosis (16.69 ± 5.85 vs 25.45 ± 5.70 n=42 p<0,001) (11/42 patients within normal range N.R.), after 6 months treatment (17.55 ± 5.74 vs 24.83 ± 4.72 n=48 p<0.001)(21/48 N.R.), 18 months treatment (18.10 ± 5.49 vs 23.65 ± 5.23 n=21 p<0,01) (11/21 N.R.), in relapse patients ($17 \pm 6,07$ vs $25,40 \pm 3,92$ n=15 p<0,001 (5/15 N.R.) and even in case of remission for 2 years after treatment withdrawal (20.01 ± 4.61 vs 24.82 ± 6.56 n=22 p<005 (11/12 N.R.); OKT4/OKT8 ratio was significantly supranormal in all patients except those in remission. A progressive increase of T cells essentially due to OKT8 cells was observed during treatment,which reached significance (p<0.05) only between diagnosis and remission groups. Similarly OKT4/OKT8 ratio was significantly lower in remission than in diagnosis patients (2.23 ± 0.97 vs 2.95 ± 1.37 p<0,05). In conclusion OKT8 cells increased progressively with treatment course but as a group they never reached control levels even in patients in remission with however a normalisation of individual values in 50 % of these patients.

259 PREDICTION AND PREVENTION OF POSTPARTUM DEVELOPMENT OF PRIMARY HYPOTHYROIDISM IN HASHIMOTO'S DISEASE. N. Amino*, Y. Iwatani, H. Tamaki, H. Mori, M. Aozasa, M. Mori, O. Tanizawa, Y. Kumahara and K. Miyai, Department of Laboratory Medicine, Osaka University Medical School, Osaka 553, Japan.

For establishing a method for prediction of postpartum development of hypothyroidism, various parameters were measured in 40 patients with Hashimoto's disease during and after delivery. Age, goiter size, thyroid function tests, the titers of antithyroid antibodies, and the peripheral lymphocyte counts in early pregnancy in patients who developed postpartum hypothyroidism (group A) were compared with those who did not develop hypothyroidism (group B). Only the titer of microsomal antibody (MCHA) was found to be significantly different in the two groups. All patients with MCHA titers of $2^{11} \times 10$ or more developed hypothyroidism. Postpartum hypothyroidism recurred in all 8 patients who had previous postpartum hypothyroidism and the time when hypothyroidism occurred after delivery and the severity of hypothyroidism were almost the same in the two consecutive episodes in each patient. For prevention of postpartum development of hypothyroidism prednisolone therapy was started immediately after delivery in two patients with Hashimoto's disease, who had high MCHA and previous postpartum hypothyroidism. Development of postpartum hypothyroidism was delayed for 2 months in one patient and prevented in another patient by steroid therapy for 1 month and 2 months, respectively. Conclusion: Development of postpartum hypothyroidism could be predicted by MCHA titer and previous history and could be prevented by short-term steroid therapy immediately after delivery.

260 THE ROLE OF SUBUNIT SIALIC ACID IN THE THYROTROPIC AND GONADOTROPIC ACTIVITY OF hCG. S.M. Amir*, M.F. Randall, S.H. Ingbar, Beth Israel Hospital, Boston, Mass. U.S.A.

Removal of sialic acid (SA) from highly purified hCG (hCG-p) alters its interactions with both thyroid and testis. To determine the roles of SAs in the individual subunits of hCG-p, α- and β-subunits were dissociated, desialylated (DSA) with neuraminidase, and were recombined in various combinations. The recombinants studied were: intact α + intact β (α-β); DSAα-β; α-DSAβ; and DSAα-DSAβ. The following aspects of trophic function were studied: In rat testis, ability to inhibit binding of ^{125}I-hCG (I) and to enhance cyclic AMP in Leydig cells (II); and in human thyroid membranes, ability to inhibit binding of ^{125}I-bTSH (III) and to inhibit adenylate cyclase stimulation induced by bTSH (IV). Results obtained were as follows:

Function	Activity compared with that of native hCG-p			
	α-β	DSAα-β	α-DSAβ	DSAα-DSAβ
I	=	=	=	↑
II	=	=	↓	↓
III*	—	↑	↑↑	↑↑↑
IV*	—	↑	↑	↑↑

* activity of native hCG-p too low to measure

Conclusions: Subunit SAs are not critical to testis-binding of hCG, but β-subunit SA is required for full biologic activity. SAs in both subunits inhibit thyroid-binding, and their removal, especially from the β-subunit, bestows activity as a TSH antagonist.

261 FLUCTUATION OF SEX STEROID BINDING PLASMA PROTEIN IN GRAVES' DISEASE.

N. Aoki*, Y. Maruyama, Y. Ohno, M. Imamura, T. Yamamoto, Y. Suzuki (a) and H. Hiramatsu(b), Department of Medicine and Department of Biochemistry(a), Kinki University School of Medicine, and Bellland Hospital(b), Osaka, Japan.

Sex steroid binding plasma protein (SBP) binds estrogens as well as androgens and appears to play an important role in reducing the metabolic clearance rate of androgens in circulation. Since radioimmunoassay (RIA) for SBP has been recently developed in a couple of institutes including here, a plenty of data are accummulating to elucidate pathophysiology of SBP in a variety of diseases. In the present paper, we have extensively studied on relationship of thyroid hormone levels and SBP concentrations in Graves patients with the use of RIA for SBP. Measurement of thyroid hormone levels (T3, T4) and SBP was performed for 36 hyperthyroid Graves patients (17 males and 19 females) and 29 euthyroid Graves patients(10 males and 19 females) as well as sex-and age matched controls. Male hyperthyroid patients showed 6.5 ± 0.5 μg/ml(mean ± SE) of plasma SBP contrasting 2.1 ± 0.2 μg/ml in controls ($p < 0.001$). Female hyperthyroid patients showed 6.4 ± 0.4 μg/ml for their averaged plasma SBP contrasting 3.1 ± 0.2 μg/ml in controls ($p < 0.001$). SBP levels for euthyroid patients was decreased as 3.2 ± 0.3 μg/ml for males and 3.6 ± 0.2 μg/ml for females. Correlation between T4 and SBP was observed both for males and females. Also, significant correlation was demonstrated between plasma T3 and SBP levels in both sexes. Thus, SBP levels in plasma were closely related to thyroid states showing that plasma SBP was elevated in hyperthyroid patients and decreased along with normalization of thyroid function after treatment with antithyroid drugs.

262 PATHOGENETIC ROLE OF ANTI-TSH RECEPTOR ANTIBODIES IN NONGOITROUS HYPOTHYROIDISM.

K. Arikawa*, Y. Ichikawa, T. Yoshida, T. Shinozawa, S. kawai, H. Oshima, H. Yamada, H. Tanaka, M. Homma, N. Momotani and K. Itoh, School of Medicine, Keio University and Itoh Hospital, Tokyo, Japan.

Serum IgG of 20 patients with nongoitrous hypothyroidism (NGH) were examined for TSH displacing activity (TDA) (Smith et al. 1974) and for their biological effects on thyroid adenylate cyclase (AC) (Orgiazzi et al. 1976) . TDA was measured in the presence of 10 mg/ml of IgG, where corrected %B/F (C-%B/F) lower than 82.1% (M-2SD of 60 normal subjects) was defined as TDA positive. Results. Eight (2 male and 6 female) out of 20 patients with NGH showed markedly strong TDA (C-%B/F below 21%). Except these 8, TDA was weakly positive in 2 and negative in 10 patients with NGH. The amount of IgG required for 50% inhibition of TSH binding, determined by dose-response curves, ranged from 0.06 to 5.6mg/ml in 8 patients with strongly positive TDA. None of these IgGs (5.5 mg/ml) showed any significant AC stimulating activity. On the contrary, IgGs from 7 out of these 8 patients significantly inhibited the increase of C-AMP generation induced by 9.1mU/ml of TSH ,ranging from 2.1% ($p<0.001$) to 54.5% ($p<0.01$) of the increase in the presence of normal IgG. The other 12 patients with weakly positive or negative TDA showed no inhibitory effect. The degree of inhibitory effect of IgGs on TSH stimulation of AC correlated well with their potency of TSH displacement ($r=0.90$, $p<0.01$). Among three female patients with strongly positive TDA, who were delivered of children after the onset of hypothyroidism, only a patient whose IgG showed the strongest inhibitory effect,had three children who has experienced neonatal transient hypothyroidism. Conclusion. Pathogenetic role of blocking antibodies against TSH receptor were strongly suggested in some patients with NGH.

263 AN ANTIBODY TO EYE MUSCLE IN GRAVES' OPHTHALMOPATHY. S. Atkinson*, M. Holcome, and P. Kendall-Taylor. Endocrine Unit, Royal Victoria Infirmary, Newcastle upon Tyne NE1 4LP, UK.

The pathogenesis of Graves' ophthalmopathy is unknown and the precise nature of its association with hyperthyroidism is not clear. Previous work has suggested possible autoimmune responsiveness to retro-orbital antigens. We have developed an ELISA for detection of IgG binding to retro-orbital muscle tissue. Patients with ophthalmopathy were divided into 3 groups. In group A, with active disease, ophthalmopathic IgG (OIg) was detectable in 15/24 patients (62%); in group B, patients with active ophthalmopathy receiving treatment with prednisone, 4/10 had OIg, and in group C, patients with inactive ophthalmopathy, only 1 of 9 was positive. No IgG binding occurred in 40 healthy subjects. Of 23 patients with autoimmune or nodular thyroid disease OIg binding was seen in one. OIg did not correlate with TBII, TgAb or microsomal antibody. The OIg did not interact with thyroid tissue. We conclude that Graves' ophthalmopathy is an entity distinct from autoimmune thyroid disease. A specific OIg is present in serum of patients with ophthalmopathy, which shows some correlation with the severity of the condition, but not with thyroid disease or thyroid antibodies.

264 GLUCAGON-INDUCED THYROID STIMULATING ACTION IN PERIFUSED RAT THYROID FRAGMENTS (PRTF). J.R.ATTALI*, P.VALENSI, D.DARNIS, C.WEISSELBERG, J.SEBAOUN, Dept. of Endocrinology, CHU AVICENNE, U.E.R. PARIS NORD, Bobigny - FRANCE.

Interaction between metabolic effects of glucagon (Glu) and thyroid hormones has been reported. High concentrations of plasma Glu are often found in hyperthyroidism ; in stress situations, there is marked increase in Glu secretion, as in catecholamines secretion. Catecholamines-induced thyroid stimulating action has already been reported. We used the PRTF technique to study the direct effect of Glu on the thyroid gland. R and Im indicate respectively the ratios of the average secretion per min of T4 during the 20-min stimulation period and the T4 peak to basal secretion. For a Glu concentration as low as 2.10^{-14} M, R = 1.36 $\pm$ 0.05 and is higher than the control R = 0.82 $\pm$ 0.05, $p < 0.001$ (with Krebs Ringers alone). The highest response, R = 1.62 $\pm$ 0.12, was found with Glu 2.10^{-12} M. The release peak was generally reached within the first 6 min. It increased with the Glu concentrations : Im = 1.90 $\pm$ 0.24, 2.36 $\pm$ 1.31 and 3.06 $\pm$ 0.59 for Glu 2.10^{-14} M, 2.10^{-13} M, 2.10^{-12} M respectively. Theophylline alone (1mM) induced a slight response : R = 1.05 $\pm$ 0.21, Im = 1.51 $\pm$ 0.29 and the release peak xas also reached early. Simultaneous perifusion of 1mM Theophylline with Glu 2.10^{-14} M and 2.10^{-13} M enhanced the peak : Im = 2.29 $\pm$ 0.46 and 2.82 $\pm$ 0.66 respectively, but not the one with Glu 2.10^{-12} M. in conclusion, physiological Glu concentrations are capable of stimulating T4 secretion. The fact that a thyroid response to Glu occurs as early as with Theophylline and that Theophylline potentiates the Glu effect for low concentrations but not for the highest one suggest that Glu acts on the thyroid gland like it does on the liver, by activating the adenyl-cyclase system. In addition, the role planed by Glu in inducing thyrotoxicosis should be clarified.

265 ENVIRONMENTAL IODINE INTAKE AFFECTS THE RESPONSE TO METHIMAZOLE THERAPY.

F. AZIZI*, Taleghani Medical Center , Beheshti Univ., Tehran, Iran.

The response to Methimazole therapy was evaluated in 18 patients with Graves' disease residing in an area of mild iodine deficiency (Tehran) and in 18 patients residing in an area of iodine sufficiency (Boston). Free T4 index (FT4I; N: 5-16) and free T3 index (FT3I; N: 75-220) before and four weeks after administration of Methimazole 10mg three times daily were as follows:

	Tehran		Boston	
Therapy	FT4I	FT3I	FT4I	FT3I
Before	22.9±4.8	489±124	23.8±5.2	512±250
After	4.9±4.3	117±58	17.0±4.1	368±152

In patients residing in Tehran, four weeks after such therapy, FT4I was normal in 9 (<6.3 in 6), above normal in one, and subnormal in 8 (44%). In 4 of 8 patients with subnormal FT4I, serum TSH was also above normal and clinical findings of hypothyroidism were evident. Methimazole 10mg twice daily was then given to 15 patients with Graves' disease residing in Tehran. FT4I was 22.7±6.8, 12.1±2.5, 10.8±2.8 and 6.0±4.3, before, 8, 14 and 28 days after treatment respectively. Corresponding FT3I values were 415±90, 196±36, 162±44 and 117±46. At 28 days, FT4I was subnormal in 7(46%), of which one had increased TSH. These results indicate that treatment with recommended textbook doses of Methimazole may cause hypothyroidism in patients with Graves' disease residing in areas of iodine deficiency, probably due to inadequate hormone stores in their thyroid gland.

266 INHIBITION OF IODINE METABOLISM IN THYROID CELLS BY PHORBOL ESTERS AND EPIDERMAL GROWTH FACTOR (EGF).

* L.K. Bachrach, M.C. Eggo and G.N. Burrow, Banting & Best Dept. of Medical Research, and Dept. of Medicine, University of Toronto, Toronto, Canada. M5G 1L7

Both EGF and biologically active phorbol esters not only promote growth in a variety of cell types but may also stimulate or inhibit differentiated function. Phorbol esters have been shown to interact with EGF by altering the affinity of EGF receptors. We studied the interaction of EGF and the potent phorbol ester 4B phorbol 12B myristate 13 acetate (PMA) in primary ovine thyroid cells grown in serum-free defined medium. Under similar conditions, EGF (10^{-9}M) stimulated thymidine incorporation and inhibited iodine uptake by 88% within 20-30 h through a reduction in both trapping and incorporation of ^{125}I. Growth of the cells for 24 h in 1-1000 ng/ml PMA did not stimulate thymidine incorporation but did increase protein synthesis in a dose dependent manner with a maximal stimulation at 100 ng/ml. Preincubation for 2-24 h with PMA also caused a 91% inhibition of iodine uptake. At a maximally effective concentration (100 ng/ml) PMA suppressed iodine metabolism more than EGF (10^{-9}M). The combination of PMA and EGF had a synergistic inhibitory effect on iodine uptake. PMA also rapidly altered EGF binding in a dose dependent manner; following a 2h preincubation with 100 ng PMA, ^{125}I-EGF binding was reduced to 20% of control. Tumor-promotor phorbol esters are thought to modulate cellular growth through pathways that converge with those utilized by other growth factors. Our data indicate that in the thyroid phorbol estors are also potent inhibitors of differentiated functions similar to EGF.

267 CORRELATION OF THYROID SUPPRESSIBILITY AND DETERMINATION OF THYROTROPIN BINDING INHIBITING ANTIBODIES (TBIAb) AT THE END OF ANTITHYROID DRUG TREATMENT IN PATIENTS WITH GRAVES'DISEASE. Badenhoop, K., Finke, R., Hensen, J., Bogner, U., Kotulla, P., Koppenhagen, K., Schleusener, H.*, Thyroid Research Group, Klinikum Steglitz, Berlin, West-Germany.

To reevaluate the significance of TBIAb for recognition of regained thyroid suppressibility we investigated the correlation of suppressed 123-J-uptake and TBIAb in 55 patients with Graves' disease at the end of antithyroid drug treatment. All 55 patients were positive for TBIAb before treatment. They received a one year course of antithyroid drug treatment with methimazole. One week before discontinuing therapy 3 mg thyroxine were administered, a week later a 2 hour 123-J-uptake was measured, TBIAb were determined and the therapy was stopped. Correlation of TBIAb and thyroid suppressibility was found in 39 patients (27 TBIAb negative with suppressibility, 12 TBIAb positive with no suppressibility). Patients were then followed up in 2-month - intervals up to 10 months. They were classified: remission: positive TRH-test, relapse: negative TRH-test and/or elevated thyroid hormone levels. Remission or relapse could not be predicted by either tests or in combination. Relapse occured 75 % of all patients after 10 month follow up independently of the outcome of TBIAb measurements and suppression tests. This study suggests a correlation of TBIAb and thyroid suppressibility in Gravens' disease patients. The predictive value of both tests is poor. The small number of patients does not allow decisive conclusions and larger groups are necessary to answer this question.

268 STUDIES ON THE MECHANISM OF ACUTE INHIBITION OF THYROIDAL SECRETION BY IODINE. N. Bagchi*, B. Shivers and T. R. Brown, Department of Medicine, Wayne State University, Detroit, Michigan 48201.

Iodine in excess is known to acutely inhibit thyroid hormone secretion. In the present study we have characterized the time course of the iodine effect in vitro and investigated the underlying mechanisms. Labeled thyroid glands were cultured in medium containing mononitrotyrosine, an inhibitor of iodotyrosine deiodinase. The rate of hydrolysis of labeled thyroglobulin was measured as the proportion of labeled iodotyrosines and iodothyronines recovered at the end of culture and was used as an index of thyroid hormone secretion. NaI added in vitro acutely inhibited both basal and TSH-stimulated thyroglobulin hydrolysis. The effect of iodide was demonstrable after 2h and was maximal after 6h. Iodide abolished the dibutyryl cAMP induced stimulation of thyroglobulin hydrolysis. Iodide required organic binding of iodine for its effect but new protein or RNA synthesis was not necessary. The inhibitory effects of iodide and lysosomotropic agents such as NH_4Cl and chloroquin on thyroglobulin hydrolysis were additive suggesting different sites of action. Iodide added in vitro altered the distribution of label in prelabeled thyroglobulin suggesting increased coupling in the molecule. These data indicate that 1) the iodide effect occurs progressively over a 6h period, 2) iodide exerts its action primarily at a post cAMP, prelysosomal site and 3) the effect requires organic binding of iodine, but not new RNA or protein synthesis. Our data are consistent with the hypothesis that excess iodide acutely inhibits thyroid hormone secretion by increasing the resistance of thyroglobulin to proteolytic degradation through increased iodination and coupling.

269 SERUM THYROGLOBULIN ESTIMATION IN THE FOLLOW-UP OF TREATED METASTATIC DIFFERENTIATED THYROID CARCINOMA (M.D.T.C.).

L. Baldet*, C. Jaffiol, C. Lasfargues, H. Collet and C. Papachristou, Dept. of Endocrinology and C.P.L., Hôpital St. Eloi, 34059 Montpellier Cédex - France.

To evaluate serum thyroglobulin (Tg) estimation in the management of MDTC, serum Tg and TSH were measured both on and off thyroxine for three years in 12 patients who had undergone total thyroidectomy for thyroid cancer (6 papillary, 3 follicular, 3 mixed) and radiation for metastases. Results were related to clinical data, ^{131}I-body scans (B-S), radiological findings and treatment. Tg was measured by RIA (sensitivity 3 ng/ml) and Tg antibody-positive sera were excluded. Eight patients (Gp I) had functioning metastases and were treated by ^{131}I, four (Gp II) with negative B-S by surgery and external irradiation (two cases) or surgery alone (2 cases with chest metastases). In Gp I : Tg fell dramatically with disappearance of metastases in three patients, remained elevated with persistence of metastases (B-S) despite suppression with T4 in four patients, and became undetectable despite active bone metastases in the remaining case. In Gp II : Tg remained elevated in three patients (two with untreated metastases, one despite lymph node surgery) and decreased slightly in the remaining one despite recurrence of metastases. Conclusions : 1) Tg correlates well with behaviour of functioning metastases 2) Tg may provide the main means of monitoring therapy of non-functioning metastases 3) Tg secretion is not suppressed by thyroxine in all cases.

270 EVIDENCE FOR A T SUPPRESSOR CELL DEFECT IN GRAVES' DISEASE.

K. Banovac*, D. Neylan, A. Claflin** and M. Zakarija, Departments of Medicine and Surgery**, University of Miami School of Medicine, Miami, FL.

Hyperthyroidism of Graves' disease is due to the action of an autoantibody (thyroid-stimulating antibody, TSAb). There is speculation that this reflects a suppressor T cell (Ts) defect. To test this we measured peripheral B cell secretion of TSAb (assay=increase in cAMP in human thyroid cells *in vitro*). Patient C's serum IgG gave a linear TSAb response of 167-644% with 5-500ug IgG per ml. C's B and T cells were separated by rosetting as were normal (N) T cells. Combinations of cells were incubated for 7 days over functioning rat thyroid (FRTL) cells (provided by Dr. L. Kohn) in monolayer cultures (20,000 cells/microtiter well). FRTL cells respond to TSAb and were presumed to provide an antigenic stimulus. The medium was assayed for TSAb and positive results ($P < 0.025$) were obtained with C's B + C's T cells (172%) and C's B + irradiated (to kill T_S cells) NT cells (159%); media from various other mixtures of cells gave no significant responses (95-128%). Total IgG in media was measured by solid phase radioimmunoassay and there was no pattern related to the cell mixture. IgG binding to human thyroid cell and guinea pig fat cell membranes by ELISA showed no significant difference dependent upon cell mixture. Presumably all combinations of cells resulted in predominant secretion of non-TSAb IgG. However, from the data given above, TSAb equivalent to that in about 5 ug serum IgG was apparently secreted by C's B cells when incubated with C's T cells or NT irradiated cells. These data support a concept of defective T_S activity underlying TSAb production in Graves' disease.

271 **FUROSEMIDE (Fr) IS A COMPETITIVE INHIBITOR OF PLASMA BINDING OF T_4 AND T_3**

J.W. Barlow*, C-F. Lim, V. Stevens, D.J. Topliss, K.N. Wynne, J.R. Stockigt
Ewen Downie Metabolic Unit, Alfred Hospital, Melbourne 3181, Australia

In some patients with low T_4 (<30 nM) during severe non-thyroidal illness (NTI) we have found a circulating, heat-stable, dialysable inhibitor of ^{125}I T_4 plasma binding which coincides with Fr given in high doses (800-2400 mg/day) for oliguric renal failure. Time-course studies showed that high-dose Fr coincided with a very rapid decline in T_4 with half-life <24 h. Inhibition of ^{125}I T_4 binding in serum diluted 1:10 varied directly with circulating Fr concentrations from 1-300 µg/ml; this effect was reproduced by Fr added to normal serum in vitro. The inhibitory effect diminished with serum dilution, as described for low affinity competitors. Relative to T_4, on a molar basis, more than 1000-fold Fr excess was required to produce equivalent inhibition of ^{125}I T_4 binding in serum diluted 1:10. Fr was about 10-fold more potent in inhibiting ^{125}I T_3 than ^{125}I T_4 binding. Fr, 0.01, 0.1 and 1 µg/ml, added to 1:10,000 dilution of normal serum in barbitone pH 8.6, inhibited ^{125}I T_4 binding to 82.3±1.9, 49.6±2.6, and 17.3±1.7% B/B_0 respectively ($\bar{x}$±SD, n=4). At 1:10,000 serum dilution, Scatchard analysis of ^{125}I T_4 binding, with and without Fr, 0.1 µg/ml, showed a decrease in affinity from K_d 21 pM (-Fr) to 64 pM (+Fr) without a change in capacity, demonstrating competitive inhibition. These findings suggest that Fr, a drug frequently used in oliguric patients with NTI, inhibits plasma T_4 and T_3 binding and may alter clearance of these hormones.

272 RELEVANCE OF A CIRCULATING IMMUNE COMPLEX ASSAY (CIC) TO DISTINGUISH BETWEEN PATIENTS WITH AUTOIMMUNE THYROID DISEASES AND HEALTHY CONTROLS (ELISA, C_{1q}, Anti-C_{1q}, IgM, IgG). R. Baur, J. Schartmann, R. Göber and H. Schleusener,* F.U. Berlin, Klinikum Steglitz, Dept. of Endocrinology, Hindenburgdamm 30, 1 Berlin 45, West Germany

There is good evidence that CIC might be involved in the pathogenesis of a variety of autoimmune diseases. Graves' disease is considered to develop sui generis. The measurement of certain immunological parameters describes a pertubation of the immune system. To measure CIC, we developed an ELISA which takes advantage of one of the properties of C_{1q} to bind CIC consisting of $IgG_{1,2,3}$ and/or IgM. Microtiter plates (NUNC) were coated with C_{1q} or anti-C_{1q}, incubated with BSA and washed. After serum incubation, the possible adherence of CIC is measured via antiglobulin-conjugated phosphatase and PNPP. The assay's limitation appears at about 1 µg/ml AHG. It differentiates between sera, the absorbancies are to be found over the total absorbancy range (0.0-2.0 at 4.05 nm) with respect to all 4 parameters (C_{1q}, anti-C_{1q}, IgG, IgM) and it shows dependency on serum concentrations. The measured AHG-equivalents are dependent on free C_{1q}-concentration in the serum. In spite of the possibilities of the assay to strongly differentiate between single sera (n=400), no distinction could be made between control group (blood donors), Graves' patients and subgroups. The items to characterize the subgroups were: TBII, exophthalmus, treatment and duration of treatment. We conclude from these results that the presence of CIC does not necessarily indicate a pathological phenomenon and might also be interpreted as an individual regulatory system in order to maintain a subtle homoeostasis of globulins, antiglobulins and antigens.

273 RABBITS IMMUNIZED WITH TSH PRODUCE THYROID-STIMULATING ANTIBODIES. G.N. Beall*, B. Rapoport, I.J. Chopra, D.H. Solomon, and S. Kruger, Harbor-UCLA Medical Center and UCLA Center for Health Sciences, Los Angeles, and VA Hospital and University of California, San Francisco.

We immunized rabbits with TSH to investigate the hypothesis that such immunization could result in production of thyroid-stimulating autoanti-idiotypic antibodies to anti-TSH. Groups of 6 animals each received hTSH, hTSHβ, bTSH (Thytropar), or human serum albumin (hSA). The production of cyclic AMP by cultured thyroid cells was used to assay thyroid-stimulating immunoglobulin (TSI) in the serum. Serum from periodic bleedings was radioassayed for thyroxine (T_4) and anti-hTSH. Antibodies to human thyroid membranes (hTM) were detected by binding to hTM of antirabbit gamma globulin and ^{125}I-protein A. TSI appeared in the serum of many rabbits following immunization, most notably in serum obtained 100 days following the sixth booster TSH immunization. At that time, TSI activity equivalent to 6 to 18 μU TSH/1.5 mg IgG was present in 2 of 6 hTSH, 2 of 6 hTSHβ and 2 of the 4 surviving bTSH-immunized animals. Control (hSA-immunized rabbits) serum TSI was 4.3±0.4 (mean ± SD). TSI was greatest in bTSH-immunized rabbits, declined gradually with subsequent bleedings, did not correlate with anti-hTSH, and increased linearly with increasing amounts of IgG. Serum T_4, which was similar in all groups, did not change after immunization. No animal developed hypothyroidism. TSH-immunized rabbits developed antibodies capable of binding to hTM. Conclusion: Immunization of rabbits with TSH produced antisera containing TSI. This finding, together with the previous demonstration of anti-TSH in TSI-containing serum, provides support for the notion that the TSI of Graves' hyperthyroidism could be an antiidiotype to anti-TSH.

274 INHERITED CONGENITAL GOITER IN MICE. W. G. Beamer*, E. M. Eicher and L. J. Maltais. The Jackson Laboratory, Bar Harbor, ME USA 04609

Congenital goiter (cog) is a new recessive mutation on Chromosome 15 that has been recovered in AKR/J mice. cog/cog mice can be recognized two weeks after birth by reduced body size and enlarged thyroids. Mutant mice are characterized by mild growth retardation, reduced fertility, mild anemia (cog: 44.3 ± 0.9; +: 49.4 ± 1.0% RBC), low serum T4 (cog: 1.9 ± 0.8; +: 6.4 ± 1.7 ug/dl) and T3 (cog: 39.5 ± 3.4; +: 104.1 ± 13.3 ng/ml), 3-fold enlargement of thyroids at 7-8 weeks and 25- to 50-fold enlargement at 30 weeks, and goiter suppressible by feeding a diet supplemented with 0.025% desiccated thyroid powder. Light and electron microscopy revealed that cog/cog thyroids have rudimentary sized follicular lumena, colloid that stains poorly with PAS, and thyrofollicular cell hypertrophy and hyperplasia. Studies of fetal mutant glands indicated a significant deficiency in uptake of 125-I (cog: 1053 ± 84; +: 4171 ± 393 cpm/thyroid) despite the fact that fetal glands were significantly larger. Studies with young adult mutant mice showed that they were able to incorporate normal amounts of 125-I/mg thyroid and that the iodine was retained when challenged with a perchlorate discharge test. Based upon these data, our working hypothesis is that the cog gene induces a metabolic error in thyroglobulin production, leading to goitrogenesis. This study was supported by NIH.

275 DECREASED RECEPTOR-BINDING OF BIOLOGICALLY INACTIVE TSH IN CENTRAL HYPOTHYROIDISM: ENHANCEMENT OF TSH BINDING AND ACTIVITY AFTER CHRONIC TRH TREATMENT. P. Beck-Peccoz*, S. Amr, M.M. Menezes-Ferreira, G. Faglia and B.D. Weintraub, NIADDK and NICHHD, NIH, Bethesda, Md., USA and Chair of Endocrinology, University of Milan, Italy.

Previous studies have suggested that certain cases of idiopathic central hypothyroidism (CH) might result from the secretion of TSH forms with low bioactivity. To investigate the nature of such forms we purified serum TSH by immunoaffinity chromatography from 7 patients with apparent CH (5 idiopathic, 2 pituitary tumor) and 10 controls with primary hypothyroidism; TSH immunologic activity (I) was measured by radioimmunoassay, receptor-binding (R) by inhibition of ^{125}I-bTSH binding to human thyroid membranes, and bioactivity (B) by stimulation of adenylate cyclase in these membranes. The diagnosis of CH was based on low T_4, normal or slightly elevated TSH (I), normal thyroid response to exogenous bTSH, and absence of antithyroid antibodies. Patients with CH showed a strikingly decreased ratio of R/I ($<$ 0.15) compared to controls (0.6-2.7) and a similarly decreased B/I ($<$ 0.2 vs 2.8-5.6). After acute intravenous TRH (200 μg) the TSH (I) response was prolonged and exaggerated, but R/I and B/I normalized in only 1 of 4 patients. However, after 4-6 weeks of oral TRH (40 mg/d) there was increased serum T_4 and TSH (I) as well as normalization of both R/I (0.7-0.9) and B/I (3.1-3.7) in all 4 patients. We conclude that in both idiopathic and neoplastic CH, TSH bioactivity is decreased because of impaired binding to its receptor; chronic TRH corrects both these TSH abnormalities and restores euthyroidism. These data imply that TRH regulates not only TSH secretion but also its specific molecular and conformational features necessary for hormone action.

276 THYROXINE-BINDING GLOBULIN (TBG) AND OUTCOME OF GRAVES' DISEASE (Gd). S. Benvenga*, F. Vermiglio, R. Melluso and F. Trimarchi[1], Institute of Clinica Medica and [1]Chair of Semeiotica Medica I, University of Messina, Italy.

Since within a given series only a fraction of patients with untreated Gd has subnormal serum TBG levels, we first try to relate differences in basal TBG concentration to the outcome of the illness. Twenty-seven hyperthyroid patients suffering from Gd (age 39±16 yrs, m±SD; 21 females) had serum TBG (RIA) levels significantly reduced in comparison with 24 age- and sex-matched euthyroid controls (19.19±2.98 vs 22.8±4.0 ug/ml, $p<0.01$). A TBG concentration minus 1SD (18.8 ug/ml) the mean of controls was considered as a low value and was found in 11/27 (41%) individuals who included 2/7 of the subjects with a preceding history of Gd (pGd). Only one male and one female had TBG levels < 2SD from control mean: the first remained in remission, while the second relapsed. TBG levels were independent from the initial thyroid antibody pattern and were not statistically lower in males than in females (17.45±2.20 vs 19.64±3.04). Patients were followed up over 36±8 months and 12 relapsed after the conventional (12-18 months) methimazole treatment. Among the 11 subjects with low serum TBG, future euthyroid (E) had T3/T4 ratio significantly higher than future relapsing (R) (36.8±11.2 vs 21.9±4.0, $P<0.05$). In these patients T3/T4 ratio allowed a good separation of outcomes as it was >30 in 6 E individuals and <30 in 5.4 of whom relapsed. On the contrary in patients with pGd the risk of further relapse appeared associated with normal serum TBG concentration.

277 POTENTIATION BY NALOXONE AND INHIBITION BY LOPERAMIDE OF THE ACTH RESPONSE TO CRF, IN MAN.

F.Cavagnini*, C.Invitti, °P.Velio, °A.Bozzani, °P.Bianchi, E.E. Polli, 1st Medical Clinic, °3rd Medical Pathology, University Milan, Italy.

Opioid peptides inhibit ACTH secretion in humans. However, whether their effect is primarily mediated at pituitary or hypothalamic level is uncertain. To clarify this issue, four healthy men, 35-53 yr, underwent, on three separate occasions, three tests: (a) ovine corticotropin releasing factor (CRF), 1 μg/Kg iv at 11 a.m. (b) CRF plus naloxone, an opiate receptor antagonist, 4 mg iv plus 4 mg infused over 4 hrs (c) CRF plus loperamide, a peripheral opiate agonist, 16 mg given p.o. 2½ hrs before CRF. Blood samples for ACTH and cortisol estimation by RIA were obtained before and for 4 hrs after drug injection. Results were evaluated by the ANOVA. The ACTH response to CRF was enhanced by naloxone and inhibited by loperamide, with a significant difference resulting between the mean ACTH secretory areas observed under the two drug treatments: 3376 ± 658.51 S.E.M. pg/4 hrs vs 1156 ± 513.84 pg/4 hrs, $p < 0.01$, respectively. The cortisol response to CRF was also significantly ($p < 0.02$) potentiated by naloxone but, paradoxically, also by loperamide: mean integrated values in the three tests were 39.4 ± 9.77, 73.4 ± 11.42 and 71.5 ± 8.68 μg/dl, respectively. The loperamide result may be accounted for by an increased adrenal sensitivity to ACTH, secondary to the blunting of ACTH secretion caused by previous administration of the opioid. In all, these results demonstrate that in man opioid peptides inhibit ACTH secretion by a direct action at pituitary level. This does not exclude that they may also act at a suprapituitary site.

278 EXPRESSION OF PROOPIOMELANOCORTIN (POMC)-LIKE GENE IN MALE REPRODUCTIVE TISSUES.

C.-L.C. Chen, J.P. Mather, P.L. Morris and C.W. Bardin* The Population Council and the Rockefeller University, New York, NY 10021, USA

Adrenocortico tropin (ACTH), β-endorphin and the melanocyte stimulating hormone (MSHs), which are products of a common precursor, proopiomelanocortin (POMC) are present in a variety of tissues other than the pituitary. Recently, immunoreactive POMC-derived peptides have also been detected in the reproductive tracts. In this report, we have demonstrated that POMC-like gene is expressed in the male reproductive tissues. Messenger RNAs were extracted and POMC-like mRNAs were determined by Northern blot analysis using a cloned DNA probe complementary to rat pituitary POMC mRNA. The POMC-like mRNAs were detected in both epididymis and testis. The cellular localization in testis was established by showing POMC mRNA in Leydig cell lines (TM_3 and I10A) but not in the mouse Sertoli cell lines (TM_4). The hybridizing species of POMC-like mRNA in the testis, epididymis, and the mouse Leydig cell lines were approximately 150 bases shorter than those in the pituitary or hypothalamus. Similar results have been found in some regions of rat brain. POMC-like mRNAs from amygdala and cerebral cortex were smaller in size as compared to those in pituitary or hypothalamus. We have found that POMC-like mRNAs in the testis, epididymis or Leydig cell lines were the same size as those detected in amygdala nucleus. The concentration of POMC-like mRNA in the testis is almost as high as that in the hypothalamus. In conclusion, the presence of POMC-like mRNAs in the male reproductive tissues indicates that POMC-derived peptides may be synthesized locally in the Leydig cells and epididymis.

279 IMMUNOREACTIVE α-N-ACETYL ENDORPHIN IN RAT SPERMATOGONIA AND SPERMATOCYTES.
C. Cheng, J. Clements*, S. Lolait and J.W. Funder, Medical Research Centre, Prince Henry's Hospital, Melbourne, Australia 3004.

Immunoreactive-β-endorphin (ir-βEP) has been previously demonstrated in rat testis (BBRC 95:618, 1980; Endocrinology 110:2204, 1982). We have confirmed these findings and localized N-acetyl endorphin(s) (N-Ac-EP) in the adult male rat testis by radioimmunoassay and immunohistochemistry. Antisera used were anti-βEP (R44) which recognizes βEP_{1-31}, βEP_{1-27} and their N-acetylated forms equivalently, but not α-EP or γ-EP; and anti-N-Ac-βEP_{1-27} (R92) which recognizes the N-Ac forms of βEP_{1-31} (100% on a molar basis), βEP_{1-27} (100%), α-EP (11%), γ-EP (12%) but not the non-acetylated forms of these peptides (<1%). Intense staining, which could be abolished by pre-absorption with excess N-Ac-βEP_{1-27}, was seen with R92 (anti-N-Ac-βEP_{1-27}) in spermatogonia and primary spermatocytes. As previously found, only Leydig cells stained specifically with anti-βEP. Testicular levels of ir-N-Ac-EP (7.1±1.3 pmol N-Ac-βEP_{1-27}/g tissue, or 65±12 pmol N-Ac-αEP/g tissue, mean±SD, n=18) were substantially higher than ir-βEP levels (0.58±0.12 pmol/g tissue). Given our antisera specificity this ir-N-Ac-EP activity is not N-Ac-βEP_{1-31} or N-Ac-βEP_{1-27}, but probably smaller N-Ac-EP fragment(s), e.g. N-Ac-αEP or N-Ac-γEP. Though chemical identities remain to be established, these data demonstrate another tissue where extensive processing of POMC combined with N-acetylation would appear to be a cell-specific post-translational modification. The significance of this processing, its potential utility as a marker of stages of spermatogenesis, and its possible physiological roles remain to be established.
Supported by the National Health & Medical Research Council of Australia.

280 β-ENDORPHIN IN GENETICALLY HYPOPROLACTINEMIC RATS.
H.Cohen+, I.Sabbagh and J.Bertrand. INSERM-U.34. Hôpital Debrousse. 69322 Lyon Cedex 05. France. Institut Pasteur. Lyon. France.

It has been reported that β-endorphin is involved in the regulation of tonic, stress- or suckling- induced prolactin (PRL) secretion. In the aim to evaluate the relation between endogenous β-endorphin and PRL, β-endorphin levels were measured by a specific RIA in extracts of whole brain, hypothalamus, anterior and posterior pituitaries and plasma. This study was made in normal Sprague-Dawley rats and in a derived strain of genetically hypoprolactinemic rats (IPL nude). In IPL nude female (diestrus) post-pituitary β-endorphin contents (in ng/organ) were significantly ($p < 0.001$)lower in IPL rats than in normal, while the values observed in other extracts (ng/organ) and plasma (ng/ml) were similar (Table). In IPL male rats, post-pituitary β-endorphin contents were also significantly reduced compared to normal ones, but that of anterior pituitary were increased. This increase is likely explained by the fact that anterior pituitary weights are significantly greater in IPL nude rats than in normal.

Mean+SEM	Plasma	Ant.Pituit.	Post-Pituit.	Hypothalamus	Whole brain
IPL (6)F	0.67±0.04	1460±191	1090±53	93±24	186±34
normal(6)F	0.55±0.1	1720±163	3960±244	48±13	172±15

These results further support the concept that β-endorphin levels of anterior and posterior pituitaries were submitted to differential control as reported (Nature 1983, 305,237). The present data, together with our previous reports suggest that post-pituitary β-endorphin and PRL in IPL rats are regulated in the same way by the same factor, probably dopamine.

281 PLASMA IMMUNOREACTIVE β-ENDORPHIN (iβE) AND ACTH IN THE DIAGNOSIS OF CUSHING'S DISEASE (CD).
P.M. Copeland*, D.B. Carr, B. Kliman, M. Harding, R.N. Kjellberg and M. Rosenblatt, Mass. General Hospital, Boston, MA 02114

Although CD is caused by excessive secretion of ACTH, diagnosis by direct assay of ACTH is usually uncertain. We investigated iβE as an improved alternative test for CD using an anti-β-endorphin antiserum having nearly equimolar reactivity with β-lipotropin. Single 8 AM plasma levels of ACTH and iβE were measured in 22 consecutive patients with CD, 4 with Nelson's syndrome (NS), and 24 normal healthy volunteers. ACTH was assayed using either the Amersham or CIS commercial kits and also with the West antibody applied to plasma extracts. Determinations of either ACTH or iβE separated patients with NS from those with CD. The ACTH values of patients with CD, however, showed considerable overlap with normal controls: 5 of 19 patients with CD were in the normal range (mean ± 2SD) using a commercial kit, 7 of 22 using the West antibody. In contrast, measurement of iβE showed only 1 of 22 patients with CD in the normal range ($\chi^2 = 3.87$, $p<.05$ vs. commercial kits; $\chi^2 = 5.50$, $p<.02$ vs. West antibody). After an overnight or 2-day low dose dexamethasone test, plasma ACTH decreased 6 to 62% in 6 of 9 patients with CD but 3 patients showed a 50 to 57% increase. In contrast, plasma iβE showed a 29 to 63% decrease in all 9 patients tested. The variance of the percent reduction for iβE was significantly less than for ACTH (F statistic = 19.83, $p<.01$). In conclusion, iβE was more accurate than ACTH for the diagnosis of CD and showed more consistent reduction after dexamethasone suppression. Together with plasma cortisol measurements, single 8 AM plasma iβE levels may serve to distinguish patients with CD from normals.

282 NUCLEUS TRACTUS SOLITARIUS (NTS) DEAFFERENTATION ELIMINATES ACTH RESPONSE TO HYPOTENSIVE HEMORRHAGE.
D.N. Darlington*, J. Shinsako and M.F. Dallman. Dept. of Physiology, UCSF, San Francisco, CA, 94143 USA.

Hypovolemia and hypotension are potent stimuli for ACTH release. These stimuli can activate both peripheral and central receptors that control release of pituitary ACTH. Peripheral receptors located in the heart and vasculature send cardiovascular signals to the NTS via the vagus and glossopharyngeal nerves. Cells in the NTS project to the paraventricular nucleus through multiple pathways for control of ACTH release. Central receptors are not well understood and ill defined. To test the theory that hypotensive hemorrhage leads to ACTH release by activation of peripheral and not central receptors, plasma ACTH was measured before and twenty minutes after hypotensive hemorrhage (15% of blood volume/1min, blood volume estimated as 7% of body wgt.) in two groups of pentobarbital anesthetized Sprague-Dawley rats. One group received sagittal knife cuts lateral to the NTS in an attempt to interrupt cardiovascular afferents entering the NTS region (NTS deafferentation). The second group had all surgery except medullary cuts. Successful NTS deafferentation was checked by elimination of the bradycardia induced by elevating arterial pressure with phenylephrine (5-10ug). Sham rats had an intact reflex. Successful NTS deafferentation eliminated the increase in ACTH during hypotensive hemorrhage (4.0±48 pg/ml, n=7) as compared to sham animals (239±97 pg/ml, n=6). These data support the theory that peripheral and not central receptors are involved in the release of ACTH during hypotensive hemorrhage in pentobarbital anesthetized rats. This study was supported by HL29714.

283 IN VITRO CELL FREE TRANSLATION OF RAT ADRENAL MESSENGER RNA CODING FOR TWO ACTH-INDUCED PROTEINS. A. Dazord*, D. Langlois-Gallet and J.M. Saez, INSERM U. 162, Hôpital Debrousse, 69322 Lyon Cedex 05, France.

Protein markers induced by hormones are the necessary probes to study hormone regulation of gene expression. We have previously shown that ACTH was able to induce two of these markers, one in the cytosol of the rat adrenal : protein E (Dazord et al, Biochem. J. 176, 233-239, 1978), another in the mitochondrion protein M (Dazord et al, Biochem. Biophys. Res. Commun. 98, 885-891, 1981). In this study using in vivo ACTH treated rats, protein E, and M antibodies we show that :

1) ACTH affects both the amount of adrenal mRNA and its translational activity.
2) The translation of protein E is increased by the hormone.
3) Protein E is the major translational product after 4 hrs of ACTH treatment.
4) Protein M is also translated.
5) The precise MW and Pi of both proteins E and M are determined ; protein E has the same molecular weight in vivo in the adrenal as in the translation assay. But there is a discrepancy for protein M, suggesting post-translational modifications.

284 RADIOIMMUNOASSAY OF PLASMA β-ENDORPHINS AND β-LIPOTROPINS(βLPH) IN PRIMARY ADRENAL INSUFFICIENCY AND IN PITUITARY CUSHING DISEASE-CORRELATIONS WITH ACTH PLASMA LEVELS. D.Dewailly*, A.Reuter Y.Vrindts-Gevaert, A.Racadot, P.Fossati, P.Franchimont.
Service d'Endocrinologie et de Diabétologie, CHU, Lille, France.
Service de Radioimmunologie, CHU, Liège, Belgium.

In order to document further the function of the corticotroph in pathological situations with exagerated ACTH secretion, we have used very sensitive antisera against βendorphin and βLPH. ACTH, βendorphin and βLPH levels are concomitantly elevated in all plasma from 8 patients with primary adrenal insufficiency and from 6 patients with corticotropic adenoma. In the 26 samples from the first group, βendorphin is strongly correlated with ACTH and βLPH (r=.83 and .62, respectively) but the correlation between ACTH and βLPH is weak (r=.44). In the 32 samples from the patients with Cushing disease, strong correlations are found between ACTH and βendorphin, ACTH and β LPH, and β endorphin and β LPH (r=.83, .82 and .74, respectively). The slope of the linear regression line between βendorphin and βLPH is 3.69, in good agreement with their molecular ratio. In 5 patients from the last group, I.V. injection of Lysine Vasopressine (LVP) releases higher quantities of β LPH than ACTH (mean delta ± sem: 447±56 vs 143±27 pg/ml, $p<0.05$). LVP elicites βLPH and βendorphin responses in all patients while insulin induced hypoglycemia is uneffective in 80 % of them. In conclusion, sensitive RIA of βendorphin and β LPH afford useful and reliable tools for clinical investigation of pituitary and adrenal disorders.

285 INVESTIGATION OF METHIONINE-ENKEPHALIN AND BETA-ENDORPHIN LEVELS IN BRAIN, PANCREAS, AND ADRENALS OF DB/DB MICE. F. Ellyin*, J. Greenberg, G. Pullen, S. Singh, A. Snyder and R. Sethi. VA Medical Center and Chicago Medical School, North Chicago, Illinois 60064, USA.

Enkephalin and other opioid peptides have been shown to influence insulin secretion. To study their role in the pathogenesis of diabetes mellitus, we have determined Methionine-enkephalin (M-enk) and Beta-endorphin (B-end) immunoreactivity in selected tissues of db/db mice, a strain which is predisposed to develop diabetes mellitus. M-enk and B-end were determined by radioimmunoassay in hypothalamus, pituitary, pancreas and adrenals from db/db mice and controls at 8 weeks of age. Plasma immunoreactive insulin and glucose levels were monitored simultaneously. In hypothalamus and pituitary, the levels of M-enk (13.2 $\pm$ 2.2 and 1.7 $\pm$ 0.19 ng/mg protein respectively) were higher than in control tissues (9.3 $\pm$ 0.79 and 1.1 $\pm$ 0.077 ng/mg protein respectively), but this difference was statistically significant only in the pituitary. M-enk levels in pancreas and adrenal glands were similar in db/db mice and controls. There appeared to be no significant difference between db/db and control mice in the levels of B-end in any of the tissues tested although pituitary B-end levels were elevated slightly (11.8 $\pm$ 3.6 ng/mg protein in db/db vs 6.5 $\pm$ 0.59 ng/mg protein in controls). The significance of this finding with respect to the etiology of diabetes mellitus is highly speculative at present. M-enk levels in the hypothalamic-pituitary axis of the db/db mouse are abnormal and warrent further investigation.

Supported by the Veterans Administration.

286 EFFECTS OF LIPOPROTEIN ON STEROID SYNTHESIS AND SECRETION BY ADRENOCORTICAL ZONAL CELL TYPES. V.H. Black* and R.I. Brody, Dept. of Cell Biology, New York University Medical Center, New York, NY

Most studies of lipoprotein effects on steroidogenesis by the adrenal have utilized the mixed cell population of the whole gland. This study has examined the effect of exogenous lipoprotein on the synthesis and secretion of steroids by separated zona glomerulosa (ZG) and zona fasciculata (ZF) cells under baseline and ACTH-stimulated conditions.

Total incorporation of ^{14}C-acetate into cholesterol oleate, free cholesterol and secreted steroid was greater and was more affected by LDL in ZG than in ZF cells. In presence of LDL, incorporation into cholesterol oleate increased in ZG cells, but was little affected in ZF cells. Incorporation into free cholesterol plus secreted steroid was suppressed by LDL in both cell types. The effect of LDL was greater for ZG cells in the absence of ACTH and for ZF cells in the presence of ACTH.

Despite their capacity for endogenous synthesis, ZG cells required LDL in order to achieve secretion similar to that in controls, both with and without ACTH, while ZF cells required LDL only in the stimulated state. When the cultures were treated with mevinolin, an inhibitor of the rate limiting step in cholesterol biosynthesis, there was greater inhibition of both synthesis and secretion by ZG than by ZF cells.

These results suggest that in ZG cells, although newly synthesized cholesterol contributes to steroid production, particularly in absence of LDL, exogenous lipoprotein is essential for maximum secretion. ZF cells, on the other hand, are less sensitive to LDL, and must depend more heavily on intracellular cholesterol stores. (Supported by NIH HD 04005, AG 01468)

287 EFFECT OF DEHYDROEPIANDROSTERONE ON ERYTHROCYTE GLUCOSE-6-PHOSPHATE DEHYDROGENASE ACTIVITY IN VIVO AND IN VITRO. G. Boccuzzi*, A.°Bosia, G.°Niort, E. Brignardello and L. Bonino, Fisiopatologia Endocrina,°Chimica e Propedeutica Biochimica, Università di Torino, 10126, Torino, Italia.

The erythrocytes were incubated with increasing concentrations of dehydroepiandrosterone (DHA) (from .5 to 100 µg/dl). Glucose-6-phosphate dehydrogenase (G-6-PD) activity, reduced glutathione (GSH) and NADPH were determined before and 5, 10, 15, 30, 60 and 90 min after addiction of DHA to the buffer. DHA inhibits human erythrocyte G-6-PD activity even at concentration of 1.5 µg/dl, i.e. usually observed in plasma after stimulation with ACTH. The maximum inhibition (30%) was reached after ten minutes and disappeared after 60 min. Higher concentrations did not greatly enhance inhibition through it lasted longer. This inhibition leads to a decrease in intracellular NADPH. Glutathione reductase, wich empoys this cofactor to reduce oxidized glutathione, is blocked, so that the concentration of GSH is also diminished. In vivo studies were performed in ten normal subjects. They received 250 ug of synthetic ACTH i.v. Plasma DHA, erythrocyte G-6-PD activity, GSH and NADPH were determined before and 30, 60, 90, 120 and 150 min after the injection. ACTH caused a significant fall in red cell G-6-PD activity. NADPH and GSH also fall in step with the rise in plasma DHA. No changes in G-6-PD activity were noted in two subjects with a poor DHA response to ACTH.

288 EFFECTS OF STEROID HORMONES ON THE TRANSITION OF ADRENAL CHROMAFFIN CELLS INTO NEURITES. J. W. Brown*, A. Carballeira and L. M. Fishman, V.A. Medical Center and Department of Medicine, University of Miami School of Medicine, Miami, Florida, 33125 U.S.A.

The chromaffin cell-to-neurite transition described by Unsicker in cultures of fetal rat adrenal medullary cells was studied in chromaffin cells derived from human pheochromocytomas (PC) and from the normal bovine adrenal medulla (C). Neurite outgrowth was observed in primary cultures of both types of neural crest-derived cells, but PC underwent redifferentiation earlier (5-7 days) and more extensively (ca. 80 %) than C (15-20 days; ca. 5-8 %) and were more susceptible to the potentiating effects of nerve growth factor. The presence (10^{-5} M) of steroids with glucocorticoid (GC) activity (dexamethasone, corticosterone and cortisol) consistently inhibited the morphologic redifferentiation of both C and PC cells into neurites and increased cell size and the occurrence of large vesicles, while GC precursors (11-deoxycortisol [S] and 11-deoxycorticosterone [DOC]) failed to prevent or modify these morphologic changes. In preliminary studies, sex steroids (17β-estradiol and testosterone) stimulated neurite transition. Preincubation with GC resulted in as much as 16-fold increases in norepinephrine and 5-fold increases in epinephrine content, as well as enhanced steroid metabolizing capacity (ca. 4-fold rise in 11β-hydroxylase activity). These biochemical effects were mimicked partially by S and DOC, possibly as a result of 11β-hydroxylation by chromaffin cells of these precursors and their conversion into active GC. Steroid hormones thus have important effects on both the morphological and functional differentiation of adrenal chromaffin cells.

289 CHANGING INTRA-ADRENAL CONCENTRATIONS OF STEROIDS AFFECT RELATIVE ACTIVITIES OF 3β-HYDROXYSTEROID DEHYDROGENASE AND 17,20-DESMOLASE AND THUS REGULATE ADRENAL ANDROGEN PRODUCTION. G. C. Byrne, Y. S. Perry and J.S.D. Winter*, Department of Pediatrics, University of Manitoba, Winnipeg, Manitoba, R3E OW1, Canada.

We found that intra-adrenal concentrations of most steroids are 2-10 times higher in adults than in infants, and reach levels (10^{-7}-10^{-5} M) which might influence steroidogenic efficiency. Since 3β-HSD and 17,20-desmolase act on 17OH-pregnenolone to determine relative DHA and cortisol production during human development, we studied their kinetics in adrenal microsomes from 6 kidney donors (12-40 yr) and the effect of varying steroid concentrations on their activities. There was no age-related change in K_m for 3β-HSD (0.1-0.5 μM) or desmolase (0.2-1.7 μM). At all ages V_{max} for 3β-HSD (3-8 nmol/mg/min) exceeded that for desmolase (0.3-1.4 nmol/mg/min). Physiological intra-adrenal concentrations (10^{-6} M) of progesterone, 17OH-progesterone, 11-desoxycortisol, corticosterone, androstenedione and testosterone caused >20% inhibition of 3β-HSD, with no effect on desmolase. Estradiol and estrone caused >95% inhibition of 3β-HSD with only minimal impact on desmolase. Kinetic analysis showed competitive and non-competitive inhibition with K_i values of 10^{-7}-10^{-5} M. These data demonstrate that ambient steroids can render 3β-HSD rate-limiting and permit desmolase to compete for 17OH-pregnenolone substrate. This phenomenon provides a rational explanation both for the relative 3β-HSD deficiency of the human fetus and the increased C-19 steroid production during adrenarche.

290 DISTRIBUTION OF DEHYDROEPIANDROSTERONE AND ITS SULFATE IN DIVERSE SPECIES. J.J. Byrne*, R.K. Ringer, R.A. Aulerich, Dept. OB-GYN, SUNY, Downstate Medical Center, Brooklyn, New York 11203 and College of Physicians and Surgeons of Columbia University, New York, New York 10032 and Dept. of Animal Science, Michigan State University, East Lansing, Michigan 48824

The present study was undertaken to examine and compare the relationship of dehydroepiandrosterone (D) and dehydroepiandrosterone sulfate (DS) among a number of animal species of both genders. The purpose was to find suitable non-primate alternate models for fundamental DS investigations. Serum concentrations of D & DS were determined by RIA after samples were partitioned, extracted and chromotographed. Some species had no detectable D or DS among them both male and female sheep, rabbits, chickens, turkeys and the sow. Some had D but no DS. This group included male and female ferret (0.07 ng/ml), dog (0.12 ng/ml) and guinea pig (0.25 ng/ml). The mink, fox and rat had both D & DS serum levels which differed with gender. In this group male mink D was 0.25 ng/ml while female D was 0.07 and DS 8.5 ng.ml for both. Male fox D was 0.15 ng/ml female was 0.07 ng/ml, DS was 6 ng/ml and 7.3 ng/ml respectively. Rat D was 0.06 ng/ml while DS averaged 6.3 ng/ml. Large differences in basal levels of DS were seen with maturation in Rhesus monkeys. From neonatal levels of 116 ng/ml DS dropped to 70 ng/ml at 1 yr. By 2 yrs. they averaged 83 ng/ml and at full maturity (ages 6-7 yrs.) DS had increased to 117 ng/ml. During these years, D remained constant at 1.17 ng/ml. In conclusion, there seems to be a relationship between DS levels and the passivity of the animals.

291 SERUM DEOXYCORTICOSTERONE (DOC) AND ALDOSTERONE IN CUSHING'S SYNDROME.
J. Cassar*, S. Loizou, K. Mashiter and G.F. Joplin, West Middlesex University Hospital and Royal Postgraduate Medical School, Hammersmith Hospital, London W12 OHS, England.

We assayed serum DOC and aldosterone in Cushing's syndrome due to pituitary dependent adrenal hyperplasia (4 patients), adrenal adenoma (4 patients) and ectopic ACTH production (2 patients, carcinoid in lung and appendix) and also the response of these steroids to dexamethasone and metyrapone. Serum DOC was high (>565 pmol/l) in all the patients with Cushing's disease, the patients with ectopic ACTH secretion and 2 of the 4 patients with adrenal adenoma. Dexamethasone lowered (mean of 699 to 373 pmol/l) serum DOC in the patients with adrenal hyperplasia which was pituitary dependent or due to ectopic ACTH secretion (mean of 1512 to 545 pmol/l); two patients with adrenal adenoma showed no significant change while two showed a paradoxical rise in DOC levels (mean of 626 to 1216 pmol/l). All showed an increase in DOC levels following metyrapone. Basal serum aldosterone was within normal limits (144-434 pmol/l) in all but 1 patient (ectopic ACTH secretion 484 pmol/l). After dexamethasone serum aldosterone decreased in 1 patient with Cushing's disease and in both with ectopic ACTH secretion (the former 370 to 195 pmol/l, the latter mean of 387 to 324 pmol/l). In patients with adrenal adenomas 2 patients showed no response whilst 2 patients showed a paradoxical increase in aldosterone levels (mean of 348 to 508 pmol/l). All patients showed some decrease in circulating levels of aldosterone on metyrapone. These results suggest that there is an overproduction of DOC in most of the patients with Cushing's syndrome.

292 EFFECT OF CORTICOTROPIN (ACTH) ON MOVEMENT OF STEROL CARRIER PROTEIN WITH CHOLESTEROL TO ADRENAL MITOCHONDRIA FOR STEROIDOGENESIS.
Orla M. Conneely, Denis R. Headon, Anne McMahon, Carol D. Olson, Frank Ungar and Mary E. Dempsey,* Depts. Biochem., Univ. Galway, Ireland, and Univ. Minnesota, Minneapolis, MN, USA.

Sterol carrier protein (SCP) is an abundant, ubiquitous protein (M_r 14,200) with multifunctional roles in lipid metabolism and transport. These properties plus its unusual turnover (t 1/2 < 1 hr) led to studies probing possible functions of SCP in rat adrenal steroidogenesis. The level of SCP was quantitated by a specific immunochemical assay. SCP is a major adrenal protein (>100 μg/mg protein), present in cytosol (60%) and inner mitochondrial membrane (35%). ACTH administration *in vivo* causes increased movement of SCP with cholesterol to the inner mitochondrial membrane. To observe accumulation of SCP and cholesterol the presence of aminoglutethimide, an inhibitor of steroidogenesis, is required. Adrenal SCP also undergoes a dramatic diurnal variation in amount. However, the apparent low abundance of adrenal *versus* liver and intestine mRNA, measured by translation *in vitro* or hybridization with a cDNA probe, suggested the bulk of adrenal SCP arises from uptake. Direct evidence for movement of SCP from blood was obtained using homogeneous ^{35}S-SCP. Our findings support the occurrence of a rapid adrenal pathway for enhanced uptake of SCP and movement of SCP with cholesterol to the inner mitochondrial membrane in response to ACTH *in vivo*.

293 HUMAN LEYDIG CELL X MOUSE ADRENAL CELL Y-1 HYBRIDS : cAMP STEROID AND CELL GROWTH RESPONSE TO ACTH AND 8-BrcAMP. A.Crozat , J.M.Saez and C.Finaz.
INSERM-U. 162. Hôpital Debrousse. 69322 Lyon Cedex 05. France.

In an attempt to analyse the interaction between genomes of different steroïdogenic cells we have prepared hybrids between mouse adrenal cell line Y-1 and human Leydig cells. 6 independent hybrids were analysed for hormone receptors and for the cAMP and steroid response to ACTH, hCG, 8-BrcAMP or Forskolin (F): 1) all hybrids has lost hCG receptors at their ability to produce testosterone ; 2) compared to Y-1, ACTH-induced cAMP production was high in 2, similar in other 2 and very low in 2 hybrids. In the last group, the response to F was maintened, but the synergetic effects of ACTH and F, which was observed in Y-1 and in the other hybrids, was lost; 3) ACTH- and 8-BrcAMP- induced 20α-dihydroprogesterone production was retained by 4 hybrids, but lost by the other two. However the latest hybrids had an enhanced capacity to produce pregnenolone when compared to Y-1 cells ; 4) ACTH-induced cell growth inhibition was negatively related with ACTH-induced cAMP production. Since hybrids contained one or two mouse genomes and retained variable human chromosomes, the results suggest that the extinction or the enhancement of murine genes is the fact of a regulation by human chromosomes.

294 AGE-RELATED CHANGES IN ZONAL CONCENTRATIONS OF STEROIDS IN HUMAN ADRENAL CORTEX. Z. Dickerman and J.S.D. Winter*, Department of Pediatrics, University of Manitoba, Winnipeg, Manitoba, R3E 0W1, Canada.

Concentrations of cortisol, 11-desoxycortisol, 17OH-progesterone, progesterone, corticosterone, aldosterone, 17OH-pregnenolone, dehydroepiandrosterone, androstenedione and testosterone were assayed in serial 100-250 μ zonal plane sections from 38 frozen adrenal glands.

Mean Adrenal Cortex Steroid Concentrations (μmol/L)

Age	n	F	S	17Prog	Prog	B	Aldo	17-preg	DHA	And	Test
0 days	5	3.7	0.4	7.5	2.7	0.8	.06	1.2	0.5	0.7	.06
1-30 days	14	8.4	0.4	6.1	3.2	2.2	.08	0.6	0.1	0.8	.07
2-48 mos	8	7.4	0.8	3.7	3.9	3.1	.07	0.4	0.2	0.8	.04
8-19 yr	5	8.6	1.9	3.7	2.4	4.7	.05	1.2	0.7	1.5	.08
29-68 yr	5	55.4	2.3	8.3	5.3	16.7	.34	1.6	0.7	2.5	.16

At all ages there was a centripetal gradient for all steroids, with 2-5 times higher levels in the innermost zone. All values were 10-100 times higher than in plasma; DHA and androstenedione levels parallelled age-related changes in secretion. Concentrations of most steroids were 2-10 times higher in adults than in infants, and reached concentrations (10^{-7}-10^{-5} M) that can influence steroidogenic enzyme activity. Analysis of product/substrate ratios suggested that adrenarche is accompanied by a decline in 3β-HSD relative to the activities of 17,20-desmolase and other enzymes. These data suggest that steroid concentrations in the zona reticularis are imposed by the centripetal adrenal blood flow and increase with age and adrenal size. They support the thesis that adrenarche may result from steroid-induced inhibition of 3β-HSD relative to 17,20-desmolase.

295 EVIDENCE OF A SELECTIVE DECREASE IN B-CELL FUNCTION ASSOCIATED WITH HUMAN AGING. M. Chen*, and D. Porte Jr., Seattle VA Medical Center, University of Washington, Seattle, WA, USA.

Insulin responses to glucose have been quite variable in older subjects. Recently we have described a new method for assessing changes in islet cell responsiveness to glucose by measuring the slope of glycemic potentiation (ΔAIRa/ΔG) of the acute insulin responses to 5 g arginine pulses. In this method, the mean increase of 2-5 min insulin response to arginine above pre-stimulate insulin) at 3 different plasma glucose (G) concentrations ranging from 80-300 mg/dl is tested. Conventional intravenous glucose tolerance test (IVGTT) to 20 g glucose pulse was also performed to determine the 2-5 min acute insulin response to glucose (AIRg) and glucose disappearance rate (Kg) as an index of glucose tolerance. 8 old (age 67-82) and 8 young (18-36) normal weight, healthy male volunteers were tested. We found that ΔAIRa/ΔG was significantly decreased in the old (1.4 ± 0.2, mean ± SEM) vs. young (2.7 ± 0.3, $p < 0.01$). This 48% reduction in B-cell function in the aged was correlated with Kg measured during the IVGTT ($r = 0.75$, $p < 0.01$). When B cell function was evaluated during IVGTT and expressed as AIRg, no difference was observed between old (83 ± 14 μU/ml) and young (89 ± 10). Since ΔAIRa/ΔG has been shown to correlate closely with maximal B cell responsiveness, the decrease in ΔAIRa/ΔG suggests a possible loss of synthetic or secretory capacity. We conclude that (1) slope of potentiation derived from acute insulin response to non-glucose stimuli at two or more glucose concentrations can be abnormal while first phase insulin to glucose is intact. (2) Aging is associated with decreased B-cell function as assessed by the slope of glycemic potentiation.

296 REFRACTORINESS OF AGED FEMALE BUT NOT MALE RATS TO THE PROLACTIN(PRL) LOWERING EFFECT OF GABA AGONISTS. D.Cocchi*, J.Apud°, A.Penalva, G.Racagni° and E.E. Müller. Dept.Pharmacology and °Dept. Pharmacology and Pharmacognosy, University of Milan, Milan, Italy.

The existence of a tubero-infundibular GABAergic system which inhibits PRL secretion is well established. Muscimol(M), a potent GABA agonist, reduced significantly basal PRL levels in young(3 months) male and female rats. The drug, at the same dose(2 mg/kg ip or iv), inhibited basal PRL levels in aged (24-27 months)male rats but was completely ineffective in old females. Since, in contrast to males, most of the aged female rats beared a PRL-secreting adenoma, we investigated the possibility that the tumor had altered the kinetic characteristics of GABAergic receptors on the lactotrophs, rendering them refractory to M. In fact, M administration, as in aged female rats, had not changed the high basal PRL levels of young rats bearing an estrogen induced PRL-secreting adenoma. Evaluation of the kinetic characteristics of pituitary binding sites for GABA showed that of the two populations of receptors present in the normal pituitary(low and high affinity), the adenomatous tissue exhibited only the low affinity receptors.
These data indicate that the altered PRL responsiveness to GABA agonists of aged female rats is due to the presence of a developed (in most of them) or developing PRL-secreting adenoma with ensuing disappearance of the high affinity GABA receptors mediating the inhibition of PRL secretion.

297 SOMATOMEDIN BINDING AND ACTION IN FIBROBLASTS FROM AGED AND PROGERIC SUBJECTS.

C.A. Conover*, L.A. Dollar, R.G. Rosenfeld, and R.L. Hintz, Department of Pediatrics, Stanford University, Stanford, California, USA

Aging is associated with altered cell metabolism and diminished growth potential, which have been ascribed to decreased cellular responsiveness to serum mitogens. We have previously reported that somatomedin C (SM-C) is an important mitogen for cultured human fibroblasts and that its effect is markedly enhanced by low concentrations of human hypopituitary serum (HHS). To investigate the role of SM-C in aging, we studied SM-C binding and action in fibroblasts (passage 10-13) from 4 control (7-24 yrs) subjects, 4 aged (60-78 yrs) subjects, and 1 progeric subject. In 5 experiments, SM-C (50 ng/ml) stimulated ^{3}H-thymidine incorporation (^{3}H-thd incorp) 5 to 16-fold in control, 4 to 17-fold in aged, and 4 to 11-fold in progeric cells. The presence 0.25% HHS, which alone had no mitogenic effect, magnified SM-C's effect 11 to 40-, 8 to 37-, and 8 to 31-fold in control, aged, and progeric cells, respectively. These ^{3}H-thd incorp results were clearly supported by cell replication studies. Dose response curves for SM-C stimulation of ^{3}H-thd incorp were not significantly altered in aged or progeric cells. Half-maximal responses were seen at 5-15 ng/ml for all cell lines. In addition, binding of ^{125}I-SM-C was virtually identical in all cell lines with 50% displacement at 5 ng/ml SM-C. These data demonstrate that fibroblasts from aged and progeric subjects have normal SM-C binding, and are capable of full response to the mitogenic effect of SM-C, both alone and in combination with low concentrations of HHS. Thus, the diminished replicative potential in aging does not appear to be due to generalized alterations in SM-C receptors or to decreased sensitivity to SM-C.

298 EFFECTS OF AGING ON NOCTURNAL LH, TESTOSTERONE, AND PROLACTIN LEVELS AND THEIR RELATIONSHIP TO NPT.

*Cunningham, G.R., Thornby, J.I., Aydin, A., Sohmen, T., and I. Karacan, Departments of Medicine, Cell Biology, and Psychiatry, VA Medical Center and Baylor College of Medicine, Houston, Texas 77211 U.S.A.

The effect of aging on nocturnal LH, testosterone (T) and prolactin (PRL) levels and the relationship of these parameters to nocturnal penile tumescence (NPT) have been studied in 17 healthy men. Ten men were from 40 to 50 years of age (Group I) and 7 men ranged from 60 to 70 years of age (Group II). Each man was a normal volunteer and none complained of sexual dysfunction or was using medication known to influence sleep, NPT or the endocrine parameters under evaluation. Screening hemograms and chemistries were also normal. Subjects underwent continuous polygraphic recording of sleep and NPT and blood sampling every 20 minutes throughout the night. The mean±SE serum levels of each hormone for Group I and II, respectively were: T - 534.6±49.6 vs 534.8±53.3 ng/dl: LH - 41.9±3.0 vs 44.7±2.1 ng/ml (LER-907); and PRL 16.7±2.1 vs 17.4±3.1 ng/ml. Some men in each group had T levels <250 ng/dl but all were >200 ng/dl. PRL values exceeded 20 ng/ml in some men in each group, but all concentrations were <50 ng/ml. Each subject had at least one episode of NPT, and the total duration of NPT in the groups were similar. LH, T and PRL levels were not increased significantly during NPT as compared with values during non-NPT intervals. Furthermore, episodic secretion of LH was not related to REM sleep. We conclude that aging in healthy men between 60 and 70 years of age was not associated with changes in NPT or nocturnal LH, testosterone or PRL levels and no definite relationship existed between NPT and these endocrine parameters in healthy men.

299 ISOLATION AND CHARACTERIZATION OF mRNA AND cDNA ENCODING RAT ATRIAL NATRIURETIC FACTOR (ANF).

M. Chamberland*, M. Nemer, AND J. Drouin, Institut de recherches cliniques de Montréal, H2W 1R7, Canada.

Extracts of rat atrial muscle contain peptides that possess natriuretic, diuretic and smooth muscle relaxant activities. These peptides are localized in secretory-type granules in atrial but not ventricular cardiocytes. Recently, a family of active and related peptides was isolated from rat atria and their amino acid sequence was determined. Homologous peptides of 21 to 33 amino acids having different length amino terminal sequences show the greatest activity in in vivo assays. The complete structure of these peptides and their precursor form is best deduced from sequence analysis of cloned cDNA encoding rat atrial natriuretic factor (ANF). Rat atrial poly A+ RNA was used to construct atrial cDNA libraries using AMV reverse transcriptase. Clones containing cDNA copies for most of rat ANF mRNA were obtained by screening. A complete nucleotide sequence for rat ANF mRNA was obtained by DNA sequence analysis of these clones. The cloned ANF sequences provide probes for the study of ANF gene structure and regulation of ANF gene expression in normal and diseased tissues.

300 ATRIAL NATRIURETIC FACTOR INHIBITS THE EFFECT OF ANGIOTENSIN II, ACTH AND POTASSIUM ON ALDOSTERONE SECRETION BY ISOLATED RAT ADRENAL GLOMERULOSA CELLS.

L. Chartier*, G. Thibault, R. Garcia and E.L. Schiffrin. Clinical Research Institute of Montreal, Quebec H2W 1R7.

Atrial natriuretic factor (ANF) is a peptide isolated from the atria of rats with a powerful natriuretic and vasodilator activity. The synthetic 8-33 fragment of ANF (M.W. 2862) has the full natriuretic and vasodilating properties of the natural parent compound. Since ANF inhibits the effects of angiotensin II on vascular smooth muscle, we have tested the action of the synthetic 8-33 ANF on basal and stimulated secretion of aldosterone by isolated rat adrenal glomerulosa cells. ANF did not affect basal aldosterone output. ANF inhibited aldosterone secretion stimulated by 10^{-8} M angiotensin II with an IC_{50} of 2.6×10^{-9} M. The IC_{50} of ANF on aldosterone secretion stimulated by 2.9×10^{-10} M ACTH was 2.1×10^{-9} M. Aldosterone secretion stimulated by 15 mM potassium was similarly inhibited by ANF. We conclude that ANF is a non-specific inhibitor of stimulated aldosterone output. The relationship between this *in vitro* effect and the *in vivo* natriuresis induced by ANF remain to be elucidated. Supported by the Medical Research Council of Canada.

301 CIRCADIAN RHYTHMS OF URINARY ALDOSTERONE (UA), SODIUM (UNa), POTASSIUM (UK), CREATININE (UC) AND VOLUME (UV) IN CLINICALLY HEALTHY SUBJECTS (CHS) UNDER A MILD REDUCTION (MR) IN DIETARY SALT (DS) OR BODY WEIGHT (BW).

P. Cugini[1], D. Scavo[1], P. Lucia[1], G. Murano[1], C. Letizia[1], M. Lisanu[1], R.F. Gillum[2], J.Y. Lee[2], F. Halberg[3], Y. Koga[4]; [1]I Pat. Med., Rome Univ., Italy; Labs [2]Physiol. Hyg. and [3]Chronobiol. MN, Un., USA; [4]Inst. Cardiovascul. Dis., Kurume Univ., Japan.

The effects of MR-DS(-30 mEq/24h) and MR-BW(-2Kg) on CR of UA, UNa, UK, UC and UV have been investigated in 9 CHS. MR-DS is associated with 1. the 24h excretion rate (ER) decreased for UNa, UK and UV, increased for UA and UC; 2. the extent of circadian variation (ECV) lowered for UNa, UK and UV, amplified for UA and UC; 3. the crest of temporal phase later for UK, UA, UC and UV, earlier for UNa. MR-BW is associated with a more pronounced decrease in 24 h ER for UNa and UK, and in ECV for UNa. Peculiar events are 1. the 24h ER decreased for UA, increased for UNa; 2. the ECV increased for UV, decreased for UC. Such effects may have a practical resonance for laboratory follow-up in subjects asked to reduce DS and/or to loss BW with the aim of preventing cardiovascular risk.

302 REDUCED AFFINITY OF THE RENIN-ANGIOTENSINOGEN INTERACTION IN HUMAN PREGNANCY.

C.R. Daniels, V. Eisen and J.D.H. Slater* The Cobbold Laboratories, The Middlesex Hospital Medical School, London W1N 8AA, U.K.

Reported changes in the renin-angiotensin system during pregnancy include a moderate rise in plasma renin activity (PRA) and a pronounced rise in the plasma concentration of the angiotensinogen and inactive renin (IR). Using a new, fully autologous assay system (Daniels et al, 1982), we have now estimated the parameters of the Michaelis-Menton equation, Km and Vmax from the kinetics of the interaction of purely endogenous components. During pregnancy the Km increased from 0.51 ± 0.08 μM (mean ± SD; n=10) in the first trimester, to 0.67 ± 0.13 μM (p<0.02; n=5) in the second and to 1.17 ± 0.34 μM (p<0.001; n=13) in the third. This increase of Km was correlated positively (r=0.80) with the corresponding angiotensinogen concentrations which rose from 1.88 ± 0.42 μM (mean ± SD), to 3.12 ± 0.75 μM (p<0.01) and to 4.45 ± 0.73 μM (p<0.001). The Km values were not correlated with (a) the measured PRA (b) the calculated reaction rates in either undiluted plasma or at infinite substrate concentration (Vmax) or (c) the plasma concentration of IR which was already high in the first trimester and did not increase thereafter. After activation of the plasma IR with trypsin the high Km values in the second and third trimesters were reduced to 0.53 ± 0.24 μM and 0.57 ± 0.15 μM respectively. These values are close to those found in non-pregnant individuals.

This increase of Km during pregnancy serves to limit the increase of plasma angiotensin II concentration which would otherwise be expected. (Ref. Daniels et al (1982) J. Physiol. 325, 63P).

303 INTERACTIONS BETWEEN ADRENAL ZONA GLOMERULOSA AND MEDULLA ENABLE INHIBITORY EFFECTS OF CATECHOLAMINES ON ALDOSTERONE SECRETION IN PRIMARY CO-CULTURE OF BOVINE ADRENAL CELLS. A. De Léan* and K. Racz, Institut de Recherches Cliniques de Montréal, Montréal, Québec, H2W 1R7, Canada.

We have previously reported that enzymatically dispersed bovine adrenal subcapsular cells cultured for three days display a predominant stimulatory beta-adrenergic response to catecholamines. Since the medulla constitutes a potential intra-adrenal source for catecholamines, we have studied in vitro the interaction of medullary with subcapsular cells. When subcapsular cells are co-cultured with medullary cells for three days, the stimulatory effect of (-)isoproterenol is lost, while angiotensin II and ACTH stimulatory effects on aldosterone production are preserved. Co-culture of medullary and subcapsular cells in proportions varying from 1/10 to 1/1 results in a progressive homologous desensitization of the beta-adrenergic stimulation. In contrast with its weak beta-adrenergic stimulatory effect in pure subcapsular cells, dopamine leads to a 20 to 50% inhibition of angiotensin II-stimulated aldosterone production in subcapsular cells co-cultured with medullary cells. No influence of dopamine on the basal level of aldosterone secretion was observed in this co-culture system. The results indicate that catecholamines exert a predominant beta-adrenergic stimulatory effect only in subcapsular cells cultured in the absence of medullary cells. Coexistence of both adrenal cell types leads to homologous desensitization of the beta-adrenergic response and discloses an inhibitory influence of catecholamines on aldosterone secretion. The results suggest potential intra-adrenal modulatory interactions of medullary catecholamines on aldosterone production.

304 THE ROLE OF POTASSIUM AND ACTH IN THE RESPONSE OF ADRENAL RENIN TO NEPHRECTOMY. Y. Doi, K. Baba, K. Hashiba, K. Atarashi, R. Franco-Saenz, and P. J. Mulrow,* Departments of Medicine, Nagasaki University and Medical College of Ohio, C.S. 10008, Toledo, Ohio 43699, USA.

Adrenal renin concentration increases markedly by 24 hours after nephrectomy (nepex). A high potassium (K) diet for 5 days also increases adrenal renin (5.3 $\pm$ 0.53 to 39.8 $\pm$ 5.7 S.E. ng/mg Prot/hr). Since serum K increases post nepex, we studied the effect of the anion exchange resin Kay exalate (K-ex) on the response to nepex. After nepex, K-ex lessened the rise in serum K from 8.6 $\pm$ 0.28 to 6.3 $\pm$ 0.17 mEq/L and suppressed the adrenal renin response from 115 $\pm$ 6.6 to 31 $\pm$ 3.7 ng/mg Prot/hr. The adrenal renin of the control rats was 5.1 $\pm$ 0.46 (serum K 4.8 $\pm$ 0.14 mEq/L). Plasma ACTH was elevated several fold after nepex but K-ex treatment did not lower it. (Control ACTH 126 $\pm$ 21 pg/ml, nepex 826 $\pm$ 51.1 vs nepex + K-ex 901 $\pm$ 34.5). The pituitary via ACTH also played a role in the response. Hypox before nepex abolished the response (hypox alone 3.41 $\pm$ 0.35 vs hypox + nepex 2.94 $\pm$ 0.46. However, hypox + nepex + ACTH restored the response to 70 $\pm$ 13 (nepex controls for these experiments - 83.7 $\pm$ 7.5). ACTH alone could not reproduce the effect since hypox + ACTH only raised the level to 18.5 $\pm$ 2.3. In summary, nephrectomy is a potent stimulus to adrenal renin. Both K and ACTH are involved in the mechanism. ACTH plays an important but permissive role, while K is a potent stimulus to adrenal renin.

305 ELEVATED CRYOACTIVATABLE RENIN IN PATIENTS WITH TYPE 1 DIABETES.

P.L. Drury*, Dept. of Endocrinology, St Bartholomew's Hospital, London, UK.

Increased inactive renin has been reported in diabetic patients with nephropathy. Cryoactivatable renin was measured in 40 normal subjects (Group 1) and in 49 patients with Type 1 diabetes, 18 free of all complications (Group 2) and 31 with proliferative retinopathy (Group 3). Samples were taken after 1h of supine rest (0830h) and after 4h ambulation (1230h); all subjects were on free sodium intake and no drugs but insulin. Active renin concentration (AR) was measured before, and total renin (TR) after, cryoactivation of serum for 30 days at -4°C, using excess sheep substrate and calibrated with MRC renin 68/356. Inactive renin (IR) is TR - AR.

	Mean age (years±SD)	Sex (M:F)	Median renin concentration (mU/l) AR	TR	IR	%age IR (Mean IR/TR)
Group 1	37.8 ± 13.9	26:14	21.8	127.0	110.0	76.7 ± 14.9
Group 2	38.8 ± 11.1	12:6	15.4	380.5*	342.7*	93.6 ± 4.6*
Group 3	37.4 ± 8.7	20:11	22.8+	795.0*+	765.3*+	93.6 ± 5.9*

*p<0.0001 versus Group 1; +p<0.05 versus Group 2 (Mann-Whitney U-test).

Results above show supine AR to be 48% greater in Group 3 than Group 2 but neither is significantly different from Group 1. Median supine TR was 3 to 6-fold greater in Groups 2 and 3 than in Group 1 (p<0.0001) and two-fold greater in Group 3 than in Group 2 (p<0.04). The increase is due to a 3 to 7-fold increase in IR. Similar results were found in the erect position. Conclusion: Cryoactivatable renin is markedly elevated in Type 1 diabetes, and is further raised in the presence of microvascular disease.

306 ALDOSTERONE UNRESPONSIVENESS TO ANGIOTENSIN II IN DEXAMETHASONE-SUPPRESSIBLE HYPERALDOSTERONISM (DSH).

F.Fallo°,N.Sonino,D.Armanini,T.Luzzi,F.Pedini, C.Pasini,F.Mantero.Institute of Semeiotica Medica,University of Padua,Italy.

A family with 9 siblings in which 3 sibs have been shown to have DSH was studied.Two brothers (23 and 35 y.o.) and their sister (19 y.o.) presented with classical signs of primary aldosteronism. They also showed normal cortisol,lack of p.aldosterone(Aldo)postural response,exaggerated Aldo response to ACTH 4 h infusion.No significant change of Aldo during Angiotensin II (AII) infusion at incremental rates was found:from 13.2 to 7.9 ng/100 ml(maximal peak value),from 10 to 6.3,from 38.6 to 49.5.Adrenal scinti- and CT scan and venography,performed in two,showed bilateral hyperplasia.Dexamethasone (Dex) 2 mg/d for 2 days caused a marked decrease of p. and u.Aldo and rise of PRA in all.After prolonged Dex administration (2 mg/d for 4 weeks) PRA rose to normal/supranormal range,while p. and u.Aldo maintained within low/normal levels.Blood pressure normalized in two. No restoration of Aldo response to AII infusion on Dex,tested at 3 and 14 days (from 3 to 5.2 ng/ 100 ml,from 4.3 to 4,from 14.4 to 21.2) was observed in any of them. Two other sibs (37 and 40 y.o.) were found hypertensive with normal baseline data;however,both showed Aldo hyperresponsiveness to ACTH. Finally,4 brothers are normotensive:in two of them Aldo response to ACTH was tested and found to be normal. Family pedigree is consistent with an autosomal dominant transmission. HLA typing showed the same aplotype (A3,B35) in the hypertensive sibs. Low Aldo compared to PRA levels and Aldo unresponsiveness to AII infusion during Dex show functional impairement,at least temporary,of zona glomerulosa. These findings support the hypothesis that Aldo may arise from zona fasciculata in this disorder.

307 ENDOCRINE AND BRAIN STUDIES IN SEXUALLY AGGRESSIVE MEN. J. Bain*, R. Langevin, S. Hucker, G. Wortzman and M. Ben-Aron, Clarke Institute of Psychiatry and Mount Sinai Hospital (Toronto M5G 1X5), University of Toronto, Canada.

The etiological bases for sexually aggressive acts are not clearly understood. Because there are few controlled investigations, this study was undertaken to determine whether hormonal factors, among others, are related to dangerous sexual acts, since androgens in particular have been thought to be associated with aggressive behaviour. Forty men were studied: 20 controls (offences other than rape) and 20 men convicted of rape or attempted rape (9 sadists, 11 non-sadists). These men underwent extensive psychological and psychiatric evaluation. None had a history of endocrine disease. All had CT scans of the brain. Three blood samples were drawn at 15 min. intervals for the assay of testosterone (T), androstenedione, dehydroepiandrosterone sulfate (DHEA-S), LH, FSH, estradiol, prolactin and cortisol (C). Suitable blood results were obtained on 16 controls, 6 sadists and 9 non-sadists. Although not significant, there was a trend for the non-sadists to have the highest T and C levels. Controls had a mean T of 786 µg/dl, non-sadists-917 and sadists-793. Mean C levels were: controls-16.67 µg/dl, non-sadists-19.70, sadists-13.77. Of the 9 sadists who had a CT scan of the brain, 5 demonstrated a right temporal lobe abnormality while neither non-sadists nor controls did. These findings suggest that hormones other than T, such as the adrenal hormone, DHEA-S, may be important in sexual aggression, and that some men who exhibit sexually aggressive behaviour may have organic brain pathology. Whether the brain lesion and hormonal findings are related remains to be determined.

308 DIFFERENTIAL EFFECT OF NEONATAL GONADECTOMY AND TESTOSTERONE TREATMENT ON PROCEPTIVE AND RECEPTIVE SEXUAL BEHAVIOR IN THE FERRET. M.J. Baum*, E.R. Stockman, M.S. Erskine, S. Callaghan, L. Lundell, and C. Gallagher, M.I.T. Department of Nutrition and Food Science, Cambridge, MA. U.S.A.

Male ferrets were castrated either 5, 20, or 35 days after birth. Females were ovariectomized on day 5 and then implanted s.c. with testosterone capsules (low or high dose) over postnatal days 5-20 or 20-35. Control females were ovariectomized on day 5 or 35 and received no hormone. In adulthood control females showed dose-dependent reductions in approach latencies to a stud male when tested in a runway while receiving estradiol benzoate (EB: 0, 5, 10, and 15 µg/kg). No such reduction occurred in males castrated on day 35, whereas the approach latency functions of males castrated on day 20 or day 5 fell between the extremes of the male and female ferrets gonadectomized on day 35. The approach latency functions of all groups of females given testosterone neonatally resembled those of control females. Thus it appears that proceptive defeminization normally occurs in male ferrets in response to the action of testicular hormone over a prolonged period which begins prior to day 5. All male and female ferrets in the study showed equivalent, dose-dependent, EB-induced increments in acceptance behavior in response to the neck grip of a stud male. Thus receptive defeminization seems not to occur in this carnivore in response to perinatal sex steroid exposure. This research was supported by U.S. Public Health Service grants HD-13634 and K02-MH00392.

309 BONE SCINTIGRAPHY IN HYPERPARATHYROIDISM /HPT/. M. Gembicki* and J. Kosowicz, Department of Endocrinology, Medical Academy, Poznan, Poland.

Bone scintigraphy was performed in 5 cases of HPT and compared with scintiscans of patients with Cushing's syndrome /6 cases/, Turner's syndrome /8 cases/ and post menopausal osteoporosis /6 cases/. The patients with HPT had typical clinical and biochemical symptoms; computerized tomography revealed the presence of parathyroid tumours which were confirmed at surgery. Bone scintigraphy was performed 4 h following injection of 99m-Tc-MDP "Osteolite" /NEN/ with the use of Magnascanner 1000 /Picker/. In HPT the scintigraphy revealed a symetric increased accumulation of the tracer in the cranial vault, in the clavicles and costal cartilages. In addition there were irregular areas of excessive isotope uptake in the shafts and metaphyses of affected long bones. On the other hand, the isotope accumulation in both kidneys was drastically reduced. Three to 6 months after surgical removal of parathyroid tumours bone scintigraphy indicated that bone abnormalities completely disappeared. In other patients with osteoporosis of hormonal origin /Cushing's or Turner's syndrome, climacterium/ did not show the above described abnormalities in bone scintigraphy. Conclusions: patients with HPT show on bone scintigraphy abnormalities which differ from those seen in other patients with osteoporosis and which regress following surgical removal of parathyroid tumours.

310 MECHANISM OF PRESSOR EFFECTS BY ANGIOTENSIN IN THE NUCLEUS TRACTUS SOLITARIUS OF RATS. Rod Casto* and M. Ian Phillips. Dept. of Physiology, Univ. of Florida, Gainesville, Fl. 32610 USA.

When angiotensin II (AII) is injected into the cerebral ventricles a pressor effect is seen which consists of two distinct components; one from pituitary release of vasopressin, and another due to central activation of the sympathetic nervous system (SNS). We have recently reported that micro-injection of AII into the nucleus tractus solitarius (NTS) results in a dose-related rise in mean arterial pressure (MAP) in urethane-anesthetized rats. To investigate the contribution of the SNS in the pressor response seen with injections of AII into the NTS, we used the short-acting ganglion blocker, hexamethonium chloride, to inhibit sympathetic activation. Five minutes following hexamethonium (20 mg/kg, i.v.) treatment, 500 ng of AII was injected into the NTS. There was a significant reduction ($P<0.001$) in the magnitude of the response (4.7 ± 1.1 mmHg) compared to AII controls (15.5 ± 1.6 mmHg). Thirty minutes after ganglionic blockade, AII injections were repeated. In this case there was no significant difference in the response (15.0 ± 1.3 mmHg) compared to AII controls. Reports of high levels of angiotensin converting enzyme (ACE) in the NTS led us to investigate if injection of angiotensin I (AI) into the NTS would have a similar effect. Injection of AI (1000 ng) into the NTS leads to a small increase in MAP compared to AII. The results of the present study indicate that a) the pressor response by AII in the NTS is largely due to sympathetic activation, not hormonal mechanisms since sympathetic blockade severely attenuated the response, and b) AI produces a similar but far less potent pressor response when injected into the NTS.

311 BRAIN PROLACTIN: CHARACTERIZATION BY RIA, GEL CHROMATOGRAPHY, AND BIO-ASSAY.

N. Emanuele*, T. Hagen, C. Beer, D. Martinson, P. Gout, G. Baker, L. Kirsteins and A. M. Lawrence, Hines VA Hospital, Hines, IL 60141, USA; Loyola Univ. Med. Ctr., Maywood, IL 60153, USA; Wood VA Med. Ctr., Wood, WI 53193, USA; and Cancer Control Agency, Vancouver, V5Z3J3, Canada.

Prolactin (Prl) may have important effects on the mammalian brain. Immunoreactive prolactin (iPrl) and specific Prl receptors have been demonstrated in the CNS. Prl modulates electrical activity of single neurons, augments CNS dopamine turnover, and influences a variety of animal behaviors. We report the first quantitative, immunologic and biologic analysis of this activity from rat brain. iPrl was detected in all brain areas examined ranging from 402 ± 23 pg/mg in the hypothalamus to 29 ± 3 pg/mg in the caudate. iPrl was demonstrated in brains from long-term hypophysectomized rats. Chromatography on Sephadex G-75 revealed virtual co-elution of hypothalamic and pituitary iPrl, and serial dilutions of brain extract displaced I-125 Prl from antibody in a manner parallel to pituitary Prl. In addition, extract from the hypothalamus and extrahypothalamic areas of the brain was active in the rat Nb_2 node lymphoma cell bioassay for pituitary Prl. Conclusions: 1) iPrl is widely distributed in the rodent CNS, 2) Chromatographic, immunologic, and biologic analyses show molecular similarity to pituitary Prl, and 3) The presence of brain-based iPrl, after removal of the pituitary, implies *in situ* synthesis of Prl in the CNS, findings that complement identification of mRNA for Prl in the rat brain.

312 AN IMPROVED NON-HPLC 1α,25-DIHYDROXYVITAMIN D BINDING ASSAY

M R Bye, M J O'Sullivan, P M Baxendale, J I Hulme, and G L Guilford*, Tritium Products Department, Amersham International plc, Forest Farm, Whitchurch, Cardiff, UK.

The steroid hormone 1α,25-dihydroxyvitamin D, a metabolic product of vitamin D, is a major regulator of mineral metabolism. Elucidating the role of vitamin D has been hampered by the lack of a straightforward, reliable assay for 1α,25-dihydroxyvitamin D, its active metabolite. Conventionally, techniques used to quantitate 1α,25-dihydroxyvitamin D have required extensive sample purification including HPLC before the final assay. A simplified sample purification procedure for 1α,25-dihydroxyvitamin D has been described recently (Mallon *et al* (1980) Arch.Biochem.Biophys. **201**, 277-285). We present data which supports the validity of this purification procedure. We have also combined this simplified non-HPLC sample purification procedure with a considerably improved binding assay protocol. The resultant 1α,25-dihydroxyvitamin D assay offers significant advantages of convenience over those hitherto employed in this field.

313 REACTIVE HYPERPARATHYROIDISM IN PATIENTS TREATED FOR HYPERCALCEMIA OF MALIGNANCY. J. Carmichael*, M. Antos, R. Kremer and D. Goltzman, Departments of Medicine, McGill University and Royal Victoria Hospital, Montreal, H3A 1A1, Canada.

A subset of patients with malignancy and hypercalcemia develop concomitant hypophosphatemia, reduced renal phosphate threshold, increased fractional calcium excretion and elevated nephrogenous cyclic AMP excretion. Baseline levels of circulating bioactivity in a cytochemical bioassay for parathyroid hormone (PTH) are generally elevated, whereas immunoreactive PTH, measured with a variety of sequence-specific radioimmunoassays are low normal or undetectable. We have examined the effect of reducing hypercalcemia in 3 such patients, one with bronchogenic carcinoma and two with hypernephromas. Levels of serum calcium, cytochemical bioactivity, and immunoreactive PTH (employing an antiserum recognizing primarily the carboxyl region of the molecule) were measured sequentially after administration of either salmon calcitonin, 100 MRC units subcutaneously, or mithramycin, 20 µg/Kg intravenously. Reductions of serum calcium were accompanied by at least a 3-fold rise in immunoreactive PTH and at least a 4-fold increase in bioactivity. Gel chromatographic analysis suggested that the increase in circulating bioactivity was due to release of the major glandular form of PTH. The results indicate the development of reactive hyperparathyroidism as hypercalcemia is acutely treated in patients with malignancy. To date calciuric agents have been the mainstay of hypercalcemic therapy in this disorder. Our study emphasizes the importance of the use of hypocalcemic agents which inhibit skeletal resorption, to prevent potential worsening by reactive hyperparathyroidism of the already compromised osseous status of these patients.

314 PARATHYROID HORMONE EFFECT ON CHICKEN RENAL BRUSH BORDER MEMBRANE PHOSPHATE TRANSPORT. N. B. Clark* and J. Larry Renfro, Biological Sciences Group, University of Connecticut, Storrs, CT. 06268 USA.

Renal clearance studies showed that parathyroidectomy (PTX) stimulated renal phosphate reabsorption within 90 min in 3 wk old chicks. Subsequent parathyroid hormone (PTH) infusion caused net phosphate secretion. Kidneys were taken for brush border membrane (BBM) preparations 3 h after PTX or sham operations and 1 h after PTH or saline injections thus yielding four categories of PTH status: PTX/saline, sham/saline, PTX/PTH, and sham/PTH. Efficacy of PTX and PTH was confirmed by examination of serum calcium concentrations. A 100 mM NaSCN gradient, out>in, caused concentrative phosphate uptake by BBM from sham/saline animals. Concentrative uptake was not produced by 100 mM KSCN, out>in; pH 7.4 in vs. pH 5.4 out; or 100 mM NaCl out=in. Removal of endogenous PTH (PTX/saline) significantly stimulated Na-dependent phosphate uptake compared to sham/saline. PTH infusion significantly depressed Na-dependent phosphate uptake in PTX/PTH and sham/PTH groups compared to sham/saline and PTX/saline. Na-dependent, concentrative glucose uptake was present and unchanged by PTH. Kinetic analysis, based on 5sec uptakes, showed that both apparent affinity and Vmax for Na-dependent phosphate transport was decreased by PTH treatment. The data suggest that PTH influences avian renal phosphate excretion at least in part through a Na-dependent phosphate transport system in proximal tubule BBM. This study was supported by National Science Foundation Grants PCM 81-04037 and PCM 80-03452 and the University of Connecticut Research Foundation.

315 AN ULTRASTRUCTURAL STUDY OF THE SECRETORY CYCLE OF THE PARATHYROID GLAND OF THE EUROPEAN STARLING *Sturnus vulgaris*

J.A. Cole* and N.B. Clark, The Biological Sciences Group, The University of Connecticut, Storrs, CT 06268

The avian parathyroid gland (PTG) has been extensively studied in domestic birds such as the chicken but relatively few wild species have been examined. This study was undertaken to extend previous work on the fine structure of the starling PTG and to determine if annual cyclical changes occur in the fine structure of the gland. Low magnification electronmicrographs were analyzed for the relative areas (R_a) of the nucleus, cytoplasm, lipid and intercellular spaces (ICS) and were graded for 12 subcellular characteristics indicative of PTG activity. There was no change in the R_a of the nucleus during the year. The R_a of the cytoplasm was maximal Nov-Jan and declined to a minimum May-July. The R_a of the ICS was minimal Nov-Jan and maximal May-July. The R_a of lipid was maximal Nov-Jan and minimal May-July. Lysosomes were numerous Nov-Apr and were often associated with lipid Feb-Apr. RER and polysomes were dispersed Nov-Jan and were aggregated in parallel cisterns and rosettes respectively Feb-July The Golgi complex was most prominent Feb-Apr but was not particularly large at any time of the year. Secretory granules were rare but were most frequently encountered Feb-Apr near the plasma membranes of the lateral margins of the cell, the vascular pole and occasionally in the capillary endothelium. This study indicates that the starling PTG undergoes morphological changes suggestive of cycles in secretory activity. The PTG appears most active Apr-July during what is considered the breeding season of the animal. This morphological evidence suggests that the PTG may be important in reproductive periods in birds. Support: NSF Grant PCM81-04037

316 LATE INCREASE IN SERUM $1,25(OH)_2D$ ONE MONTH AFTER SURGERY FOR ADENOMATOUS HYPERPARATHYROIDISM.

P. D'Amour*, F. Gilbert, M. Gascon-Barré, J.-M. Boutin, J. Havrankova, R. Matte, R. Bélanger, R. Poisson, Centre de Recherches Cliniques, Hôpital St-Luc, Montreal, Canada.

We have studied the stages of the recovery of the parathyroid function after surgery for a single parathyroid adenoma. Phosphocalcic metabolism was assessed through measurement of various parameters at regular time intervals. Ten patients were followed for one month and 6 for 80 days. PTH, and urinary cAMP were measured by radioimmunoassays and $1,25(OH)_2D$ by a radioreceptor assay. Results (Mean±SEM) are summarized in the following table.

Day	Ca_s (mg %)	PO_{4s} (mg %)	PTH (pg/ml)	$1,25(OH)_2D$ (pg/ml)	$cAMP_u$ (nmol/ 100 ml GF)	Ca_u (mg/ 100 ml GF)	PO_{4u} (mg/ 100 ml GF)
-1	11.8±.3	3.2±.3	364±51	61.8±7.9	3.9± .7	.268±.028	.644±.042
1	8.8±.2	3.2±.3	42±16	35.9±4.3	2.4± .2	.187±.030	.151±.062
4	8.7±.3	4.4±.4	104±17	41.5±4.7	2.4± .4	.109±.023	.433±.045
15	9.1±.2	3.7±.3	125±20	37.6±3.8	2.7± .8	.082±.019	.538±.071
27	9.7±.2	3.9±.3	143±23	57.7±5.1	2.8± .4	.075±.022	.590±.040
55	9.6±.2	3.9±.3	133±27	58.3±4.3	3.3± .4	.078±.016	.579±.064
80	9.8±.2	3.2±.2	139±50	44 ±7.7		.079±.026	.596±.074

After a short period (3 days) of relative hypoparathyroidism, the recuperation of the parathyroid function was complete by day 27, as reflected by stable values for serum calcium, phosphorus and PTH. Serum $1,25(OH)_2D$, which had decreased after surgery, increased to pre-op. values between day 27 and 55. This increase could not be related to serum phosphorus or PTH, to urinary cAMP or to changes in diet. Its signification remains to be elucidated but could be related to the correction of the mild bone disease in these patients.

317 CALCITONIN GENE TRANSCRIPTION IS INCREASED BY TUMOR PROMOTING PHORBOL ESTERS IN CULTURED HUMAN MEDULLARY THYROID CARCINOMA (MTC).

A.deBustros*#, S.B.Baylin#, C.L.Berger#, B.A.Roos+, S.S.Leong§ and B.D.Nelkin#. #The Johns Hopkins Medical Institutions, Baltimore, Md. 21205, +Case Western Reserve University, Cleveland, OH 44106, §Roswell Park Memorial Institute, Buffalo, NY 14263.

In addition to acting as tumor promoters, phorbol esters can alter differentiation of cultured cells. The TT line is a unique human MTC line that produces large amounts of calcitonin. We found that the phorbol esters 12-0-tetra-decanoylphorbol-13-acetate (TPA-1.6 to 160 ηM) and 12,13-dibutyrate (PDBU-200 to 2000 ηM) caused within 6 hours: (1) a marked change in cell morphology, (2) a 2-to-4-fold stimulation of calcitonin secretion, (3) a 2-to-4-fold increase in the level of calcitonin mRNA. Actin mRNA levels were unchanged whereas myc oncogene mRNA levels were decreased. These changes were sustained after 48 hours. When nuclei were isolated from cells treated with TPA or PDBU for 3 hours, they showed a 2-fold increase in calcitonin specific nascent RNA thus showing that accumulation of calcitonin mRNA was due to increased transcription. Actin gene transcription was unchanged. Biologically inactive phorbols failed to produce any of the above changes. Thus, tumor promoting phorbol esters selectively increase calcitonin gene transcription. Their effect on cell morphology suggests that perturbation of the cell membrane with subsequent secretion of calcitonin provides a cytoplasmic trigger to transcription. The differential effect of the phorbol compounds on the expression of 3 genes suggests that they can be used to switch the differentiation program of cultured human MTC cells.

318 VITAMIN D METABOLISM IN BREAST-FED CHILDREN AND THEIR MOTHERS.

H.J. Degenhart*, S.M.P.F. de Muinck Keizer, T. Hoogenboezem and H.K.A. Visser, Dept. of Paediatrics, Erasmus University Rotterdam, Univ. Hosp. Rotterdam/Sophia Children's Hosp., The Netherlands.

In a longitudinal study focused on calcium homeostasis in the neonatal period, 41 healthy pregnant Caucasian women and (after birth) their children participated. With informed consent venous blood samples were drawn at 36 wks gestation. At birth cord blood and simultaneously maternal venous blood was obtained. Subsequently venous blood from mothers and children was drawn at 2-4 wks interval, up to 6 months. Breast milk samples were obtained during the same period. Rickets was not observed in the children. Their Ca levels were stable and in the normal (age-matched) reference range. Serum parameters used also included 25-OH-vit.D (25); 1,25-di-OH-vit.D (1,25); 24,25-di-OH-vit.D (24,25); 25,26-di-OH-vit.D (25,26); PTH, calcitonin, Mg, P, alk.fosfatase. Breast milk was assayed for free and glucuronated vit.D metabolites. Main results and conclusions: 1. Maternal levels at birth and cord blood levels of (25); (1,25); (24,25) and (25,26) were all correlated at a highly significant level. In later samples this correlation disappeared. 2. Maternal (1,25) levels decreased from 11.2 ± 2.9 (mean ± SEM; ng/100 ml) 4 weeks an te partum to 1.7 ± .3 (2-3 weeks post-partum (p.p.)). Infants reached a maximum in the 2nd week p.p. (6.2 ± .8). 3. In the presence of normal maternal (24,25) levels (1.1 ± .2; ng/ml), 8 weeks p.p. the infants' (24,25) disappeared (<.1). 4. Breast milk (25)-glucuronide was undetectable. Free (25) was present (ca 1% of maternal serum values). Free (1,25) was present (≤1pg/ml).

319 IN VITRO METABOLISM OF 25-HYDROXYVITAMIN D_3 [25-$(OH)D_3$] BY ISOLATED HUMAN DECIDUAL CELLS. E.E. Delvin* and A. Arabian. Genetics Unit, Shriners Hospital, McGill University, Montreal, H3G 1A6, Canada.

Our understanding of the foeto-maternal inter-relationship in terms of vitamin D metabolism and of the foeto-placental contribution to the hormonal control of the foetal mineral homeostasis is limited. Lester et al. (Science 204:1311, 1979) have shown that, in the rat, the foeto-placental metabolism of calcidiol (25-OHD_3) was independent of that of the mother. Weissman et al. (Nature 281:317, 1979) have demonstrated, in organ culture, the conversion of 25-OHD_3 into 1,25-$(OH)_2D_3$ by human decidua. We have attempted to elucidate the source of the 25-OHD_3-1α-hydroxylase. Term decidual tissue was incubated for 110 min at 37°C with collagenase (Clostridium hist.) followed by an additional 10 min in presence of DNAse (bovine pancreas) in Eagle's Minimum Essential Medium (MEM) containing 10 mM HEPES buffer at pH 7.40. The digested material was filtered through nylon mesh and the resulting suspension centrifuged at 4°C for 20 min at 800 g in a discontinuous Percoll gradient. Cells were collected, washed from the colloid and set into culture in MEM containing streptomycin, penicillin and Fungizone[r]. After 18 hours, 25-hydroxy [26(27)-methyl-^{3}H]cholecalciferol (6 nM) and varying amounts of unlabeled 25-OHD_3 were added and the incubation pursued. Cells and media were extracted with diethyl ether and extracts purified by HPLC. Metabolites were identified by co-chromatography with pure standards, periodate oxidation and receptor binding. The enzyme activity, selectively observed in two cell populations (s.g. 1.0452 and 1.0578), was directly related to cell number and to time. The apparent Km and Vmax in combined cells were 108 ± 13 nM and 3.0 ± 0.9 pmol/h/10^6 cells respectively (m ± s.d.). These results establish that cells isolated from term human decidua are able to hydroxylate 25-OHD_3. The physiologic relevance of this function remains however to be determined.

320 PHOSPHORYLATION OF A PROTEIN IMMUNOLOGICALLY-RELATED TO PARATHYROID SECRETORY PROTEIN IN MULTIPLE ENDOCRINE TISSUES. G. Bhargava*, T. Lu and L. M. Sherwood, Departments of Medicine and Biochemistry, Albert Einstein College of Medicine, Bronx, New York

We have recently reported that bovine parathyroid secretory protein (PSP) is actively phosphorylated, with the degree of phosphorylation being inversely related to calcium concentration (PNAS 80:878, 1983). PSP is closely related immunologically to adrenal chromogranin A and to a similar protein in multiple endocrine tissues. We have now extended our studies of phosphorylation to include the bovine adrenal medulla, pituitary, pancreas, thyroid and small intestine. In extracts of each tissue there was a distinct 68,000 dalton band on SDS gel electrophoresis in the position of PSP. When this band was eluted from the gel, it caused displacement in the radioimmunoassay for PSP, with the displacement curve being parallel to that of PSP. The relative concentrations of this protein in various tissues were as follows: adrenal medulla > pituitary > pancreas > small intestine > thyroid. Incubation of a homogenate of each tissue with ^{32}P-labeled ATP for two minutes showed active phosphorylation of the protein in each. cAMP caused no enhancement of PSP phosphorylation in the parathyroid, whereas calcium inhibited phosphorylation in the parathyroid and thyroid and appeared to enhance it in the intestine. Although the function of this protein is still unknown, its active phosphorylation, release from secretory granules and relationship to calcium suggest that it may play an important role in the regulation of hormone secretion. This study was supported by USPHS grant AM28556.

321 HYPERCALCEMIA AND HYPERCALCIURIA IN RATS BEARING THE MStT/W15 PITUITARY TUMOR. H.E. Carlson*, A.S. Brickman, L.J. Deftos, R.L. Horst, Harry Truman, Sepulveda and San Diego VA Hospitals, Columbia, MO, and Sepulveda and LaJolla, CA, and National Animal Disease Center, Ames, IA.

Since prolactin (PRL) and growth hormone (GH) are both believed to influence mineral metabolism in various animal species, we studied the effects of chronically elevated serum GH and PRL (2-5 μg/ml each) on mineral metabolism in female Wistar-Furth rats bearing the MStT/W15 transplantable pituitary tumor. 24-hr urine excretion of calcium and magnesium was elevated in the tumor-bearing rats (Table). Total and ionized serum Ca were both elevated, as was total serum Mg (2.36±0.08 in controls vs. 2.64±0.06 in tumors). Serum and urine PO_4 were not changed. Serum PTH was slightly but significantly higher in the tumor-bearing animals, as was serum $1,25(OH)_2D$ (Table shows mean ± SE).

	Urine Ca	U-Mg	S-Ca	Ion. S-Ca	PTH	$1,25(OH)_2D$
Control	2.9±0.2	4.8±0.5	10.1±0.1	2.53±0.01	927±35	29±6
Tumor	10.2±0.7	6.7±0.5	11.9±0.1	2.88±0.05	1172±78	70±13

Starvation reduced both hypercalcemia and hypercalciuria, suggesting that these are largely dependent on dietary calcium rather than bone resorption. Dexamethasone 0.5 mg/day for 4 days did not lower serum Ca. The parathyroid dependence of the hypercalcemic state was further shown by a fall in serum Ca to 5.8±0.2 after parathyroidectomy of tumor-bearing rats. Conclusion: rats bearing the GH- and PRL-secreting MStT/W15 pituitary tumor manifest hypercalcemia and hypercalciuria along with elevated serum PTH and $1,25(OH)_2D$. Elevated GH may be responsible for these abnormalities by stimulation of PTH secretion (Endocrinology 98:1289, 1976).

322 HORMONAL INFLUENCES ACTING ON SOLID OVARIAN CARCINOMA TISSUES AND OVARIAN CARCINOMA CELLS SUSPENDED IN ASCITIC FLUID.
Ch. Bieglmayer+, K. Schieder, Ch. Nowotny.
2nd Department of Obstetrics and Gynecology, University of Vienna, Spitalgasse 23, A-1090 Vienna, Austria

Steroid hormone receptors of ovarian carcinoma tissues or tumor cells suspended in ascitic fluid were measured by the DCC-method and sucrose gradient centrifugation, respectively. A human tumor colony forming assay (HTCFA) was set up whenever possible. In vitro colony formation during continuous exposure to tamoxifene and medroxyprogesterone acetate was compared to untreated controls. Sex steroids, steroids from the adrenal cortex, pituitary hormones, placental hormones and an ovarian carcinoma marker, Ca 125, were measured in ascitic fluid and serum samples by radioimmunological methods. Hormone levels from both specimen were comparable, exhibiting the typical patterns of postmenopausal women. Beta-HCG and HCS could be detected in more than half of the ascitic fluid samples. In serum samples Ca 125 levels were lower than in the ascitic fluid. Differences between biochemical analysis of hormone receptors and hormone sensitivity in the HTCFA may result from the use of different samples for the assay (e.g. receptor analysis from solid tumor, HTCFA set up from cells suspended in ascitic fluid) or from selection modes acting on colony forming cells.

323 THE RELATIONSHIP OF THE ANTIESTROGENIC EFFICACY OF LY156758 TO ITS PHARMACOKINETICS AND METABOLISM FOLLOWING ORAL ADMINISTRATION TO ADULT OVARIECTOMIZED RATS. L. J. Black*, N. V. Owen and T. D. Lindstrom, The Lilly Research Laboratories, A Division of Eli Lilly and Company, Indianapolis, IN 46285, USA.

One hour after a single oral dose of LY156758 (8 mg/kg) the plasma levels of LY156758 glucuronide were 4 times that of unchanged LY156758, and both compounds were nearly undetectable by 12 hours. When ^{3}H-estradiol was administered continuously from Alzet osmotic pumps (4 µg/kg/day), an 8 mg/kg oral dose of LY156758 once each day inhibited uterotropic activity to as great an extent as the same daily dose delivered continuously by osmotic pumps. Both treatments completely blocked uterine accumulation of ^{3}H-estradiol in vivo.

Three daily oral administrations of a lower dose of LY156758 (825 µg/kg) maximally inhibited the uterotropic action of 1.7 µg/kg estradiol injected concomitantly, s.c. Free LY156758 was not detected in the plasma (less than 1 ng/ml), while considerable LY156758 was present as the glucuronide conjugate. A direct correlation between the oral dose of LY156758 administered and the reduction of uterine ^{3}H-estradiol accumulation or uterotropic activity was observed.

LY156758 was conjugated following oral administration and rapidly cleared within a few hours as was free LY156758. The presence of LY156758 glucuronide was associated with potent antiuterotropic activity, and prolonged blockade of uterine uptake of ^{3}H-estradiol.

324 INTERACTION BETWEEN MELATONIN (Mel) AND UNDERFEEDING IN SUPPRESSING 7,12-DIMETHYLBENZANTHRACENE (DMBA)-INDUCED MAMMARY TUMORIGENESIS. D. Blask*, S. Hill, M. Orstead, and J. Massa, Dept. of Anatomy, Univ. of Arizona, Tucson, Arizona.

Either chronic Mel treatment or severe underfeeding inhibits the development of DMBA-induced mammary tumors in rats. We studied the interaction between chronic Mel treatment and chronic, mild (30%) underfeeding in order to determine whether the combination of these factors is more effective than either treatment alone in inhibiting DMBA-induced mammary tumorigenesis. Female rats, injected with DMBA, were fed a semipurified diet and four weeks later assigned to one of the following groups: 1) Fullfed (FF)-Saline (S), 2) FF-Mel, 3) Underfed (UF)-S or 4) UF-Mel. Mel (250 µg) was injected sc every day in the late afternoon. UF rats received 70% of the daily food intake of the FF groups. Mel injections and underfeeding were continued for 14 weeks. The cumulative tumor incidence was 100% for FF-S, 87% for both FF-Mel and UF-S and 62% for UF-Mel. The total number of tumors was 305 for FF-S, 217 for FF-Mel, 102 for UF-S and 48 for UF-Mel. The mean tumor diameter was 4.84 ± 0.41 for FF-S, 4.26 ± 0.44 for FF-Mel, 2.20 ± 0.25 for UF-S and 1.71 ± 0.38 for UF-Mel. The percentage of complete tumor regressions was 3.3 for FF-S, 10.1 for FF-Mel, 13.7 for UF-S and 20.8 for UF-Mel. These data indicate that Mel together with underfeeding is more effective than either treatment alone in inhibiting mammary tumorigenesis. Supported by NIH grant #R01 5 R23 CA27653-02.

325 PROPERTIES OF A PROLACTIN-DAUNOMYCIN (PRL-D) CONJUGATE WITH INTACT HORMONE SPECIFICITY.

H.C. Blossey*, B. Gaier, F. Kohen, Department of Hormone Research, The Weizmann Institute of Science, Rehovot 76100, Israel.

Since a considerable amount of human and experimentally induced rat breast cancers express the prolactin (PRL) receptor, a PRL-D conjugate was synthesized by coupling periodate oxidized daunomycin to the lysine residues of ovine PRL (oPRL). The properties of the oPRL moiety in the conjugate was analyzed with liver plasma membranes and cultured granulosa cells derived from estradiol and pregnant mare serum gonadotropin treated immature female rats. ^{125}I-oPRL had a K_d of 6 x 10^{-10}M in both systems. Ovine PRL-D had a K_d of 5 x 10^{-9}M in competition experiments. The ^{125}I-oPRL-D conjugate had a K_d of 8.8 x 10^{-9}M in the rat liver system. When cultured granulosa cells were exposed to daunomycin alone at a concentration of 5 x 10^{-7}M the intrinsic fluorescence of the drug was visible at the nuclei of the cells whereas exposition of the conjugate resulted in fluorescence of the cytoplasm. The latter effect was time and dose dependent and could be suppressed by an excess of unconjugated oPRL. The cytoplasmic fluorescence was observed only in vital cells. These data suggest that the affinity of the oPRL-D conjugate to the PRL receptor is nearly unimpaired and that the conjugate is concentrated by PRL receptor containing cells. These characteristics of the conjugate allow to evaluate the possibility of using internalization mechanisms to introduce cytotoxic drugs into cancer cells.
H.C.B. is a fellow of the MINERVA and Minna-James-Heinemann-Foundation. This work was supported by the Schilling Foundation.

326 SELECTION AND CHARACTERIZATION OF A BREAST CANCER CELL LINE RESISTANT TO ANTIESTROGENS.

D.A. Bronzert*, G.L. Greene†, R.B. Dickson and M.E. Lippman. Medicine Branch, National Cancer Institute, Bethesda, MD 20205 and †Ben May Labs, University of Chicago, Chicago, IL 60637.

We have selected and cloned a variant of the MCF-7 breast cancer cell line (LY 2) that is resistant to LY 117018 (LY), a potent antiestrogen that inhibits cell growth at concentrations as low as 10^{-10}M. The cell line was selected by increasing the concentration of LY in the growth media in a stepwise manner from 10^{-8}M to 10^{-6}M as the cells became resistant. LY 2 has been cloned in soft agar and carried for over 50 passages with no change in resistance. Other antiestrogens such as tamoxifen and 4OH-tamoxifen no longer inhibit cell proliferation in LY 2. The cell line has retained its growth response to estradiol. However, in a whole cell assay, the LY 2 cell line has only 43,000 sites/cell of estrogen receptor while under comparable conditions, MCF-7 cell line has 156,000 sites/cell. [^{3}H] estradiol binds with the same affinity at 4°C to cytosolic estrogen receptors from both MCF-7 and LY 2 cells. In addition, LY 117018 competes for [^{3}H] estradiol binding with the same K_i. Using an antiestrophilin antibody and SDS gel-Western blot analysis, immunoreactive estrogen receptor is compared in 33% ammonium sulfate precipitated cytosol from MCF-7 and LY 2 cells. While MCF-7 cells shows a single characteristic 69K species, no immunoreactive estrogen receptor is detected in LY 2. Another estrogen response in the MCF-7 cell line is the induction of progesterone receptor. The LY 2 cell line fails to show this induction and no detectable progesterone receptor can be measured. By further characterizing this cell line, we hope to better understand antiestrogen resistant breast cancer.

327 FREE ESTRADIOL,SEX HORMONE BINDING GLOBULIN,BREAST CANCER AND BREAST CANCER RISK.

P.F.Bruning*,J.M.G.Bonfrèr,M.de Jong-Bakker and A.A.M.Hart.
The Netherlands Cancer Institute,1066 CX Amsterdam.

It has been shown by Siiteri et al.(Banbury Report no.8,Cold Spring Harbor Lab.1981,pp.87-101) that despite a normal serum concentration of estradiol(E2), the percentage of non protein bound or free E2, which is supposed to be biologically active, is abnormally high in breast cancer patients. Using the same centrifugal-ultrafiltration method of Hammond et al.(J.Biol. Chem.255:5023,1980) we have measured free E2 in heparinized plasma from 58 premenopausal women:a.at high familial risk for breast cancer (n=20),b.with benign breast disease(n=10),c.cured for T1NoMo breast cancer at least 6 months ago (n=17),d.normal controls matched for age,parity and Quetelet index (n=11).SHBG was measured as ^{3}H-dihydrotestosterone binding capacity.Free E2 and SHBG were also measured in the serum of e.mainly postmenopausal breast cancer patients (n=40) and f.matched control cancer patients (n=70). We could confirm a very good inverse correlation between log free E2% and log SHBG (p <0.0001).The regression lines for groups a.-d.were identical. The regression lines for groups e. and f.were also identical and ran parallel to those for groups a.-d.though significantly lower.

Group	a.	b.	c.	d.	e.	f.
mean ± s.d.	1.78	1.84	1.86	1.70	1.59	1.43
Free E2%	± 0.28	± 0.34	± 0.39	± 0.54	± 0.41	± 0.40
SHBG	35.9	31.6	33.9	47.1	43.4	41.8
mmol/l	± 11.3	± 10.3	± 12.1	± 20.6	± 28.2	± 15.4

We could not find any significant difference in free E2 or SHBG between women at risk,women with benign breast disease,patients cured for early breast cancer or having breast cancer before or after menopause and matched controls.

328 A 250-K CELLULAR PROTEIN IS INDUCED BY PROGESTINS IN THE MCF7 AND T47D HUMAN BREAST CANCER CELL LINES.

D. Chalbos* and H. Rochefort,
Unité d'Endocrinologie Cellulaire et Moléculaire (U 148) INSERM, 60 rue de Navacelles, 34100 Montpellier, France.

While progestins modulate the growth and function of mammary cancer cells, no convenient induced protein has been described allowing the study of the regulation of gene expression by progestins in continuous cell lines. We have studied the effect of R5020, a synthetic progestin, on the cellular proteins of two human breast cancer cells (T47D and MCF7), using sodium dodecyl sulfate-polyacrylamide gel electrophoresis. R5020 stimulated the synthesis, as measured after [^{35}S]-methionine labeling for 4 hours, and the accumulation, as shown by silver staining, of a protein of molecular weight 250,000 (250-K). The increase of the labeled 250-K protein was observed as soon as 3 hours after treatment and its accumulation was maximal after 3 days where the 250-K protein represents ≅6 % of the total cellular proteins (≅1 μg/150,000 cells). This response was not observed in 2 estrogen receptor negative cell lines (BT20 and T47D clone 8). It was obtained by physiologically active concentrations of progestins (R5020, progesterone, medroxyprogesterone acetate) but not by estradiol or dexamethasone. 5α-dihydrotestosterone behaved as a weak agonist. The induction of the 250-K protein was inhibited by Cordycepin, Actinomycin D and R486, a progestin antagonist, but not by flutamide, an androgen antagonist. We conclude that the 250-K protein is specifically induced by progestin *via* the progesterone receptor. The abundance, specificity and rapidity of induction indicate that the 250-K protein is a good probe to study the mechanism of action of progestins in cell culture.

329 DEPO-PROVERA SUPPRESSES PROGESTERONE RECEPTOR AND DNA SYNTHESIS IN THE EPITHELIAL-STROMAL COMPLEX OF THE RABBIT ENDOCERVIX.

B.S. Chilton*, K.L. Gettys, M.G. Newman and C.J. McAllister, Anatomy Department, Medical University of South Carolina, Charleston, S.C. 29425, U.S.A.

The effects of a contraceptive dose (2.14 mg/kg) of Depo-Provera were studied in estrous rabbits 7 days after an intramuscular injection. The concentration (mean±SEM) of cytosol progesterone receptor in the epithelial-stromal complex of the endocervix was 23.1±2.3 pmol/g tissue for estrous animals, with 12% of the total receptor in the nuclear fraction (3.1±0.4 pmol/g tissue). The concentration of cytosol progesterone receptor in the uterine endometrium was 75.8±7.6 pmol/g tissue, with 9% of the total receptor in the nuclear fraction (7.6±1.9 pmol/g tissue). Depo-Provera reduced the concentration of cytosol progesterone receptor (12.0±0.3 pmol/g tissue) in the epithelial-stromal complex of the endocervix 50%, but 23% of the total receptor was retained in the nuclear fraction (3.5±0.7 pmol/g tissue). In the uterine endometrium the concentration of cytosol progesterone receptor was significantly reduced ($p<0.01$) to 8.5±0.1 pmol/g tissue, and 20% of the total receptor was retained in the nuclear fraction (2.1±0.3 pmol/g tissue). Depo-Provera depressed cell-free DNA synthesis (mean±SEM). For estrous rabbits, DNA synthesis averaged 33.5±5.1 DPM/μg DNA for the epithelial-stromal complex of the endocervix, and 16.5±3.5 DPM/μg DNA for uterine endometrium. After Depo-Provera treatment these values were reduced 3-fold to 9.7±0.9 DPM/μg DNA (endocervix) and 5.7±0.5 DPM/μg DNA (uterus). Thus it is apparent that Depo-Provera suppressed progesterone receptor synthesis and DNA synthesis in the rabbit endocervical epithelial-stromal complex and in the uterine endometrium. NIH Grant HD-16676.

330 THE EFFECT OF INSULIN, GLUCAGON, CORTICOSTERONE AND CORTISONE ON THE GLUCOSE CARRIERS OF EHRLICH ASCITES TUMOUR CELLS.

Y. M. Choy*, K. P. Fung and C. Y. Lee, Department of Biochemistry, The Chinese University of Hong Kong, Shatin, N.T., Hong Kong.

The effects of different glucose-regulatory hormones on the glucose carrier densities of Ehrlich ascites tumour cells were studied. Tumour cells, harvested from mice bearing 7 day-old tumour were incubated with hormones in phosphate buffered saline supplemented with 3.2 mM $CaCl_2$, 1.5 mM $MgSO_4$, 6.1 mM pyruvate, 6.7 mM fumarate, 6.1 mM glutamate and 0.56 mM glucose for 60 min. at 37°C. Glucose carriers of tumour cells were identified by the density of glucose-reversible binding sites for cytochalasin B on the cells. Addition of insulin at 0.05 unit/ml or 0.5 unit/ml did not affect glucose carrier density. Glucagon at $5x10^{-3}$ mg/ml caused a 35% significant reduction in carrier density as compared with control. Similarly, the addition of corticosterone ($25x10^{-3}$ mg/ml) and cortisone ($25x10^{-3}$ mg/ml) caused significant reduction in carrier density by 34% and 36% respectively comparing with control. The dissociation constant (Kd) of cytochalasin B binding on the tumour cells were not affected by the addition of various hormones throughout incubation. The present data demonstrate that except insulin, glucagon, corticosterone and cortisone can cause reduction in glucose carrier density of Ehrlich ascites tumour cells and both hormones will not cause qualitative changes in turnover and affinity for substrate of the glucose carrier molecules throughout incubation. This study was supported by World Health Foundation (Hong Kong).

331 STEROID RECEPTORS IN HUMAN SPINAL CORD TUMORS. G. Concolino*, C. Conti, G. Liccardo°, and R. Giuffrè°, Istituto di Clinica Medica V - Università di Roma "La Sapienza", °Istituto di Clinica Neurochirurgica - Università di Roma "Tor Vergata", Rome, Italy.

To explain the sex and age related incidence of various primary spinal cord oncotypes and to study the hormone sensitivity of some of these tumors cytoplasmic and nuclear estradiol (ER) and progesterone (PR) receptors were evaluated in 40 primary spinal cord tumors (16 neurinomas, 2 neurofibromas, 9 meningiomas, 11 ependymomas and 2 astrocytomas). The method employed was the exchange assay at low temperature in the presence of sodium thiocyanate or sodium molybdate respectively for ER and PR. Threshold values were 3 fmoles/mg protein for ERc and PRc, 50 fmoles/mg DNA for ERn and 100 fmoles/mg DNA for PRn. Dissociation constants from Scatchard plot analyses were in favour of high affinity bindings. Regardless of oncotypes examined the incidence of both ER and PR was higher in male than in female patients (77.22% vs 45.45% for ER, 87.50% vs 73.33% for PR) and the overall occurrence of PR was higher than that of ER (80.66% vs 57.50%). Therefore the endocrine influence on the growth of these CNS tumors and the possibility of a hormonal treatment as a form of adjuvant therapy to neurosurgery should be taken into consideration.
This work was supported in part by a grant of C.N.R. (Italy), special project "Control of Neoplastic Growth", contract N° 8200280.96

332 SOME CHARACTERISTICS OF NUCLEAR BINDING BY ESTROGEN RECEPTORS LIGANDED WITH ESTRADIOL (ER) OR MONOHYDROXYTAMOXIFEN (AER). Connie L. Cushing*, Robert A. Bambara and Russell Hilf, Department of Biochemistry, University of Rochester Medical Center, Rochester, New York 14642 USA

Studies were undertaken to elucidate the nuclear interactions of estrogen receptor complexes which were liganded with either estrogens or anti-estrogens. Experiments were designed to determine the biochemical actions of the anti-estrogens at this cellular site. A nuclear binding assay *in vitro* was developed. Initial characterization of this assay showed that specific binding of partially purified uterine ^{3}H-ER displayed complex binding curves, which exhibited more than one binding plateau, suggesting the presence of more than one class of sites. Partially purified receptor liganded with monohydroxytamoxifen, which was used in the assay under identical conditions, also exhibited complex binding curves. Scatchard analysis of the initial binding plateau, (0 to 1000 picomoles ^{3}H receptor complex/mg DNA) obtained from ^{3}H-ER and ^{3}H-AER nuclear interactions, suggested that the affinity of ER and AER for these sites was similar. However, the number of nuclear acceptor sites binding AER was approximately 50% lower than that observed for ER. Experiments characterizing the dissociation kinetics of ER and AER complexes from nuclei are being conducted to further investigate the molecular basis of these apparent differences in their nuclear binding properties. (Supported by NIH grants CA 29324, 5 T32 GM 07102 and ACS, FRA220.)

333 CHANGES IN CIRCULATING T4 DURING ADMINISTRATION OF EXOGENOUS T3: A NEW THYROID SUPPRESSION TEST. J.M. Boutin*, R. Matte, P. D'Amour, F. Gilbert, R. Bélanger, J. Havrankova and R. Chartrand, Hop. St-Luc, Un. of Montreal.

Recent studies have shown the usefulness of suppression test in revealing autonomy of the thyroid gland in apparently euthyroid patients with blunted TSH response to TRH. To avoid the problems inherent to the use of radioiodine uptake we studied changes in serum T4 during T3 administration as a thyroid suppression test. 13 normal subjects, 8 hyperthyroid patients and 13 patients with normal T3 and T4 and blunted TSH response to TRH (ΔTSH<1.5μU/ml) were studied. All received a daily dose of 50 μg of T3 for 21 days and serum T4 was measured on days 0, 14 and 21. In normal subjects, T4 decreased from 8.5 ± 0.6 μg/dl to 4.0 ± 0.3 and 3.2 ± 0.3 μg/dl ($p<0.0005$) on days 14 and 21. In hyperthyroid patients with basal T4 of 17.8 ± 1.4 μg/dl T4 did not change after 2 weeks and by the third week had fallen only to 15.8 ± 1.9 μg/dl ($p<0.0125$). In the group with blunted TSH response to TRH basal T4 (9.8 ± 0.4 μg/dl) did not change after two weeks and by the third week fell to 8.6 ± 0.7 μg/dl ($p<0.01$). The decline in T4 in this group and in hyperthyroid patients was similar but significantly less ($p<0.001$) than in normal subjects. According to the 95% confidence limits of our results, a decline in serum T4 of more than 35% on the 14th day or 45% on the 21st day of T3 administration, clearly differentiates normal subjects from those with autonomous thyroid function. This new and simple test should become useful in daily practice for certain clinical situations where assessment of thyroid autonomy is important and TRH stimulation test impractical.

334 FREE THYROXINE (FT_4) AND FREE TRIIODOTHYRONINE (FT_3) DURING PREGNANCY. R.G. Brodows*, and N.P. Kubasik, The Genesee Hospital, Rochester, NY 14607

A number of recent reports indicate confusion regarding the "true" concentration of free thyroid hormones during pregnancy. We measured FT_4 and FT_3 throughout gestation using new commercially available direct FT_4 and FT_3 RIA kits (Diagnostic Products Corp., Los Angeles, CA 90045) that use the radiolabeled thyroid analog technique. We compared these results with total T_4 and T_3, T_4/TBG and T_3/TBG ratios, the FT_4 and FT_3 indices, TBG, and TSH for 71 females in the first, second, or third trimester of pregnancy. Our "normal ranges" for FT_4 and FT_3 were established from testing over 1400 nonpregnant healthy subjects. The following table summarizes some of our findings (mean±SE):

	T_4 (ug/dl)	FT_4 Index	FT_4 (ng/dl)	T_3 (ng/dl)	FT_3 Index	FT_3 (pg/ml)
Normals (range)	4.5-12.5	1.5-3.3	0.6-1.7	68-170	23-46	1.7-4.3
1st trimester	10.2±.4	2.7±.07	1.1±.04	128±6	33±1.1	3.4±.14
2nd trimester	10.9±.3	2.2±.06	0.8±.03	143±10	29±1.7	3.3±.22
3rd trimester	11.0±.4	2.2±.08	0.7±.03	179±5	33±0.9	3.0±.11

The FT_4 and the T_4/TBG ratio fell significantly during gestation, with some values below normal limits during the third trimester. The FT_4 index, however, remained in the normal range. In contrast, the FT_3, T_3/TBG ratio, and the FT_3 index showed no change during the course of gestation. Total T_4 and T_3 increased during gestation while TSH was constant. Our data confirm that the free fraction of thyroxine is decreased during late pregnancy and suggest the euthyroid state is most likely maintained due to normal concentrations of Free T_3.

335 ANDROGENS AND TeBG IN IDIOPATHIC HIRSUTISM : CLINICAL CORRELATION AND RESPONSE TO ANTIANDROGEN THERAPY. B. Burnand*, F. Gomez, W. Rosner, S. Kahn, F. Rey, G. Chiodoni, Division d'Endocrinologie, CHUV, CH-1011 Lausanne, Switzerland and St. Luke's-Roosvelt Hospital Center and Columbia University, New York, USA.

In order to study which androgens and/or TeBG correlated better with clinical hirsutism score and its response to antiandrogen therapy, 26 young non obese women with idiopathic hirsutism (IH), "hormonal" hirsutism score (HHS) above 7, were studied. Plasma and urinary steroids and plasma TeBG were measured on the 8th cycle day and correlated with HHS. TeBG was inversely correlated with HHS ($r=-0.435$, $p<0.01$), whereas androgens correlated positively in the following order: 24-hour urinary 17KS/creatinine (u17KS, $r=0.615$, $p<0.001$), plasma DHEA-s ($r=0.536$, $p<0.001$), calculated free testosterone (fT, $r=0.514$, $p<0.001$), total testosterone (tT, $r=0.325$, $p<0.05$), and androstenedione ($r=0.301$, $p<0.05$). The evolution of plasma steroids and TeBG was observed during cyproterone acetate-ethinylestradiol (CPA-EE2) treatment in the reverse cycle sequence up to 9 months. There was a rapid increase of plasma TeBG (+245 %, $p<0.0005$), and a simultaneous decrease of fT (-86 %, $p<0.005$), tT (-47 %, $p<0.0005$), and androstenedione (-41 %, $p<0.0005$). At the same time, HHS showed a significant decrease (-44 %, $p<0.0025$) which correlated best with the decrease of fT. Plasma DHEA-s failed to show any significant reduction during treatment. These data suggest that although adrenocortical androgen secretion is most often increased in IH, the clinical improvement during CPA-EE2 treatment is mainly due to the increase of TeBG and the decrease of fT.

336 ELEVATED PROGESTERONE (P) IN CONGENITAL ADRENAL HYPERPLASIA (CAH) ALTERS LH SECRETORY DYNAMICS. Stephen Burstein*, E. Turkington and R.L. Rosenfield, Univ. of Chicago, Depts. of Peds. & Med., Chicago, IL, USA.

To determine the pathophysiology of amenorrhea in CAH, we examined 24-h secretion profiles for LH before and after controlling P levels with dexamethasone (DEX). We studied 2 patients whose androgens, but not progestins, were well-controlled (Ob Gyn 56:208, 1980). Case 1 was a 19.3 year old girl with irregular menses (menarche 11.7 years). On 50 mg cortisol daily androgen levels were normal, e.g., mean testosterone (T) 54 ng/dl, but P (mean 1200 ng/dl) and 17-hydroxyprogesterone (17-OHP) (9500 ng/dl) were elevated throughout the day. Substitution of DEX, 0.75 mg daily, normalized P (94) and 17-OHP (97). DEX clearly changed the 24-h LH secretory profile: the number of peaks increased (12 to 24), the mean peak LH increased (47.8 ng LER-907/ml to 85.9, p of logs <0.02), and integrated LH secretion increased 1.7 times (5.3×10^4 ng·min/ml to 9.0×10^4). Monthly menses ensued. Case 2 was a 7.9 year old premenarchal girl with a bone age of 12.5. On 60 mg cortisone daily all 24-h mean androgen levels were normal, e.g., T 11, but P (268) and 17-OHP (480) were elevated due to a peak in the early morning. Substitution of DEX, 0.2 mg hs, abolished the early morning P peak and normalized mean P (94); menarche followed one month of DEX. DEX converted the LH secretory pattern from one with reversed diurnal augmentation in mid-afternoon to one with normal pubertal sleep-spikes. The number of LH peaks (10 v 9), the mean LH peak height (35.9 v 56.4), and integrated LH secretion (5.0×10^4 v 4.1×10^4) did not change. Conclusions: 1. Elevated progesterone alone can cause amenorrhea in CAH by altering gonadotropin secretory dynamics for stage of puberty. 2. Even transient, mild elevations of progesterone can cause clinically important changes in the pattern of LH secretion in women with CAH.

337 EVALUATION OF PREVALENCE OF CARDIOVASCULAR AUTONOMIC NEUROPATHY IN FEMALE LATIN AMERICAN DIABETIC AND NON-DIABETIC PATIENTS.

C. Callegari*, P. DePrat de Alfonso, A. Chacin de Bermudez, Universidad de Carabobo, Valencia, Venezuela and Harbor-UCLA Medical Center, Torrance, CA

To assess some of the diabetes associated autonomic and peripheral nervous disorders in female Latin-American patients, we studied 87 diabetic (age range 18-84) and 67 non-diabetic (age range 19-82) patients. Examinations were conducted to assess peripheral neuropathy (loss of sensation, deep reflexes, etc.) and five bedside tests of cardiovascular autonomic dysfunction were applied (beat-to-beat heart rate variation during deep breathing, heart rate and arterial blood pressure to standing, Valsalva maneuver, and arterial blood pressure to hand grip). There were significant differences between diabetics and non-diabetics in the prevalence of abnormalities at physical exam ($p<0.01$); diabetics had between two and ten fold more peripheral neuropathy than non-diabetics. When absolute numbers were used to compare the bedside tests between the two groups, there were no significant differences. However, when results were divided into categories (normal, borderline and abnormal) according to the literature, twice the prevalence of peripheral neuropathy was found in diabetics vs non-diabetics; the borderline percentages were similar in both groups. With the exception of heart rate to standing, a slight but significant correlation between duration of diabetes and absolute values of the other tests was found. Even though the sample studied was heterogeneous in age and type of diabetes, our results are comparable with earlier reports. Conclusion: Aging may affect autonomic and peripheral nerve function, but earlier dysfunction is observed in patients with Diabetes Mellitus.

338 PLASMA ACTH AND αMSH RESPONSE TO EXOGENOUS CORTICOTROPHIN-RELEASING FACTOR (CRF) IN A GROUP OF PATIENTS SUFFERING FROM NELSON'S SYNDROME.

[1]E. A. Campbell*, [2]A. Thody, [3]A. R. H. Altaher, [4]R. R. Abraham, [4]V. Wynn, [1]B. Gillham and [3]M. T. Jones, Departments of [1]Biochemistry and [3]Obstetrics and Gynaecology, St. Thomas's Hospital Medical School, [4]Alexander Simpson Laboratory for Metabolic Research, St. Mary's Hospital, London, and [2]Department of Dermatology, University of Newcastle-upon-Tyne.

This study formed part of a larger investigation to determine whether the pituitary tumours in a group of patients with Nelson's syndrome were derived from corticotroph or melanotroph cells. Eight patients were tested on different days with either 100 μg synthetic oCRF or saline as a single intravenous injection. Blood samples were taken over a period of 2 hours and plasma levels of ACTH, αMSH and CRF measured by radioimmunoassay. Following injection, plasma CRF levels reached a maximum during the first 10 minute collection period. Thereafter they declined throughout the course of the experiment but were still elevated at the end of the 2 hours. The time course of this decay varied from patient to patient. Mean basal plasma ACTH in these patients ranged from 240 ± 30.5 to 7166.6 ± 726.4 pg/ml. All eight patients demonstrated an increase in plasma ACTH following oCRF injection. In two patients values had returned to pre-treatment values by the end of the 2 hours. Plasma ACTH in the remaining patients was still elevated and, in some cases, still rising when compared to saline control values. In contrast, all patients examined so far demonstrated low plasma αMSH values which did not rise in response to CRF. Therefore, the present data demonstrate that these adenomas arise from corticotrophs rather than melanotrophs.

339 CLINICAL AND SOCIAL BENEFITS OF THYROID NODULE ASPIRATION. A.Carpi*, A.Nicolini, I.Marchetti, M.R.Metelli, G.Di Coscio.Nuclear Medicine Service and Institute of Pathological Anatomy. University of Pisa and City Hospital, Via Roma, Pisa, Italy

Since 1972 we face the clinical problem of thyroid nodule. Before April 1980 131I thyroid scan was used to suspect a cancer therefore all the hypofunctioning nodules which did not markedly reduce after 6 months of thyroid hormone therapy were excised. After April 1980 cytological and histological examinations are routinely performed by fine needle aspiration (FNA) and aspiration needle biopsy (ANB). Surgery is advised only when cytohistological findings show or suspect a cancer. From 1972 to April 1980 1,140 pts aged 14 to 79 years (87.2% women, 12.8% men; 72.6% single nodule, 27.4% multiple) were operated. Postoperative histological findings were: benign nodule in 1,105 (96.9%) pts, cancer in 35 (3.1%) pts. From April 1980 to now 1,475 pts, aged 14 to 79 yrs.(87% women,13% men; 73.6% single nodule, 26.4% multiple) were submitted to FNA or to FNA+ANB. Aspiration specimens do not contain any useful element for diagnosis in 153 pts (10.3%).Aspiration diagnoses were: benign nodule (1338), suspected cancer (65),cancer (19). Operation was performed in the 84 pts with diagnosis of cancer or of suspected cancer and also in 54 pts with diagnosis of benign nodule for advice other then ours. Postoperative histological findings were: 46 cancers (3.1%) 92 benign nodule (96.9%). Therefore four years routine use of thyroid nodule aspiration reduced the number of operations from 142 to 34.5 per year and increased the number of cancers found from 4 to 11.5 per year. Reduction of useless operations made possible to use surgery for diseases more important than the thyroid ones in our University Hospital.

340 HLA-DR IN CHINESE PATIENTS WITH THYROTOXICOSIS

SH Chan, PPB Yeo, JS Cheah*, KF Lui, GB Wee, AC Thai, and P Lim. WHO Immunology Centre and Department of Medicine, Faculty of Medicine, National University of Singapore, Singapore General Hospital, Outram Road, Singapore.

We have previously reported HLA-A and B locus association in Chinese patients with thyrotoxicosis in Singapore. This association is with BW46. In this paper we investigated the HLA locus A and B association in 195 Chinese patients with thyrotoxicosis compared to 330 normal subjects. In addition, 72 thyrotoxicosis patients were typed for HLA-DR locus and the comparison group consisted of 37 normal subjects.

The association of BW46 with Chinese thyrotoxicosis was confirmed. The frequency of BW46 was observed in 93/195 (47.7%) patients compared to 70/330 (23.9%) controls. (X^2 = 31.4, Pc $<$.001; RR = 2.9).

The frequencies of DRW9, DRW5, DRW8 were increased in patients compared to controls. However, in only DRW9 was this difference significant after correction. DRW9 was observed in 32/72 (44.4%) patients compared to 10/38 (26.3%) controls (X^2 = 8.04; Pc$<$.05; RR = 6.4). DRW9 is in linkage disequilibrium with BW46 in normal Chinese subjects. The higher relative risk seen with DRW9 than with BW46 suggested that the association is stronger with the DR locus than the B locus.

341 PHEOCHROMOCYTOMA, CLINICAL AND BIOCHEMICAL FEATURES. Chávez-Lara B, Olguín Almada R, Serrano PA, Sánchez-Torres G, Posadas-Romero C. Instituto Nacional de Cardiología Ignacio Chávez. Mexico City, Mexico.

In patients with clinical manifestations of sympathetic hyperactivity, specific laboratory testing must be done to stablish the diagnosis of pheochromocytoma. We report a retrospective study of 66 patients. Among 43 women and 23 men, whose age-range was 7 to 63 years, hypertension was paroxismal in 66% and sustained in 26%. The most frequent symptoms were headache, palpitations and generalized sweating. The observed complications were hyperglycemia (59%), cerebrovascular accident (17%), myocardial infarction (8%) and renal artery stenosis (4%). Only one patient had neurofibromatosis and 7 women were pregnant. The tumor was malignant in 6 cases. Urinary catecholamines gave 2, 4 and 12% false negative results for noradrenaline, adrenaline and VMA determinations, respectively. Total plasma catecholamines were within normal range in 3.6% of the cases. Administration of clonidine to 3 patients (0.3 mg,p.o) resulted in blood pressure decrease with no changes in plasma catecholamines. Computarized tomography was the most reliable test for the localization of the tumor (88%). Follow up of 30 patients from 2 to 15 years showed that 25 remained normotensive after surgery while 5 required antihypertensive therapy. Ten out of the 66 patients died for causes related to the tumor.

These data emphasize the relevance of proper diagnosis and therapeutic management of the pheochromocytoma patient.

342 PINEALECTOMY EFFECTS ON HORMONAL PROFILES. C.L. Chik*, A. Talalla and G.M. Brown, McMaster University, Hamilton, Ontario, Canada L8N 3Z5.

Pinealectomy increased LH secretion while attenuating the nocturnal rise of PRL in rams, Barrell and Lapwood, 1978. We report here a case where changes in hormonal profiles were observed post-pinealectomy. A 47 year old female presented with symptoms of increased intracranial pressure. Her only endocrine complaint was postmenopausal flushing. Radiographic investigation by CT scan showed obstructive hydrocephalus from an axial midline cyst in the pineal region. Endocrine testings showed high morning basal LH at 67 IU/L and FSH at 76 IU/L. PRL was 8 ug/L. Post 100 ug LHRH IV stimulation, LH increased to 228 IU/L and FSH increased to 107 IU/L. Daytime melatonin levels by RIA were not detectable. Nighttime melatonin levels at 0200 and 0400 hours were 77 and 107 pg/ml. Surgical removal of the cystic mass revealed an ependymal cyst and normal pineal tissue. Post-pinealectomy, the nighttime melatonin rise was abolished at 2 weeks, 4 months and 9 months after the operation. 9 months post-operation, morning basal LH was increased 50% to 100 IU/L and FSH was unchanged at 70 IU/L. Morning basal PRL was 3 ug/L. Post LHRH stimulation, LH increased to 350 IU/L and FSH increased to 106 IU/L. 24 hour LH secretory profile showed pulsatility. However, 24 hour PRL secretion showed no fluctuation from the baseline value of 3 ug/L other than the PRL level of 11 ug/L measured. at 0530 hour. These changes in LH and PRL secretions are considered to be related to her pinealectomy.

343 THE EFFECT OF PULSATILE INTRAVENOUS ADMINISTRATION OF GNRH ON GONADOTROPHIN SECRETION IN POLYCYSTIC OVARIAN DISEASE. Herjan J.T. Coelingh Bennink*, Han W. Weber, George P.J. Alsbach and Jos H.H. Thijssen, Department of Obstetrics, Gynecology and Reproductive Endocrinology and Department of Clinical Endocrinology, State University Hospital AZU, Utrecht, the Netherlands.

Induction of ovulation by pulsatile intravenous administration of GnRH has been demonstrated by our group in anovulatory women with polycystic ovarian disease (PCOD). To study the mode of action of this treatment the effect of GnRH on gonadotrophin serum levels has been investigated in 8 infertile women with PCOD. GnRH was administered pulsatile intravenously by a portable rollerpump. The pulse-interval was 90 minutes. The dosage GnRH was 10 microgram per pulse for two weeks and 20 microgram per pulse thereafter. Treatment was monitored by basal body temperature, endocrine parameters and ultrasound. Before treatment, the first day of treatment and once a week thereafter gonadotrophin-levels were measured every 20 minutes for periods of 12 hours in 3 women and for periods of 6 hours in 5 women. Ovulation was induced in 5 from 8 women and one of them became pregnant. Before treatment the gonadotrophin peak interval (GPI) appeared to be shortened compared to figures from the literature (45-70 minutes versus 90 minutes). During GnRH treatment the GPI increased to 90 minutes, the mean FSH-levels did not change and the mean LH-levels increased significantly as well as the LH pulse amplitude.
Conclusion: In women with PCOD the LH pulse frequency is normalized and the LH pulse amplitude is increased by pulsatile intravenous administration of GnRH but ovulation does not always occur.

344 INDUCTION OF OVULATION BY PULSATILE INTRAVENOUS ADMINISTRATION OF GNRH IN POLYCYSTIC OVARIAN DISEASE. Herjan J.T. Coelingh Bennink*, Han W. Weber, George P.J. Alsbach and Jos H.H. Thijssen, Department of Obstetrics, Gynecology and Reproductive Endocrinology and Department of Clinical Endocrinology, State University Hospital AZU, Utrecht, the Netherlands.

Fifteen infertile anovulatory women with polycystic ovarian disease (PCOD) were selected for treatment with GnRH because other methods of induction of ovulation had failed or had been complicated by hyperstimulation. GnRH was given pulsatile intravenously by a portable rollerpump for a period of at least four weeks. The pulse-interval was 90 minutes. The dosage GnRH was 10 microgram per pulse for two weeks and 20 microgram GnRH per pulse thereafter. Treatment was monitored by basal body temperature, endocrine parameters and ultrasound.
In 15 women 42 treatment courses were carried out. Ovulation occurred in 29 courses (69%) in 10 women. In 4 from 29 ovulatory cycles luteal insufficiency occurred. During treatment the menstrual cycle was regular (26-35 days) in 5 women and irregular (>35 days) in 5 women. Treatment failed in 5 women for a variety of reasons such as anovulation and luteinization of unruptured follicles developing in cysts. Eight women became pregnant with viable singleton pregnancies. Pregnancy occurred at the first ovulation in 3, at the second ovulation in 2 and at the third ovulation in 3 women. Serious side-effects did not occur.
Conclusion: By pulsatile intravenous administration of GnRH ovulation may be induced in women with PCOD in whom other methods of induction of ovulation have failed.

345 NON-SHBG BOUND TESTOSTERONE AS A MARKER FOR HYPERANDROGENISM.

D.C. Cumming*, S.R. Wall, Depts of Ob/Gyn and Medicine (Div of Endocrinol), University of Alberta, Edmonton, Alberta, T6G 2G3.

Recent evidence has suggested that the biologically active testosterone included both free and albumin bound fractions while SHBG bound steroid dissociates less readily. To examine testosterone distribution among serum binding proteins, we obtained single blood samples from 17 normal controls (NC), 20 regularly menstruating but hirsute women (H-R) and 20 oligo-amenorrheic, hirsute women (HO/A). Each serum sample was analyzed for total testosterone (T), by RIA, SHBG-Binding Capacity (SHBG-BC) by protein precipitation with 50% saturated $(NH_4)_2SO_4$ and albumin (ALB) by colorimetry. Non-SHBG bound (Tu(c)) and free (Tf) testosterone and T/SHBG ratio were then calculated. Non-SHBG bound testosterone (Tu(m)) was also measured using differential protein precipitation. There were significant differences among the groups in all variables studied (all $p<0.05$) except ALB. Despite similar methodology measurement of Tu(c) and Tu(m) did not produce identical results, perhaps because of inaccuracies in the binding equation. There was considerable overlap between normal (control mean ±2 Std Dev) and abnormal except in Tu(m) where only 3 H-R and 2 HO/A subjects were in the normal range. The relative increases in Tu by both methods are much greater than would be anticipated from the differences in T, Tf or SHBG. These data suggest that with higher T levels, ALB becomes increasingly important in T binding. Therefore, Tu may be the optimal marker to distinguish hyperandrogenic women. Supported by UAH Special Services and Research.

346 HORMONES IN LEPROSY.

R.J.Dash*, Bhushan Kumar & B.N.Datta
Departments of Endocrinology, Dermatology and Pathology. Postgraduate Institute of Medical Education & Research, Chandigarh, India.

Circulating LH, FSH, PRL, GH, TSH, T4, T3, Testosterone estradiol-17 B and cortisol in the basal and following intravenous bolus injections of GnRH (50 ug), TRH (100 ug) and cryst. insulin (0.1 U/kg bw) were estimated in 25 lepromatous, 10 tuberculoid and 15 dimorphous leprosy patients and 20 age and sex matched controls. The hormone variations were largely confined to alterations in testicular function and were more marked in lepromatous leprosy (60%) followed by border line (36%) and tuberculoid (13%) leprosy. Consequently the LH, FSH and PRL were elevated in the basal state and were hyperstimulated following GnRH and TRH bolus. Testicular biopsies revealed changes of advanced testicular atrophy with leprous granuloma and such patients had increased incidence of impotency, sterility and gynaecomastia. No significant alterations in thyroid hormones, TSH response to TRH, basal cortisol, and its increment following insulin hypoglycemia were observed in leprosy. The data suggest direct involvement of testes in leprosy.

(Supported by PGI Research Fund and WHO)

347 EVOLUTION OF MULTIDOMAIN NEUROPEPTIDE PRECURSORS : VERTEBRATE NEUROHYPOPHYSIAL HORMONES AND NEUROPHYSINS.

J. Chauvet*, M.T.Chauvet, D.Hurpet and R.Acher, Laboratory of Biological Chemistry, University of Paris VI, 96 Bd Raspail 75006 Paris (France)

Neurohypophysial hormones and neurophysins have been shown to be fragments of common multidomain precursors. Because all vertebrate neurohypophysial hormones are nonapeptides and all neurophysins have 93-95 residues, a precise processing was preserved in the course of evolution. Ten vertebrate neurohypophysial hormones and twelve mammalian neurophysins have been characterized to date ; they can be classified into two lineages of multidomains precursors ending, in placental mammals, with the oxytocin/VLDV-neurophysin and the vasopressin/ MSEL-neurophysin tandems. Cyclostomes, the earliest vertebrates, have in contrast to other species a single hormone. It is assumed that a duplication of an ancestral gene gave rise to the two main lines of precursors. An additional duplication of the vasopressin precursor gene has now been observed in several Australian and American marsupials leading to lysine vasopressin and phenypressin for the first, to lysine vasopressin and arginine vasopressin for the latter. The vasopressin precursor gene is composed of 3 exons: A (signal peptide, vasopressin, neurophysin 1-9), B (neurophysin 10-76) and C (neurophysin 77-95, copeptin). When bovine and rat precursors are compared in this respect, the homology is 83 % for exon A, 96 % for exon B and 60 % for exon C. The multidomain precursor is a composite protein, each domain having its own rate of evolution.

348 CIRCULATORY IODOTHYRONINES IN SNAKES.

K.W. Chiu* & C.C. Wong, Department of Biology and Department of Physiology, The Chinese University of Hong Kong.

An attempt was made to measure circulatory iodothyronines in snake serum. Serum T_4, T_3, rT_3 and even rT_2 were measured with direct methods by using 8 anilino-naphthalene-1-sulphonic acis (ANS), thimerosal, and barbital buffer to minimize the problem of protein binding in the radioimmunoassay. The assay conditions were optimized with different amounts of ANS to get a maximum specific binding and a minimum non-specific binding under similar incubating condition. Measurement of iodothyronines were based on standard curves constructed with known amounts of respective iodothyronines and hormone free serum from the same species. Serum rT_3 in pool sera in 5 species of snakes, namely, Naja naja, Ptyas korros, Elaphe taeniura, Elaphe radiata & Ptyas mucosa were 68, 43, 31, 61, 54 & 61 ng/dl respectively. Serum T_4 from the same samples were 24, 78, 56, 37, 36 & 43 ng/dl. Serum T_3, the most active natural occurring iodothyronine were found to have a value of 5.4, 6.1, 3.1, 4.5 & 6.1 ng/dl. rT_2 serum levels were found to be extremely low, close to the detecting limit of the assay at 2.0 ng/dl. Further measurements of these iodothyronines in individual snake, sera revealed as expected great variations of serum T_4 & T_3 values ranging from undetectable to 6.8 ug/dl for T_4 and undetectable to 56 ng/dl for T_3. Interestingly, rT_3 seems to be the dominant circulatory iodothyronine in snakes. This may indicate that inner ring deiodination of thyroxine is the main pathway for thyroxine metabolism in snakes.

349 BREEDING SEASON EFFECTS ON THE PROSTATE AND EPIDIDYMIS OF THE BRUSH-TAIL POSSUM (TRICHOSURUS VULPECULA). J.D. Curlewis and G.M. Stone*, Department of Veterinary Physiology, University of Sydney, Sydney, 2006, Australia.

To gain some information on the mechanism(s) responsible for the dramatic increase in weight of the prostate, but not the epididymis, of this marsupial species during the breeding season, cytosol androgen receptor concentration, the plasma and tissue level of testosterone (T) and 5α-dihydrotestosterone (5α-DHT) and in vitro tissue T metabolism were measured within and outside the breeding season. Receptor concentration in the prostate only was significantly higher ($P<0.01$) in breeding season animals. Plasma levels of T and 5α-DHT were elevated, but not significantly so, in the breeding season; however overall the correlation of each with prostatic weight was poor (co-efficients of 0.62 and 0.57 respectively). T was the major plasma androgen, while 5α-DHT predominated in both tissues. In the prostate the concentration of both steroids, expressed in terms of tissue DNA, was significantly higher ($P<0.05$) in breeding season animals. Although the pattern of in vitro T metabolism changed with season, to yield an increased formation of androstanedione in both tissues, the level of 5α-reductase activity in the prostate was always low. The results indicate that although 5α-DHT is the likely active androgen in the prostate it may be formed elsewhere. Part of the explanation for the increased growth of the prostate in the breeding season appears to be a change in receptor concentration coupled with elevated tissue and possibly plasma androgen level.

350 EFFECT OF PROGESTERONE UPON ADENYLATE CYCLASE ACTIVITY AND cAMP LEVELS ON BRAIN AREAS. Collado, M.L.*, Cruz, M.L. and Beyer, C. Unidad de Investigacion Biomedica, Centro Medico Nacional del Instituto Mexicano del Seguro Social. Mexico D.F. 03020, MEXICO.

Estrogens (E) induce lordosis behavior through a mechanism involving protein synthesis in the brain, while progesterone (P), as suggested by recent reports, acts upon the membrane adenylate cyclase-cAMP system increasing the nucleotide brain levels in E primed rats. However, this last effect of P on brain tissues has not been directly proved. Thus, this work is aimed to determine the changes induced by P in adenylate cyclase activity and cAMP levels in brain areas involved in the integration of sexual behavior. Wistar adult female rats were ovariectomized and 3 weeks later were primed with 4 μg of estradiol benzoate, after 44 hours they were injected with 4 mg of P. The control group was injected with oil. Tests for lordosis behavior were conducted 1, 2 and 4 hours after P administration. Animals were sacrified by decapitation and the enzyme activity and cAMP concentration were assayed in: preoptic area, ventromedial hypothalamus and cerebral cortex. Our results shown a significant increase in both enzyme activity and cAMP levels at 2 and 4 hours after P administration in all the brain areas studied. These data suggest that the facilitatory effect of P on lordosis behavior involves a direct or indirect activating mechanism of this steroid upon the adenylate cyclase enzyme which results in a intraneuronal cAMP enhancement.

351 EFFECTS OF THYROID HORMONE ON CYCLIC NUCLEOTIDE METABOLISM AND LIPOLYSIS IN 3T3-L1 ADIPOCYTES.

M. L. Elks* and V. C. Manganiello, National Heart, Lung, and Blood Institute, NIH, Bethesda, Maryland.

Effects of agents whose actions are mediated by cAMP are enhanced in hyperthyroid and reduced in hypothyroid states. After incubation of mature, cultured 3T3-L1 adipocytes for 10 days in medium containing 10% serum from a thyroidectomized calf (T_3, 81 pg/ml; T_4, 1 ng/ml), basal lipolysis in these hypothyroid cells was lower than that in cells (euthyroid) incubated in the same medium with added T_3 (1.5 ng/ml), and sensitivity to isoproterenol was less. Cells incubated for 10 days with 10 ng/ml of T_3 (hyperthyroid) exhibited higher basal lipolysis and enhanced responsiveness to submaximal, but not maximally effective, concentrations of isoproterenol. cAMP content, with or without isoproterenol (2 min), was lower in hypothyroid and higher in hyperthyroid than in euthyroid cells. Although basal particulate cAMP phosphodiesterase (PDE) activity was increased ~ 40% in hypothyroid adipocytes and reduced ~ 30% in hyperthyroid adipocytes, acute increases in particulate cAMP PDE activity produced by either insulin or isoproterenol were not affected by thyroid status. Soluble cAMP PDE activities were similar in hypo-, hyper-, or euthyroid adipocytes. The changes in basal particulate cAMP PDE activities could account in part for the differences in cAMP content, lipolysis, and isoproterenol responsiveness of cells in different thyroid states. The relatively homogenous population of cultured 3T3-L1 adipocytes may be a useful system in which to investigate further effects of thyroid hormones and other agents which require a prolonged period of time to exert their biological actions.

352 DIRECT CYTOCHEMICAL LOCALIZATION OF THE REGULATORY SUBUNIT (R) OF THE cAMP-DEPENDENT PROTEIN KINASE (PK) AND THE PK INHIBITOR PROTEIN (PKI)

W. H. Fletcher, S. Van Patten, H-C Cheng and D.A.Walsh*. Dept of Biological Chemistry, University of California, Davis, and Division of Biomedical Sciences, University of California, Riverside, USA.

Cytochemical localization of the catalytic subunit (C) of PK, identified with a FITC-PKI, have revealed the kinetics of its dissociation and subsequent localization to discrete subcellular compartments (J.Cell Biol. 93:719). We have sought to assess PKI and R under similar *in vivo* circumstances and report here developement of a direct cytochemical method to detect these proteins at subcellular resolution. A C probe (FC) was prepared by the FITC derivatization of holoenzyme in the presence of Mg.ATP with subsequent separation of subunits by DEAE. FC retained full catalytic activity and equivalent binding of PKI and R. Cells were fixed at -30° C in anhydrous acetone, rehydrated at 4° C, and then incubated with FC and Mg.ATP and plus or minus cAMP for 16h at 4° C. In the absence of cAMP the expected binding of RC is to endogeneous R and PKI, with cAMP it binds to PKI alone. A 20-fold excess of native C eliminated FC binding. With Reuber H-35 cells and unstimulated cultures, R, not associated with endogeneous C, appeared to be mainly confined to the nucleolus although some was observed in the cytoplasm. 5 min exposure to 8BrcAMP caused abundant cytoplasmic R. Less PKI was found in the controls but the subcellular distribution was the same. Longer stimulation led to detectible qualitative but not quantative changes in PKI and R. We conclude that FC is a reliable probe capable of localizing PKI and R.

353 CALCITONIN GENE PRODUCTS IN LEUKAEMIA. C.J. Hillyard*, P.A. Hill, S.I. Girgis, I. MacIntyre. Chemical Pathology, Royal Postgraduate Medical School, Hammersmith Hospital, LONDON W12 OHS. UK.

The calcitonin gene encodes a peptide family contained in two precursors: the calcitonin (CT) precursor in which katacalcin (KC) and an N-terminal peptide flank the main product and the calcitonin gene-related peptide (CGRP) precursor which has a C-terminal tetrapeptide and an N-terminal peptide similar to the corresponding portion of the CT precursor (Amara et al 1982). We have set up a radioimmunoassay for CGRP and this has been used, together with the existing assays for CT and KC, to screen plasma from patients with a variety of solid carcinomas and leukaemias. Circulating CGRP was found in patients with lung and prostate carcinomas and in all patients with myeloid leukaemias and myelofibrosis. Patients with myeloid leukaemias were found to have levels more than tenfold higher (5.28 ± 0.52 μg/l) than the normal controls (<0.3 μg/l). We have shown previously that patients with myeloid leukaemias have raised immunoreactive CT levels but i-CGRP levels are markedly higher than CT (0.58 ± 0.14 μg/l) and KC (0.24 ± 0.04 μg/l). There are no correlations between the levels of any of these peptides. This contrasts with medullary thyroid carcinoma where CT and KC are produced in equimolar amounts (r=0.98). It thus appears that ectopically produced calcitonin gene products may be processed in a different manner from C-cell peptides. These differences may have diagnostic importance. This study is supported by the Leukaemia Research Fund.
ref: Amara SG, Jonas V, Rosenfeld MG, Ong ES, Evans RM. Nature 298 240, 1982.

354 **Possible Control of Implantation by the Inhibition of Progesterone Initiated Endometrial Estrogen Sulfurylation.** S.C. Brooks*, J. Corombos, M.G. Battelli and D. Saunders. Dept. of Biochem., Wayne State Univ. School of Medicine, Detroit, Mich., USA.

Implantation of the blastocyst is facilitated by the secretory differentiation of the endometrium. Progesterone (Pg) controls this differentiation phenomenon via its receptor mechanism only if estrogen's activity is attenuated. The *in situ* metabolic deactivation of estrogens in human and porcine secretory endometrium is accomplished through progesterone's induction of estrogen sulfotransferase (Meyers et. al Biol. Reprod. 28 1119, 1983) which forms estrogen-3-sulfates, an ester incapable of binding to the estrogen receptor. Utilizing G-200 and chromatofocusing columns, we have purified this enzyme from endometrium of Pg treated pigs and found it to be highly specific for estrogens. This soluble enzyme has a M.W. of 82,000, a pI of 6.1, and a Km < 20 nM. The substrate specificity and affinity of this endometrial estrogen sulfotransferase is far greater than that of other known sulfotransferases. Estrogen sulfotransferase was absent in proliferative endometrium. Knowledge of the reaction transition state aided the design of specific inhibitors of estrogen sulfurylation. Several such compounds, 4-nitro-and 4-fluoroestrone 3-methyl ether and 4-fluoro-1,3,5(10) estratriene-17B-01, actively block estrogen sulfurylation without demonstrable binding to the estrogen receptor. *In vivo* and *in vitro* these compounds are capable of increasing the nuclear uptake of endogenous levels of estrogen via the receptor mechanism in secretory endometrium. Such inhibitors would be expected to prolong proliferative endometrium in the presence of postovulatory Pg. Supported by the NICHHD of the NIH.

355 EFFICACY OF AN ANTIPROGESTERONE STEROID (RU 38486) BY DIFFERENT ROUTES OF ADMINISTRATION IN THE RAT.

C.C. Chang, S.J. Segal and C. Wayne Bardin, The Population Council, New York, N.Y. and The Rockefeller Foundation, New York, N.Y.

RU 38486 is a steroid with high affinity to progesterone (P) and glucocorticoid receptors that has been shown to anatagonize the effects of P on deciduoma formation (DCR) and on pregnancy maintenance. In the present study, we assessed the effects of this compound by different routes of administration. A test system was developed in which pseudopregnant rats were ovariectomized, adrenalectomized and given a cotton pellet subcutaneously (s.c.) on day 4; administration of P (2 mg) and cortisol (C) (0.375 mg) s.c. maintained pseudopregnancy and inhibited granuloma formation around the cotton. RU 38486 was given either orally s.c. or intravaginally (v) to P and C treated rats from day 4 through day 7. A dose of 4 mg/kg/day of RU 38486 given orally exerted both anti-P and anti-C activities as evidenced by inhibition of DCR by blockade of C induced reduction of thymus weight and by prevention of C induced reduction of granuloma formation. A lower dose of RU 38486 was required by the s.c. or v routes to produce inhibition of P action (e.g., 1.0 mg/kg/day by s.c. or 2.0 mg/kg/day by v). Unexpectedly these doses did not interfere with C action. In the rat, implantation was completely inhibited by a single dose of RU 38486 given on day 6 of pregnancy by either oral (16 mg/kg) or i.m. (4 mg/kg) or s.c. (6 mg/kg) or v (12 mg/kg) routes. Conclusion: (1) in rats the anti-C but not anti-P activity of RU 38486 is dependent upon the route of administration and (2) RU 38486 exerts its most potent antifertility effect following i.m. or s.c. injection.

356 LATE EFFECTS OF AN ACOUSTIC STIMULATION ON CORTICOSTERONE LEVEL IN MICE PREVIOUSLY STIMULATED DURING PRE OR EARLY POSTNATAL LIFE.

Ph. Bourgeois*, P. Bourgeois, D. Molin, M.C. Busnel, * Laboratoire d'Ecophysiologie, Faculté de Sciences 76130 Mt St Aignan, France; Laboratoire de Physiologie Acoustique INRA-CNRZ, 78350 Jouy-en-Josas, France.

Since high intensity sound influences the gestation and the development of young mice, we have studied the effect of an acoustic stimulus (5 KHz, 105 dB) on 21-day-old mice (corticosteroid levels were used as a test of stress). Three groups of mice were given the same stimulus at regular intervals during their pre or postnatal life (from conception to birth; from birth to Day 9 -onset of audition; from Day 9 to Day 21 -weaning). Those frequencies best heard by the animal were also those which proved to be the most stressful. However, the mice reacted in a lesser degree to this acoustic stress than to any other psychophysiological stress, such as early separation from the mother or change of environment. Although the acoustic stimulus given to all the mice on Day 21 did not increase significantly the corticosteroid level in mice pretreated from Day 9 to Day 21, it did however cause a 3 or 4-fold increase of the corticosteroid level in mice pretreated from conception to birth or from birth to Day 9; the same increase was observed in a control group treated on Day 21 for the first time. In conclusion, it seems that a sound accomodation appears concurrently with the onset of audition.

357 FETAL ADRENAL CORTISOL SYNTHESIS FROM PROGESTERONE: FETAL VS. DEFINITIVE ZONE.

C. Branchaud*, L. Lipowski and Y. Lefebvre, McGill University - Montreal Children's Hospital Research Institute and Hôpital Notre Dame - Université de Montréal, Montreal, H3H 1P3, Canada.

Because the human fetal adrenal (HFA) is deficient in 3β-hydroxysteroid dehydrogenase activity, it has been assumed that cortisol (F) is formed from circulating progesterone (P_4) during fetal life. Tracer incorporation studies have supported this view. We have recently shown that the fetal zone (FZ) of the HFA over 5 days in explant culture exhibits a much greater capacity to utilize substrate amounts of P_4 to form F than does the definitive zone (DZ). In order to examine the nature of this difference more closely, short-term (4 hrs) incubation studies of explants of the separated zones of early 2nd trimester HFA's were carried out in the absence of fetal bovine serum and in the absence or presence of 3000 ng/ml of P_4. The findings confirm those of the culture studies, i.e. in the presence of P_4, F production by the FZ was increased up to 200 fold. The DZ response was 10 times less. On the other hand, there was an accumulation of 17α-hydroxy P_4 in the DZ but not the FZ medium in the presence of P_4. ACTH had no effect on either F or 17α-hydroxy P_4 production from P_4 by either zone. These results suggest 1)that the DZ of the early 2nd trimester HFA is deficient in 21-hydroxylase activity but that the FZ possesses the necessary enzyme systems to form F from P_4, and 2)that ACTH has no short-term effect on the enzymes involved in this part of the F biosynthetic pathway.

Supported by the Medical Research Council of Canada.

358 EFFECT OF STREPTOZOTOCIN ON FETAL LAMBS IN LATE GESTATION

M. Brinsmead* and J. Falconer, Faculty of Medicine, University of Newcastle, N.S.W. 2308 Australia.

Diabetogenic and toxic effects of streptozotocin ($) were assessed by the intravenous administration of 60-260 mg/kg (estimated body weight) to 7 fetal lambs (3 singletons and 4 twins) after 110 days of gestation. Controls (4 twins) received 2-5 ml of citrate buffer (pH4.4). Doses were repeated 2-3 times weekly and fetal arterial blood assessed daily for pH, pO_2, PCO_2, Hb and O_2saturation. Insulin response was assessed by weekly challenge with glucose (55 mg/min infused intravenously) for 3 hours.

One fetus, receiving 300 mg $/kg over 3 days, died 6 days after the first dose but 3 fetuses survived equivalent or greater doses and there was no evidence that the drug causes hypoxia or acidosis. Insulin responses to glucose challenge were observed in fetuses which had received $<$110 mg$/kg (n=8). Little or no insulin response occurred in 6 instances where fetuses received $>$125 mg $/kg. However, in one fetus receiving 250,275 and 280 mg $/kg a significant insulin response was observed on each of 3 occasions. The weight of livers from all fetuses treated with $ was low but kidney, brain and total body weights were not significantly affected.

We conclude that fetal lambs in late gestation tolerate streptozotocin doses of up to 300 mg/kg, that $>$125 mg/kg can render them insulin deficient but not reliably (1 failure in 6) and that this drug affects liver weight without abolishing insulin response to a glucose challenge.

Supported by our Faculty's Research Committee.

359 SULFATASE DEFICIENCY DETERMINED BOTH IN PLACENTA AND CULTURES OF FORESKIN FIBROBLASTS OF A NEWBORN. J.A. Canick*, L.R. Brown, D.R. Coustan, N.M. Clifford, J. Kredentser, and D. Tulchinsky. Depts. of Path and Obs. Gyn., Women & Infants Hosp., Brown Univ., Providence, RI 02908, and Dept. of Obs. Gyn., Brigham & Women's Hosp., Boston, MA 02115.

A case of placental sulfatase deficiency was suspected on the basis of extremely low serial levels of serum unconjugated estriol (<3ng/ml) during the third trimester and normal amniotic fluid DHEA sulfate (0.08μg/ml). The placenta was obtained at delivery and a portion processed for measurement of sulfatase activity. The newborn's foreskin was obtained one day after delivery, the cells dispersed by trypsin digestion and placed in culture. Third generation fibroblast cultures were used to determine the presence or absence of sulfatase activity. Using the 10,000g supernatant of the affected placental homogenate, we could detect no enzymatic conversion of either ^{3}H DHEA sulfate or ^{3}H estrone sulfate to their respective hydrolysis products. By contrast, in control supernatants, both sulfatase activities were easily measured, with estrone sulfatase 4x higher than DHEA sulfatase (50 vs 12 pmol/min/mg prot.). When the same ^{3}H substrates were added to fibroblast cultures from the affected fetus, neither hydrolysis product could be detected upon sampling the culture medium during a 24h period. In control cultures run at the same time, the ^{3}H hydrolysis products were easily measured and were produced in the same ratio as in the placenta (estrone sulfatase=1085 fmol/culture/24h; DHEA sulfatase=277 fmol/culture/12h). These results demonstrate that in a case of placental sulfatase deficiency, the foreskin can be used to confirm the diagnosis.

360 ADENYLATE CYCLASE ACTIVITY IN NEOCORTEX AND FETAL ZONE MEMBRANE FRACTIONS OF THE HUMAN FETAL ADRENAL GLAND. Bruce R. Carr*, Cecil H. and Ida Green Center for Reproductive Biology Sciences and the Department of Obstetrics and Gynecology, University of Texas Health Science Center, Dallas, Texas 75235, U.S.A.

Whether peptide hormones other than $ACTH_{1-24}$ may be responsible for the difference in size or rate of steroidogenesis of the fetal zone (FZ) as compared to the neocortex (NC) of the human fetal adrenal gland remains controversial. In the present investigation, the activity of adenylate cyclase in membrane fractions of separated zones of the human fetal adrenal gland was determined. Basal adenylate cyclase activity was 3-5 fold greater in NC than in FZ membrane fractions. The addition of ACTH stimulated adenylate cyclase activity in both zones but to a greater (2 to 3-fold) degree in NC than in FZ membrane fractions. Adenylate cyclase activity was also more sensitive to ACTH (10^{-10} M) in NC fractions than was the FZ (10^{-6} M). In addition to $ACTH_{1-24}$, the effect of other ACTH-related peptides on the activity of adenylate cyclase in the separated zones of the adrenal gland was investigated. 16K fragments (1-36), γ_3-MSH, α-MSH, β-endorphin and leu-enkephalin did not stimulate adenylate cyclase activity in either zone. Met-enkephalin stimulated adenylate cyclase activity only slightly in both zones. It is concluded that basal and $ACTH_{1-24}$-stimulated adenylate cyclase activity is greater in NC than in FZ membrane fractions. In addition, the results of the present investigation do not suggest that other ACTH-related peptides increase steroidogenesis by stimulating adenylate cyclase activity in the human fetal adrenal gland.

361 PREMATURE OPENING OF THE DEVELOPMENTALLY PROGRAMMED α_{2u} GLOBULIN GENE DOMAIN BY 5-AZACYTIDINE. B. Chatterjee*, D. Majumdar, C.V.R. Murty and A.K. Roy, Oakland University, Rochester, MI 48063, U.S.A.

The conformation of the chromatin domain for the α_{2u} globulin gene manifests age-dependent changes in the sensitivity to pancreatic DNAase I. In male rats, the α_{2u} globulin gene domain exists in the DNAase I resistant form up to 22 days of age after which it shows an enhanced sensitivity to DNAase I and this sensitivity is maintained throughout the life of the animal. However, a male rat does not begin to synthesize α_{2u} globulin until about 35 to 40 days of age, and the synthesis of this protein ceases at senescence (>750 days). The present communication reports that the α_{2u} globulin gene domain can be prematurely opened (DNAase I sensitive) as early as 9 days of age by treating 1-day-old male animals with a single injection of 5-azacytidine, a drug known to induce expression of developmentally silent genes through demethylation of cytidine residues. Nuclei isolated from rat liver were digested with increasing concentrations of DNAase I and the isolated DNA was subjected to EcoRI restriction cleavage. Southern blotting of the electrophoretically separated EcoRI-cleaved DNA, followed by hybridization with a ^{32}P-labeled cloned α_{2u} globulin cDNA probe showed that the α_{2u} globulin gene domain of the 5-azacytidine injected rats is four- to five-fold more sensitive to DNAase I as compared to the α_{2u} globulin gene of control animals of the same age. These results indicate that methylation of critically located cytidine residues may play a determinant role in the conformational change that is a prerequisite for α_{2u} globulin gene expression. Supported by the NIH.

362 NEONATAL EXPOSURE TO ANDROGEN IMPRINTS THE RESPONSIVITY OF HEPATIC SOMATOGENIC RECEPTORS TO SEX STEROIDS IN ADULT RATS. Christopher H.K. Cheng*[a], Karl W.K. Tsim[a] and Raphael C.K. Pak[b], Departments of Biochemistry[a] and Pharmacology[b], The Chinese University of Hong Kong, Shatin, N.T., Hong Kong.

A high level of somatogenic receptors was found in membranes from adult female rat liver whereas the level in the male was low. Castration of adult rats decreased and increased the receptor level in female and male animals, respectively, to a neutral level. Administration of estradiol benzoate (0.05 μmol/kg on alternate days s.c. for 9 days) to adult castrated female rats increased the somatogenic receptor level by approximately 3 fold whereas these animals were non-responsive to testosterone (2.5 μmol/kg/day s.c. for 9 days) treatment. Administration of estradiol to adult castrated male rats also increased the somatogenic receptor level, but to a much less extent. In addition, the receptor level of these animals was decreased by testosterone treatment. This sexually dimorphic pattern in adult rats appears to be determined neonatally. Neonatal castration of male rats (within 24 h after birth) completely changed the hepatic response system to the female pattern in adulthood. Replacement of testosterone (1.45 μmol at day 1 and day 3 after birth) to these rats restored the male pattern. Exposure of intact female rats neonatally to testosterone changed the response pattern to the male type in adulthood. Estrogen derived from neonatal androgen is probably responsible for these observations since diethylstilbestrol administered neonatally (1.45 μmol at day 1 and day 3 after birth) to intact female rats and to neonatally castrated male rats also produced the same effects as testosterone. This study was supported by the Chinese University of Hong Kong.

363 AETIOLOGICAL FACTORS IN THE HYPOGLYCAEMIA OF INFANTS OF DIABETIC MOTHERS.
CL Clarson*, GJM Ievaarwerk, GW Chance and CJ Hurst. St. Joseph's Hospital University of Western Ontario, London N6A 5B8 Canada.

We have examined the effect of several factors on the development of neonatal hypoglycaemia in the infants of 16 overt (IDM) and 8 gestational (IGDM) diabetic mothers. Maternal glycosylated haemoglobin levels (HbA_{1c}) and cord glucose (CG), insulin (CI) and C-peptide (CCP) levels at delivery, and gestational age, birthweight and type of maternal diabetes were determined. Neonatal glucose (G) and insulin (I) were measured at 2 hrs., following an oral glucose load (OGTT) and every 12 hrs. for 4 days. The mean HbA_{1c} in the 16 mothers of the IDM (8.4 1%) was higher ($p<0.05$) than in the 8 mothers of IGDM (7.6 1%). The mean CG in the two groups were similar (6.8 3.8 vs 5.9 2.8 mmol/L) but both CI and CCP were higher ($p<0.05$) in the IDM. Two hours after birth the mean G was lower in the IDM (1.9 0.8 vs 3.1 1.0 mmol/L; $p<0.01$). Seven of the IDM, but none of the IGDM, became hypoglycaemic (G <1.7 mmol/L). The glucose response to OGTT was less in the IDM ($p<0.05$) while the I/G ratio was higher ($p<0.01$). Hypoglycaemia did not occur after 12 hours of age while the I/G ratio remained significantly higher in the IDM until 4 hrs. of age and became identical after 48 hrs. The 2 hr. G correlated inversely with CI ($r = -0.41$; $p<0.05$) and CCP ($r = -0.48$; $p<0.05$) but not with CG or HbA_{1c}. Both CI and CCP correlated positively with CG. There was no effect of gestational age or birthweight. In conclusion, neonatal hypoglycaemia: 1 - occurred only in IDM; 2 - was evident by 2 hrs. and did not recur after 12 hrs; 3 - correlated inversely with glucose-induced cord hyperinsulinism.

364 THE ERYTHROTROPINS, NEW ERYTHROID CELL STIMULATING FACTORS EXTRACTED FROM HUMAN AND BOVINE FETAL TISSUES.
L.F. Congote, Endocrine Laboratory, Royal Victoria Hospital and Department of Medicine, McGill University, Montreal, H3A 1A1, Canada.

A sensitive bioassay system based on the measurement of thymidine incorporation into trichloroacetic acid-insoluble materials in erythroid cell suspensions from fetal calf liver led to the isolation by reversed-phase and gel permeation high pressure liquid chromatography (HPLC) of two small peptides from fetal calf intestine (Biochem. Biophys. Res. Commun. 115:477, 1983). The names Erythrotropins I and II (EPI and EPII) have been suggested for these 3500 dalton factors, which have a very similar amino acid composition but different retention times in reversed-phase HPLC. ET I and II stimulate thymidine incorporation and globin chain synthesis in cell cultures of calf liver cells and act synergistically with erythropoietin (EP) in cultures of rat liver cells. At least one of these factors seems to be secreted from the intestine or other tissues into the fetal circulation. Fetal bovine serum has large amounts of a factor which is very similar if not identical to ET I, because of its amino acid composition, molecular weight and retention time in reversed-phase HPLC. Human cord blood serum contains a factor similar to bovine ET I, whereas a factor similar to ET II can be extracted from fetal intestine of human fetuses obtained following therapeutic abortions. It is concluded that human and bovine tissues have factors acting on erythroid cells with physical and biological properties different from those of EP. This study was supported by the MRC.

365 DIRECT AND INDIRECT EFFECTS OF INSULIN (I) AND GH ON GROWTH OF FETAL RAT TISSUES. P. Cooke*, L. Higa and C. Nicoll, Dept. of Physiology-Anatomy and Cancer Research Lab., University of California, Berkeley, CA 94720 USA.

We previously reported that paws from fetal rats grow and differentiate normally when transplanted under kidney capsules of intact syngeneic hosts. Growth of transplants (TP) was inhibited in hypophysectomized (HX) or diabetic (D) hosts, and was restored by GH or insulin (I) therapy, respectively. We investigated whether these hormones restored growth of the fetal tissue by direct or indirect effects. Diabetic or HX hosts received bilateral TP of paws from 14-15-day fetuses. I or GH, respectively, was infused for 7 days into the left renal artery by means of a catheter attached to an osmotic minipump. This system allows the left TP to be exposed directly to high local levels of the infused hormone. If it acts directly, the left kidney TP should show preferential growth. If the infused hormone acts indirectly, TP growth in both kidneys should be equal. Insulin infusion at 2U/kg/day stimulated growth of the left TP without affecting that of the right. At 6U/kg/day the I restored TP growth nearly to normal on the left and had a slight effect on the right. Since the infused TP were directly exposed to supraphysiological concentrations of I, and since growth restoration close to normal was observed only when systemic effects were evident, I appears to act both directly and indirectly to restore growth of fetal TP. GH stimulated TP growth in a dose-dependent manner, but growth was equal in both kidneys with three different doses of GH (0.1, 0.3 and 1.0 μg/g/day). Thus, GH may act only indirectly to promote TP growth, possibly through metabolic effects in the hosts and/or by stimulating somatomedin secretion. Supported by NIH grant HD 14661.

366 TUMOR PROMOTING PHORBOL DIESTER ACTION LEADS TO THE PHOSPHORYLATION OF THE EGF RECEPTOR AT DISCRETE SITES. Roger J. Davis* and Michael P. Czech, University of Massachusetts Medical Center, Worcester, MA 01605

Addition of phorbol diesters to human A431 epidermoid carcinoma cells causes an inhibition of the high affinity binding of EGF. Analysis of the phosphorylation state of the EGF receptor isolated from [^{32}P] phosphate labeled cells demonstrates that phorbol diesters increase the net incorporation of phosphate into the receptor. Most of the increase is due to phosphoserine with a small increase in phosphothreonine. The sites of phosphorylation were examined by exhaustive digestion of the receptor with trypsin to yield a complex mixture of phosphopeptides which were analysed by HPLC. Phosphopeptides were first separated by chromatography on a μBondapak C-18 reverse phase column equilibrated with 0.1% TFA and eluted with n-propanol. Fractions were then further resolved by ion-exchange chromatography with a Partisil-10 SAX column. A number of differences between the trypsin digested receptor from control and phorbol diester treated cells were noted. In particular most of the increase in the phosphorylation state of the receptor due to phorbol diesters could be accounted for by a single fraction which eluted at 8% n-propanol from the C-18 column. Ion-exchange HPLC of this fraction resolved it into 3 peaks, the second of which was increased two-fold by phorbol diester treatment of cells. Analysis of this peak by thin layer chromatography and electrophoresis indicates that it is a single phosphopeptide. Phosphoserine was the only phosphoamino acid detected after partial acid hydrolysis. These data demonstrate that phorbol diesters promote the phosphorylation of the EGF receptor on a distinct tryptic peptide site or sites, an effect which may be related to potentiation of EGF action by these agents.

367 DIFFERENTIAL CHANGES IN CIRCULATING SOMATOSTATIN (SS) RELATED PEPTIDES IN MAN AFTER EATING. J.W. Ensinck*, E. Laschansky, R. Vogel, B.H. Francis, Department of Medicine, University of Washington.

Posttranslational processing of pro-SS differs amongst SS secreting cells in brain, pancreas, and intestinal tract. At least two bioactive SS peptides [SS28 and SS28(15-28)] are secreted into the circulation. To measure them, we have generated two antisera recognizing specific regions of SS28. Antiserum AS-10, interacting with SS28 and SS28(15-28), was used for radioimmunoassay (RIA). Antiserum F4 interacting with SS28 was conjugated to agarose and used as an immunoabsorbent. Healthy young men (N=10), patients with total gastrectomy (N=2), and total pancreatectomy (N=2) were studied after an overnight fast. Blood was withdrawn before and up to 4h after intake of liquid formula or a mixed meal (700 KCal). Plasma adjusted to pH 3 was passed through Sep-Pak and adsorbed peptides eluted with methanol: 5mM TFA (80:20). The reconstituted eluate was filtered through the column of agarose-F4 conjugate. SS28(15-28), which passed through the immunoadsorbent, and SS28, which was retained and eluted with acid, was measured by AS-10 RIA. In normal men, mean basal levels of SS28 (15-28) were 10 pg/ml and did not change after nutrient intake. Mean basal levels of SS28 were 15 pg/ml and a 2 fold increase occurred 2-4h after food. In gastrectomized and pancreatectomized patients, levels and pertubations of SS28 were either similar to normals or exaggerated and in the gastrectomized subjects, shifted earlier. We conclude that SS28, but not SS28(15-28), rises in the circulation after eating and the major source of circulating SS28 is the small intestine. We propose that SS28 acts as a traditional hormone to modulate peptide release during nutrient absorption.

368 PATHOLOGICAL ROLE OF GASTRIC INHIBITORY POLYPEPTIDE IN THE HYPERINSULINAEMIA OF OBESE HYPERGLYCAEMIC (ob/ob) MICE. P.R. Flatt*, C.J. Bailey, P. Kwasowski, T. Page and V. Marks. Division of Nutrition and Food Science, Department of Biochemistry, University of Surrey, Guildford, UK, and Department of Biological Sciences, University of Aston, Birmingham, UK.

Gastric inhibitory polypeptide (GIP) is a component of the enteroinsular axis. To evaluate the regulation of plasma GIP and its role in the hyperinsulinaemia of adult obese hyperglycaemic (ob/ob) mice, GIP and insulin were determined after fasting and refeeding, and after administration of GIP, different nutrients and insulin to 18h fasted mice. Plasma GIP and insulin were markedly elevated in ob/ob mice. Values were suppressed by fasting and promptly restored by refeeding. Intraperitoneal injection of GIP to mimic postprandial concentrations evoked a marked but transient insulin response which was protracted in the presence of rising hyperglycaemia. Orally administered fat, glucose and amino acids raised GIP concentrations with a particularly strong effect of fat. Fat produced only a small elevation of insulin under conditions of basal hyperglycaemia, but this was greatly enhanced at higher glucose concentrations. Intraperitoneal injection of insulin up to 100 U/kg failed to suppress either basal, fat-stimulated or glucose-stimulated GIP release. The results demonstrate that hypersecretion of GIP in adult ob/ob mice provides a powerful glucose-dependent insulinotropic stimulus. Hypersecretion of GIP appears to result in part from a defective feedback inhibition by insulin on the GIP-secreting intestinal K-cells.

369 46,XX TRUE HERMAPHRODITISM : PRESENCE OF Y-DNA SEQUENCES AND POSSIBLE PREFERENTIAL INACTIVATION OF THE PATERNALLY DERIVED X CHROMOSOME. C. Boucekkine*, F. Latron, B. Nafa, M. Casanova, M. Fellous, M. Benmiloud. Service d'Endocrinologie, CPMC, Alger, Algérie. Laboratoire d'Immunogénétique, Institut Pasteur, Paris, France.

With regard to the pathogenesis of 46,XX true hermaphroditism (T.H.) four main hypothesies are taken into consideration : a cryptic presence of the Y chromosome, translocation of a Y-male determining material, X-Y interchange, deletion or inactivation of X chromosomal genes controlling the testis determination. In order to determine which of these explanations would apply in a case of T.H. we analysed the familial transmission of three X-markers e.g. the glucose-6-phosphate deshydrogenase, 12 E7 and Xg^a antigens. Likewise we looked for Y-DNA sequences by hybridization procedures. The patient was a 20 year-old phenotypic male presenting with a gynecomastia and hypogonadism. The hormonal investigations revealed high concentrations of FSH and LH and a low level of testosterone. The karyotype was 46,XX on blood leucocytes. The laparotomy disclosed an ovotestis in the right bursa and a testis in the left bursa. H-Y antigen was present at a low level on peripheral lymphocytes. G6PD phenotypes studied by the starch gel electrophoresis of red cell lysates and lymphocytes were AB in the mother, B in the father and A in the propositus. On the other hand, the father was Xg (a+) and expressed high levels of 12 E7. The mother and the affected child were Xg (a-) and expressed low levels of 12 E7. Some Y specific bands were present in the genome of the patient. These results support the contention that there was an inactivation of the Xg^a, 12 E7 and H-Y regulatory genes located on the Xp22.3→pter segment of the paternally derived X chromosome.

370 SODIUM IONS MODULATE THE AFFINITY OF THE LUTEINIZING HORMONE/ CHORIOGONADOTROPIN (LH/CG) RECEPTOR. K. Buettner and M. Ascoli*, Division of Endocrinology, Vanderbilt Medical School, Nashville, Tennessee, 37232, U.S.A.

Previous studies from many laboratories have shown that, although LH and CG bind to the same receptor, the affinity of CG is higher than that of LH from several mammalian species. Although this difference in affinities has been ascribed to differences in the structure of the hormones, one must also consider the possibility that other factors are involved. We now report that Na^+ regulates the affinity of this receptor. Using intact cultured Leydig tumor cells (designated MA-10) or membranes isolated from these cells, competition binding experiments were done with ^{125}I-hCG and increasing concentrations of ovine LH (oLH) or human CG (hCG) in isotonic buffers containing NaCl (121 mM) or an iso-osmolar concentration of several NaCl substitutes (N-methyl-D-glucamine, choline, sucrose, or tetramethylammonium chloride). Our results show that in NaCl the affinity of oLH is about 5 times lower than that of hCG. In buffers containing a NaCl substitute, however, the affinity of oLH increases about 5-fold, and the affinity of hCG does not change. Thus, in the absence of NaCl, the affinities of oLH and hCG are identical. We also show that the affinities of human LH, deglycosylated hCG, and a hybrid of oLHα-hCGβ are not affected by NaCl; but the affinity of a hybrid of hCGα-oLHβ is increased when NaCl is absent. These studies show that the different affinities of oLH and hCG for the LH/CG receptor are not entirely due to the different structures of the hormones, and that Na^+ modulates the affinity of this receptor for oLH but not that of hCG.

Supported by the NIH (CA-23603).

371 ASSESSMENT OF FSH ACTIVITY PRESENT WITHIN AND SECRETED FROM PITUITARIES OF CYCLIC AND OVARIECTOMIZED (OVX) HAMSTERS. J.L. Cameron* and S.C. Chappel, Dept. Ob-Gyn, Univ. Pennsylvania, Philadelphia, PA 19104 and Dept. Pediatrics, Univ. Michigan, Ann Arbor, MI 48109.

Multiple forms of FSH exist within pituitary tissue. These forms differ in plasma halflife, receptor binding and bioactivity. The present studies were designed to determine if changes in the type of secreted FSH occurred as a function of hormonal milieu. Pituitaries were obtained on each day of the estrous cycle or after ovx and bisected. One half was solubilized while the other was incubated for 3h (±LHRH) and then solubilized. FSH content was assessed in all tissue and medium samples by RIA and radioreceptor assay (RRA). LHRH stimulated releases of FSH with the greatest observed from diestrous II and proestrous tissue. RRA/RIA of secreted FSH was greatest from tissue collected at these times. FSH RRA/RIA was greatest for medium samples (although ratios were similar for basal and LHRH-exposed samples) and least in tissue samples obtained at the end of culture. FSH immunoactivity was 10X greater in medium and tissue samples from ovx animals compared with intact, although FSH RRA/RIA were much lower. We conclude that: 1)FSH forms with greater RRA/RIA are released during culture compared with that remaining in the gland; 2)Acute LHRH exposure affects the amount but not the RRA/RIA of secreted FSH, although that ratio was highest for samples obtained during times of enhanced LHRH sensitivity; 3)FSH present within and secreted from pituitaries of ovx hamsters exhibits a lower RRA/RIA than corresponding samples obtained from cyclic animals. These results suggest that the endocrine status of the animal influences the RRA/RIA of secreted FSH, and therefore the stimulus intensity presented to the ovaries. (Supported by NIH Grant # HD 14742).

372 ABSENCE OF CHORIONIC GONADOTROPIN mRNAs IN THE RAT PLACENTA. F.E. Carr*, W.W. Chin, and J.F. Habener, Laboratory of Molecular Endocrinology, Massachusetts General Hospital and Howard Hughes Medical Institute Laboratories, Harvard Medical School, Boston, MA.

Placental chorionic gonadotropin (CG), one of the four glycoprotein hormones, has been well characterized in only a few mammals. While the presence of a luteotropic factor in the rat placenta has been suggested by the detection of bioactivity and immunoactivity similar to the α and β subunits of human CG, no specific gonadotropin-like molecule has yet been isolated. We investigated the potential presence of mRNAs encoding for both the α and β subunits of a gonadotropin-like molecule using cloned α and β cDNAs derived from rat placental and pituitary mRNA. RNA was prepared from placentae of timed-pregnant (7-21d) and from normal and ovariectomized rat pituitaries of Sprague-Dawley rats. The presence of subunit specific mRNAs was determined by blot hybridization analyses at high and low stringencies using subunit cDNA probes. Our results indicated no detectable hybridizable bands at any gestational stage with either of the cDNA probes with 10 μg of total RNA from rat placentae. However, with as little as 1 μg of normal pituitary and 0.1 μg of stimulated pituitary total RNA, single bands were detected with each of the α and LHβ cDNA probes. Moreover, with 5 μg of placental poly(A+) RNA, a 250-fold enrichment, no detectable bands were obtained from 7-11, 13-15, or 18-21 days of gestation. The pituitary bands were still detectable in the presence of placental mRNA. We conclude that mRNAs encoding proteins structurally homologous to rat LH subunits are absent in the rat placenta.

373 PRESENCE OF AN O-LINKED OLIGOSACCHARIDE ON THE LARGE FREE α-SUBUNIT OF HUMAN CHORIONIC GONADOTROPIN (hCG). Laurence A. Cole*, Fulvio Perini and Raymond W. Ruddon, Departments of Internal Medicine and Pharmacology, University of Michigan Medical School, Ann Arbor, Michigan 48109, U.S.A.

Previously, ours and other laboratories have shown that trophoblast cells produce a free α-subunit in addition to the hCG αβ dimer. Free α was shown to be larger than that combined (hCGα) and unable to associate with β-subunit to form hCG. To compare the free and combined forms of α, we examined those produced by the JAr line of choriocarcinoma cells. Free α and hCGα, biosynthetically labeled with radioactive amino acids and sugars, were purified using immobilized antibodies. The JAr free α (mol wt 25,000 by electrophoresis), hCGα (mol wt 23,000), and urinary α standard were each digested with trypsin, and fragments separated on Bio-Gel P4 and examined by amino acid analyses and by their sensitivity to glycosidases and abilities to bind peanut lectin. Whereas JAr hCGα tryptic peptides coeluted with those of urinary α standard, the free α tryptic digest lacked a peptide eluting in the position of hCGα residues 36-42. Instead, additional fragments of greater molecular size were found. These fragments contained 2 prolyl and 1 leucyl residue as expected for residues 36-42, but also contained sialyl, galactosyl and N-acetylgalactosaminyl/galactosaminyl residues as found in O-linked oligosaccharides of the type on β-subunit. The presence of this type of oligosaccharide on free α peptide 36-42, presumably at the potential O-glycosylation site, -pro-thr-pro-, was also indicated by its ability to bind peanut lectin. Removal of peptide 36-42 from free α and hCGα by trypsin treatment ablates their size difference on gel filtration. This study was supported by USPHS Grant CA-32949 from NCI.

374 PATTERNS OF LUTEINIZING HORMONE SECRETION DURING THE MIDCYCLE SURGE IN NORMAL WOMEN. R.L. Collins, S.A. Brody*, D.L. Loriaux, and G.R. Merriam. DEB, NICHD, NIH, Bethesda, Maryland 20205 USA.

In some animal species, the frequency of LH pulses increases during the midcycle LH surge. It is unclear if this occurs in normal women, and fixed-frequency GnRH treatment can induce LH surges in amenorrheic patients. To evaluate midcycle gonadotropin secretion patterns, 7 women underwent venous sampling for 24 h on cycle day 6, and for 24-72 h during the LH surge. Follicular development was monitored by daily serum estradiol and ovarian sonography. Midcycle sampling was begun when E_2 values plateaued or ovarian follicle size approached 20 mm. Samples were collected q 20 min for LH and FSH, q 60 min for progesterone (P_4), and q 6h for E_2. LH patterns were characterized by a computer method (PULSAR). Mean LH was 42.4 ± 9.5 (SE) mIU/ml at midcycle, and 7.3 ± 1.2 on day 6. LH pulse frequency during the surge (15.1 ± 1.4 /24 h) was not significantly greater than the frequency on day 6 (13.1 ± 1.6; n.s.), although mean pulse amplitude increased 5-fold (22.3 ± 5.0 vs. 4.7 ± 0.9 mIU/ml, $p<0.05$). Three subjects did show higher frequencies at midcycle, up to 19/24 h; this may be a "magnification" effect, in which small LH variations were amplified into significant peaks. P_4, initially below assay detectability, increased prior to the initiation of the surge. The time intervals between successive pulses during the surge remained constant or increased, suggesting that the P_4-mediated slowing of LH pulse frequency, which is striking in the late luteal phase, may begin as early as the LH surge. We conclude that the midcycle LH surge in normal women is primarily due to increased pulse amplitude rather than to a change in pulse frequency; and that P_4 elevation begins prior to the LH surge and could affect its timing.

375 BLOCKADE OF THE SPONTANEOUS MIDCYCLE LH SURGE BY A PROGESTERONE ANTAGONIST.
R.L. Collins*, B. Kreitmann-Gimbal, O.L. Kreitmann and G.D. Hodgen, PRB, NICHD, NIH, Bethesda, MD 20205, USA.

Recent studies in normal cycling women demonstrate that the preovulatory progesterone (P_4) rise begins as much as 12 hours prior to the initiation of the midcycle LH surge. Although the exact role of P_4 at midcycle is disputed, it may influence the timing, duration, and/or amplitude of the LH surge. To investigate this putative role of P_4, a progesterone receptor antagonist, RU 486 (Roussel-Uclaf, Paris), was administered to four normal adult cynomolgus monkeys. The anti-progesterone was given (5 mg/day, im) on days 10-12 of the menstrual cycle. Femoral blood for RIA of FSH, LH, PRL, E_2, P_4 was obtained daily under ketamine anesthesia from D8 of treatment cycle until D2 of subsequent menses. Daily menstrual records were kept. One monkey menstruated within 48h after receiving RU 486. She had had a spontaneous LH surge prior to RU 486 treatment, as evidenced by rising plasma P_4 and corpus luteum formation. Three preovulatory monkeys failed to manifest an LH surge, despite familiar elevations of serum estradiol ($>$ 200 pg/ml), suggesting the emergence of a dominant follicle; plasma P_4 remained $<$ 0.4 ng/ml. An attenuated LH rise ($\sim$ 2 fold above basal) occurred 11.7 $\pm$ 0.8 day after RU 486 treatment, without an intervening increase in plasma P_4. The intermenstrual interval (75.4 $\pm$ 9.7 days) was significantly lengthened ($p < 0.05$) when compared to pretreatment control cycles (31.33 $\pm$ 1.5 days). We conclude that preovulatory P_4 may be required for full expression of a timely midcycle LH surge. Although the mechanisms remain obscure, P_4 may augment estrogen positive feedback, thereby facilitating the timing, duration and amplitude of the preovulatory LH surge.

376 DNA PROBES FOR DEMONSTRATING GONADAL STEROID CONTROL OF THE MESSENGER RNAs ENCODING LH AND FSH SUBUNITS.
R. Counis*, M. Corbani, M. Schmitt-Ney and M. Jutisz , Laboratoire des Hormones Polypeptidiques, CNRS, 91190 Gif-sur-Yvette, France.

Using translation of rat and ovine pituitary mRNAs in a cell-free system, we and others have previously shown that α, LHβ and FSHβ subunits are synthesized as precursors, encoded by separate messengers. Recently, we obtained evidence for hormonal control of these mRNAs. In order to further investigate this problem, 15-16 base long oligodeoxynucleotides (ODNs) were chemically synthesized and used as probes for characterizing and quantifying the respective mRNAs. The required nucleotide sequence of the ODNs was deduced from the aminoacid sequences of specific and highly conserved regions in the polypeptide chains of the corresponding subunits. Hybridization with ^{32}P-labeled ODNs allowed identification of a single mRNA for each subunit α, LHβ and FSHβ. The size of the corresponding mRNAs was estimated to be respectively 820, 640 and 680 bases. Further, cDNAs, reverse transcribed from gonadectomized rat and ovine poly-(A^+)mRNAs have been cloned and oligodeoxynucleotides used to screen the cDNA libraries. Cloned cDNAs were characterized and used in turn to investigate the hormonal control of the gonadotropin subunit mRNAs. Using both ODN and cloned cDNA probes, we quantitatively determined the amount of each specific mRNA present in the pituitaries of normal and castrated animals. Our data demonstrate that gonadectomy induces the increase of intracellular levels of all 3 specific mRNAs, thus suggesting regulation by gonadal steroids on the level of gene expression.

377 INSULIN-INDUCED HYPOGLYCAEMIA AND LH RELEASE IN THE EWE. Alison D. Crump and R.G. Rodway*, Department of Animal Physiology and Nutrition, The University of Leeds, Leeds LS2 9JT U.K.

It has been suggested that the reduced fertility seen in cattle and sheep at times of nutritional or metabolic stress may be caused, at least in part, by the low blood glucose concentrations of such animals. In the present experiment we have studied the release of LH in anoestrous ewes made hypoglycaemic by the infusion of insulin. Eight mature seasonally anoestrous ewes were used in a total of 28 trials. Either saline (n=17) or insulin (n=11) was infused into the jugular vein for 48h periods. The insulin infusion rate was increased approximately every 8h (initial rate 120mU/min;final rate;314mU/min) in order to maintain a constant level of hypoglycaemia. Mean glucose concentrations over the 48h period were 4.43±0.07mM(control) and 2.44±0.07mM(insulin). Oestradiol(1μg/kg,sc) was given either 8h or 16h after the start of the infusion to trigger an LH peak. Blood samples were collected every 30min via jugular catheters during the expected time of the LH peak. Neither the time from oestradiol injection to the LH peak (15.9±0.6h,control);(15.2±0.5h,insulin) nor the mean peak height (62.9±9.0ng/ml,control); (67.8±9.6ng/ml,insulin) was affected by insulin infusion. However the number of animals not giving an LH peak in response to oestradiol was significantly greater in the hypoglycaemic group (1/17 controls;5/11 insulin,$p<0.001$).Plasma concentrations of non-esterified fatty acids (238±23μeq/l(control);403±49μeq/l(insulin)) and cortisol (20.9±3.0nM(control);69.1±8.4nM(insulin)) were both increased by insulin infusion.

378 DISTRIBUTION OF EPIDERMAL GROWTH FACTOR (EGF) RECEPTORS IN THE RAT OVARY.
J.-G. Chabot*, J. Guy, R. St-Arnaud, P. Walker and G. Pelletier, MRC Group in Molecular Endocrinology and Laboratory of Endocrinology and Metabolism, CHUL, Quebec G1V 4G2, Canada.

Since specific and high affinity receptors for EGF were recently characterized in total rat ovarian homogenate and since EGF may also play a role in the control of ovarian steroidogenesis, we felt it of interest to accurately identify the cell types containing EGF receptors in the rat ovary. For this purpose, in vivo radioautographic localization of EGF receptors was performed at different time intervals (2 to 60 min) after intravenous injection of [^{125}I]EGF into adult female rats at random stages of the estrous cycle. The localization of EGF receptors was also performed in vitro by incubating [^{125}I]EGF with frozen sections of rat ovary. In both cases, the ovaries were processed for light microscope radioautography. After in vivo injection, specific labeling was found in the cells of the theca interna of follicles at different stages of development and in the cells of the corpus luteum. Primordial and primary follicles did not show any significant labeling. In both corpora lutea and follicles, the distribution of silver grains in the same cell types was uneven. In vitro, a positive radioautographic reaction was observed in the same cellular elements as found in vivo, with the additional labeling of the granulosa cells of growing follicles. Control experiments indicated that the radioautographic labeling was due to specific interaction of [^{125}I]EGF with its receptor. These results clearly indicate that EGF receptors are present in luteal, thecal and granulosa cells, and provide support for the inhibitory role of EGF on gonadotropin-induced steroidogenesis in the ovary.

379 SOMATOMEDINS AND INSULIN STIMULATE THYMIDINE UPTAKE INTO CULTURED FETAL RAT CELLS.

C.J. Crace*, D.J. Hill and R.D.G. Milner, Department of Paediatrics, Clinical Sciences Centre, Northern General Hospital, Sheffield, S5 7AU, U.K.

Under- and over-secretion of insulin are associated with disturbances in insulin-like growth factor (IGF) production and with abnormal fetal growth. We have therefore studied the effects of insulin, somatomedin-C and multiplication-stimulating activity (MSA) on radiothymidine uptake into myoblasts and fibroblasts obtained from thigh muscle of rats from 19 days gestation to postnatal day 1. Cells were isolated with dispase, and the two cell types were separated by addition of cytochalasin B, which causes myoblasts to detach from the dish. Myoblasts were replated once and used prior to myotube formation, while fibroblasts were passaged twice before use. Cells were exposed to insulin or IGF for 16 h, after which a 4 h pulse of thymidine was added. In the absence of exogenous hormones there was a significant age related increase in thymidine incorporation by myoblasts from day 19 to postnatal day 1. Dose-related stimulation of ^{3}H-thymidine uptake was shown by myoblasts from 21-day fetuses to all three peptides; significant increases being observed at 10^{-5} U/ml insulin and 100 ng/ml partially purified somatomedin-C (30 U/MG), and half-maximal response at 5-10 ng/ml MSAIII-2. Fibroblasts were unresponsive to insulin at concentrations up to 10^{-1} U/ml, but their responses to IGFs were not different from those of myoblasts. These direct actions of insulin and related peptides on fetal rat muscle cells at physiological concentrations support evidence that they are fetal growth factors.

380 INSULIN ALTERS EARLY CHICK EMBRYO DEVELOPMENT APPARENTLY ACTING THROUGH A NON METABOLIC PATHWAY.

F. de Pablo*, E. Hernandez and J.A. Gomez, Endocrinology and Biochemistry Services. H. S. Cruz y S. Pablo. Barcelona, Spain.

Classically, Insulin has been considered a teratogen for young embryos in vertebrates, although its mechanism of action had not been elucidated. We studied the effects of purified insulins on chick embryos at differentiation stages and we compared them with the effects of Proinsulin, Desoctapeptide insulin (DOP) and Multiplication Stimulating Activity (MSA), which have very little metabolic activity while they have significant growth effects. Embryos at 48 h of development were windowed and injected with 0.05 to 50 µg/embryo of the different peptides. At 96 h, mortality and abnormal growth appeared to be dose-dependent. Indexes of lethality (LD_{50}) and total embryos affected (ED_{50}) were derived from the dose-response curves:

	LD50 µg/emb.	%	ED50 µg/emb.	%
Insulin (pork & beef)	0.7	100	0.4	100
Proinsulin (pork & beef)	1.2	59	0.6	66
DOP (pork)	38	2	7	6
MSA	0.4	176	0.2	204

The magnitude and relative potencies were what we expect when these peptides act through a growth type receptor (IGF/MSA). In the surviving embryos 5 µg of insulin decreased the content of DNA, RNA and proteins to about 50% of that in control embryos. Proinsulin was slightly less potent. 5 µg of MSA increased DNA in the embryos two fold with a minor effect in RNA and protein content. The effects of insulin were not corrected by injecting glucose simultaneously. These data suggest a possible role for insulin in early embryo differentiation mediated by a MSA type of receptor.

381 THE B-DOMAIN OF INSULIN-LIKE GROWTH FACTOR I (IGF-I) IS INVOLVED IN THE BINDING OF IGFS TO THEIR CARRIER PROTEINS.

M. A. De Vroede*, S. Joshi, P. G. Katsoyannis, S. P. Nissley and M. M. Rechler. NIADDK, NICHHD and NCI, National Institutes of Health, Bethesda, MD and Mt. Sinai School of Medicine, New York, NY, USA.

Although the IGFs are highly homologous to insulin, IGF carrier proteins and Type II IGF receptors discriminate between these polypeptides, interacting specifically and exclusively with the IGFs. To define the molecular basis for this specificity, we have prepared hybrid molecules that combine the A chain of bovine insulin and a chemically synthesized B chain of human IGF-I. IGF carrier protein from normal rat serum was resolved from endogenous IGF by acid gel filtration (Sephadex G-50, 1M acetic acid), neutralized, and used in a competitive binding assay with ^{125}I-labeled MSA (rat IGF-II). Radioligand binding was inhibited 50% by 1.2 ± 0.3 ng/ml of rat IGF-II (n=3), but was not inhibited by porcine insulin at 10 μg/ml. By contrast, the IGF-I-insulin hybrid molecule gave full and parallel inhibition [ED_{50} 4 ± 1 ng/ml (n=2)]. The hybrid molecule also inhibited ^{125}I-MSA binding to partially purified carrier proteins from human serum and BRL 3A cell conditioned media albeit with lower potency (70-85% inhibition at 10 μg/ml); insulin at 10 μg/ml gave no significant inhibition. Neither the IGF-I-insulin hybrid nor insulin at 5-10 μg/ml inhibited ^{125}I-MSA binding to Type II IGF receptors on rat liver membranes, placental membranes, or chondrosarcoma cells. CONCLUSIONS: Hybrid molecules in which the insulin B chain is replaced by the B domain of IGF-I interact with IGF carrier proteins but not with Type II IGF receptors. The binding site for the carrier proteins may be formed at least in part by the B domain.

382 PLATELET RELEASE REACTION AFTER GROWTH HORMONE REPLACEMENT THERAPY IN GROWTH HORMONE DEFICIENT PATIENTS.

R. Delius, J. Lazerson, J. Harrison and M. Connors*, Department of Pediatrics, University of California, Davis, California 95616, USA.

The lack of atherosclerotic disease in growth hormone (GH) deficient subjects as well as in diabetic patients with concurrent GH deficiency has been a repeated observation. These findings suggest that GH may be involved in the underlying pathophysiologic mechanism of atherosclerosis. The purpose of this study was to examine the possibility that this lack of atherosclerotic disease is related to a decreased platelet-vessel wall interaction. Twenty children with GH deficiency had their platelet-vessel wall interaction studied before and one month after GH replacement therapy. Factor VIII activity was determined by procoagulant, related antigen and ristocetin cofactor assays. Plasma levels of beta thromboglobulin (BTG) and platelet factor 4 (PF4), a measure of platelet α granule release, were assessed by RIA. Prostacyclin stimulating factor (PSF) production was assayed through its biologic activity in the aortic ring model. Prostacyclin (PGI_2) levels were determined by RIA of its metabolic end product, 6 keto α PG. No significant differences were found in factor VIII activities, PSF, PGI_2 formation or PF 4 levels. A dramatic increase was noted in BTG levels (94.0 ng/ml ± 47.3 vs. > 195 ng/ml), indicating in vivo activation of the platelet release reaction after GH treatment. This suggests that in GH deficient patients, the platelets appear capable of interacting with the vessel wall, but may lack the stimulus for α granule release, including platelet derived growth factor. This may explain the decreased incidence of atherosclerosis in patients with GH deficiency.

383 EVALUATION OF MURINE PLACENTAL DEGRADATION AND TRANSFER OF ^{125}I-αEPIDERMAL GROWTH FACTOR (EGF). R.P. DiAugustine*, M. Rosch, and R.M. Pratt, Lab. Reprod. and Devel. Tox., Natl. Inst. Environ. Health Sci., Research Triangle Park, NC 27709, USA

A study was undertaken to assess the placental degradation and transfer of maternally administered epidermal growth factor (EGF), since this peptide has been postulated to play a role in embryonic and fetal growth. Prior to iodination, mouse EGF was purified to homogeneity (αEGF) by HPLC. Approximately 5 ng of ^{125}I-αEGF (∿ 10^6cpm) was injected intravenously into 10,13, or 17d pregnant CD-1 mice; radioactivity in plasma, placentas, and conceptuses was measured up to 2h following injection. The time-course revealed an initial rapid clearance of ^{125}I-αEGF (t ½ < 1 min) in maternal plasma with a second peak at 30 min. Gel filtration (G-10, G-50) revealed that by 5 min radioactivity was associated with free ^{125}I and with material much larger than EGF. No degradation of ^{125}I-αEGF occurred following direct incubation with maternal plasma. Placental radioactivity had an initial phase of decay between 1-5 min followed by a second peak at 30-60 min. Aqueous extracts of lyophilized placentas removed 1,5,15, and 30 min after injection revealed radioactivity co-eluting predominantly with ^{125}I-αEGF at 1 min but shifting to fragments of lower m.w. in 5-15 min and mostly free ^{125}I by 30 min. Uptake of radioactivity into conceptuses did not occur until about 15 min and only free ^{125}I was detected in extracts of whole conceptuses obtained 15 min to 2h after injection. Our results indicate that placentas rapidly degrade blood-borne ^{125}I-αEGF. It is also apparent that free ^{125}I, and not ^{125}I-αEGF or its fragments, crosses the placenta.

384 ISOLATION OF GROWTH PROMOTING PEPTIDES FROM SERUM FREE CONDITIONED MEDIA OF MCF-7 HUMAN BREAST CANCER CELLS. R.B. Dickson*, K.K. Huff and M.E. Lippman. Medical Breast Cancer Section, Medicine Branch, NCI, NIH, Bethesda, Maryland 20205.

Experiments were carried out to evaluate the possible role of autocrine hormones in the growth of human breast cancer. Serum free conditioned medium (IMEM + 10^{-9}M E_2 + 2mg/l transferrin + 2mg/l fibronectin) from MCF-7 cells was characterized for growth promotion and for known growth factors. After removal of transferrin and fibronectin by affinity chromatography and E_2 by extensive dialysis against charcoal, conditioned medium (CM) was capable of growth promotion of MCF-7 cells using two assays: ^{3}H-thymidine incorporation into DNA after 24 hrs, and increasing cell number and DNA content after 3-7 days. CM from E_2-treated cells had greater growth promoting capacity than from untreated control cells, and after concentration it could stimulate cell growth to the same extent as E_2. CM also contained immunoreactive IGF-1/SmC and EGF receptor binding activity using ^{125}I-EGF and A431 cells as a receptor source (suggestive of TGFα). At neutral pH, 88% of the ^{3}H-thymidine-incorporation activity of CM adsorbed to DEAE-Sephadex, while only 48% adsorbed to CM-Sephadex. After chromatography of CM on Sephacryl S-200 (pH 7.2) ^{3}H-thymidine incorporation activity was observed in several peaks ranging from 3500-60,000 MW. 99% of ^{35}S-cysteine-labeled secreted proteins traveled from 20,000-70,000 MW, well separated from 60% of ^{3}H-thymidine incorporation activity which migrated from 3500-20,000 MW. These data are consistent with at least a portion of the growth promoting activity of estradiol in human breast cancer being mediated by secreted growth factors.

385 INFUSION OF EPIDERMAL GROWTH FACTOR REDUCES THYROXIN SECRETION FROM THE FETAL SHEEP THYROID M. Dolling*, M.J. Waters†, G.C. Carmichael and G.D. Thorburn, Dept of Physiology, Monash University, Clayton, 3168, Vic, and †Dept of Physiology, University of Queensland, St. Lucia, 4067, Qld., Aust.

EGF is able to stimulate mitosis in a variety of tissues, but also has effects which are apparently not related to cell division such as inhibition of gastric acid secretion. EGF infusion into fetal sheep resulted in a rapid decline in plasma concentrations of T_4 and an increase in TSH. It was not known whether this effect was due to a stimulation of mitosis and hence dedifferentiation of thyroid cells, or whether it was a direct inhibition of thyroid cell function. Fetuses were infused for four days and thyroids were analysed for TSH receptor content.

Thyroid	Mean Receptor Content	Affinity (high component)
Saline (n=6)	4.7±1.4 pmoles/g wet wt	1.13±0.33 M^{-1}
EGF treated (n=9)	4.0±1.2 pmoles/g wet wt	1.18±0.30 M^{-1}

Receptor content (per gram) and receptor affinity were unchanged, however gland weight doubled after EGF treatment, hence total receptor content was significantly higher. Histological examination of thyroids from EGF treated fetuses showed more large follicles ie. increase in colloid stores. Autoradiography with I^{125} EGF showed marked uptake of EGF into follicle cells, (no uptake with 1000x excess of unlabelled EGF). Analysis of fetal plasma samples showed that both TSH and T_4 rapidly returned to normal on completion of the infusion. T_4 is known to increase EGF levels in skin and stimulate EGF synthesis in the submandibular gland. Our results suggest that there is a direct inhibition by EGF on T_4 release by thyroid cells. This work was supported by a grant from the Australian Wool Research Trust Fund.

386 MODIFICATION OF cAMP AND GROWTH HORMONE (GH) BY PHOSPHOLIPID METABOLIC ENZYME INHIBITORS AND A PHORBOL ESTER. PL Canonico*, RM MacLeod, MJ Cronin, University of Virginia School of Medicine, Charlottesville, Virginia, USA.

The relative importance of several phospholipid pathways in cAMP metabolism and GH release was determined by using cultured anterior pituitary cells through an indirect, pharmacological approach. The diglyceride lipase inhibitor RHC 80267 (30-100 µM) did not affect basal, but tended to enhance GH releasing factor (GRF)-stimulated cAMP levels and markedly inhibited basal and GRF-stimulated GH release. The phospholipase A_2 inhibitor (PLA_2-I) quinacrine (30 µM) increased cellular cAMP content while decreasing GH release, whereas bromophenacylbromide (10-100 µM), another PLA_2-I, reduced cAMP content and enhanced GH release. Indomethecin, which reduces cyclooxygenase activity, affected neither cAMP levels nor GRF-enhanced GH release; this drug (30-100 µM) reduced basal GH release. The lipoxygenase inhibitors nordihydroguaiaretic acid and BW-755c both reduced basal and GRF-stimulated GH release in a concentration dependent manner. The potent protein kinase C activator, phorbol myristate acetate (1-100µM) progressively stimulated cAMP accumulation and GH release. These results suggest that phospholipid metabolism, through both the cyclooxygenase and lipooxygenase pathways, contributes to basal GH secretion, while the lipooxygenase route predominates in GRF-stimulated GH release in vitro. Interestingly, cAMP metabolism can be dissociated from GH release with some of these probes, indicating an action distal or lateral to the cAMP-generating system. Finally, a phorbol ester can profoundly enhance both cAMP levels and GH release, reinforcing the possible contribution of diacylglycerol to these processes by way of protein kinase C activity. [Supported by CA07535, RCDA 1K04NS500601, HD18409 and AM221125.]

387 EFFECT OF A SINGLE AND REPEATED ADMINISTRATION OF HUMAN GROWTH HORMONE RELEASING FACTOR ON PLASMA GROWTH HORMONE LEVELS IN PATIENTS WITH GROWTH HORMONE DEFICIENCY.
K. Chihara* and T. Fujita, Third Div., Dept. of Med., Kobe Univ. Sch. of Med., Kobe 650 Japan

Human growth hormone releasing factor, hGRF(1-44)NH_2 was repeatedly admistered for 5 consecutive days to 10 children with growth hormone (GH) deficiency (GHD); 8 patients had idiopathic GHD, 2 others had GHD secondary to a germinoma. Practically, a single bolus iv injection test of hGRF(1 μg/kg BW) was performed the day before and the day after treatment with a daily 1 h iv infusion of hGRF (2 μg/kg BW) for 3 days. In 6 idiopathic GHD dwarfs, the mean ± SE peak values after a first bolus, 2.3 ± 0.6 ng/ml were not different from those after insulin-induced hypoglycemia and arginine infusion, whereas the significant GH responses to hGRF with the peak of 8.9 ± 1.0 ng/ml occurred on a second day of hGRF infusion. The second bolus iv injection of hGRF on the fifth day caused a small increase in plasma GH with the peak of 3.6 ± 1.2 ng/ml, not significantly different from those after the first hGRF bolus in the idiopathic GHD dwarfs. In 4 GHD children (2 germinoma, 2 idiopathic cases), a first bolus iv injection of hGRF resulted in a significant increase of plasma GH with the peak values of 8.2 ± 0.9 ng/ml. The slightly greater GH peaks were observed during hGRF infusions, but the plasma GH responses to the second hGRF bolus were rather smaller than those to the first bolus injection. These findings suggest that a single bolus or repeated administration of hGRF may be of value for the diagnosis of GH deficiency of hypothalamic origin. This work was supported by the grants from the Japanese Ministry of Health and Welfare, and from the Japanese Ministry of Education, Science and Culture.

388 ON THE ROLE OF HYPOTHALAMIC SOMATOSTATIN, GRF AND CNS NEUROTRANSMITTERS IN THE AUTOFEEDBACK INHIBITION OF GROWTH HORMONE (GH) SECRETION IN RATS.
S. Conway* and L. Krulich, Univ of Texas Health Sci Center, Dallas, Physiology Dept.

In the present work we studied the roles of hypothalamic somatostatin, GRF and CNS neurotransmitters in the autofeedback inhibition of endogenous GH secretion by exogenous GH. Intraventricular (IVT) administration of purified rat GH (20 μg) to conscious, unrestrained male rats inhibited activation of GH, but not TSH by clonidine (clon) (50 μg/kg iv) given 1 or 3 hrs later. This inhibition was not abolished by pretreatment with antiserum to somatostatin (kindly provided by Dr. A. Arimura) and conversely administration of GH did not alter the GH response to synthetic GRF (250 ng/kg i.v.) and TRH (150 ng/kg i.v.). Blockade of NE synthesis with FLA-63 (15 mg/kg i.p.) did not alter either the GH response to clon or the inhibiting effect of GH on the clon-stimulated GH release. Blockade of DA receptors with either pimozide (0.6 mg/kg s.c.) or spiroperidol (0.2 mg/kg s.c.) abolished the inhibiting effect of GH on the clon-activated GH release. Furthermore, the GH and TSH responses to clon were suppressed by the DA receptor agonist, piribedil (3.0 mg/kg s.c.). The inhibiting effect of GH was also removed following administration of atropine (2.5 mg/kg vi, multiple doses). These results suggest that 1) the inhibitory effect of GH on its own secretion is not due to an enhanced release of hypothalamic somatostatin but rather to inhibition of GRF release 2) the inhibiting mechanism seems to involve the central dopaminergic and cholinergic systems. Supported by NIH grant HD07062.

389 CARBOHYDRATE (CHO) AND INSULIN (I) METABOLISM IN IDIOPATHIC HYPOPITUITARISM: EFFECTS OF CHRONIC HUMAN GROWTH HORMONE (HGH) TREATMENT (Rx). G. Costin* and M. Kogut, Depts. of Peds., Univ. of So. Calif. Sch. of Med., Los Angeles, Calif., and Wright State Univ. Sch. of Med., Dayton, Ohio, USA.

To assess the long term effects of HGH Rx on CHO and I metabolism in growth hormone deficiency (GHD), we measured glucose (G) and I after oral G tolerance tests (OGTT) in 39 patients (pts) before and yearly up to 10 yrs after HGH Rx (.06-.1 U/kg, I.M., t.i.w.). Pts and controls (C) were grouped by age: group (gr) 1, 1½-4 yrs; gr 2, 5-9 yrs; gr 3, 10-18 yrs. Before HGH Rx mean fasting (F) G in gr 1 and 2 were significantly less than in age matched C ($p<.025$); FG $\lessapprox$ 60 mg/dl were noted in 4 pts in gr 1 and 1 pt in gr 2. Reactive hypoglycemia occured frequently in gr 1 while abnormal elevations of G at 1 and 2 hrs during OGTT were noted in gr 2 and 3. Mean FI was significantly less in gr 2 and 3 than in C ($p<.025$); the area under the I curve and the insulinogenic index (I/G) were significantly less in all pts than in C ($p<.05$). During HGH Rx there was a progressive correction in CHO abnormalities, however, new evidence of CHO intolerance was noted in 6 of 10 pts at 4 to 10 yrs of HGH Rx and 1 pt developed a diabetic OGTT. After 5 yrs of HGH Rx the area under the G curve in gr 1 was significantly greater than basal ($p<.05$); the area under the I curve and the I/G were significantly greater than basal in all pts ($p<.05$). In 2 pts in gr 1, after 8 and 10 yrs of Rx, mean FG and I, the area under the G and I curves, and the I/G were significantly greater than basal and age matched C levels ($p<.005$). The data indicate that: 1) CHO abnormalities and insulinopenia associated with GHD are corrected by HGH Rx, and 2) chronic HGH Rx may induce CHO intolerance and hyperinsulinemia, most likely due to insulin resistance.

390 CALORIE DEFICIENCY CAUSES REDUCED PROTEIN UTILIZATION: EFFECTS ON GROWTH RATE AND SERUM GROWTH HORMONE, SOMATOMEDIN, THYROXINE, FREE THYROXINE INDEX, TRIIODOTHYRONINE AND CORTICOSTERONE LEVELS. T. Cree and D. Schalch*, University of Wisconsin Hospital, Madison, WI, USA.

We have previously shown in the rat that growth rate and serum somatomedin insulin-like growth factor (IGF) correlate better with protein utilization than with either total calorie or protein intake (Clin Res 31:775A, 1983). To further examine this hypothesis, we pair fed an experimental group of rats (n=23) a diet containing 76% of the total calories but isonitrogenous with respect to the 25% casein diet fed controls (n=23). The significantly different growth rates of control (3.6 gm/d) and calorie-restricted (2.2 gm/d) animals were approximately linear for the duration of the experiment; sera were obtained from 3 groups of age-matched and 2 of weight-matched rats sacrificed on days 9, 16 and 23 of the study. While serum GH did not vary as a function of age, weight or diet, total IGF and IGF-I showed strong correlations with body weight ($r=0.93$, $p<0.01$, and $r=0.67$, $p<0.01$, respectively). Calorie-restricted rats had depressed levels relative to controls of T_4 (3.5 vs 4.9 µg/dl, $p<0.001$), free thyroxine index (1.8 vs 2.2), and T_3 (107 vs 135 ng/dl, $p<0.001$). In contrast, corticosterone levels were virtually identical in the control (201 ng/ml) and experimental (202 ng/ml) groups. We conclude that, in agreement with our previous study of qualitative protein malnutrition, serum total IGF and IGF-I, while dissociated from GH levels, appear to reflect anabolic utilization of dietary protein as manifest by lean tissue accretion. Moreover, serum T_4, free thyroxine index, T_3 and corticosterone appear to reflect adaptations to the utilization of total energy in conjunction with growth.

391 ORAL GLUCOSE ATTENUATES THE GROWTH HORMONE RESPONSE TO HUMAN PANCREATIC GROWTH HORMONE RELEASING FACTOR. R.R. Davies*, D.G. Johnston, and S. Turner, Department of Medicine, Royal Victoria Infirmary, Newcastle upon Tyne, UK.

The ability of oral glucose ingestion to suppress growth hormone (GH) release induced by human pancreatic growth hormone releasing factor (hpGRF 1-44) was evaluated in 5 normal subjects. Two males and three females aged 24 to 35 years were studied on three occasions. On one occasion, they received oral glucose 75g, and blood samples for glucose and GH estimation were taken at 15 min intervals for 60 min before and 180 min after glucose ingestion. On a second occasion, hpGRF 1-44, 10 µg, was given as an intravenous bolus 60 min after glucose ingestion. Finally, hpGRF 1-44, 10 µg, was given alone and blood samples were taken at 15 min intervals for 120 min prior to and 120 min following injection. After oral glucose alone, blood glucose concentrations rose to a peak of mean ± SEM, 6.7 ± 0.3 mmol/l, 30 min after glucose ingestion. All subjects showed suppression of GH levels by 30 min with the lowest mean value at 75 min, 0.7 ± 0.2 mU/l. With hpGRF 1-44 in the absence of glucose, the maximal GH response occurred at 90 mins, 24.7 ± 8.0 mU/l. With combined administration of oral glucose and intravenous hpGRF 1-44 the peak GH response occurred 75 min after hpGRF 1-44 injection and was attenuated to 9.4 ± 3.0 mU/l. This data demonstrates that oral glucose ingestion partially suppresses the GH release induced by hpGRF 1-44 and suggests that oral glucose inhibits GH release from the pituitary by a mechanism other than by inhibiting the release of growth hormone releasing factor from the hypothalamus. This study was supported by the Wellcome Trust.

392 DOSE-DEPENDENT RELEASE OF GROWTH HORMONE AND PROLACTIN IN HUMANS BY FENTANYL WITH PSYCHOMETRIC EVALUATION. *Th. Dukal[1], M. Hoehe[2], A. DOENICKE[1], N. Matussek[2]. 1 Anaesth. Dept., Surg. Clinic and Policlinic, University of Munich, 2 Neurochem. Dept., Psychiatric Hospital, University of Munich.

Whereas there is sound evidence that opiates increase the concentration of Prolactin (PRL) in plasma both in animals and in humans, contradictory data have been reported regarding the effect of opiates on Growth Hormone (GH) release in humans. To further investigate this endocrine effect, we examined the dose-related effect of Fentanyl (FE) on GH and PRL release. 14 healthy volunteers received saline (S) or FE (0.1, 0.2, 0.25 mg/70 kg) i.v. according to a randomised block design. For the estimation of hormone plasma levels blood samples were collected at different time points after FE up to 2 hrs. A psychometric test battery (PTB), a visual analogue scale, as well as subjective and objective symptoms were evaluated during the trial. All subjects exhibited a dose-dependent increase of PRL plasma levels following FE treatment. Specifically, plasma PRL levels increased from 200 ± 55 µIU/ml following S injection to 782 ± 150 µIU/ml and 1371 ± 644 µIU/ml with injections of 0.1 and 0.2 mg/70 kg FE, respectively. Whereas PRL levels increased with injection of 0.1 mg/70 kg FE, GH levels were modified only after injection of 0.2 mg/70 kg (S injection: 0.7 ± 0.1 ng/ml; 0.2 mg/70 kg FE: 4.9 ± 1.6 ng/ml; 0.25 mg/70 kg FE: 7.33 ± 0.8 ng/ml). These data suggest different mechanisms for the modulation of GH and PRL by opiates. The correlation between the effect of FE on GH release and the performance on PTB will be discussed.

393 DIRECT VISUALIZATION OF BINDING AND INTERNALIZATION OF HUMAN GROWTH HORMONE IN CULTURED HUMAN LYMPHOCYTES. R. Eshet, S. Peleg and Z. Laron*, Institute of Pediatric & Adolescent Endocrinology, Beilinson Medical Center, Petah Tikva, Tel Aviv University Medical School, Israel.

THe distribution of human growth hormone (hGH) receptor complexes on IM-9 cultured lymphocytes was studied using fluorescein and ^{125}I labelled hGH (F-hGH and ^{125}I-hGH). The cells labelled with F-hGH were visualized with a sensitive video intensification microscopic system which permitted direct observation of the location of the fluorescent hormone on the surface of the living lymphocytes. At 4°C F-hGH bound diffusely to the cell surface and remained dispersed but following incubation for 30 minutes at 37°C the hormone receptor complexes aggregated into patches on the cell surface and formed a single cap on one pole of the cell. Progressive internalization into the cell was demonstrated at 37°C with ^{125}I-hGH. It is hypothesized that the aggregation and internalization of the hGH receptor complexes are associated with the action and degradation of the hormone and probably also with the mechanism of down-regulation of the receptors.

394 **NUCLEAR METABOLITES OF ^{3}H-TESTOSTERONE IN THE RHESUS MONKEY BRAIN: MALE-FEMALE COMPARISONS.** **Robert W. Bonsall* and Richard P. Michael, Department of Psychiatry, Emory University School of Medicine and the Georgia Mental Health Institute, Atlanta, Georgia 30322, U.S.A.**

It has been proposed that local aromatization of testosterone (T) to estradiol (E_2) in the brain has a role in the action of T on sexual behavior in both sexes. To investigate this possibility in the primate brain at the biochemical level, we have studied the metabolites of ^{3}H-T that accumulated in cell nuclei from a variety of brain and peripheral structures in 2 adult male and 2 adult female rhesus monkeys gonadectomized 5-6 days before the experiments. A bolus of ^{3}H-[1,2,6,7]-T (5-5.7 mCi) was injected intravenously 30 min before death. Brains were rapidly removed and samples were immediately chilled. Nuclei were isolated, mixed with carrier steroids and extracted with ether. Extracts were chromatographed by reverse-phase hplc. Eluates, monitored at 206 nm to detect the carrier steroids, were collected in 1 ml fractions for measurement of radioactivity. In both sexes, E_2 was a major form of radioactivity in nuclei from hypothalamus, preoptic area and amygdala (4.3-24 dpm/ug DNA) while testosterone predominated in the pituitary (8-10 dpm/ug DNA in males, 2.7-3.5 dpm/ug DNA in females). In nuclei from seminal vesicles, prostate, glans penis and clitoris (but not uterus), dihydrotestosterone (20-90 dpm/ug DNA) was the major metabolite. The lower level of ^{3}H-T in the pituitary of the female was the only consistent difference between the sexes. We conclude that local steroid metabolism may have a significant role in the behavioral actions of T but that it does not explain the differences in the behavioral effects of T in the two sexes. Supported by U.S.P.H.S. Grant MH 19506.

395 PREGNENOLONE (P) METABOLISM IN THE RAT BRAIN.
C. Clarke*, A. Groyer, E.E. Baulieu and P. Robel, CNRS ER125 and INSERM U 33, Lab. Hormones, 94270 Bicêtre, France.

We have characterized pregnenolone (P) and its sulfate ester in the rat brain (C. Corpéchot et al. Brain Res. 270:119, 1983). We proposed that their formation or accumulation in the rat brain depended on in situ mechanisms unrelated to the peripheral endocrine gland system. Incubation of rat brain minces with ^{3}H-P yielded ^{3}H-progesterone (P4) and saponifiable lipoidal derivatives of P (PL).

	Percent conversion of ^{3}H-P per incubation						
	HT	OB	AMY	COR	CER	C6	L 929
	(0.6 µM ^{3}H-P, ∿ 100 mg tissue, 3 h)					(0.2 µM ^{3}H-P, 10^{7} cells, 24 h)	
P4	1.3	0.9	0.8	0.0	0.0	0.6	0.2
PL	1.4	1.5	1.1	0.2	0.0	1.8	0.0

The yield of P4 and PL per 100 mg tissue was in the ∿ 1 % range in hypothalamus (HT), amygdala (AMY), olfactory bulbs (OB) and other regions of the brain, with the exception of the cerebellum (CER) and the frontal cortex (COR), where very little metabolism was observed. The rat glioma C6 cell line also formed measurable amounts of PE and PL, whereas mouse L 929 fibroblasts did not. It was concluded that pregnenolone may affect the brain by metabolism to the sex hormone progesterone.

396 CHARACTERISTICS OF 17β-HYDROXYSTEROID DEHYDROGENASE IN HUMAN ENDOMETRIUM AND ADRENAL CORTEX WITH RESPECT TO ADRENAL ANDROGEN METABOLISM.
R.C. Bonney,* M.J. Reed and V.H.T. James. Dept. of Chemical Pathology, St. Mary's Hospital Medical School, London, W2 1PG U.K.

Our previous studies have demonstrated that 5-androstene-3β,17β-diol (ADIOL), a weak androgen with oestrogenic properties, and the metabolically related dehydroepiandrosterone (DHA) are present in human endometrium and that concentrations increase 4-fold during the secretory phase without any corresponding increase in the plasma. In order to obtain information about the origin of ADIOL in endometrium we studied the enzyme 17β-hydroxysteroid dehydrogenase with an aim to determining whether ADIOL arises from DHA or vice versa. We subsequently compared the characteristics of the enzyme of endometrium with that of the adrenal cortex. In both endometrium and adrenal cortex the metabolism of ADIOL to DHA is linear with time and with increasing enzyme concentration. The preferred cofactor is NAD and the Km values for ADIOL were 3.3uM (endometrium) and 56uM (adrenal cortex). In endometrium, DHA was not metabolised to ADIOL in the presence of either NADH or NADPH whereas in the adrenal cortex, the reaction proceeded in the presence of NADPH (kM for DHA:50uM) but not NADH. Our findings suggest that the enzyme of endometrium differs from that of the adrenal cortex. The study also indicates that ADIOL present in endometrium does not arise from the metabolism of DHA but that increased secretory phase concentrations are more likely to be due to the presence of a progesterone dependent binding protein or receptor. Whether this steroid has any significance in the physiology or pathology of the endometrium has yet to be established.

397 INVOLVEMENT OF THE GLYCOPEPTIDES OF HCGα IN THE INHIBITION OF ADENYLYL CYCLASE ACTIVITY (AC) IN RAT CORPORA LUTEA. F. O. Calvo* and R. J. Ryan, Dept. Cell Biology, Mayo Medical School, Rochester, MN 55905

Previously we have shown that asparagine-linked glycopeptides (GP) of hCG inhibit the hCG-stimulated AC activity in rat corpus luteum (CL) membranes. Our present studies examine the GP of hCGα, fetuin, bovine γ globulin (IGg) and eight synthetic oligosaccharides that vary in size and branch structure (a gift of H. Lönn, Stockholm). Fetuin GP were isolated as described (JBC 254:789,1979) with a further purification step. The γ globulin and hCGα were reduced and carboxymethylated, digested with trypsin and pronase and purified by gel filtration and/or con A affinity chromatography. Purification was followed by assays for sialic acid and/or neutral sugars. Protease activity was not present in the final product. There was no cross-reactivity of the hCGα-GP, IGg-GP or fetuin GP when tested in a hCG-RIA or RRA. The relative potencies were <0.001% at 200μg GP/ml, the highest concentration tested. The GP of hCGα, IGg, or fetuin were tested in an AC assay in which the GP were preincubated for 10 min at RT with CL membranes and then coincubated with 100 ng hCG/ml for 20 min. While the GP of fetuin and IGg had no effect on the hCG stimulated AC activity at 200 μg GP/ml the GP of hCGα inhibited the AC activity in a dose-response manner. The inhibition by the GP of hCGα at 1, 50, and 200μg/ml when compared to hCG without GP was 54.55, 75.0, and 84.74%, respectively. None of the oligosaccharides had any effect on AC activity at 200 or 500μg/ml. These results suggest that there is a high degree of specificity in the hCG-GP inhibition of hCG-stimulated AC and provide indirect evidence for the involvement of a membrane lectin in the activation of the luteal AC system.

398 HYPERRESPONSIVENESS TO PULSATILE GnRH IN HYPERPROLACTINEMIC WOMEN MAY ANTAGONIZE THE POSITIVE FEEDBACK ACTION OF ESTROGEN ON LH SECRETION.
P. Belchetz* and S. Weldon, Department of Medicine, University of Liverpool P.O. Box 147, Liverpool L69 3BX, U.K.

LH levels were monitored in 8 hyperprolactinemic women at 15 min intervals for 6 h, then estradiol benzoate (E_2B) 1mg administered intramuscularly, and LH and E_2 levels measured on the next 4 days. 4 women - basal prolactin 932 to 15300 mU/l (normal <600 mU/l) - displayed pulseless LH secretion and no positive feedback. 4 women - basal prolactin 914-2900 mU/l - exhibited regular LH pulses and more than doubled basal LH levels after E_2B. Subsequently GnRH was administered subcutaneously by a portable syringe driver. This was programmed to deliver doses ranging from 13 to 21μg at hourly intervals in one, and 2 hourly intervals in 7 subjects for 5 days. LH levels were monitored every 15 min for the first 6 h, E_2B 1mg administered I.M. and LH and E_2 levels measured over the remaining 4 days. LH responses while receiving GnRH were unrelated to the earlier observations. 3 subjects receiving the highest doses showed exaggerated LH responses, sometimes falling before E_2B given, and LH was suppressed post E_2B in 2 while the 3rd sustained higher LH levels for only 24 h after E_2B. Positive feedback patterns with LH levels >double basal values 48-72 H post E_2B were seen in 5 subjects receiving lower doses of GnRH, of whom 2 displayed exaggerated responses to GnRH prior to E_2B. It is concluded that pulsatile GnRH may induce exaggerated LH responses associated with defective positive feedback response to E_2 in hyperprolactinemic women. This work was supported by a Grant from Mersey Regional Health Authority and Ayerst Laboratories.

399 THYROID HORMONE FEEDBACK EFFECTS ON HYPOTHALAMIC NUCLEAR DISTRIBUTION OF SOMATOSTATIN (SRIF) AND TRH.
M. Berelowitz,* J. Pollack and L. A. Frohman, Div. of Endocrinology, Univ. of Cincinnati Coll. of Med., Cincinnati, Ohio.

Previous studies suggest that TSH secretion is influenced by feedback effects on hypothalamic TRH and SRIF. Both peptides are present throughout the hypothalamus and exert numerous functions. Thus, only those peptide-containing neurons in TSH regulatory centers should be responsive to perturbations of thyroid status. Triiodothyronine-treated (T_3 Rx) and untreated thyroidectomized (Tx) rats and sham-operated controls (Eu) were studied 4 and 7 weeks post-Tx. TRH and SRIF were measured in 2N HAc extracts of microdissected hypothalamic nuclei. No changes in hypothalamic nuclear TRH or SRIF content were seen at 4 wk despite elevated serum TSH levels. At 7 wk post Tx TRH content was reduced in median eminence (-50%,p<.01) and in periventricular (-55%, p<.01) and anterior hypothalamic nuclei (-62%, p<.01) compared to Eu. TRH content in median eminence and periventricular nucleus was restored in T_3 Rx rats (NS vs Eu). SRIF content was reduced in median eminence (-50%, p<.01) and retrochiasmatic (-66%, p<.01), anterior hypothalamic (-43%, p<.01), arcuate (-55%, p<.05) and dorsomedial nuclei (-61%, p<.01) of Tx rats and was restored by T_3 Rx in median eminence and dorsomedial nucleus. These studies demonstrate reduction of TRH only in nuclei comprising the thyrotropic area and of SRIF only in nuclei within the hypophysiotropic SRIF pathway. The median eminence was depleted of both peptides and T_3Rx repleted nerve endings before nuclear content. The late occurrence of these changes following Tx suggests that hypothalamic TRH and SRIF play a modulatory role in pituitary TSH regulation in contrast to the more rapid and direct effects of T_3.

400 ULTRADIAN FLUCTUATIONS OF PLASMA CORTISOL ARE ENTRAINED BY REPEATED I.V. INJECTIONS OF CRF IN NORMAL MAN.
M. Beyloos*, D. Désir, D. Bosson, J.R.M. Franckson and G. Copinschi, Free University of Brussels, Belgium.

The mode of secretion of CRF (continuous or pulsatile) is not known. In man, single bolus injections of CRF at various times of the day elicit dose-dependent stimulation of ACTH and cortisol secretion. We performed repeated intravenous injections of ovine CRF (25 μg) at 4-hour intervals for 25 to 49 hours in 3 normal male volunteers. Blood samples were obtained at 15-minute intervals for plasma cortisol determinations. Hormonal profiles obtained during periods of repeated CRF administration were compared to control profiles obtained one week earlier in the same subjects. A plasma cortisol response to CRF was observed after each bolus injection. Mean 24-hour concentrations of cortisol were slightly increased by repeated CRF administration (70 ± 15 ng/ml vs 98 ± 8 ng/ml in control and CRF studies respectively). The cortisol response to CRF averaged 99 ± 35 ng/ml (range : 27 to 167 ng/ml). The circadian variation of basal cortisol secretion was not influenced by CRF injections. No circadian periodicity of the cortisol response to CRF was detected. The number of endogenous secretory episodes was markedly reduced after one day of repeated CRF injections, so that ultradian fluctuations of plasma cortisol became mainly synchronized on exogenous CRF pulses. Our data suggest that ultradian activation of the pituitary-adrenal axis can be entrained by intermittent CRF injections.

401 LONG-TERM EXPOSURE OF CULTURED RAT ANTERIOR PITUITARY CELLS TO RAT HYPOTHALAMIC GRF ALTERS SOMATOTROPIC RESPONSIVENESS TO GRF.

L.M. Bilezikjian* and W.W. Vale. Peptide Biology Laboratory, The Salk Institute, La Jolla, CA.

Continuous exposure of target cells to a peptide hormone is generally associated with an altered responsiveness to subsequent challenge with the hormone. In order to determine whether desensitization is also a feature of somatotropic response to GRF, the effect of long-term exposure of cultured rat anterior pituitary cells to GRF was investigated. Somatotropic responsiveness to GRF was monitored by measuring GH release and cAMP levels after a 1-hour incubation with synthetic replicates of rat hypothalamic GRF. In control cells, EC_{50}'s for rhGRF-stimulated GH release and cyclic AMP production were 40 ± 3.8 (n=7) and 230 ± 24 (n=3) pM rhGRF, respectively. Maximal stimulation of GH release corresponded to a 6-7-fold increase above basal (0.32 ± 0.02 μg GH/ml/h). Pretreatment of cells with 500 pM rhGRF for 24 hours caused significant depletion of cellular GH; 2.85 ± 0.16 and 0.47 ± 0.04 μg GH/dish for control and pretreated cells, respectively. These cells, though, still responded to rhGRF in a dose-dependent manner and exhibited diminished sensitivity to the peptide with a 7.5-fold shift of the EC_{50} to a value of 300 ± 35 pM rhGRF. The EC_{50} for forskolin-stimulated GH release, on the other hand, was not altered. Since GH pools were depleted, cyclic AMP production was also investigated as another index for cell responsiveness. Pretreatment with 500 pM rhGRF did not alter maximal cyclic AMP production but increased the EC_{50} by 2.5-fold. These results suggest that the attenuation of somatotropic responsiveness to GRF is, in part, due to depletion although it may also represent desensitization.

402 GNRH ANTAGONIST-MEDIATED SUPPRESSION OF TESTICULAR FUNCTION IN MONKEYS.

F. Bint Akhtar*, G.F. Weinbauer and E. Nieschlag, Max Planck Clinical Research Unit for Reproductive Medicine, Steinfurter Straße 107, D-4400 Münster, F.R. Germany.

The effects of chronic administration of a GnRH antagonist, a potential means of male fertility control, on reproductive function of adult cynomolgus monkeys (M. fascicularis) were evaluated. The antagonist, (Ac-D-p-Cl-Phe^1,D-p-Cl-Phe^2,D-Trp^3,D-Arg^6,D-Ala^{10}-GnRH, Org 30276), was injected s.c. daily at a dose of 1 mg/kg body weight for 9 weeks. Serum testosterone (T) levels decreased from 16.0 ± 1.3 nmol/l to 2.3 ± 0.9 nmol/l within 24 h and remained low throughout treatment (1 - 5 nmol/ l), while bioactive LH became undetectable. The serum LH response following GnRH injection (50 μg i.v.) was blunted during antagonist treatment whereas the T-response was abolished. Testicular volumes started to decline after 2-3 weeks and were reduced to approximately 25 % of control volumes after 9 weeks. The ejaculates obtained at the end of treatment were azoospermic or contained only few dead sperm. On histological examination, spermatogenesis was severely disrupted. Only spermatogonia, Sertoli cells and occasional pachytene spermatocytes were present. A few round and elongated spermatids were seen in one animal. In summary, GnRH antagonist treatment rapidly decreased serum LH and T and disrupted spermatogenesis in this primate species. Although testicular function can also be suppressed by high doses of GnRH agonists, the antagonist achieves the same effect more rapidly and dispenses with the initial stimulatory phase accompanying agonist treatment. (We are grateful to Dr. A.V. Schally and ORGANON for providing the antagonist).

403 INDUCTION OF CONCOMITANT RELEASE OF LH AND PROLACTIN BY PULSATILE INTRAVENOUS ADMINISTRATION OF LH-RH IN PATIENTS WITH POLYCYSTIC-OVARY-SYNDROME (PCO-S).

M.H. Birkhäuser*, P. Huber, I. Werner-Zodrow and M. Mall-Haefeli, Div. of Endocrinology, Universitäts-Frauenklinik, Kantonsspital, 4031 Basel, Switzerland.

The present study intended to induce follicular growth in amenorrhoic or anovulatory patients suffering from PCO-S. We tried to correct the inaccurate endogenous frequency of LH-RH-pulsatility by chronic i.v. pulsatile administration of exogenous LH-RH (20 µg every 90 min.). 6 treatment cycles have been performed in 4 women aged from 24 to 31 yrs. For each patient, serum values of LH, FSH and Prolactin were measured every 6 min. for a period of 5 h, 7.30 - 12.30 a.m., before and during pulsatile LH-RH administration. Without treatment serum LH-pulsatility varied between 42 and 76 min. During pulsatile administration of LH-RH LH adopted the frequency of the pump (Zyklomat[R]). FSH did not present any particular pattern. Prolactin which had not shown any regular pattern before treatment, showed a highly characteristic pulsatile pattern concomitant to that of LH in 3 treatment cycles; in one more cycle, the frequency of Prolactin pulsatility was twice that of LH. In the cycles where no follicular maturation could be induced by LH-RH administration no regular Prolactin pulsatility appeared. These data bring some evidence that in PCO-S induction of ovulation by pulsatile LH-RH administration might require simultaneous modification of the LH and Prolactin release.

404 STUDIES IN CONSTITUTIONALLY TALL ADOLESCENTS: SOMATOSTATIN DECREASE ASSOCIATED WITH GROWTH HORMONE INCREASE AFTER TRH INJECTION.

M. Garcia Blanco*, D. Evain-Brion. Inserm U 188, Paris

11 adolescents referred for excessive height prediction were studied. Somatostatin-like immunoreactivity (SLI) and GH levels were measured during saline infusion and after TRH injection (200 µg/m2). SLI was measured after extraction on Sep Pak cartriges by RIA with antibody against 14 cyclic somatostatin. Basal plasma levels (mean ± SEM) were 1.7 ± 0.8 ng/ml for GH, 12.4 ± 2 pg/ml for SLI. No significant changes occurred during a 2 hour saline infusion. 9 subjects received TRH. 4 did not show significant changes of plasma GH (1.8 ± 0.9 ng/ml) nor SLI (10.4 ± 1.7 pg/ml), though the effect of TRH was evidenced by prolactin increase. In 5 patients TRH injection induced a sharp increase of GH within 10 to 60 minutes (mean peak values 18.4 ± 5.4 ng/ml). In these same subjects the SLI levels dropped significantly by 50% after TRH, from 18.7 ± 3.9 pg/ml to 9.8 ± 2.8 pg/ml. These 5 subjects undergone bromocriptine treatment 5 mg/day. After 3 months of treatment the paradoxical rise of GH and the drop in SLI levels after TRH injection were suppressed. It is thus hypothesized that the GH release after TRH in tall adolescents is due to a decreased inhibitory effect of somatostatin at the pituitary level.

405 INHIBITION OF GnRH RELEASE IN VIVO AND IN VITRO BY 4-AMINOPYRAZOLOPYRIMIDINE. M. S. Blank*, M. Ching, K. J. Catt and M. L. Dufau, Endocrinology and Reproduction Research Branch, NICHD, NIH, Bethesda, MD 20205.

The inhibitor of hepatic lipoprotein release, 4-aminopyrazolo-(3,4-d)-pyrimidine (4-APP), has been shown to lower testosterone production via decreased pituitary gonadotropin secretion rather than through decreased cholesterol availability (Endocrinology 112:1973, 1983). Serum LH levels are reduced by more than 75% in male rats treated with 4-APP, but pituitary stores of LH and the gonadotropin response to exogenous GnRH are maintained in spite of a reduction in pituitary GnRH receptors which is consistent with hypothalamic GnRH deficiency. The present studies were undertaken to examine the mechanism by which 4-APP inhibits GnRH secretion and/or release. Intact, adult male or two-week ovariectomized female rats were injected daily with 25 mg/kg 4-APP for three days. Both sexes showed lowered basal serum levels of LH and complete absence of the elevations in serum LH normally elicited by the opiate antagonist, naloxone. In pituitary portal plasma collected from male rats, GnRH was significantly elevated by naloxone treatment, confirming that naloxone acts at the level of hypothalamic GnRH release. However, naloxone stimulation of GnRH secretion into portal blood was absent in rats treated with 4-APP. In vitro, the potassium-induced release of GnRH from perifused medial basal hypothalami was reduced by 57% in 4-APP-treated male rats. These data indicate that 4-APP has an inhibitory effect on the mechanism of GnRH release, and that analysis of its actions should clarify the processes involved in neurohormone secretion.

406 *CALCIUM-DEPENDENT PULSATILITY OF LHRH RELEASE FROM RAT HYPOTHALAMUS IN VITRO.* *J.P. Bourguignon* and P. Franchimont, Pediatric Department and Radioimmunoassay Laboratory, University of Liège, Hôpital de Bavière, B 4020 Liège, Belgium.*

Retrochiasmatic hypothalamus (RCH) were removed from 50-day-old male rats and their LHRH release in vitro was studied for 3 h. Each incubation chamber contained a single RCH in 0.5 ml Dulbecco's Modified Eagle's Medium (DMEM) containing 1.25 mM calcium. The medium was renewed every 7.5-min period. In these serial samples, the release of LHRH from the RCH was measured by a highly sensitive RIA. The mean recovery of synthetic LHRH from the incubation system was 94 % with a coefficient of variation of 14%. The viability of RCH in vitro was assessed by the increased release of LHRH in response to the depolarizing agent, veratridine (20 to 50 μM). In control conditions, 36 RCH were studied for a cumulative period of 86 h ; the mean interval calculated between pulses was 0.85 h. In the presence of 2.4 or 4.8 mM EGTA for a cumulative period of 48 h, 16 RCH showed a mean interval of 3.0 h between pulses. With 20 mM EGTA, 1 pulse was observed from 5 RCH during a cumulative 15-h period. In control conditions, the mean increase of LHRH release from 10 RCH in response to 50 μM veratridine was 14.1 pg/7.5 min. In the presence of 20 mM EGTA, the mean response was blunted (1.5 pg/7.5 min). The responsiveness to veratridine was recovered (21.6 pg/7.5 min) using control DMEM.

In conclusion, the in vitro pulsatile release of LHRH from the hypothalamus, either spontaneous or in response to veratridine, is calcium dependent.

407 MULTIPLE RECEPTORS MEDIATE GH RELEASE. C.Y. Bowers*, F.A. Momany, G.A. Reynolds and O. Sartor, Tulane Medical School, New Orleans, LA, 70112 and Memphis State University, Memphis, TN, 38152, USA.

A new hexapeptide, His-DTrp-Ala-Trp-DPhe-LysNH$_2$(GHRP), has been developed which has potent and specific actions on GH release both *in vitro* and *in vivo*. This peptide was developed without reference to hpGRF by a combination of bioactive and conformational data. GHRP has activity in rats, lambs, calves, and monkeys, indicating a lack of species specificity. Despite hpGRF-like activity, our data suggests that a different somatotroph receptor is involved. Interactions between GHRP, hpGRF29/40/44, and a kappa opiate agonist 2549 have been studied in the rat. Repeated GHRP injection down regulates GH release but does not change the hpGRF response. In addition the maximal GH response to hpGRF can be increased by simultaneous GHRP injection. 2549 has a synergistic effect on both hpGRF and GHRP responses while hpGRF and GHRP effects are only additive. 2549 and GHRP easily down regulate while hpGRF does not. 2549 down regulation does not down regulate GHRP or hpGRF. *In vitro* results support the *in vivo* data in that GHRP and hpGRF responses are additive and during periods of down regulation with GHRP, hpGRF is fully active. 2549 is not active *in vitro* because of its extrapituitary site of action. In conclusion, indirect evidence suggests that the pituitary somatotroph has multiple agonist receptors. It is possible that several endogenous ligands with GH releasing activity have yet to be identified. Supported by NIH AM 06164.

408 CORTICOTROPIN-RELEASING FACTOR (CRF) STIMULATES OXYTOCIN SECRETION INTO SYSTEMIC CIRCULATION. T.O. Bruhn*, S.W. Sutton and W.W. Vale. Peptide Biology Laboratory, The Salk Institute, La Jolla, CA.

Oxytocin was recently demonstrated to be secreted in response to stressful stimuli in the rat. In this study, we investigated whether CRF, the predominant regulator of adenohypophyseal ACTH and β-endorphin release, stimulates neurohypophyseal hormone secretion. Rat CRF was administered intracerebroventricularly (icv) 5-7 days after the implantation of lateral ventricle cannulae. Rats were handled daily and experiments were performed under minimum stress conditions. In both male and female rats, the icv injection of 0.75 nmoles CRF elevated plasma oxytocin (OT) levels 2.4-3.5-fold as measured 5 min after the injection. Plasma vasopressin (AVP) concentrations were not affected by the treatment. When rats were exposed to ether vapor for 3 min and sacrificed 2 min later, similar elevations in plasma OT were found without changes in AVP levels. In another set of experiments, male rats were pretreated with 0.75 ml CRF antiserum (-20 min) given peripherally, while CRF (0.75 nmoles) was injected centrally. The antiserum completely blocked the ACTH response without affecting the OT response. This suggests that CRF acts at a level inaccessible to the CRF antiserum, perhaps on magnocellular neurons of the paraventricular and/or supraoptic nucleus to modulate oxytocin secretion. Pretreatment with dexamethasone (20 μg,ip,-4h) blocked the ACTH response to icv CRF (0.75 nmoles), but did not modify the plasma OT elevation, suggesting that the observed OT release in response to CRF is not steroid sensitive. Neither pretreatment modified AVP release. We conclude that CRF may play a role in the control of neurohypophyseal oxytocin secretion in the rat.

409 CORTICOTROPIN-RELEASING FACTOR- (CRF) LIKE PEPTIDE OF THE BRATTLEBORO RAT BRAIN : IMMUNOLOGICAL DISTRIBUTION AND QUANTITATIVE EVOLUTION UNDER VARIOUS EXPERIMENTAL CONDITIONS. A. Burlet*, M.C. Tonon, M. Chapleur, F. Dreyfuss, P. Tankosic and C. Burlet, Groupe de Neuroendocrinologie, Faculté de Médecine, BP 184, 54505 Vandoeuvre-les-Nancy, France.

In the Brattleboro (DI) rat, genetically unable to synthezise vasopressin (VP), several anomalies of the corticotrope function were described and, following the authors, attributed to either the lack of VP or the reduced activity of the hypothalamic CRF. We report light and electron immunological observations and radioimmunoassays of the CRF-like peptide in the DI rats, using specific sera prepared against the ovine 41-CRF. In basal conditions, the CRF content of the hypothalamus was lower in DI rats than in Long Evans (LE) rats. But, the chronic treatment of DI rats by a structural analogue of VP restored a normal hydric balance and increased the hypothalamic CRF content. In treated DI rats, CRF was stained in two distinct systems: a hypothalamo-infundibular system carrying CRF only and a hypothalamo-neurohypophysial system containing simultaneously CRF, oxytocin and neurophysin-oxytocin. In LE and heterozygous DI rats, both CRF systems were totally different from the parvo- and magnocellular VP systems. A distinct evolution of each CRF system could be induced by bilateral adrenalectomy, total hypophysectomy or injections associating dexametha sone, chlorpromazine and pentobarbital. These data confirmed that the perturbations of the corticotrope function were due to the lack of VP in the DI rats and that the infundibular and neurohypophysial CRF systems were respectively implied in the secretion of the adenohypophysial ACTH and intermediate peptides.

410 APPARENT BIPHASIC RESPONSE OF SOMATOSTATIN TO THYROID HORMONE BY FETAL RAT CEREBRAL CORTEX CELLS IN CULTURE. L.Cacicedo* and F. Sánchez-Franco Hospital Ramón y Cajal,Servicio de Endocrinologia,Madrid 34,Spain.

The relationship between somatostatin(SRIF) and thyroid hormone (TH) is controversial. Release of SRIF from hypothalami of hypothyroid rats was demonstrated to be decreased. More recent studies have shown a direct inhibitory effect of triiodotironine(T_3) and thyroxine(T_4) on SRIF-like immunoreactivity(SRIF-LI) in cerebral cortex cells.The present work was designed to clarfy the role of TH on SRIF regulation. Cortical(C) and hypothalamic(H) tissues from 17 days fetal rats were mechano-enzimatically dispersed and cells cultured in a serum supplemented MEM medium. After seven days media were removed and serum free medium with or without T_3 and T_4 was added for 48 hr.In Ç cells T_3 has a biphasic effect on SRIF-LI, with a significant increase at the lowest concentration tested(10^{-11}M) and a significant inhibition at 10^{-8}M and 10^{-7}M in both media and intracellular content. Total SRIF-LI (cells+media): control 1.66±.04, T_3(10^{-11}M) 2.48±.09, T_3(10^{-8}M) 1.40±.15, T_3(10^{-7}M) .44±.06 (ng/plate). Treatment with T_4 was associated with a dose dependent decrease of SRIF-LI in response to concentrations of 10^{-9}M and 10^{-8}M but it was not evident a stimulatory effect at the smallest concentrations. Exposure of H cells to TH resulted in a similar decline of SRIF-LI secretion at the highest concentrations tested (10^{-9}M and 10^{-8}M).In contrast to the biphasic effect of T_3 on SRIF-LI secretion this hormone produced a dose dependent inhibition of total protein content in C and H cells between concentrations of 10^{-12}M and 10^{-8}M. These results indicate that SRIF-LI secretion by C and H cells is stimulated by low T_3 and depressed by high T_3 and T_4 concentrations. The opposite effect of low T_3 on SRIF-LI and proteins suggest a specific effect of TH on SRIF regulation.

411 MOLECULAR WEIGHT OF A PUTATIVE LHRH PRECURSOR SYNTHESIZED IN CELL FREE SYSTEM.

J.L. Charli*, S. Cohen, L. Díaz de León, R.O. Millar+, A. Arimura° and P. Joseph-Bravo, Centro de Investigación sobre Ingeniería Genética y Biotecnología, UNAM, Cd. Universitaria APDO. POSTAL 70228, 04510 México, D.F., México. +U. of Capetown Med. Sch., South Africa. °Veterans Adm. Hosp. New Orleans, La. USA.

In order to understand the regulatory mechanisms that rule the biosynthesis of LHRH, some studies have demonstrated the existence of higher molecular weight forms in hypothalamus. We have looked for the molecular weight of a precursor of LHRH once it is translated from rodent hypothalamic mRNA. Poly A^+ RNA isolated from rat or mice hypothalami was translated in a cell free rabbit reticulocyte lysate in the presence of ^{35}S-met or ^{3}H-pro. The translation products were subjected to immunoprecipitation using several antisera against LHRH. We used Arimura's # 419, 744 and 743 whose antigenic determinant is for the center part of the molecule. However, no signal was obtained. The only antibody that was able to show a signal over the noise, displazable with cold LHRH was Millar's Ab # 1076. The signal was very low suggesting either low affinity for the precursor or low LHRH mRNA levels. Following purification of the immunoprecipitate by Protein A-Sepharose chromatography, a SDS-urea-PAGE demonstrated the existence of a 60 000 dalton polypeptide which is not seen when using normal rabbit serum. This was observed after pooling the translation product of 40-60 µg of mRNA. These results suggest that the primary translation product for the hypothalamic LHRH precursor is a 60 000 dalton polypeptide.

This study was supported by grant # ICCBXNA-001926 from CONACyT.

412 GROWTH HORMONE RELEASING FACTOR(GRF)IN CHILDREN WITH GROWTH HORMONE(GH) DEFICIENCY:POSSIBILITY FOR A NEW "ARCUATE NUCLEUS SYNDROME".

P.Chatelain*[1], G.Sassolas[2], N.Catbeh[3], M.David[3], T.Philip[4] R.Gilly[3], L.David[3], A.Ruitton[1], and R.François[3] I=INSERM U 34, hop.Deb-rousse, 2=Cent.Med.Nucl., 3=Dépt.Pédiatrie, Univ.Cl.Bernard, 4=Cen. L.Bérard.LYON.FRANCE.

In order to explore the pathophysiology of GH deficiency,synthetic I-44-GRF,generously provided by R.Guillemin-The Salk Inst.- was given I.V. bolus(I ug/kg/b.w.)to 22 children with severe growth failure due to GH deficit.Patients included 4 with Idiopathic Isolated GH deficit,3 with Idiopathic Multiple hormone deficit,II with Brain tumor,I with a midline defect,I with Histiocytosis X,I with acquired post-head trauma GH deficit,and I with the "Arcuate Nucleus Syndrome".2 patients only displayed a lack of GH response to GRF compared to classical provocative test response:the patient with a midline defect and the one with post-trauma ,both with pan-hypopituitarism.In the 20 others, GRF induces a GH peak not less than 2.5 up to 5 time greater than with "classical" test.One 8.y.o. patient,a former 35 week premature,with severe growth failure,pronounced hyperphagia without obesity both of early post-natal onset,shows a dramatic GH peak(88ng/ml) after GRF.We believe this patient has a defect of the Arcuate Nucleus,involved in both hunger controle and GRF secretion,and propose to name it "the Arcuate Nucleus Syndrome". GRF,of excellent clinical tolerance,provides useful informations on the diagnosis of GH deficiency and its etiology.

413 ACUTE RISE IN CIRCULATING LUTEINIZING HORMONE (LH) LEVELS AFTER PITUITARY STALK SECTION: EVIDENCE FOR FACTOR(S) THAT INHIBIT LH SECRETION?

M. Ching*, M. S. Blank, K. J. Catt and M. L. Dufau, Endocrinology and Reproduction Research Branch, NICHD, NIH, Bethesda, Maryland 20205, U.S.A.

It is generally accepted that interruption of portal blood flow to the pituitary will result in a decline in circulating LH levels suggesting that facilitative influences predominate in gonadotropin release. However, in most studies dealing with this question, LH levels were measured hours or days after stalk section. The present experiments examined the acute effects of pituitary stalk section on LH secretion. Adult male rats (n = 59) were anesthetized with Althesin, ip, and the pituitary stalk or portal veins transected 70 min later. In one group (PVS) only the vessels were severed while in a second group (SS) the entire stalk was cut. No cuts were made in a third group (IN). In the PVS group 88% of animals showed increases in plasma LH (2-14 fold, $P<0.05$) within 20 min after cutting the portal veins. LH levels remained elevated (2-7 fold, $P<0.05$) over the next 10-40 min in 80% of rats. In the SS group LH was elevated ($P<0.05$) at 5 and 120 min but not at 10, 30, and 60 min after stalk section. Rats in the IN group failed to exhibit elevations in LH levels. Bromocriptine (5 mg/kg, sc) prevented the rise in LH levels 5 or 45 min after stalk section. Naloxone (2 mg/kg, iv) administered 5 min before stalk section further elevated LH levels ($P<0.02$) in 100% of PVS rats. These results suggest the existence of yet unidentified regulatory factor(s), possibly related to endogenous opiates and/or dopamine, whose influence on LH release is normally masked by the action of GnRH.

414 THE EFFECT OF SALT DEPRIVATION ON THE RESPONSE TO CORTICOTROPHIN RELEASING FACTOR (CRF) IN MAN.

J. Conaglen, E.A. Espiner, R.A. Donald*, J. Livesey and M.G. Nicholls, Department of Endocrinology, The Princess Margaret Hospital, Christchurch, New Zealand.

It has been reported that the action of CRF can be potentiated by a number of factors including angiotensin II (AII). As the physiological importance of AII remains in doubt, we studied the response to CRF in five normal males after 5 days on a low salt (10 mmol Na^{+}) diet, and compared the responses with those obtained on an unrestricted salt intake. The responses to CRF or diluent alone without salt restriction were also compared in a double-blind randomised trial. All subjects received 200µg ovine CRF in Haemaccel/saline diluent or diluent alone at 0800h as a 1 minute infusion. At least one week was allowed between repeat tests in the same subject. Responses in plasma hormone concentrations were assessed by the change of the mean of the 15, 30, 60, 90 and 120 minute values from the 0 minute value, and significance was evaluated by the paired t test. Salt restriction resulted in urine sodium excretion of <10 meq/24h in all subjects with a significant increase in plasma renin ($p<0.02$), angiotensin II ($p<0.05$) and plasma ($p<0.01$) and urine aldosterone ($p<0.005$). The responses to CRF in plasma ACTH ($p<0.01$) cortisol ($p<0.005$) and aldosterone ($p<0.05$) which had been observed on the unrestricted salt diet were not significantly altered by salt restriction. It is concluded that a rise in plasma angiotensin II, under the conditions of this study does not potentiate the action of CRF on ACTH, cortisol or aldosterone secretion.

415 GONADOTROPIN RELEASING HORMONE (GnRH) STIMULATED LUTEINIZING HORMONE (LH) RELEASE: RELATIVE ROLES OF INTRA- AND EXTRACELLULAR CALCIUM P. M. Conn[1,2]*, D.C. Rogers[2], and M.D. Bates[2], Departments of Pharmacology, Univ. of Iowa[1], Iowa City, Iowa 52242, and Duke Medical Center[2], Durham, NC 27710 U.S.A.

Gonadotropin releasing hormone (GnRH) stimulates pituitary gonadotropin release by a Ca^{2+} dependent mechanism. Indeed, while it is clear that Ca^{2+} fulfills the requirements of a second messenger, the relative roles of Ca^{2+} derived from intra- and extracellular sources have never been identified. In the present study we have used a specific Ca^{2+} ion channel blocker, methoxyverapamil (D600) to block entry of extracellular Ca^{2+} into pituitary cell cultures in order to determine if intracellular Ca^{2+}, whether derived from external or internal sources, could support continued release. Studies at a wide range of GnRH concentrations in both static (i.e. "well" cultures) and dynamic (i.e. perifused cultures) indicate that blockade of Ca^{2+} entry into the gonadotrope (in the presence of continued occupancy of the GnRH receptor by the releasing hormone) results in very rapid (min) termination of luteinizing hormone (LH) release. Additionally compounds which stabilize intracellular Ca^{2+} (preventing its mobilization) such as TMB-8, mersalyl acid, and dantrolene (Dantrium) did not alter the potency or efficacy of GnRH in stimulating LH release. These observations suggest that LH release in response to GnRH is tightly coupled to Ca^{2+} mobilized from extracellular sources. Termination of access to this pool also results in termination of release. The data are consistent with a model in which GnRH occupancy of its receptor regulates a plasma membrane Ca^{2+} ion channel which regulates functional Ca^{2+} mobilization from extracellular sources. (Supported by NIH HD13220, HD00337 and the Mellon Foundation.)

416 PLASMA AND CEREBROSPINAL FLUID (CSF) CONCENTRATIONS OF ACTH, β-ENDORPHIN AND CORTICOTROPIN RELEASING FACTOR (CRF) DURING EXPERIMENTAL STRESS AND GLUCOCORTICOID SUPPRESSION. P. Avgerinos, W. Gallucci, S. Paul, P. Skolnick D. Loriaux, G. Chrousos, E. Oldfield, J. Harwell, R. Post, and P. Gold. BPB & CNSB, NIMH; LBC, NIADDK; DEB, NICHD; SNB, NINCDS; VRB, DRS; NIH, Bethesda, MD 20205, USA.

To evaluate the relationships between the hypothalamic-pituitary-adrenal (HPA) axis and the CSF concentrations of ACTH, β-endorphin and CRF, we administered the ethyl ester of β-carbolene-3-carboxylic acid (β-CCE) or dexamethasone to male adult sheep. The former compound is known to act via benzodiazepine receptors and to elicit an anxiety-like syndrome accompanied by a marked rise in plasma cortisol. We determined cortisol, ACTH, β-endorphin and CRF responses in plasma and CSF before and after an iv bolus injection of β-CCE (1 mg/kg). The same experiment was repeated using normal saline instead of β-CCE for control purposes. Plasma and CSF cortisol, ACTH, β-endorphin and CRF concentrations were also measured after an overnight dexamethasone suppression or following a four-day period of 12-hourly high dose dexamethasone administration. Plasma cortisol and ACTH levels rose markedly after intravenous β-CCE. Plasma CRF remained undetectable (<25 pg/ml). There was no increase in CSF ACTH and β-endorphin. There was a ~10% rise in CSF CRF. A marked drop in plasma cortisol was noted following dexamethasone suppression. However, there was no change in CSF ACTH, β-endorphin or CRF. We conclude: 1) CRF is present in measurable amounts in sheep CSF, 2) β-CCE and dexamethasone cause marked changes in plasma but not in CSF ACTH and cortisol, 3) the small increase in CSF CRF after β-CCE might reflect a rise of hypothalamic CRF, which may be responsible for β-CCE-induced stimulation of the HPA axis.

417 EFFECT OF ARCUATE NUCLEUS LESIONS ON GONADOTROPIN AND GROWTH HORMONE SECRETION IN THE MONKEY. B.B. Bercu*, D.P. Friedman, M. Mishkin, and B.E. Spiliotis, Pregnancy Research Branch, NICHD and Laboratory of Neuropsychology, NIMH, NIH, Bethesda, MD, U.S.A. 20205

Hypothalamic areas controlling gonadotropin secretion have been studied in female but not in male monkeys. Here, we have performed lesion studies aimed at involving only the arcuate nucleus in order to determine its role in the neuroregulation of gonadotropin (Gn) and growth hormone (GH) secretion. Five castrate, adult, male cynomologous monkeys had lesions performed either by aspiration under direct visualization or by radiofrequency stimulation done under stereotactic control. The animals were fitted with a mobile vest and tether which allowed blood to be withdrawn through a femoral venous catheter at frequent intervals (5 or 15 min up to 12 h) without anesthesia and without disturbing the animals. Pulsatile secretory studies were done before and after the surgical procedures. LH was measured by bioassay and LH, FSH, prolactin and GH by radioimmunoassay. The extent and effectiveness of each lesion was evaluated by examination of coronal sections that had been stained with thionin or by immunohistochemical techniques using specific antiserum raised against GnRH and GH releasing factor. These anatomical findings were correlated with biochemical pulsatile secretory data. Gn and GH levels were reduced below the sensitivity of the assay in those animals with complete bilateral arcuate nucleus lesions. On the other hand, Gn and GH secretory pulses were either partially preserved or altered in animals without complete destruction of the arcuate nucleus. Our data suggest that the arcuate nucleus plays a major role in neuroregulatory control of both Gn and GH secretion.

418 AN HOMOLOGOUS RIA FOR HUMAN RELAXIN C-PEPTIDE. G.D. Bryant-Greenwood and F.C. Greenwood*, Department of Anatomy and Reproductive Biology and Pacific Biomedical Research Center, University of Hawaii, Honolulu, Hawaii 96822.

Sufficient quantities of human relaxin (RLX) are not available as yet to develop homologous RIAs, whether by isolation, chemical synthesis or by the rDNA technique. The structure of the coding region of a human prepro-RLX gene has been elucidated by Dr. P. Hudson and his colleagues. The amino acid sequence (104 residues) of the C-peptide shows 65 sequence homologies with the C-peptide of porcine pro-RLX. An homologous RIA for human RLX C-peptide could provide an index of RLX secretion, both in human and porcine plasma and the antiserum also used to study processing of prepro-RLXs. Accordingly, a sequence of 14 amino acids (79-92) of human RLX C-peptide was synthesized (Peninsula Labs). The homogeneity of the purified peptide was confirmed by amino acid analysis, TLC and high-voltage paper electrophoresis. The peptide was readily soluble and its single tyrosyl residue (90) readily and directly iodinated by the chloramine-T method to specific activities in the range of 90 μC/μg. The labelled peptide showed no significant binding to a number of antisera raised to purified porcine RLX. An antiserum to the peptide was raised in rabbits by conjugating the peptide to bovine serum albumin, followed by intradermal injections, bleeding at 2 months and boosting thereafter. This forms the basis of an homologous RIA for the quantitative measure of the C-peptide, and of pro-RLX, in a survey of plasma and follicular fluid samples from women in different phases of the reproductive cycle.

419 RELAXIN IN THE PREGNANT BABOON: EVIDENCE FOR LOCAL PRODUCTION IN REPRODUCTIVE TISSUES.

V. Daniel Castracane, Joseph Lessing +, Steven Brenner+ and Gerson Weiss +*. Southwest Foundation for Research and Education, San Antonio, TX. and +NYU School of Medicine, New York, NY, USA

We have examined the nonluteal production of relaxin in the pregnant baboon. In experimental animals (n=5), the corpus luteum-bearing ovary had been removed in early prenancy (day 25-30) and untreated pregnant baboons served as controls. Peripheral plasma levels of relaxin were reduced to undetectable levels immediately following surgery. In both groups of baboons, peripheral uterine and ovarian vein blood samples and amniotic fluid were collected immediately prior to hysterotomy, which was performed late in pregnancy (day 139-142). Following hysterotomy, samples of reproductive and control tissues were obtained (placenta, decidua, myometruim, fetal membranes and omentum). Relaxin concentration was determined in all samples using an antiporcine relaxin radioimmunoassay. In unilaterally oophorectomized pregnant baboons, peripheral plasma levels of relaxin were below the limits of detection (< 159 pg/ml) over 100 days following corpus luteum removal, while levels in control pregnant baboons were >1000 pg/ml. Relaxin levels in uterine vein plasma in both groups were comparable to peripheral plasma levels in each group. Relaxin concentration in amniotic fluid of both groups was below the limits of detection (< 159 pg/ml). Significant concentrations of relaxin were found in decidua, placenta and myometruim in those pregnant baboons in which the corpus luteum-bearing ovary had been removed over 100 days earlier. This, together with the absence of a relaxin gradient in uterine vein plasma and undetectable relaxin levels in amniotic fluid, is taken as a strong indication of local production of relaxin in reproductive tissues without contribution to peripheral plasma levels.

420 INFLUENCE OF THE FREQUENCY OF GONADOTROPIN-RELEASING HORMONE (GnRH) ADMINISTRATION ON OVULATORY RESPONSES IN WOMEN WITH HYPOTHALAMIC ANOVULATION (H.A.) AND POLYCYSTIC OVARIAN SYNDROME (P.C.O.).

J. Bringer*, B. Hedon, C. Jaffiol C. Cristol, S. Nicolau, A. Orsetti, N. Bressot, J.L. Viala, J. Mirouze. Endocrinologie, Hôpital Saint Eloi, 34059 Montpellier - France.

In an attempt to optimize GnRH treatment of anovulation, we compared the effect of intravenous GnRH administration at 3 various pulse-intervals (p.i.) during 46 cycles from 10 to 25 days in 22 anovulatory patients with HA (15 patients, 31 cycles) or PCO (7 patients, 15 cycles). Reason for GnRH treatment was sterility resistant to clomiphene citrate in all patients with PCO and in 10 women (26 cycles) with HA. In HA, p.i. of 64, 90 and 128 min. were selected in 6, 13 and 12 cycles respectively. In PCO 7 cycles were performed with 90 min. and 8 with 128 min. p.i. Doses per pulse (8.4 ± 1.3 µg) were not different with the frequency used. Follicular development was monitored by ultrasonographies and by daily enzymatic determination of the urinary estradiol (E_2) and estrone (E_1). Luteal phase was assessed by three measurements of plasma progesterone (P) performed on days 3, 6 and 9 after ovulation. In HA, ovulations were achieved in 26 of the 31 cycles (83 %). The results were not different with frequency and 4 of the 10 sterile women conceived : 2 with 90 min. p.i., one with 64 and one with 128 min. p.i. The means of the preovulatory follicle diameters, urinary E_1E_2 preovulatory peaks, durations of luteal phase and P levels were unrelated to the frequency. In PCO, ovulation occured in 2 of the 7 cycles with 90 min. p.i and in 4 of the 8 cycles with 128 min. p.i. Three pregnancies were obtained with 128 min. p.i. Further studies are needed to confirm if the 128 min. p.i; increase effectiveness of GnRH in PCO.

421 THE RESPONSE OF HUMAN ENDOMETRIOID IMPLANTS TO THE STEROID R 2323 : A HISTOLOGIC AND ULTRASTRUCTURAL STUDY.

F. Cornillie*, G. Vasquez and I. Brosens, Department of Obstetrics and Gynecology, U.Z. St. Rafaël-Gasthuisberg, Katholieke Universiteit te Leuven, Belgium.

Midcycle administration of the steroid Gestrinone (R 2323) results in an abnormal differentiation of the endometrial glandular cells. Its biological activities on endometrioid tissue however, remained unknown. Therefore a morphologic study was performed before and after 4 months of R 2323 treatment (2 or 3 times 2.5 mg/week) in 12 patients with laparoscopically proven moderate endometriosis (AFS II - III). All tissues were fixed in phosphate-buffered (0.1 M; pH 7.2) 2.5 % glutaraldehyde at 4°C and processed according to routine schedules. During first and/or second look laparoscopies 80 biopsies were sampled and 257 semithin sections were studied. After treatment with R 2323 there was a marked decrease in the total number of glands encountered. However, in four out of nine patients with two biopsies the number of glands was slightly increased while in another four it was dramatically decreased, two of these latter being free of glands after treatment. In only one patient the number of glands remained unchange After treatment, endometrioid glandular cells were cuboidal to low columnar demonstrating a positive nucleo-cytoplasmic ratio. Mitoses were absent. Some epithelial cells revealed apical granules which correspond to lysosomes. In few other cells lipid vacuolation was found. In contrast with pre-treatment findings, glycogen stores were only seldom recovered. Dilatations of the perinuclear and endoplasmic reticulum cisternae were frequent findings. In conclusion, these results demonstrate an inhibition of glandular proliferative and secretory activities of endometrioid glands in response to R 2323.

422 FAILURE OF THE ENDOMETRIUM CAPACITY TO RETAIN CIRCULATING PROGESTERONE (P_4) IN WOMEN WITH HISTORY OF HABITUAL ABORTION(HHA).

V.Cortés-Gallegos*, J.Gordillo-Fernández and I.Sojo. División Fisiología Gonadal y Hospital Gineco-Obstetricia, CMN., IMSS., México 73, D.F., CP 03020, Mexico City.

Previous study from our laboratory (Obstet Gynecol 49: 705, 1977) showed that patients with HHA had lower than normal P_4 levels in the luteal phase, suggesting a method for evaluating the treatment of such problems. Nevertheless, neither the oral supplement of the natural hormone nor the capacity of the endometrium to retain the circulating P_4 has been contemplated; therefore, in ten fertil women (FW) and in six with HHA, plasma (ng/ml) and endometrium (ng/g, wet tissue) P_4 concentrations were simultaneously measured (Fertil Steril 30:66, 1978), between the +6 and +10 ovulatory days. The values obtained ($\bar{x}\pm SD$) were as follows: FW vs HHA=8.7±1.6 vs 4.0±1.5 (plasma= $P<0.005$); 17.2±3.5 vs 0.09±0.01 (endometrium=$P<0.001$). HHA after 600 mg of orally administered P_4/d/10d after BBT rise= 11.5±4.3 (plasma) vs 0.11±0.04 (endometrium). These results suggest a failure of the endometrium capacity to retain the presence of pharmacologic circulating P_4 and this observation could be an endometrial defect of the progesterone receptor.

423 THE COUNTERACTING EFFECTS OF CIGLITAZONE AND DEXAMETHASONE IN FAT TISSUE METABOLISM. A.Y. Chang*, B.M. Wyse and B.J. Gilchrist, Diabetes and GI Diseases Research, The Upjohn Co., Kalamazoo, MI 49001, USA.

Ciglitazone, 5-[4-(1-methylcyclohexylmethoxy)benzyl]-thiazolidine-2,4-dione, lowers blood glucose and plasma insulin in obese-hyperglycemic and hyperinsulinemic animals such as ob/ob, db/db and KKA^y mice, but it is inactive in normal or insulinopenic diabetic animals. Its major modes of action are to ameliorate the insulin-resistant state by increasing insulin sensitivity and responsiveness in the adipocytes and to preserve β-cell granulation in the pancreatic islets. It is well documented that glucocorticoid is elevated in the obese-hyperglycemic animals and dexamethasone treatment induces insulin resistance. Although ciglitazone lowers blood glucose, it has no effect on the hyperglucocorticoid state in the ob/ob mice. Chronic injection of dexamethasone in the lean littermates induced increases in pancreatic insulin and glucagon contents and epididymal and brown adipose tissue weights but it caused no change in non-fasting blood glucose level. Adipose tissue isolated from dexamethasone-treated mice showed decreased basal and insulin-stimulated glucose oxidation and conversion into lipids. Oral administration of ciglitazone reversed dexamethasone-induced changes in adipose tissue weights and glucose metabolism but it did not lower dexamethasone-induced increases in pancreatic insulin and glucagon contents. Ciglitazone alone showed no effect on any of these parameters but the combined administrations of ciglitazone and dexamethasone elicit a hypoglycemic effect in the lean mice. The data indicate that ciglitazone has a counteracting effect on dexamethasone-induced changes in adipose tissue metabolisms.

424 EFFECTS OF VITAMIN A PALMITATE ON STREPTOZOTOCIN AND ALLOXAN-INDUCED DIABETES MELLITUS IN THE RAT. B.S. Chertow,* M.D. Webb, N.G. Baranetsky, W.I. Sivitz, and D.L. Thompson, Department of Medicine, Marshall University, and Medical Service, VA Medical Center, Huntington, West Virginia, United States.

Vitamin A interacts with membranes and affects membrane permeability and transport, which may influence the development of streptozotocin (SZ) and alloxan-induced diabetes. To determine whether retinyl palmitate (vit A) protects the beta cell from SZ and alloxan, we injected SZ, 60 mg/kg or alloxan, 100 mg/kg with or without varying doses of vit A ip or by tail vein (tv). Plasma glucose (PG, mg/dl) was measured for over 4 weeks. Mean PG ± SEM for the period were:

I SZ 60 mg/kg, ip		II SZ 60 mg/kg, tv			III Alloxan 100 mg/kg,ip	
Control	vit A ip 2.7 mg/kg	Control	vit A tv 10mg/kg	vit A tv 16mg/kg	Control	vit A ip 2.4 mg/kg
528±32 (5)	225±83†† (5)	480±32 (6)	335±12† (5)	354±27† (5)	239±10 (7)	150±13††† (7)

†p<.05, ††p<.01, †††p<.001 for vit A vs control; ( ), number of rats

In conclusion, vit A palmitate treatment, perhaps by its effect on membranes, lessens the severity of both SZ- and alloxan-induced diabetes. Vit A status may be important in the development of chemically-induced diabetes.

425 EFFECTS OF CONTINUOUS SUBCUTANEOUS INFUSION VERSUS MULTIPLE INJECTIONS ON INSULIN RECEPTORS IN IDDM. J.L. Chiasson*, L. Lecavalier, J. Havrankova, J.L. Petit, L. Germain, D. Bedard and P. Hamet, Clinical Research Institute of Montreal, Montreal, H2W 1R7, Canada.

The purpose of the present study was to compare continuous subcutaneous infusion (CSII) (Auto-Syringe AS6MP) versus multiple injections (MI) (Pen-Pump) in the treatment of IDDM and to assess the effect of glucose control on monocytes insulin receptors. Each diabetics (n = 8) were treated 2 months by MI (HS Ultra-Lente and AC boluses of Regular) and 2 months by CSII in a randomised fashion. Pre-study AC/PC blood glucose levels were 199/265 mg/dl and improved to 124/156 mg/dl during MI and to 115/151 mg/dl during CSII. Glycosylated hemoglobin before the study was 10.1% and decreased to 8.8 and 8.3% during MI and CSII respectively. The specific ^{125}I-insulin binding to circulating monocytes in a group of non obese control (n = 17) was 4.6%. In our poorly controlled diabetics during conventional therapy, the ^{125}I-insulin binding was decreased to 3.7% ($p < 0.025$). This was not significantly affected by MI despite good glucose control (4.0%). With CSII, however, good glucose control was associated with normalization ^{125}I-insulin binding to monocytes (4.7%). The affinity of the insulin receptors was normal before the study and was not affected by either MI or CSII. In conclusion, these observations demonstrate that in IDDM, 1) intensive therapy by MI and CSII resulted in similar good glucose control, but, 2) only CSII resulted in normalization of monocytes insulin receptors.

426 EFFECT OF SUCROSE MEAL ON GLUCOSE TURNOVER IN IDDM AND ITS MODULATION BY ACARBOSE. J.L. Chiasson*, L. Lecavalier, A. Martineau, P. Falardeau, Clinical Research Institute of Montreal, Montreal, H2W 1R7, Canada.

In IDDM we have studied the effect of sucrose meal on glucose gut absorption, glucose turnover, and insulin requirement and its modulation by a disaccharidase inhibitor, Acarbose. After an overnight fast the subjects were "hooked up" to the artificial pancreas (Biostator) to maintain normoglycemia. Glucose turnover was measured by using the stable isotope d5-D-glucose and gut absorption by trace labeling the glucose moiety of sucrose with ^{14}C. Each subject (n = 3) was studied during a sucrose meal of 75 g with and without Acarbose 100 mg. Blood glucose and insulin requirement were recorded by the Biostator for 120 minutes. Free plasma insulin was measured by radioimmunoassay. The mean basal glucose level was 81 mg/dl and increased to 129 and 200 mg/dl after 75 g of sucrose with and without Acarbose respectively. The area under the curve for blood glucose was 1.0 and 1.6 g/dl and for free plasma insulin 149 and 209 μU/ml. The total insulin requirement was 5.5 and 13.2 units. The mean basal total glucose production (Ra) was 99 mg/min and increased to 175 and 238 mg/min after the sucrose meal with and without Acarbose respectively. The glucose gut absorption was 36.8 g after 75 g of sucrose and decreased to 18.5 g after Acarbose treatment. At least 20% of the absorbed glucose was taken up by the liver. It is concluded that in IDDM 1) Acarbose will decrease a) blood glucose excursion and insulin requirement and b) total glucose production in response to a sucrose meal, and, 2) this effect of Acarbose is due to a decrease in glucose gut absorption.

427 EFFECT OF CONTINUOUS SUBCUTANEOUS INSULIN INFUSION VERSUS MULTIPLE INJECTIONS ON DIABETIC COMPLICATIONS IN IDDM. J.L. Chiasson*, F. Ducros, M. Poliquin-Hamet, D. Lopez, L. Lecavalier and P. Hamet, Clinical Research Institute of Montreal, Montreal, H2W 1R7, Canada.

The purpose of the present study was to compare continuous subcutaneous insulin infusion (CSII) (Mill-Hill Infusor) versus multiple injections (MI) (Medi-Jector) in the treatment of IDDM and to assess the effect of glucose control on nerve conduction and proteinuria. Each diabetic (n = 12) was treated 3 months by CSII and 3 months by MI (HS Ultra-Lente and AC boluses of Regular) in a randomised fashion. Pre-study pre-prandial/post-prandial (AC/PC) glucose levels were 147/215 mg/dl and improved to 108/138 mg/dl during CSII and to 115/139 mg/dl during MI with M-values of 48, 11 and 10 and HbA_{1c} of 12, 9 and 8.7% respectively. This good glucose control with either CSII or MI resulted in an increase in sural nerve conduction from 42.9 to 45 m/sec and in a decrease in proteinuria from 1.9 to 0.5 g/24 h. The 24 h insulin dose was 45 units before the study, 44 units during CSII and 56 units during MI. Having free choice, half of the patients opted for continued treatment with the Mill-Hill pump and half with the Medi-Jector. Conclusion: 1) Treatment with either CSII or MI was well accepted and resulted in similar good glucose control; 2) this good glucose control resulted in improved nerve conduction and proteinuria; and 3) MI required 20% more insulin than CSII to achieve similar glycemic control.

428 TARGET CELLS FOR 1,25-DIHYDROXYVITAMIN D_3 (1,25-D_3) IN DEVELOPING PANCREATIC ISLETS. S.A. Clark*, W.E. Stumpf, M. Sar, H.F. DeLuca† Department of Anatomy, University of North Carolina, Chapel Hill,NC and †Department of Biochemistry, University of Wisconsin, Madison,WI, USA.

Autoradiographic studies have demonstrated that islets have target cells for 1,25-D_3. In the present combined immunocytochemical-autoradiographic studies a significant nuclear accumulation (p<0.01) of ^{3}H-1,25-D_3 was seen in immunostained autoradiograms in insulin-positive cells,but not in somatostatin or glucagon cells. Pretreatment with 1,25-D_3 prevented nuclear accumulation,while pretreatment with 25-hydroxyvitamin D_3 (25-D_3) did not prevent nuclear accumulation of ^{3}H-1,25-D_3. Islet cells concentrated ^{3}H-1,25-D_3 similarly with or without 25-D_3 pretreatment. The nuclear uptake of 1,25-D_3 by islet cells in vivo and in vitro was also similar. In contrast,islet cell nuclei showed no nuclear concentration of ^{3}H-25-D_3. In cells of fetal islets specific nuclear uptake of ^{3}H-1,25-D_3 was observed as early as 18 days of gestation;about 5% of islet cells showed low,but significant,uptake of ^{3}H-1,25-D_3. The number of labeled cells and the nuclear uptake increased during islet development: the labeling index increased to 40% in 1-2 dayold rats,and the nuclear uptake of ^{3}H-1,25-D_3 by islets was similar between neonatal and mother rats. Quantitative results indicated that insulin cells selectively accumulate 400-900 fmol of 1,25-D_3/mg DNA. We conclude that insulin cells of islets are targets for 1,25-D_3 action in fetal and adult islets, suggesting that in addition to affecting insulin release, 1,25-D_3 may also affect differentiation of islet B-cells. Supported by NSF grant PCM8200569.

429 THERAPEUTIC EFFECTS OF DEHYDROEPIANDROSTERONE (DHEA) ON GENETIC DIABETES IN MICE. D. L. Coleman, E. H. Leiter*, and N. Applezweig. The Jackson Laboratory, Bar Harbor, ME 04609 and Progenics Inc., New York, NY 10036

DHEA fed at 0.4% in the diet is known to have marked beneficial effects on the development of the diabetes-obesity syndrome in C57BL/Ks diabetic (db) mice. The large effective dose suggested that some product or DHEA metabolite may be the active factor(s). We found that feeding 0.1% of either of the two 5β (cis) reduced metabolites, α-hydroxyetiocholanolone (α-ET) and β-hydroxyetiocholanolone (β-ET) were equally as effective as 0.4% DHEA. The two 5α (trans) reduced metabolites, androsterone and epiandrosterone were ineffective at 0.1%. Another potential DHEA metabolite estradiol (E_2) was therapeutic when fed at 0.005% in the diet or injected (S.C. 100 μg/wk). When suboptimally therapeutic doses of E_2 (5-20 μg/wk) were combined with diets containing non-therapeutic amounts of either ET, a marked potentiating effect was seen with normalization of the hyperglycemia and prevention of islet destruction being produced by as little as 0.025% of β-ET or 0.05% of α-ET. The ability of these 5β reduced steroids to maintain islet integrity and prevent development of most diabetes symptoms suggested that these metabolites were not merely inactive end-products of steroid metabolism but were physiological effectors in their own right. The synergism observed when both ETs are combined with E_2 suggested a mechanism whereby DHEA may be producing its beneficial effects. These studies were supported by NIH, JDF, and the Kroc Foundation.

430 THERMOGENESIS IN ALLOXAN DIABETIC RATS. D. A. Craddock*, and M. K. Yousef. Desert Biological Research Center, University of Nevada, Las Vegas, Nv. 89154.

Voluminous literature has accumulated on thermoregulation of "healthy" animals during exposure to various environmental stresses. However, similar work on responses of animals with major "chronic" disease to thermal stress has received little attention. The question of a possible link between diabetes and maintenance of homeothermy remain to be open for investigation. The following experiments were designed to measure any anomalous thermoregulation in alloxan diabetic (AD) rats during acute exposure to heat and cold. Thermoneutral zone (TNZ) of the AD rats as compared to their controls was measured at ambient temperature (Ta) ranging from 8 to 40C. At TNZ the AD rats had lower rate of oxygen consumption (VO_2) and rectal temperature (Tre) than the control. Both groups increased their (VO_2) curvilinearly as Ta decreased below 24C. The Tre decreased significantly in the AD rats as Ta declined. Above a Ta of 33C, the AD rats increased their Tre and VO_2, however the control rats showed similar responses only when Ta was above 36C. Exposure of the AD rats and their control to a Ta of 42C for 6 hr. showed that the AD rats were much less heat tolerant than the controls. During exposure of these two groups of rats to a Ta of -2C for 8 hr. Tre declined 2-3C in the AD group as compared to 1.0-1.5C in the control group. Changes in tail skin temperature was not significantly different between the AD and control rats suggesting the adequacy of the peripheral vascular reactivity to thermal stress in these animals. In conclusion, the data suggest that diabetic rats can tolerate acute exposure to cold more successfully than to heat.

431 ALTERATIONS OF PHOSPHOLIPID METABOLISM IN THE DIABETIC RAT.

A.Q. Dang, F.H. Faas* and W.J. Carter. Dept. of Medicine, VA Medical Center and Univ. of Arkansas for Medical Sciences, Little Rock, AR 72206 USA

Since hepatic microsomal fatty acid composition is altered in streptozotocin (SZ) diabetic rats, this study was done to determine the effects of diabetes on the synthesis and degradation of glycerophospholipids.

Enzymes (Acyl-CoA)	Controls (n)	Diabetic (n)	Insulin Tx (n)
†GPAT (Oleoyl-CoA)	62.2 ±3.0 (4)	*80.9 ±5.2 (4)	60.8 ±2.6 (5)
†GPCAT (Arachidonoyl-CoA)	64.5 ±3.8 (4)	*94.9 ±6.5 (4)	64.9 ±2.9 (5)
††Phospholipase A_2	0.53±0.10 (8)	*0.36±0.07 (8)	*0.71±0.12 (8)
†Lysophospholipase	3.16±0.45 (4)	*1.61±0.33 (4)	3.44±0.63 (5)

†Enzyme activity (nmoles/mg/min); ††nmoles/mg/hr; *p < .01 exp. vs control. SZ-diabetes significantly increased the activity of the liver microsomal enzymes which synthesize phospholipids such as acyl-CoA:1-acyl-Sn-glycerol 3-phosphate acyltransferase (GPAT) (30%) and acyl-CoA:Sn-glycerol 3-phosphorylcholine acyltransferase (GPCAT) (47%). However, diabetes decreased the activity of enzymes which degrade phospholipids such as mitochondrial phospholipase A_2 (32%) and cytosol lysophospholipase (49%). Insulin treatment (10-12 U/day) for 3 days corrected these enzymatic alterations. Since microsomal GPAT and GPCAT have higher activity toward unsaturated than saturated fatty acids, the increase of these enzyme activities coupled with the decreased phospholipase A_2 and lysophospholipase in diabetes indicates that diabetes enhances the formation of hepatic unsaturated fatty acid containing glycerophospholipids. These results combined with the previously reported decrease of fatty acid desaturase activity may explain the altered phospholipid fatty acid composition in diabetes.

432 INFLUENCE OF INSULIN AND SUBSTRATE CONSUMPTION ON THE LEVEL OF SPECIFIC CARDIAC MESSENGER RNAs.

W.H. Dillmann* and A. Barrieux, Division of Endocrinology and Metabolism, U.C.S.D., San Diego, California, U.S.A.

In 4 week diabetic (D) rats 7 cardiac mRNAs are decreased and 6 mRNAs are increased compared to cardiac mRNAs in normal (N) rats. D mRNA pattern reverts to N after 4 weeks of 3 U of long-acting insulin (I)/day. In order to determine whether I exerts fast, direct effects or secondary effect on mRNAs due to changes in substrate consumption, 4 week D rats received 2 U regular I i.v. and were killed 1.5, 3, 5, 12 and 24h after I. Other D rats were placed on 25 mg of methyl palmoxirate (MP)/kg/day for 4 weeks in order to inhibit long-chain fatty acid oxidation. The abundance of individual mRNA species was determined by in vitro translation of RNA, separation of labeled peptides by two-dimensional gel electrophoresis, visualization by fluorography and quantitation by photometry. One specific mRNA (106) increased 20-fold in D, decreased to N within 1.5h after I and returned to the D level 24h after I. In contrast, 2 other mRNAs (247 and 257) which show no response to I after 24h were normalized by MP. Plasma I was not changed by MP (D = 6±3 uU/ml), D+MP = 7±2 uU/ml, N = 68±9 uU/ml). Conclusion: 1. Diabetes induces changed in 13 specific cardiac mRNAs which show different response patterns to insulin. 2. The level of 1 mRNA (106) which is markedly elevated in D hearts responds to I within 1.5h. 3. Long-term MP to D rats leads to normal levels of 2 mRNAs (247 and 257) in D in the absence of changes in I levels. 4. D-induced changes in cardiac mRNA levels seem to result from direct effects of I itself and from secondary I effects resulting from changes in cardiac substrate consumption.

433 THE EFFECT OF HYDROCHLOROTHIAZIDE (HCTZ) AND PROPRANOLOL (PROP) ON INSULIN SECRETION AND GLYCEMIC CONTROL IN HYPERTENSIVE TYPE II DIABETICS.

A. Dornhorst*, S. Powell and J. Pensky. Departments of Medicine and Pathology, Case Western Reserve University, Cleveland, Ohio, USA.

Hyperglycemia occurs with both HCTZ and PROP but the mechanisms remain controversial. This study examines the effects of therapeutic doses of these drugs given alone and in combination on fasting sugar (FBS), glycosylated hemoglobin (HbA1c) and 24 hr urinary C-peptide (UCP), the last being an estimate of daily insulin secretion. Ten type II diabetics were studied in a randomized cross-over trial with treatment periods lasting 3 weeks separated by 1 week washout. A no treatment period served as control. FBS, potassium (K) and UCP were measured weekly and HbA1c was measured at the beginning and end of each treatment period.

	CONTROL	PROP	HCTZ	HCTZ+PROP	p
FBS mg%	187.9	212.8	253.3	294.7	<.0005
%Δ FBS	-6.31	15.13	25.68	49.57	<.0005
%Δ HbA1c	0.95	0.02	8.38	14.72	<.001
UCP ug/g creat.	53.15	54.81	51.09	55.06	NS

HCTZ+PROP produced a significantly greater increase in both HbA1c and FBS compared to either drug alone. HCTZ effects were significantly greater than PROP. These drugs did not alter UCP. Three patients had a consistent fall (>0.5 meq/l) in K while taking HCTZ but there was no difference in FBS, HbA1c and UCP between these patients and the others. The combination of HCTZ and PROP may have synergistic effects in causing deterioration of glycemic control. These drugs act through mechanisms other than inhibition of daily insulin secretion and which are independent of K.

434 EFFECTS OF NALOXONE ON HORMONAL AND METABOLIC RESPONSES TO INSULIN-INDUCED HYPOGLYCEMIA.

K.M.A. El-Tayeb*, P.L. Brubaker, H.L.A. Lickley and M.Vranic. Depts. of Physiology, Surgery and Medicine, University of Toronto, Canada.

Insulin hypoglycemia is a powerful stimulus to the nervous system for the release of counterregulatory hormones. We have examined hormonal and metabolic responses to hypoglycemia and the role of endogenous opiates in the counterregulatory mechanisms. Insulin (7mU/kg-min x 70min) was infused with or without the opiate antagonist naloxone (2mg/kg bolus, 33 ug/kg-min) in six normal dogs. During insulin infusion alone, plasma glucose decreased by 59±4mg/dl (p < .001), due to an increase in glucose disappearance of 4.2±.6mg/kg-min (p < .001). This was partially counteracted by an increase in glucose production of 2.3±0.6mg/kg-min (p < .02). As glucose levels plateaued at 43±4mg/dl, glucagon rose from 132±41 to 405±101pg/ml (p < .02), epinephrine from 75±14 to 2433±506pg/ml (p < .01), and ACTH, β-endorphin and cortisol rose concurrently from basal levels of 24±6pg/ml, 47±21pg/ml and 2.1±0.5ug/dl to 389+118 (p < .05), 259±46 (p < .02) and 9.1±1.7 (p < .02), respectively. Interestingly when naloxone was given with insulin, there was a much earlier response of the counterregulatory hormones. When plasma glucose fell to 71±7mg/dl (a drop of only 25±4mg/dl), epinephrine, glucagon, β-endorphin and cortisol had risen significantly by 215±53pg/ml (p < 0.01), 83±31pg/ml (p < 0.05), 47±18pg/ml (p < 0.05), 4.1±1.5ug/dl (p < 0.05). There were also greater integrated glucagon (p < .01) and cortisol (p < .02) responses during insulin infusion with naloxone. We conclude that a blockade of endogenous opiates sensitizes the counterregulatory responses to hypoglycemia. We speculate that opiate receptors may be involved in regulation of the set point for glucose in the brain.

435 DUAL ACTION OF PROGESTINS ON UTEROGLOBIN GENE EXPRESSION IN THE RABBIT UTERUS.

J. Biro*, T. Torkkeli, H. Isotalo, C.-L. C. Chen and O.A. Jänne, The Population Council and The Rockefeller University, New York, NY 10021

Progesterone and other progestins stimulate acutely the synthesis of rabbit endometrial uteroglobin (Ugl), at least in part, by increasing the rate of Ugl gene transcription. On the other hand, prolonged progestin treatment is known to depress endometrial functions. The purpose of this work was to compare acute and chronic effects of two different progestins, progesterone (P) and medroxyprogesterone acetate (MPA), on Ugl gene expression, and to relate these actions to changes in uterine progesterone receptor (PR) concentrations. Ugl content was measured by RIA, Ugl-mRNA concentration by Northern-blot analysis, and cytosol and nuclear PR levels by exchange assays. Daily administration of P (1 mg/kg body wt) or MPA (0.5 mg/kg) for 3-5 days elicited a 2,000-fold increase in uterine fluid Ugl concentration which, however, declined sharply to values that were 1/50th of the maximal Ugl concentration on day 15. Similar changes occurred in the uterine tissue Ugl content. Ugl-mRNA accumulation peaked on days 3-5 (a 10-fold relative increase) and then subsided to one-fifth of the maximal values on prolonged treatment. Quantitatively, P and MPA elicited very similar changes in Ugl and Ugl-mRNA concentrations. Both P and MPA depressed cytosol and nuclear PR concentrations by 3 days with MPA decreasing the receptor values more than P. However, even after the prolonged treatment, the receptor concentrations remained clearly measurable. Conclusions: (1) Short-term progestin treatment stimulates Ugl gene expression while continued steroid administration reverses this effect, and (2) Changes in the PR concentrations do not explain this dual action of progestins. (HD-16105).

436 STEREOCHEMICAL COMPLEMENTARITY OF REPRODUCTIVE STEROID HORMONES AND DNA: EVIDENCE THAT STEROIDS CAN HAVE DIRECT, STEREOSPECIFIC INTERACTIONS WITH DNA.

E.D. Bransome, Jr.*, L.B. Hendry, M.S. Hutson, A.F. Lehner, T.G. Muldoon and V.B. Mahesh, Departments of Medicine and Endocrinology, Medical College of Georgia, Augusta, Georgia, 30912, USA.

Two important questions about the action of steroid reproductive hormones have not yet been answered: what is the basis for constraints on hormonal activity and why are affinities of binding to specific protein receptors (the moieties purported to interact specifically with DNA) sometimes inconsistent with potency? Our approach to these questions has involved the study of the molecular structure of steroid hormones and of nucleic acids. In our analysis of published xray data, we discovered that the most active natural products, estradiol, testosterone, and progesterone, are stereochemically complementary to partially uncoiled DNA. These hormones were accomodated best between T-A and G-C base pairs, each forming hydrogen bonds to the sugar-phosphate backbone of DNA in a manner stereochemically unique to each type of hormone. Known antagonists have stereochemically complementary features similar to the respective active hormones but either have different hydrogen bonding characteristics (e.g. estrogens vs androgens) or possess structural features which protrude from the cavities between DNA base pairs (e.g. tamoxifen, RU 486). These findings suggest that the mechanism of steroid hormone action may involve direct, stereospecific interaction of DNA with steroids in concert with activated "receptor" proteins. Our prediction that the TpG sequence will be found in transcriptional control sites is consistent with sequence data recently reported by others.

437 GLUCOCORTICOID INHIBITION OF GLUCOSE TRANSPORT IN RAT ADIPOCYTES.

C. Carter-Su* and K. Okamoto, Dept. Physiology, Univ. of Mich. Med. School, Ann Arbor, MI 48109, USA.

The ability of glucocorticoids to alter glucose transport in isolated rat adipocytes was investigated. Hexose transport was directly assessed using 3-O-methylglucose rather than glucose or 2-deoxyglucose. A maximally effective dose of dexamethasone (dex) (10^{-7} M) inhibits transport up to 80%, acts as early as 15-30 min after addition, and is totally effective within 60-90 min. Transport inhibition requires both mRNA and protein synthesis. When actinomycin D (actin D) (10 μg/ml), which has little or no effect on basal transport, is added up to 15 min after dex, it completely blocks the ability of dex to inhibit transport. However, it alters only slightly the ability of dex to inhibit transport when added 45 or more min after dex. Cycloheximide (cyclo) (10 μg/ml) also completely prevents dex inhibition of transport when added 15-60 min after dex. It differs from actin D in that it prevents complete inhibition of transport by dex when added as little as 15 min prior to assay. Thus, although dex effects on transport are normally maximal by 90 min, cyclo still can prevent dex expression when added 145 min after dex. These data, in conjunction with glucose transport labeling studies, are consistent with the following: 1)Glucocorticoids inhibit glucose metabolism in rat adipocytes by decreasing glucose transport, 2)Transport inhibition by dex requires mRNA synthesis 15-45 min after hormone addition, 3)Transport inhibition also appears to require continuous synthesis of a fast acting ($<$15 min) and rapidly turning over protein which causes a decrease in the number of glucose transport proteins in the plasma membrane.

438 BIOCHEMICAL AND QUANTITATIVE ELECTRON MICROSCOPE AUTORADIOGRAPHIC (EM-AR) STUDIES ON ^{125}I-HUMAN CHORIONIC GONADOTROPIN (^{125}I-hCG) INTERNALIZATION IN BOVINE LUTEAL SLICES.

N. Chegini* and Ch. V. Rao, Depts. of Ob/Gyn and Biochem., University of Louisville, Louisville, KY 40292, USA

Luteal slices of well preserved morphological and biochemical integrity were used in investigating the fate of ^{125}I-hCG following initial binding to cell surface receptors. Biochemical approach, which involved isolation of purified fractions from slices preincubated with 0.1 nM ^{125}I-hCG, revealed specific radioactivity not only in plasma membranes (PM), but also in nuclei (N), lysosomes (LY), rough endoplasmic reticulum (RER) and Golgi (G). Marker enzyme analyses and EM examination of the fractions revealed that neither PM nor cross contamination could explain the presence of radioactivity in various organelles. The radioactivity was found to be an intact and macromolecular bound ^{125}I-hCG. The ^{125}I-hCG degradation products (~ 15%) were found in the medium. The internalization and intracellular binding of ^{125}I-hCG was ligand and tissue specific and dependent on incubation time and temperature. The EM-AR approach, after three step mask analysis which corrects for radiation spread, revealed the presence of silver grains not only on PM but also on N, LY, RER and G. The grain distribution in the intracellular organelles was ligand and tissue specific and dependent on time and temperature of incubation. In summary, both biochemical and EM-AR approaches agree that a) while ^{125}I-hCG does not internalize at 4°, considerable internalization takes place at 22° and 38° and b) internalized ^{125}I-hCG associates with N, LY, RER and G with the highest concentration in G. Support - NIH HD 14697

439 REVERSIBLE PREACTIVATION OF PURE ADENYLYL CYCLASE (AC) REGULATORY COMPONENTS N_s AND N_i WITHOUT SUBUNIT DISSOCIATION. J. Codina* and L. Birnbaumer Dept. of Cell Biology, Baylor College of Medicine, Houston, TX 77030, USA.

Pure N_s and N_i, subunit composition: $\alpha\beta\gamma$, are each of 95 kDa in mass and 4.2S. Treatment of N_i with 10 mM Mg^{2+} and 10 uM GMP-P(NH)P or GTPγS (G) at 32.5°C for 10 min changes its S from 4.2 to 2.2. This agrees with dissociation of α_i subunit from $\beta\gamma$ complex (both of 40 kDa). If Mg^{2+} and G treated N_i is cooled to 4°C it changes to 3.2S. This correlates with a calculated mass of 80 kDa after correction for detergent binding and indicates subunit reassocaition. Both 2.2S N_i and 3.2S N_i have G bound, as seen by [^{35}S]GTPγS binding. Bound G can be released by addition of EDTA. This leads to reformation of 4.2S N_i, indistinguishable from control. N_i can be recycled, for readdition of Mg^{2+} to 4.2S N_i, formed from 3.2S N_i, leads to reformation of 3.2S N_i. Treatment of N_s with 50 mM $MgCl_2$ and 10 uM G for 40 min at 32.5°C leads to a change in its S from 4.2 to 2.2. This agrees with dissociation of α_s from $\beta\gamma$ complex. This state is not temperature dependent. Removal of the Mg^{2+} and reduction of the ionic strength at 3% Lubrol PX, changes its S from 2.2 to 3.2, indicating reassociation of subunits. Both the 2.2S N_s and the 3.2S N_s reconsitute cyc^- S49 AC in the absence of G in the medium and are therefore preactivated forms of N_s. Removal of Mg^{2+}, reduction of ionic strength plus a decrease of Lubrol PX to 0.5%, leads over a 24 hr period at 4°C to a partial deactivation of N_s. which is correlated with quantitative re-formation of 4.2S N_s as seen by reconstitution of cyc^- S49 AC in the presence but not absence of G. It is concluded that N_s and N_i can be affected by Mg^{2+} and G reversibly and that N_s and N_i can exist in a preactivated form without subunit dissociation.

440 CONSTRUCTION OF A HYBRID HORMONE GENE AND ITS EXPRESSION IN VITRO. N.E. Cooke*, S.M. Rosenshine, and S.A. Liebhaber, University of Pennsylvania, Philadelphia, Pennsylvania 19104.

The peptide hormones growth hormone (GH) and prolactin (Prl) differ in structure and spectrum of biological activity. The structural basis of their bioactivities and the mechanisms which mediate their actions on target cells need to be further defined. Although GH and Prl share similar secondary structures as defined by their disulfide bonding, their primary structures are quite divergent (23% amino acid homology). The genes encoding GH and Prl are identically organized. To begin to define the structural regions which differentiate the activity of these two polypeptides, we have exchanged corresponding exons of the Prl and GH genes to construct a new gene which encodes a human GH protein in which amino acids 32 to 71 are substituted with amino acids 39 to 74 of rat Prl. We have subsequently introduced this gene via an SV40 viral vector into a monkey kidney cell line (CV1-p) and have demonstrated its expression as a stable protein product of 22,000 daltons. This experiment supports the general feasibility of constructing hybrid hormone genes by genetic recombination and demonstrates that such hybrid genes can be used to synthesize stable hybrid proteins for subsequent physiological investigation. This approach should allow the design of specific deletions and/or recombinations with these genes to define better the structure-function relationships among these hormones.

441 CHARACTERIZATION OF THREE ESTROGEN REGULATED FORMS OF RAT UTERINE GLUCOSE-6-P DEHYDROGENASE.
A. Cummings* and K.L. Barker, Dept. Biochem., Texas Tech Univ. Health Sci. Ctr., Lubbock, TX 79430, U.S.A.

Amounts of glucose-6-P dehydrogenase (G6PD) in rat uterus are regulated by estradiol (E) at four molecular levels: increased mRNA; increased mRNA translation rate; decreased G6PD degradation; and an increased rate of processing of a "putative" pre-G6PD. SDS-PAGE of radiolabeled uterine G6PD revealed three immunoreactive proteins (A,B, and C) with molecular weights of 60-65,000, 57,000, and 42,000, respectively. A,B, and C were tentatively identified as precursor, predominant, and nascent peptide forms of G6PD based on the E-dependent kinetics of A,B, and C synthesis, the association of C and A with ribosomes, and the E-dependent accumulation of B but not A and C after longer labeling times (Donohue et al. Biochim. Biophys. Acta 658:356, 1981 and 739:148, 1983). The present study examined amino acid sequence homologies among A,B, and C. Uterine proteins were labeled with ^{3}H- or ^{35}S- methionine. ^{35}S-A, ^{35}S-B, and ^{35}S-C were isolated by precipitation with anti-G6PD and SDS-PAGE, and each was indially co-digested with authentic ^{3}H-(met)-G6PD (protein B) using papain. Resultant peptides were resolved by IEF-PAGE. A,B, and C have 6 methionine containing peptides in common, both A and C have 2 peptides not present in B, and B has 1 peptide not present in A or C. The sequence homology and immunoreactivity indicate that A,B, and C are related to G6PD while the presence of 2 additional peptides in A and C suggests that these peptides may be derived from a common N-terminal leader sequence which is removed from A to produce B. Sequence data for the N-terminus of proteins A and C should identify the sequence specificity of the E-dependent G6PD processing mechanism. (Supported by NRS HD-06387 and NIH HD-16236)

442 PHORBOL ESTERS STIMULATE PHOSPHOLIPID METABOLISM IN RAT GRANULOSA CELLS.
John S. Davis*, Leigh A. West, Robert V. Farese, VA Hospital and Dept. of Medicine, Univ of South Florida College of Medicine, Tampa, FL, USA 33612

Perturbation of membrane phospholipid metabolism is an early consequence of the tumor promoting phorbol esters. Recent reports also suggest that phorbol esters can regulate cellular activity by activation of calcium and phospholipid dependent protein kinase (C-kinase). These studies were carried out to determine whether phorbol esters alter phospholipid metabolism in granulosa cells. Granulosa cells were incubated in medium containing $^{32}PO_4$ in the absence (control) or presence of LH or 12-O-tetradecanoyl-phorbol-13-acetate (TPA). Phospholipids were extracted and purified by two dimensional TLC. In 60 min incubations, TPA (100nM) increased ^{32}P incorporation into total cellular phospholipids (120%), while LH had no effect. In controls, phosphatidylcholine (PC) contained the majority of the radioactivity (83%); phosphatidylethanolamine (PE) and phosphatidylinositol (PI) each contained approximately 5% of the radioactivity. TPA (100nM) markedly increased ^{32}P incorporation into PC (70%), PE (123%) and phosphatidic acid (PA, 182%). TPA reduced labeling of PI and the polyphosphoinositides by 35% and 20%, respectively. LH (1ug/ml) only increased labeling of PA (42%) and PI (75%). Effects of TPA on ^{32}P incorporation into PC and PE were demonstrated within 30 min and appeared to be maximal at TPA concentration of 20nM. In contrast to LH, phospholipid metabolism in TPA-treated cells is shunted away from the phosphoinositides. These results suggest that in addition to interaction with a receptor protein (C-kinase) membrane lipids are also involved in the cellular response to phorbol esters. Supported by NIH HD-17939 and the Veterans Administration.

443 DIETARY FAT COMPOSITION DIFFERENTIALLY ALTERS HORMONE SENSITIVE ADENYLATE CYCLASE ACTIVITIES IN RAT LIVER WITHOUT CONCOMMITANT CHANGES IN RECEPTOR NUMBER. E.M. Dax*, J.S. Partilla, M.A. Piñeyro and R.I. Gregerman. Gerontology Res. Ctr., Natl. Inst. on Aging , N.I.H. at Baltimore City Hospitals, Baltimore, MD 21224. U.S.A.

Glucagon(glu) stimulated hepatic adenylate cyclase activity(AC) is reduced in rats fed diets containing only saturated fats. We investigated if changes in the composition of dietary fat affected glu receptor:AC relationships and if the β-adrenergic system were similarly affected. Three groups of rats were fed synthetic diets for 4 weeks after weaning: 10% corn oil (w/w), 10% coconut oil, or 8.5% coconut oil with 1.5% corn oil (essential free fatty acid replete). Hepatic glu and β-adrenergic receptors were characterized and quantitated using [^{125}I Tyr^{10}] monoiodoglu and [^{125}I] pindolol(p). No change was observed in EC_{50} of AC activation for either glu or isoproterenol(Iso) or Kd of binding.

	AC Activity(nmol/mg/10min)			Receptors(fmol/mg)	
Diet	Basal	Iso [10^{-5}M]	Glu [10^{-5}M]	[^{125}I]p	[^{125}I]Glu
Corn	1.00±.03	2.74±.12	9.81±.94	6.3±.9	450±45
Coconut	0.93±.06	2.07±.19[a]	5.27±.30[a,b]	6.6±.4	614±34[a,b]
coco/corn	0.84±.03	2.14±.13	7.52±.74	5.5±.3	430±25

Repeated measure ANOVA and multiple range testing $p<.05$; a, corn vs coco b, coco vs coco/corn.

The results demonstrate that dietary fat compostion differentially alters receptor:AC relationships in two distinct hormone activated systems of the same membranes.

444 RELATION OF GLUCAGON (G) AND OTHER NONTHYROIDAL HORMONES TO RESTING HYPERMETABOLISM (RH) AFTER BURN INJURY (BI). R.A. Becker*, G.M. Vaughan, R. Unger, M.G. Ziegler, T.M. Siler-Khodr, B.A. Pruitt, Jr., and A.D. Mason, Jr., U.S. Army Institute of Surgical Research, Fort Sam Houston, TX 78234; Univ. Texas Health Science Centers at San Antonio and Dallas, TX; and Univ. California Medical Center at San Diego, CA, U.S.A.

The endocrine/metabolic basis for resting hypermetabolism (RH) in febrile nonthyroidal illness is not yet understood. Burn injury (BI) is associated with hyperthermia and RH, and one index of severity is total burn size (TBS, % body surface). After overnight fasting and recumbency, resting metabolic rate (MR, O_2 consumption) was measured weekly and plasma was sampled for determination of glucose (GLSE), total cholesterol (CHL), triglycerides, insulin, glucagon (G), somatostatin, growth hormone, norepinephrine (NE), epinephrine, and cortisol (F), in 28 burned men, TBS 2-85%, 17-23 years old, including 8 controls with minimal injury (TBS ≤ 7.5%). MR was elevated in proportion to burn size ($p < 0.001$) mainly in the first week then declined toward normal. Two multiple regression analyses (validated by random partitioning of data) determined which plasma variables independently reflected residual variation in MR: without TBS entered as a variable, high MR was associated with elevated GLSE, F, and G, and low CHL (cumulative $r^2 = 0.79$, $n = 62$); with TBS entered, high MR was associated with greater TBS, elevated NE and again high G and low CHL ($r^2 = 0.83$). Conclusions: resting hypermetabolism, likely related to the elevated calorigenic hormones NE and F, also appears independently related to elevated plasma glucagon which suggests a calorigenic role for glucagon in burn injury. This involves marked changes in metabolism not only of glucose but also of cholesterol.

445 IMMUNOCYTOCHEMICAL LOCALIZATION OF THE MITOCHONDRIAL UNCOUPLING PROTEIN IN RAT BROWN ADIPOSE TISSUE. M. Cadrin*, M. Tolszczuk, and L. Bukowiecki. Laval University, Med. Sch., Dept. Physiol., and Laboratory of Physical Activity Sciences, Québec, G1K 7P4, Canada.

Recent studies have shown that brown adipose tissue plays an important role in the regulation of energy balance and that it represents the major anatomical site of norepinephrine-induced thermogenesis in homeotherms. Brown adipose tissue mitochondria possess an uncoupling protein localized in their inner membrane that confers on them an unusual capacity for substrate-induced thermogenesis. The presence of this protein in rat brown adipose tissue was demonstrated using both immuno-histo and cyto-chemical techiques, the peroxidase-anti-peroxidase (PAP) method and the coloid gold labelling method. The results indicated that the distribution and localization of the uncoupling protein across brown adipose tissue are not uniform. Confirming and extending previous biochemical investigations showing that the presence of the uncoupling protein was specific to brown adipose tissue, this study revealed that, in brown adipose tissue itself, the uncoupling protein appeared to be confined only to one type of cell, "typical" brown adipocytes. No staining was detected in pericytes, endothelial or interstitial cells. It is concluded that the presence of the uncoupling protein represents an excellent criterion for identifying brown adipocytes. Immunohistochemical techniques will certainly represent a powerful tool for studying brown adipocyte function and differentiation. This study was supported by the MRC and the LABSAP.

446 INTERSPECIFIC DIFFERENCES IN BETA-AND ALPHA$_2$-ADRENOCEPTOR INTERPLAY IN THE REGULATION OF LIPOLYSIS. C.Carpene, M.Berlan and M.Lafontan*Inst.Physiol.UPS, ERA412CNRS, 31400 TOULOUSE, France.

It is well established that postsynaptic α_2-adrenoceptors exist concomitantly with β-adrenoceptors in white fat cells of various species.Physiological amines have a strong lipolytic effect in hamster and dog fat cells and a weaker effect in human and rabbit adipocytes.The lipolytic(β-effect) and antilipolytic(α_2-effect) of epinephrine(EPI) and norepinephrine(NEPI) have been compared in hyperresponsive and hyporesponsive fat cells to test the functional balance between β-and α_2-response.EPI is the major stimulant of hamster and human α_2-receptors as opposed to NEPI;its antilipolytic action(with 10μM propranolol)is clearly different from that of NEPI in the fat cells of both species incubated with adenosine deaminase.Moreover,EPI alone promotes a clear antilipolysis in human fat cells while exerting a lipolytic effect in hamster in similar conditions.EPI has a higher affinity for human than hamster α_2-adrenoceptors.Concerning β-adrenergic response, EPI is less lipolytic than NEPI.However,EPI has a higher affinity for β-sites in hamster than in human fat cells.To conclude,studies of the lipolytic responses of these two kinds of fat cells to EPI and NEPI reveals that EPI-dependent inhibitory effects are stronger in human fat cells,in which EPI has a higher affinity for α_2-than β-sites.An opposite observation was done in hamster fat cells,EPI has a higher affinity for β-than α_2-sites.Finally,the α_2-adrenoceptors have probably an important regulatory rôle in human fat cells while they are less efficient in the control of hamster fat cell lipolysis; the β-effect being predominant in this species.

This study was supported by CNRS and INSERM (CRL & PRC grants)

447 PRODUCTION OF MONOCLONAL ANTIBODIES TO HUMAN TRANSCORTIN. USE IN A RADIOIMMUNOASSAY. D. Faict * and P. De Moor, Laboratory of Experimental Medicine, Minderbroedersstraat 10, B-3000 Leuven, Belgium.

The technique of somatic cell fusion offers the opportunity to produce virtually unlimited quantities of homogeneous antibodies. By fusion of Sp2/0 Ag14 myeloma cells and spleen cells from a mouse immunised with human transcortin, we obtained five hybrids secreting antibodies to transcortin. The hybrids were detected by radioimmunoassay and cloned by limiting dilution. One antibody belonged to the IgG_{2a} subclass, the others were of the IgG_1 type. The association constants ranged from 3×10^8 l/mol to 4×10^{10} l/mol. The antibodies were used in a RIA of transcortin. Although the most sensitive RIA (detection limit : 0.23 ng/tube) was obtained with a high affinity antibody, an antibody of moderate affinity was more suitable for the measurement of transcortin in serum, since it allowed a lower dilution of the serum samples. The detection limit of the latter assay was 24.0 ng/tube and the mid-range 267.0 ng. Intra-assay coefficients of variation were 2.5% for a serum pool containing 41 mg/l transcortin and 2.9% for a pool with a transcortin concentration of 90 mg/l. Interassay coefficients of variation for the same pools were 7.1% and 9.1%. After serial dilution of a serum sample, the expected amount of transcortin was recovered. There was a good agreement between the transcortin values obtained by this assay and by radial immunodiffusion ($r = 0.976$; $n = 99$). These results indicate that monoclonal antibodies to human transcortin provide a useful reagent for a RIA of this protein.

448 SELECTION AND CHARACTERIZATION OF ANTI-hGH MONOCLONAL ANTIBODIES. F. Gomez*, G. Pirens, J. Closset and G. Hennen. Endocrinologie Expérimentale et Clinique, Université de Liège, Institut de Pathologie, C.H.U. B23, B-4000 Liège, BELGIQUE.

Biozzi-strain mice were immunised with a highly purified preparation of 20K variant of hGH. Spleen-cells were fused with SP2/0Ag14 myeloma cells. Clone productions were screened for specificity toward 20K and 22K hGH and for the affinity constant of antibody-antigen reaction. For the selected monoclonal antibody, Ka was 1,2.1011 L/M using GH 22K variant as both tracer and reference preparation. No cross reactivity was found with PRL and other pituitary hormones; hPL reactivity was 0.002 per cent that of hGH. According to these antibody characteristics, a highly sensitive RIA system was developed, and used for specific GH measurement in human serum. Using logit-log co-ordinates, the slope of the standard curve was -1.059 and the minimum detected dose was 0.5 µUI/ml. Excellent correlation was found between assay data in this system and those of a conventional RIA method using specific polyclonal rabbit antiserum. The International Reference preparation (66/217) could adequately be used to calibrate the Mab system since the internal 22K GH standard and the international one were equally well recognized by the monoclonal antibody.

We thank Dr Biozzi and J. Smal for gift of mice and antigen, C. Schaus and C. De Ricker for active cooperation, Ms Marrai, Pirard and Mottard for technical aid, Executive Regional Wallon and Techland S.A. for research funding.

449 ONTOGENIC STUDY OF HYPOTHALAMIC-PREOPTIC SUPRACHIASMATIC SEROTONERGIC RECEPTORS AND SEROTONIN INDUCED PROLACTIN RELEASE IN RATS.

D.Becú de Villalobos and C.Libertun*, Instituto de Biología y Medicina Experimental Obligado 2490, 1428 Buenos Aires, Argentina.

The development of hypothalamic-preoptic suprachiasmatic (HPS) seroto nin 1 receptors of 4-6, 12-16, 26-28 and 36-38 day old female rats was studied in correlation with the PRL releasing effect of 5-HT. A specific 5-HT receptor was quantified at the first postnatal week (B Max: mean 8.0, confidence limits 6.9-9.0 fmol/mg tissue; Kd: 4.7:0.7 nM). Receptor densi ty increased with advancing age. At 26-28 days B Max was 16.5 (11.9-24.0) fmol/mg tissue ($p < 0.05$), Kd 5.3:0.7 nM. On the other hand, 5 and 10 mg/kg of 5-HT were ineffective in altering serum PRL in 4-6 days old females. By 12 days the higher dose released PRL significantly and from then onwards the response increased. As a sex difference in the 5-HT modulation of PRL release have been documented by our laboratory (Endocrinology 110:1879, 1982), the hyperprolactinemic effect of 5-HT in correlation with serotonin binding in HPS of 28 day old female and male rats was studies. Though the PRL increment achieved by 5-HT, 5 or 10 mg/kg, was higher in the male than in the female (14 vs 5 ng/ml and 50 vs 24 ng/ml for each dose respective ly), serotonin binding was not significantly different between sexes. This data indicate: 1.A specific binding site for 5-HT in HPS is present from the first postnatal days; from then onwards a gradual increment in B Max is observed. In correlation, 5-HT shows a PRL releasing effect that increa ses with age. 2.At 28 days, no clear differences in B Max or Kd are pre sent in 5-HT binding between male and female rats, though PRL levels attained after 5-HT are higher in the male. Supported by the CONICET.

450 EFFECTS OF INTRAVENTRICULAR INFUSION OF NOREPINEPHRINE ON LUTEINIZING HORMONE RELEASE: RECEPTOR SPECIFICITY.

H. Bergen*, D. Choo and P.C.K. Leung, Dept. of Ob/Gyn. and of Physiology, University of British Columbia, Vancouver, Canada.

We have reported previously that infusion of norepinephrine (NE) into the third ventricle of ovariectomized adult rats inhibits pulsatile luteinizing hormone (LH) secretion. The receptor specificity of this adrenergic action is not clear, as both α- and β-adrenoceptor agonists can induce the response. In this study we examined the effects of administration of specific α- and β-adrenergic blockers on the intraventricular NE-induced inhibition of LH release. Unanaesthetized long-term ovariectomized rats with intra-atrial cannulae were bled at 10 min intervals, 1 hour before and 2 hours after intraventricular NE infusion (0.06 moles in 2 μl over 2 min). In one experiment, the rats were injected intraperitoneally with phenoxybenzamine (1.5 mg/100 g b.w.), propranolol (0.6 mg/100 g), or an equal volume of saline (as controls) 1.5 hours before NE infusion. In another experiment, intravenous injections of phenoxybenzamine (1.0 mg/100g), or propranolol (0.5 mg/100 g) or saline were given 1 hour before NE administration. Immediately following intraventricular infusion of NE, the control rats showed a decrease in mean blood LH level of ca. 20% ($p<0.05$). Likewise, in the propranolol treated groups, intraventricular NE caused a 22-30% decrease in the mean LH levels ($p<0.01$). By contrast, mean blood LH levels actually increased slightly following NE infusion in the rats injected with phenoxybenzamine, ($p<0.05$). These data suggest that the hypothalamic α-adrenoceptor may be more involved in the inhibition of pulsatile LH release by NE in ovariectomized rats. (Supported by the BCHCRF and the MRC of Canada)

451 POSSIBLE ROLE OF MEMBRANE PHOSPHOLIPIDS IN THE MECHANISMS OF HORMONE SECRETION. A.C. Bonetti*, G. Calderini, E. Galbiati and G. Toffano, Fidia Research Laboratories, Dept. of Biochemistry, Abano Terme, Italy.

Recent evidences indicate the importance of phosphatidylinositol (PI) turnover in the stimulus-secretion coupling in many endocrine organs, particularly the anterior pituitary gland, where the PI cycle appears to be involved in the mechanisms controlling the release of selected hormones. Brain cortex phosphatidylserine (BC-PS) has been shown to be able to stimulate the dopaminergic system in the CNS and to inhibit prolactin secretion in humans as well as in animals. We have investigated the effect of BC-PS on PI turnover in rat pituitary, both in vivo and in vitro. Treatments with BC-PS significantly decrease PI turnover, without affecting other membrane phospholipids metabolisms. In vitro incubation of the glands with micromolar (0.5 μM to 10 μM) concentrations of BC-PS produces inhibitory effects on PI turnover similar to those obtained with dopamine (DA) in the same conditions. Experiments with thyrotropin releasing hormone (TRH) and dopaminergic drugs suggest a possible common mechanism and/or site of action for DA and BC-PS. During aging an unbalance occurs in the hormonal systems and this phenomenon appears to be due to an impairment of hypothalamic control mechanisms. In particular an impairment of the tubero-infundibular dopaminergic neurons seems to be responsible for the high prolactin levels found in the aged rat. Therefore the effect of BC-PS on PI turnover in the pituitary has been examined during aging too. Biochemical data as well as functional correlates (release of hormones from the pituitary) are presented.

452 MORPHOLOGICAL EVIDENCE FOR CELLULAR INTERACTIONS BETWEEN SEROTONINERGIC TERMINALS AND VIP AND GABA-ERGIC ELEMENTS IN RAT SUPRACHIASMATIC NUCLEUS. O. Bosler*, A. Beaudet and M. Tappaz, CNRS, INP 08, B.P. 71, 13277 Marseille Cedex 9, France, Montreal Neurological Institute, 3801 University Street, Montreal, Quebec H3A 2B4 and INSERM U 171, 8, Av. Rockefeller, 69373 Lyon Cedex 2, France.

Cellular relationships between serotonin (5-HT) and vasoactive intestinal polypeptide (VIP) or GABA neurons were investigated by combined radioautographic and immunocytochemical techniques in the suprachiasmatic nucleus (SCN) of rats pretreated with a monoamine oxydase inhibitor and injected in the lateral ventricle with 10^{-5} -10^{-4}M (^{3}H)5-HT. In light microscopic radioautographs prepared from sections reacted with an anti-VIP antibody, (^{3}H)5-HT-labeled axons were found to run in-between and often alongside nerve cell bodies and dendrites showing VIP-like immunoreactivity in the ventral half of the SCN. In sections reacted with an anti-glutamate decarboxylase (GAD) antibody, (^{3}H)5-HT-labeled axonal varicosities were intermingled with GAD-positive varicose axons which formed an extensive plexus throughout the nucleus. In the electron microscope, (^{3}H)5-HT-accumulating terminals were distinct from their immunoreactive congeneers and were frequently seen in direct apposition to VIP immunoreactive perikarya and dendrites as well as to GAD immunoreactive varicosities. While providing a morphological support for functional 5-HT/VIP and 5-HT/GABA interactions in the SCN, these data should be of potential value in determining the neurochemical mechanisms subserving 5-HT mediated regulation of circadian rhythmicity of pituitary hormones secretion. Supported by CNRS (France) and MRC (Canada).

453 ENHANCEMENT OF PLASMA CATECHOLAMINE (CA) RESPONSE TO INSULIN HYPOGLYCAEMIA BY NALOXONE.

P. Bouloux*, N. Lytras, A. Grossman, P. Drury and G.M. Besser, Department of Endocrinology, St. Bartholomew's Hospital, London, UK.

Much evidence suggests a close interaction between endogenous opioids and the sympathoadrenal system in man. The nature of this interaction has been investigated during hypoglycaemia by evaluating the effect of opiate blockade by naloxone on the plasma CA response to intravenous insulin. 8 normal males were studied after an overnight fast. At weekly intervals, the individual effects of saline, naloxone (8mg bolus + 2.5mg/hr), insulin (0.15U/kg) and naloxone plus insulin were studied. Treatments were randomised by latin square design, and administered double blind. Blood was sampled at frequent intervals for 90 mins for assay of catecholamines (HPLC/ECD), cortisol, aldosterone (both RIA) and potassium. Neither saline nor naloxone altered basal plasma CA but naloxone significantly enhanced the plasma noradrenaline and adrenaline response to hypoglycaemia (insulin alone: noradrenaline Δ 0.9±0.26nmol/l, adrenaline Δ 5.02±1.1nmol/l; naloxone + insulin: noradrenaline Δ 1.7±0.18nmol/l, adrenaline Δ 12.3±3.1nmol/l). Naloxone caused a rise in basal **cortisol** and aldosterone levels (plasma cortisol Δ -32±27nmol/l after saline, 34±24nmol/l after naloxone. Plasma aldosterone Δ -5±22pmol/l after saline, 170±70pmol/l after naloxone) but did not alter the cortisol or aldosterone responses following hypoglycaemia. Potassium fell during hypoglycaemia, this fall being accentuated in the presence of naloxone (insulin: potassium Δ -0.65±0.15mmol/l, naloxone + insulin:Δ -0.98±0.1mmol/l). These data provide evidence for an inhibitory modulation of endogenous opioids on the sympathoadrenal response to insulin hypoglycaemia in man. PB is an MRC Training Fellow.

454 *CHOLINERGIC PARTICIPATION ON GROWTH HORMONE AND PROLACTIN SECRETION AFTER PHYSICAL EXERCISE, CLONIDINE, ARGININE AND PLACEBO IN MAN.*

F.F.Casanueva, L.Villanueva, J.Cabranes, J.Cabezas-Cerrato, A.Fernández-Cruz. Endocrinology Unit,School of Medicine, Madrid and Compostela University. Inst.U.Iberoamericano Endocrinología,Metabolismo,Nutrición.Santiago de Compostela. SPAIN.*

To assess the role of acetylcholine (Ach) on the hypothalamic regulation of growth hormone (GH) and prolactin (PRL) paired test were performed in 22 volunteers with and without the muscarinic receptor blocker atropine, 1 mg/ml im, administered 15 min before.As the table shown atropine completely blocks (p<0.05) GH secretion under the three tests employed, without alter PRL secretion by arginine or the GH and PRL basal levels.*

n	*Stimulus*	*Atropine*	*GH peak ng/ml*	*PRL ng/ml*
6	Arginine 30 g/30 min	---	16.6±5	16±3.1
6	" "	Yes	0.9±0.1 *	14±3
6	Clonidine 300 μg po	---	11.8±2.7	8±2
6	" "	Yes	1.2±0.2 *	11±4
5	Ph exercise 80W x 20 min	---	19.4±4.9	---
5	" "	Yes	2.0±0.9 *	---
5	Saline	---	2.0±1	5±2
5	"	Yes	1.0±0.5	5±3

The results suggest that Acetylcholine is a neurotransmitter of highly relevance on GH regulation in man.

455 THE EFFECT OF HMG AND FOLLICULAR FLUID PROTEINS ON 3-BETA-OL-DEHYDROGENASE (3B-OL) ACTIVITY IN MICROSOMES FROM CULTURED HUMAN GRANULOSA CELLS. DA Battin*, GS diZerega, Livingston Lab, Ob/Gyn, USC, LA, CA 90033.

Previously, we reported the identification of a protein fraction (OP) isolated from both human and porcine follicular fluid, which inhibited FSH induced granulosa cell aromatase activity, FSH induction of LH receptors, and hMG augmented rat ovarian weight gain. Recently, we found that OP stimulated 3B-OL activity in cultured porcine granulosa cells. To further investigate the actions of OP, granulosa cells were obtained from patients undergoing oocyte aspiration for in vitro fertilization. Freshly obtained granulosa cells were washed then divided into 10 ml aliquots (500,000 cells per aliquot). Each aliquot was cultured at 37C with either 0, 167, or 500 ug/ml OP and with either 0 or 10 mIU/ml hMG (1:1 FSH:LH). After 48 hours in vitro the cells were separated from the spent media, mechanically lysed, and the cell wall debris removed by centifugation (10,000g). A mircosomal fraction was obtained from the cytoplasm by centifugation at 100,000g. The microsomal fraction was re-suspended in media 199 (2 ml) with 10^{-5}M pregneolone, 5 mM NAD^+, then incubated at 37C. After 2 hours the reaction was stopped (57C for 30 min) and concentrations of progesterone in the spent culture media, cytoplasm, and microsomal fractions determined by radioimmunoassay. Progesterone concentrations are expressed in ng per 500,000 granulosa cells. Progesterone levels in the spent culture media fraction slightly increased when cells were cultured with 167ug/ml OP (1941$\pm$121 ng vs control: 1201$\pm$62 ng, $p<0.05$), then decreased with 500ug/ml OP (1046$\pm$145 ng). The cytoplasm fraction contained elevated levels of progesterone with both the 167ug/ml and 500ug/ml dose of OP (33$\pm$1 ng and 23$\pm$4 ng respectively vs control: 20$\pm$2 ng, $p<0.01$). The microsomes from control cultures produced 3.3$\pm$0.1 ng progesterone. This increased to 3.7$\pm$1.0 ng with 167ug/ml OP and to 4.6$\pm$1.3 ng with 500ug/ml OP ($p<0.05$). When 10 mIU/ml hMG was added to the cultures, microsomes produced 1.4$\pm$0.2 ng progesterone ($p<0.05$). OP increased the progesterone production by microsomes in cultures with hMG, 7.3$\pm$1.0 ng with 167ug/ml OP and 4.1$\pm$0.1 ng with 500ug/ml OP ($p<0.01$). In conclusion, OP altered 3B-OL activity in whole human granulosa cells, their secretory products, and their microsomal fractions. When added together with hMG, OP produced a biphasic response in 3B-OL activity. Thus OP may be an important regulator of human granulosa cell luteinization. (HD-00401)

456 MICROTUBULES, CALCIUM AND THE CONTROL OF GRANULOSA CELL STEROIDOGENESIS.
J.A.Carnegie* and B.K.Tsang, Reproductive Biology Unit, Depts. of Obstetrics & Gynecology and Physiology, University of Ottawa, Ottawa Civic Hospital, 1053 Carling Avenue, Ottawa, Ontario, Canada, K1Y 4E9.

We have previously demonstrated that the calcium-calmodulin system is involved in the FSH-regulation of progesterone production by rat granulosa cells in vitro. We have also shown this stimulation by FSH to be sensitive in culture to the microtubule-depolymerizing agent, colchicine. Calcium influences microtubule depolymerization in many cell types. In this study, we have further investigated a possible relationship between calcium, microtubules and the control of ovarian steroidogenesis by monitoring the effects of two microtubule-depolymerizing agents (colchicine and nocodazole) and one which stabilizes the tubulin polymers on progesterone production by granulosa cells (isolated from 30-day-old estradiol-17β-pretreated rats) stimulated in vitro by FSH (NIAMDD oFSH-13, 0.1 ug/ml) or the ionophore A23187 (0.5 ug/ml), an agent known to facilitate calcium transport across cell membranes. Low concentrations of colchicine (0.003-0.05 µM, $p<0.05$) or nocodazole (0.01 µM, $p<0.01$) enhanced FSH-stimulated progesterone production but higher concentrations [4-256 µM (colchicine) and 10-100 µM (nocodazole)] were inhibitory. The inhibition of steroidogenesis by nocodazole was not accompanied by a reduction in [^{3}H]-leucine incorporation into proteins. Taxol (10 µM) also reduced FSH-stimulated progesterone production by about 55%. In contrast, progesterone production in response to A23187 was unaffected by colchicine (0-256 µM) or taxol (0-10 µM). These findings suggest that while microtubules may be involved in the steroidogenic response of granulosa cells to FSH, their control may be independent of the calcium-requiring FSH-regulated events in the steroidogenic process. (Supported by MRC of Canada).

457 CONTROL OF RAT OVARIAN FOLLICULAR INHIBIN PRODUCTION BY PMSG AND hCG.

Ronald Carson* and Victor Lee, Medical Research Centre, Prince Henry's Hospital, Melbourne, Australia, 3004.

Studies in sheep and rats indicate that follicular inhibin content is related directly to the extent of follicular development and suggest that preovulatory follicles are the major source of inhibin *in vivo*. In this study, inhibin content and production by rat ovarian follicles during the antral phase of development and after luteinization has been examined. Rats were injected with either saline or PMSG (20IU ip) on the morning of day 23 (D23). A group of PMSG-treated animals was also administered a luteinizing dose of hCG (10IU iv) at 0800h on D25. All animals were killed at 1200h and the 5 largest follicles on each ovary isolated and pooled for each animal. Groups of 5 follicles were then either immediately frozen (t_0) or incubated for 4h (t_4) in M199 or M199+hCG (1 or 10IU/ml). Prior to bioassay of inhibin activity, follicular homogenates were treated with charcoal to remove steroids. Injection of PMSG was associated with significantly increased follicular inhibin content (t_0) and production *in vitro* (t_4-t_0) when compared to follicles isolated from saline-treated animals. Treatment of PMSG-primed rats with a luteinizing dose of hCG 4h prior to isolation of follicles resulted in significantly reduced follicular inhibin content and production *in vitro*. In contrast, the addition of hCG to incubation medium did not alter inhibin production *in vitro*. Increased inhibin content (t_0) and production *in vitro* (t_4-t_0) is associated with the transition of follicles from small antral to preovulatory and further exposure to hCG *in vitro* is without effect. Luteinization of preovulatory follicles results in reduced follicular inhibin content and completely abolishes inhibin production *in vitro*. Supported by N.H. & M.R.C.

458 ESTROGEN CONTROL OF CORPUS LUTEUM FUNCTION IN PREGNANT RATS.

V. Chandrashekar* and R.E. Falvo, Medical Physiology and Pharmacology, School of Medicine, Southern Illinois University, Carbondale, IL.62901,USA

To evaluate the role of estrogen on progesterone (P) secretion by the corpus luteum (CL) of pregnant rats, aminoglutethimide phosphate (AGP) was used to block the aromatization of androgens to estrogens. Pregnant rats were divided equally into three groups (n=6/group). Group 1: controls, injected with acetate buffer; Group 2: treated with AGP in acetate buffer, 7.5 mg/100g BW; Group 3: treated with the same dose of AGP plus estradiol-17β (E_2), 100 μg/rat. Acetate buffer or AGP was administered twice and E_2 once daily from days 12-14 of gestation. Blood samples were drawn by cardiac puncture and serum levels of P determined by RIA. The findings are as follows:

Treatment	% Pregnant	Serum progesterone (ng/ml) Before treatment	Serum progesterone (ng/ml) After treatment
Controls	100	61 ± 8.6*	75 ± 15.2
AGP	17	67 ± 13.9	7.9 ± 1.7
AGP + E_2	100	65 ± 5.9	65 ± 10.5

* Mean ± SE.

P secretion by the CL is essential for pregnancy maintenance. Since AGP treatment reduced P levels, whereas AGP + E_2 treated rats retained normal P concentrations and carried viable fetuses to term, our data indicate that estrogen is luteotropic in pregnant rats.

459 VASOACTIVE INTESTINAL PEPTIDE (VIP) STIMULATES STEROID BIOSYNTHESIS BY CULTURED RAT GRANULOSA CELLS. J. Ben Davoren* and Aaron J.W. Hsueh, Department of Reproductive Medicine, University of California, San Diego, La Jolla, CA 92093, USA.

VIP and VIPergic nerve fibers are abundant in the female genital tracts of several mammalian species, including humans. *In vivo* administration of VIP to rabbits results in increased plasma progesterone, suggesting a possible ovarian action of VIP. We have investigated the direct effects of synthetic porcine VIP on rat granulosa cell steroidogenesis *in vitro*. The cells were obtained from immature hypophysectomized, estrogen-primed rats, and cultured in a serum-free medium for 24 hours in the presence of varying amounts of VIP. Medium steroids were then determined by specific radioimmunoassay. VIP dose-dependently stimulated pregnenolone, progesterone, 20α-hydroxypregn-4-en-3-one, and estrogen production with a minimum effective dose of $\sim 10^{-9}$M and an ED_{50} of $\sim 3\times10^{-8}$M. Maximal steroid production induced by VIP was 20-25% that seen with maximal FSH stimulation. VIP appears to act at least partly through cyclic AMP-dependent processes; addition of a phosphodiesterase inhibitor (0.1mM 3-isobutyl-1-methylxanthine) significantly potentiated the VIP stimulation of granulosa cell steroidogenesis. In contrast to VIP, the closely related gastrointestinal peptides secretin and glucagon had no effect on steroid synthesis. These results indicate that VIP exerts a specific action on granulosa cells to increase estrogen and progestin production. The observed direct effects of VIP, coupled with its identification in the female reproductive system, suggest that this gastrointestinal hormone may play a neural or paracrine role in the physiological regulation of ovarian activity.

460 THE EFFECT OF THYMOSIN FRACTION 5 (TSN5), LH AND FSH ON OVARIAN DYSGENESIS IN THYMECTOMIZED (TX) MICE. L. De Angelo*, A. Kaikis-Astaras, and S.D. Michael, Dept. Biol. Sci., Univ. Center at Binghamton, SUNY, Binghamton, N. Y. 13901.

Our previous studies have shown that Tx at 3 days of age in (C57Bl x A/J)F_1 mice results in accelerated reproductive aging. By 60 days of age, the ovaries of these mice are reduced in weight, occupied mostly by interstitial cells, and usually devoid of follicles, oocytes and corpora lutea. Further, Tx-3 females have delayed vaginal openings (VO) and reduced levels of circulating LH and FSH (Biol. Reprod. 22: 343, 1980). The purpose of the present study was to attempt to prevent or retard ovarian dysgenesis with exogenous gonadotropins or TSN5. TSN5, a family of thymic polypeptide hormones, is a potent immunopotentiating preparation which has been able to reconstitute a number of immune functions in humans and animals. Groups of intact, sham Tx-3 and Tx-3 females were treated between 3-10 days of age then sacrificed at 60 days of age for evaluation. Only a dose of 4 mg/kg of TSN5 restored VO to that of the control mice, while both TSN5 and the gonadotropins increased ovarian weights to near control levels. However, only TSN5 treatment maintained normal ovarian morphology. The data demonstrate that replacement with this thymic hormone preparation can overcome the adverse effects on ovarian development caused by Tx-3.

461 STUDIES ON FOLLICULAR ATRESIA: THE INTERPLAY OF GONADOTROPINS AND GONADAL STEROIDS ON LYSOSOMAL ENZYME CATHEPSIN-D OF RAT GRANULOSA CELL. N. Dhanasekharan and N.R. Moudgal*, Cent.for Adv.Study in Reprod.Biol., Lab.of End. Biochem., Ind.Instt. of Sci., Bangalore 560012, India.

We recently reported on the changes that occur during follicular atresia in the lysosomal enzyme activities and gonadotropin receptors of granulosa cells (GC). (Mol.Cell.Endocrinol. 33,97,1983). In the present study using PMSG primed 21 day female rats, the increment in GC cathepsin-D activity and inhibition of steroidogenesis (indices of atresia) brought about by PMSG antiserum (a/s) was arrested by simultaneous injection of FSH or LH Injection of cyanoketone or clomiphene citrate with FSH/LH prevented this 'rescue' thus suggesting a role for estrogen (E_2) in inducing atresia. Administration of E_2 alone to the PMSG+a/s group prevented atresia, cathepsin D activity being held at normal levels. However, E_2 injection could not restore the functionality of these GC. The injection of 5 -dihydrotestosterone (DHT), 48h after PMSG priming, induced atresia as noted by an increase (55%) in cathepsin-D. As exogenous injection of FSH with DHT could prevent the atretic effect, suggesting that DHT is not having a direct effect on atresia of GC. Determination of androgen (A):estrogen (E) ratio in the GC at different times (0-168h) following a PMSG injection showed that while A:E ratio was lower at 48h it increased from 96h and this was concomitant with the induction of cathepsin-D. As early as 60h after PMSG injection E_2 production was reduced by 93%, cathepsin-D activity was beginning to raise while A level remained unchanged. These observations strongly support the idea that lack of E_2 rather than an increase in A is the cause of atresia. (Supported by Ind.Counc.of Med.Res., New Delhi).

462 EFFECT OF ESTRADIOL-17β (E_2) ON FOLLICULOGENESIS IN RHESUS MONKEYS: DOSE-DURATION RELATIONSHIPS. D. J. Dierschke*, R. J. Hutz and R. C. Wolf, Wisconsin Regional Primate Research Center, University of Wisconsin, Madison, Wisconsin 53715-1299 U.S.A.

We demonstrated previously (Biol. Reprod. 25:332, 1981) that E_2 (4 capsules), administered s.c. for 24 or 48 hr from day 6 of the menstrual cycle, induced atresia of the preovulatory follicle (confirmed by morphology and hormonal patterns) in every animal. Present objectives were to determine if this represents an all-or-none effect, and to identify possible "partial atresia" along with resulting effects on luteal function. Cyclic females (n=32) were treated with 4, 2, 1 or 0.5 capsules for 24, 12 or 6 hr. Each capsule increased peripheral concentrations of E_2 by ∿100 pg/ml. Four capsules for 12 hr and 2 or 1 capsule for 24 hr induced atresia in essentially all animals while lesser treatments produced variable results. Half-capsules for any of the durations tested were ineffective in inducing atresia, although ovulation of the original follicle was delayed, i.e., "partial atresia", in 2 of 9 animals so treated. Where atresia was induced, follicular phases were extended ∿8 days, permitting development of a "substitute" follicle. Luteal phases, resulting from ovulation of the original or substitute follicle, were of normal duration. However, corpora lutea were deficient in progesterone secretion in ∿50% of all animals treated, regardless of dose or duration of E_2 treatment. Since evidence of "partial atresia" was rare, we conclude that the atretogenic action of E_2 in this experimental situation is probably all-or-none, exerted directly on the ovary or indirectly through the pituitary; however, subsequent luteal activity may be modified due to altered folliculogenesis. Supported by NIH HD17370.

463 EFFECT OF THE SEX-STERIODS ON URINARY EXCRETION OF VASOPRESSIN IN THE RAT. J.T. Crofton*, P.G. Baer, D.P. Brooks, and L. Share. Dept. of Physiology, UTCHS, Memphis, TN 38163, USA.

Plasma vasopressin concentration was 2.5X, and the 24 h urinary excretion of vasopressin ($U_{ADH}V$) 2X greater ($p<0.01$) in male than female Wistar rats. In an attempt to determine the role of sex-steroids in this difference, $U_{ADH}V$, used as an index of vasopressin secretion from the posterior pituitary, was examined in intact (I) 7-8 wk old male and female rats and in 7-8 wk old male and female rats that were gonadectomized (GX) at 3 wks of age. GX rats were injected s.c. twice over 4 days with vehicle (V), or with depot forms of estradiol (E), progesterone (P), E and P combined (E+P), or testosterone (T). 24 h after the second injection, urine was collected for 24 h for the measurement of $U_{ADH}V$. $U_{ADH}V$ in I males was 7.9 ± 0.7 (S.E.) mU/day. Gonadectomy reduced vasopressin excretion ($p<0.05$) to 5.8 ± 0.8 mU/day. $U_{ADH}V$ in GX males treated with E, P, or E+P was similar to that in GX males and was subtantially lower ($p<0.01$) than values observed in I males. T restored $U_{ADH}V$ in GX males to levels observed in I males. $U_{ADH}V$ was not different when I females, GX females or GX females treated with E, P, or E+P were compared. T, however, increased ($p<0.01$) $U_{ADH}V$ in GX females 2.5X above values observed in I females. Thus, it appears that the female sex-steroids have little or no effect on urinary vasopressin excretion, whereas T plays a stimulatory role. Whether this effect of T is due to increased vasopressin release or a difference in the renal handling of vasopressin remains to be determined. (Supported by USPHS grants HL-12990, HL-19209 and HL-23548).

464 THE EFFECTS OF TESTOSTERONE AND ITS MAJOR METABOLITES ON THE VASOPRESSIN INNERVATION OF THE BRAIN. G.J. De Vries and W. Duetz, Netherlands Institute for Brain Research, IJdijk 28, 1095 KJ, Amsterdam.

Vasopressin (VP) fibers have been reported to innervate various areas in the brain, where VP probably acts as a neurotransmitter. The major sites of origin of the fibers seem to be the paraventricular nucleus, the suprachiasmatic nucleus and the bed nucleus of the stria terminalis (De Vries and Buijs, Brain Res. 273 (1983) 307). The projections of this latter nucleus to the lateral septum and the lateral habenular nucleus are sexually dimorphic with the VP fiber density being higher in male than in female rats (De Vries et al., Brain Res. 218 (1981) 67). After castration of adult male rats, all projections of this nucleus showed a gradual decrease in VP fiber density over a period of 15 weeks to a point where hardly any fibers were found. The original fiber density could be restored by testosterone replacement therapy within four weeks. To determine whether testosterone has to be metabolized before it causes this effect castrated rats were implanted with estrogen (E), dihydrotestosterone (DHT) or a combination of these steroids. DHT alone appeared to be without any effect. E restored the original fiber density, but the staining of the individual fibers was weaker than in normal males. Only the combination of E and DHT was able to restore the original male type of innervation. No effects of hormonal manipulations were found in the VP projections of the paraventricular and the suprachiasmatic nucleus. Ovariectomy of female rats resulted in the same changes in the VP fiber pathways, as did castration in males.

465 LOCALIZATION AND CHARACTERIZATION OF VASOPRESSIN BINDING SITES IN THE AMYGDALA OF THE RAT BRAIN.

D. Dorsa*, F. Petracca, D. Baskin, and L. Cornett. GRECC, VA Med. Center and Univ. of Wash., Seattle, WA and Dept. of Physiology, Univ. of Ark. for Med. Sci., Little Rock, AR, USA.

Vasopressin-containing neurons have been shown to innervate several extra hypothalamic brain structures including the amygdala. We have used autoradiographic and radioligand binding techniques to localize and characterize putative receptors for arginine^8-vasopressin (AVP) in this region of the rat brain.

When brain slices were incubated with ^{3}H-AVP (S.A. - 55 Ci/mMole) and placed in contact with a tritium sensitive film, an intense concentration of specific (displaceable by 1 μM cold AVP) binding sites was identified which included the central and medial amygdaloid nuclei. We then studied binding of ^{3}H-AVP to membranes prepared from amygdala tissue from the brains of 120 male Sprague-Dawley rats. Binding of ^{3}H-AVP was saturable, of high affinity (K_d = 0.49 ± 0.06 nM, n = 3) and reversible. Unlabeled AVP potently displaced labeled AVP from binding (K_i = 0.43 ± 0.09, n = 3) as did the vasopressin pressor antagonist (1-ß-mercapto-ß, p-cyclopentamethylene proprionic acid) 2-(0-methyl) tyrosin-AVP (M-AVP) (K_i = 0.32 ± 0.06, n = 3). Lysine^8-vasopressin was 8 times less potent than AVP and oxytocin and did not compete for binding significantly even in the μM concentration range. Since pressor antagonists such as M-AVP are not potent competitors for binding to antidiuretic vasopressin receptors, these results suggest the existence of a pharmacologically distinct class of receptors for AVP in the medial aspects of the amygdalar region of the rat brain.

This work was supported by the Veterans Administration, NIH Grant NS 20311, and NSF Grant IISP 8011447.

466 EFFECT OF VERAPAMIL UPON THE VASCULAR AND RENAL ACTIONS OF VASOPRESSIN IN MAN.

L. Favre* and M.B. Vallotton, Division of Endocrinology, University Hospital, CH-1211 Geneva, Switzerland.

Vasopressin (AVP) is assumed to act at vascular and renal sites upon two different receptors. To examine the role of calcium in its action, AVP was infused in six normal females (1 ng/kg/min for 2 hours after a 2-hour control period) alone on day 1 and with a concomitant verapamil (V) infusion (3.6 μg/kg/min for 4 hours) on day 2. Urine volume, osmolality, prostaglandins E_2 and $F_{2\alpha}$ were determined for 2-hour periods. V increased heart rate but did not influence mean arterial pressure (MAP). The slight MAP rise induced by AVP (+ 2.1±1.1 mmHg;±sem) was reversed by V (-2.2±0.7 mmHg, $p< 0.01$). By contrast the changes in urinary osmolality (+411±72 mmol/kg and in urinary volume (-600±31 ml) under AVP were not modified by V (+411±33 mmol/kg,ns; -711±91 ml,ns). V did not change basal excretion of PGE_2 (25±9 vs 36±5 ng/2h) and $PGF_{2\alpha}$ (44±5 vs 45±13 ng/2h). The trend of AVP to release PGE_2 (+36±21 ng/2h) was enhanced by V (+83±29 ng/2h, $p<0.05$), whereas $PGF_{2\alpha}$ response was unchanged (+68±15 vs 81±13 ng/2h,ns). In conclusion, calcium-channel blockade by V reduced AVP pressor effect without affecting antidiuresis and renal PG stimulation, suggesting that calcium-dependent mechanisms are involved in the vascular but not in the renal action of AVP.

467 HYPERTENSION AND VASOPRESSIN SECRETION IN CORONARY ARTERY SURGERY.

M.L. Forsling*, S. Hawkins, W. Aveling and T. Treasure, Departments of Physiology, Anaesthetics and Surgery, The Middlesex Hospital Medical School, London, W1P 6DB.

Post-operative hypertension is a frequent occurrence with coronary artery surgery, a systolic pressure in excess of 130 mm Hg (mean 153±2.9 (SE) mm Hg) being seen in 60 consecutive cases in this hospital. Of the possible contributory causes vasopressin (AVP) could be important as there is increasing evidence that vasopressin contributes to blood pressure regulation and plasma hormone levels are known to be elevated during cardiopulmonary bypass. A study was therefore performed on the pattern of AVP secretion in a group of patients aged 30-65 years undergoing routine coronary artery surgery. Arterial blood pressure, right atrial pressure and urine flow were recorded and 12 blood samples taken at various intervals during and after the operation. Plasma AVP was determined using a sensitive specific radioimmunoassay. Induction of anaesthesia and skin incision had no significant effect on vasopressin concentrations which were initially 0.8±0.26 pmol/l. However following sternotomy concentrations were elevated into the pressor range reaching a mean of 66.8±18.5 pmol/l. A further increase was seen after the start of pulsatile bypass. Concentrations remained elevated throughout the course of surgery and for the following 6 h. By 6h after surgery the concentrations had fallen only to 43.7±6.0 pmol/l. Over the course of surgery there was no significant correlation between arterial blood pressure and plasma vasopressin concentrations. However blood pressure was significantly elevated 2h after bypass and in the concentrations observed AVP could play a role.

468 PITUITARY AND PINEAL FUNCTION PRE- AND POSTOPERATIVELY IN PRIMARY HYPERPARATHYROIDISM.

K. Brismar*, S. Werner and L. Wetterberg. Dept. of Endocrinology*, Karolinska Hospital and Dept. of Psychiatry, S:t Görans Hospital, Stockholm. Sweden.

Prolactin and cortisol secretion interact with both the parathyroid and the pineal gland function. Melatonin is reported to be a marker for affective disorders, which often accompany primary hyperparathyroidism, thus the pineal gland may also interact with the parathyroid function. To investigate the role of the pituitary and pineal glands in regulating the parathyroid hormone (PTH) secretion, we studied the diurnal secretion of cortisol, prolactin and melatonin in primary hyperparathyroidism before and after operation. After the removal of a parathyroid adenoma all patients became normocalcemic and melatonin and cortisol secretion diminished significantly while the diurnal secretion patterns were unchanged. Prolactin levels were not changed. The pre-operatively mean levels of S-cortisol and S-melatonin were high compared to the expected levels. Since cortisol and melatonin levels were normalized after the removal of the PTH-adenoma, a primary disorder of these hormones can not be the cause of primary hyperparathyroidism. In vitro- studies have shown that Ca^{++} stimulates the activity of the pineal gland and the adrenal response to ACTH. Thus, this study suggests that the moderately increased levels of circulating Ca^{++} enhanced the synthesis of both cortisol and melatonin most probably by a direct effect on the adrenal and pineal glands. However, it is not excluded that Ca^{++} also interferes with those CNS monoamines regulating the ACTH and melatonin but not prolactin secretion.

469 SEASONAL ALTERATION OF THE 24 HOUR PLASMA MELATONIN PROFILE IN MAN. J. Ehrenkranz*, Columbia U. College of Physicians, N.Y.

The secretion of melatonin in man is sensitive to acute changes in artificial lighting; whether the naturally occurring annual cycle in day length is associated with changes in plasma levels of melatonin is not known. This study characterized the 24 hour profile of melatonin in a group of northern Labrador Eskimo living almost exclusively under natural lighting conditions and exposed to markedly variable day night lengths through the year. Four adult male subjects were studied at four times during the year: March, July, October, January. Blood samples were taken at 2 hourly intervals from 1000 to 2200 hours and at hourly intervals from 2200 to 1000 hours. Subjects were not exposed to any artificial light during the sampling period. Melatonin was measured using a radioimmunoassay validated for human plasma. To exclude interassay variability, all samples from an individual were assayed in a single batch. Statistics were performed using analysis of variance. Both the daily pattern of melatonin secretion as well as the mean 24 hour plasma melatonin concentration varied throughout the year. In July, peak daytime melatonin levels equalled those seen at night, while in January the daytime peaks were less than those seen at night. Mean 24 hour levels of melatonin were greater in March than at other times of the year. This study demonstrates that alteration of both the circadian profile as well as integrated 24 hour levels of plasma melatonin occur seasonally in man.

470 RESULTS OF TRANSSPHENOIDAL ADENOMECTOMY FOR CUSHING'S DISEASE RELATED TO THE PATHOLOGY. C. W. Burke*, C. B. T. Adams and M. M. Esiri, Endocrinology, Neurosurgery and Neuropathology, Radcliffe Infirmary, Oxford. England.

Good results (25 of our 30 patients completely relieved of ACTH excess) can be obtained by adenomectomy in Cushing's Disease and Nelson's syndrome but some problems remain. We attempt to relate these to four types of pathology in the "adenoma"; A, clumps of large polygonal ACTH+ve cells with Crookes cells elsewhere; B, diffuse sheets of smaller ACTH+ve cells variably staining; C, mass of small ACTH+ve cells sandwiched between anterior and posterior pituitary; D, ACTH+ve cells scattered throughout normal looking gland. Problems: (a) 8 of 10 cured with steroid dependence <2 year had A or D type pathology, while 3 of 7 cured with B pathology and 2 of 4 with C pathology were dependent >2 years. The relation between intermediate-lobe hyperplasia and steroid-dependence merits further study. (b) The small (10%) loss of function other than ACTH was equally spread between A, B, C and D. (c) 20/26 cases were GH-deficient post-op; this was unrelated to A, B, C or D or to surgical findings. (d) Our 5 failures were 2 with B and one each A, C and D, but 3 had previous DXR and 1 was invasive. (e) We find more permanent diabetes insipidus (4/30) than with other pituitary disease; this also is unrelated to A, B, C or D or surgical findings.

Our results agree with previous hints that Cushing's disease may be heterogeneous, and more critical studies are needed.

471 REGULATION OF GROWTH HORMONE (GH) SECRETION BY INSULIN-LIKE GROWTH FACTORS (IGF) I AND II IN HUMAN AND RAT PITUITARY CELLS IN VITRO. GP Ceda*, AR Hoffman, DM Wilson, LA Dollar, RL Hintz and RG Rosenfeld. Depts. of Medicine and Pediatrics, Stanford University, Stanford, CA 94305 USA.

The somatomedins (SM), IGF-I and II, inhibit GH secretion by a long loop negative feedback mechanism. We have recently demonstrated the presence of specific membrane receptors for IGF-I, IGF-II and insulin on cultured pituitary cells derived from normal rats, from a human somatotropinoma and from a rat pituitary tumor line (GC). To confirm the biological significance of these receptors, we assessed the ability of insulin and a partially purified, insulin-free SM preparation to inhibit GH secretion by these cultured anterior pituitary cells and compared this potency with the percent of specific binding for IGF-I, IGF-II and insulin. Cells were cultured (300-500 K/well) in the presence of SM (equivalent of 0.3 nM IGF-I and 0.2 nM of IGF-II) or insulin (10 nM) for 4 hours, and the medium then assayed for GH by radioimmunoassay.

Cell type	Specific binding (%)/well			Inhibition of GH secretion (%)	
	IGF-I	IGF-II	Insulin	SM	Insulin
Normal rat	1.2	11.8	0.3	35	0
GC tumor	8.9	1.4	10.2	20	33
Human tumor	5.0	9.3	0.3	47	Not done

Moreover, the simultaneous addition of SM with growth hormone releasing factor (GRF, 10^{-7} M) completely prevented the increase in GH secretion from normal rat and human somatotropinoma cells elicited by GRF alone. These data indicate that 1) the presence of insulin and SM receptors on cultured rat pituitary cells reflect the ability of these peptides to modulate GH secretion and 2) GH secretion from human somatotropinoma cells may be inhibited by SM.

472 SEXUAL DIMORPHISM OF PITUITARY GONADOTROPES DURING POSTNATAL DEVELOPMENT IN THE RAT. H.T. Chen* and J.D. Neill. Dept. of Physiology & Biophysics, Univ. of Alabama in Birmingham, AL 35294

In the present study we applied both the reverse hemolytic plaque assay for studying luteinizing hormone (LH) secretion from single cells and LH immunocytochemistry (ICC) to conduct quantitative studies of the sexual differences in the gonadotrope population during the postnatal period. Pituitary glands from both sexes at different ages were mono-dispersed with trypsin. The cells were incubated in Cunningham chambers in the presence of 10^{-7}M gonadotropin-releasing hormone (GnRH) for measurement of the fraction of cells secreting LH (plaque assay) and the mean amount of LH secreted/gonadotrope (plaque assay), or attached to slides for measurement of the fraction of cells containing LH (ICC). In female rats the fraction of LH secreting cells increased from ∿3% at 5 days of age to ∿10% by 15 days and remained at this level through day 40. It then fell to ∿5% in the adult at proestrus. These data matched closely with the results from ICC. The fraction of cells secreting LH was ∿5% in male rats at 10-20 days of age and was ∿2% in adult males. The fraction of LH containing cells demonstrated by ICC at these ages did not show the sex differences observed in the fraction of cells secreting LH. The mean amount of LH secreted/gonadotrope showed sex differences beginning at 10-20 days of age with larger amounts in females than in males. These results demonstrate that in the female all LH containing cells also secrete LH, whereas in the male at certain developmental stages only half of the gonadotrope population secretes LH in response to GnRH.

473 GONADOTROPIN-SECRETING PITUITARY TUMOR MASQUERADING AS EARLY OVARIAN FAILURE
D. M. Cook*, H. D. Paxton, P. J. Snyder, Oregon Health Sciences University, Portland, OR 97201 and University of Pennsylvania, Philadelphia, PA 19104.

A previously healthy 34 year-old white female presented with amenorrhea and postmenopausal symptoms of eight months' duration. Basal luteinizing hormone (LH) and follicle stimulating hormone (FSH) concentrations in plasma (mIU/ml) were markedly elevated and estradiol (pg/ml) was low. Because of headaches a CT scan was performed demonstrating a pituitary tumor. Preoperative gonadotropin responses to LHRH (Table), estradiol, bromocriptine and TRH were consistent with primary ovarian failure rather than tumor autonomy. Other anterior pituitary hormones were normal by appropriate testing.

LHRH 100 ug I.V.	Preoperative			Postoperative		
	LH	FSH	Estradiol	LH	FSH	Estradiol
Basal	95	134	<10	16	22	101
Peak	264	291	<10	63	44	94

Following tumor removal at surgery the patient's gonadotropin levels fell dramatically and normal menstrual periods resumed. Chromatography of preoperative plasma on G-100 Sephadex revealed LH and FSH immunoreactivity near LH and FSH standards and could not be accounted for by βLH, βFSH or α subunits. The uniqueness of this case lies in the demonstration of reversible amenorrhea in a clinical setting consistent with primary ovarian failure. No single theory adequately explains the data. The elevated LH, FSH and chromatography pattern are consistent with biologically inactive but immunologically reactive hormone. This hypothesis however fails to account for the low estradiol.

474 EFFECTS OF GONADAL STEROIDS ON SUBSTANCE P (SP) CONTENT IN THE ANTERIOR PITUITARY. R. Coslovsky*, R.W. Evans, L.E. Braverman, S.E. Leeman and N. Aronin, University of Massachusetts Medical School, Worcester, MA, 01605.

SP is an undecapeptide present in the central and peripheral nervous systems, gastrointestinal tract and anterior pituitary (AP). We have recently reported a 4-fold increase in immunoreactive SP in the AP of thyroidectomized (TX) male rats. It was noted that the SP content in the AP was 2-3 fold higher in male (M) as compared to female (F) rats (M, 768±183 fmol/mg protein vs F, 206±124; $p < 0.01$), suggesting a possible role of gonadal steroids in the regulation of SP in the AP. Rats were ovariectomized (OVX) and 14 days later AP-SP content was significantly increased (OVX, 410±57 vs control, 106±13; $p < 0.001$). Treatment of OVX rats with estradiol (E_2), 2 μg/rat/day for 5 days, restored values to normal. In contrast, orchiectomy failed to affect AP-SP content. Adrenalectomy did not alter AP-SP in either M or F rats. The daily administration of E_2 to F rats (2 μg/rat for 14 days) decreased AP-SP content (E_2, 122±20 vs control, 293±34; $p < 0.02$). In order to determine whether E_2 could prevent the rise in AP-SP caused not only by OVX but also by TX, E_2 (2 μg/rat/day for 13 days) was administered to F rats beginning the day after OVX and TX. The marked rise in AP-SP content observed 14 days after TX and OVX (TX+OVX, 1382±196 vs OVX, 282±54; $p < 0.001$) was attenuated by E_2 treatment (TX+OVX+E_2, 245±37 vs TX+OVX, 1382±196; $p < 0.001$). Conclusion. The content of SP in the AP is decreased by E_2 administration, suggesting that gonadal steroids may play a role in modulating the synthesis and/or release of SP. E_2 also prevents the marked rise in AP-SP that occurs in TX animals, indicating that E_2 affects the increased pool of AP-SP by mechanisms which are independent of thyroid hormone.

475 PERTUSSIS TOXIN (PT) ACTIONS ON DISPERSED AND CLONAL RAT ANTERIOR PITUITARY CELLS.

M. Cronin*, A. Rogol, R. MacLeod, W. Evans, M. Thorner, G. Myers and E. Hewlett. Univ. of Virginia Sch. Medicine, Charlottesville, VA., U.S.A.

Bordetella pertussis bacteria synthesize a PT protein that appears to covalently modify hormone-receptor coupling to the adenylate cyclase system in many eukaryotic cell types. We have applied this toxin to endocrine cells to study concurrently (in most instances) the effects of PT on cellular cAMP metabolism and specific hormone release. In primary cultures of anterior pituitary cells, PT significantly reduces the ability of dopamine agonists to inhibit basal, vasoactive intestinal peptide-, forskolin- and cholera toxin-stimulated cAMP levels and prolactin release. In the somatotroph, PT potentiates growth hormone (GH) releasing factor- and prostaglandin E_2-stimulated cAMP accumulation and GH release, but attenuates the ability of somatostatin to reverse these actions. In the gonadotroph, PT increases the efficacy of gonadotrophin releasing hormone-amplified luteinizing hormone release. Some of these responses can also be measured in clonal cells derived from pituitary tumors. In the GH_4C_1 clone, PT reverses the somatostatin-induced inhibition of cholera toxin-evoked cAMP accumulation. In the 235-1 clone, PT increases prostaglandin E_1- cholera toxin- and forskolin-stimulated cAMP levels while having no apparent effect on cell growth. The actions of PT can be prevented with an antibody against PT protein. However, once the PT effects are established, they last for days *in vitro*. It is suggested that the PT protein acts on a highly conserved, constitutive component(s) that is obligatory for transducing inhibitory hormonal messages, and is at least permissive for the expression of stimulatory hormone receptors that are coupled to adenylate cyclase. (Supported by RCDA 1K04NS500601, NS18409, AM32632, CA07535 & HD00439.)

476 INCREASED PROLACTIN RELEASE AFTER SEQUENTIAL TRH AND METOCLOPRAMIDE ADMINISTRATION IN PRIMARY EMPTY SELLA.

L.De Marinis,A.Mancini*,C.Anile, G.Maira,and A.Barbarino. Institutes of Internal Medicine,Division of Endocrinology, and Neurosurgery,The Catholic University School of Medicine Rome, Italy.

Recent studies have documented that in normal subjects dopaminergic antagonist drugs induced considerable additional PRL secretion when injected during TRH infusion.This observation suggests that prolonged TRH infusion is not capable of depleting the pituitary PRL stores. We have studied the PRL response to sequential stimulation with TRH and metoclopramide in normal subjects and patients with primary empty sella (PES). Metoclopramide (MCP,10 mg p.o.) was administered 60 min after the injection of 200 µg TRH i.v. In normal subjects after TRH injection PRL levels increased sharply,with peak values occurring at 30 min.PRL levels decreased gradually to normal values after 60 min.Although a similar pattern of response was observed in patients with PES,after 60 min PRL values were still elevated. Following MCP administration a greater PRL increment($p < 0.001$) was present at 60 min in patients with PES than in normal subjects. These data indicate that MCP exerts its action even on recently stimulated lactotropes and suggest that an altered dopaminergic regulation of PRL secretion is present in patients with PES. The nature of this alteration awaits further clarification.

477 HYPOTHALAMIC-ADENOHYPOPHYSEAL ORIGIN OF REPRODUCTIVE FAILURE FOLLOWING INFECTION WITH THE PARASITE TOXOPLASMA GONDII. J.A. Dias* and W. Stahl, Dept. of Biochemistry, Albany Medical College and Division of Laboratories and Research, New York State Dept. of Health, Albany, NY 12208, USA.

Female albino mice (Nya:NYLAR) were infected with the Cornell strain of Toxoplasma gondii (T. gondii) at 8-10 weeks of age. After six months, infected mice failed to cycle and vaginal smears revealed a diestrus cytology. Body weight of control and infected animals were not different ($P < 0.01$). Infected mice were treated with either saline or 20 ng of D-Leu^6-des-Gly-NH$_2$-Pro-ethylamide (D-Leu^6) three times a day for 3 days. Infected animals treated with D-Leu^6 had greater pituitary weight ($P < 0.01$), ovarian weight ($P < 0.01$) and uterine weight ($P < 0.025$) than infected animals treated with saline. In addition, a change in vaginal cytology from diestrus to estrus, metestrus and protestrus of the D-Leu^6 treated animals was observed. The infected and uninfected animals both had the same basal levels of serum luteinizing hormone (LH). However, infected animals exhibited a decreased pituitary responsiveness (LH released) when examined at 60 ($P < 0.025$) and 120 min ($P < 0.01$) following intraperitoneal administration of D-Leu^6. The etiology of reproductive failure appears to involve the readily releasable pool of pituitary LH since basal LH is similar in both groups. This study demonstrates that infection of mice with T. gondii results in infertility. This infertility appears to involve a dysfunction of the hypothalamic-adenopophyseal axis following parasitosis.

Supported in part by NIH-HD-16675.

478 VASOACTIVE INTESTINAL PEPTIDE (VIP) INCREASES PROLACTIN mRNA CONTENT IN GH3 CELLS. A.J. Carrillo*, T.B. Pool and Z.D. Sharp, Department of Cellular and Structural Biology, The University of Texas Health Science Center, San Antonio, TX 78284

This experiment was designed to determine if the stimulation of prolactin secretion by VIP is associated with an increase in prolactin mRNA production. GH3 cells were incubated in 2ml of Ham's F-10 medium with heat inactivated serum (10% fetal calf and 2.5% horse), 10ug/ml gentamicin sulfate and 10^{-5}M Bacitracin with the following hormones: VIP ($2x10^{-7}$M, $2x10^{-8}$M and $2x10^{-9}$M), TRH ($2x10^{-7}$M), dexamethasone sulfate, (Dex) ($2x10^{-7}$M) and VIP + Dex (both $2x10^{-7}$M). 25 hrs. later the media were removed and frozen for prolactin determination (RIA). The cells were counted, lysed and the cytoplasm processed for prolactin mRNA determination using the cytoplasmic dot hybridization techniques with a prolactin ^{32}P-cDNA. The three different concentrations of VIP resulted in a dose response increase in cytoplasmic prolactin mRNA content with $2x10^{-7}$M producing a two-fold increase when compared to controls. TRH resulted in an increase in prolactin mRNA content that was equivalent to that stimulated by $2x10^{-7}$M VIP. Dex resulted in a significant reduction of prolactin mRNA content however, VIP ($2x10^{-7}$M) reversed the inhibitory effect of Dex and increased the content of prolactin mRNA to a level comparable to that achieved after $2x10^{-8}$M VIP alone. Prolactin secretory rates after these various hormone treatments were parallel to those observed on prolactin mRNA content. These results suggest that VIP, like TRH and Dex, influences prolactin secretion by altering the concentration of prolactin mRNA. Supported by NIH Grant NS15454 and Texas State Funds OR004.

479 PROLACTIN DYNAMICS IN LONG DISTANCE RUNNERS WITH AND WITHOUT MENSTRUAL DYSFUNCTION. Frank E. Chang*, Stephen R. Richards, Moon H. Kim, William B. Malarkey, Depts. of Ob-Gyn and Endocrinology, Ohio State University, Columbus, Ohio 43210

Long distance runners have a high incidence of oligo-amenorrhea. In order to study the possible role of PRL in contributing to this menstrual dysfunction, we have studied eumenorrheic and oligo-amenorrheic runners who averaged 25-40 miles/week as well as non-running controls during the mid-follicular phase of their cycles. Serum PRL was determined by assaying samples acquired hourly over a 24-hour period. The following day they received a dopamine infusion (0.004μg/kg/min. for 180 mins.) which produced physiologic serum dopamine levels to explore potential differences in dopaminergic tone.

SUBJECTS	MEAN 24 hr.* PRL (ng/ml + S.E.)	DOPAMINE INFUSION* MAX CHANGE FROM BASELINE
Controls (n=5)	13.6 ± 2.2	-41.0%
Eumenorrheic (n=7)	14.4 ± 1.7	-46.5%
Oligo/Amenorrheic (n=9)	16.2 ± 1.5	-49.0%

(* ANOVA - no difference between groups)

In conclusion, normal 24 hour PRL secretion and normal PRL responses to dopamine in oligo-amenorrheic runners suggest that PRL didn't play a major role in the menstrual dysfunction seen in these runners.

480 DECREASED SECRETION OF rPLI IN THE HYPOPROLACTINEMIC IPL NUDE RAT. H. Cohen*[1], M.C. Robertson and H.G. Friesen, [1]Inserm U34 Hopital Debrousse, 69332, Lyon, France and Dept. of Physiology, University of Manitoba, Winnipeg, Manitoba, Canada R3E 0W3.

The IPL nude rat is characterized by a total lack of lactation, even though the mammary gland develops normally during pregnancy. We have previously reported that male and female rats are hypoprolactinemic regardless of whether serum samples are measured by RIA or by bioassay (BA). Moreover,the PRL BA/RIA ratio is decreased, indicating that circulating PRL is less bioactive in the IPL nude rat than in normals. In this study, we report the values of serum placental lactogens measured in IPL nude rat compared to normal rat. Groups of 8 female pregnant IPL or normal rats were decapitated at different days of gestation, the day of sperm detection being designated day 0. The two forms of placental lactogens were measured by the Nb2 lymphoma cell bioassay, while rPLII was also estimated by RIA. At day 11, rPLI values were 2997 ± 353 and 5775 ± 372 ng/ml respectively in IPL nude compared to normal rats. This difference is highly significant ($p < .01$). The rPLII values as measured by RIA or Nb2BA were found to be similar in IPL nude and normal rats. Thus the secretion of PRL as well as the larger form of placental lactogen (rPLI) in the IPL nude rat is deficient. These results suggest that a common genetic regulatory defect leads to a deficiency of secretion of both a placental and pituitary lactogenic hormone and may imply a chromosomal linkage of the two lactogenic hormones.

481 HORMONAL REGULATION OF PROLACTIN RECEPTORS IN PORCINE MAMMARY TISSUE. M.H. Dehoff*, R.J. Collier, F.W. Bazer, R.R. Kraeling, Dairy and Animal Science Dept., University of Florida, Gainesville, Florida 32611 and USDA Russell Research Ctr., Athens, Georgia 30603.

Two trials examined relationships between hormone and PRL receptor (R) concentrations, and mammary development in pigs. In Trial I blood and mammary tissue samples were taken from 3 gilts each on day (d) 15,30,45,60,75, 90,105 and 112 of pregnancy, parturition (dP) and d 4 of lactation (dL). The R were determined from radioreceptor assays utilizing $[^{125}I]$oPRL. Available R corrected to gram of tissue wet weight (fM/gWW) were 26.4, 156.7 and 347.9 ($P<.01$) for periods d 15-45, d 60-90 and d 105-dL, respectively. Total estrogens (E) rose at d 30 (3.1 ± 1.4 ng/ml) then declined on d 45 and began to rise at d 60 to a second peak (21.4 ± 1.6 ng/ml) on d 112. Progesterone varied little (25 ± 5.0 ng/ml) until a dramatic drop at d 112 associated with dP. Mean PRL remained below 15 ng/ml through d 105; values increased to 87.2,62.0 and 37.3 ng/ml for d 112, dP and dL respectively. Available R in Trial I resemble patterns of E and metabolic activity of mammary tissue (Kensinger et al. 1982, J. An. Sci. 54:1297). Trial II utilized 3 control (C) and 3 treatment (T) pseudopregnant pigs on d 60,90 and 112. T received 5 mg 17β-estradiol valerate daily from d 45 through last sample day; C received corn oil vehicle. Mean wet weight of a single gland was greater in T than C (436.4 vs 156.0 g). Available R were higher on d 60 and 90 in T than C (228.1 vs 26.6, 355.9 vs 85.0 [fM/gWW]), but not different on d 112, likely due to higher circulating PRL in T on d 112 ($P<.01$). Mammary growth in the pig is associated with increased R and estrogen may be involved in regulation of mammary R during pregnancy.

482 PATTERNS OF PROLACTIN (PRL) RELEASE CAUSED BY AGENTS THAT AFFECT CALCIUM, PROTEIN KINASE C AND CYCLIC AMP. D. Delbeke*, I. Kojima, P.S. Dannies, and H. Rasmussen, Depts. of Pharm. & Internal Med., Yale School of Medicine, New Haven, Conn., USA

We have investigated the time course of PRL release using TRH, TPA (12-O-tetradecanoylphorbol-13-acetate, which activates protein kinase C), A23187 (an ionophore that mobilizes Ca^{++}), forskolin (which activates adenylate cyclase) or a combination of these agents. We cultured the pituitary tumor cell strain GH_4C_1 on cytodex beads, and perifused the cells. Release was measured at 2 min intervals. TRH (100 nM) increased PRL release within 2 min 3- to 5-fold above basal levels; the rate of release decreased to normal within 30 min. TPA (50 nM) caused a 2-fold release within 4 to 6 min, that was sustained for 30 min or more. A23187 (20 uM) caused only a small and transient response; combined TPA and A23187 induced release similar to that caused by TRH. Forskolin (1 uM) also had little effect by itself, but potentiated release caused by either combined TPA and A23187 or by TRH. In the presence of forskolin, release of PRL was sustained. These data are consistent with a model in which 2 branches of the Ca^{++} messenger system participate in the action of TRH: a calmodulin branch largely responsible for the initial phase of response, and a C-kinase branch responsible for the sustained phase of secretion. Forskolin, by regulating the cAMP content of the cell, determines the set point around which the Ca^{++} messenger system operates. These data are similar to those found in adrenal glomerulosa cells (BBRC 116: 555, 1983) and pancreatic islets (BBRC 117: 444, 1983).

483 PROLACTIN INHIBITS OVARIAN STEROIDGENESIS BEYOND C-AMP IN RAT.
R. Demura*, T. Suzuki, T. Yamaguchi, K. Jibiki, E. Odagiri, H. Demura and K. Shizume. Dept. of Internal Medicine, Tokyo Women's Medical College, Tokyo, Japan.

Inhibitory effect of prolactin on ovarian steroidgenesis has been demonstrated in man, but it is still controversial in rat. Adult female rats were made hyperprolactinemic by injecting 0.5 mg/kg/day of domperidone (D) s.c. for 3 weeks and subjected to the studies. Estrous cycle became ambiguous in D group. Short term incubation of chopped whole ovarian tissues demonstrated that estradiol (E_2) and progesterone (P) secretion in D group during 30 min period was not different under basal condition but the increase of E_2 and P to 10 IU of HCG was suppressed to 66 % of normal control at proestrous stage. C-AMP and GMP production was not different in 2 groups at any conditions. Ovine prolactin, 10 IU, did not affect E_2, P and C-AMP production from normal proestrous ovaries, chopped and incubated as above, under basal condition, but reduced the response of E_2 and P to 10 IU of HCG to 72 % of control without influencing C-AMP production.Ovarian content of DHEA, androstenedione, testosterone, E_2 and E_1 was decreased to 55-83 % of normal, while that of progesterone and 17-OH prog. was the same. It was suggested from above results that prolactin also has inhibitory effects on ovarian steroidgenesis in rat mainly through decreased production of androgens and this effect may not be mediated C-AMP.

484 DEFECTIVE CENTRAL NERVOUS DOPAMINERGIC SYSTEM IN RATS WITH ESTROGEN-INDUCED PITUITARY TUMORS.
T. Di Paolo*, P. Falardeau, G. Pelletier and N. Barden, Department of Molecular Endocrinology, Laval University Hospital Center, Quebec, G1V 4G2, Canada.

Prolactin (PRL)-secreting tumors represent the majority of hormone-secreting pituitary adenomas, but it is uncertain whether a central nervous system (CNS) disturbance or autonomous lactotroph growth and function is the most important aspect of their pathogenesis. We have studied dopamine (DA) metabolism in rats bearing estradiol-induced PRL-secreting pituitary tumors recently characterized as a model for human prolactinoma (Endocrinology 110: 590, 1982). Female rats were injected at 3-week intervals with 2 mg estradiol valerate (EV) or with diluent. EV first induced hyperplasia and then, 10 weeks after, adenomatous changes in the pituitary gland were seen. Concurrently, there was a striking rise in plasma PRL concentrations, up to 3 μg/ml at 35 weeks. Inversely, there was a progressive reduction of DA and dihydroxyphenylacetic acid (DOPAC) in the median eminence and arcuate nucleus while dopaminergic nuclei in the nigro-striatal, meso-limbic and meso-cortical pathways were not affected. The ratio DOPAC/DA in the median eminence and arcuate nucleus was unchanged after 1 week, it then progressively decreased and was significantly lower after 10 weeks of estradiol. Anterior pituitary weight increased progressively while its DA concentration (expressed per pituitary, per mg of tissue, or per mg of protein) decreased during estradiol treatment. In the neurohypophysis, DA concentrations were unchanged while DOPAC decreased progressively. Our data suggest that rats with primary estrogen-induced PRL-secreting tumors have a defect in the CNS-DA neurotransmission. (Supported by the MRC).

485 A RAT MODEL FOR THE SEPARATION OF DIFFERENT PROLACTIN RELEASE MECHANISMS.
K.D. Döhler*, B. Jarzab, C.C. Wong and A. von zur Mühlen, Dept. Clinical Endocrinology, Medizinische Hochschule, 3000 Hannover, W. Germany.

A number of endogenous and exogenous stimuli are known to activate the release of prolactin. Very little is known, however, about the detailed central nervous and pituitary mechanisms involved in this process, and whether different stimuli (e.g. suckling, stress, proestrus) may activate prolactin release via the same or via different central nervous mechanisms. We recently discovered one strain of rats, the BS/Ztm rat, which may function as a useful model for the separation of different prolactin release mechanisms. In contrast to other strains of rats the BS/Ztm rat does not release prolactin in response to stress (i.e. cage transport, handling or ether vapor); corticosterone release in response to stress, however, is normal. The inability to release prolactin in response to stress seems to be an isolated defect in this rat strain, since storage of prolactin in the pituitary gland and release of prolactin in response to TRH or to dopamin antagonists is normal. Furthermore, female BS/Ztm rats are able to lactate, and they show normal release of prolactin in the afternoon of proestrus and in response to estrogen treatment. In search for localization of this defect in the mechanism of stress-dependend prolactin release we observed that, in contrast to Sprague-Dawley rats, BS/Ztm rats did not release prolactin in response to the serotonin precursor 5-hydroxy tryptophane or to CRF. The results indicate that prolactin release in response to stress is activated by a different mechanism than prolactin release in response to other stimuli. The stress-induced mechanism of prolactin release seems to include serotonin and/or CRF and is defective in the BS/Ztm rat.

486 DEMONSTRATION OF A DIRECT ARTERIAL BLOOD SUPPLY TO THE ANTERIOR PITUITARY GLAND OF RATS WITH ESTROGEN INDUCED PROLACTIN SECRETING TUMORS.
K.A. Elias* and R.I. Weiner, Dept. OB/GYN and Reprod. Sci., UCSF, San Francisco, CA

We have previously reported that microspheres are able to reach the anterior pituitary (AP) of rats with prolactin (PRL) secreting tumors induced by estradiol (E_2). This observation is consistent with a direct arterial blood supply to the AP since microspheres are too large to transverse capillaries and thus are trapped in arterioles. We have confirmed and expanded this observation using a vascular cast technique. Fischer 344 rats were ovariectomized and implanted with 1 cm E_2 filled or empty silastic capsules. After 26 or 63 days rats were anesthetized and injected with $2x10^6$, 15 μ microspheres in the left ventricle of the heart. Rats were perfused via the aorta with Microphil, a cast material. Dissection of the AP of E_2 treated animals (N=6) from a ventral approach revealed numerous arteries entering the gland. Microspheres were trapped in the terminal branches of these arteries. These new arteries were observed to originate from the basilar, internal carotid, posterior communicating and anterior cerebral arteries. In 3 control rats no arteries were observed to enter the AP while in one a small artery was seen. These results demonstrate that E_2 induced tumorigenesis of the AP is associated with development of a direct arterial blood supply. These arteries carry systemic blood with low levels of dopamine thus regions supplied by them would escape from dopaminergic inhibition. We hypothesize that removal of dopaminergic inhibition in concert with estrogenic stimulation results in tumor formation. Supported by NIH grants HD08935 and HD06243.

487 MORPHOLOGICAL STUDIES ON MICROVASCULATURE OF MICRO- AND MACROPROLACTINOMAS
A.Erroi, A.Spada*, M.Bassetti, G.Giannattasio CNR Center of Cytopharmacology, Department of Pharmacology and Chair of Endocrinology, School of Medicine, University of Milan, Milano, Italy

The microvasculature of 9 micro- and 9 macroprolactinomas has been studied by means of morphological techniques (light and electron microscopy and morphometry). The main difference found between micro- and macroadenomas was related to the frequency of capillaries, which was higher in micro- than in macroprolactinomas (51.5 vs 9.3 capillaries/0.1 mm^2 of tissue section). The abnormalities observed in human adenomas by others (thikening, swelling and bledding of the endothelium, loss of fenestration, multilayer basement membrane etc.) were found in micro- and macroprolactinomas. In both types of tumor the capillaries were mature and in all tissue sections sprouting capillaries were very rare. From these data one could infer that, due to the low growth rate of capillaries, in macroprolactinomas the microvasculature cannot keep up with the parenchymal cell proliferation. The different frequency of capillaries in micro- and macroprolactinomas could have important consequences: in fact, because of the different blood supply which reaches micro- and macroprolactinomas, the concentration of the factors which regulate prolactin secrètion could be, at cell level, very different in the two types of tumor.

488 EFFECT OF ATRIAL NATRIURETIC FACTOR (ANF) ON URINARY PROSTAGLANDINS IN THE RAT.
J. Gutkowska*, G. Thibault, R. Garcia, M. Cantin and J. Genest, Clinical Research Institute of Montreal, Montreal, Quebec, H2W 1R7, Canada.

The presence of a powerful diuretic and natriuretic peptide in atrial specific granules has received ample confirmation. Forty female Sprague Dawley rats were anesthetized with pentobarbital and a bladder and intrajugular vein catheter were installed. The animals received an infusion of 5% dextrose (2.1 ml/hr) before the assay and during the collection period. After a preassay period, the animals were injected with an acid extract of the right and left atrium of one rat in 1 ml of Krebs fluid. Urine was collected in preweighted vials for two 20 min period, one before the assay and the other immediately following the injection of ANF. PGE_1 and PGE_2 were measured in urine by specific immunoassays (Desjardins-Giasson et al., Prostaglandins 24:105, 1982). Urinary PGE_2 excretion during the preassay period was 73.3 ± 1.7 pg/min and increased to 2550.2 ± 237.0 pg/20 min after the injection of ANF. PGE_1 excretion went from 200.5 ± 19 pg/min to 422.4 ± 45.7 pg/20 min after the injection of ANF. Although indomethacin does not alter the diuresis induced by ANF (Keeler, R., Can. J. Physiol. Pharmacol. 60:1078, 1982), the present results indicate that injection of the peptide is followed by a significant increase in the urinary excretion of both PGE_1 and PGE_2. This study was supported by the MRC group grant.

489 THE USE OF LONAZOLAC (LON) AND INDOMETHACIN (IND) AND ITS INFLUENCE ON OVUM TRANSPORT (OT) IN THE RABBIT. H. Khalil; T. Vancaillie and W. Schlegel. Univ.-Frauenklinik, 4400 Münster, W-Germany.

The cyclo-oxygenase and the prostaglandin-15-hydroxydehydrogenase were selectively inhibited by IND and LON by continuous intrauterine or single vaginal applications. 9 series of 3-4 does were primed with 25 IU hMG per kg. In 6 series an Alzet osmotic minipump (Model 2ML1) was inserted with its outlet into the right uterine horn. The 3 treatment regimen were: 1) vehicle, 2) IND: 100 ug/h, and 3) LON: 100 ug/h infused. 3 days later ovulation was induced by 100 IU hCG iv, followed by artificial insemination. In 3 series without pump, 1 mg of drug or placebo were vaginally applied. Both oviducts were divided into 3 equal parts - isthmus (I), ampullo-isthmic junction (AIJ) and ampulla (A) - and flushed separately, 27 hours after insemination in 3 series (P) with and 3 series (V) without pump, 51 hours after insemination in the 3 remaining series (P^{o}). The ovum recovery (OR) expresses the relation of the sum of ova to the number of corpora lutea, the relative ovum recovery (ROR) the proportion of ova recovered in a particular part of the oviduct, related to the OR. The results of the 3 control series (C) indicate an inhibition of OT due to the surgery itself (OR-C-V: 75.3%, P: 1.6%). IND abolishes the inhibiting effect of the manipulation, moreover it enhances the OT (ROR-I-IND-P^{o}: 94.0% vs ROR-I-C-P^{o}: 40.1%). The latter effect is also apparent in the V series (ROR-I-IND-V: 5.0% vs ROR-I-C-V: 0.3%). LON treatment in the P^{o} series resulted in a ROR comparable with the control series (ROR-I-LON-P^{o}: 36.1%). But the relative higher dose applied in the V series, provoqued a marked enhancement of the OT (ROR-I-LON-V: 26.5%). In conclusion, our data indicate that prostaglandins are actively involved in the OT, particularly at the level of the isthmus.

490 ISOSEXUAL PRECOCIOUS PUBERTY ASSOCIATED WITH TEMPORAL ARACHNOID CYST. S.M. Corsello°, G.De Rosa, C.Di Rocco and M.Caldarelli, Institutes of Endocrinology and Neurosurgery, Catholic University School of Medicine, Rome, Italy.

Although various intracranial diseases can be associated with isosexual precocious puberty, the combination arachnoid cyst-pubertas precox is very unusual and only eleven cases have been reported to date.

We recently observed a male with true isosexual precocity secondary to a left temporal arachnoid cyst. The boy was admitted at 11 years of age, with a 3-year hystory of precocious puberty, seizure disorder and psychomotor impairment. On admission body weight was 57 kg, height was 160 cm and the stage of sexual development was P-5 according to Swerdloff criteria. Bone age was interpreted as 16 years. RIA determination of basal serum levels of the following hormones showed a male adult pattern: Testosterone 3,9 ng/ml; Androstenedione 1,45 ng/ml; DHEAS 920 ng/ml; 17-OH-Progesterone 1,7 ng/ml; FSH 6,9 mIU/ml; LH 14,3 mIU/ml. A mature pattern of gonadotropin release was also found after LHRH stimulation (100 µg i.v.): FSH 7,6 at 30' and LH 43,2 at 30'.TeBG binding capacity was 0,73µgDHT/dl,as in adult controls.Neuroradiological study(CT scan,left carotid arteriography,RISA cisternography)showed a cyst in the left polar temporal region communicating whit optic and chiasmatic cisternae. At surgery the diagnosis of arachnoid cyst was confirmed. A cysto-peritoneal shunt was inserted and a complete regression of the lesion was noticed at the follow-up examination.

491 A MIXED HETEROZYGOTE FOR LATE-ONSET AND CLASSICAL FORMS OF CONGENITAL ADRENAL HYPERPLASIA (21-HYDROXYLASE DEFICIENCY).

R. Couch* and J.S.D. Winter, Department of Pediatrics, University of Manitoba, Winnipeg, Manitoba, R3E 0W1, Canada.

We have previously described (Am J Med 68:441, 1980) a family with late-onset CAH and established by HLA typing that the defect appeared to be allelic with classical CAH. With steroid therapy the proband began to ovulate and became pregnant, producing a female infant with normal genitalia. The infant's basal serum 17OH-progesterone remained elevated (12.5-16.5 nM) during the first 2 months, although her serum testosterone was normal. Investigation at age 5 months showed: normal growth and bone maturation; normal urine 17KS (4.0 μmol), cortisol (30 nmol) and 17OHCS (4.1 μmol); a normal serum cortisol response, but a markedly excessive 17OHP response (58.0 nM at 30 min) to ACTH stimulation; and suppression of serum 17OHP (2.5 nM), cortisol ($<$30 nM) and urinary steroids by dexamethasone. ACTH testing of the father and paternal grandfather showed responses which suggested they were heterozygous for classical CAH. HLA typing of the entire family showed concordance between the genotype and ACTH response, and suggests this infant is a mixed heterozygote for the late-onset and classical forms of CAH. She may therefore be at risk for later premature adrenarche, hirsutism or virilization.

492 DEVELOPMENTAL PATTERN OF 5-ANDROSTENE-3β, 17β-DIOL (DIOL) IN HUMAN.

E.de Peretti[+], M.J.Asensio, E.Mappus and M.G.Forest. INSERM-U.34.Hôpital Debrousse. 69322 Lyon Cedex 05. France.

Plasma Diol was measured by specific RIA after celite column chromatography in 223 normal boys and girls 1-17 year old and in 36 adult volunteers. Results in mean±SD are given in ng/dl. In adults, Diol levels were significantly ($p < 0.001$) higher in males (148±47) than in females (73±14). In children, plasma Diol, low in the first 5 years of life (10±4), rose steadily until the 13th year of life with no sex difference (40±12). A significant positive correlation ($r = 0.75$) was found between Diol and either DHA or DHAS. In pubertal children (13-18 year old), plasma Diol continued to rise with age but did so more rapidly in boys than in girls. Plasma Diol was extremely low in prepubertal children with adrenal insufficiency (AI) ($<$ 5) but rose in parallel with Testosterone (T) in boys with AI during pubertal development. In normal prepubertal boys, plasma Diol rose 5 fold (21±1 to 114±44) after hCG stimulation test (1500 IU x 7/48 h), ten times less however than T (13±11 to 626±365). A positive correlation ($r = 0.74$) was found between Diol and T. No rise was observed in 4 agonadal boys. In 3 boys (3-8 year) with precocious puberty, plasma levels of both Diol and T were in the adult range. In conclusion, the temporal pattern observed in normal children together with the other data presented here, suggest that plasma Diol is mainly of adrenal origin before puberty; the testis contribute significantly (≃ 40 %) to the plasma pool of Diol in pubertal or adult males.

493 PROGESTERONE RECEPTOR-OVALBUMIN GENE INTERACTION: A BINDING SITE IDENTIFIED ADJACENT TO THE PROMOTER,
J. G. Compton*, K. Townsley, W.T. Schrader, and B. W. O'Malley, Department of Cell Biology, Baylor College of Medicine, Houston, TX 77030 U.S.A.

In previous reports we have shown that purified progesterone receptor A from chicken oviducts preferentially binds DNA fragments containing the 5'-flanking sequences of target genes. An analysis of receptor binding to DNA fragments from a series of deletion DNA constructions containing progressively shorter ovalbumin 5'-flanking sequences indicates that selective receptor binding requires elements between -77bp and -222bp upstream from the gene. Direct interaction of receptor A with the DNA has been observed by DNaseI footprinting. In solution, receptor effects on coding strand cleavage extend between -78bp and -240bp and appear to be grouped into several, nearly contiguous regions protected (-78:-96, -117:-139, -205:-240) or protected and enhanced (-145:-154, -176:-187) cleavages. On filters, where single protein-DNA complexes (1:1) predominate, protein effects on DNaseI cleavage are seen primarily between -155bp and -190bp. Surprisingly, experiments to date with the non-coding strand show few comparable effects. The location of this in vitro receptor binding site(s) coincides with the sequence requirements for progesterone induction of transcription of an ovalbumin-β-globin fusion gene in chicken oviduct cells. This suggests that progesterone action in target cells is mediated, at least in part, by receptor binding adjacent to the promoter of affected genes. Supported by HD-07857 and HD-07495.

494 MELATONIN-INDUCTION OF ESTROGEN RECEPTOR HORMONE BINDING ACTIVITY IS ASSOCIATED WITH INHIBITION OF E_2-STIMULATED GROWTH OF MCF-7 HUMAN BREAST CANCER CELLS.
DN Danforth Jr.,* L Tamarkin, and ME Lippman. National Cancer Institute, and the National Institute of Child Health and Development, NIH, Bethesda, Maryland, 20205, USA.

We have previously shown that melatonin (M) enhances the ER hormone binding activity of human breast cancer cells in vitro (Nature 305:323, 1983). Enhancement is rapid, requires protein synthesis, and persists for at least 5 hours in the presence of melatonin. We now report the activation and growth stimulation properties of ER in M treated cells. The cytosolic ER sediments at 8S in low salt sucrose density gradients (SDG). Unoccupied nuclear ER (R_n) sediments at 4.4S in high salt SDG. R_n is salt extractable, and following binding to ^{3}H-estradiol at 0^oC in 0.4M KCL binds to DNA cellulose to an extent equivalent to R_n from control cells. M, given alone or simultaneously with E_2, did not alter the growth rate. When given either 4 or 24 hours prior to E_2 a 25% reduction in growth was observed after 6 days of incubation with 10^{-11}M E_2. This effect was overcome by 10^{-10}M E_2. M induced ER thus has normal sedimentation properties and capacity for activation and translocation but may weakly antagonize an estrogen stimulated process. Subtle conformational changes in the receptor, including alteration of the chromatin acceptor site, must be considered. These observations may have important implications for understanding the mechanism of hormonal regulation of cellular activity.

495 RADIOCHEMICAL DETERMINATION OF STEROID RECEPTOR CONTENT OF FROZEN SECTIONS[1]

A. De Goeij*, M. Volleberg, G. Hondius and F. Bosman. Department of Pathology, University of Limburg, P.O.B. 616, Maastricht, The Netherlands.

A method for the measurement of steroid receptors has been developed for sections of calf and rat uterus and human mamma carcinoma samples. Unfixed frozen sections are mounted on coverslips, dried and incubated with radio-labeled ligands. For estrogen receptors (ER) 0.1-8 nM [^{3}H]- or[^{125}I] -Estradiol ± excess DES was used and for progesterone receptors (PR) 0.1-8 nM [^{3}H]- R5020 + 10 fold dihydrotestosterone ± excess R5020. Parallel sections were used for determination of protein and DNA and for histological staining. After incubation of the sections the overlay buffer was assayed for the presence of soluble ER and PR. The sections were washed and section-bound SR was quantified by direct liquid scintillation counting of the coverslips. Scatchard analysis showed the presence of specific binding sites with limited capacity and high affinity (Kd 0.2-2 nM). The soluble fraction represented usually 40-60% of the total receptor content. The steroid specificity of the ligand binding was found to be characteristic for ER and PR resp. Tissue specificity was demonstrated by a very low level of specific ligand binding to sections of rat skeletal muscle, spleen and intestine, and by a moderate level in rat liver. An excellent correlation has been found for receptor assay on cytosol and sections prepared from calf and rat uterus. Preliminary results on human mamma tumor samples show a less significant correlation presumably due to a high degree of heterogeneity in these samples. It is concluded that this method allows quantification of total steroid receptor content in relatively small amount of tissue samples.

[1] Supported by grant RL 82-2 from the Dutch Cancer Foundation KWF.

496 ESTROGEN DEPENDENT INDUCTION OF UNSATURABLE ESTROGEN BINDING SITES (E_2R) IN THE NUCLEAR FRACTION OF MATURE NON OVARIECTOMIZED AND ESTROGEN PRIMED OVARIECTOMIZED RAT UTERUS.

R. De Hertogh *, I. Vanderheyden and E. Ekka. Endocrinology and Nutrition Unit, University of Louvain, School of Medicine, Brussels, Belgium.

Type II nuclear E_2R have been reported in mature ovariectomized and immature rat uterus after estrogen administration. In this study mature non ovariectomized and ovariectomized estrogen-primed rats were administered 20 µg estradiol (E_2) by intraperitoneal route (ip) 60 minutes prior to sacrifice and the uterine nuclear E_2R were measured by an exchange technique in the presence and absence of reducing agents in the buffer. The results obtained showed that in the absence of mercaptoethanol a preliminary saturation plateau was reached (type I sites) at concentrations lower than 12 nM of $E_2{}^3H$, followed by a non-saturable binding up to 80 nM of $E_2{}^3H$. The latter type of binding was also encountered in non-injected rats, although to a lesser-extent. The estrogen bound to these sites was only sightly exchangeable at 4°C. The effect of saturation was observed in the "non-specific" moiety by increasing concentrations of diethylstilbestrol up to 8000 nM. In conclusion, in the absence of mercaptoethanol a second type of E_2R of non-saturable capacity was observed in the nuclear fraction of mature non-ovariectomized and estrogen-primed ovariectomized rat uterus, which was further amplified after an acute ip administration of E_2.

497 CHANGES IN THE DEPENDENCY OF PITUITARY AND UTERINE PROGESTIN RECEPTORS ON ESTRADIOL DURING THE ESTROUS CYCLE. B.N.Díaz-Chico*, J.Gómez, J.C.Díaz-Chico and A.Sosa. Dept.of Physiology. Colegio Universitario.Apdo.550.Las Palmas. Canary Islands.Spain.

It has been demonstrated that 17βEstradiol (E2) induces the cytosolic Progesterone Receptor (cPR) synthesis in reproductive tissues and also that both plasma E2 and cPR content fluctuates during the estrous cycle. The dependency on E2 of cPR in uterus and anterior pituitary during the estrous cycle has been studied here in acutely ovariectomized (ovx) rats at noon of metaestrous (Me), diestrous (De) and proestrous (Pe), with or without E2 replacement. The cPR were measured by means of ^{3}H-R5020 exchange and the dextran-coated charcoal method. The uterine content of cPR was low in Me (64 fmol/mg protein (p.)), increasing in De, reaching its highest value in Pe (237 fmol/mg p.) and decreasing in estrous (Es). Twenty four hours after ovx in De or Pe, the cPR content decreased significantly. The injection of 5 µg E2/kg 1 h after ovx increased the cPR content 24 h later in the uterus of the ovx in Me and De rats, but not in those ovx in Pe. The anterior pituitary content of cPR was low in Me (10.7 fmol/mg p.) and De, increasing in Pe (58 fmol/mg p.) and lowering in Es. The rats ovx in Me or De did not show any change in their cPR content 24 h later, either injected with vehicle alone or with E2. Those ovx in Pe showed a cPR decrease that was reversed by E2. The cPR content of both tissues reaches its highest value following the upper plasma E2 level on the Pe morning. However, the uterus showed a dependence on E2 during De, whereas pituitary did not. This situation was inverse for both tissues in Pe. These results show the existence of different mechanisms of cPR regulation by E2 in uterus and anterior pituitary.

498 NON QUANTITATIVE RECOVERY IN THE NUCLEAR FRACTION OF THE DEPLETED CYTOSOL ESTROGEN RECEPTOR COMPLEXES (E_2R) IN UTERUS OF MATURE NON OVARIECTOMIZED AND ESTROGEN-PRIMED OVARIECTOMIZED RATS AFTER INTRA-PERITONEAL INJECTION OF ESTRADIOL. E. Ekka *, I. Vanderheyden and R. De Hertogh - Endocrinology and Nutrition Unit - University of Louvain, School of Medicine, Brussels, Belgium.

In ovariectomized rats acutely injected with estradiol (E_2) translocation of E_2R from the uterine cytosol to the nucleus has been shown to be quantitative. In this study translocation of E_2R to the nuclear fraction in mature non-ovariectomized and ovariectomized estrogen-primed rats were analysed. 20 µg of E_2 in saline were injected intraperitoneally to the animals and one hour later the E_2R in the cytosol and nuclear fractions were assayed by an exchange technique in Tris-EDTA-Mercapto-ethanol buffer (TEM) at pH 7,4. The results showed an 85 % recovery of the depleted cytosol E_2R in the nuclear fraction of ovariectomized rats whereas only 50 % were recovered in the mature non-ovariectomized and ovariectomized estrogen-primed rats. Depending on the temperature and time of incubation, 20 to 40 % of the recovered nuclear E_2R were present as soluble complexes in the incubation medium and recuperated with hydroxylapatite. Saturation experiments in TEM showed a plateau from 12 nM $E_2{}^3H$ onwards up to 80 nM. The Kd values computed for the three groups were of the order of 2×10^{-9}M. In conclusion, E_2 administration to mature non-ovariectomized or ovariectomized estrogen-primed rats did not result in a quantitative recovery in the uterine nuclear fraction of E_2R depleted from the cytosol.

499 ANDROGEN BINDING IN NUCLEAR MATRIX OF HUMAN GENITAL SKIN FIBROBLASTS. T.R. Brown* and C.J. Migeon Pediatric Endocrine Labs, Johns Hopkins University, Baltimore, MD 21205

Specific sex-steroid binding sites are associated with the salt-insoluble nuclear matrix (NM) from which lipids, histones and chromatin have been extracted. Intact cultured human genital skin fibroblasts (GSF) incubated (37C,1h) with saturating concentrations (2nM) ^{3}H-dihydrotestosterone (DHT), translocate approximately 50% of total cell androgen receptor (AR)-steroid complexes to the nucleus. Within nuclei from normal GSF strains (n=6), 28-49% of specific AR binding is associated with NM. Scatchard analysis of specific DHT binding in NM following an in vitro exchange assay (0C,24h), revealed saturable (B_{max}=4.4 fmol/μg matrix DNA), high affinity (K_d=0.6 nM) binding (r = -0.96). Cell free in vitro incubations (0C,1h) of cytosol AR-DHT with nuclei and NM in the presence of 0.15 M KCl, resulted in 40-60% of specific nuclear binding associated with NM. GSF from two unrelated patients with receptor positive complete androgen insensitivity (CAIS,AR+), both with abnormal K_d values for DHT but only one expressing thermolability (42C) of DHT binding, exhibited normal (~50%) nuclear binding of DHT with 35% and 45% of it localized to NM. GSF from a patient with CAIS,AR- had no specific DHT binding in nuclei or NM. In summary, NM contain specific, high affinity, saturable sites for AR binding in GSF, which may be associated with nuclear "acceptor" sites, and do not appear to be abnormal in cells from patients with CAIS,AR+. (Supported by NIH grant AM-00180.)

500 A NATURAL MODEL IN WHICH ESTROGEN RECEPTORS ARE EXCLUSIVELY NUCLEAR. G.V. Callard* and P. Mak, Biology Dept., Boston Univ., Boston, MA 02215, U.S.A.

Although the generally accepted model of estrogen action includes a two-step receptor translocation mechanism, we recently observed that estrogen receptors (ER) in the dogfish (Squalus) testis were limited to the nuclear compartment (Endocrine Soc. Abstr. #103, 1983). Moreover, these were both occupied and unoccupied. Further investigations were conducted to resolve this paradox. Saturation analysis, competition studies, and sucrose gradient centrifugation demonstrated that Squalus ER resembled classical mammalian ER in all respects. By contrast, DNA cellulose affinity chromatography revealed a receptor with an exceptionally high NaCl resistance (elution maximum: 550 mM for Squalus vs 200 mM for rodents). High affinity for nuclei in situ was confirmed by homogenizing tissues in buffers ranging from 0 to 1000 mM KCl. A graded, quantitative redistribution of ER from the nuclear to the cytoplasmic compartment was observed (50% maximal: 430 mM). Increased buffer volume also affected ER redistribution but adjustment of molarity with urea was ineffective. Properties of the testicular ER were confirmed in Squalus oviduct. The DNA/nuclei-adhering characteristics of Squalus ER may represent an adaptation to the high body fluid osmolarity which is found in marine elasmobranchs (1010 mOsm), since ER from a freshwater elasmobranch (Potamotrygon) which osmoregulates at 308 mOsm had DNA-adhering characteristics more closely resembling mammalian ER (elution maximum: 220 mM NaCl) and was detectable in cytosol of low salt buffers. The Squalus model supports the view that the tendency for nuclear ER to be extracted into cytosol during tissue processing is dependent on its affinity for DNA/nuclei. (HD-16715; NSF PCM82-08248)

501 EFFECT OF CHRONIC ETHANOL INGESTION ON ANDROGEN METABOLISM AND MECHANISM OF ACTION IN RAT EPIDIDYMIS. K.W. Chung*, Department of Anatomical Sciences, University of Oklahoma College of Medicine, Oklahoma City, Oklahoma U.S.A.

The present study was carried out to examine ethanol-induced changes in androgen metabolism and molecular processes in androgen actions in rat epididymis. Young adult male King-Holtzman rats matched for body size were maintained for 5 months on a liquid diet containing 36% of its calories as ethanol or isocaloric maltose-dextrin. Androgen binding was measured in cytosol of the epididymis by sucrose density gradient centrifugation and by charcoal assay. The epididymis of ethanol-fed rats contains androgen receptors which migrate at 8S in a sucrose gradient. This organ contains a significantly reduced concentration (1.1×10^{-14} moles/mg protein) of androgen receptor sites, compared to controls (4.6×10^{-14} moles/mg protein), with slightly reduced affinity ($K_d = 1.6 \times 10^{-9}$M) for dihydrotestosterone (DHT). Since conversion of testosterone to the more potent metabolite DHT is an essential step in many target organs, it was important to investigate whether ethanol alters testosterone metabolism in the epididymis. Homogenates of epididymides from controls and ethanol-fed rats were incubated with ^{3}H-testosterone for 2 hours and testosterone and DHT were isolated by thin layer chromatography and quantitated by reverse isotope dilution. Formation of DHT from testosterone by epididymis was reduced in ethanol-fed rats as compared to control rats, indicating an adverse effect of ethanol on epididymal 5α-reductase. These findings suggest that ethanol inhibits the action of androgens in target cells by interfering with binding of androgen to receptors and transformation of testosterone to DHT which are essential steps in the mechanism of action.

502 SYNTHESIS OF C21-OIC ACID ESTERS OF TRIAMCINOLONE ACETONIDE AND BINDING TO HEPATIC GLUCOCORTICOID RECEPTORS. J. Gorsline,*[1] M.R. Sherman[2] and H.L. Bradlow,[1] [1]The Rockefeller University and [2]Sloan-Kettering Institute, New York, NY 10021 USA.

The C21-oic acid esters of glucocorticoids such as prednisolone have significant local anti-inflammatory activity and minimal systemic side effects (J. Steroid Biochem. 14, 1325, 1981). As triamcinolone acetonide (TA) is a more potent glucocorticoid than prednisolone, we have synthesized the methyl and ethyl C21-acid esters of TA and assessed their affinities for the glucocorticoid receptor in rat liver cytosol. Synthesis involved three steps: 1) oxidation of TA with methanolic cupric acetate to form the C21-aldehyde, 2) further oxidation with methylene blue and KCN to obtain the C21-acid, and 3) reaction with diazomethane in methanol or ethanol to yield the methyl or ethyl ester of the C20-keto, C21-acid of TA, respectively. Purity of the products was monitored by thin layer and high performance liquid chromatography, and the structures were confirmed by nuclear magnetic resonance and mass spectrometry. The ability of these esters to inhibit the binding of [^{3}H]TA to the rat liver receptor was studied in cytosols containing 20 mM Na_2MoO_4. The amount of competitive binding during a 2-h incubation at 4°C was evaluated by chromatography on Sephadex LH-20 in aqueous buffer. The apparent dissociation constants of the methyl and ethyl esters of TA acid from the hepatic receptor were comparable to those of TA. The demonstration that these modifications of the side chain of TA do not alter its affinity for the glucocorticoid receptor suggests that these derivatives may be useful therapeutically. (Supported by NIH grants AM07313, CA28392 and CA22795).

503 ANALYSIS OF GLUCOCORTICOID-RESISTANT HUMAN LEUKEMIC CELLS BY SOMATIC CELL HYBRIDIZATION. J. M. Harmon*, K.A. Baione and E. B. Thompson, Department of Pharmacology, Uniformed Services University of the Health Sciences and Laboratory of Biochemistry, National Cancer Institute, Bethesda, MD, USA.

Glucocorticoid-resistant mutants isolated from the glucocorticoid-sensitive human leukemic cell line CEM-C7 can be divided into three phenotypes: i) those with almost no steroid binding activity; ii) those whose steroid-receptor (SR) complexes are unstable during attempted activation but which are stabilized by sodium molybdate; and iii) those whose SR complexes are unstable during attempted activation but are insensitive to molybdate. To determine if these phenotypes represent different mutations within the receptor itself, or reflect alterations in other components modifying receptor function, somatic cell hybrids were constructed between resistant mutants and wild-type cells as well as between various classes of resistant cells. Hybrids were analyzed for growth inhibition, induction of glutamine synthetase (GS) and SR content. Hybrids constructed between wild-type cells and any of the resistant phenotypes were growth inhibited in the presence of steroid, displayed normal levels of GS induction and contained a quantity of SR equal to the sum of the SR concentration of the parents. Hybrids constructed between various classes of resistant cells were not growth inhibited, displayed no GS induction and also contained the sum of the SR concentration of the parents. Thus, each phenotype is recessive and there is no complementation between phenotypes. We conclude that the three phenotypes are the result of different mutations within the receptor itself, and do not represent the presence of dominant inactivating factors or the absence of positive regulatory components.

504 MOUSE GLUCOCORTICOID RECEPTOR IMMUNOAFFINITY PURIFICATION USING A MONOCLONAL ANTIBODY. R. W. Harrison* and B. Gametchu, Endocrinology Div., Vanderbilt University School of Medicine, Nashville, TN, 37232, U.S.A.

We have reported production of a stable mouse hybridoma clone, BuGR1, producing antibody which recognizes the rat and mouse (but not human) glucocorticoid receptor. A total of 3 distinct IgG-producing clones have now been stabilized. All three antibodies are directed towards identical or overlapping antigenic sites, since unlabeled BuGR2 or BuGR3 can prevent binding of labeled BuGR1 to the receptor. We have used BuGR1 antibody in two protocols to purify the AtT-20 mouse pituitary tumor cell glucocorticoid receptor. In protocol 1, the antibody in crude medium was reacted with dexamethasone 21-mesylate-labeled cytosol and the resulting receptor-antibody complexes bound to protein A Sepharose. After washing, the bound complex was eluted using 0.58% acetic acid. In protocol 2, BuGR1 antibody was reacted with protein A Sepharose and the resulting complexes covalently linked by a cross-linking reagent. The affinity gel was mixed with labeled cytosol, then washed and eluted with 3 M NaSCN, pH 5. Both protocols resulted in receptor yields of 35-50%. Analysis of the purified material by SDS polyacrylamide gel electrophoresis consistently showed that both protocols result in a major radioactive band of 97,000 M.W. and a minor labeled band of ~50,000 M.W. Protein silver staining showed bands at 97,000 and 50,000 M.W. only (protocol 2) or bands at 97,000, 50,000, and 20,000 M.W. (protocol 1). The 20,000 M.W. band and part of the 50,000 M.W. band seen in protocol 1 result from coelution of antibody. Both protocols are being used to purify the intact receptor, as well as fragments after enzymatic digestion, in order to further determine the structure of the steroid binding domain of the receptor and the antigenic site identified by the BuGR1 antibody. In conclusion, immunoaffinity chromatography is a facile method for large-scale purification of the mouse glucocorticoid receptor.

505 EVIDENCE FOR A MINERALOCORTICOID EFFECT OUTSIDE OF THE CLASSIC ALDOSTERONE RECEPTOR SYSTEM WITH THE REDUCED METABOLITES OF ALDOSTERONE.

C.E. Gomez-Sanchez*, J.S. Smith, M.W. Ferris and E. Gomez-Sanchez. Dept. of Internal Medicine, Univ. of South Florida College of Medicine and the J.A. Haley Hospital, Tampa, Florida 33612 USA.

Reduced metabolites of aldosterone have been shown to have antinatriuretic and kaliuretic effects. We have studied the ability of five reduced metabolites of aldo to compete with (^{3}H)-aldo and (^{3}H)-dexamethasone for binding to the mineralocorticoid (Type I) and glucocorticoid (Type II) receptors of the kidney using adrenalectomized rat renal slices and cytosol respectively. 5α-Dihydroaldo had 18.9% the ability to compete with (^{3}H)-aldo for binding to the cytoplasmic receptor of adrenalectomized rat renal slices in comparison to unlabelled aldo. Its antinatriuretic potency varies between 7-17%. Its ability to compete with (^{3}H)-dex for binding to the renal glucocorticoid receptor is only 1.9% in comparison to unlabelled dex. The relative competitive activity of 3α5α-tetrahydroaldo, 3β5α-tetrahydroaldo and 3β5β-tetrahydroaldo with (^{3}H)-aldo to adrenalectomized rat renal slices cytosol was 10%, 1.26% and 0.05% respectively in comparison to aldo. Their reported mineralocorticoid activities (antinatriuresis) are 2-3%, 0.1-0.4% and 0.15% respectively in comparison to aldo. The most important aldo metabolite 3α5β-tetrahydroaldo showed negligible competitive activity for the renal corticoid Type I or Type II receptors. However, this compound has weak but clear cut mineralocorticoid activity which cannot be explained by a mechanism involving the classic renal mineralocorticoid receptor.

506 INSULIN RECEPTOR METABOLISM IN HEPATOMA CELLS : BASAL AND HORMONE ACTIVATED RECEPTOR DEGRADATION.

J. Capeau* , C. Flaig-Staedel, M.J. Blivet, J.P. Beck & J. Picard. Laboratoire de Biochimie, INSERM U.181, Faculté de Médecine Saint-Antoine, 75571 Paris Cédex 12 and Institut de Physiologie, Université Louis Pasteur, Strasbourg, France.

Insulin receptor processing was studied in cultured Zajdela hepatoma cells (ZHC), a highly insulin responsive cell line. In the presence of tunicamycin (TM), the insertion into plasma membranes of newly synthesized underglycosylated receptors was precluded. For receptor catabolism, the basal receptor half-life was of 7 h. This turnover was markedly slowed down when cells were either briefly preincubated with dansylcadaverine, chloroquine or cycloheximide, or treated for 24 h with TM. The effect of these agents was then tested upon the insulin-induced receptor down-regulation (DR) process. This phenomenon, which was easily revealed in ZHC, was shown to result from an increased rate of receptor degradation. When ZHC were briefly treated with dansylcadaverine, chloroquine, actinomycin D or cycloheximie, DR was inhibited. Similarly, it disappeared after a 24 h incubation with TM, although receptors remained functional when testing insulin's action upon glycogen synthesis. These results indicate that receptor degradation, both basal and activated by insulin leading to the down-regulated state, was altered under similar experimental conditions. The effects of dansylcadaverine or chloroquine reveal that endocytotic pathways were involved in these processes. The results obtained when mRNA, protein or glycoprotein synthesis was inhibited, indicate that (a) cellular glycoprotein(s) and (a) short-lived protein(s) were necessary for the receptor processing, in both cases. These data led us to postulate that basal and insulin-activated receptor degradation may occur in the same way within the cell.

507 IMPLICATION OF GLYCOPROTEINS OF THE COMPLEX N-LINKED TYPE IN THE INSULIN STIMULATION OF GLUCOSE AND AMINO ACID INTRACELLULAR METABOLIC PATHWAYS IN RAT ADIPOCYTES. G.Cherqui, M.Caron, J.Capeau & J.Picard* . Laboratoire de Biochimie. INSERM U.181, Faculté de Médecine Saint-Antoine, Paris, France.

The abilities of lectins specific for D-mannose (concanavalin A, con A), N-acetyl-D-glucosamine (wheat germ agglutinin, WGA), D-galactose (ricinus communis agglutinin I) to mimick the effect of insulin on glucose and amino acid intracellular metabolic pathways in rat adipocytes were examined. {3-^{3}H} glucose conversion into ^{3}H-lipids and L-{U-^{14}C} leucine incorporation into ^{14}C-proteins were studied under conditions where neither insulin nor lectins had an effect on membrane transport processes. 1) When glucose transport was rate-limiting (0.5 mM-glucose), lectins, like insulin, increased lipogenesis 2.4 fold. 2) When passive diffusion of glucose was amplified (10 mM-glucose), lectins, like insulin, increased lipogenesis 1.8 fold even when cytochalasin B (50 μM) completely blocked glucose transport. 3) Con A and WGA, like insulin, activated L-{U-^{14}C} leucine incorporation into fat-cell proteins by 1.5 fold while ineffective on α-aminoisobutyric acid uptake or ^{14}C-protein degradation. 4) Peanut or soybean agglutinins, specific for O-glycosyl-proteins, neither altered insulin binding nor mimicked insulin effects. 5) Monosaccharide competitors specifically inhibited lectin effects. 6) Insulin and lectin maximal effects were not additive and were abolished in neuraminidase-treated fat cells. Thus, insulin stimulates glucose and amino acid intracellular metabolic pathways through cell surface glycosylated entities containing oligosaccharides of the complex N-linked type. It is suggested that these effector entities are a part of, or are closely linked to, the insulin receptor macromolecule.

508 CHARACTERIZATION OF INSULIN BINDING AND STIMULATION OF 2-DEOXY D-GLUCOSE UPTAKE BY INSULIN IN GLIAL CULTURES FROM RAT BRAIN. D.W. Clarke, F.T. Boyd, Jr.,* M.S. Kappy, and M.K. Raizada, Departments of Physiology and Pediatrics, University of Florida, Gainesville, FL, USA 32610.

Previous studies have shown that neuronal and glial cultures prepared from the brain contain insulin specific receptors although the physiological role of these receptors is still unclear. This study was undertaken to investigate characteristics of glial insulin receptors and the effects of insulin which may be mediated through that receptor. Glial cells were established in culture by dissociating individual cells from one-day-old rat brain with trypsin and plating the cells in DMEM with 10% FBS. Cells were transferred once and used for experiments when confluent. Binding of ^{125}I-insulin to glial cells was specific, time- and pH dependent. Porcine, human and chicken insulins competed as expected for ^{125}I-insulin binding while structurally unrelated peptide hormones failed to compete for binding. ^{125}I-Insulin dissociated from glial cells with a $T_{1/2}$ of 8 min. Scatchard analysis provided a curvilinear plot with K_e of 6.4 x 10^{8} M^{-1} and K_f of 0.3 x 10^{8} M^{-1}. There were 7.7 x 10^{4} binding sites/cell. Incubation of glial cultures with insulin caused a time- and dose dependent stimulation of 2-deoxy D-glucose uptake. Maximal stimulation of 190% was observed with 20 nM insulin and the ED_{50} was 4 nM. This effect of insulin was due to an increase in V_{max} without affecting Km. These results indicate that insulin specific receptors are present on glial cells and mediate a classical physiological effect of insulin typical of peripheral cell types. Supported by NIH grant HD 16722.

509 SPECIFIC ALTERATIONS OF LIVER VASOPRESSIN RECEPTOR SITES IN OB/OB, DB/DB MICE AND FA/FA RATS. Cl. Chevillard‡ B. Cantau and G. Guillon. Montpellier (France)

Selective lacks of vasopressin (VP) receptors and glycogen phosphorylase activity were observed in the liver of ob/ob, whereas VP receptors present in the kidney membranes were coupled to adenylate cyclase activation. To know if these alterations are genetically linked to a lack of V_1 receptor type or secondary to obesity and/or hyperinsulinemia, we have studied 1) the binding of ^{3}H-VP on kidney and liver plasma membranes of diabetic db/db mouse and obese fa/fa rat, in which the hyperinsulinemia patterns are extremely different during postnatal development ; 2) the contractile responses to VP and phenylephrine (PHE) in ob/ob, db/db and fa/fa isolated tail artery. The number of db/db liver VP receptor was 5 or 20 % of control values at 9 and 30 weeks. In fa/fa liver membranes VP receptors were decreased only by 50 % in the 30 week old animals. No difference appeared in VP kidney receptors between fa/fa, db/db and their respective controls, whatever their age. The contractile responses of the tail artery to VP and PHE were identical in ob/ob, db/db, fa/fa to that of their control. These results suggest that the lack of liver VP receptor was not due to a defect in V_1 receptor genetic expression. The decrease or lack of VP receptor was specific for liver and appeared to parallel the levels of hyperinsulinemia in the 3 mutants studied.

510 EVIDENCE FOR ARGININE^8 VASOPRESSIN RECEPTOR SUBTYPES IN RAT RENAL MEDULLA AND DORSAL HINDBRAIN. L.E. Cornett* and D.M. Dorsa, Dept. of Physiol. & Biophys., UAMS, Little Rock, AR, USA; VA Med. Center, Seattle, WA, USA.

Arginine^8 vasopressin (AVP) has a variety of actions both in the periphery and the central nervous system. AVP receptor subtypes have been postulated based on whether calcium (V_1 receptor) or cyclic AMP (V_2 receptor) serve as second messengers. Using (^{3}H) AVP and synthetic vasopressin analogues in radioligand assays we provide further evidence for AVP receptor heterogeneity. (^{3}H) AVP bound saturably and with high affinity to renal medulla (K_d=1.8±0.3nM; B_{max}=238±44fmol/mg prot) and dorsal hindbrain (K_d=0.9±0.2nM; B_{max}=25.2±2fmol/mg prot). Analogues tested included two pressor antagonists, [1-(β-mercapto-β,β-cyclopentamethylenepropionic acid, 2-(O-methyl) tyrosine] arginine vasopressin (d(CH)$_5$Tyr (Me)AVP); deamino penicillamine, 2-(O-methyl) tyrosine arginine vasopressin (dPTyr(Me)AVP); a selective antidiuretic, deamino arginine vasopressin (D-AVP); and lysine vasopressin (LVP). The rank order of potency in competing with (^{3}H) AVP in renal medulla was AVP (K_i=1.9±0.6nM)≅D-AVP (K_i=2.9 ±0.7nM) > d(CH_2)$_5$Tyr(Me)AVP (K_i=16.4±5.0nM) ≅ dPTyr(Me)AVP (K_i=16.1±6.4nM) > LVP (K_i=58.1±11nM) and in dorsal hindbrain was AVP (K_i=0.4±0.1nM) ≅ d(CH_2)$_5$Tyr(Me)AVP (K_i=0.6±0.2nM) ≥ dPTyr(Me) AVP (K_i=1.7±0.6nM) > D-AVP (K_i=3.5±1.1nM) > LVP (K_i=13.9±9nM). Oxytocin and pressinoic acid did not compete at concentrations up to 100 nM. In conclusion, our data suggests that AVP binding sites in renal medulla and dorsal hindbrain may represent different receptor subtypes. As yet it is unclear whether the dorsal hindbrain AVP binding site is best classified as a V_1 receptor or alternatively as a third receptor subtype. Supported by NSF ISP8011447.

511 AFFINITY CROSSLINKING OF VIP TO SPECIFIC BINDING SITES IN RAT LIVER PLASMA MEMBRANES.

A. Couvineau and M. Laburthe*, CNRS ERA 494, INSERM U.55, Hôpital Saint-Antoine, 75012 PARIS, FRANCE

The cleavable cross-linking reagent dithiobis (succinimidyl) propionate (DTSP) is used to investigate the molecular nature of VIP binding sites in rat liver plasma membranes. Solubilization of membranes covalently labeled with ^{125}I-VIP followed by SDS-PAGE analysis yields a major Mr 51,000 component and a minor Mr 89,000 component. Labeling of the two components is specific since it is completely abolished by incubation of membranes with 0.1 μM native VIP while not affected by 1 μM glucagon or octa CCK. The same doses of native VIP (10^{-11} - 10^{-7} M) reduce the labeling of Mr 51,000 and 89,000 components. The VIP agonists, PHI and secretin, are also active but with a 1/10 and 1/100 lower potency than VIP, respectively. The guanine nucleotide GTP (10^{-6} - 10^{-3} M) inhibits the labeling of the two components. Assuming one molecule of VIP bound per protein, two rat liver membrane proteins with Mr of 48,000 and 86,000 are identified as VIP binding sites. The functional and/or structural relationship between the two proteins remains to be elucidated. Furthermore it must be noticed that the Mr of VIP binding proteins in rat liver membranes contrast markedly with those previously identified in rat intestinal epithelial membranes i.e. a Mr 73,000 protein for the high affinity binding site and a Mr 33,000 protein for a low affinity binding site (Laburthe et al. Eur. J. Biochem in press 1984). Whether these structural discrepancies are related to different biological functions of VIP binding sites in the two tissues remains to be elucidated

(Supported by INSERM, CRL 827017)

512 SPECIFIC BINDING SITES FOR CORTICOTROPIN-RELEASING FACTOR IN RAT PERIPHERAL TISSUES AND THEIR MODULATION IN VITRO BY ETHANOL.

J.R. Dave*, J.C. Bisserbe and R.L. Eskay, Laboratory of Clinical Studies, National Institute on Alcohol Abuse and Alcoholism, Bethesda, Maryland - 20205, U.S.A.

The objective of this study was to determine if rat peripheral tissues possessed specific binding sites for Corticotropin-releasing factor (CRF). Using ^{125}I-rat CRF, specific binding sites for CRF were identified in adrenal, ventral prostate, spleen, liver, kidney and testis of adult male SD rats. The microsomal membrane fraction exhibited higher CRF binding capacity than the crude homogenate in adrenal, prostate and liver. The binding of CRF was saturable and time- and temperature-dependent, with a maximal binding achieved at 25 min and 4°C. Scatchard analysis of the CRF binding data revealed the existence of two classes of binding sites. One class had an apparent K_a of 0.008 nM and lower number of binding sites (23 pmol CRF/mg protein), whereas, the other class had a lower affinity (apparent K_a of 0.001 nM) and higher number of binding sites (76 pmol/mg protein). The existence of specific CRF binding sites was also supported by inhibition-analysis and by autoradiographic studies using 10μ sections of adrenal gland. Addition of ethanol to membrane preparations produced dose-related, biphasic modifications in CRF binding. Our data suggest the existence of specific binding sites for rat CRF in rat liver, kidney, adrenal, spleen, testis and ventral prostate. Furthermore, ethanol-induced changes suggest that CRF binding sites are dependent on the physical state of the membrane.

513 INTERACTION OF RECOMBINANT BOVINE SOMATOTROPIN WITH HEPATIC RECEPTORS.
LUIS S. HARO*,[a] ROBERT J. COLLIER,[b] and FRANK J. TALAMANTES[a]. [a]Biology Board of Studies, Thimann Laboratories, University of California, Santa Cruz, CA 95064 and [b]Department of Dairy Science, University of Florida, Gainesville, FL 32611.

In order to study the physiological ontogeny and biochemistry of somatogenic receptors in bovine tissue we have developed a homologus radioreceptor assay. The assay parameters and methodology for preparation of membrane receptors were optimized to give a maximum of specific binding to recombinant bovine growth hormone, because the use of conventional techniques allowed less than 1.5% of the labeled somatotropin to be specifically bound. Bovine somatotropin was iodinated by a lactoperoxidase method. Hepatic membranes were prepared by homogénization in 10 mM sodium phosphate, 300 mM sucrose, with 1 mM phenylmethylsulfonyl fluoride, 10 mM ethyleneglycol-bis-(B-aminoethylether)N,N'-tetraacetic acid, 10 mM ethylenediaminetetraacetic acid, Trasylol at 100 units/ml, and pH 9.0 to inhibit proteinase activity, then subjected to differential centrifugation. The binding of bovine somatotropin to hepatic receptors was both time and temperature dependent. 48% of the labeled hormone was specifically bound in 24hr at 25°C. A pH maximum for the specific binding of bovine somatotropin occured at pH 7.8. Binding of labeled somatotropin to hepatic receptors was not completely reversible; only 60% of the hormone dissociated after 74hr. The K_d at equilibrium was 3.9×10^{-12} M. Bovine somatotropin was effectively displaced by human, ovine, and porcine somatotropins but not by bovine and ovine prolactins. The hepatic receptors are thus somatogenic .(Supported by UCSC FRC, NIH RR-08132 and Monsanto Co. grants).

514 IDENTIFICATION OF A SPECIFIC GROWTH HORMONE BINDING PROTEIN IN RABBIT LIVER CYTOSOL.
A.C. Herington* and S.I. Ymer, Medical Research Centre, Prince Henry's Hospital, Melbourne, Australia 3004.

We have recently identified in solubilized preparations of pregnant female rabbit liver a growth hormone (GH) binding protein (M_r 100-124,000) that is not detected by the widely used polyethylene glycol (PEG) precipitation method (Endocrinology (1984) in press). Thus, we have re-examined the possibility that a similar soluble GH binding protein might be present in the intracellular cytosol fraction of rabbit liver. Gel filtration on Ultrogel AcA34 of i) an incubation mixture of ^{125}I-human GH and pregnant rabbit liver cytosol (200,000 g supernatant) or ii) cytosol alone (followed by incubation of column fractions with ^{125}I-hGH), revealed a prominent specific GH binding protein of M_r ~100,000. The binding species was detectable by a standard charcoal separation procedure but not by PEG precipitation. The GH binding protein had similar binding characteristics to those of classical membrane-bound GH receptors - in particular, the kinetics of association and dissociation, binding affinity (2.5×10^9 M^{-1}) and specificity for somatotrophic but not lactogenic hormones. There appears to be equivalent amounts of GH binding protein in the cytosol and in the membrane fraction. A similar binding protein has been observed in cytosol from nonpregnant and male rabbit liver as well as at much lower concentration in rabbit muscle, heart and kidney cytosol. This is the first report of a GH binding protein in cell cytosols and its existence raises important questions regarding its origin and its potential physiological role in the mechanism(s) of action of GH.
Supported by the National Health & Medical Research Council of Australia.

515 RADIORECEPTOR ASSAY (RRA) FOR CATECHOLAMINE IN URINE SAMPLES.
H. Bessho*, G.Matsumoto, H. Kikuoka, M. Nishi, H. Honda, K. Iwo and K. Miyamura, Division of Endocrinology, Department of Internal Medicine, Wakayama Medical School, Wakayama 640, Japan.

We investigated RRA for catecholamine, in favor of its advantages which indicated not only biological activities to stimulate β-adrenergic receptor but also tissue sensitivities and structure-function relationships. In methods, 150 μl of incubation medium containing 10^{-9} M (-)-[^{3}H]-dihydroalprenolol ([^{3}H]DHA), 100 μg of crude fat cell membrane protein and several competitors in 50 mM Tris-HCl buffer with 10 mM $MgCl_2$ (pH 7.4, 37° C) were incubated for 12 min at 37°C with shaking. [^{3}H]DHA bindings were saturable by increasing the concentrations of [^{3}H]DHA or membrane protein and revealed stereospecificity. Half-maximally inhibitory concentrations determined were as follows; (-)-adrenalin: 5.9 x 10^{-7} M (108 μg/L), (-)-noradrenalin: 4.6 x 10^{-7} M, (-)-isoproterenol: 4.6 x 10^{-8} M, and dopamine: 3.4 x 10^{-4} M. Urine samples below pH 6.4 or above pH 7.4 inhibited or accelerated [^{3}H]DHA binding, respectively. Urine samples more than 60 mg/dl nonspecifically inhibited [^{3}H]DHA bindings in relation to the concentrations. Therefore, urine samples stored under acidic condition were adjusted to pH 7.1 and urine proteins above 50 mg/dl were removed by filtration within 30 min. The values determined by radioreceptor assay could be termed β-receptor reactive catecholamine (β-RRCA). Hydrolysis of conjugated catecholamine by boiling acidified urines elevated the values of β-RRCA, indicating little biological activities of conjugated catecholamines.

516 BETA-ADRENERGIC RECEPTORS IN HUMAN AND RAT LEFT VENTRICLE:COMPARISON OF SUBTYPE HETEROGENEITY DELINEATED BY DIRECT RADIOLIGAND BINDING.M.Bevilacqua* T.Vago,R.Meroni,R.Dagani,E.Malacco,C.Santoli and G.Norbiato,Endocrine Unit, Internal Medicine and Cardiothoracic Surgery Departments,Osp L Sacco(Vialba) Via GB Grassi 54,20157 Milano and Drug-cell Interaction Study Center(DISC) Via Pisacane 34A,Milano, ITALY

Human ventricular tissue (papillary muscles obtained during open heart surgery,n=8) and rat left ventricles (Sprague-Dawley male rats,n=32),were assayed to identify beta-adrenergic receptors.Saturation experiments and Scatchard analysis with ^{3}H-dihydroalprenolol were used to obtain B_{max} and K_D,whereas the relative proportion of beta1 and beta2 subtypes were determined by the use of competition radioligand binding and computer modeling techniques (RECEPT),employing the subtype selective agents atenolol (beta1 selective) and ICI 118,551 (beta2 selective).Rat left ventricles contained 37.8 f moles/mg of protein of beta receptors,with a K_D=1.67 nM,beta1 receptors being 78.5±2% and beta2 21.5±1.5%.Human left ventricles contained 46 f moles/mg of beta receptors,with a K_D=2.74 nM,beta1 receptors being 73.2±1.5% and beta2 26.8±0.5%.
We conclude that human left ventricles contain a high proportion of beta2 receptors (about 25%),which may contribute to the inotropic effect of catecholamines;furthermore the population of human beta receptors is similar in affinity,total number and subtype heterogeneity to that of rat ventricle.

517 STEROIDOGENESIS BY THE PREPUBERTAL RHESUS MONKEY OVARY IN VITRO.
Bruot, B.C.*, M. Gearing, P.I. Musey, M.E. Wilson, and D.C. Collins, Kent State University, Kent, OH, Yerkes Primate Research Center, and Emory University School of Medicine/VA Med. Center, Atlanta, GA 30033.

Numerous results suggest a very low level of ovarian steroidogenic activity in the prepubertal primate. The objective of this study was to determine the secretion of estradiol-17β (E_2) and progesterone (P) by the prepubertal rhesus monkey ovary in vitro. Ovaries were removed from six immature females between 286-363 days of age. Ovaries were quartered and placed in 1 ml of 25 mM HEPES buffered supplemented minimum essential medium (MEM) and incubated at 37°C under 95% air/5% CO_2 for 48 hr. Ovaries showed a mean release $\pm$ SE of 887 $\pm$ 374 pg E_2/mg ovary over the 48 hr. This release rate was not significantly altered by the addition of 100 ng LH or 1 mmole $(Bu)_2$cAMP. The addition of 100 mmole P or androstenedione did not affect the release of E_2. Prepubertal rhesus monkey ovaries incubated without substrate released 299 $\pm$ 35 pg P/mg ovary. This release was not affected by the addition of LH or $(Bu)_2$cAMP. The addition of 0.8 mg lipoprotein to the medium significantly increased the secretion of P to 650 $\pm$ 221 pg/ng ovary. The effect of the lipoprotein on P was further enhanced by the addition of $(Bu)_2$cAMP (1462 $\pm$ 165). These results suggest that ovaries from prepubertal rhesus monkeys have minimal steroidogenic activity. The failure of LH but not $(Bu)_2$cAMP to increase lipoprotein-argumented P release suggests that no LH receptors, but adequate lipoprotein receptors were present. The inability of androstenedione or P to enhance E_2 secretion suggests that a cellular component necessary for aromatase activity is absent. Supported by VA Project 1517-001.

518 CHARACTERIZATION OF INSULIN RESISTANCE IN POLYCYSTIC OVARIAN DISEASE (PCO).
R.J. Chang*, M. Geffner, D. Golde, N. Bersch, R. Bergman, and S. Kaplan, Depts. of OB-GYN, Peds, Med and Physiol, UCLA and USC, LA, CA.

We have previously shown that non-obese PCO patients are insulin resistant. To characterize this insulin resistance 6 non-obese PCO and 6 weight-matched controls were studied in regards to 1) growth promoting action of insulin; 2) insulin-dependent glucose disposal; and 3) insulin receptor binding. Diagnosis of PCO was based on the presence of hirsutism and oligo-amenorrhea with elevated serum testosterone, androstenedione and LH. The ability of insulin to stimulate cell growth was assessed by an in vitro bioassay of red cell colony proliferation from peripheral blood erythroid precursors. To evaluate in vivo glucose disposal all subjects after an overnight fast had blood drawn at frequent intervals following an intravenous glucose (0.3 gm/kg) load for determination of glucose and insulin levels. First- and second-phase insulin secretion and insulin sensitivity were assessed by the minimal modeling technique of Bergman. Monocyte insulin receptor binding was measured in each subject. The results show that mean red cell colony proliferation in the presence of physiological amounts of insulin in PCO (13% increase from baseline) was significantly less than that seen in normal subjects (92% increase). Insulin sensitivity (glucose disposal) in PCO was markedly impaired compared to normal women in the presence of similar first- and second-phase rates of insulin secretion. In PCO monocyte insulin receptor binding was indistinguishable from that of controls. The data indicate that expression of insulin resistance in non-obese PCO includes: 1) cell growth promoting activity; 2) glucose disposal by tissue. Normal receptor binding in PCO suggests that insulin resistance is due to a postreceptor defect.

519 INHIBITION OF UTEROGLOBIN GENE EXPRESSION BY AN ANTIPROGESTIN, RU38486.
C.-L.C. Chen*, C.-C. Chang, C.W. Bardin and O.A. Jänne, The Population Council and The Rockefeller University, New York, N.Y.

RU38486(RU), a 11β-substituted 19 norsteroid, has high affinity for uterine progestin receptor and antagonizes the endometrial proliferation induced by progesterone (P). In this work, we have used RU to study its antiprogestin effect on the expression of uteroglobin (Ugl) gene that is regulated by progestins in the rabbit endometrium. Administration of P (1mg/kg/day, S.C.) for 3 days caused a dramatic increase in Ugl content, (at least 400 fold) as determined by radioimmunoassay and the level of its mRNA, (10-15-fold) as measured by dot blot or Northern blot analysis using a cloned Ugl cDNA as a hybridization probe. The induction of Ugl gene expression by P could be inhibited by RU. A significant decrease in both Ugl content (70%) and its mRNA level (43%) was observed when RU (0.3 mg/kg/day, S.C.) and P (1 mg/kg/day, S.C.) were given concomitantly to the rabbits for 3 days. RU completely antagonized the stimulatory effect of P if the ratio of RU to P was 1:1. Administration of RU (3mg/kg/day) alone for 3 days did not increase Ugl or Ugl mRNA concentrations over control values. The antiprogestin activity of RU was also demonstrated in the rabbits whose Ugl level had been elevated by a prior P treatment. A profound suppression of Ugl gene expression was detected after administration of RU for 3 days. In conclusion, RU exerts an inhibitory effect on the Ugl gene expression induced by P.

520 INDUCTION OF MENSES BY RU 38486 DURING EXTENSION OF THE LUTEAL PHASE BY EXOGENOUS hCG.
H.B. Croxatto*, A.M. Salvatierra & I. Spitz. Consultorio de Planificación Familiar, Santiago, Chile and The Population Council, New York, USA.

Trophoblast hCG maintains high progesterone secretion from the corpus luteum preventing endometrial bleeding in early pregnancy. This situation can be mimicked by exogenous hCG given in the luteal phase and was used in this study to examine the effects of the antiprogesterone RU 38486. Twelve, normally cycling, previously sterilized women volunteered to participate. Two extended luteal phases, one with hCG alone and one with hCG + RU 38486, separated by two resting cycles, were studied in each woman. The order was alternated from one subject to the next. In each cycle serial blood samples were collected around midcycle for the assay of LH. The day of the LH peak was designated Day 0. Treatment began on day 9 and consisted of one im injection of hCG per day x 7 days, during which the dose was progressively increased from 500 to 15000 IU per day. When RU 38486 was tested, 50 or 100 mg were given orally every 12h x 8 times begining with the fourth hCG injection. Blood samples were collected daily for the assay of gonadotropins, progesterone, estradiol and cortisol. All vaginal blood losses were recorded. The LH peak-bleeding interval was 20-23 days and 13-15 days in cycles treated with hCG alone or hCG + RU 38486 respectively. Estrogen and progesterone blood levels at the onset of bleeding were low in the first group and high in the second. Cortisol levels increased during treatment with RU 38486. No untoward reactions were recorded. These results are consistent with the blockade of endometrial progesterone receptors with RU 38486 and indicate that this effect is not prevented by exogenous hCG at doses which simulate the early pregnancy profile.

521 HYPERANDROGENIA AFTER PORTOCAVAL SHUNT IN FOUR GIRLS WITH FAMILIAL HYPERCHOLESTEROLEMIA.

F. DAIROU, G. TURPIN, J. TRUFFERT, JL de GENNES, I. MOSCHOWICZ MF WRIGHT et H. BISMUTH
Service d'Endocrinologie-Métabolisme, Hôpital de la Pitié, 83 bd de l'Hôpital 75013 PARIS (France)

A portocaval shunt (PCS) has been carried out in four girls (13,5-15-19 and 22 years old) for homozygous familial hypercholesterolemia. All four patients presented cutaneotendinous xanthomatosis ; three of them had severe ischemic heart disease and in one case a coronary by pass has been necessary before PCS. Two were LDL receptor negative (less than 2% of normal) and two were LDL receptor defective (about 5% of normal). All these 4 girls had completed their puberty before PCS and ovarian function and sexual hormonal levels were normal. After PCS all four girls presented an amenorrhea which lasted 3, 6, 8 and 30 months, without galactorrhea without hirsutism, clinical regression of sexual characteristics. In all cases we observed a biologic hyperandrogenia : plasma levels of testosterone ranged between 2 fold and 5 fold normal value. $\Delta 4$ androstenedione : 2 and 3 fold normal value. Plasma estradiol was normal in all cases, as well as prolactin, and basal gonadotrophin. Pituitary response to LHRH was normal. Testosterone metabolic clearance rate was low in one case and normal in two others. Hyperandrogenia seems to be related to decreased hepatic catabolism. Mechanism of amenorrhea remained unclear.

522 ANDROGENS IN GENETIC MALES WITH A DELETION OF THE LONG ARM OF CHROMOSOME 18 (18q-syndrome). F. Chasalow*, S. Blethen, and K. Taysi. Dept. of Pediatrics, Washington University, St. Louis, MO, 63110, USA

18q-syndrome is characterized by growth and mild to severe mental retardation, facial dysmorphism, and abnormalities of genitalia. In genetic males, genital abnormalities vary from testicular ectopia, small penis to severe hypospadias resulting in ambiguous genitalia in the newborn. We have studied 3 patients who have the deletion of the long arm of chromosome 18 distal to band q21. In 2 adolescent boys dehydroepiandrosterone sulfate (DS) levels were low compared to those observed in age-matched controls (90 and 60 μg/dl vs normal of >200 μg/dl). In a newborn genetic male, cord blood levels of both DS (20 μg/dl vs 100 ± 15 μg/dl) and total androgen sulfates (44 μg/dl) were low as was the infant's serum DS at 4 days of age (30 μg/dl vs 105 ± 30 μg/dl). Serum testosterone was <20 ng/dl (200 ± 40 ng/dl) and increased to only 50 ng/dl (normal >300 ng/dl) after a 4 day course of HCG. An incubation of testicular tissue from this patient with [1,2-^{3}H]progesterone and 17-hydroxy[4-^{14}C]progesterone showed formation of 17-hydroxy[1,2-^{3}H] progesterone but no further conversion of 17-hydroxyprogesterone to androgens. Conclusion: Decreased androgen synthesis seems to be a feature of 18q-syndrome. The defect appears to be in the steroid-17,20-lyase. It is possible that the structural gene for steroid-17,20-lyase or a regulatory gene for that enzyme is located on the long arm of chromosome 18, distal to band q21.

523 NON-STEROIDAL MODULATORS OF PROSTATIC FUNCTIONS AS DEFINED BY IN VITRO STUDIES.

S. Chevalier*, G. Bleau, K.D. Roberts and A. Chapdelaine. Maisonneuve-Rosemont Res. Center and U. of Montreal, Quebec, Canada.

To test the hypothesis that humoral components, other than sex steroids, might regulate specific prostatic functions, fetal bovine serum and dog serum were fractionated by gel filtration and evaluated for their ability to induce the attachment and spreading of canine prostatic epithelial cells in monolayers as well as their subsequent proliferation and differentiation. Cell attachment required components which were found in a 55-65 Kd fraction of fetal bovine serum, but absent in dog serum. Plating in the presence of fibronectin, collagen, laminin, polylysine, cycloheximide and steroids or in Primaria dishes did not alter the efficiency of attachment. Dog serum was more potent than human, guinea pig, hamster or fetal bovine serum to stimulate cell proliferation. No growth occurred in cultures supplemented with cycloheximide. The effect of dog serum on cell growth was due to two fractions of 200 Kd and 1-2 Kd. Cell differentiation, as monitored by intracellular accumulation of lipid droplets and an increase in acid phosphatase activity were also regulated by dog serum. A 300 Kd component was responsible for the accumulation of lipid droplets and this process was not altered by the presence of cycloheximide. The increase in acid phosphatase activity was due to the de novo synthesis of a major form of the enzyme and was inhibited by cycloheximide. Thus, several functions of prostatic epithelial cells which are controlled in vivo by steroids, are regulated in vitro by non-steroidal components present in the circulation. (Supported by MRC, FRSQ and FCAC).

524 MONOCLONAL ANTIBODY TO MCF-7 CELL LINE ESTROGEN-REGULATED PROTEIN RECOGNIZES ESTROGEN DEPENDENT LEYDIG CELL PROTEIN: AN IMMUNO-CYTOCHEMICAL STUDY.

D. R. Ciocca* and M. L. Dufau. LARLAC-CONICET, P.O. Box 855, Mendoza, Argentina, and Mol. Endo. Section, ERRB, NICHD, Bethesda, MD, 20205, U.S.A.

A Mr 28,000 E_2-regulated protein isolated from MCF-7 human breast cancer cells has been detected by monoclonal antibodies (MAbs) in human E_2 target organs, tumors and cell lines. (Adams et al Cancer Res. 43:4297, 1983). Also, a 27,000 Mr protein was demonstrated in the rat Leydig cell (LC) after E_2 and hCG treatment in vitro. The hCG effect occurred through increased E_2 production (Nozu et al, J. Biol. Chem. 256:12875, 1981). In this study we explored the cross-immunological identity of these proteins. Isolated LCs, and paraffin sections of testes from control rats, or rat treated with E_2 or hCG, in the presence or absence of tamoxifen, or cultured rat and human LCs treated in vitro, were analyzed by indirect immunofluorescence and the avidin-biotin peroxidase complex techniques using MAb to MCF-7 E_2-protein (provided by Dr. W. McGuire). The LCs from rat and human showed specific immunofluorescence and immunostaining upon incubation with MAb and the reaction was observed in the cytoplasm. LCs after exposure with E_2 or hCG showed the highest immunostaining/fluorescence intensity and this was reduced markedly by tamoxifen treatment. No reaction was associated with other testicular cells, and LCs exposed to preadsorbed MAb showed no reaction. We have demonstrated that the E_2 regulated protein from human cell lines and that of the rat LC share immunological similarities, showing cross-species specificity, and that this protein is present in the cytoplasm of the rat and human LC. The MAb used in this study is a valuable probe for studies on further characterization of the LC protein.

525 Functional properties of the naturally soluble adenylate cyclase from rat testis. T. Braun, Department of Physiology, Northwestern University Medical Center, Chicago, Illinois, USA.

The adenylate cyclase (AC) of germ cells, in contrast to AC of somatic cells, is not coupled to commonly known hormonal receptors. Experimental evidence thus far available also suggest that the mode of regulation and the regulatory components associated with the germ cell AC are probably different from those known to be involved in the regulation of somatic AC. In an attempt to identify potential physiological modulatory factors and the mechanism of their interaction with the germ cell AC, we have undertaken its purification from rat testis. The AC has been purified by a 5-step procedure (up to about 45,000-fold) using ion-exchange, gel-exclusion and ATP-affinity chromatography. In the course of purification the properties of the AC has been monitored at different stages of purity. The purified AC, like the AC in the unpurified state, is unresponsive to guanyl-5'-yl imidodiphosphate, fluoride and gonadotropic hormones. Forskolin a diterpene derivative, known to activate AC from a variety of somatic cells, had no effect (in a concentration range of 10^{-9}-10^{-4} M) on the activity of the germ cell AC either in unpurified cytosolic preparations, or on the activity of the purified AC. The germ cell AC is markedly inhibited by adenosine in a dose-dependent manner. However, adenosine inhibition of the purified AC occurs only in the presence of BSA in the assay medium. Thus, it appears that interaction of the purified AC with BSA, [probably taking the place of a yet unidentified cytosolic component(s)], is required to render is susceptible to inhibition by adenosine. This work was supported by a grant from NICHD HD-10006.

526 MORPHOLOGIC AND BIOCHEMICAL ANALYSIS OF HUMAN CRYPTORCHID TESTES. J.P. Buch*, P.W. Fletcher, and W.J. Cromie, Departments of Urology and Biochemistry, Albany Medical College, Albany, New York, 12208, U.S.A.

Experimental animal models of cryptorchidism, especially in the rat, have been well studied in terms of testicular morphologic changes. More recently, investigators have also begun to examine animal models in regards to changes in local hormonal-biochemical physiology. However, comparatively little such data has been presented from naturally occurring cryptorchidism in the human. In the present study testicular tissue obtained from patients undergoing surgical treatment for cryptorchidism, either orchiopexy or orchiectomy, was subjected to morphologic and biochemical analysis. Several consistent morphologic changes were noted in the testes of post-pubertal patients with long standing cryptorchidism. These findings include: 1) increased vacuolization and lipid accumulation within Sertoli cells; 2) absence of more mature testicular germ cell forms; 3) predominantly Leydig cell atrophy, with occasional evidence of hyperplastic cells; 4) increased proportions of collagen within the interstitium; and, 5) thickening and infolding of the basement membranes of the seminiferous tubules. By comparison, the prepubertal testes showed few of these changes. Preliminary results from analysis of adenylate cyclase activity in cryptorchid parients and controls indicate that basal activity is uneffected by testis location or duration of nondescent. In conclusion, the basement membrane changes that we have observed have not been presented elsewhere, and ultimately reflect a change in the nature of the blood-testis barrier in these individuals.

527 hCG REGULATION OF ANDROGEN BINDING PROTEIN (ABP) IN THE IMMATURE RAT TESTIS AND EPIDIDYMIS. ACUTE EFFECTS. S. Cigorraga*, E. Chaler, S. Campo and M.A. Rivarola. CEDIE, Hospital de Niños, Buenos Aires, Argentina.

Sertoli cells secrete most of their ABP into tubular lumen, from there it is transported to the epididymis where it is taken up by epithelial cells. Reports on androgen acute effects on ABP levels, have been challenged since Tindall et al reported that this effect might be an artifact due to the ability of testosterone (T) to stabilize ABP "in vitro". We have recently shown the presence of ABP in a particulate fraction of testes (ABPtm), which probably represents ABP before being secreted. We have studied ABP levels in testis (ABPtm and ABPtc) and epididymis (ABPec) 1 and 4 h after hCG(10 U ip) administration to 18-day-old rats (homogenization buffer containing 350 nM T). Results expressed as per cent untreated control (C) were as follows; ABPtm:1 h=101 $\pm$ 3% (n=3), 4 h=71 $\pm$ 19% (n=6), $p < 0.001$; ABPtc:1 h=97 $\pm$ 6% (n=6), 4 h=77 $\pm$ 8.5% (n=6) $p < 0.005$; ABPec:1 h=170 $\pm$ 26% (n=4) $p < 0.002$, 4 h=161 $\pm$ 28% (n=4) $p < 0.05$ (paired t test). ABPec was also studied 1 h after hCG administration in animals in which steroidogenesis was blocked by previous administration of 1 mg Aminogluthetimide (A), ABPec; C=138 $\pm$ 43 (n=8), A + hCG=165 $\pm$ 10 (n=2), hCG=250 $\pm$ 63 (n=5) fmoles/mg protein. These results suggest that acute hormonal stimulation of Leydig cells induced ABP secretion from testes to epididymis which is independent of an "in vitro" stabilizing effect on ABP.

528 EARLY EXPOSURE TO FSH AUGMENTS TESTICULAR GROWTH BUT NOT SPERM PRODUCTION IN HYPOGONADOTROPIC HYPOGONADISM. R.V. Clark* and R.J. Sherins, Developmental Endocrinology Branch, NICHD, Bethesda, Maryland, 20205, USA.

Treatment of men with complete, isolated hypogonadotropic hypogonadism (IHH) with hCG induces full virilization and initiates spermatogenesis. Completion of spermiogenesis and a sperm positive ejaculate are acheived by subsequent addition of FSH as hMG. We hypothesized that co-administration of hCG and hMG from the start of therapy would augment the testicular response. We tested this by giving either hCG alone (2000 iu, tiw) or hCG plus hMG (FSH, 75 iu, tiw) to 30 men with IHH. Changes in testis size and sperm output are below (mean $\pm$ SEM), grouped by initial testicular size, A $\leq$ 3ml, B $\geq$ 4ml. Sperm positivity indicates $\geq$ 2 million sperm per ejaculate.

	A basal	24 months	sperm	B basal	24 months	sperm
hCG	2.0±0.2ml	5.4±0.5ml	0/7	7.3±1.1ml	15.6±2.2ml	4/8
hCG/hMG	2.2±0.3	9.1±0.7	2/9	6.5±0.9	14.8±1.2	5/6
	NS	$p<0.01$	NS	NS	NS	NS

Testicular growth plateaued after 15-18 months of therapy. Patients with small testes had significantly greater testicular growth when treated with hCG/hMG than with hCG alone, 4-fold vs 2-fold, but sperm production was poor with either regimen. In patients with testes $\geq$ 4ml, final testicular size and sperm output were significantly greater with either therapy than in men with small testes. Pretreatment biopsy showed that testicular size correlated with the degree of germinal maturation. This suggests initial testis size reflects endogenous gonadotropin stimulation, and only testes $\leq$ 3ml are associated with complete IHH. We conclude that testicular size before treatment predicts response to exogenous therapy, and that early exposure to FSH (hMG) augments testicular growth but not sperm production.

529 SPECIFIC EFFECTS OF HIGHLY PURIFIED FSH ON THE TESTIS OF IMMATURE HYPOPHYSECTOMIZED RATS. J. Closset* F. Hamoir and G. Hennen. Endocrinologie Expérimentale et Clinique, Université de Liège, Institut de Pathologie, C.H.U.B23 B-4000 Liège, BELGIQUE.

The action of FSH on LH receptor development has been reappraised using the model of, and referring to, the initial observations of Ketelslegers et al. Porcine FSH has first been extensively purified and made LH free by immunosorption chromatography. Hypox. rats (24 days old, 10 per dose) were treated with increasing doses (from 2 to 128 μg) of FSH once a day for 7 days until sacrified. Maximum specific binding of LH to testicular tissue homogenate increased with FSH doses, this resulting from an increase in total number as well as in the affinity of the binding sites. Testis size improved, the germinal epithelium exhibiting evident maturation even at low doses of FSH. Despite these changes, testosterone levels in the blood remained undetectable and prostate weight was unaffected. FSH did not affect liver, adrenal, lung, thyroid or kidney tissues. Prostate acini appeared significantly modified compared to controls. Fragments of testicular tissue from FSH treated rats incubated in a HCG rich medium responded in testosterone production with sensitivity greater than that of the controls. The effects specially attributed to FSH are 1. on the tubular compartment, resulting in germinal maturation 2. priming of the interstitial cells which gain in the receptor content and affinity for LH and brings the interstitial tissue to a level of responsiveness to LH stimulation.

530 LEYDIG CELL DYSFUNCTION IN THE PUBERTAL RAT FOLLOWING TESTICULAR IRRADIATION. J.I. Delic[1]*, J.H. Hendry[1], I.D. Morris[2] and S.M. Shalet[3], [1]Department of Radiobiology, Paterson Laboratories; [3]Department of Endocrinology, Christie Hospital, Manchester, U.K., and [2]Department of Pharmacology, Medical School, University of Manchester, Manchester, U.K.

Irradiation of the testes during cancer therapy has been reported to cause Leydig cell dysfunction, particularly in children (Brauner et al. 1983, New Engl.J.Med. 309, 25). We have evaluated the effect of single acute doses (1-20 Gy) of 300 kVp x-rays administered locally to the testes of pubertal Wistar rats (4-5 weeks old). Measurements of serum LH and testosterone (T) were made, together with counts of Leydig cells and the in vitro measurement of LH receptors. Leydig cell dysfunction was observed at 2 weeks after doses of 5 Gy and above, as evidenced by reduced serum T concentrations, though LH was unchanged. By 8 weeks, some recovery of serum T was observed, though it was still depressed after 10 and 20 Gy. Serum T had recovered after all doses by 24 and 36 weeks, but progressive Leydig cell dysfunction was observed as evidenced by the increased secretion of LH after 15 or 20 Gy at 24 weeks and 10 to 20 Gy at 36 weeks. Leydig cell numbers and LH receptors were reduced at all times and doses where hormone changes indicated dysfunction, suggesting cell loss as a major mechanism. The threshold dose for dysfunction appeared to be about 5 Gy, similar to that observed in the adult rat, but the progressive dysfunction was the reverse of the recovery with time that we have previously reported in the adult rat (Delic et al. 1983, Br.J.Radiol. 56, 900). These results give support to the clinical observations in humans that the Leydig cell in the young animal may be more sensitive to cytotoxic insult than in the adult.

531 ARE ANTIMICROSOMAL AND ANTITHYROGLOBULIN PRODUCTION UNDER DIFFERENT CONTROL MECHANISMS? P.Benveniste*, B.E.Wenzel, A.Khalil, V.V.Row and R.Volpé, Department of Medicine, The Wellesley Hospital, University of Toronto, Toronto, Ontario, Canada.

Using optimal lymphocyte culture conditions ($2x10^6$ MNC/ml in Falcon tubes for 7 days at 37°C) for detection of spontaneous thyroid autoantibody production in vitro, and ELISA detection systems for antithyroglobulin (aTg) and antimicrosomal (aM) antibodies, we detected spontaneous production of these antibodies in all of 35 Hashimoto's thyroiditis (HT) mononuclear cell culture supernatants. Correlation was found only between serum aM detected by haemaglutination and in vitro aM antibody production, but not for aTg. As M antigen is apparently confined to the thyroid follicular cell, it seems unlikely that M-sensitized lymphocytes are re-stimulated in the periphery; therefore spontaneous aM production can be accounted for, either by plasma cells released from the thyroid gland, or by a T-dependent mechanism in which T-helper cells are activated enough to provide signals for blast transformation without requiring M antigenic presence, or by both mechanisms. Thus spontaneous production of aM in the periphery is a consequence of the cellular interactions taking place within the thyroid gland. The correlation between serum aM and in vitro aM production favours such a view. Conversely aTg production follows a different pattern. All elements necessary for a secondary response are present in the periphery. The lack of correlation between serum aTg and in vitro spontaneous aTg production suggests that the peripheral compartment is contributing to total aTg production. This system provides a tool for further studies of the immunoregulation of spontaneous antibody production.

532 EFFECTS OF ESTROGENS ON THE ABNORMAL THYROID STIMULATOR (TDI) IN PATIENTS WITH GRAVES' DISEASE. B. Bertrand, L. Contreras*, S. Rodriguez, J. A. Andrada and A. A. Zaninovich, Endocrine Research Lab., Nuclear Medicine Center, Hospital de Clínicas and Medical Research Institute, Univ. of Buenos Aires, Argentina.

Estrogen treatment decreased thyroid gland release in patients with Graves' disease (Zaninovich et al. J Clin Endocrinol Metab 49: 533, 1979), whereas alleviation of thyrotoxicosis during pregnancy and the postpartum recurrence of the disease were associated with changes in serum TDI and antimicrosomal (MCA) and antithyroglobulin (TgA) antibodies (Yabu et al. J Clin Endocrinol Metab 51: 1454, 1980). This work studied the effect of estrogens on serum TDI, MCA and TgA that could explain the estrogenic depression of thyroidal release. A thyrotropin (TSH) receptor antibody assay (R.S.R.Limited, Cardiff, England, normal range -8 to +8 %) was utilized. In 14 untreated patients with Graves' disease the mean inhibition of TSH binding to solubilized TSH receptors was 38.5 ± 14.3 (S.D.) % in basal samples and 35.5 ± 19.3 % after 10 days of treatment with pharmacological doses of estrogens (25 mg Dienestrol daily). The high levels of MCA (1:3657 2880) and TgA (1:828 700) were not altered by that treatment. In 11 control subjects the mean serum TDI was -4.5 ± 3.2 %. The data rule out an effect of estrogen on serum TDI, allowing the contention that the estrogenic inhibition of thyroidal secretion may be effected through blocking of the stimulatory action of TDI on thyroidal release.

533 CYTOTOXICITY IN HASHIMOTO'S THYROIDITIS. U. Bogner, H. Schleusener*, and J.R. Wall, Klinikum Steglitz, *Free University Berlin, Berlin, West-Germany and McGill University, Montreal General Hospital, Montreal, Quebec, Canada.

Antibody-dependent cell-mediated (ADCC) and natural killer (NK) cell mediated cytotoxicity against human thyroid cell targets were measured, using a chromium release assay, in patients with Hashimoto's thyroiditis (HT). In ADCC assays 51 Cr labelled thyroid cells were preincubated with patients' sera, washed and incubated with peripheral lymphocytes from normal subjects at an effector: target (E:T) ratio of 25:1 for 18 hrs. In NK assays labelled thyroid target cells were incubated with patients' lymphocytes at various E:T ratios in the absence of serum for 4 hrs. Supernatents were collected and counted in a gamma counter. Cytotoxicity was expressed as % specific release of 51 Cr from the target cells.

In ADCC mean $\pm$ SD specific lysis in patients with HT was 27.3 $\pm$ 6.1%, compared to 10.6 $\pm$ 4.7% in normals ($p < 0.0005$). A positive correlation between cytotoxicity and titers of microsomale antibodies (Mab) ($r = 0.78$, $p < 0.0005$) and titers of thyroglobulin antibodies (Tab) ($r = 0.59$, $p < 0.005$) was shown. While addition of Tab positive IgG to 2 normal sera did not influence cytotoxicity, enhanced lysis was found with a Mab positive IgG added to the same sera. NK mediated cytotoxicity was 18.3 $\pm$ 14.3 % in patients with HT, compared to 3.6 $\pm$ 2.1 % in normals ($p < 0.01$) at an E:T ratio of 50:1. The present data demonstrates that ADCC and NK activity play an important role in the immunomechanisms of patients with HT. This study was supported by a grant of NATO.

534 THE USE OF ANTI-IDIOTYPIC ANTIBODIES TO STUDY THE INTERACTION OF TSH WITH ITS RECEPTOR. R. Briones-Urbina and N.R. Farid*, Thyroid Research Laboratory, Health Sciences Centre, St. John's, Newfoundland A1B 3V6, Canada

In an attempt to investigate the nature of the interaction of TSH with its receptor we have raised anti-idiotypic (anti-id) antibodies by immunizing rabbits with rat monoclonal antibodies specific respectively for the α and β subunits of TSH. Only the β subunit specific monoclonal inhibited ^{125}I-TSH binding to thyroid plasma membranes although both monoclonals inhibited TSH driven adenylate cyclase activation. Neither of the two anti-id antibodies alone nor combinations thereof were capable of inhibiting ^{125}I-TSH binding to thyroid plasma membrane. The combination however, did stimulate adenylase cyclase to an extent comparable to 200 mU/ml TSH. α subunit specific anti-id antibodies (as normal rabbit IgG) had no effect, anti-β anti-id alone had minimal influence in promoting ^{131}I incorporation into thyrocytes and the organization of these cells into follicles. By contrast the combination of anti-id antibodies promoted these two biological activities to an extent comparable to that of 100 mU/ml TSH. Lastly, whereas the combination of α and β subunit specific anti-ids bound to the TSH holoreceptor band (M_r200,000) on protein blots of thyroid plasma membrane, neither anti-id antibody alone interacted with that band. This study stresses the dissociation of ^{125}I-TSH displacement and adenylate cyclase activation. These results favor a model of interaction of TSH with the receptor where each one of its subunits delivers a separate signal to the receptor; the β subunit apparently delivers the hormone specific signal and the α subunit acts as anchorage or maintains a favourable conformation for the β subunit.

535 BIOSYNTHESIS AND TURNOVER OF THE THYROTROPIN (TSH) RECEPTOR - EVIDENCE FOR POSITIVE REGULATION BY TSH. R. Briones-Urbina* and N.R. Farid, Thyroid Research Laboratory, Health Sciences Centre, St. John's, Newfoundland A1B 3V6, Canada.

The TSH receptor (TSH-R) is an M_r200,000 heterotetrameric glycoprotein which is specifically recognized by anti TSH-idiotypic antibodies. We have used these antibodies to study the rate of biosynthesis and turnover of TSH-R and the influence of TSH upon these parameters. 1 x 10^7 cultured porcine thyroid cells were labeled with 40 μCi [^{3}H] leucine from 15 min to 6 h in the absence or presence of bTSH (50-500 mU/ml) added at different stages of culture. TSH-R turnover rate was studied by labeling the cells for 3 h and chasing the cold medium from 2 to 96 h. At the end of the incubation periods, cells were lysed with 1.5% SDS. Protein blots of cell lysates resolved on 5-15% SDS-PAGE were incubated with anti-idiotypic antibody for 15 h and bound antibody visualized by enzyme-linked specific antibody and chromophore. The holoreceptor (M_r200,000), TSH-R subunit as well as unrelated peptide bands were cut and counted. [^{3}H] leucine incorporation was different from background within 30 min. of labeling, was maximal by 3 h and decreased beyong 6 h. Preincubation of cells with bTSH increased receptor labeling (in parallel with other cellular proteins) in a dose-dependent manner up to 100 mU/ml beyond which it declined. TSH-R had a half life of 5 h in control cultures, 7 h when TSH was included during labeling and 12 h when TSH was maintained throughout the procedure. We conclude that TSH modulates its receptor by accelerating its synthesis and prolonging its half-life. Our observations account for persistent thyroid stimulation by Graves' IgG leading to hyperthyroidism.

536 SOME CHARACTERISTICS OF THE SECOND INTERNATIONAL REFERENCE PREPARATION (IRP) OF TSH, HUMAN, FOR IMMUNOASSAY. A.F. Bristow*, N. Sutcliffe, C. Ayling and R.E. Gaines Das. National Institute for Biological Standards and Control, London NW3 6RB, UK.

The Second IRP for human TSH (coded 80/558), established in 1983, replaces the current immunoassay and bioassay standards, the first IRP (68/38) and MRC Research Standard A (63/14) respectively, and is described in this report. The bulk TSH used for the 2nd IRP was prepared in the laboratory of Dr A.F. Parlow and donated to the World Health Organization by the National Pituitary Agency of the USA. The material, extracted from human pituitary glands which were fresh-frozen post-mortem, had in vivo biological activity of 5.5 IU/mg and immunoactivity of 4.5 IU/mg. Levels of LH and FSH were 194 IU/mg and 82 IU/mg respectively, contamination with free subunits was negligible and the TSH preparation showed 5 molecular charge variants following electrophoresis. The bulk TSH was freeze-dried and ampouled and further evaluated by collaborative study in which 22 laboratories in 9 countries participated. The study revealed a difference in the stabilities of biological and immunological activites, and the ampouled material was judged to be sufficiently stable at -20°C to serve both as immunoassay and bioassay standards. Within- and between-assay variation, parallelism and assay of clinical serum samples were all acceptable. With the agreement of participants, the preparation in ampoules coded 80/558 was, with the authorization of the ECBS of WHO, established as the 2nd IRP for TSH, with a defined potency of 37 mIU/ampoule.

537 A STRUCTURAL COMPARISON OF TSH RECEPTORS FROM DIFFERENT SPECIES AND TISSUES BY PHOTO-AFFINITY LABELLING. P.R.Buckland and B. Rees Smith. Endocrine Immunology Unit, Department of Medicine, Welsh National School of Medicine, Heath Park, Cardiff U.K.

TSH receptors from porcine, human and guinea pig thyroid and from guinea pig fat have been covalently crosslinked to ^{125}I-labelled TSH and the molecular weights of the TSH-TSH receptor complexes compared. Highly purified bovine TSH (70U/mg) was coupled to the photo-reactive crosslinking reagent N-hydroxysuccinimidyl-4-azidobenzoate (HSAB) and labelled with ^{125}I. This preparation was incubated with detergent solubilised TSH receptors and the product photolysed to covalently crosslink the ^{125}I-labelled HSAB-TSH to its receptor. The TSH-TSH receptor complexes were analysed by SDS polyacrylamide gel electrophoresis with and without reduction by mercaptoethanol. Autoradiography of dried gels was carried out and bands due to the TSH receptor crosslinked to ^{125}I-labelled TSH could be seen in addition to those due to TSH and its subunits. Analysis of the relative molecular masses (M_r) of the crosslinked complexes and correction for the contribution made to the M_r by TSH indicated that all four TSH receptors examined contained two subunits of differing M_r linked by disulphide bridges: porcine thyroid 45600 and 26500; human thyroid 49900 and 32300; guinea pig thyroid 59900 and 30500 and guinea pig epididymal fat 57200 and 32000. Mild trypsin treatment of the cross-linked TSH-TSH receptor complexes from the four tissues removed a polypeptide chain from the larger of the two subunits reducing the M_rs in each case: porcine thyroid reduced by 7200 to 38400; human thyroid reduced by 6400 to 43700; guinea pig thyroid reduced by 8800 to 51100 and guinea pig epididymal fat reduced by 13900 to 43300. In the case of human and porcine receptors analysed under non-reducing conditions, removal of this polypeptide by trypsin treatment resulted in the loss of the disulphide linked second subunit. These results indicate that TSH receptors from different species and tissues are similar but not identical.

538 IODIDE ADMINISTRATION ENHANCES THYROTROPIN RESPONSIVENESS TO TRH DURING FASTING: EVIDENCE FOR NORMAL PITUITARY FEEDBACK REGULATION. K.D. Burman*, R.C. Smallridge, L. Wartofsky, Department of Clinical Investigation, Walter Reed Army Medical Center, Washington, D.C., USA 20307.

Fasting in humans is associated with diminished ΔTSH to TRH. The purposes of the present study were to: 1) reassess basal TSH levels and TRH responsiveness during fasting utilizing a highly sensitive RIA (sensitivity 0.3 µU/ml; normal range .66-2.98 µU/ml) (Nichols Institute, Los Angeles, CA) and 2) determine if normal feedback regulation is maintained during the fasting state. 8 control subjects (C) and 6 iodide-treated (I) subjects (262 mg/d) were studied in the fed state and on day 10 of fasting. T3, T4, and TSH were measured by RIA, and Free T4 (FT4) and Free T3 (FT3) by equilibrium dialysis. Statistical significance of results (mean ± SD) was assessed by paired t tests.

	Basal TSH (µU/ml)		TSH 20' After TRH	
	Fed	Fast	Fed	Fast
Control	2.0 ± 0.8	1.6 ± 0.9*	14.7 ± 9.9	8.8 ± 6.4*
Iodide	1.4 ± 0.5	2.9 ± 1.6**	12.6 ± 6.1	17.3 ± 7.1

Compared to respective fed period; * $p < .01$; ** $p < .025$

Free and total T3 decreased during fasting in both groups. Total T4 was unchanged between the fed and fasted periods in the two groups. That FT4 (ng/dl) rose significantly during fasting (2.3 ± 0.2 vs 2.7 ± 0.3, $p < .01$) in C but was unaltered in I (1.9 ± 0.3 vs 2.1 ± 0.5) suggests an etiologic role of FT4 in blunting TSH. The abolition by I of fasting-related changes in TSH further suggests that normal pituitary feedback regulation is maintained during fasting.

539 VARIANT PREALBUMIN: ANOTHER CAUSE OF EUTHYROID HYPERTHYROXINAEMIA.
P.G.H. Byfield*, M.R.A. Lalloz and R.L. Himsworth, Endocrinology Research Group, Clinical Research Centre, Harrow, Middlesex HA1 3UJ, UK.

Six unrelated euthyroid subjects have been identified in whom serum total T4 and total rT3 levels are raised whilst total T3 levels are normal. T3 resin-uptake is normal and thus a calculated free thyroxine index is greater than normal although free T4 and free T3 levels (Amerlex method) are within normal limits. These results contrast with euthyroid hyperthyroxinaemia due to variant albumin when rT3 need not be high but free T4 is always spuriously high when measured by the Amerlex analogue-tracer method. Reverse-flow electrophoresis of trace-labelled sera showed an increased carriage of T4 and rT3 on prealbumin (42% and 20%) compared with normals (20% and zero) suggesting increased affinity for the compounds. Equilibrium dialysis experiments on pure prealbumin confirmed a raised affinity for T4 (5.5×10^{8} l.mole^{-1}, normal 7.0×10^{7} l.mole^{-1}). Affinity for rT3 was 1.3×10^{6} l. mole^{-1} whereas that of the normal protein was unmeasurable. The charge and molecular size of the variant protein were shown to be unchanged from normal. We therefore propose a non-polar amino acid substitution in the binding site for T4. Negative co-operativity appears to be retained in the variant since the T4-binding capacity of the protein in serum determined directly, or indirectly by Scatchard analysis of binding data, is normal. It is not known if all four subunits have been modified; if not then polymorphism in prealbumin will have been demonstrated in the human as in the rhesus monkey.

540 THE PERFUSED GUINEA PIG PLACENTA: A MODEL TO DEMONSTRATE ACUTE IN VIVO EFFECTS ON PLACENTAL IODOTHYRONINE 5 DEIODINASE.
M. Castro*, S. Alex, R. Matys, S. Fang, L. Braverman, and C. Emerson, Univ. Mass. Med. Sch., Worcester, MA, USA.

Homogenates of rat, guinea pig (g.p.) and human placenta contain potent inner ring 5-deiodinase activity (5-D) toward T_4 and T_3. We have employed a one-pass perfusion system of g.p. placenta to study the acute effect of potential modulating agents on T_3 5-D *in vivo*. One fetal umbilical artery and vein of a pregnant g.p. is cannulated under general anesthesia and the placenta perfused for 120 min through the fetal umbilical artery with tracer ^{125}I-T_3 (0.14 nM) in KH buffer. Fractions of effluent are collected from the umbilical vein catheter and analyzed for ^{125}I labeled T_3, 3,3'-T_2 (T_2) and 3'-T_1 (T_1) by HPLC. Steady state levels of the % distribution of the ^{125}I labeled iodothyronines were reached by 20 min (T_3, 60.5 ± 6.2%; T_2, 19.6 ± 6%; T_1 9.3 ± 0.5%; n=5; mean ± SE). A marked reduction in the generation of T_2 and T_1 occurred when iopanoic acid (IA, 1 mM) was added to the perfusate from 40 to 80 min (T_3, 97.1 ± 1.3%; T_2, 1.8 ± 0.9%; T_1, undetectable). Values returned to baseline after IA perfusion was discontinued (81-120 min). The addition of 140 nM unlabeled T_3 to the perfusate also decreased T_2 and T_1 generation from ^{125}I-T_3. PTU (3mM) had no effect on 5-D. Conclusions: Guinea pig placental inner ring deiodination of T_3 can be demonstrated *in vivo* by a one-pass perfusion system. *In vivo* 5-D is inhibited by IA and an excess of unlabeled T_3. The present system provides a unique model to further evaluate the role of placental 5-D on thyroid hormone kinetics during pregnancy.

541 EFFECT OF T_3 ON PROTEIN TURNOVER IN CULTURED CARDIAC MYOCYTES.
W.J. Carter*, W.S. Benjamin and F.H. Faas, VA Medical Center and Univ. of Arkansas for Medical Sciences, Little Rock, AR, USA.

Since systemic actions of T_3 increase cardiac work, direct effects of T_3 on myocardial protein turnover may be obscured in the intact animal. Also T_3 may have a disproportionate effect on the turnover of specific protein fractions. For these reasons, the effect of T_3 on the turnover of total cellular protein, actin, and the myosin heavy chain (HC) fraction were measured in cultured cardiac myocytes from chick embryos. Fractional synthesis rates were measured by a dual isotope accumulation method, and degradation rates by release of labeled amino acids from prelabeled cell protein. During the initial 3 days exposure to 10^{-8}M T_3, the fractional synthesis rate of total cell protein increased 13-14%, the degradation rate did not change, and the rate of protein accumulation increased 30-50%. After 4 to 5 days T_3 exposure, both protein synthesis and degradation increased so that protein accumulation was no longer stimulated. A similar pattern of change in myocardial protein turnover occurred in response to T_3 treatment in intact animals. After 5 days exposure to 10^{-8}M T_3, the fractional synthesis rate of total cell protein was increased 10.4 ± 2.4%, actin, 12.8 ± 2.8%, and myosin HC, 26.8 ± 4.4%. Since T_3 exposure increased actin content 38 ± 7.6%, and myosin HC content only 12 ± 8.3%, myosin HC degradation as well as synthesis appears to be increased relative to actin. The increased turnover of the myosin HC fraction may be related to the change in myocardial isomyosins that occurs in response to T_3. This study was supported by the VA and NIH.

542 IS THERE A THYROTOXIC CARDIOMYOPATHY IN CHILDREN?
A. Cavallo*, H. D. Fawcett, A. Casta, W. J. Wolf and M. L. Nusynowitz, Departments of Pediatrics and Division of Nuclear Medicine, UTMB, Galveston, Texas, USA.

Assessment of cardiac complications related to thyrotoxicosis (T) in adults is often hampered by possible underlying cardiovascular disease. To determine the role of T alone in the development of cardiac complications we studied 8 children, ages 8-17 y, with untreated Graves' disease and without congenital or previously acquired heart disease. All had elevated serum thyroxine (T4) and triiodothyronine (T3). Left ventricular (LV) function was evaluated by M-mode echocardiography at rest and radioangiocardiography at rest and during exercise. Echocardiographic evidence for increased myocardial contractility was present in all by at least one of the following criteria: high LV shortening fraction, increased velocity of circumferential fiber shortening, or decreased ratio LV pre-ejection period/LV ejection time. Mean LV radionuclide ejection fraction (EF) was $.68 \pm .08$ at rest. During exercise, EF increased by .05 to .10 in 4 patients, but it increased by only .03 in one and decreased by .03 to .08 in 3. The correlation coefficient between ΔEF (exercise EF minus resting EF) and T4 was $r = -.87$ and between ΔEF and T3, $r = -.93$. The increase in EF during exercise in 4 patients is in keeping with the expected response in normals, but the response observed in the other 4 patients indicates decreased LV reserve. Our data confirm that T increases myocardial contractility; however, diminished LV reserve observed in 4 of 8 children without underlying heart disease suggests thyrotoxic cardiomyopathy. Furthermore, severity of T, by T4 and T3 levels, may be a determining factor in occurrence of cardiomyopathy.

543 ESTROGEN AND ANDROGEN RECEPTORS IN HUMAN THYROID TISSUE P.K. Chaudhuri,* R.A. Prinz, L. Skowron, L. Sandberg, Dept. of Surg. Loyola Univ. at Med. Center, 2160 South First Avenue, Maywood, Illinois 60153

Clinical and experimental evidence suggest that estrogen (E_2) and androgen (AND) may influence the behavior of thyroid lesions. As an initial study to evaluate the effect of these hormones, we assayed the incidence and distribution of cytosolic receptors for E_2 and AND in thyroid lesions. 28 specimens for estrogen receptor (ER) and 22 specimens for androgen receptor (AR) were assayed. All assay were performed by protamine sulfate precipitation technique and analyzed by method of scatchard. 2,4,6,7, ^3H E_2 and 17 methyl ^3H methyltrienolone (R1881) was used for ER and AR assay respectively. Triamcinolone acetonide was incorporated in AR assay to reduce non-specific binding. A receptor content (RC) of 1 fmol/mgm cytosol protein was taken as positive. Selected tissue specimens were analyzed by sucrose density gradient.

RECEPTOR	DISTRIBUTION(#Pos/#Assayed)				BINDING PARAMETER		
	Carcinoma	Adenoma	Goiter	Norm Thy.	Rc(fmol/mgm)	Kd(10^{-10}M)	Type
Estrogen	5/5	5/6	2/10	3/7	38.4±9.9	.36±.09	4.1S
Androgen	3/4	3/4	/8	4/6	16.8±5.9	.22±.06	6S

No significant binding of steroid was observed to TSH, L-Thyroxine or Bovine thyroglobulin. Our data suggest that normal and neoplastic thyroid tissue contains cytosolic ER and AR. These receptors are comparable to the receptors demonstrated in other estrogen and androgen dependent tissue raising the possibility that physiologic androgenic and estrogenic milieu may influence the growth of thyroid lesion accounting for difference in incidence and survival among male and female patients with thyroid disease.

544 Thyroid hormone secretion and metabolism in vitiligo.
M. Chaya*, T. Mitsuma, K. Sahashi, K. Murakami, E. Chaya and K. Sasada, Fourth Department of Internal Medicine, and Department of Dermatology, Aichi Medical University, Nagakute, Aichi, Japan.

Thyroid hormone secretion and metabolism in vitiligo were studied. 72 cases of vitiligo were divided into five groups, namely, general type (47), localized type (5), segmental type (5) and photosensitizer type (15). Total & free thyroxine (T_4, FT_4), total & free 3,3',5-triiodothyronine (T_3, FT_3), 3, 3',5'-triiodothyronine (rT_3), 3,3'-diiodothyronine (3,3'-T_2), thyrotropin (TSH) and thyroxine binding globulin (TBG) were measured by radioimmunoassay. Anti-thyroglobulin antibody (TGHA) and anti-microsomal antibody (MGHA) were determined by commercial available kits. Plasma T_4, T_3 and 3,3'-T_2 levels were significantly lower in general type, comparing with control. In localized type and photosensitizer type plasma T_3 was also significantly lower. Plasma FT_4 was significantly higher in segmental type. However, plasma FT_3, rT_3, TSH and TBG did not differ from those of the control. TGHA or MGHA was possitive in 38.3 % cases of general type, 21.4 % cases of photosensitizer type and in 20 % cases of segmental type, but not in localized type. The present findings suggest that some abnolmality of thyroid hormone secretion, metablism and immunological abnolmality may exist in vitiligo.

545 ROLE OF THE THYROID HORMONE BINDING INHIBITOR (THBI) IN THYROID FUNCTION ABNORMALITIES OF NONTHYROID ILLNESSES (NTI) I.J. Chopra*, T.S. Huang, A. Beredo, D.H. Solomon, UCLA School of Medicine, Los Angeles, CA 90024

Using the competitive ligand binding assay (CLBA, J.C.E.&M., 4/1984), we detected THBI in ether extracts of sera of 60% of ICU patients using 1 sample/patient (n=25) and in 88% using multiple samples (n=17). THBI levels varied up to 4-fold on different days. Mortality rate and mean serum T_4, T_3 and albumin were similar in THBI pos. and THBI neg. patients. However, low T_4 tended to be more frequent in THBI-pos. (10/15) than THBI neg. patients (3/10) ($P<0.1$). Dialyzable fraction of T_4 (DFT_4) was significantly higher in THBI pos. than THBI neg. patients (0.11±0.02 vs. 0.054±0.004%, $P<0.05$). THBI and DFT_4 were correlated significantly ($r=0.55$, $P<0.02$). In NTI patients, residual serum after ether extraction had reduced DFT_4 (0.135% to 0.069%); in normals there was no change. Addition of evaporated ether extract of NTI serum to normal serum increased DFT_4 from 0.025% to 0.14%; extract of normal serum had little or no effect. Addition of fatty acids (arachidonic, linoleic and linolenic, ∿0.2mM) to normal serum increased DFT_4 by 137 to 381% but increased resin uptake of T_3 (RT_3U) only by 13-34%. Arachidonic acid or ether extract of pooled NTI serum reduced T_4 binding activity of TBG, albumin or prealbumin in the CLBA. THBI activity of arachidonic acid in CLBA was 3.7 fold higher in the presence of 1.7mg than 5mg albumin/tube. Conclusions: i) THBI inhibits all three T_4 binding serum proteins; ii) THBI contributes importantly to high DFT_4 and to the discrepancy between DFT_4 and RT_3U in NTI; iii) THBI may contribute to low T_4 of NTI but it is multifactorial; iv) low serum albumin in NTI may enhance activity of THBI.

546 THYROID GLAND FUNCTION IN PATIENTS TREATED WITH AMIODARONE. L. Contreras, O. J. Degrossi and A. A. Zaninovich*, Endocrine Research Laboratory, Nuclear Medicine Center, Hospital de Clínicas and Deutsches Hospital, Buenos Aires, Argentina.

Amiodarone contains 75 mg iodine/200 mg of active drug. Thus a maintenance dose of 400 mg/day supplies 1000 times the daily iodine need. We studied production rates of thyroxine (T4) and thyroid gland release in 8 patients treated with 200-800 mg of amiodarone during 1-5 years. The kinetics of ^{131}I-T4 were measured by the semilogarithmic regression slope of plasma PB^{131}I and thyroidal release slopes by the daily plasma ratios of ^{127}I-T4:^{131}I-T4. Amiodarone slowed fractional turnover (8.0 ± 1.3 -S.D.- versus 11.4 ± 2.0 %/day in 5 normal subjects $P<0.005$) production rate (152 ± 75 vs 200 ± 29 ug/day, NS) and thyroidal release slopes (0.063 ± 0.033 vs 0.104 ± 0.030, NS). Five acutely treated normal subjects (400 mg/day during 8 days) had no changes during a paired study. The data failed to show significant effects of amiodarone on thyroidal secretion, albeit with a slight depression. On the other hand, in over 500 hyperthyroid or hypothyroid patients treated in our Clinics in the past 3 years, 14 had Graves' disease and 5 had hypothyroidism induced by 1 month to 5 years treatment with amiodarone. There was a prevalence of thyrotoxicosis in males (10 males, 4 females) and hypothyroidism in females (4 females, 1 male). None of the patients were from endemic goiter areas. Those with hyperthyroidism had no goiter or 0+ and only 1 patient had exophthalmos.

547 EFFECTS OF AMIODARONE ON CHILDHOOD THYROID FUNCTION (TF). D.C. Costigan*, D. Daneman, P. Hesslein, F.J. Holland, Dept. of Pediatrics, U. of Toronto, Hosp. for Sick Children, Toronto, Canada.

Normal TF is very important in childhood. We thus evaluated TF in 15 children ($\bar{X}$ age 11.7yr, range 0.5-19.5yr) treated with amiodarone(A), a potent anti-arrhythmic. A effects TF (i) by competitive inhibition of 5'monodeiodinase and (ii) through its high iodine(I) content. Three patients developed hypothyroidism; 2 required L-T4 therapy. One developed persistent hyperthyroxinemia, but was clinically euthyroid. In the remaining 11, characteristic alterations were seen in TF: significant increases in serum T4 (93±7 to 138±11 nmol/L, $p<0.01$); TSH (4±0.4 to 7±17 mU/L, $p<0.005$), and Δmax TSH post TRH stimulation (16±3 to 28±5, $p<0.05$); and decrease in rT3 (239±49 to 50±71, $p<0.02$). The latter are seen as a compensatory response of the hypothalamic-pituitary axis to A. The hypothyroidism is likely a response to the high I content of A, with failure of the compensatory mechanisms. The 20% incidence of hypothyroidism is higher than that reported in A-treated adults. Knowledge of the effect of A on TF is important since in 1 case, a 1 yr old girl, hypothyroidism went undetected, presenting as isolated developmental delay. This case emphasizes the need for serial TF testing and an adequate knowledge of the possible changes in TF seen with A-therapy.

548 BIOASSAY AND RECEPTOR ASSAY FOR THE ASSESSMENT OF THYROID STIMULATING ANTIBODIES IN UNEXTRACTED SERUM. F. M. Creagh, F. Hashim, W. Perkins, B. Rees Smith. Endocrine Immunology Unit, Dept. of Medicine, Welsh National School of Medicine, Cardiff.U.K.
Thyroid stimulating antibodies in unextracted serum have been measured by a) their ability to inhibit receptor purified 125-I-labelled TSH binding to detergent solubilised porcine TSH receptors and b) stimulation of cyclic AMP production by porcine thyroid cells in culture. Using the receptor assay (50 µl neat serum incubated with 50 µl receptors followed by 100 µl labelled TSH, with bound and free being separated by polyethylene glycol precipitation) 28 out of 28 thyrotoxic Graves' patients studied had readily detectable antibodies. In contrast, 14 patients euthyroid after antithyroid drug treatment had been discontinued showed low or undetectable levels of receptor antibody in all but one case. Thus the level of TSH receptor antibody measured tended to reflect the activity of the underlying disease. Comparison of assays using neat sera and immunoglobulin concentrates showed good agreement ($r = 0.94$). In the bioassay, isolated porcine thyroid cells were cultured for 48 hrs. (500,000 per well). The medium was then replaced with 300 µl low sodium Hanks BSS containing test serum (100 µl heat activated) or immunoglobulin concentrate (1.25 mg) both of which had been dialysed against low sodium Hanks. After 2 hours incubation, the cyclic AMP released into the medium was measured. In the absence of serum, basal cyclic AMP levels were 4.9 ± 1.3 pmol/well and in the presence of 10 µU bovine TSH 18 ± 1.5 pmol/well (mean ± SD of 8 separate assays). With individual normal sera, released cyclic AMP levels ranged from 2.5 - 15.8 pmol/well (mean ± SD 8.9 ± 4.6, n = 12). Sera from 14 out of 18 (77 %) thyrotoxic Graves' patients caused cyclic AMP levels to increase significantly ($p < 0.05$) above the level observed in the presence of pooled normal human serum control. Immunoglobulin concentrates of these 18 sera gave similar results ($r = 0.95$). TSH receptor binding activity was also measured in the patients' dialysed serum and was positive in all 18. Quantitatively stimulation of cyclic AMP production and inhibition of TSH binding showed the same trend and the relationship between the two parameters was highly significant ($r = 0.75$).

549 SYNGENEIC CO-CULTURES OF ISOLATED THYROID CELLS AND PERIPHERAL T CELLS FROM PATIENTS WITH GRAVES' DISEASE. T.F. Davies*, M. Platzer and S.H. Roman, Department of Medicine, Mount Sinai School of Medicine, New York, New York, USA.

We, and others, have shown that Ia (DR) antigens are present on the surface of stimulated human thyroid cells. Therefore, the use of allogeneic thyroid membrane preparations for the demonstration of T cell autosensitization may lead to erroneous results. To overcome this problem, we have employed a system utilizing thyroid cell monolayers initiated following thyroid surgery and co-cultured with syngeneic T cells. Antigen-induced blastogenesis was monitored using 24 hr. ^{3}Hthymidine uptake. Control experiments with 5-day cultured normal thyroid cells from tissue around benign adenomata showed no evidence of syngeneic T cell autosensitization, although both phytohemmagglutinin (PHA) and allogeneic cells induced blastogenesis. Human thyroid cells alone could not be induced to take up ^{3}Hthymidine even in the presence of bTSH. In 3 of 4 experiments with Graves' thyroid cells there was significant induction of syngeneic T cell blastogenesis with a mean stimulation index of 220%. Both PHA and allogeneic cells were able to induce a much larger response indicating that the experimental conditions were not limiting. These data show that patients with Graves' disease possess circulating T cells which exhibit a modest degree of autosensitization to syngeneic thyroid cell surface antigens, a phenomenon not demonstrable in normal individuals.

550 HUMAN-HUMAN B CELL HYBRIDOMAS FROM IN-VITRO STIMULATED LYMPHOCYTES OF PATIENTS WITH AUTOIMMUNE THYROID DISEASE. E. DeBernardo*, S.H. Roman and T.F. Davies. Department of Medicine, Mount Sinai School of Medicine, New York, N.Y., USA.

Human-human B cell hybridomas have been established using lymphocytes of patients with Hashimoto's thyroiditis and Graves' disease. Peripheral mononuclear cells (PMC) were co-cultured with either PWM (0.5%) or Staph. aureus (0.003%) for 48 hrs, or employed directly, and fused with an HGPRT negative human myeloma cell line (Gm-4672) using PEG (40%). Developing hybridomas were screened by ELISA's for human IgG, IgM and antibodies to thyroglobulin (Tg) and thyroid microsomal (M) antigen. Hybridoma formation was only observed after prior mitogen stimulation of PMC and was optimal with a PMC:Gm ratio of 1:1. The amounts of antibody produced by IgM and IgG secreting hybridomas were similar (50-500ng/ml). PMC from patients with Hashimoto's thyroiditis exhibited significantly greater hybridoma production than PMC from patients with hyperthyroid Graves' disease and specific antibody secretion was observed to be predominantly IgM.

Disease	Fusions	% Hybridomas	% Hybridomas with anti-Tg	% Hybridomas with anti-M
Hashimoto's	(n=3)	50.5	13.8	3.2
Graves'	(n=4)	7.5	7.0	7.0

These data establish critical criteria for the production of human thyroid autoantibody secreting hybridomas and their subsequent clonal analysis.

551 RELATION OF MORBIDITY AND MORTALITY OF THYROID CANCER TO CLINICAL STAGE AND TREATMENT. L.J. DeGroot*, M. McCormick, F. Straus, and E.L. Kaplan. Thyroid Study Unit, Department of Medicine, The University of Chicago, Chicago, IL.

We have analyzed therapy of 265 patients with thyroid cancer (ca) followed on average 9 yrs. Survival, recurrences, and complications were related to histology, stage, extent of surgery, neck dissection, and ^{131}I ablation. Deaths from papillary-follicular (P-F) ca were 2%, 0%, 12%, 33% in Stages I-III. In 91 Stage I P-F ca, recurrences were more frequent in lobectomy compared to near total thyroidectomy ($p < .05$), and in patients not given ^{131}I ablation ($p < .01$), independent of extent of surgery. Recurrence correlated with tumor size but not multifocality. Cervical adenopathy did not affect outcome. Recurrence or death in Stage III P-F correlated with tumor size, capsular invasion, and multifocality. Some Stage IV P-F survived with mets 2-40 years. In F ca, stage correlated with age and tumor size. The only death in Stage I or II F ca occurred in a patient not ablated with ^{131}I. No patient with Stage I or II P-F or F ca < 2 cm given near total resection and ^{131}I ablation has died from ca. All 12 patients with medullary ca are alive, although 8/12 have residual. Postoperative ^{131}I thyroid ablation failed to reduce CT. All patients with anaplastic ca died in 1-30 months. Intentional single recurrent nerve (RC) section occurred in 2.7%, and unintentional RC section in 3.8%. Hypoparathyroidism occurred in 3.9% of all patients, but in 1/119 patients operated by one surgeon. Freedom from recurrence in P-F ca, and specifically in Stage I tumors, was best in patients receiving more extensive operations and ^{131}I ablation. These results can be achieved with very low complication rates. Results of ^{131}I therapy in Stage IV patients were highly variable, primarily in relation to tumor ^{131}I uptake, but bone metastasis carried a poor prognosis.

552 CRONOPHYSIOLOGICAL VARIATIONS OF TRIIODOTHYRONINE (T3) KINETICS. O.J.Degrossi,* T.Watanabe, A.A.Zaninovich, M.Cabrejas and N.Altschuler. Biolog.Appl. Dment.,Atomic Ener.Commission and Endr.Res.Lab. Clin.Htal.Bs. Aires.

We reviewed 68 studies of T3 kinetics in a group of euthyroid subjects(6-83 years old,37 males).The single i.v. injection method employing less than 0.5 µCi b.w. of 125-I-T3(100-150 mCi/mg) was utilized. Maximum activity used up to 15 years of age was 10 µCi. An age dependent distribution volume (V) was observed up to 60years old subjects;V increased from 15.5 l $\pm$ 3.4 ($\bar{x}$; s.d.) below 10 years of age up to 40.9 l$\pm$ 7.6 in adults (55% b.w. in both groups) and decreased to 20.9 l$\pm$2.8 (30% b.w.) over 60 years ($p <$ 0.01).Plasma half-time(t 1/2) increased with age,from 18.5 h$\pm$ 3.3 below 15 years old subjects to 32.9 h$\pm$ 9.9 in middle age subjects and to 36.8 h$\pm$ 11.2 over sixty years. The production rate (R) showed a decrease with age When PR was expresed in µg/d/kg b.w.,two exponential curves were found,the first one with a fast decrease representing subjects below 15 years old and the second with a slow decrease for subjects over 15 years of age ($PR = 1.01\ e^{-0.1447ag} + 0.614\ e^{-0.0173ag}$).PR decreased from 0.74µg/d/kg b.w.$\pm$ 0.17 below 15 years of age to 0.39 $\pm$0.17 in adults and to 0.14µg/d/kg b.w. $\pm$0.03 over sixty years old subjects ($p < 0.01$).

Previous work suggested that a diminution on extrathyroidal thyroxine (T4) convertion to T3 was the main factor for the decrease of serum T3 values observed in elderly subjects. Our findings suggest that factors other than T4 convertion to T3 may participate in this observed decrease in serum T3 in the elderly.

553 N-TERMINAL PROOPIOCORTIN (N-POC) PEPTIDES ARE INVOLVED IN ADRENAL REGENERATION IN THE RAT

F. Estivariz, Centro de Estudios Endócrinos, Universidad Nacional de La Plata, 1900, La Plata, Argentina.

In order to establish wether N-POC peptides play a role in the mechanisms controlling the rapid regeneration of the adrenal cortical parenchyma after complete adrenal enucleation in the rat, we have administered either anti-N-POC serum, anti ACTH serum or normal rabbit serum (NRS) to bienucleated rats. Adult male rats 9 and 16 days post enucleation (PE) were distributed in six groups which received 100 µl daily of either of the mentioned sera subcutaneously for 5 days. After the last serum injection at 14 and 21 days respectively, each animal was injected intraperitoneally with colchicine (1 µg/g body weight) and sacrificed 6 hours later. Adrenal glands were removed, weighed, fixed and processed for light microscopical examination. Mitotic figures were counted in at least three sections per adrenal and mitotic indexes were calculated. Relative adrenal weights of anti-N-POC-treated groups at 14 and 21 days PE were lower than anti-ACTH or NRS-treated groups but differences were not statistically significant. Adrenal mitotic indexes of anti-N-POC-treated animals were 38% and 25% lower than NRS controls at 14 and 21 days PE respectively, the differences were highly significant. Anti-ACTH serum treatment only significantly lowered mitotic indexes in about 10% respect to NRS groups at 21 days PE. It is concluded that N-POC peptides may play an important role in the regeneration of the adrenal cortex after bienucleation in the rat. This study was supported by the Consejo Nacional de Investigaciones Científicas y Técnicas de la Republica Argentina.

554 CHARACTERISTICS OF RELEASE OF ACTH, β-LPH AND β-ENDORPHIN FROM PERIFUSED OVINE PITUITARY CELLS STIMULATED BY CRF PULSE TRAINS.

M.J. Evans*, J.T. Brett, R.P. McIntosh, J.E.A. McIntosh, H.K. Roud, J.H. Livesey and R.A. Donald, Dept of Endocrinology, The Princess Margaret Hospital, Christchurch, and Dept of Obstetrics & Gynaecology, Wellington Clinical School of Medicine, University of Otago at Wellington, New Zealand.

We have shown that each pulse of synthetic corticotrophin-releasing factor (CRF) stimulates a highly correlated pulsatile release of ACTH, β-endorphin immunoreactivity and β-lipotrophin from dispersed, perifused ovine pituitary cells. Here we report changes in the dynamics of release of these hormones when the stimulating CRF pulse period and width are varied. After 24h culture, sets of 14 identical dispersed cell samples were loaded into computer controlled columns and stimulated with 200ng CRF/ml continuously or with trains of pulses varying in width from 2-16 min and in period from 10-160 min over 10h. Cell hormone responses were analysed by radioimmunoassay. We found that a) hormone release was maximal at initial application of each pulse. Response then declined slowly, becoming desensitized as stimulation continued. b) Longer periods between pulses of constant width increased both response per pulse and response height ($p < .001$). c) Maximal total release over 10h occurred at stimulation periods in the region 20-80 min and depending on pulse width/pulse period. Similar characteristics are found also in LH release stimulated by GnRH pulse trains (McIntosh & McIntosh, J Endocr 98, 411, 1983). In summary, perifused ovine pituitary cells display particular sensitivity to abrupt changes in levels of these stimuli, but have an inherent lag time before responding optimally to subsequent signals.

555 SUBNORMAL ACTH SECRETION AFTER NEUROINTERMEDIATE LOBECTOMY (NIL-X) IN THE RAT IS RELATED TO STIMULUS MODALITY, NOT INTENSITY. K. Fagin*, C. Cascio, M. Dallman, Dept. of Physiology, UCSF, San Francisco, CA 94143 USA.

After NIL-X surgery, rats have elevated basal plasma ACTH and corticosterone (B) levels and attenuated increases in these after NEUROTROPIC (noise, novelty), but not INTEROCEPTIVE (hemorrhage, surgery), stimuli (Endocrinology 110:289A). This occurs in spite of normal perceptual capacity (Neuroscience 8:53A) and is not due to negative feedback by chronically high B (Endocrinology 112:148A). Since in control (NIL-C) rats plasma ACTH after interoceptive stress is twice that after neurotropic stress, we tested the hypothesis that the subnormal ACTH response of NIL-X rats to the latter is due to its low intensity rather than its modality. Male Sprague-Dawley NIL-X (n=9) and NIL-C (n=5) rats were instrumented with femoral artery cannulas chronically exteriorized from the cage for 15 days for use without being handled. All rats received each of the following: noise, low, and high, doses of hypoglycemia, an interoceptive stimulus. RESULTS: NIL-C and NIL-X rats had identical dose-related profiles of plasma glucose and B after intra-arterial injection of saline, or insulin at 0.1 and 0.5 IU/kg body weight when fasted overnight. Plasma ACTH levels after low and high doses of insulin were approximately 150 pg/ml and 2-2.5 fold this level, respectively, in each group. After metal-rattling noise, plasma ACTH levels in these NIL-C rats increased from 55 ± 5 to 237 ± 51 pg/ml, but did not increase in the NIL-X rats (from 69 ± 4 to 87 ± 17 pg/ml, $p>0.10$). CONCLUSION: NIL-X rats have normal ACTH responses to a low intensity stimulus that is interoceptive in modality. Thus, in NIL-X rats the subnormal ACTH response to neurotropic stimuli is due to the modality of the stimulus rather than to the relatively low intensity. (Grants AM28172, AM07265).

556 A DOPAMINE-2 RECEPTOR MECHANISM STIMULATES THE RELEASE OF IMMUNOREACTIVE β-ENDORPHIN (iβ-END) FROM THE RAT PARS DISTALIS IN VIVO. J.M. Farah*, and G.P. Mueller, Dept. Physiol., USUHS, Bethesda, MD 20814 USA

Although corticotrophs of the pars distalis (PD) are not directly influenced by dopamine *in vitro*, results of our recent *in vivo* studies suggest that, in addition to well-established dopaminergic inhibition of pars intermedia (PI) iβ-END release, dopamine may also regulate PD iβ-END release. We examined this possibility further by determining the effects of dopaminergic agonists on plasma levels of total iβ-END, as well as β-lipotropin (β-LPH), the molecular form of iβ-END secreted exclusively by the PD. Apomorphine, an agonist of D-1 and D-2 dopamine receptor subtypes, dose-relatedly increased circulating levels of total iβ-END up to 4-fold as compared to control values. Gel chromatography revealed that apomorphine consistantly increased the form of plasma iβ-END resembling β-LPH nearly 8-fold, whereas β-END-sized peptides in plasma were decreased by 30%. These reciprocal changes in the major molecular forms of circulating iβ-END, as well as increases in plasma levels of total iβ-END, were mimicked by the D-2 agonist, LY 141865, but not by the D-1 agonist, SKF 38393. These observations suggest that D-2 receptor stimulation evokes the release of PD iβ-END while simultaneously decreasing PI release of iβ-END. Consistent with this interpretation, the LY 141865-induced release of iβ-END was prevented by pretreatment with sulpiride, a D-2 antagonist, and also by dexamethasone, an inhibitor of PD corticotrophs. Together these findings suggest that dopamine neurons exert a stimulatory influence over corticotropin releasing factor as well as inhibitory control over PI release of iβ-END and both processes are mediated via D-2 receptors.

557 PRODUCTION OF MONOCLONAL ANTIBODIES TO HUMAN β-ENDORPHIN. Ivy Fettes*, S. Kuzniak, Dept. Medicine, Univ. of Toronto, Toronto, Canada.

The hybridoma methodology of Köhler and Miltstein has been used to produce monoclonal antibodies to human β-endorphin (β_h-END). Spleen cells from Balb/C mice immunized with synthetic β_h-END were fused with the myeloma spleen cell line SP 2/0. The desired hybrids were selected with HAT medium containing the nucleotides hypoxanthine and thymidine and the folic acid antagonist aminopterin. The hybrid supernatants were tested for β_h-END antibody production by the Elisa technique (enzyme linked immunosorbent assay). Those cell populations producing antibodies to β_h-END were cloned by limiting dilution to obtain single cell colonies. Positive clones were cultured and expanded by production of ascites in mice. The ascitic antibodies were subtyped for immunoglobulin identification (Boehringer-Manheim) and purified on a protein A-Sepharose column. Five monoclonal antibodies to human β-endorphin thus produced were found to be IgG_1. Antibody specificity and usefulness in Endocrine assessment will be described and compared with the polyclonal antibody in current use.

558 TRANSCRIPTIONAL REGULATION OF PRO-OPIOMELANOCORTIN GENE EXPRESSION. J.-P. Gagner* and J. Drouin, Institut de Recherches Cliniques de Montréal, 110 Ave des Pins O., Montréal H2W 1R7, Canada.

Pro-opiomelanocortin (POMC) is the protein precursor to ACTH, β-lipotropin, β-endorphin and the melanotropins. We have isolated by molecular cloning from a rat genomic DNA library about 30 Kb of DNA containing the entire POMC gene. The three exons of the gene and about 600 bp of presumed regulatory upstream sequences have been sequenced. Southern blot analyses suggest that there is only one POMC gene in the rat. Glucocorticoids decrease steady-state POMC mRNA levels only in the anterior lobe of the pituitary but not in the intermediate lobe. In order to determine if this effect is due to regulation at the level of transcription, we have measured the effect of dexamethasone (DEX) treatment of adrenalectomized rats on POMC transcription rates by incorporation of ^{32}P-labelled UTP into transcripts of isolated pituitary nuclei. The labelled RNAs encoding POMC and actin (an internal control) were quantitated by filter hybridization. We found that DEX inhibits by 10 to 20-fold the POMC transcription rate in parallel with the decrease of plasma ACTH levels. This effect occurs within 30 min and is specific for the anterior pituitary. Actin transcription rates are not affected. Further transcription experiments using nuclei prepared from primary cultures of anterior pituitary cells show that POMC transcription rate is enhanced by corticotropin-releasing factor (CRF) and reduced by DEX both in the presence and absence of CRF. Basal POMC transcription rates are similar in cultured cells and in intact rats. These experiments indicate that DEX and CRF act directly on POMC transcription in addition to their documented effect on POMC peptide release. (Supported by the MRC and NCI of Canada).

559 CALCITONIN, ANALGESIA AND ENDOGENOUS OPIOIDS. R.C. Gaillard*, L. Gauthey, V. Boerlin+ and A.F. Muller, Clinique Médicale, University Hospital, CH-1211 Geneva 4, Switzerland, and Experimental Therapeutic Department+, Sandoz Ltd, Basle, Switzerland.

Calcitonin has been reported to possess an analgesic effect. The aim of this study was to evaluate this analgesic effect and to establish whether it can be attributed to changes in peripheral levels of endogenous opioids. Normal volunteers and cancerous patients with pain due to bone metastases were investigated. Thirteen normal volunteers received, double-blind, i.v., 100 IU of synthetic salmon calcitonin Sandoz, or an equivalent volume of 0.9% NaCl. Plasma ACTH, β-endorphin and met-enkephalin levels were measured in samples collected at regular intervals. Twenty patients with chronic pain due to bone metastases were investigated in a double-blind, parallel group comparison of salmon calcitonin and placebo over a period of 5 to 12 days. Blood samples for measuring β-endorphin and met-enkephalin were collected the first and the fifth day. Pain intensity was assessed daily by a visual analogue scale and a verbal rating scale. No significant variations in β-endorphin and met-enkephalin levels were observed in either group. β-endorphin levels however were higher in the patient group. Pain intensity diminished and general condition improved in the calcitonin group, but these changes were not statistically significant when compared with the placebo group. In conclusion, peripherally injected calcitonin, in our study, was unable to produce changes in peripheral endogenous opioids, nor to produce a significant analgesic effect in patients with bone metastases.

560 EFFECT OF CLONIDINE ON PLASMA BETA ENDORPHIN AND CORTISOL LEVELS IN OPIATE-ADDICTED SUBJECTS. I. Gil-Ad, J. Bar-Yoseph, Y. Smadja, M. Zohar and Z. Laron*, Beilinson Med. Ctr., Petah Tikva & Abarbanel Mental Hospital, Bat Yam, Tel Aviv University, Israel.

The effect of clonidine, a central alpha-2-adreno receptor agonist, on plasma beta endorphin (beta EP) and cortisol secretion was studied in 10 opiate-addicted subjects, 8 on metadone and 2 on mixed narcotic drugs (8 males and 2 females aged 21-37 yrs), and in 10 control subjects aged 15-33 yrs. Clonidine (0.075 mg/m^2 p.o.) was administered in the morning 12-18 hrs after the last opioid drug administration. Basal morning beta EP levels were lower in addicted than in control subjects (3.3 ± 0.7 vs. 6.0 ± 0.9 pmol/l) and increased following clonidine in addicted subjects to reach normal values; in the controls clonidine did not modify plasma beta EP levels. Basal morning cortisol levels were higher in addicted subjects as compared to control subjects (21.0 ± 3.6 ug/dl vs. 13.0 ± 1.2 ug/dl mean ± SEM). Clonidine induced a 20% decrease in plasma cortisol in addicted subjects whereas in control subjects there was a 50% decrease. It is hypothesized that in addicted subjects there is an impaired activity of endogenous opioid peptides leading to alterations in plasma cortisol secretion. In conclusion, clonidine probably relieves narcotic withdrawal symptoms by decreasing the central noradrenergic activity and stimulating beta endorphin secretion.

561 CHARACTERISATION AND BIOACTIVITY OF N-PRO-OPIOMELANOCORTIN FRAGMENTS FROM TUMOURS ASSOCIATED WITH CUSHING'S SYNDROME. Ann C. Hale*, Sally J. Ratter, G.M. Besser and Lesley H. Rees, Departments of Chemical Endocrinology and Endocrinology, St. Bartholomew's Hospital, London, EC1A 7BE, U.K.

The molecular forms of pro-opiomelanocortin (POMC)-derived peptides in extracts of pituitary and ectopic ACTH secreting tumours have been characterised by acid-dissociating Sephadex G75 chromatography. In pituitary microadenomas associated with Cushing's disease, predominant peaks of 1-39 ACTH, 1-76 N-terminal pro-opiocortin (N-POC), β-LPH, γ-LPH and β-endorphin were observed. However, extracts of ectopic tumours contained, in addition to these major peaks, a peak eluting at a molecular weight of 22K, with both γ-MSH and ACTH immunoreactivities. This 22K fragment was also observed in the chromatographic profile of tumour tissue from three patients with large, invasive pituitary tumours, and biochemical characteristics of the ectopic ACTH syndrome. The bioactivity of 22K MSH/ACTH and 1-76 N-POC, isolated from tumour tissue, was investigated using the perfused isolated rat adrenal cell column. 22K ACTH was equipotent (on a molar basis), with 1-39 ACTH, in inducing steroidogenesis. Both aldosterone and corticosterone were secreted in a linear, dose-dependent manner (10^{-11}-10^{-9}M). During a constant perfusion of 22K ACTH, (10^{-11}M) the response of both steroids to 1-39 ACTH was potentiated. This potentiation effect was not observed during perfusion of 1-76 N-POC (10^{-9}M). The characterisation of 22K MSH/ACTH in ectopic tumours and atypical pituitary tumours suggests that it is this peptide which may be responsible, both through its own bioactivity and its potentiation effect on 1-39 ACTH, for the hypokalaemia usually associated with the ectopic ACTH syndrome.

562 DEOXYCORTICOSTERONE (DOC) -PRODUCING ADRENOCORTICAL CARCINOMA : TWO CASES OPERATED ON WITH LONG TERM REMISSION AND IN VITRO STUDY.
R. DOUMITH*, Y. TOUITOU and J. CABANE. Hôpital de la PITIE, 83 bld de l'Hôpital, 75013 PARIS, FRANCE.

We report two patients with adrenal tumors revealed by hypermineralocorticism. The hormonal picture was particular because only the levels of DOC (6000 and 24000 pg/ml, respectively) and to a lesser degree of 11-deoxycortisol (S) (2 and 3 µg/dl, respectively) were high . Plasma Aldosterone and renin values were low . Plasma cortisol (F) and sex hormone levels were in the normal range. The malignant nature of these tumors was proved by hepatic metastases in one case and by local extension, cytologic study and weight (640g) in the other one. The histologic aspect suggested a glomerular origin for these tumors. Both could be operated on with success allowing a reversal of the hormonal abnormalities and a disease-free survival of five and two years, respectively (the patient with hepatic metastases underwent a right hepatectomy at the same time and was then given o,p'-DDD). Incubations were performed in vitro, using tritiated Progesterone,DOC, Corticosterone(B), 17 hydroxy-Progesterone and S as precursors according to a protocol previously published (Touitou, et al., J. Steroid Biochem;1978, 9, 1217). The conversion rates of S to F and DOC to B were markedly reduced (about 2 % for each synthesized steroid) in one tissue, suggesting a 11 β-hydroxylase deficiency. In the other tissue they reached 11 %, a figure which can be considered as low when compared with "normal" human adrenals.
The two patients are rare cases of DOC-producing adrenocortical carcinoma from both in vivo and in vitro study.

563 ACTH-DEPENDENT STIMULATION OF STEROIDOGENESIS AND TETRAHYDROBIOPTERIN BIOSYNTHESIS IN ADRENAL CORTICAL CELLS IN CULTURE. D.S. Duch*, J.H. Woolf, M.P. Edelstein and C.A. Nichol, The Wellcome Research Laboratories, Research Triangle Park, NC 27709, U.S.A.

The adrenal cortex contains high levels of tetrahydrobiopterin (BH_4) and GTP cyclohydrolase (GTP-CH), the initial enzyme in the *de novo* biosynthetic pathway for BH_4. Although BH_4 is the cofactor for aromatic amino acid hydroxylations in tissues which synthesize monoamines, the role of BH_4 in the adrenal cortex is unknown. Abou-Donia *et al.* (Endocrinology 112, 2088, 1983) have shown that the administration of ACTH *in vivo* elevated both BH_4 and GTP-CH levels in rat adrenal cortex. The role of ACTH in the regulation of BH_4 biosynthesis was studied using Y-1 adrenal cortical tumor cells in culture. ACTH produced increases in GTP-CH and BH_4; stimulation was dependent on the source of ACTH. Synthetic $ACTH_{1-24}$ was more potent than porcine ACTH. BH_4 biosynthesis was increased at the same concentration which caused maximum stimulation of steroidogenesis. Smaller fragments of the ACTH molecule (1-4, 1-10, 1-17 and 11-24) were inactive at concentrations up to 100-fold higher than $ACTH_{1-24}$. Other peptides derived from the pro-opiomelanocortin molecule, either alone or in combination with submaximal doses of ACTH, also had no effect on BH_4 biosynthesis. The increase in BH_4 biosynthesis in response to ACTH was dependent on cell density, stimulation being higher at lower cell densities, but was independent of length of time in culture. The lack of ACTH stimulation at high cell density was not due to steroids produced by the cells, since addition of cell extracts or other steroids had no effect on ACTH-dependent stimulation of BH_4 biosynthesis at low cell densities The agreement of these results with the effects of ACTH on the adrenal cortex *in vivo* indicates that Y-1 cells in culture can be used as a model system for studying the regulation of BH_4 biosynthesis and its functions in the adrenal cortex.

564 LOW SHBG AND NORMAL ESTRADIOL/TESTOSTERONE RATIO IN OBESE CHILDREN. L. Dunkel, R. Voutilainen *, and R. Sorva, Children's Hospital, University of Helsinki, Finland.

In adults sex-hormone binding globulin (SHBG) levels are positively correlated with the serum estrogen/androgen ratio. Little is known about SHBG regulation in prepubertal children. Serum estradiol (E_2) and testosterone (T), and serum capacity to bind dihydrotestosterone (SHBG) were assessed in 20 obese children (9 boys) with relative body weight (RBW) 135-205 % and in 41 children (18 boys) with RBW 75-120 %. Ten of the obese and 14 of the normal children were prepubertal. The E_2 and T levels and E_2/T ratio were similar in obese and normal prepubertal children, whereas the SHBG level was significantly lower in the obese. In prepuberty the mean SHBG was 30.0 (range 14.5-63.7) nmol/l in obese children and 98.6 (63.0-187.5) nmol/l in normal children ($p< 0.001$). The difference was the same at all stages of puberty.In prepubertal children SHBG was not correlated with E_2, T or the E_2/T ratio. A strong negative correlation was found between SHBG and RBW in all 61 children studied ($r= -0.79$, $p< 0.001$), even in normal prepubertal children ($N=27$, $r= -0.48$, $p< 0.01$). In obese adult males low serum T, and low SHBG but high E_2 have been found. One explanation put forward is that defective estrogen receptors permit unopposed androgen action, resulting in lower SHBG production. The present study suggests that the estrogen/androgen ratio does not explain the negative correlation between SHBG and RBW in prepuberty, when E_2 and T levels are low. It is postulated that some weight-related factors, thus far unknown, regulate SHBG levels in childhood independently of the estrogen/androgen ratio.

565 EFFECT OF ALDOSTERONE INFUSION ON ADRENAL COMPENSATORY HYPERTROPHY IN THE RAT. N. E. Dunlap* and W. E. Grizzle, Departments of Internal Medicine and Pathology, University of Alabama in Birmingham, and Veterans Administration Medical Center, Birmingham, Alabama 35294

We have reported that infusion of aldosterone at 85 ng/100 g body weight-hour (ng/wh) blocks the compensatory growth of the remaining adrenal gland following unilateral adrenalectomy in rats or hamsters. We now report that in the rat continuous infusion of aldosterone via Alzet pumps at a rate above 55 ng/wh blocks adrenal compensatory hypertrophy (ACH) and that ACH is not blocked when the infusion rate is reduced to or below 35 ng/wh. ACH also is blocked when infusion of aldosterone is postponed until 16 hours after unilateral adrenalectomy, but not if infusion of aldosterone is begun 30 hours after unilateral adrenalectomy. Continuous infusion of aldosterone at a blocking dose beginning 10 days prior to unilateral adrenalectomy and continuing until animal sacrifice did not block ACH. This result is consistent with an experiment in which animals were maintained on very low sodium diets for three weeks prior to unilateral adrenalectomy. Although endogenous levels of aldosterone in these animals reached levels much higher than those achieved by continuous infusion of aldosterone, ACH was not blocked. We conclude that 1) continuous infusion of aldosterone at a rate at or above 55 ng/wh beginning less than 16 hours after unilateral adrenalectomy blocks ACH, and 2) if either aldosterone is infused or endogenous aldosterone is elevated beginning 10 days or more prior to unilateral adrenalectomy, compensatory adrenal hypertrophy is no longer blocked by aldosterone; and thus, ACH appears to "escape" the blocking action of aldosterone.

566 **DISTINCT HLA-B ANTIGEN ASSOCIATIONS FOR THE SALT-WASTING AND SIMPLE-VIRILIZING FORMS OF CONGENITAL ADRENAL HYPERPLASIA DUE TO 21-HYDROXYLASE DEFICIENCY.** B. Dupont, R. Virdis, A.J. Lerner, M.S. Pollack, C. Nelson, M.I. New*. Sloan-Kettering Institute For Cancer Research; Cornell University Medical College, New York, N.Y. 10021 U.S.A.

The salt-wasting (SW) and simple-virilizing (SV) forms of congenital adrenal hyperplasia (CAH) due to 21-hydroxylase deficiency (21-OH def) are both autosomal recessive defects of gene(s) closely linked to the HLA-B locus. HLA-antigen associations with CAH have been described, of which an increase in Bw47, Bw60(40) and Bw51(5) and an decrease in B8 have been confirmed in several studies. We now demonstrate that some of these HLA antigen associations are characteristic of the SV form of the disease; others are characteristic of the SW form, and some are common to both forms. We have studied the complete HLA genotypes in 150 Caucasian families of patients with CAH: 83 North American Caucasian families, 40 Italian, 11 Yugoslavian and 16 Swiss. A total of 76 patients with SV and 74 with SW were studied and the HLA antigens of the patients were compared with the HLA antigens on the non-affected parental HLA haplotypes.

HLA-B	Gene Frequencies			
Antigen	Total CAH	SV	SW	Control
B5	0.122	0.183	0.062	0.072
B14	0.038	0.070	0.007	0.028
B40	0.090	0.028	0.151	0.052
Bw47	0.045	0.028	0.062	0.004
B8	0.024	0.014	0.034	0.064

The B5 and B14 antigens were selectively increased among patients with SV ($\chi^2 = 8.84$, $p < 0.0005$ and $\chi^2 = 6.28$, $p < 0.025$, respectively). The B40 was increased in SW ($\chi^2 = 11.7$, $p < 0.001$). In contrast, Bw47 was increased in both SV and SW ($\chi^2 = 7.43$, $p < 0.01$) and B8 was decreased in both disease forms ($\chi^2 = 4.19$, $p < 0.05$).

These data strongly suggest that SV and SW 21-OH-def CAH are due to different mutational defects in the 21-OH locus.

567 SYMPATHETIC ADRENAL DENERVATION DECREASES ADRENAL BLOOD FLOW WITHOUT ALTERING THE CORTISOL RESPONSE TO HEMORRHAGE(HEM). W.C. Engeland*, M.P. Lilly, and D.S. Gann, Brown Univ/RI Hospital, Providence, RI 02902, USA.

We have reported that the cortisol(F) secretory response to small hem may occur without an ACTH response, suggesting that a non-ACTH factor increases sensitivity to ACTH. To test whether or not adrenal sympathetic innervation is required for the adrenocortical response to hem, awake dogs were studied following unilateral adrenal sympathetic denervation. Bilateral adrenal vein cannulae were placed to permit measurement of F and epinephrine(E) secretion rates(by HPLC) and adrenal blood flow(BF). Plasma ACTH(A) was measured by RIA and A presentation rate(APR) was calculated (APR=AxBF). Dogs were bled 10% or 20% of blood volume/3min. Denervation inhibited E ($p<0.001$) and decreased BF relative to the intact adrenal($p<0.05$) prior to and following hem. Plasma ACTH did not change following 10% hem but increased ($p<0.01$) following 20% hem. Following either hem, APR to the denervated adrenal was decreased($p<0.05$) relative to the intact adrenal. However, there was no difference in the F response between the denervated and the intact adrenal to 10% or to 20% hem. Resting adrenal sensitivity to ACTH was tested by measuring the F response to iv ACTH(0.5,1.0,2.5 and 5.0mU). Adrenal sensitivity (estimated by slope(m) of log-dose response curves) was greater for the intact compared to the denervated adrenal(m= 18.98vs12.65; $p<0.05$). Denervation decreases BF and consequently, APR without altering the F response to hem. However, sensitivity to ACTH is not increased by denervation. These findings suggest that the full F response to hem requires a potentiating mechanism that is neither ACTH nor adrenal sympathetic neural input. Supported in part by NIH AM26381.

568 INHIBITION OF ADRENAL 11β-HYDROXYLASE BY KETOCONAZOLE IN NORMALS AND IN PATIENTS WITH CUSHING'S SYNDROME. D. Engelhardt*, H.G. Dörr, H.J. Karl, D. Knorr, Departments of Internal Medicine II and Pediatrics, University of Munich, Munich, FRG

Ketoconazole (K), an antifungal agent, induced a clear-cut fall of serum cortisol (F) in a patient with Cushing's syndrome by an adrenal adenoma and inhibited biosynthesis of F in tissue slices of this tumour (Engelhardt et al., Klin Wschr 1983,61,373). Searching for the step where K blocks F biosynthesis, we investigated basal and ACTH stimulated serum levels of F and of 11-desoxycortisol (S) as well as serum ACTH levels before and during oral K (200 mg every 5 hrs for 25 hrs) in 4 patients with Cushing's syndrome and in 3 controls. In addition, the influence of K (10-40µg/ml) on the transformation of 3H-17α-OH-progesterone (P) to 3H-S and 3H-F as well as of 3H-S to 3H-F was examined in slices of hyperplastic adrenal tissue from 1 patient. Oral K induced a rise of S but not of F so that the quotient S/F raised more than after ACTH, an indication for at least partial inhibition of adrenal 11β-hydroxylase by K itself and not by endogenous ACTH stimulated 10-100 fold during K administration.K inhibited the transformation of 3H-P to 3H-F but not to 3H-S in adrenal slices so that the quotient 3H-S/3H-F raised 20 fold with raising in vitro concentrations of K. A 100 fold increase of the quotient 3H-S/3H-F could also be found after incubation of adrenal slices with 3H-S with increasing concentrations of K. In conclusion, the in vivo and in vitro data advocate that ketoconazole inhibits cortisol biosynthesis by blocking adrenal 11β-hydroxylase activity in patients with Cushing's syndrome as well as in normals.

569 ACTH AND CORTISOL RESPONSES TO DEXAMETHASONE SUPPRESSION IN PATIENTS WITH CUSHING'S DISEASE. V.S. Fang*, M.L. Graybeal and R.L. Landau, Department of Medicine, The University of Chicago, Chicago, IL 60637, USA.

We previously reported that normal subjects respond to orally administered 1 mg dexamethasone (DEX) with disproportionately greater suppression in cortisol than ACTH. We recently investigated the ACTH and cortisol responses to DEX in three patients with Cushing's disease. Venous blood samples were collected at 30-min intervals for 24 h. Plasma ACTH and cortisol were measured by sensitive RIA procedures. All 3 patients had 24-h hypercortisolemia with inappropriately high plasma ACTH. Diurnal rhythm was apparent in all. After low dose DEX, 0.5 mg q 6 h for 2 days, a small, transient rise of AM ACTH secretion was observed on the second day with little change in total 24-h ACTH secretion. Plasma cortisol, however, was consistently suppressed during the same period. Patients responded to subsequent high dose DEX, 2 mg q 6 h for 2 days, with a uniform suppression of both ACTH and cortisol in spite of the persistence of rhythmic variations. In one patient tested with 4 mg DEX q 6 h for 2 days, only slight further suppression of ACTH but no more suppression of cortisol could be demonstrated. To explain this "paradoxical" rise of ACTH in response to low dose DEX, we suggest that 1) DEX directly inhibits cortisol secretion at the adrenal gland in the presence of ACTH; 2) pituitary tumors appear relatively resistant to DEX while remaining sensitive to cortisol feedback. We conclude that disparity in ACTH and cortisol responses to DEX is a common observation in patients with Cushing's disease. Partially supported by NIH grant to CRC, No. RR-55.

570 *SCINTIGRAPHIC IMAGING AND THERAPY OF PHAEOCHROMOCYTOMA WITH 131-I-METAIODOBENZYLGUANIDINE.* *M. Fischer*, B. Winterberg and H. Vetter, Medizinische Klinik und Poliklinik, University of Münster, FRG.*

During a 2 years period we studied 100 patients with clinical suspicion of phaeochromocytoma. Scintigraphy with 131-I-metaiodobenzylguanidine (131-I-MIBG) was performed 1-5 days after tracer administration with a computer assisted gamma camera. In 25 of these patients an increased secretion of catecholamines was proven biochemically. Scintigraphy localized an intraadrenal phaeochromocytoma in 18 patients, in 2 an adrenomedullary hyperplasia and in 3 patients a malignant phaeochromocytoma. In 2 patients with an intraadrenal lesion and increased catecholamines scintigraphy was negative, whereas in one patient scintigraphy under alcohol excess was positive. A control scintigraphy 11 months later showed a normal tracer uptake. In 2 patients with malignant phaeochromocytoma and metastases of soft tissue and bone and in one patient with an intraadrenal phaeochromocytoma, who could not be operated because of an catecholamine-induced myocarditis, we started a treatment with 131-I-MIBG. In splitted doses of 65-210 mCi uptil now total doses of 365-435 mCi were given. The therapeutic effect was controlled by clinical follow up, catecholamine secretion and in 2 patients by determination of tumor size by computed tomography. Our results document that scintigraphic imaging with 131-I-MIBG is a valid and reliable method for noninvasive localization of phaeochromocytomas with a sensitivity and a specificity of more than 92%. By treatment with 131-I-MIBG we observed a reduction of tumor size by about 10-61% in 2 patients with metastatic phaeochromocytoma, but no response in a patient with intraadrenal primary phaeochromocytoma.

571 **AGE-RELATED MORPHOLOGICAL CHANGES IN THE HYPOTHALAMO-NEUROHYPOPHYSEAL SYSTEM DURING OSMOTIC STRESS AND SUBSEQUENT REHYDRATION** I. Davies*, A.P. Fotheringham & C. Roberts, University of Manchester, Geigy Unit for Research in Aging, Withington Hospital, Nell Lane, MANCHESTER, UK

There is a decline in water conservation in the aging mammal and it has been suggested that the decreased responsiveness of the hypothalamo-neurohypophyseal system (HNS) is responsible. Neurons of the supraoptic nucleus (SON) from normally hydrated, osmotically loaded and osmotically loaded/rehydrated animals of male C57BL mice at 6 or 28 months of age were examined using quantitative morphological techniques. Osmotic loading was effected by the addition of 3% NaCl in the drinking water. The data were analysed using an analysis of variance. The volumes of hormone containing neurosecretory granules and Golgi bodies in the SON cell were not significantly different between the two age groups. However, the surface area of the rough endoplasmic reticulum (RER) per unit volume of the SON neuron was significantly reduced in the old age group under osmotic stress. Furthermore, the relative volume of the mitochondrial compartment in the old, osmotically challenged animals was similar to that in young animals. However, the number of mitochondrial profiles found in the cells from old osmotically challenged animals did decrease significantly. During the osmotic challenge, the concentration of lipofuscin within the SON cell decreased but was restored to control levels during rehydration. There was also a significant age/time interaction in the lipofuscin variable between the two age groups. We conclude that the neurons from this part of the HNS can produce hormone at the same concentration throughout the period of life-span studied despite defects iin other aspects of cellular function.

572 INFLUENCE OF AGE AND SEX ON STEROID CONCENTRATION IN DIFFERENT TISSUES IN HUMANS. J.P. Deslypere* & A.Vermeulen. Dept. of Endocrinology, Academic Hospital, GENT,Belgium.
We previously reported the effect of age on androgen concentration in skin and striated muscle in men. In this study we report the effect of age on androgen concentration (testosterone (T), DHT, 5α androstanediol (Adiol), Δ4 androstenedione (Δ4 Adion)) in other male tissues as well as in female tissue. Males: Total androgen concentration (T + DHT + Adiol) was significantly higher in heart muscle (HM) than in striated muscle (SM) or in thigh skin, but lower than in sexual skin (scrotum-pubis). In lung tissue total androgen concentration was significantly higher than in HM, but lower than in sexual skin. In both organs total androgens decrease significantly with age. As far as individual androgens are concerned, tissue sequence was for T: lung>HM>scrotal skin>pubic skin>thigh skin>SM; for DHT: scrotal skin >pubic skin>lung>HM>SM; for Adiol: scrotal skin>pubic skin>lung>HM>SM; for Δ4 Adion: lung>HM>scrotal skin>pubic skin>thigh skin>SM. In lung all androgens decreased significantly with age, while in HM only T and Δ4 Adion were significantly lower in elderly men. The Adiol/DHT and the Adiol+DHT/T ratios in HM decreased significantly with age. Female: Total androgen concentration was significantly higher in sexual skin (labia, clitoris, pubic skin) than in thigh skin and SM, and shows an age dependent decrease in all skin tissues but not in SM. As to individual androgens, tissue sequence was for all androgens and for the DHT+Adiol/T ratio: labia>clitoris>pubic skin >thigh skin>SM. All androgens decreased significantly with age in skin tissue but not in SM. In comparison to males, total androgens were lower in females in all tissues. In conclusion: in both sexes most androgens decrease with age.

573 EFFECTS OF CHRONIC FOOD RESTRICTION (CFR) AND AGING ON RAT ADIPOCYTE METABOLIC ACTIVITIES AND HORMONAL RESPONSIVENESS. M. DiGirolamo*, D. Crandall, S.K. Fried, M. Nickel, and J.O. Hill, Department of Medicine, Emory University School of Medicine, Atlanta, GA, USA.

To dissect the influence of age vs adiposity on fat cell (FC) metabolism and responsiveness to insulin (I) and epinephrine (E), we subjected rats to variable degrees of CFR. Male Wistar rats were fed, at 3 mo of age, either ad lib or in restricted amounts (75% or 50% of ad lib) and killed at 3,6,12,18,24 mo of age, in the fed state (90 min after last meal). FC suspensions ($1\text{-}2 \times 10^5$ FC/ml) were incubated in KRB with 4% BSA and 6mM glucose; ^{14}C-glucose metabolism, glycerol release, lipoprotein lipase activity (LPLa) were expressed per FC. The lipolytic effect of E (5μg/ml) and the lipogenic and antilipolytic effects of I (0 to 1 mU/ml) were examined in each group. Basal glucose conversion to fatty acids declined rapidly with age and remained low (<5%) both in ad lib and CFR rats. In ad lib, basal glyceride synthesis increased until 12 mo and then progressively declined; CFR reduced basal glyceride synthesis but preserved relative response to I which slowly declined with age. CFR totally prevented the decline in lipolytic response seen with age in ad lib fed rats. In contrast, the antilipolytic effect of I declined with age regardless of the rats' nutritional status. LPLa declined with severe CFR, but moderate CFR maintained LPLa in the fed state close to that of ad lib rats in spite of a smaller FC size. We conclude that adipocyte lipolytic responses are altered by obesity but not by age, whereas age leads to a decline in glucose metabolism, insulin responsiveness, and LPLa which can be partially prevented by CFR.

574 SALIVA AND PLASMA TESTOSTERONE FOLLOWING ORAL TESTOSTERONE UNDECANOATE ADMINISTRATION IN NORMAL AND ELDERLY MEN. F. Franchi, D. Barletta, G.F. Argenio, G.P. Bernini, S. Bianchi and M. Luisi, Endocrine Research Unit of the C.N.R., Pisa University, 56100 Pisa, Italy.

Since salivary testosterone reflects the unbound moiety of the steroid in plasma and consequently the fraction of testosterone available to target tissues, the pharmacokinetics and therapeutic effectiveness of orally administered testosterone undecanoate was assessed by measuring testosterone in plasma and saliva. Matched saliva and plasma samples were obtained from 10 normal men (25-40 yrs) and 12 elderly men (62-76 yrs) with the so-called "climateric syndrome", before and at hourly intervals after the administration of 120 mg testosterone undecanoate (TU). In all the subjects the administration of 40 mg TU three times daily was repeated for 16 weeks. Following TU, plasma and salivary testosterone showed parallel rises. The absorption pattern was similar in the normal and elderly groups, in whom a decrease of clinical negative symptomatology was observed. The absorption curves showed a high interindividual variability in the time when maximum concentrations were reached, as well as in the maximum values themselves. These data show that TU is well absorbed from the gut and releases significantly elevated amounts of testosterone which is available to target tissues, without the accumulation phenomenon. This study was supported by CNR, Roma).

575 ISOLATION AND GC/MS CHARACTERIZATION OF A POSSIBLE NEW MARKER FOR PRIMARY ALDOSTERONISM. T. Fisher*, P. Bubel, K. Lichtwald, P. Vecsei. Dept. of Pharmacology, University Heidelberg, FRG.

Urine from patients with 1°aldosteronism and control persons were chromatographed on a reverse phase HPLC column using a gradient with acetonitrile and water. The 80 fractions from each HPLC run were assayed using tetrahydroaldosterone antibodies. The patients showed strong tetrahydroaldosterone antibody crossreactivity (∼17µg/24h, tetrahydroaldosterone equivalents n=12) in an unpolar region of the HPLC run where only a small amount of tetrahydroaldosterone antibody crossreactivity (∼0.6µg/24h, tetrahydroaldosterone equivalents, n=10) was found in the urine of normal subjects. This fraction was studied using various other antibodies to help elucidate the structure. From the crossreactivities it was found that the structure should show similarities to tetrahydroaldosterone and to etiocholanolone. This fraction was also treated to form the methoxime:tetramethylsilane derivative and injected on a GC/MS (Finnigan 4021 GC/MS with a J&W DB-1 fused silica capillary column). Two spectra were observed with the possible structural features indicated by the antibody crossreactivities. These are: 3-hydroxy-11,18; 18,21-diepoxy pregnane with mass spectral fragments at m/z 404 (parent), 389,360,270,260,241 and 175 and 19-nor-3, 17-dihydroxy-11, 18-epoxy-5ß-androstane with mass spectral fragments at m/z 436 (parent) 421,360,246,270,256 and 241. Evaluation of the GC/MS results from different patients and urine extracts indicated a greater importance of the latter compound. Work to further isolate these compounds using two separate HPLC systems is in progress.

576 CALCIUM-DEPENDENCE OF SEROTONIN-MEDIATED ALDOSTERONE SECRETION AND DIFFERENTIAL EFFECTS OF CALCIUM ANTAGONISTS. A. Ganguly* and T. Hampton, Dept. of Medicine, University of South Florida College of Medicine and V.A. Hospital, Tampa, Florida, USA.

Serotonin is known to stimulate aldosterone (ALDO) secretion. To investigate if serotonin-induced ALDO secretion requires calcium (CA), as for other stimuli, we incubated collagenase-dispersed rat zona glomerulosa cells in calcium-free medium or in medium containing varying concentrations of CA. The effect of serotonin (ST) on ALDO production (ng/10^6cells) are shown (mean ± SEM):

N = 5	No CA	0.2mM CA	0.5mM CA	1.8mM CA
Control	21.9 ± 0.6*	42.0 ± 1.4	36.8 ± 2.0	31.0 ± 1.7
ST 10^{-8}M	25.2 ± 1.0*	45.3 ± 4.5	53.0 ± 4.1	49.9 ± 2.0
ST 10^{-7}M	32.4 ± 0.7*	84.4 ± 3.5	105.7 ± 6.2	108.7 ± 4.8

We then examined the effects of 3 different calcium-channel blockers - verapamil (VP), nifedipine (NF), and dilitiazem (DL) - on ST-mediated ALDO production (mean ng/10^6 cells):

N = 4 or 5	Control 1.8mM CA	+VP 10^{-5}M	Control 1.8mM CA	+NF 10^{-5}M	+DL 10^{-5}M
ST 10^{-8}M	69.8	23.9*	103.3	76.5	84.1
ST 10^{-7}M	182.6	25.0*	212.9	192.5	206.5

The results suggest that ST-mediated ALDO secretion requires the presence of CA and can be markedly inhibited by VP (*$p < 0.01$) but not significantly by equimolar concentration of NF or DL. The latter may reflect different potency or mode of action of NF and DL.

577 DOPAMINERGIC MODULATION OF PLASMA ALDOSTERONE IN THE LUTEAL PHASE OF THE NORMAL MENSTRUAL CYCLE .

R.Garcia-Robles*, L.Ruilope, J.Tovar, A.Hurtado, R.Santirso, J.Parada, J.L. Rodicio, J.Sancho. Ramón y Cajal & 1º de Octubre Hospitals & Dept.Exptl. Endocrinol.,Universidad Complutense, Madrid, Spain.

A situation of relative hyperaldosteronism has been described in the luteal phase of the normal menstrual cycle. There is also evidence of a hyperresponse of prolactin(PRL)to TRH administration in the same situation. Both findings could be related through a diminution of dopaminergic control of both hormones. A group of 8 normotensive female volunteers with regular menstrual cycles in the absence of any medication has been studied during two menstrual cycles receiving in the second one Lisuride(0.025 mg/8h) a dopamine agonist drug. The following tests have been performed in every half of both cycles: a) response of PRL to TRH administration, b) responses of PRA and plasma aldosterone(PA) to furosemide (40 mg. orally) plus 1 hour of ambulation, c) the response of PRA, PA and plasma potassium, cortisol and PRL to metoclopramide (10 mg iv) administration. In the first menstrual cycle an augmented response of PRL a)($p<0.05$)together with an increased response of PA in b) ($p<0.05$) and c)($p<0.05$) in the luteal phase were found. With Lisuride administration no difference in the response of PRL a) and of PA in b) were found in the first and second phases of the menstrual cycle whilst a higher response of PA ($p<0.01$) to c) was observed.

We conclude that the increase of aldosterone normally observed during the luteal phase of the menstrual cycle is,at least partly, conditioned by a diminished dopaminergic control of its secretion.

578 DOPAMINERGIC MODULATION OF ALDOSTERONE, 18-OH-CORTICOSTERONE AND PROLACTIN SECRETION IN PATIENTS WITH PRIMARY ALDOSTERONISM.

E. Gláz*, R. Kiss, I. Varga, K. Rácz and M. Kárteszi, Second Department of Medicine, Division of Endocrinology, Semmelweis University,Budapest,Hungary

We have studied the regulation of aldosterone /Ald/ and 18-OH-corticosterone /18-OH-B/ secretion in patients with aldosterone producing adenoma /APA/ and idiopathic adrenal hyperplasia /IHA/.Our earlier results suggested that dopaminergic agonists and antagonists might regulate aldosterone secretion /Gláz et al. 1979,1980/, therefore it seemed worth studying the modulatory effect of dopaminergic system in primary aldosteronism. Plasma prolactin /PRL/ level, as an index of the actual activity of dopaminergic system, Ald and 18-OH-B concentrations were determined in 5 APA, 5 IHA and 25 control patients submitted to an acute dopamine depletion by administrating 10 mg metoclopramide /Mc-test/ before and after a long-term treatment with dopamine agonist bromocriptine /Br/, 5 mg per day. Mc-test significantly increased Ald, 18-OH-B and PRL secretion, however, the extent of stimulation was different. The highest hormonal increments were found in APA, and only in these patients PRL vs Ald, as well as PRL vs 18-OH-B correlated positively /r=0,883, p 0.02; r=0,762, p 0,05/. Bromocriptine treatment significantly inhibited Ald, 18-OH-B and PRL secretion induced by Mc in all groups, however the basal level of Ald, 18-OH-B and PRL decreased only in APA. Our results indicate that on the basis of specific dopaminergic modulation of mineralocorticoid secretion one can differentiate the two types of primary aldosteronism.

579 INHIBITION OF RENIN SECRETION BY VASOPRESSIN IS BLOCKED BY RENAL DENERVATION. L.C. Gregory* and I.A. Reid. Dept. of Physiology, University of California, San Francisco, CA 94143.

Previous studies have shown that the inhibition of renin secretion by vasopressin (AVP) in conscious dogs is related to vasoconstrictor activity and may be a reflex response mediated by the renal nerves. The aim of the present experiments was to determine if the suppression of plasma renin activity (PRA) by AVP is blocked by renal denervation. AVP (1.0 ng/kg/min) was infused i.v. for 45 min in seven conscious dogs before and after bilateral renal denervation. For comparison, the effect of angiotensin II (AII) (5 ng/kg/min) was also studied. Before denervation, AVP suppressed PRA from 7.9 $\pm$ 1.8 to 3.8 $\pm$ 0.8 ng/ml/3 h ($p<0.01$). There was no significant change in mean arterial pressure (MAP) (110 $\pm$ 5 to 113 $\pm$ 7 mm Hg) but heart rate (HR) decreased (77 $\pm$ 7 to 60 $\pm$ 5 beats/min, $p<0.01$). AII suppressed PRA from 7.5 $\pm$ 2.3 to 2.5 $\pm$ 0.7 ng/ml/3 h ($p<0.01$), increased MAP (106 $\pm$ 3 to 134 $\pm$ 6 mm Hg, $p<0.01$) but did not change HR (75 $\pm$ 6 to 82 $\pm$ 7 beats/min). One to three weeks following renal denervation, PRA had decreased from 6.7 $\pm$ 1.3 to 2.9 $\pm$ 0.5 ng/ml/3 h ($p<0.01$) and renal norepinephrine was undetecable. AVP produced cardiovascular changes similar to those before denervation but did not suppress PRA (3.1 $\pm$ 0.8 to 2.8 $\pm$ 0.9 ng/ml/3 h, $p> 0.05$). AII, however, suppressed PRA from 2.9 $\pm$ 0.6 to 1.5 $\pm$ 0.4 ng/ml/3 h ($p<0.01$). These data indicate that in conscious dogs, the suppression of PRA by AVP is blocked by renal denervation and support the hypothesis that the suppression is a reflex response to vasoconstriction. Supported by NIH AM07265 and HL29714.

580 PRO-OPIOMELANOCORTIN-DERIVED PEPTIDES AND IDIOPATHIC HYPERALDOSTERONISM. G. Griffing, T. McIntosh, B. Berelowitz, *M. Hudson, R. Salzman, R.C. Pedersen, A.C. Brownie, and J.C. Melby, Evans Memorial Department of Clinical Research and the Department of Medicine, University Hospital and Boston University School of Medicine, Boston, Massachusetts 02118; and the Department of Biochemistry, State University of New York at Buffalo, Buffalo, New York 14214.

An aldosterone-stimulating factor has been previously isolated from the urine of patients with idiopathic hyperaldosteronism (IHA). This putative factor may be related to POMC-derived peptides, which have aldosterone stimulating properties. The present study evaluated plasma IR-ACTH, β-endo and IR-γ-MSH levels in patients with IHA (n=10) and essential hypertension (EH, n=9). Hormonal measurements were obtained at timed intervals on a fixed electrolyte intake (sodium 128, potassium 80 mEq/day). Plasma β-endo was pre-incubated with cepharose-bound anti-β-lipotropin prior to RIA.

	0800 h (fmol/ml)			1200 h (fmol/ml)				
	β-Endo	IR-γ-MSH	ACTH	β-Endo	IR-γ-MSH	ACTH	(µg/d)	(µg/d)
IHA	44 ± 9*	101 ± 16†	9 ± 1	51 ± 9*	117 ± 30†	8 ± 1	38 ± 7	253 ± 34*
EH	16 ± 1	66 ± 19	8 ± 1	22 ± 8	73 ± 16	7 ± 1	32 ± 5	101 ± 10

(*$p < 0.05$) (†$0.1 < p < 0.05$)

The results demonstrated that aldosterone secretion rates (ASR) were elevated in IHA together with both β-endo and IR-γ-MSH at 0800 h (supine) and 1200 h (upright). ACTH and urine free cortisol (UFC), however, were not different. These data support the hypothesis that excess production of POMC-derived peptides may function as a secretogogue(s) for aldosterone in IHA.

581 A RAPID METHOD TO DISTINGUISH GLUCOCORTICOID SUPPRESSIBLE HYPERALDOSTERONISM FROM OTHER PATIENTS WITH AN ANOMALOUS POSTURAL RESPONSE OF PLASMA ALDOSTERONE. C.E. Grim,* M.H. Weinberger, A. Ganguly, Hypertension Research Center, Indiana University, Indianapolis, IN 46223.

Among patients with primary aldosteronism, an anomalous postural response of plasma aldosterone (PA) has been observed in those with an aldosterone producing adenoma (APA) and also in patients with glucocorticoid suppressible hyperaldosteronism (GSH). Since GSH can be treated effectively with glucocorticoids while APA is best treated by surgery, it is important to identify the former to avoid invasive studies and unnecessary surgery. A 4 to 6 week course of glucocorticoid therapy has previously been utilized to separate these variants, however this may be hazardous in some patients with APA and severe hypertension. As a rapid method to separate these syndromes we examined the effect of oral administration of 1.0mg dexamethasone (DEX) given at midnight and 0.5mg at 6 am on supine PA values obtained at 8 am in 9 patients with APA and 6 with GSH, all of whom demonstrated the anomalous postural response. The mean PA the morning after DEX was 27.7 $\pm$ 18.9ng/dl(SD) in APA and 2.8 $\pm$ 1.2 in GSH ($P < .001$). After overnight DEX all patients with GSH had a PA of < 4.5. In contrast, all patients with APA had a PA of > 7 ($P < .001$). The PA response to DEX is a rapid way to distinguish GSH in patients with the anomalous postural response of PA, thus avoiding 4-6 weeks of glucocorticoid therapy in patients who may have severe hypertension and will also avoid unnecessary invasive localization studies, such as adrenal vein blood sampling and/or surgical exploration in GSH.

582 THE EFFICACY OF DEXAMETHASONE SUPPRESSION ADRENAL SCINTIGRAPHY IN THE LOCALIZATION OF ABNORMAL ADRENAL FUNCTION IN PRIMARY ALDOSTERONISM (PA). M.D. Gross*, B. Shapiro, R.J. Grekin, J.E. Freitas, Divisions of Nuclear Medicine and Endocrinology and Metabolism, University of Michigan and the VA Medical Centers, Ann Arbor, Michigan 48109.

Dexamethasone suppression (DS) adrenal scintigraphy is an accurate noninvasive method to localize and distinguish adrenal adenomas (A) from bilateral adrenal hyperplasia (BAH) in PA. Previous studies have used varying DS regimens with variable success of localization. The present study was performed with a constant dose and duration of DS to establish the efficacy of this technique in PA. Eighty patients with PA (48 with A, 32 with BAH) were studied with DS, 4mg/day, for 7 days prior to the injection of 1 mCi I-131-6B-iodomethylnorcholesterol (NP-59) and for 5 days post NP-59. Adrenal images were obtained on days 3 through 5 after NP-59. On this DS regimen normal adrenal imaging is seen no earlier than 5 days post NP-59 (J.Clin.Endocrinol. Metab.54:477,1983). The diagnosis of A was confirmed by adrenalectomy in 47 and by adrenal vein sampling (AVS) in 1. BAH was confirmed by AVS in 27 and at operation in 5. Early unilateral adrenal imaging (< 5 days post NP-59) was seen in 46 of 48 patients with A and in 2 with BAH. Early bilateral imaging (< 5 days post NP-59) was seen in 29 of 32 with BAH. In 3 patients (2 of A and 1 of BAH) adrenal activity was seen late (> 5 days post NP-59). The specificity for A was 93% (30/32), while both the sensitivity (46/48) and predictive accuracy (46/48) of a localizing scan for A were 96%. Thus, using a uniform DS regimen NP-59 adrenal scintigraphy can be used to accurately portray the abnormal adrenals in PA, localize A and distinguish A from BAH.

583 NEUROPEPTIDE Y (NPY) AND HUMAN PANCREATIC POLYPEPTIDE (hPP) STIMULATE FEEDING IN THE RAT. J.T. Clark*, W.R. Crowley and S.P. Kalra. Department of OB/Gyn, University of Florida College of Medicine, Gainesville, FL 32610 U.S.A.

Neuropeptides have been implicated in the central control of feeding behavior. In view of the recent demonstrations of immunoreactive product for pancreatic polypeptides (including hPP and NPY) in cell bodies and fibers of cortical, limbic and hypothalamic areas, we examined the effect of two sequential (65 min apart) intraventricular (III) injections of hPP (2 or 10 μg/rat), NPY (2 or 10 μg/rat) and saline (3 μl/rat) on daytime feeding in ovariectomized rats treated with estradiol benzoate (30 μg) and progesterone (15mg) 48 hr previously. hPP stimulated feeding in all rats (n=13) in a dose-related manner. Total food intake after 2 μg hPP was 0.65 ± .43g, and after 10 μg hPP was 1.22 ± .53g. Latency to feeding response was 26.7 ± 3.0 min for the 2 μg dose, and 20.4 ± 4.2 min for 10 μg. All animals treated with NPY ate after each injection, but the response was more dramatic, in terms of intake and latency, than that seen after hPP. Rats treated with 2 μg NPY (n=6) initiated feeding in 14.5 ± 4.9 min and ate 2.59 ± .42g after the first injection. Following the second injection the latency was 12.3 ± 2.9 min and food intake was 2.17 ± .28g. Rats treated with 10 μg NPY (n=7) initiated feeding within 22.1 ∓ 2.8 min of the initial injection and ate 1.84 ± .46g. After the second injection, the latency was 11.1 ± 2.1 min and food intake was increased to 3.33 ± .48g. Only 3/14 saline-treated rats ate after either injection (latency: 29 min; intake 0.37g/rat). These data demonstrate that (1) pancreatic peptides, in general, can stimulate feeding in the rat and (2) NPY, an endogenous hypothalamic neuropeptide in the rat, is highly potent and, therefore, it may play a physiological role in the regulation of appetite by the brain. (Supported by NIH HD08634).

584 VASOACTIVE INTESTINAL PEPTIDE (VIP) HAS INHIBITORY EFFECTS ON STRESS-MOTIVATED BEHAVIOURS. G.A. Cottrell*, H.D. Veldhuis, W.H. Rostene[1] and E.R. de Kloet, Rudolf Magnus Institute for Pharmacology, University of Utrecht, 3521 GD Utrecht, The Netherlands and [1] Unit 159 of Neuroendocrinology, INSERM, Paris, France.

Vasoactive intestinal peptide (VIP), a gut peptide, is also present in several areas of the central nervous system, and a high concentration of VIP is found in the hippocampus. Within the rat hippocampus, VIP modulates 5-hydroxytryptamine (5-HT1) receptors while corticosterone modulates 5-HT synthesis rate, 5-HT1 receptors and VIP levels. The interaction of 5-HT and corticosterone in the hippocampus is known to regulate neural mechanisms underlying stress-responsiveness, learning and memory. It is possible that VIP also participates in the control of these brain functions. We tested this hypothesis by studying the effect of VIP on exploration of a novel environment and retention behaviour in footshock motivated tasks. Male wistar rats were implanted with a plastic cannula in the lateral ventricle. In an open field test, VIP had no effect on ambulation, though 10 ng did decrease one aspect of exploration (free rearing). Retention in a step-through passive avoidance task was inhibited by 10 and 30 ng VIP injected 1 h before the retention test. Extinction of pole-jumping active avoidance behaviour was facilitated by 10 and 100 ng VIP. In summary, VIP produces inhibitory effects on behaviour in 3 different tasks. VIP could be interacting with the hippocampal - 5-HT - corticosteroid system to produce these effects. This study was supported by INSERM.

585 THE EFFECT OF DOPAMINE ON THE SECRETION AND METABOLISM OF ALDOSTERONE C.S. Hanson* and R.D. Brown, University of Oklahoma Health Sciences Center and Veterans Administration Hospital, Oklahoma City, Oklahoma 73190, USA

Studies suggest that dopamine (DA) modulates the secretion rate (SR) of aldosterone (A). This has been inferred from the increases in serum A following administration of the dopamine antagonist metoclopromide (MCP). However, no studies have investigated the effect of DA on the metabolic clearance rate (MCR) of A. To investigate this 7 male subjects were infused with DA (4 μg/kg/min). After one hour, a 5 mg bolus of MCP was administered followed by an infusion at 110 μg/min for 45 minutes. The SR of A was calculated from the MCR and serum A values.

	Syst BP	P	Serum A ng/dl	MCR l/24h	SR ug/24h
Basal ± (S.E.)	114.50 ± (2.62)	58.86 ± (2.00)	3.02 ± (0.44)	1591.11 ± (98.79)	47.64 ± (4.49)
DA ± (S.E.)	145.29 ± (3.89)	69.14 ± (1.73)	5.50 ± (0.93)	1447.47 ± (73.48)	80.43 ± (15.53)
DA + MCP ± (S.E.)	140.71 ± (2.64)	70.00 ± (1.86)	12.06 ± (2.45)	1428.80 ± (94.21)	168.83 ± (38.29)

There were no significant changes in the MCR of A. Although the SR of A rose during DA infusion, it was not significant. However, during the DA+MCP infusion there was a significant ($p = 0.03$) increase in the SR of A. In conclusion, the administration of DA does not affect either the MCR or SR of A. In contrast, administration of MCP causes a significant rise in the SR of A without affecting the MCR of aldosterone.

586 NEUROHUMORAL AND METABOLIC RESPONSES TO CHRONIC INTRACEREBROVENTRICULAR ANGIOTENSIN II (IVT AII) INFUSION IN TRAINED, CONSCIOUS DOGS. M. Fujimaki*, T. Eguchi and E. L. Bravo, Research Division, Cleveland Clinic Foundation, Cleveland, Ohio, 44106, U.S.A.

Acute IVT AII infusions produce natriuresis, increase arterial pressure, drinking, ACTH and ADH release, and decrease plasma renin activity (PRA). The present study assessed the effects of chronic IVT AII infusion in trained, conscious dogs on normal dietary sodium. Isotonic saline (n=7) or AII (n=8), 0.3 μg/μl saline, was infused (10 μl/hr) continuously into the lateral cerebral ventricle for 7 days using osmotic minipumps. Drinking behavior, aortic pressure, serum sodium (Na) and potassium (K), PRA, plasma aldosterone (PA), ADH, ACTH and cortisol responses were determined before, during 6 days of infusion, and 7 days after. Chronic IVT AII infusion increased water intake (5013 ml/dog/7 days) and decreased serum sodium (Δ4.4 ± 1.6 mEq/L, $p < 0.05$). No significant changes in arterial pressure, K, PRA, PA, ACTH or cortisol were noted. ADH remained normal (4.4 ± 1.0 pg/ml) despite decreases in serum Na. When water intake was fixed at control levels (600 ml/day) serum Na did not change. Intracerebroventricular saline had no effect on any of the above parameters. Results indicate that during chronic IVT AII infusion, 1) neurohormonal and cardiovascular responses differ from acute infusions, 2) dipsogenic and pressor responses are dissociated, and 3) water retention is sustained by increased drinking and continued ADH release despite reduced serum Na.

587 CENTRAL B-ENDORPHIN PROCESSING IN TEMPERATURE ACCLIMATED ANIMALS. A. P. Han*, T. P. Davis and M. K. Yousef. Dept. Biol. Sci. Univ. of Nevada, Las Vegas, Nv. 89154 and Dept. of Pharamacology Univ. of Arizona, College of Med., Tucson, Az. 85724.

Characterization of the metabolism of B-endorphin (BE) in the brain of thermally stressed animals has not been addressed. The objective of this study was to measure the central processing of BE by membrane bound enzyme homogenates to specific α and γ-type endorphin (E) fragments. Two species of desert rodents, Peromyscus maniculatus and P. truei were acclimated to heat (35C), cold (5C) and thermoneutral zone (TNZ) (28C) for 5 weeks. Temperature acclimated animals were sacrificed and the brains were immediately removed and frozen for analysis of BE and its processing using reversed phase HPLC. The data demonstrated that metabolism of BE is faster in desert species than in Sprague Dawley laboratory rats. In heat and cold acclimated animals, BE was metabolized at a slower rate than at TNZ. The decreased metabolism of BE was greater in P. truei, (heat tolerant) than in P. maniculations, (heat-intolerant) during heat acclimation. In both species membrane bound metabolism of BE was reduced more in heat than in cold. Based on the hypothesis that an alteration in the homeostatic balance of α:γ E may result from thermal stress, we measured the ratios of α/γ E in both species. Our data showed that the α/γ E ratio at 35°C or 5°C was not altered in the heat tolerant P. truei when compared against the TNZ but was altered in P. maniculatus. In general, the data suggest that central processing of BE may be of importance to thermal tolerance in mammals.

588 INCREASED UNBOUND 1,25-DIHYDROXYVITAMIN D LEVELS IN PATIENTS WITH THE NEPHROTIC SYNDROME. J.F. Dunn*, L.S. Akright, C. Smagula, D. Fetchick, and N.D. Adams. Department of Medicine, University of Texas Health Science Center at San Antonio, Texas 78284, USA.

1,25-dihydroxyvitamin D (1,25$(OH)_2$D) circulates bound to serum proteins including vitamin D-binding protein and albumin. Since current evidence suggests that only that portion of 1,25$(OH)_2$D which is not bound to serum proteins is biologically active, we examined unbound 1,25$(OH)_2$D concentrations in patients with decreased binding protein levels secondary to the nephrotic syndrome. Total 1,25$(OH)_2$D extracted from serum samples was measured by a competitive protein-binding assay. The percent unbound 1,25$(OH)_2$D was measured by ultrafiltration of undiluted serum at 37°C using a modified polypropylene Amicon micropartition system. Results are shown in the table below:

1,25$(OH)_2$D	Total (pM)	% Unbound	Unbound (pM)
Normal (n=10)			
Mean±S.D.	85±16	0.15±0.03	0.13±0.02
Range	62-111	0.098-0.20	0.10-0.16
Nephrotic Syndrome (n=5)			
Mean±S.D.	56±29	1.26±1.49	0.40±0.37
Range	21-85	0.27-4.81	0.12-1.0

While patients with the nephrotic syndrome tended to have lower total 1,25$(OH)_2$D concentrations, their unbound 1,25$(OH)_2$D concentrations were normal or increased due to an increase in the percent unbound fraction. We conclude that measurement of unbound 1,25$(OH)_2$D levels is improtant in the evaluation of disease states characterized by abnormal levels of 1,25$(OH)_2$D or its serum binding proteins.

589 FUNCTIONAL CONSEQUENCES OF AMINO-TERMINAL MUTATIONS IN THE LEADER SEQUENCE OF PREPROPARATHYROID HORMONE. M. Freeman*, J. Hellerman, A. Rapoport, R. Mulligan, J. Potts, Jr. and H. Kronenberg, Endocrine Genetics Unit and Department of Medicine, Massachusetts General Hospital, Boston, Massachusetts 02114, U.S.A.

Parathyroid hormone (PTH) is initially synthesized as a larger precursor, preproPTH, containing a 25 amino acid leader or pre sequence. To evaluate the role of the amino terminal portion of the leader sequence in the processing of preproPTH, mutations in the cDNA sequence encoding this hormone were made. Taking advantage of the fact that preproPTH has methionines at positions one, seven, eleven, and fourteen, Bal 31 nuclease was used to produce deletion mutants that encoded peptides missing the first six, ten, or thirteen amino acids, respectively, of the precursor. Native preproPTH and these mutants were then introduced into rat pituitary GH4 and murine 3T3 fibroblasts via a retroviral vector. Cells were labeled with [^{35}S]-methionine, using a "pulse-chase" protocol. PTH-related peptides were immuno-precipitated from cell extracts and characterized by fluorography after polyacrylamide gel electrophoresis. The mutant lacking only the first six amino acids of the pre sequence behaved like the normal precursor: it was processed to proPTH and PTH, and the PTH was secreted into the medium bathing the cells. The precursors lacking ten and thirteen amino acids were rapidly degraded in the cells without conversion to proPTH or PTH; no PTH-related peptides were secreted. Thus the first six amino acids of preproPTH have no apparent role in directing preproPTH along the secretory pathway; part or all of the next four residues are absolutely required for leader sequence function.

590 SURGICAL STRATEGY FOR RECURRENCE OF PARATHYROID CARCINOMA. Y.Fujimoto*, T. Obara, Y. Ito, T. Kodama and M. Nobori, Department of Endocrine Surgery, Tokyo Women's Medical College, Shinjuku, Tokyo, 162 JAPAN

Parathyroid carcinoma is a rare disease in Western countries and its prognosis is mostly poor because of high recurrence rate accompanied by its intolerable marked hypercalcemia. However, in Japan, unequivocal parathyroid carcinoma comprises as high as 5% of all primary hyperparathyroidism and most patients show rather less malignant clinical course. Thus far we accumulated a variety of new experiences in individual patients. In order to determine the surgical treatment of choice at the recurrence, a retrospective review was carried out on our 6 cases. The surgical managements performed and the results are as follows; (A) a wide local re-resection was done in 4 patients. Two have shown successive recurrences after multiple surgical trials and the other 2 are eucalcemic after once and twice reoperations, respectively. (B) One patient, who showed widely spread lymph node metastases without a local recurrence, received dissections of the neck and upper mediastinum and has been eucalcemic for the past one year. (C) One patient who had pulmonary metastasis underwent removal of metastatic lesions and has been well with mild hypercalcemia for the past 3 years. In conclusion, surgical treatment is useful for a control of hypercalcemia due to recurrence or metastasis of parathyroid carcinoma. When hypercalcemia recurs within 3 years after the initial operation, an aggressive surgical management for local recurrences, lymph node metastases, or even hematogenous metastases should be performed at the first occasion of reoperation. Thallium-201 scanning proved to be useful for a preoperative localization of recurrent or metastatic lesions.

591 INTERRELATIONSHIPS BETWEEN CIRCULATING VITAMIN D METABOLITES IN NORMOCALCIURIC AND HYPERCALCIURIC RENAL STONE FORMERS AND IN PATIENTS WITH PRIMARY HYPERPARATHYROIDISM.

M. Gascon-Barré*, P. D'Amour, L. Dufresne and J.-P. Perreault, Hôpital St-Luc, Université de Montréal, Montreal, Canada.

Plasma 25(OH)D, 24,25(OH)$_2$D and 1,25(OH)$_2$D were studied in 5 groups (normocalciuric (NSF), absorptive hypercalciuric with high 1,25(OH)$_2$D (AH-I) or normal 1,25(OH)$_2$D (AH-II), renal hypercalciuric (RH) and primary hyperparathyroidism (PHP)) of renal stone formers while on a diet containing 1000 or 300 mg Ca/day. The results indicate that on the 1000 mg Ca diet, all pts had normal 1,25(OH)$_2$D except 20% of pts with AH-I, and PHP where the 1,25(OH)$_2$D were elevated. 25(OH)D and 24,25(OH)$_2$D were within the normal range in all pts while on the 1000 mg Ca diet; on the low Ca diet, 25(OH)D decreased significantly in pts with AH-II and RH. 24,25(OH)$_2$D were not affected by the low Ca diet. 1,25(OH)$_2$D increased significantly during dietary Ca restriction in all groups but most particularly in AH-II, RH and PHP. When the relationship obtained on both diets between the 25(OH)D conc. and the 25(OH)D/1,25(OH)$_2$D conc. ratio was compared, it suggested that the increase in the 1,25(OH)$_2$D during Ca restriction was due, in all groups, to an increase in the capacity of the 25(OH)D-1 hydroxylase or to an increase in the t 1/2 of the circulating 1,25(OH)$_2$D but not to an increase in the affinity of the enzyme for its substrate. On a normal diet, only NSF and AH-I pts had plasma 1,25(OH)$_2$D compatible with their urinary Ca excretion. These results indicate that renal stone formers are able to adapt themselves to Ca restriction as shown by highly significant increases in the circulating 1,25(OH)$_2$D on a low Ca diet. In AH-II and RH, this was accompanied by significant decreases in substrate conc. suggesting an increased turnover rate of the 25(OH)D-1 hydroxylase in these pts during dietary Ca restriction.

592 ISOLATION AND IDENTIFICATION OF HUMAN CALCITONIN GENE RELATED PEPTIDE (h-CGRP) FROM MEDULLARY THYROID CARCINOMA.

S.I. GIRGIS*, H.R. Morris, M.Panico, T. Etienne, J.R. Tippins and I. MacIntyre. Department of Chemical Pathology, Royal Postgraduate Medical School, London W12 OHS and Department of Biochemistry, Imperial College, London, SW7 2AZ, UK.

Recently it has been reported that the rat calcitonin gene encodes a novel 37 amino acid peptide (r-CGRP), thought to be produced in nervous tissue after tissue specific RNA Processing (Amara et al, Nature 298, 240 1982; Rosenfeld et al, Nature 304, 129, 1983). Until now there has been no evidence that a similar peptide is present in man. Here we report the isolation of a related human peptide (h-CGRP). An antibody was raised against Tyr^0-r-CGRP$_{28-37}$ and used to detect immunoreactive material in extracts of human medullary thyroid carcinoma (MTC) tissue. A homogeneous peptide reacting with the antibody, was obtained from 15g of MTC tissue. The tissue was acid extracted (Bennett et al, Biochem.J. 175, 1139, 1978) and the supernatent adsorbed to water c-18 sep-pak cartridge which were eluted with methanol 80%, TFA 1%. The lyophilised extract was purified on a column of Sp-sephadex c-25 using a linear gradient from 0 to 1 molar Nacl in 30% acetic acid. Immunoreactive CGRP eluted as a single peak which was rechromatographed by HPLC on spherisorb 5µ ODS column using a gradient of 40-90% methanol, 0.2% TFA.The i-CGRP peak corresponded with the major U.V. absorbing peak at 210 nm. This material was then used for structural studies by a novel mass spectrometric approach, FAB mapping. (Morris et al, B B R C, 1983, in press). Furthermore i-CGRP was present in plasma from 20 patients with MTC and in 7 MTC tissue suggesting that the tissue distribution may differ from that in the rat.

593 IMMUNOLOGICAL PROPERTIES OF SYNTHETIC HUMAN PARATHYROID HORMONE. J.H.Gleed, G.N. Hendy*, T. Kimura, S. Sakakibara and J.L.H. O'Riordan, Department of Medicine, The Middlesex Hospital, London W1, U.K., Peptide Institute, Protein Research Foundation, Osaka 562, Japan.

We have investigated the immunological properties of two new synthetic forms of human parathyroid hormone (hPTH 1-84), one with aspartic acid (hPTH 1-84 Asp 76) and the other with asparagine (hPTH 1-84, Asn 76) at residue 76 in homologous region-specific labelled antibody assays using antisera raised against native hPTH 1-84. The assays were specific for either the amino-terminus (1-34), the mid-region (28-54), the mid-region (44-68) or the carboxy-terminus (53-84). In the amino-terminal and mid-region-specific assays both polypeptides showed similar reactivity. However in the carboxy-terminal assay, hPTH 1-84 (ASP 76) was less reactive than, and non-parallel to, hPTH 1-84 (Asn 76). Synthetic hPTH 53-84 (Asp 76) behaved identically to synthetic hPTH 1-84 (Asp 76) whereas hPTH 53-84 prepared from native hPTH 1-84 was more reactive and reacted identically to native hPTH 1-84. In all assays the behaviour of native hPTH 1-84 was parallel to that of synthetic hPTH 1-84 (Asn 76), although less reactive by 2.5-4-fold. Thus, the native human hormone might have undergone some change which impairs its immunoreactivity. It is shown here that deamidation at residue 76 caused a marked loss of immunoreactivity in a carboxy-terminal specific assay. As nucleotide sequencing of the messenger RNA and gene encoding human parathyroid hormone indicated that residue 76 is asparagine, future immunoassays for human parathyroid hormone should be based on synthetic hPTH 1-84 having asparagine at residue 76.

594 THIAZIDE ASSOCIATED HYPERCALCEMIA UNMASKS HYPERPARATHYROIDISM

S. Gordon*, A. Lyon, So. Calif. Permanente Med. Group, San Diego, CA 92120

Twenty patients found on routine physical examination to be hypercalcemic while on thiazide diuretics were studied. Measurements of serum calcium (Ca), parathormone (PTH), 24 hour urine Ca (24 Ca), and Urine Ca/creatinine ratio (Ca/Cr) were made at monthly intervals on thiazide, furosimide, and no diuretic. On thiazide Ca was highest, PTH most frequently elevated, 24 Ca and Ca/Cr depressed. Furosimide also increased Ca despite increasing 24 Ca. The degree of elevation of Ca on thiazide was positively correlated with elevated PTH and persistence of elevated Ca and PTH off diuretics. Five of seven patients with Ca over 11 on thiazide demonstrated this association. Conversely, 9 of 20 patients with lesser degrees of hypercalcemia on thiazide were normocalcemic off diuretics. Of this subset, 3/9 had elevated PTH on thiazide and 1/9 had elevated PTH at baseline. Similar correlations, of a lesser degree, occurred with furosimide. Ca/creat. correlated with PTH better than 24 Ca in all periods. Our conclusion is that thiazides unmask hyperparathyroidism that may not be apparent in the baseline state.

595 ESTIMATION OF INTACT PARATHYROID HORMONE (PTH)(1-84) IN NORMAL, HYPERCALCAEMIC AND HYPERPARATHYROID SERA AND SERA OF PATIENTS WITH CHRONIC RENAL FAILURE. Hackeng, W.H.L.*, Lips, C.J.M., Laboratory for Endocrinology, Bergweg Hospital, Rotterdam and Dept. of Internal Medicine, University Hospital, Utrecht, The Netherlands.

Determination of intact PTH(1-84) in sera using one anti-PTH antibody is always disturbed by the presence of multiple circulating PTH fragments which results in lack of specificity and sensitivity. We report the clinical results of a two-step immunochemical method for estimating serum intact PTH(1-84).§ The first step involves extraction and concentration of serum with antibodies against N-terminal PTH coupled to a solid phase. In the second step the initial PTH immuno-extract is analyzed with a sensitive midregion immunoassay in at least two dilutions. Intact PTH can thus be detected in virtually all normal subjects. In addition, the results show a significant discrimination between normal, hyperparathyroid and non-hyperparathyroid hypercalcaemic sera. Unlike the total PTH activity (intact PTH together with all fragments), the PTH(1-84) activity in sera of most of the patients with chronic renal failure are normal. There is a strong indication that an elevated PTH(1-84) level correlates well with the presence of renal osteodystrophy. PTH(1-84) activity in sera obtained through venous catheterization gives much more certainty about the localization of abnormal parathyroids. EDTA-stimulation and Ca^{++}-suppression tests give at least a 3-fold better response. Summarized, the PTH(1-84) assay is a new valuable tool in studying patients with possible parathyroid disorders.

§ Estimation of biologically active intact PTH in normal and hyperparathyroid sera by sequential N-terminal immunoextraction and midregion radioimmunoassay, Lindall A.W., et al., J Clin Endocr Metab 1983:57:1007-1014.

596 THE EFFECT OF CALCIUM, VITAMIN D AND PARATHYROID HORMONE ON THE RAT UTERINE ESTROGEN RECEPTOR. S. Epstein*, S. Thomas, Albert Einstein Medical Center, York & Tabor Roads, Philadelphia. PA 19141, U.S.A.

We investigated the effect of calcium, $1,25(OH)_2D$ and parathyroid hormone (PTH) on the rat uterine estrogen receptor (E_2). Sprague-Dawley rats were divided into four groups (A, B, C, D). Group C was fed a calcium deficient diet, underwent surgical thyroparathyroidectomy followed by PTH injections. Group B and Group D were also fed a calcium deficient diet, underwent sham operations and Group D was administered $1,25(OH)_2D$ while Group B received placebo injections. Group A acted as a control group, eating a normal diet, undergoing a sham operation and being injected with a placebo. Ionized calcium (Ca++) was serially measured in all groups and the animals were sacrificed after eight days of injections and the affinity and capacity of the uterus and fallopian tubes to bind estrogen measured in vitro by RIA The results revealed that Ca++ fell dramatically in Group C and rose in Group D. Group C and Group D had altered E_2 receptor affinity. However, binding capacity of the E_2 receptor was changed only in Group C. These results demonstrate that hypocalcemia, and not PTH deficiency, effects the binding capacity of the rat uterine estrogen receptor.

597 BORN RESORPTION STIMULATING FACTOR IN ADULT T CELL LEUKEMIA. T.Fujihira*, S,Eto, K.Sato, S.Oda, S.Chiba and H.Suzuki,First Dept. of Internal Med., Univ. of Occupational & Environmental Health, Kitakyushu, Fukuoka, Japan. Second Dept. of Internal Med., Tokyo Women's Medical College, Tokyo, Japan.

Adult T cell leukemia (ATL) is known to be frequently associated with hypercalcemia, but, the mechanisms responsible for hypercalcemia in this disorder are not fully understood. We have recently experienced two male patients (25 yr, 36 yr) with ATL diagnosed on typical leukemic cells with grooved and folded nucleus, surface marker, anti-ATLA etc. Serum calcium levels of these patients were 16.4, 21.4 mg/dl, respectively, with no radiological evidence of bone destruction. Peripheral blood leukemic lymphocytes from these patients were purified by Ficoll-Hypaque method and cultured at a concentration of 1.5 x 10^6 cells/ml for 3 days in F-10 medium supplemented with 10 % fetal calf serum. Supernatant media from cell culture were bioassayed for bone resorption stimulating activity (BRSA) by an assay based on the release of ^{45}Ca from pre-labeled fetal mouse forearm bones in organ culture according to Raisz's method. The supernatant media of each patient showed marked BRSA which is non-dialysable by using dialysis-membrane of molecular weight cutoff of 3,500. PTH or Prostaglandins were not detectable in supernatant media of leukemic cell culture. In one patient, BRSA was assayed twice at intervals and proved to be decreased to normal levels, when the patient was in remission with normal levels of calcium (8.3 mg/dl). These results suggest that hypercalcemia observed in patients with ATL is due, in part, to born resorption stimulating factor which is produced by leukemic T cell lymphocytes.

598 **EFFECTS OF KETOCONAZOLE ON TESTOSTERONE BIOSYNTHESIS IN SHORT TERM CULTURES OF DISPERSED RAT TESTICULAR CELLS.** **R. De Coster*, Laboratory of Endocrinology, Department of Life Sciences, Janssen Pharmaceutica, B-2340 Beerse, Belgium**

Ketoconazole induces a dose-dependent inhibition of basal and hCG stimulated testosterone (T) production by freshly dispersed rat testicular cells. Fifty procent decrease of control T production are obtained at final medium drug concentrations of 2.10^{-7} M (basal) and 5.5 10^{-7} M (hCG stimulated). Between 10^{-7} M and 5.10^{-6} M ketoconazole induces a rise of progesterone (to 170 % of its control) value and of 17α-hydroxyprogesterone (to 260 % of its control value) in the supernatant as well as in the cell extract. A slight decrease of stimulated cyclic AMP production is only detected at drug concentrations of 10^{-5} M. The inhibition of T synthesis is totally reversible by washing the cell. The addition of mevalonic acid (9.10^{-3} M), of cholesterol lipoproteins (150 µg ml^{-1}) and of pregnenolone (3.10^{-6} M) do not overcome the block. These data confirm that ketoconazole, at final medium concentration of 10^{-7} to 5.10^{-6} M inhibits <u>in vitro</u> T biosynthesis by acting on the cytochrome P 450-dependent C17-20 lyase enzyme. At high dose, other enzymes seem to be affected, probably the cytochrome P 450-dependent ones of the cholesterol side-chain cleavage.

599 PROSTAGLANDIN SYNTHASE DEPENDENT METABOLISM OF DIETHYLSTILBESTROL STRUCTURAL ANALOGS. G.H. Degen* and K. Sivarajah, Inst. Toxicology, Univ. Wuerzburg, Fed. Rep. Germ.; NIEHS, Research Triangle Park, N.C., U.S.A.

Syrian hamster embryo (SHE-) cell cultures are neoplastically transformed by the synthetic estrogen diethylstilbestrol (DES) and by some structural analogs (McLachlan et al.,Cancer Res. 42,3040,1982). Prostaglandin synthase (PGS) dependent metabolism of DES occurs in these cells (Degen et al., ibid 43,992,1983). PGS is known to have two integral enzyme activities: a cyclooxygenase and a peroxidase that metabolizes certain compounds during cooxidation. In an attempt to correlate PGS mediated metabolism with transforming activity, DES, tetrafluoro-DES (TF-DES), dimethylstilbestrol (DMS),hexestrol (HES), Z,Z-dienestrol (Z,Z-DIES), E,E-dienestrol (E,E-DIES), DES-monomethylether (M-DES),and DES-dimethylether (DM-DES) were tested as substrates for PGS in vitro. Oxygraph studies showed that DES analogs that undergo net two electron oxidation (DES, TF-DES, DMS) and analogs that can undergo one electron oxidation (HES, Z,Z-DIES, E,E-DIES, M-DES) stimulated arachidonic acid dependent oxygen consumption (PGS-cyclooxygenase activity). PGS-peroxidase mediated products (the dien- metabolites of DES, TF-DES and DMS) were identified by HPLC and GC/MS. Evidence for the formation of quinones and phenoxyradicals as reactive intermediates during cooxidation will also be presented. DM-DES was not a substrate for PGS in vitro and was not found to transform SHE-cells in culture. In conclusion, with the exception of E,E-DIES, synthetic estrogens known to transform SHE-cells with varying potency were found to be substrates for PGS in vitro. Reactive intermediates such as phenoxyradicals and quinones and stimulation of prostaglandin synthesis may play a role in this process.

600 INTRACELLULAR LOCALIZATION OF SEX STEROID BINDING PLASMA PROTEIN IN HUMAN BREAST CANCER. H. Degrelle*, J. Tardivel-Lacombe, M. Egloff, L. Benhallassa. Faculté de Médecine, 45, rue des Saints Pères, 75006 PARIS, France.

The human sex steroid binding plasma protein (hSBP) is a glycoprotein, MW ≃ 80.000, which specifically binds testosterone, 5α-dihydrotestosterone and estradiol with high affinity and low capacity. Various reports have suggested that hSBP may enter target tissues of androgens and estrogens and therefore, may not be exclusively localized in the plasma. In this report, we attempted to demonstrate the presence of SBP inside human mammary carcinoma cells, using monospecific antibodies against the homogeneous protein. Pure SBP was obtained from a pool of late pregnancy human serum by a five step conventional procedure and was used for rabbit immunization. Semi-thin sections of tissue were prepared from surgical pieces of human mammary carcinomas and were processed by the fluorescent double antibody technique. Dark controls were simultaneously carried out to rule out autofluorescence and other non specific interactions. The protein appears to be located in the cytoplasm and the membrane of the carcinoma cells, but no fluorescence was found in the nucleus. The consequence of the localization of hSBP in human breast cancer will affect our thinking about the role of this protein in the hormonodependence of breast cancer which could be more extensive that a simple control of the unbound concentration of estradiol in plasma.

601 AMINOGLUTETHIMIDE THERAPY IN BREAST CANCER: RELATIONSHIP OF BLOOD LEVELS TO DRUG RELATED SIDE EFFECTS.

*L.M. Demers, A. Boucher and R. Santen, Division of Endocrinology, M.S. Hershey Medical Center, Hershey, PA

Aminoglutethimide (AG) is now an established agent for inducing a "medical adrenalectomy" in patients with breast cancer. Although no serious toxicity to the drug has been reported, a number of annoying symptoms do occur in some patients including lethargy and the development of a skin rash. It has been suggested that the expression of symptoms may be related to the acetylator status of the patient and that a buildup of n-acetyl aminoglutethimide (NAG) the major metabolite could be responsible for these symptoms. Using HPLC, we have examined the blood levels of AG and NAG in patients with breast cancer and compared the levels to the expression and frequency of drug symptoms. 43% of patients examined were considered slow acetylators in that 92% of the drug remained unacetylated irrespective of the doses ranging from 500 to 1000 milligrams. There was no significant correlation between acetylator status (rapid versus slow) and the frequency of drug symptoms noted. In contrast there was a significant correlation between the level of AG itself found in the blood and the frequency of symptoms. 80% of patients with blood levels exceeding 12 ug/L had drug related symptoms while only 36% of patients with levels below 8 ug/L showed symptoms ($\chi^2 p<0.05$). 67% of patients with NAG levels in excess of 4 ug/L had symptoms. These studies indicate the presence of slow and rapid acetylators of aminoglutethimide in a breast cancer population and the importance of determining blood levels of the drug to minimize the onset of drug symptoms in some patients without losing drug efficacy.

602 1,25-DIHYDROXYVITAMIN D_3 INHIBITS COLONY FORMATION BY CANCER CELLS IN SOFT AGAR: A DIRECT CORRELATION WITH THE VITAMIN D HORMONE RECEPTOR.

C. Donaldson*, S. Marion, J. Pike and M. Haussler, Department of Biochemistry, University of Arizona Health Sciences Center, Tucson, Arizona, USA.

1,25-Dihydroxyvitamin D_3 (1,25$(OH)_2D_3$) has recently been shown to be a natural antineoplastic agent. We studied the influence of this hormone on the clonogenic growth of cancer cells in soft agar and correlated its effects with 1,25$(OH)_2D_3$ receptor concentration. Cells were plated in a 0.33% agar containing culture medium overlaid on a 0.5% agar containing base. Both layers contained 10 nM 1,25$(OH)_2D_3$ or 0.1% ethanol vehicle. After 14 days at 37°C, 100-1000 colonies $\geq$ 50 µm in diameter (approx. 30 cells) were scored in 35 mm plates, utilizing a computerized colony counter. The receptor in each cell line was determined via whole cell incubation with 2 nM 1,25$(OH)_2[^3H]D_3$, followed by receptor quantitation with DNA cellulose chromatography. Inhibition of colony formation by 1,25$(OH)_2D_3$ displayed a direct correspondence with the 1,25$(OH)_2D_3$ receptor copy number found in at least eight tested cell lines, including human neuroblastoma IMR-32 (< 100 copies receptor/cell and no significant inhibition of colony forming ability), human bladder EJ (1400 copies and 21% inhibition), human melanoma G-361 (1900 copies and 55% inhibition) and rat osteosarcoma ROS 17/2.8 (17,500 copies and 72% inhibition). This correlation between 1,25$(OH)_2D_3$ receptor number and inhibition of anchorage-independent growth by the hormone may represent a receptor-mediated reversion from the malignant to a more normal phenotype. Current studies include the attempted isolation of 1,25$(OH)_2D_3$-resistant clones, enabling us to further define the mechanism of this phenomenon.

603 CYTOSOLIC ESTROGEN AND PROGESTIN RECEPTORS IN UTERUS AND MAMMARY GLAND OF MICE TREATED NEONATALLY WITH TESTOSTERONE. M. Edery*, K.T. Mills and H.A. Bern, Department of Zoology and Cancer Research Laboratory, University of California, Berkeley, CA 94720, U.S.A.

The neonatal mouse is a useful animal model for analyzing the possible reproductive consequences of transplacental exposure of the human fetus to sex hormones, particularly estrogens. Both androgen and estrogen treatments of neonatal mice result in abnormal changes in the female reproductive tract and mammary gland. Inasmuch as estrogen receptors (ER) and progestin receptors (PR) are present in the normal female reproductive tract and mammary gland, we have examined the levels of these receptors after neonatal androgen exposure. After neonatal treatment with testosterone (5 µg daily for five days starting within 18 h after birth), in the uterus the ER levels are significantly lower at 40, 60, 120 and 180 days by 65%, 61%, 42% and 41%, respectively, than in the controls. The PR levels are lower, but not significantly so, at 40 days and significantly lower (by 35%) at 60 days; at 120 and 180 days the PR levels are not significantly different from controls. In the mammary gland from neonatally androgenized mice, both ER and PR levels are significantly lower (48% and 37%, respectively) than in controls at 40 days of age but not at older ages. The data indicate that although neonatal testosterone exposure results in significantly lower ER and PR levels in the uterus and mammary gland at young ages, the differences disappear or become less prominent (uterine ER) with time. (Aided by NIH grant CA05388).

604 IMMUNOMODULATORY EFFECT OF BOVINE PTH EXTRACT ON PERIPHERAL BLOOD LYMPHOCYTE RESPONSE TO PLANT MITOGENS. A. Elias*, B. Sharma, T. Kyaw and L. Valenta, University of California, Irvine, Irvine, California, U.S.A. and Endocrine and Diabetes Clinic of No. County, Oceanside, California, U.S.A.

Human peripheral blood lymphocytes (PBL) isolated by the Ficoll-Hypaque technique were incubated with (^{3}H) thymidine and various concentrations of bovine parathyroid extract (PTH) and PTH plus different concentrations of plant mitogens (PHA, Con-A, PWM). The results are expressed as stimulation indices (SI). SI = cpm cultures with PTH or PTH + mitogen/cpm in lymphocyte cultures alone. PTH stimulated (^{3}H) thymidine uptake by PBL at concentrations of 0.25 µg/0.2 ml (SI = 1.18 $\pm$ 0.22 at 0.05 µg/0.2 ml vs. 1.44 $\pm$ 0.43, $p < 0.03$), but markedly inhibited (^{3}H) thymidine uptake at PTH concentrations of > 1 µg/0.2 ml (SI at 1.5 µg/0.2 ml = 0.43 $\pm$ 0.21, $p < 0.03$). A similar biphasic response (stimulation at PTH concentrations of 0.25 - 0.5 µg/0.2 ml and inhibition at concentrations > 1 µg/0.2 ml was seen when PBL were cultured with PTH and PHA. In contrast, PTH inhibited, in a dose-dependent manner, (^{3}H) thymidine uptake by PBL when the cells were stimulated with Con-A (0.25 - 2 µg/0.2 ml). Stimulation indices with Con-A + PTH and PWM + PTH at concentrations of 0.25 µg/0.2 ml were 0.86 $\pm$ 0.14 and 0.88 $\pm$ 0.21, respectively. At PTH concentration of 2 µg/0.2 ml, stimulation indices with Con-A + PTH and PWM + PTH were both 0.01 $\pm$ 0.01 ($p < 0.001$). Our observations suggest that the immunomodulatory effect of PTH on PBL is due to PTH itself or to some other factor in the extract. In view of the common embryonic origin of the parathyroid glands and the thymus, the possibility that thymic hormones or thymic hormone-like factors are involved in the immunomodulatory process cannot be excluded.

605 SPECIFIC NUCLEAR ESTROGEN UPTAKE AND REGRESSION IN HUMAN BREAST CANCER.

*A.G. Fazekas and J.K. MacFarlane, Dept. of Surgery, McGill University, The Montreal General Hospital, Montreal, Quebec, H3G 1A4, Canada.

In order to improve the characterization of hormone dependent carcinomas a new test was developed to measure specific nuclear estrogen uptake (SNEU) by incubating at 30° washed tumor nuclei in the presence of cytosol and ^{3}H estradiol with and without an estrogen competitor, followed by isolation of nuclei, receptor extraction and quantitation of specifically bound estradiol. A systematic study of 600 human breast cancers for cytosolic estrogen (ERC) and progesterone (PgRC) receptors and SNEU revealed that a significant proportion (24%) of ERC rich tumors has no SNEU activity. This could explain the failure of endocrine therapy in many ERC rich tumor bearing patients. A number of these patients (40) were investigated for their responses to endocrine therapy. In patients with positive ERC and SNEU, the response rate was 100% while cases with negative ERC and SNEU did not respond at all. This was higher than the response rate (86%) of patients with positive cytosolic estrogen and progesterone receptors belonging to the same group. Results indicate that the assay of SNEU could be a better indicator of endocrine dependency than the measurement of cytosolic receptor activity.

606 EFFECT OF DIABETES AND FASTING ON THE GLUCOSE CARRIERS OF EHRLICH ASCITES TUMOUR CELLS.

K. P. Fung*, Y. M. Choy and C. Y. Lee, Department of Biochemistry, The Chinese University of Hong Kong, Shatin, N.T., Hong Kong.

The effect of blood glucose concentration on the glucose carrier densities of Ehrlich ascites tumour cells were studied *in vivo*. Glucose carriers of Ehrlich ascites tumour cells were identified by the density of glucose-reversible binding sites for cytochalasin B on the cells. Mice were induced diabetes by streptozotocin (200 mg/kg body weight) injection three days before the inoculation of 10^7 tumour cells. On 7-days post-transplantation, 45% significant reduction of glucose carrier density on tumour cells was observed in diabetic tumour-bearing mice as compared with control. The dissociation constant (Kd) of cytochalasin B binding on the tumour cells remained relatively unchanged in both groups. Tumour bearing mice were also fasted for 1½ and 2½ days post-transplantation. A 30% and 130% significant increases in glucose carriers on tumour cells were observed in tumour-bearing mice fasted for 1½ and 2½ days respectively with no change in Kd, as compared with control. The tumour size decreased both in diabetic and fasting mice. Since in both diabetic and fasting tumour cells the change in glucose carrier closely parallelled in a reverse manner to the change of blood glucose concentration, it is suggested that blood glucose might be a regulator for the glucose carrier on the tumour cells. The tumour size and qualitative change in affinity for glucose (Kd value) need not be invoked. This study was supported by World Health Foundation (Hong Kong).

607 STIMULATORY EFFECT OF ADRENAL STEROIDS ON UTERINE WEIGHT AND PROGESTERONE RECEPTORS IN THE RAT. P. Gagnon*, P. Poyet, J. Simard, A. Bélanger, and F. Labrie, MRC Group in Molecular Endocrinology, CHUL, Québec G1V 4G2, Canada.

There is convincing evidence that adrenal steroids, especially androst-5-ene-3β,17β-diol (Δ^5-diol) could play a role in estrogen-dependent diseases, especially breast cancer. Since estrogens are known to exert a specific stimulatory effect on LHRH-induced LH release in rat adenohypophysial cells in culture, we have studied the effect of a 48-h preincubation with Δ^5-diol on this parameter. The adrenal steroid causes an approximately 3-fold increase in LH release at an ED_{50} value of 2 nM. When Δ^5-diol is administered at the daily dose of 0.3 mg for 2 weeks to ovariectomized rats, a 150-250% increase (over control) of uterine weight and concentration of progesterone receptors is observed, the effect of the steroid being not affected by simultaneous treatment with the pure antiandrogen Anandron. Dehydroepiandrosterone (DHEA), on the other hand, injected at the twice daily 2.0 mg dose, causes a similar increase in uterine weight which is 50% prevented by simultaneous treatment with the antiandrogen. Treatment with DHT (0.5 mg), Δ^4-androstenedione (1.0 mg) or androstane-3β,17β-diol, on the other hand, causes an increase in uterine weight which is completely prevented by the antiandrogen while no effect of these androgens is observed on the level of uterine progesterone receptors, a typical parameter of estrogenic activity. The present data show that Δ^5-diol can exert potent estrogenic stimulatory effects at both the adenohypophysial and uterine levels, thus supporting the potential role of this and related adrenal steroids in estrogen-dependent cancers.

608 IMMUNOHISTOCHEMICAL DETECTION OF THE ESTROGEN-REGULATED 52,000 mol wt PROTEIN IN PRIMARY BREAST CANCERS BUT NOT IN NORMAL UTERUS. M. Garcia[*+], G. Salazar-Retana[+], G. Richer[§], F. Capony[+], B. Pau[§] and H. Rochefort[+], + INSERM U 148 (60, Rue de Navacelles) ; § Centre de Recherche CLIN-MIDY ; 34100 Montpellier, France.

An estrogen-regulated glycoprotein of molecular weight 52,000 (52 K protein) is released by metastatic breast cancer cells in culture. In order to test directly the distribution of this protein in primary breast cancers and others human tissues, murine monoclonal antibodies (MAbs) 52 K protein have been generated, their specificity assessed by immunoprecipitation and Western immunoblotting techniques. Six purified MAbs were selected to immunostain frozen tissue sections by the peroxidase-anti-peroxidase method. In 15 out of 18 breast cancer specimens, a specific and heterogeneous immunostaining was observed in the cytoplasm of 1 to 30 % of cancer cells, but not in connective tissue. Experiments with myeloma medium or negative control MAb showed the specificity of the staining. Preliminary evidence suggest that the tissular 52 K protein is correlated with the estrogen receptor content. No reactivity was observed in normal uterus collected at different periods of menstrual cycle, indicating that it is not a marker of all estrogen responsive tissues. These studies are now extended to other normal and cancer human tissues. This is the first report on the presence of the 52 K estrogen regulated protein in the cytoplasm of some primary breast cancer. Immunohistochemical and radioimmunological techniques will allow to test the clinical usefulness of the 52 K protein as an additional marker for predicting the hormone-dependency of breast cancer.

609 PROLONGED PULSATILE LRH TREATMENT:DEVELOPMENT OF A NEW TEST TO ESTIMATE THE FUNCTIONAL CAPACITY OF THE GONADOTROPHS. H.A. Delemarre-van de Waal, J. Schoemaker, Acad. Hosp. of the "Vrije Universiteit",Amsterdam, Netherlands.

It is generally agreed that a single dose LRH test does not inform us reliably about the gonadotrophic function in contrast to prolonged pulsatile LRH treatment. Valk et al.(1980) observed an exaggerated response, especially of LH to LRH a few days after LRH withdrawal in hypogonadotropic patients. This observation might be used to study the gonadotrophic capacity. 27 hypogonadotropic children with various endocrine disorders were pretreated with LRH, every 96 min 20µg/1.73m² iv,for 7 days. On day 7 as well as either 4 or 7 days after LRH withdrawal (day 11/14) a LRH test was performed The patients were divided into 2 groups: a those patients, who showed an increase of their sexsteroid level during LRH treatment (21) and b those without such an increase (6). We considered this increase an indication of an intact gonadotrophic function. On day 7 basal gonadotropin levels as well as the LH response had increased compared to the basal state in gr. a, in contrast to the patients of gr. b. However there was no significant difference between the peaks of either LH or FSH of both groups on day 7. On day 11/14 basal gonadotropin levels had returned to the low original range in all patients. The geom. mean of peak LH of gr. a was 43.7 U/l(13.3-171), of gr. b 13.1 U/l(5.6-30) (P 0.01). 2 out of 6 patients of gr. b showed no LH response whatsoever. FSH peak levels did not differ between both groups. We conclude that 1. the absent gonadotropin increase on day 7 in 4 pt of gr b was caused by a functional defect, while 2 pts suffered from an organic defect of the gonadotrophs 2.prolonged pulsatile LRH treatment followed by a LRH test within 4-7 days may give more information about the functional capacity of the gonadotrophs and therefore may be useful as diagnostic tool.

610 ISOLATED ACTH DEFICIENCY IN ASSOCIATION WITH EMPTY SELLA SYNDROME. R. DelGrande* and R. Kleinmann, West Virginia University Medical Center, Charleston Division, Charleston, WV, USA.

A 62 yr-old woman, G4, P4, previously hypertensive and obese, was admitted to a psychiatric unit for evaluation of depression. She had a 1 yr history of weakness, anorexia and weight loss. The blood pressure was 110/60 on no drugs; she was anemic and hyponatremic. T4 was 14.6 µg/dl, TSH 8.8 µU/ml (normal <7.3). A dexamethasone test for depression showed "normal" suppression of cortisol (1.1 µg/dl at 24 h). 2 wks later an AM cortisol was 1.5 µg/dl. Pituitary function was evaluated following IV regular insulin, .15U/kg, 500 µg TRH and 100 µg LHRH. Serum glucose fell to 34 mg/dl. The patient was taking doxepin at the time of the test.

	ACTH pg/ml	Cortisol µg/dl	GH ng/ml	PRL ng/ml	TSH µU/ml	T3 ng/dl	LH mIU/ml	FSH mIU/ml
Baseline	28	2.3	1.0	79	7.5	119	18	51
Peak response	23	5.3	13.0	190	11.9	143	>100	77

250 µg ACTH (Cortrosyn) was then infused over 8 h daily for 3 days. Serum cortisol rose to 25.9 after the first and 57.5 after the third infusion. Sella tomograms showed symmetrical enlargement with bowing of the floor. Computed tomography showed fluid density in the sella and no tumor. Doxepin was stopped. After 6 wks of hydrocortisone, 30 mg/d, the patient felt well. Her appetite had returned, weight was increasing and the anemia and hyponatremia had resolved. T4 was 9.8 µg/dl, TSH 6.3 µU/ml, prolactin 15.5 ng/ml. In conclusion, (1) a patient with isolated ACTH deficiency and empty sella is described, and (2) increased serum TSH, as occurs in Addison's disease, may also occur with isolated ACTH deficiency.

611 CLINICAL AND HORMONAL RESPONSE TO ETHINYL OESTRADIOL AND DESOGESTREL (MARVELON) IN HIRSUTE WOMEN. P. Dewis*, P. Petsos, M. Newman, D.C. Anderson, Department of Medicine, University of Manchester, Hope Hospital, Salford, U.K.

Some available combined oral contraceptive agents are unsuitable for the treatment of hirsutism, since although they suppress endogenous gonadotrophins and so ovarian androgen production, they contain a progestogen that is itself androgenic. Marvelon which contains 30 μg Ethinyl Oestradiol (EE2) and 150 μg desogestrel, does not suffer from this drawback. We have therefore assessed its value in 15 hirsute women, six of them oligomenorrhoeic, treated for 7 months. Mean ± SE of androgen-dependent hair growth rate, assessed photographically, fell significantly from 0.31 ± 0.12 to 0.26 ± .01 at 4 and 0.25 ± .01 mm/day at 7 months ($p < 0.001$). Ten of the 15 patients reported definite subjective improvement. Marvelon was associated with the expected marked rise in SHBG concentration, identical to that seen with 30 μg EE2 alone. By 4 months there were significant falls in serum levels of androstenedione and LH throughout the cycle, but not for 5α androstan 3α 17βdiol, 5α dihydrotestosterone or testosterone. Calculated free T levels however were suppressed to 58% of control. We conclude that this preparation is a suitable oral contraceptive for treatment of hirsute women.

612 ANOMALOUS GLUCOSE AND INSULIN RESPONSES TO FASTING IN INSULINOMA PATIENTS: CAVEATS FOR DIAGNOSIS. R. Dons*, J. Hodge, B. Ginsberg, M. Brennan, P. Cryer, I. Kourides and P. Gorden, Diabetes Br., NIH and Naval Hospital Bethesda, NMCNCR, Bethesda, MD.

The diagnosis of an insulinoma can usually be made by obtaining simultaneous glucose and insulin values during prolonged supervised fasting. We encountered two patients with insulinomas who had unusual glucose and insulin secretory dynamics in response to prolonged fasting. In order to establish the diagnosis, studies in addition to supervised fasting were required. In patient 1, very low insulin values persisted throughout three separate fasts without a steady rise in the insulin/glucose (I/G) ratio. In this patient, diazoxide therapy was associated with higher glucose levels, but little change in insulin values. In patient 2, a rising I/G ratio during a fast returned to normal after a documented catacholamine surge following a transient hypoglycemic episode. Provocative testing with tolbutamide and leucine elicited markedly different insulin secretory responses from the two patients. While patient 1 had an elevated proinsulin of 53-57%, patient 2 had a near-normal value of 23%. Localization of a pancreatic mass with arteriography and a surgical cure with removal of the insulinoma was accomplished in each case. Continuous intraoperative glucose monitoring revealed a steady rise in glucose after resection of the tumor from patient 1 consistent with the successful operation. We conclude that, rarely, anomalous results will be obtained during a supervised fast of patients with an insulinoma and that the use of a broader range of diagnostic tests will be necessary to make the correct diagnosis.

613 D,L-THREO-3,4-DIHYDROXYPHENYLSERINE (DOPS) RAISES MEAN ARTERIAL BLOOD PRESSURE (MABP) AND NOREPINEPHRINE (NE) EXCRETION IN A PATIENT WITH REFRACTORY IDIOPATHIC ORTHOSTATIC HYPOTENSION (IOH). D. Einhorn*, L. Landsberg and J.B. Young, Beth Israel Hospital, Boston, MA 02215, USA.

IOH is characterized by loss of functional peripheral sympathetic nerves, low supine and upright plasma NE levels, symptomatic postural hypotension and increased MABP responsiveness to NE infusion. DOPS (Sumitomo, Japan), a synthetic amino acid precursor of (-)-NE that is absorbed in the gut and metabolized to NE, has been used in orthostatic hypotension secondary to familial amyloidosis. We therefore examined the effect of DOPS in a female with severe IOH who had failed conventional therapies including L-DOPA, clonidine, and yohimbine. Her medications consisted of fludrocortisone, nortriptyline, metoclopramide, 18 gram NaCl diet, KCl 160 meq/d, and support stockings. In the basal state, supine MABP was 96 ± 6 mmHg (Mean ± SEM), sitting was 51 ± 7, and standing was <20. Basal pulse was 62 ± 4 beats per minute (without postural change). Basal 24 hour urinary excretion of NE was 2.34 ug, epinephrine 1.4 ug, and dopamine 129.4 ug. Over the first 8 hours following DOPS 300 mg orally, supine MABP increased to 121 ± 5 and prolonged sitting was tolerated with MABP 91 ± 7. Brief standing was tolerated at 5-8 hours after DOPS with MABP 80 ± 12. Pulse was unchanged. 24 hr urinary NE excretion increased to 447.2 ug. There was no effect on the excretion of epinephrine or dopamine. The increase in MABP and NE excretion following DOPS was dose dependent. The MABP effects of DOPS began at 2 hours after oral ingestion and peaked at 4-5 hours. Although the MABP effect of DOPS was largely dissipated by 8 hours, the urinary NE excretion remained 20 to 30 times higher than basal values at 12-24 hours following DOPS. The major side effect was increased supine hypertension. The effect of DOPS was sustained through 4 weeks of daily use. DOPS appears to be a novel oral agent for the management of IOH.

614 TERTIARY HYPERALDOSTERONISM (THA): A NEW ENTITY. A. EL-KHODARY and F. MONTALBANO*, Providence Hospital, Washington, D.C. 20017, U.S.A.

The evolution of Idiopathic Hyperaldosteronism (IHA) is unknown. A hypertensive, hypokalemic 64 year old black male diagnosed to have IHA in 1973, developed an aldosterone producing adenoma (APA) over the ensuing ten years. IHA was diagnosed in 1973, confirmed in 1975 based on: persistent elevation of urinary aldosterone (UA), physiologic fluctuations in plasma renin activity (PRA) in response to low/high salt diet; UA was 68-47 mcg/24 hr and PRA varied from 2.3-0.9 ng/ml/hr respectively. Plasma aldosterone (PA) and PRA increased in the upright position, 40.1-167.4 ng/dl and 1.33-2.17 ng/ml/hr respectively; left adrenal vein PA was 410 ng/dl when right hepatic and iliac vein PA were 10 and 100 ng/dl respectively. The patient responded initially to spironolactone. Hypertension and hypokalemia became progressively resistent to therapy. Reinvestigation in 1983 revealed a right adrenal mass, persistent elevation of UA with undetectable PRA levels irrespective of salt intake or posture. PA response to posture was variable, however, there was a paradoxical rise of PA in response to overnight and following ten days Dexamethasone suppression, 110-248, 392-1040 ng/dl respectively. PA dropped from 190 to 12 ng/dl and UA from 93 to 1 mcg/ 24 hrs immediately following the removal of a right adrenal macroadenoma with subsequent normalization of blood pressure and serum potassium. The data indicate that an APA evolved from an IHA (THA), the hormonal biodynamics of this type of APA are different from primary adenomas. The significance of the paradoxical PA response to Dexamethasone suppression in the pathogenesis and diagnosis of THA needs further evaluation.

615 RATIOS OF FSH/LH SECRETION IN TIMED URINARY SPECIMENS: A SIMPLE MEASURE OF PUBERTAL DEVELOPMENT. E.C. Ewen*, M.P. Warren and J. Brooks-Gunn, St. Luke's-Roosevelt Hospital, New York, New York, USA

Nocturnal pulsatile release of LH and to some extent FSH has been noted in early puberty. With maturation this phenomenon reportedly disappears. The study of gonadotropin patterns in puberty is cumbersome and prohibitive due to large amounts of samples needed and inconvenience obtaining nighttime samples. We obtained nocturnal and daytime timed urine samples from 72 girls in Tanner stages of 1 - 5 of pubertal development and measured LH and FSH in a acetone extract by radioimmunoassay. Ratios of FSH/LH in day and nighttime samples were compared to stages of sexual maturation. Girls in stages 1 and 2 of breast development had higher daytime FSH/LH ratios with a mean ratio of 5.04, significantly higher than fully mature stage 4 and 5 with a mean ratio of 2.9 $p < .05$. Nocturnal ratios decreased with sexual maturation reflecting a rise in LH secretion at night and occasional reversals in ratios were seen. The mean ratio of FSH/LH secretion was significantly higher in the day when compared to night samples at all stages of physical development ($p < .05$ - $p < .001$). The patterns described above were also consistent when analyzed according to the stages of pubic hair development. These data suggest that the rise in FSH seen in early puberty can be discerned by timed urinary specimens and that LH nocturnal spurting occuring in puberty leading to lowered FSH/LH ratios at night can also be analyzed by this method. Further investigation is needed to examine the applicability of FSH/LH in timed urinary specimens as a guideline in assessing pubertal development.

616 TREATMENT OF MCCUNE-ALBRIGHT SYNDROME (MAS) WITH A LUTEINIZING HORMONE - RELEASING HORMONE ANALOG AND WITH TESTOLACTONE. C. Foster*, O. Pescovitz, F. Comite, T. Shawker, D. Loriaux and G. Cutler Jr., NICHD, and Diagnostic Radiology, NIH, Bethesda, MD 20205 USA.

Six 1-8 year old girls with MAS were treated with 4 µ/kg/d SC of a long-acting analog of luteinizing hormone-releasing hormone, D-trp^6-pro^9-NEt-LHRH (LHRH$_a$) which has been shown to suppress serum gonadotropins in true precocious puberty. Five girls, who before treatment had prepubertal nocturnal and LHRH-stimulated serum gonadotropins, had no decrease in plasma estradiol or serum gonadotropins and no cessation of menses after 8-12 weeks of therapy. Serial ultrasound examinations revealed fluctuating ovarian cysts. Ovarian volumes by ultrasound correlated with plasma estradiol ($p<0.05$). The sixth girl, who before treatment had nocturnal and LHRH-stimulated gonadotropins in the pubertal range, responded to LHRH$_a$ therapy with suppression of serum gonadotropins and plasma estradiol, cessation of menses and, after one year of therapy, regression of secondary sexual characteristics. This girl was the oldest patient studied and had a bone age (13 y) in the range when normal puberty occurs. Two of the five girls who did not respond to LHRH$_a$ were treated with the aromatase inhibitor, testolactone at a dose of 40 mg/kg/d for 8 weeks. Menses ceased in both girls and plasma estradiol available for one of the girls fell from 79 to less than 15 pg/ml. These data indicate that precocious puberty in most girls with MAS does not respond to LHRH$_a$ therapy. Testolactone shows promise for suppressing estrogen secretion and pubertal progression in these girls. A trial of LHRH$_a$ therapy may be warranted in the occasional girl with MAS who has pubertal serum gonadotropins.

617 HORMONAL AND CLINICAL EVALUATION OF CENTRAL NERVOUS SYSTEM (CNS) GERMINOMA IN CHILDHOOD. K. Fujieda*, N. Matsuura, H. Fujita, Department of Pediatrics, Hokkaido University School of Medicine, Sapporo, Japan.

Clinical manifestations and endocrine functions were evaluated in 27 patients with CNS germinoma in order to develop a diagnostic strategy. Patients were divided into three groups according to the tumor site: Group A consisted of 21 patients with tumors in sellar region; Group B had 4 patients with tumors in pineal region and 2 with tumors in both pineal and suprasellar region; Group C had 2 patients with tumors in basal ganglia and 1 with tumors both in basal ganglia and suprasellar region. Diabetes insipidus, or a presenting sign, was observed in all group A patients but in none of Groups B and C. Five of Group A also had adipsia. Elevation of plasma β-HCG and α-fetoprotein was present, respectively, in 3 (2 in Group A, 1 in Group C) and 2 (1 in Group B and 1 in Group C). Impaired GH secretion was observed in 18/18 of Group A and 3/4 of Group B. Abnormal TSH response to TRH along with delayed response was noted in 14/20 of Group A and low or no response in 5/20 of Group A, 1/4 in Group B and 1/2 of Group C. Impaired gonadotropin secretion was observed in 20/21 of Group A, 2/4 of Group B and 1/2 of Group C. Circadian rhythm in serum cortisol was impaired in all except 1 (1/10) of Group A, but in none of Groups B and C. These findings indicate that 1) Abnormality of endocrine function depends on the tumor site; 2) Germinoma in sellar region produce more severe pituitary dysfunction; 3) Tumor markers are often present; 4) Signs of precocious puberty due to HCG are observable in males with germinoma in both pineal and basal ganglia; 5) Hypothalamo-pituitary dysfunction is early and universal, and thus helpful in early diagnosis and follow up.

618 STUDY ON THE RELEASE AND SYNTHESIS OF HUMAN PITUITARY GONADOTROPINS BY UTILYSING "PRIMING EFFECT" OF LH-RH. Kazuki Fukuoka*, Tsunehisa Makino, Tsuneo Yokokura, Bao-Liang Lin, Hiroaki Suekane, Mamoru Takahashi and Rihachi Iizuka, Department of Obstetrics and Gynecology, School of Medicine, Keio University, Tokyo, Japan

To observe not only the function of releasing but also of the synthesizing of the anterior pituitary hormones, LH-RH two step test was introduced for this study. Blood samples were obtained from 20 women with ovarian dysfunction and other 20 women with regular menstrual cycle. One hundred micrograms of synthetic LH-RH was administrated intramuscularly twice at 60 minutes interval and serum gonadotropins were measured by radio-immunoassays. The evaluation of this new test was performed as follows; Δ_1=30(60) min. value - 0 min.value, Δ_2=90 (or 120,180) min. value - 60 min.value, $\Delta_1\Delta_2$ ratio=Δ_2/Δ_1. Δ_1 was the value of gonadotropin which was released by first LH-RH, while Δ_2 was presumed as the value including newly synthesized gonadotropin. Simultaneous alteration of these parameters was observed between the values of native gonadotropins and their subunits in normal women but no correlation was detected in Δ_1 and Δ_2 values of ovarian dysfunction. Thus LH-RH two step test suggests the possibility to differentiate pituitary function in both normal and abnormal subject. The results, we obtained, also suggest that double administration of LH-RH is a more useful method to observe the endocrinological function of the pituitary gland than by single administration of this hypothalamic peptide.

619 ABNORMAL ACTH RESPONSES TO CRF IN AFFECTIVE ILLNESS AND ANOREXIA NERVOSA

P.W. Gold*, G.P. Chrousos, P.C. Avgerinos, C. Kellner, A. Roy, R.M. Post, H. Schulte, W. Gallucci, H. Gwirtsman, and D.L. Loriaux. NIMH and NICHD, NIH Clinical Center, Bethesda, Maryland 20205, USA.

To explore the possible mechanism(s) of the sustained hypercortisolism seen in psychiatric patients with depression and anorexia nervosa, we administered synthetic ovine CRF (oCRF)(1 ug/kg at 2000h) to 15 healthy controls, 24 drug-free patients with affective disorder (10 depressed, 6 manic and 8 recovered) and 4 chronically underweight patients with anorexia nervosa. Bloods were drawn at -15, 0, +15, +30, +60, +90, +120, +150 and +180 min for IR-ACTH, cortisol, and IR-CRF determinations. The following responses were noted (mean ±1 SE; * $p<0.02$, patients vs controls)

Groups	Basal F	Peak F	Net F Area	Basal ACTH	Peak ACTH	Net ACTH Area
	ug/dl	ug/dl	ug/dl/h	pg/ml	pg/ml	pg/ml/h
Controls	1.6±0.3	15.6±3.5	1922±166	8.3±1.1	30.0±2.5	2138±278
Depressed	3.8±0.4*	13.8±2.1	1463±283*	7.4±1.4	20.2±3.1*	1101±218*
Manics	3.2±1.1	13.9±2.6	2182±351	7.5±1.3	23.2±3.6	1765±505
Recovered	1.7±0.2	15.3±3.0	2132±258	7.5±1.5	26.5±2.5	2482±360
Anorexics	13.6±3.4*	19.8±4.4	768±425*	8.0±0.6	17.7±5.0*	690±400*

Although the MCR for CRF was similar in the controls and all four patient categories, the net ACTH responses were significantly reduced in the depressed and anorexia nervosa groups, both of whom showed elevated basal cortisol levels. This suggests that the corticotroph cell in these patients responds normally to the negative feedback effects of cortisol. Thus, hypercortisolism in these disorders may reflect excessive secretion of CRF, a peptide which is known to play an important role both in the behavioral and physiological components of the stress response in laboratory animals.

620 FIRST CASE ON THE COEXISTENCE OF TWO SOLITARY PANCREATIC ISLET TUMORS: MALIGNANT GLUCAGONOMA AND BENIGN INSULINOMA.

Y.GORIYA*, M.KATSURA, K.BANDO, R.KAWAMORI, M.SHICHIRI and H.ABE, First Department of Medicine, Osaka University Medical School, Osaka, Japan

Two solitary pancreatic islet tumors, glucagonoma and insulinoma, were found in a 59 year-old female who had symptoms of fasting hypoglycemia and hepatomegaly without typical skin lesions or hypoaminoacidemia. Plasma insulin in frequent samplings and various stimulations did not show quite high concentrations or exaggerated responses, whereas plasma glucagon remained elevated from the fasting state around the level of 500 pg/ml and exaggerated after stimulations. A hypervascular tumor was found in the pancreatic tail and hypovascular tumors were also found in the liver and the right kidney by selective angiography. During the operation, a tumor, 17 mm in diameter, was found in the tail and another pancreatic tumor, 15 mm in diameter, which could not be detected preoperatively, was found in the body. In histological examinations, it was revealed that tumor of the tail contained many β-granules whereas tumors of the body and the metastasis contained many α-granules both by the specific staining with Aldehyde-Fuchsin and Grimelrius and by electronmicroscopy. Immunohistological examination using peroxidase-antiperoxidase method also confirmed above results. From these observations, it was concluded that benign symptomatic insulinoma and malignant asymptomatic glucagonoma with metastasis to liver, kidney, lung, thyroid, uterus and bones which had been confirmed by autopsy resided independently in a single pancreas.

621 RESPONSES TO ANALOGUES OF GROWTH HORMONE-RELEASING HORMONE (GHRH) IN NORMALS AND PATIENTS WITH GH DEFICIENCY (GHD). A. Grossman*, N. Lytras, M.O. Savage, M.A. Preece[+], D.H. Coy[o] and G.M. Besser, Department of Endocrinology, St. Bartholomew's Hospital, London, UK, [+]Institute of Child Health, London, UK, and [o] Department of Medicine, Tulane University, New Orleans, Lo,USA.

Growth hormone-releasing hormone-(1-40) and (1-44) have been shown to be potent stimulators of GH release in normal subjects, and in some patients with GH deficiency. We have compared GHRH-(1-40) with its shorter congener GHRH-(1-29)NH_2 in two groups of normal subjects in the dose range 10-200μg/subject. Analysis of variance revealed a significant effect of dose in the range 10-100μg for both compounds (n=5); 200μg produced no additional increase in GH secretion (n=7), and there was no significant difference between GHRH-(1-40) and GHRH-(1-29)NH_2 at any dose. Twenty patients aged 5-20y with GHD were given 200μg GHRH-(1-40) or (1-29)NH_2 as an iv bolus, and GH sampled for 120 min. Fourteen had idiopathic GHD, while 6 had hypothalamic tumours. Significant increases in serum GH (peak>10mU/l) were seen in 8 patients - 6 with idiopathic GHD, one germinoma and one histiocytosis X. Only one patient with idiopathic GHD who had not been previously treated with GH failed to respond. Neither a higher dose of GHRH (500μg), nor single GHRH infusions (20μg/hr for 4hr), further increased GH in the non-responders. Patients tested with both GHRH-(1-40) and (1-29)NH_2 showed similar peak responses. It is concluded that 1. GHRH-(1-29)NH_2 is a potent stimulus to GH release in normal subjects, peak release being seen at 50-100μg per subject; 2. Most children with untreated idiopathic GHD respond to GHRH acutely, suggesting a hypothalamic defect in endogenous GHRH.

622 THE MECHANISMS OF HIGH BLOOD PRESSURE OF PATIENTS WITH CUSHING'S SYNDROME M.Handa*,T.Saruta,H.Suzuki,Y.Igarashi and K.Kondo.Dept of Internal Med. Keio University Hospital and Jiichi Med. School, Tokyo,Japan.

The mechanisms of high blood pressure of patients with Cushing's syndrome were investigated by the measurments of humoral factors and pharmacological maneuver.Nine patients who were all verified by the surgery as having adenoma were used. Plasma renin activity(PRA),plasma renin concentration(PRC),plasma renin substrate(PRS),plasma cortisole(PC),plasma aldosterone(PA) and plasma catecholamines(PCS)and urinary kallikrein(UK) and urinary prostaglandin E2(PGE2) were measured and compared from the normal values. PRS,PRC and PC increased:(1327±41 vs 981±78 ng/ml,5.8±0.4 vs 7.2±0.4 u/ml and 189±17 vs 85±16 ng/ml).On the other hand, UK and PGE2 decreased: (276±60 vs 828±13 n mol/day and 15±1 vs 40±4 ng/day). PRA,PA and PCS did not show any significant differences. [1-Sar,8-Ile] angiotensin II(ANGIIA) (300ng/kg/min) were infused and captopril (37.5 mg/day) were given orally. Captopril reduced blood pressure(174±17/111±3 to 142±8/94±6 mmHg), however, ANGIIA rather increased(178±10/110±8 to 198±13/121±10). The smaller doses of angiotensin II(5.3±0.1 ng/kg/min) and norepinephrine(0.13±0.01 ug/kg/min) increased diastolic blood pressure(20 mmHg) compared to those of patients with essential hypertension(6.6±0.4 and 0.18±0.02, respectively). From our experiments, the possible mechanisms by which elevates blood pressure of patients with Cushing's syndrome are 1. partial involvement of the R-A-S,2.enhanced pressor responses to the vasoactive substances and 3. suppression of depressor systems.

623 A UNIQUE GLUCOCORTICOID RECEPTOR FOUND IN GILL AND GUT OF TELEOST FISH. J. A. DiBattista*, A. Z. Mehdi and T. Sandor, Hôpital Notre-Dame, Montréal, Canada, H2L 4K8.

It is widely recognized that corticosteroids modulate electrolyte exchange through teleost gill and gut epithelia. We describe here a high affinity-low capacity cytoplasmic glucocorticoid receptor (GR) system present in the eel and quite different from those of other vertebrates. Unlike the latter types, the fish receptor does not bind to DNA but translocates to homologous nuclei *in vitro*. The molecule shows no surface charge alterations following heat activation. Its sedimentation coefficient (s) is 6.7S, Stokes radius (Rs) is 6.8 nm and molecular weight (Mw) 240K Da. These are significantly lower than values suggested for other, molybdate-stabilized vertebrate GR (s~9S, Rs~8 nm, Mw~310K Da). The fish receptor shows extraordinary stereospecificity in that of the natural adrenal steroids, only cortisol binds with high affinity. Cortisone, corticosterone, aldosterone, deoxycorticosterone are without binding capacity. Preliminary studies indicate that hydroxylation at positions C-11, C-17 and C-21 are absolute requirements for binding. It is possible that the piscine GR is an ancestral form of the vertebrate GR and as such, its study can give insight into GR evolution. This study was supported by the MRC.

624 ABERRATION IN PREGNANCY DEVELOPMENT FOLLOWING INDUCTION OF ESTRUS BY PMSG DURING THE NONBREEDING SEASON OF THE CAMEL (*C. DROMEDARIUS*). E. Elias*, E. Bedrak[+] and D. Cohen, Isan Center for Comparative Medicine, Blaustein Institute and [+]Department of Biology, Ben-Gurion University of the Negev, Beer-Sheva 84105, Israel.

The camel, whose habitat is the harsh arid desert, is a seasonal breeder. Its breeding season is relatively short and accompanies the winter months followed by a long nonbreeding season (NBS). The objective of the present study was to elucidate whether the endocrine balance existing during the NBS could be altered to render fertile mating and successful pregnancy. Overcoming this problem is of great economic importance since the camel, because of its unique characteristics, could become the major source of animal protein for desert-dwelling man. Estrus was induced in multiparous camels during the NBS by an IM injection of PMSG (7000 IU). Pregnancy was confirmed by determination of serum levels of progesterone (P) along with rectal palpation. The results suggest that PMSG: 1) induces multiple estrus periods which last 2-3 days with 5-10 day intervals between two consecutive heat periods; 2) enhances the development of multiple (6-9) mature follicles. Ovulation did not occur in sterile mating. Fertile mating (as determined on day 50 following last service) is associated with an approximate 2 and 15-35 fold increase in serum levels of estradiol and P, respectively. However, probable resorption of fetus occurs around day 60 of pregnancy and is accompanied by a sharp decline in serum levels of P. It is concluded that: 1) mating is indispensable for ovulation and 2) resorption of fetus is probably associated with malfunctioning of the corpus luteum.

625 Prostaglandins level in blood and oviduct with special reference to the physiological activity of the reproductive tract in immature turkeys during development.
A. El-Badry*, F.B.S. Wehaish, W.S.Mohamed and S.F. El-Mougy. Department of physiology, Faculty of veterinary medicine, Zagazig University, Egypt.

This study was made to indicate the level of thromboxane B_2, PGF_{11}, $PGF_{2\alpha}$ and PGE in the blood and oviduct of immature turkeys. Blood samples were collected starting from 3 months of age until 5 months of age for hormonal determination in the plasma. Samples from different regions of the oviduct were also taken for measuring the level of hormones in the oviduct. The radioimmunoassay technique was used for hormonal determination. The level of thromboxane B_2, PGF_2, and PGE were increased in the plasma with the development of the birds as they reached their highest level in 5 months old birds. The concentrations of thromboxane B_2, PGF_2, and PGE in the oviduct were different from one part to other, whenever the highest level of the hormones were in the isthmus and uterus. The gradual increase in plasma and oviduct prostaglandins during the development of the reproductive tract give a further evidence that these substances are involved in the reproductive process.

626 GUANINE NUCLEOTIDES AND SODIUM IONS MODULATE THE SENSITIVITY OF ANTERIOR PITUITARY DOPAMINE RECEPTORS TO DOPAMINE AGONISTS AND ANTAGONISTS.
S.R. George*, M. Watanabe and P. Seeman, Depts.of Medicine and Pharmacology University of Toronto, Toronto, Ontario, Canada

Although we confirmed that the dopamine receptor of the porcine anterior pituitary (AP) has high-and low-affinity states for agonists, we have firm evidence that antagonists recognize these two states with equal affinity. The AP dopamine receptor is negatively coupled to adenylate cyclase and we have examined the effects of guanine nucleotides (GN) and sodium ions (Na^+) on this system. Interactions of the receptor with antagonists were affected by both Na^+ and GN: Na^+ increased the affinity of the receptor for the antagonist spiroperidol (2-3 fold) with an increase (10-30%) in the numbers of sites detected; GN did not affect antagonist affinity but greatly increased ($\geq$ 50%) the number of available sites. The effect of GN and Na^+ to increase the density of D_2 receptors was found to be due to endogenous agonist occupation of sites, as this phenomenon could be abolished with GN preincubation or extensive washing and could be exaggerated by addition of exogenous agonist. Agonist interactions with the receptor were also affected by Na^+ so that the proportion of receptors having high-affinity for dopamine was reduced while the proportion having low-affinity was increased concomitantly. Thus Na^+ facilitated a conversion of the agonist high-affinity form to the low-affinity form and decreased the affinity of both states of the receptor for agonist. GN effects were additive to that of Na^+ and resulted in a uniform population of sites with low-affinity for agonist. Thus, Na^+ and GN have important modulatory effects on the dopamine receptor of AP, as is expected of receptor systems inversely coupled to adenylate cyclase.

627 CHANGES OF HORMONE-SENSITIVE ADENYLATE CYCLASE IN UMR-106 CLONED RAT OSTEOSARCOMA CELLS MAINTAINED FOR LONG PERIODS IN CONTINUOUS CULTURE. G.E. Gutierrez*, G.R. Mundy and M.S. Katz, Department of Medicine, University of Texas Health Science Center and Audie Murphy VA Hospital, San Antonio, Texas 78284, USA.

We have examined the adenylate cyclase (AC) system in a cloned cell line (UMR-106) derived from a rat osteosarcoma and have compared hormone-sensitive AC activities in cells of early passages (<50) with those of cells maintained in continuous culture for > 2 years (late passages). -Fold stimulations (ratio of stimulated:unstimulated activities) of AC by parathyroid hormone (PTH;4x10^{-6}M), salmon calcitonin (CT;3x10^{-7}M), isoproterenol (ISO;10^{-4}M), and prostaglandin E_2 (PGE_2;10^{-5}M) during early and late passages were as follows:

	PTH	CT	ISO	PGE_2
Early passages	35.2±3.3 (SE)	1.1±0.0	11.5±1.6	14.0±1.7
Late passages	35.6±5.5	4.8±0.9	2.8±0.5	19.0±2.9
p values	N.S.	<.001	<.001	<.05

In both early and late passages, stimulation of AC by PTH, CT, and ISO was dependent on agonist concentration, with half-maximal stimulation at 4x10^{-7}M PTH, 10^{-10}M CT and 2x10^{-6}M ISO. Fluoride (5mM) stimulation of AC and enhancement of PTH- and PGE_2-stimulated AC activities by GTP (10^{-4}M) were similar during early and late passages, implying no change of the nucleotide regulatory and catalytic components of AC. These results suggest that UMR-106 cells cultured for long periods acquire CT receptors functionally linked to AC but lose functional beta-adrenergic receptors. To our knowledge, this is the first example of a cloned cell line in which spontaneous changes of hormone- and catecholamine-sensitive AC occur during long-term culture.

628 REGULATION OF THE ADENYLATE CYCLASE SYSTEM IN RAT OVARIAN MEMBRANES: ROLE OF REGULATORY GUANINE NUCLEOTIDE COMPONENTS. Lars Hedin* and Sten Rosberg, Dept of Physiology, University of Göteborg, Sweden.

The hormone-sensitive adenylate cyclase (AC) is in many tissues regulated by two distinct guanine nucleotide regulatory binding proteins. The stimulatory component (N_s) is not only involved in hormonal stimulation of AC but also in the stimulation by stable GTP analogues, fluoride and forskolin. The inhibitory component (N_i) has been demonstrated in simple cell systems (e g platelets and S49 lymphoma cells), where stable GTP-analogues can decrease basal and forskolin-stimulated AC activity (Seamon and Daly, J Biol Chem 257, 11591, 1982; Jakobs and Schultz, Proc Natl Acad Sci USA, 80, 3899, 1983). The present study was performed to study the eventual existence of a N_i component in an endocrine organ, the ovary.

Membranes from prepubertal rat ovaries were assayed for AC activity as earlier described (Hedin and Rosberg, Mol Cell Endocrinol 33, 69, 1983). AC activation by forskolin and fluoride was tested in the presence of different stable analogues of GTP.

Gpp(NH)p inhibited both forskolin and fluoride stimulated AC activity at low concentrations, while at higher concentrations a stimulatory effect was seen. Another analogue, Gpp(CH)p, gave a similar pattern. GTPγS, on the contrary, did not inhibit under any of the conditions tested.

These results implicate that the rat ovarian membranes posses a N_i component, analogously with other cells systems. Furthermore, it is evident that this N_i component is activated at much lower concentrations of the GTP analogues than the N_s component. The physiological implications of this N_i component in the ovary remains however to be elucidated.

629 AFFINITY-PURIFIED ECTOPIC FREE hCGβ-LIKE MATERIAL FROM HUMAN CERVICAL CARCINOMA CULTURE FLUID (CASKI CELL LINE) DOES NOT COMBINE WITH STANDARD hCGα. R. O. Hussa*, L. A. Cole, H. G. Fein, and R. A. Pattillo, Medical College of Wisconsin, Milwaukee, WI 53226, USA (ROH, RAP), Univ. Michigan Med. Sch., Ann Arbor, MI 48109, USA (LAC), and Walter Reed Army Institute of Research, Washington, D. C. 20307, USA (HGF).

This study was undertaken to determine whether CaSki hCGβ-like material, which apparently lacks the carboxy-terminal peptide (CTP), combines with standard hCGα, after the CaSki-β has been purified so as to avoid contamination with hCGβ dissociated from intact hCG. Confluent CaSki cultures, in 140 roller bottles (850 cm^2), were incubated in serum-free Waymouth's medium (no butyrate) for three 48-hr intervals. The pool of serum-free medium (38 liters) was clarified by centrifugation and concd. 100X by ultrafiltration. The ultrafiltrate contained 96 μg hCGβ immunoreactivity by core-directed H2 RIA, and 43 μg hCGβ by CTP-directed R525 RIA, giving (by difference) 53 μg of CTP-free hCGβ. The dialyzed, lyophilized concentrate was affinity purified; CaSki-β is the fraction not bound by either anti-hCGα·Sepharose or anti-[hCGβ]CTP·Sepharose but bound by anti-[hCGβ] core·Sepharose and eluted with 4M guanidine·HCl. After final desalting and lyophilization, CaSki-β (99% CTP-free) was tested for its ability to combine with standard hCGα (Endocrinology 101:225, 1977). Under conditions where >80% of standard hCGβ combined with standard hCGα, CaSki-β showed no combination, even after 58 hr of incubation with hCGα. CaSki-β co-migrated with standard hCGβ on gel filtration (Bio-Gel P100), verifying that CaSki-β had not been degraded during purification. Thus, the ectopic hCGβ-like immunoreactive material from CaSki cells does not combine with hCGα. This work was supported by NCI Grant No. CA23357, DHHS.

630 CONTROL OF OVULATION BY HORMONAL MEASUREMENTS IN NORMAL AND INDUCED OVULATORY CYCLES. Y. Chikhaoui* (1), N. Boucekkine (1), F. Chitour (1), P. Cristol (2), B. Descomps (2) and A. Crastes de Paulet (2).
1 - Service d'Endocrinologie HCI-ANP, Alger - Algérie. 2 - INSERM U.58, 60, Rue de Navacelles 34100 - Montpellier - France.

Urinary estrogens (Estrone-E1 and Estradiol-E2) content has been shown to be a good indicator of impending ovulation. The purpose of this work was the control of ovulation in normal women and in patients seeking remedy for infertility. The control of ovulation is very important mainly in artificial insemination and in vitro fertilization. Furthermore the gonadotrophins therapy must be regulated in view to avoid hyperstimulation. We used an accurate and specific routine enzymatic assay of estrogens. Follicle maturation (occured spontaneously or after HMG or clomiphene therapy) was followed up by daily evaluation of E1 + E2 and LH in urine and E2 and LH in plasma. In some patients, follicle development and ovulation were also controlled using ultrasound. The pattern of E1 + E2 variations in urine can be considered as a good index of estrogen secretion. 3 or 4 days before the LH peak, the mean value of urinary estrogens concentration was twice as much as that of follicular phase. The preovulatory peak of urinary E1 + E2 was observed 12 to 36 hours before the LH peak, giving a useful indication for an imminent ovulation. The knowledge and the follow up of the estrogens urinary levels allowed us to modulate the HMG dose and to decide of the HCG administration.

631 CIRCULATING IMMUNE-COMPLEXES (CIC) IN SEX HORMONE USERS PRESENTING WITH VASCULAR THROMBOSIS.

M. COIBION(1), J.L. NIZET(1), J.Cl. HENDRICK(2), Ch. HANSSEN(3), R. LAMBOTTE(1) and U.J. GASPARD(1*), Dept of OB/GYN, (2)RIA Lab, State University of Liege, 4020 Liège, Belgium, (3)Verviers Hospital, Belgium

Beaumont et al (Atherosclerosis 44:343,1982) have claimed to observe high serum levels of CIC, potentially containing antiethinylestradiol(EE) or other antisteroid antibodies(AB) in oral contraceptive and in sex steroid(SS) users, particularly in case of vascular thrombosis. We further investigated this possibility with the Beaumont precipitation technique and with an original specific method in 6 healthy control subjects not using SS and in 20 female SS ever-users presenting with vascular thrombosis. Serum samples were incubated with 3HEE, submitted to $(NH_4)_2SO_4$ precipitation and the precipitate was counted for radioactivity (RA) according to Beaumont. Additional aliquots of the same 3HEE incubated samples were precipitated by polyethyleneglycol(PEG), chromatographed on protein A-sepharose columns and the CIC-containing eluted fractions were submitted to spectrophotometry and RA counting. Elevated levels of CIC were observed in 1 male control and in 3 patients after spectrophotometry. However, no 3HEE RA was detected in the isolated CIC. By contrast, both $(NH_4)_2SO_4$ precipitation(Beaumont's technique) and also PEG precipitation yielded high levels of immunoglobulins+albumin with an elevated amount of 3HEE RA in the precipitate, in 8 samples originating either from healthy controls *not* using SS or from thrombotic women. In conclusion, CIC containing antiEE ABs cannot be detected with a specific assay technique in thrombotic SS ever-users. Our study also demonstrates the lack of specificity of Beaumont's method.

632 INVESTIGATION OF A 'DIRECT' RADIOIMMUNOASSAY (RIA) FOR MEASUREMENT OF 17-HYDROXYPROGESTERONE (17-OHP) IN NEONATAL BLOOD SPOT SAMPLES.

A.J. Currie, A.M. Ross and A.M. Wallace*. Endocrine Section, Department of Pathological Biochemistry, Royal Infirmary, Glasgow, U.K.

Large-scale screening for congenital adrenal hyperplasia (CAH) using 'Guthrie' card blood spot samples is hampered by expensive and time-consuming solvent extraction prior to RIA of 17-OHP. We have developed an alternative 'direct' (non-extraction) method which used a 6 mm blood spot sample, a ^{125}I tracer and an antibody encapsulated within semipermeable nylon microcapsules. Levels of 17-OHP obtained were 22 ± 19 nmol/l blood (n = 3567) and 29 ± 23 nmol/l (n = 158) for term and pre-term respectively. Between batch precision was 10% (at the upper cut-off of 50 nmol/l 17-OHP). Lower values were obtained if solvent extraction was performed prior to RIA (upper limit of normal 25 nmol/l). Blood spots (n = 233) with 17-OHP levels > 50 nmol/l ('direct' assay) were further evaluated by solvent extraction prior to RIA to exclude CAH. Neonates with confirmed CAH all had 17-OHP levels (extraction blood spot assay) of > 50 nmol/l (mean > 300 nmol/l, n = 7). The present data suggests that although the 'direct' assay lacks the specificity of measurement after solvent extraction, it is a valuable screening procedure for CAH which is currently used to screen all neonates in the West of Scotland.

633 DEXAMETHASONE SUPPRESSION OF GROWTH HORMONE (oGH) RESPONSE TO SYNTHETIC GROWTH HORMONE-RELEASING FACTOR (GRF-44-NH_2) IN THE OVINE FETUS AND LAMB.

L. Cuttler*, C.A. Egli, S.L. Kaplan, M.M. Grumbach, Department of Pediatrics, University of California San Francisco, San Francisco, CA USA

Glucocorticoids suppress the secretion of GH in response to provocative stimuli in vivo, but the site of action is not known. We previously showed that GRF is a specific secretagogue of GH in the ovine fetus and neonate, its effect decreasing with advancing gestational age (GA). We have now studied the effect of dexamethasone (DEX) on GRF-induced oGH secretion in 5 chronically-catheterized ovine fetuses (GA 104-139d) and 4 neonatal lambs (2-34d). Following a baseline period, each animal received DEX 0.2 mg/kg iv, half as a bolus and half over 3.5 h. Two hours after the DEX began, GRF 1 μg/kg was administered as an iv pulse. For controls, animals were studied with saline alone and GRF. The response to GRF was expressed as the incremental change (Δ) in both peak oGH (ng/ml) and integrated oGH area (ng·min/ml) over baseline values. In lambs, the ability of GRF to stimulate oGH release was dramatically reduced by pretreatment with DEX. Incremental peak oGH fell from 52.8 ± 9 (mean ± SE) in the saline controls to 3.2 ± 2 ng/ml following DEX ($p<.03$); Δ oGH area was sharply reduced from 16.6 ± 4.3 to 1.4 ± 0.8 ng·min/ml ($p<.04$). In contrast, in fetuses Δ peak oGH response to GRF was 177 ± 24 ng/ml with saline and 100 ± 44 ng/ml following DEX (N.S.); Δ oGH area (55 ± 25) was also not altered by DEX (42 ± 31 ng·min/ml) (N.S.). These results suggest: 1) In the neonatal lamb, acute exposure to DEX inhibits the ability of the pituitary somatotrope to release oGH in response to GRF. 2) The discrepancy in the suppressant effect of DEX on oGH release in the fetus and neonatal lamb may be a consequence of maturation of pituitary responsiveness.

634 DEVELOPMENT OF IMMUNOREACTIVE INSULIN IN THE FETAL BOVINE PANCREAS.

J.B. D'Agostino*, J.B. Field and M.L. Frazier. Diabetes Research Laboratory, St. Luke's Episcopal Hospital, Baylor College of Medicine, Houston, TX 77225 USA

Although maturation of the fetal endocrine pancreas has been studied in a number of species, the bovine pancreas has not been thoroughly characterized. The aim of this study was to characterize the development of immunoreactive insulin (IRI) in the fetal bovine pancreas. Pancreatic IRI was acid-extracted, and both pancreatic and serum IRI quantitated by radioimmunoassay. Standardization of IRI for wet tissue weight revealed that first trimester concentrations were similar to those seen in the adult (8.2 ± 0.7 and 5.9 ± 1.7 U/g pancreas, respectively). IRI increased progressively during gestation attaining 39.2 ± 6.5 U/g pancreas in the third trimester which was approximately seven-fold higher than that seen in the adult. Normalization of pancreatic IRI concentrations for acid-soluble protein resulted in a significant decrease in IRI between the mid-second (0.39 ± 0.03 U/mg protein) and third (0.22 ± 0.03 U/mg protein) trimesters, presumably due to dilution of the endocrine pancreas at this time by the rapidly growing exocrine pancreas. IRI was also detectable in fetal sera from all three trimesters. In contrast to the profile for pancreatic concentrations of IRI during fetal development, serum concentrations of IRI remained constant throughout gestation at approximately 20 μU/ml. We conclude: 1) that the endocrine pancreas is functional with respect to insulin biosynthesis during all three trimesters of development in the bovine fetus; and 2) that pancreatic, but not serum concentrations of IRI increase progressively as development proceeds.

635 THE EFFECTIVENESS OF FSH LEVEL DOSAGE IN AN AMBIGOUS CASE OF PRENATAL CHROMOSOME DIAGNOSIS

L. Dalprà, M. Castagni, G. Nocera, M.G. Tibiletti, G. Riboni, S. Agosti

III Clinica Ostetrica e Ginecologica, Università di Milano.

One of the problems which faces us in prenatal chromosome diagnosis is the presence of maternal cells in amniotic fluid cell cultures. According to the data reported in literature its frequency is less than 0.5%. We are going to describe one of our cases in which a discrepancy emerged between the prenatal diagnosis of the chromosomal sex and the phenotipic sex. A primigravida woman of 40 years requested prenatal diagnosis because of advanced age. The karyotype analysis performed on amniotic fluid at 17 weeks of gestation showed a 46,XX chromosome constitution. At 32 weeks the ultrasound examination revealed the external genitalia of a normal male. The FSH level dosage of this case was performed by means of RIA on amniotic fluid stored for other purposes. The FSH value (5 mU/ml) corresponded to the FSH level range found in a control group of amniotic fluid samples with a 46,XY karyotype. Looking back we can conclude that only maternal cells grew in this case. This means that no fetal cells were able to reproduce. At birth the chromosome analysis carried out on the peripheral blood cells showed a 46,XY Karyotype. We will discuss the effectiveness of the FSH dosage in prenatal chromosome diagnosis.

636 EFFECTS OF PHOTOPERIOD AND ORCHIECTOMY ON THE POSTNATAL INDUCTION OF PLASMA SEX STEROID-BINDING PROTEIN (SBP) IN THE MALE LITTLE BROWN BAT. D. A. DAMASSA* AND A. W. GUSTAFSON, Department of Anatomy and Cellular Biology, Tufts University Schools of Medicine, Boston, Massachusetts, 02111, USA.

The little brown bat (*Myotis lucifugus lucifugus*) possesses an SBP which, like that of primates, not only exhibits high affinity for both testosterone (T) and estradiol (E2) but also shows a striking postnatal rise in plasma concentrations. Similar increases can be induced experimentally when immature male bats are aroused during the latter half of hibernation and maintained at 25C under a long photoperiod. To examine the role of gonadal steroids in this induction, SBP was measured in castrated (C) and intact (I) males removed from hibernation; effects of photoperiod and timing of arousal (early vs. late hibernation) were also studied. Although E2 remained low in all groups and castration abolished the post-arousal rise in plasma T, plasma SBP levels increased in both intact and castrated bats. SBP was low in hibernating controls (10±2 nM, mean ± SE), but was markedly elevated in males aroused from hibernation either early (I: 158±51; C: 134±33) or late (I: 228±17; C: 256±43) when maintained on a long photoperiod (16L:8D) for three weeks. Likewise, castration had no effect on plasma SBP levels in bats maintained on a short photoperiod (8L:16D). However, the short photoperiod itself inhibited the SBP rise during early hibernation (I: 44±22; C: 58±20) but not during late hibernation (I: 271±5; C: 231±19). Thus, the post-arousal increase in SBP appears to be independent of gonadal secetions but, during the first half of hibernation, can be influenced by photoperiod. Supported by the NICHHD, Grant nos. HD16535 and HD00485.

637 THE EFFECTS OF STEROIDS AND GONADOTROPINS ON IN-VITRO PLACENTAL CONVERSION OF PREGNENOLONE (P_5) TO PROGESTERONE (P_4). N.P. Das, F.S. Khan-Dawood and M.Y. Dawood*, Department of Obstetrics and Gynecology, University of Illinois College of Medicine, Chicago, Illinois 60612, U.S.A.

To determine factors controlling placental conversion of P_5 to P_4, mitochondrial preparations of placental cotyledon removed at term elective cesarean section (n=38), were incubated with 0.05 μCi of ^3H-P_5 at 37^{0}C x 30 min. The reaction was terminated by extracting with diethyl ether: ethyl acetate (1:1, v/v) and using P_4, P_5 and ^{14}C-P_4 for recovery. The converted products were separated by thin layer chromatography, identified and radioactivity counted. Protein content in mitochondrial preparation was measured. P_5-P_4 conversions were 68.4, 75.1, 79.5, 83.1 and 94.7% for 5,10,15,30 and 60 min. of incubation respectively. Optimal conversion was reached when mitochondrial preparations had 2.5 - 3.0 mg protein/ml. Using mitochondrial preparations containing 2.5 -3.4 mg protein/ml and an incubation time of 30 min., 50-1000 ng of luteinizing hormone (LH) and 5-500 IU of human chorionic gonadotropin (hCG) did not affect P_5-P_4 conversion compared to controls. In contrast, estradiol (E_2), estriol (E_3), P_4 and testosterone (T) inhibited P_5-P_4 conversion. With E_2, 10,50 and 500 μg inhibited conversion to 50.1,25.3 and 14.6% respectively; with E_3, 50,500 and 2500 μg inhibited conversion to 71.2,43.9 and 20.6% respectively; with P_4, 20,50 and 500 μg inhibited conversion to 74.6,59.5 and 35.5% respectively; with T, 10,50 and 500 μg inhibited conversion to 70.2,37.8 and 13.2% of controls. Our findings indicate that placental Δ^5, 3β-hydroxysteroid dehydrogenase converting P_5-P_4 is suppressed by E_2,E_3,P_4 and T in a dose dependent manner but is unaffected by LH and hCG.

638 SEROTONIN CONTENT OF RABBIT LUNG AND SMALL INTESTINE DURING PERINATAL DEVELOPMENT. V. de Bock*, K. Yoshizaki and S. Solomon, Dept. of Medicine, Obstetrics & Gynecology & Biochem. McGill University and the Endocrine Laboratory, Royal Victoria Hospital, Montreal, P.Q., Canada. H3A 1A1.

Using immuno staining techniques it was previously found that serotonin (5HT) is present in endocrine-like cells in the rabbit fetal lung and small intestine from early pregnancy onward. Using reversed phase HPLC and electrochemical detection the 5HT content of fetal lung and fetal small intestine (18, 28 and 30 days gestation) and from the newborn was determined. In this study lung and intestine were extracted with $HClO_4$ and the extract loaded onto a Bio-Rex 70 column. After elution with HCOOH the samples were injected onto the HPLC column. 5HT was detected in lung and intestine at 18 days gestation. In lung the 5HT content increased steadily from days 18 to days 28 and 30, decreased at birth and then rose again to day 10 after birth. In the intestine the 5HT content also increased till term but fell on the first day postpartum and stayed the same until day 10 of life. These results are shown below as 5HT-ng/mg protein.

Age (days)	18	28	30	(Newborn) 1	(Newborn) 10
Lungs mean(SE)	80 (-)	380 (40)	800 (130)	190 (60)	640 (90)
Intestines mean(SE)	90 (-)	2080 (390)	3820 (290)	3040 (320)	2900 (240)

It can be concluded that 5HT in the lung and intestine is found early in pregnancy and that the content in small intestine is always much higher than in lung. After birth the intestine 5HT concentrations stay the same, but the lung 5HT concentrations increase up to 10 days after birth.

639 NEONATAL GONADAL STEROID TREATMENT AND GROWTH IN THE FEMALE RAT. L. R. DePalatis* and R. A. Madison, Central Research Bioproducts Laboratory, Dow Chemical Company, Midland, MI 48640

Testosterone proprionate (TP) treatment of female rats during the neonatal period is known to effect a sex reversal of various reproductively related parameters. Administration of TP, an aromatizable androgen, during the neonatal period has also been shown to cause a significant stimulation of growth in female rats. In this study, a single injection of 200 µg estradiol benzoate (EB) or 1000 µg TP on day 4 resulted in a significant stimulation of body weight in female rats through adulthood. On the other hand, a single injection of 500 µg of the non-aromatizable androgen, 5α-dihydrotestosterone proprionate (DHTP) was ineffective in altering body weight during the course of the study. The final body weights (80 days of age) of the 4 groups were: control=201.6$\pm$4.6g, DHTP=203.7$\pm$5.8g, EB=243.8$\pm$3.2g, TP=233.6$\pm$3.5g. The velocity of growth was similarly affected by the respective steroid treatments. The levels of various metabolic hormones were determined after termination of the experiment but no definite correlations with body weights could be made. We conclude that neonatally administered TP and EB but not DHTP can result in the stimulation of growth in the female rat. It is therefore hypothesized that the conversion of aromatizable androgens to estrogens during a critical neonatal period is responsible for the growth enhancement in this rat model.

640 **SYNTHESIS OF PUTATIVE OESTRADIOL RECEPTOR OR PRECURSOR *IN VITRO*, DIRECTED BY mRNA ISOLATED FROM NEONATAL RAT BRAIN.** E.B.R. de Silva, I. Adcock* and B.D. Greenstein, Department of Pharmacology, St. Thomas's Hospital Medical School, London SE1 7EH, UK. Liu Shi Fan, Shanghai Institute of Planned Parenthood Research, No. 4, 2200 Lane, Xie Tu Road, Shanghai, China.

As part of a study dedicated to the elucidation of oestrogen-mediated sexual differentiation of the rat brain, we have already reported that polyadenylated RNA (mRNA) appears to direct the synthesis of [^{3}H]oestradiol-binding activity in a rabbit reticulocyte lysate system *in vitro* (de Silva, Shi Fan and Greenstein, 1983). The [^{3}H]oestradiol-binding activity may represent oestrogen receptor since the binding could be suppressed by addition of excess unlabelled diethylstilboestrol (DES) to the incubation. In further studies we have found that whereas the oestrogen receptor is soluble in the cytosol, the DES-suppressible [^{3}H]oestradiol-binding activity in the lysate appears to be associated with particulate matter. Therefore the binding activity may represent a receptor precursor which is later released into the cytosol, or it is possible that the mature oestrogen receptor is particle-bound and solubility in cytosol is an artifact of homogenisation.

This work was supported by St. Thomas' Hospital Research Endowments Fund.

de Silva, E.B.R., Shi Fan, L. and Greenstein, B.D. (1983). J.Physiol., **343**, 38P.

641 ESTROGEN, PROGESTERONE, & GLUCOCORTICOID - BINDING PROTEIN(BP) INTERACTIONS IN MID TRIMESTER AMNIOTIC FLUID(AF).

M.I. Evans*, G.P. Chrousos, D. Rodbard, J.W. Larsen Jr., R.C. Staton, J.D. Schulman, and B.C. Nisula. Med Genetics CC, DEB LTPB, NICHD NIH Bethesda, Md. & OB GYN George Washington U., Wash. D.C.

The purpose of this study was to examine the interactions of steroids and their BP's - both specific with high affinity [testosterone-estradiol binding globulin (TEBG) and cortisol binding globulin (CBG)] and albumin (A) with low affinity in midtrimester AF. We studied these interactions in 419 amniocentesis specimens obtained at 17-18 weeks gestation and applied our model (JCEM 53:58,1981) to calculate bound(B) and unbound(UB) fractions. E1,E2,E3,Prog,17OHProg,S,and F were measured by RIA, TEBG and CBG by Concanavalin A Sepharose precipitation with Scatchard plot analysis, and A by automated immunoprecipitate analysis. The data were grouped by fetal sex (cytogenetic analysis). Means are shown in in pg/ml.

LIGAND	N	Tot Conc.	TEBG(B)	CBG(B)	A(B)	UB Conc	%UB
E2(m)	53	53.67	29.57	.0121	18.55	7.538	14.1
E2(f)	52	54.40	27.40	.0127	19.49	7.495	13.8
Prog(m)	50	43,300	493.9	6693	25,680	10,430	24.1
Prog(f)	54	46,700	510.6	7338	28,060	10,790	23.1
F(m)	49	31,500	85.70	20,230	1225	9959	31.6
F(f)	54	31,000	81.02	20,280	1224	9418	30.4

No sex differences were found in all parameters measured. Compared to plasma, AF steroid concentrations are lower, but the %UB of E1,E2, E3,Prog, 17OHProg, S, and F are markedly increased. We conclude that developmental differences between male and female fetuses are not manifested in steroid levels or their distribution among various BP in AF.

642 HYPOTHYROID-INDUCED ALTERATIONS IN GASTRIN RELEASE IN RATS.

G. H Greeley, Jr.*, T. Dinh, A. Spannagel, J.C Thompson. Dept. of Surgery, The University of Texas Medical Branch, Galveston, Tx, 77550

The objectives of this study were to examine the influence of hypothyroidism on gastrin (G) secretion, antral G replenishment, and relative concentrations of different molecular forms of antral G. Table I shows serum G levels (pg/ml) before and after I.V. bombesin (BBS) in fed, 4-wk thyroidectomized (thyrx) rats. On a separate day, serum was obtained before and after food ingestion from 24 hr fasted thyrx rats. Results. (*= p<.05 vs controls)

Serum G	N	Basal	10 min. After BBS	Gastrin Increment
Controls	6	198±17	392±26	193±13
Thyrx	6	70±12*	129±32*	62±21*
Serum G	N	Basal	15 min after Food	60 min after Food
Controls	6	59±6	170±9	157±15
Thyrx	6	44±3*	128±16*	79±13*

The time course of antral G replenishment in thyrx rats was identical to controls. Antral G levels in fasted thyrx and controls were 2.7±3 and 2.5±4μg/g tissue, respectively. Continuous access to food for 120 hr resulted in replenishment of antral G stores in thyrx (6.23±1.1) and controls (5.6±6 μg/g). Chromatography of antral G revealed: (control) 97.3±3.0% G-17 and 2.0±4.0% G-34; (thyrx) 89.6±7.0% G-17 and 10.4±7.0% G-34. Conclusions. Hypothyroidism caused: 1) decreases in basal G release after BBS and food; 2) a decrease in the concentration of G-34 and an increase in the concentration of G-17 in the antral mucosa, and 3) no change in antral replenishment of G after food.

643 BOMBESIN LIKE IMMUNOREACTIVITY IN MAMMALIAN FOLLICULAR FLUID.

J.Hansky* and C.Soveny. Department of Medicine, Monash University, Prince Henry's Hospital, Melbourne, Australia.

Bombesin a tetradecapeptide, first isolated from the skin of the European frog, B.Bombina, has been found to be widely distributed in the mammalian nervous, respiratory and digestive systems. We have developed a sensitive, specific radioimmunoassay for measurement of bombesin like immunoreactivity BLI (1) and have explored the distribution of BLI in various mammalian tissues including ovary and testis. Follicular fluid was harvested from the ovaries of sheep and human, and BLI measured in unextracted fluid by radioimmunoassay. Samples of follicular fluid were further concentrated and subjected to chromatography on 1X100 cm Sephadex G50 columns to determine molecular size of the BLI. Human follicular fluid contained 427 $fmol.ml^{-1}$ of BLI and eluted predominantly at the region of Gastrin releasing peptide (27 amino acids) with a small amount as tetradecapeptide. Sheep follicular fluid contained 6.7 $pmol\ ml^{-1}$ and also eluted in the same position as human fluid BLI. The finding of significant amounts of BLI in ovarian follicular fluid suggests a role for this peptide in aspects of ovarian function, perhaps as a peptidergic neurotransmitter. Further studies to determine changes in BLI concentrations during the menstrual cycle together with studies during pregnancy, lactation, parturition or menopause are required to elucidate the possible role of this peptide in ovarian physiology.

(1) Soveny, C. and Hansky, J. Regulatory Peptides 3:325, 1982.

644 STRUCTURE OF A GENE ENCODING A PRECURSOR OF HUMAN VASOACTIVE INTESTINAL PEPTIDE (VIP).

S.J. Horovitch, J.F. Habener and R.H. Goodman, Division of Endocrinology, Tufts-New England Medical Center and Lab Molec. Biol., Mass. General Hospital, Boston, MA

To determine the structure of the gene encoding VIP, we have isolated two recombinant bacteriophages from a human genomic library by hybridization with a cDNA derived from an islet cell tumor. The cDNA library was screened with synthetic oligonucleotides encoding the amino acids Lys-Gln-Met-Ala, and a recombinant plasmid encoding VIP was isolated and sequenced. This plasmid contained the entire pre-pro VIP coding sequence as well as portions of the 3' and 5' untranslated regions. The sequence of the islet cell tumor pre-pro VIP is identical to that found by Itoh, et al in a human neuroblastoma. Northern blot analyses detected a single pre-pro VIP mRNA of 1900 nucleotides which, therefore, consists mostly of untranslated sequences. The 5' untranslated region of islet cDNA is 484 bases long, considerably longer than that of most eukaryotic mRNAs. To characterize the 5' end of the cDNA, we analyzed this region by Northern blot hybridizations and S-I nuclease mapping. The predominant VIP mRNA was found to extend only 60 bases upstream from the initiater AUG codon. Southern blot hybridizations indicated that the sequence further upstream in the cDNA is represented in multiple copies in the human genome, and raises the possibility that our cDNA may represent an mRNA precursor. To establish whether this repetitive sequence is represented in the VIP gene, we have screened a human genomic library and have isolated two hybridizing bacteriophage clones. The degree of hybridization of the cDNA to these clones suggests that one may represent the VIP gene and the other may encode another member of the VIP multigene family.

645 BONE MINERAL CONTENT OF THE CENTRAL SKELETON IN PATIENTS WITH TURNER'S SYNDROME. S. Fleming*, J. Harrison and C. Cowell, Depts Ob and Gyn and Medicine, Toronto General Hospital, Toronto, M5G 1L7, Canada.

Turner's Syndrome (TS) has been associated with a reduced phalangeal cortical width and reduced forearm and os calcis bone mineral content as measured by photon absorptiometry. This apparent demineralization has been termed osteoporosis although it has not been associated with an increased fracture rate. In order to test the relationship between osteoporosis and TS, 42 patients with TS aged 17 - 38 (24.9 ± 6.5), 32 normal control individuals aged 16 - 35 (25.7 ± 5.3) and 36 osteoporotic females aged 55 - 78 (66 ± 6) were studied. All patients with TS had had a spontaneous menarche (N=4) or at one time received estrogen replacement therapy (N=38). The total bone mineral content of the central third of the skeleton (the area most susceptible to osteoporotic fracture) was measured in all individuals using in vivo neutron activation analysis and expressed as the Calcium Bone Index (CaBI) which normalizes for body size (Harrison et al, Investigative Rad; 14:27-34, 1979). The CaBI of the patients with TS (1.004 ± 0.162) was not significantly different from that of the control females (0.96 ± 0.13) and was significantly greater ($p<0.001$) than that of the oesteoporotic females (0.69 ± 0.09). In the patients with TS there was no significant correlation between CaBI and age, years since age 13 of estrogen deprivation or karyotype. The data does not support an association between osteoporosis of the central skeleton and TS. It is proposed that the demineralization previously reported in the appendicular skeleton of patients with TS is apparent rather than real due to the failure to normalize the data for skeletal size.

646 GONADOTROPIC HORMONE CORRELATES OF HIBERNATION IN THE TURKISH HAMSTER, *MESOCRICETUS BRANDTI* J.M. Darrow*, L. Yogev, B.D. Goldman, Worcester Foundation for Experimental Biology, Shrewsbury, MA 01545, USA.

Previous studies demonstrated that the 4-6 month hibernation season of Turkish hamsters can be interrupted by the administration of exogenous gonadal steroids, particularly testosterone. We now examined circulating follicle-stimulating-hormone (FSH) and prolactin (PRL) in intact males serially sampled at 3-week intervals throughout hibernation (at 6°C, LD10:14). As in room temperature controls, mean serum FSH levels of the hibernating group declined to baseline (<100ng/ml) by 2 weeks of short-day exposure, remained low for 20 weeks, then rose to levels >200ng/ml by 24 weeks, when gonadal regrowth became evident. Individuals showed high FSH values as early as 10 weeks before the end of hibernation and in most cases, prior to measurable increases in testis size. These elevated values were evident only in hibernators sampled during bouts of spontaneous arousal from torpor, not during bouts of torpor. In contrast, PRL levels remained low (<5 ng/ml) throughout hibernation (whether hamsters were sampled during arousal or torpor), then underwent an abrupt, 10-fold increase within 3 weeks after the end of hibernation. These data suggest that increased levels of FSH occurring during bouts of arousal may be involved in the gonadal stimulation which precedes emergence from hibernation. This may represent a mechanism which helps to ensure that hibernation will terminate in approximate synchrony with the achievement of reproductive competence.
This study was supported by Grant No. HD 15912.

647 ARREST OF THE HYPOTHALAMIC GnRH PULSE GENERATOR DURING PROTEIN/CALORIE (P/C) DEPRIVATION IN CASTRATED MALE RHESUS MONKEYS.

A.K. Dubey*, J.L. Cameron, R.A. Steiner and T.M. Plant. Depts of Physiology, Univ Pittsburgh Sch Med, PA 15261, and Univ Washington, Seattle, WA 98195 USA.

In many species, P/C malnutrition is often associated with reproductive dysfunction, and it has been postulated that certain metabolic substrates or hormones may therefore play a crucial role in the maintenance of gonadal activity. To determine the locus of action of P/C deprivation on the H-P-G axis and to pin-point its metabolic sequelae, 10 orchidectomized rh monkeys (3 1/2-5 yr) were maintained on low P/C (164 Kcal/day) for 20-30 days and the effects of this nutritional insult on gonadotropin (GTH) secretion and metabolism were monitored. In approximately 50% of the monkeys, P/C deprivation resulted in dramatic declines in plasma GTH from open-loop control concentrations (LH-150 ng/ml; FSH-100 ng/ml) before P/C deprivation to undetectable levels (LH $<$ 11 ng/ml; FSH $<$ 3 ng/ml) 6-19 days later. In the remaining monkeys GTH secretion was only marginally suppressed. In both groups, the mean changes in plasma insulin (75% ↓), glucose (30% ↓), cortisol (200% ↑) and in BW (20% ↓) during P/C deprivation appeared similar and, to date, we have failed to identify a metabolic concomitant of low P/C induced inhibition of GTH secretion. In the animals in which GTH secretion was abolished by P/C deprivation it was possible to fully restore plasma LH & FSH to control levels by 'physiologic' GnRH replacement (chronic intermittent iv infusion at 0.1 μg GnRH/min for 3 min every h). These results in castrates graphically demonstrate that nutritional insults on GTH secretion can be mediated exclusively at the hypothalamic level via interruption of GnRH secretion. Supported by NIH grants HD16851, HD12625 and HD08610.

648 THE EFFECT OF ETHANOL FEEDING ON THE MICROHETEROGENEITY OF PITUITARY LUTEINIZING HORMONE.

M. A. Emanuele*, S. Hojvat, N. Emanuele, E. Bermes, L. Kirsteins and A. M. Lawrence, Depts. of Med., Clin. Chem. and Biochem., Loyola Univ. Med. Ctr., Maywood, IL 60153, USA; and Research and Med. Services, Hines VA Hospital, Hines, IL 60141, USA.

In order to study the impact of ethanol feeding on pituitary luteinizing hormone (LH) levels, hormone microheterogeneity, and LH release, 30 female oophorectomized rats were fed either a diet containing 36% ethanol or an isocaloric diet without ethanol for 15 days. All rats were given 50 μg of estradiol SQ to provide a uniform steroid milieu, and to induce an LH surge, and were sacrificed 48 h later. Total levels of pituitary and serum immunoreactive LH (iLH) were identical between ethanol and control groups, as were Sephadex gel chromatographic profiles. When pituitary LH was analyzed by isoelectric focusing on Agarose gel, 6 distinct immunoreactive peaks were observed at pI's 3.5-4.0, 5.0-5.4, 6.2-6.5, 7.4-7.5, 8.0-8.2, and 8.5-8.9. Ethanol-treated animals exhibited an 8-fold increase in acidic LH species pI (3.5-4.0) and, similarly, more iLH was determined at pI (7.4-7.5) compared to controls ($p < 0.01$). However, at pI's (8.0-8.2) and (8.5-8.9), more basic points in the gel, an increased iLH level was observed in controls over alcoholics ($p < 0.01$). Conclusion: Short-term ethanol feeding in the female rodent does not cause quantitative differences in pituitary iLH levels or steroid-induced LH release. However, qualitative changes are present on isoelectric focusing with a shift to the less mature species of pituitary LH isohormone noted in the ethanol fed animal compared to controls.

649 OVARIAN STEROID REGULATION OF PULSATILE LH RELEASE DURING THE INTERVAL BETWEEN THE MORNINGS OF DIESTRUS 2 (D2) AND PROESTRUS IN THE RAT.
R.V. Gallo*, R.E. Leipheimer, and A. Bona Gallo, Physiology Section, Biological Sciences Group, and Department of Biobehavioral Sciences, University of Connecticut, Storrs, CT. USA

The influence of ovarian steroids on pulsatile LH release in the D2-proestrous interval was examined. Four groups of rats were bled continuously for 3h between 09:30-12:30h at a rate of 75 µl whole blood/6 min: 1) D2; 2) Sham ovariectomy (OVX) on D2 and bled on proestrus; 3) OVX on D2, implanted with empty or oil-filled capsules, and bled 24h later; and 4) OVX on D2, implanted with estradiol (E_2) capsules, and bled 24h later. Between D2 and proestrus there was no change in mean blood LH levels, LH pulse amplitude, or pulse frequency. During this interval plasma E_2 levels increased from 13 ± 1 to 42 ± 9 pg/ml, and progesterone levels decreased from 27 ± 3 to 13 ± 2 ng/ml, reflecting the decline of the corpus luteum on D2. OVX on D2 increased mean blood LH levels 2.5-fold vs values on proestrus due to a 3.5-fold elevation in LH pulse amplitude and an 80% increase in pulse frequency. E_2 levels fell in these rats to 8 ± 1 pg/ml. Restoration of physiological proestrous levels of E_2 (57 ± 3 pg/ml) significantly reduced the increase in mean blood LH levels by lowering pulse frequency to proestrous values, and by causing a 50% reduction in pulse amplitude. However LH pulse amplitude and therefore mean blood LH levels were still higher than values on proestrus. Thus far these data demonstrate that ovarian E_2 exerts a restraining effect on both LH pulse amplitude and frequency between the mornings of D2 and proestrus.
Supported by NIH HD17728.

650 THE EFFECT OF CHRONIC ANDROGEN TREATMENT ON GONADOTROPHIN RESPONSES IN INTACT FEMALE TRANSSEXUALS.
H.H. Goh*, S.S. Ratnam, Department of Obstetrics and Gynaecology, National University of Singapore, Kandang Kerbau Hospital for Women, Singapore.

In an earlier study we have shown that longterm oestrogen treatment to males can feminise their gonadotrophin responses. As a sequel to this study we were interested to know what effect longterm androgen therapy to females might have on the gonadotrophin responses. We have therefore studied female transsexuals before and after chronic androgen therapy given for at least six months to masculinise their body habitus before undergoing surgical "change of sex."

Subjects were assessed for the gonadotrophin responses to gonadotrophin releasing hormone at different time periods of the menstrual cycle: 3-5, 7-8, 12-14, and 20-24 days. After six months of androgen treatment, subjects were assessed for the acute effects of oestradiol valerate on sex steroid hormone levels and gonadotrophin responses to gonadotrophin releasing hormone. The results showed that gonadotrophin responses vary at different time periods of the menstrual cycle. After six months of androgen treatment, an acute dose of oestradiol was shown to increase baseline levels of LH and amplify the effect of GnRH on gonadotrophin release. This pattern is similar to those found in the late follicular and luteal phases and suggests that androgen treatment for six months did not change the gonadotrophin responses in female transsexuals.

651 RAPID REGULATION OF mRNAs ENCODING THE SUBUNITS OF RAT LUTEINIZING HORMONE (LH) BY GONADAL STEROIDS.

S.D. Gharib*, W.W. Chin, S.M. Bowers, and J.F. Habener. Laboratory of Molecular Endocrinology, Massachusetts General Hospital and Howard Hughes Medical Institute Laboratories, Harvard Medical School, Boston, MA.

We are studying the regulation of luteinizing hormone (LH) mRNA biosynthesis by gonadal steroids. The α and β subunits of LH are encoded by separate genes. In order to measure subunit mRNA levels in the pituitary gland, we have recently isolated and characterized cloned cDNAs representing the precursors of the α and LH β subunits. Ovariectomized or orchiectomized rats (Sprague-Dawley, 200-225g) were replaced three weeks postoperatively with a single subcutaneous dose of estradiol benzoate (2μg/100g bw) or testoterone propionate (100μg/100g bw) in sesame oil, respectively. Animals were sacrificed at 0hr and 24hr. Levels of LH were determined in serum by RIA and levels of subunit mRNAs were determined by blot hybridization analyses of total RNA in the pituitary gland using cloned subunit specific cDNAs. In ovariectomized rats, serum LH fell to 20% of 0hr values and the levels of subunit mRNAs fell to 30-35%. In orchiectomized rats, the serum LH fell to 25% of 0hr values and the levels of subunit mRNAs fell to 50-65%. We conclude that replacement doses of gonadal steroid hormones produce rapid declines in the levels of the subunit mRNAs that parallel the decreases in the serum LH. Thus, the effect of the gonadal steroids on the regulation of subunit mRNAs occurs, at least in part, at the levels of transcription and/or RNA stability.

652 BETA-HCG IN BREAST CYST FLUID.

R.B. Greenblatt* and V.B. Mahesh, Department of Endocrinology, Medical College of Georgia, Augusta, GA 30912.

The breast is thought to be primarily as a target organ but the possibility that glandular epithelium could produce certain hormones bears consideration. Almost half of the 50 cyst fluid samples obtained from 24 women had β-hCG values greater than 5 miu/ml. Of the other polypeptides studied (FSH, LH, PRL, TSH), only TSH was consistent though slightly elevated. In one patient with a recurrent gross cyst, high β-hCG values were obtained on 5 samplings ranging from 82 to 194 miu/ml. Biologic activity of the cyst fluid was determined by injecting immature female rats. A positive ovarian hyperemia test suggested that the fluid had hCG-like properties. β-hCG obtained from human breast cyst fluid was also identified by parallelism with authentic hCG in the radioimmunoassay. Other investigators (Srivatava et al., Braunstein et al.) found hCG present in breast cyst fluid but did not attempt to prove biologic activity. Since serum β-hCG was < 5 miu/ml in every instance, it would appear that high concentrations of β-hCG in cyst fluid represents the production of this hormone de novo and may indicate that the cells lining the cysts have lost their capacity to repress the production of this polypeptide inherent in all cells.

653 QUANTITATION OF FSH BETA SUBUNIT IN RAT ANTERIOR PITUITARY CELL CULTURES.
H.E. Grotjan, Jr.*, B.A. Keel and A.S. Berkowitz, Dept. Physiol. & Pharm., U.South Dakota School of Medicine, Vermillion, SD 57069 and U.Texas Medical School, Houston, TX 77225, U.S.A.

We have recently demonstrated that rat anterior pituitary cell cultures contain and release uncombined rLHβ at a rLHβ/rLH molar ratio of ∿ 0.04. This series of experiments was performed to quantitate intracellular and secreted FSHβ. Rat anterior pituitary cells were established in culture for 4 days. The medium was changed and cells were incubated for an additional 6 or 24h. Some 6h cultures were stimulated with 10^{-7} M GnRH. FSHβ in cell extracts and medium was quantitated with a heterologous radioimmunoassay (RIA) employing anti-rFSHβ and hFSHβ-#2 as the standard and hormone for idoination. rFSH was quantitated with a homologous RIA. FSHβ was non-detectable (< 0.018 ng/100,000 cells) in the medium from unstimulated or GnRH-stimulated cultures. This translated to a FSHβ/rFSH molar ratio of < 0.01. Cell extracts, for the most part, contained detectable quantities of FSHβ which translated to FSHβ/rFSH molar ratios of 0.05, 0.04, 0.35 and 0.21, respectively, in 4 day (time = 0), 6h basal, 6h GnRH-stimulated and 24h basal cultures. These results suggest that rat anterior pituitary cells contain detectable FSHβ but that minimal quantities of FSHβ are released. Furthermore, GnRH appears to increase intracellular FSHβ but does not appear to induce the release of uncombined FSHβ. Supported by NIH HD12006 and HD18879 as well as Robert A. Welch Foundation AU-931.

654 STUDIES ON THE IDENTITY OF A ∼40 K SOMATOMEDIN BINDING PROTEIN IN AMNIOTIC FLUID AND SERUM.
S. Drop*, D. Kortleve, J. D'Ercole, Dept. of Pediatrics, Erasmus University Rotterdam, The Netherlands, and University of North Carolina, Chapel Hill, U.S.A..

A specific double antibody radioimmunoassay (RIA) was developed for a ∼40 K somatomedin binding protein (SMBP), purified from midgestational human amniotic fluid (AF) and termed amniotic fluid binding protein (AFBP). ^{125}I-Sm-C (300,000 cpm) and AF as well as cord serum and serum of an acromegalic and pregnant patient were cross-linked in the presence of 0.5 mM disuccinimidylsuberate (DSS). Aliquots were reacted with rabbit anti-AFBP antibody and anti-rabbit 2nd antibody. The precipitates were solubilized, boiled and loaded on an SDS polyacrylamide gel. Autoradiography of the gels showed a ∼40 K band, most densely in AF, followed by cord, pregnancy and acromegalic plasma. Preterm AF (± 25 µg prot.) was subjected to the cross-linking procedure in the presence of unlabeled SM-C. Up to 250 ng SM-C was required to obtain full displacement. Cord serum was chromatographed on Sephadex G-200 at neutral pH. ∼150 K protein fractions were pooled and concentrated. Acidification did not increase AFBP concentration of this pool. Rechromatography of the 150 K pool at pH 2 did not result in an increment of ∼40 K AFBP-RIA activity.

Since AFBP antibody recognizes one species of SMBP in human AF and postnatal serum, we conclude that ∼40 K SMBP in AF and serum may well be identical. AFBP cannot be generated from ∼150 K SMBP by simple acidification. The elucidation of a relation between ∼150 K and ∼40 K SMBP in serum requires further study.

655 CHARACTERIZATION OF RECEPTORS FOR INSULINLIKE GROWTH FACTOR (IGF)-I IN HUMAN PITUITARY GLAND. N. Emoto*, T. Tsushima, K. Wakai, H. Murakami and K. Shizume. Department of Internal Medicine, Tokyo Women's Medical College and the Institute for Growth Science, Tokyo 162, Japan

Recently, it has been reported that IGF-I inhibits GH secretion by acting on hypothalamus or by interacting with pituitary somatotrophes, suggesting the presence of IGF-I receptors on pituitary gland. Human pituitary glands were obtained at autopsy and homogenated in 0.3 M sucrose. The homogenate were sequentially centrifuged, and the 100,000 x g pellet was used as receptor preparation because of the highest binding activity in the fraction. IGF-I was purified from Cohn fraction IV of human plasma. The binding of ^{125}I-IGF-I was time- and temperature-dependent and reached maximum within 3 h at 20°C. Specific binding was approximately 7 % per 100 μg protein of membranes. Binding was dose-dependently inhibited by unlabeled IGF-I,with half maximal displacement occurring at 10 ng/ml. MSA-II also inhibited IGF-I binding, but potency was only 1/50 compared with IGF-I. Porcine insulin and proinsulin displaced ^{125}I-IGF-I only at the high concentrations more than 1 μg/ml. SRIF and hpGRF were without effect. Scatchard plot of the binding data was curvilinear and Kd vaue was 1.5 nM for the high affinity binding sites. One anti-insulin receptor autoantibody blocked binding of ^{125}I-IGF-I partially. Treatment with trypsin, heating or dithiothreitol significantly reduced the binding activity of receptors. Receptor activity solubilized with Triton X-100 eluted as a macromolecule (300K) on a column of Sepharose 6B. SDS-PAGE of ^{125}I-IGF-I crosslinked pituitary membranes revealed a 130 K subunit. Thus, characteristics of pituitary IGF-I receptors were similar to those reported for human placenta.

656 ISOLATION AND CHARACTERISATION OF SOMATOMEDIN A FROM HUMAN PLASMA G. Enberg*, M. Carlqvist, H. Jörnvall and K. Hall. Department of Endocrinology and Departments of Biochemistry II and Chemistry I, Karolinska Institutet, S-104 01 Stockholm, Sweden.

The polypeptide somatomedin A (SMA) originally proposed to be a more neutral polypeptide than insulin-like growth factor 1 (IGF-1), has been isolated from human plasma. By a new purification procedure, not utilizing acid-ethanol extraction, both SMA and insulin-like growth factor 2 (IGF-2) were purified to homogenity. The chromatography system consisted of six steps. Step one to four was controlled by a microcomputer, facilitating the processing of larger amounts of plasma. The fractions containing SMA were monitored by the placenta radioreceptorassay (RRA-SMA) and the radioimmunoassay (RIA-SMA) for SMA.

The first column of CM-Affigel Blue adsorbed the majority of RRA-SMA, while approximately two thirds of the other serum proteins passed through. After desalting RRA-SMA was found in the albumin fraction eluted by 1.4 M NaCl. RRA-SMA was separated free from both albumin and NaCl by gelchromatography on Sephadex G50M. The separation between SMA and IGF-2 was achieved on two cation-exchange columns, but not in the final HPLC step.

The amino acid composition and sequence analysis of SMA, disclosed no significant dissimilarities to the known structure of IGF-1. An isoelectric point of 8.0 was determined by chromatofocusing. The present results do thus not support the original proposal of SMA, being a neutral polypeptide different from IGF-1.

657 ACTIONS OF RAT INSULIN-LIKE GROWTH FACTOR-II ON MYOBLASTS: A SINGLE MOLECULE ACTING VIA TWO RECEPTORS?

J. R. Florini*, D. Z. Ewton, S. L. Falen, J. F. Regan, and R. Lau. Biology Dept., Syracuse University, Syracuse, NY. 13210 USA

In the past few years, we have reported that rat Insulin-like Growth Factor-II (rIGF-II, formerly designated Multiplication Stimulating Activity) stimulates many aspects of growth and differentiation in cultured muscle cells. Improvements in our production and purification capabilities now make it possible for us to quantitate interrelationships among the various actions of rIGF-II on L6 myoblasts. We find that the same molecular species (based on molecular exclusion chromatography on Fractogel TSK HW-55, confirmed by reverse-phase HPLC on a C-18 column and SDS gel electrophoresis) is active in the routine chick embryo fibroblast assay, in displacing ^{125}I-labeled hormone from L6 cells, and in stimulating amino acid (AIB) uptake, cell proliferation, and (under appropriate conditions) differentiation to form postmitotic myotubes. The concentration dependencies of the various processes are strikingly different; half-maximal stimulation of AIB uptake is at 5 nM, but for proliferation and differentiation it is at 50 nM. These differences suggest that these processes are mediated by different receptors, possibly uptake by the type II and proliferation/differentiation by the type I IGF receptor. (Supported by grants from the USPHS and the Muscular Dystrophy Association)

658 ASYMMETRIC DISTRIBUTION OF INSULIN AND IGF RECEPTORS IN RENAL PROXIMAL TUBULAR CELLS.

J. R. Gavin, III* and M. R. Hammerman, Washington University School of Medicine, St. Louis, Missouri, USA.

The effects of insulin (Ins) on renal proximal tubular cells are thought to be mediated by hormone binding to specific receptors localized predominantly in the basolateral membranes. Since Ins and insulin-like growth factor (IGF) receptors frequently coexist in mammalian cells and often mediate similar biologic responses, we examined isolated basolateral (BLM) and brush border (BBM) membranes for the presence of IGF receptors. ^{125}I-labeled Ins, IGF I or IGF II was incubated with BLM and BBM (75-150 μg) under various conditions in the absence and presence of competing ligands. While Ins binding to BLM was 14 to 20-fold greater than to BBM, IGF II binding was only 30-40% greater in BLM than in BBM. The ratios of Ins/IGF II bound were 8-10 and 0.6-1.5 for BLM and BBM, respectively. These quantitative relationships were found both in intact and detergent-treated membranes, suggesting that receptor inaccessibility did not account for the observed differences. BLM and BBM bound much less IGF I than IGF II. IGF I binding was inhibited by IGF II, but not by IGF I, and was not affected by insulin-receptor antibody, suggesting that binding of IGF I was to an IGF II receptor. Consistent with these findings was the demonstration of Ins and IGF II, but not IGF I, effects on protein phosphorylation in BLM. We conclude that specific Ins and IGF II receptors are asymmetrically located in BLM and BBM. These findings are compatible with the concept of different functional roles for Ins and IGF II in renal cells. (Supported by NIADDK grants AM05105, AM27600 and the JDF)

659 SOMATOMEDIN C (SMC) PLASMA CONCENTRATIONS IN GROWTH DEFICIENCY: CORRELATION BETWEEN RADIOIMMUNO (RIA) AND RADIORECEPTOR (RRA) ASSAYS. D. Giannella-Neto*, E. Martin Spencer, B.L. Wajchenberg and B.B. Mendonça, Hospital das Clínicas, São Paulo, Brazil and Laboratory of Growth and Development, Children's Hospital of San Francisco, USA.

SMC was determined by a specific double antibody RIA and by an human placental membrane RRA in plasma samples obtained from 17 patients (13M, 4F; aged 7.67 to 20.25 yr) with constitutional growth deficiency and normal GH dynamics (group I), 11 patients (7M, 4F; aged 10 to 21 yr) with isolated GH deficiency without treatment (group II) and 7 patients (6M, 1F; aged 11.5 to 19.42 yr) with isolated GH deficiency on longstanding hGH treatment 24 h after the last injection. The best correlation was fitted by a geometric regression in all 3 groups, showing coeff. of correlation (r) of 0.69 ($p<0.001$), 0.81 ($p<0.01$) and 0.93 ($p<0.001$), respectively. There were significant differences between the r of groups I vs. III and groups II vs. III but not between the slopes of all 3 curves. There were significant differences between means of groups I and II both by RIA (140.9 ± 32.5 vs. 43.1 ± 11.83 ng/ml) and RRA (291.1 ± 68.2 vs. 104.0 ± 32.4 ng/ml) ($p<0.05$) with t 0.05 greater for RIA than RRA (2.42 vs. 2.13) but not between the means of groups II and III both by RIA (43.1 ± 11.8 vs. 35.7 ± 11.2 ng/ml) and RRA (104.0 ± 32.4 vs. 85.8 ± 16.4 ng/ml). The present data demonstrate that both methods correlate well and that RIA seems to differentiate better patients with constitutional growth deficiency from those with isolated GH deficiency without treatment but they are unable to differentiate isolated GH deficiency patients on and without treatment. A probable explanation could be the lack of increased caloric intake despite the use of hGH injections. This work was supported by CNPq (No.101748-82).

660 SOMATOSTATIN AND CALCITONIN PROMOTE CALCIUM METABOLISM IN THE MANTLE EDGE AND NEURITE OUTGROWTH IN NEURONS OF A GASTROPOD. Y. Grimm-Jørgensen* and M. Ducor, University of Connecticut Health Center, Farmington, CT 06032. U.S.A.

Somatostatin (SS)- and calcitonin (CT)-like material is found in the brain and hemolymph of gastropods and it has been postulated that the SS-like material serves as a growth factor in these animals. SS and CT have similar effects on the function of some vertebrate tissues. We wanted to determine whether synthetic SS and salmon CT can alter the metabolism of 2 gastropod tissues known to be under the trophic control of endogenous growth factors. Gastropod growth hormone stimulates Ca^{++} metabolism in the mantle edge which is responsible for shell growth. Ca^{++} release by *in vitro* incubated mantle edge tissue was quantitated by measuring the fluorescence emitted by the Ca^{++} sensitive dye Quin II added to the incubation medium. SS and CT (10^{-9}M) significantly increased Ca^{++} efflux mimicking the effect of crude growth hormone-containing extracts. Neurite outgrowth by *in vitro* cultured dissociated gastropod neurons is dependent on the presence of factors secreted by brain tissue. CT and SS (10^{-8}M) increased the percentage of neurite-containing cells 2.2 and 1.7 fold and increased the number of cells with sprouting neurites per dish ∿2 fold hereby mimicking the action of the endogenous growth factors. These results indicate that SS and CT can serve as growth factors in 2 gastropod tissues and suggest that the endogenous SS- and CT-like materials are growth hormones. It is possible that SS and CT also promote growth and differentiation in embryonic tissues of "higher" animals. Supported by grant AM 20929 from NIH.

661 BINDING OF MULTIPLICATION STIMULATING ACTIVITY (MSA) AND MSA-STIMULATED PHOSPHORYLATION IN BASOLATERAL MEMBRANES FROM DOG KIDNEY. M.R. Hammerman* and J.R. Gavin III, Washington University School of Medicine, St. Louis, MO, 63110, USA.

Early physiologic actions of insulin and insulin-like growth factors (IGFs) are thought to be initiated by binding of these peptides to insulin or IGF responsive tissues, followed by phosphorylation of specific hormone receptors. Both insulin and IGF bind to renal membranes, suggesting functional roles for these peptides in kidney. The present studies further characterize the interaction of MSA/IGF II with its renal receptor. We measured binding of [^{125}I] IGF II and MSA-stimulated phosphorylation of basolateral membranes (BLM) isolated from proximal tubular cells of dog kidney. Specific binding of [^{125}I] IGF II was half maximal at 10^{-9} M MSA and was not inhibited by hGH, IGF I, insulin, or anti-insulin receptor antibodies. Concentration-dependent MSA-stimulated phosphorylation of a 135,000 M_r protein band was demonstrated in autoradiograms of SDS-polyacrylamide gels from BLM suspensions. Insulin increased phosphorylation of this band only in the presence of MSA, while a 92,000 M_r band was consistently phosphorylated with insulin alone. Incubation of BLM with anti-insulin receptor antibodies reduced Coomassie blue staining of the 135,000 M_r band in gels and reduced ^{32}P in autoradiograms, suggesting that the band may be the alpha subunit of the insulin receptor. We conclude that receptor-mediated MSA-stimulated phosphorylation of BLM may reflect a process by which biological actions of IGF II are mediated in vivo. Our data suggest that insulin and IGF II may interact by regulating protein phosphorylation. (Supported by NIADDK Grants AM27600 and AM20579)

662 INHIBITORY EFFECT OF BROMOCRIPTINE ON HUMAN FIBROBLASTS GROWTH IN VITRO. D. Evain Brion*, E. Binet. Inserm U 188, 75014 Paris - France.

Addition of bromocriptine mesylate 1 nM to 100 nM inhibits in a dose-dependent manner the growth of normal human fibroblasts in culture media supplemented with 10% fetal calf serum. Bromocriptine 10 nM also decreases the potentiation of fibroblasts growth by fibroblast growth factor (0.3 µg/ml). As soon as after 18 h of treatment, bromocriptine 10 nM strongly inhibits the thymidine incorporation into the DNA of human fibroblasts growing in 10% fetal calf serum. Bromocriptine causes a similar decrease of thymidine incorporation, approximately 70%, irrespective the cells are stimulated by fibroblast growth factor, epidermal growth factor or 10% fetal calf serum. These results suggest a direct inhibitory effect of bromocriptine upon cell growth. This effect would give some insight into unexplained clinical facts, such as clinical improvement of acromegaly with out decrease of somatomedins, or accelerated bone maturation in the tall adolescents we treated with bromocriptine.

663 EFFECTS OF HUMAN PANCREATIC GROWTH HORMONE (GH) RELEASING FACTOR (hpGRF)-40 ON SERUM GH, PROLACTIN (PRL), LUTEINIZING HORMONE (LH), FOLLICLE-STIMULATING HORMONE (FSH) AND SOMATOMEDIN C (SC) IN NORMAL WOMEN DURING THE MENSTRUAL CYCLE. W.S. Evans*, J.L. Borges, M.L. Vance, D.L. Kaiser, A.D. Rogol, R. Furlanetto, J. Chitwood, and M.O. Thorner. University of Virginia Medical Center, Charlottesville, VA and Children's Hospital of Philadelphia, Philadelphia, PA, USA.

To document the effects of hpGRF-40 on anterior pituitary hormone release in women, and to examine the effects of the gonadal hormone environment on such release, we administered intravenously vehicle or 3.33 ug/kg of the peptide during the early follicular (EF), late follicular (LF), and luteal (L) phases of the menstrual cycles of 9 women. Mean ($\pm$ SEM) integrated serum levels of GH (ng/ml/h) above baseline were higher after hpGRF-40 compared to after vehicle during the EF (16 $\pm$ 11.6 vs 1.4 $\pm$ 2.7; p=0.0053), LF (10.7 $\pm$ 11.7 vs 1.6 $\pm$ 1.3; p=0.0488) and L (13.4 $\pm$ 19.5 vs -1.8 $\pm$ 2.4; p=0.0486) phases of the cycle; however, no differences in the levels of GH achieved in response to hpGRF-40 were detected when results during the EF, LF and L phases were compared. Serum SC levels measured 24 h after hpGRF-40 administration were higher than after vehicle during all phases of the cycle (n=5). hpGRF-40 did not stimulate the release of PRL, LH or FSH (n=5). We conclude that hpGRF-40 selectively stimulates the release of GH but that, at the dose tested, hpGRF-40-stimulated GH release does not vary as a function of the gonadal hormone environment. Supported by HD-00439, AM-23632, HD-13197 and RR-847.

664 PHOSPHORYLATION OF PROTEINS IN A PARTIALLY PURIFIED PREPARATION OF LIVER RECEPTORS IS REGULATED BY HUMAN GROWTH HORMONE (GH). T. J. Fields and J. P. Hughes*, Department of Life Sciences, Indiana State University, Terre Haute, IN 47809.

Since protein phosphorylation is an intrinsic function of receptors for several substances involved in regulation of cellular growth, we have examined the possibility that rabbit GH and/or prolactin receptors also contain intrinsic kinase activity. Receptors solubilized from rabbit liver membranes were purified by affinity chromatography using a two-step procedure: 1) hGH coupled to agarose beads and 2) organomercurial agarose. The receptor preparation was preincubated with hGH (20 μg/ml) for 10 min at 22 C and phosphorylation was initiated by addition of [γ-^{32}P]ATP. Aliquots of the reaction mixture removed at 1, 15 and 60 min were examined by sodium dodecyl sulfate-gel electrophoresis and autoradiography. No GH effect was observed at 1 and 15 min; however, after 60 min, hGH stimulated phosphorylation of proteins which migrated with apparent mol wts of 23,000 and 40,000 daltons. It is unlikely that the 23,000-dalton protein is hGH because the position of the phosphorylated protein did not correspond to that of a hGH standard when the two proteins were electrophoresed in adjacent lanes. The 40,000-dalton protein also has not been identified; however, the mol wt of this protein is similar to that reported for the rabbit prolactin receptor. These results suggest that activation of rabbit GH and/or PRL receptors stimulates protein phosphorylation under *in vitro* conditions.

665 EFFECTS OF SOMATOSTATIN-14,-28 AND SOMATOMEDIN C ON RAT HYPOTHALAMIC GROWTH HORMONE-RELEASING FACTOR (rhGRF) STIMULATION OF GROWTH HORMONE IN VITRO. J. Fukata* and J.B. Martin, Dept. of Neurology Massachusetts General Hospital, Boston, MA 02114.

Somatostatin (SS)-14,-28 and somatomedin C (SMC) are considered to be the principal inhibitory factors to regulate the functions of the somatotroph at the pituitary level. We examined the effects of these peptides on the function of rhGRF in stimulating GH in cultured rat anterior pituitary cells. Pituitary cells obtained from 150-170g male CD rats were incubated for 24 hours in a serum-free medium with 30pM triiodothyronine and 5 nM dexamethasone before treatment. After 4 hours test incubation with rhGRF or the other peptides, GH levels in cells and media were determined by radioimmunoassay. 0.01-3nM rhGRF stimulated the release of GH dose-dependently to 660% of control. Concurrently, rhGRF decreased intracellular GH levels and increased the total amount of GH (cells and media). SS-14 (0.1nM-1nM) antagonized the three effects of 3nM rhGRF. Either synthetic SMC(25-500ng/ml) pretreatment for 24 hours or SS-28 (1-10nM) suppressed the releasing effect of rhGRF without significant changes on the total GH levels. Simultaneously, decrease of intracellular GH levels by rhGRF were antagonized by SMC or SS-28. These findings suggest that rhGRF stimulates both release and synthesis of rGH and the releasing effect is more predominant than the synthesizing effect; SS-14 blocks both of these effects of rhGRF. SS-28 and SMC appear to antagonize only the releasing effect of rhGRF under these conditions.

Supported by U.S.P.H.S. Grant No. AM26252. Synthetic SMC was donated by Dr. C.H.Li.

666 SUSPECTED PARTIAL GROWTH HORMONE (GH) DEFICIENCY. EFFECT OF ETHINYL-ESTRADIOL (EE) ON GH RESPONSE TO EXOGENOUS STIMULI. P.E. GARNIER*, M. ROGER, P.CANLORBE and J.C. JOB. Fondation de Recherche en Hormonologie and Hôpital St.Vincent de Paul, PARIS, France.

GH secretion was studied in 90 dwarf children (mean-3.5 SD) aged from 2 to 16 years (64 males and 16 females) before and after EE 100 µg/day for 3 days. At least 2 stimulation tests using insulin, arginine and/or ornithine were performed before EE and one after. In 12 out of 18 short endocrinologically normal controls, the GH responses, which were normal at first, increased after EE. 21 cases had a documented GH deficiency resulting from a known cause, gross hypothalamo-pituitary lesion, breech delivery, familial hypopituitarism or multiple idiopathic pituitary defect, GH response ranged from non detectable (ND), level to 7.6 ng/ml before EE and from ND to 9.4 ng/ml after, the mean ± SD peak GH values being 3.6 ± 2.3 ng/ml before and 3.4 ± 2.5 ng/ml after. 51 without prior evidence of pituitary deficiency had a GH peak response below 10 ng/ml (mean 6.1 ± SD 2 ng/ml) before EE. Among them,36 with increased GH response after EE, from at least 11 to 45 ng/ml (mean 19 ± SD 8.1 ng/ml) were considered as short normal. In 15 others the GH response was still below 10 ng/ml after EE (mean 7.1 ± SD 2.4 ng/ml). That lead to suspect an isolated GH deficiency. Treatment with hGH was allowed for 10 out of these 15 and induced a significant increase of their growth rate from mean ± SD 3.7 ± 0.9 to 7.9 ± 2.0 cm/year, thus supporting the diagnosis of GH deficiency. It may be suggested that EE priming is useful to distinguish GH deficiency in short patients having low or bordeline response to stimulation tests.

667 CHANGES IN GROWTH HORMONE BINDING AND METABOLIC EFFECTS OF GROWTH HORMONE IN RAT ADIPOCYTES FOLLOWING HYPOPHYSECTOMY.

I. Gause*, S. Edén, O. Isaksson, M. DiGirolamo and U. Smith, Dept of Physiology and Dept of Medicine II, University of Göteborg, Sweden.

Adipocytes from normal and hypophysectomized (hx) rats specifically bind growth hormone (GH). In the present study, changes in GH-binding and GH responsiveness after hx were studied. Various times after hx of male rats (130-150g), adipocytes were prepared by mild collagenase digestion (0.5 mg/ml, 60 min at 37C) and the effects of GH on glucose oxidation and glucose incorporation into lipids were studied in both tissue and cells. GH binding was measured in cell aliquots using ^{125}I-hGH.

With careful handling of the cells similar metabolic responses to GH (and insulin) in the tissue and the cells were observed. Six hours after hx, GH binding was unchanged (3-5 % specifically bound/10^5 cells). Thereafter, (1,3,7 and 14 days after hx) binding progressively declined and was only about 25% of that of cells from sham-operated animals 14 days after hx. Six and 24 hours following hx, the effect of GH on glucose oxidation was increased, probably reflecting loss of refractoriness to GH. Thereafter, the metabolic effects of GH progressively decreased in parallel to the loss of GH binding.

These results suggest that the pituitary, directly or indirectly, is necessary for the maintenance of GH binding sites in adipose tissue and that these binding sites are related to the insulin-like effect of GH. The study was supported by Nordisk Insulinfond and Svenska Diabetesförbundet.

668 THE USE OF PERCOLL GRADIENTS IN COMBINATION WITH SHORT-TERM CULTURE FOR THE SEPARATION OF SOMATOTROPHS AND LACTOTROPHS FROM THE OVINE ANTERIOR PITUITARY

J.J. Gomm*, K.P. Ray and M. Wallis, Biochemistry Laboratory, University of Sussex, Brighton, Sussex BN1 9QG, U.K.

Previous attempts have been made to purify the cell types present in the anterior pituitary gland based on differences in cell density. Various methods, including isopycnic centrifugation in gradients of Ficoll, dextran, bovine serum albumin and Percoll have been employed. Hall et al. (1982), using a 25-80% hyperbolic Percoll gradient, purified a fraction of cells which consisted of 90% somatotrophs from the rat anterior pituitary gland. Attempts to use a similar Percoll gradient for the purification of sheep somatotrophs have been less successful. This may be due to the high proportion of lactotrophs present in this gland (as identified by immunofluorescent staining) and the apparently similar densities of lactotrophs and somatotrophs. When lactotrophs are removed from the inhibitory influence of the hypothalamus, they secrete prolactin at a rapid rate with consequent degranulation (Ray and Wallis, 1982). A period of culture (24-48 hours) was therefore employed to deplete these cells of their hormone content, after which time they were fractionated on 50 or 55% sigmoidal Percoll gradients. A differential shift in the peak density of the lactotrophs from 1.075 to 1.065 g/ml, as compared to the somatotrophs, was observed. This provides a basis for the separation of the two cell types, and its use in the purification of somatotrophs and lactotrophs from the sheep anterior pituitary is being explored further.

Hall,M., Howell,S.L., Schulster,D. & Wallis, M. (1982) J.Endocr.94,257-266.
Ray,K.P. and Wallis,M. (1982) Mol.Cell.Endocrinol. 27, 139-155.

669 STUDIES ON THE ROLES OF GROWTH HORMONE RELEASING FACTOR (GRF) AND SOMATOSTATIN (SRIF) IN GENERATION OF THE ULTRADIAN RHYTHM OF GROWTH HORMONE SECRETION. W. Gurd*, N. Ling, S. Trudel and G.S. Tannenbaum, McGill Univ.-Montreal Children's Hosp. Res. Inst., Montreal, Quebec H3H 1P3, Canada.

Growth hormone (GH) secretion in the rat is characterized by an endogenous ultradian rhythm with major peaks of GH secretion occurring at regular 3-4 h intervals; in the intervening trough periods plasma GH levels are undetectable. The recent discovery of GRF peptides provides a powerful tool to investigate the mechanisms governing the rhythmic secretion of GH. In the present studies freely-moving chronically cannulated rats were iv administered 10 μg of either rat hypothalamic (rh)GRF or human pancreas (hp) GRF during both peak (1100 h) and trough (1300 h) periods of GH secretion. Administration of both peptides at 1100 h resulted in 3-5 fold increases in plasma GH 5 min post injection. However, the mean peak GH response to rhGRF (1845±298 ng/ml) was significantly ($P < 0.01$) greater than that to hpGRF (821±115 ng/ml). In contrast, injection of the GRF peptides at 1300 h had only a minimal effect on plasma GH and there was no significant difference in the mean GH response to rhGRF (387±155 ng/ml) versus hpGRF (192±68 ng/ml). Neutralization of endogenous circulating SRIF with a specific antiserum to SRIF permitted a marked GH response at 1300 h to both rhGRF (3127 ±349 ng/ml) and hpGRF (1154±285 ng/ml) with the former being significantly greater ($P < 0.01$). Taken together these results suggest that rhGRF may be a more potent GH secretagogue than hpGRF in the rat. Furthermore, the findings provide support for the hypothesis that SRIF is secreted episodically to inhibit pituitary GH release and that its interaction with the phased release of GRF provides for integration of the ultradian GH rhythm as observed in the peripheral blood.

670 EFFECTS OF INSULIN AND 2-DEOXYGLUCOSE ON THE ADRENOCORTICAL FUNCTION IN INTACT AND INDOMETHACIN PRETREATED MALE RATS. A. P. Corcos, J. Weidenfeld and I. Chowers*, Lab of Exp.Endocrinology, Dept. of Neurology, Hadassah Hebrew Univ. Hosp., Dept. of Int.Med., Bikur Cholim Hosp.,Jerusalem,Israel.

Adrenocortical (AC) function can be activated by either insulin induced systemic hypoglycemia or by 2-deoxyglucose (2DG) induced cytoglucopenia. We have previously demonstrated that insulin induced AC activation may be mediated by sites located inside the hypothalamus; whereas the response to 2DG is mediated by extra-hypothalamic sites. The molecular mechanisms involved in mediation of these responses have not been ascertained. In the present study we examined the role of prostaglandins (PG) in the stimulatory effects of insulin and 2DG upon AC function. Adult male rats were given a single SC injection of indomethacin (IM:5mg/100gBW) or vehicle (v). After 15h, either insulin (0.1u/100gBW) or 2DG(40mg/100gBW) were injected (IP) and 1h later they were decapitated and trunk blood was collected for corticosterone (CS) and glucose determinations. Hypothalamic and adenohypophyseal PGE_2 were reduced by approximately 70% in IM treated rats. In v-treated animals insulin and 2DG elevated serum CS by approximately 6-fold; blood glucose levels were 2 and 9mmol/l. respectively. In IM pretreated rats the CS response to 2DG was abolished while a full CS response to insulin was observed; blood glucose levels were similar to those found in v-pretreated animals. These results suggest that central PG are important for the mediation of the AC response to 2DG, but not for the hyperglycemic effect of this drug. In contrast the AC response to insulin induced hypoglycemia is probably not mediated by central PG. These data support our previous finding,demonstrating that activation of the AC axis in the response to insulin and to 2DG depends on two different mechanisms.

671 EFFECTS OF THYROIDECTOMY ON MITOCHONDRIAL ENZYME ACTIVITIES AND NUCLEAR RNA SYNTHESIS IN BRAIN REGIONS OF ADULT MONKEYS.

A. Dembri*, J.P. Clot, O. Michel, M. Baudry and R. Michel. Collège de France, Paris & FRH, Fresnes, France

The adult brain has long been considered as refractive to thyroid status, but recently it has been clearly established that rat cerebral cortex was sensitive to thyroid hormones. Here the subcellular effects of thyroidectomy (T) on liver and well defined parts of monkey brain were analyzed. 4-year old monkeys (Macaca Fascicularis) were surgically thyroidectomized(Tx) and used 20 days after T. The activities of succinate oxidase, succinate cyt c reductase and Mg^{++}-ATPase were measured in mitochondria isolated from liver and 5 brain regions. In Tx group, these enzyme activities decreased in all brain structures and liver. The highest reduction(30%) was found in cerebral cortex(Cx) and hippocampus. Cerebellar(Cbl) and striatal activities were reduced by about 20%. A smaller decrease(15%) was observed in thalamus(Th). The effects of T on in vitro RNA synthesis was followed in Cx, Cbl and Th by measuring nucleolar and nucleoplasmic RNA polymerase activities. As in liver the 2 nuclear enzyme activities dropped significantly by 40% in the 3 analyzed regions. Replacement therapy with T_3(1µg/kg/day) or T_4(5µg/kg/day), administered immediately after T for 20 days using osmotic minipumps, maintained mitochondrial and nuclear activities at normal levels in both liver and brain structures. In conclusion, our results demonstrate that adult monkey brain is responsive to thyroid hormones. The reduction in mitochondrial energetic metabolism is due to a decrease in the respiratory chain activity and in the phosphorylation capacity. The decreased RNA polymerase activities suggest that replacement of protein components in the brain depends on thyroid secretion.

672 ANTIESTROGEN ACTION IN UTERINE CELL CULTURES.

Carolyn Campen*, V. Craig Jordan, and Jack Gorski, Depts. of Biochemistry, Animal Sciences and Human Oncology, Univ. of Wisconsin-Madison, Madison, WI, U.S.A.

Primary cell cultures derived from immature rat uteri respond to 17β-estradiol (E2) in a dose-dependent fashion with an increase in the amount of progesterone receptor (PgR). Six triphenylethylene derivatives were tested in this system to determine their estrogenic and/or their antiestrogenic activity in vitro. Tamoxifen (1 µM) was fully antiestrogenic when incubated with 0.1 nM E2 and was nonestrogenic at 0.1 nM - 10 µM. Monohydroxytamoxifen (OH-Tam) and Ly117018 were each fully antiestrogenic at 1 µM against 1 nM E2 and both were nonestrogenic at 1 pM - 1 µM. The inhibition of the E2-induced increase in PgR by 1 µM OH-Tam was reversible with 100 nM - 1000 nM E2, which suggests that the inhibition is competitive and not a cytotoxic effect of OH-Tam. Metabolite E (ICI 77949) and cis-Tamoxifen elicited a dose-dependent increase in PgR at 1 nM - 1 µM and both were full agonists. Bisphenol was a partial agonist at 1 nM - 1 µM and was a partial antagonist in the same range against 1 nM E2. Paradoxically, antiestrogens are generally agonists of several uterine estrogenic endpoints in vivo, which might be due to in vivo metabolism. However, these results in the uterine cells are analogous to those found using similar antiestrogens in primary pituitary cultures. Therefore, these results support the model of antiestrogen action where the position of a dimethylaminoethoxy side chain (or similar structure) and of a phenolic hydroxyl group are important in determining the antiestrogenic activity and potency of a compound. Supported by NIH grants 1T32 HD07259-01, CA32713 and HD08192.

673 THYROID HORMONE STRUCTURE-ACTIVITY RELATIONSHIPSHIPS: AN UNUSUAL CONFORMATION OF A METHYLENE-BRIDGE 3,5-DIIODO THYROID HORMONE ANALOGUE. Vivian Cody*, Medical Foundation of Buffalo, 73 High St., Buffalo, NY 14203 USA.

It has been shown that a bridging oxygen is not an absolute requirement for thyromimetic activity as CH_2- and S-bridged thyroxine analogues show high activity. To determine the effects of CH_2-bridge substitution on thyroid hormone conformation, the X-ray crystal structures of two CH_2-bridge hormone analogues were determined. The bulk of the 3,5-iodines causes the diphenyl ether rings to adopt a skewed (Φ/Φ' = $\pm 90^\circ/0^\circ$) or twist-skewed (Φ/Φ' = $\pm 108^\circ/\pm 28^\circ$) conformation, with a bridge angle of 120°. In the structure of 3,5-diiodo-(3-isopropyl-4-methoxybenzyl)benzylchloride, the conformation is twist-skewed (Φ/Φ' = $-100^\circ/27^\circ$) and the bridge angle is 115°; similar to that observed for its carbonyl bridge analogue. However, in the structure of methyl-3,5-diiodo-(3-isopropyl-4-methoxybenzyl)benzoate, the conformation is twist (Φ/Φ' = $82^\circ/62^\circ$) and the bridge angle is 112°. The CH_2 bridge distances are 1.52 A in both structures and are 1.396 A for the thyroid hormones. This is the first observation of a twist conformation for a 3,5-diiodo hormone analogue. As a consequence of this unusual conformation, there is a short intramolecular contact, I5...H2'= 3.07A. This distance is 4.09A in the twist-skewed CH_2-bridge analogue and 3.62 A for the active hormone structures. These results are so unusual that, if this analogue should prove to be active, then the role of the diphenylether conformation in hormone-receptor binding will have to be reevaluated. This research supported in part by AM-51051.

674 LOW-DOSE DOPAMINE INFUSION INHIBITS SUBMAXIMALLY STIMULATED TSH SECRETION IN MAN. J.M.C. Connell,* G.C. Inglis, S.G. Ball, G.H. Beastall,# D.L. Davies†, MRC Blood Pressure Unit and +Gardiner Institute, Western Infirmary and #Department of Biochemistry, Royal Infirmary, Glasgow.

Hypothalamic dopamine (DA) released into hypophyseal portal capillaries directly inhibits prolactin (PRL) secretion from the anterior pituitary gland: the role of DA in control of TSH is less clear. Although previous studies in man have suggested that basal TSH levels fall during DA administration, circulating plasma DA concentrations during the majority of such intravenous (IV) infusion studies (4 µg/kg/min) are far in excess of DA levels in hypophyseal capillary blood of experimental animals. We have examined the effect of a lower rate of DA infusion, which gives peripheral plasma DA concentrations similar to those found in rat portal capillaries (Connell et al 1983, Clin Endocrinol 18, 527), on basal and submaximally stimulated (TRH) concentrations of TSH and PRL. Six normal males were given DA (0.1 µg/kg/min) or placebo infusions for 165 min on separate days. A bolus of TRH (7.5 µg) was given IV at +90 min, followed by TRH infusion (750 ng/min) for 45 min. Basal concentrations of TSH and PRL were not affected by DA. In all subjects TRH caused a small increase in TSH which was partially inhibited by DA (peak 5.73±0.85 mU/l v 4.58±1.09, mean ± SEM, $p < 0.05$). PRL response to TRH was inhibited by DA (peak 620±164 mU/l v 234±96, $p < 0.01$). In 6 normal female subjects DA infusion (0.1 µg/kg/min) inhibited basal PRL but not TSH secretion. These findings are consistent with a direct physiological action of DA on the pituitary causing inhibition of TSH and PRL release secondary to TRH stimulation.

675 Ca^{++} INVOLVEMENT IN $hpGRF_{44}$ STIMULATED GH RELEASE IN VITRO.
M.D. Culler*, N. Obara and A. Arimura, Lab. for Molecular Neuroendocrinology and Diabetes, Tulane University Hebert Research Center, Belle Chasse, LA, USA

Calcium (Ca^{++}) is believed to be an important factor for the release of growth hormone (GH) from the anterior pituitary. The following study examines the involvement of Ca^{++} in 44-residue, human pancreatic growth hormone-releasing factor ($hpGRF_{44}$) stimulated release of GH in rat anterior pituitary cell cultures. After 4 days in culture, the cells were exposed to Krebs-Ringer bicarbonate buffer (containing 2.5 mM Ca^{++}:0.5 $\mu Ci\,^{45}Ca^{++}$/ml) with 0.05% glucose and 0.25% BSA (KRBG), either alone or containing 10 nM $hpGRF_{44}$ for 1, 2, 4, 8, 16, 32 or 64 min. At the appropriate time, the KRBG and cells from each culture were collected to determine GH concentration and intracellular $^{45}Ca^{++}$content. Addition of 10 nM $hpGRF_{44}$ to the cultures resulted in a significant increase in the intracellular content of $^{45}Ca^{++}$ at 16 min and a significant increase in GH secretion by 32 min, as compared to cultures exposed to KRBG alone. From 16 min through 64 min, the intracellular $^{45}Ca^{++}$content of both control and $hpGRF_{44}$-treated cultures increased in a linear and parallel manner, although the $^{45}Ca^{++}$content of $hpGRF_{44}$-treated cultures remained significantly higher. These results indicate that $hpGRF_{44}$ stimulated increased Ca^{++} uptake between 8-16 min following exposure, which preceeded or, at least, coincided with the observed increase in GH release. The addition of verapamil, a proposed blocker of Ca^{++} influx, or Co^{++}, a competative Ca^{++} antagonist, inhibited 10 nM $hpGRF_{44}$ stimulated GH release in a dose-related manner, but had no effect on basal GH release. The elimination of Ca^{++} from the KRBG also inhibited $hpGRF_{44}$ stimulated GH release. These results demonstrate that Ca^{++} is required for hpGRF44 stimulated GH release.

676 CORTICOTROPIN-RELEASING FACTOR (CRF)-LIKE IMMUNOREACTIVITY IS DECREASED AFTER STRESS AND AFTER ADRENALECTOMY IN RAT MEDIAN EMINENCE.
J.Čulman,* J.M.Saavedra, M.Niwa, A.Israel, M.C.Tonon, and H.Vaudry. Laboratory of Clinical Science, NIMH, Bethesda, Md. 20205, USA.

Corticotropin Releasing Factor (CRF), after its release from median eminence (ME) stimulates secretion of ACTH from anterior pituitary. In addition, CRF fibers of hypothalamic origin occur in posterior pituitary (Burlet et al, 1982; Saavedra et al, 1984). We determined CRF-like immunoreactivity by RIA in rat ME and posterior pituitary after manipulations which increased secretion of ACTH: bilateral adrenalectomy (7 days after surgery) and acute (150 minutes) or repeated (150 minutes daily for 7 days) immobilization stress. Adrenalectomized rats showed a marked (-76%) decrease in ME CRF (from 8.8±1.2 to 2.1±0.5 ng/mg p, $p<0.01$). On the contrary, posterior pituitary CRF levels were increased (0.38±0.03 to 0.48±0.05 ng/mg p) although the results were not statistically significant. After acute immobilization, ME CRF content was decreased by 32% (from 9.7±1.1 to 6.6±0.6 ng/mg p, $p<0.01$). ME CRF was also decreased after repeated stress (-40%, to 5.9±1.3 ng/mg p, $p<0.02$) when compared to control rats. Conversely, repeated, but not acute, stress produced an increase (+ 369%, from 0.45±0.05 to 1.6±0.6 ng/mg p, $p<0.01$) in posterior pituitary CRF. These results are consistent with previous data of decreased CRF in ME after adrenalectomy, but suggest that this depletion might be of longer duration than previously reported. Our data also suggest a role of posterior pituitary CRF fibers of brain origin in the regulation of the stress response.

677 CORTICOSTERONE AND CATECHOLAMINE ELEVATION DURING CONTINUOUS INTRACEREBROVENTRICULAR INFUSION OF CORTICOTROPIN-RELEASING FACTOR (CRF) IN THE RAT.
J. Cunningham*, P. Meara, R. Lee, H.H. Bode, Ped. Endocrine Unit,Shriners Burns Instit., Mass. Gen. Hosp. and Harvard Med. Sch., Boston, MA U.S.A.

Intracerebroventricular (icv) bolus injection of CRF has been shown to elicit acute stress responses such as proopiomelanocortin and corticosterone(B) secretion, release of norepinephrine(NE) and epinephrine(EPI) and a rise in O_2 consumption. We studied the effects of continuous icv infusion of CRF to determine if these acute responses could be chronically sustained. CRF(5 or 20ug/day) or saline(S) was continuously infused icv for 6 days using an Alzet^R minipump(n=5rats/group). On day 1, saline was infused in all groups to measure surgical stress. RESULTS: In controls, daily urinary B excretion remained basal after day 1. In contrast, B excretion peaked($p<0.01$) on day 3 of 5ug CRF(0.60ug/d vs 0.23 basal) or 20ug(0.43ug/d vs 0.20). Thereafter, a progressive decline occurred despite continued CRF infusion. Urine NE(807ng/d) and EPI(80ng/d) were basal on day 3 of S infusion. NE rose significantly from 990ng/d(day 1) to 1350 or 1213ng/d($p<0.05$) on day 3 in 5 or 20ug groups, respectively. A 75% rise in EPI was seen on day 3 with 20ug CRF. EPI did not rise with 5ug CRF.Reduced weight gain(1.8g/d) and small adrenals(37±2.5mg) occurred on 5ug while rats on 20ug gained normally(4.8g/d) and had enlarged adrenals(47±1.4mg vs 43±1.4 in S). No significant differences in resting O_2 consumption were observed with either dose. These results show that chronic continuous central elevation of CRF mediates both hormonal(B) and neuronal(NE,EPI) responses seen in chronic stress. The dampened response to icv CRF over time suggests possible desensitization which may not be seen during prolonged pulsatile CRF administration.

678 EFFECT OF GRF 1-44, SOMATOSTATIN, AND CYCLOHEXIMIDE ON GH SECRETION FROM HUMAN SOMATOTROPHINOMAS IN CULTURE.
M. Daniels*, S.J. Turner, D.B. Cook, D. Mathias, P. Kendall-Taylor, G. Teasdale, and M.C. White. Royal Victoria Infirmary, Newcastle on Tyne and Southern General Hospital, Glasgow, UK.

Human somatotrophinoma cell cultures were separately obtained by enzymic dispersal from 7 pituitary tumors and maintained for up to 28 days. Studies were performed over 4h incubations between day 3-27 using a minimum of triplicate cultures for each experimental variable. Statistics were determined using Student's t test. GRF 100 ng/ml significantly ($p<0.02$) stimulated GH secretion from all 7 tumors (36-231% > control). Dose response studies (1-100 ng/ml) on 5 tumors showed a minimum effective dose of 1 ng/ml (3 tumors), and 10 ng/ml (2 tumors). Somatostatin (SRIF)(10 ng/ml) completely blocked the stimulatory effect of 1 and 100 ng/ml GRF on GH secretion from 4 tumors thus studied, but only inhibited basal GH secretion from one. During a subsequent 4h recovery period cultures previously exposed to GRF with SRIF showed an increased ($p<0.05$) GH secretion. In a further study, cultures from one tumor pretreated with cycloheximide (CH) 10 µg/ml to block protein synthesis, were subsequently incubated with CH (10 µg/ml) and GRF (100 ng/ml) either alone or in combination. CH alone suppressed ($p<0.01$) GH secretion, whilst GRF with CH stimulated ($p<0.001$) GH secretion, but only to 53% of that observed in cultures incubated with GRF alone. These data show GRF stimulates GH secretion from human somatotrophinomas in a dose dependent manner, that this stimulation is blocked but not abolished by SRIF, and suggest that some part of the stimulatory action is mediated via de novo protein synthesis.

679 COMBINED ANTERIOR PITUITARY TESTING WITH FOUR HYPOTHALAMIC RELEASING HORMONES IN NORMAL SUBJECTS AND PATIENTS WITH PITUITARY DISORDERS.

C.R. DeBold*, W.R. Sheldon, Jr., G.S. DeCherney, D.P. Island, M.O. Thorner, W.S. Evans and D.N. Orth, Depts. of Medicine, Vanderbilt University, Nashville, Tennessee and University of Virginia, Charlottesville, Virginia, USA

To determine the feasibility of administering simultaneously four hypothalamic releasing hormones as a single test of the release of all known anterior pituitary hormones, we gave ovine corticotropin-releasing hormone (1 µg/kg body wt), human pancreatic growth hormone-releasing hormone-(1-40) (1 µg/kg), gonadotropin-releasing hormone (100 µg), and thyrotropin-releasing hormone (200 µg) as successive 20-sec iv infusions at 9 a.m. to 11 normal men, 11 normal women in early follicular phase of the menstrual cycle, and 8 patients with various hypothalamic-pituitary disorders. Peak increments (mean ± SEM) in circulating hormone concentrations and peak time (range) during the 120 min after the infusions in normal subjects were:

	Men	Women	Time of Peak
ACTH (pg/ml)	46 ± 9.0	41 ± 7.4	10 - 60 min
Cortisol (µg/dl)	9.2 ± 1.2	9.8 ± 1.4	30 - 120
GH (ng/ml)	18 ± 5.7	58 ± 21** ($p < 0.05$)	15 - 90
PRL (ng/ml)	41 ± 4.3	93 ± 17**	10 - 30
FSH (mIU/ml)	2.7 ± 0.7	2.8 ± 0.3	45 - 90
LH (mIU/ml)	21 ± 3.5	12 ± 2.3**	15 - 45
TSH (µU/ml)	12 ± 1.6	16 ± 4.9 (n=3)	15 - 30

Hormone concentrations almost always reached or were near their peak by 60 min. No unusual or dangerous side effects were observed. This test has proved useful for evaluating pituitary hormone status in the 8 patients thus far studied. In conclusion, the simultaneous administration of these 4 hypothalamic releasing hormones provides a short, safe and practical test of combined anterior pituitary function.

680 SOMATOSTATIN (SRIF) RADIOIMMUNOASSAY (RIA) AFTER GEL FILTRATION AND HPLC.

E. De Palo°, D. Paccagnella, C. Crivellaro, L. Marchioro, R. Vettor and G. Federspil, Istituto di Semeiotica Medica, Università di Padova, Italy.

A series of SRIF extraction methods was proposed but so far only insatisfactory results was obtained. In order to study a more precise, rapid and simple extraction method useful to identify plasma SRIF we performed:

A) Extraction was obtained with octyl silica cartridges outlined in: a) sample application (2 ml) after H_2O and CH_3CN washing; b) plasma components weakly bound elution with H_2O; c) SRIF elution with 0.5 ml of CH_3CN : TFA 10 mM in phosphate 0.1 M pH 4.5 CH_3CN 25.5% 50 : 50 , and lyophilization. The recovery HPLC assayed was about 70% in ageement with other extraction methods.

B) HPLC separation on Ultrasphere Octyl (4.6x150 mm Column) - Eluent: sodium phosphate 0.1 M pH 4.5 and CH_3CN 25.5% final. SRIF elution time was 20 min with 1600 psi and elution rate 1 ml/min.

C) RIA was performed employing phosphate buffer (50 mM pH 7.4; BSA 0.5%; EDTA 2.5 g/l; Aprotinine $5x10^5$ U/l; NaN_3 0.2 g/l), ^{125}I-Tyr^1-SRIF (1000µCi/ug; 2-4 µCi/tube) 100 µl, rabbit antiserum anti-SRIF (final dil. 1/8000) 100 ul, reconstituted lyophilized sample 300 µl, 72 h at 4 °C incubation time and Charcoal (20 mg/ml) 500 µl.

In conclusion our preliminary data showed that extraction with octyl silica cartridge, HPLC and RIA could be useful in SRIF determination.

681 HISTIDYL-PROLINE DIKETOPIPERAZINE {CYCLO (HIS-PRO)}: A NEW NEUROHORMONE UBIQUITOUSLY PRESENT IN THE HUMAN GASTROINTESTINAL (GI) TRACT E. Diamanti-Kandarakis*, T. Iriuchijima, and J. Wilber, LSU Medical Center, New Orleans, Louisiana.

Cyclo (His-Pro){C(H-P)} is an endogenous neurohormone which is derived from thyrotropin-releasing-hormone (TRH) by limited proteolysis. C(H-P) has a number of biological properties, including inhibition of gut cholesterol synthesis and suppression of food intake. Because C(H-P) has been found by us to be present in the rat gastrointestinal (GI) tract, we wondered if C(H-P) were present also in the human GI tract. To explore this question, human GI tissues obtained at post-mortem examination from 8 patients free of GI disease were extracted with 0.4 M perchloric acid. Supernatants were neutralized with $KHCO_3$, lyophilized, and resuspended in buffered saline for C(H-P) concentrations by specific radioimmunoassay. C(H-P) was found in all GI structures and mean C(H-P) concentrations were 95 fold those of TRH. Such human GI C(H-P)-like immunoreactivity exhibited identity immunologically with synthetic C(H-P) and co-chromatographed with ^{3}H-C(H-P) during High Performance Liquid Chromatography (HPLC). Highest concentrations of C(H-P) were found in stomach (599±102 pg/mg protein) and caecum (462±121), and lowest concentrations were observed in esophagus (127±26) and ileum (171±30 pg/mg protein). Intermediate C(H-P) concentrations were found in all other GI regions which were not statistically distinguishable, ranging from 204±83 (rectum) to 294±73 (duodenum). Conclusions: 1) C(H-P) activity, identical to synthetic C(H-P), is present throughtout the human GI tract 2) C(H-P) is a new human gut neurohormone which may modulate gut functions, like its precursor TRH, by paracrine and/or endocrine mechanisms.

682 ACTH AND CORTISOL RESPONSIVENESS TO CORTICOTROPIN-RELEASING FACTOR (CRF) IN PSEUDOHYPOPARATHYROIDISM. R.W.Downs*, H.M.Schulte, G.P.Chrousos, M.A.Levine, and A.M.Spiegel, Department of Medicine, Medical College of Virginia, Richmond, VA 23298, and the National Institutes of Health, Bethesda, MD, USA.

A deficiency of the adenylate cyclase coupling protein (Ns) has been demonstrated in some patients with pseudohypoparathyroidism (PHP), and probably accounts for resistance to multiple hormones in these patients. Since corticotropin-releasing factor (CRF) and ACTH stimulate cAMP production in target cells as part of their mechanism of action, we tested the response to CRF in patients with PHP who have low Ns activity. 5 patients and 15 normal volunteer controls received 1 ug/kg ovine CRF as an iv bolus at 8pm, and the subsequent ACTH and cortisol responses were measured for 180 minutes. At 15 min after CRF injection, plasma ACTH was higher in patients with PHP than in controls (36.8 ± 6.6 vs. 23.3 ± 2.7, mean ± SEM, $p<.05$). ACTH levels peaked at 15 min in the group with PHP, but controls peaked later, at 30 min after injection of CRF. The higher 15 min ACTH was accompanied by a higher 15 min cortisol response in the PHP group (12.2 ± 1.6 vs. 6.1 ± 0.9, $p<.01$), and cortisol levels peaked at 30 min in the PHP group, compared to 60 min in controls. Despite the earlier peak responses for both ACTH and cortisol in PHP, total area under the response curves for both ACTH and cortisol were similar for the two groups. We conclude that deficiency of the adenylate cyclase coupling protein in PHP causes no major defect in hypothalamic-pituitary-adrenal function, but that the observed early response to CRF may possibly indicate a subtle disorder of CRF or ACTH action upon target cells in PHP.

683 PITUITARY AND GONADAL RESPONSES TO GRADED DOSES OF LH-RH IN BULLS.

M.J. D'Occhio* and B.P. Setchell, Department of Animal Sciences, Waite Agricultural Research Institute, Glen Osmond, 5064, South Australia.

The capacity of the anterior pituitary (A.P.) and testes in bulls to respond to graded doses of luteinizing hormone-releasing hormone (LH-RH) was assessed relative to endogenous profiles of LH and testosterone (T) secretion. On separate days, adult bulls (705±9kg,mean±SEM,n=4) received an i.v. bolus of either 1,5,10,50 or 100ng LH-RH/kg body weight and blood samples were taken at -40,-20,0,10,20,30,40,60 and 120 min. Endogenous profiles of LH and T were determined by bleeding animals at 20-min intervals from 0600 to 1800 h. The amplitudes of spontaneous LH and T peaks were 2.6±0.5 and 12.8±2.0 ng/ml, respectively. Respective peak LH and T responses (ng/ml) to LH-RH were as follows: 1ng LH-RH(3.0±0.7; 13.6±1.1); 5ng LH-RH(8.0±1.2; 15.2±1.7); 10ng LH-RH(11.1±2.3; 16.6±2.6); 50ng LH-RH (19.2±2.8; 13.8±2.4); 100ng LH-RH(19.1±4.7; 12.7±1.8). A dose of 1ng/kg LH-RH produced LH and T responses which were comparable in amplitude to spontaneous peaks in the respective hormone. There was a progressive increase in the LH response to doses of LH-RH between 1 and 50ng/kg; corresponding T responses remained constant. The capacity of the A.P. to release amounts of LH 8 to 10 times in excess of those secreted during spontaneous peaks suggests that (1) hypothalamic LH-RH is a limiting factor in gonadotropin secretion and (2) there exists a releasable store of LH in the A.P. In contrast to LH release, the androgenic response of the testes to varying amounts of gonadotropin is determined largely by prevailing steroidogenic activity.

This study was supported by a grant from the Davies Bequest.

684 REGULATION OF POMC GENE EXPRESSION BY CRH AND GLUCOCORTICOIDS IN PRIMARY RAT PITUITARY CULTURES.

J.H. Eberwine, J. Jonassen, M.J. Evinger, and J.L. Roberts*, Dept. Biochem. and Cntr. for Repro. Science, Columbia U., NY 10032.

Corticotropin releasing hormone (CRH) and glucocorticoids have profound stimulatory and inhibitory effects, respectively, on pro-opiomelanocortin (POMC) peptide secretion from rat pituitary primary cultures. Using an in vitro nuclear runoff assay to measure the active state of transcription of the POMC gene, we have investigated the effects of these two hormones separately and together on POMC gene transcription in anterior (AL) and intermediate (IL) lobe pituitary primary cultures. CRH (10^{-9}M for AL, 10^{-8}M for IL) rapidly stimulates 10-15 fold POMC transcription in both lobes with a maximum at 30 min. Glucocorticoids (dexamethasone (DEX) 10^{-7}M) have a five fold inhibitory effect within 20-30 min. on POMC transcription only in the AL; there is little effect in the IL. The response of POMC gene transcription in the AL to various combinations of CRH and DEX was complex. The response was dependent upon the length of time the cells were in the presence of the first hormone that was added, as well as the length of time the second hormone was present. For example, if DEX was given to the cultures long enough to inhibit CRH stimulated POMC release (i.e. at least 20 min.), the CRH mediated stimulation of POMC transcription was blunted. These results suggest that POMC secretion is coupled in some way to POMC gene transcription.

685 PITUITARY GROWTH HORMONE (GH) RESPONSE TO GROWTH HORMONE RELEASING-FACTOR (GRF-44) DIFFERS DURING THE MENSTRUAL CYCLE. C.A. Egli*, B.P. Hauffa, S.L. Kaplan, M.M. Grumbach, Department of Pediatrics, University of California San Francisco, San Francisco, CA

GH levels post-ambulation are higher in normal women than in men and show a distinct midcycle peak. We investigated the GH response to GRF during the menstrual cycle in 7 healthy, resting, ovulatory women (21-33 yr), randomly starting each subject's study at 1 of 3 times: follicular (F=d4-7), mid (M=d12-17), or luteal (L=d19-23). Basal plasma GH concentrations did not differ significantly during the cycle (F=2.3 ± 1.1, M=0.7 ± 0.24, L=1.67 ± 0.96 ng/ml, mean ± SE, n=7). GH secretory response to a 1 μg/kg IV bolus of GRF was significantly less in the luteal phase than in the midcycle or follicular phases as determined by peak GH level (F=20.9 ± 5.6, M=22.3 ± 6.2, L=10.4 ± 1.2 ng/ml, mean ± SE, p<.05 M vs L and F vs L). In addition, integrated GH area post-GRF was lower at L than at M (F=1,023 ± 557, M=1,630 ± 556, L=596 ± 72.7 ng·min/ml, mean ± SE, p<.05 M vs L; F vs L NS). While results at the midcycle and follicular phases did not significantly differ using either parameter, 5 of 7 women responded maximally at midcycle by both peak GH and integrated GH areas post-GRF. Ovulation was established on the basis of rises in basal body temperature and increases in plasma luteinizing hormone and estradiol values midcycle (p<.01), while substantial elevations in plasma progesterone occurred in the luteal phase in all subjects (p<.01). Conclusions: 1) GH response to GRF differs during the menstrual cycle in normal women, with significant decreases in luteal responses when compared to the midcycle or follicular phases. 2) These findings suggest that gonadal steroids may modulate sensitivity to GRF at the pituitary somatotrope level.

686 SEQUENTIAL ADMINISTRATION OF AN INTRANASAL LHRH AGONIST AND ORAL PROGESTAGEN FOR INHIBITION OF OVULATION AND CONTROL OF UTERINE BLEEDING IN NORMAL WOMEN. N.Faure,* A.Lemay, F.Labrie and A.T.A.Fazekas. Endocrin. of Reprod., St-François d'Assise Hospital, Quebec and Molec.Endocrin.,C.H.U.L., Quebec, Canada.

Increasing intranasal doses of 100, 200 and 300 μg of [D-Ser(TBU)^6-des-Gly-NH_2^{10}] LHRH ethylamide (buserelin HOE 766) were administered every 12 hours and compared to a 400 μg dose given daily. 8 normally cycling women per group were treated for 2 periods of 21 days separated by a pause of 7 days. 5 mg of medroxyprogesterone acetate (provera) was added orally on days 17 to 21. A mean 2 to 3 fold increase in serum LH was maintained during the first 2 weeks of LHRH agonist administration in any of the 4 dosage groups. Serum FSH levels were increased during the first 3 days of treatment and decreased to normal or below starting levels during the remaining treatment period. Serum gonadotropins returned to normal levels during the pause. A wide range of interindividual variation was found in serum estradiol of each group. The surface areas under treatment curves were compared to the mean of the 4 normal pre and post-treatment control cycles.Values above the superior limit increased from 25% at 100 ug dosing to 66% at 300 ug dosing. At 400 ug once daily 66% of the treatment cycles had total estradiol values below the inferior limit of control normal range. In all 4 groups, serum estradiol were in the early follicular range during the pause. All the women had 2-5 days of light to moderate bleeding during the pause. Breakthrough bleeding occurred in 5 cycles in the 300 ug group while it happened only once or twice in the other groups. It is hoped that an appropriate and practical dosage regimen will maintain estradiol in a more physiological range.

687 REPEATED ADMINISTRATION OF SYNTHETIC HUMAN PANCREAS GROWTH HORMONE RELEASING FACTOR (HPGRF-44) STIMULATES GH SECRETION IN NORMAL MAN

J.P. Felber*, I. Lancranjan, D. Vouillamoz, P. Marbach, Division d'Endocrinologie et Biochimie Clinique, CHUV, Lausanne, Clinical and Preclinical Research Dept., Sandoz Ltd, Basle, Switzerland.

The secretory pattern of GH secretion in normal man is episodic whereas short children with a growth rate below -2 standard deviation have irregular GH secretion with few peaks of low amplitude if any. Therefore, it is reasonable to suspect that GRF if used therapeutically may require administration several times a day. A study was conducted to examine the effect of repeated administration of GRF-44 in 6 normal young male volunteers who received in a randomized order at 3-day interval either placebo or GRF-44 as an iv repeated bolus (at 9 am, 12 am, 3 pm). At 1 pm a standard lunch was given. Venous blood was withdrawn through an indwelling canula from 8 am to 6 pm to measure GH, insulin and glucose plasma levels. Although GH secretory spikes were found during the day of placebo administration these were not related to the injection of placebo. Conversely GRF-44 selectively stimulated GH secretion with mean peak concentrations of 19.9 $\pm$ 11.3, 7.9 $\pm$ 4.4 and respectively 16.1 $\pm$ 8.0 ng/ml occurring between 15 to 60 min after each iv bolus of GRF-44. GH response to the last GRF-44 bolus was not suppressed by the high glucose plasma levels which followed lunch and occurred between 2 and 3 pm. The concentrations of blood glucose and plasma insulin stimulated by lunch were unaffected by GRF-44. The above results suggest that GRF holds promises for a new therapeutic approach of children with growth deficiency.

688 IMMUNOCHEMICAL PROPERTIES OF (Glu^8) LUTEINIZING HORMONE RELEASING HORMONE (CHICKEN LHRH) by H.M. Fraser*, R.J. Sterling°, P.J. Sharp°, P.L. Taylor, W. König,+ and J. Sandow+. MRC Reproductive Biology Unit, Edinburgh, EH3 9EW, UK.°ARC Poultry Research Centre, Roslin and +Hoechst A.G. Frankfurt.

Mammalian luteinizing hormone releasing hormone (m LHRH) and chicken LHRH (ch LHRH) are believed to differ by substitution of Glu^8 in the chicken decapeptide. To study the immunochemical properties of chLHRH we produced antibodies to the synthetic peptide in 5 rabbits. All 5 antisera bound ^{125}-I-labelled chLHRH but not labelled mLHRH. This ability of the antibodies to chLHRH to recognise the difference between Glu^8 and Arg^8 in mLHRH was confirmed by the establishment of a radioimmunoassay using one of the antisera. Extracts of rat hypothalamus and synthetic mLHRH failed to displace binding, while hypothalamus of chicken, dove, grouse and turkey, together with plasma obtained from venous sinus encircling the pituitary in chickens or peripheral blood, all demonstrated parallel displacement in the radioimmunoassay. The antibody demonstrated cell bodies and nerve terminals immunohistochemically in the anterior hypothalamus and external layer of the median eminence respectively in the hen. HPLC of hypothalamic extracts or chicken plasma extracts generally revealed one or more immunoreactive peak in addition to the one corresponding to chLHRH. These results confirm the existence of Glu^8 LHRH in the bird. The nature of the additional immunoreactive component is currently being investigated.

689 SOMATOSTATIN IN THE RAT GLOMERULUS: SECRETION AND FUNCTIONAL IMPLICATION.
S. Fujibayashi*, G. Aponte, T. Yamada and K. Kurokawa Medical and Research Servises, VA Wadsworth Medical Center and Dep. of Medicine, UCLA School of Medicine, Los Angeles, CA 90073, USA.

Increasing data indicate that somatostatin may modulate renal function. Studies in toad bladder revealed the presence of somatostatin in bladder epithelia and its modulating effect as a local hormone on vasopressin action. The present study was performed to investigate the role of somatostatin in mammalian kidney. In 4 μm kidney section, 4 to 5 somatostatin-containing cells were observed in each glomerulus, using avidin-biotin-peroxidase-conjugate. Somatostatin-containing cells were not found except in the glomerulus. Rat kidney extracts contained significant amount of somatostatin, measured by radioimmunoassay (360 ± 50 fM / kidney). Upon Sephadex G-50 column chromatography, somatostatin-like immunoreactivity in kidney extracts comigrated with authentic $somatostatin_{1-14}$. Further to determine a possible role of somatostatin, we examined factors affecting somatostatin release using a perifusion system of isolated glomeruli. A mixture of essential amino acids stimulated somatostatin release with 2.2-fold increase. In contrast, vasopressin, angiotensin II, epinephrine, and prostaglandin E_2 (PGE_2), agents known to act directly on the glomerulus, had no effect. Our studies showed the presence of somatostatin-containing paracrine cells in the glomerulus and stimulation of its release by amino acids. Since recent studies showed that amino acids cause glomerular hyperfiltration, and that somatostatin infusion inhibits the amino acid-induced hyperfiltration, these results suggest a possible link between somatostatin and amino acids in regulation of glomerular function.

690 CONTINUOUS INTRAVENOUS INFUSIONS OF GROWTH HORMONE-RELEASING FACTOR 1-44 NH_2 (GRF-44) IN NORMAL MEN: PITUITARY RESPONSES AND PHARMACOKINETICS.
M. C. Gelato*, O. Pescovitz, W. Nixon, R. D'Agata, F. Cassorla, D.L. Loriaux, and G.R. Merriam. DEB, NICHD, Bethesda, Md. 20205.

Bolus injections of GRF-44 stimulate a rapid release of GH in man. We compared these effects to those of continuous infusions of GRF-44 in normal men. Five resting, fasted subjects aged 24-32 received 1 μg/kg/h GRF-44 for 4h, followed immediately by a 1 μg/kg iv bolus. GRF plasma levels were measured by RIA, using an antiserum raised in rabbits to a GRF-BSA conjugate. GH levels were measured at 20 min intervals during a 2h baseline period, the 4h infusions, and for 3h after the bolus doses. During infusions, GRF levels averaged ~5 ng/ml, corresponding to a plasma metabolic clearance rate of ~350 L/day. GH levels rose progressively, reaching a maximum of 34 ± 13 (SE) ng/ml at ~80 min following the start of the infusions; this is similar to the peak value following a maximally effective bolus dose (1 μg/kg). GH concentrations then fell despite continued elevations in GRF levels. In some subjects there was a smaller second GH rise. The final bolus doses of GRF stimulated only a slight elevation of plasma GH (ΔGH 3.1 ± 1.8 ng/ml), a much lesser response than seen in subjects without prior infusions (33 ± 8 ng/ml). GH levels did, however, remain above basal values throughout the sampling period. Conclusions: GRF-44 is cleared relatively slowly from plasma. Peak responses to infusions are similar to those after bolus doses. The response is not sustained; later smaller peaks may represent either release of a second pool of GH or coincident endogenous secretion. The GH response to a GRF bolus is attenuated after GRF infusions. This could be due to receptor desensitization, counterregulation, or depletion of releasable GH stores.

691 GROWTH HORMONE RELEASING HORMONE 1-40-OH (GHRH) IS A PROLACTIN (PRL)-RELEASING FACTOR. J.A. Goldman*, M.E. Molitch, M.O. Thorner, J. Rivier, W. Vale, and S.R. Reichlin. Endocrine Division, Tufts-New England Medical Center, Boston, MA, University of Virginia School of Medicine, Charlottesville, VA and Neuropeptide Laboratory, Salk Institute, La Jolla, CA.

To determine the effect of GHRH on PRL secretion, we carried out single bolus and 6 hr infusions in 5 normal men. IV bolus(1.0 to 3.3 μg/kg) caused a small increase in PRL in 4 of 5 subjects (increment 0.9 to 4.6 ng/ml), but the differences from control were not significant by statistical test, (p>.05). Each subject was then infused with GHRH(10 ng/kg/hr) causing no change in PRL in 4 and a slight elevation in the fifth. At 5½ hours of infusion, each subject received a bolus injection of 3.3 μg/kg of GHRH. PRL rose from 6.1 ± .08 to 11.3 ± 2.0 ng/ml (mean ± SEM)(p<.05). Seven patients with active acromegaly were also studied, of whom two were hyperprolactinemic. After a bolus injection of 3.3 or 1.0 μg/kg of GHRH, mean PRL rose from 26.1 ± 8.3 to 33.1 ± 10.3 with a clear rise in each patient. This was a mean increase of 30.5 ± 5.3% (p<.01). The 2 hyperprolactinemic patients showed parallel changes in GH and PRL during both GHRH stimulation as well as spontaneous peaks. Summary and conclusions: 1.GHRH causes a small rise in serum prolactin when given as an IV bolus; 2.Continuous infusion of GHRH has no effect on serum prolactin but sensitizes the response to a GHRH injection; 3.GHRH raises serum prolactin in patients with acromegaly, and in those with associated hyperprolactinemia it may originate from the neoplastic tissue.

692 MORPHINE AND NOREPINEPHRINE MODULATION OF HYPOTHALAMIC UNIT RESPONSES TO MICROIONTOPHORETICALLY APPLIED LHRH AND MIF. S.A. Chepurnov, N.E. Chepurnova and G.K. Ketiladze, Faculty of Biology, Lomonosov Moscow State University, Moscow, USSR.

The effects of microiontophoretic application of LHRH and MIF, norepinephrine (NE) and morphine on the hypothalamic units activity (medial preoptic area) were studied in male rabbits. About 80% of all examined neurons responded to MIF and LHRH, mainly by facilitation (75% of responding neurons to MIF and 65% to LHRH). NE appeared to have inhibitory modulating action on MIF induced effects: when MIF was applied against the background of NE or during their simultaneous application the number of inhibitory responses increased. But NE decreased the number of inhibitory reactions of neurons to LHRH. Since the peptides effect might be mediated via opiate receptors, its action was examined against the background of morphine application. MIF and LHRH applied after morphine results in an increase of the number of nonresponsive units. During simultaneous application MIF and morphine, LHRH and morphine, the number of nonresponsive units increased to 54% and 30% respectively as compared with obtained during the application of the peptides only. The modulating actions of morphine were antagonized by i/v administration of naloxone. These results are consistent with the hypothesis that the opiate receptors and NE system play role in the central effects of MIF and LHRH. The corresponding of reactivity hypothalamic neurons of medial preoptic region to the responses amygdaloid neurons to these peptides (Chepurnov et al., 1980, IV Int. Congress Endocrinology, Melbourne, Abstr. p. 376) seems to imply that baso-lateral limbic circuit of brain may participate as sensitive component in the feedback control mechanisms of gonadotropins and melanotropin.

693 ANATOMICAL LOCALIZATION OF CORTICOTROPIN-RELEASING-FACTOR ACTIVITY (CRFa) IN THE HUMAN HYPOTHALAMUS. C.A. Favrod-Coune*, H. Langevin, R.C. Gaillard, M.C. Jacquier, W. Dolci and A.F. Muller, Department of Medicine, University Hospital, CH-1211 Geneva 4, Switzerland.

Understanding of the neuro-endocrine structures regulating the secretion of ACTH has markedly increased in the past few years, but data on the human being have remained relatively scarsed. We have measured the CRFa and vasopressin (VP) concentration in 12 areas of 8 hypothalami obtained from routine autopsies in a general hospital (Processing and dissection was performed according to a previously published technique, H. Langevin and L.L. Iversen, Brain 103 : 623-638 (1980)). CRFa was determined using perfused isolated rat anterior pituitary cells and measuring ACTH secretion. VP and ACTH were measured by radioimmunoassay. CRFa was found in all the areas and nuclei of the hypothalami. Paraventricular, supraoptic and infundibular nuclei had very similar high CRFa, while VP concentration differed strongly among them. In the other nuclei, CRFa was 2 to 5 times lower. VP concentration was low in all of them, except the anterior area, where, like in the median aminence, VP/CRFa ratio was 3 to 5 times higher than in the other areas. These results suggest that, in contrast to data obtained in animals by immunohistochemistry, CRFa is dispersed throughout the human hypothalamus. They show that our technique provides suitable material for the study of the biological activity of peptides in the human hypothalamus, thus allowing comparison with animal data and study of pathological conditions.

694 EVIDENCE THAT THE OVARIAN HORMONE RELAXIN PROMOTES LIVE BIRTHS IN THE RAT. Sandra J. Downing* and O. D. Sherwood, Department of Physiology and Biophysics, University of Illinois, Urbana, IL 61801, U.S.A.

Relaxin (R) reduces myometrial activity and induces cervical softening during pregnancy, and thus may be important for ensuring live births. The necessity for relaxin at parturition was studied by determining length of gestation, duration of delivery and fetal survival in four groups of pregnant rats. Gp C (n=8) intact control rats received vehicle injections daily from day 9 (D9). The rats were checked hourly for labor from 1200 h D22 and were observed continuously during delivery. Gp OPE (n=10) rats were ovariectomized on D9 and given progesterone (P) implants and daily estrogen (E) injections to mimic P and E levels of intact rats. The P implants were removed late on D21. Gp OPER (n=9) rats were treated as gp OPE but also received twice daily injections of highly purified porcine R to mimic R levels of intact rats. Gp OPR (n=8) rats were treated as gp OPER but did not receive E. For gp C rats, length of gestation was 535.4±2.1 h, duration of delivery was 94±18 min and fetal survival was 71.6±10.5%. Gestation was prolonged ($p<0.01$) in gps OPE (552.5±4.1 h) and OPR (551.0±5.3 h). Delivery was also prolonged in gp OPE (960 min) but not in gp OPR (140±36 min). Fetal survival was reduced ($p<0.001$) in gps OPE (0.7±0.7%) and OPR (13.8±10.5%). With combined R and E treatment (gp OPER), length of gestation (525.3±2.1 h), duration of delivery (128±29 min) and fetal survival (71.8±7.1%) were not different from controls. It is concluded that R in combination with E is probably important for ensuring normal parturition and a high incidence of live births in rats.

695 CLONING OF RAT PLACENTAL LACTOGEN (rPLII). M.L. Duckworth*, K. Kirk and H.G. Friesen, Dept. of Physiology, University of Manitoba, Winnipeg, Manitoba, Canada R3E OW3.

Two forms of placental lactogen are expressed in the rat: rPLI, molecular weight (M.W.) 40-50K, which peaks in serum at Day 12 of pregnancy, and rPLII, M.W. 22K, which peaks at Day 18 of pregnancy. Although human placental lactogen has been extensively studied, there is little information on the structure and regulation of the rPL gene(s). In order to facilitate our studies on rPLII, we have made a cDNA library from Day 18 placental mRNA, using the standard techniques of G-C tailing and cloning into the PstI site of plasmid pAT153. We have isolated a cDNA clone, pRP52A, which is 740 base pairs long, and whose sequence appears to represent approximately 0.5% of the clones in the library. Using hybrid select translation, we have shown that this clone codes for a protein approximately 25K M.W. which can be processed in vitro by dog pancreatic microsomes to a M.W. of 22K. Using a hybridot technique to analyse RNA isolated from different days of pregnancy we have shown that the transcription of the pRP52A gene is turned on rapidly at Day 12 of pregnancy and increases a further 3-4 fold up to Day 18. This corresponds to the initial appearance of low levels of rPLII in serum and placental tissue beginning Day 12. Northern blot analysis of the RNA shows hybridization to one band of approximately 930 nucleotides. Hybridization of pRP52A to cDNA clones of hPRL, hPL, rPRL and rGH at non-stringent conditions shows homology with rPRL and hPRL, but not rGH or hPL. This would suggest that unlike hPL, rPLII is more closely related to PRL than GH.

696 A NEW SUCCESSFUL TREATMENT FOR INFERTILE WOMEN WITH POLYCYSTIC OVARIAN SYNDROME. J.R.T. Coutts, M.P.R. Hamilton*, W.P. Black, M. Haxton and R. Fleming, Departments of Obstetrics and Gynaecology and Midwifvery*, University of Glasgow, Glasgow, Scotland, U.K.

Although many infertile women with oligomenorrhea associated with elevated LH and androgen levels (polycystic ovarian syndrome) ovulate on anti-estrogen therapy (e.g., clomiphene citrate) a significant percentage of such patients do not become pregnant despite long term clomiphene citrate therapy. Ovulation induction of this latter infertile group using exogenous gonadotrophins has shown poor success rates in terms of pregnancies and a high incidence of side effects (ovarian enlargement, etc.). In this study a new approach to the treatment of such long term clomiphene failures was adopted.

Six patients in whom ovulation induction using exogenous gonadotrophins alone had been tried without pregnancy were treated with a Gn-RH agonist (Hoe 766, Hoechst U.K. Ltd; 5 x 100 µg/day intranasally) to suppress their endogenous pituitary gonadotrophin release. While maintaining this pituitary suppression, follicle growth and ovulation were induced using conventional exogenous gonadotrophin regimens. Five patients conceived rapidly without the side effects of premature luteinisation and ovarian enlargement that were associated with their treatments without pituitary suppression. This combined therapy allows better and more successful clinical management of these infertile patients.

697 OVULATION INDUCTION WITH ENDOGENOUS GONADOTROPHIN SUPPRESSION IN INFERTILE WOMEN WITH NORMAL MENSTRUAL RHYTHM. R. Fleming, M.P.R. Hamilton*, M.C. Macnaughton and J.R.T. Coutts, Departments of Obstetrics and Gynaecology and *Midwifery, University of Glasgow, Glasgow, Scotland, U.K.

Infertile women with normal menstrual rhythm may show a number of ovarian hormone profile abnormalities on analyses of daily plasma samples; the most common of these abnormalities is poor progesterone (P) surge (deficient luteal phase). Treatment of this condition must recognise that the patient has active gonadotroph function. A Gn-RH analog (Hoe 766, Hoechst U.K. Ltd., 5 x 100 μg daily intranasally) has been used in these patienets to suppress endogenous LH and FSH concentrations and induce hypogonadotrophic hypogonadism. The Hoe 766 treatment was maintained through follicular growth and ovulation induction with exogenous gonadotrophins (HMG and HCG respectively). Assessment of follicular growth was monitored by daily plasma estradiol (E_2) analyses and appropriately timed ovarian ultrasonography. The aim was to achieve a follicular diameter (FD) of 20 mm in 1, 2 or 3 follicles prior to HCG administration. Seven of ten patients who had shown a poor P surge during their investigation cycles conceived on this treatment. Patients showing no hormonal abnormality (n = 4) have also been subjected to this treatment regime and so far none has conceived. These results show that the poor P surge is involved in the aetiology of infertility, and that this treatment is an effective method allowing greater clinical control of ovarian function than other regimens.

698 PROGESTERONE SECRETION IN OVULATORY CYCLES INDUCED BY PULSATILE LH-RH. S Franks*, H S Jacobs, J Adams, W P Mason and Z Van der Spuy, Department of Obstetrics and Gynaecology, St Mary's Hospital Medical School, London W2 1PG and The Middlesex Hospital, London W1 8AA.

The purpose of this study was to examine the function of the corpus luteum and its dependency on gonadotrophin support in women in whom ovulation (confirmed by ultrasound) was induced by pulsatile low dose LH-RH therapy. Data were analysed from 16 conception cycles (CC) and 20 ovulatory, non-conception cycles (NCC) induced by LH-RH delivered by a portable automatic pulsatile pump (NIMR, Mill Hill) at a dose of 15 μg every 90 minutes throughout the cycle. The mean length of the luteal phase (timed from the LH surge; day 0) was 13.4 ± 0.8 (SD) days in NCC. There was no difference in serum progesterone (P) levels between CC and NCC on any day up to day +8; thereafter there was the expected increase in P in CC. Follicular growth, as judged by ultrasound and serum oestradiol levels, was similar in NCC and CC. Peak P concentration in NCC was 53.4 ± 9.3 (SE) nmol/l. Serum concentrations of LH and FSH in the luteal phase of NCC were comparable with those in spontaneous ovulatory cycles despite continuation of LH-RH therapy every 90 minutes. In three NCC patients with normal follicular growth, LH-RH therapy was stopped 1, 3 and 5 days after ovulation. Serum P levels fell and menstruation occurred 2 days later in each case. These data demonstrate that 1) luteal function in LH-RH induced cycles is indistinguishable from that in spontaneous ovulatory cycles 2) progesterone concentrations in the early luteal phase are similar in CC and NCC 3) maintenance of the corpus luteum is dependent on gonadotrophin secretion until at least day 5 after ovulation.

699 MEASUREMENT OF FREE INSULIN IN SALIVA. Angela Fairney*, I. Godsland and V. Wynn, Departments of Chemical Pathology and Metabolism, St. Mary's Hospital Medical School, London W2 1PG U.K.

Methods for measuring free steroids in saliva are well established, but the lack of similar assays for peptide hormones has prevented the easy quantitation of free biologically active insulin in patients with diabetes melitus. An assay for insulin in saliva has been established by adapting a routine radioimmunoassay used for serum. The immuno reactive insulin detected in saliva has been studied by gel filtration on G 50 Sephadex and the elution profiles of ^{125}I insulin, insulin standard added to saliva, plasma insulin and immuno reactive insulin in saliva compared. Paired samples of saliva and plasma for insulin assay were also collected from patients during oral glucose tolerance tests and I.V Tolbutamide tests. The intra and interassay coefficients of variation for the salivary insulin assay were 12% or less and the lower limit of sensitivity was 4.2 uU/ml. The elution profiles of insulin added to saliva, plasma insulin and immuno reactive insulin in saliva coincided exactly with that of ^{125}I insulin, and there was a significant correlation of salivary insulin with plasma total insulin in the basal samples ($R = 0.63$, $p = 0.02$). However, on stimulation with glucose or Tolbutamide there was a variable response with a marked divergence of the values of the paired salivary and plasma insulin values in some patients. These studies show that insulin is present in saliva and suggest that salivary insulin estimations may be used to monitor free insulin concentrations in diabetic patients.

700 INSULIN RECEPTOR AND POSTRECEPTOR EFFECTS OF METFORMIN IN NON-INSULIN DEPENDENT DIABETES MELLITUS (NIDDM). I.G. Fantus and D. Zura, McGill University, Montreal, Quebec, Canada, H3A 2B2.

Metformin (M) is a biquanide oral hypoglycemic used in the treatment (Rx) of NIDDM. To define whether its glucose (G) lowering effects are mediated via alterations of insulin (I) receptors, oral glucose tolerance tests (OGTT) and insulin binding (IB) studies to monocytes were performed before and after 7 days of M Rx (2 G/day) in 10 subjects with poorly controlled NIDDM (fasting plasma glucose (FPG) >140 mg/dl). All subjects responded to Rx with a fall in G, fasting and throughout the OGTT (FPG, Mean ±SEM, 199±15 vs 158±16, Pre-M vs Post-M, $p < .001$) and no change in fasting serum I (FSI)(uU/ml) (15.7±2.4 vs 16.6±2.0, pre-M vs post-M) or in I response to G. When IB was examined 5 subjects (Group 1) had low IB and each had a >50% increase after M, while 5 subjects (Gp 2) had normal IB and <20% change. (% specific tracer IB/10^7 cells, Gp 1 pre-M vs post-M, 2.81±0.40 vs 5.79±1.13, $p<.02$: Gp 2 pre-M vs post-M, 5.84±0.52 vs 5.78±0.50, NS). However both Gps had similar lowering of G post-M (FPG, Gp 1 200±29 vs 155±32, $p<.02$; Gp 2 197±14 vs 162±13, $p<.02$) and no change in I. The increase in IB in Gp 1 was associated with an increase in receptor affinity and binding capacity and the % increase in IB correlated with the decrease in FPG ($r=0.866$, $p<.05$). There was a linear correlation between pre-M and post-M FPG for all 10 subjects described by the equation: Post-M FPG = pre-M FPG − 41($r=0.923$, $p < .001$). We conclude that 1)M acts predominantly at a postreceptor site to lower G, 2)this response is independent of pre-Rx IB status, 3)M Rx increases IB in subjects with NIDDM with low IB without altering I, and 4) the G lowering response to M may be predictable in most subjects with NIDDM.

701 MANAGEMENT OF PREGNANT INSULIN DEPENDENT DIABETES MELLITUS (IDDM) PATIENTS BY CONVENTIONAL THERAPY, SELF-MONITORING AND SUBCUTANEOUS INSULIN INFUSION PUMP. D. Feldberg*, J. Goldman, D. Dicker, N. Samuel, M. Karp and G. Faiman, Dept. of Obstetrics and Gynecology, Hasharon Hospital, and Institute of Adolescent Endocrinology, Beilinson Medical Center, Petah-Tiqva, Israel.

The importance of strict diabetic control in pregnant insulin-dependent patients is well documented. Three groups of diabetic pregnant patients and a control group were compared during the years 1975-1983: a) Group I - 20 women managed by "conventional" insulin therapy. Mean blood glucose was 148 $\pm$ 23 mg%. Five patients (25%) developed PIH and 3 had IUGR (15%). Fifteen (75%) delivered by C/S. Mean birth weight of neonates was 3723$\pm$162 g, and 10 (50%) developed neonatal hypoglycemia. Groups II and III included 36 patients managed by self blood glucose monitoring (SBGM) and by means of subcutaneous insulin infusion pumps (SIIP). Parameters for diabetic control were mean blood glucose, glycosylated Hb, M value, MAGE and C-peptide. b) Group II - 25 patients treated by SBGM. Mean blood glucose was 121$\pm$18 mg%. Three women (12%) developed PIH. Ten women (40%) were delivered by C/S. Mean birth weight of neonates was 3431$\pm$176 g, and 4 (16%) developed hypoglycemia. c) Group III - 11 highly selected, severe, type I (juvenile) diabetic patients treated by SIIP. Mean glucose values were 106$\pm$11 mg%. Three women (27%) developed PIH. Five patients (45%) delivered by C/S. Mean birth weight was 3216$\pm$161 g, and no hypoglycemia occurred. d) Group IV - control group of 20 nondiabetic pregnant women. No congenital malformations were observed in Groups II-III. SBGM with SIIP is an excellent method of management of diabetic pregnant women in selected cases.

702 Preparation and Biological Activity of Amino-Terminal Semisynthetic Derivatives of Glucagon. K.C. Flanders* and R.S. Gurd, Medical Sciences Program and Dept. of Chemistry, Indiana University, Bloomington, IN 47405, USA.

His-1 of glucagon is necessary for the full expression of hormone binding to hepatic receptors and activation of adenylate cyclase. To assess the importance of the imidazole ring, this His was replaced with Ala or Phe. This was accomplished by N-hydroxysuccinimide-active-ester couplings of the N^{α}-t-butyloxycarbonyl amino acids to (des-His^1)N^{ε}-acetimidoglucagon. The reactions were performed in dimethylformamide in the presence of 1-hydroxybenzotriazole. The deprotected products were purified to homogeneity by cation-exchange chromatography. To demonstrate that this semisynthetic strategy can yield a peptide with full biological activity, N^{ε}-acetimidoglucagon was regenerated from the (des-His^1)analog. Both the original and regenerated N^{ε}-acetimidoglucagons were equipotent with native glucagon with respect to receptor binding affinity and biological potency. (Phe^1)-, (Ala^1)-, and (des-His^1)N^{ε}-acetimidoglucagons were all partial agonists achieving 85, 55, and 35%, respectively, of the maximal adenylate cyclase stimulatory activity exhibited by N^{ε}-acetimidoglucagon. By contrast, the concentrations of these analogs required for half-maximal activation of adenylate cyclase were 27, 2, and 6%, respectively, of that for N^{ε}-acetimidoglucagon. Each derivative also showed a similar decrease in binding affinity, as assessed by the displacement of [^{125}I]glucagon from rat liver plasma membranes. This suggests that the decreased biological potencies of the analogs resulted from decreased receptor affinity. These results indicate that the aromatic nature and hydrogen bonding capability of the imidazole ring of His-1 are necessary for full expression of glucagon binding and transduction. (Supported by USPHS Grants AM-21121 and HL-14680).

703 PROPOSED CRITERIA FOR THE SCREENING AND THE DIAGNOSIS OF GESTATIONAL DIABETES ADAPTED FOR EACH TRIMESTER OF PREGNANCY.

J.C. Forest,* J. Alain, Maria Garrido-Russo, A. Bédard, G. Hamel, A. Lemay, J.L. Dubé, Dept. of Medical Biochemistry, Medicine and Obstet.-Gynecol., Hôpital Saint-François-d'Assise, Québec G1L 3L5, Canada.

So far little information has been published concerning the establishment of reference values for an optimal screening test and the Oral Glucose Tolerance Test (OGTT) at each trimester of pregnancy that would take into account the physiologic changes in the glucoregulation. We have established reference values for OGTT in a group of 200 normal pregnant women. Fasting serum glucose did not differ significantly between the trimesters. The values at 60 and 120 min were significantly different for the 5th, 50th and 95th percentiles between each trimester. For the 180 min readings those of the third trimester were significantly higher than those of the other trimesters. The interpretation of OGTT must therefore take into account the time of pregnancy. As screening test, glycemia 1 h post ingestion of 50 g of glucose was compared to glycemia 1 h post 100 g glucose in terms of sensitivity and specificity at each trimester (N = 1212) using our reference values for the diagnosis of gestational diabetes. Screening for gestational diabetes was found to be superior with the 100 g glucose loading dose. When a cut off value of 7.7 mmol/L (140 mg/dl) was used for the 1 h glycemia, overall sensitivity was found to be 100% and the specificity 55%. A new screening and diagnostic protocol is proposed using the 100 g-OGTT. If the 1 h glycemia value is less than 7.7 mmol/L the test is terminated. If glycemia is above that value, OGTT is continued on a three hour period and reference values of the appropriate trimester are used for the diagnosis of gestational diabetes.

704 LOWER PREVALENCE OF DIABETES AND POLYCYSTIC OVARIES AMONG FORMER COLLEGE ATHLETES COMPARED TO NON-ATHLETES.

R.E. Frisch,* G. Wyshak, N.L. Albright, T.E. Albright and I. Schiff, Harvard Center for Population Studies, 9 Bow Street, Cambridge, MA 02138, U.S.A.

The prevalence (lifetime occurrence) of diabetes, and independently, polycystic ovary disease (PCO), among athletic women compared to comparable non-athletic women has not been reported heretofore, as far as we know. We report the prevalence of diabetes, and PCO among 5,400 college alumnae, 2,622 former college athletes and 2,778 non-athletes (controls), ranging in age from 21 to 80 yr. Data are from a self-administered, detailed questionnaire on medical and reproductive histories, physical characteristics, diet and activity. Of the athletic alumnae, 83% had begun training in high school or earlier, compared to 25% of the controls. The prevalence of diabetes for the total sample is one percent (52/5400); the prevalence of PCO is also one percent (55/5400). The athletes had a significantly lower prevalence of diabetes 0.6% (15/2,622) compared to that of the controls, 1.3%, (37/2,778), RR=2.3, $P < 0.01$, although athletes and controls had similar percentages of family history of diabetes, 13.6% and 12.8% respectively. The athletes also had a significantly lower prevalence of PCO, 0.5% (12/2,622) compared to that of the controls 1.5% (43/2,778) RR=3.4, $P < 0.01$. Among the athletes and controls with PCO, 25% (3/12) and 26% (11/43), respectively had a family history of diabetes. The athletes were leaner than the controls at all ages up to 70 yr. We conclude that women with long term athletic training are significantly less at risk of diabetes and, independently, of PCO. This research was supported by the Advanced Medical Research Foundation.

705 LACK OF A-CELL HYPERRESPONSIVENESS IN THE EARLY PHASE OF TYPE I DIABETES.
O.P. Ganda*, S. Srikanta, R.E. Gleason, J.S. Soeldner and G.S. Eisenbarth, Joslin Diabetes Center, Boston, Mass., U.S.A.

The essentiality of glucagon in the pathogenesis of diabetes (DM) remains a controversial issue. We have previously demonstrated a selective loss of insulin release in response to IV glucose which progresses over years and precedes overt type I DM. In six pre-type I diabetics (age 10-26 yr), each having anti-islet antibodies and/or elevated Ia+ T cells, we studied glucagon release in response (Unger's 30K antibody) to IV arginine (460 mg/kg over 40 min) and to oral glucose (100 g) at a time of impaired (n=5) or normal (n=1) oral glucose tolerance. The first-phase insulin release to IV glucose was absent in each subject. The glucagon (pg/ml) responses to arginine were as follows:-

								Normals*	
Patient #	1	2	3	4	5	6	Mean$\pm$SE	(Mean$\pm$SE)	p
Basal	0	5	0	0	15	45	11$\pm$7.2	30$\pm$4.9	ns
Peak	110	120	120	210	190	220	162$\pm$20.6	301$\pm$17.2	<.01

* n=30; Age range, 24-69 yr.

The glucagon nadir after oral glucose studied in 3 patients (#1,3,4) was completely suppressed to 0 in each. Thus, in individuals prior to complete B-cell destruction, a diminished rather than an exaggerated A-cell secretory response was observed. The hyperglucagonemia of overt type I DM is most likely the consequence of complete B-cell destruction, whereas the diminished glucagon release in the pre-type I diabetic phase may be secondary to "insulitis" which occurs prior to total B-cell loss.

706 CHRONIC ADMINISTRATION OF DEHYDROEPIANDROSTERONE REDUCES PANCREATIC B-CELL HYPERPLASIA AND HYPERINSULINEMIA IN GENETICALLY OBESE RATS. T.S. Gansler*, S. Muller†, and M.P. Cleary°, *Dept. of Path. & Lab. Medicine, Univ. of Penn., Phila., Pa., †Dept. of Nutrition & Food Sciences, Drexel Univ., Phila., Pa., and °The Hormel Institute, Univ. of Minn., Austin, MN, USA.

The Zucker obese (fa/fa) rat is a model of hypertrophic/hyperplastic obesity. These rats develop marked hyperinsulinemia, insulin resistance, and pancreatic B-cell hyperplasia. In the present study, chronic (20 weeks) administration of the 17-ketosteroid, dehydroepiandrosterone (DHEA), to obese Zucker rats significantly ($p<0.05$) decreased body weight by 37%, combined retroperitoneal and parametrial fat pad weight by 40%, serum insulin concentration by 80% and pancreatic insulin content by 36%. Morphometric examination of pancreatic islets revealed that DHEA treatment reduced the median cross-sectional islet diameter by 12% ($p<0.05$) and caused a shift in the islet size histogram toward an increased proportion of small (diameter <200 μm) islets. DHEA treatment also prevented development of the histopathologic changes usually seen in obese Zucker rats (loss of trabecular islet architecture, proliferation of fibrous tissue, presence of intra-islet ductules, and B-cell degranulation). DHEA treatment of lean Zucker rats also reduced ($p<0.05$) body weight, fat depot weight, islet size and pancreatic insulin content without significant changes in serum insulin concentration. These data indicate that DHEA treatment inhibits insulin release and B-cell proliferation. Whether this is due to a direct effect on the pancreas or to improvement of peripheral insulin sensitivity remains to be determined.
(Supported by the Hormel Inst., NIH, and the American Heart Association)

707 IMPORTANCE OF PRE-ADRENALECTOMY LEVEL OF INSULIN(PALI) IN HORMONAL RESPONSE TO ADRENALECTOMY IN DOGS. C. Gauthier*, M. Vranic and H.L.A. Lickley, Departments of Physiology, Surgery and Medicine, University of Toronto and Women's College Hospital, Toronto, Ontario, Canada.

We studied the effects of adrenalectomy on insulin(IRI) and counter-regulatory hormone secretion and glucose kinetics before and during the infusion of cortisol and/or epinephrine to re-establish physiological levels. Eighteen hrs after the last iv injection of hydrocortisone sodium succinate plasma cortisol and epinephrine were undetectable,glucose production,clearance and concentration were normal and norepinephrine levels doubled($p<.02$). Three distinct patterns were observed: Dogs with a PALI smaller than 7 mU/L responded with a larger than 40 pg/ml increase in glucagon(IRG) but no change in IRI. A 40±3 pg/ml increase in IRG with no change in IRI was observed for PALI between 7-12 mU/L. The IRI and IRG levels fell in the animals with a PALI higher than 12 mU/L following adrenalectomy,the drop in IRI being 10 times that of IRG on a molar basis.A 4-hr infusion of cortisol re-established a circulating level of 2.2±.1 µg/dl and returned IRG to its pre-adrenalectomy(PA) level of 127±29 pg/ml.Glucose production and clearance declined by 25±11%($p<.05$) with no change in IRI. A 90-min infusion of epinephrine re-established normal levels of 113±6 pg/ml with no change in glucose kinetics. The simultaneous infusion of cortisol and epinephrine increased plasma IRI by 30±12%($p<.05$),though glucose kinetics again did not change. Conclusions:(1) PALI sets the direction and magnitude of changes in insulin and glucagon which compensate for the lack of adrenal hormones, maintaining normal glucoregulation. (2) The infusion of cortisol at its basal secretion rate returns glucagon to its PA level and (3) the simultaneous infusion of cortisol and epinephrine returns insulin to its PA level.

708 DEPRESSED GLUCOSE UTILIZATION AND REDUCED PLASMA INSULIN DURING PROLONGED EUGLYCEMIC CLAMP. S. S. P. Gebhart*, J. R. Brennan, W. G. Blackard, Department of Medicine, Medical College of Virginia, Richmond, Virginia, U.S.A.

Exogenous insulin administered as a bolus or as a primed infusion has been shown to suppress endogenous insulin release. This study demonstrated that at low insulin infusion rates with blood glucose maintained slightly above fasting values, plasma insulin levels fell out of proportion to C-peptide levels. Six healthy volunteers were subjected to a euglycemic clamp (Biostator clamp algorithm) for 16 hours. The blood glucose was maintained at 94 mg/dl and regular insulin was infused at a rate of 2 mU/kg/min. The plasma insulin level achieved was variable but the pattern of glucose utilization, plasma insulin and plasma C-peptide were consistently altered in all subjects. Although dextrose utilization (mg/kg/min) was 15% higher during hour 2 & 3 of the infusion than during the initial control hour, utilization had returned to baseline by hour 4 and decreased to 30% below the first hour's utilization by hour 6 through 16. Plasma insulin levels showed a similar progressive decrease, falling 20 to 40% despite maintenance of baseline C-peptide levels. Erythrocyte insulin receptors were not down-regulated after the 16 hour insulin infusion. The decreased dextrose utilization found in this study during a prolonged euglycemic insulin clamp appeared to be the result of lowered insulin levels, suggesting either increased insulin clearance or defective endogenous insulin release.

709 CORRELATIONS BETWEEN HUMORAL AND CELLULAR IMMUNE RESPONSES TO INSULIN (I) TREATMENT (Rx) AND METABOLIC CONTROL IN DIABETES MELLITUS (DM).
J.Goldman*, D. Ownby, R. Vukmirovich and J. McCullough, Department of Medicine, Henry Ford Hospital, Detroit, MI 48202, U.S.A.

Treatment of DM with animal I's frequently results in humoral and/or cellular immunity to I. To determine whether these two types of immune responses are correlated to each other and/or to the degree of metabolic control, we have studied 10 subjects with DM type 2 and 6 subjects with DM type 1. Humoral responses to I Rx were assessed by measurement of I antibody (Ab) (high and low affinity classes) binding affinities (K_1,K_2) and capacities (C_1,C_2,C_{total}) with beef (B) and pork (P) I. Cellular immunity to I was assessed by ^{3}H-thymidine uptake (TU) of peripheral mononuclear cells cultured with B and P I for 5,7 and 9 days. TU was expressed as the ratio of maximal insulin stimulated over control TU. Metabolic control was assessed by the level of stable, total glycosylated hemoglobin (GHgb). Significant linear correlations were found between B TU and B K_1 (high affinity I Ab) in DM type 1 (r=0.82, p=0.04), and P TU and P K_1 r=0.51, p=0.04) in the overall group of patients. Otherwise, there appear to be no significant correlations between P and B TU, K_2, C_1,C_2,C_{total} and GHgb. The data suggest that cellular immunity to I Rx may correlate with the affinity of high affinity I antibodies, a molecular species similar to the antigen specific surface receptors of regulatory T lymphocytes involved in both cellular and humoral immune responses to heterologous antigens.

710 **PEPTIDE INHIBITION OF INSULIN DEGRADING ENZYME.**
E.E. Gordon*, and J. Wilson, Methodist Hospital and Indiana University Medical School, Indianapolis, IN 46206 (U.S.A.)

Insulin degrading activity (IDA) released from isolated tubules and slices of rat renal cortex exhibits the characteristics of a sulfhydryl enzyme with a Km of 8.6×10^{-8}M and a specific activity of 3.56 ± 0.32 fmoles insulin degraded/µg protein/20 min. Addition of bovine serum albumin (BSA) to the assay medium results in a concentration dependent inhibition of ^{125}I-insulin conversion to trichloracetic acid (TCA) soluble ^{125}I labeled fragments with a Ki of 5.6×10^{-5}M. When 10^{-3}M to 10^{-11}M ^{125}I-albumin is incubated with the enzyme preparation, there is no breakdown of the albumin as determined by the release of radioactivity into the TCA soluble fraction. When 10^{-3}M to 10^{-11}M azoalbumin is incubated with the enzyme preparation, there is no release of dye into the TCA soluble fraction as determined by absorption at 440 nm. However, incubation of either ^{125}I-albumin or azoalbumin with 100 µg trypsin/ml results in appreciable albumin degradation. The specificity of the BSA effect on IDA was determined by examining the inhibitory effect of a series of proteins on IDA. At equimolar concentrations, the inhibitory activity of human serum albumin > α casein > γ globulin > α globulin > BSA > sheep serum albumin > porcine serum albumin > protamine > ovalbumin. In summary, the IDA released from rat renal cortex does not degrade, but is inhibited by BSA; this characteristic is shared by a number of other peptides. These findings suggest that the soluble IDA of tissues may be regulated (inhibited) by the high intracellular protein concentration.

711 TISSUE-SPECIFIC REGULATION OF RAT LIVER MALIC ENZYME mRNA BY TRIIODOTHYRONINE (T_3) AND DIET: A HYBRIDIZATION ANALYSIS.

B. Dozin, M.A. Magnuson, and V.M. Nikodem*, NIADDK, NIH, Bethesda, MD, USA 20205.

The cytoplasmic level of the rat liver malic enzyme (ME) activity is modulated by T_3 and diet. Using the ME cDNA recently cloned in our laboratory, hybridization experiments were carried out to quantitate the induction of ME mRNA. Normal rats were injected daily with T_3 (15 µg/100 g B.W., i. p.) or kept on high carbohydrate diet (CHO) for 10 consecutive days. Hybridization of $[^{32}P]$ labeled ME cDNA with poly$(A)^+$ RNA derived from normal and induced livers showed an increase in the ME mRNA concentration by 11 and 7 fold above the basal level in T_3 and CHO treated rats, respectively. ME activity was increased to the same degree. After a single injection of T_3 (200 µg/100 g B.W., i.p.) there was a lag period of 6 hr before ME activity and ME mRNA rose reaching a maximal induction at 48 hr (9 and 16 fold above the basal level, respectively). Northern analysis of poly$(A)^+$ RNA prepared from T_3 treated rats revealed two hybridizable mRNAs for ME (2,700 and 4,500 nucleotides, respectively). When these two mRNAs were separated on an agarose gel and then used to direct protein synthesis by *in vitro* translation, products corresponding to the full size of ME were detected. Southern analysis of genomic DNA suggests that both ME mRNAs are transcribed from a single gene. Although ME activity and ME mRNA were found in other tissues (brain, kidney, spleen, heart, testis and lung) the induction by T_3 was observed in none of them but liver. These quantitative hybridization data provide direct evidence for tissue-specific regulation of ME at a pretranslational level.

712 GIP AND PANCREATIC GLUCAGON ARE cAMP-INDUCING HORMONES IN THE HUMAN GASTRIC CANCER CELL LINE HGT-1

Shahin EMAMI, Anne-M. Lhiaubet and Christian GESPACH, INSERM U.55, Hôpital Saint-Antoine, 75012 Paris, France.

Gastric Inhibitory Peptide: GIP (EC_{50}=8x10^{-9} M, 5-fold stimulation), pancreatic glucagon (EC_{50}=1.7x10^{-8} M, 17-fold) and porcine or chicken Vasoactive Intestinal Peptide: VIP (EC_{50}=2.5x10^{-9} M, 14-fold) are shown to activate the cAMP generating system in HGT-1 cells. The three hormones interact on distinct receptor sites, as shown by combinations of GIP, glucagon and VIP or by selective disappearance of receptor activities after long-term culture (6 days) of HGT-1 cells with the hormones. Other peptides structurally related to the secretin-glucagon family (somatostatin-14 Growth hormone Releasing Factor: GRF), to neurotensin (pancreatic polypeptide and the peptide having N-terminal tyrosine and C-terminal tyrosine: PYY), or to gastrin (cholecystokinin) are either ineffective or very weak agonist (GRF). GIP or pancreatic glucagon are ineffective on the human colonic cell line HT-29, indicating the gastric specificity of the effect of GIP and glucagon in transformed gut epithelial cells. This implies that GIP and (pancreatic-entero) glucagon peptides interact directly on distinct receptor sites in human gastric cells and that these hormones could regulate gastric secretion directly. These properties account for the enterogastrone activity of GIP and indicate that the secretion of somatostatin (an inhibitor of acid secretion) by the gastric D-cells could be regulated by GIP *via* a cAMP-dependent mechanism.

713 EFFECTS OF MICROCOCCAL NUCLEASE AND TRYPSIN ON THE RELEASE OF ANDROGEN RECEPTORS COVALENTLY BOUND TO THE CHROMATIN OF RAT PROSTATES. J.A.Foekens*, P.S.Rennie, H.Cheng and N. Bruchovsky, Cancer Control Agency of B.C., 2656 Heather Street, Vancouver, British Columbia, Canada, V5Z 3J3.

To isolate the chromatin acceptor sites for androgen receptors, experiments were performed involving fixation of androgen receptors to chromatin in situ with 0.5% (w/v) formaldehyde for 1 h at 4°C in 50 mM TES-buffer (pH 8.0). The fixed chromatin was centrifuged at 20,000xg for 15 min, suspended by brief sonication in 50 mM Tris-buffer (pH 8.0), made to 0.6 M NaCl, and labelled by isotope-exchange assay with ^{3}H-dihydrotestosterone for 20 h at 4°C. Analysis with CaCl gradients revealed specific binding in the chromatin density regions, whereas no peak of radioactivity corresponding to free androgen-receptor complexes was observed after glycerol gradient centrifugation. Extensive digestion of chromatin with micrococcal nuclease immediately after fixation resulted in the appearance of a small amount of 3s androgen receptor in the glycerol gradients. However when nuclease digestion was followed by mild digestion with trypsin (10 µg/ml , 1 h at 20°C) all of the bound radioactivity (approximately 13,000 molecules/nucleus) was recovered as 3s androgen-receptor complexes. After trypsin treatment alone, specific binding was associated with 3s androgen receptors and with several more rapidly sedimenting forms. Since androgen receptors can be fixed to prostatic chromatin in situ, and largely released by trypsin, we conclude that peptide linkages are required to maintain the structural integrity of the chromatin acceptor site. (Supported by the National Cancer Institute of Canada).

714 INFLUENCE OF PROLONGED HYPOTHYROIDISM ON SYNTHESIS OF SPECIFIC PROTEINS IN CARDIAC AND SOLEUS MUSCLES OF THE RAT. J. Gagnon*, M.A. Ho-kim, P.A. Rogers and R.R. Tremblay, Dept. of Medicine & LABSAP, Laval Un., Qué.,Can.

Changes in thyroid hormone levels are known to affect the physiological properties of both cardiac and skeletal muscles; these modifications in contractility and/or velocity of shortening have been correlated with protein muscle composition. To further elucidate the relationship between chronic hypothyroidism and protein synthesis in both cardiac and skeletal muscles, surgical thyroidectomy (TH-X) was performed in male Sprague-dawley rats. Six months later, polyribosomes were isolated from heart and soleus muscles of TH-X and normal age-matched control (N) rats and subsequently translated in mRNA-dependent rabbit reticulocyte lysates. The [^{35}S] methionine-labelled "in vitro" synthesized polypeptides were resolved by fluorography after two-dimensionnal electrophoresis. These were compared to fractionated soluble enzyme and high salt extractable peptide counterparts from the corresponding TH-X and N rat tissues. Compared to the actual "in vivo" peptide composition, an increase in the template activity of a mRNA coding for a 30K dalton polypeptide was observed when isolated from TH-X rat soleus. This polypeptide was tentatively identified as phosphoglycerate mutase by reference to proteins markers. Furthermore, polyribosomes from TH-X rat heart directed to a greater extent the synthesis of a 55K dalton mRNA believed to code for β-desmin. These results indicate that long term TH-X exerts a selective effect on the template activity of a limited number of specific mRNAs in muscle tissue. This study was supported by MRC and FCAC.

715 EFFECT OF STEROID HORMONES ON cAMP PRODUCTION AND β ADRENERGIC RECEPTOR CONCENTRATION IN SMOOTH MUSCLE CELLS GROWN IN CULTURE.

S. Gallant* and J.F. Moran, Departments of Pathology and Biochemistry, School of Medicine, State University of New York at Buffalo, N.Y. USA

The catecholamines isoproterenol, epinephrine, and norepinephrine stimulate, in a dose-dependent manner, cAMP accumulation in rat aortic smooth muscle cells in culture. The increment in cAMP is blocked by propranolol. The order of potency observed is Iso > Epi >> Norepi which is suggestive of β2 adrenergic receptor activity. Incubation of cultures with corticosterone induces a marked potentiation (151±1.1 vs 377±3.6 p mol/mg protein) of catecholamine mediated increases in cAMP accumulation. The potentiation by corticosterone is observed after a lag phase of several hours and is near maximum at 24 hours. The effect is dose-dependent, with an ED_{50} of approximately $5x10^{-8}$M, and both the sensitivity and maximum response to catecholamines are increased. Deoxycorticosterone also effectively potentiates catecholamine increases in cAMP. Progesterone and estradiol are less effective while aldosterone, 18-OH-DOC and testosterone are without apparent effect. Smooth muscle cells exposed to 1 μM corticosterone for 24 hrs exhibited a greater than 2-fold increase in the number of β adrenergic receptors (83 vs 184 f mol/mg protein) as determined by Scatchard analyses of $[^{125}I]$ L-cyanopindolol binding to plasma membrane preparations. The apparent Kd (5 pM) was not significantly altered by steroid treatment. The results demonstrate that steroids modulate vascular smooth muscle cAMP production brought about by catecholamines and that the mechanism of this potentiation, at least in part, can be explained by an increase in the number of β adrenergic receptors. (Supported by NIH Grant HL 25256)

716 HOMOLOGOUS DESENSITIZATION OF VIP AND HISTAMINE H_2 RECEPTORS IN THE HUMAN GASTRIC CANCER CELL LINE HGT-1

Christian Gespach, Shahin Emami, Claudine Boissard and Gabriel Rosselin. Unité INSERM U.55, Hôpital Saint-Antoine, 75012 Paris, France

Desensitization (the loss of drug or hormone response after exposure of cells to those agents) has been demonstrated for a variety of ligands including glucagon, insulin, TSH, LH, FSH, prostaglandins, opiates, catecholamines and carbachol. Up to now, there are no data available for such mechanism after Vasoactive Intestinal Peptide (VIP) or histamine. 1) HGT-1 cells which possess both VIP and histamine H_2 receptors similar to those evidenced in human gastric glands is therefore a suitable model for this study. Cultured HGT-1 cells were incubated at 37°C in MEM medium, during one hour, in absence (controls) or in presence of VIP (10^{-7} M) or histamine (10^{-3} M). Then this medium was eliminated and the cells were washed in the culture flask with PBS (x 2), harvested after EDTA treatment and washed again (x 4) in KRP buffer. VIP or histamine H_2 receptor activity was then evaluated by measuring cAMP generation in HGT-1 cells incubated with IBMX (1 mM) and 1% BSA. 2) VIP treatment resulted in a considerable decline of the subsequent cAMP generation capacity after VIP (10^{-10}-10^{-7}M), while the histamine effect (10^{-7}-10^{-3}M) remains unchanged. Histamine treatment resulted nearly in a complete loss of the cAMP response to histamine, while the potency and the efficacy of VIP was not affected. 3) Our data indicate for the first time that short-term exposure of HGT-1 cells to VIP or histamine results in homologous desensitization of VIP or histamine H_2 receptor activity. This phenomenom could be involved in the physiological regulation and pharmacological control of the gut epithelial cell function.

717 A NEW REGULATORY PROTEIN FOR ADENYLATE CYCLASE?

John C. Gordon and Melvin Blecher*, Department of Biochemistry, Georgetown Univ. Med. Ctr., Washington, D.C. 20007 (USA).

We have identified in water-soluble extracts of rat liver and cloned RL-PR-C rat hepatocytes a protein factor that markedly enhances basal, isoproterenol-activated, and cholera toxin (CT)-activated adenylate cyclase (AC) of rigorously-washed hepatocyte plasma membranes (PM), in the absence of exogenous GTP, and using GTP-free ATP in the AC assay. The protein factor (Mr=35,000) has been purified about 250-fold from crude liver cytosol by sequential gel filtration and ion exchange chromatographies. As the factor, cooperatively with GTP, greatly enhanced the ability of CT to ADP-ribosylate (from ^{32}P-NAD) the 46K and 48K subunits of the guanine nucleotide regulatory protein (G-protein) of the AC complex, its is likely that this is the site of action of the new factor. As the factor did not bind detectable amounts of added ^{3}H-GTP, it is unlikely to be a GTP reservoir; it also did not shift the GTP dose-effect curves in several AC activation systems. As the factor was uninfluenced by Ca^{++} and EGTA, and because of its size, it is unlikely to be calmodulin. Other experiments suggest that the factor is lost from PM to the washings during the typical preparation of "clean" PM. We postulate that the factor is a peripheral PM protein, probably contiguous to the G-protein, that is a member of the family of regulatory proteins for hepatic AC. Supported by a B.R.S.G. from the University.

718 HORMONE SENSITIVE REDOX SYSTEMS IN PLASMA MEMBRANE. C. Grebing*, H. Löw, and F.L. Crane, Dept. of Endocrinology and Metabolism, Karolinska Institute, Stockholm, Sweden, and Dept. of Biological Sciences, Purdue University, W. Lafayette, Indiana, USA.

A hormone sensitive, protontranslocating transmembranous NADH-dehydrogenase has been found in the plasma membrane from rat hepatocytes, adipocytes and human erythrocytes. The present results represent experiments with isolated rat adipocytes. The plasma membrane potential (ψ_p) was estimated from the distribution of the lipophilic cation triphenylmethylphosphoniumion ($TPMP^+$) in the presence of selective mitochondrial inhibitors. The cellular ATP content was determined simultaneously with ψ_p. The Na^+/K^+-ATP-ase inhibitor, ouabain, was without effect on ψ_p. However, a pronounced depolarization was observed in the presence of the H^+/Na^+-ATP--ase inhibitor amiloride and the H^+/K^+-ATP-ase inhibitor omeprazol. The protonophoric uncoupler, FCCP, resulted in a ψ_p of approximately zero. Ionophores, exchanging H^+ with Na^+ or K^+, (monensin and nigericin), resulted in a pronounced hyperpolarization. Glucagon and noradrenalin had an effect resembling that of the protonophores, i.e. a marked depolorization. The hyperpolarization caused by insulin, previously reported by Cheng et al (J Biol Chem 256, 649, 1981) was slight and mainly dependent on the glucose concentration. The results suggest a contribution of protontranslocating ATP-ases to ψ_p. These ATP-ases together with the transmembranous dehydrogenase might function in the protonization of the plasma membrane. The energy conserved in such a gradient could be used for transport of cations, glucose and amino acids. The mechanism of hormone action at the cell surface would be to modify the proton movement in the plasma membrane. Supported by the Swedish Medical Research Council and the Wenner-Gren Foundation.

719 INTERACTIONS OF ANGIOTENSIN II (AII) RECEPTORS WITH CATIONS, GUANYL NUCLEOTIDE (GN) BINDING PROTEIN AND ADENYLATE CYCLASE (AC) IN THE ADRENAL GLOMERULOSA CELL.

J. P. Harwood*, G. Aguilera, C. Grewe and K. J. Catt, ERRB, NICHD, NIH, Bethesda, MD; and FDA, Washington, D.C., U.S.A.

Although the action of AII on aldosterone production is calcium-mediated and independent of cAMP, the ability of GN to reduce AII binding suggests a relationship between the AII receptor and AC in the adrenal glomerulosa cell. We therefore analyzed the effects of cations and GN on receptor binding of AII agonist and antagonist analogs, and the effects of AII agonists on AC activity in rat adrenal glomerulosa. Binding affinity for ^{125}I-AII was increased 20-fold by 140 mM Na, 5 mM Mg, or 5 mM Ca. These cations reduced receptor binding of the antagonist ^{125}I-[Sar^1,Ala^8]AII, and also that of the superagonist ^{125}I-[Sar^1]AII, with potency ratio Na>Ca>Mg. Addition of 0.1 mM Gpp(NH)p reduced AII binding by 20% in the absence of cations, by 35% with Na or Mg alone, and by 60% with Na plus Mg. In contrast, Gpp(NH)p did not inhibit binding of [Sar^1,Ala^8]AII or [Sar^1]AII in the absence of cations or with Na alone, but caused 40% inhibition with Na plus Mg. When the effects of AII on AC were evaluated by direct enzyme assay, by cellular cAMP production, and by [^{3}H]adenosine prelabeling, only a slight inhibition of basal and ACTH-stimulated activity was observed. These data indicate the importance of cations in the GN inhibition of AII binding, and show that the differential effects of cations and GN on AII analog binding are more related to the [Sar^1] residue than to the agonist/antagonist properties of the peptides. We suggest that the GN binding protein that is functionally associated with the AII receptor may mediate AII action by mechanism(s) other than its inhibitory effect on the AC system.

720 FAMILIAL HOMOZYGOUS HYPERCHOLESTEROLEMIA(FHH): EFFECTS OF CONTINUOUS INTRAGASTRIC FEEDING(CIF).

D. Daneman*, E. Regelink, V. Rose, Dept. of Pediatrics, U. of Toronto, Hosp. for Sick Children, Toronto, Canada.

Recent data suggests that CIF may reduce circulating cholesterol(C) concentrations in FHH. We report the effect of CIF in 2 FHH children unresponsive to drug therapy: A: 5yo boy (receptor negative); B: 15yo girl (receptor deficient-15%). CIF was administered as Vivonex(V) to supply daily caloric & fluid requirements through a nasogastric tube. Total C(TC), LDL-C, HDL-C, and triglycerides were measured 3 times at baseline, & after 12,36,72hr, 10 & 14d of CIF. In A, CIF was discontinued for 4hr/d after 7d & completely at 14d. In B, at 3wk CIF was changed to 10-12hr nocturnal(N) IF for a further 5wk to provide 1/3 of total daily caloric needs. A low C diet was given during the day. CIF led to a maximum decrease in i) TC of 10% (772-692 mg/dL) at 7d in A, & 24% (567-427) at 3wk in B; ii) LDL-C: 12% in A (709-623); 23% in B (516-400); iii) HDL-C: 71% in A (14-4) and 51% in B (31-15). In A, stopping CIF for 4hr/d for 4d led to return of all levels to baseline. In B, NIF kept TC, LDL-C & HDL-C levels at 85,84 & 77% of baseline. We conclude that CIF led to a small but definite drop in all C-components in both FHH patients. The response varied greatly & May be dependent on receptor status. The lowering of HDL-C may negate potential benefit of C/NIF. The mechanism of C-lowering in these patients is unexplained.

721 SKELETAL MUSCLE METABOLISM AND ENERGY BALANCE: RELATIONSHIP TO NaK PUMP ACTIVITY. M. De Luise*, University of Melbourne, Department of Medicine, Repatriation General Hospital, Heidelberg, Victoria, Australia.

To investigate the role of cellular thermogenesis in skeletal muscle as a determinant of energy balance, three animal models of altered energy balance were studied. Mouse soleus muscle energy utilization was measured in vitro as the rate of oxygen consumption; concurrently the activity of the NaK pump, a biochemical mediator of cellular thermogenesis, was determined so the ouabain-sensitive rate of potassium uptake by the muscles. In a normal strain of mice induction of hyperthyroidism by i/p injections of T_3 resulted in a 56.4% increase in food intake, a 15.5% gain in body weight, a 12.3% increase in soleus muscle O_2 consumption and a 30.1% increase in NaK pump activity. When compared to a non-obese strain, soleus muscles from the genetically obese NZO mouse were found to have a reduction in both O_2 consumption (20.75±0.76 vs 25.13±0.95 nl O_2/min/mg muscle, n=6, $p<0.01$) and NaK pump activity (0.519±0.039 vs 0.770±0.030 nmole K/min/mg muscle, $p<0.02$). Carbohydrate overfeeding in normal mice, induced by supplementing their usual diet with a 10% sucrose solution for one week, resulted in a 20% increase in caloric consumption, a 4% increase in body weight, an increase in soleus muscle O_2 consumption (31.50±1.19 vs 28.81±1.68 nl/min/mg muscle, n=10g, $p<0.05$) and an increase in NaK pump activity (0.962±0.035 vs 0.810±0.038 nmole K/min/mg muscle, $p<0.01$). It is concluded that changes in skeletal muscle thermogenesis may well contribute significantly to alterations in whole body energy balance and that the NaK pump is a potential biochemical mediator of such changes.

722 HYPERALIMENTATION CHANGES LIPID COMPOSITION OF ERYTHROCYTE MEMBRANES. H. Doorenbos*, J.J.van Doormaal, F.A.J.Muskiet and W.J.Sluiter.Div. of Endocr. and of Clin.Chem. Univ. Hosp. Groningen, The Netherlands.

The function of cellular membranes may be influenced by variation in their lipid composition. As lipid synthesis is absent in erythrocytes alterations in their membrane result from exchange with plasma lipids. The extent of change in a short time was studied by decreasing the supply of exogenous and endogenous fatty acids. Ten healthy men (ages 23-47) fasted during 18 hours. Nasogastric drip carbohydrate hyperalimentation (Nutrical[R]) was started at 8.00 a.m. and continued during 48 hours. Twice the estimated basal energy requirement (3150-3670 kcal per 24 hours) was given. After this, fasting was resumed during 7 hours.
Triglycerides, phospholipids, total and unesterified cholesterol, ratio phospholipids/unesterified cholesterol and FFA fell and glucose (from 4.17 ± 0.09 to 5.49 ± 0.24 mmol/l, $p \leq 0.01$) and insulin (from 16.4 ± 2.0 to 122.3 ± 14.2 μE/l, $p \leq 0.01$) rose. In the erythrocyte membrane cholesterol and total fatty acids fell ($p < 0.01$). The absolute amount of linoleic acid and oleic acid decreased steadily. The relative amount of saturated fatty acids increased ($p < 0.01$). After resumed fasting glucose (4.06 ± 0.12 mmol/l, $p < 0.01$) and insulin (19.0 ± 1.8 μE/l, $p < 0.01$) returned to but did not reach base line level. In the erythrocyte membrane linoleic acid (nmol/10^8 ery) continued to fall (mean ± SD. 7.758 ± 0.166 → 6.443 ± 0.182; $p < 0.01$).

Conclusion: during short term carbohydrate hyperalimentation an evident change in erythrocyte lipid composition was observed.

723 CHARACTERISTICS OF CLONOTYPE ANTIBODY PREPARED FROM POLYCLONAL ANTIBODY TO HORMONES BY ISOELECTRIC FOCUSING AND CHROMATOFOCUSING TECHNIQUES.
K. Miyai*, Y. Endo, N. Hata and K. Ichihara, Department of Laboratory Medicine, Osaka University Medical School, 1-1-50 Fukushima, Osaka 553, Japan.

The IgG fraction of rabbit anti human thyrotropin (hTSH) antibody was fractionated by agarose isoelectric focusing in the range of pH 3 to 10. Protein staining showed that the polyclonal IgG separated into more than 20 bands. The characteristics of the antibody in these fractions were analyzed by Scatchard plot analysis and examination of cross reactivity with human chorionic gonadotropin (hCG) by double antibody radioimmunoassay. The affinity constant of the initial anti h-TSH-IgG was $1.9x10^{10}M^{-1}$ and the constants of the fractions ranged from $6.4x10^{9}M^{-1}$ to $3.1x10^{10}M^{-1}$. The cross-reactivities with hCG of the fractions ranged from 0.21 to 6.6% and there was a good correlation between the pI's of the antibody fractions and their cross reactivities. The IgG fraction of rabbit anti thyroxine (T_4) antibody was fractionated by the chromatofocusing technique with the Pharmacia Fast Protein Liquid Chromatography (FPLC) system. The column was equilibrated with 25 mM diethanolamine-HCl (pH 9.5) and material was eluted with diluted "Polybuffer 96" (pH 6.0). The eluate was collected in 8 fractions, which were examined by Scatchard plot analysis on radioimmunoassay. The highest affinity constants were calculated as $2.5x10^{9}M^{-1}$ for the initial anti T_4 IgG and $2.4x10^{9}$-$6.0x10^{9}M^{-1}$ for the fractions.

These data suggest that clonotype antibody with different characters can be separated from polyclonal antibody to hormones and applied in radioimmunoassay.

724 EXPERIMENTAL PRODUCTION BY THE HYBRIDOMA TECHNIQUE OF ANTIBODY TO THE TSH RECEPTOR (TSH-R): PROBLEMS AND SUCCESS. D. Neylan*, A. Claflin**, M. Zakarija and J. M. McKenzie. Departs. of Medicine and Surgery**, Univ. Miami Sch. of Medicine, Miami, FL.

Production of hybridomas that secrete antibodies, e.g. to human thyroid cell membrane components, is now a standard procedure. Problems lie in screening for individual antibodies. Inhibition of ^{125}I-TSH to TSH-R has been used. We tested a preparation of guinea pig fat cell membranes for this but found large variation due in part to products of disintegrating cells and to the many media required at different stages. Therefore, for 230 hybridomas that produced Ig, we used solid phase ELISA assays to test for IgG binding to human thyroid or guinea pig fat cell membranes. Some IgG bound to both membranes but those positive for anti-microsomal (anti-M) (4) and anti-thyroglobulin (anti-Tg) (39) antibodies bound only to thyroid membranes. IgG from 7 hybridomas, negative for anti-M and anti-Tg, bound to both thyroid and fat; binding was inhibited by addition of TSH, e.g. (#150) binding to fat cell membranes, O.D. 767% of control; plus TSH, 200% control. For thyroid stimulation (increase in cAMP in human thyroid cells in vitro), we dissolved precipitated protein from one hybridoma (#150) in assay buffer at 1/10 the original vol.; 1:128 dilution of this increased cAMP 218%. Lesser dilutions were non-stimulating or even inhibitory. Conclusions: errors may occur in producing antibodies to TSH-R if vagaries of the screening and specific assays are not controlled. With the procedures outlined an antibody to the TSH-R that was capable of stimulating human thyroid cells in culture was produced.

725 RELATIONSHIP BETWEEN HYPOTHALAMIC CATECHOLAMINERGIC ACTIVITY AND PLASMA LH LEVELS IN OVARIECTOMIZED, POSTPARTUM RATS. JM Catelli, AT Townsend, DN Marple and CH Rahe*. Department of Animal and Dairy Sciences, Agricultural Experiment Station, Auburn University, Alabama 36849

The present study was conducted to determine the relationship between suppression of plasma LH during the postpartum (PP) period and hypothalamic catecholaminergic activity (HCCA) in female rats. Charles River derived, CD strain rats were designated to suckled (S) or non-suckled (NS) PP groups and bred whereas virgin rats served as controls. Virgin rats were ovariectomized (OVX) on day 1 of diestrus while S and NS rats were OVX on day 1 PP. Litters were removed or standardized to 8 pups on the day of parturition. All rats were sacrificed by decapitation on day 5 or 20 post-OVX/PP. Brains were subjected to 10 sec microwave irradiation, rapidly frozen in liquid nitrogen and stored at -80C. Trunk blood was collected for quantitation of LH by RIA. Eight catecholamines or metabolites were quantitated from six microdisected hypothalamic regions using HPLC with EC detection. As expected, LH levels were depressed following parturition. Moreover, suckling continued to suppress plasma LH levels during late lactation. Highest levels of HCCA were observed in long-term OVX virgin rats, particularly in the SCN and ME regions. HCCA was increased in the SCN, ME and AHY regions of S compared to NS rats. The results of this study demonstrate that HCCA is modulated in response to OVX and S. Furthermore, alterations in plasma levels of LH in response to OVX and S may reflect localized changes in HCCA.

726 INFLUENCES OF DOPAMINE (DA), NOREPINEPHRINE (NE), AND DES-GLY^{10} [D-ALA^{6}] LUTEINIZING HORMONE-RELEASING HORMONE ETHYLAMIDE (LHRH-A) ON IN VITRO GONADOTROPIN (GTH) RELEASE BY GOLDFISH PITUITARY. J. P. Chang*, D. S. MacKenzie and R. E. Peter, Department of Zoology, University of Alberta, Edmonton, Alberta, T6G 2E9, Canada.

Trypsin-DNAse-dispersed goldfish pituitary cells, cultured for 3 days, or freshly prepared goldfish pituitary fragments, were placed in perifusion columns, each containing a layer of Bio-carrier beads, and perifused with a Hepes-Hanks solution. In both systems, gonadotrophs continued to secrete GTH into the perifusate spontaneously. After the establishment of basal secretion rates, perifusion of dispersed pituitary cells with 5 and 500 nM DA, or pituitary fragments with 50 and 100 nM DA, decreased the amount of GTH released into the perifusate. Perifusion with 500 nM DA also abolished the GTH release-response to challenges of 10 nM LHRH-A in both perifusion systems. Perifusion of pituitary dispersed cell or fragment preparations obtained from sexually regressed goldfish with 50 nM NE consistently increased the amount of GTH released into the perifusate; however, pituitary preparations from sexually mature goldfish did not respond to NE. These results provide *in vitro* evidence for the presence of direct DA inhibition of spontaneous GTH release, blockade by DA of GTH-releasing hormone actions, and NE stimulation of GTH secretion in goldfish. These results also suggest that the action of NE is seasonal. This study was supported by AHFMR.

727 NEURAL SUBSTANCE P (SP) DEFICIENCY IN DIABETIC NEUROPATHY. R. Clements*, S. Leeman and N. Aronin, Universities of Massachusetts and of Alabama, Worchester, Massachusetts and Birmingham, Alabama 35294, U.S.A.

We previously demonstrated a markedly diminished concentration of radioimmunoassayable SP in the peripheral nerves of the legs of patients with diabetic neuropathy. Since the release of SP from certain sensory nerve terminals is thought to mediate the cutaneous flare in response to noxious stimuli to the skin, we compared the size of the flare following the forearm intradermal injection of substances that cause the release of endogenous SP (histamine, 10 ng and capsaicin, 100 ng) or of synthetic SP (3 ng) in age- and sex-matched controls, non-neuropathic diabetics and severely neuropathic diabetics. While the cutaneous flare in response to injection of authentic SP was not statistically different in the two diabetic groups, it was decreased in the neuropathic diabetics compared to the controls ($p < 0.05$). Responses to histamine and capsaicin were profoundly reduced in the neuropathic diabetics when compared to controls or to non-neuropathic diabetics (p values all < 0.005). These findings suggest that diabetics with neuropathy may have a generalized deficiency of SP in their cutaneous nerve terminals that accounts, in part, for their diminished cutaneous responses to certain noxious stimuli.

	Cutaneous Flare (cm^2)		
Study Group	Histamine	Capsaicin	Substance P
Non-diabetic controls (11)	48.0 ± 11.7	47.9 ± 8.8	46.8 ± 12.7
Non-neuropathic diabetics (11)	43.1 ± 5.4	65.6 ± 11.9	36.3 ± 8.9
Neuropathic diabetics (24)	10.6 ± 1.9	15.3 ± 2.8	15.7 ± 3.4

728 EVIDENCE FOR A NECESSARY INVOLVEMENT OF ADRENALINE IN BOTH THE PREOVULATORY SURGE AND THE PULSATILE RELEASE OF LUTEINIZING HORMONE IN RATS. C.W.Coen*, A.Simonyi and M.I.K.Fekete, Department of Human Anatomy, Oxford University,U.K. and The Institute of Experimental Medicine, Budapest, Hungary.

LY 87130 is a potent inhibitor of brain phenylethanolamine N-methyltransferase (PNMT), the enzyme which catalyses the conversion of noradrenaline to adrenaline (A) (Fuller et al., Brain Res. 190: 215,1980). The preovulatory surge of luteinizing hormone (LH) in rats normally occurs at 18.00h (lights 06.00-20.00h) on the day of pro-oestrus. In a manner dependent upon the dose/number of treatments, LY 87130 administered to pro-oestrous rats either leads to an occurrence of the surge at 24.00 instead of 18.00h or blocks the LH surge at both times and prevents ovulation; the incidence and timing of the surge of follicle stimulating hormone are affected in an identical fashion. The treatments with LY 87130 do not disturb the occurrence of the prolactin surge. Comparable effects on the incidence and timing of the LH surge occur after treatment with SKF 64139, another PNMT inhibitor, or clonidine, a drug which inter alia suppresses the turnover rate of hypothalamic A (Coen & Coombs, Neuroscience 10: 187, 1983). A pulsatile pattern in the release of LH is apparent in sequential blood samples taken from cannulated rats every 6 minutes. The amplitude of the pulses is increased in the absence of oestrogen but attenuated during the oestrous cycle except at the time of the LH surge when the frequency and amplitude of the pulses are enhanced (Gallo, Biol. Reprod. 24: 100, 1980). The pulsatile release of LH in ovariectomized rats is blocked by treatment with LY 87130 at a dose which also prevents the pro-oestrous surge and ovulation. It is proposed that the pulsatile release of LH is a necessary condition for the preovulatory surge and that these pulses are dependent upon A-containing neurons.

729 DELAYED APPEARANCE OF DIFFERENTIAL AUDITORY PATHWAY LABELING IN RAT BRAIN AFTER INTRAVENOUS (IV) ^{125}I-THYROXIN (T_4^*) IS STRONGLY CORRELATED WITH THE TIME COURSE OF IN SITU CONVERSION TO LABELED TRIIODOTHYRONINE (T_3^*).

Crutchfield, F. L., McNamara, M. B., Gordon, F. L. and Dratman, M. B.*
VA Medical Center and The Medical College of Pennsylvania, Phila., Pa.

Previous studies have shown marked concentration of high specific activity (SA) T_3^* in rat central auditory systems (AUD) with time-dependent shifts in labeling patterns indicating movement of hormone from AUD nuclei through relevant axons to terminal field projections at AUD relay centers. To obtain further information about the T_3-specificity of the AUD uptake and transport process, thaw-mount film autoradiograms of serially sectioned (20 mμ) rat brains obtained 1, 3, 24 and 48 h after IV high SA T_4^* were prepared by exposing the sections to high sensitivity film for 30 days. RESULTS: Although no delay in brain uptake of the hormone was noted, there was a marked delay in differential localization in AUD, with distinctive labeling patterns comparable to those seen early after T_3^* appearing gradually over the 48 h period of observation. As noted after T_3^*, the visual (Retino-Striate cortex) projection pathways showed little predilection for T_4^* or its labeled metabolites. Parallel biochemical studies confirmed that the appearance of T_3^* in brain after IV T_4^* was due to in situ conversion; T_3^*/T_4^* in whole brain and synaptosomes respectively increased from .34 and 1.62 at 3 h after T_4^* to .81 and 2.5 at 48 h. CONCLUSION: The marked thyroid hormone dependence of AUD is specific for T_3 rather than T_4. Supported by funds from VA Medical Research Service and NSF Grant #BNS 8210354.

730 HIGHLY SENSITIVE TLC-SPECTROFLUORIMETRIC METHOD FOR SPECIFIC ASSAY OF INDOLEAMINES AND RELATED COMPOUNDS. A.de Leiva*,J.Serrano,J.M.Arqué and R.Segura.Endocrinology Service and Dept. of Physiology,Hosp. de la Santa Cruz y San Pablo and Univ. Autónoma de Barcelona,SPAIN. (Grants from CAICYT and FISS).

Individual 5-hydroxyindoles(5-hydroxytryptophan,5-HTP,5-hydroxytryptophol,5-HTPol,5-hydroxytryptamine,serotonin,5-HT, N-acetylserotonin,NAS,5-hydroxyindole acetic acid,5HIAA)and 5-methoxyindoles(5-methoxytryptamine,5-MT,5-methoxytryptophol,5-MTPol,N-acetyl-5-methoxytryptamine,melatonin,MEL,5-methoxyindole acetic acid,5MIAA)were simultaneously isolated and quantified,after condensation with o-phthaldialdehyde in 3-6 M HCl,followed by separation in silica gel TLC plates developed with a mixture of 1-penthanol:1-propanol:methanol:formic acid: 0.5 mol/liter HCl(58:30:1:0.5:10).5-methoxyindoles were recognized by the bluish color of the emitted fluorescence(366 nm); 5-hydroxyindoles despicted an orange fluorescence.The final introduction of the TLC plates in a saturated enviroment of ammonium leads to a specific assay for 5-hydroxyindoles (pinkish fluorescence at 525 nm);the fluorescence for methoxyindoles vanishes.Distinct Rf values and minimal detectable doses (MDD) for each compound are shown:

COMPOUND	Rf	MDD	COMPOUND	Rf	MDD	COMPOUND	Rf	MDD
5-MT	.18	.30ng	NAS	.38	.80ng	5-HTPol	.63	.85 ng
MEL	.23	.25ng	5-MTPol	.43	.40ng	5-MIAA	.68	2.0 ng
5-HT	.27	.60ng	5-HTP	.48	2.0ng	5-HIAA	.82	4.0 ng

731 FSH STIMULATES THE PRODUCTION OF A MOLECULE WHICH TRIGGERS THECA/INTERSTITIAL CELL CYTODIFFERENTIATION. C.A. Dyer* and G.F. Erickson, Dept. Repro. Med., Univ. California, San Diego, La Jolla, CA 92093 U.S.A.

Based on our understanding of ovarian theca-interstitial cell (TI) differentiation, the process is believed to be under LH control. In this report, we provide surprising evidence that a granulosa substance, generated in response to FSH, can transform undifferentiated TI cells into fully functional androgen producing cells in a manner similar to LH induction. When collagenase dispersed ovarian cells from immature hypox. rats were cultured in defined medium with increasing amounts of NIAMDD-oFSH-14, there was a dose-dependent (ED_{50}= 30 ng/ml) stimulation of androstenedione (Δ^4) production. The amount of Δ^4 produced with a maximum dose of FSH was $\geq$ than that produced by a maximum dose of LH or hCG. Inductions of Δ^4 production were obtained by four different types of highly purified FSH (provided by Dr. Papkoff). These and other data show that the results are not due to contaminating LH in the FSH preparations. If a pure population of granulosa cells was cultured with FSH for 2 days, the spent media (after dialysis) induced maximal Δ^4 production when applied to cultures of TI cells. This response was not due to FSH carryover. No Δ^4 response was obtained from spent media of control (non-FSH-treated) granulosa cell cultures. In summary, we have found that FSH can induce the differentiation of TI cells in a manner like that obtained with LH. The mechanism seems to be that FSH stimulates granulosa cells to release a molecule which interacts with TI cells causing them to differentiate into active Δ^4 producing cells. This finding opens for future investigation the issue of intraovarian regulation of steroidogenesis.

732 EVIDENCE FOR CHLOROQUINE INDUCED REDISTRIBUTION OF LH/hCG RECEPTOR. G.T. Faircloth*, J.J. Pehrson, H. Kawamura, E.A. Rorke and J.L. Vaitukaitis, Departments of Medicine and Physiology, Boston University School of Medicine, Boston, MA 02118, U.S.A.

In previous studies of chloroquine treated rats, significantly more free LH/hCG receptor was present in the ovarian membrane fraction of chloroquine treated rats but significantly less hCG bound to that membrane fraction relative to that of controls. To ascertain whether receptors present in the membrane fraction of pseudopregnant ovaries were functional, rats were treated with chloroquine 6 hours prior to injection with 1 μg (12.8 IU) hCG intravenously and groups of animals sacrificed intermittently for the next 18 hours. Ovarian cyclic AMP-dependent protein kinase (CDPK) activity, cytosolic cAMP and progesterone levels were determined prior to and after hCG stimulation. A mouse Leydig cell assay determined hCG bioactivity. When compared to untreated controls, the chloroquine treated rats had significantly less intracellular accumulation of cAMP and progesterone as well as a less marked change in CDPK activity. No significant difference in hCG binding affinity was observed for LH/hCG receptors present in ovarian plasma membrane harvested from either control or chloroquine treated rats. For the first several hours after hCG stimulation, ovarian hCG bioactivity present in cytosol harvested from the control group exceeded that for the chloroquine treated rats. However, 6 hours after hCG injection, bioactive cytosolic hCG activity was greater among the chloroquine treated animals. The foregoing observations strongly suggest rearrangement of functional ovarian plasma membrane LH/hCG receptors in chloroquine treated pseudopregnant rats.

733 INDUCTION OF SYNTHESIS OF CHOLESTEROL SIDE-CHAIN CLEAVAGE CYTOCHROME P-450 (P-450_{scc}) AND ADRENODOXIN (ADX) BY FSH, 8-BROMO CYCLIC AMP (8-Br-cAMP) AND LOW-DENSITY LIPOPROTEIN (LDL) IN GRANULOSA CELLS. B. Funkenstein*, M.R. Waterman, and E.R. Simpson, Cecil H. and Ida Green Center for Reprod. Biol. Sci., Univ. of Texas Health Science Center, Dallas, TX 75235, U.S.A.

The influence of FSH, 8-Br-cAMP and LDL on the synthesis of P-450_{scc} and ADX was studied in confluent bovine granulosa cells by means of radiolabeling cellular protein with [^{35}S]methionine followed by immunoisolation, SDS-polyacrylamide gel electrophoresis and autoradiography. Treatment of granulosa cells with FSH or 8-Br-cAMP resulted in an increased rate of synthesis of these proteins as early as 12 h. The effect of FSH on P-450_{scc} synthesis was concentration-dependent (maximum rate at 250 ng/ml). LDL also stimulated the synthesis of both proteins when added to cells maintained in lipoprotein-poor serum either alone or in combination with FSH or 8-Br-cAMP. FSH, 8-Br-cAMP and LDL also stimulated progesterone producton by cultured granulosa cells. By using an immunoblotting technique, P-450_{scc} and ADX could be detected in freshly obtained granulosa cells, but their contents were much lower than in the corpus luteum. The results of the present study suggest a possible role for LDL in the process of cytodifferentiation of granulosa cells into luteal cells in vivo. The concentration of LDL in follicular fluid is very low. Following ovulation, the follicle becomes vascularized and thus the granulosa cells are exposed to high levels of LDL, allowing for the provision of substrate cholesterol, and stimulation of the synthesis of enzymes involved in cholesterol side-chain cleavage, namely, P-450_{scc} and ADX.

734 DIRECT EVIDENCE FOR IN VIVO TRANSFER OF HCG FROM PLASMA MEMBRANE TO LYSOSOMES IN RAT OVARY. A. Gilligan*. G. T. Faircloth and J. L. Vaitukaitis, Departments of Medicine and Physiology, Boston University School of Medicine, Boston, MA 02118, U. S. A.

Pseudopregnant rats pretreated with the lysosomotropic agent, chloroquine (CQ), and stimulated with hCG have significantly higher cytosolic hCG levels than those of controls for the first 1-2 hours after injection. To better characterize those observations, plasma membrane (PM) and lysosomal vesicles were separated with a self generated Percoll gradient and separation confirmed by specific enzyme markers. Pseudoprenant rats were treated with CQ and injected with 1.0 µg (12.8 IU) hCG intravenously 6 hours later. Rats were sacrificed 0.5, 2, 4 and 6 hours after hCG and appropriate ovarian homogenization fractions applied to Percoll gradients. Membrane bound hCG potentially present in each gradient fraction was dissociated at pH 3.0 and subjected to radioimmunoassay. Although hCG bound to control PM 30 minutes after hCG injection was significantly greater among control rats, lysosomal associated hCG levels were at the limit of assay sensitivity for both CQ and control groups. Lysosomal hCG was 1/3 lower at 2 hours among CQ treated rats. Although a marked increase in PM and lysosomal hCG was observed among controls between 4-6 hours after hCG stimulation, hCG present in those fractions were 50% lower among CQ rats. The ratios of hCG associated with PM and lysosomal vesicles differed at all time points for both groups. Ovarian lysosomal hCG metabolism is both an early and late event after hCG stimulation. Increased cytosolic hCG levels observed among CQ rats soon after internalization reflect altered lysosomal function and possibly CQ-induced altered internalization.

735 SYNTHESIS OF CATECHOL ESTROGENS IN THE PORCINE OVARY. James M. Hammond*, Roscoe M. Hersey, Michael Walega, and Judith Weisz, Depts. of Medicine and OB/GYN, The M.S. Hershey Med. Ctr., The PA State Univ., Hershey, PA 17033

The ovary is not only the major site of estrogen biosynthesis but also an estrogen target tissue. Thus, the routes and products of local estrogen metabolism may be doubly significant. We evaluated the capacity of the porcine ovary to convert estradiol (E_2) to the catechol estrogens, 2-hydroxyestradiol (2-OH-E_2) and 4-hydroxyestradiol (4-OH-E_2). With a product-isolation assay (Hersey et al., Endocrinology 109: 1912, 1981), we found significant production of 2- and 4-OH-E_2 in the follicular wall. The reaction was linear with time and with ovarian protein concentration and was dependent on temperature, pH, and NADPH or NADH. The K_m for production of 2- and 4-OH-E_2 were similar (7 and 5 x 10^{-6} M, respectively). However, the V_{max} was higher for 2-OH-E_2 than for 4-OH-E_2 (129 vs. 29 pmol/mg/40 min). Enzymic activity, assessed at 10 μM E_2, was highest in the walls of preovulatory follicles (108 ± 32 pmol/mg protein/40 min for 2-OH-E_2; 27.6 ± 9.2 for 4-OH-E_2, n=12), with approximately equivalent activity in theca and granulosa. The activity was at least 5-fold lower in immature follicles and corpora lutea, and it was undetectable in interstitium and cumulus. Conclusions: 1) The preovulatory porcine follicle can metabolize estradiol to catechol estrogens. 2) The striking compartmentalization of this activity within the ovary suggests a dependence on ovarian cytodifferentiation; this may explain the apparent lack of ovarian activity in previous reports. 3) Since the cells in the preovulatory follicle respond to both catecholamines and estrogens, the catechol estrogens could play a local regulatory role.

736 CHRONOLOGICAL BIPHASIC ACTION OF LUTEINIZING HORMONE(LH) ON PROGESTATIONAL FUNCTION OF RAT CORPORA LUTEA. I. Hashimoto*, M. Kawaminami, K. Mutoh and H. Wakuri, Laboratories of Veterinary Physiology and Anatomy, Kitasato Universtiy School of Veterinary Medicine and Animal Sciences, Towada, Aomori 034, Japan.

Since proestrous rats have peak LH concentrations which are about 10 times that required for ovulation, the role of periovulatory LH release for progesterone(P) secretion from newly formed corpora lutea(CL) was examined. In the 4-day cyclic rats blood P increased from 0400 h on estrus(E) to 2300 h on early diestrus(D_1) and then decreased to 1800 h on late diestrus(D_2). A single iv injection of human CG(hCG; 5 IU) at 1500 h on proestrus(PE) did not alter P secretion on D_1. After a single iv injection of either hCG(5 IU) or antiserum against ovine LH(A-LH;0.3 ml) at 1900 h on PE, ovulation occured normally by 1000 h on E, but no increase in P was observed on D_1. Daily ip injection of A-LH from 0800 h on E, however, resulted in a marked increase in P from E to D_2 in the hCG-treated rats but not in the A-LH-treated rats. The daily A-LH injection from 0000 h on E did not alter P secretion in the hCG-treated rats. These findings suggest (1) that tonic level of LH secreted after ovulation suppresses CL's P secretion and (2) that the 2nd half of LH surge, at the least, increases CL's potential ability to secrete P and, at the same time, it increases CL's sensitivity to the suppressing effect of LH on their P secretion. The suppressing effect was also demonstrated in the intact 4-day cyclic rats; the daily A-LH injection from 0800 h on D_1 prolonged CL's P secretion. Administration of indomethacin into the ovarian bursae(0.5 mg/rat) replicated the effect of the daily A-LH injection in both the intact and the hCG-treated rats. Therefore, the suppressing effect of LH on CL's P secretion is assumed to be mediated by intra-ovarian(presumably intra-luteal) production of prostaglandins.

737 RESTORATION OF LUTEAL CELL FUNCTION IN PGF2α-TREATED RAT OVARY.
DeAnna D. Hatmaker* and Thomas T. Chen, Department of Zoology, University of Tennessee, Knoxville, Tennessee 37916, U.S.A.

Prostaglandin $F_{2}\alpha$ has been shown to cause luteolysis in many species, including the rat. Few drugs/hormones are capable of reversing its action. Conflicting evidence exists as to the in vivo vs. in vitro effect of PGF_2 on luteal function. The purpose of this study is to determine the functional state of cultured luteal cells previously exposed in vivo to a luteolytic dose of $PGF_{2}\alpha$. PMSG/hCG-primed 25-day-old female rats were treated with PGF_2 on Day 7 (D.0=day of PMSG). Thereafter, ovaries and trunk blood were collected for cell culture and steroid determinations. Cells were collagenase-dissociated and cultured for up to nine days. Progesterone (P4), estradiol (E2), and 20α-dihydroprogesterone (20α-DHP) were assayed in spent media and in extracted sera. LH binding capacity and total DNA were also determined on cultured cells over this period. Within 1 h of $PGF_{2}\alpha$ treatment, serum P4 fell precipitously by 80%, while 20α-DHP levels rose fourfold within 24 h. When ovaries were removed and cultured within 24 h following $PGF_{2}\alpha$ treatment, the ability of luteal cells to produce P4 was significantly impaired. However, if the ovaries were removed later than 24 h, luteal cells exposed to $PGF_{2}\alpha$ were capable of producing more P4 than controls. LH receptors and 20α-DHP levels correlated well with P4 values. E2 levels were low throughout the culture period. These results show that even 24 h after $PGF_{2}\alpha$ injection, when the luteolytic process is well underway in vivo, the process of luteolysis can be reversed and, the functional state of luteal cells can be restored when the cells are cultured under more favorable conditions. (Supported by NIH grant HD-14505)

738 THYMIC REGULATION OF PRIMATE FETAL OVARIAN-ADRENAL DIFFERENTIATION.
D.L. Healy*, J. Bacher and G.D. Hodgen, Pregnancy Research Branch and Veterinary Resources Branch, NICHD, NIH, Bethesda, MD 20205 U.S.A.

Premature ovarian failure and ovarian neoplasia have been reported with thymic aplasia or neonatal thymectomy in lower mammals. Our aims were to examine the ovarian and endocrine sequelae of primate fetal thymectomy. Fetal thymectomy was performed in 39 rhesus monkeys (including 7 sham operations), between days 59-103 of gestation (median 89 days; term gestation 167 days). All neonates (5 thymectomy; 2 sham; 5 intact controls) were sacrificed within 2 days of birth to determine organ weights and to harvest plasma for measurement of FSH, LH, PRL, estradiol (E_2), cortisol, dehydroepiandrosterone sulfate (DHEAS) and a thymic peptide, thymosin α_1, concentrations by radioimmunoassay. Fetal thymectomy decreased individual ovarian (7.1 ± 0.9 mg per 100 g body weight vs. 11.4 ± 2.0 mg per 100 g; mean ± SE; $P < 0.05$) and combined adrenal gland weight (102.8 ± 28.2 mg per 100 g vs. 157.6 ± 35.3 mg per 100 g; $P<0.05$) compared with sham and non-operated operated controls. Quantitative ovarian morphometry from 5 thymectomized newborns (n=8 ovaries), and 7 controls (n=7) showed that fetal thymectomy markedly depleted total ovarian germ cell number (118,431 ± 11,308 vs. 424,639 ± 39,249; $P < 0.001$). By contrast, the percentage of primary follicles increased following fetal thymectomy (6.1 percent vs. 1.2 percent; $P < 0.01$). Fetal thymectomy elevated FSH (7.8 ± 1.1 μg/ml vs. 4.2 ± 0.5 μg/ml; $P < 0.05$) but decreased PRL concentrations (24.5 ± 3.3 ng/ml vs. 76.3 ± 11.2 ng/ml; $P < 0.05$). We conclude that fetal primate thymectomy results in aberrant oogenesis. The data indicate physiological communications exist between the nascent immunological and endocrinological systems.

739 THE MODE OF THE TRANSMISSION OF THE SUCKLING STIMULUS THROUGH THE SPINAL CORD.

T. FUKUOKA*, H. NEGORO, K. HONDA, T. HIGUCHI
Dept. Physiol., Fukui Medical School, Fukui 910-11, Japan

The effects of lesions of the spinal cord on the milk-ejection reflex were studied in anesthetized rats. All lesions were made between C6 and C7 vertebrae and milk ejection was monitored by recording intramammary pressure. First, in rats with bilateral lesions, the 3 h suckling test with 5 pups on each side was performed. The incidence of milk ejection in Group2 with the section of the dorsal funiculus and in Group4 with the combined section of the dorsal and ventral funiculi was 11/13 (84.6%) and 12/14 (85.7%), respectively, and was not significantly different from 9/11 (81.8%)in Group1 with sham operation. In contrast, Group3 (N=12) with the section of the lateral funiculus displayed no milk ejection. Secondly, in 10 rats with unilateral section of the lateral funiculus, bilateral suckling with 10 pups (5 pups on each side) and unilateral suckling (both ipsilateral and contralateral to the lesion) with 5 pups were consecutively performed. Milk ejection was induced in 100 %, 0 % and 50 %, respectively, by bilateral, ipsilateral and contralateral suckling, respectively. There was a significant difference in the incidence of milk ejection between these three sucklings. These results suggest that the suckling stimulus is transmitted through the lateral funiculus mainly in an ipsilateral manner and partly in a contralateral manner.

740 LACK OF EFFECT OF A GRADED OXYTOCIN (OXY) INFUSION ON CARBOHYDRATE METABOLISM IN NORMAL MAN.

V. Geenen, J.J. Legros*, A. Luyckx, P. Lefebvre. Psychoneuroendocrine and Diabetes Units, CHU-B23, University of Liège, Sart Tilman, B-4000 Liège, Belgium.

Infusion of OXY (50-500 μU/kg/min) into normal dogs was found to cause a rise of plasma insulin and glucagon levels, accompanied by a prompt increase in glucose production followed by an increase in overall glucose uptake (Altszuler and Hampshire, 1981). Knudtzon (1983) reported an acute and rapid effect of OXY (0.3 μg) on plasma insulin levels 2 min. after IV administration in fed rabbits, without significant change of glucagon or glucose levels. A graded OXY infusion was performed in 6 normal male volunteers (aged 24-28, mean weight of 76.6 ± 6.4 kg) with successive rates of outflow (16, 32, 64 and 128 mIU/min) every 30 min. As the following table shows, no apparent effect on plasma insulin, glucagon or glucose levels could be evidenced (values expressed as mean ± SEM).

Time	OXY outflow(mIU/min)	Glucose(mg%)	Insulin(μU/ml)	Glucagon(pg/ml)
- 30	Basal	83.7 ± 0.9	6.7 ± 1.0	103.1 ± 21.6
0	Basal	87.0 ± 1.5	6.4 ± 0.6	97.8 ± 27.7
30	16	85.6 ± 1.8	6.4 ± 0.9	102.6 ± 29.8
60	32	83.8 ± 2.3	5.5 ± 0.4	108.2 ± 30.1
90	64	83.1 ± 3.0	5.4 ± 0.5	118.7 ± 31.8
120	128	87.8 ± 3.1	6.6 ± 0.7	102.2 ± 21
150	0	88.3 ± 2.6	5.2 ± 0.3	84.6 ± 30.6

From these data, we can conclude that it seems to exist some species differences in the metabolic effects of OXY.

741 DYNORPHIN(1-8) BINDS TO OPIATE-KAPPA-RECEPTORS IN THE NEUROHYPOPHYSIS AND IS INVOLVED IN THE REGULATION OF VASOPRESSIN-RELEASE. R. Gerstberger* and N. Barden, MRC Group in Molecular Endocrinology, CHUL, Québec, G1V 4G2, Canada.

The existence of multiple opiate receptors in bovine and rat posterior pituitary and the binding of endogenous opioid peptides to these receptor subtypes were investigated using radioreceptor assay (RRA) and autoradiography. Saturation kinetics with ^{3}H-etorphin (binding to mu, sigma and kappa subtypes) revealed a high and a low affinity site (K_D: 1.2 nM and 7.1 nM). Various specific agonists for each receptor subtype were used, in a concentration range from 10^{-12} to 10^{-5}M, to displace ^{3}H-etorphin (2 nM) from its binding sites. 1) Cold etorphin led to a clearly biphasic release of labelled ligand. 2) The mu-specific agonists DAGO and Morphiceptin did not displace etorphin while the sigma-specific agonists DADLE and DSTLE as well as beta-endorphin displaced etorphin from its low affinity site only. 3) Ketazocine, believed to be kappa-specific, showed a similar displacement pattern to etorphin. 4) Dynorphin (1-8), a kappa-specific agonist which is found in the same nerve terminals of the neural lobe as vasopressin displaced ^{3}H-etorphin from its high affinity binding site. Film-autoradiography of thaw-mounted sections with 2 nM labelled etorphin alone and in the presence of cold etorphin (10^{-6}M) or dynorphin (10^{-8}M) demonstrated that dynorphin displaces 30% of the labelled ligand, a value similar to that found with the RRA-technique. After exposure to dynorphin (1-8) cultured rat neurointermediate lobes showed a stimulation of vasopressin release into the medium. This study indicates that dynorphin (1-8) regulates vasopressin-release via interaction with opiate kappa receptors.

742 OXYTOCIN STUDIES IN THE GUINEA PIG HYPOTHLAMO-NEUROHYPOPHYSEAL COMPLEX(HNC) IN ORGAN CULTURE. Ichigen Haginiwa*, Tsunehisa Makino, Hideaki Suzuki, Kazumi Nakazawa, Kazumi Ui, Masato Sugawara and Rihachi Iizuka, Dept. of Obstetrics and Gynecology, School of Medicine, Keio University, Tokyo,Japan

The Guinea Pig HNC, including paraventricular and supraoptic nuclei, was removed and cultured in Eagles's MEM for 7 days at 37°C in 95% air and 5% CO_2. The amount of Oxytocin (OT), released from the HNC into the culture medium each day over 20-minutes-period was measured by specific radioimmunoassay. The amount of oxytocin release from HNC was constant except the day of operation. The hypothalamus or the pituitary were cultured on the same condition as the HNC. The hypothalamus released significantly less, the pituitary released more OT than the HNC did. The content of OT in the hypothalamus and the pituitary remained constant during the culture period of the HNC. They showed no difference between the sexes. Synthetic OT, hypothalamic or the pituitary extracts were eluted separately by ion-exchange chromatography. The elution patterns were almost the same. The neurosecretary cells were almost intact histologically throughout the culture period under light microscopy. The administration of 100mM KCℓ on the HNC in culture showed increase of OT release. The administration of Prostaglandin $F_{2}\alpha$ on the HNC showed sequential increase of OT release. But the administration of Prostaglandin D_2 and E_2 on the HNC failed to increase. The administration of Progesteron and Estrogen on the HNC showed increase of OT release. These results suggest that the cultured HNC can be a useful in vitro model for studies of OT dynamics and OT release will be effected by Prostaglandin or steroid hormones.

743 DIFFERENTIAL CHANGE IN HYPOTHALAMIC AND EXTRAHYPOTHALAMIC OXYTOCIN CONTENTS OF BRATTELBORO DI RAT FOLLOWING 1-DEAMINO-8-D-ARGININE VASOPRESSIN ADMINISTRATION. J. Haldar*, G. Nilaver and E. A. Zimmerman, Dept. of Biological Sciences, St. John's University and Dept. of Neurology, College of Physicians & Surgeons of Columbia University New York NY

Brattleboro DI rats have high urine flow, low urine osmolality and elevated plasma oxytocin (OT) level. Prolonged vasopressin administration changes both the urine osmolality and urine flow to almost normal levels. In the present study we report the effect of 1-deamino-8-D-arginine vasopressin (DdAVP) administration on (i) plasma OT level (ii) extrahypothalamic OT contents of different brain regions of DI rats. Experiments were conducted in 6 Long Evans controls, 7 DI controls and 8 DI rats with DdAVP treatment. Oxytocin content was measured in acid homogenized brain samples by bioassay and/or RIA. Plasma samples were assayed by RIA following Sep-pak extraction. DdAVP was administered SC by osmotic minipumps (Alzet 2001) in a dose of 50 ng/kg/day for two weeks. At the end of the treatment there was an increase of urine osmolality, decrease of urine flow and plasma OT level. However, following DdAVP administration, while pituitary OT levels increased, OT levels of hypothalamus, pons, medulla, midbrain, hippocampus, frontal cortex and cervical, thoracic and lumber regions of the spinal cord decreased. Immunocytochemical data further demonstrated a reduction in OT staining in the anterior part of the PVN in DdAVP treated animals. These results suggest that one of the sources of the extrahypothalamic OT in DI rats is PVN. Supported by NIH Grant # HD 13147

744 EFFECTS OF PINEALECTOMY OR CONSTANT ILLUMINATION ON PLASMA TESTOSTERONE,LH RESPONSIVENESS TO LH-RH AND HYPOTHALAMIC LH-RH IN ADULT MALE RATS. M.Fèvre-Montange*, M. Pugeat, C. Brebant and J. Tourniaire, *INSERM U.197, Fac.Méd. A.Carrel and Clinique Endocrinologique, Hôp. Antiquaille, Lyon, France.

The pineal gland exerts an inhibitory effect on gonadal activity but the mechanisms of this action have not been clearly resolved. This study examined the effect of suppression of melatonin secretion by pinealectomy or constant illumination on hypothalamo-pituitary gonadal axis in adult male rats. It was performed in pinealectomized (PX) or sham operated (SPX) and control rats (lights on 7am-7pm) and in normal rats under continuous illumination (LL).Three weeks later, plasma testosterone (T) and LH were measured in basal condition ; the LH response after IV injection of LH-RH (50ng) was measured on pooled samples (15,30,45 minutes). Hypothalamic LH-RH content was measured 24 hours later by radioimmunoassay. In PX rats (n=22), LH increased from 49±7 to 125±5 ng/ml after LH-RH injection and did not differ from the SPX group (n=20)(36±5 to 127±12 ng/ml). T level was significantly higher in PX animals than in SPX rats:383±37 vs 217±26 ng/100 ml. Hypothalamic LH-RH content is not modified by pinealectomy. In rats maintained under LL (n=9) basal LH (37±22 ng/ml) did not differ from the control (28±7 ng/ml). The LH response to LH-RH is significantly decreased (95±18 vs 137±63 ng/ml). T concentration is not modified while hypothalamic LH-RH content is significantly increased (12.7±3.4 vs 9.5±3.5 ng). The lack of melatonin secretion induced by pinealectomy or constant illumination has not the same effect on gonadal axis. Pinealectomy seems to affect essentially the gonads while constant illumination probably acts at a supra-hypothalamic level.

745 SHORT TERM PHOTOPERIOD EFFECTS ON LH AND PRL LEVELS AND OVARIAN HISTOLOGY IN CHARLES RIVER LSH/SsLAK FEMALE HAMSTERS. U. Hauser* and B. Benson,
University of Arizona, Tucson, Arizona, 85724, U.S.A.

The inbred hamsters utilized in these experiments were shown to cease ovarian cyclicity after two to four weeks of short photoperiod (Hauser and Benson, 1984). After regular cyclicity was established in a long photoperiod (LP, 14L:10D), forty-two animals were transferred to a short photoperiod (SP, 8L:16D) on day one (D1) of the cycle; ten animals remained as LP controls. Groups of eight animals were sacrificed after 4, 8, 12 and 16 days of SP on D1 between 0600 hrs and 0730 hrs (lights on = 0600 hrs) and sera, pituitaries and uteri were saved. LP animals were sacrificed on D1 while SP-acyclic (SP-AC) animals were sacrificed at 4-5 weeks. PRL levels, determined by RIA, were significantly lower as early as eight days of SP treatment, were reduced to 9.83 ± 1.61 ng/ml after 16 days (controls = 19.83 ± 2.83 ng/ml) and fell to 2.13 ± 0.44 ng/ml in SP-AC animals. Pituitary PRL content did not change in cycling SP animals, but were depressed from 38.42 ± 4.49 in controls to 7.36 ± 0.87 ng in SP-AC animals. No effect of SP treatment was noted on serum LH levels yet pituitary content increased from 30.16 ± 7.67 μg (LP controls) to 64.5± 6.23 μg (SP-AC) after the animals became acyclic. During 16 days of SP exposure, uterine weights dropped from 349.6 ± 8.09 to 281.0 ± 11.15 mg, and were reduced to 88.17 ± 3.89 mg in SP-AC animals. Compared with LP controls, fewer corpora lutea were observed in cycling animals after 16 days of SP exposure (5.42 ± 0.36 vs. 7.57 ± 0.52/ovary). These results suggest that PRL levels are reduced early after SP exposure and fewer follicles reach full maturation, eventually leading to the cessation of cyclicity.

746 PEPTIDE HORMONES REGULATE IONIC CONDUCTANCES IN CLONAL PITUITARY CELLS. B. Dufy* and J.L. Barker,
Lab. Neurophysiology, Univ. of Bordeaux II, France, and Lab. Neurophysiology, NINCDS, Bethesda, Md., U.S.A.

Previously we have found that brief application of thyrotropin releasing hormone (TRH), which stimulates prolactin release from GH3/6 cells, induces a rapid, hyperpolarizing response and increase in conductance lasting 10-30 seconds followed by the appearance of spontaneous action potential activity, which is sustained for a minute or more. In contrast, somatostatin (SRIF) suppresses prolactin release and action potential generation. We have used voltage clamp techniques to study the ionic conductances resident in these cells and the mechanism of action of the peptides on the excitability of GH3/6 cells. TRH induces an initial outward (K^+) current response and increase in membrane conductance at the level of the resting membrane potential and a depression of Ca^{2+} current evoked during depolarizing commands. These effects coincide temporally, lasting for 10-30 seconds, and are followed by sustained attenuation of a transient-type K^+ current. Since the latter functions to dampen the rate of action potential generation, depression of its expression probably accounts for the appearance of spontaneous action potential activity. These effects of TRH on Ca^{2+} and K^+ conductances are likely related to sequential changes in free intracellular Ca^{2+} reported to occur following TRH exposure. Conversely, SRIF promotes the activation of the transient-type K^+ conductance, thereby dampening action potential activity. These effects of the peptides on membrane excitability correlate well with their actions to regulate prolactin release.

747 IN VIVO PERFUSION OF THE ANTERIOR PITUITARY IN FREELY MOVING RATS.
E. M. Düker*, W. Wuttke, Dept. of Reproductive Biology, German Primate Center, 3400 Göttingen, FRG.

Stereotaxic implantation of the tip of a push-pull cannula into the anterior pituitary allows focal perfusion of the pituitary after recovery of the rats. Catecholamines or prolactin and LH can be measured in 15 min perfusate fractions. Intrapituitary prolactin and LH release can be stimulated by TRH or LRH respectively, and always parallels changes in blood concentrations of these hormones. Catecholamines measured in the perfusates under TRH or LHRH stimulation did not change. Systemic treatment of rats with the dopamine (DA) receptor blocking drug Sulpiride (10 µg / 100 g b.w.) results in a prompt increase in intrapituitary prolactin release rates and in blood prolactin levels without concomitant changes in catecholamine concentrations in systemic venous blood. DA concentrations in the pituitary perfusates, however, increased within 15 - 60 min following Sulpiride treatment. Norepinephrine, but not epinephrine, often paralleled the pattern observed for DA. It is concluded that intrapituitary perfusion utilizing the push-pull cannula technique is a powerful tool in the study of short-term dynamic interactions between catecholamine and prolactin release in unanesthetized, freely moving animals.

748 PITUITARY AND GONADAL INFLUENCE ON FATTY ACID COMPOSITION OF LECITHIN IN RAT SERUM. S Edén*, J-O Jansson and A Svanborg, Dept of Physiology and Geriatrics and Long-Term Care Medicine, University of Göteborg, P O Box 33031, S-400 33 Göteborg, Sweden.

Changes in the fatty acid (FA) composition of lecithin (L) reflect the activity of different synthetic pathways of L in the liver, which in turn are affected by gonadal steroids. It was investigated how gonadal steroids and the pituitary interacts in the control of the FA composition of L in rat serum. Male and female rats, 30-40 days old, were gonadectomized (GX) and/or hypophysectomized (HX). After 1-2 weeks, the rats were killed and the FA composition of L in serum was analyzed as described by Gustavson et al (Scand J Clin Lab Invest 33 Suppl 137:63-70, 1974). Female rats had higher proportions of stearic and arachidonic acid, and lower proportions of palmitic and linoleic acid as compared to male rats. While there was no effect of GX of female rats on the FA composition of L, GX males showed a partial "feminisation" that was completely reversed by testosterone enanthate (0.5 mg/kg/day). Also in intact and GX female rats testosterone treatment resulted in a "masculine" FA composition of L. HX of female rats caused a "masculinisation" of FA that was not reversed by treatment with estradiol valerate (0.1 mg/kg/day). There was no effect of HX of male rats on the FA composition of L.

It is concluded that testosterone "masculinizes" the FA composition of L in rat serum. The "feminine" FA composition of L seems to be dependent on an intact pituitary. It might be speculated that testosterone acts inhibitory on pituitary factor(s) that are responsible for "feminisation" of the FA composition of L in serum.

749 EFFECTS OF GONADECTOMY AND ESTRADIOL BENZOATE (EB) ADMINISTRATION IN MALE RATS BEARING A PITUITARY GRAFT SINCE DAY 5 OF LIFE. A.I. Esquifino* and J.A. F. Tresguerres, Chair Extpl. Endocrinology, Dept. Physiology, Fac. Medicina, Univ. Complutense, Madrid-3, SPAIN.

Five days old male rats of the Wistar strain were grafted with a pituitary (PG) of litter-mate donnors under the pectoral muscles or sham operated (C) to be used in this study. Plasma prolactin (PRL) and LH were measured by specific RIA methods using reagents from NIH. Gonadectomy was performed at 90 days of life and EB (100 µg. s.c.) administration (12 a.m.) was done 14 days after gonadectomy. Basal plasma PRL levels at 90 days of age were found to be higher in PG than in C rats ($P<0.01$). Basal LH levels on the contrary were depressed in PG animals ($P<0.01$). After gonadectomy, a decrease in PRL levels was observed in both groups but still mantaining PG rats higher levels than C ($P<0.05$). LH levels were raised in both groups but the increase was less marked in PG animals. After EB administration a higher PRL increase was detected in C than in PG animals ($P<0.05$). LH levels in C rats showed the well known negative feedback effect after EB administration whereas a pulsatile response was detected in PG rats, with negative feedback in the morning and a positive one in the afternoon. All these data suggest that neonatally induced hyperprolactinaemia was able to modify LH secretion in the adult age.

This work has been possible through CAICYT nº 4290.

750 CELLS WITH POSITIVE IMMUNOSTAINING FOR ONE OR MORE ADENOHYPOPHYSIAL HORMONES IN NULL CELL ADENOMAS OF THE HUMAN PITUITARY. C. Ezrin*, E. Horvath, N. Ryan and K. Kovacs, Div. of Endocrinology, Cedars-Sinal Medical Center, UCLA, Los Angeles, CA 90048, USA: Dept. of Pathology, St. Michael's Hosp., University of Toronto, Toronto, Ont. M5B 1W8, Canada.

Advances in immunocytology and electron microscopy led to a new pituitary adenoma classification which hinged on hormone content, ultrastructural characteristics and cytogenesis. Based on histologic, immunocytologic and ultrastructural study of more than 800 surgically-removed human pituitary adenomas, it became apparent that all 5 adenohypophysial cell types can give rise to tumors. Approximately 75% of adenomas contained GH, PRL, ACTH, TSH, FSH and /or LH and consisted of appropriate cell types. About 25% of pituitary adenomas, however, were unassociated with clinical and biochemical evidence of hormone excess and lacked immunocytologic and ultrastructural markers permitting the disclosure of their cellular derivation. These tumors, termed null cell adenomas, invariably possessed cytoplasmic secretory granules and organelles necessary for hormone synthesis and release. Using the sensitive avidin-biotin-immunoperoxidase comples technique, it was apparent that many of these tumors contained a few single cells or varying numbers of small cell groups which showed positivity for one or more adenohypophysial hormones, most often β-TSH, β-FSH, -LH and/or α-subunit. The presence of hormones in a few adenoma cells may represent genuire tumor cell heterogeneity,pluridirectional differentiation, or gradual dedifferentiation. How to classify those pituitary adenomas which are mainly immunonegative but show focal positivity for one or more adenohypophysial hormones remains to be established. (Supported in part by Grant MA-6349 of the MRC of Canada)

751 EVIDENCE THAT THE SIZE OF THE RELEASABLE POOL OF FSH IS DETERMINED SOLELY BY EXTRAPITUITARY FACTORS. W. Findley*, Dept. Ob/Gyn, Baylor College of Medicine, and Reproductive Research Lab., St. Luke's Episcopal Hospital, Houston, TX 77030.

A variety of studies have indicated that only a small portion of the pituitary content of FSH is released in response to maximum stimulation by gonadotropin releasing hormone (GnRH). (See Endocr. Rev. 4:179, 1983.) The purpose of this study was to determine if the relatively small size of this "releasable pool" is due, at least in part, to an intrinsic pituitary factor. Rat anterior pituitary cell cultures were exposed to media with or without 1 uM GnRH for various intervals. The FSH content of the media and cell lysates was measured using a radioimmunoassay with less than 0.04% crossreactivity with purified rat LH (I-5, NIAMDD). In the presence of GnRH, there was a rapid release of 2006 $\pm$ 87 ng FSH RP-1/culture within the first 4 hours. During the next 4 hours, the rate of release leveled with a total of 2242 $\pm$ 69 ng/culture released by the end of 8 hours, compared to 277 $\pm$ 13 ng/culture in the absence of GnRH. During the same period, the intracellular content of the stimulated cultures declined from 1952 $\pm$ 74 ng/culture to 303 $\pm$ 25 ng/culture, while that of the unstimulated cultures rose slightly to 2157 $\pm$ 25 ng/culture. Thus, rat pituitary gonadotropes are capable of releasing over 75% of the total FSH present during a 4 hour exposure to GnRH. Because the total FSH increases, presumably via synthesis of new FSH (Mol. Cell. Endocrinol. 12:53, 1978), the amount released is actually equivalent to the entire cellular content initially present. It is therefore concluded that the relatively small releasable pool observed in previous studies is not the result of an intrinsic limitation on pituitary FSH release. It may instead reflect modulation by steroids, inhibin, or down regulation of GnRH binding.

752 KALLIKREIN GENE EXPRESSION IN THE RAT ANTERIOR PITUITARY. P.J. Fuller*, J.A. Clements, P.L. Whitfeld and J.W. Funder, Medical Research Centre, Prince Henry's Hospital, Melbourne, Australia 3004.

Glandular kallikrein is one of several serine proteases involved in post-translational processing of biologically active peptides. The report of "kallikrein-like" activity in the rat neuro-intermediate lobe (N-IL) and its possible involvement in the processing of pro-opiomelanocortin (Endocrinology 112:1194, 1983) led us to explore the expression of the gene(s) in the pituitary, using a plasmid containing a rat pancreatic kallikrein cDNA insert generously provided by Dr. Ray MacDonald (Dallas). Northern blots of polyadenylated RNA from rat liver, kidney, anterior pituitary (AP) and N-IL were hybridized with the ^{32}P labeled plasmid; tissue sections were hybridized with the 620 bp cDNA insert by the method of Hudson et al (Endocrinology 108:353, 1981). Hybridization confirmed the presence of kallikrein mRNA in kidney and its absence from liver. Positive hybridization was seen for the AP-derived poly A RNA; the size ($\sim$1.0 kb) was identical to kidney poly A RNA run in parallel. Total RNA from rat N-IL showed significant hybridization not at 1 kb but to a larger species ($\sim$4.5 kb), possibly representing an unprocessed gene transcript. Hybridization histochemistry confirmed these results with a characteristic cortical pattern in the kidney, hybridization in the anterior pituitary and non in the N-IL. These findings suggest that the previously reported kallikrein activity in N-IL is due to some other, non-kallikrein serine protease; in contrast, kallikrein may have a physiological role in limited precursor proteolysis in the anterior pituitary gland. Supported by the National Health & Medical Research Council of Australia.

753 NUCLEAR MAGNETIC RESONANCE (NMR) IMAGING OF THE PITUITARY GLAND - UTILITY IN TUMOR LOCALIZATION.

B. Glaser*, M. Sheinfeld, †Y. Benmair, †S. Stoker, §N. Kaplan. Inst. of Endocrinology, Kupat Holim, Carmel Hospital, Haifa; §Rakah Inst. of Physics, Hebrew University, Jerusalem, Israel.

Recent technical advances in NMR scanning have improved spacial resolution so that the pituitary gland can now be readily visualized in 3 planes -- without the interference of bone artifacts or the need for contrast enhancement or ionizing radiation. We have evaluated the utility of NMR scanning in identifying pituitary lesions using a prototype Gyrex 5000 unit (Elscint, Herzliya, Israel). Fifteen healthy volunteers and 15 patients were studied. Normal pituitary dimensions computed from the CRT monitor, were -- sagittal 7-12 mm; vertical 7-9 mm; transverse 7-9 mm; calculated volume 0.28-0.41 cm^3. The optic chiasm and suprasellar area were well visualized, allowing sensitive evaluation of suprasellar extention. Pituitary tumors were readily visualized in 7 patients with large adenomas documented by X-ray computed tomography (CT), 2 of these had suprasellar extension. In two patients with enlarged radiolucent sella on CT and normal pituitary functions, the "empty sella" syndrome was confirmed. Four CT negative patients -- one with Cushing's disease and 3 with hyperprolactinemia had 2-5 mm intrasellar lesions with normal pituitary dimensions. One patient with idiopathic recent onset diabetes insipidus had a mildly enlarged nodular pituitary suggestive of tumor, but no suprasellar involvement. One patient with hyperprolactinemia and 1° hypothyroidism had a normal scan. Conclusion: NMR imaging of the pituitary provides a powerful non-invasive tool for the visualization of pituitary micro- and macroadenomata. †NMR Unit, Elscint, Herzliya, Israel.

754 ANTERIOR PITUITARY DOPAMINE RECEPTORS IN RATS WITH ESTROGEN-INDUCED PITUITARY TUMORS.

P. Falardeau*, G. Pelletier & T. Di Paolo, Dept. of Molecular Endocrinology, Laval University Hospital Center, Quebec, G1V 4G2, Canada.

Prolactin (PRL)-secreting tumors represent the majority of hormone-secreting pituitary adenomas in man, but it is uncertain whether a central nervous system disturbance or autonomous lactotroph growth and function is the most important aspect of their pathogenesis. We have studied dopamine (DA) receptors in rats bearing estradiol-induced PRL-secreting pituitary tumors recently characterized as a model for human prolactinoma (Endocrinology 110: 590, 1982). Female rats were injected at 3-week intervals with 2 mg estradiol valerate (EV) or with diluent. After 10 weeks, adenomatous changes in the pituitary gland were seen and plasma PRL concentrations reached 1 μg/ml. Anterior pituitary weights were increased significantly in the tumors compared to controls while the affinity and the density of DA receptors (expressed per mg of tissue or per mg of protein) as assessed by [^{3}H]spiperone binding remained unchanged. However, the DA receptor concentration per pituitary is significantly elevated. Bromocriptine (BROM) is commonly and successfully used for treatment of human prolactinomas. BROM administration (2.5 mg/kg for 1 month) to control rats and rats bearing estrogen-induced pituitary tumors was studied. BROM induced a 65% decrease in the density of DA receptors without any change in affinity both in normal pituitaries and in tumors. Concurrently, plasma PRL concentrations, elevated in the tumor bearing rats, were decreased to control values following the BROM treatment. Our data suggest that rats with primary estrogen-induced PRL-secreting tumors have normal pituitary DA receptors.
(Supported by the NCI).

755 DIFFERENT HORMONAL PATTERNS IN PATIENTS WITH PRL SECRETING TUMOR AND HYPER-PROLACTINAEMIC PCO SYNDROME. P. Falaschi^, A. Rocco, P. Pompei and G. Frajese, Dept. of Clinica Medica V, University of Rome, 00161 Rome, Italy.

HyperPRL represents one of the most common conditions of infertility in woman. To our experience hyperPRLs related to PRL adenomas (PRLa) and to polycystic ovary (PCO) are the more frequent. In fact about 30% of patients with PCO present hyperPRL. In the majority of cases PRL levels higher than 100-200 ng/ml with clear skull x-ray alterations (confirmed by CAT) reveal a PRLa. The diagnostic problem is present when PRL levels are 30-60 ng/ml and there is no evidence of skull x-ray alterations or positive CAT.In such condition it is necessary to identify if hyperPRL is of tumoral or functional origin for a correct therapeutic approach. We studied 104 and 35 patients with PRLa and hyperPRL PCO to evidentiate the different hormonal parameters (results in the table). There are several parameters able to discriminate the two forms of hyperPRL. It is important, without evident skull x-ray alterations, to differentiate tumoral and PCO hyperPRL. A correct diagnosis will be useful in recovering normal ovarian function and fertility in patients with these different pathologies.

	PRL	FSH	LH	T	E2	E1	A	DHEAS	LH to GnRH	PRL to TRH	DMP	NFS	Response to Clomiphene
PCO	↑	→ ↓	↑↑	↑	→ ↓	↑	↑	↑	↑↑	↑↑^	→↑	→	+
PRLa	↑↑↑	→ ↓	→↓	→↓	↓	↓	→	→ ↑	↓→ ↑	↓^	↓^	↓^	−

↑:increase - →:unmodified - ↓:decrease - ^:as a group - DMP:domperidone - NFS:nomifensine

756 PROLACTIN EXTRACTED AT HIGH pH IS READILY RELEASED FROM THE ANTERIOR PITUITARY AND LESS SENSITIVE TO DOPAMINE INHIBITION. P.R. Findell* and B. Benson, Department of Anatomy, Univ. of Arizona, Tucson, AZ 85724.

Homogenization of male rat anterior pituitaries (AP) at high pH (10.0) extracts significantly more prolactin (PRL) than at neutral pH. We have tested whether this difference in extractability is modified by chronic (8 wks) or short term (4 days) hyperprolactinemia (HypPRL) produced by ectopic AP transplants. In situ AP from chronic or short term HypPRL male rats and their age-matched, sham-operated controls were homogenized at pH 7.4 or pH 10.0, or were incubated at 37.5°C for 60 or 120 minutes with or without Dopamine (10^{-7} or 10^{-5}M).

	PRL in µg/mg pituitary, mean ± SEM		
	Chronic HypPRL	Short term HypPRL	Controls
PRL extracted @ pH 7.4	1.10 ± 0.15	1.45 ± 0.16	2.30 ± 0.24
PRL extracted @ pH 10.0	1.10 ± 0.25	2.86 ± 0.34	3.51 ± 0.30
PRL release 60 min.	0.18 ± 0.04	0.34 ± 0.03	0.36 ± 0.02
PRL release 120 min.	0.20 ± 0.04	0.53 ± 0.04	0.57 ± 0.02

Chronic HypPRL resulted in the loss of the additional PRL extractable at pH 10.0 and a significant ($p<0.01$) decrease in PRL released into the incubation media. Dopamine (10^{-7} or 10^{-5}) was also significantly more effective (68% and 72%) in suppressing PRL release from these AP ($p<0.05$). No difference in AP responsiveness to dopamine was observed in short term HypPRL. These data suggest that the additional pH 10.0 extractable PRL represents a separate pool of PRL which is readily released from the AP and which is less sensitive to dopamine inhibition. Supported by NIH Grant #HD-08759.

757 INFLUENCE OF NALOXONE ON PROLACTIN SECRETION INDUCED BY FENFLURAMINE IN MAN.

C.Foresta, G.Scanelli, A.Tramarin, N.Sicolo°, G.Federspil and C.Scandellari
Istituto di Semeiotica Medica-Cattedra di Patologia Medica III-Università di Padova,Italy.

It is known that central serotoninergic neurons exert a modulatory role in the regulation of prolactin release from the anterior pituitary. The activation of central serotoninergic pathways, in fact, stimulates prolactin secretion by the pituitary gland. The mechanisms regulating prolactin secretion also include opiate receptors. It has been demonstrated that exogenous and endogenous opiates stimulate prolactin secretion in a dose-dependent fashion. To ascertain whether there is a relationship between serotoninergic and opioidergic control of prolactin secretion, we investigated the effect of naloxone, a specific opioid antagonist, on prolactin secretion in normal men, after treatment with fenfluramine, drug which induces a release of 5-HT and inhibits its reuptake. The study was carried out on 5 normal men, aged 21 to 25 yrs. To all subjects were given, in a randomized fashion at 7 day intervals: placebo and 0.9% saline in infusion for 5 hours; fenfluramine (60 mg orally) and saline, in infusion for 5 h; fenfluramine and naloxone (30 mg over 5 h). Blood samples were taken at 30-min. intervals for 5 h. In all subjects, fenfluramine induced an increase in prolactin plasma levels ($p<0.05$ at 180 and 300 min., $p<0.01$ at 240 min. versus placebo). The prolactin response to fenfluramine was found to be lower during naloxone infusion ($p<0.01$). The mechanisms by which serotonin exerts its stimulatory effect on prolactin secretion is not entirely clear. Our results suggest that serotonin may also affect prolactin secretion by stimulating hypothalamic opioid system.

758 ON THE CONTROLLING MECHANISMS OF THE TWO TYPES OF PROLACTIN SURGES DURING PSEUDOPREGNANCY IN RATS.

S. Furudate* and I. Hashimoto, Department of Laboratory Animal Science, Kitasato University School of Medicine, 1-15-1 Kitasato, Sagamihara, Kanagawa 228, Japan.

During pseudopregnancy(PSP) induced by cervical stimulation, two surges of PRL are observed, the nocturnal surge st dawn and the diurnal surge in the evening. In order to clarify difference(s) in the controlling mechanisms of the two types of PRL surges, an attempt was made to correlate changes in serum and pituitary PRL contents and in PRL release during 2 h's incubation of the pituitary with turnover rates of dopamine(DA) and norepinephrine(NE) in the preoptic-anterior hypothalamus(PAH) and in the mid-posterior hypothalamus(MPH) on days 5-6 of PSP. At the nocturnal surge, pituitary PRL contents decreased significantly from 0000 h to 0300-0600 h and the *in vitro* PRL release from the pituitary was significantly less at 0300-0600 h than at 0000 h. Contrarily, during the diurnal PRL surge, both the pituitary PRL contents and the *in vitro* PRL release remained unchanged at high levels. The turnover rates of DA in the hypothalamus were inversely correlated with serum PRL levels at the diurnal surge when a significant increase in serum PRL was accompanied by not only marked decrease in turnover rates of DA in PAH but also a slight decrease in turnover rates of the amine in MPH. No significant decrease occured in the turnover rates of DA in either PAH or MPH at the nocturnal surge. There was no obvious correlation between turnover rates of NE in the hypothalamus and serum PRL levels at either PRL surge. These findings suggest that the decreased turnover rates of DA in the hypothalamus and PRL synthesis in the pituitary are involved in the diurnal surge, and it is most probable that the nocturnal PRL surge occurs, under control of hypothalamic PRL-releasing factor, without any significant synthesis of PRL in the pituitary.

759 LATENT HYPERPROLACTINAEMIA AND CORPUS LUTEUM FUNCTION. I. Gerhard* and B. Runnebaum, Department of Endocrinology, Women's Hospital, University of Heidelberg, D-6900 Heidelberg, FRG.

Within a prospective study of infertility patients the connection between latent hyperprolactinaemia and corpus luteum function has been analysed after clarification of tubal, andrological and immunological factors. In 120 women with biphasic cycles and normal basal hormone concentrations (FSH, LH, prolactin, testosterone, DHAS, thyreoid gland function) the TRH test for prolactin (Pr) was performed in the early follicular phase and the metoclopramide test (met) in the luteal phase. In addition, during the hyperthermic phase repeated determinations of progesterone (P) and estradiol-17ß (E_2) were performed. Diagnostics were completed by an endometrium biopsy (EB) and ß-hCG measurement premenstrually. The following results were obtained: 1. Significantly higher Pr concentrations in the luteal phase ($p=0.002$). 2. Pr response 3 to 4 times higher after met than after TRH. 3. No correlation between P concentrations for one thing and Pr or E_2 for another. 4. Significant positive correlation between E_2 and Pr 30 minutes after met ($p=0.01$). 5. Compared to infertile patients and women with abortions, women with spontaneous gestation and delivery ($n=30$) had significantly lower Pr concentrations with and without stimulation and higher P/E_2 ratios ($n=0.01$), however no difference in the basal P and E_2 concentrations and in the dating of the EB. Calculation of the P/E_2 ratio and Pr after met allowed the best prognostics and subtile treatment.

760 BROMOCRIPTINE INDUCED DECREASE OF PROLACTIN (PRL) IS FOLLOWED BY AN INCREASE OF FSH AND LH IN HEMODIALYZED CHRONIC UREMIC MEN. R. Giannella*, P. Carpano Maglioli, R. Quadri, M. Manenti, M. Varengo, G. Bellomo and D. Fonzo, Patologia Medica E, Istituto di Medicina Interna, via Genova 3, 10126 Torino, Italy

To evaluate the influence of PRL on pituitary function in chronic renal failure, the effect of long term bromocriptine (BCR) treatment on PRL and gonadotropin levels was studied in 7 hyperprolactinemic and 5 normoprolactinemic hemodialyzed uremic men. All patients had impotence, reduced libido and/or infertility. Drugs acting on pituitary-gonadal axis were avoided. Four of the normoprolactinemic and only one hyperprolactinemic patient dropped out because of postural hypotension. BCR treatment was followed by a significant decrease of PRL after 15, 30, and 310 days. FSH levels showed a continuous increase during treatment with statistical significance after 310 days. The elevated basal LH levels rose further reaching a maximum after 30 days. Testosterone levels and sperm analysis at 90 days did not show any significant modification. From our data it appears that gonadotropin levels in hemodialyzed chronic uremic men are partially inhibited by the elevated PRL levels as implied by the increase after long term BRC treatment.

761 REGULATION BY CA^{2+} OF PROLACTIN AND GROWTH HORMONE GENE EXPRESSION IN PRIMARY RAT PITUITARY CELL CULTURES.
G.G. Gick*, and F.C. Bancroft, Molecular Biology and Virology Department, Sloan-Kettering Institute, New York, N.Y. 10021.

We have demonstrated previously that Ca^{2+} (0.4 mM) specifically stimulates prolactin (PRL) RNA sequences in rat pituitary tumor (GH_3) cells incubated in serum-free medium (J. Biol. Chem. 258:4618). The regulation by Ca^{2+} of PRL and growth hormone (GH) mRNA and transcription in primary cultures of rat pituitary cells was investigated. Incubation of these cultures in serum-free medium with 0.4mM Ca^{2+} yielded no significant increase in PRL mRNA. Assays with arsenazo III of Ca^{2+} in this medium yielded values in the range of 10-40 uM. Incubation of cells with 50 uM EGTA for 3 days yielded decreases in PRL and GH mRNA of 33- and 7-fold, respectively, relative to untreated controls. These decreases were prevented by simultaneous addition of Ca^{2+} to 50 uM, and partially reversed after 6 days by addition of Ca^{2+} after 3 days. Hence the EGTA affects were due to removal of Ca^{2+}, but were not due to total inactivation by EGTA of pituitary cells producing PRL and GH mRNA. Transcription of these genes was assayed by the nuclear run-on procedure. Transcription of the PRL and GH genes in cells incubated 4 days without EGTA was greater by 6.9- and 2.7-fold, respectively, than in cells incubated with 50 uM EGTA. Thus, in normal rat pituitary cells, Ca^{2+} stimulates mRNA levels and transcription of PRL and, to a lesser extent, of GH. Supported by a grant from NIH.

762 **TESTING AS TO ESTROGEN-INDUCED PROLACTINOMAS IN MALE-TO-FEMALE TRANSSEXUALS.**
Louis Gooren*, H. van Kessel and W. Harmsen-Louman, Hospital of the Vrije Universiteit, Amsterdam, the Netherlands (P.O. Box 7057).

Transsexuality in the male requires long-term estrogen treatment with the potential risk of inducing prolactinomas. We report on 142 subjects, treated with 100 µg ethinyloestradiol/day. Duration of treatment: 12-96 months. The upper limit of normal for a male in our lab= 0,30 U/l. In 13 subjects prolactin (PRL) was > 1.0 U/l, in 12: > 0,75, in 42: > 0,50, in 45: >0,25, in 30: < 0,25 U/l. In ten subjects galactorrhea (PRL 0,40-1,5 U/l). We tested whether subjects with high PRL levels differ from those with lower PRL levels in their regulation of PRL secretion, in other words are more tumor prone. The sensitivity to a dopamine infusion of 0,1 µg/kg/min for 1 h, followed by 1,0 µg/kg/min for 1 h was measured in 6 subjects (PRL > 1,0) (A) and in 6 subjects (PRL < 0,5) (B). No difference was found. Further,the response to an inhibitor of central dopamine synthesis, monoidotyrosine (MIT) was measured in the two groups (JCEM 56: 692,1983); this was significantly smaller in group A, suggestive for a loss of hypothalamic dopamine control. Further it was noted in 23 subjects, with PRL > 0,75 U/l, that these values dropped to levels < 0,40, three weeks after withdrawal of E treatment. Conclusion: in our population so far no conclusive evidence for induction of prolactinomas. A small group (13/142) might be at risk.

763 UTERINE EPITHELIAL CELLS SECRETE PROLACTIN INHIBITORY ACTIVITY. William C. Gorospe* and Marc E. Freeman, Biological Science, Florida State University, Tallahassee, Florida 32306

The non-pregnant uterus may secrete a prolactin (PRL) inhibitory factor. We have demonstrated that uterine extracts will specifically inhibit PRL release, in a dose-dependent fashion, from cultured pituitary cells. The purpose of the present study was to determine what specific cell type(s) within the uterus contains and secretes this PRL inhibitory activity (PIA). Suspensions of isolated epithelial, stromal and myometrial cells were prepared by differential enzymatic disaggregation of uteri from ovariectomized rats and cultured for 24h in serum-free Dulbecco's Modified Eagles Medium. The integrity and population purity of the isolated cells were determined by Trypan blue exclusion and histological examination, respectively. Spent media were recovered from each uterine cell culture and placed in culture with monolayers of anterior pituitary cells for 24h. Media were collected and PRL concentrations assayed. PRL levels were unaffected by spent media obtained from either stromal or myometrial cells. However, media recovered from cultured epithelial cells induced a significant dose-dependent suppression of PRL release. These findings confirm our earlier observations that the uterus contains a PIA and that this activity is secreted by the epithelial layer. Supported by the NIH, HD-11669.

764 COMPARATIVE STUDIES ON THE KINETICS OF PROSTAGLANDIN E_2 IN THE HUMAN THYROID TUMOR. C.Kikuchi*, M.Miyakawa, M.Ota, T.Aoki and A.Sato, Department of Surgery, Azumi Hospital, Nagao 399-86, Japan.

Biochemical evidence has accumulated concerning the potential role of prostaglandins (PGs) in the intracellular regulatory system, suggesting that determination of PG synthesis and metabolism may clarify the causes underlying some neoplasm. We, consequently, have undertaken an investigation on blood (drawn directly from the carotid artery and the inferior thyroid vein) and tumor tissue prostaglandin E_2 (PGE_2) levels in individuals with various thyroid tumors. The patients were divided according to the proved histology into 3 groups; Group I (colloid adenoma or cyst), Group II (trabecular or tubular adenoma) and Group III (papillary or follicular carcinoma). The values for PGE_2 of the arterial blood were consistently lower than those of the blood from the thyroid vein. PGE_2 concentrations in the venous blood of Group I, II, III were 3.11±1.43 ng/ml (mean ±SD), 3.99±0.61 ng/ml and 6.63±3.19 ng/ml, respectively, disclosing highly significant difference among each group ($p<0.001$). The venous-arterial difference in the concentrations of PGE_2 for Group I, II and III were 0.63±0.32 ng/ml, 1.72±0.29 ng/ml, 3.51±1.75 ng/ml respectively, and the difference was significant at 0.1% level. Tumor tissue PGE_2 levels of Group II were twice as much as those of Group I, whereas those of Group III disclosed an amount of more than three times those of Group I. Thus, it is clear from these data that elaboration of PGE_2 in the thyroid carcinomas extremely exceeds that of benign thyroid tumors. Our observations furthermore indicate potential malignancies of the trabecular and tubular adenomas which have been believed to be benign tumors so far.

765 SUPPRESSION OF PROSTACYCLIN PRODUCTION BY INSULIN IN CULTURED BOVINE ENDOTHELIAL CELLS. R.G. Larkins*, and A. Chrisanthou, University of Melbourne Department of Medicine, Royal Melbourne Hospital, 3050, Australia.

It has been suggested that systemic hyperinsulinemia may predispose to atherosclerosis. Theoretically, decreased production of prostacyclin (PGI_2) by endothelial cells of arteries could favor platelet adhesion,with release of platelet derived growth factor, smooth muscle proliferation and ultimately development of atherosclerosis. This study was designed to see whether exposure of endothelial cells to insulin affects PGI_2 production. Endothelial cells were digested from bovine aorta and established in culture. After subculture, they were grown to confluence, and cultured for 16 h at glucose concentrations 3.3, 11 and 33 mmol/l, and insulin concentrations of 0, 0.5, 10 and 40 ng/ml, in RPMI 1640. A final incubation in Krebs Ringer bicarbonate buffer containing 10 mmol/l Hepes, 0.1% bovine serum,and the appropriate insulin and glucose concentration for 120 min was performed. Supernatant fluid was assayed for 6-keto-$PGF_{1\alpha}$, the stable metabolite of PGI_2. The results were normalized for cell number. No significant difference in cell number between the groups was detected. Glucose had no significant effect on PGI_2 production. Insulin at 10 ng/ml (50.8±11.4% of control, $p<0.01$, n=12) and 40 ng/ml (54.2±7.0% of control, $p<0.005$, n=12) significantly inhibited prostacyclin production. As systemic plasma insulin levels in obese type II diabetics and insulin-treated type I diabetics would frequently be of the order of 10 ng/ml, the observed inhibitory action of insulin on production of PGI_2 by endothelial cells may be relevant to the in vivo situation and could play a role in the susceptibility of diabetic subjects to atherosclerosis.

766 ASSESSING SERTOLI CELL FUNCTION IN THE RABBIT BY MEASUREMENT OF SERUM ANDROGEN BINDING PROTEIN. N. Escobar* and N.A. Musto, The Population Council, New York, NY 10021

We have shown previously that Sertoli cell activity in neonatal rats can be assessed by serum measurements of androgen binding protein (ABP), a secretory product of this cell. This activity is characterized by steadily increasing serum rABP levels in the prepubertal rat. Then at 20 days of age, concomitant with complete closure of the blood testis barrier (BTB), serum rABP decreases rapidly (10- to 20-fold) to adult levels. In other species, for example the human, the presence in blood of sex steroid binding protein (SBP), a protein sharing similar physical and immunological properties with ABP, this problem is more complex. Using the rabbit as a model, we have taken advantage of the observation that rbSBP, but not rbABP, is completely bound by Concanavalin A (ConA) Sepharose. Following ConA Sepharose extraction of rbSBP, the rbABP in serum of 6 to 30 week old male rabbits was measured by a rbSBP RIA which cross reacts 100% with the testicular protein. The results of this study show the 6 week old male rabbit to have high levels of rbABP in blood which remain elevated until 19 weeks and then rapidly decrease to reach undetectable levels at 24 weeks. Thus as early as 6 weeks of age, the rabbit testis is sufficiently developed for the Sertoli cell to actively produce rbABP. Furthermore, the rapidly declining rbABP levels in blood between 19 and 24 weeks of age indicate closure of the BTB at this time.

767 PITUITARY-GONADAL FUNCTION IN KLINEFELTER'S SYNDROME BEFORE AND DURING ADOLESCENCE. C. Faiman*, J.A. Salbenblatt, A. Robinson and J.S.D. Winter, University of Manitoba, Winnipeg, Manitoba, Canada and University of Colorado, Denver, Colorado, U.S.A.

Serum concentrations of FSH, LH, testosterone (T) and estradiol (E_2) were determined at intervals before and during pubertal development in 40 individuals with Klinefelter's syndrome (KS: 47,XXY karyotype), of whom 27 had been detected in neonatal cytogenetic screening programs. A second group of 22 chromatin negative male siblings served as a control group for comparison with our previously published age-specific normal hormone values. In subjects with KS, prior to the appearance of secondary sexual changes, basal serum hormone concentrations and acute responses to stimulation with gonadotropin releasing hormone and human chorionic gonadotropin were not significantly different from normal. The timing of the onset of clinical puberty was normal. Early pubertal patients showed initial testicular growth and normal serum T levels; serum FSH and E_2 concentrations were significantly elevated. By mid-puberty, the subjects were uniformly hypergonadotropic and their testicular growth had ceased. After age 15, serum T concentrations remained in the low-normal adult range. Serum E_2 levels remained high irrespective of the presence or absence of gynecomastia. During early pubertal development, in spite of a primary testicular defect, subjects with KS show relatively normal T production at the expense, however, of elevated gonadotropin levels. These, in turn, may lead to disproportionately enhanced E_2 production and the common occurrence of gynecomastia. These findings suggest that early T therapy might suppress gonadotropins and thus prevent the gynecomastia.

768 DIFFERENTIAL LH RESPONSE TO CLOMIPHENE (C) IN HYPOGONADOTROPIC HYPOGONADISM (HH) AND DELAYED PUBERTY (DP) FOLLOWING PULSATILE INTRANASAL LH-RH ADMINISTRATION. H Fideleff*, O. Levalle, G. Aszenmil, H. Boquete, J.Ross, B. Espínola, A. Guitelman. Servicio de Endocrinología. Hosp. Alvarez, Aranguren 2701, Bs. As., Argentine.

Difficulties to differentitate HH from DP are well-known; this study evaluates a possible sensitivity modification of gonadostat to C, following pulsatile intranasal LH-RH administration in DP. Seven male patients (HH: 3; DP: 4) were studied. Serum LH, FSH and testosterone (T) by RIA and Bio-LH were determined: 1)before and after 8 days C therapy, 2) before and after 10 days LH-RH therapy and 3) before and after a 2nd C test. Basal gonadotropins maintained prepuberal values and did not alter after first C stimulation in both groups. After LH-RH, LH-RIA increased slightly in HH ($\bar{x}\pm SE$): 4.3 ± 1.1 to 12.8 ± 2.7; in DP: 5.8 ± 0.9 to 10.5 ± 0.7 mUI/ml. HH hormonal values did not change after 2nd C stimulation while in DP patients serum LH-RIA raised significantly (5.8 ± 0.7 to 12.6 ± 1.1). In 3 out of 4 DP, T increased slightly after LH-RH administration.

These results suggest that pulsatile LH-RH therapy could induce LH response to 2nd C stimuli in DP, but not in HH, possibly due to congenital LH-RH defficiency in this pathology. Bio-LH did not change probably because the pituitary responds only with LH secretion of low biological activity while a more prolonged LH-RH application could alter this situation. Possible effect of T on gonadostat sensitivity and direct effect of LH-RH on the central nervous system could be considered.

769 UTERINE PROGESTIN RECEPTOR/PROTEIN ANALYSIS BY PROTEIN BLOTTING.

P.D. Feil* and J.R. Vance. Depts. of Biol. Chem. and Medicine (Endocrinology) The M.S. Hershey Med. Ctr., The PA State University, Hershey, PA 17033

Antibodies against the progestin receptor (PR) were produced in a guinea pig. Since only a partially purified rabbit uterine receptor preparation was employed as antigen, it was necessary to determine the number of proteins recognized by this antiserum. Protein blotting to nitrocellulose paper followed by autoradiographic detection of antigen:antibody complexes with ^{125}I-Protein A (I-peak) revealed 5-12 bands depending upon the uterine preparation employed. Two prominent I-peaks were seen in cytosol and nuclear extract with MW ~ 85,000 and 120,000. Several procedures were utilized in an attempt to determine which band(s) represented PR. Isoelectric focusing and SDS studies revealed similar migration properties for I-peaks (85 K and 120 K) and ^{3}H-progestin prelabeled receptor (2D gel). When a partially purified receptor preparation was photoaffinity labeled with ^{3}H-R5020, the 2 major and 1 minor band (~ 68 K) of ^{3}H correlated with the I-peaks. Modulation of uterine proteins by steroid treatment provided interesting comparisons. Uterine cytosol from immature or ovariectomized rabbits revealed the presence of the 2 major I-peaks, which were absent in spleen, liver, and intestinal preparations. Following increasing progesterone administration, the 2 major cytosol and nuclear bands varied in concert with a direct binding assay. Several minor I-peaks decreased or shifted following treatment, suggesting that they were hormonally responsive and/or due to receptor metabolism. Conclusion: Modulation of uterine proteins, including PR, can be followed by protein blotting.

770 HUMAN DECIDUAL DEVELOPMENT IN EARLY PREGNANCY: CHANGES IN NUCLEAR PROGESTERONE (P) RECEPTORS AND PLASMA P AND ESTRADIOL (E_2) LEVELS.

P. Feng*, L-Z. Zhang, Dept. OB/GYN, 3rd Teaching Hospital, Beijing Medical College, Beijing, China.

Nuclear P receptors were determined after 0.6M KCl extraction in endometrium during the normal menstrual cycle (n=6) and in decidua obtained by suction curettage in the 5th to 10th week of normal pregnancy (n=59). Plasma P and E_2 levels were determined by RIA, and morphological changes in decidua were evaluated by light microscopy. 10 cases of early pregnancy with vaginal bleeding were also studied. Results showed that nuclear P receptor concentration in the decidua rose gradually between the 5th and 10th weeks, and significantly at the 7-8th week, when decidua were thicker with marked proliferation and hypertrophy accompanied by significant increases in plasma E_2 levels. Cytosolic P and E_2 receptors and nuclear E_2 receptors were low. In the 3 cases with little vaginal bleeding, all 3 parameters were normal; in the other 7 cases with either heavy vaginal bleeding or expulsion of tissue fragments, nuclear P receptor concentration and plasma P and E_2 levels remained low, and decidua showed degenerative changes. These studies indicate that nuclear P receptors of human decidua in early pregnancy are mainly distributed in the nuclei and that their content was proportional to decidual development. Since normal decidual function is important in the maintenance of pregnancy, the use of analogs to block or to occupy P receptor sites provide a potential effective method for interrupting pregnancy in its early stage.

771 PROGESTERONE ABBREVIATES THE NUCLEAR ACCUMULATION AND RETENTION TIME OF THE ESTROGEN-RECEPTOR COMPLEX (RnE) IN THE RAT OVIDUCT. B. Fuentealba* and M. Nieto. Endocrinology Lab., Fac. Biological Sciences, Pontificia Universidad Católica de Chile. Casilla 114-D. Santiago, Chile.

Exogenous estradiol (E_2) induces accelerated egg transport through the oviduct of pregnant rats, with a latency of 12 hours. Simultaneous administration of progesterone (P) inhibits this estrogen induced accelerated transport of embryos. In order to examine the antagonism of these hormones in the earlier part of their action, nuclear estrogen binding sites were measured in rat oviducts between 0 and 12 hours after treatment with E_2 (1ug); E_2 + P (1ug + 5mg) or vehicle (0.2ml oil) given s.c. on day 1 of pregnancy. Estrogen binding sites were measured in oviductal crude nuclear pellet by the 3-H-estradiol exchange assay in the presence of 1 mM dithiotreitol at 0, 1, 3, 7 or 11 after treatment.

RnE levels remained unchanged at 0.8 pmol/mg DNA in the control group and presented a transitory elevation in the hormone treated groups. The maximum quantity of RnE which accumulated in the nuclear fraction was the same in both hormone-treated groups (3pmol/mg DNA) but the temporal distribution was different. The highest level was observed at 3 h in the E_2 treated group and at 1h in E_2 + P treated group. Following these peak levels, RnE complex concentration decreased and reached basal levels, in E_2 and E_2 + P treated groups, at 7 and 3 h respectively.

These data indicate that progesterone treatment induces an earlier accumulation and disppearance without affecting the peak levels of the RnE complex.

This work was supported by Grants DIUC 9/79 and RF 80007.

772 PROGESTERONE RECEPTOR (PR) IN THE CHICK OVIDUCT : IMMUNOHISTOCHEMICAL STUDY WITH ANTIBODIES TO DISTINCT RECEPTOR COMPONENTS. J.M. Gasc, J.M. Renoir, C. Radanyi, I. Joab, P. Tuohimaa and E.E. Baulieu*, INSERM U 33, Lab. Hormones, 94270 Bicêtre, France.

Immunohistochemical studies were carried out using antibodies raised against the 8S-PR, its (progesterone binding) B-subunit and its (non-progesterone binding) 90K protein constituent. An immunoperoxidase technique with biotinylated secondary antibodies and the avidin-biotin complex was employed. PR was detected not only in well characterized target tissues (glands and luminal epithelium), but also in stromal cells, mesothelium and smooth muscles. Studies with the different antibodies, together with controls performed by presaturation of antibodies with purified 8S-PR, B-subunit, and 90K protein, revealed in cell nuclei the presence of a B- and/or A-subunit-like antigen (cross-reactivity of the antibodies with A and B does not allow a distinction between the 2 subunits). No difference was observed in the subcellular distribution of A and B whether the animals received or not progesterone. The 90K protein was revealed in both cytoplasm and nuclei. The distribution of A and/or B mainly or exclusively in the cell nuclei in absence of progesterone leads to reevaluate the concept of translocation of PR from cytoplasm to nucleus as a prerequisite for progesterone action.

773 FURTHER CHARACTERIZATION OF STEROID RECEPTOR-TRANSFORMING FACTOR FROM MATURE RABBIT EPIDIDYMIS. W.J. Hendry III* and B.J. Danzo, Depts. of Ob/Gyn and Biochemistry, Vanderbilt University, Nashville, TN, 37232, U.S.A.

Having identified a macromolecular factor in the epididymis of sexually mature rabbits which induces a discrete reduction in the sedimentation coefficient of cytosolic estrogen receptors, and having determined that this process is inhibited by molybdate and leupeptin, we endeavored to further characterize the transformation process. Since leupeptin, a thiol-protease inhibitor, inhibits several receptor-active proteases, we tested the influence of sulfhydryl-modifying reagents on epididymal factor-induced transformation of rabbit uterine estrogen receptors. Iodoacetamide (10mM) and N-ethylmaleimide (10mM) did not, while sulfhydryl-reducing agents (monothioglycerol, 12 mM; dithiothreitol, 5mM) did inhibit transformation. Other reagents (Ca^{2+}, 10mM; Mg^{2+}, 10mM; ATP, 1mM), known to influence the activity of various receptor-active proteases, had no effect on the transformation process. Hypertonic buffers extracted the factor from the myofibrillar debris of homogenized epididymides, but little activity was recovered in extracts of partially purified epithelial nuclei from the same tissue. Under hypotonic and hypertonic conditions, native estrogen receptor sedimented at 9-10S and 4-5S, respectively; whereas epididymal factor-transformed receptor, similar to the "mero-receptor," sedimented at 2-3S. Transformed estrogen receptor, like "mero-receptor," did not bind to soluble DNA. Our results indicate that the epididymal factor resembles receptor-active proteases present in other tissues, but also has characteristics that are unique, or have not been investigated in other systems. Supported by NIH grant HD 08295 and a grant from the Andrew W. Mellon Foundation.

774 PURIFICATION OF PROGESTERONE RECEPTOR IN RABBIT UTERUS. N. Ide*, T. Tamaya, S. Ishihara and H. Okada, Dept. of OB/GYN, Kyoto Pref. Univ. Med., Kyoto 602, Japan.

Progesterone receptor (PR) in rabbit uterus was studied for purification. PR was stabilized with molybdate as 8S in cytosol, ammoniumsulfate precipitate and fractions by DEAE chromatography or affinity chromatography. A new steroid affinity resin [medroxyprogesterone acetate(MPA)-BSA-Sephadex] has been invented, and can be successfully used to partially purify the non-transformed species of the PR. The usefulness of the fast protein liquid chromatography (FPLC) technique was determined. A molybdate-stabilized, non-activated form of the PR from the cytosol of estrogen-stimulated rabbit uterus has been purified to homogeneity by a several-step procedure. Purification was achieved by ammonium sulfate precipitation, MPA-BSA-Cellurose chromatography and FPLC. The receptor was obtained in 10% yield with a specific activity for [^{3}H] promegestone binding of 500 pmole/mg protein. The pure receptor migrated as a single band on SDS-gel electrophoresis, with a M.W. of 100,000.

775 ANDROGEN RECEPTORS IN CALF UTERINE CYTOSOL: R1881 DISSOCIATION KINETICS AND DNA-CELLULOSE BINDING. W. de Boer*, L.M. Lindh, A.O. Brinkmann, E. Mulder and H.J. van der Molen, Dept. of Biochemistry II, Erasmus University, Rotterdam, The Netherlands.

Calf uterine cytosol contains an androgen receptor (AR), which binds R1881 with a high affinity (K_d=0.15 nM) in the presence of 2.5 μM triamconoloneacetonide. Sodium molybdate (10 mM) stabilizes the AR as was shown by an increase in R1881 binding from 55 to 114 fmol/mg protein. The AR sedimented as an 8S or 4S molecule on low and high salt sucrose density gradients respectively. AR prepared with molybdate was fairly stable during incubation at 25°C and showed fast dissociation kinetics (k= 0.064 min^{-1}). AR prepared without molybdate was less stable at 25°C, but showed 30-fold slower dissociation kinetics (k=2.2 x 10^{-3} min^{-1}). Identical kinetics were obtained after precipitation of the molybdate-stabilized AR with ammonium sulphate (0-40%). The fast dissociating AR (with molybdate) did not show significant DNA-cellulose binding activity at 0°C (1.5%). Cytosol AR prepared without molybdate as well as the molybdate-stabilized AR precipitated with ammonium sulphate, showed an increase in DNA-cellulose binding activity (50-70%). The bound AR was eluted from the DNA-cellulose at 0.2 M NaCl.
We conclude that the uterine cytosol AR can exist as a fast dissociating, non-DNA-binding form and as a slowly dissociating, DNA-binding form. Molybdate prevents the formation of the activated, DNA-binding form.

776 NEONATAL IMPRINTING OF 8S-HEPATIC ANDROGEN BINDING PROTEIN IN RAT LIVER. D. Decker, T. Saunders and D. Levinson*, Michael Reese Hospital, Lake Shore Drive at 31st Street, Chicago, Illinois 60616.

Recent results using the synthetic androgen methyltrienolone, R1881 have demonstrated an 8S-hepatic androgen binding protein which is male specific, capable of nuclear translocation and absent in the Tfm rodent (Decker and Levinson, Endocr. Suppl, #227:137, 1983). The results of the present study indicate that expression of R1881-androgen binding sites (ABS) in liver cytosol of the adult male rat depends upon exposure to androgen during a brief critical period of neonatal life. Male rats castrated on day 30 exhibit concentrations of hepatic ABS similar to those of intact males which reach a peak at 65 days (castrate, 25.7 fmol/mg prot; control, 26.4 fmol/mg prot). Further, castration or hypophysectomy of mature males does not alter the peak level of hepatic ABS. However, ABS are absent in immature rats of either sex, adult females, or males castrated on day 2 of life regardless of testosterone (T) replacement prior to sacrifice at 65 days. Treatment of neonatal male castrates with T or dihydrotestosterone (DHT) on days 2, 4, 6 and 9 restores the concentration of ABS to those of adult intact males (castrate, 18.2 fmol/mg prot; control, 20.8 fmol/mg prot). Neonatal T or DHT treatment of females ovariectomized on day 45 results in development of ABS in the adult which is 50% of the intact male whereas, ovariectomy on day 45 and T treatment in the adult have no effect, the female or basal pattern in retained (neonatal androgen treatment, 10.3 fmol/mg; adult androgen treatment, 0.7 fmol/mg prot). These results suggest that important sex differences in hepatic function defined as sexual dimorphism in adult rats are determined by the hormonal environment during a critical period shortly after birth.

777 ANDROGEN RECEPTOR IN MALE RAT LIVER. PK Eagon*, JE Willett, SM Seguiti, BJ Rogerson. VA Med Center and Univ. of Pittsburgh, Pgh., PA 15261, USA.

Mammalian liver of both sexes is responsive to sex steroid hormones. Male rat liver cytosol contains androgen receptor (AR) which binds ^{3}H-MT (methyltrienolone, 17β-hydroxy-17α-methyl-4,9,11-estratriene-3-one) with high affinity (Kd=1.1±0.4nM), a capacity of 9.3±1.6 fmol/mg protein (range 2.3-18.8, n=12), and specificity for androgens. Heparin-Sepharose resin retains 50% of ^{3}H-MT binding activity in triamcinolone acetonide (TA)-blocked cytosol. Gel filtration chromatography of ^{3}H-MT labeled cytosol containing protease inhibitors, sodium molybdate (Mo) and TA on Sephadex G100 or Biogel A-0.5m separates a low molecular weight species (26Å) and a large species voided by the resin. The latter species elutes as a 54Å protein on Biogel A-1.5m. Cytosolic AR (cAR) is unstable; 50% of binding is lost in 48h even with Mo, dithiothreitol (DTT) or glycerol present. Castration results in temporary enhancement of cAR at 48h post surgery, followed by a decline to undectable levels at 30d. A decline in the activity of an androgen-dependent cytosolic estrogen binding protein parallels the loss of AR. cAR is not detectable before 90d of age. Several methods for quantitation of nuclear AR have been compared to standard exchange conditions (SEC), i.e., incubation of washed nuclei with 10nM ^{3}H-MT for 1h at 30°. Inclusion of 0.4M NaSCN enhances binding 4-fold, but DTT with or without mersalyl does not. Incubation of nuclei with 10nM ^{3}H-MT at 4° overnight enhances binding 5-6 fold over SEC. Inclusion of DTT with or without mersalyl is less effective, resulting in a 2-3 fold increase over SEC. NaSCN is not effective under these conditions since its use results in partial release of AR into the supernate.

778 ALTERATIONS IN STEROID RECEPTORS IN RAT BULBOCAVERNOSUS/LEVATOR ANI MUSCLES (BCLA) AFTER DENERVATION OR CASTRATION. B.J.Hughes[x], M.Rybczyńska, A.Lämmel and M.Krieg, Dept.Clinical Chemistry, Medical University Clinic, Hamburg, FRG.

Alterations in protein degradation or synthesis associated with muscle atrophy may be related to alterations in glucocorticoid (GR) and androgen (AR) receptor function. We have performed castration or unilateral denervation to induce atrophy of the androgen-sensitive BCLA. BCLA was removed 15 days after denervation (DEN) of the right part of BCLA or castration (CAS) for comparison with the innervated (INN) left part of BCLA or sham-operated rats (SHAM). Receptor analyses were performed with cytosol using charcoal adsorption or agar-gel electrophoresis. To standardize assay conditions rats used for ^{3}H-DEX binding were adrenalectomized 3 days prior to sampling; noncastrated rats were castrated 20 h prior to determination of ^{3}H-R 1881 binding. Under our experimental conditions the interassay CV was less than 9% for both assays. Binding parameters were calculated according to Scatchard. No differences in K_D were observed for GR or AR between groups. GR were increased after DEN compared to INN (86 vs 40 fmoles/mg prot; $p < 0.0003$) or CAS (86 vs 52 fmoles/mg prot; $p < 0.0025$). In contrast, AR were not altered after DEN but increased after CAS compared to SHAM (15 vs 9.3 fmoles/mg prot; $p < 0.001$) or DEN (15 vs 11 fmoles/mg prot; $p < 0.01$). Cytosolic protein was constant following all treatments. In conclusion, the data obtained may reflect a stronger response for BCLA to denervation than to castration if GR concentration is taken as a parameter for catabolic processes, or may reflect different mechanism underlying the two types of atrophy. Supported by SFB 34"Endocrinology".

779 IMMOBILIZATION OF GLUCOCORTICOID RECEPTOR COMPLEX ON ACTIVATED THIOL-SEPHAROSE 4B.

T.Idziorek,B.Sablonnière,V.Dumur,P.Formstecher*and M.Dautrevaux,Laboratoire de Biochimie structurale,Faculté de Médecine, 59045 LILLE, France.

Rat liver glucocorticoid receptor is believed to bear at least two accessible sulphydryl groups since the sulphydryl reagents not only inhibit the binding of glucocorticoids to the cytosolic receptor but also the activation of preformed hormone-receptor complex.Thus we have studied the interaction of the [^3H] Triamcinolone acetonide-glucocorticoid receptor complex with Activated thiol-Sepharose 4B,(Pharmacia). [^3H]TA-receptor complex partially purified by protamine sulfate precipitation was submitted to gel-filtration to remove any added thiols and then adsorbed at 20°C on the activated thiol column equilibrated in thiol-free buffer.After washing with the same buffer,elution was performed in presence of 10mM mercaptoethanol.Both excluded and retained peaks were analyzed by high performance size-exclusion chromatography on TSK G3000 SW column.Bound radioactivity was found in the latter peak only, which was eluted with an apparent MW of 54 KD.Pretreatment of the [^3H] TA-receptor complex by N-ethylmaleimide 3mM before loading on the activated thiol column resulted in complete exclusion of the bound radioactivity.Similarly [^3H] TA-receptor complex highly purified by affinity chromatography could be retained on the same matrix at 0°C.Thus the activated thiol column appeared to afford the first direct evidence of sulphydryl group presence on the native receptor itself.

780 GLUCOCORTICOID REGULATION OF HEPATIC GLUCOCORTICOID RECEPTORS IN VIVO AND ITS RELATIONSHIP TO INDUCTION OF TYROSINE AMINOTRANSFERASE (TAT) ACTIVITY.

M. Kalimi*, J.R. Hubbard, D.P. Poppas and T.A. Shirwany, Dept. Physiology and Biophysics, Medical College of Virginia, Virginia Commonwealth Univ., Richmond, Virginia, 23298, U.S.A.

Regulation of rat hepatic glucocorticoid receptors (GR) was studied using our newly developed exchange assay (Kalimi and Hubbard, Endocrinology 113:1161, 1983). Adrenalectomy (ADX) caused a significant increase in GR binding, with optimal binding 24-48h after surgery. Injection of 1 mg dexamethasone or corticosterone into $\sim$ 300 g ADX rats caused a rapid decline in GR binding. GR levels were depressed 80-90% in less than 15 min after hormone treatment, and remained low for $\sim$ 24h. 48h after glucocorticoid administration significant GR binding was regenerated, and complete binding was recovered by 72h. Regenerated GR binding could be re-depressed by a second injection of hormone. Similar results were obtained using normal (not ADX) rats. Induction of TAT activity (measured 2h after a second injection of glucocorticoid) correlated with GR levels. Thus 1 mg dexamethasone or corticosterone greatly enhanced liver TAT activity in ADX rats (not hormone treated) and in ADX rats injected 72 h previously with 1 mg glucocorticoid hormone. Enhancement of TAT activity was lowest 16-24 h after the first hormone injection (when receptor levels were extremely low). These results indicate that glucocorticoids reversibly down-regulate hepatic receptors, and that induction of liver TAT activity by glucocorticoid hormones is dependent on GR levels.

781 MINERALOCORTICOID RECEPTOR ACTIVITY IN INTACT RAT RENAL CYTOSOL.
M.M. Holbrook*, S.L. Dale, and J.C. Melby, Evans Memorial Department of Clinical Research and the Departments of Medicine and Physiology, University Hospital and Boston University School of Medicine, Boston, Massachusetts 02118.

Present methods for determining mineralocorticoid activity employ either the rat kidney slice or cytosol preparation. Both procedures utilize adrenalectomized rats. When employing the cytosol preparation, exogenous steroid is added to saturate non-aldosterone (aldo) receptors (type II). Occupancy of the type II receptors by basal steroid levels in the intact rat on high salt intake with measurement of the displacement of aldo from the aldo receptor was utilized in the present procedure. Saline-drinking intact rats were sacrificed by nitrogen (N_2) suffocation and a kidney cytosol high-speed supernatant (HSS) was obtained following preparation of a 600 x g homogenate in 0.1 M TRIS/HCl, 0.25 M sucrose, 0.1 M sodium molybdate buffer, pH 7.4. The displacement of labelled aldo by unlabelled aldo (0-200 pg) was compared in intact and adrenalectomized rats sacrificed as above. A linear relationship was observed in both cases when the free to bound steroid ratio was plotted against pg unlabelled aldo added; however, a steeper slope was observed in the N_2 sacrificed rats ($Y = 0.090X + 6.85$ versus $Y = 0.041X + 2.60$). Activities of various steroids obtained at 50% displacement of labelled aldo were determined in the intact and adrenalectomized rat. Values expressed as percent of aldo were found to be consistently lower in intact rats.

782 IN VIVO ENDOCYTOSIS OF ^{125}I-INSULIN IN HEPATOCYTES OF CHLOROQUINE-TREATED RATS.
Javier Cruz*, B.I. Posner, and J.J.M. Bergeron, Departments of Anatomy and Medicine, McGill University, Montreal, Quebec, H3A 2B2.

The in vivo binding and internalization of ^{125}I-insulin has been previously demonstrated in hepatocytes (1980, Journal of Cell Biology 80, 427). In this study in vivo binding and internalization of ^{125}I-insulin was studied (2,10,20 and 45 min after IV injection of labeled hormone) in chloroquine-treated rats and compared to that in rats not so treated. Chloroquine increased retention of radioactivity in the liver but electron microscope radioautography revealed that such retention was not due to accumulation of labeled hormone in lysosomes since no difference in the intracellular distribution of radioactivity was found. Over 30 morphologically distinct structures > 200 nm in diameter were examined for associated radioactivity. Up to 30% of total grains were associated with oval 0.6 μm diameter lipoprotein-containing vesicles, up to 10% with large vesicles (0.4 μm diameter) having a densely stained often indented delimiting membrane and containing one or two 0.04 μm diameter vesicles, while less than 5% of total grains associated with large (> 1 μm) lysosomes containing undegraded material. In all cases close to 50% of examined grains were far (> 6 half-distances) from all examined structures presumably reflecting insulin in transit between the cell membrane and the structures described. In conclusion, chloroquine causes an intracellular accumulation of radioactivity but not by a preferential accumulation in secondary lysosomes. In hepatocytes, insulin is internalized to various clearly recognizable lipoprotein-filled intracellular elements.

783 EFFECTS OF LYSOSOMOTROPIC AGENTS ON THE SUBCELLULAR DISTRIBUTION OF INSULIN RECEPTORS IN RAT LIVER. B. Desbuquois*, S. Lopez and H. Burlet, INSERM U 30, Hôpital des Enfants-Malades, 75015 Paris, France.

Chloroquine (Clq), a lysosomotropic agent, has recently been shown to inhibit the processing of ^{125}I-insulin taken up by rat liver in vivo, leading to accumulation of undegraded ligand in Golgi (G) and lysosomal (L) fractions (Posner et al., J. Biol. Chem. 257: 5789, 1982). The effects of Clq (4 mg/100 g BW ip) alone or in association with quinacrine (Qui) on the subcellular distribution of insulin receptors in livers of control and insulin-injected rats have now been examined. In control rats, Clq and Qui treatment decreases insulin receptor number in plasma membranes (PM) and, reciprocally, increases receptor number in G and L fractions (% change, about 20, 20-60 and 80-120, respectively); receptor number in the total particulate fraction is unaffected. Such treatment also increases by 4-6 fold the content of immunoreactive insulin in G fractions. As previously reported (Desbuquois et al., J. Biol. Chem. 257: 10852, 1982), the injection of native insulin (25 µg/100 g BW iv) decreases by 2-fold insulin binding to PM and increases by 4-5 fold insulin binding to G fractions; insulin treatment also causes a marked accumulation of insulin in G fractions. These changes achieve maximum by 10-40 min and undergo reversal in 2 h. In insulin-injected rats, Clq and Qui treatment does not affect the early changes in the subcellular distribution of insulin receptors, but retards the restoration of the initial receptor distribution as well as the loss of insulin from G fractions. It is suggested that Clq and Qui do not affect the intracellular translocation of insulin receptors induced by insulin, but interfer with the recycling of intracellular and/or internalized receptors.

784 FAMILIAL INSULINRESISTANT DIABETES SECONDARY TO A STRUCTURAL DEFECT OF INSULIN-BINDING-SITES. M. Dreyer*, J. Kühnau, U. Siemers and H. W. Rüdiger, Dep. Internal Med., University of Hamburg, Martinistr. 52, 2000 Hamburg 20, West-Germany

Insulin binding studies on erythrocytes, monocytes and cultured fibroblasts from 3 sibs with insulinresistant diabetes and acanthosis nigricans revealed a complete lack of the high affinity receptor component but a normal number of total binding sites. ^{125}I-insulin was covalently cross-linked to the insulin binding protein of fibroblasts in culture obtained from these patients and controls using Disuccinimidyl-suberate as a crosslinker. Autoradiographic analysis after discontinous SDS-PAGE disclosed a labelled band with a MW of about 400 K representing the intact tetrameric receptor protein (ß-α-α-ß). The patients' receptor protein moved consistantly slower compared to controls. Under reducing conditions (50 mM Dithiothreitol) the α-subunit was found in the region of about 125 K, again moving slower in patients. The ß-subunit appeared as a 98 K protein in both groups. We conclude from these data that these patients with an inherited form of insulinresistant diabetes may have a structural defect of their insulin receptor which causes a reduced affinity of insulin binding. The defect might be located in the α-subunit of the insulin receptor which seems to be responsible for insulin binding in vivo.

785 BINDING SITES FOR ARGININE-VASOPRESSIN AND RELATED PEPTIDES IN RAT BRAIN: A QUANTITATIVE AUTORADIOGRAPHIC STUDY. E.R. de Kloet*, A. Biegon[1], Th.A.M. Voorhuis, F. Rotteveel and J.P.H. Burbach, Rudolf Magnus Institute for Pharmacology, University of Utrecht, Vondellaan 6, 3521 GD Utrecht, The Netherlands and [1]Department of Isotopes, Weizmann Institute of Science, Rehovot, Israel.

Binding sites for arginine-vasopressin (AVP) were detected after in vitro incubation of brain sections, autoradiography with LKB Ultrofilm and computerized densitometry of the film images. The largest density of ^{3}H-AVP labeled sites was observed in the olfactory nucleus, lateral septal nucleus, ventral hippocampus, central amygdaloid nucleus, medial geniculate nucleus, and nucleus tractus solitarii. These brain regions contain nerve terminals of the AVP peptidergic system and respond to AVP or smaller AVP fragments in brain biochemistry, electrophysiology and behavior. Hypothalamic, thalamic, cortical (except the entorhinal cortex), cerebellar and striatal regions had low densities of AVP binding sites. Binding sites for AVP were found in large amounts in kidney and in pituitary. Two selective antagonists of the AVP effect on blood pressure, dPTyr(Me)AVP and d$(CH_2)_5$ Tyr(Me)AVP competed for ^{3}H-AVP binding in the brain with an IC_{50} in the 10^{-7} - 10^{-8} molar range. Recently it was found that a metabolite of AVP in brain, pGluAVP$_{4-9}$ and its derivative [pGlu^{4}, Cyt^{6}]AVP-(4-8) was far more potent than AVP on behavior and displayed a more selective central action, suggesting the presence of subclasses of AVP binding sites in the brain. Such subclasses are being characterized in brain and in peripheral AVP receptors, using autoradiography and kinetic analysis of AVP binding to membrane fractions.

786 CORTICOTROPIN-RELEASING FACTOR (CRF) RECEPTORS IN RAT BRAIN: AUTORADIOGRAPHIC LOCALIZATION. E.B. De Souza*, M. Perrin, J. Rivier, W. Vale and M.J. Kuhar. Dept. of Neurosci., Johns Hopkins Univ. Sch. of Med., Balto., MD 21205 and Peptide Biology Lab, The Salk Institute, La Jolla, CA 92138, USA.

A 41 amino acid peptide that fulfills the criteria of a physiological CRF has been isolated from ovine hypothalami, characterized, and synthesized. This peptide is a potent stimulus to the release of proopiomelanocortin-derived peptides from anterior and intermediate lobes of the pituitary. In addition, there is increasing pharmacological and immunohistochemical evidence that CRF acts as a neuromodulator in brain. Recently, we have identified and localized high affinity CRF receptors in anterior and intermediate lobes of rat pituitary (De Souza et al., Brain Res., in press, 1984), and in anterior lobe of human pituitary. In the present study, we have used the radioiodinated analog of ovine CRF (oCRF), Nle^{21}, ^{125}I-Tyr^{32}-CRF (^{125}I-CRF), to identify, characterize, and map receptors for CRF in rat brain sections by an in vitro labeling light microscopic autoradiographic method. The binding of ^{125}I-CRF to rat brain sections was saturable and of high affinity. Rat CRF, oCRF and its biologically active analog Nle^{21}, Tyr^{32}-CRF exhibited similar potencies in inhibiting ^{125}I-CRF binding. The biologically weaker analogs, oCRF(1-39)-NH_2 and oCRF(1-22)-OH were less potent displacers and the unrelated peptide arginine vasopressin was minimally effective. Rat brain autoradiograms showed high concentrations of ^{125}I-CRF binding in cerebral cortex, with lower concentrations in olfactory tubercle, striatum, amygdala, cerebellum and specific nuclei in thalamus, hypothalamus and brain stem. In summary, our demonstration of CRF receptors in discrete areas of rat brain supports a physiological role for endogenous CRF in regulating activity of the central nervous system.

787 COUPLING OF SOMATOSTATIN RECEPTORS TO ADENYLATE CYCLASE IN BRAIN AND PITUITARY. J. Epelbaum*, E. Moyse, P. Leblanc, C. Kordon and A. Enjalbert, Unité 159 de Neuroendocrinologie INSERM, 2ter rue d'Alésia, 75014 Paris (F).

Specific binding sites for $somatostatin_{14}$ and $somatostatin_{28}$ have already been characterized in the rat brain and pituitary. Using ^{125}I-N-Tyr-$somatostatin_{14}$ and ^{125}I-N-Tyr-$somatostatin_{28}$ as ligands, the kinetics and pharmacological properties of somatostatin binding sites in both tissues are similar. Subcellular localization studies reveal that ^{125}I-N-Tyr-$somatostatin_{14}$ binding sites are mainly located on plasmic or synaptosomal membranes in the pituitary and the cortex respectively. In both tissues and with both ligands, somatostatin binding is sensitive to guanine nucleotides. Using ^{125}I-N-Tyr-$somatostatin_{14}$ as a ligand, GTP is the most potent guanine nucleotide, followed by GDP and GMPPNP whereas ATP, ADP, AMP, cAMP, GMP and cGMP are inactive. Guanine nucleotides convert the high affinity form of the somatostatin receptor to a lower affinity state, since they increase the dissociation rate of ^{125}I-N-Tyr-$somatostatin_{14}$ binding without affecting the association rate. These results are strongly suggestive of a coupling between somatostatin receptors and adenylate cyclase in the brain and the pituitary. Indeed somatostatin inhibits basal adenylate cyclase activity in adenohypophyseal homogenates. The effect is more pronounced in female than in male rats, an observation which could reflect different ratios of adenohypophyseal cell types in both sexes. In conclusion, ^{125}I-N-Tyr-$somatostatin_{14}$ and ^{125}I-N-Tyr-$somatostatin_{28}$ binding sites appear negatively coupled with adenylate cyclase in both brain and pituitary.

788 AUTOANTIBODY TO BOVINE TSH DETECTED IN SERUM OF PATIENTS WITH AUTOIMMUNE THYROID DISEASES. S.Eto*, T.Fujihira, S.Ohnami and H.Suzuki, First Dept. of Internal Med., First Dept. of Surgery, University of Occupational and Environmental Health, Kitakyushu, Fukuoka, Japan

In the assay of TSH receptor antibody (TRAb by Smith's kit: expressed by % inhibition of TSH binding), abnormally low levels of TRAb were detected in the sera of two patients with Hashimoto's thyroiditis (-173, 175 %, respectively) and one patient with Graves' disease (-73 %). To determine if this phenomenon is due to the presence of autoantibody to bovine TSH (bTSH), the present studies were undertaken as follows. After each patient's serum and ^{125}I-bTSH were incubated overnight at 24°C, this mixture was used in following procedures. The fraction precipitated by 15 % PEG was highly labeled (bound with ^{125}I-bTSH) and this binding was completely inhibited by adding cold bTSH, but not inhibited by human TSH. In the gel-filtration experiment on Sephadex G 200 column (1.0 x 30 cm,PBS,pH 7.4), the peak of eluted radioactivity was found just behind void volume and this peak was shifted to the area of ^{125}I-bTSH by adding cold bTSH. Autoradiography following immunoelectrophoresis against anti-human Igs revealed that the high label corresponded to the precipitating line specifically against anti-IgG. This bTSH-binding protein disappeared in patient with Graves' disease after 2yrs. of MMI treatment, when the levels of TRAb was increased up to 73 %. In conclusion, this bTSH-binding protein found in patients with autoimmune thyroid diseases was proved to be autoantibody to bTSH (IgG type). The pathogenic or clinical significance of this antibody and the posibility of anti-idiotype antibody related to TSH receptor antibody remain to be elucidated.

789 A FRAGMENT OF THE TSH-RECEPTOR WITH BINDING SITES FOR BOTH TSH AND TSH-RECEPTOR ANTIBODIES.
Eirian Davies Jones* and Bernard Rees Smith. Endocrine Immunology Unit, Department of Medicine, Welsh National School of Medicine, Cardiff CF4 4XN. U.K.

Antibodies which bind to the TSH-receptor and stimulate thyroid function are present in the sera of patients with hyperthyroid Graves' disease. A water soluble protein released during freezing and thawing of human thyroid homogenates reversibly binds these antibodies and abolishes their thyroid stimulating properties as measured by mouse bioassay. This hydrophilic molecule has been designated LATS absorbing activity or LAA. A new assay for LAA based on the measurement of TSH-receptor antibodies by radioreceptor assay has been developed and data obtained with this new method compared favourably with results from the bioassay. The properties of LAA have been investigated further using the new assay. Fractionation of LAA on Sephacryl S-300 resolved the activity into two peaks; a minor peak containing approximately a third of the applied activity eluted in the void volume of the column and the remaining activity co-eluted with the 4S fraction of thyroid protein. The 4S LAA was heat labile (56°C 30 min). Both crude LAA and LAA, partially purified on Sephacryl S-300, were retained specifically on affinity chromatography columns of Sepharose-TSH (60-70U/ml) under the same conditions that attained binding of detergent solubilised receptors to the column. No binding of either crude or partially purified LAA was observed to columns of Sepharose-hCG, Sepharose-normal IgG or Sepharose-bovine serum albumin. The affinity of TSH for LAA was weak relative to the affinity of the hormone for the detergent solubilised receptor since affinity chromatography columns containing lower concentration of TSH (1U/ml) could retain only the receptor. Application of both crude and partially purified LAA to Sepharose-concanavalin A demonstrated the glycoprotein nature of the molecule. These results strongly suggest that LAA is a fragment of the TSH receptor, which contains binding sites for both TSH and TSH-receptor antibodies. The mechanism of formation of LAA is unknown at present but proteolytic fragmentation of the receptor by thyroid protease released during freezing and thawing of human thyroid membranes is a likely possibility.

790 MONOCLONAL ANTIBODY AGAINST HORMONE BINDING DOMAIN OF RABBIT MAMMARY PRL RECEPTORS.
M. Katoh*, M. Brochu, J. Djiane and P.A. Kelly. Lab. Molecular Endocrinology, Royal Victoria Hospital, Montreal, H3A 1A1, CANADA and Laboratoire de Physiologie de la Lactation, INRA, 78350 Jouy-en-Josas, FRANCE.

We have previously developed polyclonal antibodies against rabbit mammary PRL receptors and established the PRL-like biological effects of this antibody on rabbit mammary explants. In order to further clarify the significance of the PRL binding domain in the receptor molecule, we attempted to produce a monoclonal antibody specific to this domain. Partially purified rabbit mammary receptor prepared by CHAPS solubilization and oPRL-agarose affinity chromatography were used as the antigen, and the inhibition of ^{125}I-oPRL binding to microsomes was employed as a criteria of the antibody activity. One hybrydoma (M 110) was found to inhibit binding and ascites fluid was prepared followed by IgG purification on a protein A-sepharose column. This antibody completely inhibited ^{125}I-oPRL binding to mammary microsomes at 120 nM with a ED_{50} value at 0.4 nM (32 ng), which was comparable to that by unlabeled oPRL. M 110 IgG also completly inhibited binding in microsomes from rabbit kidney, adrenal, ovary and pig mammary gland and by 80% in rabbit liver. PRL binding to microsomes from rat liver, adrenal, ovary and the human breast cancer cell line (T-47D), however, were not affected. Iodinated antibodies (^{125}I-mAb) showed similar binding characteristics to ^{125}I-oPRL. Namely, ^{125}I-mAb binding to rabbit mammary microsomes was effectively competed for only by lactogenic hormones with a comparable ED_{50} value to that for ^{125}I-oPRL. ^{125}I-mAb binding was observed only in tissues in which PRL binding was inhibited by this antibody. These findings indicate that this monoclonal antibody is specific to the oPRL binding domain, but that some species differences exist.

791 PROTECTION OF NUCLEAR 3,5,3' TRIIODOTHYRONINE RECEPTORS (nR) FROM INACTIVATION IN VITRO. J. Brtko* and L.J. DeGroot, Thyroid Study Unit, Department of Medicine, The University of Chicago, Chicago, IL U.S.A.

During purification of nR, it is necessary to protect nR from "spontaneous" degradation. We studied the effect of organic solvents (ethanol 10% v/v, butanol 5% v/v, glycerol 10% v/v), inhibitors of proteolytic or nucleolytic activity (aprotinine, soybean trypsin inhibitor, parahydroxymercuribenzoate, 0.1 mM, EDTA, 5mM), diamines (spermine, spermidine), and γ-globulin as nonspecific protein on triiodothyronine (T_3) binding parameters. Ka and MBC were tested by Scatchard analysis. 0.5 ml of nR fraction prepared by extraction with 0.3 M KCl from rat liver nuclei, with or without a chemical agent, was tumbled at 20°C for 16 hours. Binding data of the fresh nR were MBC=2.03±0.18 pmol mg^{-1}; Ka=2.39±0.62 x 10^9 $lmol^{-1}$. A 30% diminution of MBC without change of Ka was found without chemical agent after 16 hrs at 20°C. Incubation of nR in the presence of glycerol (10%) maintained the MBC and Ka with no reduction. A similar protective effect was found with spermine (2 mM) and γ-globulin (40 μg ml^{-1}). Spermidine (2mM) or PMSF (0.1 mM) had no protective effect. Ethanol (10%) and butanol (5%) caused a significant decrease of MBC. Soybean trypsin inhibitor decreased Ka without a significant change in MBC. The protective effect of glycerol was demonstrated during glycerol gradient (2-15%) centrifugation (40000 RPM, 16 hrs). Near 100% yield of nR with 2-3 fold purification was achieved. In conclusion, triiodothyronine nR in 0.3 M KCl nuclear extracts maintain their binding parameters (MBC, Ka) even at 22°C after 16 hrs in the presence of glycerol (10%), spermine (2 mM) or γ-globulin (40 μg ml^{-1}). Characteristics of glycerol (viscosity and protective effect) may be advantageously utilized in initial purification of nR by gradient centrifugation.

792 RECEPTORS FOR Δ^9-THC IN THE RAT BRAIN. D.K. Das* and W.B. Essman, Long Island Jewish-Hillside Medical Center, New Hyde Park, N.Y. 11040 and Queens College, of the City University of N.Y., Flushing, N.Y. 11367.

Molecular mechanisms for the central action of marijuana (M) and its major biologically active ingredient, Δ^9-tetrahydrocannabinol (THC) have been sought in several areas. This is particularly appropriate where M has produced hormonal effects or hormones have changed the effect of M. After M inhalation THC can be found in the brain in concentrations comparable to the neurotransmitters, suggesting possible receptor sites modulating the effects. Rats exposed to either marijuana (15 min) with delivery of 1.07±0.04 μg of THC/g. of marijuana or to air in the same Walton Upright Smoking Machine showed evidence of cognitive and physiological effects. Brain concentration of THC after M inhalation, persisting for at least 3 days was highest in the hippocampus (5.37±1.52 μg/mg protein). Using ^{3}H-THC (50 mCi/mMole), binding to membrane fractions from control rats, was measured for the hippocampus (37.9 fMoles/mg protein) with a K_D=12.15. Such hippocampal binding was greatest for presynaptic membranes. These THC binding sites were shown to be specific, saturable, and regulated by pH and temperature maxima. Displacement of specifically bound THC was effected by Δ^8-THC>cannabinol>cannabidiol> cannabigerol. Marijuana exposure (0.428 mg in smoke) increased specific THC binding sites in the hippocampus by 3 days after exposure. Present findings support specific Δ^9-THC receptors in the rat hippocampus capable of being altered by marijuana exposure, and modifiable by hormonal agents.

793 *BROMOCRIPTINE PRODUCES A STRIKING DECREASE OF THE PLASMATIC ANDROGENS IN IDIOPATHIC HIRSUTISM.* *J.Devesa*, R.Pérez Fernández, L.Lima, A.Pandiella, J.A.Mato, J.Cabezas-Cerrato. Inst.Univ.Iberoamericano Endocrinología,Metab.Nutr. Faculty of Medicine, Santiago de Compostela University. SPAIN.*

Hyperprolactinemia in women has been reported to result in androgenic plasma pattern abnormalities, that are corrected with the normalization of prolactin levels. We have studied the effect of bromocriptine treatment in hirsute normoprolactinemic women, in order to fully investigate the relationship between prolactin and androgens. Seven women, aged 16-24 years, with Idiopathic Hirsutism and normoprolactinemia were studied before and after bromocriptine treatment, 5 mg/day per os. All studies were conducted in the follicular phase of the menstrual cycle. Student's t test were used for analysis of data. After one month on treatment, plasma concentrations of Testosterone, 17-OH progesterone, Androstenedione and Testosterone/SHBG ratio, showed a significative decrease ($p < 0.01$) in all the women studied. Plasma concentrations of Cortisol, FSH, LH, Estradiol, DHEA-S and SHBG were similar before and during Bromocriptine treatment. Urinary Cortisol also did not change. The present data support the hypothesis about a specific hormone, other than ACTH and Prolactin, stimulating the reticular adrenal zone. Dopaminergic agonists may be a new and succesfull treatment in idiopathic hirsutism, acting on the release of this putative hormone.

794 *LOW T3-SYNDROME AND HIGH TeBG BINDING CAPACITY IN ANOREXIA NERVOSA.*
B. Estour, M. Pugeat, F. Lang, H. Dechaud, P. Pellet and H. Rousset, Service de Médecine Interne, Hôpital Bellevue, 42023 Saint-Etienne and INSERM U34 69321 Lyon, France.*

It is known that in humans administration of oestrogens and/or triodothyronine (T3) increases plasma testosterone-binding globulin (TeBG) concentration. A Low-T3 syndrome and a low estradiol (E2) concentration are generaly observed in women with anorexia nervosa. In this report the binding affinity and capacity of TeBG was measured on plasma from 10 patients with anorexia nervosa, by a solid phase method previously described (Steroids,31: 681, 1978). On the same samples the concentration of thyroxine (T4), T3, testosterone (T) and E2 were measured by radio-immunoassay. The results were compared with those of normal women in early follicular phase (n=27) and with hyperthyroid women (n=52). The data showed a low T3 concentration (74±13 vs 120±20nm/l in controls (X±SD) and a low E2 concentration (2.56±1.46 vs 3.78±1.96 ng/dl) in patients with anorexia nervosa. In these patients the T4 levels and the T levels were within the normal range. Surprisingly the TeBG binding capacity was greater than two SD of the control value (1.21±0.31 ug/dl) in 7 out of the 10 anorexic patients. For these 7 patients the range of TeBG binding capacity (2.08-3.63 ug/dl) was in the range of our hyperthyroid patients (2.01-12.68 ug/dl). The TeBG binding affinity was not different between the groups. IN CONCLUSION : Our results show that the observed increase in TeBG binding capacity in anorexic patients was not associated with an increase in T3 or E2 values, suggesting that factors other than thyroid and sex-steroid hormones influence TeBG in anorexia nervosa.

795 PROGESTERONE KINETICS, PLASMA, AND URINARY METABOLITES IN THE CYNOMOLGUS MONKEY: ASSESSMENT OF AN ANIMAL MODEL. M.C. Frederiksen*, H.V. Braasch, R.T. Chatterton, Jr., Department of Obstetrics and Gynecology, Northwestern University School of Medicine, Chicago, Illinois, 60611, USA

The cynomolgus monkey, smaller and easier to handle than the Rhesus monkey, is increasingly being used in reproductive endocrinology. To investigate the manner in which this species handles progesterone we administered 4-^{14}C-progesterone intravenously to 2 cycling female monkeys in luteal phase and sampled blood and urine over a 24-hr period. ^{14}C-Steroids were identified by chromatographic and recrystallization techniques. The time-course of progesterone concentration in plasma was analyzed in a 3 compartment open mammillary model with the aid of the SAAM-23 computer program. Progesterone had a volume of distribution of 6.4 ± 0.8 L or 1.75 ± 0.3 L/kg, compatible with high affinity protein binding. The plasma elimination clearance was found to be 0.22 ± 0.11 L/min or 0.06 ± 0.03 L/kg/min. The major metabolite in plasma was 20α-hydroxy-4-pregnen-3-one. Only 6.2% of ^{14}C-products in urine were extractable into ethyl ether; of these 2.3% was ^{14}C-progesterone. Conjugated metabolites in urine, fractionated by TLC, were 24% sulfates, 19% glucuronides, and 52% a more polar conjugate. About 35% of conjugated metabolites could bind to an antiserum that is specific for ring D and the C_{17} side-chain of pregnane-3α, 20α-diol. Pregnanediol was identified as 37% of ^{14}Csteroids liberated from conjugates by acid hydrolysis. In comparison to the human, progesterone clearance is slower in the cynomolgus monkey, but the pattern of metabolites is closer to the human than other primates with pregnanediol being measureable as a major metabolite by RIA, and, therefore, the cynomolgus may be preferred to other primates for reproductive studies.

796 AROMATASE ACTIVITY IN HUMAN FORESKIN FIBROBLASTS: BIPHASIC RESPONSE TO DEXAMETHASONE. M.Fujimoto, G.D.Berkovitz*, T.R.Brown, and C.J.Migeon, Pediatric Endocrine Labs, Johns Hopkins University, Baltimore, MD 21205

Aromatase activity of human foreskin fibroblasts (FF) can be determined by analysis of (^{3}H)H_2O released upon conversion of (1-^{3}H)androstenedione (A) to estrone. FF were incubated (37C, 3-6h) with (1-^{3}H)A (12.5-200nM) plus 5μM progesterone. In FF from 5 newborns (NFF) and 5 adults (AFF), the K_m was 23nM (12-52) and the V_{max} was0.55 pmol/mg protein/h (0.19 -1.41). The mean V_{max} for AFF (0.89 pmol/mg prot/h) was higher than the V_{max} for NFF (0.31 pmol/mg prot/h). The induction of aromatase activity by dexamethasone (Dex) was studied in 3 AFF and 3 NFF strains preincubated with MEM containing 15% fetal bovine serum (FBS) ± Dex (250nM) for 12 h. Cells were incubated with MEM containing (1-^{3}H)A (150nM) and P (5μM) for an additional 3 h. Mean activity was 7.3 pmol/mg prot/h (4.7-11.0) in cells pretreated with Dex compared to 0.75 pmol/mg prot/h (<0.1-2.0) in the absence of Dex. In FF the stimulatory effect of Dex did not require FBS in the preincubation media. Half maximal stimulation of aromatase activity was achieved by 2.7nM Dex. When cells were preincubated (0-72 h) with 250nM Dex, aromatase activity followed a biphasic curve with peak levels at 12 h followed by a gradual decline of enzyme activity to baseline levels. This pattern persisted even if fresh media containing Dex was replaced every 12 h. In summary: 1) aromatase activity in FF can be determined by (^{3}H)H_2O generation, 2) the apparent K_m is 23nM and the V_{max} ranges from 0.19 to 1.41 pmol/mg prot/h, 3) mean activity in AFF is higher than in NFF and 4) aromatase activity can be induced by Dex but exposure for periods of >12 h results in a diminution of activity suggesting the presence of a repressive factor.

797 STIMULATION OF LUTEAL ANDROGEN AND ESTROGEN BIOSYNTHESIS: EVIDENCE FOR LH REGULATION OF 17α-HYDROXYLASE AND 17,20 LYASE ACTIVITIES. G. Gibori, D.C. Johnson, R. Sridaran & I. Khan*. Dept. of Phys. & Biophys., Coll.Med., U.of Illinois, Chicago, IL., & Dept. of OB/Gyn., U. of Kansas, Kansas City, KS.

Luteal cells of pregnant rats possess an active aromatase system yet they are considered to possess weak 17α-hydroxylase and 17,20 lyase systems and to depend on exogenous testosterone (T) for estradiol (E) biosynthesis. Recent investigations have indicated that sustained treatment with low levels of hCG increases luteal production of both T and E. In this investigation we sought to determine the time course of hCG action and to find out whether LH plays a direct role in the induction/activation of the enzymes responsible for the conversion of progesterone (P) to E. HCG (3IU) was administered to day 14 pregnant rats and the capacity of luteal cells to secrete T and E was determined 0,0.5,2,4,12 and 24h later. There were no increases in luteal cell production of either steroid until 12h after hCG administration when a 40 fold increase in the synthesis of both steroids was observed. HCG stimulated T and E without enhancing P production, indicating that P substrate is not a rate limiting step for T biosynthesis. To determine whether the locus of hCG action is on the 17α-hydroxylase and/or 17, 20 lyase enzymes, 3IU of hCG were administered to rats daily between days 12-14 and both enzyme activities were determined. HCG enhanced 17α-hydroxylase and 17,20 lyase activity 2.5 and 40 fold respectively. These results demonstrate that LH acts on luteal cells of pregnant rats to stimulate 17α-hydroxylase and 17,20 lyase. LH appears to stimulate the synthesis of these enzymes rather than activate existing enzymes since a delay of 12h is observed between hCG administration and the first observable increase in T and E production. Supported by HD11119.

798 EFFECTS OF PHOSPHOLIPASES ON MEMBRANE BOUND Δ^4 STEROID 5α-REDUCTASE ACTIVITY (5α-R) FROM THE RAT EPIDIDYMIS. G.M.Cooke* and B. Robaire, Centre for the Study of Reproduction, Departments of Pharmacology and Ob/Gyn, McGill University, Montreal Que. H3A 1A1, Canada.

5α-R, the enzyme that converts testosterone (T) to dihydrotestosterone, is essential for epididymal function. It is found in both the nuclear and microsomal membranes of this tissue. The present investigations were done to determine the importance of the membrane structure to 5α-R activity. Modification of membrane phospholipid was achieved using phospholipases. Phospholipase A_2 (A_2) removes a fatty acid residue from phospholipids, whereas phospholipase C (C) removes the phosphate/polar group. 5α-R activity was measured radiometrically in KRP buffer pH 6.9 with NADPH (0.5 mM) and T (25-500nM); when included, phospholipases were added at concentrations of 2, 5 or 10 units/ml. Both phospholipases caused a time dependent decrease (30-40%) in nuclear and microsomal 5α-R activity which plateaued by 120 min. Furthermore, the Km_{app} and $Vmax_{app}$ of the nuclear and microsomal 5α-Rs were differentially altered by A_2 and C. The Km_{app} of the nuclear 5α-R was increased two fold by C, but not affected by A_2, and the $Vmax_{app}$ was decreased by both C (40%) and A_2 (33%). In the case of the microsomal 5α-R, A_2 and C increased the Km_{app} two fold, but A_2 did not affect the $Vmax_{app}$ whereas C decreased the $Vmax_{app}$ by 33%. Thus, 1) the phosphate/polar group of phospholipids is involved in determining the affinity (Km_{app}) of both 5α-Rs investigated, and 2) fatty acid residues of phospholipids are apparently not involved in determining nuclear 5α-R activity (Km_{app}), but may have a protective role for the 5α-Rs in both subcellular compartments ($Vmax_{app}$). Supported by MRC of Canada and FRSQ.

799 AGE-RELATED TESTOSTERONE (T) METABOLISM AND BIOLOGICAL EFFECT IN MALE RABBIT CARTILAGE TISSUE AND CELLS. M.T. Corvol*, S. Bok, L. Tsagris, A. Carrascosa, R. Rappaport, INSERM U.30, Hôpital des Enfants-Malades, 75015 PARIS, France.

Androgens play in cartilage an important role in skeletal growth but their mechanism of action is unknown. In the present work, using thin layer and celite column chromatographies, and recrystallization methods, the metabolism of $[1,2,6,7-^3H]$-Testosterone ($[^3H]$-T) was assessed in epiphyseal cartilage tissue and cultured chondrocytes derived from pre-per and post pubertal male rabbits. Among the newly formed metabolites observed, $[^3H]$ -dihydrotestosterone ($[^3H]$-DHT) was shown to be the sole metabolite which accumulated in the cells. $[^3H]$-T was metabolized into $[^3H]$-DHT much more rapidly in chondrocytes originating from prepubertal animals (10-40 day old), as compared to pubertal (40-80 day old) and post pubertal (more than 90 day old) animals. The half maximal rate of DHT formation occurred at a substrate concentration of 0.4 uM, a value similar to that reported for DHT formation in other androgen target organs. We also examined the biological effect of T and DHT on 35 sulfate incorporation into proteoglycans synthesized by the chondrocytes cultured from animals at corresponding different ages. A stimulating effect was observed when T or DHT were added to cartilage cells from pubertal animals only, with a maximum effect at 10^{-9} M and 10^{-11} M concentration respectively. These results show that 1/ T has a stimulatory effect on cartilage metabolism in vitro, 2/ This effect is probably mediated by its metabolic transformation into DHT and 3/ it seems to be related to the age of the animal.

800 EFFECTS OF ESTROGEN THERAPY ON IN VITRO ANDROGEN METABOLISM IN HUMAN EPIDIDYMIS. M.A. de Larminat*, M.H. Vazquez, E. Gurpide and J. Blaquier, Inst. Biol. & Med. Exp., Buenos Aires, Argentina, and Dept. Obstet. Gynecol. & Reprod. Sci., Mount Sinai Sch. Med., New York, N.Y., USA

Androgen-dependent epididymal function is controlled through mechanisms involving regulation of the number of intracellular androgen receptors and modulation of NADPH: 5 -reductase activity, required to convert testosterone (T) and androstenedione (A) to the active metabolite 5 -dihydrotestosterone (DHT). We are now reporting quantitative patterns of androgen metabolism in human epididymides obtained from 10 patients undergoing orchidectomy as treatment for prostatic carcinoma. Five of these patients have received estrogen therapy (2.5 mg DES/d) for 3 months or longer. Minced epididymal specimens were superfused with mixtures of ^{3}H-T and ^{14}C-A in balanced salt solution and concentrations of isotopically labeled T, A and the 5 -reduced metabolites DHT, androstanedione, 3 ,17 -androstanediol and 3 ,17 -androstanediol were measured in tissue and superfusate at the steady state. These data indicated that the output of 5 -reduced metabolites was significantly lower in the estrogenized epididymis (3600 vs 410 pmol $g^{1}h^{-1}$). Estrogen treatment also resulted in a marked shift of androgen metabolism from the oxidative to the reductive direction, as evidenced by the ratio of concentrations of labeled T and A and by the higher proportion of androstanediols among the 5 -reduced metabolites. Similar results were obtained from "batch" incubations of tissue fragments. These findings suggest an antiandrogenic effect of estrogens mediated by the inhibition of 5-reductase activity.

801 HORMONAL AND SURGICAL TREATMENT (Rx) OF UNI-AND BILATERAL CRYPTORCHIDISM.

S. de Muinck Keizer*, F. Hazebroek, H. Visser, J. Molenaar and S. Drop, Dept. of Pediat. & Pediat. Surgery, Erasmus Univ. Rotterdam, the Netherlands.

Pilotstudy: 22 healthy boys (age 3-12 yrs) with 26 undescended testes were treated with LH-RH nasal spray (HOE 471) 400 µg t.i.d.; 28 days. Whenever a second Rx course proved unsuccessful after a 4 wk interval, orchidopexy was performed. Complete descent was found in 16/26 testes (60%; n=13 boys). For 8 boys 2 Rx courses were necessary. Subsequently, a double blind placebo controlled (dbpc) study was initiated. The following data were obtained from 58 boys (age 6-12 yrs): descent occurred in 25/76 testes (30%; n=20 boys; success group), 3 testes descended during placebo Rx. 10 boys needed 2 courses. 38 boys in whom hormonal Rx proved unsuccessful (failure group) underwent surgery. Anatomical findings in 40 boys: an obstructed inguinal canal was most commonly found (50%). In all other cases, anatomical anomalies of epidydimis (28%), or a wide open processus vaginalis (25%) were present. The pretreatment response of LH/FSH to LH-RH (50 µg i.v.) and of testosterone to HCG (1500 U i.m.) was similar in boys with either uni- or bilateral cryptorchidism as well as in the success and failure group, except for a significantly ($p < 0.05$) higher peak LH value in the failure group. After Rx: the LH response to LH-RH increased significantly only in the success group; the FSH response decreased in the success and failure group and significantly more in the success group. We conclude that the success rate of HOE 471 treatment in a dbpc study and in an open study vary by 50%! Pretreatment hormonal serum values do not assist in the prediction of the outcome. FSH decrease after Rx will be subject of further study. However, failure to respond to hormonal Rx makes it very likely that an anatomical anomaly exists, requiring surgery.

802 DIRECT EFFECT OF THE GnRH ANALOG D-Trp^6-Pro^9-NEt-GnRH ON RAT TESTICULAR STEROIDOGENESIS.

Rosario D'Agata*, Abraham K. Munabi, Veronica Mericq, Marie C. Gelato, Barry D. Albertson, D. Lynn Loriaux and Fernando Cassorla. DEB, NICHD, NIH, Bethesda, MD, USA, and University of Catania Medical School, Sicily, Italy.

The GnRH-analog D-Trp^6-Pro^9-Net-GnRH ($GnRH_a$) inhibits rat testicular testosterone secretion. To determine whether $GnRH_a$ decreases serum testosterone concentrations solely by inhibiting gonadotropin secretion or, in addition, by directly inhibiting testicular testosterone biosynthesis, we examined the effects of $GnRH_a$ on the activities of 5 key testicular steroidogenic enzymes. Thirty hypophysectomized, gonadotropin replaced rats were treated for 7 days with either $GnRH_a$ (1 µg sc/day) or saline. The $GnRH_a$ treated animals exhibited a significant decrease of serum testosterone when compared to the control group (498 ± 37 ng/dl vs 2044 ± 105 ng/dl, mean ± SEM, $P<0.001$). 17-hydroxyprogesterone serum levels were also decreased in the $GnRH_a$ treated rats (61 ± 6 ng/dl vs 93 ± 7 ng/dl, $P<0.005$), while serum progesterone levels were similar in both groups of animals. These changes in steroid concentrations were associated with decreases in the microsomal enzyme activities of 17-hydroxylase (37 ± 9 vs 654 ± 41 pmol/mg protein/min, $P<0.001$), 17,20-desmolase (103 ± 9 vs 522 ± 47 pmol/mg protein/min, $P<0.001$), 3 β-hydroxysteroid dehydrogenase (1.7 ± 0.02 vs 4.1 ± 0.1 nmol/mg protein/min, $P<0.001$), aromatase (95 ± 7 vs 228 ± 6 pmol/mg protein/min, $P<0.001$) and 17-ketosteroid reductase (167 ± 9 vs 290 ± 18 pmol/mg protein/min, $P<0.01$) in the $GnRH_a$ treated animals. We conclude that $GnRH_a$ can inhibit directly rat testicular testosterone biosynthesis.

803 hMG IN THE TREATMENT OF CRYPTORCHIDISM.
G.De Rosa°, S.Della Casa, S.M.Corsello, F.Colabucci and A.Rossodivita, Institutes of Endocrinology and Pediatrics, Catholic University School of Medicine, Rome, Italy.

Recent experimental data lead to hypotesize that FSH may play an important role in the descent of the testes either directly or by modulating the LH action on Leydig cell. 15 prepubertal cryptorchid boys (10 unilateral and 5 bilateral cryptorchids), 2-7 yrs old (mean age 4,6 yrs) were treated with human Menopausal Gonadotropin (hMG), which chiefly possesses FSH activity, at the dosage of 40 IU x 3/week im for 6-8 weeks. An additional treatment with hMG 40 IU x 3/ week im plus human Chorionic Gonadotropin (hCG) 500 IU/ week was carried out for the following 4 weeks in the non responders. Clinical examination, sonographic evaluation and RIA determination of Testosterone, estradiol, FSH and LH were performed before, during (4th and 6th week) and after therapy. Testicular response to hCG was evaluated before and at the end of the treatment. After hMG therapy a complete descent of the testes into the scrotum was achieved in 7 patients (47%) of whom 2 bilateral and 5 monolateral cryptorchids. After the following administration of hCG, a positive response was observed in 2 other bilateral cryptorchids of the 8 non responders. In any case, ultrasonography showed an increase in testes size and various degrees of gonad migration through the inguinal canal. No significant hormonal modification occurred. No virilizing effect was seen. These findings suggest that hMG is useful in the treatment of cryptorchidism or itself or by increasing testicular sensitivity to hCG.

804 DYNAMICS OF STEROIDOGENESIS OF ISOLATED RAT ADRENAL AND TESTICULAR CELLS IN A MULTICHANNEL SUPERFUSION SYSTEM.
C.M. Feek*, B.C. Williams, A.M. Wallace, C.E. Gray and C.R.W. Edwards, Departments of Medicine, Western General Hospital, Edinburgh EH4 2XU, and Pathological Biochemistry, Royal Infirmary, Glasgow G4 OSF, Scotland.

We have adapted a previously reported isolated cell superfusion system to investigate the interaction between isolated rat adrenal and testicular cells in the secretion of sex steroids. The system has advantages of using ten parallel columns simultaneously, allowing data to be analysed with adequate precision, and specific direct radioimmunoassays for the steroids progesterone, 17α-hydroxyprogesterone, androstenedione, testosterone and corticosterone. The between column variation in steroidogenesis (mean ± SD) for a mixed population of cells was 15.4 ± 6.7% for testosterone, 20.3 ± 12% for corticosterone, 25.1 ± 28.5% for progesterone, 32.4 ± 15.1% for androstenedione and 34.2 ± 15.2% for 17α-hydroxyprogesterone in response to the administration of ACTH over the dose range 1-100 pg/ml. Using this multichannel superfusion technique we have discovered a major interaction between isolated adrenal and testicular cells. When adrenal or testicular cells alone are stimulated by ACTH negligible amounts of androstenedione and testosterone are produced. When both cell types are present and ACTH administered, there is a tenfold increase in adnrostenedione and testosterone secretion. Stimulation of adrenal cells with ACTH and perfusion of the adrenal eluate through testicular cells also stimulates testosterone production. This finding suggests that an unidentified adrenal product can modulate the control of testosterone secretion by the rat testis *in vitro*.

805 RAT EPIDIDYMAL ANDROGEN BINDING PROTEIN IS INCREASED BY 20α-HYDROXY-4-PREGNEN-3-ONE.

K.E. Friedl*, S.R. Plymate and B.L. Fariss, Dept of Clinical Investigation, Madigan Army Medical Center, Tacoma, WA, 98431,USA.

An in vivo investigation of the biological activity of 20α-hydroxy-4-pregnen-3-one (20αOHP) in the testis was conducted with rats (250-300 gms) receiving daily intramuscular injections of 1-5 mgs 20αOHP for 3 weeks. The rationale for this study was based on previous in vitro studies which demonstrated the endogenous production of 20αOHP from progesterone by the rat seminiferous tubules and the suppression of 17α-hydroxylase activity by 20αOHP. Rats receiving 5 mgs 20αOHP demonstrated a significant three-fold increase in plasma 20αOHP over control animals and a significant 50% increase in epididymal rat androgen binding protein (rABP), 12 hours after the last injection. A direct action of 20αOHP on the testis is supported by the absence of any significant change in rLH or rFSH levels in spite of a significant decrease in intratesticular and plasma testosterone concentrations. Daily treatments with 1 mg of progesterone also significantly increased rABP (+25%) and caused a decrease in rLH, rFSH and intratesticular testosterone. This is particularly interesting because the increase in rABP was associated with a significant conversion of progesterone to 20αOHP representing a three-fold increase in plasma 20αOHP compared to control animals (controls = 4.0 ±0.2; progesterone treated = 12.1 ±1.0 ng/ml). Plasma 20αOHP concentrations had an inverse correlation with intratesticular testosterone concentrations. This study indicates that in addition to the in vivo reduction of testosterone production by the testis, 20αOHP directly increases epididymal rABP.

806 EFFECT OF GOSSYPOL ON THE MODULATION OF TESTOSTERONE PRODUCTION IN YOUNG MALE RATS.

T. Fukaya*, Y. C. Lin, Y. Rikihisa and T. DeSanto, VA-MD Regional College of Veterinary Medicine, VPI&SU, Blacksburg, VA 24061, USA.

Pre-weaning male rats caged with their dams were used in an attempt to resolve reported varying conclusions regarding the in vivo effects of gossypol on synthesis and secretion of testosterone in some mammalian species. Previously, we had demonstrated that under the stimulation of human chorionic gonadotropin (HCG) testosterone production in 15-day-old rats was 2-10x higher than at ages 5, 10, 20, 25 and 30 days. Therefore, 2 days prior to sacrifice at day-15 of age, 4 groups of rats were administered i.m. saline (controls), HCG (20 IU twice daily), gossypol acetic acid (GP) in 10% EtOH (25 mg/kg/daily) and a combination of HCG and GP. At sacrifice, blood samples and testes were collected for testosterone measurement by radioimmunoassay. The avg. serum testosterone concentrations in control, HCG, GP and HCG+GP treated animals were 1.97±0.33, 18.08±1.11, 0.87±0.20 and 5.33±0.99 ng/ml, respectively; the avg. testicular testosterone levels were 1.97±0.40, 18.39±1.94, 1.05±0.26 and 9.34±1.30 ng/mg protein, respectively. Both serum and testicular testosterone values in GP and HCG+GP treated rats were significantly lower than values of control and HCG-treated rats. Our results indicate that: 1) GP is capable of decreasing testosterone production in the testes of young rats. 2) The testicular responsiveness to HCG stimulation with testosterone production in young rats can be drastically reduced by treatment with GP. 3) This in vivo model will be useful for studying testicular function during the early stages of development. Supported by NIH Grants HD 17627 and HD 16883.

807 ACTION OF OVARIAN STEROIDS ON TSH AND PRL SECRETION IN PREGNANT RATS.
R.P. Deis* and A.M. Rastrilla. Laboratorio de Reproducción y Lactancia, CONICET. Casilla de Correo 855, 5500 Mendoza, Argentina.

In the present study we have examined the effect of ovariectomy, / luteectomy and ovarian hormones on TSH and prolactin (PRL) release in preg nant rats. A significant increase in serum PRL was observed 8, 16, 24 and 30 h. after ovariectomy performed on day 18 of pregnancy. After 36 and / 48 h. however, PRL values were similar to the control rats. Luteectomy on the same day of pregnancy induced a similar rise but values were signifi-/ cantly higher at 24 h. when compared with the ovariectomized groups. In / the sham operated rats the release of TSH seems to occur in a phasic form/ with maximal values 16 and 36 h. after surgery. After ovariectomy serum/ TSH concentration showed a similar pattern but at 36 h. TSH level was significantly lower when compared to the sham group. In luteectomized rats,/ serum TSH was measured only 8, 16 and 24 h. after surgery. The mean serum concentration was significantly higher than the sham and ovariectomized / values. The administration of estrogen (1 µg) to sham operated and / ovariectomized pregnant rats, 12 h. after surgery, induced 12 h. later, a/ significant increase in serum TSH values in both groups. Estrogen induced PRL release only in the ovariectomized rats. It was concluded that TSH secretion is not affected by progesterone but it is stimulated by estrogen / and that PRL release only occured in the absence of progesterone, and probably not mediated by TRH.

808 MORPHINE STIMULATION OF TSH SECRETION IN MAN.
L.Devilla*, A.Pende, A.Morgano, N.R.Musso, G.Lotti, Cattedra Semeiotica Medica R ISMI, Viale Benedetto XV, 6 16132 Genova ITALY.

The aim of this study was to elucidate the role of opioid system in the control of TSH secretion in humans by using morphine, an opioid agonist, and naloxone, an opioid antagonist. The intravenous administration of 10 mg. of morphine chloridrate caused a prompt increase in serum TSH in both normal subjects (70% increase with respect to basal values) and hypothyroid patients (40% increase with respect to basal values). Previous administration of naloxone (4 mg. i.v.) completely abolished the morphine induced TSH increase. These data demonstrate that morphine stimulatory effect on TSH secretion is specifically mediated by opioid receptors. However naloxone alone did not produce TSH modifications in all subjects. This may fit well with the hypotesis of a minor role of endogenous opioid tone in the control of TSH secretion. In normal volunteers pretreatment with morphine caused a 60% increase of TRH-induced TSH release, whereas naloxone showed no effect. The morphine effect on TRH-induced TSH secretion suggests a direct action of morphine on pituitary TSH release. Another hypothesis is that the morphine effect could be mediated via the reduction in dopamine concentration of pituitary stalk blood previously demonstrated by experimental studies in rats.

809 SUBCELLULAR LOCALIZATION OF IMMUNOREACTIVE THYROID STIMULATING HORMONE (IR-TSH) IN RAT HYPOTHALAMUS. W. DeVito*, T. Spearman#, and G. Hedge, Depts. of Physiol. and Biochem.#, West Virginia Univ., Morgantown, WV, USA.

IR-TSH is stored in a releasable pool in the hypothalamus (HYP) and its presence is not dependent on pituitary (PIT) TSH. To determine whether HYP IR-TSH is associated with specific organelles, we compared the subcellular localization of IR-TSH in PIT and ventral and dorsal HYP tissue. Tissue homogenates from hypophysectomized (HYPOX), thyroidectomized (TX) and intact rats were centrifuged (150x g, 10', 4 C) and supernates were layered onto continuous sucrose (SUC) density gradients (0.3 to 2.0 M) and centrifuged at 100,000 x g max for 16 hr. IR-TSH in PIT supernates from intact and TX rats showed peaks with densities similar to those reported for PIT TSH secretory granules (1.65 and 1.55 M SUC, respectively). Both ventral and dorsal HYP supernates showed IR-TSH peaks at 0.4 M, and second peaks at 1.25 and 1.45 M SUC, respectively. In all tissues the high density IR-TSH peak was associated with the lysosomal enzyme, β-glucuronidase. High density IR-TSH peaks in ventral supernates from TX and HYPOX rats overlapped with plasma membrane fractions (1.05 M SUC). The high density IR-TSH peak in the dorsal supernate from TX rats was at 1.5 M SUC, and this peak from HYPOX rats was at 1.8 M SUC. Incubation of HYP or PIT tissue for 2 hr with ^{125}I-TSH resulted in a large cytoplasmic peak at 0.45 M SUC, and a small peak at 0.95 M SUC. CONCLUSIONS: HYP IR-TSH occurs in two peaks, one of which coincides with PIT TSH secretory granules. These peaks are maintained after HYPOX. (AM 21348, 07017.)

810 CARDIAC FUNCTION IN SHORT-TERM HYPOTHYROIDISM
K. Donaghue*, I. Hales, R. Cooper, A. Edwards, S. Allwright, S. Grant, A. Morrow, E. Wilmshurst. Royal North Shore Hospital, Sydney, Australia.

Reversible cardiac abnormalities occur in long-standing hypothyroidism. Those reported included reduced cardiac output, prolongation of the pre-ejection period of systole, thickening of the interventricular septum and a reduction in the left ventricular ejection fraction (LVEF) both at rest and during exercise. The study was designed to assess the effect of acute hypothyroidism on the heart. Ten patients were studied (mean age 45.8 years: range 33-64 years). No patient had symptomatic or known heart disease. All had total thyroid ablation for thyroid cancer and were proven to have no functioning thyroid tissue. Rest and exercise radionuclide gated blood pool scans (GBPS) and resting 2D echocardiography were performed while each patient was receiving thyroid hormone replacement and then repeated 10 days after ceasing triiodothyronine. Mean TSH level at the time of the second study was 86.5 μIU/ml (range 20.7 - 228.4 μIU/ml). Two patients had an abnormal exercise GBPS (i.e. the LVEF failed to rise by at least 5%) while euthyroid. Of the remaining 8 patients three had abnormal exercise responses when hypothyroid. In addition another 2 patients were found to have minor changes in left ventricular (LV) dimensions on echocardiography, when hypothyroid. After only 10 days hypothyroidism at least 3 of 8 patients developed reversible changes in LV function. It is not clear by what mechanism this effect occurs but its occurrence may be relevant to the clinical risks of even short duration hypothyroidism.

811 EFFECT OF TSH ON INTRACELLULAR PROTEIN TRANSPORT IN THYROID FOLLICLE CELLS.
L.E. Ericson*, V. Johanson and T. Öfverholm, Dept. of Anatomy, University of Göteborg, S-400 33 Gothenburg, Sweden.

TSH stimulates exocytosis of protein into the follicle lumen but an effect on earlier steps of intracellular protein transport is unknown. The redistribution of labeled protein in thyroid follicles in normal and T_4-treated (2 d) rats was studied by quantitative EM autoradiography 1, 1.5, 2, 3, 4.5 and 6 h after ^{3}H-leucine. The half-life of labeled, exportable protein was determined by regression analysis using an one-way flow, 3-compartment model based on first order kinetics. In normal rats the half-life of exportable protein in the compartment "ER-Golgi" was 32 min and in the compartment "exocytotic vesicles" 16 min. In the absence of TSH in T_4-treated rats the corresponding half-lives were considerably longer, 73 and 48 min. TSH (100 mU) given to T_4-treated rats 1.5 or 3 h after ^{3}H-leucine and 20 min or 1.5 h before fixation stimulated exocytosis as reflected by a decrease of half-life of labeled protein in "exocytotic vesicles" to about 7 min. In addition, TSH increased the transfer of protein out from the compartment "ER-Golgi" in which the half-life of exportable, labeled protein decreased from 73 min to 25-33 min. Combination of kinetic data on exocytotic vesicles with stereological measurements indicated that the apical plasma membrane was exchanged by addition of new membrane from exocytotic vesicles in 80 min in normal rats and in 130 min in T_4-treated rats. The present data demonstrate that TSH influences the rate of intracellular protein transport by a stimulation of exocytosis as well as by a stimulation of the transfer of protein out of the endoplasmic reticulum-Golgi apparatus.

812 THE OPTIMAL DOSE OF THYROXINE ASSESSED BY THE TRH-TEST DEPENDS ON THE INDIVIDUAL DEGREE OF THYROID AUTONOMY AND AGE.
P.Erne*, J.J. Staub, A. Ryff, Y. Fleig, J. Girard Dept. of Medicine, University of CH-4031 Basle.

In order to assess the optimal dose of thyroxine replacement and suppressive therapy in simple goiter and thyroid cancer, we measured basal TSH, T4 and T3 and the TSH response to 40mg of oral TRH as described previously (JCEM 46:26, 1978). 53 patients with overt hypothyroidism, 17 with preclinical hypothyroidism, 22 with simple euthyroid goiter and 22 patients treated for thyroid cancer (total thyroid ablation) comprised our study group. The individual doses of thyroxine were monitored by repetitive oral TRH-testing and adjusted accordingly. - The mean thyroxine dose of $128.5 \pm 34 \mu g/d$ ($\bar{x} \pm SD$) in overt hypothyroidism was significantly higher than in preclinical hypothyroidism ($101.5 \pm 24 \mu g/d, p < 0.01$). The mean suppressive dose ($184.6 \pm 47 \mu g/d$) in treated thyroid carcinoma was significantly higher than in simple goiter ($119.3 \pm 26 \mu g/d$, $p < 0.001$). In the group of patients with overt hypothyroidism the necessary thyroxine replacement dose decreased with age (below 40y $\bar{x}$ was 150µg/d; 40-65y $\bar{x}$ was 131µg/d; over 65y $\bar{x}$ was 108.9µg/d: differences significant). In all groups of patients the individual doses showed a wide variation and the dose did not relate to bodyweight or to body-mass-index. - Our data suggest that the individual degrees of autonomous thyroid function determine in part the dose of thyroxine necessary for replacement or suppression. They may further support evidence for a decreased need of thyroxine or a diminished TRH-receptor sensitivity to exogenous TRH with advancing age.

813 ANTAGONISTIC EFFECTS OF EPIDERMAL GROWTH FACTOR (EGF) AND THYROTROPIN (TSH) ON THYROGLOBULIN SYNTHESIS IN CULTURED OVINE THYROID CELLS. J.E. Errick, M.C. Eggo and G.N. Burrow, Banting & Best Dept. of Medical Research and Dept. of Medicine, University of Toronto, Toronto, Canada. M5G 1L7

EGF stimulates growth in ovine thyroid cells in culture and inhibits a number of aspects of differentiation like iodine trapping and incorporation. TSH stimulates differentiated function but has relatively little effect on growth. Neither TSH nor EGF significantly affected thyroglobulin synthesis in thyroid cell cultures plated at a density of 2.5 X 10^5 cells/cm^2. However, when the cells were plated at 10^3 cells/cm and maintained for 3 weeks in medium supplemented with insulin (10 ug/ml), hydrocortisone (10 nM), transferrin (5 ug/ml), somatostatin (10 ng/ml), and glycyl-histidyl-lysine (10 ng/ml), plus 0.5% calf serum, a nearly confluent monolayer of thyroid follicular cells was obtained. The addition of TSH (100 uU/ml) stimulated thyroglobulin synthesis, demonstrated both by immunoprecipitation of ^{35}S-methionine labelled cultures and indirect immunofluorescence. No fluorescence was visible at 2 or 4 days after the addition of TSH, but intense fluorescence was seen by 7 days. A similar time course was noted with ^{125}I-incorporation. Thyroglobulin production increased from 0.06% of total protein synthesis to 3.7% of the total by 7 days. When EGF (10^{-9}M) was added with TSH, thyroglobulin production was only 0.57% and this was confirmed by immunofluorescence. These data suggest that extensive proliferation of thyroid cells in the absence of TSH results in an undifferentiated population that can be induced to synthesize thyroglobulin in the presence of TSH and this action can be blocked by EGF.

814 LOCALIZATION OF BOVINE THYROTROPIN AND ANTIBODIES IN THYROID DISEASES IN PORCINE THYROCYTES USING IMMUNOCYTOCHEMISTRY. G.E. Fåhraeus-van Ree*, T.M. Scott and N.R. Farid, Thyroid Research Laboratory, Health Sciences Centre, St. John's, Newfoundland, A1B 3V6, Canada.

Localization of receptor-bound bovine thyrotropin (bTSH) and immunoglobulins G from sera of patients with Graves' (G-IgG) or Hashimoto's (H-IgG) disease in porcine thyrocytes was studied at structural and ultrastructural levels by the double antibody immuno-enzyme method. Porcine fragments were fixed or kept in organ culture in a hormone-free medium or in a medium with bTSH for 3-4 days. Enzymatically isolated thyrocytes were cultured in primary monolayer in a hormone-free or in a bTSH-enriched medium for 7 days. Follicular cells in explants and monolayers cultured in bTSH-enriched medium contain a number of intracellular Periodic Acid Schiff (PAS)-positive colloid droplets (phagosomes) and give a weak to moderate immuno-reaction to anti-bTSH and a strong reaction to G-IgG and H-IgG in comparison to the immunoglobulins of the controls. The precipitate is particularly found at surface membranes of the microvilli, the phagosomes, and around the nuclei. Follicular cells cultured in the absence of bTSH contain less phagosomes and show almost no immuno-reaction to anti-bTSH but a moderate reaction to G-IgG and H-IgG. Preincubation of these fixed cells with bTSH leads to a strong reduction of the immuno-reaction to G-IgG but does not affect the reaction to H-IgG. The morphological results indicate that G-IgG and H-IgG interact with the same cellular sites as bTSH and that H-IgG are directed towards a different epitope on the TSH receptor than the TSH and G-IgG binding sites.

815 IMMUNOLOGICAL SIMILARITY BETWEEN TWO COMPONENTS OF AFFINITY LABELLED NUCLEAR T3 RECEPTOR IN RAT LIVER. R. Faure*, J. Ruel and J.H. Dussault, Thyroid Research Unit, Dept of Endocrinology and Metabolism, CHUL, Québec, G1V 4G2, Canada.

Thyroid hormone action appears to be mediated by the binding of triiodothyronine to a chromatin associated protein. In order to bring further evidence for this mechanism we isolated the receptor from rat liver nuclei using ^{125}I labelled bromoacetyl T3 (BrAcT3) as an affinity probe. Salt extracted receptor was dialysed and submitted to SDS PAGE. Autoradiography revealed two bands, one major (MW: 57000 d) and one minor (MW: 47000 d) which were decreased by 40% when a 1000 fold excess of unlabelled T3 was added. Great similitude was observed in the S. Aureus V8 protease digestion products of each band. Rabbits were immunized with either the major or the minor component. The presence of antibodies was tested with the Hybridot BRL apparatus using as antigens total nuclear extract, major bands and minor bands. Two rabbits injected with the major band and one with the minor band were found positive for each antigen, thereby demonstrating the immunologic similarity of both receptor bands. Electrophoresis of the nuclear extract and transfer onto nitro cellulose paper confirmed the result showing the appearance of two bands at positions corresponding to the receptor bands when incubated with the positive antisera.

Conclusion: Labelling of rat nuclear extract with BrAcT3 revealed the presence of two receptor bands with the same antigenic properties and similar peptide maps. Further studies are needed to elucidate the origin and the significance of these T3 receptor bands.

816 LONG-TERM MONOLAYER CULTURE OF A TSH- AND GH-SECRETING PITUITARY ADENOMA: RESPONSE TO T_3, DEXAMETHASONE (DEX), HYPOTHALAMIC FACTORS, AND NEUROTRANSMITTERS. H.G. Fein*, I. Richmond, and R.C. Smallridge. Depts of Medicine and Surgery, Walter Reed Army Medical Center & Institute of Research, Washington, D.C. 20307 USA.

A 49 y.o. woman with acromegaly (GH: 44-76 ng/ml) and TSH-induced hyperthyroidism (T_4 18.3 µg/dl, Free T_4 3.6 ng/dl, TSH 4.8 uU/ml, thyroid stimulating antibody negative) underwent transsphenoidal removal of an intrasellar macroadenoma. A portion of the adenoma was minced, trypsinized and plated in 13 microwells at 5.4 X 10^5 cells/well. Initial secretion was brisk (TSH = 72.3 ± 2.6 uU/well/day, GH > 250 ng/well/day) but gradually declined. Nevertheless, hormone secretion continued for more than 50 days. As with preoperative *in vivo* studies, TSH secretion was not stimulated *in vitro* by 10^{-6}M TRH. TSH secretion was likewise not significantly suppressed by 3 or 6 h of 10^{-7}M dopamine or 10^{-8}M SRIF or by 5 days of 10^{-7}M T_3 or 10^{-7}M DEX. However, TSH was suppressed 69.4 ± 14.3% by 3 h exposure to 10^{-5}M acetylcholine with 10^{-5}M physostigmine (A/P; p<0.0005 vs control wells). *In vitro* GH secretion was not altered by TRH, GH-releasing hormone (hpGRF-44, 10^{-9}M to 10^{-7}M), or hpGRF with TRH, but was suppressed by dopamine (77.9 ± 9.1%, p<0.025), SRIF (74.8 ± 13.6%, p<0.05) and A/P (86.8 ± 3.6%, p<0.01). Atropine (10^{-6}M) blocked the suppression of TSH by A/P but had no effect on A/P suppression of GH. These atropine effects suggest that cholinergic regulation of TSH may be mediated in humans through muscarinic sites, while regulation of GH may be through nicotinic receptors. The *in vitro* TSH and GH responses to all these agents suggest that these secretory adenomas may have a partial loss of the receptor or post-receptor mechanisms generally found in human or animal pituitary models.

817 TRIIODOTHYRONINE (T_3) PRODUCTION BY THE PERFUSED KIDNEY IS REDUCED BY DIABETES BUT NOT BY FASTING. D.C. Ferguson*, M. Hoenig, and A.S. Jennings, Dept. of Pharmacology, Cornell University, Ithaca, N.Y. 14853, and Dept. of Medicine, University of Pennsylvania, Philadelphia, PA 19104 USA.

Both fasting (F) and diabetes mellitus (DM) lead to reductions in serum T_3 in rat and man. Renal homogenate studies have demonstrated no change in T_3 production (T_3P) from thyroxine (T_4) during F, while there have been no studies of renal T_3P during DM. Both conditions were studied in rat kidneys perfused for one hour at 37°C, pH 7.4. Studies were performed using two perfusion media designed to create a wide difference in free T_4 (FT_4) concentration. Basal kidney T_3 concentrations fell to 35 and 38% of control after 3 days of F and 5 days of streptozotocin (STZ)-induced DM, respectively, in parallel with changes in serum T_3. However, in F, there was no significant change in perfused kidney T_4 uptake (T_4U), T_3P, or T_4 to T_3 conversion rate (CR). However, DM decreased T_3P to 56 and 70% of that of insulin-treated controls (I) at low and high perfusate FT_4 concentrations, respectively ($p<0.005$). T_3P in I was not different from that in a group not treated with STZ demonstrating that the reduction was insulin-reversible and not attributable to STZ. The decrease in T_3P in DM was attributable to a diminished CR as T_4U did not differ between groups. The relative reduction in renal T_3P during DM was not as great as decreases in basal kidney T_3, serum T_3, or T_3P by perfused liver in our previous studies (T_3P in DM was ∿20% of I). We conclude that renal T_3P is decreased in DM in contrast to F, and that the relative decrease is less than that in hepatic T_3P during DM. We postulate that the absent or smaller decrease in renal T_3P in these conditions reflects less exposure to intraportal factors.

818 AUTOREGULATION OF TSH SECRETION VIA DOPAMINE IN VITRO. S.M.Foord*, C.Dieguez J.R.Peters, R.Hall and M.F.Scanlon. Department of Medicine, Welsh National School of Medicine, Heath Park, Cardiff CF4 4XN, Wales, United Kingdom.

TSH and PRL secretion by 3 day primary cultures of male rat anterior pituitary (AP) cells is inhibited by the neurotransmitter dopamine (DA). The specificity of the inhibition is the same as shown by DA receptors in live AP cells and in particulate preparations of AP glands. We have found that the dopaminergic inhibition of TSH secretion by AP monolayer cultures is dependent on the amount of TSH accumulated in the culture medium. Within 4hrs of replacing the culture medium on 3 day AP cultures with fresh medium the dopaminergic inhibition of TSH secretion could be completely abolished whereas the effects of TRH or somatostatin were unaffected. Total DA receptor binding to the cells, analysed upon the culture dish or as a particulate preparation, was similarly dependent on 'old' culture medium (a 50% fall in receptor number being measured when 'fresh' medium was replaced). Exogenous purified TSH (up to 30U/mg) and Graves' IgG mimick endogenous TSH to the same extent and with similar ED_{50}s (0.I-ImU determined by porcine thyroid cell bioassay using Thytropar as a standard). Heat treated TSH, hCG, insulin, glucagon, ACTH and PRL were without effect on either DA receptor binding or TSH inhibtion by DA. The dopaminergic inhibition of PRL secretion was not medium or hormone dependent. The data suggest the presence of a mechanism whereby TSH may control its own secretion. Full expression of this control pathway in vivo would be dependent on the integrity of the tuberoinfundibular dopaminergic system and the hypophyseal portal circulation.

819 EFFECTS OF RADIOIODINE TREATMENT ON THYROID ^{127}I CONTENT (TIC)
P. Fragu*, M. Schlumberger, C. Parmentier, Institut Gustave-Roussy - 94805 Villejuif Cedex France.

The aim of this study was to analyse the short and long term effects of ^{131}I treatment for Graves' disease on TIC and the relationship between it and hormonal status. The short term effects were studied in 9 patients assessed serially for 5 to 26 months after treatment. TIC decreased in all patients and became undetectable in 8 cases within 4 months. This fall was parallel to those of T_3 and T_4 and was not prevented by the administration of large doses of iodine. In 4 patients this decrease was irreversible and they became clinically hypothyroid. In the 5 others, it was partly reversible and simultaneous to a normalisation of T_3 T_4 TSH levels. The long term effects have been studied in 38 patients treated from 1.5 up to 22 years before. 16 patients with normal TSH level (< 8 µU/ml) had a low TIC (3.2 ± 3 mg). Furthermore patients with normal TRH test had a TIC twice fold higher (4 ± 3.9 mg) than that of patients with increased response to TRH (2.4 ± 1.7 mg). The 22 others patients had elevated TSH levels, 11 had undetectable TIC. There was only a close positive relationship between TIC and T_4 (r = 0.60). The T_3/T_4 ratio in patients with undetectable TIC (20.5 ± 7.9) was higher than that of the other patients (14.6 ± 3.2). These data confirm that there is a fast turnover of intrathyroid ^{127}I.

820 SERUM CONCENTRATIONS OF CALCITONIN (Ct) IN THYROID DISEASES.
A.Franke* and K.Oeff, Department of Nuclear Medicine, Klinikum Steglitz, Free University of Berlin, D-1000 Berlin 45, F.R.G.

Serum levels of Ct were measured by radioimmunoassay in 1437 patients subjected to diagnostic and therapeutic procedures for thyroid diseases. Significant alterations in the distribution of serum values of Ct were observed in patients categorized according to thyroid size, cytology, clinical disease entities, and current thyroid function. Thyroid morphology, Pap staging of cytological smears, and current treatment of thyroid disorders yielded no significant changes in the concentrations of Ct. The present data demonstrate that a functional relationship exists between different cell types in the thyroid gland as well as between thyroid hormones and Ct.

821 Peripheral K Lymphocytes in Subacute Thyroiditis in Relation to Immunosuppressive Acidic Protein

H. Fukazawa*, T. Sakurada, K. Tamura[1], M. Yamamoto, K. Yoshida, S. Saito, N. Ishida[1], and K. Yoshinaga, Dept. of 2nd Int. Med. and Dept. of Bacteriol[1]., Tohoku Univ. Sch. of Med., Sendai, Japan.

We have reported that the immunosuppressive acidic protein (IAP), a type of α_1-acid glycoprotein, is increased in the acute phase of subacute thyroiditis (SAT) (Excerpt Medica 605, 453, 1983). The present work was undertaken to estimate antibody-dependent cell-mediated cytotoxicity (ADCC) activity (percentage of peripheral K cells) in SAT and Graves' hyperthyroidism (HT) by the plague-forming cell technique. Inhibition rate of K-cells from a normal subject was investigated by incubating the K-cells with sera of SAT and HT and purified IAP. The percentages of K-cells of patients with SAT in acute and recovery phases were 2.4 ± 1.8% (mean ± S.D., n=19) and 5.0 ± 1.7% (n=12), respectively. The former was significantly lower than the latter. The value in acute phase showed siginificantly decrease against that of normal control (6.8 ± 3.0%, n=25). The percentage of K-cells of HT, 2.8 ± 2.2% (n=16), was also significantly lower than that of normal. The percentages of K-cells were significantly lower in acute phase of SAT and in HT than in sex-matched controls. Inhibition rates of K-cells by 13 sera from SAT in acute and recovery phases were 68 ± 21% and 38 ± 23%, respectively, which were significantly higher than those in 13 normal sera, 15 ± 19%. The inhibition rate was significantly higher in the acute phase than in the recovery. The sera from 10 patients with HT also inhibit K-cells. A dose-related inhibition of K-cells by purified IAP was observed. It was suggested that, in the serum of SAT, there are some factors, such as IAP, which inhibit K-cells.

822 SUBCHRONIC EXPOSURE OF CULTURED HUMAN THYROID MONOLAYER CELLS TO THYROID-STIMULATING IgGs ALTERS SUBSEQUENT STIMULATION WITH TSI OR TSH.

Y.Fukue * H.Uchimura, T.Mitsuhashi, K.Kubota, N.Kuzuya, A.Ikeda, S.Okano,** Y.Kanaji **, and F.Takaku; Third Department of Internal Medicine, Faculty of Medicine, University of Tokyo, Hongo, and Kanaji Hospital**,Kitaku,Tokyo,Japan.

Thyroid responsiveness to repeated exposure of TSH or IgGs is controversial. We studied cAMP responses in human thyroid cutured cells after subchronic exposure (4d) to IgGs from untreated Graves' patients and subsequent stimulation with TSH or thyroid stimulating IgGs (TSI). Graves' tissues were obtained at surgery. After enzymatic dispersion, cells were suspended in Ham's F-12, seeded $1.5x10^6$cells and cultured with or without IgG(1mg) for 4 days. Cells were then stimulated with IgG 10mg for 2hr or bovine TSH 100mU for 30min and intracellular cAMP was measured by RIA.IgGs were prepared by Protein A Sepharose and high TSI activities were ascertained by our standard cAMP assay using human thyroid monolayer cells. After bTSH stimulation, cAMP responses were greater in IgG-pre-exposed cells than in non-exposed cells. Responses were also greater in bTSH pre-exposed cells than in non-exposed cells after IgG stimulation. When homologous IgG pre-exposed cells were stimulated with homologous IgG (tissue and IgGs from same patient), cAMP responses in 5 such patients were as great or greater as found when using different thyroid cells. When heterologous IgGs were employed under the same conditions, 11 of 15 showed no response. No specific interrelationship between pre-exposed IgG and IgG used in subsequent stimulation was observed. Results suggest the site/s of action of TSI may be different from that of TSH and specific interrelationship between the patient's thyroid cells and TSI may exist in Graves'disease.

823 ENHANCED GOITROGENICITY OF RESORCINOL IN THE GUNN RAT WITH UDP-GLUCURONYL TRANSFERASE (UDP-GT) DEFICIENCY. E. Gaitan*, R. C. Cooksey and J. S. Legan, University of Mississippi Medical School and VA Medical Center, Jackson, MS 39216.

Resorcinol (R), a monomeric derivative of flavonoid humic substances in the natural environment, as well as an abundant by-product in waste-water effluents of coal-conversion processes, is known to possess antithyroid and goitrogenic properties. However, these activities are short-lived probably because the rapid conjugation and excretion of R with glucuronic acid. To test this hypothesis Gunn rats (G), devoid of UDP-GT and normal Wistar rats (W), were compared in their thyroidal responses to orally administered R-(10 and 100 µmol/day) for one month. Rats, 80 g initial b.w. were fed on a low-iodine diet. Thyroid weight (mg/100 g rat) was similar in the control groups (N=5 ea) (W=16.8 $\pm$ 2.1 SD vs G=18.6 $\pm$ 1.7, NS), but it was significantly greater in Gunn rats given R (W=R-10:17.6 $\pm$ 4.2 and R-100:21.3 $\pm$ 6.6 vs G=R-10: 22.8 $\pm$ 2.6, p<.02 and R-100:28.1 $\pm$ 3.2, p<.05). Same was observed with thyroid 125-I uptake (% at 3h) (W=Control:59 $\pm$ 8 vs G=55 $\pm$ 4, NS; W=R-100:55 $\pm$ 9 vs G=65 $\pm$ 3, p<.05). Yet, the control Gunn's thyroid was less efficient than the W's thyroid to organify 125-I (I/MIT&DIT) (W:.39 $\pm$ .05 vs G:.67 $\pm$ .03, p<.005) and to form T_3&T_4 (%) (W=7.8 $\pm$ 0.3 vs G=6.3 $\pm$ 0.3, p<.005). The antithyroid effect of R was evident in both W and G rats by dose-response increments in MIT&DIT/T_3&T_4 and decrements in % T_3&T_4. Results demonstrate significant enhancement of the goitrogenic activity of R in Gunn rats. Whether this is only due to lack of UDP-GT and/or other strain differences needs to be determined.

824 EVIDENCE THAT CHOLERA TOXIN (CT) STIMULATES THE THYROID WITHOUT DIRECT BINDING TO THYROTROPIN RECEPTOR (TSH-R). A. Garcia. Dept. of Medicine, Faculty of Medicine, Autonomous University of Barcelona, Barcelona, Spain.

CT is a potent stimulator of adenylate cyclase in many tissues, including the thyroid. Since it also has been reported both to enhance and inhibit the binding of TSH to the TSH-R and potentiate thyroid stimulation by TSH and thyroid-stimulating antibody the relation of CT to the TSH-R is unclear. We therefore conducted studies with ^{125}I-CT, ^{125}I-TSH and preparations of TSH-R from human thyroid and guinea pig fat cell membranes. There was specific, saturable binding of ^{125}I-CT to particulate and Triton-N101-solubilized thyroid and fat cell membranes; Ka using particulate thyroid membranes was $5.26 \times 10^9 M^{-1}$. With particulate thyroid or fat cell membranes, unlabelled TSH, 1-1000 mU/ml, did not affect binding of ^{125}I-CT. Unlabelled CT apparently inhibited binding of ^{125}I-TSH to either thyroid or guinea pig membranes but this was found to be due to the buffer (Tris-EDTA-NaN_3-NaCl) in which the CT was supplied; dialyzed CT, free from buffer, had only a slight ($\simeq$ 25%) enhancing effect on ^{125}I-TSH binding at 10 uM and was not inhibitory at lesser concentrations. Functioning rat thyroid (FRTL) cells, provided by Dr. L. Kohn, were stimulated (increase in cAMP) linearly by dialyzed CT in concentrations up to 0.1 uM and by TSH (maximum effect obtained with 5mU/ml). Unlabelled CT (1-1000 uM) had no effect on ^{125}I-TSH binding to intact FRTL cells although the binding was inhibited by either cold TSH or human IgG containing thyroid stimulating antibody obtained from Graves' disease sera. These data indicate that the effects of CT on thyroid function do not reflect direct interaction with the receptor for TSH.

825 SIMULTANEOUS ASSESSMENT OF TSH RECEPTOR ANTIBODY ACTIVITY AND THYROIDAL STIMULATION OF IODINE ORGANIFICATION BY GRAVES' IMMUNOGLOBULINS.

J. Ginsberg*, G. Shewring, and B. Rees Smith, Endocrine Immunology Unit, Department of Medicine, Welsh National School of Medicine, Cardiff, U.K.

To determine the relationship between TSH receptor antibody activity (TRAA) and thyroid stimulation, 53 Graves' IgGs were assessed in a radioreceptor assay for TRAA and a bioassay simultaneously. Of the patients studied, 15 were untreated with thyrotoxicosis and 38 were treated; 6 of whom had relapsed. TRAA was based on the ability of the Graves' IgG to inhibit the binding of radiolabelled TSH to its receptor (Shewring and Rees Smith, 1982). The bioassay employed measured the stimulation of iodine organification in cultured porcine thyroid cells by Graves' IgGs (Plannels et al., 1975; Ginsberg et al.,1983). TRAA positivity occurred if >20% inhibition was produced. A IgG was considered stimulatory if organification > x + 2 S.D. of 6-8 normal control IgGs was achieved. The following results were obtained:

	TRAA POSITIVE	TRAA NEGATIVE	
BIOASSAY POSITIVE	23	6	= 29
BIOASSAY NEGATIVE	13	11	= 24
	36	17	= 53

These data suggest that: (1) Neither assay was uniquely more sensitive in detecting the presence of Graves' IgG, (2) The Graves' IgGs tested exhibited agonist, partial antagonist, and super-agonist properties. We conclude that Graves' IgGs have different capacities for TSH receptor activation. J.G. was supported by a MRC Canada Fellowship.

826 GRAVES' DISEASE OPHTHALMOPATHY (GO) TREATED BY INTENSIVE PLASMA EXCHANGE.

D. Glinoer*, M. Schrooyen, G. Sand, J. Etienne, and R. Winand. Hospitals Saint-Pierre and Baviere, Universities of Brussels and Liege, Belgium.

Nine female patients (32-76 yrs) with severe, progressive GO (grade 3 to 6, ATA classification) were treated by plasmapheresis (PP). A total of 10 liters of plasma was exchanged in 4 sessions, over 8 days. Thereafter, 7/9 patients received immunosuppressive therapy. The effects of PP were evaluated by an "ophthalmopathy index" for 6 ocular parameters, derived from Donaldson et al. (JCEM, 1973). Numerical scores from 0 (no injury) to 3 (marked injury) were compared before PP and 4-8 days after PP (highest possible score : 18/18) :

Patient N°	1∅o	2*o	3*	4∅o	5*o	6∅o	7*	8∅	9∅o
before PP	13	7	9	6	11	3	17	11	9
after PP	6	3	6	3	7	3	9	7	7

(*) acute GO (≤ 1 to 6 months); (∅) GO present since ≥ 1 yr; (o) patients with previous corticosteroid treatment with poor response or recurrence.

An excellent or good response was obtained in 8/9 patients. The best positive effects were on soft tissue, proptosis, intraocular pressure and, most important, on sight loss. The least positive effects were on cornea and extraocular muscle, even though there was a significant reduction in the size and density of extraocular muscles as estimated by CT-scans. In conclusion, intensive plasma exchange provides an effective and prompt improvement in acute and chronic progressive ophthalmopathy. We suggest that PP (followed by immunosuppression) can be used as the first therapeutic approach to severe Graves' ophthalmopathy.

827 TRIIODOTHYRONINE (T_3) INDUCES A RAPID Ca^{2+}-DEPENDENT STIMULATION OF MEMBRANE TRANSPORT PROCESSES & Ca^{2+} FLUXES IN MOUSE KIDNEY CORTEX.

A. Goldstone*, H. Koenig, C.Y. Lu, C.P. Barsano & J.J. Trout, Neurology, Biochemistry & Endocrinology Svcs, VALMC & Neurology, Biochemistry & Center for Endocrinology & Metabolism, NUMS, Chicago, IL 60611

The thyroid hormone triiodothyronine (T_3) elicits a rapid (<5 min) stimulation of endocytosis, hexose transport & amino acid transport in mouse kidney cortex slices from hypothyroid but not euthyroid mice. This uptake is concentration dependent & is maximal at .45-45 nM. Peroxidase cytochemistry utilizing horseradish peroxidase (HRP) demonstrated the T_3 induced HRP uptake is restricted to proximal tubules. The absence of these rapid membrane responses in Ca-free medium & the total lack or negligible response to rT_3 (4.5 nM) or T_4 (450 nM) indicate Ca^{2+}- & T_3 receptor-dependence. 4.5 nM T_3 rapidly stimulates $^{45}Ca^{2+}$ influx (<30 sec) & $^{45}Ca^{2+}$ efflux (<30 sec). Rates of Ca^{2+} influx & efflux, & of endocytosis, hexose & amino acid transport are significantly greater in euthyroid than in hypothyroid kidney cortex. These results suggest that the rapid changes in hexose & amino acid transport, endocytosis & Ca^{2+} fluxes involve a direct receptor-mediated response of the plasma membrane to T_3 & a resultant increase in cytosolic $[Ca^{2+}]$. (Supported by the VA & NIH grants NS 14700, NS 18047 & HL 26835)

828 PURIFICATION AND CHARACTERIZATION OF A NEW THYROXINE BINDING PROTEIN (nTBP) FROM HUMAN SERUM.

S.Grimaldi, F. Carlini, C. Carducci, R. Dominici, M. Andreoli* F. Monaco, Thyroid Center C.N.R. c/o II Clinica Medica Policlinico Umberto I-Rome, Italy

Human serum TBG purified by affinity chromatography on T_4 agarose, followed by ion exchange and gel filtration chromatography often contains variable amounts of another protein with molecular weight on SDS elettrophoresis of 27000 dalton. nTBP was separated from TBG by differential elution from T_4 agarose. The proteins retained on the column were eluted with a gradient of T_4 from 10^{-11} to 10^{-6}M; TBG was recovered at 10^{-9}M and nTBP at 10^{-8}M. By chromatofocusing nTBP is eluted at pI = 5.3 and Tbg at pI = 4.7. By equilibrium dialysis an affinity constant for T_4 of 2.0 10^{-7} and 8.0 10^{-8} was measured respectively. Double immunodiffusion with both antisera showed no identity pattern between the two proteins. These data indicate that TBP is a thyroxine binding protein different from TBG for immunochemical properties, molecular weight and affinity constant for T_4. In conclusion the presence in normal human sera of a new T_4 binding protein has been demonstrated; its possible role in some thyroid status (i.e. TBG deficiency) needs further studies.

829 EFFECT OF ANGIOTENSIN II (AII) INFUSION ON THE PLASMA ACTH MORNING PEAK AND ON ACTH RESPONSE TO CRF. H. Haller, J. Hensen, V. Bähr and W. Oelkers*, Dept. of Medicine, Klinikum Steglitz, Freie Universität Berlin, Germany.

Cerebroventricular application of AII triggers ACTH release. Systemic infusion of AII was reported by one group to acutely suppress ACTH secretion, while others found evidence for ACTH stimulation by high endogenous AII levels.
We studied the effect of AII on ACTH and cortisol in 2 conditions: 1) 6 normal men received AII (5 ng/kg/min) or sham infusions in randomized sequence between 3 a.m. and 7 a.m. 2) 6 other normals received the same dose of AII or sham infusions between 4:30 p.m. and 8 p.m., and CRF (100 µg bolus) was injected i.v. at 5 p.m. In both studies, plasma ACTH and cortisol were measured by RIA in short intervals.
Results: 1) AII had no effect on the onset of the early morning peak of ACTH and cortisol. Mean ACTH peak levels reached during AII infusion (85 ± SEM 36 pg/ml) were insignificantly higher than in the sham study (56 ± 23 pg/ml). Peak levels of cortisol were 451 and 414 mN/l resp.
2) After CRF, ACTH increased from 14 ± 4 pg/ml to 53 ± 16 pg/ml with AII infusion and from 13 ± 5 to 46 ± 16 pg/ml with sham infusion. Cortisol rose from 304 to 955 nM/l with AII and from 344 to 1077 nM/l with sham infusion.
Thus, AII may exert, if anything, a slight enhancing effect on ACTH release, but not on cortisol. All differences between the AII and sham infusion experiments were insignificant.

830 BENZODIAZEPINE INHIBITION OF PITUITARY β-END RELEASE AND ANXIETY IN HUMANS UNDERGOING ORAL SURGERY. K.M. Hargreaves*, R.A. Dionne, S. Maiewski, and G.P. Mueller. NAB, NIDR, NIH and Dept. of Physiology, Uniformed services University of the Health Sciences, Bethesda, MD 20205 USA

This double blind study evaluated the effects of iv diazepam (0.3 mg/kg) or placebo on pituitary β-END release in 24 conscious patients undergoing surgical removal of impacted third molars. This model allows determination of immunoreactive beta-endorphin (iβ-END) responses to anticipatory anxiety in the absence of pain (pre-op) and to surgical stress (intra-op) when anxiety is dramatically increased but pain is low due to local anesthesia. The level of pain was assessed by a visual analog scale (VAS); levels of anxiety were estimated by the Spielberger State Trait Anxiety Index (STAI) and a separate VAS. Mean pre-op anticipatory anxiety compared to baseline measures taken at least 1 week earlier, increased significantly on both the VAS (6.8 to 25.7, $p<.01$) and STAI (31.2 to 40.0, $p<.01$), while plasma levels of iβ-END, as measured by RIA after Sep-Pak extracttion, did not change. The surgical procedure was associated with further increases in mean anxiety (to 44.2 on VAS, $p<.01$; to 48.0 on STAI, $p<.01$) and a 72% elevation ($p<.01$) in circulating levels of iβ-END over pre-op values. Diazepam pretreatment prevented the intra-op increases in both anxiety and plasma iβ-END. Neither group differed in their perception of small levels of pain. These findings suggest that anxiety of the intensity experienced during surgical stress, constitutes a stimulus for pituitary iβ-END release in humans.

831 PRESENCE OF ACTH-POTENTIATING FACTORS IN PORCINE THYMUS. S. Iida*, Y. Itoh, M. Gomi, K. Moriwaki and S. Tarui, The Second Department of Internal Medicine, Osaka University Medical School, Fukushima-ku, Osaka, Japan 553.

We have noted that acid extracts of rat and porcine anterior glands and thyroid enhanced corticosterone production of isolated rat adrenal cells in response to low concentrations of ACTH-(1-24). Designated ACTH-potentiating factor(s) (APF), it possessed no biological activity by itself. We demonstrate the presence of the activity in porcine thymic extract. Extraction was done in 0.1N acetic acid after boiling the thymus. Purification of the factors with small molecular weights was performed using reversed-phase high performance liquid chrmatography following gel filtration and cation-exchange chromatography. Dispersion of rat adrenal cells followed the method of Sayers, et al., and corticosterone production was measured by competitive protein-binding assay. ACTH-potentiating activity was judged by comparing the biological ACTH activities exerted by the addition of thymus extract in the presence of a known amount of ACTH-(1-24). The factors were acidic and heat stable in nature, and were present in heterogeneous forms having various molecular weight. Potentiation of ACTH by partially purified factors was dose-dependent. Loss of the APF activity of purified fractions by treatment with carboxypeptidase Y indicated their peptide nature. Since, even in the presence of bacitracin at a concentration to prevent ACTH degradation, the enhancement of ACTH-induced steroidogenesis by the factors was observed, the existence of potentiating mechanisms other than inhibition of ACTH proteolysis was indicated.

832 METHIONINE-ENKEPHALIN, LEUCINE-ENKEPHALIN, METHIONINE-ENKEPHALIN-ARG^6-GLY^7-LEU^8 AND METHIONINE-ENKEPHALIN-ARG^6-PHE^7 IN GUINEA PIG CENTRAL NERVOUS SYSTEM AND PITUITARY. Y. Ikeda*, M. Ijima, T. Suzuki, T. Nakazawa, K. Nakao+, T. Yoshimasa+, M. Sakamoto+, M. Suda+, N. Morii+ and H. Imura+. Dept. of Neuropsychiatry, Fujita-Gakuen Univ. Sch. of Med., Aichi and +2nd Div., Dept. of Med., Kyoto Univ. Sch. of Med., Kyoto, Japan.

Analysis of cloned cDNA for preproenkephalin A from the adrenal medulla revealed that this precursor contains four copies of methionine-enkephalin(Met-Enk) and one copy each of leucine-enkephalin(Leu-Enk), methionine-enkephalin-Arg^6-Gly^7-Leu^8(Met-Enk-Arg-Gly-Leu) and methionine-enkephalin-Arg^6-Phe^7(Met-Enk-Arg-Phe). We previously showed the existence of these four opioid peptides in whole brains of guinea pig, rat and golden hamster in a molar ratio similar to that contained in proenkephalin A(Ikeda et al. BBRC, 107, 656, 1982). In this study, we have examined extracts from various parts of the guinea pig brain, spinal cord and pituitary using HPLC and gel filtration coupled with RIAs for these opioid peptides. In the central nervous system, the ratios of contents of these opioid peptides in various regions of the brain are almost constant and similar to the ratio of these peptides contained in proenkephalin A. Gel filtration revealed no big forms. These results indicate the almost completed processing of proenkephalin A in various parts of guinea pig brain. In the neurointermediate pituitary, the content of Leu-Enk was much higher than the other three opioid peptides. Gel filtration revealed the presence of big forms of Leu-Enk without any big forms of the other opioid peptides. These results suggest that Leu-Enk is synthesized from proenkephalin B, or neo-endorphin/dynorphin precursor, besides proenkephalin A in the guinea pig neurointermediate pituitary.

833 CHARACTERIZATION OF PRO-OPIOMELANOCORTIN mRNAs IN PITUITARY LOBES AND HYPOTHALAMUS. L. Jeannotte*, P. Burbach and J. Drouin, Institut de Recherches Cliniques de Montréal, 110 Ave des Pins O., Montréal, Qué. H2W 1R7, Canada.

The pro-opiomelanocortin (POMC) gene is expressed in the anterior and intermediate lobes of the pituitary and in some brain regions mostly in the arcuate nucleus. The regulation of POMC gene expression and the processing of POMC are different in the two pituitary lobes. For instance, glucocorticoids decrease transcription rates and steady-state POMC mRNA levels only in the anterior pituitary but not in the intermediate lobe. We have cloned 30Kb of rat genomic DNA containing this gene and we have determined the DNA sequence of its three exons and upstream presumed regulatory sequences. Southern blot analyses indicate that there is only one POMC gene in the rat. The tissue-specific regulation of POMC expression prompted us to precisely define the transcription unit of this unique gene in three tissues where it is expressed. Northern blot analyses indicate that, in rats and pigs, POMC mRNAs of similar size are found in the anterior and intermediate pituitary lobes but that the hypothalamic POMC mRNA is slightly larger. The transcribed portion of POMC mRNAs were shown to be the same in the three tissues using a full-lenght cDNA probe in S1 mapping experiments. Digestion of poly A^+ RNA isolated from these tissues with RNAase H in the presence of oligo $(dT)_{12-18}$ suggests that the size difference between hypothalamic and pituitary POMC mRNAs is due to different lenghts of poly A tails. Taken together, these data support the idea that the unique POMC gene is transcribed in the same way in these different tissues where evidence indicates that control of transcription is specific for each tissue. (Supported by the MRC of CANADA).

834 WHAT IS THE ROLE OF GLYCOSYLATION OF PRO-OPIOMELANOCORTIN (POMC) IN THE PARS INTERMEDIA OF THE MOUSE? B.G. Jenks*, A.G.H. Ederveen and A.P. van Overbeeke, Dept. of Zoology, Cath. Univ., Nijmegen, The Netherlands.

The functional significance of glycosylation(s) of POMC has not been established. Using the antibiotic tunicamycin to block glycosylation, we have compared the processing of glycosylated and non-glycosylated POMC in the pars intermedia of the mouse. Non-glycosylated prohormone was processed to correct cleavage products; no evidence of random proteolysis was found. Tunicamycin also had no effect on release of the peptides. The mouse pars intermedia synthesizes two forms of POMC: 34K and 30.5K (K = 1000 daltons). Both are glycosylated in the γ-MSH region. The 34K-prohormone has an additional glycosylation in the corticotropin-like-intermediate lobe peptide (CLIP) region. Thus, processing of 34K-POMC yields glycosylated CLIP while the 30.5K-prohormone gives non-glycosylated CLIP. Using these two CLIPs as "markers" to follow the release of peptides derived from the two prohormones, the question was approached whether the occurrence of two forms of POMC might be indicative of a compartmentalization (e.g. two cell-types). In pulse-chase experiments the two CLIPs were released at the same rate during a 7-h chase-incubation. Moreover, dopamine equally inhibited the release of these two peptides. The results suggest that the CLIPs are likely sequestered within the same secretory granules. In conclusion, glycosylation apparently plays no role in the processing or release of POMC peptides, nor is there evidence that the differences in glycosylation of the POMCs lead to packaging in different cellular compartments. Possibly, glycosylation has a function following release of the peptides.

835 INTERACTION BETWEEN STIMULUS INTENSITY AND CORTICOSTEROID (CS) FEEDBACK IN THE CONTROL OF CORTICOTROPIN (ACTH) SECRETION. M. Keller-Wood*, J. Shinsako and M.F. Dallman, Dept. Physiol., UCSF, San Francisco, CA,USA.

These studies were performed to examine the relationship between stimulus intensity and CS feedback in the control of ACTH scretion. In each of 5 conscious dogs, saline or ACTH (20,50,500 ng/min) were infused for 40 min and insulin (.05,.1,.5 U/kg) was injected at 120min. Plasma ACTH levels were measured after insulin injection by RIA. ACTH infusions increased plasma CS to 6.2±0.6, 8.4±0.7 and 9.5±0.5 ug/dl. ACTH infusions did not alter the degree of hypoglycemia produced by insulin injections. In the saline-infused dogs peak and integrated ACTH responses were related to the degree of hypoglycemia; peak ACTH levels after .05, .1 and .5 U/kg insulin were 254±73, 514±76 and 752±62, respectively. 20 ng/min ACTH inhibited integrated ACTH responses to .05, .1 and .5 U/kg insulin by 62±18, 56±21 and 55±11%, and peak levels by 49±16, 33±12 and 42±10%, respectively. 50 ng/min ACTH inhibited integrated ACTH responses to .05, .1 and .5 U/kg insulin by 94±17, 84±10 and 91±5%, and peak levels by 72±8, 75±8 and 84±3% respectively. 500 ng/min ACTH inhibited integrated ACTH responses to .1 and .5 U/kg insulin by 104±5 and 103±1%, and peak levels by 90±2 and 93±1%, respectively. The degree of inhibition of ACTH was the same for a given prior CS feedback signal regardless of the intensity of hypoglycemia (by ANOVA). Therefore, the ACTH response was proportional to the stimulus intensity divided by the feedback dose. Thus, CS exert a modulatory, rather than a simple subtractive, effect on ACTH secretion. The results also suggest that the CS-insensitivity of the responses to some stimuli is not the result of the high intensity of these stimuli since even the response to .5 U/kg insulin was inhibited by CS. This work was supported by NIH.

836 RELIABLE TESTING OF ACTH RESERVE WITH AN IMPROVED RADIOIMMUNOASSAY FOR PLASMA ACTH. B.Kliman* and C. Bagul, Endocrine Unit, Mass. General Hospital, Boston, MA, 02114 and Damon Biotech, Needham Heights,MA 02194.

Current tests of ACTH reserve which rely on assays of either plasma cortisol (F) or 11-deoxy-cortisol (S) are subject to variables of adrenal gland response, metabolic clearance rates of steroids and serum protein binding. These factors can be eliminated by an efficient ACTH assay using a new kit produced by Damon Biotech, with features of high sensitivity, resistance to heparin, second antibody separation and rapid overnight incubation. Normal subjects (40) had 8 AM ACTH of 29.5 ± 21.8 pg/ml (mean ± SD) with intra-assay CV of 10% and inter-assay CV of 15%. We compared ACTH assays to RIA plasma F at 30 min. intervals during insulin tolerance tests (ITT) or to RIA plasma S at 8 AM after an oral dose of 2.5 gm Metyrapone at midnight (MET) for subjects with a variety of test responses. In 18 ITTs, F peaked at 60 to 90 min., whereas ACTH peaked at 30 to 60 min. In 14 normal ITTs with F=20 ug/dl or above, ACTH rose 402% above control and 12 values exceeded normal limits. In the same ITTs, the mean ratio of F peak to control was 202% with 11 values above the normal range. In 4 subnormal ITTs, ACTH fell in two, reached only 30 pg/ml in one and rose 355% in one with F=19.4 ug/dl. In 8 MET tests with S=7.5 or above, ACTH was 25-460 pg/ml. In 3 equivocal MET tests with S below 7.5 but F=10 to 15 ug/dl, ACTH was 86-116 pg/ml. From these results, we conclude that reliable testing of ACTH reserve is achieved by ITT or MET stimulation in conjunction with this improved, convenient RIA for plasma ACTH.

837 STEROIDOGENIC EFFECTS OF PROOPIOMELANOCORTIN (POMC)-DERIVED PEPTIDES ON RABBIT ADRENOCORTICAL CELLS.

J. Kolanowski[+], N. Ortega, M. Chrétien[§] and J. Crabbé. Dept. Physiol., Univ. Louvain, Brussels (Belgium) and Clin. Res. Inst. Montreal (Canada)[§].

The postulated stimulatory influence of POMC-derived peptides on adrenocortical steroidogenesis was evaluated by incubation of dispersed rabbit adrenocortical cells in the presence of various concentrations (from 10^{-12} to 10^{-5} M) of the N-terminal portion of POMC (NT), γ lipotropin (γ LPH), β-endorphin (β End) or corticotropin tetracosapeptide (ACTH). The net maximal steroidogenic response was comparable for NT and ACTH, averaging respectively (per 10^5 cells and 2-h incubation) 40.8 and 45.8 pmol for aldosterone and 1.37 and 1.45 nmol for corticosterone. However, while the maximal effect of ACTH was elicited at 10^{-9} M concentration of the peptide, the same concentration of NT only barely stimulated steroidogenesis ; the concentration of NT had to be raised to 10^{-5} M in order to obtain the full steroidogenic effect. The steroidogenic activity of γ LPH and β End was much smaller than that of ACTH and occurred only at concentrations higher than 10^{-7} M. None of these POMC-derived peptides stimulated adrenal androgen production or modified the steroidogenic response of adrenocortical cells to ACTH. It appears therefore unlikely that these POMC-derived peptides are involved in the physiological regulation of adrenocortical secretion.

838 EFFECTIVENESS OF DIFFERENT KREBS CYCLE INTERMEDIATES (KCI) IN SUPPORTING MITOCHONDRIAL STEROID ENZYMES FROM VARIOUS ADRENAL TISSUES.

L.M. Fishman*, A. Carballeira, J. Brown and C. Bertetta. V.A. Medical Center and Department of Medicine, University of Miami School of Medicine, Miami, Florida 33125, U.S.A.

Our previous studies have shown that adrenal medullary mitochondria possess an 11β-hydroxylase (11βOH) but, unlike the cortex, show no cholesterol cleavage enzyme (CCE) activity. Potential sources of reducing equivalents in support of these reactions in normal and pathologic specimens of cortex and medulla have been examined by comparing the effects of supplementation with NADPH and with KCI. Using ^{14}C-DOC as substrate, the effectiveness of individual KCI (isocitrate, succinate, fumarate or malate, 10 mM each) in supporting 11βOH compared with NADPH (=100) was: Cortex: normal (rat, bovine) 75-112; human adenomas (n=4) and carcinomas (n=2) 50-95. Medulla: normal (bovine) 65-103, except succinate 0-6; pheochromocytomas (n=8) 0, for all KCI. In studies of ^{14}C-cholesterol incubated with either normal or neoplastic cortical mitochondria, KCI in no instance could replace exogenous NADPH in support of CCE. Chromaffin tissues from various sources showed no CCE, irrespective of whether NADPH or KCI was used. These data are consistent with the observation that histochemical assays for succinic dehydrogenase in the adrenal demonstrate an unreactive medulla enveloped by a strongly positive cortex. The ability of succinate to support 11βOH in the adrenal cortex and its failure to do so in chromaffin cells thus represents another difference between these enzyme activities in the two tissues. These studies also demonstrate that cortical mitochondria may use different sources of reducing equivalents for the support of CCE and 11βOH.

839 USEFULNESS OF HIGH PRESSURE LIQUID CHROMATOGRAPHY(HPLC)IN THE SEPARATION OF MINERALOCORTICOIDS PRIOR TO RADIOIMMUNOASSAY(RIA). R.Garcia-Robles*, B.Penna-Lisboa, J.Tovar,L.M.Ruilope, A.Hurtado, H. de la Calle, J.L. Rodicio, and J.M.Sancho. Serv. Endocrinology Centro "Ramón Y Cajal". Madrid, Spain. UKE Eppendorf Hormon Labor Frauen K.L. Hamburg Deutschland. Serv. Nephrology C.S. "1º de Octubre". Madrid. Spain.

The usefulness of HPLC in the process of separation of minieralocorticoid pathway components for the ulterior quantification by specific RIA has been tested. The system consisted in a HPLC Perkin-Elmer Series-3, equipped with a Perkin-Elmer ultraviolet detector, model LC-65T, and two Watters Fatty Acid columns conected in serie. The column effluent was typically monitored at 240 n.m. As mobil phase acetonitrile: water(25:75) was used and volumes of 100 µl were injected manually. Several conditions were checked and the best one was: Flow rate of 0.5 ml/min. , pressure 14.2±2.1 (SD) MP, temperature 22±3ºC. With these conditions the time of development of the separation process was 200 min. The peaks of mineralocorticoids appearance were 24 min. for 18-OH corticosterone, 30 min. for aldosterone, 34 min. for cortisol, 57 min. for 18-OH DOC, 74 min. for corticosterone, and 200 min. for DOC. The identification of the peaks was performed by the addition of internal standards-H^3. The final recovery of samples was higher than 75 per cent. A close correlation for aldosterone and cortisol measured by RIA, with and without prior HPLC separation was found. We conclude that HPLC is a reliable and quick method for the separation of mineralocorticoids prior to their quantification by RIA methods.

840 SYNTHESIS OF 18-HYDROXYCORTISOL IN BEEF ADRENAL SLICES. E.P. Gomez-Sanchez*, C.E. Gomez-Sanchez, M.W. Ferris, M.F. Foecking. Dept. of Internal Medicine, Univ. of South Florida College of Medicine and the J.A. Haley Hospital, Tampa, Florida 33612 USA.

The purpose of the study was the localization of the production of 18-hydroxycortisol and its correlation to the production of other steroids within the adrenal gland. Small blocks (2 x 5 x 5 mm) were cut from freshly collected beef adrenals and 0.2 mm slices parallel to the capsule with a McIlwain tissue slicer. Each slice was incubated in 0.5 ml of M-199 medium for 2 hr at 37 C. Aldosterone, cortisol, corticosterone, and 18-hydroxycorticosterone were measured by RIA using specific antibodies. A specific RIA for 18-hydroxycortisol was developed using an antibody which showed negligible cross reactivity with cortisol, aldosterone, and corticosterone and 4% with 18-OH-B for these measurements. A total of eight sets of 8-14 slices were incubated. As expected, aldo and 18-OH-B were preferentially formed in the outer 3 slices, but small but measurable amounts were formed in deeper slices. Cortisol was produced in small concentrations in the first outer slice (274 ± 54 ng/mg protein) and increased in deeper slices (1777 ± 311 ng/mg protein). Corticosterone and 18-OH-F production was fairly uniform throughout the beef adrenal slices. These studies suggest that 18-hydroxylation of cortisol occurs throughout the adrenal cortex. It is not known whether the same enzyme is involved in the 18-hydroxylation of both cortisol and corticosterone.

841 THE PATTERN OF PLASMA "FREE" DHEA AND DHEA-S STIMULATION TO FOUR ACTH REGIMENS. G. Griffing*, J. Allen, and J.C. Melby, Evans Memorial Department of Clinical Research and the Department of Medicine, University Hospital, Boston, Massachusetts 02118.

The origin and time course of DHEA and DHEA-S stimulation to ACTH is controversial. These studies sought to compare four ACTH regimens on the stimulation of plasma "free" DHEA and DHEA-S. Fourteen young men underwent five study periods: (1) control; (2) α1-24 ACTH, 40 U IV; (3) α1-18 ACTH (D-Ser^1, Lys^{17}, Lys^{18}), 0.4 mg IV; (4) 1-39 ACTH, 40 U IM; and (5) α1-18 ACTH (D-Ser^1, Lys^{17}, Lys^{18}), 0.4 mg IM. Plasma and urine was collected at timed intervals for hormonal measurements over 72 hours. ACTH 1-18 IV had the most potent and prolonged corticotropic effect (measured by plasma cortisol, 17-OHCS, and cortisol secretion rates), lasting up to 24 hours. ACTH 1-39 and 1-18 IM were corticotropic up to 12 hours, and ACTH 1-24 IV was corticotropic only up to one hour. Free DHEA increased acutely with all of the ACTH regimens ($p < 0.05$), but declined to normal with ACTH 1-24 IV at 12 hours and with the remaining ACTH regimens at 24 hours. DHEA-S, on the other hand, did not rise acutely at one hour, but it did rise at 12 and 24 hours with ACTH 1-18 IV, 1-18 IM, and 1-39 IM ($p < 0.05$). Thus, these ACTH regimens induced an acute but transient increase in DHEA-S. These data suggest that ACTH induction of DHEA sulfurylation is a delayed step, possibly occurring in the extra-adrenal tissues. These results also demonstrate that the synthetic ACTH analogue, α1-18 ACTH, is a potent adrenal androgen secretogogue.

842 ANTAGONISTS TO ALDOSTERONE BLOCK ITS EFFECT ON ADRENAL COMPENSATORY HYPERTROPHY IN THE RAT. W. E. Grizzle* and N. E. Dunlap, Departments of Pathology and Internal Medicine, Veterans Administration Medical Center and University of Alabama in Birmingham, Birmingham, Alabama 35294

It has been proposed that the growth of the remaining adrenal gland following unilateral adrenalectomy is controlled primarily by a neural mechanism. We and others have reported results that make an alternate theory, i.e. regulation of adrenal compensatory hypertrophy by the glucocorticoid-ACTH negative feedback system, unlikely. Also, we have reported that continuous infusion of aldosterone (ALDO) blocks adrenal compensatory hypertrophy. We extend these observations by reporting that administration of deoxycorticosterone (DOC) or of corticosterone at dosages exceeding the mineralocorticoid activity of the blocking dose of ALDO does not block adrenal compensatory hypertrophy. Also, administration of either spironolactone or dexamethasone does not block adrenal compensatory hypertrophy. When either dexamethasone or corticosterone is administered concomitantly with a blocking dose of ALDO, adrenal compensatory hypertrophy is blocked. In contrast, when either spironolactone or DOC is given together with the blocking dose of ALDO, adrenal compensatory hypertrophy is not blocked. We conclude that 1) some substances with mineralocorticoid activity do not block adrenal compensatory hypertrophy, and 2) if certain substances with ALDO receptor activity are given together with ALDO, they reverse the blocking action of ALDO on adrenal compensatory hypertrophy.

843 ENDOGENOUS OPIATES MODULATE THE PLASMA EPINEPHRINE RESPONSE TO SUBMAXIMAL EXERCISE IN MAN. A. Gustafson*, P. Farrell, T. Garthwaite, and R. Kalkhoff, Medical College of Wisconsin and University of Wisconsin-Milwaukee, Milwaukee, Wisconsin 53226, USA.

Endogenous opiates may regulate the neuroendocrine response to stress. To examine their influence on the sympathoadrenal response to exercise, the effects (mean±SE) of intense isotonic exercise on plasma catecholamines were studied in 5 men after oral administration of placebo or 50 mg naltrexone, an opiate-receptor antagonist. Subjects were young (21-26 yr), healthy (54±4 ml/kg·min $\dot{V}O_2$ max), and lean (10±2% body fat determined by hydrostatic weighing). After an overnight fast and beginning 120 min after naltrexone or placebo given 2 weeks apart, blood samples were obtained sequentially after 10 min sitting on cycle ergometer, 10, 20 and 30 min of exercise at 70% $\dot{V}O_2$ max, 10 min further sitting, and 20 min supine bedrest. On placebo and naltrexone days, baseline sitting plasma epinephrine (E) as well as plasma norepinephrine (NE), lactate, heart rate and blood pressure did not differ. Catecholamine levels peaked at 30 min of exercise and diminished in recovery. Naltrexone E values (363±52 pg/ml at 30 min) significantly exceeded by almost 2-fold the placebo E response (191±18 pg/ml at 30 min) both during and after exercise ($P<0.05$). This was accompanied by greater plasma glucose concentrations during exercise and recovery and a higher heart rate at 30 min exercise with naltrexone ($P<0.05$). During exercise and recovery no differences in blood pressure or concentrations of NE and lactate were observed. We conclude that naltrexone in man exaggerates the plasma E response to submaximal exercise. This effect suggests that endogenous opiates modulate adrenomedullary function during aerobic exercise.

844 RECOVERY OF THE HYPOTHALAMIC-PITUITARY ADRENAL (HPA) AXIS FOLLOWING CHRONIC STEROID THERAPY. P. Hartzband,* L. Sorger and A. Van Herle, UCLA School of Medicine, Los Angeles, CA., USA.

The hypothalamic-pituitary adrenal (HPA) axis was assessed in patients maintained for various lengths of time (4 wks-20 yrs) on replacement doses of prednisone (5-7.5 mg/day) following prior therapy with high dose corticosteroids. Three groups of subjects were tested using ACTH stimulation, insulin tolerance test (ITT) and single dose metyrapone: I, subjects with inflammatory or allergic disorders (n=12); II, subjects on replacement therapy with prednisone after suprasellar or sellar tumor resection, and otherwise normal residual pituitary function (n=6); III, normal control subjects on no prednisone therapy (n=8).

Group	Basal Cortisol (F) ug/dl ± SEM	Basal DHEA-S ug/ml ± SEM	post ACTH peak F ug/dl ± SEM	post ITT peak F ug/dl ± SEM	post metyrapone Compound S ug/dl ± SEM
I	6.5 ± 0.9	1.5 ± 0.2	19.0 ± 1.8	19.7 ± 1.9	7.8 ± 1.1
II	8.8 ± 1.5	1.6 ± 0.2	27.2 ± 4.1	23.2 ± 3.7	5.5 ± 1.2
III	10.4 ± 1.6	3.7 ± 0.4	31.8 ± 1.3	27.7 ± 1.8	12.6 ± 1.7

The mean basal F level and the peak F (post-ACTH and post-ITT) was lower ($p <0.001$ and $p <0.005$) in Group I than in Group III. Group II F values were not significantly different from Group III. Post metyrapone Cpd-S levels were significantly lower in prednisone treated subjects (I and II) than in Group III ($p <0.05$ and $p <0.005$). In summary after reduction of pharmacologic doses of steroids to replacement doses of prednisone significant suppression of the HPA axis persists. The metyrapone test detects more subtle degrees of HPA axis suppression than ACTH and ITT and is the test of choice. Suppressed DHEA-S levels don't rule out a normal HPA axis.

845 PROLACTIN AND ADRENAL ANDROGENS. K. Higuchi*, H. Nawata, T. Maki, M. Higashijima, K. Kato, and H. Ibayashi, Third Department of Internal Medicine, Faculty of Medicine, Kyushu University, Fukuoka 812, Japan.

The role of prolactin in the secretion of androgens by the adrenal was investigated in vivo and in vitro. In women with hyperprolactinemia without dysfunction of pituitary-adrenal axis, significant correlation between serum prolactin and dehydroepiandrosterone sulfate (DHEA-S)($r=0.47$, $P<0.05$, $n=35$) and between serum prolactin and dehydroepiandrosterone (DHEA)($r=0.50$, $P<0.05$, $n=35$) were found. But no significant correlation between serum prolactin and androstenedione was observed. Long term administration of sulpiride to normal women caused increase in both serum prolactin and DHEA-S, while acute elevation of serum prolactin by bolus injection (i.v.) of domperidone did not cause increase in serum DHEA-S levels.

A technique of monolayer culture of human adrenal cells was used in order to study the direct effect of prolactin on adrenal androgen secretion.

The daily secretion rates of DHEA-S, DHEA, androstenedione and cortisol were determined. In the absence of ACTH, prolactin alone had no effect on the steroid secretion for 7 day-culture period. ACTH caused increase in daily steroid secretion. Prolactin, when administered in combination with ACTH, potentiated the effect of ACTH on DHEA-S and DHEA but not on androstenedione and cortisol secretion on seventh day in culture.

DHEA-S secretion significantly increased as a function of prolactin concentration in the presence of ACTH. These results indicate that prolactin has direct effect on adrenal androgens secretion from adrenal cells in the presence of ACTH. The site of action of prolactin was suggested to be the partial inhibition of adrenal 3β-hydroxysteroid dehydrogenase.

846 FUNCTIONS OF THE ADRENAL CORTEX IN AN INTACT GLAND PERFUSION SYSTEM
J.P. Hinson*, G.P. Vinson, B.J. Whitehouse+ and G.M. Price+, Department of Biochemistry, St Bartholomew's Hospital Medical College, Charterhouse Square, LONDON EC1M 6BQ; +Department of Physiology, Queen Elizabeth College Campden Hill Road, LONDON W8 7AH

Adrenocortical function was studied in the rat using an in situ perfused preparation which allows the study of steroid production by the intact gland under precisely controlled experimental conditions. Modified medium 199 at 37°C was used as perfusion medium (3.6mM K^+), supplied at constant pump speed, and the steroid content of ten-minute samples was determined by RIA and glc. Results are presented as stimulation ratios (S.R.) (experimental/control values). The system was used to study aldosterone (aldo) secretion. Aldo production was stimulated by several effectors; 5.4mM K^+ (S.R. 2.7 ± 0.3, n=8) serotonin 10^{-5}M (S.R. 2.48 ± 0.33 n=5); $ACTH_{1-24}$, 10^{-9}M (S.R. 3.51 ± 0.6, n=6), all given as constant infusions. A bolus injection of 1pg of angiotensin II amide (AII) stimulated aldo (eg. S.R. 2.1) as does a bolus of 100ng αMSH (eg. S.R. 2.69) in normal rats, although in sodium restricted rats aldo stimulation was seen with as little as 1ng αMSH (eg. S.R. 1.57). Cyclic AMP (bolus of 35μg) also stimulates aldo (S.R. 1.8). Specific glomerulosa effectors (eg. AII and K^+) had only an inconsistent effect on corticosterone release: αMSH stimulated corticosterone only at high concentrations. In the perfusion system corticosterone is a more specific marker of fasciculata function, and aldosterone of the glomerulosa than in cell suspensions and the system offers a more physiological means of studying adrenocortical function.

847 LONG-TERM OVARIECTOMY DOES NOT MODIFY THE AGE-ASSOCIATED REDUCTION IN HYPOTHALAMO-HYPOPHYSEAL β-ENDORPHIN CONCENTRATIONS IN THE FEMALE RAT. S.M. Gabriel*, J.W. Simpkins and W.J. Millard. University of Florida, Gainesville, FL and Harvard Medical School, Boston, MA.

Persistent hyperprolactinemia as well as reproductive senescence in the female rat are associated with a decline in levels of β-endorphin in the medial basal hypothalamus (MBH). Since the hyperprolactinemia of senescence is ovarian dependent, we investigated the possibility that ovariectomy at the time of sexual maturation could prevent the age-related decline in MBH β-endorphin activity. Young (2-3 months old) rats were ovariectomized and, like intact controls, were allowed to age to 15-16 months. The young controls for these old constant estrous (CE) and ovariectomized rats were 2-3 month old rats on the day of estrus or 2 weeks after ovariectomy, respectively. Also, a group of 15-16 month old rats were ovariectomized and killed 2 weeks later. As expected, serum PRL levels increased 2-fold with age and this increase was prevented by ovariectomy at 2-3 months of age or was reduced acutely after ovariectomy. In old CE rats, β-endorphin concentrations were reduced by 48% in the MBH, 46% in the anterior pituitary, 24% in the neurointermediate lobe of the pituitary and 42% in the serum. Except for the serum, long-term ovariectomy was ineffective in modifying β-endorphin concentrations. Similarly, acute ovariectomy in old CE rats was ineffective in modifying β-endorphin concentration in any of the tissues examined. Collectively, these data suggest that the persistent alteration in the secretion of ovarian steroids or PRL, associated with constant vaginal estrus, is not responsible for the age-related decline in β-endorphin concentrations. (Supported in part by AG02021 to JWS).

848 **AGE-RELATED DECREASE IN THE RENAL RESPONSE TO VASOPRESSIN.** C. Goddard* & I. Davies, University of Manchester, Geigy Unit for Research in Aging, Withington Hospital, Nell Lane, MANCHESTER, UK

Elderly patients often manifest disorders of fluid and electrolyte balance, possibly predisposed by an age-related decrease in urine concentrating ability. This is possibly due to a decreased plasma vasopressin (AVP), but may also be due to a reduced renal response to AVP. Plasma AVP was measured in 9 dehydrated elderly patients, 11 healthy young and 12 healthy elderly control subjects. The response of isolated renal medullary cells to AVP in terms of cAMP output in aging C57BL/Icrfa^t mice was taken as an index of renal response. Plasma AVP in the elderly control subjects was higher than the young controls (range 3.7-6.9 pmol/l vs 2.4-5.1 pmol/l; Kruskal-Wallis rank sums z = 3.29, p = <0.001), despite similar plasma osmolalities (corrected for the osmotic contribution of urea). The elderly patients' AVP (range 6.9-30.0 pmol/l) was higher than the elderly controls (z = 4.16; p = < 0.001). Renal cell cAMP responses to increased concentrations of AVP was studied in animals of 6,12,18,24,29 and 35 months of age. Basal cAMP output was similar but the threshold dose of AVP increased from 10^{-11}M (6,12,18 months) to 10^{-10}M (24,29,35 months). The dose response curve in 35 month old mice was to the right of those for the other age groups with the ED_{50} increased from $9.4 \pm 0.37 \times 10^{-11}$M (6 months) to $3.1 \pm 1.6 \times 10^{-10}$M (35 months). Maximum cAMP output at 10^{-9} AVP was also reduced in the same animals (stimulated: basal ratio, 51.22 ± 19.12 at 6 months; 11.50 ± 6.02 at 35 months). The results suggest that the dehydration which often accompanies accute illness in the elderly is not primarily a consequence of inadequate plasma AVP and that a lack of renal response to AVP could play a role with increasing age.

849 COPULATORY ACTIVITY OF OLD MALE RATS WITH TESTOSTERONE REPLACEMENT.
H.K. Hsü and M.T. Peng*, Departments of Physiology, Kaohsiung Medical College and National Taiwan University, Kaohsiung 800 and Taipei 100, China.

Various parameters of male sexual behavior were examined in intact and castrated testosterone(T)-treated male rats of various ages ranged from 3 to 27 months of age. Serum T levels were controlled by subcutaneous implantation of different sizes of T-filled silastic capsules, thereby avoiding effects of alterations in serum T in advancing age on copulatory behavior and focusing on possible changes in central sexual behavior control mechanisms of aged animals. In intact male rats, copulatory activity declined gradually from 18 months of age and no ejaculation was observed in all rats over 22 months of age. When serum T levels were maintained 1.1-1.5 ng/ml, rats showed good copulatory activity up to 21 months of age. Elevation of serum T levels to 2.6-2.9ng/ml did not improve the activity in 3- to 4-month old rats but improved mounting and intromission in 24- to 26- month old rats. When serum T levels were maintained 0.7 ng/ml for 6 months from 4 months of age, rats showed as good copulatory activity as intact rats. Even serum T levels were maintained 3.0 ng/ml for 6 months from 18 months of age, copulatory activity still declined gradually. These results indicate that the copulatory activity of male rats in response to T declines in advancing age and this phenomenon is not due to long term decrease of serum androgen level in old age.

850 PREVENTION OR DELAY IN ONSET OF LUPUS ERYTHEMATOSUS (LE) IN NZB/NZW F_1 MICE BY DEHYDROISOANDROSTERONE.
John Lucas*, Paul C. MacDonald, and M. Linette Casey, Cecil H. and Ida Green Ctr. for Reprod. Biol. Sci., Univ. of Texas Southwestern Med. Sch., Dallas, TX

Other investigators find that the C_{19}-steroid, dehydroisoandrosterone (DHA), acts to prevent spontaneous and carcinogen-induced neoplasias in mice, the spontaneous occurrence of autoimmune hemolytic anemia in mice, the spontaneous occurrence of diabetes mellitus in rats, and to prevent obesity despite normal food consumption in genetically obese rats. For this reason and because essential fatty acid-free diets prevents the morphological changes of LE in NZB/NZW f_1 mice, we investigated the possibility that (1) DHA is esterified with free fatty acids; and, (2) that DHA may act to prevent the development of the pathological manifestations of LE. We found that DHA in kidney tissue of lupus mice is esterified with fatty acids. We then evaluated the effect of parenterally administered DHA or orally administered DHA in attenuating the pathological manifestations and the mortality rate due to lupus. In the animals treated with DHA by injection, the mortality rate at 12 months was 60% whereas in the control group it was 100% (n = 10 each group). In the animals given DHA orally, the mortality rate at 9 months was 0% (n = 25) compared with 50% (n = 24) in controls. Importantly, the rate of weight gain in both groups was the same. We conclude that DHA acts to prevent the development of LE in the mice and prolongs life by a mechanism independent of failure of weight gain. We cannot, at this time, exclude the possibility that DHA acts by way of conversion to a potent androgens, which are known to attenuate the severity and early onset of LE in these mice.

851 CONCENTRATIONS OF IMMUNOREACTIVE TONIN IN RAT SUBMANDIBULAR GLAND AND SALIVA AND ITS SECRETORY MECHANISM. Y. Hirata*, M. Tomita and M. Ikeda, Hypertension-Endocrine Div., National Cardiovascular Center Research Institute, Osaka 565, Japan.

Tonin, an enzyme of the serine protease family, isolated from rat submandibular gland (SMG), cleaves renin substrate and angiotensin (A) I to form AII directly. However, its physiological functions remain obscure. We have developed specific RIA for rat tonin to examine the concentrations of tonin in SMG and saliva of male and female rats and to study the mechanism by which tonin is secreted from the dispersed cells of male rat SMG in vitro. SMG and saliva of normal adult males contained far more (x11 and x5, respectively) concentrations of tonin than those of normal adult females. Its SMG contents of castrated males fell to those of normal females, while its contents of testosterone-treated females reached those of normal males. Its SMG content of immature males was very low, but increased dramatically after 6 weeks of age. Norepinephrine, epinephrine and phenylephrine significantly stimulated secretion of tonin from dispersed SMG cells in a dose-dependent manner (1 - 100 μM), whereas isoproterenol did not; the stimulatory effect was abolished by phentolamine, but not by propranolol. Carbamycholine, histamine, serotonin, dibutylyl cyclic AMP, methyisobutylxanthine, and AII had no effect on its release. These data indicate the sexual dimorphism of the rat SMG with respect to tonin concentrations; its synthesis is under androgenic control and increases with age. Tonin is secreted into saliva of which concentrations reflect SMG content. Secretion of tonin is predominantly stimulated by α-adrenergic agents. (We thank Dr. J. Genest for his kind supply of rat tonin.)

852 REGULATION OF ANGIOTENSIN II RECEPTORS AND STEROIDOGENESIS BY POTASSIUM IN RAT ADRENAL GLOMERULOSA CELLS. T. Hirota*, K. Fujita, K.J. Catt and G. Aguilera, ERRB, NICHD, NIH, Bethesda, MD 20205, U.S.A.

Potassium (K) has important regulatory actions in the adrenal glomerulosa cell, including direct stimulation of aldosterone (aldo) secretion, potentiation of the actions of angiotensin II (AII), and up-regulation of AII receptors. To further investigate the interaction between K and AII, we analyzed steroid production and AII receptors in rat adrenal glomerulosa cells cultured with selected concentrations of K. After 2 to 18 hr culture with 7.5 or 10 mM K, AII receptor concentration was increased by 20 to 50% compared with control cells cultured with 4.5 mM K, without change in receptor affinity. Despite the increase in AII receptors, maximum AII-stimulated aldo production was decreased by 40 and 80% after culture with 10 mM K for 2 and 4 hr, respectively. Comparable decreases in K-, ACTH- and 8-Br-cAMP-stimulated aldo production were observed, indicating that the site of inhibition is at a post-receptor level. Measurement of pregnenolone formation in the presence of cyanoketone revealed that AII-, ACTH-, K- and 8-Br-cAMP-stimulated pregnenolone production were also decreased by 40% after preincubation of the cells with K. Comparable inhibition of steroidogensis was observed following preincubation of the cells with 10 nM AII or 100 nM ACTH. These results demonstrate that steroid production by the adrenal glomerulosa cell can be desensitized after in vitro stimulation, by inhibition at a step prior to pregnenolone formation. It is also evident that K can up-regulate adrenal AII receptors in vitro, without relation to its actions upon steroidogenesis.

853 THE EFFECT OF LONG-TERM SPIRONOLACTONE TREATMENT ON SODIUM PUMP ABNORMALITIES OF RED BLOOD CELLS /RBC/ IN BARTTER'S SYNDROME:

K. Horký* and V. Schreiber, Lab. Endocr. and Metab. Charles University Fac. of Medicine, Prague, Czechoslovakia.

To elucidate the possible sodium transport alteration across the cell membranes in Bartter's syndrome and its influecing by spironolactone treatment, Na^{+}-K^{+}-ATPase activity was studied by means of radioactive 86-Rb influx into the RBC of 9 pts. with Bartter's syndrome prior to and after a 4 weeks spironolactone treatment /200-300 mg/day/. As compared with 9 controls the untreated pts. with Bartter's syndrome had a more than 5 times higher ouabain-sensitive 86-Rb uptake by the RBC. The spironolactone treatment led to the decrease of this high influx almost to the control values. Serum of pts. with Bartter's syndrome incubated with healthy RBC distinctly increased their 86-Rb influx. None of the studied known humoral factors as aldosterone, renin, prostaglandin, or changes of the serum potassium were responsible for these abnormalities. Even though it is not possible to explain the accurate mechanism of the high 86-Rb uptake by pts. RBC on the basis of our results, the participation of an endogenous humoral anti-digoxin-like activity could not be excluded. The changes of sodium transport in the RBC of pts. with Bartter's syndrome could be a part of a much more generalized disturbance in the transport mechanisms and so participate in the pathogenesis of this disease.

854 ROLE OF CALCIUM IN EFFECTS OF Na INTAKE ON ALDOSTERONE RESPONSE TO ANGIOTENSIN II.

T. Howland, G.H. Anderson, Jr., D.H.P. Streeten, SUNY-Upstate Medical Center, Syracuse, NY 13210, USA.

We have reported that the increased plasma aldosterone (Aldo) responsiveness to angiotensin II (AII) on a low-sodium (Na) diet is blocked by nifedipine (Clin. Res. 31:328A, 1983). Further studies of this phenomenon are reported here. Like nifedipine, diltiazem, 60 mg po, reduced the low-Na-induced increase in responsiveness to AII in 9 normal subjects. The slope of the regression of AII infusion rate (3, 6, and 9 ng/kg/min, each for 20 minutes) vs plasma Aldo concentration was less ($p < .05$) on a 10 mEq than on a 200 mEq Na diet. The similar effects of the 2 drugs suggest that Ca movements mediate the increased Aldo response to AII on a low-Na diet. AII was then infused in 5 normal subjects, prior to, and during the third hour of, Ca gluconate infusion (7 mg/kg/h) on 200 and 10 mEq Na diets:

CHANGES IN PLASMA ALDOSTERONE, ng/dl (mean $\pm$ SE)

	before calcium			after calcium		
AII (ng/kg/min)	3	6	9	3	6	9
high Na	3.7$\pm$1.5	8.5$\pm$1.9	13.0$\pm$2.0	7.2$\pm$2.4	14.4$\pm$3.6	15.9$\pm$2.4
low Na	3.8$\pm$1.2	11.7$\pm$2.1	19.1$\pm$3.0	11.9$\pm$2.1	19.0$\pm$3.1	29.3$\pm$3.5

The slope of AII infusion rate vs plasma Aldo after calcium infusion on the low-Na diet (3.2$\pm$.4) was significantly greater ($p < .05$) than the slope before Ca infusion (2.2$\pm$.6). There was no significant difference on the high-Na diet. Conclusion: The increased Aldo responsiveness to AII on a low-Na diet is inhibited by nifedipine and diltiazem, and enhanced by raising the serum Ca concentration. This further supports the concept that Aldo sensitivity to AII on a low-Na diet is mediated by Ca movements.

855 SIGNIFICANT DIFFERENCES IN RENIN(R) AND ANGIOTENSINOGEN(AGN) LEVELS IN DISCRETE BRAIN REGIONS OF SPONTANEOUSLY HYPERTENSIVE (SHR) AND NORMOTENSIVE (WKY) RATS.

T. Inagami*, M. Naruse, K. Naruse, J.D. McKenzie and K. Shizume. Vanderbilt University School of Medicine, Nashville, TN 37232, USA and Tokyo Women's Medical College, Tokyo 162, Japan

Although a possible role for the brain R-angiotensin (A) system in the etiology of hypertension in SHR was suggested, the quantatative evaluation of R in the brain has not been reported. We investigated regional distribution of R and AGN in the brain of SHR and WKY. Approximately 150, 10-week-old male rats of both strains were killed 24hrs after nephrectomy. The brain were frozen on dry-ice and cryosectioned serially (300um). Micropunches of the following areas were made: septal nucleus (SN), medial preoptic nucleus (MPN), anterior hypothalamic nucleus (AHN), amygdaloid nuclei (AN), caudate-putamen (CP), globus pallidus (GP), periaqueductal central gray (PCG), paraventricular and periventricular nuclei (PAV, PIV), hippocampus (HP), cerebellar cortex (CC), and frontal cortex (FC). R activity in the extracts was determined by RIA of AI generated at pH 7.0 with nephrectomized rat plasma. The difference before and after preincubation with anti-renin antibody was defined as specific R activity. AGN concentration was determined by incubating the extract with excess rat R. Specific R activity was significantly lower in SHR vs WKY in HP, CP, GP, HA, SFO, PCG, and FC and significantly higher in anterior and posterior pituitaries. AGN was significantly elevated in SN, MPN, PAV, AN, HP, CP, GP, CC, and FC of SHR compared to WKY. These results suggest alterations in the R-A system of the brain play an important role in the pathogenesis of hypertension in SHR. Supported by NIH grants HL-24112 and HL-14192.

856 αMSH STIMULATED ALDOSTERONE SECRETION, MECHANISM OF ACTION

D. Kem* and R. Schiebinger, Endocrinology, Hypertension and Metabolism Section, University of Oklahoma, Oklahoma City, OK, USA 73190

αMSH shares the first 13 amino acids of ACTH and stimulates aldosterone (A) secretion. This may be mediated through the ACTH receptor and adenylate cyclase activation. However, αMSH 10^{-6}M does not stimulate corticosterone secretion from rat fasciculata cells. Additionally, the A response to αMSH differs markedly from that to ACTH. The 50% maximal stimulatory concentration of αMSH is $5x10^{-8}$M, for ACTH is $5x10^{-11}$M, and the maximal A production by αMSH is 30% of ACTH. We have used dispersed rat adrenal glomerulosa cells to examine the hypothesis that αMSH activates adenylate cyclase by binding to the ACTH receptor. Nifedipine markedly inhibits angiotensin II and potassium (calcium-dependent) stimulation but not cAMP-stimulated A secretion. Nifedipine 10^{-4}M inhibits αMSH and ACTH stimulated A secretion by only 10% and 30% respectively suggesting a cAMP-dependent mechanism. Cyclic-AMP measurements were made at the maximal stimulatory concentration of αMSH 10^{-6}M. These were compared to ACTH 10^{-10}M stimulation which gives a similar A response. There was no increase above basal for both αMSH and ACTH. Corticotropin inhibitory peptide (CIP) at 10^{-6}M inhibited ACTH ($5x10^{-10}$M) stimulated aldosterone secretion by 67%. αMSH 10^{-7}M stimulated aldosterone secretion was not inhibited by CIP 10^{-6}M but higher concentrations of CIP were not feasible. A dose response curve of αMSH 10^{-9} to 10^{-6}M was not shifted to the right by CIP $1.4x10^{-6}$M suggesting that αMSH may not stimulate A via the ACTH receptor. We conclude: 1) αMSH stimulation is not mediated by a calcium-dependent mechanism, 2) These data are compatable with adenylate cyclase activation but we cannot exclude a unique non calcium channel dependent pathway, and 3) αMSH stimulation may not occur via the classical ACTH receptor.

857 EFFECTS OF RAT ATRIAL NATRIURETIC FACTOR (rANF) ON OXYGEN CONSUMPTION IN RAT KIDNEY MITOCHONDRIA. N. Kohashi,* N. Trippodo, A. MacPhee, E. Frohlich, and F. Cole. Alton Ochsner Medical Foundation, New Orleans, LA 70121.

Since active cation transport is partially dependent upon oxidative phosphorylation in the kidney, we studied the effect of rANF on oxygen consumption (OC) in isolated kidney mitochondria. Purified rANF was prepared from acetic acid extracts gel filtered into low (LMW) (3-10K dalton) and high (HMW) (10-30K dalton) molecular weight fractions. OC was measured in the presence of 7 mM succinate, 250μM ADP, and ~4 units (U) of LMW or HMW. The respiratory control index (RC) and ADP/O ratio were used as indices of mitochondrial integrity. Four U caused maximum natriuresis in bioassay rats. The difference in rate of OC due to the addition of saturating ADP in the presence of saturating succinate was 610.9$\pm$82.2 ($\bar{x}\pm$S.D.) nl O_2/mg protein/min in the control. This rate decreased to 371.5$\pm$41.5 in the presence of LMW ($p<0.05$), and to 521.4$\pm$131.3 in the presence of HMW ($p<0.05$). RC was 3.8$\pm$0.5 in the control, decreased to 2.4$\pm$0.2 in the presence of LMW ($p<0.05$) and unchanged (3.5$\pm$0.7) in the presence of HMW. ADP/O was 2.6$\pm$0.4 in the control, increased (4.1$\pm$0.5) when exposed to LMW ($p<0.05$) and unchanged (2.9$\pm$0.6) when exposed to HMW. RC and ADP/O were unchanged in the presence of trypsin-treated (natriuretically inactive) LMW and an equal amount of similarly prepared ventricular protein extract. Furosemide (FU) completely blocked OC after ADP addition. Angiotensin II (AII) and vasopressin (VP) inhibited RC (3.4$\pm$0.5, $p<0.05$, 3.1$\pm$0.4, $p<0.05$, respectively) and increased ADP/O (3.4$\pm$0.4, $p<0.001$, 3.6$\pm$0.9, $p<0.01$, respectively). These data demonstrate that LMW has a direct subcellular effect on OC in the kidney similar to that of AII and VP, that rANF and FU, though both natriuretic, affect mitochondrial OC differently in rat kidney, and that LMW is more potent than HMW in its effect on mitochondrial OC. Supported in part by NIH HL-29952.

858 CHLORIDE AND RENIN DEPENDENT HYPERTENSION. T. A. KOTCHEN*, C. E. OTT, J.H. DOWNS, B. J. HOLTZCLAW, Depts. of Medicine and Physiology, University of Kentucky, Lexington, Kentucky.

We have previously shown that renin release is inhibited by selective chloride (without sodium) loading in the intact Sprague-Dawley rat on a low NaCl diet. This study was undertaken to determine if selective Cl^- loading would lower PRA and hence blood pressure in a model of renin dependent hypertension: 1-kidney, 1-clip hypertension in Sprague-Dawley rats on a low NaCl diet. In the experimental (Exp) group (n=16), selective Cl^- loading was achieved by adding 1.5% glycine chloride to the chow at the time of clipping. Pair-fed control (Con) animals (n=16) were treated identically except no glycine chloride was added. During the five weeks after clipping, blood pressure increased ($p<0.001$) comparably in Con (115 mmHg $\pm$ 2 SE to 166 $\pm$ 9) and Exp (115 $\pm$ 1 to 160 $\pm$ 10) animals; weight gain was also comparable. Net five week Cl^- balance of Exp (17.3 mEq $\pm$ 1.2) was greater ($p<0.001$) than Con (-6.7 $\pm$ 0.4). In intact animals (2-kidneys, no-clip) of similar age and weight, on a low sodium chloride diet, blood pressure (125 $\pm$ 2) was lower ($p<0.001$) than Con or Exp animals. Elevated arterial pressure of both Con and Exp animals was responsive to captopril. At sacrifice, PRA of Con (7.2 ng/ml/hr $\pm$ 1.4) and Exp (9.4 $\pm$ 1.3) animals did not differ. Renal renin content also did not differ (1231 U/g $\pm$ 126 vs 999 $\pm$ 165). Selective Cl^- loading also did not lower blood pressure in animals with 2-kidney, 1-clip hypertension. Thus, in contrast to the normal kidney, selective Cl^- loading did not inhibit renin release from the ischemic kidney and did not lower arterial pressure in these renin dependent models of hypertension.

859 PARADOXICAL EFFECT OF LUTEINIZING HORMONE-RELEASING HORMONE(LHRH) ON SEXUAL BEHAVIOR. C. Dudley* and R. Moss, Dept. Physiol., UTHSCD, Dallas, TX 75235

LHRH potentiation of sexual behavior in the estradiol-benzoate (EB) primed female rat is paradoxical in that it facilitates receptivity but also produces resistive behaviors which are not normally observed in EB-progesterone(P) primed animals. To investigate the motivational state of EB-LHRH treated animals, sexual preference tests were conducted in a choice box apparatus where time spent in close proximity to four stimulus animals was measured. The stimulus animals were a proestrus female (PF), an ovariectomized female(OF), a sexually active male(SM), and a castrated male(CM). Experimental females were ovariectomized, tested with and without EB-P priming, and subsequently implanted with third ventricular cannula, primed with EB and tested following infusion of LHRH or saline. Sexual receptivity was expressed in terms of the lordosis to mount ratio(L/M). Without hormone therapy, females avoided proximity to SM and exhibited a preference for PF and CM. EB-P treatment (L/M=1.00) drastically elevated preference for SM over all other choices. Infusion of either LHRH (L/M=.97) or saline (L/M=.31) in EB primed animals resulted, in both cases, in a preference for SM. This preference was higher than that obtained with no hormone therapy but significantly lower than that produced by EB-P priming. In fact, preference for SM was slightly higher in saline infused animals than in LHRH infused animals indicating that the elevation in preference for SM was due to EB priming alone. Thus, LHRH, unlike P, elevates receptivity without creating a condition in which preference for SM is heightened over that produced by EB alone. The increase in resistive behaviors noted in LHRH animals may reflect a deficiency in "sexual motivation." NIH #HD11814.

860 5α-DIHYDROTESTOSTERONE (DHT) INHIBITS LORDOSIS BEHAVIOR INDUCED BY PULSED INJECTIONS OF ESTRADIOL (E_2) PLUS PROGESTERONE (P) IN OVARIECTOMIZED RATS. M.S. Erskine* and M.J. Baum, Dept. Nutrition & Food Sci., Massachusetts Institute of Technology, Cambridge, MA 02139 U.S.A.

The present studies examined the possibility that DHT inhibits E_2-induced lordosis by interfering with the priming action of E_2. DHT (2.5 mg in 5% ethanol:propylene glycol) or vehicle was administered to separate groups of rats at various times before and after pulsed injections of E_2 (1 μg/injection in 10% ethanol at 0 and 6 h); P (0.5 mg in oil) was administered to all rats at 20 h and testing for behavioral receptivity occurred at 24 h. As previously reported, the two E_2 injections plus P were effective in inducing moderate levels of receptivity (mean Lordosis Quotient = 45). Females given DHT at -12h, -3h, +3h, and at both -3 and +3h all showed significantly suppressed lordosis behavior below control levels. Additional groups were given E_2 only or E_2 followed by DHT at +8 or +20h; receptivity was also reduced in animals given DHT at these times. Mean serum levels of DHT measured by RIA were 24.9 ng/ml 30 min after an injection of 2.5 mg DHT and declined gradually to 0.6 ng/ml by 12 h. In a final experiment all three doses of DHT (0.5, 1.0, and 2.5 mg) administered at -3h significantly suppressed lordosis responsiveness. These data demonstrate that DHT, when given as early as 12 h before and as late as 20 h after the first injection of E_2, inhibits the expression of estrous behavior, and suggest that DHT's action on lordosis is independent of and overrides that of E_2.

Supported by HD16746 awarded to M.S.E.

861 ORAL VERSUS INTRAVENOUS APD (3-AMINO-1-HYDROXYPROPYLIDENE-1-BISPHOSPHONATE) FOR THE TREATMENT OF PAGET'S DISEASE OF BONE. H.K. Ibbertson*, T.R.C. Fraser, I.M. Holdaway, M. Rutland, A. King, G. Dodd, D. Wattie, Section of Endocrinology, Department of Medicine, School of Medicine, Auckland, N.Z.

50 patients with moderate to severe Paget's disease of bone have been treated with oral (n=34) or intravenous (IV) (n=16) APD and followed for at least 6 months. The oral dose was 5, 7.5 or 10 mg/kg/day for 6 months and the IV dose was 0.25 mg/kg/day in a 2 hour infusion on 5 or 10 successive days. In both treatment groups there was an early and rapid reduction in log mean urine calcium (uCa) and log mean urine hydroxyproline (uHP) and a later fall in serum alkaline phosphatase. The responses were more rapid following IV APD; the mean nadir for uCa and uHP being 2 weeks compared with 6 weeks for the oral group. The uHP fell to within 10% of normal in 18/34 and 3/16 patients in the oral and IV groups respectively and remained suppressed for at least 6 months after therapy was stopped. In contrast the initial reduction in uCa was not sustained and rose to normal or near normal within this period. This change occurred in some patients despite persisting elevation of serum parathyroid hormone and 1-25$(OH)_2D_3$ levels. In both groups there was a significant reduction in osteoclast numbers ($p=<0.01$) without an increase in osteoid indices. Bone scintigraphy showed a mean 50% reduction in counts following treatment and healing of osteolytic bone lesions was demonstrated in matched x-rays. Intravenous therapy is unattended by side-effects and it is anticipated that biochemical remission will be secured in most patients with moderate or severe Paget's disease by further adjustment of APD dosage.

862 ACTH AND CORTICOSTERONE RESPONSES TO SYNTHETIC CORTICOTROPIN RELEASING FACTOR AND ARGININE VASOPRESSIN IN SPONTANEOUSLY HYPERTENSIVE AND NORMOTENSIVE RATS. T. Hattori*, K. Hashimoto, K. Murakami, K. Fujino and Z. Ota, Third Department of Internal Medicine, Okayama University Medical School, Okayama 700, Japan

It has been reported that spontaneously hypertensive rats (SHR) show hyperresponsiveness to stress. We examined the responsiveness of ACTH and corticosterone (compd. B) to corticotropin releasing factor (CRF) and arginine vasopressin (AVP) in SHR and normotensive Wister Kyoto rats (WKY). Untreated SHR and WKY were decapitated at 6 and 11 weeks of age, and basal ACTH and compd. B levels were measured. Experimental animals were treated with chlorpromazine (CPZ, 1 mg/100g sc) at 0 time, morphine HCl (M, 1 mg /100g sc) at 3 hr and nembutal (N, 2.5 mg/100g ip) at 3 hr and 15 min to eliminate endogenous CRF secretion. Blood samples were collected from the jugular vein at 4 hr, and then synthetic ovine CRF or AVP was adminstered intravenously. Blood samples were collected at 4 hr 20 min. Serum ACTH level did not differ between the two untreated strains, but serum compd. B levels were higher in SHR. In CPZ-M-N treated WKY, an ACTH and compd. B response was absent to 0.05 ug - 0.15 ug/100g AVP but there was a small response to 0.25 ug/100g AVP. ACTH and compd. B showed greater responses to CRF. But in CPZ-M-N treated SHR, the basal ACTH level was reduced and ACTH and compd. B responses to CRF were weaker than those in WKY. However, AVP at 0.05 ug - 0.25 ug/100g induced dose related ACTH and compd. B responses, and the responses were much greater than those in WKY. These results suggest that a hypersensitivity to AVP exists in the SHR anterior pituitary. The reduced ACTH basal level and the response to CRF in CPZ-M-N treated SHR might be ascribed to the feedback effect of elevated compd. B.

863 HISTIDYL-PROLINE DIKETOPIPERAZINE, CYCLO(HIS-PRO): A POSSIBLE ANTIDIPSOGENIC FACTOR IN THE RAT BRAIN.
H. Ishihara*, M. Mori, M. Murakami, I. Kobayashi and S. Kobayashi. Division of Endocrinology, First Department of Medicine, Isesaki Hospital, Gunma University, School of Medicine, Maebashi 371, Japan

An influence of cyclo(His-Pro), a biologically active metabolite of TRH, on water intake was examined in the conscious rats. Adult male rats were exposed to water deprivation, but fed freely, for 48 h, and varying doses of TRH or cyclo(His-Pro) were administered to the animals through the cannulae implanted into the lateral ventricle. Although injection of 0.03 n mol TRH caused no change in water intake, TRH in the doses of 3 and 30 n mol suppressed the ingestion of water. Intracranial injection of 0.3 n mol cyclo(His-Pro) led to a significant inhibition of water intake (cyclo(His-Pro), 7.2 $\pm$ 1.8 ml/30 min and 11.6 $\pm$ 1.7 ml/60 min vs saline, 15.8 $\pm$ 1.3 ml/30 min and 17.4 $\pm$ 1.4 ml/60 min, $p<0.01$). This inhibition was observed in the dose-dependent manner of cyclo(His-Pro) (0.3-30 n mol). Rat brains possessed a specific receptor for TRH, but cyclo(His-Pro) did not significantly interfere with its binding. In conjunction with evidence that cyclo(His-Pro) is present throughout the rat brain (Brain Res 231: 451, 1982), the present study implies that cyclo(His-Pro) may be involved in acting as an intrinsic factor of antidipsogen, which is not mediated through TRH receptor, in the rat brains.

864 CHARACTERIZATION AND INSULIN STIMULATION OF GLUCOSE TRANSPORT IN THE OSTEOBLAST.
TJ Hahn* and LR Halstead, Wadsworth VA Medical Center, UCLA School of Medicine, Los Angeles, California.

To investigate the mechanisms of hormonal control of glucose metabolism in the osteoblast, we examined *in vitro* regulation of hexose uptake in a purified osteoblast preparation. 5 mm diameter punch sections were obtained from the cartilage-free frontal portions of the calvaria of 3-day old rats, and the periosteum was removed. The resulting sections contained greater than 95% osteoblast-like cells based on histologic criteria and elimination of calcitonin-stimulatable cAMP generation. Sections were incubated for 24 hours at 37 in BGJb medium and then transferred to modified glucose-free Krebs-Ringer bicarbonate buffer. Active uptake of the non-metabolizable glucose analogue ^{3}H-2-deoxy-D-glucose (^{3}H-DG) was examined at 25 . Uptake of ^{3}H-DG (0.1 mM) was linear with time over 60 min., temperature-sensitive, and stereospecific. ^{3}H-DG transport demonstrated a saturable mechanism with a Km (2.2 mM) similar to that observed in other tissues. ^{3}H-DG uptake was rapidly stimulated by both concanavalin A (10-50 uM) and insulin (0.5 nM-1uM), with maximal insulin effect observed at 50 nM. Insulin stimulation of ^{3}H-DG transport was associated with an increase in transport Vmax with Km remaining constant. Both basal and insulin-stimulated ^{3}H-DG uptake were reversibly inhibited by cytochalasin B (50uM). These studies provide the first demonstration that the osteoblast possesses an insulin-stimulated hexose transport system with characteristics similar to those found in other insulin-sensitive tissues.

865 RECEPTORS FOR 1α,25-DIHYDROXYCHOLECALCIFEROL IN RAT PITUITARY CELLS.

E. HAUG*, M. Kriz and K.M. Gautvik, Hormone Laboratory, Aker Hospital, Oslo, and Institute of Physiology, University of Oslo, Oslo, Norway.

Recent studies have demonstrated the importance of prolactin (PRL) and growth hormone (GH) in the regulation of 25-hydroxycholecalciferol-1α-hydroxylase activity. We have previously shown that 1α,25-dihydroxy-cholecalciferol (1α,25-$(OH)_2D_3$) reduces PRL and GH production by a clonal strain of rat pituitary tumor cells (GH_3) (Haug et al. 1982, Mol Cell Endocrinol 28:65). Cytosol fractions prepared from GH_3 cells were incubated with $|^3H|$1α,25-$(OH)_2D_3$ (0.1-6 nM) at 0^oC for 3 h prior to sucrose gradient (5-20%) centrifugation (vertical-tube rotor, 3 h, 4^oC, 250 000 x g). In high salt (300 mM KCl) gradients the GH_3 cells possessed stereospecific 1α,25-$(OH)_2D_3$ binding components with a sedimentation coefficient of 3.7S, while in salt-free gradients the 3.7S complex was transformed to a ∿6S form. Scatchard analysis of the binding data indicated one single class of high-affinity binding sites (K_d ∿0.3-0.6 nM, B_{max} ∿50-100 fmol/mg protein). Treatment of the GH_3 cells with corticosterone (10^{-6} M) and 17β-estradiol (10^{-6} M) increased 1,25-$(OH)_2D_3$ receptor concentration 1.5-2 fold without altering receptor affinity. Isoelectric focusing localized most of the binding of $|^3H|$1α,25-$(OH)_2D_3$ to a peak with an isoelectric point of 6. The 1α,25-$(OH)_2D_3$ receptor of the GH_3 cells therefore has all the properties of the vitamin D_3 receptor found in normal rat tissues.

866 THE POLYMORPHIC HUMAN CALCITONIN GENE IS LOCATED ON CHROMOSOME 11.

J.W.M. Höppener*, P.H. Steenbergh, A.H.M. Geurts van Kessel, H.S. Jansz and C.J.M. Lips, Institute of Molecular Biology, Laboratory of Physiological Chemistry and Department of Internal Medicine, University Hospital, State University, Utrecht, Department of Cell Biology and Genetics, Erasmus University, Rotterdam, The Netherlands.

Calcitonin (CT) is a 32-aminoacid polypeptide hormone (MW 3,500 daltons), secreted by the C-cells of the thyroid gland in mammals. The major function of CT in mammals is to protect the skeleton during periods of calcium stress. Recombinant-DNA-research has revealed that CT is produced by proteolytic processing of a much larger precursor protein which is formed by translation of mRNA molecules, previously transcribed from the CT gene. We have studied the chromosomal localization of the human CT gene. A recombinant plasmid, containing a nucleotide sequence complementary to human CT mRNA, was used as a molecular probe for hybridization with DNA, isolated from human-rodent somatic cell hybrids. These hybrids contain in addition to the entire rodent genome, only a specific subset of human chromosomes. The human CT gene was found only in DNA from hybrids containing the p14→qter region of human chromosome 11. Restriction enzyme digestion and Southern blot analysis of human genomic DNA indicate the possible existence of (a) CT related pseudo-gene(s). Additional analysis of human genomic DNA showed that the CT gene has a polymorphic site for restriction endonuclease Taq I. The allele frequencies (0.34 and 0.66 respectively) support that this polymorphism occurs with such frequency to be suitable for gene linkage studies. This investigation was supported by the foundation for Medical Research (FUNGO) and the Queen Wilhelmina Cancer Fund (KWF).

867 REGULATION OF TRANSCRIPTION OF THE HUMAN PARATHYROID HORMONE GENE.
T. Igarashi*, J. Hellerman, R. Gaz, J.T. Potts, Jr. and H. Kronenberg, Endocrine Genetics Unit and Department of Medicine, Massachusetts General Hospital, Boston, MA 02114, USA.

Weaver et al have shown that two closely spaced TATA sequences determine two initiation sites for the transcription of the bovine parathyroid hormone (PTH) gene. To see whether this unusual pattern is conserved in the human gene, we hybridized human parathyroid adenoma mRNA with cloned human PTH DNA and used S1 nuclease analysis to determine the mRNA's 5'-ends. We found two clusters of initiation sites, each approximately 30 base pairs away from the human gene's two TATA sequences. To analyze further the use of these two initiation sites and also to determine the functional importance of other sequences in the promoter region of the PTH gene, we have constructed a plasmid linking the PTH promoter region to the *E. coli neo* gene, encoding resistance to the antibiotic, G418. This plasmid was introduced into rat pituitary GH4 cells using an electroshock technique developed by H. Potter. GH4 cells allow us to study whether vitamin D and intracellular calcium regulate the PTH gene, since these cells contain vitamin D receptors, and since secretogogues can alter the cells' intracellular concentrations of calcium. The electroshock method was used because standard transfection methods cannot be used with GH4 cells, and attempts to use retroviral vectors led to genomic rearrangements. Colonies newly resistant to GH18 were selected. They express the *neo* gene, presumably using the PTH promoter. We are now analyzing the initiation of PTH gene transcription using these colonies.

868 EFFECT OF CALCITONIN ON PHOSPHORYLATION OF RAT LIVER CYTOSOLIC PROTEINS.
M. Inaba*, H. Morii, Y. Nishizawa, N. Hamada, J. Yamakawa, Y. Ohnishi, M. Yukioka+ and A. Inoue+, The Second Department of Internal Medicine and +Department of Biochemistry, Osaka City University Medical School, Osaka 545, Japan.

Since it had been reported that calcitonin (CT) had stimulatory effects on glucose production in hepatocyte, we investigated the effect of CT on phosphorylation of cytosolic proteins in rat liver. Cytosolic proteins were phosphorylated by endogenous protein kinase with [γ-^{32}P]ATP, followed by sodium dodecyl sulphate polyacrylamide gel electrophoretic and autoradiographic analyses. A single subcutaneous administration of CT (salmon CT; 1,000 mU/head) stimulated phosphorylation of at least 2 proteins in rat liver cytosol, with molecular weights of 67,000 and 93,000. The stimulation of 67,000-Mr protein phosphorylation was both cyclic AMP- and Ca^{++}-independent. The effect was clearly evident by 3 min, with phosphorylation decreasing to control level by 30 min. The stimulation of 93,000-Mr protein phosphorylation was Ca^{++}-dependent and it could be inhibited by 50 μM naphthalenesulfonamide (W7), indicating that Ca^{++}-calmodulin is involved in phosphorylation of the protein (phosphorylase ?). It was not until 30 min that the stimulation was evident. CT could not influence phosphorylation of 61,000-Mr protein (pyruvate kinase ?), which was a major protein phosphorylated in a cycic AMP-dependent manner. These data demonstrated that CT exerts its action in rat liver through the process of protein phosphorylation, and that the effect cannot be accounted for by a pathway dependent upon cyclic AMP.

869 THE TWO-HIT THEORY OF NEOPLASIA: IMPLICATIONS FOR THE PATHOGENESIS OF HYPERPARATHYROIDISM. C.E. Jackson* and K.A. Greenawald, Division of Clinical Genetics, Department of Medicine and the Department of Pathology, Henry Ford Hospital, Detroit, Michigan, 48202, U.S.A.

Knudson's two-hit or two-mutational-event hypothesis for the initiation of neoplasia suggests that two somatic mutations are necessary for initiation of sporadic neoplasms and that a genetic plus a somatic mutation are required for hereditary neoplasms. Glucose-6-phosphate dehydrogenase (G-6-PD) studies of parathyroid tumors of 11 heterozygotes with hyperparathyroidism (HPT), including 1 with hereditary HPT, have shown both A & B isoenzymes. These findings suggest multicellular development of parathyroid tumors and are compatible with tumors being manifestations of either non-neoplastic hyperplasia or a genetic first mutational event. Parathyroid carcinoma may be the result of a second mutation in cells made susceptible by previous genetic or somatic mutations. Comparison of the age of onset of parathyroid cancer in families with hereditary HPT with that of sporadic parathyroid cancer from the literature reveals a generally younger onset with hereditary HPT compatible with the two-hit theory. Consideration of these age of onset and G-6-PD findings suggests that hyperparathyroidism may result from either non-neoplastic or mutational-induced processes even though no histological distinctions have yet been observed between the hyperplasia associated with these two different processes. The multicellular development of the parathyroid tumors is consistent with generalized non-neoplastic effects of cellular growth factors as the likely cause of most non-hereditary tumors causing hyperparathyroidism. Supported by USPHS grant #CA22595.

870 AUTO-ANTIBODIES AGAINST MID-C/MID-REGIONAL PTH (MID-C-PTH/MID-PTH) IN AN UREMIC PATIENT. H. Jüppner*, R. Baethke[+] and R.D. Hesch, Kinderklinik and Abt. Klinische Endokrinologie, Medizinische Hochschule Hannover, 3 Hannover and Peter Friedrich Ludwigs Hospital[+], 29 Oldenburg, West-Germany

Antibody production against injected hormone preparations is well established. Auto-antibodies (auto-Ab) against endogenous peptides without prior antigenic exposure are only reported for Insulin and Glucagon. We studied a patient with terminal renal insufficiency who developed auto-Ab against endogenous PTH. MID-C-PTH was determined by selective radioimmunoassay (RIA) using 43-68(Tyr)hPTH as tracer, bound and free hormone was separated by double-antibody. Initial concentration of MID-C-PTH was 3375 (normal: 100-300 pg/ml), 2105 after initiation of dialysis, increasing to 5835 during the following 3 years. Intact PTH (measured by RIA using an Ab against 28-48 hPTH and 28-48(Tyr)hPTH tracer) was initially within the normal range (100-400 pg/ml), then gradually increased to 749. Ca, PO_4 and AP were constantly normal. 125I 43-68(Tyr) and 42-55(Tyr)hPTH were specifically bound to the patients native plasma and the IgG-fraction. In contrast to native 43-68 and 42-55 intact PTH failed to displace either tracer. Binding of radiolabelled 1-34, 28-48(Tyr), 62-68(Tyr) and 70-84(Tyr)hPTH was less than 2%. Maximal binding of 43-68(Tyr)hPTH to native plasma was 61% three months after initiation of regular hemodialysis, binding subsequently decreased inversely related to the increase of MID-C-PTH and intact PTH. Since the patient had no signs of hyperparathyroid bone disease (AP, X-ray studies, and bone histology without evidence of fibroosteoclasia) we conclude that this auto-Ab against MID-PTH was protective against the osteoclast stimulating activity of PTH, implying that MID-PTH has biological activity.

871 MID-C-REGIONAL PTH (MID-C-PTH): DIAGNOSTIC IMPORTANCE. H. Jüppner* and R.D. Hesch, Kinderklinik and Abt. Klinische Endokrinologie, Medizinische Hochschule Hannover, 3 Hannover 61, West-Germany.

The selective determination of MID-C-PTH using antibody G III, 125I 43-68 (Tyr)hPTH tracer and 44-68 hPTH standard has been used as a routine methode for more than three years. The diagnostic importance and clinical implications are subsequently summarized. 94.5 - 335.2 pg/ml represents the normal range (2 SD-range). Coefficient of variation in 180 separate assays is 15.7 (% SD of the mean) for control serum K23 (mean ± SE: 258.8 ± 4.6), 10.3 for P10 (478.9 ± 5.6) and 11.8 for P9 (1135.4 ± 15.1). Patients with histologically proven parathyroid adenomata and normal renal function had MID-C-PTH levels of 567.5 ± 358.6 (mean ± SD), those with impaired renal function 1632.1 ± 781.6; calcium was 3.10 ± 0.42 mmol/L, and 3.26 ± 0.61 respectively. Alkaline phosphatase activity and phosphate were normal in more than 50% of the patients. Thus the diagnosis of autonomeous hyperparathyroidism (auto HPT) can reliably be based on the determination of MID-C-PTH, calcium and creatinine. After successful renal transplantation creatinine and MID-C-PTH decrease simultaneously; high levels of MID-C-PTH despite normal graft function indicate auto HPT. The index (AP x PTH)(U x $\mu g/L^2$) is an importante parameter to characterize biochemically the course of renal osteodystrophy. Low turnover osteoidosis: 88.7 ± 49.0 (mean ± SD) - treat with reduced bath calcium or even desferrioxamine to avoid pathological fracture due to osteopenia. Stabile combination of osteoidosis and fibroosteoclasia: 291.2 ± 160.0 - no change in dialysis treatment. Early phase of osseous HPT: 1938.7 ± 1012.4 - try low dose $1.25(OH)_2D_3$ treatment. Severe osseous HPT: $>$5000 (U x $\mu g/L^2$) - auto HPT: parathyroid ectomy recommended.

872 IN VITRO BONE METABOLISM IN OSTEOPOROSIS (OP), OSTEOMALACIA (OM) AND PRIMARY HYPERPARATHYROIDISM (HPT). E. Keck*, T.B. West, H.K. Kley and H.L. Krüskemper, Med. Universitätsklinik C, Moorenstr. 5, 4000 Düsseldorf, F.R.Germany

We adapted our procedure for incubating trabecular bone to study smaller bone samples of 5o mg from patients with various bone diseases. Control samples were obtained from the femoral heads of 12 patients aged between 66 and 78 years, 1♂, 11♀, who underwent hip replacement for coxarthrosis. Medium concentrations before and after 6 h incubation were for calcium (Ca) 1.82 + o.13 and 1.25 + o.16, magnesium (Mg) o.8o + o.06 and o.68 + o.o5, phosphate (PO_4^{-3}) 1.o6 + o.o8 and 1.o3 + o.17 mmol/l and alkaline phosphatase activity (aP) not detectable and 2o + 16 U/l. In trabecular bone obtained by iliac crest biopsy from 13 patients with clinic and histologic evidents for OP no significant differences in net electrolyte movements or aP activity could be observed. In patients with OM due to non tropical sprue (7), renal insufficiency (1) and dietary vitamin D deficiency (1) net movements of Ca and Mg were similar to controls, however, a release of PO_4^{-3} (1.47 + o.6o, $p<$ o.oo5) into the medium was observed accompanied by an enhanced rise of aP activity (42 + 4o). An increased net uptake of Ca was observed in 3 of 7 experiments after addition of 12o pg/ml $1,25(OH)_2D_3$ and in 3 of 3 experiments after addition of 5 ng/ml $24,25(OH)_2D_3$ to incubation medium. In 8 out of 9 patients with HPT a net release of Ca was observed compared to controls, while the other parameters were not affected. Addition of calcitonin (1o ng/ml) in 5 experiments led to a partial suppression of Ca release in four. Thus we have demonstrated typical patterns of in vitro electrolyte movements in various bone diseases.

873 CALCIUM METABOLISM IN DIABETES MELLITUS. N. Krishnamra*, L. Limlomwongse and P. Soogaroon, Mahidol University, Faculty of Science, Department of Physiology, Rama VI Rd., Bangkok 10400, Thailand.

This study aims to investigate the relationship of diabetes mellitus (DM), insulin and alterations in plasma calcium (Ca) and phosphate (PO_4) in fasted thyroparathyroidectomized (TPTX), parathyroidectomized (PTX)and intact diabetic rats. Insulin (5 U/kg BW, im) resulted in a marked drop in plasma PO_4 in every group within 1 hr which was due to insulin-stimulated uptake of PO_4 into cells. The plasma Ca remained normal in intact DM 2 hr after insulin when compared to saline control (10.0±0.1 mg/dl). In TPTX diabetics, plasma Ca increased from 7.8±0.2 to 10.7±0.4 mg/dl (P< 0.001) and 10.4±0.5 mg/dl (P<0.001) 2 and 4 hr respectively after insulin, while plasma PO_4 decreased from post-TPTX level of 8.3±0.5 to 4.3±0.7 (P< 0.001) at 2 hr. However, in PTX diabetics, plasma Ca remained at a hypocalcemic level of 7.9±0.3 mg/dl, while plasma PO_4 dropped from post-PTX level of 7.7±0.5 to 3.9±0.4 mg/dl (P<0.001) at 2 hr. The plasma Ca seemed to respond to insulin independently of PO_4. The rate of Ca removal from plasma as indicated by ^{45}Ca disappearance was slower in both TPTX and PTX diabetics after insulin as compared to TPTX diabetics control, whereas the rate of bone ^{45}Ca uptake and bone ^{45}Ca release in 2 hr were not affected. Thus, Ca raising effect of insulin, a consequence of slower removal of Ca from plasma was not due to insulin action on bone. The site of insulin-mediated hypercalcemia is being investigated.

874 MEASUREMENT OF URINARY IMMUNOREACTIVE HUMAN N-TERMINAL FRAGMENT OF PRO-OPIOMELANOCORTIN IN PATIENTS WITH LUNG CANCER. L. Gaspar*, F. Gilbert, J.S.D. Chan, N.G. Seidah and M. Chrétien, Laboratories of Biochemical and Molecular Neuroendocrinology, Clinical Research Institute of Montreal, H2W 1R7, Canada.

We have previously demonstrated that determination of plasma immunoreactive NH_2-terminal (IR-hNT) of pro-opiomelanocortin (POMC) could be a useful parameter for diagnosis and follow-up of patients with lung cancer. In the present study we investigated the urinary level of IR-hNT in normal subjects and patients with pulmonary carcinoma. 24h urine samples were dialyzed and IR-hNT material was extracted by Sep-Pak C_{18}-cartridges (Waters) using propanol/trifluoroacetic acid solvent system. In urine of healthy volunteers (N=13) the IR-hNT level was 49.9±13.9 (mean±SEM) pg/ml creatinine. In patients with histologically proven lung cancer (N=34), the urinary IR-hNT was 119.2±63.2 (mean±SEM) pg/mg creatinine ($p < 0.001$). When urinary measurements are compared to plasma levels of IR-hNT, more patients had elevated values in their urine samples (83% vs 76%). When both urine and plasma results were analyzed together, 94% of patients had increased values. Results indicate that the radioimmunoassay of urinary hNT may provide an improved tool for diagnosis and surveillance of patients with pulmonary carcinoma. This study was supported by the National Cancer Institute of Canada and the Medical Research Council of Canada (PG-2). L.G. is a recipient of fellowship from the Cancer Research Society, Inc.

875 ANDROGEN RECEPTOR CONTENT OF BIOPSIED HUMAN PROSTATE IS HETEROGENEOUS.
Lester S. Gorelic*, Robert W. Klipper, and Sydney A. Shain, Southwest Foundation for Biomedical Research, San Antonio, Texas

We used saturating dose analysis with methyltrienolone, 15 nM cytoplasmic (R_c) or 10 nM nuclear (R_n), to develop a microassay (45 µl total volume) for quantitation of androgen receptors in human prostate specimens of ≤100 mg. We eliminated possible assay protocol bias by demonstrating that values of R_c simultaneously determined in split preparations using our standard assay, 220 µl (≥100 mg tissue), and the microassay, 45 µl, were identical in 8/10 trials, whereas values for R_n were identical in 10/10 trials. Subsequent patient analyses were performed in triplicate. All biopsy specimens were obtained during open surgery. Microassay analyses of multiple specimens from the same patient for R_c showed 1.6- to 15-fold differences among individual values in 50% (8/16) of patients. R_n values for these cases showed 2.6- to 22-fold differences in 53% (8/15) of patients. Multiple specimen standard assay analyses of R_c for another series showed 1.3- to 4.8-fold differences in 27% (7/26) of patients, whereas R_n values for these cases showed 1.4- to 4.6-fold differences in 28% (7/25) of patients. All differences were statistically significant, $P < 0.05$. Heterogeneity of human prostate androgen receptor content is most apparent when multiple small, ≤100 mg, samples are analyzed from the same biopsy specimen. As might have been anticipated, frequency of detected heterogeneity is decreased when multiple large, ≥100 mg, specimens are analyzed. Our studies suggest that the prognostic utility of androgen receptor determinations performed on single small specimens may be limited. (Supported in part by USPHS grant CA 23668 from the DHHS.)

876 ADENYLATE CYCLASE IN HUMAN OVARIAN CANCERS: SENSITIVITY TO GONADOTROPINS AND NONHORMONAL ACTIVATORS. P. Graves*, E. Surwit and R. Stouffer. Depts. of Physiology and Ob-Gyn, Univ. of Arizona, Tucson, Arizona USA 85724.

Many of the effects of the gonadotropic hormones, FSH, LH and CG on the ovary are mediated by the activation of adenylate cyclase (AC) in target cells. To establish whether ovarian cancers have a gonadotropin-sensitive AC system, 20000g particulates prepared from ovarian tumor biopsies of 13 women were analyzed for their ability to convert α^{32}P-ATP to ^{32}P-cAMP. Under control conditions, ten tumors exhibited AC activity similar to that observed in normal ovaries from estrogen-primed or pseudopregnant rats. Incubation with the GTP analog, guanyl-5'-yl imidodiphosphate (50 µM), and NaF (10 mM) markedly enhanced cAMP production 6.0 ± 2.6 and 6.4 ± 3.3 fold ($\bar{x} \pm$SE, n=10), respectively. Tumors of epithelial (n=10) or germinal (n=2) origin failed to exhibit additional AC activity when incubated in the presence of GTP and human (h) FSH (NIH-FSH-S1, 10 µg/ml) or hCG (CR123, 10 µg/ml) over that with GTP alone. In contrast, a granulosa cell-theca cell (GC-TC) tumor exhibited a significant increase in the presence of GTP and FSH(147.6 pmol cAMP), compared to GTP alone (50.0 pmol). The concentration of FSH required for half-maximal stimulation of AC in the GC-TC tumor and in ovaries from estrogen-primed rats was comparable (1.6 vs 1.7 µg/ml). Addition of CG failed to enhance AC activity in the GC-TC tumor. Thus, ovarian tumors contained an active AC system which was acutely responsive to nonhormonal activators. Although AC from the GC-TC tumor was stimulated by FSH, the more common ovarian tumors of epithelial origin did not demonstrate any capacity to respond to gonadotropins. Therefore, the epithelial tumors may not be target tissues for the gonadotropins. NIH CA 33336

877 MEDROXYPROGESTERONE ACETATE TISSUE LEVELS AND 17-ß-HYDROXYDEHY= DROGENASE ACTIVITY IN RATS WITH DMBA-INDUCED MAMMARY TUMOR.

A.Grieco*,E.Strocchi,F.De Cicco N.,C.M.Camaggi,S.Dell'Acqua,P. Beghelli,S.Biondi,C.Barone,F.Pannuti, and G.Gambassi.Ist.Pat. Medica e Ist. Clin. Ostetrica e Ginec. Un. Cattolica Rome.Ist. Chim. Org. Un. Bologna; Div.Oncologia Osp.Malpighi,Bologna-Italy

High-dose Medroxyprogesterone acetate(MAP)induces objective tumor response in 25-45% of patients with metastatic breast can= cer. The mechanism of its antitumor action is still under deba= te. 20 female Sprague-Dawley rats with DMBA-induced mammary tu= mor,were treated with 100 mg/kg/PO of MAP for 7 days. The ani= mals were sacrified at different times after the last admini= stration. Plasma, tumor and tissue samples were collected and analyzed for MAP concentration by a specific gas-chromatographic method and for 17-ß-hydroxydehydrogenase(17ßHDS) activity in subcellular fraction. Higher levels of MAP were found in the li= ver, uterus and ovary samples and were 0.3 mcg/gr. 24 hours af= ter the last administration. 17-ß-HDS activity, MAP level-rela= ted, was higher in microsomial fraction and lower in nuclear fraction, cytosol and 800xg surnatant phase. These data seem to confirm the MAP antiestrogenic action, expressed by transforming the very active Estradiol in the less active Estron.

878 GLUCOCORTICOID AND GESTAGEN EFFECTS OF MEDROXYPROGESTERONE ACETATE (MPA).

Grill H.-J., Manz B., Kreienberg R., Melchert F., Heubner A. and Pollow K.*, Universitätsfrauenklinik, Abt. f. Experimentelle Endokrinologie, Mainz, F.R.G.

High dose MPA treatment gains increased importance in hormonal treatment of mammary carcinomas. Besides its known gestagen effects were clinical and biochemical data found resembling marked glucocorticoid effects in 30 patients under high dose MPA treatment over 3 months. MPA binds with relative binding affinities (RBA-values) of 1.15 better to the progesterone receptor than R5020 (1.0), but shows also an RBA of 0.29 to the glucocorticoid receptor (dexamethasone 1.0, cortisol 0.45). Another sensitive test system for glucocorticoid potency is the inhibition of mitogen induced blastogenesis of normal peripheral blood lymphocytes. The inhibitory activity of MPA is 13% of the activity of hydrocortisone and ranges in the same order of magnitude as other synthetic glucocorticoids (e.g. fluorocortulon, prednisolone). Clinical glucocorticoid effects: Most obvious was the increase in body weight (9/30 <10%, 9/30 <20%, 5/30 <30%). Other effects were elevated oral GGT values (19/30), increase in blood lymphocytes, erythrocytes and thrombocytes (19/30) as well as psychological alterations.

879 EFFECT OF PHENOBARBITAL ON THYROID TUMORIGENESIS IN HYPOPHYSECTOMISED RATS TREATED WITH N-BIS(2-HYDROXYPROPYL)-NITROSAMINE. Y. Hiasa , N. Konishi*, Y. Kitahori, T. Shimoyama and A. Miyashiro, 1st Dept. of Pathology, Nara Medical University, Kashihara, Nara, 634, Japan.

The effect of phenobarbital (Pb) on the development of thyroid tumors in hypophysectomised (H.S.) rats initiated by N-bis(2-hydroxypropyl)nitrosamine (DHPN) was studied by histological and biochemical methods. Sixty-four male Wistar rats and 64 H.S. male Wistar rats were divided into 4 groups respectively. A single dose of 250 mg DHPN per 100 g B.W. was injected with i.p. into rats in Groups 1 and 2. Commercial diet containing 500 ppm Pb was given to animals in Groups 1 and 3 from week 2 to 20 for 19 weeks as experimental diet. All animals that survived for 20 weeks were killed with ether. Blood was collected for 5 nonfasted rats in each groups for assay of T4 and T3 in serum by radioimmunoassay. Serial sections for histological studies were made of the thyroid gland of all animals. Incidences of thyroid tumor were 62% (10/16) in non H.S. rats given Pb and 0% in other groups. Pb decreased the serum concentration of T3 in non H.S. rats but did not effect on it in H.S. rats. Pb promoted the development of thyroid tumors in non H.S. rats but not in H.S. rats. It was suggested that Pb does not promote directely the development of thyroid tumor and TSH increased by Pb promotes the development of thyroid tumors.

880 PROMOTING EFFECT OF BUTYLATED-HYDROXYTOLUENE (BHT) AND PROPYLTHIOURACILE (PTU) ON THYROID TUMORIGENESIS IN RATS TREATED WITH N-BIS(2-HYDROXYPROPYL)NITROSAMINE. Y. Hiasa*, N. Konishi, Y. Kitahori, T. Shimoyama and A. Miyashiro, 1st Dept. of Pathology, Nara Medical University, Kashihara, Nara, 634, Japan

The effect of butylated-hydroxytoluene (BHT) and propylthiouracile (PTU) on development of thyroid tumors in rats initiated by N-bis(2-hydroxypropyl)nitrosamine (DHPN) was studied by biochemical and histological methods. A total of 120 6 weeks old male Wistar rats were divided into 6 groups. A single dose of 250 mg DHPN per 100 g B.W. was injected with i.p. into rats in Groups 1, 2 and 3. Commercial diet containing 3000 ppm BHT was given to animals in Groups 1 and 4 and commercial diet containing 1500 ppm PTU was given to animals in Groups 2 and 5 from week 2 to 20 for 19 weeks as experimental diet. All animals that survived for 20 weeks were killed with ether. Blood was collected for 5 nonfasted rats in each groups for assay of T4 and T3 in serum by radioimmunoassay. Serial sections for histological studies were made of the thyroid gland of all animals. Serum concentration of T3 was decreased by PTU but not by BHT. Incidences of thyroid tumors were 35% (7/20) in rats given DHPN and BHT, and 100% (20/20) in rats given DHPN and PTU, but 0% in other groups. It was confirmed that BHT and PTU promotes the development of thyroid tumors in rats initiated by DHPN.

881 REGULATION OF INSULIN RECEPTORS IN CULTURED CELLS. I.M. Holdaway*, K.G. Mountjoy and G.J. Finlay, Department of Endocrinology, Auckland Hospital, and Cancer Research Laboratory, School of Medicine, Auckland 1, New Zealand.

Although a wide variety of tumours contain insulin receptors (IR) it is uncertain whether tumour IR levels can be down-regulated by exogenous insulin or up-regulated by oral hypoglycaemic agents as can IR in normal tissues. The effects of insulin, metformin (MET) and glibenclamide (GLIB) have been studied in cell cultures of breast (MCF-7, T-47D) and colon (HCT-8) tumours, and compared with responses in human diploid fibroblasts. Down-regulation of IR was seen in fibroblasts after 4h exposure to 10^{-9}M insulin, in HCT-8 at 10^{-5}M insulin and the breast lines showed no down-regulation up to 10^{-5}M insulin. The lack of down-regulation in the tumour cell lines did not appear to be due to decreased internalisation of insulin-IR complexes. MET and GLIB did not affect basal IR levels in any tissue, but 10^{-5}M MET significantly impaired insulin-induced down-regulation of IR in fibroblasts. Neither MET nor GLIB at levels up to 10^{-5}M and 10^{-6}M respectively influenced IR levels in any of the tumour cell lines during exposure to insulin. The biological response to insulin was tested in parallel with binding studies, and ^{3}H-leucine incorporation into protein was stimulated at $\geq 10^{-7}$M insulin in T-47D and MCF-7 cell lines. After exposure to insulin levels which down-regulated receptors in normal cells the tumour lines still showed a biologic response to insulin. These data indicate that tumour IR are less readily regulated by external agents than IR in normal tissues, and these findings may have implications in both tumour biology and cancer management.
This study was supported by the New Zealand MRC.

882 ANTIBODY-RECOGNIZED BINDING OF I-125-LABELED 11beta-METHOXY-17alpha-IODOVINYL-ESTRADIOL (I-125-MIVE2) TO ESTROGEN RECEPTOR (ER) IN OVARIAN CARCINOMAS IN WOMEN. J.A. HOLT*, R.E. GIBSON, G.L. GREENE and R.C. REBA. Dept Obstet Gynecol and the Ben May Laboratories, University of Chicago, Chicago, IL 60637 and Sect Radiopharmaceut Chem, George Washington University Medical Center, Washington, D.C. 20037 USA.

A radiohalogenated derivative of Moxestrol, I-125-MIVE2, has been developed as a prototype compound for the imaging and potential therapy of ER-rich breast cancers (Gibson et al., J Nuc Med 24:P49. 1983). We now report that I-125-MIVE2 binds to the ER, which is found in amounts greater than 500 fmoles/g wet wt in more than 50% of epithelial ovarian carcinomas (OVCA) of women. We used monoclonal antibodies H222, H226 (Abbott Laboratories) and D547, all raised against human breast cancer ER, to identify the I-125-MIVE2 binding protein by sedimentation velocity analysis in sucrose gradients. The fact that both diethylstilbestrol and estradiol but not testosterone, cortisol or progesterone competed for binding at 0.1-100 fold molar excesses confirmed that the I-125-MIVE2 binding moiety in OVCA is ER; the Ka of I-125-MIVE2 for OVCA ER is 1.1×10^{-10}M. Because ER survives chemotherapies in OVCA (Holt et al., Soc Gynec Oncol, 1984), MIVE2 radiolabeled with alternative isotopes, e.g., I-123, Br-80 & -80m and F-18, should prove useful in monitoring disease progression by imaging and may offer novel treatment modalities by radiocytotoxicity delivered via the receptor-seeking ligands. (Supported by CA-27476, CA-18675, The Mothers' Aid Research Fund of CLIH, ACS BC-86, CA-02897, UCCRF Women's Board, Abbott Laboratories).

883 HETEROGENEITY OF AXC RAT PROSTATE ADENOCARCINOMA AS ESTABLISHED BY CLONALLY DERIVED CELL LINES.

Rachel I. Huot*, G. Con Smith and Sydney A. Shain, Southwest Foundation for Biomedical Research, San Antonio, Texas

Heterogeneous parental cultures of LSC-AXC rat prostate cancer cells: LSC-AXC-C/O, maintained on culture medium; LSC-AXC-D/O, maintained on medium containing 10^{-7} M 5α-dihydrotestosterone (5α-DHT); and LSC-AXC-T/O, maintained on medium containing 10^{-7} M testosterone (T), were used to isolate clonally derived cell lines. Eight tumorigenic, hypotriploid, clonal cell lines were selected for detailed evaluation. All were found to possess features characteristic of secretory epithelium as judged by light and electron microscopy. All cell lines contained abundant 5α-reductase activity; however, metabolite distribution was variable and cell line specific. Total 5α-reductase activity varied 10-fold between cell lines. All cell lines contained secretory prostatic acid phosphatase; however, relative secretory isoenzyme content varied twofold. There was no consistent effect of maintenance on T- or 5α-DHT-containing medium on 5α-reductase or acid phosphatase activities in these cell lines. Cells maintained on T-containing medium had the highest androgen receptor content, whereas those maintained on 5α-DHT-containing medium had the lowest receptor content. Total androgen receptor content (mean ± SD) for C, D, and T cells respectively was 131 ± 61, 43 ± 32, and 274 ± 96 fmol/100 μg DNA. Differences between means were significant ($P < 0.05$). If androgen receptor content is an index of hormonal responsiveness, our studies suggest that high intracellular levels of 5α-DHT may direct prostate carcinoma cells toward hormone independence. (Supported in part by USPHS grant CA 30116 from the DHHS.)

884 CIRCULATING HORMONE LEVELS IN MICE BEARING HYPOPHYSEAL GRAFTS: DEVELOPMENT OF PITUITARY ADENOMAS, MAMMARY CARCINOMAS AND ADENOMYOSIS UTERI.

R.A. Huseby, Michigan Cancer Foundation, Detroit, Michigan 48201.

Serum prolactin (PRL), growth hormone (GH), and progesterone (Pr) levels were determined* at intervals up to 18 mos following the ectopic grafting of a single hypophysis to 4 wk old female mice of 2 inbred strains and their F_1 hybrids all lacking expression of MuMTV. Although by the third week PRL levels ($\bar{x}$ 45ng/ml) had reached those reported on days 5-8 of pregnancy with these reagents, the premature increase in Pr was only to the level ($\bar{x}$ 3.7ng/ml) seen in normal adult females in diestrus. Four weeks later, Pr levels had tripled in F_1 but were unchanged in Balb/c recipients, and it was determined that there were no differences in PRL levels whether male or female donors had been used. By 6 mos, PRL levels had increased in C3H and F_1 recipients ($\bar{x}$ 85ng/ml) but had fallen slightly in Balb/c ($\bar{x}$ 25ng/ml), while GH had become slightly elevated in the latter. Adenomyosis had become evident in the C3H and F_1 animals. Mammary cancers that differed histologically from those usually occurring in mice expressing MuMTV developed in 74% of mice by 18 mos of age. Sixteen of 17 hybrid animals over 14 mos of age had adenomatous grafts 5 to 11mm in greatest diameter. Serum PRL levels ranged from 1.6 to 20 x 10^3ng/ml dependent upon the size of the adenoma, but only one tumor secreted excessive amounts of GH. The development of prolactinomas was much less marked in aged Balb/c. After 1 yr of age, adenomyosis became less conspicuous, probably due to declining ovarian function.

*RIA's graciously performed in the laboratory of Dr. F. Talamantes, University of California, Santa Cruz.

885 AN AUTOMATED ENZYME INHIBITION ASSAY FOR ESTIMATION OF UNSATURATED THYROXINE BINDING PROTEIN ON THE DU PONT aca® DISCRETE CLINICAL ANALYZER†.
T. P. Hartz, Jr.*, W. L. Collinsworth, C. T. Hodges and A. A. Jarvis, E. I. du Pont de Nemours & Company (Inc.), Clinical and Instrument Systems Division, Wilmington, DE 19898 USA

A fully automated enzyme inhibition assay and calibration system has been developed for the Du Pont aca® discrete clinical analyzer for estimation of the relative level of unsaturated binding sites on thyroxine binding proteins, predominantly thyroxine binding globulin. The assay employs a thyroxine-phosphonate conjugate to both mimic the action of thyroxine with regard to protein binding and to inhibit the activity of acetycholinesterase (AChE). In the presence of a serum sample, the activity of AChE is directly proportional to the level of unsaturation of thyroxine binding protein. Results of the assay are reported in terms of percent uptake, a derived unit reflecting the approximate magnitude of results obtained with conventional radiometric thyronine uptake assays. Field evaluation results demonstrate different reference intervals for males (26.5 - 38.1%) and females (19.1 - 33.5%). Diagnostic agreement between the results from the thyronine uptake (TU) assay for the aca® discrete clinical analyzer and radiometric assays was reached for greater than 95% of the patient samples tested.

†registered trademark of E. I. du Pont de Nemours and Company, Inc.

886 ALTERATION OF THYROIDAL ^{131}I UPTAKE AFTER ^{131}I TREATMENT FOR HYPERTHYROIDISM.
Robert C. Heath, Ved V. Gossain* and David R. Rovner, Department of Medicine, Michigan State University, East Lansing, Michigan, USA.

^{131}I uptake by the thyroid gland (RAIU) is frequently utilized for evaluation of patients with thyroid disease. Many factors in addition to primary thyroid disease can influence the RAIU, but the effect of therapeutic doses of ^{131}I on subsequently obtained RAIU has not been well described. From our records of the previous 8 years, we have identified 26 patients previously treated with ^{131}I for hyperthyroidism who also had clinical evaluation, a serum thyroxine (T4) level measurement and ^{131}I uptake obtained at approximately the same time. These evaluations were done six months to 1 year after ^{131}I therapy. In 5 patients, 24 hour RAIU was increased (normal 10-35%), but all these patients were clinically euthyroid and their serum T4 levels were normal (4.5-11.5 μg/dl). In three other patients, the RAIU was discrepant with the clinical picture. One patient was hyperthyroid clinically, with elevated T4 (14.5 μg/dl), but RAIU was within normal limits (23%). He subsequently required retreatment with ^{131}I. Another patient was clinically euthyroid, had a normal T4 (11.5 μg/dl), but low 24 hr. RAIU (6%) suggested hypothyroidism. However, 5 months later, he had elevated TSH (21 μIU/ml) and became clinically hypothyroid. Finally, another hypothyroid patient with low T4 (2.3 μg/dl) had normal 24 hr. RAIU (28%). We were unable to identify other factors which might have influenced RAIU measurements. These findings suggest that following treatment with ^{131}I, RAIU becomes diagnostically unreliable in as many as 30% of patients (8/26).

887 TREATMENT OF HYPERTHYROIDISM IN COMMUNITY HOSPITALS. Robert C. Heath, Ved V. Gossain and David R. Rovner*, Department of Medicine, Michigan State University, East Lansing, Michigan, USA.

Despite several reports from major medical centers, the treatment of hyperthyroidism remains controversial. We report here our experience with the treatment of hyperthyroidism in University Affiliated Community hospitals. 144 patients with documented hyperthyroidism were seen during 1972-82 at the Michigan State University Clinical Center. As a community based program, most patients received therapy from community based radiotherapists and surgeons. Sufficient followup was available on 119 patients (82%). There were 92 women and 27 men. The age range at the time of diagnosis of hyperthyroidism was 12 to 75 years. The etiology of hyperthyroidism in these patients was Grave's disease 94, toxic multinodular goiter 11, Hashimoto's thyroiditis 6, iatrogenic 5 and subacute thyroiditis 3. Of 105 patients with Grave's disease and toxic multinodular goiter, 68 (65%) were treated with ^{131}I; 19 (18%) had surgery and 18 (17%) were treated with drugs alone. The average dose of ^{131}I was approximately 9 millicuries. Two-thirds of the patients treated with ^{131}I were rendered euthyroid by a single dose whereas about 1/3 (22 patients) required an additional dose. Among those treated with ^{131}I, about 40% (28 patients) have become hypothyroid. Of 19 patients treated with surgery, 6 became hypothyroid (31%) and in 3 (16%), hyperthyroidism recurred. Hypoparathyroidism developed in one patient (5%) and no patient developed recurrent laryngeal nerve damage. No serious complications were noted in patients with drugs alone. These data suggest that despite a significant incidence of hypothyroidism (40%), ^{131}I remains the preferred treatment of patients with hyperthyroidism and can be safely carried out in community hospitals.

888 CLINICAL EVALUATION OF ASPIRATION BIOPSY CYTOLOGY FOR CHRONIC THYROIDITIS. M. Hieda*, A. Ishihara, T. Sasho, Y. Shiokawa and R. Ariwa[1]. Dept. of Internal Medicine, Juntendo University and [1]Tokyo Metropolitan Okubo Municipal Hospital.

Aspiration biopsy cytology was performed in 3330 cases of thyroid diseases during the period of January 1975 to September 1983. Among them, 929 cases (27.9%) were chronic thyroiditis, which represents a high incidence compared with other facilities. Criteria of chronic thyroiditis by aspiration biopsy cytology are hyperplasia of small follicular cell with many lymphoid cell and oxyphilic change in follicular cells, lymphoid cells, plasma cells and reticulum cells. The diagnostic significane of aspiration biopsy cytology in chronic thyroiditis can be stated as follows:

1) As for the correlation between the cytological findings and the thyroid function or thyroid antibodies, the following conclusin were obtained:
   i) There is a negative correlation between the number of lymphocytes and T_7 levels (thyroid function) in chronic thyroiditis.
   ii) There is a positive correlation between the number of oxyphilic cells or lymphocytes and the titer of the microsome test in chronic thyroiditis.
2) 29 cases were diagnosed as chronic thyroiditis in 88 cases of diffuse goiter with negative thyroid test and microsome test.
3) Diagnosis of chronic thyroiditis among nodular goiter.
4) Aspiration biopsy cytology is of great value for the diagnosis of Hashitoxicosis. This correct diagnosis is very important for the treatment.
5) Aspiration biopsy cytology for exophthalmos with euthyroid state and non-diffuse goiter revealed the finding of chronic thyroiditis.

889 INAPPROPRIATE SECRETION OF ACTH IN NELSON'S SYNDROME ASSOCIATED WITH TESTOSTERONE PRODUCING HYPERPLASTIC OVARIAN NODULES. H.P. Higgins*, S.L. Asa and K. Kovacs, Departments of Medicine and Pathology, St. Michael's Hospital, University of Toronto, Toronto, Ontario, Canada.

Hyperplasia of extraadrenal steroid producing tissue is a rarely reported complication of Nelson's syndrome. We present the case of a 30-year-old woman who had undergone bilateral adrenalectomy at age 11 and 13 for treatment of hypercorticism. Subsequently, she developed Nelson's syndrome and a pituitary tumor was resected at age 16 and 27. Morphologic investigations including electron microscopy revealed a densely granulated corticotroph cell adenoma of the pituitary containing immunoreactive ACTH and other fragments of proopiocortin. At age 30, the patient complained of virilization. Serum testosterone was elevated at 500 ng/ml, plasma ACTH measured 3200 pg/ml. Serum cortisol while on replacement therapy was 3.6 μg%. Dexamethasone administration lowered serum testosterone to 100 ng/ml and plasma ACTH to 530 pg/ml; addition of hCG induced a rise in serum testosterone to 230 ng/ml. Bilateral salpingoophorectomy was performed and multiple ovarian hilar nodules were found. They were composed of large steroid producing cells showing ultrastructural evidence of stimulation: well developed smooth endoplasmic reticulum and numerous spherical mitochondria with tubulovesicular cristae. Reinke crystals were not identified. A microscopic tubular androblastoma was also found in one ovary. Postoperatively, serum testosterone fell to the normal range. It can be concluded that ACTH overproduction in Nelson's syndrome may induce proliferation of ACTH responsive extraadrenal tissue capable of steroid synthesis and, by stimulating testosterone secretion, result in virilization.

890 AN OPTIMIZED ASSAY FOR THE DETERMINATION OF SERUM THYROXINE USING THE DU PONT aca® DISCRETE CLINICAL ANALYZER†, C. T. Hodges*, W. L. Collinsworth, T. P. Hartz, Jr., A. A. Jarvis, D. M. Obzansky and P. M. Tuhy, E. I. du Pont de Nemours & Company (Inc.), Wilmington, DE 19898

A new assay and calibrator for the determination of total serum thyroxine (T4) have been optimized for use on the Du Pont aca® discrete clinical analyzer. The assay is based on an enzyme inhibition immunoassay technology. A combination of sodium salicylate and 8-anilino-1-naphthalenesulfonic acid is used to release T4 from binding proteins. A thyroxine-phosphonate conjugate competes with serum thyroxine for anti-thyroxine antibody added in the assay. The residual thyroxine-phosphonate conjugate then irreversibly inhibits some of the acetylcholinesterase present in the assay. The remaining acetylcholinesterase activity is then measured using the substrate acetyl-β-(methylthio)choline iodide and the developer 5,5′-dithiobis-(2-nitrobenzoic acid) (DTNB). Orphenadrine hydrochloride is used to inhibit endogeneous serum pseudocholinesterase activity. The concentrations of all active components were optimized to provide greatest sensitivity and stability and minimize serum matrix effects. This method requires 60 μL of serum with no pretreatment, is rapid (7 min.) and fully automated. The T4 assay gives a correlation slope of 1.03 and intercept of -0.1 μg/dL with a r=0.962 when compared to an RIA assay. Within-run precision estimates of 4.3% CV and 1.6% CV were obtained at the 5.4 μg/dL and 11.8 μg/dL levels respectively. This gives estimates of total analytical error of 0.51 μg/dL and 0.63 μg/dL at the 5.4 μg/dL and 11.8 μg/dL levels respectively.

†registered trademark of E. I. du Pont de Nemours and Company, Inc.

891 *TESTOSTERONE METABOLISM OF SCALP HAIR ROOTS IN 5α-REDUCTASE DEFICIENCY.* *M.B. Hodgins, Dermatology Department, Glasgow University, Anderson College Building, Dumbarton Road, Glasgow, G11 6NU, Scotland.*

In four male pseudohermaphrodites, 5α-reductase deficiency was demonstrated by analysis of testosterone metabolism in fresh genital skin slices. Cultured genital skin fibroblasts were unsuitable for the detection of 5α-reductase deficiency, due to very low rates of testosterone conversion in some normal foreskin fibroblast cell lines. For family studies of 5α-reductase deficiency, scalp hair follicles were chosen as a convenient tissue in which to measure testosterone metabolism. 5α-Reduction of testosterone was readily demonstrated in anagen hair roots plucked from the scalps of 4 normal men and 4 normal women (rate of conversion 4 to 29 pmol testosterone reduced /h/mg DNA, 17-oxosteroid metabolites predominating), but was slower than in genital skin, where 5α-dihydrotestosterone was the major metabolite. In scalp hair roots from two pairs of siblings with typical 5α-reductase deficiency, the rates of testosterone 5α-reduction (3 to 25 pmol/h/mg DNA) were similar to normal values. This suggests that 5α-reductase activity in hair follicles differs in its genetic control from the enzyme activities in genitalia and liver.

892 METYRAPONE AND PITUITARY IRRADIATION AS PRIMARY TREATMENT FOR CUSHING'S DISEASE. T.A.Howlett*, P.L.Drury, L.H.Rees, A.E.Jones and G.M.Besser, Departments of Endocrinology, Chemical Endocrinology and Radiotherapy, St Bartholomew's Hospital, London EC1A 7BE, U.K.

22 patients (16F 6M; 15-61 years) with pituitary dependent Cushing's disease (CD) have been treated with metyrapone (MET), to lower and maintain cortisol production within the normal range, followed by external pituitary irradiation (RT)(4500cGy in 25 fractions over 35 days; 3 field technique using 4MeV linear accelerator) with the intention of reducing excessive ACTH secretion in the long term. MET (1-4G/day) effectively normalised cortisol production and resulted in clinical remission of CD in all patients; worsening of hirsuties (7 patients) was the only unwanted effect. Six patients were able to stop all treatment 6 months to 10 years after RT (mean 4.4 ± 3.5 years). Cyclicity of CD was common and necessitated adrenalectomy or medical adrenolysis with op'DDD in 6 patients. At review 1 to 11 years after RT (mean 5.8 ± 3.0 years): 6 patients are off all cortisol-lowering drugs (40% of patients who were >4 years after RT); 12 patients continue treatment, but with progressive dose reduction in 8 (MET alone - 7; MET + op'DDD - 3; op'DDD alone - 1; bromocriptine - 1). Four patients required adrenalectomy, one subsequent hypophysectomy for enlarging tumour. Anterior pituitary function: 1 hypothyroid (3 years), 1 cortisol deficient (4 years), no others require any pituitary replacement; 3 patients have had successful pregnancies. Conclusions : MET can control CD in the long term. RT results in amelioration of CD in the majority of patients and complete remission in some, although often after a delay of a number of years.

893 INCREASED CIRCULATING INACTIVE RENIN IS AN EARLY MANIFESTATION OF DIABETIC NEPHROPATHY. W.A. Hsueh*, J. Mainelli and W. Uyehara, Section of Endocrinology, LAC/USC Medical Center, Los Angeles, California.

Patients with diabetic nephropathy and hyporeninemic hypoaldosteronism have increased plasma levels of inactive renin. To determine whether inactive renin (IR) is elevated early in diabetic renal disease and to study factors which may control IR production, we measured upright active and inactive renin concentration in 67 patients ages 19-80 with Types I and II diabetes mellitus. Duration ranged from new onset to 30 years. No patients were ingesting drugs known to affect renin. A simultaneous 24 hr urine was collected. Patients were divided into 4 groups based on creatinine clearance (C_{cr}). Active renin levels were similar among the groups and in the normal range:

Group	n	$C_{cr}/1.73m^2$	Active Renin ng/ml/hr (mean $\pm$ SE)	Inactive Renin ng/ml/hr (mean $\pm$ SE)	% with Proteinuria
I	5	0.60	6.8$\pm$1.8	29.0$\pm$3.8	100
II	11	60-90	10.6$\pm$1.7	47.0$\pm$8.6	80
III	36	90-150	13.6$\pm$3.8	69.3$\pm$8.2	56
IV	15	150	7.7$\pm$1.7	28.6$\pm$6.8	93

In II and III, IR was increased above normal (range 7-37ng/ml/hr) and above I and IV ($p<0.001$). Eight patients in III had elevated IR, but no significant proteinuria (<150mg/24h). IR did not correlate with degree of retinopathy, neuropathy, fasting blood sugar or hemoglobin A-I-C. We conclude that the first manifestation of diabetic nephropathy can be either a rise in plasma IR or a supranormal C_{cr} with proteinuria. These changes may not be interdependent, and measurement of both may be useful in recognizing early diabetic nephropathy.

894 LH AND FSH PULSATILITY IN HYPOTHALAMIC AMENORRHEA(HA). D.M.Hurley*, R.Brian, H.G.Burger, MRC, Prince Henry's Hospital, Melbourne, Australia.

To assess gonadotrophin releasing hormone (GnRH) pulsatility in HA, LH and FSH pulse frequency and amplitude were determined by radioimmunoassay of 20 minutely blood samples obtained from 14 HA patients during 4 hours and were compared with values obtained from 7 healthy women studied in the early follicular phase (EF). HA patients fell into 3 groups, based on mean LH and FSH levels: group I: low LH and FSH (n=2); group II: low LH, normal FSH (n=5); group III: normal LH and FSH (n=7). Results are shown as mean ± SEM.

	Normal EF	HAI	HAII	HAIII
LH - mean level (IU/L)	2.6-5.4	<0.2-1.4	0.2-1.4	3.1-5.3
- pulses / 4 hour	3.2±0.3	0^{c}	1.3±0.3^{b}	2.1±0.3^{a}
- mean pulse ampl. (IU/L)	2.5±0.2	0^{c}	0.9±0.2^{c}	2.1±0.3^{NS}
FSH- mean level (IU/L)	3.9-6.7	0.7-1.2	3.4-5.8	2.9-6.1
- pulses / 4 hour	2.4±0.2	1.0±0.5^{NS}	1.7±0.5^{NS}	1.7±0.4^{NS}
- mean pulse ampl. (IU/L)	1.1±0.1	0.3±0.03^{b}	0.9±0.2^{NS}	1.1±0.2^{NS}
E_2 - (pmol/L)	274±40	208±28	153±27	310±65

a:$p<0.05$;b:$p<0.01$;c:$p<0.0005$ compared to normal EF value.NS=not significant

These results suggest a reduction in GnRH secretion which is greatest in group I, intermediate in group II and least in group III patients. The results are best explained by a reduction in both frequency and amplitude of GnRH pulses or by a selective reduction in amplitude, resulting in an apparent reduction in frequency because of failure to identify small pulses. FSH pulse frequency was higher than LH pulse frequency in groups I and II and may be a better index of GnRH pulse frequency in these patients with relatively high FSH:LH ratios. * Supported by the NH & MRC of Australia.

895 GROWTH ENHANCEMENT BY DOPAMINERGIC (DA) THERAPY IN CHILDREN WITH INTRA-UTERINE GROWTH RETARDATION (IUGR). C.A. Huseman* and M. Sibilia, Department of Pediatrics, University of Nebraska Medical Center, Omaha, NE 68105, USA.

In a previous study we observed stimulation of growth velocity in hypopituitary children by DA therapy alone. The purpose of our present study was to determine if DA therapy could prove useful in stimulating endogenous GH release and growth in children with IUGR. Effect of DA on LH, FSH, gonadal steroid, cortisol, T_4, and TSH was also examined. Six prepubertal children (4 girls, 2 boys, BA 2-4y) were divided into 2 study groups. Grp 1 (n=3) received L-Dopa (L-D) 15mg/kg po every 6h for 6mo. Grp 2 (n=3) received bromocriptine (BCT) 1.25mg po every 12h for 6mo. A GnRH test, 2.5ug/kg IV bolus and 25ng/kg/96min/24h as IV pulses, was done pre and after 6mo of DA. LH & FSH responses to GnRH were determined at 15min intervals 1h before and 3h post bolus and for two 2h periods during pulses. Testosterone (T) in boys, estradiol (E_2) in girls, and Somatomedin C (SMC) were measured in 4 samples at 2h intervals. GH was measured in samples drawn every 15min during each study period. Results: 1) Growth rate (cm/y±SE) in Grp 1 increased from $\bar{x}$: 5±1 to 7±0.1, an increase of 50-80%; Grp 2 from 4±1 to 8±0.5, an increase of 43-160%. Peak and mean GH values increased significantly ($p<0.05$) in 5 of 6 subjects. Mean GH values (ng/ml±SE) were 5±1 pretherapy and 20±4 during DA therapy. SMC values increased significantly in 3 children. 2) L-D or BCT had no significant effect on basal or GnRH induced LH & FSH secretion in most children. T, E_2, cortisol, T_4, and TSH did not change from pretherapy values of 8±1(SE)ng/dl, 20±3pg/ml, 13±1ug/dl, 6±1uU/ml, respectively. Conclusions: Dopaminergic therapy alone is effective in inducing linear growth and increased GH secretion in IUGR children without affecting LH, FSH, gonadal steroid, cortisol, T_4 or TSH secretion.

896 SIMULTANEOUS QUANTITATIVE MEASUREAMENT OF VARIOUS STEROIDS USING HIGH RESOLUTION GASCHROMATOGRAPHY-MASS SPECTROMETRY (GC/MS) AND ITS CLINICAL APPLICATION. K.Ichimura*, Y.Shiki, S.Kusano, S.Ameniya, H.Yamanaka, K.Chiba, K.Saito, T.Shinozuka, Y.Nozaki, K.Ohyama and K.Kato, Dept. of Ped. School of Med., Keio Univ., 35 Shinanomachi, Tokyo, 160 Japan.

In this study, we established the method of the quantitative measureament of native adrenal steroids with GC/MS equipped with capillary column (cross-linked methyl silicone 25m x 0.2 mm I.D., 0.11μm thin film). 1 ml of serum sample containing 5-α-cholestane as internal standard(IS) was elicited by organic solvent using extrelunt column®. The solvent was evapolated by dried N_2 gas, then steroids of these samples were derivatized by n-butylboronic acid, o-methylhydroxylamine and trimethyl-silylating agents, and were finally applied to GC/MS. The intensities of molecular ions were used for the calculation of the serum concentration of steroids. The molecular ion peaks of steroids were obtained at m/z460(17-hydroxyprogesterone;17OHP), m/z470(11-deoxycortisol;S), m/z417(pregnenolone;PL), m/z372 (progesterone;PT), m/z558(cortisol;F), m/z389(dehydroepiandrosterone; DHEA), m/z371(estorone;E1), m/z416(estradiol;E2), m/z389(testosterone;T), m/z344(androstenedione;A) and m/z372 (IS). The sensitivities of the GC/MS method were less than 5pg/one shot of each sample. The coefficients of variations of accuracies and precisions in this GC/MS method were less than 7% of each steroid. In 2 fresh cases of congenital adrenal hyperplasia of simple type, the basal steroid levels obtained by GC/MS method were shown as 2.34, 2.63ng/ml for PT, 64.5, 25.0ng/ml for 17OHP, 1.31, 1.33ng/ml for S, 25.5, 16.9ng/ml for F, 4.19, 3.21ng/ml for DHEA, 2.2, 0.58ng/ml for T, 32.4, 27.4pg/ml for E1 and 20.0, 11.1pg/ml for E2, respectively. These results implied the usefulness of our system in clinical standpoint. Moreover, our assay takes only 3 hrs. This showed it saves much time in comparrison with the consuming time of radioimmunoassay system.

897 INDUCTION OF OVULATION WITH PULSATILE INTRAVENOUS INJECTIONS OF GONADOTROPIN-RELEASING HORMONE (GnRH) R.P.S. Jansen*, D.J. Handelsman and L.M. Boylan, Departments of Obstetrics and Gynaecology and of Endocrinology, Royal Prince Alfred Hospital, Sydney 2050, Australia.

Studies have shown that GnRH is released into the hypophyseal portal venous system in a pulsatile manner; that GnRH has a half-life of only a few minutes in the circulation; and that either increasing the frequency of pulses much above 1 per 60 minutes or administering long-acting GnRH-analogs desensitizes the pituitary and abolishes response. Using an intravenous pulsatile (q90m, 2.5-5ug/pulse) GnRH regimen up to ovulation, followed by hCG 1500 U i.m. every 4 to 5 days for 3 doses to support the luteal phase after stopping GnRH, we have induced ovulation (a) in 5 of 5 cycles studied in 2 patients with primary amenorrhea (with one singleton pregnancy), and (b) in 17 of 17 cycles studied in 10 patients with weight-loss-related, clomiphene-resistant secondary amenorrhea (with 6 singleton and 2 twin pregnancies). The mean duration of the follicular phase was longer in patients with primary amenorrhea (16 ± 1.9 days [mean $\pm$ S.E.]) than with secondary amenorrhea (11.5 ± 0.5 days) ($P < 0.01$). Life table analysis of the pooled results (n=12 patients; T=22 cycles; C_T=9 conceptions) indicates a monthly probability of pregnancy $\hat{f}=0.41$. Intravenous GnRH regimens are particularly effective for ovulation induction in primary and severe secondary hypothalamic amenorrhea, but more work on optimum dosage for individual patients is needed (and is underway); preliminary observations suggest that 2.5ug/pulse is sufficient in most patients with secondary amenorrhea, but that more than 5ug/pulse may be needed for optimum results in primary amenorrhea.

898 A URINARY STEROID STUDY OF CONGENITAL ADRENAL HYPERPLASIA (CAH) DUE TO AN 11β-HYDROXYLASE DEFICIENCY (11β-HD). G.E. Joannou*, Biochemistry Department, Royal Prince Alfred Hospital, Camperdown, Sydney, 2050, Australia.

The identification and role of 3α,15β,17α-trihydroxy-5β-pregnan-20-one [I], in perinatal diagnosis of CAH was first reported in a urinary study of neonates by gas chromatography-mass spectrometry [G.E. Joannou, *J steroid Biochem.* 14(1981)901-12]. A similar study is reported here for the diagnosis of CAH in a pregnant woman who had previously given birth to two male sibs affected with 11β-HD. The male children were 9 and 12 years' old when first presented for study. Antenatal diagnosis of 11β-HD based on maternal urinary levels of 3α,17α,21-trihydroxy-5β-pregnan-20-one (THS) throughout pregnancy, did not show any significant disparity from normal pregnancies until after the 27th week of gestation when THS levels of 0.4mg/24h rose to 8.16mg/24h urine by the 36th week and exponentially to 32.7mg/24h one week before birth. The urinary levels of THS in the affected male newborn were greatly diminished (0.67mg/24h). The results on antenatal cortisol disfunction may be the first direct evidence obtained so far on the onset of foetal cortisol synthesis since lack of feedback control between ACTH and foetal cortisol accentuated the exact timing of the process. Two significant steroid hydroxylations have emerged in this study, viz., the 15β-hydroxylation of progesterone metabolites in perinatal and 18-hydroxylation of 17-ketosteroids in pre-pubertal CAH. The former has been considered an exclusive function of the foetus. The identification of I in the urinary extracts of the newborn and its possible implication in antenatal diagnosis of CAH, is highlighted by the fact that diagnosis of this syndrome has so far been based on steroid determinants common to both the foetal and maternal compartments.

899 ENDOGENOUS TOTAL TISSUE CORTISOL/ETC/IN PERIPHERAL TISSUES/PT/AND ADRENALS OF GUINEA-PIGS AFTER NARCOSIS/N/AND HEATBURN SHOCK/HBS/

A.T.A.Fazekas*[1] E. Kramer[2] A.Zentai[2] A.K.Fazekas[1] and A.G.Fazekas[1] Exp.Surgery, McGill University Montreal[1] and Medical Faculty, University of Ulm, Germany[2]

Since endogenous total tissue corticosteroids/ETC/are still neglected in shock or stress we have studied ETC concentration/measured by competitive protein binding and confirmed by RIA/in 8 peripheral tissues, plasma and adrenals in 48 adult female colored guinea-pigs 1/2,3 and 6 hours after 3-5 minutes ethylether narcosis/EN/and after HBS induced by II-III degree heatburn of 25-30% of body surface. Total ETC concentration/expressed in µg/100g/ of untreated guinea-pigs/taken as 100%/were as follows: liver 12.4±0.7 /SEM/ kidney 9.6±1.21, spleen 1.2±0.17, muscle 1.3±0.11, lung 3.0±0.41, heart 2.1±0.25 cerebrum 0.6±0.11, cerebellum 0.7±0.17, adrenals 909.3±90.2, plasma 10.25±1.56 Compaired to untreated level 1/2hour after EN ETC values/in %/increased significantly to peak level/li:308, ki:547, spl:533, mu:453, lu:543, he:595, Cer:833, cereb:728, adr:435, pl:694/and subsequently decreased upto 6 h with values between 108 and 246%. During HBS an enormous increase and accumulation of ETC was observed peaking at 3h/values in % of control/li:4201, ki:4947, spl:2858, mu:4584, lu:4303, he:4219, ce:4150, cereb:4414, adr:390, pl:1118/which declined 6h after, remaining still between 1070 and 1855% except adrenals/280%/and plasma/483%/. Our results showed: during stress or shock PT are capable to take up and concentrate a 28-49 times higher amount of corticosteroids than under normal conditions. The 7.7-11.9 times larger increase of ETC in PT related to the 2.4-3.0 times higher increase in adrenals and plasma in HBS compared to EN stress may be in correlation with the uptake capacity of corticosteroid receptors in PT and with the intensity of shock indicating the importance of ETC measurement beside receptor analysis.

900 BIOCHEMICAL AND BIOLOGICAL CHARACTERIZATION OF RABBIT AND HEIFERS EMDOMETRIAL CELLS IN CULTURE.

M.A. Fortier*, M. Boulanger, R.D. Lambert, M.A. Sirard and C. Bernard. Génétique moléculaire (Reproduction), CHUL, Québec, G1V 4G2, Canada.

Epithelial and stromal cells were isolated from endometrium by trypsin and trypsin-collagenase-DNase digestion respectively. Dispersed cells were grown in RPMI 1640 supplemented with 10% fetal calf serum (FCS) whole or steroid depleted by dextran-charcoal (DC) treatment. The cells reached confluency after 7 to 8 days in culture while growth monitored by protein and DNA content, proceeded for 2 days past confluency. Growth rate was higher in whole serum than in DC treated serum. Control rate could be recovered in DC groups by adding increasing doses of sex steroids. Epithelial cell growth was maximally stimulated by 1 nM progesterone and unaffected by estradiol 1 nM to 1 µM while stromal cell growth was optimal with 100 nM estradiol and unaffected or inhibited by progesterone 1 nM to 1 µM. The cultures were stable for 3 weeks in the rabbit and 7 to 8 weeks in heifers. Trials of spermatozoa capacitation were also performed on the cells. Capacitation was evaluated by *in vitro* fertilization of rabbit tubal oocytes or bovine follicular oocytes. A 17 h incubation of rabbit spermatozoa (0.5×10^6 cells/ml) on stromal cells enhanced both fertilization and cleavage rates. Preliminary results in the bovine have shown fertilization and cleavage after capacitation over the cells under conditions where there was no fertilization in the control. Our results suggest that endometrial cells in culture have physiological and functional properties similar to their *in vivo* counterpart and should prove useful in reproductive biology to study gametes-and embryo-genital tract interactions.

901 Comparative Structural Analyses of Corticosteroid Binding Globulin. E.A. Kato and R.W. Kuhn*, Department of Obstetrics, Gynecology & Reproductive Sciences, University of California, San Francisco, CA 94143.

Plasma samples from a variety of species were analyzed using the polyacrylamide gel electrophoresis (PAGE) technique of Ferguson and sucrose density centrifugation to determine native molecular weight estimates for their CBG-like binding proteins. The following molecular weight estimates were obtained: guinea pig (58,600); rat (54,000); dog (44,000); sheep (57,500); human (60,000); cynamologous monkey (53,500); squirrel monkey (120,000); and turtle (60,000). In addition, CBG was purified to homogeneity from the sera of human, guinea pig, and rat. Molecular weight estimates for the purified proteins as determined by SDS-PAGE were consistent with the above results. Westphal and coworkers have previously demonstrated that purified human CBG consists of two distinct molecular variants when carefully analyzed by PAGE. We have confirmed these results and in addition have found that the purified rat and guinea pig proteins display similar heterogeneity. This suggests that CBG's from a variety of species may consist of more than a single electrophoretic variant. HPLC-tryptic peptide maps of the purified proteins appear nearly identical for the rat and human proteins and are very similar for the guinea pig CBG. Only the three least hydrophobic peptides of the guinea pig protein are different from those of the other two species. Antibodies have been generated against the purified proteins and have been used to assess similarities between the proteins from these three species. Despite their marked similarities in physical characteristics, no cross reactivity between species has been detected. (Supported by HD-10328).

902 THE EFFECTS OF GONADOTROPINS IN VITRO ON OOCYTE MATURATION AND CYCLIC NUCLEOTIDE CHANGES IN THE HAMSTER. C. J. Hubbard*, Department of Anatomy, University of South Dakota School of Medicine, Vermillion, SD 57069.

A possible association between oocyte maturation and inverse changes in adenosine 3':5' cyclic monophosphate (cAMP) and guanosine 3':5' cyclic monophosphate (cGMP) has been described previously by this researcher in hamster graafian follicles following gonadotropin stimulation *in vivo* (Life Sci. 33:1695-1702, 1983). In the present study incubations of whole hamster graafian follicles with ovine LH (NIAMMD oLH-24, 1ng-1μg/ml) produced increases in cAMP and declines in cGMP which were dose dependent. Oocyte maturation occurred after 6 hours incubation time in groups which showed a rise in the cAMP/cGMP ratio that was significantly higher than the controls (incubation in plain medium). Both ovine and rat FSH (NIAMMD-oFSH-14; rat FSH-B-1) also stimulated a rise in the cAMP/cGMP ratio and oocyte maturation but only at the highest dose used (10μg/ml). Ovine FSH was also a more potent stimulator of cAMP than was rat FSH. When follicles were incubated with methylisobutyl xanthine (0.2 mM MIX) plus LH (10μg/ml) oocyte maturation was inhibited. Though the cAMP/cGMP ratio rose significantly, cGMP levels never declined as they did when follicles were incubated with LH or FSH alone. cAMP levels were also much higher than those seen in the LH or FSH incubations. These data confirm our previous studies *in vivo* which indicated that inverse changes in cAMP and cGMP which produce a rise in the cAMP/cGMP ratio may be related to oocyte maturation in the hamster.

903 THE EFFECT OF SEVERAL HORMONES ON THE CYCLIC 3',5'- NUCLEOTIDE PHOSPHODIESTERASE IN RAT KIDNEY.
K. Iwase*, A. Nagasaka, K. Miura, K. Kawase, H. HIDAKA°, H. Isaji, A. Nakai, T. Aono, T. Ohyama and H. Nakagawa, Fujita-Gakuen Univ. and °Mie Univ. School of Medicine, Toyoake, Aichi 470-11,Japan.

Kidney function is regulated by several hormones which act through cyclic nucleotide metabolism. We investigated cyclic AMP- and cyclic GMP-phosphodiesterase(cAMP-PDE and cGMP-PDE respectively) activities in the rat kidney and also the effect of several hormones affecting kidney function on these enzyme activities in vitro. Rat kidney cortex(C) and medulla(M) were homogenized in 50mM Tris-HCl buffer, pH 7.5, containing 0.32M sucrose and fractionated. PDE activity was measured using the two-step assay system. Substantial activity was present in all of the fractions and most of the activity existed in the soluble fraction. The effect of $1\alpha,25(OH)_2D_3(D_3)$, parathyroid hormone, antidiuretic hormone(ADH), calcitonin(CT), angiotensin II and trichrolomethiazide on cAMP-PDE and cGMP-PDE purified by Sepharose 6B column chromatography was examined. D_3 activated cAMP-PDE activity and did not affect cGMP-PDE activity. The concentrations of D_3 producing 50% activation of cAMP-PDE activity were 5.0×10^{-11}M(C) and 6.7×10^{-10}M(M). CT and ADH inhibited both cAMP-PDE and cGMP-PDE activities. The concentrations of CT producing 50% inhibition of cAMP-PDE activity were 4.0×10^{-5}M(C) and 3.3×10^{-7}M(M), and those of cGMP-PDE activity were 1.0×10^{-5}M(C) and 1.0×10^{-4} M(M). Concerning ADH, the concentrations required for 50% inhibition of cAMP-PDE activity were 5.3×10^{-6}M(C) and about 1.0×10^{-3}M(M), and those of cGMP-PDE activity were 5.3×10^{-3}M(C) and 5.3×10^{-8}M(M). The data described here imply that these hormones may control kidney function through cyclic nucleotide metabolism by affecting cAMP-PDE and/or cGMP-PDE activity.

904 ESTROGEN AFFECTS HORMONE-SENSITIVE ADENYLATE CYCLASE IN CULTURED MYOMETRIAL CELLS.
J.F. Krall, N. Jamgotchian, and S.G. Korenman*, Dept. of Medicine, UCLA San Fernando Valley Program, VA Medical Center, Sepulveda, CA 91343, USA.

Isoproterenol (ISO) and other β-adrenergic catecholamines have relaxing effects on myometrium. Sex steroids have a profound effect on uterine motility and on sensitivity to ISO. We investigated the interaction between estradiol (E_2) and ISO using primary culture of cells from 21 day old rat myometrium. These cells had many properties of uterine smooth muscle including an elongated spindle shape and receptors for prostaglandin $F_{2\alpha}$, carbachol, and ISO as shown by the effects of these agonists on $^{45}Ca^{+2}$-efflux and adenylate cyclase (AC). Treatment with 1nM E_2 stimulated culture growth as evidenced by a 2.2 ± 0.4-fold (mean $\pm$ S.E., n=4) increase in acid insoluble ^{3}H-thymidine incorporation after but not before 11 days of continuous exposure to E_2 in RPMI 1640 medium with 10% charcoal extracted fetal calf serum where E_2 was replenished every 4 days and no breakdown occurred with incubation. Basal AC activity was unchanged in cells grown in E_2 vs. controls, 100 ± 18 vs. 125 ± 10 pMoles cAMP/mg.min respectively but GTP stimulated AC was markedly reduced ($p < 0.01$) 147 ± 30 vs. 286 ± 55 pMoles/mg.min ($p < 0.01$) and hormone stimulated AC (GTP+ISO) reduced to 344 ± 43 vs. 514 ± 81 pMoles/mg.min ($p < 0.01$). As with AC from myometrium, GTP binding is an essential step in coupling the ISO-receptor with the AC catalytic subunit (C) in these cultured cells. E_2 treatment therefore seems to have specific effects on AC proximal to C, perhaps at the level of the GTP requiring coupling step. The capacity of E_2 to modify β-adrenergic catecholamine-dependent AC *in vitro* may shed light on the sex-steroid sensitivity of contractility that exists *in vivo*.

905 EVIDENCE OF ECTOPIC PRODUCTION OF THE ACTH-PRECURSOR BY HUMAN MEDULLARY THYROID CARCINOMA. C.J.M. Lips*, P.H. Steenbergh, J.W.M. Höppener and H.S. Jansz, Department of Internal Medicine, Institute of Molecular Biology and Laboratory of Physiological Chemistry, State University, Utrecht, The Netherlands.

Ectopic production of one or several peptide hormones has been reported to occur in a number of neoplasms, e.g. oatcell carcinoma of the lung, pancreatic islet cell carcinoma and medullary thyroid carcinoma (MTC). In the case of MTC, usually producing calcitonin (CT), ectopic production of ACTH may lead to Cushing's syndrome. The incidence in patients with MTC was estimated to be about 3%. This is in contrast with the high degree of coincidental histochemical localization of both ACTH and CT demonstrated in MTC. We investigated the production of the ACTH precursor proopiomelanocortin (POMC) by MTC. Messenger-RNA from 8 patients was isolated and screened by Northern blot analysis. All tumours were found to contain mRNA hybridizing to a CT specific probe. However, POMC related sequences were detected only in two cases. Compared with the POMC mRNA occurring in the human pituitary gland, the size of the RNA hybridizing to the POMC specific probe was longer in the MTC metastases of our patients. Copy-DNA complementary to mRNA from one of the metastases was cloned in pBR322. From this MTC library two plasmids were isolated containing inserts which proved to be completely homologous to a sequence of 190 nucleotides from the 3'-end of human pituitary POMC mRNA. It was concluded that the presence of mRNA encoding POMC in MTC implies that the tissue is capable of producing this peptide. The POMC gene is expressed in MTC, possibly due to a derepression mechanism. Expression occurs, however, only in a small percentage of cases.

906 ON THE ROLE OF HAMSTER ANDROGEN-INDUCED EPIDIDYMAL PROTEINS IN SPERM MATURATION. P.Cuasnicu, M.G.Echeverria, A.Piazza, L. Pineiro, J.Blaquier*.Instituto de Biologia y Medicina Experimental, Buenos Aires 1428, Argentina.

We intend to demonstrate that the increase in zona pellucida binding (ZPb) and fertility of spermatozoa during maturation is partly due to their interaction with androgen-dependent epididymal proteins (EP). Epididymal tubules were cultured for 24-48h. Addition of 2uM dihydrotestosterone (DHT) to the medium stimulated the synthesis of several proteins whose electrophoretic mobility was coincident with those of EP previously shown in vivo. These proteins could also be extracted from spermatozoa contained in the stimulated tubules. The ZPb of these spermatozoa was significantly greater than controls (5.51 vs 0.87 sperm/egg respectively, $P<0.001$). The effect was lost when cyproterone acetate (4 uM) or cycloheximide (20 uM) were added together with DHT (0.79 and 0.72 sperm/egg respectively). A fraction enriched in EP (3-fold) was obtained from normal hamsters and when added to the medium (1 mg/ml) significantly increased ZPb of contained sperm (0.55 vs 2.73 sperm/egg in control and EP treated cultures, respectively, $P<0.02$) Equal amount of protein prepared from epididymides of castrated hamsters (EPc) was unable to produce this effect. EP also increased the fertility of distal corpus sperm when present (1.6 mg/ml) in the fluid used for in vivo artificial insemination (13% vs 24% fertilized oocytes in control vs EP exposed sperm, $P< 0.01$). The effect was also observed in in vitro fertilization tests (25% vs 45% fertilized eggs in control vs EP exposed sperm, $P< 0.05$). These effects were not elicited by EPc. We propose that EP participate in the development of ZPb and fertility during maturation in the epididymis.

907 EFFECT OF LEVONORGESTREL RELEASING IUD ON ENDOMETRIAL ESTRADIOL AND PROGESTERONE RECEPTORS IN MONKEY. Farooq, A*, Dileep Kumar and Vijay Kumar, Department of Reproductive Biology, All India Institute of Medical Sciences, NEW DELHI-110029, India.

In order to investigate the mechanism of contraceptive action of levonorgestrel (Ng) administered in utero from a 24 mm long silastic capsule (i.d. 1.57 mm, o.d. 2.41 mm and release rate of Ng 7.2 μg/day) attached to a small polyethylene-T, estradiol receptors (ER) and progesterone receptors (PR) were measured in endometrium. The Ng-IUD and a plain IUD without any Ng was inserted into the uterine cavity of treatment and control group of monkeys, respectively. After a period of 6 months, 4 monkeys from each group were hysterectomized in follicular (FP, day 8 to 12) and luteal phase (LP, day 20 to 24), endometrium homogenized in Tris-HCl 10 mM (pH 7.4, EDTA 0.5 mM, thioglycerol 12 mM) and cytosolic ER and PR estimated by radioreceptor assay. The ER concentration in FP and LP was 271 ± 37 and 67 ± 8 in the Ng group whereas it was 939 ± 85 and 336 ± 18 f mol/mg protein in the control group. The PR concentration in FP and LP was 23 ± 9 and 18 ± 7 in the Ng group whereas it was 403 ± 27 and 89 ± 12 f mol/mg protein in the control group. The present data demonstrate that Ng released in the uterus from an IUD inhibits the action of endogenous estradiol and progesterone by suppressing endometrial ER and PR and may, thereby, render the endometrium unsuitable for embryo implantation. (Supported by the Indian Council of Medical Research, New Delhi)

908 IMMUNOREACTIVE INSULIN IN OVINE MILK. J. Falconer*, R. F. Sheldrake and J. S. Robinson, Faculty of Medicine, University of Newcastle. Newcastle. NSW 2308, Australia.

Many hormones have been detected in the milk of various mammals usually at concentrations similar to, or lower than, plasma levels. Little is known of whether these hormones are important for the process of lactation or for the neonate. We have measured immunoreactive insulin in milk obtained from sheep. Immunoreactive insulin was measured using an RIA with ovine insulin (Eli Lilly, Indianapolis) as tracer and standard (1 ng of this standard was equivalent to 24 μU of porcine insulin). Samples were obtained from two groups of sheep. In the first, 4 sheep were sampled daily for 2 to 10 days post partum (pp). The concentration of insulin in milk was very high on day 1 pp (98 ± 44 ng/ml, n = 4) and declined rapidly over the first 6 days of lactation ($6.6 \pm$ Q.1 ng/ml on day 6 pp, n = 3) although concentrations were still high in relation to normal plasma concentrations (0.5 - 2ng/ml). In the second group milk samples with paired plasma samples were obtained from 19 ewes sampled at various stages of lactation including post-weaning. The insulin content of milk was always higher than plasma (ratio milk: plasma ranging from 1.9 to 111). The concentration of prolactin in milk was lower than in plasma in 14 out of 18 of these pairs of samples. This data indicates that insulin is specifically concentrated in ovine milk.

It is suggested that insulin in milk may alter glucose metabolism in the neonate in addition to any possible effects on the function of the mammary gland.

909 MATERNAL FACTORS REGULATE MIDGESTATIONAL PROGESTERONE SECRETION IN THE MOUSE. R. FitzGerald and M. Barkley*, Department of Animal Physiology, University of California, Davis, CA 95616, USA.

The maintenance of mouse pregnancy depends on the continuous secretion of luteal progesterone. At midgestation pituitary stimulation of luteal function is relinquished to placental factors by unknown mechanisms. We have studied the relative luteotropic roles of maternal and fetal-placental secretions at midgestation in strains of mice known to differ in maternal levels of progesterone (P). The genotype of the embryo and dam were varied by performing reciprocal blastocyst transfers in strains with high (line S1) or low (line G) maternal P levels. Intraline blastocyst transfers were performed to provide experimental controls. Plasma samples for the radioimmunologic determination of P were collected following decapitation on days 8, 9, or 10 of pregnancy (day 0 = day of vaginal plug). Although the duration of gestation is correlated with the genotype of the embryo ($p < 0.05$), maternal levels of P are consistent with the genotype of the dam ($p < 0.05$) regardless of the number of fetuses present. On day 9 maternal P levels in S1 recipients of S1 embryos (intraline transfers) = 29.6 ± 1.8 ng/ml; P levels in G recipients of G embryos = 12.5 ± 4.8 ng/ml; in S1 recipients of G embryos P = 24.7 ± 1.2 ng/ml; and in G recipients of S1 embryos P = 14.8 ± 1.2 ng/ml. These results provide the first evidence that at midgestation the setpoint for luteotropic stimulation of the ovary is determined by factors derived from the mother rather than the fetus. This study was supported by HD 00394.

910 DEXAMETHASONE INDUCES ORGAN-SPECIFIC DEVELOPMENTAL PROTEINS (fsa, fsb) IN RAT LUNG FIBROBLASTS. J. Floros*, D.S. Phelps and B.T. Smith. Department of Pediatrics, Harvard Medical School, Boston, MA, 02115.

Glucocorticoids enhance fetal lung maturation. Previous studies with whole lung have shown that specific proteins are induced by these hormones. Several glucocorticoid effects on fetal lung epithelia require the presence of mesenchyme. Since the lung consists of multiple cell types, further understanding of glucocorticoid effects on fetal lung requires study of individual cell types. Using two-dimensional gel electrophoresis, we have examined the synthesis and secretion of ^{35}S-methionine labeled proteins by fetal rat lung fibroblasts in the presence and absence of glucocorticoid. Two proteins, fsa and fsb, are induced by dexamethasone, whereas over 100 other secreted proteins detected in this system are unaffected under these conditions. Fsa and fsb are organ specific in that they are not secreted or induced by dexamethasone in fibroblasts from fetal rat liver, skin or kidney. They are induced only during prenatal and early postnatal life but not during adult life. Fsa and fsb are not induced by a variety of other hormones, including dihydrotestosterone, tri-iodothyronine, estradiol-17β or an analogue of progesterone (17,21-dimethyl-19-nor-pregna-4,9-diene-3,20-dione). These data demonstrate that during lung development in the rat, the synthesis and secretion of specific proteins (fsa and fsb) are regulated in the mesenchyme by glucocorticoids.

(Supported by the American Lung Association and by NIH HL-27372)

911 PRENATAL TREATMENT OF CONGENITAL ADRENAL HYPERPLASIA (CAH) DUE TO 21-HYDROXYLASE DEFICIENCY. M.C.Forest+ and M.David. INSERM-U.34 and Endocrine Clinic Hôpital Debrousse. 69322 Lyon Cedex 05. France.

Six at risk mothers were started on either cortisol (F) (n =1) or dexamethasone (Dex) (n =5) before 9 Wks'gestation. Karyotype, HLA-typing, amniotic fluid (AF) levels of 17-OH-Progesterone (OHP), Estriol (E_3) and F were determined at 16-18 Wks: only 2 females were CAH affected. Treatment was stopped in the other 4. In the families of the 2 CAH fetuses, the first CAH sib. had severely masculinized genitalia (stage IV and IV-V). Mother n°1 received oral F (40 mg from 9 to 18 Wks, then 50 mg until term): mother n°2 received Dex (0.5 mg qid from 5 Wks to term). Steroids are given in ng/dl. 1) Maternal adrenal suppression was documented by drastic fall in plasma DHA and F. 2) Transplacental passage of F was shown by high AF levels of F at 18 Wks (2391). 3) Fetal adrenal suppression: in case n°1, it was not achieved at 18 Wks as shown by maternal E_3 (465) or AF level of OHP (981), but was partial at term (near normal E_3 in AF = 364); it was complete in case n°2 low normal AF levels of OHP (49) and E_3 (103) at 16th Wks, lack of rise in maternal E_3 (25-60 at 4-32 Wks). 4) Proof of severe form of CAH was obtained after birth, before treatment: case n°1 plasma OHP = 21,510 on day 1; in case n°2, OHP normal on day 1 rose to 11,320 on day 6. 5) Clinical results: in child n°1 (stade II), clitoral size decreased with age; she is now 4 yrs and no surgery will be needed. Child n°2 had normal genitalia. The 6 pregnancies were uneventfull and all newborns normal. In conclusion, fetal adrenal suppression can be achieved by a simple oral maternal treatment. Dex is more effective than F. This treatment may prevent *in utero* virilization in CAH female fetus.

912 MATURATION OF SOMATOTROPES IN FETAL RAT PITUITARIES: ANALYSIS BY REVERSE HEMOLYTIC PLAQUE ASSAY (RHPA) & IMMUNOCYTOCHEMISTRY (ICC). L.S. Frawley*, J. Hoeffler & F.R. Boockfor, Zool. Dept., Iowa State Univ., Ames 50011 USA

Considerable radioimmunological and immunocytochemical evidence indicates that somatotropes first appear within pituitaries of fetal rats during the last few days of gestation. However, the temporal relationships between hormone production and secretion by somatotropes and the onset of responsiveness of these cells to secretagogues is not understood. In the present study we investigated these aspects of somatotrope development by using an RHPA to detect individual GH-secreting cells in cultures of fetal pituitaries and ICC to identify GH-containing cells in the same cultures. Trypsin-dispersed pituitary cells from fetal rats on days 18-21 of gestation were cultured for 24 hr and subjected to ICC and RHPA for GH. Growth hormone-containing cells rose from undetectable levels on day 18 to 19.9%, 21.7% and 24.9% of all cultured cells on days 19, 20 and 21, respectively. The proportion of GH-secreting cells as determined in long-term (2 hr) plaque assays was 21.9% and 23.2% for days 20 and 21, respectively, but only 12.8% for day 19 cells. Thus, many cultured cells from day 19 fetuses contained but did not secrete GH. While growth hormone-releasing factor (1 x 10^{-7}M) had no effect on the percentage of GH plaque-forming cells in long-term incubations, the secretagogue enhanced (to approximately the same degree in day 19-21 groups) the rate of plaque development (196.1 $\pm$ 27.2%, $\bar{X} \pm$ SEM, of control value) and the size of plaques formed (165.3 $\pm$ 4.8% of control) in short-term (45 min) incubations. These results demonstrate that somatotropes appear within an extremely narrow time-frame during development and suggest that GH production, secretion and responsiveness to secretagogues evolve sequentially. (Supported by NIH Grant AM-33943 to LSF)

913 OVINE PLACENTAL LACTOGEN (oPL) INHIBITS cAMP- AND CALCIUM-MEDIATED GLYCOGENOLYSIS IN FETAL RAT HEPATOCYTES. M. Freemark* and S. Handwerger, Dept. of Pediatrics, Duke Medical Center, Durham, N.C., U.S.A. 27710

Recent studies from this lab have demonstrated that oPL stimulates glycogen synthesis in fetal rat hepatocytes. To examine further the actions of oPL on glycogen metabolism in fetal liver, hepatocytes from 20 day rat fetuses were treated with oPL or diluent for 20-60 minutes. The cells were then exposed to glucagon, isoproterenol or dibutyryl cAMP (dBcAMP), which increase intracellular cAMP, or to the ionophore A23187, which increases cytosolic free calcium. In diluent-treated cells, glucagon (1nM), isoproterenol (1uM), dBcAMP (0.1mM) and A23187 (1uM) each inhibited ^{14}C-glucose incorporation into glycogen by 42-51% ($p<0.01$). However, when cells were treated with oPL (1ug/ml) as well as these glycogenolytic agents, glycogen synthesis was inhibited by only 6-15% ($p<0.01$). Higher concentrations of oPL (>2ug/ml) stimulated glycogen synthesis even in the presence of glucagon or A23187, though to a lesser degree than did oPL alone. OPL (5ug/ml) alone had no effect on phosphorylase a activity (Pa) but inhibited the stimulation of Pa by glucagon (1nM) or A23187 (1uM) by 71 and 30% ($p<0.02$). The effects of oPL (5ug/ml) on glycogen synthesis were abolished by incubation of cells with cycloheximide (50 uM). These studies suggest that the action of oPL on glycogen synthesis occurs at a site distal to the cytosolic accumulation of cAMP and calcium and depends upon protein synthesis. OPL may contribute to fetal hepatic glycogen storage in late gestation by both stimulating glycogen synthesis and antagonizing the glycogenolytic actions of glucagon and catecholamines. NIH grants HD07447 and HD06301.

914 STUDY ON THE SUCCESSIVE CHANGE OF BLOOD TSH, T4, T3, FT4, FT3 AND TBG IN PREMATURE INFANTS - INVESTIGATION ON 76 SAME INDIVIDUALS, Y. Fuse[1]*, N. Uga[1], T. Fujii[1], Y. Fuse[2], K. Inoue[2] and M. Irie[2], 1) Perinatal Center, 2) First Dept. of Med., Toho Univ. School of Med., Tokyo, 143 Japan.

76 low birth weight infants less than 2500g at birth were selected for the study. Cord blood, venous or capillary blood were taken at the time of hospitalization, and once weekly until 40 to 42 weeks, then once monthly. TSH and T4 were measured using filter paper blood spots, and T3, FT4, FT3 and TBG were measured using serum by RIA. Birth weight range was 480 to 2499g, average 1601g, and gestational ages were 22 to 43, average 31 week. Birth weights include less than 1000g (12 cases), 1000 to 1499 (17), 1500 to 1999 (24) and 2000 to 2499 (23). 20 cases of normal infants were studied as the control. In low birth weight infants, most cases showed high TSH values more than 10 μu/ml, and clear surge was observed in 6 cases. During time course, TSH showed large variability within normal range. T4 was average 1.4 ug/dl at 23 week (w), 4.2 at 28w, 5.6 at 32w, 7.7 at 36w and reached 10.3 at 40w. T3 was also low, average 0.3 to 0.9 ng/ml from birth to 32w, reaching 10.3 at 40w. There was no significant change of FT4 and FT3 following day of life, FT4 ranged 0.9 to 2.0 ng/dl, FT3 ranged 1.0 to 5.5 pg/ml. TBG was low from birth to 29w, average value being less than 20 μg/ml, then increased to 20 to 25 μg/ml. Among 12 cases less than 1000g weight, 7 cases died. Most of these cases showed T4 less than average at the time of death, thus this decrease appeared to be related to the mortality.

915 PERINATAL REGULATION OF ORNITHINE TRANSCARBAMYLASE (OTC) IN RAT LIVER. II-EFFECTS OF GLUCOSE, ACTINOMYCIN D AND INSULIN IN NEONATAL LIVER.
C. Gautier*, M. Belbekouche and R. Vaillant. Groupe de Recherches "Régul. Métaboliques, ERA CNRS 891, Fac. Sciences, Univ. Haute Normandie, 76130 Mont-Saint-Aignan, France.

Repeatedly supplementing glucose after birth (25 mg every two hours) abolishes postnatal increase in ornithine transcarbamylase activity. Immunoreactive OTC remains at the level found in 21.5 day-old foetuses and plasma insulin level increases as measured 24 hours later. A single administration of actinomycin D (3 µg) does not affect this activity. When glucose and actinomycin D are administered in association at birth or 13 hours after birth, actinomycin D overcomes the inhibitory effect of glucose on enzyme activity and decreases insulinemia to the level found in normal neonates. Insulin supply (40 mU) 20 hours after birth to neonates which previously received glucose and actinomycin D, decreases enzyme activity and increases plasma insulin level. It is concluded that the postnatal rise in OTC activity is bound to the normal decrease in insulinemia. Furthermore, the paradoxical effect of actinomycin D on enzyme activity might be due to an inhibition of insulin synthesis or insulin release.

916 PERINATAL REGULATION OF ORNITHINE TRANSCARBAMYLASE (OTC) IN RAT LIVER. I-EFFECTS OF CORTISOL AND ACTINOMYCIN D IN FOETAL LIVER.
C. Gautier* and R. Vaillant. Groupe de Recherches "Régul. Métaboliques", ERA CNRS 891, Fac. Sciences, Univ. Haute Normandie, 76130 Mont-Saint-Aignan, France.

Ornithine Transcarbamylase (OTC ; EC 2.1.3.3), located in mitochondrial matrix, catalyses the second step of urea synthesis in rat liver. Its activity appears on day 16.5 of gestation, regularly increases during late foetal period and presents a marked rise 24 hours after birth. OTC was purified from beef liver by affinity chromatography and a rabbit immunserum against OTC was obtained. Quantitation of immunoreactive OTC was performed according to the Mancini method. OTC level is detected on day 16.5 and increases ten fold five days later on day 21.5. Supplementing cortisol on day 18.5 significantly decreases enzyme level (32%) and enzyme activity (42%) three days later. Moreover, actinomycin D supply (2 µg) on day 18.5 significantly increases enzyme activity and decreases foetal insulinemia (about 42%) one day later. This paradoxical effect of actinomycin D on OTC activity might be due to the decrease in an intrauterine repressor. The high plasma insulin level might act as inhibitor of enzyme rise in normal foetuses.

917 THE APPEARANCE OF AROMATASE ACTIVITY IN NEWBORN RAT OVARIES IS REGULATED BY EXTRAGONADAL FACTORS. F. W. George* and S. R. Ojeda, Departments of Cell Biology and Physiology, The University of Texas Health Science Center at Dallas, Southwestern Medical School, Dallas, Texas, USA.

In order to gain insight into the factors regulating the appearance of aromatase activity in the ovary, we have cultured newborn rat ovaries from the day of birth for three days in a serum-free defined medium. At the end of the culture period aromatase activity was assessed by incubating the tissue fragments (3 ovaries; 0.06-0.1 µg protein) with 0.5 µM [1 β-^{3}H]testosterone for 1 h at 37°C in an atmosphere of 95% O_2/5% CO_2 and measuring the amount of ^3H_2O formed. Aromatase activity in rat ovary in situ increased from a baseline level of <0.5 pmol/h/mg protein at birth to >4 pmol/h/mg protein by 3 days after birth. In contrast when cultured in serum-free medium for 3 days after birth, the ovaries failed to develop aromatase activity. The addition of oFSH (100 ng/ml), oLH (100 ng/ml) or the combination of the two hormones failed to induce aromatase activity in cultured ovaries. However, dibutyryl cyclic adenosine monophosphate (0.1-1 mM) and prostaglandin E_2 (2.8 µM) induced a 5-9 fold increase in aromatase activity in the cultured ovaries. More significantly, the diterpene stimulator of adenylate cyclase, forskolin (50 µg/ml) increased aromatase activity 4-fold indicating that the inability of isolated ovaries to develop aromatase activity was due to the absence of an external stimulus and not to an inherent deficiency of the gland. We conclude that the development of aromatase activity in the newborn rat ovary is dependent on extragonadal factor(s), and that cyclic adenosine monophosphate-mediated events are involved in the induction process. (Supported by NIH grants AM03892 and HD-09988-07)

918 EXERCISE-INDUCED HPP SECRETION IN NORMALS AND DIABETICS. Th.Hossdorf[+],E.Zierden and H.Wagner,Medizinische Universitäts-klinik,Abt.B,Domagkstr.3,4400 Münster,BRD.

HPP secretion in man seems to be mediated by vagal,extravagal cholinergic as well as ß-adrenergic stimulation,like muscular exercise.In order to examine ß-adrenergic function in diabetics HPP serum levels were measured by radioimmunoassay(HPP and BPP standard preparation,Antiserum to HPP,generously donated by R. E.Chance,Ely Lilly Co.)in 6 longterm diabetics(aged 20 to 42 years,diabetes duration 10 to 16 years) and in 6 regularly training sportsmen of the same ageduring bicycle labour, starting at 50 watt.Every 10 min.labour increased for 25 w up to 250 or 300 w.For HPP determination blood was drawn twice before and 5 min.after each time labour increased, as well as twice after the test stopped.Basal HPP values didn't vary in both groups:normals:($\bar{x}$+sem)126,00±18,74pg/ml;diabetics:120,12±11,69 pg/ml HPP.In healthy sportsmen HPP levels increased to ($\bar{x}$±sem) 264,00±51,87 pg/ml HPP at 250 w(p<0,01).No change of HPP serum levels could be detected in diabetics.
The obove stated results suggest that ß-adrenergic stimulation of HPP secretion in diabetics may be disturbed.Diminished HPP secretion after ß-adrenergic stimulation in longterm diabetics may be based on decreasing function of the autonomous nervus system caused by longterm disturbance of carbohydrate metabolism.

919 SOMATOSTATIN SECRETION FROM MONOLAYER CULTURES OF RAT ANTRAL CELLS. N. Jacovidou*and Y.C. Patel, Fraser Labs, McGill University, Royal Victoria Hospital, Montreal, Quebec H3A 1A1, Canada.

In the present study we have established monolayer cultures of rat antral cells and characterized them as an in vitro system for studying somatostatin (SLI) secretion. Cells isolated by tryptic digestion of antra from 2 week old rats were plated in 35 mm Petri dishes (5 x 10^6/dish) where they attached within 24 h and grew as monolayer clusters of glandular cells containing within them scattered SLI-positive immunofluorescent cells. Extracts of the scraped cells showed by RIA (Table) a high content of SLI for 96 h followed by a sharp decline associated with detachment and fibroblast overgrowth. Secretion experiments were performed on day 2 by incubating groups of 4 dishes for 4 h with 1 ml control medium (medium 199 + 0.5% fetal calf serum) or medium containing test substances. Basal release of SLI from the cultures was 82.5 ± 12 pg/ml/h and increased significantly to 123 ± 11 ($P < 0.01$) and 113 ± 7.7 ($P < 0.05$) following exposure to 1 ug/ml glucagon or secretin respectively. Released SLI (basal and stimulated) was stable in the medium for >10 h and when assayed in serial dilutions showed parallelism with synthetic S-14. SLI in cell extracts eluted from Sephadex G-50 columns (in 6 M urea) as one major peak (97% of SLI) corresponding to S-14 (KD=0.75) and a minor peak (3% of SLI) of Mr=14K. Released SLI consisted of the same two molecular forms in the same ratio as present intracellularly. Monolayer cultures of antral cells should provide a powerful in vitro system for further studies of gastric somatostatin synthesis and secretion.

Day	SLI in Cells ng/ml (n=4)
1	6.4 ± 0.2
2	6.3 ± 0.8
3	3.2 ± 0.2
4	1.8 ± 0.1
5	0.9 ± 0.02
6	0.7 ± 0.05
7	0.7 ± 0.01

920 GROWTH HORMONE RELEASING FACTOR (GRF) LIKE IMMUNOREACTIVITY IS PRESENT IN HUMAN GASTRIC AND DUODENAL MUCOSA. T.Kobayashi*, S. Sawano, T. Itoh, K. Kosaka, H. Okumura and S. Ohashi, Dept. Endocrinology and Metabolism, Toranomon Hosp.; Okinaka Memorial Inst. for Med. Res; Asahi Life Inst. for Adult Diseases; Teikoku Hormone MFG. Co., LTD.; and Res. Inst. for Polymers and Textiles, Tokyo 105, Japan.

The presence of GRF like immunoreactivity was examined in human gastrointestinal (GI) tissues, which had been sampled from fresh operative specimens. The samples from body and antrum of the stomach and the duodenum were homogenized in 2N acetic acid containing 0.1% β-mercaptoethanol. The supernatant from each extract was lyophilized to dryness. The GRF content of each sample was measured by RIA for GRF-44 using a specific antiserum (G52-6). Bouin-fixed and paraffin-embedded samples from each GI tissue were processed for the immunohistochemical examination according to the PAP or indirect method. In the RIA system of GRF, the extracted samples from the gastric antrum and duodenum displaced the radioiodinated GRF in a parallel manner with synthetic GRF-44. The mean content of GRF in the gastric antral and duodenal mucosa was 245 and 71 pg/mg protein, respectively. GRF like immunoreactivity was found in many cells of the gastric antrum, but only in a few mucosal cells of the duodenum. The GRF-containing cells characteristically opened to the glandular lumen of the stomach and duodenum. We could not find GRF-cotaining cells in the gastric body. The GRF like immunoreactivity in the gut was abolished by pretreatment of the antiserum with synthetic GRF-44. The presence of GRF like immunoreactivity in human GI tract suggests that GRF may play some roles on the nutrient homeostasis through endocrine or paracrine mechanism.

921 CENTRAL REGISTRATION OF FAMILIES WITH A GENETIC PREDISPOSITION TO CANCER IN ENDOCRINE ORGANS. Geerdink, R.A.*, Lips, C.J.M., Department of Internal Medicine, University Hospital Utrecht, Utrecht, The Netherlands.

In several inherited tumor syndromes patients and close relatives realize that the main advantage of periodic screening consists of tracing and removing tumors in a stage when cure is still possible. An example of such a disease is the multiple endocrine neoplasm syndrome type 2. This well-known clinical syndrome is characterized by the autosomal dominant inheritance of the predisposition to medullary thyroid carcinoma in combination with intra- and extra-adrenal phaeochromocytoma. A pilot study with this syndrome as the focus is currently performed in The Netherlands. One way to solve the practical problems involved might be to have the administrative work organized centrally and to decentralize the main screening work. A registration center, supervised by a multi-hospital committee was set up in the University Hospital in Utrecht. Personal data, results of investigation, diagnosis and results of treatment of patients are recorded of patients as well as personal data and screening results of all first degree relatives. The advantages of a central system, including the continuity of periodic screening, free choice of physician and specialist, and optimal coverage, clearly counterbalance the disadvantages, the most important of which is the risk of invasion of the privacy of both patients and relatives. After two years of study, it is concluded that there is a need for central coordination and registration and for decentralized investigation of those individuals with a genetic predisposition to tumor development, provided that both detection in an early stage and effective treatment are possible.

922 EFFECTS OF 2-METHOXYESTRONE ON GONADOTROPINS IN THE HUMAN. Alireza Guerami*, M. Linette Casey, John C. Porter, and Paul C. MacDonald, Cecil H.and Ida Green Center for Reprod. Biol. Sci. and the Depts. of OB-Gyn and Biochem., Univ. of Texas Southwestern Med. Sch., Dallas, TX.

The results of studies in the human and rat are suggestive that catechol estrogens modulate gonadotropin secretion. However, the MCR of catechol estrogens is extraordinarily high (12,000-80,000 L/24 h) presumably due to extensive metabolism of catechol estrogens in the vascular compartment by the action of the catechol-O-methyltransferase in erythrocytes. Thus, the presumed biological effects of catechol estrogens, including the modulation of gonadotropin release might be related to methylated derivatives of catechol estrogens rather than to catechol estrogens per se. The MCR of 2MeO-E1 is 1246 ± 137L/24 h (mean ± SEM, n = 5) in men and women, a value that is markedly less than that of catechol estrogens and thereby appreciable levels of 2MeO-E1 may be in blood. Therefore, we infused 80 µg of 2MeO-E1 in 6% ethanol solution for 4 h into 3 premenopausal women, 1 postmenopausal woman and 2 men. Serum from the blood samples obtained every 20 min for 2 h prior to, and 4 h after the commencement of the infusion was assayed for LH and FSH. We found a 18-60% decrease in LH levels in women at the end of 4 h of infusion, but no change in FSH levels. 2MeO-E1 infusion in men did not affect the serum gonadotropin levels. We suggest that methylated derivatives of catechol estrogens, directly or after the in situ demethylation may modulate serum LH levels in women.

923 BIOLOGICALLY ACTIVE HCG IS PRODUCED IN VITRO BY LHRH-STIMULATED HUMAN TROPHOBLASTIC CELLS. J.F. Guévin*, S.Bélisle, J.G. Lehoux, D.Bellabarba, Sherbrooke, Faculty of Medicine, P.Q., Canada, J1H 5N4

Ongoing studies in our laboratory have demonstrated specific binding of LHRH to human trophoblast. In order to assess the physiological significance of this binding, we studied the production of hCG from midterm and term placentas. Viable human trophoblastic cells were obtained after enzymatic digestion and purification over a Percoll gradient. Dose-response curves were subsequently conducted by incubations with LHRH (10^{-10} M to 10^{-6} M) as well as with synthetic agonists and antagonists of LHRH. HCG was measured immunologically and biologically in the intra and extracellular milieux. Compared to baseline, LHRH and its agonists induced a net synthesis of immunologically and biologically active hCG which was maximal at 1×10^{-7} M of LHRH. Parallel incubations with TRH, oxytocin and LHRH antagonists had no effect. Isobutyl-methyl Xanthine, in a dose-response manner, and dbcAMP also increased hCG production. The synthesis and liberation of immunoassayed hCG was much greater at midterm (414.6 ± 49 and 165.8 ± 24 mU/ml) than at Term(8 ± 17 and 63.8 ± 16.1 mU/ml) and this was paralleled in the bioassays (midterm : 5.9 ± 0.86 and 0.85 ± 0.09 ng Testosterone/200,000 cells /3 hours, Term :2.54 ± 0.29 and 1.34 ± 0.06 ng T/200,000 cells/3 hours). Prolonged incubations with LHRH showed a decrease in hCG production without evidence of LHRH or hCG degradation in the milieu, suggesting a desensitization of the LHRH receptor. These results suggest a biological role for LHRH in the regulation of hCG production. Supported by MRC Canada.

924 GROWTH FACTOR/GONADOTROPIN INTERACTIONS IN FSH-DEPENDENT LH RECEPTOR INDUCTION: PLATELET-DERIVED GROWTH FACTOR (PDGF) PREPARATIONS CONTAIN SEPARATE MITOGENIC AND DIFFERENTIATION-ENHANCING ACTIVITIES. Elizabeth B. Gunn* and David W. Schomberg, Depts. of Physiology and Obstetrics and Gynecology, Duke University Medical Center, Durham, NC 27710

The differentiation of ovarian granulosa cells is critically dependent upon the induction of LH receptors by FSH, a process which can be modulated by PDGF *in vitro*. Further purification of PDGF preparations by column chromatography (Bio-Gel P60) results in the separation of two activities - a mitogenically active component (P60-PDGF, defined by increased DNA synthesis in BALB-3T3 cells) and a differentiation-modulating fraction (DMF, defined by enhancement of FSH-dependent LH receptor induction in cultured granulosa cells isolated from intact, immature, estrogen treated rats). In all preparations tested (n=5) DMF activity was located in column fractions devoid of mitogenic activity (MW 21,000). Further comparison of P60-PDGF and the DMF activities shows that P60-PDGF has no statistically significant effect on either the levels of media cAMP (stim/cont=1.0 ± 0.1, $\bar{x} \pm SE$, n=10) or 125-I-hCG binding (stim/cont=0.8 ± 0.1), of 6-day monolayers following 3-day exposure to various doses of P60-PDGF and 50 or 250ng/ml FSH. In contrast, the DMF consistently increased 125-I-hCG binding (as much as 18-fold over FSH alone) in a dose-dependent manner. However, this was not always reflected in the media cAMP levels. These results indicate that the DMF activity may consist of components which modulate both cAMP-dependent and putative cAMP-independent actions of FSH. Further studies with more highly purified preparations of the DMF will be necessary to resolve these questions.
(Support: Grant No. HD11827, NICHHD)

925 IN VITRO REGULATION OF OVINE PITUITARY GLYCOPROTEIN HORMONE ALPHA SUBUNIT mRNA BY 17β-ESTRADIOL. S. H. Hall* and W. L. Miller*, Department of Biochemistry, Box 7622, North Carolina State University, Raleigh, NC 27695-7622, U.S.A.

In vivo investigations with sheep have previously demonstrated that levels of mRNA for pituitary glycoprotein hormone alpha decrease with 17β-estradiol (E_2) treatment. The present study with dispersed ovine pituitary cell cultures showed that E_2 causes a similar reduction in translatable alpha mRNA levels in vitro. Total RNA was translated in a wheat germ system labelling proteins with [^{35}S]cysteine. Alpha mRNA was quantitated with a two-cycle immunoprecipitation using affinity purified antibody raised to the reduced carbamylmethylated alpha subunit. This assay measured alpha protein from 0.9% of total incorporation of cysteine down to 0.03%. In a time-course experiment, ovine pituitary cultures were treated 0, 1, 2, 3, 4, 5, 6, 7, or 8 days with 10^{-9} M E_2. Secreted alpha protein and translatable alpha mRNA declined to 12% and 8.4% of control values, respectively, and both decreased with a $t_{1/2}$ of about 55 hours. In a dose-response experiment, cultures were treated with 10^{-12} M to 10^{-8} M E_2 continuously for 8 days. The decreases in secreted alpha protein and alpha mRNA activity paralleled one another with the midpoint of the dose-response curves near 3 X 10^{-11} M E_2 in both cases. While it may be possible for E_2 to decrease alpha mRNA in vivo by a secondary mechanism such as through the hypothalamus, our data indicate that 17β-estradiol can act directly at the pituitary to reduce alpha mRNA and thus the secreted alpha protein. (Supported in part by NIH Grant HD 10773)

926 ALTERATIONS IN LUTEINIZING HORMONE SECRETION IN ADULT MALE AND FEMALE RATS FOLLOWING FETAL EXPOSURE TO ALCOHOL. Robert J. Handa*, Robert F. McGivern and Roger A. Gorski. Lab. of Neuroendo. and Br. Res. Inst., Dept. of Anat. UCLA and Dept. of Psych., Harbor Med. Ctr., Los Angeles, CA 90024.

LH secretion was characterized in adult male and female rats which were exposed to ethanol (ETOH) in utero. Pregnant dams were fed a nutritionally controlled diet containing 35% ETOH derived calories or an isocalorically matched control diet (Bioserv) from day 14 of gestation until parturition. Fetal alcohol exposed (FAE) and pair fed (PF) pups were weaned at 21 days of age and group housed by treatment and sex. At 150 days of age FAE and PF males and females were gonadectomized (gx). 14-15 days after gx a 5mm silastic capsule filled with crystalline extradiol 17B (E) was implanted subcutaneously. 72 hrs after E a single injection of progesterone (2 mg) was administered. Intra-atrial cannulae were inserted just prior to the time of E administration and blood samples were taken immediately before E and throughout the following 3 afternoons. Prior to E treatment, LH titers were significantly less (p 0.01) in both FAE males and females as compared to PF controls. Afternoon LH surges were significantly depressed (p 0.01) in FAE females versus PF females. No males showed afternoon LH surges. Subsequently, the episodic nature of LH secretion was characterized in a second group of PF and FAE animals gx'd 14-15 days previous. FAE animals exhibited a decreased pulse amplitude as well as a decreased baseline versus PF animals. There were no alterations in pulse frequency. These data suggest that fetal exposure to alcohol results in developmental alterations in the mechanisms controlling LH secretion. Supported by HD 01182

927 STIMULATION OF LH RELEASE BY PHORBOL ESTER: ENHANCEMENT BY CALMODULIN ANTAGONISTS AND REDUCTION BY A POTENT GnRH ANTAGONIST. M. Iwashita*, G. Aguilera, and K. J. Catt. ERRB, NICHD, Bethesda, MD 20205, U.S.A.

The actions of GnRH on LH release in cultured rat pituitary cells are inhibited by calcium channel antagonists and calmodulin antagonists, and are reproduced by high concentrations of A23187. However, the ability of 12-O-tetradecanyl-phorbol-13-acetate (TPA) to stimulate LH release at low concentrations (0.1 nM) and with up to 50% of the efficacy of [D-Ala^{6}]-des-Gly^{10}-GnRH-N-ethylamide (GnRHa) at 10 nM indicates that protein kinase C could also be involved in LH release. In analyzing the role of these mechanisms in LH release by cultured rat pituitary cells, we observed two new findings of interest. First, calmodulin antagonists increased the LH response to TPA: 10 μM pimozide or W7 doubled the LH release elicited by 10 pM to 1 μM TPA, although these antagonists reduced GnRHa-stimulated LH release by 50%. Second, the potent GnRH antagonist [Ac-D-p-Cl-Phe^{1,2},D-Trp^{3},D-Lys^{6},D-Ala^{10}]GnRH not only completely inhibited GnRHa-stimulated LH release, but also reduced the effect of TPA by 50%. These results support the involvement of both calmodulin and kinase C pathways in Ca-mediated LH release and suggest that inhibition of calmodulin binding renders cytosolic Ca more available for activation of kinase C. The inhibition of TPA-induced LH release by a GnRH antagonist suggests that kinase C causes phosphorylation and activation of the GnRH receptor, via a conformational change that is prevented when the receptor is locked into its inactive state by the tightly bound antagonist.

928 Effect of injecting synthetic LHRH and its antiserum on serum Chorionic Gonadotropin (CG) levels in the bonnet monkey *Macaca radiata*. A. Jagannadha Rao* and N.R. Moudgal, ICMR Cent. for Advan.Res. in Reprod.Biol., Dept. of Biochem., Ind.Inst. of Sci., Bangalore-560012, India.

In vitro studies with human placenta has suggested that it produces a chorionic gonadotropin releasing hormone which stimulates the release of hCG (Biol.Reprod.25,353,1981). In the present study we have examined the *in vivo* effect of synthetic LHRH on serum monkey chorionic gonadotropin (mCG) of the pregnant bonnet monkey using a specific radioimmunoassay validated to measure mCG. The injection of 50-100 ug of LHRH i.v. to pregnant monkeys (between days 20-40 of gestation)caused a rapid increase in mCG levels reaching peak values by 45-60 min. The effect of LHRH was more pronounced when mCG was still in ascending phase (days 20-33 gestation) compared to when mCG levels were naturally declining (days 35-50 gestation) Injection of LHRH antiserum during early pregnancy in bonnets caused a transient decrease in serum mCG levels. This effect though might be depended upon the amount, affinity and cross-reactivity of antibody injected, does corroborate that placental LHRH could be one of the factors involved in regulating CG secretion in non-human primates. Supported by grants from Ind. Council of Medical Research and Family Planning Foundation, New Delhi and WHO, Geneva.

929 ISOLATION AND CHARACTERIZATION OF THE GENE ENCODING THE β SUBUNIT OF RAT LUTEINIZING HORMONE. J.L. Jameson*, W.W. Chin, A.S. Chang, A.N. Hollenberg and J.F. Habener. Laboratory of Molecular Endocrinology, Mass General Hospital, Harvard Medical School, and Howard Hughes Medical Institute Laboratories, Boston, MA.

Luteinizing hormone (LH) consists of two different subunits, α and β, which are encoded by separate genes. We are studying the mechanisms by which gonadal steroids regulate these genes. We used a recombinant plasmid containing rat LH cDNA, previously cloned and characterized in our laboratory, to analyze blots of rat genomic DNA by in situ hybridization techniques indicating the presence of only a single gene encoding LHβ. The same cDNA probe was used to detect and isolate the chromasomal gene encoding LHβ from a bacteriophage Charon 4A library of rat genomic DNA. Restriction enzyme mapping and sequence analyses indicate that the isolated fragment is 3.8 kb in length containing the entire transcriptional unit as well as 2.0 kb of 5'-flanking sequence and 1.0 kb of 3'-flanking sequence. There are three exons and two introns. The positions of the two introns are the same as previously reported by other laboratories for human chorionic gonadotropin (CG) with intron 1 located between codons -16 and -15 of the signal sequence and intron 2 located between codons 41 and 42. The conservation of intron locations between rat LH and human CG indicates a strong selective pressure on the gene structure. We are currently studying regulation of expression of the LHβ gene following its introduction into eukaryotic cell lines.

930 IDENTIFICATION OF SOMATOMEDIN (Sm) AND ITS RECEPTORS IN DEVELOPING CORTICAL NEURAL CELLS IN CULTURE. Victor K.M. Han,* A. Joseph D'Ercole and Jean M. Lauder, Departments of Pediatrics and Anatomy, University of North Carolina School of Medicine, Chapel Hill, NC 27514, U.S.A.

A specific monoclonal antibody against Somatomedin C/Insulin like growth factor I (Sm-C/IGF I) [5% crossreactivity with IGF II, 1% with multiplication stimulating activity (MSA), and none with insulin at 10^{-6}M] and a highly sensitive immunocytochemical technique (Avidin-Biotin method) were used to stain Sm-C/IGF I in primary monolayer neural cell cultures obtained from cortical precursor regions of 15-day gestation fetal rats. Cultures were maintained in Eagle's basal medium containing 10% fetal calf serum and stained after 7 and 15 days. After 7 days the cytosol of all undifferentiated neuroepithelial and glial cells, stained in a granular pattern. Staining was absent in the nuclei, and in neurons it extended partially into the neurites. As differentiation occurred (at 15 days in culture) the staining of neurons and their neurites became more intense, and that of the glial cells less so. Specificity was confirmed by showing that micromolar concentrations of pure Sm-C blocked staining completely. Equimolar concentrations of MSA, but not insulin, had an identical effect. That the Sm identified by this technique has a biologic action in the fetal brain is supported by receptor studies. Using both affinity labeling with the chemical cross-linker disuccinimidyl suberate and autoradiography of ^{125}I-Sm-C bound to cultured neural cells, the presence of type I and type II IGF receptors has been verified. The specific Sm identified in this study remains to be established, but the results suggest that Sm is involved in the stimulation of brain growth.

931 EVIDENCE FOR PHOSPHORYLATION OF THE TYPE II INSULIN-LIKE GROWTH FACTOR (IGF) RECEPTOR IN CULTURED CELLS. J. F. Haskell*, S. P. Nissley, M. M. Rechler, N. Sasaki, L. A. Greenstein, and L. Lee, NCI and NIADDK, National Institutes of Health, Bethesda, MD, 20205, USA.

The β subunit of the Type I IGF receptor has been shown to be phosphorylated (J. Biol. Chem. 258, 9581, 1983). We asked whether the Type II IGF receptor is also phosphorylated. Monolayer cultures of cells (rat embryo fibroblasts, BRL 3A2 rat liver, and H35 rat hepatoma) were cultured in the presence of $[^{32}P]H_3PO_4$ for 2½ hrs to label the ATP pool. Rat IGF-II (1 μg/ml) was then added and after 5-30 min the cell monolayers were washed and solubilized with 1% Triton X-100. Glycoproteins were purified using wheat germ lectin Sepharose columns and analysed by $NaDodSO_4$/polyacrylamide gel electrophoresis and autoradiography. The patterns of glycoprotein phosphorylation were similar for the 3 cell types. Among the labeled bands was a species with the same size as the Type II receptor (Mr ≃ 250K with reduction, Mr ≃ 200K without reduction). The intensity of this band did not appear to increase with IGF-II treatment of the cells. Importantly, the Mr=250/200K species bound to an IGF-II Sepharose column. After washing the column extensively with neutral buffer, the Mr=250/200K component was eluted with a low pH, high salt buffer. We have been unable to demonstrate phosphorylation of a Mr=250/200K species using $[\gamma-^{32}P]$ATP together with solubilized receptors purified with wheat germ Sepharose, whereas the Type I receptor (Mr=98/>300K) was phosphorylated. CONCLUSIONS: The Type II IGF receptor is phosphorylated in intact cells in culture; phosphorylation could not be demonstrated in cell-free preparations. In contrast to Type I IGF receptor phosphorylation which is IGF-I dependent, Type II receptor phosphorylation does not appear to be IGF-II dependent.

932 RAT MAMMARY MITOGENIC ACTION OF PROLACTIN, SOMATOMEDIN AND LIVER FACTORS. N. Hebert*, E.M. Spencer and C.S. Nicoll, Dept. of Physiology-Anatomy and Cancer Research Lab., University of California, Berkeley, CA 94720 and Children's Hospital, San Francisco, CA 94119, USA.

Previous work has shown that insulin-like growth factors (IGF), including somatomedin-C (SM-C), act synergistically with PRL to promote growth of the mucosal epithelium of the pigeon crop sac *in vivo* (Anderson *et al*., *In*: Insulin-like Growth Factors/Somatomedins, E.M. Spencer, ed., 1983). We have investigated whether IGF, liver factors or PRL are mitogenic on rat mammary epithelium. Rats at 14-17 days of pregnancy were hysterectomized to eliminate placental lactogens, and their mammary glands (MG) were removed about 18 hr later. The MG were cut into explants that were incubated for 6 hr in medium 199 containing ^{3}H-thymidine (T) and test substances. Human SM-C (100 ng/ml) or rat PRL (10 and 100 ng/ml) doubled the incorporation of ^{3}H-T into DNA but bovine proinsulin (100 ng/ml) was inactive. Secreted hepatic factors were obtained by incubating slices of rat liver in medium 199 for 4 hr. The medium was diluted to a final concentration of 10 mg liver equivalent/ml and used for incubation with MG explants. Medium from male or virgin female liver did not stimulate ^{3}H-T incorporation; however, medium from pregnant rat liver doubled ^{3}H-T incorporation and that from lactating rats showed a 50% increase. Thus, the pregnant rat liver secretes a mammary mitogenic factor and the liver from lactating rats secretes less of this factor. Although SM-C can mimic the action of the liver mitogen, they may not be the same because male and virgin female liver lack mitogenic activity. Measurement of SM-C levels in medium should clarify this. Supported by NSF grant PCM 8203583 and NIH grant HD 14506.

933 THE PHYSICAL NATURE OF SOMATOMEDIN BIOACTIVITY RELEASED FROM ISOLATED FETAL RAT MYOBLASTS. D.J. Hill*, C.J. Crace, A.T. Holder and R.D.G. Milner, Department of Paediatrics, University of Sheffield, Children's Hospital, Sheffield, S10 2TH and Institute of Child Health, Guildford Street, London, WC1, U.K.

Somatomedins may regulate growth and differentiation in utero. We have shown that isolated fetal rat myoblasts release somatomedin-C-like immunoreactivity and somatomedin bioactivity and here report their characteristics after gel filtration. Bioactivity, measured by radiothymidine or radiosulphate uptake by fetal rat cartilage explants, and immunoreactivity eluted with an apparent molecular weight of 40-60K when myoblast-conditioned culture medium was chromatographed on Sephadex G200 at pH 7.5 Chromatography on Biogel P10 at pH 3.5, conditions favouring a dissociation of somatomedins from binding proteins, resulted in two discrete peaks of immunoreactivity, the first eluting with the void volume (>18K daltons) and the second co-eluting with radiolabelled somatomedin-C (7-8K). Bioactivity was associated with the latter. The void volume peak from P10, but not the 7-8K peak, possessed somatomedin binding activity and when rechromatographed on G200 eluted in the 40-60K position. The 7-8K peak of immunoreactivity from P10 produced a dose-dependent increase in radiothymidine uptake by fetal rat myoblasts in vitro. Results suggest that at neutral pH the bioactive fetally-derived somatomedin is specifically bound to carrier protein. At acid pH this complex incompletely dissociated releasing free somatomedin peptides of 7-8K daltons. This material had anabolic actions on cultured fetal myoblasts suggesting a paracrine role in vivo.

934 STRUCTURAL SIMILARITIES BETWEEN THE LIVER IGF BINDING PROTEINS (BPs) AND THE SERUM IGF BPs FOUND IN THE > 100 K AND THE 40-60 K MATERIAL. P. Hossenlopp*, S. Hardouin, D. Seurin and M. Binoux INSERM U 142, Hôpital Trousseau, 75012 Paris, France.

Results of our competitive binding studies have suggested the production by the liver and the presence in the serum of two IGF BPs with similar mol. wt., one having a greater affinity for IGF I and the other a greater affinity for IGF II (J. Clin. Endocrinol. Metab. 1982, 55, 600). After incubating rat liver culture medium with ^{125}I IGF I, [IGF-BP] complexes covalently bound by dimethylsuberimidate were analyzed by SDS-PAGE and autoradiography. Two forms of ~ 37 and 40 K were observed, which were more easily identified under non-reducing conditions. Incubation of the same material with increasing concentrations (1-30 ng/slot) of unlabeled IGF I (generous gift of Dr R. Humbel, Zürich) resulted in a progressive disappearance of the two bands which, at the lower concentrations, was more efficient for the 37 K complex. Similar bands were revealed by SDS-PAGE under reducing conditions when studying [IGF-BP] complexes from human liver culture medium or from the 40-60 K serum material isolated by gel filtration at neutral pH. A 3rd minor band was observed. The migration pattern of the > 100 K serum material could not readily be analyzed, due to the excess of endogenous IGF. But, this was made using SDS-PAGE under non-reducing conditions followed by electrophoretic transfer to nitrocellulose, incubation with ^{125}I IGF I and autoradiography. Two forms of BP (~38 and 42 K) migrated from both the 40-60 K and the > 100K serum material. A 3rd form (~34 K) migrated from the 40-60 K material. Conclusion : 1) The liver synthesizes two forms of BPs with close mol. wts.. 2) BPs with similar mol. wts. are present in the serum, both in the 40-60 K and the > 100 K material.

935 SECRETION OF IMMUNOREACTIVE IGF-1/SmC BY CULTURED BREAST CANCER CELLS IN SERUM FREE MEDIUM. K.K. Huff*+, M.E. Lippman+, E.M. Spencer†, and R.B. Dickson+. +Medical Breast Cancer Section, Medicine Branch, NCI, NIH, Bethesda, MD 20205, and †Children's Hospital of San Francisco, San Francisco, CA 94118.

A study was carried out to evaluate the possible production of IGF-1/SmC by human breast cancer cells in culture and establish the effects of 17β-estradiol (E_2). Four human breast cancer cell lines were used: estrogen responsive MCF-7 and ZR-75-1, and estrogen unresponsive MDA-231 and Hs578T. After 3 days of culture in serum free medium, conditioned medium was collected and aprotinin added. IGF-1/SmC was determined by RIA before and after extraction with EtOH/HCl. IGF-1/SmC could only be detected after EtOH/HCl extraction implying all cell lines secreted IGF-1/SmC and a binding protein: MCF-7 2.1 ng/ml, 91.3 pg/ug DNA; ZR-75-1 2.8 ng/ml, 166 pg/ug DNA; MDA-231 4.9 ng/ml, 209 pg/ug DNA; Hs578T 16.8 ng/ml, 1540 pg/ug DNA. No significant increase in levels of IGF-1/SmC were detected in the conditioned medium from the MCF-7 or ZR-75-1 cells after E_2 treatment (10^{-9}M, 5 days). Treatment of MCF-7 cells with authentic IGF-1/SmC increased their growth rate after 4 days. 1 nM (7.6 ng/ml) IGF-1/SmC increased DNA 1.4x and cell number 1.3x, while 5 nM (38 ng/ml) IGF-1/SmC increased DNA 1.9x and cell number 1.7x. Since serum free conditioned medium from MCF-7 breast cancer cells is mitogenic for MCF-7 cells in culture, it is possible that the immunoreactive IGF-1/SmC in conditioned media may contribute to the proliferation of these and other breast cancer cells in a autocrine fashion.

936 STIMULATION OF MAMMARY EPITHELIAL CELL GROWTH IN VITRO: INTERACTION OF EGF AND MAMMOGENIC HORMONES. W. Imagawa*, Y. Tomooka, and S. Nandi. Cancer Research Lab. and Dept. of Zoology, Univ. of Calif., Berkeley, Ca. 94720

A serum-free, primary cell culture system was used to examine the direct effects and interactions of mammogenic hormones and epidermal growth factor (EGF) on the growth of mouse mammary epithelial cells. Epithelial cells were isolated by collagenase dissociation and cultured within collagen gels in Ham's F12:Dulbecco's MEM (1:1) containing insulin (10ug/ml), liposomes, trace elements, trypsin inhibitor, and antioxidants. In the absence of EGF, progesterone(P, 10^{-6}-10^{-8}M) or ovine prolactin(PRL, 1 ug/ml) stimulated the growth of cells from mature virgin mice 2-4X over controls cultured in basal medium only. P and PRL synergized in stimulating growth 3-17X. Estradiol-17B(10^{-7}-10^{-10}M)alone did not stimulate growth or synergize with P and/or PRL. EGF(10 ng/ml) alone stimulated growth to the same extent as the combination, P+PRL. EGF at 1 but not 10 ng/ml, when combined with P and PRL could additively stimulate growth. Pregnancy reduces the growth response to P and PRL but not to EGF. Corticosterone, deoxycorticosterone (DOC), and aldosterone but not cortisol could synergize with PRL in stimulating the growth of cells from mature virgin mice. However, only DOC could stimulate growth in the absence of PRL. These results show that the hormonal stimulation of growth in vitro can be obscured by EGF, that the relative growth response to mammogenic hormones and EGF may depend on the degree of differentiation of the cells, and that mineralocorticoids may stimulate ductal growth. Supported by NCI grants CA 05388 and CA 09041.

937 EPIDERMAL GROWTH FACTOR (EGF) IN GUINEA PIG. Y. Imai*, T. Nagano and F. Matsuzaki, The Third Department of Internal Medicine, Faculty of Medicine, University of Tokyo, Tokyo, Japan

Since little is known about guinea pig EGF, we studied its tissue distribution and physical characteristics. EGF activity was measured by a receptor assay using mouse EGF as a standard and particulate fraction of male mouse liver as a receptor. Salivary glands, the richest sources in EGF in mice and rats, contained about 0.6 μg/g tissue, which is less than 0.1% of that found in male mouse submaxillary glands. Remarkable sexual dimorphism of EGF levels in salivary glands as seen in mice was not observed. Interestingly, guinea pig prostate glands contained the highest concentration of EGF (40.8±8.9 μg/g tissue, Mean ± SEM) among other tissues tested. This level is about 100-fold higher than that of mouse and rat prostate glands. Twenty four hr urinary excretion of EGF in female guinea pigs was about 26 μg and was 3-fold higher than that of males. This difference is also significant when values are standardized with urinary creatinine. Such a big sexual difference in urinary EGF was not observed in rats, mice or humans. On gel filtration of prostate extracts on Sephadex G-50, a peak of activity was recovered in the region where human EGF migrates. Isoelectric focusing of the extracts revealed that the pI was 4.7 which was slightly different from those of mouse and human EGFs. The present data demonstrate that prostate glands are rich in EGF of guinea pig and urinary excretion of EGF is higher in female guinea pigs than in males, indicating that the regulatory mechanism for EGF production and release is different in the guinea pig from other species.

938 THE TRANSCRIPTION AND PROCESSING OF A REPETITIVE DNA SEQUENCE IN THE RAT GROWTH HORMONE GENE. A. Gutierrez-Hartmann,* I.L. Lieberburg, D. Colby, D.G. Gardner, and J.D. Baxter, Metabolic Res. Unit and Dept. of Biochem. Biophys., Univ. of Calif., San Francisco, CA. 94143

The 2nd intron (I_B) and 3' flanking region (3'FR) of the rat growth hormone (rGH) gene contain large repetitive DNA (RD) structures consisting of 2 rat RD families. The 1st family is the same as the hamster type 2 repeats and the 2nd (TR;66% homologous) is a truncated version of the first. Also, many rat genes expressed specifically in the brain contain TR, thus TR may serve as a brain-specific identifier sequence. Thus, by defining the transcription of TR DNA, our understanding of brain- and pituitary-specific gene expression may be advanced. Cell-free transcription of the rGH gene results in 14 products of 175-970 nucleotides (nt) transcribed by RNA Polymerase III (Pol III), but not Pol II, from I_B and 3'FR RD. Interestingly, TR sequences are present only as downstream structures in the 2 overlapping transcription units mapped to the I_B RD cluster, implying TR promoter inactivity. Apparently, such inactivity is due to a single base change in the TR promoter. Furthermore, rGH gene RD products are processed in frog oocytes to yield a discrete 73 nt RNA, whose fingerprint is most consistent with the identifier (TR) sequence. These data suggest: 1) pituitary genes can have DNA structural features characteristic of brain-specific genes; 2) these structures can be independently expressed by Pol III, even though they are located in the middle of a gene usually transcribed by Pol II; 3) the transcripts of these structures can extend past the RD, yet can be processed precisely to yield the identifier (TR) sequence. Therefore, these structures are candidates for regulation of brain- and pituitary-specific functions.

939 THE ROLE OF ENDOGENOUS DOPAMINE ON PLASMA GROWTH HORMONE SECRETION IN PATIENTS WITH ACROMEGALY. K. Hanew*, S. Sato, A. Sasaki, Y. Shimizu, O. Murakami and K. Yoshinaga, Department of Medicine, Tohoku University School of Medicine, Sendai 980, Japan

The role of endogenous dopamine (DA) on plasma GH secretion was studied using DA-receptor blockers (sulpiride and domperidone) in 12 patients with active acromegaly. After intramuscular administration of 100 mg sulpiride, 3 out of 12 patients showed distinct increases (293-766%) in their plasma GH (cases 1-3: sulpiride-responders). The GH increases far exceeded the ranges of physiological fluctuation in two cases studied (case 1 & 3). After domperidone (10 mg, iv) administration, case 3 showed a quite similar GH increase as after sulpiride. Plasma GH responses to TRH and DA-receptor blockers were examined in two cases (#2 & #3) pre- and postoperatively. Although the GH level normalized in both cases after the hypophysectomy, clear GH increases to either TRH or sulpiride were observed in case 2 throughout the study, whereas GH increases induced by TRH, sulpiride, and domperidone disappeared completely in case 3 after the operation. Further, in this case the so-called paradoxical response to L-dopa observed before the operation reverted to normal postoperatively. The three sulpiride-responders showed paradoxical GH decreases following the administration of L-dopa or DA. However, the basal plasma PRL levels and the responses to sulpiride in these 3 cases were not homogeneous. These results indicate that endogenous DA has a tonic, but not maximal, inhibitory effect on GH secretion in some cases of acromegaly, and that tumorous somatotrophs are the critical factor for such inhibition. Further, the sensitivities of somatotrophs and lactotrophs to DA appeared to be heterogeneous in acromegalic patients.

940 CATCH-UP GROWTH FOLLOWING TRANSFER FROM 3 TIMES WEEKLY i.m. INJECTION TO DAILY s.c. ADMINISTRATION OF HGH MONITORED BY KNEMOMETRIC TECHNIQUE IN GROWTH HORMONE DEFICIENT CHILDREN. M.Hermanussen*and W.G.Sippell, Endocrine Unit, Univ.Dept. of Pediatrics, Kiel, W-Germany, and I.M.Valk, Univ.Dept. of Anatomy,Embryology and Physical Anthropology, Nijmegen, The Netherlands.

It is now possible to study growth effects in short intervals of only a few days by knemometry. This novel and non-invasive technique (Valk et al., GROWTH XLVII,53-66,1983) measures the exact distance between heel and knee in sitting children. During the measurement the child is placed on a chair which can be moved forewards and backwards. The sitting position can be recorded exactly for identical positioning in following measurements. When the child feels totally comfortable, lower leg length is measured by repeated crosswise movements of the child's knee under the measuring board. The highest distance reached is diplayed electronically. Each single measurement consists of 6 independent estimations of which the median is recorded. The SD of 6 estimations is below 0.1 mm. Using this method we studied immediate changes of growth rates after transfer from alternating (3 times weekly) i.m. injections to daily s.c. administration of hGH in 7 growth hormone deficient children, age 5 to 22 yrs. All had been treated with pituitary hGH for 6 months to 7 yrs before the study. They were measured for periods of 72 to 162 days up to 23 times before and up to 13 times after transfer of application. In all cases we detected increased growth rates 30 to 127 days after transfer, mean growth rates under i.m.-treatment being -0.0148 mm/d (no growth) to 0.0703 mm/d, followed by growth rates of 0.0465 mm/d to 0.0835 mm/d under daily s.c.-treatment. In conclusion, daily s.c. application of hGH induces catch-up growth after transfer from alternating i.m. administration.

941 BROMOCRIPTINE ENHANCES OR UNMASKS THE THYROTROPIN-RELEASING HORMONE-INDUCED GROWTH HORMONE RELEASE IN ACROMEGALY. H.M. Heshmati*, G. Turpin, S. Jambart, M. Roger and J.L. de Gennes, Department of Endocrinology, Hôpital de la Pitié, 75013 Paris, and Fondation de Recherche en Hormonologie, 94260 Fresnes, France.

In order to study the effect of bromocriptine (Br) on the thyrotropin-releasing hormone (TRH)-induced growth hormone (GH) release in acromegaly, TRH (200 µg, iv) was administered alone or 150 min after the acute administration of Br (2.5 mg, orally) to 8 patients (5 males, 3 females) with GH adenoma (2 had mixed adenoma: GH + prolactin). Plasma GH and prolactin (PRL) were measured by radioimmunoassay before (2 baseline determinations) and 15, 30, 60 and 90 min after TRH administration (day 1), and before and 60, 120, 150, 160, 170, 180 and 190 min after Br administration (day 2). Significant response of GH or PRL to TRH or Br was defined as a variation of more than 50 % above or below the basal values. Basal GH and PRL were 19 ± 14 ng/ml (mean ± SD) and 23 ± 30 ng/ml respectively. Under TRH alone, the mean increments of GH and PRL were 11 ± 14 ng/ml and 24 ± 9 ng/ml respectively. GH increased significantly in 4 patients and PRL in 7. On day 2, during the first part of the test (Br alone), GH decreased significantly in 2 patients and PRL in 4. After the injection of TRH, the mean increments of GH and PRL were 21 ± 15 ng/ml and 6 ± 7 ng/ml respectively. GH increased significantly in 6 patients (2 had a higher increment than day 1, 2 were new TRH responders), and PRL in 6 (5 had a lower increment than day 1). It is concluded that in some acromegalic patients, acute administration of Br prior to TRH injection may enhance or unmask the abnormal GH increment under TRH, while the PRL increment is diminished. The interpretation of this phenomenon needs further investigation.

942 EVALUATION OF SECRETOGOGUES FOR GROWTH HORMONE RELEASE IN ANESTHETIZED AND CONSCIOUS DOGS, P. A. Hofker*, R. H. McIntosh, R. W. Deacon, A. H. Surve, and L. D. Boyajy, Sandoz, Inc., E. Hanover, NJ USA 07936

Potential secretogogues of canine growth hormone (cGH) were evaluated in male Beagle dogs (7-15 kg) 1) to develop a model of sustained cGH release suitable for testing increasing doses of SRIF-like inhibitors; and 2) to test long acting inhibitors on a chronic basis. Na pentobarbital (P) (35 mg/kg IV, n=36) produced release of cGH to plasma peaks of 15-50 ng/ml (basal: 2-8 ng/ml) within 15-30 min. cGH levels returned to baseline values 60-90 min after anesthesia induction. In P anesthetized animals after cGH levels returned to baseline, L-Dopa (D) (50 mg/kg IV, n=59) elicited cGH release of 60-90 min duration with plasma peaks of 20-50 ng/ml (basal: < 1-2 ng/ml) 15-30 min after drug. Sustained cGH plasma levels of 20-100 ng/ml (basal: 3-8 ng/ml) were produced for periods of 2-6 h in anesthetized dogs by infusion of D (0.75-2 mg/kg/min IV, n=4) or morphine (M) (1,2,4,8, and 16 mg/kg SC at 1 h intervals, n=2). Trials with apomorphine infusion (1.7-800 µg/kg/min IV, n=6) showed inconsistent results. In the conscious animal, clonidine (C) (12-15 µg/kg IV, n=154), D (50 mg/kg IV, n=4) and M (8 mg/kg SC, n=30) all produced cGH release of 60-90 min duration with plasma peaks of 12-50 ng/ml (basal: 0-3 ng/ml) 10-40 min post-injection. Hypoglycemia (20-40 mg/dL) induced by insulin (0.4 IU/kg IV, n=4) failed to evoke a cGH release. Conclusions: 1) sustained cGH release by D or M is not a usable model due to variations in levels 2) chronic use of C is highly satisfactory, and produced the most quantitatively consistent cGH release, reproducible for periods up to 1.25 yr. M and D were less suitable for chronic use because of gradual decline in the magnitude of responses and adverse effects.

943 PLASMA GH RESPONSES TO hpGRF-44 IN NORMAL CHILDREN WITH SHORT STATURE BY IV BOLUS AND IV INFUSION.
N. Honda*, K. Takano, N. Hizuka, K. Shizume, M. Miyakawa, K. Asakawa and N. C. Ling. Department of Medicine, Tokyo Women's Medical College, Tokyo 162, Japan.

The effect of synthetic human pancreatic growth-hormone-releasing factor (hpGRF-44) was studied on the GH secretion in normal children with short stature. A total of 100 males and 40 females, aged 4-18 years, were in this group.

After a single iv bolus injection of 2 μg GRF/kg BW, mean plasma GH level peaked at 30 min with the value of 31.8 ± 2.4 (±SE) ng/ml (N=140). There were no sexual and age differences on plasma GH responses between them. The overall plasma GH response was greater than that of insulin-induced hypoglycemia and was similar to that of glucagon-propranolol test.

During a constant GRF infusion (2.5 μg/min) for 180 min (N=3), plasma GH levels reached a peak at 60-120 min with a mean value of 69.1 ± 14.3 ng/ml and then declined gradually. Similary, constant infusion of GRF for 90 min, together with an iv bolus injection of GRF (2 μg/kg) administered at 0 and 90 min (N=5), elicited a prompt rise of plasma GH after the first bolus but no significant elevation of GH after the second bolus. In contrast, when two iv bolus injections of GRF (2 μg/kg) were given at 0 and 90 min (N=4), respectively, significant elevation of plasma GH was found after each bolus. Side effects were very rare in children.

These results suggest that GRF is useful for evaluating pituitary GH reserve in children with short stature and that under the constant infusion of GRF the pituitary experiences a down-regulation after the initial peak of GH response, possibly due to desensitization to GRF.

944 GROWTH HORMONE RESPONSE TO THYROTROPIN-RELEASING HORMONE IN DIABETES.
T. Ieiri*, N. Banba, T. Emoto, M. Kiyota, Y. Hashigami, M. Ishikawa, H. Kobori, Y. Mochizuki and S.-I. Shimoda, Department of Endocrinology, Internal Medicine, Dokkyo University School of Medicine, Mibu, Tochigi 321-02, Japan.

We previously reported that growth hormone(GH) increasing responses after L-DOPA and after arginine were diminished in diabetes. Some recent reports indicate that thyrotropin-releasing hormone(TRH) stimulates GH release in some patients with diabetes. In the present study, a significant negative correlation between the net increases of serum levels of GH after TRH and after arginine in non-insulin-dependent diabetes was described. TRH(500 μg iv) test was carried out in 26 patients with diabetes and 9 controls. Arginine(0.5 g/kg of body weight div for 30 min.) infusion test also was carried out in 22 out of 26 patients with diabetes. Increased GH response to TRH in diabetes(defined response as a rise at least twice the base line and a peak absolute value above 5 ng/ml) was seen in 6 out of 26 patients, 5 males and 1 female, including 3 patients without diabetic retinopathy. Two diabetic patients with proliferative retinopathy were included in GH-non-responders to TRH. The correlation coefficient between the net increases of GH to TRH and that to arginine was -0.657(n=22, statistically significant at the level of $p < 0.01$). These results suggest that the GH releasing mechanism in diabetes is abnormal and that paradoxical GH increasing response to TRH is observed in low responders to the ordinary provocation tests such as arginine.

945 EPIDERMAL GROWTH FACTOR (EGF) STIMULATES GH SECRETION FROM SUPERFUSED RAT ADENOHYPOPHYSEAL FRAGMENTS. H. Ikeda*, T. Mitsuhashi, K. Kubota, N. Kuzuya and H. Uchimura, The Third Department of Internal Medicine, Faculty of Medicine, University of Tokyo, Hongo, Bunkyo-ku, Tokyo, Japan.

Epidermal growth factor (EGF) is one of the growth factors which has been isolated from the submandibular glands of male mice. Recently, it has been reported that EGF stimulates PRL synthesis and release in cultured rat pituitary tumor cells, GH_3 and GH_4C_1. In the present study, we have examined the effects of EGF on GH, PRL and TSH release from normal rat pituitaries, using a superfusion technique. Adenohypophyseal fragments were obtained from adult female Sprague-Dawley rats by mincing anterior pituitary glands into 30-40 pieces which were then packed into a small chamber (0.2 ml) supported by Bio-gel P2 and perfused with Dulbecco's modified Eagle's medium with 10% horse serum. EGF (8-500 ng/ml) was perfused for 5 or 10 min and TRH (100 nM) was perfused for 1 min. Concentrations of pituitary hormones in the effluents were measured by RIA. GH concentrations in the effluents increased immediately after the addition of EGF. The increases of GH release induced by EGF were dose-related (8-50 ng/ml). PRL or TSH release was not affected by EGF. TRH markedly stimulated TSH and PRL release, but did not significantly affect GH release. These results indicate 1) that EGF selectively stimulates GH release from normal rat anterior pituitary in vitro, and 2) that EGF may play a role in GH secretion in the rat.

946 INSULIN BINDING IS DECREASED IN THE OLFACTORY BULB OF TWO GENETICALLY OBESE RAT MODELS. D.P. Figlewicz*, T. Hunt, D.L. Dorsa, H. Ikeda, L.J. Stein, D.G. Baskin, S.C. Woods, and D. Porte, Jr., University of Washington, Seattle, WA 98195, U.S.A.

Genetically obese Zucker fatty and Wistar fatty rats become obese in an early dynamic phase of growth and maintain excess adiposity throughout life. Previous studies from this lab have implicated insulin as a central modulator of food intake and body weight. Since both Zucker and Wistar fatties exhibit hyperinsulinemia and elevated CSF insulin levels at 4 mo., we measured insulin binding in the brain to assess whether binding (and hence reception) of insulin is altered. Insulin binding to membranes from liver, olfactory bulb (OB), medial (MH) and lateral hypothalamus (LH), and cerebral cortex (C) was measured following a 4-hr incubation at 25°C, pH 8. "Specific binding" was defined as binding of 0.1 nM ^{125}I-insulin minus binding of ^{125}I-insulin in the presence of 1000 nM insulin. Insulin binding by livers of both fatty models was decreased compared to lean controls (9 vs. 32 fmol/mg protein in Wistars; 90 vs. 150 fmol/mg protein in Zuckers). Insulin binding was also decreased in the OB of both fatty models (7 vs. 17 fmol/mg protein in Wistars; 32 vs. 52 fmol/mg protein in Zuckers). Binding was not different in fatty vs. lean Wistar MH; LH; or C (12 vs. 16; 16 vs. 13; or 8 vs. 8 fmol/mg protein) nor in fatty vs. lean Zucker MH; LH; or C (21 vs. 22; 13 vs. 8; or 11 vs. 10 fmol/mg protein). These findings suggest that insulin may be regulated in some brain areas by endogenous insulin levels. The decrease of insulin binding in the OB, an important site for regulation of food intake in the rat, may reflect an impaired reception of insulin feedback and may contribute to the hyperphagia and subsequent obesity of these animals.

947 CENTRAL NERVOUS ACTIVATION FOLLOWING PITUITARY STALK STIMULATION, AS SEEN USING 2-DEOXY-D-GLUCOSE IN RATS.
M.C.HARRIS*, D.BANKS, †J.K.McQUEEN & J.S. YOUNG. Dept. of Physiology, The Medical School, Birmingham and†MRC Brain Metabolism Unit, Edinburgh, U.K.

Within the hypothalamic paraventricular nucleus (PVN) there is a population of neurones that is synaptically activated by stimulation of the pituitary stalk. Some of those neurones project caudally and others rostrally, but nothing is known of their functions. In a preliminary study we have used ^{14}C-2-deoxyglucose (DOG) to locate the brain areas influenced by the synaptically activated PVN neurones. In anaesthetised rats the pituitary stalk was stimulated electrically with biphasic 1ms pulses of up to 1mA and at 50Hz. Stimulation was started 45min before the I.V. injection of DOG (16.7µCi/100g B.W.), and was continued for a further 45min after the injection. In control animals stimuli were applied to the peripheral end of the stalk following section close to the median eminence. As expected, stimulation activated both the supraoptic and PV nuclei as well as the median eminence. Outside the hypothalamus, however, activation seemed to be confined to the nucleus of the tractus solitarius in the medulla oblongata; there was no obvious activation in the spinal cord or the rostral forebrain. This suggests that the oxytocin and vasopressin-containing PVN neurones to the spinal cord and other medullary nuclei have no direct functional connection with the neurohypophysis. This work is supported by the SmithKline Foundation.

948 NEUROPEPTIDE Y, A VASOCONSTRICTOR PEPTIDE, CIRCULATES IN PATIENTS WITH ADRENAL MEDULLARY PHAEOCHROMOCYTOMA.
R. Corder*, P.J. Lowry, P.C. Emson§, and R.C. Gaillard†. Protein Hormone Unit, St. Bartholomew's Hospital, London EC1, UK. §MRC Neurochemical Pharmacology Unit, Cambridge, UK. †Dept. of Medicine, University Hospital, Geneva, Switzerland.

Neuropeptide Y (NPY), a 36 amino acid peptide was originally purified from porcine brain. We have identified NPY-like immunoreactivity in human adrenal medullary phaeochromocytoma tissue. This NPY-like immunoreactivity has been purified to homogeneity from the pooled extracts obtained from 16 human adrenal medullary tumours (total tissue wet wt. 1607g). Chemical characterization has shown it to be the authentic peptide. Recent studies of adrenal medullary phaeochromocytoma from four patients revealed tumour concentrations of NPY-like immunoreactivity of 0.32, 1.91, 2.51 and 0.22 nmole/g. When plasma from the latter two patients was subjected to Sephadex G-75 gel filtration chromatography large amounts of NPY-like immunoreactivity were found, eluting predominantly in the position of authentic NPY. Total immunoreactivity obtained after gel filtration chromatography of the plasma samples from these patients indicate circulating concentrations of NPY-like immunoreactivity of 320 and 440 fmol/ml respectively, compared to levels in normal plasma, subjected to the same procedure, of <10 fmol/ml. Neuropeptide Y has been shown to have vasoconstrictor actions in other species. NPY released with catecholamines from adrenal medullary phaeochromocytoma during hypertensive crises may potentiate the vasoconstrictor actions of noradrenaline and contribute to some of the diverse cardiovascular symptoms occurring in patients with tumours of this type. A direct plasma assay for NPY may be useful in the diagnosis of phaeochromocytoma.

949 EFFECTS OF RLX ON THE MICROCIRCULATION. A.Del Mese[+], R.Casali, G.P.Novelli, F.Petrucci and M.Bigazzi, Servizio Anestesia, Ospedale Poggiosecco, INRCA ed Istituto Anestesia e Rianimazione, Università degli Studi, Firenze, Italy

The clinical improvement of Reynaud disease during pregnancy has been attributed to the increased relaxin (RLX) level in blood. Therefore we investigated the effect of pure porcine RLX standard (NIH) and a partially purified human decidual RLX on the microcirculation "in vivo". The study was performed on the mesocaecum of Wistar male rats,according to the Zweifach method (1948),modified by Novelli (1981) under direct microscope observation. Porcine RLX, 30-60 GPU, or human RLX, 20-40 μg,were locally applied to avoid systemic interferences,before and after local stimulation of norepinephrine (NE) 0.1 mlx 10^{-13} and 10^{-7}. The results were recorded separately by two observers. Porcine RLX induces rapid dilatation of the veins of rat mesocaecum in a dose-related manner. The size of arteriolae was increased only with higher doses and to a lesser degree. The arteriolas and capillary flows id not change, while the venular flow was progressively reduced. The observed effects were substained and disappeared with tissue wash-out. The RLX effects were removed by addition of NE,conversely high doses of RLX were able to oppose the NE vasospasm and showed RLX action. We may conclude that RLX is able to affect locally the microcirculation through an action on the smooth muscle,mainly on the venulae; such effect seems to be antagonized by NE.

950 PROLACTIN (PRL) AND TSH RESPONSE TO TRH DURING CHRONIC ADMINISTRATION OF D-TRP^6-LH-RH IN MEN WITH PROSTATIC CARCINOMA (PC). D.Gonzalez-Barcena*. P.L. Perez, S. Ureta, H. Berea, A. Graef, M. Becerril, A.M. Comaru-Schally and A.V. Schally. Hosp.Especialidades, CM La Raza, Mexico 07870 and V.A. Hospital and Tulane Univ. Sch. Med. New Orleans, LA 70146.

A successful palliation of advanced PC by LH-RH agonists was first reported in men in 1982 (PNAS 78:1658,1982). Acute injection of superactive long-acting agonist D-TRP^6-LH-RH causes a marked elevation of LH and FSH but, paradoxically, chronic administration induces a state of "biochemical castration". In order to obtain more data on the effects of chronic administration of D-TRP^6-LH-RH, the serum PRL and TSH response to TRH (20 mg orally) was studied before and after 1,2 and 3 months of therapy in 10 patients with PC-stage D2. Resting TSH (3.1 ± .2 mUI/ml) and PRL (15 ± 2.7 ng/ml) remained unchanged during the therapy. After TRH, TSH increased in 5 patients (13.3 ± 2.15), but 5 did not respond. However, at 2 and 3 months, all patients released TSH post TRH. Pre-therapy, the PRL response to TRH was 53.5 ± 16.3 ng/ml. This response was maintained at 1,2 and 3 months. Basal GH and Cortisol pre and during the analogue therapy remained within normal values. These results show that chronic administration of D-TRP^6-LH-RH seems to selectively block the pituitary-gonadal axis. This represents another advantage in using LH-RH agonists for the therapy of PC.

951 IMMUNOCYTOCHEMICAL LOCALIZATION OF SOMATOSTATIN-28(1-12) IN THE RAT HYPOTHALAMUS.

J. Guy*, R. Benoît and G. Pelletier, MRC Group in Molecular Endocrinology, CHUL. Québec, G1V 4G2, Canada and Laboratories for Neuroendocrinology, The Salk Institute for Biological Studies, La Jolla, CA 92037.

Somatostatin-28 (SS28) is considered as the precursor of somatostatin-14 (SS14) and also of the remaining NH_2-terminus of SS28, namely the dodecapeptide SS28(1-12) which has been recently characterized (Benoît et al., PNAS 79, 917, 1982). In order to study the cellular and subcellular localization of SS28(1-12) in the rat hypothalamus, we have conducted a light and electron microscopic immunocytochemical study using both the peroxidase-antiperoxidase and the immunogold techniques. Several antisera which selectively recognize one or more of these three somatostatin-related peptides were used. Using serial paraffin sections, it was observed that SS28(1-12) was contained in the same neuronal cell bodies which also contain SS28 and SS14. These neurons were exclusively located in the periventricular nucleus. All the antisera studied also strongly stained terminals in the external zone of the median eminence. At the electron microscopic level, the three peptides were localized exclusively in the dense core vesicles of cell bodies, axons and terminals. These morphological data indicate that SS28(1-12) and SS14 have the same precursor SS28 and suggest that the processing of the precursor occurs in the cell body. They also support the hypothesis that these somatostatin-related peptides are released simultaneously under appropriate stimulatory conditions.

952 PHARMACOKINETICS OF SUBCUTANEOUS (SC) AND INTRAVENOUS (IV) GONADOTROPIN RELEASING HORMONE (GnRH).

D.J. Handelsman*, R.P.S. Jansen, L.M. Boylan, Departments of Endocrinology and Obstet. & Gynec., Royal Prince Alfred Hospital, Sydney, Australia.

Pulsatile IV GnRH has been used to induce normal gonadal function in hypogonadotropic individuals but deficient responses are reported with SC delivery. We compared the pharmacokinetics of SC and IV GnRH in 14 hypogonadotropic subjects (11 women, 3 men; age 29.6±1.9 [mean±SEM]; 3/14 anosmic). Plasma GnRH was measured by radioimmunoassay after acid-methanol extraction of samples (4°C, bacitracin 1mM). Bolus studies (5 ug, IV+3 SC profiles/subject,n=6 subjects) produced earlier (median 2 vs. 10 min.) and higher (median 400 vs. 93.5) peak plasma GnRH levels than SC. Plasma GnRH levels after IV were higher between 1 and 5 minutes and returned to basal by 60 min. After SC, plasma GnRH levels were higher between 30 and 90 minutes and remained elevated at 120 mins. Plasma GnRH profiles of 5ug SC in different volumes (25,100, 250 ul) were similar. Steady-state SC infusions of GnRH (n=11 subjects) produced lower plateau GnRH levels between 2 and 6 hours than IV infusions (67.5±20.0 vs. 102.4±30.2 pg/ml) indicating irreversible loss of about 1/3 of GnRH during chronic SC infusion. Plasma GnRH profiles of patients on pulsatile GnRH pumps were damped with SC but not IV administration. We conclude that SC delivery of GnRH results in lower and delayed peaks but prolonged elevation of circulating plasma GnRH compared with IV. The altered bioavailability of SC GnRH may induce pituitary desensitization. The damping of plasma GnRH profiles may explain the difference in clinical results of SC compared with IV GnRH delivery. Supported by N.H.& M.R.C. (Australia).

953 GONADOTROPIN AND TESTOSTERONE RESPONSE TO PULSATILE GONADOTROPIN-RELEASING HORMONE (GnRH) THERAPY IN MALE PATIENTS WITH KALLMANN'S SYNDROME (KS) OR DELAYED PUBERTY (DP). J. Happ*, W. Ditscheid and U. Krause, General Nuclear Medicine, University of Frankfurt and Clinical Endocrinology, University of Mainz, Fed. Rep. Germany.

Response to subcutaneous (s.c.) pulsatile low-dose (2 µg every 2.5 hrs) GnRH therapy was studied in 3 patients with Kallmann's syndrome and a boy with idiopathic delay of puberty presenting different gonadotropin responsiveness before treatment: in standard intravenous (i.v.) GnRH tests, LH response (ΔLH) was found to be markedly decreased in 2 patients with KS whereas ΔLH was within the lower part of the normal adult range in the other 2 patients. Measurements of the serum gonadotropins during the 3-month period of treatment showed increasing gonadotropin responsiveness to the treatment in all patients: this expressed itself by increasing maximum serum gonadotropin values as well as by prolonged serum gonadotropin elevation after a single pulse dose of 2 ug GnRH s.c. However, in the 2 patients with decreased ΔLH in the routine GnRH tests before treatment, serum testosterone (T) did not increase during treatment whereas, in the 2 patients with normal ΔLH before treatment, normalization of serum T occurred during treatment. In the 2 patient without T response to the treatment, continuation of the treatment for 2 months using an increased dosage and i.v. administration (4 ug s.c. and 8 ug i.v. every 2.5 hrs) did not produce an increase in serum T either. Primary refractoriness to treatment is due to pituitary particularities and not to under-dosage; it might be overcome by long-term treatment (>6 mths).

954 BIOLOGICAL PROPERTIES OF CHICKEN LUTEINIZING HORMONE-RELEASING HORMONE([Gln^8]-LHRH) AND DEVELOPMENT OF ITS RIA SYSTEM. Y. Hasegawa*, K. Miyamoto and M. Igarashi, Department of Obstetrics and Gynecology, School of Medicine, Gunma University, Maebashi, Gunma 371, K. Kangawa and H. Matsuo, Department of Biochemistry, Miyazaki Medical College, Kiotake, Miyazaki 889-16, Japan.

We have examined the biological properties of chicken LH-RH, which has been isolated and characterized in our laboratory, using primary monolayer culture of rat anterior pituitary cells and chicken anterior pituitary cells and radioligand analysis. The ED_{50} values for mammalian LH-RH and chicken LH-RH were 0.455 nM and 18.2 nM for LH secretion, respectively, and 0.263 nM and 8.28 nM for FSH from rat pituitary cells, respectively. Relative potencies of chicken LH-RH were 2.5 % for LH and 3.2 % for FSH of mammalian LH-RH acting on rat anterior pituitary cells. On the other hand, the ED_{50} of chicken LH-RH for LH release from chicken anterior pituitary cells was 1.03nM, which indicates that the biological potency of chicken LH-RH acting on chicken pituitary cells was higher than that of chicken LH-RH acting on mammalian pituitary cells.

Highly specific antiserum against chicken LH-RH has been raised in rabbits by immunizing with chicken LH-RH-BSA conjugate. The antiserum bound 40 % of ^{125}I- labelled chicken LH-RH at final dilution of 1:500,000. Half-maximum inhibition by chicken LH-RH was obserbed at 15 pg and the minimum detectable dose was as little as 0.5 pg/tube. The antiserum possessed practically no cross-reactivity with mammalian LH-RH and chicken GnRH II. Distribution of chicken LH-RH has been determined in Japanese quail brain. The highest concentration was obserbed at hypothalamus at level of 2.98ng ± 0.33ng/100 mg wet tissue.

955 URINARY IMMUNOREACTIVE CORTICOTROPIN RELEASING FACTOR. K. Hashimoto*, K. Murakami, T. Hattori and Z. Ota, Third Department of Internal Medicine, Okayama University Medical School, Okayama 700, Japan

As measuring blood concentration of corticotropin releasing factor (CRF) is difficult, we tried measuring CRF in urine. Human and rat CRF were extracted from the urine by adsorption to Vycore glass, Florisil or silicic acid. The highest extraction rate was obtained with Florisil but non-specific substances which interfered with later radioimmunoassay were also extracted. Vycore glass extraction was generally most suitable. CRF was measured by radioimmunoassay using anti-ovine CRF serum, and human (rat) CRF was used for tracer labelling and reference preparation. Human and rat urine extracts showed four or five immunoreactive peaks on Sephadex G-50 fine chromatography. One peak coeluted with marker CRF, and the other immunoreactive peaks (smaller molecular CRF) eluted between CRF and arginine vasopressin. When synthetic CRF was injected to rats, smaller molecular CRF immunoreactivity increased. When urine was collected with 6 N HCl (urine : 6 N HCl = 100 : 1), the ratio of authentic CRF peak to smaller molecular CRF peaks increased. The total urinary CRF immunoreactivity in normal human was 15.6 -68.9 ng/day. Patients with Cushing's disease showed significantly elevated levels of urinary CRF immunoreactivity. Urinary CRF immunoreactivity increased after Metyrapone administration. These results suggest that urinary CRF immunoreactivity represents hypothalamic CRF secretion and smaller molecular CRF immunoreactivities might be degradated fragments of authentic CRF.

956 POTENCY OF GRF AGONISTS STIMULATING GH RELEASE FROM CULTURED PITUITARY CELLS CORRELATES WITH BINDING TO A PUTATIVE GRF RECEPTOR. M.L. Heiman*, M.V. Nekola, V.A. Lance, W.A. Murphy and D.H. Coy, Dept. of Medicine, Tulane University School of Medicine, New Orleans, LA, 70112 USA.

The N-terminal 29 residues [hpGRF(1-29)-NH_2 (GRF-29)] of human pancreatic growth hormone-releasing factor-(1-44) possess full intrinsic *in vitro* activity (Nature 300:276, 1982).We have tested 5 substituted analogs of this sequence for GH releasing activity in cell culture and for receptor binding to pituitary membranes. Male rat anterior pituitaries were removed and dispersed by a combination of trypsin digestion and mechanical agitation. After 4 days of culture, the monolayer of cells was stimulated with peptide for 3h. The EC_{50} values for D-Ala-2-GRF-29, D-Tyr-1-GRF-29, N-Ac-Tyr-1-GRF-29, D-Asp-3-GRF-29, GRF-29 and D-Thr-7-GRF-29 were 0.02 fM, 0.06 fM, 0.6 fM, 0.9 fM, 1.3 fM and 0.5 nM, respectively. Additionally, no stimulation by D-Trp-6-LHRH (a potent LHRH agonist), VIP or bombesin was observed at concentrations up to 10 nM. A tracer with high biological activity was used for studying receptor binding to partially purified male rat anterior pituitary membranes. This tracer was prepared by iodinating N-Ac-His-1,D-Ala-2-GRF-29, a mono-tyrosyl analog. In preliminary experiments, specific binding of this tracer to the membrane was saturable, of high affinity and reversible. Rank order of potency in competing for [125-I]-N-Ac-His-1,D-Ala-2-GRF-29 sites was D-Ala-2-GRF-29 > GRF-29 >> D-Thr-7-GRF-29 >>> D-Trp-6-LHRH, VIP, and bombesin. These data suggest that the enhanced biological activities of these analogs is due at least in part to increased receptor binding. This work was supported by NIH grant AM 30167.

957 CIRCADIAN RHYTHM OF PLASMA CORTISOL AND PITUITARY-ADRENAL RESPONSIVENESS TO CRF AND INSULIN-INDUCED HYPOGLYCEMIA (IIH).
R. Herrera*[1], A.V. Schally[1] and G. Tolis[1,3], [1]McGill University, Montreal, Quebec, Canada, [2]Tulane University School of Medicine and V.A. Medical Center, New Orleans, U.S.A. and [3]Hippokrateion Hospital, Athens, Greece.

To explore the etiology behind the circadian periodicity in plasma cortisol (F) we measured its plasma levels in 5 healthy volunteers at 0800 h and 1800 h under two experimental protocols. Subjects were given intravenously CRF (100 ug/bolus) and 4 weeks later insulin for induction of hypoglycemia. Above tests were done in a circadian manner i.e. at both 0800 h and 1800 h and blood was collected at 15 min intervals for two hours. A prompt release of F was noticed after either challenge (Table I).

Table I. Effect of CRF and IIH on cortisol release (ΔF)

	CRF		IIH	
ΔF	AM	PM	AM	PM
mean(range) ug/dl	11.3(7-14)	14 (5-29)	9.7(1-28)	23 (15-21)
%	102(94-140)	157(33-300)	72 (1-233)	512(313-850)

Peak values after CRF were reached at 15-30 min for ACTH and at 45-60 min for cortisol; these curves were shifted to the right after IIH. The brisk release of cortisol at PM following CRF or IIH suggests that the circadian attenuation of cortisol secretion at PM is not due to down regulation of pituitary or adrenal receptors to CRF and ACTH respectively but rather to a circadian periodicity in the amount of endogenously released CRF.

958 GLUCOCORTICOID MODULATION OF CORTICOTROPIN RELEASING FACTOR (CRF) DESENSITIZATION IN CULTURED RAT ANTERIOR PITUITARY CELLS.
A. Hoffman* and G. Ceda. Dept. of Medicine, Stanford University Medical Center, Stanford CA 94305 USA.

The ability of CRF to stimulate both ACTH release and intracellular cyclic AMP accumulation is rapidly and reversibly desensitized when rat anterior pituitary cells are cultured in the absence of added glucocorticoids. Since this desensitization has not been readily apparent in vivo where initial CRF exposure results in high levels of ambient glucocorticoids, we examined the effect of glucocorticoids on the desensitization process in vitro. Rat anterior pituitary cells were cultured for 3-5 days; the fetal calf serum, which was added to the incubation medium, had been treated with activated charcoal to remove endogenous glucocorticoids. Dexamethasone was then added to some culture wells 24 hours before the desensitization experiment began. Desensitization to CRF was achieved by preincubating the cells for 4 hours with varying concentrations (10^{-11}M to 10^{-8}M) of ovine CRF, washing the cells with medium alone and then re-exposing the cells to 10^{-8}M CRF. In the absence of glucocorticoid, the ED_{50} for CRF (the preincubation dose causing 50% desensitization of subsequent ACTH release) was 3×10^{-10}M, but cells which had been pre-exposed to dexamethasone desensitized less readily. With concentrations of dexamethasone $> 10^{-8}$M, no desensitization at all occurred. Similar changes in CRF desensitization were observed when cells were incubated with 10^{-8}M corticosterone, but not with 10^{-8}M estradiol, testosterone, progesterone or aldosterone. These data demonstrate that glucocorticoids profoundly alter the development of desensitization in vitro and suggest that high ambient glucocorticoid concentrations prevent the development of substantial CRF desensitization in vivo.

959 CHARACTERIZATION AND LOCALIZATION OF CORTICOTROPIN-RELEASING FACTOR RECEPTORS IN THE RAT BRAIN.
M.C. Holmes*, P.C. Wynn, R.L. Hauger, M.A. Millan, K.J. Catt and G. Aguilera, ERRB, NICHD, NIH, Bethesda, MD, U.S.A.

In addition to regulating the secretion of ACTH and related pituitary peptides, corticotropin-releasing factor (CRF) has been shown to exert direct actions within the central nervous system (CNS). To elucidate the sites of action and potential physiological roles of CRF in the CNS, we identified and characterized CRF receptors in the rat brain, and determined their anatomical distribution by autoradiographic analysis of the binding of radioiodinated Tyr-oCRF to 20 μm frozen brain sections. Specific binding of ^{125}I-Tyr-CRF to brain cortex membrane-rich particles was rapid and temperature dependent and reached equilibrium within 30 min at 22 ^{o}C. The brain binding sites were saturable and of high affinity, with Kd of 1 nM, and were selective for CRF and its active fragments. Autoradiographic localization of CRF receptors in the brain revealed a high density of sites in the olfactory bulb, primary olfactory cortex, neocortex, claustrum, lateral septal nucleus, amygdaloid complex, bed of the stria terminalis, anterior and laterodorsal thalamic nuclei, supramammilary nucleus, interpeduncular nucleus, pontine nuclei and cerebellar cortex. These studies demonstrate that specific CRF receptors are selectively concentrated in a number of physiologically relevant sites in the brain, the majority of which are related to the limbic system. Such data indicate that CRF is involved in multiple functions in the CNS, including the behavioural as well as the neurohumoral responses to stress.

960 EFFECT OF THE PEPTIDES PHI, VIP AND GALANIN ON PRL, ACTH AND GH RELEASE FROM RAT PITUITARY CELLS IN VITRO.
A-L. Hulting*, S. Werner. K. Tatemoto, V. Mutt. T. Melander. and T. Hökfelt. Dept. of Endocrinology, Karolinska Hospital, Depts. of Biochemistry and Histology, Karolinska Institute, Stockholm, Sweden.

PHI, VIP and galanin are peptides with 27, 28 and 29 amino acids, respectively, isolated from porcine intestine. PHI- and galaninlike immunoreactivity has been demonstrated in separate hypothalamic systems with nerve endings in the median eminence, a localization which suggests involvement in the regulation of anterior pituitary function.

In cultures of dispersed rat anterior pituitary cells, PHI, 10^{-8} and 10^{-7} M, stimulated PRL and ACTH release. The stimulatory effect on both PRL and ACTH decreased at 10^{-6} M. VIP caused a significant release of PRL only at 10^{-6} M and had no effect on ACTH release. Galanin exhibited no stimulatory or inhibitory effect on PRL or ACTH secretion. None of the three peptides affected the release of GH, whereas the structurally similar GRF was a potent GH releaser.

The concentrations needed to obtain a stimulatory effect on PRL release by PHI and VIP and on ACTH release by PHI, were higher than those needed for CRF to release ACTH and GRF to release GH. Galanin did not affect basal secretion of PRL, ACTH, GH, TSH, LH or FSH.

Thus, PHI appears to be a modulator of PRL as well as ACTH secretion, VIP a modulator solely of PRL release, while galanin, also present in the hypothalamus, has no effect on the release of the six anterior pituitary hormones studied.

961 CORTICOTROPIN-RELEASING FACTOR TEST IN PATIENTS WITH CUSHING'S SYNDROME BEFORE AND AFTER ADENOMECTOMY.

T. Imaki*, T. Shibasaki, M. Nakahara, A. Masuda, T. Suda, H. Demura, k. Shizume and [1]N. Ling. Department of Medicine, Tokyo Women's Medical College, Tokyo 162, Japan, [1]Laboratories for Neuroendocrinology, The Salk Institute, La Jolla, CA 92037, U.S.A.

Six patients with Cushing's disease and three with Cushing's syndrome due to an adrenal adenoma were followed up after adenomectomy to evaluate the degree of recovery of pituitary-adrenal function with corticotropin-releasing factor (CRF) test. In patients with Cushing's disease who showed high, normal or low responses of plasma ACTH and cortisol to 100 µg synthetic ovine CRF before adenomectomy, basal levels of both hormones were extremely low with no response to CRF one month after surgery and entered the normal ranges with lower normal responses to CRF 6 months after the operation. Though the recovery of function of adrenal was slightly behind that of pituitary, both functions were recuperated almost in parallel and reached the normal ranges approximately 9 months after adenomectomy. In the patients with Cushing's syndrome due to an adrenal adenoma who showed no response of both hormones before adenomectomy, ACTH reached the normal basal range with almost normal response to CRF 3 to 6 months after surgery and increased with the excessive and prolonged response in CRF test 8 months after surgery. On the other hand, only slight response of plasma cortisol induced by CRF was observed 14 months after surgery in spite of the elevation of basal value. The difference of recovery course between Cushing's disease and Cushing's syndrome due to an adrenal adenoma was considered to result from the existence of adrenal atrophy in Cushing's syndrome due to an adrenal adenoma.

962 STUDY ON THE EFFECT OF hpGRF(1-44) IN NORMAL ADULT AND IN THE PATIENTS WITH ACROMEGALY AND OBESITY

K. Inoue[1]*, T. Shimizu[1], H. Kaneko[1], S. Sawano[2] and M. Irie[1], 1)First Dept. of Med., Toho Univ. School of Med., Tokyo. 2)Dept. of Endocrinology, Toranomon Hospital, and Okinaka Memorial Inst. for Med. Res., Tokyo Japan.

Studies were performed to prove the effect of hpGRF, which was synthesized by solid phase method and showed definite in vitro and in vivo effect of GH stimulation in rats, in the same extent with commercial GRF of Peninsula Co.. 0.3, 0.5, 1.0, 2.0, 4.0, µg/kg of hpGRF and saline were injected as i.v. bolus at the fasting states in 8 normal volunteers (6 male, 2 female), and blood was drawn at 0, 5, 10, 15, 30, 60, 90, 120, 180 minutes after injection. Dose-response relationship was not clear, but 1.0 µg/kg injection showed maximal response as the average. 6 subjects showed definite response, whereas 2 showed no response in any of these doses. Reproducibility was not good in the dose of 1.0 µg/kg in responders. In 1 of 2 non-responders, insulin and arginine administration showed no response, whereas another subject showed GH response only to insulin hypoglycemia. Oral 10 mg administration of propranolol was attempted to 2 non-responders at 60 and 30 minutes before, and at the same time of hpGRF injection, but no definite increment was observed. Among 5 aged subjects over 61 year old, 3 showed no response. 4 obese subjects showed low or no response. In 11 acromegalic patients, the type of response was divided into 3 - normal, low and exaggerated responses. The good controlled group showed normal or low response, and exaggerated response with high peak values of GH was observed in the group without good clinical control.

963 THE STIMULATION OF SOMATOSTATIN (SS) RELEASE BY $hpGRF_{44}$ FROM RAT HYPOTHALAMIC CELLS AND FRAGMENTS IN VITRO.

K. Iwasaki*and A. Arimura, LMNED, Tulane University Hebert Research Center, Belle Chasse, La. 70037, USA.

Clinical evidence indicates that the administration of hpGRF occasionally fails to increase the secretion of GH in healthy humans. The action of GRF may be overcome if the secretion of SS increases. It is possible that GRF has a direct action on SS neurons, thereby stimulating SS release from the median eminence. We decided to examine if GRF stimulates SS release from cultured rat hypothalamic cells and fragments in vitro. The hypothalami of rat fetuses were collected on the 17th day of pregnancy under a dissection microscope. 40 hypothalami were collected in phosphate buffered saline, and then dispersed with 0.1% collagenase. These cells were cultured in DMEM/F_{12}/HEPES containing 10% fetal calf serum and 2.5% horse serum for 12 days at 37C under 5% CO_2/air. The cultured cells were washed with Krebs Ringer bicarbonate/glucose buffer 3X, then incubated with test samples for 1hr. SS released into the medium was quantitated by RIA.The mean basal release of SS was 12 ± 1.9pg/dish/hr. 60mM K^+ stimulated SS release 20 fold. 1, 10 and 100 nM $hpGRF_{44}$ increased SS release by 1.2, 1.4 and 1.5 fold respectively. 0.1nM $hpGRF_{44}$ was ineffective. 10nM oCRF and TRH stimulated SS release by 1.5 and 2.5 fold respectively. Neither 10 nM GnRH nor 10nM VIP increased SS release. 0.1nM to 100nM of $hpGRF_{44}$ also stimulated SS release from rat hypothalamic fragments in a dose-related manner (1.1 to 1.8 fold). A significant increase was observed only with 10 and 100nM $hpGRF_{44}$. The results of this study suggest that a high concentration of GRF may also stimulate SS release in vivo thereby obscuring GH response to GRF under certain conditions. Aided by NIH grant AM09094.

964 CENTRAL MECHANISMS INVOLVED IN THE CORTICOTROPIC RESPONSE TO ETHER-STRESS IN RATS.

G.Ixart*,B.Conte-Devolx, A.Szafarczyk,S.Arancibia,C.Oliver, and I.Assenmacher,Lab.Neuroendocrinology,ERA 85-CNRS, University of Montpellier II (G.I.,A.S.,S.A.,I.A.) and Lab.Experimental Medicine,University of Marseille (B.C-D.,C.O.), France

The CNS control of the dramatic increase in plasma ACTH and corticosterone evidenced in individual ether-stressed rats and culminating within 10-15 min post-stress was,firstly attested by the occurence of a concomitant rise in RIA-CRH-41 release measured in the median eminence locally implanted with a push-pull canula.The preeminent role of CRH in the ACTH stress-response emerged further for the demonstration that passive immunization against CRH-41 induced a depression of the hormonal response (- 60%),fairly close to that following a bilateral stereotaxic ablation of the paraventricular nuclei (PVN) (- 50%),whereas homozygous Brattleboro rats displayed a normal response. Additionally a striking inhibition of the ACTH stress-response resulted also from a pharmacological blockade of the rerotoninergic system (2 x 300 mg/kg pCPA) (-50%), or after bilateral stereotaxic lesions of the suprachiasmatic nuclei (-45%),both neuronal systems being already known to participate in the rhythmic pattern of ACTH secretion. Finally, the possible mechanisms whereby bilateral lesions of the supraoptic nuclei(SON)-which incidentally were shown to send only restrcted projections to the external median eminence-doubled the ACTH response to ether-stress, are discussed

965 GH RELEASING FACTOR (GRF) PRETREATMENT ENHANCES THE GRF INDUCED GH SECRETION IN RATS WITH THE PITUITARY AUTOTRANSPLANTED TO THE KIDNEY CAPSULE.

John-Olov Jansson* and Lena Carlsson, Dept of Physiology, University of Göteborg, P O Box 33031, S-400 33 Göteborg, Sweden

In vitro experiments have suggested that growth hormone releasing factor (GRF) not only increases the GH release but also the GH biosynthesis (Vale, Endocrinology 112,1553,1983). Preliminary case reports indicate that GRF pretreatment to patients with growth hormone (GH) deficiency might enhance the GH response to GRF (Borges et al, The Lancet ii,119,1983). The aim of the present study was to investigate the effect of long-term GRF pretreatment on the GRF induced GH release in the rat.

Male rats, 40 days old, were hypophysectomized and the pituitary was autotransplanted to the right kidney capsule. Replacement therapy with thyroxine and cortisone was given. One week after surgery the rats were prepared with a chronic intracardiac catheter. GRF (4 ug/kg) was given i v every 8 h for 3 days. Controls were given saline. On the 4th day all animals received GRF i v (4 ug/kg) and repeated blood samples were withdrawn. The animals were sacrificed 3 h after the last GRF injection and the grafted pituitaries were homogenized. Plasma and pituitary GH levels were measured by RIA. The maximum GH response to GRF was higher in the GRF pretreated group (398 ± 104 ng/ml, n=3) as compared to rats receiving saline (107 ± 10 ng/ml, n=5; $p<0.01$). There was, however, no difference in pituitary GH content between GRF and saline pretreated rats. It is concluded that chronic GRF treatment increases the GH response to GRF in the rat. Furthermore, autotranspanted pituitary grafts might be a useful model for further investigation of the long-term effects of GRF on GH secretion.

966 CLONING AND SEQUENCING OF cDNA FOR RAT CORTICOTROPIN-RELEASING FACTOR PRECURSOR AND DEMONSTRATION OF ITS mRNA IN HYPOTHALAMUS.

H. Jingami*, S. Shibahara, Y. Furutani, H. Imura and S. Numa, Department of Medical Chemistry and Second Division, Department of Medicine, Kyoto University Faculty of Medicine, Sakyo-ku, Kyoto 606, Japan.

DNA complementary to the rat hypothalamic mRNA encoding the corticotropin-releasing factor precursor (prepro-CRF) has been cloned by screening a cDNA library, constructed by the method of Okayama and Berg, with a human genomic DNA probe (Shibahara et al., EMBO J. 2, 775-779, 1983). Nucleotide sequence analysis of the cloned cDNA has revealed the primary structure of rat prepro-CRF. Blot hybridization analysis of rat hypothalamic poly(A) RNA using a cDNA probe exhibits a hybridization-positive species with an approximate size of 1300 nucleotides. The effects of adrenalectomy and steroid administration on the hypothalamic content of prepro-CRF mRNA are currently under investigation.

967 GROWTH HORMONE RESPONSE TO HUMAN PANCREATIC GROWTH HORMONE RELEASING FACTOR-44 IN RUMINANTS.
T. Johke*[1], K. Hodate[1], S. Ohashi[1], M. Shiraki[2] and S. Sawano[3] [1]National Institute of Animal Industry, Tsukuba Norindanchi P.O.BOX 5, Ibaraki 305, [2] Research Institute for Polymers and Textiles , Yatabe Higashi, Ibaraki 305, [3] Department of Endocrinology, Toranomon Hospital, and Asahi Life Institute for Adult Diseases, Toranomon Minatoku, Tokyo 105, Japan

The effects of human pancreatic growth hormone releasing factor-44 (hpGRF-44) on growth hormone(GH) secretion in cattle, goats and sheep were studied. The hpGRF-44 preparation was synthesized by solid-phase method. Single intravenous injection of 0.1, 0.25, 0.5 or 1.0 μg of hpGRF-44 per kg of bw in calves and goats significantly elevated immunoreactive circulating GH levels within 5 min($p < 0.01$). The plasma GH level increased proportionally to the dose of hpGRF-44 and reached a peak at 5 - 10 min. Intravenous injection of 0.25 μg per kg of bw to female calves, heifers, and cows significantly elevated mean GH levels from 8.5, 2.3, and 1.6 ng /ml at 0 time to peak values of 97, 26, and 12 ng/ml, respectively($p < 0.01$). The responses in calves, kids, and lambs were significantly higher than those in cows, adult goats and sheep($p < 0.05$). The plasma GH response to hpGRF-44 in the ruminants decreased with advancing age. The GH response in male calves was significantly greater than that in female calves($p < 0.01$) Similar result was also obtained in lambs. Simultaneous administration of somatostatin-14 inhibited the plasma GH response to hpGRF-44 in the male calves. These results indicate that synthetic hpGRF-44 is a potent secretogogue for bovine, caprine, and ovine GH in vivo, and suggest its usefulness for the assesment of GH secretion and reserve in the ruminants.

968 THE SOURCES OF PEPTIDERGIC INNERVATIONS OF VENTROMEDIAL HYPOTHALAMIC NUCLEUS (VMH) IN THE RAT: NEUROTENSIN (NT), CHOLECYSTOKININ-8 (CCK) AND ENKEPHPALIN (ENK).
S. Inagaki*, M. Yamano[1], M. Tohyama[1], Y. Shiotani[1], and A. Parent, Lab. of Neurobiol., Fac. Med., Laval University, Quebec, GlK 7P4, Canada, and ([1])Dept. Neuroanatomy, Inst. Higher Nervous Activity, Osaka Univ. Med. School, Nakanoshima, Kita-ku, Osaka 530, Japan.

Our previous immunohistochemical observations made in stereotaxically lesioned rats have revealed that NT-like immunoreactive fibers, which are mainly confined to the dorsomedial part of VMH, arise from the medial amygdaloid nucleus, while CCK-like immunoreactive fibers present in VMH originate from the lateral part of the dorsal parabrachial nucleus. In this report we describe the distribution and source of ENK-like immunoreactivity found in the VMH area in rat.

The leu-enkephalin antibody was raised in rabbit against synthetic leu-enkephalin conjugated with bovine thyroglobulin and the indirect immunofluorescent method was used. In rat ENK-like immunoreactive (ENI) fibers occur throughout VMH and ENI cell bodies are found in area surrounding VMH. Electrolytic lesion of paraventricular hypothalamic nucleus (PV) decrease significantly the number of ENI fibers in ipsilateral VMH. Moreover, sagittal knife cut placed lateral to PV induce a pile up of ENI in fibers on PV side, and a reduction of ENI in fibers reaching the ipsilateral VMH. The results suggest that ENI neurons located in PV innervate directly VMH through axons coursing ventrolaterally in hypothalamus. The existence of such ENI projection is further supported by the results of HRP injections into VMH.

969 THE INFLUENCE OF PRENATAL EXPOSURE TO MORPHINE ON POSTNATAL OPIATE RECEPTOR DENSITY IN RAT BRAIN. S. Iyengar* and J. Rabii, Dept. of Biol. Sci., Rutgers Univ., Piscataway, NJ 08854, USA.

Opiates have been implicated in the modulation of several neuroendocrine mechanisms. We have studied the effect of morphine sulfate exposure, during a critical period of prenatal life (days 7-12 of gestation), on opiate receptor density in several areas of the postnatal brain important to neuroendocrine function. Opiate receptor density was measured by receptor autoradiography and computerized densitometry, at postnatal ages 15 and 75 days. It was found that there was a significant increase in opiate receptor density in morphine exposed female pup brains, both at 15 and 75 days of age, in the medial preoptic area, suprachiasmatic nucleus, stria terminalis, arcuate nucleus, median eminence, ventromedial and dorsomedial nuclei and the amygdala. The brain of male pups, however, did not show any significant differences at day 15, but a decrease in the above areas at day 75. Biochemical analyses of receptor density in whole brain, in animals treated as above, showed similar results. Furthermore, a sex difference was observed in receptor density in various brain regions of the control (untreated) rats. It is suggested from these data that prenatal exposure to opiates can affect opiate receptor density in important nuclei of the brain in the offspring and, that a sex difference also exists. Supported by the Busch Memorial Fund and NIH Grant DA02227.

970 ANDROGEN SECRETION DURING EARLY PREGNANCY IN THE RHESUS MONKEY: CORRELATION WITH CHORIONIC GONADOTROPIN SECRETION. William E. Ellinwood*, Reproductive Biology and Behavior, Oregon Regional Primate Research Center, Beaverton, Oregon, USA.

During early pregnancy in rhesus monkeys, estrogen concentrations in the peripheral circulation rise and follow a temporal pattern that mimics that of chorionic gonadotropin (CG), while progesterone (P) concentrations, after an initial rise, decline and remain low until the placenta begins to secrete significant amounts of P. To examine the dynamics of androgen secretion in relationship to these phenomena, we obtained daily blood samples from six pregnant rhesus monkeys during the cycle of conception and for the first 50 days of pregnancy. Concentrations of androstenedione (A), testosterone (T), estradiol (E_2), estrone (E_1), P, and CG were determined by RIA. In all six animals, concentrations of A and T were significantly elevated by day 13 of pregnancy (Day 0 = day of mating) and reached levels 5- to 10-fold greater than those observed during the late luteal phase by days 17-18 of pregnancy. The temporal patterns of A and T concentrations were identical to those of CG and the estrogens. Between days 13 and 23 of pregnancy, concentrations of androgens and estrogens were inversely correlated with concentrations of P. Bilateral ovariectomy on day 23 of pregnancy (n = 2) reduced A and T concentrations to late luteal phase levels, indicating an ovarian source for these androgens. These data provide the first information on the dynamics of androgen secretion during early pregnancy in rhesus monkeys, and suggest that the dramatic rise in A and T concentrations is a consequence of CG stimulation of ovarian androgen synthesis. Supported by the NIH.

971 DIFFERENTIAL STEROIDOGENESIS BY CELLS OF THE EQUINE CONCEPTUS.
Goff, A.K.*, Renard, A., LaFrance, M. and Marsan, C. Centre de Recherche en Reproduction Animale, Fac. Méd. Vét., Univ. Montréal, St-Hyacinthe, Canada.

Estradiol-17β (E2) production by the equine conceptus is possibly involved in the maternal recognition of pregnancy, as in the pig. We have previously demonstrated that conceptuses (blastodermic vesicles) produce less E2 after rupture than when intact although no similar decreases occur in progesterone (P), estrone (E1) or androstenedione (A) production. This present study has examined the possibility that steroid secretion varies with embryonic cell type. Ten conceptuses, diameters 10-14 mm, were obtained transcervically 12-14 days after ovulation. After dissociation (0.25% collagenase) and separation of the embryonic cells by density using a 40% Percoll gradient, each fraction was cultured for 24h in MEM ± 10% charcoal-treated fetal calf serum. Steroids secreted into the media were measured by RIA. Results showed that the fractionated cells could be divided into two distinct types, (a) and (b). Indirect evidence suggests that these are predominantly ectodermal and endodermal cells respectively. Type (a) produced 2.4-fold more E2 than P whereas type (b) produced 185-fold more P than E2. Also, type (a) produced 11.2-fold more E2 and 47-fold less P than did type (b). Only type (b) cells made significant quantities of A. Addition of exogenous P or A increased E2 production to a much greater extent in type (a) cells than in type (b). These data show that steroid hormone secretion varies with conceptus cell type, and suggest that in the intact conceptus E2 secretion depends on an interaction between cell types.
Supported by grants from the MRC, NSERC & the Max Bell Foundation.

972 Pulsatile LH-RH substitution in hypothalamic amenorrhea.
J.P. Hanker*, L. Nieschlag and H.P.G. Schneider, University Women's Hospital and Max Planck-Clinical Research Unit for Reproductive Medicine, 4400 Muenster, Germany

In hypothalamic amenorrhea endogenous LH-RH secretion is inadequate or abolished as evidenced by impaired or absent episodic LH release. To reestablish cyclic gonadotropin secretion chronic-intermittent LH-RH substitution (12 μg/pulse i.v.) was performed on 53 hypothalamo-amenorrheic patients by means of a portable mini-pump (Auto-Syringe). In 25 patients 30 ovulatory cycles were induced by LH-RH pulses, administered once every 96 min throughout the follicular phase; 7 patients conceived and have been delivered from healthy children. In 24 patients 28 ovulatory cycles were induced by LH-RH pulses, the initial frequency of which was 4 h (for 2 days) and then increased to 3 h (for 1 day) and 96 min (for the remainder of the follicular phase). Five patients conceived and have been delivered from healthy children. In 4 patients ovulations were induced by LH-RH pulses administered once every 3 hours during the follicular phase and 2 women conceived. Luteal LH-RH support was provided in all cases, either by maintenance of pump-assisted LH-RH substitution or by LH-RH nasal-spray (200 μg once every 4 hours). Consistently luteal function was enhanced when follicular development had been initiated by frequency-varied LH-RH pulses in the beginning of therapy.

973 HORMONAL PARAMETERS IN INCIDENTAL VARICOCELES AND THOSE CAUSING INFERTILITY. R.W. Hudson, Department of Medicine, Queen's University, Kingston, Ontario, Canada K7L 6V7.

Since 8-22% of men have varicoceles, it is likely that the varicosity is not always the causative factor in those infertile men in whom they are present. We have studied the hormonal patterns of 4 groups of men with varicoceles prior to, and between 9 and 12 months after, varicocelectomy. Groups 1 (n=12) and 2 (n=8) had preoperative sperm densities of 5 ± 3 and 6 ± 3 x 10^6/ml respectively, while Groups 3 (n=10) and 4 (n=5) had densities of 19 ± 5 and 22 ± 8 x 10^6/ml. All men had normal baseline serum levels of testosterone (T), estradiol, LH, FSH and prolactin. Peak LH and FSH values (mean ± s.d.), in response to an I.V. infusion of gonadotropin releasing hormone (GnRH), and seminal plasma dihydrotestosterone (DHT) levels were 120±33, 70±6 and 0.92±0.29; 38±8, 26±6 and 2.08±0.46; 106±12, 63±17 and 1.17±0.33; and 35±9 I.U./L, 24±5 I.U./L and 2.11±0.42 nM, respectively, for Groups 1 to 4. Between 9 and 12 months following surgery, 8 men from Group 1 and 6 from Group 3 had significant improvements in sperm density (23±5 and 41±9 x 10^6/ml), respectively. Peak LH and FSH values in response to GnRH and seminal plasma DHT levels were also improved (70±6 I.U./L, 37±3 I.U./L and 1.8±0.3 nM, Group 1; 45±6; 26±4 and 1.99±0.5, Group 3). The remainder of the men in both groups and all of the men in Groups 2 and 4 had no postoperative changes in seminal or hormonal parameters. The results of this study demonstrate that the gonadotropin response to GnRH and the level of seminal plasma DHT can be used to predict the likelihood of a favourable response to varicocelectomy.

974 HISTOLOGY, ESTROGEN-, PROGESTOGEN RECEPTORS AND PREGNANCY AFTER MICROSURGICAL RECONSTRUCTION OF INDUCED HYDROSALPINGES IN RABBITS. B. Karbowski*, G. Vasquez, I. Brosens and H.P.G. Schneider, Department of Gynecology and Obstetrics of the University of Münster, Domagstr. 11, West Germany.

Damage to fallopian tubes caused by hydrosalpinges is a major reason for persisting infertility. The postoperative time course of mucosal recovery following tubal microsurgery in correlation to pregnancy rate at varying intervals of time after reanastomosis of mechanical induced hydrosalpinges in rabbits were examined. We describe the mucosal changes by light and scanning electron microscopy and measuring estrogen and progestogen receptors. Groups of rabbits were mated one to two, three to four, seven to eight weeks after surgery and were used for morphologic and receptor studies. The mucosa of hydrosalpinges showed progressive atrophy of folds, flattened epithelium, deciliation and cell desquamation. Three weeks after reanastomosis mucosal recovery was well advanced. Changes in fertility were observed. Although patency rate was 70 - 80 % and recovery of tubal damage was largely complete seven to eight weeks after microsurgical reconstruction of hydrosalpinges we did not see more than 30 % pregnancy rate. This study was supported by Deutsche Forschungs-Gemeinschaft in the Centre for Infertility Microsurgery Leuven/Belgium.

975 FACTORS AFFECTING PERIPHERAL AND AUTONOMIC NEUROPATHY IN DIABETES. A. L. Graber* and L. Graber, Vanderbilt Univ., Nashville, Tn., 37205, USA.

The effect of age, sex, cigarette smoking, serum glucose, and glycosylated hemoglobin (GHb) on neurololgical function was studied in 145 nondiabetic subjects and 173 diabetic patients. Vibratory perception threshold (VPT) in thumb and great toe was measured with a biothesiometer as an index of peripheral nerve function, and the ratio of heartbeat during expiration and inspiration (E/I ratio) was used as a measure of autonomic nerve function. VPT in both thumb and toe increases with age in normals ($R=.29$, $p=.001$), so that age-adjusted normal ranges are necessary. At all age levels from teens to seventies the mean VPT in thumb and toe was significantly higher in diabetics than in nondiabetics ($p<.05$). Multivariate analysis using stepwise regression with VPT as the dependent variable showed a significant relationship only with age, and no significant relationship with sex, cigarette smoking, serum glucose, or GHb in diabetics. The E/I ratio decreases with age in normals ($R=-0.4$, $p= .001$). The mean E/I ratio is 1.33 before age 40 and 1.12 after age 60. The mean E/I ratio in diabetics is lower than in nondiabetics at all age levels, but the difference is significant ($p<.05$) only at the 40-59 age level. Multiple regression analysis with the E/I ratio as the dependent variable showed a significant relationship only with age, and no significant relationship with sex, cigarette smoking, serum glucose, or GHb in diabetics. These data demonstrate that quantitative evidence of both peripheral and autonomic nerve dysfunction is present in diabetic patients of all ages. When the effect of age is controlled, the dysfunction does not correlate with indices of glucose control or the use of cigarettes. The factors responsible for the neurological dysfunction in diabetes are unknown.

976 ADENOSINE BLOCKS CATECHOLAMINE INHIBITION OF INSULIN ACTION IN ADIPOCYTES AT THE N_S REGULATORY PROTEIN. Allan Green* and Idania M. Alvarez, Dept. of Medicine, Univ. of Florida, Gainesville, FL 32610, U.S.A.

We have reported that catecholamines inhibit insulin-stimulated glucose transport (GT) in adipocytes. Endogenously produced adenosine blocks this catecholamine effect unless prevented from accumulating by use of adenosine deaminase (ADA). To investigate the role of cyclic AMP (cAMP) and the mechanism by which adenosine blocks the effect, we have utilized dibutyryl cAMP (DBcAMP) and agents which raise cellular cAMP levels by various mechanisms: theophylline (phosphodiesterase inhibitor) forskolin (activator of the catalytic subunit (C) of adenylate cyclase) cholera toxin (activator of adenylate cyclase at the N_S regulatory subunit) and isoproterenol (β-agonist). DBcAMP, theophylline and forskolin inhibited insulin (25 ng/ml)-stimulated GT (2-deoxyglucose uptake). IC_{50} values were 1mM, 1mM and 2 μM respectively. These agents were equally effective in the presence and in the absence of ADA (10 μg/ml). Conversely cholera toxin and isoproterenol only inhibited insulin-stimulated GT in the presence of ADA. IC_{50} values were 200 ng/ml and 30 nM respectively. These effects could not be accounted for by changes in ^{125}I-insulin binding to the cells. Conclusions: 1) Agents which raise cellular cAMP levels inhibit insulin-stimulated GT at a post-insulin receptor level. 2) Agents which act at or before the level of N_S (isoproterenol, cholera toxin) require the presence of ADA to inhibit insulin-stimulated GT. Those which act distal to N_S (forskolin, theophylline, DBcAMP) do not require ADA. This suggests that adenosine prevents or limits the interaction of N_S with C, thus preventing cAMP levels from rising sufficiently for inhibition of insulin action.

977 **FIBROSIS AND CALCIFICATION OF THE PANCREAS: T.A.I. Grillo, Faculty of Health Sciences, University of Ife, Ile-Ife Nigeria**

Fibrosis and calcification of the pancreas occur commonly in Africa. It is suggested that the pathological conditions are the result of chronic pancreatitis produced by a number of factors — malnutrition, alcoholism and ductal obstruction. These factors have been made the objectives of experiments in laboratory animals while postmortem sections of human pancreases have been reviewed. Malnutrition particularly as a result of high carbohydrate diet or kwashikor in man results in both fibrosis and calcification. In an older age group of patients alcoholism with malnutrition is another factor. Obstruction of the pancreatic duct in helmithic infestations in Africans or when produced experimentally resulted in fibrosis and calcification.
Insulin secretion is impaired in calcification of the pancreas as well as in malnutrition.

The processes of fibrosis and calcification as studied by electron-microscopy will be discussed.

978 THE EFFECTS OF HYPERGLYCEMIA ON THE HYPOTHALAMIC-PITUITARY-ADRENAL AXIS IN MAN. H.S. Grunstein* and G.A. Smythe, Garvan Institute of Medical Research, St. Vincent's Hospital, Sydney, 2010, Australia.

Hypoglycemia is a profound stimulus to the hypothalamic-pituitary-adrenal (HPA) axis and recent data indicate the responses are mediated by the neuronal activity of central norepinephrine (NE). However, there is scant data on the effects of hyperglycemia on the HPA axis and in this study we examined the effects of hyperglycemia on urinary 3-methoxy-4-hydroxy-phenethylene glycol (MHPG) (as a reflection of central NE neuronal activity), and on plasma ACTH and cortisol in 8 normal subjects. Each subject underwent 3h i.v. infusions of 20% dextrose (sufficient to increase blood glucose by 2mm/l above basal), dexamethasone 1mg/h (an agent known to reduce plasma ACTH and cortisol) or saline. Urine MHPG rose by 4±4% (mean, SEM, saline) and fell by 18±6% (dextrose) and 15±8% (dexamethasone) (both $p<0.05$ vs saline). Following saline, dextrose or dexamethasone respectively, maximal falls in plasma ACTH were 15±14%, 37±8% and 61±9% while maximal falls in plasma cortisol were 31±12%, 48±7% and 66±4%. Compared to the saline infusion significant falls in plasma ACTH and cortisol following dextrose ($p<0.05$ to 0.005) or dexamethasone ($p<0.05$ to 0.0005) were observed at multiple time points. The data reveal falls of urinary MHPG, plasma ACTH and cortisol during hyperglycemia which are similar to those seen following dexamethasone. We conclude that hyperglycemia inhibits the hypothalamic-pituitary-adrenal axis in man and suggest that glucose exerts a fundamental influence on this axis via a negative feedback effect on central NE activity. This study was supported by the NH&MRC of Australia.

979 FILTER PAPER SPOTS GLYCEMIA IN THE QUALITY CONTROL OF HOME BLOOD GLUCOSE MONITORING (HBGM) TECHNIQUES. J.P. Hallé*, E. Renaud, A. Toupin, R. Lepage, C. Hinse and G. Lalumière, Sacré-Coeur Hospital, Montréal, H4J 1C5, Canada.

Our purpose was to perform, without hospitalization, a quality control of the HBGM techniques done by diabetics at home. We instructed 22 diabetics to put a drop of blood on a stabilized filter paper and to use the following drop to measure their blood glucose with reactive strips Chemstrips BG. Filter papers were previously stabilized by soaking them in benzoic acid 3g/l to prevent glycolysis. Each patient collected 9 to 12 samples at home and mailed the filter paper along with their own HBGM results. A piece of filter paper, equivalent to 9.5 ul of blood, was punch out from each filter paper spot. After solubilization in trichloroacetic acid 2%, centrifugation and neutralization with sodium hydroxyde 1.5 N, the glycemia is measured by the glucose oxydose method (correlation 0.96, $p<0.005$, C.V. - 4.83%, stability 14 days). Using filter paper spots glycemia as a reference technique and Chemstrip B.G. as HBGM technique, the whole group of patients had a r of 0.82. Individual patients results were as follows: $r \geq 0.81$ in 12 patients; r=0.51 to 0.80 in 4 patients; $r \leq 0.50$ in 6 patients. Filter paper spots glycemia is a useful technique to identify patients, whose HBGM techniques are unreliable. This study was supported by the Quebec Diabetic association.

980 GLUCAGON AND TWO GLUCAGON-LIKE PEPTIDES ARE ENCODED BY SEPARATE EXONS IN THE RAT GLUCAGON GENE. G. Heinrich*, P.Gros, J.F. Habener, Laboratory of Molecular Endocrinology, Howard Hughes Medical Institute, Massachusetts General Hospital, Boston, MA 02114, USA.

We are investigating glucagon gene expression. The glucagon gene is a member of a gene family that includes among others, vasoactive intestinal peptide, secretin, and growth hormone releasing hormone genes. The glucagon gene is expressed in at least two tissues, gut and pancreas. We have previously demonstrated two distinct glucagon genes in anglerfish. Each gene encodes a separate pancreatic glucagon precursor whose primary structure includes glucagon and a glucagon-like peptide (GLP) arranged in tandem. The rat haploid genome in contrast, contains only one glucagon gene. Moreover rat pre-proglucagon is longer than the anglerfish pre-proglucagons. Our recent structural analysis of a cloned cDNA complementary to rat pancreatic glucagon mRNA demonstrates that rat pre-proglucagon contains an additional GLP at the C-terminus, i.e. there are glucagon and two rather than one GLPs arranged in tandem. We have now determined the structural organization of the rat glucagon gene. The transcriptional unit is 10 kilobase pair long and consists of 6 exons and 5 introns. The promoter and additional regulatory elements were identified by nucleotide sequencing and S1 nuclease mapping. Glucagon and each of the two GLPs are encoded by separate exons. The correspondence of glucagon gene organization with functional domains of the encoded polyprotein precursor, and the strong evolutionary conservation of glucagon and the GLPs is striking. Glucagon gene expression will now be investigated in normal and diabetic rats.

981 EVALUATION OF AN ANTI-PLATELET AGGREGATION INHIBITOR (TICLOPIDINE) ON DIABETIC PERIPHERAL NEUROPATHY.

H. Hosojima*, T. Kakita and S. Morimoto
Department of Internal Medicine, Kanazawa Medical University, Ishikawa, Japan.

Diabetic neuropathy is the most common and serious complication in diabetes. We evaluated the effect of an anti-platelet aggregation inhibitor (Ticlopidine) in diabetic patients with pri-neuropathy. (Method) Motor nerve conduction velocities (MCVs) and platelet aggregations before and after 12 weeks of ticlopidine treatment (300mg daily) were determined in 37 diabetic patients with impaired MCVs. (Results) Ticlopidine treatment caused no significant change in postprandial plasma glucose and a slight but insignificant decrease in hemoglobin A1c (HBA1c). MCVs in the median, ulnar, peroneal and post-tibial nerves increased significantly after the treatment, although these levels were still well below those for normal subjects. The treatment also resulted in some improvement of complaints. The ADP-and epinephrine-induced platelet aggregations decreased significant -ly after the treatment while the collagen-induced platelet aggregation did not change. When correlations between the ticlopidine-induced changes in MCVs(ΔMCVs) and those in platelet aggregations(Δplatelet aggregations), HbA1c(ΔHbA1c) and red cell 2,3-diphosphoglycerate(2,3DPG, Δ2,3DPG) were estimated, positive correlations between ΔMCVs in the ulnar, peroneal and post-tibial nerves and Δepinephrine-induced platelet aggregation were observed. Negative correlations between ΔMCVs in the median and post-tibial nerves and either ΔHbA1c or Δ2,3DPG were found.

It is suggested that treatment of ticlopidine may improve the impaired MCVs, probably by the inhibition of platelet aggregation and the improvement of tissue hypoxia, in diabetes mellitus.

982 **MAP OF PANCREATIC VENOUS INSULINEMIA IN "NORMAL" HUMAN SUBJECTS : INTEREST IN DIAGNOSTIC APPROACH OF INSULINOMAS.**

D. Houlbert*, A. Roche, J. Capeau, D. Julien, J.J. Altman, G. Friedberg, J.M. Segrestaa.
CHU Lariboisière, CHU Bicêtre, CHU St-Antoine. Paris. France.

In 30 subjects with normal glucose homeostasis, 22 of them suffering from gastrinomas, a transhepatic portal catheterism was performed and 600 blood samples were collected. Non selective staged samplings were systematically performed and the greatest number of pancreatic veins was catheterized in every case. The aim of the study was 1) to establish a map of pancreatic venous basal insulinemia in "normal" subjects 2) to determine the confidence limits to each point in order to help the localization of insulinomas. In selective sampling there is a highly significative difference (p < 0,05) between cephalic (49 µu/ml) and caudal (156 µu/ml) insulin levels (mean). A correlation was demonstrated between insulin levels of draining veins of cephalic pancreatic parenchyma and those of the portal trunk (PT) (r = 0,548 p < 0,01) and those of the superior mesenteric vein (SMV) (r = 0,621 p < 0,01). There was no correlation between splenic vein (SV) insulin and selective levels from the tail of the pancreas. Those data suggest a lamellar flow in the SV and a partial mixed, homogeneous blood in the PT and the SMV. Insulinemia above the determined confidence limits allowed the insulinoma localization in 20 other patients. Hyperselective pancreatic venous sampling is particularly adapted to the localization of insulinomas. The insulin map and the knowledge of confidence limits may allow differentiation between diffuse islet cell hyperplasia, solitary and multiple insulinomas.

983 INDICATIONS OF GLUCAGON DELIVERY PORTABLE PUMP.
D. Houlbert, J.J. Altman*, A. Lageron, G. Friedberg, J.M. Segrestaa. Hôpital Lariboisière, Hôpital Saint-Antoine. Paris. France.
Glucagon appears to be a new candidate for the increasing field of hormone pump delivery. The subcutaneous infusion of glucagon by portable pump appears to give very effective symptomatic relief from hypoglycemia with extra-pancreatic tumor. This mode of glucagon administration was proposed in 3 patients who had severe nocturnal hypoglycemic attacks. The aim of the study was 1) to specify the indications of the subcutaneous glucagon infusion 2) to specify the modes of utilization 3) to test the efficiency and the tolerance of this treatment. The subcutaneous glucagon infusion can be proposed in non beta cell tumor hypoglycemia 1) when surgery, radiotherapy and chemotherapy are impossible or ineffective. This treatment allows the patients to return home and provides an advantage over the glucose perfusion in improving the quality of life of these patients. 2) before the surgical step 3) while waiting for the chemotherapy to become efficient. The glucagon was perfused at a flow rate of from 400 µg/h to 1 mg/h every 12 hour night. Because of hepatic glucagon action it is very important to associate this treatment to an adequate diet and to stop the glucagon infusion during the day to reconstitute the glycogen overload. An hepatic histological and histoenzymological study before and under glucagon confirms this point. In the 3 cases this mode of glucagon administration was very effective and well tolerated in spite of very high glucagon levels which approach those seen in glucagonoma syndromes. This study proves that glucagon can be used in subcutaneous infusion without any inconvinience.

984 ACTIVATION BY A TUMOR-PROMOTING PHORBOL ESTER OF PROTEIN KINASE C IN PANCREATIC ISLET HOMOGENATES. C.J. Hubinont* and W.J. Malaisse, Laboratory of Experimental Medicine, Brussels Free University, Brussels, B-1000, Belgium.

The tumor-promoting phorbol ester 12-O-tetradecanoylphorbol-13-acetate (TPA) stimulates insulin release from pancreatic islets incubated in the absence of exogenous nutrient. At variance with the situation evoked by nutrient secretagogues, the secretory response to TPA is not associated with obvious changes in K^+ conductance or ^{45}Ca net uptake. In the present study, we investigated the effect of TPA upon the phosphorylation of lysine-rich histones from calf thymus as catalyzed by rat islet homogenates. The islet homogenate displayed protein kinase C activity, dependent on the simultaneous presence of phosphatidylserine, 1,3-diolein and Ca^{2+}. In the presence of phosphatidylserine but absence of diolein, TPA (20 nM) although failing to affect histone phosphorylation in the absence of Ca^{2+}, conferred Ca^{2+}-responsiveness to the protein kinase C. In the presence of phosphatidylserine and TPA, the threshold concentration for activation by Ca^{2+} was close to 0.04 µM, the Ka close to 5 µM, and the maximal velocity at least twice higher than basal value. These findings are compatible with the view that TPA stimulates insulin release by causing activation of protein kinase C, even when the cytosolic conentration of ionized Ca^{2+} remains close to its basal value.

985 EFFECT OF INSULIN ON ALTERED VITAMIN D METABOLISM IN STREPTOZOTOCIN-INDUCED DIABETES. H. Ishida*, Y. Seino, T. Taminato, S. Ishizuka and H. Imura, Second Division, Department of Internal Medicine, Kyoto University School of Medicine, Kyoto 606, Japan.

It has been recognized recently that mineral and vitamin D metabolism is altered in diabetes. In order to ascertain whether or not this alteration can be reversed by insulin, male Wistar rats were administered 60mg/kg streptozotocin (STZ) and were treated with 8U NPH and 2U Actrapid insulin daily for two weeks. Five weeks after the STZ administration, control (C), diabetic (D), and insulin-treated diabetic (I) rats were fasted overnight. Plasma Ca and Ca^{2+} in D were significantly lower than in C ($P<0.01$), and were completely reversed after insulin injection. Circulating 25-hydroxyvitamin D (25(OH)D) and 24,25-dihydroxyvitamin D ($24,25(OH)_2D$) in D were 7.0±1.1 and 2.1±0.2 (ng/ml)(M±SE), respectively, both of which were significantly lower than 13.6±1.8 and 2.7±0.2 in C ($P<0.01$ and $P<0.02$, respectively), and were also completely reversed to 17.2±2.4 and 3.0±0.3 by insulin therapy. However, plasma 1,25-dihydroxyvitamin D ($1,25(OH)_2D$) tended to be lower, but not statistically different, both in D and I compared to C. The ratio of $1,25(OH)_2D$ to 25(OH)D in D was significantly higher than in C ($P<0.02$), and was decreased after insulin therapy ($P<0.01$). Moreover, this ratio in I was also significantly lower than in C ($P<0.05$). In conclusion, the negative calcium balance and the altered vitamin D metabolism in experimental diabetes can be reversed by insulin therapy. These alterations, therefore, might be secondary to the metabolic derangement due to insulin deficiency. Furthermore, insulin seems to suppress the conversion of 25(OH)D to $1,25(OH)_2D$ in experimental diabetes *in vivo*.

986 EFFECTS OF OPIOID PEPTIDES ON INSULIN SECRETION FROM THE PERFUSED ISOLATED RAT PANCREAS. J. ISHIZUKA*, M. KOIZUMI, T. TOYOTA and Y. GOTO, Third Department of Internal Medicine, Tohoku University School of Medicine, Seiryocho 1-1, Sendai 980, Japan.

We examined effects of opioid peptides, which are dynorphin (1-17), rimorphin, porcine-leumorphin and leucine-enkephalin (leu-enk), on insulin secretion from the perfused isolated rat pancreas. Preproenkephalin B is a precursor of dynorphin, rimorphin and leumorphin. The rat pancreas was isolated using the procedure described by Grodsky et al with some modifications. KRBB which contain 4 % Dextran and 0.5 % BSA was used as a perfusate. (RESULTS) Dynorphin (4×10^{-8} M) inhibited glucose-induced insulin secretion most strongly among four peptides. But this peptide didn't inhibit GIP-induced insulin secretion. Rimorphin also inhibited glucose-induced insulin secretion, but its inhibitory effect was less than that of dynorphin and more than that of leu-enk. Porcine-leumorphin didn't inhibit the insulin secretion. (DISCUSSION) Dynorphin, rimorphin and leumorphin belong to a family of preproenkephalin B which have leu-enk at N-terminus of each peptide. The results that dynorphin and rimorphin inhibited the glucose-induced insulin secretion more than leu-enk suggest that insulin secretion is regulated by opioid polypeptide containing leu-enk and that especially, the extensive peptides of leu-enk at C-terminus potentiate it. However, porcine-leumorphin which contains rimorphin at N-terminus didn't show inhibition of insulin secretion, resulting in masking rimorphin action. It has never been proven that preproenkephalin B is synthesized in the islets. Therefore, the question remains to be solved whether leu-enk comes from preproenkephalin B.

987 MECHANISM OF REPRODUCTIVE FUNCTION DISORDERS AND ABNORMAL FERTILIZATION IN DIABETIC RATS. N. HASHIZUME* AND N. SHIMIZU, The First Department of Medicine, Teikyo University School of Medicine, Tokyo 173, Japan.

The hypothalamic, hypophyseal and ovarian functions were investigated using alloxan-diabetic Wistar-Imamichi rats with estrous cycle abnormalities. Furthermore, abnormal fertilization was examined. The rate of occurrence of estrous cycle abnormalities was 40.5% between 5-10 days after onset of diabetes. The ovary showed a reaction to administration of PMS-G. The hypophyseal reaction to LH-RH and the LH and FSH contents were no different from those of the control group. There was also no difference in the hypothalamic LH-RH content compared to that of the control group. The injection of Insulin was carried out for 10 days, 24 hours after administration of alloxan. During this period, estrous cycle abnormalities were not recognized but they appeared after discontinuation of insulin. When insulin was administered to diabetic rats with continuous diestrus, the estrous cycle recovered irrespective of the blood sugar values. Abnormal fertilization was recognized in 9.6% of the diabetic rats compared with 0.4% in the control group. From the above results, estrous cycle abnormalities of alloxan diabetes are different from those due to long standing causes, such as neuropathy, and occur at an early stage. There were no abnormalities in the ovaries and hypophysis but disturbance of the LH-RH releasing mechanism was presumed. It was found that insulin is closely involved in this disorder. Fertilization abnormalities in diabetic rats might be caused not by hyperglycemia itself, but by an estrous cycle malfunction due to diabetes.

988 STEREOCHEMICAL COMPLEMENTARITY OF THYROID HORMONES AND DNA: EVIDENCE THAT TRIIODOTHYRONINE CAN INTERACT DIRECTLY AND STEREOSPECIFICALLY WITH DNA L.B. Hendry*, T.J. Smith and E.D. Bransome Jr., Departments of Medicine and Endocrinology, Medical College of Georgia, and Veterans Administration Medical Center, Augusta, Georgia 30912, USA.

That there are rigid structural constraints on the biological activity of thyroid hormones is well established (see Table). In an effort to understand why, we have constructed molecular models of thyroid hormones and DNA, the apparent site of hormone action. The naturally occurring active hormone, T_3, was stereochemically complementary to DNA in that it was virtually accomodated by the space between base pairs and formed complementary hydrogen bonds to the sugar-phosphate backbone. Biological activity correlated with complementarity. Thus, active thyroid hormones (perhaps in concert with a proteinaceous receptor) may interact stereospecifically with DNA. Inasmuch as the active thyroid hormones are accomodated best between base pairs in the partially uncoiled sequence TpG, we predict that this site will be found in control regions sensitive to thyroid hormones, as it has been for some steroid hormones.

	COMPLEMENTARITY TO DNA		(LITERATURE)	
HORMONE OR ANALOG	BASE PAIR	H-BOND	BINDING	ACTIVITY
L-3,5,3'-triiodothyronine (T_3)	+	+	+	+
L-3'-isopropyl-3,5-diiodothyronine	++	+	+	$>T_3$
L-3,5,3',5'-tetraiodothyronine (T_4)	–	+	$<<T_3$	$<<T_3$
L-3,3',5'-triiodothyronine (rT_3)	–	+	$<<T_3$	$<<T_3$
3,5,3'-triiodothyroacetic acid	+	–	+	$<<T_3$
3,5,3',5'-tetraiodothyroacetic acid	–	–	$<<T_3$	$<<T_3$

989 AN ESTRADIOL (E_2) RESPONSIVE, CALCIUM DEPENDENT TOSYL ARGININE METHYL ESTER (TAME) HYDROLASE IN IMMATURE RAT UTERINE CYTOSOL. K. P. Henrikson* and H. W. Dickerman, Center for Laboratories and Research, New York State Department of Health, Albany, New York, 12201, U.S.A.

A calcium dependent enzyme which hydrolyzes TAME, a model substrate for trypsin-like proteases, appears in immature rat uterine cytosol after in vivo administration of E_2. TAME hydrolase activity reaches a maximum 3 h after injection of E_2 and returns to initial levels after 18 h. The increase is hormone and tissue specific. The E_2 dose-response curve for TAME hydrolase 3 h after injection shows a maximum response at 0.45 µg E_2 per animal. A maximum increase in uterine wet weight occusr at 0.1 µg per rat. TAME hydrolase is a soluble enzyme; 86% of activity occurs in the cytosol with the remaining activity distributed in the particulate fractions. The development of the enzyme is an endogeneous uterine response to E_2 rather than an artifact of plasma contamination because 1) the dose response curves for uterine wet weight (a measure of plasma infiltration) and TAME hydrolase are quite different; 2) goat antibody to rat serum inhibits plasma TAME hydrolase but not the uterine enzyme; and 3) washing of intact uteri before homogenization removes 50-70% of plasma protein contamination but does not reduce activity of uterine TAME hydrolase. The nonlinear response of the uterine enzyme activity to dilution suggests the presence of an activating factor in cytosol. Gel filtration separates the activator and the enzyme and results in a complete loss of activity which can be restored by the addition of small amounts of cytosol to the purified fractions. The nature of the activator is under investigation.

990 PERMISSIVE EFFECT OF THYROID HORMONES IN THE INDUCTION OF HEPATIC P-ENOLPYRUVATE CARBOXYKINASE. W. Höppner, W. Süßmuth and H.J. Seitz*, Institut f. Physiologische Chemie, Universität Hamburg, FRG

The purpose of the present study was to investigate the supporting effect of thyroid hormones on stimulating the synthesis of important proteins in liver cells. Therefore the induction of the main glucoregulatory enzyme, P-enolpyruvate carboxykinase (PEPck) (EC 4.1.1.32) by triiodothyronine (T3), epinephrine (Epi), dibutyryl cAMP (dBcAMP) and their interaction was measured in two different in vitro liver systems.- dbcAMP provoked within 2 h a significant increase in PEPck synthesis and activity in the isolated perfused liver from hypothyroid, fed rats. This cAMP and Epi-effect was approximately doubled when livers were taken from hyperthyroid rats. T3 per se was without effect on enzyme synthesis. Concomitantly with hormonally induced alteration in enzyme synthesis increased levels of PEPck mRNA were detected in livers from hyperthyroid rats compared to eu- or hypothyroidism. Using primary serum free cultures of hepatocytes from hypothyroid fed rats, the permissive effect of T3 on dBcAMP- or Epi-induced PEPck synthesis could be demonstrated within 4 h.

Summarizing thyroid hormones exert similar to glucocorticoids a rapid (within 4 h) permissive action on the cAMP provoked induction of hepatic PEPck predominantly by increasing PEPck mRNA activity, while T3 within this time-period was without effect.

991 STEROID-DEPENDENT DISSOCIATON OF RECEPTOR ASSOCIATED REGULATORY COMPONENTS FROM UNACTIVATED GLUCOCORTICOID RECEPTOR. T.W. Hutchens*, W.E. Gibbons, and P.K. Besch, Baylor College of Medicine and Reproductive Research Lab, St. Luke's Hospital, Houston, Texas 77030.

We have investigated the nature of cytosolic components associated with the reversible structural alterations accompanying steroid-dependent transformation (activation) of unactivated receptor to the nuclear binding form. Determination of receptor size (density gradient centrifugation and size exclusion chromatography) and surface charge (ion-exchange chromatography, isoelectric focusing and high performance chromatofocusing) demonstrated that a reduction of apparent molecular weight (300K to 56K) and increase in basicity (pI 5.5 to 7.5) accompanies transformation. Analyses of 'unactivated' steroid-receptor complexes have been impeded by the proclivity of chromatographic techniques to activate receptor. Unliganded goat mammary glucocorticoid receptor was analyzed by DEAE-cellulose and Sephacryl S-300 chromatography (±1M NaBr). Detection of receptor by post-labeling revealed size and surface ionic properties similar to those of molybdate-stabilized steroid-receptor complexes. Thus, chromatography (purification) of steroid-receptor complexes (but not unliganded receptor) can result in a decrease in size with the acquisiton of activated properties which could occur by the loss of a non-steroid-binding, receptor-associated component(s) (RAC). The unliganded receptor and the molybdate-stabilized steroid-receptor complex are similar in their large size, relatively acidic surface charge and resistance to activation. We suggest these are related properties and that the affinity of RAC for receptor is steroid-dependent. The binding of steroid reduces RAC affinity for receptor thus allowing dissociation of RAC which determines receptor activation.

992 ELECTROPHYSIOLOGICAL EFFECTS OF DOPAMINE ON ENRICHED POPULATION OF RAT MAMMOTROPHS CELLS IN PRIMARY CULTURE. J.M. Israël* and J.D. Vincent, INSERM U.176, Rue Camille St-Saëns 33077 BORDEAUX-Cedex, France.

Since it has been demonstrated that PRL-secreting cells of tumoral origin are electrically excitable, the present study was undertaken to see whether electrophysiological properties described in tumour cells also exist in non-transformed rat pituitary cells and to determine the effects of dopamine (DA) on these properties. Intracellular recordings were performed on enriched normal mammotrophs isolated from pituitaries of 14 day-old (P1) and lactating female (P2) rats. Fourty per cent of the P1 cells displayed a low resting potential (-25mV) and were inexcitable even after the cells were hyperpolarized to -60mV. Locally applied, DA was able to hyperpolarize these cells with an increase of the input resistance. This response was reversed at about 0mV. Sixty per cent of the P1 cells displayed spontaneous or triggered action potentials inhibited by Co^{2+} and Mn^{2+}. Local application of DA induced a strong hyperpolarizing response with an increase of the input resistance. This response reversed at -100mV and led to a cessation of firing. P2 cells were not spontaneously active but exhibited spikes during depolarizing pulse and after cessation of hyperpolarizing pulse ("off-spikes"). DA had no effect on the membrane resting potential and input resistance but blocked the off-spikes. Our results demonstrate that isolated pituitary cells display different electrophysiological properties depending on their origin. DA affects these properties but in a variable manner which may depend on this origin.

993 ANALYSIS OF ANDROGEN-SENSITIVITY OF RAT PROSTATE X MOUSE KIDNEY HYBRIDS. S. M. Judge*, M. M. Phillips, and S. Liao, Ben May Laboratory for Cancer Research, University of Chicago, Chicago, IL 60637, USA

Variant androgen-sensitive cell lines were produced by fusing freshly isolated epithelial cells from the rat ventral prostate with a line of murine renal tumor (RAG) cells. These hybrid cell lines can be used for genetic analysis of the mechanism of androgen action in target cells. The proliferative response of the various hybrid lines to treatment with 10 nM 5α-dihydrotestosterone (DHT) was used to classify the hybrids as either very sensitive (A+, > 40% reduction in doubling time, Dt), sensitive (A, > 10% reduction in Dt), or insensitive (A-, < 10% reduction in Dt) to androgens. The variance in the androgen-sensitivity of the hybrid cells was unrelated to the growth rate and morphology of the cells. The increased sensitivity of some hybrids to DHT in comparison to the insensitive RAG parent cells implied that some androgen-dependent regulatory processes derived from the rat prostate parent cells were expressed in these hybrids. Androgen-sensitivity was not dependent upon gene dosage because only 3-4 rat chromosomes were found in karyograms of the A+ lines. Analysis of the [^{3}H] DHT and [^{3}H] methyltrienolone binding activity of various hybrids showed little correlation of either receptor level or hormone binding affinity with the androgen-sensitivity of the cells. Furthermore, A and A- hybrids were indistinguishable by their ability to retain [^{3}H] DHT in their nuclei. These studies suggest that events distal to receptor binding are critical for a proliferative response of the hybrid cells to androgens. Regulation of these events may have a function in the discrimination of tissue-specific responses to hormonal stimulation.
Supported by grants from NIH AM 09461, CA 09183 and Amer. Canc. Soc. 151.

994 THE INTERACTION OF ANDROGEN RECEPTORS WITH NONSPECIFIC DNA. J. Kallos* and R. Buttyan, Department of Urology, Columbia College of Physicians and Surgeons, New York, New York, 10032

How do sex-steroid hormone receptors find specific DNA sites among the vast excess of nonspecific sites? Although evidence for site-specific binding of steroid hormone receptors to DNA is accumulating, androgen receptors (AR) also exhibit appreciable affinity for nonspecific DNA as shown by our DNA competition experiments. We propose that the nonspecific DNA binding may play an important role in the search for the specific binding site, possibly in a two-step binding process. The first step presumably involves the receptor binding to nonspecific sites. The second step involves a direct transfer around the DNA molecule until the specific site is reached. This mechanism may be very fast because the receptor will never leave the DNA molecule until the target site is reached. Using DNA-cellulose dissociation measurements, we describe model experiments for the facilitated transfer of AR from one DNA molecule to another. A similar mechanism may be used to locate the specific binding site by receptors in vivo. Since hormonally stimulated, actively transcribing genes seem to be associated with the nuclear matrix of target tissue, we would also suggest that this association may enhance intramolecular transfer and accelarate target location by the steroid receptor.

995 The Role of Calmodulin in Hormone-stimulated lipolysis. A. Kawai* and Y. Shimizu, The Institute for Adult Diseases, Asahi Life Foundation, Tokyo, Japan.

Our previous report revealed that a calmodulin(CaM) inhibitor, W-7 remarkedly suppressed stimulation of lipolysis by epinephrine, ACTH, MIX or DBcAMP. (7th Asia & Oceania Congress of Endocrinology, 1982).
To explore further the role of Ca^{2+}-CaM in lipolysis, studies were carried out out on the effects of CaM inhibitors on cAMP-dependent protein kinase and Ca^{2+}, Mg^{2+}-ATPase in cell extracts as well as on endogenous protein phosphorylation induced by lipolytic hormones.
Activity of cAMP-dependent protein kinase was blunted when either W-7 or antiCaM antibody (50μg/ml) was added to the assay medium.
CaM-dependence of the protein kinase was also proved by the fact that in CaM-depleted cell extracts, the protein kinase activity was markedly reduced, which was significantly restored by addition of exogenous CaM. Likewise, phospholylation of endogenous substrate proteins was inhibited in the CaM-depleted cell extracts and restored by addition of exogenous CaM to them. Furthermore, Ca^{2+}, Mg^{2+}-ATPase in microsomal fraction which is closely related to Ca^{2+} uptake in the fraction, was suppressed by either W-7 or trifluoperazine. These findings indicate that Ca^{2+}-CaM is involved in hormone-induced lipolysis by exerting stimulatory effects on activation of cAMP-dependent protein kinase in cell extracts capable of phosphorylating substrate proteins including hormone-sensitive lipase and Ca^{2+}, Mg^{2+}-ATPase.

996 ALTERATIONS IN GLUCOSE TOLERANCE AND PLASMA INSULIN LEVEL BY PROGESTOGEN IN POSTMENOPAUSAL NONDIABETIC AND DIABETIC WOMEN. K. Fukuma*, Y. Souda, T. Tanaka, I. Matsuo, K. Nakahara and M. Maeyama, Department of Obstetrics and Gynecology, Kumamoto University Medical School, Kumamoto 860, Japan.

The effect of progestogen on the blood glucose and plasma insulin levels was studied in 35 postmenopausal patients (30 nondiabetic and 5 diabetic) according to the duration of menopause. Thirty nondiabetic patients were divided into three groups (Group I, 1-10 years after menopause; Group II, 11-20 years; and Group III, 21-30 years). The progestogen Lyndiol (lynestrenol, 5.0 mg and mestranol, 0.15 mg) was administered daily for seven days. A 75 gm oral glucose tolerance test (OGTT) including plasma insulin determination was performed before and after the progestogen administration. In 14 premenopausal and 5 postmenopausal diabetic patients, no elevation of the blood glucose and plasma insulin levels after the progestogen administration was found, wherease in 30 postmenopausal nondiabetic patients the blood glucose levels at 30, 60 and 120 minutes in OGTT were significantly higher than those found before the progestogen administration. The plasma insulin levels after the progestogen administration increased at 30, 60 and 120 minutes in Group I, at 60 and 120 minutes in Group II, and at 120 minutes in Group III. These data suggest that the lack of compensatory insulin secretion in response to progestogen in postmenopausal women is probably related to the diminished β-cell reserve with aging.

997 EVIDENCE OF SUB-FRACTIONS OF HIGH DENSITY (HDL) AND LOW DENSITY (LDL) LIPOPROTEINS BY CONTINUOUS GRADIENT ELECTROPHORESIS ON POLYACRYLAMIDE GEL: CLINICAL RELEVANCE OF NEW ELECTROPHORETIC PATTERNS. P.* GAMBERT, M. FARNIER, C. LALLEMANT, A. MARTINAND, S. MEUNIER and J. M. BRUN, Groupement de Recherche sur l'Athérosclérose et sa Prévention (G.R.A.P.), Service de Médecine II, Hôpital du Bocage, BP 1542, 21034 Dijon Cédex, France.

Previous research findings (1) have shown the analytical potential of continuous gradient electrophoresis on polyacrylamide gel for separating lipoproteins according to size. Optimization of the technique permits separation of both small-sized (HDL_P) and large-sized (HDL_G) HDL sub-fractions and of LDL sub-fractions. The LDL sub-fraction distribution was shown to be subject-dependent. After cutting off the gel, solubilization and extraction, the HDL sub-fractions were determined quantatively by assaying their constituent cholesterol by gas liquid chromatography (GLC). The same assay was performed by laser densitometry. A very good correlation was shown between both methods. This contributes to the evidence that routine determination of cholesterol in HDL_P and HDL_G sub-fractions is now practicable. New electrophoretic patterns have been defined elsewhere in various clinical states (essential hypercholesterolemia, endogenous hypertriglyceridemia, etc...). These electrophoretic patterns will be presented and their clinical and diagnostic relevance further discussed.

(1) GAMBERT P., LALLEMANT C., ATHIAS A., PADIEU P., Alterations of HDL cholesterol distribution induced by incubation of human serum, Biochem. Biophys. Acta, 713, 1-9 (1982).

998 EFFECT OF CASEIN HYDROLYSATE INGESTION ON GLYCOGEN SYNTHASE ACTIVITY IN HEART, SKELETAL MUSCLE, AND LIVER IN THE RAT. M.C. Gannon* and F.Q. Nuttall, VA Medical Center, Minneapolis, MN. 55417, USA.

Glycogen synthase, the rate limiting enzyme in glycogen synthesis, exists in a physiologically active form, synthase I, and an inactive form, synthase D. We have previously shown administration of insulin or a carbohydrate meal resulted in an increase in % I in 24 hour fasted rats. Subsequently, we observed a dramatic increase in % I in fasted rats 1-2 hours after ingestion of a casein hydrolysate meal. This occurred even though casein did not stimulate a rise in insulin concentration. We were therefore interested in determining if a similar increase in % I would be observed in skeletal muscle and liver after casein. Rats were gavaged with a 50% casein hydrolysate suspension (4 g/kg) and synthase activity was measured in heart, skeletal muscle, and liver 1 or 2 hours later. In heart, the % I increased from 8% in fasted rats to 14% at 1 hr and 45% at 2 hr after gavage. In skeletal muscle the % I was ∿26% and remained unchanged following casein gavage. In liver, the % I was ∿14% in fasted rats and remained unchanged following casein gavage. Thus, the increase in % I following casein was unique to the heart. At 30 minutes after casein, synthase phosphatase activity also was increased in heart. In conclusion, oral administration of a casein hydrolysate resulted in an increase in synthase I in rat heart, but not in liver or skeletal muscle. The increase in synthase I in heart was preceded by a stimulation of synthase phosphatase activity. These effects were observed without an increase in insulin concentration, previously the only known stimulator of synthase and synthase phosphatase activity in heart.

999 THYROGLOBULIN DETERMINATION WITH MONOCLONAL ANTIBODY MINIMIZES INTERFERENCE OF AUTOANTIBODY. Shiro Noguchi, K. Kato, N. Murakami, A. Noguchi, Noguchi Thyroid Clinic & Hospital Foundation, Beppu, Oita-ken, Japan 874

Elevated thyroglobulin levels in the circulation have been observed in various thyroid disorders. The presence of autoantibody(AutoAb) against thyroglobulin(Tg) interferes immunoassay of serum Tg. A method for determination of Tg with monoclonal antibody(m-Ab) which recognize an epitope rarely reacted with AutoAb was developed. The method was consisted with polyclonal antibody(p-Ab) coated microplate, standard Tg and m-Ab-peroxydase conjugate. A sensitive AutoAb determination with the same principle as Tg determination was also developed, using Tg-coated microplate, standard AutoAb and anti-human Ig-G-peroxidase conjugate. One monoclonal antibody, 31A, was selected from 75 m-Abs reacted with Tg. With m-Ab 31A, a sensitive solid phase enzyme immunoassay for Tg was developed.
The recovery rate of added Tg with m-Ab system at AutoAb titer 25,600x was 71%, contrasting to 47.5% at 160x with p-Ab system. The upper limit of normal value of Tg in both p-Ab and m-Ab systems were 60ng/ml. Normal Tg values with p-Ab and abnormally high values with m-Ab 31A were observed in 11 of 109 patients (pts), 10%, with Graves' disease and 47 of 438 pts, 10.7% with thyroid cancer. In 90% of pts with Graves' disease pts who showed discrepancies between m-Ab and p-Ab Tg determinations were found to have Tg AutoAb by a sensitive enzyme immunoassay of AutoAb.
Conclusion: by using m-Ab 31A, it is possible to minimize the interference of AutoAb for determination of serum Tg.

1000 EFFECT OF ACTIVE VITAMIN D_3 ON HUMAN IMMUNITY IN VIVO AND IN VITRO. K. Okano*, S. Kou, M. Shimizu, Y. Nozawa, T. Kato, M. Yamamoto, H. Kida, C. Nawa, Y. Yamada, N. Sekita and K. Someya, St. Marianna University School of Medicine, Kawasaki, Japan.

Peripheral blood T lymphocyte, B lymphocyte, IgG-FcR$^+$T cell, IgM-FcR$^+$ T cell, lymphocyte blasttransformation, serum immunoglobulins and tuberculin reaction were examined before and after the oral administration of 1.5 µg/day 1α-hydroxyvitamin D_3 (1α-OHD_3) to 5 aged normal human subjects and 10 patients with senile osteoporosis for 8 weeks. OKT3$^+$T cell (pan T cell), OKT4$^+$T cell (helper-inducer T cell) and OKT8$^+$T cell (suppressor-cytotoxic T cell) were determined using monoclonal antibodies. IgG-FcR$^+$T cell was significantly increased both in the normal aged group and osteoporotic group after the administration of 1α-OHD_3. OKT8$^+$T cell tended to decrease and OKT4$^+$T cell/OKT8$^+$T cell ratio tended to increase after the administration of 1α-OHD_3 to the aged. Tuberculin reaction was negative in 5 of 9 osteoporotic patients and 1 of 5 normal subjects and enhanced in the both groups after 1α-OHD_3 administration. When peripheral blood mononuclear cells from 11 young normal adults and 5 aged human subjects were incubated in vitro with 10^{-7}-10^{-12}M 1,25$(OH)_2D_3$, 10^{-5}-10^{-10}M 24,25$(OH)_2D_3$ or 10^{-5}-10^{-10}M 1α-OHD_3, their incorporation of [^{3}H]-thymidine into the cells which were simultaneously incubated with PHA, Con A or PWM, were significantly increased by 10^{-8}-10^{-12}M 1,25$(OH)_2D_3$ and tended to be suppressed by 10^{-7}M 1,25$(OH)_2D_3$. These data imply that active vitamin D_3 influences helper T cell/suppressor T cell ratio, leading to enhancements of delayed hypersensitivity and lymphocyte blasttransformation in vivo and in vitro.

1001 CASTRATION REVERSES DIURNAL CHANGES IN IN VITRO DOPAMINE RELEASE FROM THE CORPUS STRIATUM OF INTACT MALE RATS.

D. Dluzen* and V. Ramirez, Department of Physiology and Biophysics, University of Illinois, Urbana, IL 61801.

Previous research in our laboratory had indicated a diurnal variation in the spontaneous *in vitro* dopamine (DA) release from the corpus striatum (CS) of cycling female rats which was disrupted during the proestrous-estrous phase. Here we examine whether an analagous phenomenon is present in male rats. Intact and castrate (> 30d) male rats were decapitated at 0600 and 1800 h of a 14:10 h cycle (lights on 0500 h), the CS removed and superfused *in vitro*. Perfusate samples were collected at 10 min intervals and DA levels determined. Opposite DA release rate profiles characterized the spontaneous release of this neurotransmitter when intact and castrate male rats were decapitated 1 h after lights on (0600 h - Figure A) and were reversed when decapitated 1 h before lights off (1800 h - Figure B). A similar trend in total dopaminergic activity of this system (amount released + amount remaining in CS - Figure C) was obtained. These results indicate that not only is the function of the CS in the male rat altered by castration, but that this manipulation also disrupts the diurnal fluctuations in activity of the nigrostriatal dopaminergic system of intact male rats.

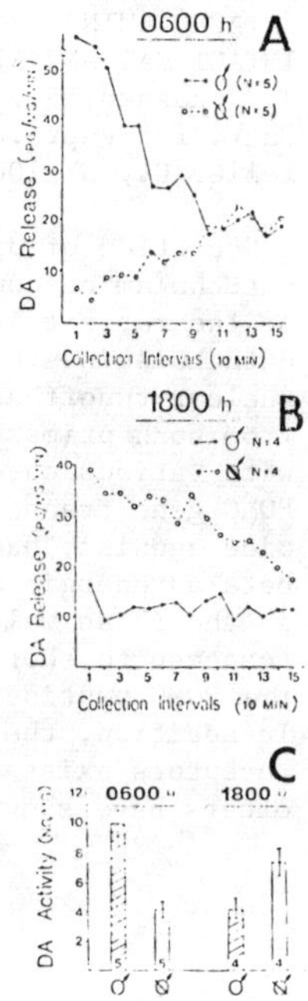

1002 GABA INCREASE AT THE LOCUS CERULEUS AREA PREVENTS THE POST-CASTRATION RISE OF LH RELEASE.*

A.O.Donoso. Laboratorio de Investigaciones Cerebrales,Facultad de Ciencias Médicas,UNC. Casilla de Correo 425,Mendoza-Argentina.

Recent evidence from our laboratory strongly suggests that brain GABA exerts an inhibitory action on LH release in the rat. The aim of the present work was to localize the effect of GABA on the acute release of LH that follows orchidectomy in rats.

Endogenous GABA levels were increased by means of microinjections of the GABA-transaminase inhibitor gamma vinyl GABA(GVG). Adult male rats were implanted stereotaxically with guide cannulas at different brain sites: at medial and dorsal preoptic areas(mPOA;dPOA), ventromedial-arcuate area(VMH-ARH), and locus ceruleus-fasciculus longitudinalis medialis area(LC). Bilateral injections(1 µl) of GVG or saline(controls) were performed immediately after castration and at 24 h later; 48 h after orchidectomy the control rats showed increased plasma LH levels. Local GVG injection on the mPOA, dPOA(20 µg) or VMH-ARH area(5 µg) produced no significant changes on plasma LH increase. In contrast, when GVG was injected on the LC area (10 µg), it prevented plasma LH levels to increase after castration.

Results suggest that GABA inhibition of the post-castration rise of plasma LH is located at mesencephalic sites. These sites are known to be the origin of the ascendent noradrenergic pathways. It seems, therefore, that this action of GABA is connected to the adrenergic system controlling secretion of LH.

* Supported by the Program LINCE of the Consejo Nacional de Investigaciones Científicas y Técnicas,Argentina.

1003 CATACHOLAMINE REGULATION OF POMC GENE TRANSCRIPTION IN PRIMARY CULTURES AND INTACT RAT ANTERIOR AND INTERMEDIATE PITUITARY LOBES. J.H. Eberwine, J. Jonassen, F.T. Dionne, M. Blum*, and J.L. Roberts, Dept. Biochem. and Cntr. for Repro. Science, Columbia U., NY 10032, and Dept. Biology, Rockerfeller U., NY 10021.

Secretion of pro-opiomelanocortin (POMC) derived peptides is under complex catecholamine control in both the anterior (AL) and intermediate (IL) lobes of the rat pituitary. In order to ascertain if there are similar effects of catacholamines on POMC gene transcription in these tissues, we have used a nuclear runoff assay to measure POMC gene transcription in nuclei isolated from both primary pituitary cultures and intact animals after treatment with various catecholamines. Haloperidol, a dopamine antagonist, stimulated POMC gene transcription in both AL and IL. 8-bromo-ergocryptine, a dopamine agonist, had inhibitory effects only in the IL. Isoproterenol, a beta-adrenergic agonist, had stimulatory effects on POMC gene transcription in the IL as well as in the AL. The rapidity of the transcriptional response to short time periods (hrs.) of neurotransmitter treatment suggest that POMC peptide secretion is coupled in some fashion to POMC transcription. In addition, the AL response to isoproterenol suggests that beta-adrenergic receptors exist and function within the anterior lobe corticotroph, as others have shown.

1004 ESTRADIOL INDUCED ALTERATION OF THE MUSCARINIC RECEPTOR IN THE PREOPTIC AREA IS RESTRICTED TO THE CRITICAL PERIOD OF THE RAT ESTROUS CYCLE. Y. Egozi* and Y. Kloog, Department of Biochemistry, The George S. Wise Faculty of Life Sciences, Tel Aviv University, Tel Aviv 69978, Israel

The muscarinic acetylcholine receptor was studied in rats following treatment with estradiol in vitro during estrous cycle. Muscarinic acetylcholine receptors in the preoptic area (POA) of the hypothalamus represent both low and high affinity sites for agonists. The proportion between them varies as a function of the estrous cycle, thus suggesting that sex hormones may modulate the muscarinic receptors. This possibility was investigated by in vitro binding studies in which POA homogenates were preincubated in the presence of estradiol (30 ng/ml) and their muscarinic properties were then examined. Binding of the muscarinic antagonist [^{3}H]-4-N-piperidyl benzilate was not affected by estradiol. However, binding of the muscarinic agonist oxotremorine was affected in a distinct manner. On the morning of proestrous, the high affinity binding sites for oxotremorine in the POA, representing 55% of total sites in control membranes, mostly disappeared after estradiol treatment and low affinity sites were detected. The same pattern was also observed at noon, but after further three hours the steroid was no longer effective. The effect of estradiol thus appears to be restricted to a specific time period which coincides with the well-known critical period in proestrous. Binding of oxotremorine to receptors in the POA was not affected by estradiol treatment on other days of the estrous cycle, nor was it affected in the POA or other brain regions of male rats. Taken together the results indicate a specific time- and sex-dependent effect of estradiol on the muscarinic receptors in the POA.

1005 INVOLVEMENT OF VALPROIC ACID ON ANTERIOR PITUITARY SECRETION. A PRESUMPTIVE ACTION OF GABA. M. GIROUD*, G. MARCHAL, F. BALEYDIER-GIROUD, J. DEGRES, G. MACK, R. DUMAS, Service de Neurologie, Hôpital Général, 3 rue du Faubourg Raines, 21033 DIJON CEDEX, FRANCE.

Anterior Pituitary Hormone secretion on 6 males and 4 women were studied before and after two months of treatment with the Gaba-Transaminase inhibitor : Valproic Acid. The drug was given at the dose of 20 mg/kg/day for Epilepsy without cerebral tumor at C.T. Scan. Pituirary function was evaluated by measurement of basal ACTH, TSH, FSH, LH, Prolactin, Cortisol, 11-desoxy-cortisol, T3 and T4. Then, LHR-stimulated LH and FSH release, TRH-stimulated TSH and Prolactin release, Metopiron-stimulated ACTH release were measured. The evaluations were always practiced 15 days after the last seizure. Serum levels of Valproic Acid were always below the toxic level of 100 mg/l. Values of basal and induced TSH, FSH and LH (males and women) were unaffected and on the other side, basal and induced Prolactin, basal and induced ACTH, were significantly decreased. These changes have already been observed in the literature. Valproic Acid, inhibiting the Gaba-Transaminase, increases the cerebral levels of Gaba, especially in hypothalamus. Gaba may act directly either at the Anterio Pituitary level, where Gaba receptors have been localized (Prolactin), or at the hypothalamic area level, through neurotransmitters (ACTH). The lack of changes for TSH, LH, FSH, showes the problem of the dual mechanism of action for Gaba (excitatory , no effect) explaining the opposed results described in the literature. Our results confirm that Gaba acts as a neurotransmitter on the hypothalamo-Pituitary axis, that Valproic Acid may study Pituitary function and treat a few neuro-endocrine diseases as Nelson's Syndrome.

1006 Plasma conjugated dopamine is abnormal in patients with functional amenorrhoea and in diabetic patients. C. Hagen*, N.J. Christensen, K. Tvede, H. Djursing, A.N. Andersen, K. Petersen, Department of Internal Medicine and Endocrinology, Herlev University Hospital, 2730 Herlev, Denmark.

The abnormal secretion of prolactin (Prl), and luteinizing hormone in women with normoprolactinaemic, normo-/hypogonadotrophic amenorrhoea with and without diabetes mellitus may be compatible with increased central and/or peripheral dopamine activity. Therefore, we measured plasma concentrations of free (f-DA) and conjugated dopamine (c-DA), Prl, gonadotrophins, oestradiol, free-norepinephrine (NE) and free-epinephrine (E), in 17 uncomplicated insulin dependent diabetic patients (8 women with amenorrhoea and 9 normal menstruating) and in 16 non-diabetics (7 with amenorrhoea and 9 normal menstruating). Basal levels of f-DA, NE and E were not different in the four groups. Plasma c-DA was significantly increased in both groups of patients with amenorrhoea as compared to their respective control groups ($p < 0.05$). Unexpectedly, we found that c-DA was significantly lower in diabetic patients as compared to controls ($p < 0.05$). The ratio f-DA/c-DA was significantly higher ($p < 0.01$) in diabetics than in non-diabetics. No significant correlations between catecholamine and pituitary hormone levels were found. These findings support our hypothesis that dopaminergic activity is increased in patients with amenorrhoea. Furthermore, our observations suggest that the sulfate conjugation capacity is reduced in diabetes mellitus, and this important detoxification mechanism could possibly be involved in the development of diabetes mellitus. This study was supported by the Danish Medical Research Counsil.

1007 POSSIBLE INVOLVEMENT OF CYCLIC AMP ON THE OVULATORY PROCESS OF THE ISOLATED PERFUSED RABBIT OVARY.

P.V. Holmes, L. Hedin, P.O. Janson, and K. Ahrén, Departments of Physiology and Obstetrics and Gynecology, University of Gothenburg, Sweden.

LH increases ovarian cyclic AMP (cAMP) formation and mediates steroidogenesis. In addition, LH initiates oocyte maturation and follicle rupture. In this study, ovine LH and IBMX, an inhibitor of phosphodiesterase, were used to elucidate a possible relationship between steroidogenesis and ovulation rate. Ovaries were surgically removed from estrous rabbits with artery and pedicle intact on a segment of aorta, this being cannulated for in vitro perfusion (Janson et al., Biol Reprod 26, 456-65, 1982). After 1 hour of perfusion, the ovaries were stimulated with 1 ug/ml ovine LH or with LH plus 0.2 mM IBMX. Medium samples were assayed for cAMP, progesterone (P4), and estradiol (E2).

Results: In both experimental groups levels of cAMP, P4 and E2 rose significantly. The cAMP response was greatest after LH plus IBMX. P4 and E2 release paralleled the cAMP production. Furthermore, ovulations were seen in both groups, the frequency being greatest after LH plus IBMX.

Conclusions: Cyclic AMP is of importance both for ovarian steroidogenesis and the ovulatory process. Forskolin, an activator of adenylate cyclase, is currently being tested in this model for its effects on ovarian cAMP and steroid release, as well as on ovulation.

1008 HOMOLOGOUS HORMONE REGULATION OF HORMONE RECEPTORS: LUTEINIZING HORMONE INCREASES ITS OWN RECEPTORS IN CULTURED RAT GRANULOSA CELLS. X.-C. Jia* and A.J.W. Hsueh. Dept. of Reproductive Medicine, Univ. of California, San Diego, La Jolla, CA 92093 U.S.A.

Luteinizing hormone (LH) receptors in granulosa cells are essential for ovulation and luteinization of ovarian follicles. We have studied the possible role of LH in the regulation of its own receptors *in vitro*. Granulosa cells, obtained from immature hypophysectomized, estrogen-treated rats, were primed with FSH for 2 days to induce LH receptors. The cells were then challenged with or without increasing concentrations of LH or hCG for an additional 2 days. LH receptor content in these cells was measured by ^{125}I-hCG binding. Without gonadotropins, FSH-induced LH receptors in these cells decreased to negligible levels (0.063 ng/2.5x10^5 cells). In contrast, LH receptors were further increased by rat LH or hCG ($\sim$15-fold) without a change in the Kd value (control: 1.22±0.22x10^{-10}M; LH: 2.55±0.55x10^{-10}M). Maximum stimulation of LH receptors was obtained with doses of 6, 10 and 2.5 ng/ml for rat LH, ovine LH and hCG, respectively, while higher doses of the gonadotropins were less effective. At all doses, minimal occupancy of LH receptors was observed. Also, the LH-induced number of LH receptors was correlated with increased responsiveness of the cells to the LH stimulation of cAMP production. Furthermore, cycloheximide, a protein synthesis inhibitor, blocked LH receptor induction by LH (46%), suggesting the involvement of protein synthesis. Thus, our data in cultured granulosa cells indicated that LH, like FSH, plays an important role during advanced stages of follicular maturation through autoregulation of its own receptors.

1009 OVARIAN STEROIDOGENESIS AND ADRENAL FUNCTION IN THE JAPANESE PATIENTS WITH POLYCYSTIC OVARY SYNDROME. Y.Kasuga*, M.Akatsuka, A.Nakayama and H.Arai, Dept. of OB/GY, Ashikaga Red Cross Hospital, 3-2100 Honjo, Ashikaga, Tochigi, 326 Japan.

Steroid hormone levels in both peripheral and ovarian blood obtained from Japanese polycystic ovary syndrome(PCO) patients were measured by RIA. Human menopausal gonadotropin(HMG) and dexamethasone(DXM) were administered to PCO patients. Elevated ovarian DHEA levels in PCO were noticed, while DHEAS levels were comparable with both normal and PCO. The concentrations of DHEA and DHEAS were decreased after wedge resections of ovary, thereafter HMG elevated the levels of DHEA in PCO. In PCO, administered DXM were decreased the levels of DHEAS in peripheral blood and HMG administrations couldn't elevate the concentrations of them. These facts denied the existence of adrenal hyperfunction in PCO patients. Markedly elevated $^4\Delta$ androstenedione and testosterone levels in both peripheral and ovarian blood were noticed in PCO. According to these data, abnormality of adrenal function in PCO patients were denied and elevated steroid levels were probably caused by the overproductions of them from polycystic enlarged ovaries in PCO.

1010 MORPHO-FUNCTIONAL CHARACTERISTICS OF MONOLAYER-CULTURED HUMAN THECAL CELLS. E.Katayama*, Y.Nakamura, K.Sugimura and R.Iizuka, Dept. of Obstetrics & Gynecology, School of Medicine, Keio University, Shinjuku-ku, Tokyo, Japan

The aim of this study was to establish monolayer culture system of human ovarian thecal cells to investigate the morpho-functional potentials of them. Theca layer was isolated and digested by collagenase-hyaluronidase solution, and dispersed thecal cells were cultured for 10 days in Falcon plastic dishes(35x10mm, $1x10^5$cells/dish). Abundant lipid droplets and 3β-hydroxysteroid dehydrogenase activity were revealed in cultured cells by various histochemical studies. It was revealed that these cells secreted Δ_4-androstenedione(Δ_4) and progesterone(P) predominantly. Δ_4 secretion was very high during the first 2 days(31.6ng/$1x10^5$cells/2days), and declined thereafter. P was secreted in moderate amounts throughout the 10 days culture period(9.0-21.3ng/$1x10^5$cells/2days), while estradiol was secreted in small amounts($\leqq$2.0ng/$1x10^5$cells/2days). To investigate the responsiveness of cultured thecal cells to gonadotropins, they were cultured with various concentrations of LH, HCG, or dibutyryl cyclic AMP (Bu_2cAMP). LH and HCG stimulated Δ_4 and P secretion in a dose-related manner. The maximal effective doses of LH and HCG were both 10ng/ml, elevating Δ_4 secretion 4.1 and 2.0 fold, respectively. Bu_2cAMP likewise stimulated Δ_4 and P secretion with the maximal effective does of 10^{-3}M, elevating Δ_4 secretion 4.4 fold. In conclusion, it was clearly convinced that these monolayer-cultured human thecal cells could maintain the morphofunctional characteristics during culture. Therefore, this culture system will provide an excellent model for further researches on the functional properties of thecal cells.

1011 IDENTIFICATION OF 19-NOR-4-ANDROSTENE-3,17-DIONE(19-NORANDROSTENEDIONE) AS A MAJOR STEROID IN PORCINE FOLLICULAR FLUID. M. Wahid Khalil*, MRC Group in Reproductive Biology, University of Western Ontario, London, Ontario N6A 5A5, Canada.

Steroid metabolites are important modulators of ovarian follicular maturation and oocyte development and follicular fluid (FF) constitutes the endocrine milieu in which these changes occur. Steroids in porcine FF obtained from follicles (2-6 mm) of pre-pubertal gilts, were purified on C18 SEP PAK, Lipidex 5000, Sephadex SP-25 and triethylaminohydroxypropyl Sephadex LH-20 (TEAP-LH-20). As many as 16 unconjugated neutral steroids were detected; we have now unambiguously identified 19-norandrostenedione as a major component (150-200 ng/ml FF) from the following chromatographic and spectroscopic data (i) Retention times (r.t.) of the FF steroid and authentic 19-norandrostenedione were identical (6.05 minutes) on C_{18} μ Bondapak column eluted with 70% methanol-water; (ii) R.T. of the underivatised FF steroid (16.92 min.) analysed by capillary gas chromatography on 5% Phenyl Methyl Silicone was similar to that of authentic 19-norandrostenedione (r.t. 16.95 min.) but shorter than that of androstenedione (17.79 min.); (iii) The r.t. of the di-O-methyloxime derivative of the FF steroid (17.34 min.) was similar to the r.t. of the authentic sample (17.40 min.); (v) The mass spectrum of the underivatized FF steroid showed intense ions at m/z 272 (molecular ion), and m/z 110; the di-O-methyloxime derivative showed ions at m/z 330 (molecular ion), m/z 299 (M^+-OCH_3) and m/z 284. The presence of endogenous 19-nor-steroids in the pig ovary is of interest in view of the demonstrated contraceptive effects of synthetic 19-nor-steroids in humans. (Supported by the Medical Research Council of Canada.)

1012 EFFECT OF VARIOUS PROGESTINS AND ANTIPROGESTINS ON GOAT OVARIAN STEROIDOGENESIS. S.M. Kharbanda*, V. Sharma, K. Murugesan, U. Verma and A. Farooq, Department of Reproductive Biology, All India Institute of Medical Sciences, NEW DELHI-110029, India.

Progesterone (P_4) and estradiol 17B (E_2) production by granulosa (G), theca (TH) and corpus luteum (CL) compartments of the goat ovary was studied in vitro. Effect of various progestins and antiprogestins on P_4 and E_2 production with and without LH, FSH, FSH and androstenedione (A) has been studied. Cells were cultured in medium 199 at 37°C for 48 hours. Basal P_4 production (per 10^6 cells) in CL was higher compared to G and TH, and basal E_2 production in TH was higher compared to G and CL Synthetic progestins Promegestone (R5020), d-Norgestrel (d-Ng), norethisterone (NET), and norethisterone acetate (NETA) stimulate P_4 and E_2 production in all the cells but do not have any significant effect. Concomitant treatment with $3x10^{-5}$M R5020 , 10^{-5}M d-Ng, 10^{-6}M NET and 10^{-5}M NETA increases significantly the FSH- stimulated production of P_4. On the other hand, these progestins significantly inhibit the FSH and A stimulated E_2 production. A potent synthetic antiprogestin R 2323 significantly inhibits the basal production of both these steroids whereas the weak antiprogestin STS 557 does not. This study revealed that progestins may have a direct effect on ovarian steroidogenesis.

1013 DIRECT EFFECTS OF GONADOTROPIN-RELEASING HORMONE(GnRH) ON STEROIDOGENESIS OF CULTURED GRANULOSA CELLS. A. Kimura*, T. Uemura and H. Minaguchi, Department of Obstetrics and Gynecology, Yokohama City University, School of Medicine, Yokohama, 232, Japan.

We have examined effects of gonadotropin-releasing hormone(GnRH) on ovarian steroidogenesis in vitro. Dietylstilbestrol primed hypophysectomized immature rats(28 days old) were autopsied and granulosa cells(1× 10 cells/ml) were incubated with PMSG(10iu/ml) and GnRH analog(D-Ser-(TBu)^6-LHRH-EA; 100ng/ml) for 48 hours. After incubation, PMSG alone stimulated estradiol (8.04±1.61 vs. 0.65±0.08ng/mg protein, p<0.01) and progesterone(1.59±0.26 vs. 0.29 ±0.03ng/mg protein, p<0.05) production by granulosa cells. But, GnRH analog inhibited this PMSG stimulated estradiol(1.92±0.27ng/mg protein, p<0.01) and progesterone(0.55 ±0.08ng/mg protein, p<0.05) production. Tracer experiments incubated with ^{14}C-pregnenolone for 24 hours demonstrated that PMSG significantly increased its conversion to progesterone(19.10±9.18 vs. 1.48±2.51%, p<0.05) by granulosa cells. However, when incubated with PMSG+GnRHA, the conversion to progesterone(7.03±3.34%, p<0.05) decreased and that to 20α-hydroxy-progesterone(3.46±2.78 vs. 1.58±0.41%, p<0.05) increased. PMSG significantly increased ^{14}C-androstenedione conversion to estradiol(28.5±7.58 vs. 1.18±0.43%, p<0.01). However, when incubated with PMSG+GnRHa, the conversion to estradiol(1.83±0.85%, p<0.01) decreased and that to testosterone(9.75±3.75 vs. 5.80±2.64%) increased.

These results suggest that GnRH acts directly on granulosa cells to stimulate 20α-hydroxysteroid-dehydrogenase and inhibit 3β-hydroxysteroid dehydrogenase and aromatizing enzyme activity.

1014 ANTI-ESTROGENS INHIBIT THE ESTRADIOL-MEDIATED ENHANCEMENT OF cAMP-INDUCED LH RECEPTOR EXPRESSION IN CULTURED RAT GRANULOSA CELLS. M. Knecht*, T. Ranta, O. Shinohara, S. Hoffmann, A. Baukal, and K.J. Catt, ERRB/NICHD, Bethesda, MD, USA

The effects of estrogens and anti-estrogens on cAMP-induced LH receptor expression were studied in granulosa cells isolated from immature diethylstilbestrol-implanted rats. In cells stimulated with choleragen (CT) for 48 h, estradiol (E_2) concentrations from 10 pM to 10 nM progressively enhanced cAMP production and LH receptor formation by 2-fold and 6-fold, respectively. E_2 also enhanced LH receptor induction by other cAMP-stimulating ligands including FSH, PGE_2, and forskolin. The stimulatory action of 8-Bromo-cAMP (5 mM) on LH receptors was also increased by E_2, indicating that part of the E_2 effect was exerted on cAMP action. Scatchard analysis indicated that E_2 increased the number of CT-induced LH receptors from 13,000 to 85,000 sites/cell with no change in binding affinity. The anti-estrogens, tamoxifen (T) and keoxifene (K) caused a concentration-dependent inhibition of E_2 action on granulosa cell differentiation. T (1 μM) reduced cAMP production and LH receptors induced by CT or FSH plus E_2 (10 nM) by approximately 50%, while K (1 μM) completely prevented E_2 action. In the absence of E_2, T (0.4 μM) amplified CT-induced LH receptors, while K had no agonist effect. Concentrations of T and K of 1 μM and above decreased cAMP content and LH receptors to levels below that stimulated by CT alone. These results demonstrate that E_2 enhances both ligand-induced cAMP production and cAMP action. The inhibitory effects of estrogen antagonists demonstrate the essential role of endogenous estrogen in cAMP-induced granulosa cell differentiation.

1015 THE MILK EJECTION REFLEX: NEURAL AND ANATOMIC CHARACTERISTICS OF AFFERENT FIBERS. E.W. Haller* and J.B. Gearns. Department of Physiology, School of Medicine, University of Minnesota, Duluth, MN 55812, U.S.A.

Episodic secretion of oxytocin in response to suckling has been well documented in the rat, but the mechanism underlying this secretory pattern remains to be identified. Since synaptic interaction in the afferent input of the milk ejection reflex could account for the pattern of activation of oxytocinergic neurons and oxytocin secretion, the present study examined electrophysiologic characteristids and anatomic distribution in spinal cord of afferent nerve fibers in mammary nerve. Electrical stimulation of this nerve in postpartum rats has been shown to result in oxytocin secretion (Mena,F. et al. Endocrinology 103:1929,1978). Electrophysiologic and norphologic experiments required isolation of an abdominal mammary nerve for measurement of conduction velocities or injection of lucifer yellow fluorescent dye. A segment of spinal cord was exposed by laminectomy either for electrode placement or subsequent (6-30 hrs. later) histologic examination. Conduction velocities measured in orthodromic or antidromic direction revealed a predominance of slow fibers (22.6 at 1-6 m/s and 36.9% at 6-21 m/s). Electron microscopic examination confirmed the presence of numerous small myelinated and unmyelinated fibers (29.8% at 6μ and 52% at 6-21μ). Fluorescent dye in spinal cord distributed mainly to three areas ipsilaterally and contralaterally in Clarke's column, and a lesser extent in the contralateral nucleus cervicalis. Our data are consistent with the conduction of primary afferent input to the spinal cord via small fibers. These distribute to synapses (both ipsi- and contralaterally) where initial modification of afferent input may result in episodic activation of hypothalamic oxytocinergic neurons. Supported gy NIH 5R01 HD13906-05.

1016 ROLE OF OSMOLALITY IN AN ANTAGONISM OF PROSTAGLANDIN (PG) E ON VASOPRESSIN (VP)-INDUCED CELLULAR cAMP IN THE CULTURED RAT RENAL PAPILLARY COLLECTING TUBULE (RPCT) CELLS. S. Ishikawa* and T. Saito, Div. Endocrinol. and Metab., Jichi Medical School, Tochigi 329-04, Japan.

In the present study a role for environmental osmolality in interaction between VP and PGE was examined in the cultured rat RPCT cells. Both VP and PGE_2 stimulated intracellular cAMP in a dose dependent manner in an isotonic medium of 300 mOsm/kg H_2O with the phosphodiesterase inhibitor. Environmental tonicity modulated the effect of VP, PGE, or both, on cellular cAMP production. Specifically, the effect of a submaximal stimulatory concentration of 10^{-9} M VP on cAMP production was enhanced by 2-fold, but the effect of 2 x 10^{-8}M PGE_1 or E_2 was markedly reduced by 1/6 or 1/3, when the cells were exposed to the hypertonic medium with 1800 mOsm/kg H_2O (NaCl and urea with 1 : 2 molar ratio) compared to the isotonic medium. The inhibitory effect of PGE_1 on the hydroosmotic action of VP was not shown under the isotonic medium. However, this was demonstrated under the hypertonic medium which pertains in the papillary tissue of the kidney, as the cellular cAMP of 438 ± 39 (n=6) induced by a combination of 2 x 10^{-8} M PGE_1 and 10^{-9} M VP was significantly less than the value of 806 ± 143 fM/ug protein/10 min (n=6) with 10^{-9} M VP alone ($p<0.05$). Similar results were obtained with 2 x 10^{-8} M PGE_2 and 10^{-9} M VP. Synthesis of [3H]PGE_2 was enhanced by hypertonicity, but not by VP, when [3H]arachidonic acid was available. These results therefore indicate that an environmental osmolality is an important factor for PGE modulating VP-induced cAMP production in the papillary collecting tubule. However, the interaction between PGE and VP via a closed feedback loop remained to be determined.

1017 SUCKLING-INDUCED RELEASE OF OXYTOCIN AND PROLACTIN IN LONG-TERM LACTATION.
J.M. Johnston and J.A. Amico*, Department of Medicine, University of Pittsburgh, Pittsburgh, PA, USA.

Both oxytocin (OT) and prolactin (PRL) are released in lactating women in response to infant suckling, but the pattern of release of PRL in long-term lactation has been more intensively investigated than that of OT. We thus serially studied 6 lactating women during 3 intervals postpartum:1-4, 5-14, and 15-24 weeks (early, middle, and late lactation, respectively). Blood for RIA of OT, PRL, and vasopressin (VP) was drawn 15 minutes (min) before and every 3 min during 15 min infant feedings. Comparisons (analysis of variance) were made between mean ($\bar{M}$) basal vs stimulated levels of hormones, and among levels of hormones in early, middle, and late lactation $\bar{M}(\pm SD)$ basal OT did not differ among early 0.72 ± 0.37 μU/ml, middle 0.64 ± 0.16 μU/ml, and late 0.64 ± 0.28 μU/ml lactation. $\bar{M}$ OT, but not VP, increased within 3 min of suckling and remained significantly elevated above basal levels during 15 min of breast feeding ($p<.0005$). The pattern of release of OT was pulsatile with 1 to 2 peaks per 15 min period. Among women, peak OT ranged from 3.82-23.2 μU/ml. $\bar{M}$ OT in response to suckling was not different among early, middle and late lactation. $\bar{M}$ PRL increased steadily in response to suckling ($p<.0075$) with maximal levels achieved at 15 min of suckling. Both basal and stimulated levels of PRL decreased from early to late lactation ($p<.009$). PRL and OT did not correlate. In lactating women, OT is released in response to infant suckling in a pulsatile pattern, independent of PRL and VP. In contrast to basal and suckling-induced levels of PRL which decrease with time postpartum, basal and suckling-induced release of OT remain unchanged from early to late lactation.

1018 PRESENCE AND CONCENTRATION OF OXYTOCIN IN MONKEY CORPUS LUTEUM THROUGHOUT THE LUTEAL PHASE OF THE MENSTRUAL CYCLE.
Firyal S. Khan-Dawood*, Edward L. Marut and M. Yusoff Dawood, Department of Obstetrics and Gynecology, University of Illinois College of Medicine, Chicago, Illinois 60612 U.S.A.

Our recent studies indicate that immunoreactive oxytocin (OT) is present in human ovarian stromal and corpus luteum tissues. To determine if OT is present in ovaries of other primates, 13 corpora lutea (CL) were removed at laparotomy during the luteal phase (LP) from 9 monkeys (Macaca fascicularis) with timed regular ovulatory cycles. Ipsilateral ovarian vein blood and peripheral venous blood were collected and measured for OT and progesterone (P) by a sensitive and specific radioimmunoassay (RIA). Serial dilution of the acetic acid extract of individual corpus luteum showed parallelism with standard OT in the RIA. Total content of OT in CL was 1.9 ± 0.5 ng (mean ± SEM) with a content of 0.4 - 0.8 ng in early LP, 1.0 - 6.2 ng in mid LP and 0.4 - 0.7 ng in late LP. OT concentrations per mg protein in the CL were 0.05 - 19.6 ng with peak concentrations of 14.7 - 19.6 ng/mg protein on day 22. Sephadex G-25 column chromatography of individual corpus luteum extract revealed a single peak similar to that of synthetic OT in the RIA. Ovarian vein blood from the same side as the CL has a significantly higher OT concentration of 161.2 ± 29.7 pg/ml on days 15-24 than 16.8 ± 3.6 pg/ml on days 25-28 ($p = <0.01$) and peripheral plasma OT levels of 23.2 ± 3.4 pg/ml ($p = <0.025$). The OT levels paralleled the progesterone levels in the ovarian vein blood. These findings indicate that OT is present and is probably produced by the monkey ovary and that it may be involved in the control of the corpus luteum.

1019 EFFECT OF MONOVALENT AND DIVALENT CATIONS ON ^3H-ARG^8-VASOPRESSIN BINDING TO THE RAT MESENTERIC VASCULATURE.
R. Larivière* and E.L. Schiffrin, Clinical Institute of Montreal, Montreal, Quebec H2W 1R7, Canada.

Vasopressin is a powerful vasoconstrictor of the mesenteric vascular bed. We have previously demonstrated the presence of high affinity, low capacity binding sites specific for ^3H-Arg^8-vasopressin in a particulate fraction of the rat mesenteric vascular bed (E.L. Schiffrin and J. Genest, Endocrinology 113:409, 1983). We have now investigated the *in vitro* effect of monovalent and divalent cations on the binding of ^3H-Arg^8-vasopressin to the same preparation. The absence of NaCl did not affect binding, but increasing the concentration to 150 mM reduced binding by 50 percent. KCl also reduced binding at concentrations of 150 mM, as did NH_4Cl. The addition of $MgCl_2$ at 1 mM increased binding 2-fold, and concentrations of up to 20 mM further increased binding 4-fold. $MnCl_2$ increased binding 3 to 10 times at concentrations of 1-20 mM. We conclude that binding of ^3H-Arg^8-vasopressin is reduced by high ionic strength but unaffected specifically by any monovalent cation. It is increased by divalent cations such as Mg and Mn, indicating the presence of a divalent cation sensitive site which is critical for the affinity of the membrane-bound receptor for vasopressin. Supported by the Medical Research Council of Canada.

1020 REGULATION OF PINEAL FUNCTION BY VASOACTIVE INTESTINAL POLYPEPTIDE (VIP)
K. Kaku*, S. Matsumura and T. Kaneko, Internal Medicine, Yamaguchi Univ. Sch. of Med., Kogushi 1,144, Ube 755, Japan

The role of vasoactive intestinal polypeptide (VIP) on the regulation of pineal functions was studied using rat dispersed pineal cells. We have characterized the specific binding site of VIP, and determined the stimulatory effects of VIP on adenylate cyclase and serotonin N-acetyltransferase (NAT) activities. Scatchard analysis of the iodinated-VIP binding to pineal cells indicated the presence of two classes of binding sites : a high affinity-low capacity site (Kd;0.8nM) and a low affinity-high capacity site (Kd;32nM). Peptide with N-terminal histidine and C-terminal isoleucine (PHI) and secretin, structurally related peptides, inhibited the tracer binding with the lower potency (1/20 and 1/100 of VIP, respectively). Norepinephrine could not inhibit the tracer binding to pineal cells. VIP stimulated cyclic AMP production of pineal cells with dose-dependency (ED_{50};1 nM). The stimulatory effects of PHI and secretin on cyclic AMP accumulation seemed to be parallel to their inhibitory potencies against the tracer binding to pineal cells. The NAT activity of pineal cells was significantly stimulated by VIP. Our data demonstrate that the pineal cell has VIP-receptors coupled to adenylate cyclase system, which is independent of β-adrenergic system. Consequently, it is strongly suggested that the pineal function is regulated through a dual (β-adrenergic and VIPergic) control system.

1021 MELATONIN FEEDING INCREASES OVULATION RATE IN EWES. D.J. Kennaway* E.A. Dunstan, T.A. Gilmore and R.F. Seamark, Department of Obstetrics, University of Adelaide, South Australia, and Kybybolite Research Centre South Australia Department of Agriculture, Kybybolite, South Australia.

In many breeds of sheep ovulation rate (OR) is highest in the middle of the breeding season, and is related to the seasonal decrease in daylength (E.A. Dunstan, Aust. J. Exp. Agric. Anim. Husb., 17, 741, 1977) Three weeks of short daylength followed by introduction of a ram and a further 6 weeks of short daylength results in up to 30% more lambs. In 9 field experiments involving 1525 Border Leicester X Merino ewes, melatonin feeding 2mg/day for 9 weeks) in late afternoon similarly increased fecundity (median 25%, range -6 to 39%). A further study of 78 BLxMo ewes compared short daylength (darkness 1600h i.e. 4h prior to natural sunset) and melatonin feeding at 1600h. Blood samples were taken at 15min intervals for 5h on day -1, day 20 and day 60, together with daily samples during the first 10 days after introduction of rams on day 21. All groups of ewes showed the typical ovarian response to the rams with oestrus and fertile mating occurring approximately 23 days after ram introduction in all groups. Lambing percentages were 92%, 146% and 131% for control, short daylength and melatonin fed groups respectively. Neither treatments altered LH pulse frequency or FSH levels prior to ram introduction although prolactin levels were markedly decreased on days 20 and 60. These results show that melatonin feeding mimics the effects of short daylength on fecundity.
Supported by grants from the NHMRC and the AMRC.

1022 INTERACTIONS BETWEEN SEX STEROIDS AND INHIBIN ON LHRH-INDUCED GONADOTROPIN SECRETION IN RAT ANTERIOR PITUITARY CELLS IN CULTURE. M. Godbout, F. Ruel*, H. Gauthier and F. Labrie, MRC Group in Molecular Endocrinology, CHUL, Québec, G1V 4G2, Canada.

We have recently purified ovarian inhibin to near-homogeneity using porcine follicular fluid as starting material. This material exerts a specific inhibitory effect on spontaneous FSH secretion but not on LH release while it inhibits the LHRH-induced release of both LH and FSH in rat anterior pituitary cells in culture. Using the same in vitro bioassay system, it has previously been demonstrated that sex steroids exert specific and differential effects on LH and FSH secretion. More specifically, all three classes of sex steroids are exclusively stimulatory on FSH secretion. On the other hand, estrogens and progestins stimulate while androgens inhibit LH secretion. When anterior pituitary cells were preincubated with inhibin and sex steroids for 48h and the LH and FSH response to LHRH was measured during a 4-h incubation, the following observations were made: all the stimulatory effects of 1.0 nM 17β-estradiol (E_2), 10 nM 5α-dihydrotestosterone (DHT), 300 nM progesterone (P), as well as the combination of E_2 + P, on LHRH-induced FSH release were completely inhibited by preincubation with 250 ng of the purified Inhibin preparation. Inhibin prevents the stimulatory effects of sex steroids on gonadotropin secretion and could well play an important physiological role in association with sex steroids in the control of reproductive functions.

1023 IDENTIFICATION AND CHARACTERIZATION OF CALMODULIN AND Ca^{2+}, CALMODULIN-DEPENDENT PROTEIN KINASE IN RAT ANTERIOR PITUITARY GLAND.

Y. Hatada*, M. Munemura, K. Fukunaga†, H. Yamamoto†, M. Maeyama, and E. Miyamoto†, Department of Obstetrics and Gynecology, and Department of Pharmacology†, Kumamoto University Medical School, Kumamoto, Japan.

Ca^{2+} plays a critical role in the release of adenohypophyseal hormones. The action of Ca^{2+} may, if not all, be mediated by calmodulin. An accumulating evidence supports that protein phosphorylation is involved in many of cellular events including stimulus-secretion coupling. In this study, we identified and characterized calmodulin and Ca^{2+}, calmodulin-dependent protein kinase in rat anterior pituitary gland. Calmodulin was purified from the cytosol. The calmodulin of the anterior pituitary gland had similar properties to brain calmodulin with respect to a M_r on SDS-PAGE and myosin light-chain kinase activation. The concentration of calmodulin was 1.18 ± 0.11 μg/mg protein in the cytosol. Ca^{2+}, calmodulin-dependent protein kinase was partially purified by DEAE-cellulose and calmodulin-Sepharose affinity column chromatography. The K_a value of the enzyme for Ca^{2+} was 3.3 μM. Trifluoperazine and chlorpromazine inhibited enzyme activity, with K_i values of 13 and 26 μM, respectively. At least 9 proteins in the membrane fraction were phosphorylated by the enzyme. The enzyme was resolved into two peaks of activity, with sedimentation coefficients of 5.5 S and 16.5 S. These results support the idea that the effect of Ca^{2+} on the release of adenohypophyseal hormones is mediated by the Ca^{2+}, calmodulin-dependent protein kinase system.

1024 PROLONGED ACTIVATION OF MUSCARINIC CHOLINERGIC RECEPTORS CAUSES DESENSITIZATION AND AN INCREASE IN FORSKOLIN-STIMULATED CYCLIC AMP SYNTHESIS AND ACTH SECRETION FROM PITUITARY TUMOR CELLS.

S. Heisler*. Unité de Biorégulation cellulaire et moléculaire, CHUL, Québec, Canada, and Département de Pharmacologie, Université Laval, Québec, Canada.

Activation of muscarinic receptors on the AtT-20/D16-16 (AtT-20) clonal line of mouse pituitary cells inhibits forskolin-stimulated cyclic AMP formation and ACTH secretion. In this study, the effect of prolonged treatment of AtT-20 cells with the muscarinic agonist, oxotremorine, was examined. Oxotremorine antagonism of forskolin-stimulated cyclic AMP formation and ACTH release was reduced by prior exposure of AtT-20 cells to oxotremorine. The response to somatostatin-14, a second antagonist of forskolin action in AtT-20 cells, was also desensitized by oxotremorine pretreatment. Additionally, prolonged oxotremorine pretreatment resulted in an increased ability of forskolin to stimulate cyclic AMP formation and to a lesser degree ACTH secretion. Sensitization of the cyclic AMP response to forskolin extended to other muscarinic agonists, was dependent on the oxotremorine concentration used and required two or more hours of pretreatment. Sensitization was blocked by cycloheximide and was reversed by the muscarinic antagonist, scopolamine, or by a 5 hr recovery period following pretreatment. A decrease in muscarinic receptor density was observed after 3-4 hr exposure to oxotremorine without any change in ligand-receptor affinity. The data suggest that oxotremorine desensitization and the apparent sensitization of adenylate cyclase are associated with muscarinic receptor activation (rather than simple occupancy) and that neither event requires prior muscarinic receptor down-regulation.
(Supported by The Medical Research Council of Canada)

1025 ROLE OF CALCIUM-ACTIVATED, PHOSPHOLIPID-DEPENDENT PROTEIN KINASE (PROTEIN KINASE C) IN GnRH ACTION.

K. Hirota*, T. Hirota, G. Aguilera and K.J. Catt, ERRB, NICHD, NIH, Bethesda, MD 20205, U.S.A.

The calcium requirement and altered phospholipid metabolism associated with GnRH-induced LH secretion suggests the possible involvement of calcium-activated, phospholipid-dependent protein kinase (C-Kinase) in GnRH action. We have studied C-Kinase activity of anterior pituitary cells and have assessed the effects on LH secretion of C-kinase activation by TPA (12-O-tetra-decanoylphorbol-13-acetate) and specific inhibition by retinal. Protein phosphorylation by rat anterior pituitary cytosol was increased in the presence of Ca^{2+} and was further enhanced by phosphatidylserine (PS) and 1,2-diolein, indicating that the C-Kinase at pituitary was similar to the enzyme from platelet and brain and its cofactor requirements. TPA was found to fully activate C-Kinase in pituitary cytosol in the presence of Ca^{2+} and PS, and also shown to cause a dose-related partial stimulation of LH secretion. Retinal inhibited C-Kinase activity in the presence of Ca^{2+} and diolein when added at concentrations greater than 10^{-5} M, with half-maximal inhibition at 2 x 10^{-7} M. In cultured pituitary cells stimulated with a maximal dose of GnRH (10 nM), we found that retinal reduced GnRH-induced LH release in a dose-dependent fashion. The maximum inhibition of GnRH-induced LH release was 47 ± 13% with 10^{-4} M retinal, a concentration at which C-Kinase activity was completely inhibited. The ability of TPA to activate pituitary and to stimulate LH secretion and the converse effects of retinal on C-Kinase and GnRH-induced LH release, indicate that C-Kinase participates in the action of GnRH upon LH secretion.

1026 RADIATION THERAPY FOR INTRACRANIAL METASTASES OF PITUITARY (CORTICOTROPHS) TUMORS.

M. Horwith*, R.E.Peterson, N.Sonino, J.Richard, N.Ertel, B.Lee, R.A.R.Fraser, R.H.Patterson Jr., N.Y. Hospital-Cornell Medical Center, N.Y.,N.Y., U.S.A.

A 13 yr. m (A),and 12 yr.f (B) were bilaterally adrenalectomized (ba) for Cushing's disease. Pt. A had 4 months previously undergone transfrontal pituitary adenomectomy (tpa) followed by ^{60}Co radiation (5400 r) to the sella. Pt. B required tpa 6 yrs. post-ba and subsequently received 5600 r α-particle radiation to the sella. Twenty-two yrs. (A) and 14 yrs. (B) post-ba, they developed clinical evidence of intracranial disease. CT demonstrated widely disseminated intracranial metastases, which on biopsy was pituitary tissue positive for ACTH by immunoflourescence. Craniotomy attempted for debulking was unsuccessful. Plasma ACTH was 2200 pg/ml (A), and 3000 pg/ml (B). Pharmacological regimens were unsuccessful in lowering ACTH levels or altering the clinical course. Whole brain ^{60}Co radiation (2400 r) was administered. Repeat CT scans and NMR demonstrated marked reduction in extent of metastatic lesions. Both patients have improved clinically; but, ACTH levels although decreased (500 pg/ml), remain above normal. Although initial radiation to the sella did not prevent development of intracranial pituitary tumor spread, whole brain radiation to the metastatic tumor was of significant benefit and suggests radiosensitivity of this tissue.

1027 DES-INDUCED PROLACTINOMAS IN THE FISCHER 344 RAT: HETEROGENEITY OF MAMMOTROPH FORM AND FUNCTION. W. C. Hymer*, K. Motter, J. M. Hatfield and G. Mansur. Department of Biochemistry, Pennsylvania State University, University Park, PA 16802.

Implantation of DES-containing (8 mg) Silastic capsules into F-344 ovx rats causes pituitary tumors (Wiklund et al., Endo. 109:1700, 1981). We studied tumor mammotrophs after separation on 1-3% BSA gradients at unit gravity. 30 x 10^6 cells prepared from 70-90 day old tumors were separated into large (Fr. I), intermediate (Fr. II) and small (Fr. III) cells (40 exps). Of the total recovered cells (88 $\pm$ 3%), 17%, 49%, 33% were found in Frs. I, II and III, respectively. Mammotrophs accounted for 86%, 86% and 72% of the large, intermediate and small cells. By EM, cells in Frs. I and II were laden with secretory granules whereas those in Fr. III were not. This observation was confirmed by laser flow cytometry (size vs 90° light scatter). After 1-4 hrs in culture, Fr. I cells released 157%, 132% and 172% PRL compared to unfractionated cells, while Fr. III cells released only 29%, 35% and 44%. However, when secreted PRL was related to intracellular PRL, Fr. III cells were most active. High PRL turnover rates in Fr. III cells were confirmed by reverse plaque assay (Neill and Frawley, Endo. 112:1135, 1983). Of the total plaque-forming cells, those in Frs. I, II and III accounted for 5, 38 and 57%, respectively. Differences in PRL forms between the three fractions were revealed on immunoblots after electrophoresis on 15% native gels and after HPLC on C-18 reverse phase columns. Conclusion: Tumor mammotrophs of different size and cytoplasmic granulation contain different hormone forms. Not all of these mammotrophs are active in culture. (Supported by USPHS CA 23248).

1028 ALTERED PRL,TSH AND GH SECRETION IN ISOLATED RETINITIS PIGMENTOSA. G.Iervasi*, M.Ferdeghini,F.Genovesi-Ebert,A.L.Guastella,M.Lotti,A.M.Wirth and R. Bianchi. Istituto di Fisiologia Clinica del CNR,Centro di Medicina Nucleare e Clinica Oculistica,Università di Pisa,Pisa,Italia.

Retinitis Pigmentosa(RP)is very invalidant,higly frequent degenerative retinal disease,sometimes associated with CNS disorders.Coinherited retinal and nigrostriatal dopamine(DA)defect in hypogalactorrhoic BW rats support a recent pathogenetic hypothesis involving retinal DA failure in RP.We studied 26 males,aged 20-56,affected by severe isolated RP;11 inpatients,aged 23-48,with traumatic corneal lesions were controls.All subjects were unmedicated and without endocrine disorders.Pts.with Moon-Biedl syndrome were excluded.TSH and GH response to TRH(200 ug iv),PRL and TSH response to Metoclopramide(Mcp,10 mg iv)and Domperidone(Dom,4 mg iv)were evaluated.PRL basal levels were 5.6$\pm$2.1 ng/ml(m$\pm$SD)in RP pts and 6.2$\pm$1.5 ng/ml in controls(NS). PRL peaks after TRH,Mcp,Dom were significantly lower than in controls respectively 26.2$\pm$6.4 vs 50.4$\pm$18.3 ng/ml($p<.001$);68.4$\pm$18.5 vs 105.2$\pm$15.3 ng/ml($p<.001$);50.2$\pm$9.4 vs 86.3$\pm$9.6 ng/ml($p<.001$).TSH basal levels were 1.3$\pm$0.8 in RP males and 1.3$\pm$0.6 uIU/ml in controls(NS).Mean TSH peak to TRH was 10.8$\pm$7.6 in RP pts. and 14.1$\pm$3.5 uIU/ml in controls(NS).Nevertheless 13/26 RP pts showed a blunted TSH response(ΔTSH<7 uIU/ml).A negative correlation was found between GH and TSH peak in the 13 pts.with the lowest Δ TSH($p<.05$).No significant increment of TSH serum levels was found after Mcp or Dom in RP males.TT_4,TT_3,fT_4,fT_3,rT_3,LH,FSH,Testosterone,Estradiol,Cortisol basal levels were in the normal limits.Our data suggest an altered hypothalamic control of pituitary secretion mainly of PRL,but also concerning TSH and GH in males with severe RP,according to results obtained in Parkinson's disease.

1029 TISSUE DISTRIBUTION AND MOLECULAR FORM OF A NOVEL PITUITARY PROTEIN IN THE RAT. H. Iguchi*, J.S.D. Chan, N.G. Seidah and M. Chrétien, Clinical Research Institute of Montreal, Montreal, Canada H2W 1R7.

We developed a sensitive and specific radioimmunoassay (RIA) for a novel pituitary protein, designated as 7B2, which has been purified from human and porcine pituitary gland using an antiserum raised against a synthetic 7B2 fragment. By employing this RIA, the highest levels of immunoreactive (IR)-7B2 were found in anterior lobe (AL) (10,400±804 pg/mg tissue, mean±SE) and neurointermediate lobe (NIL) (6,190±908). Relatively high levels were found in hypothalamus (247±27), adrenal medulla (697±83) and thyroid gland (1,368±116), while low levels ($<$ 30) were found in pancreas, ileum and colon. IR-7B2 was not detected in liver, kidney, spleen, lung, adrenal cortex and testis. Chromatographic studies of the tissue extracts on Sephadex G-100 revealed that the majority of IR-7B2 has an apparent molecular weight (MW) of 45-50K daltons. However, analysis of this 7B2 on SDS-polyacrylamide gel electrophoresis showed a smaller MW (20K). In addition, the release of IR-7B2 was induced from cultured cells of AL and NIL by high K^+ (50 mM). IR-7B2 was detected in the neurosecretory granule fraction prepared from pig NIL. These results indicate that 7B2 is a novel secretory protein. Immunocytochemical studies showed that IR-7B2 is located in AL and posterior lobe (not intermediate lobe) of pituitary gland and hypothalamus in several species. The findings reported here suggest that 7B2 is synthesized in AL and hypothalamus and that hypothalamic 7B2 is transported to posterior lobe in a manner similar to that described for vasopressin and oxytocin.

1030 PROLACTIN AND GROWTH HORMONE IMMUNOREACTIVITY IN PITUITARY MACROADENOMAS. Nandita Gupta; N. Kochupillai*; M.M. Godbole; R.K. Goulatia and P.N. Tandon, Department of Endocrinology and Neurosurgery, A.I.I.M.S., New Delhi, India.

122 large pituitary adenomas (median size = 19.2 c.c.) including 44 with clinical acromegaly were studied for their endocrine status. 80 (34 with acromegaly) of these were also studied for tumour tissue concentrations of PRL, GH, LH and TSH. The tissue concentrations measured were compared with those observed in 16 normal pituitaries. Hyperprolactinemia was present in 66.4% of the whole group and 61% of the subject with acromegaly. However, all the tumour tissues studied showed dominant PRL immunoreactivity (median concentration - 16.75 ug/mg protein). GH immunoreactivity could also be demonstrated in all the tissues, with significantly higher concentrations in tumour tissues from acromegalics. The various data suggest that all the large pituitary adenomas studied produce prolactin. This study was supported by Indian Council of Medical Research, New Delhi.

1031 PARTIAL CHARACTERIZATION OF PLASMA PROLACTIN RELEASING FACTOR-LIKE ACTIVITY (PRF-LA). T.C. Hagen,* T.L. Garthwaite, and D.R. Martinson, Wood VA Medical Center and the Medical College of Wisconsin, Milwaukee, WI.

We have previously reported that a PRF-LA is present in methanol extracts of normal human plasma (N), with similar concentrations in the plasma of pregnant subjects, but higher concentrations in plasma from subjects with pathologic hyperprolactinemia (HP). In order to further characterize this material, 100 ml of plasma from N and HP subjects were extracted, dissolved in 2 N acetic acid, and chromatographed on a 100 x 4.5 cm Sephadex G-25 column. Eluates were bioassayed for PRF-LA by incubation with acutely dispersed male rat anterior pituitary cells for 1 hour and measurement of prolactin (PRL) released in the medium. A single peak of PRF-LA was obtained with N and HP extracts. 25, 50, and 100 μl aliquots of the HP peak resulted in 282 ± 16, 322 ± 41, and 322 ± 22 ng PRL/ 2.5×10^5 cells ($\bar{X} \pm$ S.E.), respectively, compared to control cell release (137 ± 13), significant at $p < 0.002$ by analysis of variance and T-test. In separate experiments, 50 μl aliquots of the HP peak were pre-incubated with and without pronase (500 μg/ml), boiled for 10 minutes to inactivate the enzyme, and subjected to bioassay. PRL release was 199 ± 32 and 516 ± 29 ng/2.5×10^5 cells with and without pronase, respectively ($p < 0.0001$). A similar change in PRF-LA obtained with and without trypsin (50 μg/ml): 144 ± 10 and 352 ± 13 ng/2.5×10^5 cells, respectively ($p < 0.0001$). Carboxy and aminopeptidases were without effect. These results indicate that a partially purified sample of PRF-LA is inactivated by endopeptidases but not terminal peptidases, and suggest that PRF-LA from human plasma is a peptide.

1032 TREATMENT OF IDOPATHIC INFERTILITY IN COUPLES WITH NORMOPROLACTINAEMIA AND INTERMITTENT ELEVATIONS OF PROLACTIN. R.F. Harrison* R. O'Moore A.M. O'Moore TCD Dept. Ob/Gyn, Clin. Bioch. and Teacher Ed. Dublin Ireland.

No infertility cause was found in 18% of clinic Pts., although some occasionally showed premenstrual intermittent elevations of prolactin (SPr). However prolactin in the others remaining normal (NPr). In these two Gps. various modes of therapy were tried. The results are presented in terms of the Biochemical and pregnancy outlook.

1. Bromocriptine V Placebo for 6 Mths. 30 Pts., (SPr 11 NPr 19) 8 Preg. 4 Pl. 4 Br. (1 SPr). No Sig. Diffs. Biochem. except SPr Gp. not affected by Br. therapy.
2. Clomid 30 Pts.(HPr 8 NPr 22) O Pregs. O Biochem. effect.
3. Clomid + hCG V Placebo + hCG 6 Mths. X over (HPr 8 NPr 22) 6 preg. 1 Pl. + hCG 5 Cl. + hCG (3 SPr) no Sig. Diff. Biochem. except SPr Gp. not affected by Cl. + hCG therapy.
4. Clomid + Bromocriptine V Placebo 6 mths. X over. 70 Pts. (47 SPr 22 NPr) 26 Preg. 6 Pl. 20 Cl. + Br. (2 Pl. SPr 16 Cl. + Br. SPr). No Sig. Diff. Biochem. except SPr Gp. affected by active therapy. Prolactin lowered.
5. Autogenic therapy 22 Pts. to date 2 Preg. Mean Prolactin SPr Gp. Sig. higher than fertile controls and Sig. fall in Prolactin ($P<0.05$) post treatment.

1033 DIFFERENTIAL ACTION OF DEXAMETHASONE ON GROWTH HORMONE (GH) AND PROLACTIN (PRL) SECRETION DURING LONG-TERM CULTURE OF BOVINE PITUITARY CELLS. C.D.Ingram* and R.J.Bicknell, ARC Institute of Animal Physiology, Babraham, Cambridge CB2 4AT UK

Since glucocorticoid binding sites are present in GH and PRL secreting cells, we have examined the effects of dexamethasone (DEX) on the secretion of GH and PRL. Primary cultures were maintained in Dulbecco's MEM containing either L- or D-valine, a substitution known to suppress fibroblast division and maintain PRL secretion (Padmanabhan et al Mol.Cell.Endocr. 28:613,1982). GH secretion from these cells declined to less than 10% of initial rates by day 10 of culture and was unaltered by D-valine substitution. From day 5-25 DEX(10^{-7}M) caused an increasing stimulation of secretion, reaching 250-500% of control by day 25, an effect which persisted after removal of DEX. In L-valine DMEM PRL secretion declined by 80% from day 5 to 25. The presence of DEX caused an increasing inhibition of PRL secretion reaching 90% by day 25.Cells remained responsive to DEX throughout culture but its inhibitory effects were not totally reversible. In contrast,PRL secretion in D-valine DMEM was maintained for 20-25 days.Addition of DEX at various times caused a 50% inhibition that did not increase with duration of exposure and was reversed upon removal.These data suggest that 1) DEX stimulates GH and inhibits PRL secretion, effects that persist throughout chronic culture, 2) part of the inhibition of PRL may be mediated via fibroblast growth or metabolism.

1034 EFFECTS OF AN INTRACELLULAR PROLACTIN MEDIATOR ON INSULIN MEDIATOR SENSITIVE ENZYMES. L. Jarett*, S.L. Macaulay, J.O. Macaulay and L.M. Houdebine+, University of Pennsylvania School of Medicine, Philadelphia, PA and +National de la Recherche Agronomique, Jouy-en-Josas, France.

The supernatant from prolactin-treated rabbit mammary gland membranes contains a mediator (P-M) which stimulates β-casein gene transcription to a greater extent than supernatant from untreated membranes (C-M). The C-M and P-M were partially purified by ultrafiltration to yield a fraction of 500-2000 MW, similar to the fraction containing insulin-generated mediator (I-M) when partially purified by the same technique. These fractions were tested on three enzyme systems: pyruvate dehydrogenase (PDH), low Km cAMP phosphodiesterase (PDE) and adenylate cyclase (A/C), all previously shown to be altered by I-M. As has been shown for I-M, P-M stimulated basal PDH activity by 150-500% whereas C-M stimulated PDH by only 50-100%. P-M, like I-M, also suppressed A/C more than did C-M. However unlike I-M, which stimulated PDE, P-M markedly inhibited PDE. The P-M activity which affected all three enzymes was shown to be soluble in 100% ethanol (EtOH). However, I-M was insoluble in 100% EtOH. Mixtures of I-M and P-M were extracted in EtOH. I-M was again insoluble in 100% EtOH and P-M extracted into the supernatant indicating differences between the two mediators. These studies show that although there are similarities between I-M and P-M, distinct differences exist between the two types of mediator indicating they may be part of a new family of mediator molecules. Supported by NIH, JDF and Reynolds Foundation.

1035 PROLACTIN SECRETION AND BIOLOGICAL ACTIVITY IN FEMALES WITH GALACTORRHOEA AND NORMAL CIRCULATING PROLACTIN CONCENTRATIONS AT REST.

D.G. Johnston*, J. Haigh, R.W.G. Prescott, A. Heaton, R. Rowe, H. Friesen, P. Kendall-Taylor, and P.H. Baylis, Royal Victoria Infirmary, Newcastle on Tyne NE1 4LP UK, and University of Manitoba, Canada, R3E OW3.

Prolactin secretion and biological activity have been investigated in 20 females with galactorrhoea who had normal resting serum prolactin levels, and in 34 normal controls. Two patients became hyperprolactinaemic with observation for 1.5 to 8.5 years while resting prolactin stayed normal in the remaining 18 who were further studied. Menstruation was disordered in only 6 of the 18, while ovulation occurred (progesterone >20 nmol/l) in all 7 patients studied over a 5 week period. Prolactin levels over 24h were similar in patients and controls (24h mean ± SE prolactin, 288 ± 36 vs 291 ± 21 mU/l respectively) as were prolactin estimates twice weekly for 5 weeks. Prolactin responses to TRH, domperidone and hypoglycaemia were similar in patients and controls. Two different radioimmunoassays gave similar prolactin values and bioactivity was normal in the Nb2 Node rat lymphoma cell proliferation assay (basal prolactin, patients 355 ± 43 mU/l; controls 348 ± 64 mU/l). Metabolic abnormalities similar to those previously noted in hyperprolactinaemia were observed in the patients' 24h profiles. These included mild hyperglycaemia (24h mean ± SE glucose, 5.47 ± 0.08 vs 5.05 ± 0.14 mmol/l, p <0.05), elevations in circulating lactate, pyruvate and alanine and a decrease in blood glycerol. In most patients with idiopathic galactorrhoea, prolactin levels, regulation of secretion and bioactivity in vitro are normal. The galactorrhoea and metabolic abnormalities suggest increased tissue sensitivity to the lactogenic and metabolic actions of prolactin, while ovarian cyclical function is relatively spared.

1036 A PHYSIOLOGICAL ROLE FOR α-MSH AS A MODULATOR OF PULSATILE AND STRESS-INDUCED PROLACTIN (Prl) SECRETION IN THE FEMALE RAT.

O. Khorram*, J. Bedran de Castro and S.M. McCann. Dept of Physiology, Univ of Texas Hlth Sci Center at Dallas, Dallas, Texas 75235.

We have previously demonstrated that intraventricular (3rd V)(IVT) administration of α-MSH inhibits basal and stress-induced Prl release. To assess the physiological significance of these observations, we passively immunized long-term ovariectomized (OVX) rats with a specific antiserum to α-MSH. OVX rats were injected IVT with 5 µl of antiserum to α-MSH (purified IgG fraction) or NRS (IgG fraction). On the following day one blood sample was withdrawn and the animals were injected a second time with the same volume of the antiserum or NRS. Twenty-four hours after the first injection of anti-MSH plasma levels of Prl were significantly elevated (p<.05). Blood samples were withdrawn every 10 minutes for a total of 3 hours after the 2nd injection. Analysis of the 3 hr hormonal profiles indicated a significant increase in the area under the secretion curve of Prl (p<.025) and in the amplitude of Prl pulses (p<.01) after anti-MSH. The antiserum had no effect on the frequency of Prl pulses. When rats which had received two injections of anti-MSH or NRS were subjected to a 2 min ether stress, Prl levels significantly increased within 5 min in the NRS-injected rats, whereas Prl levels in the antiserum injected rats did not increase any further from the initially high baseline levels. These results support our hypothesis that α-MSH of hypothalamic origin inhibits the secretion of basal and stress-induced Prl possibly by a hypothalamic mechanism. Supported by PHS grants AM 10073 and HD 09988.

1037 EFFECT OF BROMOCRIPTINE LONG-TERM TREATMENT AND PREGNANCY ON GROWTH AND ACTIVITY OF PITUITARY PROLACTINOMA.
T. Kimura*, S. Kazeto, A. Takada, M. Asai, T. Masahashi, M. Osawa, M. Suzuki, O. Narita, and Y. Tomoda, Department of Obstetrics and Gynecology, Nagoya First Red Cross Hospital. Department of Obstetrics and Gynecology, Nagoya University School of Medicine, Nagoya, Japan.

Thirty one female patients with radiologically event prolactin (PRL) secreting pituitary adenoma (macroadenoma; 5, microadenoma; 26) were treated with bromocriptine (BC) to study the anti-proliferative effect on tumor growth. Clinical, endocrinologic, and radiologic findings were observed before, during and after long-term BC treatment. The persisting suppression of PRL secretion after BC treatment was noticed in 2 patients with large adenomas and excessively high PRL levels. Out of 31 patients, 12 patients conceived in whom growth and acrivity of adenoma was followed up by measuring PRL levels before, during and after pregnancy and lactation, since PRL levels correlated well with tumor size and activity. After the end of lactation, PRL levels declined to lower values than before attempting pregnancy in 7 patients, and restoration of menstrual cycle was observed in 2 patients. These results suggest that long-term BC treatment, may have the anti-proliferative effect on large adenomas. Moreover there is little influence on the growth and activity of adenoma during pregnancy and lactation.

1038 TRH AND DOPAMINE MODIFY ARACHIDONIC ACID RELEASE FROM ANTERIOR PITUITARY CELLS.
K Koike*, AM Judd, MJ Cronin, RM MacLeod, University of Virginia, Charlottesville, Virginia, U.S.A.

The cleavage of arachidonic acid (AA) from phospholipids and its release from anterior pituitary cells (AP) may contribute to the process of prolactin (PRL) release. To test this hypothesis, primary cultures of AP from female rats were employed. Exogenous addition of AA increased PRL release (vehicle, 657 ± 118 ng/well; 0.1 μM AA, 805 ± 87; 0.5 μM, 1330 ± 132[a]; 1.0 uM, 1403 ± 24[a]; 5.0 μM, 1758 ± 73[b]; 10 μM, 3632 ± 299[b]; [a]$P <$ 0.05; [b]$P <$ 0.01 vs. vehicle). Subsequently, we measured the release of newly-esterified AA from AP. Cultured AP were pre-incubated 90 min with ^{3}H-AA (0.25 μCi/ml, 86.6 Ci/mmol) to incorporate the AA into esterified lipids. The cells were then washed with buffer without ^{3}H-AA, and incubated 30 min with vehicle or TRH and/or dopamine (DA). The medium was extracted with ethyl acetate, applied to silica gel TLC plates and the cpm in the ^{3}H-AA band determined. TRH increased ^{3}H-AA release into the medium in a concentration-dependent manner (vehicle, 238 ± 5 cpm; 10 nM TRH, 435 ± 10[b]; 100 nM, 468 ± 10[b]; 1 μM, 512 ± 17[b]; [b]$P <$ 0.01 vs. vehicle). Basal AA release apparently was not affected by DA but 0.5 μM and 1 μM DA reduced AA release induced by 1 μM TRH (TRH alone, 512 ± 17; TRH + 1 μM DA, 359 ± 11[b]; TRH + 0.5 μM DA, 363 ± 6[b]; [b]$P <$ 0.01 vs. TRH). In conclusion,exogenously administered AA acutely stimulates PRL release from AP and TRH induces an increase in endogenous AA release that can be inhibited by DA. These findings support the hypothesis that AA or its metabolites have a correlative or stimulatory function in the process regulating PRL release. [Funded by CA-07535 (RMM), F032 CA-07137 (AMJ), HD 18409 (MJC).]

1039 STUDY ON THE HYPOTHALAMIC DOPAMINERGIC ACTIVITY IN THE WOMEN OF PREGNANCY AND NO PREGNANCY. T. KUBOTA*, Y. YADI, M. NAGAE, N. NISHI and M. SAITO, Dept. of Obstetrics and Gynecology, Tokyo Medical & Dental Univ., Tokyo 113, JAPAN.

The purpose of this study was to investigate the PRL releasing mechanism on hypothalamo-pituitary axis during pregnancy. Forty-one gravidas of 1st and 2nd trimester received 2.5mg of bromocriptine(BRC):dopamine agonist orally, 10mg of metoclopramide(MCP):dopamine antagonist intravenously(iv) and 500μg of TRH iv. Furthermore, BRC was given orally to the gravidas 60 min prior to iv injection of MCP(n=35) or TRH(n=7). These volunteered women were admitted for therapeutic abortion to our hospital. Twelve non-pregnant women were also given MCP 10mg iv. Plasma prolactin(PRL), estradiol-17β(E_2), progesterone(P), hCG, hPL and GH were measured by radioimmunoassay during 180 min after the administration of these agents.
1) The plasma PRL levels decreased significantly from 120 to 180min after BRC administration orally, and those remained significantly elevated for 180min after MCP and TRH administration iv ($p<0.001$-0.05). The releasing activity of MCP 10mg was significantly higher ($p<0.01$-0.05) than that of TRH 500μg in the gravidas. However, there were no significant difference of PRL response to these agents between 1st and 2nd trimester groups or between pregnant and nonpregnant groups. 2) The administration of these agents or acute change of plasma PRL levels had no effect on E_2,P,hCG,hPL and GH levels. 3) The PRL release from the pituitary by MCP and TRH was supressed significantly ($p<0.01$) by pretreatment of BRC in the gravidas.
We concluded that the dopaminergic activity of hypothalamus during pregnancy were maintained as well as that of nonpregnant state.

1040 MECHANISM OF FUROSEMIDE (F) INDUCED NATRIURESIS BY DIRECT STIMULATION OF RENAL PROSTAGLANDIN E_2 (PGE_2). James B. Lee* and Shigehiro Katayama, Dept.Med., SUNY at Buffalo, Buffalo, N.Y. USA

In order to clarify F-induced natriuresis, interaction of renal PGE_2 and renin-angiotensin was studied. In conscious rabbits, F administered in vivo (10 mg/kg, iv) increased $U_{Na}V$ from 10 ± 3 to 114 ± 4 μEq/kg/min (p.<.01) at 20 min and $U_{PGE_2}V$, measured by RIA, from 0.28 ± 0.04 to 1.95 ± 0.10 ng/min at 20 min both declining to control by 50 min. Plasma renin activity (PRA) rose from 6.0 ± 1.2 to 17.4 ± 2.0 ng/ml/h (p.<.01) over a period of 50 min. Animals were sacrificed 10 min following F and renal de novo in vitro papillary slice PGE_2 synthesis (P-PGE_2) determined following 30 min incubation (37° C, 95% O_2-5% CO_2). Administration of F in vivo enhanced P-PGE_2 from 39.2 ± 3.7 to 68.4 ± 6.7 ng/mg tissue. Prior administration of indomethacin (I) at 2 mg/kg iv augmented the saluretic effect of F, decreased its effect on $U_{PGE_2}V$ (1.09 ± 0.12 ng/min), abolished the rise in PRA and reduced cortical but not P-PGE_2. At 10 mg/kg, I reduced F-induced natriuresis to 74 ± 2 μEq/kg/min and eliminated the increase in renal P-PGE_2 and PGE_2 excretion. Angiotensin blockade (Sar^1-Ile^8-A II, 200 μg/kg sc) suppression of P-PGE_2 (23.5 ± 0.9) was restored by F to control. Direct addition of F to the media stimulated P-PGE_2 to 200% of controls. The results suggest that 1) F stimulates renal P-PGE_2 directly without mediation through angiotensin II and 2) the enhanced or inhibitory effect of I on F-induced natriuresis is dose-related and dependent on the degree of inhibition of P-PGE_2.

1041 EFFECT OF 5,8,11,14-EICOSATETRAYNOIC ACID (ETYA) ON THE SYSTEMIC AND UTERINE VASCULATURE IN THE PREGNANT EWE. Ronald R. Magness, Murray D. Mitchell, and Charles R. Rosenfeld*, Depts. Peds., Biochem., and Ob-Gyn., Southwestern Med. Sch., Dallas, Texas, USA.

The role of leukotrienes(L) in the maintenance of the cardiovascular system during pregnancy is poorly understood. ETYA, an inhibitor of lipoxygenase and cyclooxygenase enzyme activity, decreases both L and prostaglandin(PG) production in vitro. To examine the effects of ETYA on the cardiovascular system and plasma PG levels during pregnancy, we infused 30 [n=6] and 90 [n=2] μg of ETYA/kg•min i.v. for 20min in 6 instrumented, late pregnant sheep (133-141 days), obtaining hemodynamic measurements and blood samples at 0,3,7,15,20,30,40,100,200, and 240min. Responses to both doses of ETYA were similar. Mean arterial pressure and systemic and uterine vascular resistances rose during ETYA, attaining maximum increases of 24±4.9*, 65±2.4*, and 84±19.3%* [$\bar{X}$±SE], respectively, at 15min; cardiac output, heart rate, and uterine blood flow fell 24±5.6*, 14±4.8*, and 32±4.8*%, respectively, at 15min. These cardiovascular parameters returned to control values at 140min. Hemodynamic changes were temporally related to increases in plasma thromboxane B_2 in arterial and venous blood, increasing from 158±105 and 163±114pg/ml to 1762±1122* and 1444± 975* by 15min and returning to values of 207±79 and 108±35 by 100min, respectively. PGEM levels were unchanged; however, levels of PGFM and 6-Keto $PGF_{1\alpha}$ tended to rise during ETYA. Although ETYA inhibits PG and L production in vitro, we did not observe cyclooxygenase inhibition in vivo, but rather increases in PG's. The observed hemodynamic responses may reflect lipoxygenase inhibition and selective PG production. *p<.05.

1042 SUBCUTANEOUS AND INTRANASAL USE OF D-SER (TBU)[6] LHRH 1-9 EA[10] (HOE766) IN PRECOCIOUS PUBERTY (PP). L. Fishman, D.C. Costigan, G. Wielgosz, A. Fazekas, J. Holland*. Dept. of Pediatrics, U. of Toronto and U. of Western Ontario; Hoechst-Canada, Montreal.

We treated 10 children (7 F, 3 M) with PP, ages 2.8-9.8 yrs, for 11.8±1.8 mos (mean±SEM) using HOE766, with frequent assessment of efficacy and safety. Eight patients with central PP (3 acquired) responded to HOE766 given once daily s.c., with reduction in growth velocity (GV), LH/FSH and sex steroids. Pre-Rx, GV was 12.3±0.6 cm/yr, basal LH 17.9±0.9 and peak LH 70.6±13.0 U/L after LHRH stimulation. All had advanced bone age (BA). Post-Rx, GV was 7.2±0.8 cm/yr (p<0.002), LH 8.6±2.5 (NS) and peak LH 10.5±2.4 U/L (p<0.002). BA did not change (p>0.5). Four of these patients then received intranasal (IN) HOE766, 200 μg tid for a further 8-12 mos with no significant change in GV, BA or hormone concentrations, as compared with s.c. Rx. The minimal effective dose of s.c. HOE766 ranged from 10-30 μg/kg/day and for IN Rx, 15-30 μg/kg/day. No clinical or biochemical side effects were noted, and antibodies to native LHRH or HOE766 were not detected. Two males with familial PP failed to respond to Rx despite reduction in basal and peak gonadotropins. Conclusion: HOE766 is effective in suppression of central PP; IN therapy sustains the suppression induced by initial s.c. Rx; in up to 18 mos of Rx, no undesirable side effects have been observed.

1043 EVIDENCE FOR THE EXISTENCE OF ESTROGEN RECEPTIVE GABAERGIC NEURONS AND THEIR INVOLVEMENT IN THE PROCESS OF SEXUAL DIFFERENTIATION OF THE BRAIN.

E. Fuchs*, G. Flügge, W. Wuttke, German Primate Center, Dept. of Reproductive Biology, 3400 Göttingen, FRG.

The medial preoptic-anterior hypothalamic area (MPAH) is an important region for regulating pituitary luteinizing hormone (LH) secretion in the rat. It is known that a population of estrogen receptive neurons exists in the MPAH which utilizes GABA as neurotransmitter. This area is also known to be of importance for sexual differentiation. To test the working hypothesis if GABA or GABA agonists can mimic the effects of estrogens on sexual differentiation of the brain, Sprague Dawley rats were treated daily from day 16 of pregnancy on with muscimol (MU), a potent GABA agonist (2 mg/kg b.w.). GABA and glutamate concentrations were measured in punches of the MPAH and a number of other hypothalamic and mesolimbic structures of newborn, 5, 10, and 15 days old animals. LH levels were measured in the serum. At day 10 after birth MPAH-GABA concentrations were significantly lower in sham treated female than in sham treated male rats. An inverse sexual difference was observed in the substantia nigra. Perinatal MU-treatment abolishes the sex dependent differences at day 10. In contrast to GABA no significant differences in glutamate concentrations were found. The observed postnatal sex differences in serum LH levels were also abolished by perinatal MU-treatment. Vaginal smears taken from perinatally MU-treated animals indicate that the majority of the females showed predominantly estrous smears. These effects of the GABAergic drug are very similar to those observed after perinatal estrogen and testosterone treatment and corroborate the above outlined working hypothesis.

1044 PRECOCIOUS MENARCHE IN THE RHESUS MONKEY ASSOCIATED WITH A MICROBALLOON IMPLANTED INTO THE THIRD CEREBRAL VENTRICLE.

J.A. Germak*, D. Pang, J. Horton, Dept. of Pediatrics, Medical College of Wisconsin, Milwaukee, Wis. 53233 (USA) and Departments of Neurosurgery and Radiology, University of Pittsburgh School of Medicine, Pittsburgh, Pa. 15213 (USA).

In an attempt to simulate the precocious puberty associated with certain non-destructive cerebral aberrations(hydrocephalus, third ventricular cysts), a model was designed in which a Silastic microballoon(MB) was chronically implanted into the inferior third cerebral ventricle(3V) of the rhesus monkey via a subfrontal translamina terminalis approach. The MB is connected by a catheter to a subgaleal injection port and filled with a radiocontrast(metrizamide)solution allowing post-operative radiographic MB monitoring. In 8 prepubertal female rhesus monkeys(aged 11.8-18 months)which underwent MB placement, menarche(MEN)occurred at age 19.7±3.2 months(mean ±SD)(range 12-23 months)compared to 27.1±2.8 months(23.5-32 months) in 9 unoperated controls(P<.001). MEN occurred 0.25-9(mean 5)months after original MB placement. Serum FSH concentrations, mostly undetectable pre-MB, became elevated 0.4-3 months post-MB, while the initial rise in serum LH usually followed that of FSH(n=6). Serum estradiol attained pre-MEN concentrations of 26-65 pg/ml(n=7). Deflation of the MB in 2 monkeys corresponded to an abrupt decline in serum FSH, whereas intermittent MB inflation in 1 animal was associated with cyclic serum FSH elevations followed by MEN. Thus MB placement into the 3V is associated with precocious MEN in the rhesus monkey. The exact effect of the MB, which dilates the walls of the 3V and presumably compresses the bordering mediobasal hypothalamus, remains to be elucidated. Supported by the Andrew W. Mellon Foundation, Medical College of Wisconsin, and Milwaukee Children's Hospital.

1045 LABELLING AND TURNOVER OF POSTERIOR PITUITARY PEPTIDES IN THE GUINEA PIG.

P.M. Jones and I.C.A.F. Robinson,* National Institute for Medical Research, Mill Hill, London, NW7 1AA, U.K.

In recent studies we have used *in vivo* radiolabelling to investigate the biosynthesis of oxytocin(OT), vasopressin(AVP) and their neurophysins (NPot,NPav) in the guinea pig, and have found that some vasopressin-related NP is present in the neural lobe in a partially processed form, still bearing a C-terminal glycopeptide extension (NPGP). We have now studied the time-course of labelling of these components in the neural lobe. At different times after hypothalamic injection of ^{35}S-cysteine, neural lobes were removed and subjected to HPLC to separate the radiolabelled peptides. The results are summarised as follows:

RATIO (Mean+SEM) OF ^{35}S INCORPORATION INTO PITUITARY PEPTIDES

	2h(n=5)	8h(n=4)	2d(n=6)	4d(n=6)	8d(n=6)
AVP:OT	0.8 +.1	2.1 +.1	2.3 +.6	2.0 +.3	3.7 + 1
NPav:NPot	0.3 +.03	1.2 +.1	1.4 +.4	1.5 +.2	2.7 +.7
NPav+NPGP:NPot	0.5 +.04	1.7 +.2	1.8 +.4	2.0 +.2	3.4 +.9
NPav:NPGP	1.4 +.2	2.8 +.5	3.2 +.4	3.5 +.2	5.1 +.5

The AVP system appears to label more slowly than the OT system, taking >8 days for the AVP:OT ^{35}S ratio to approach the ratio for total AVP and OT content, found by RIA (5.6+.5). The NPav:NPGP ratio also rises with time, suggesting that some of the NPGP may be further processed into NPav in the neural lobe.

1046 DYNAMICS OF ACTIVATION AND TRANSLOCATION OF ESTROGEN AND PROGESTERONE RECEPTORS IN UTERINE TISSUES OF THE VERVET MONKEY (CERCOPITHECUS AETHIOPS PYGERETHRUS) AND MAN.

T. Klein, H. Potgieter, N. Savage* and J.J. van der Watt, Nucor Institute of Life Sciences, Faculty of Medicine, University of Pretoria, Pretoria 0002, R.S.A. and *Department of Medical Biochemistry, Faculty of Medicine, University of the Witwatersrand, Johannesburg 2000, R.S.A.

It is presently accepted that the ∿5S estradiol-receptor complex of the uterine cell's nucleus is derived from the cytosol by some unknown process which can be stimulated by a temperature change in the *in vitro* incubation conditions (0-4°C to 30°C). This transformation process, accepted to imply a characteristic shift in the conformation of the cytosolic complex, appears to be an essential pre-requisite for the binding of the complex to the nuclear chromatin. Estrogen (ER) and progesterone receptors (PR) of the Vervet monkey have been shown to be stabilised by 10mM sodium molybdate, while the translocation of the complexes to intact uterine nuclei was only slightly decreased (15-20%) in the presence of molybdate. Maximum translocation of the labelled complexes was found to be 55-60% in the absence of sodium molybdate. On 10-35% sucrose density gradients, marked differences were seen in the gradient profiles of the complexes in the presence or absence of sodium molybdate and/or high and low ionic strength gradients, following reincubation at 30°C for varying time intervals. The dynamics of normal Vervet monkey uterine receptor activation and translocation was compared to that in normal and abnormal human uterine tissue.

1047 CHANGES IN OVIDUCT PROGESTERONE RECEPTOR CORRELATE WITH PLASMA STEROIDS IN A SEASONAL BREEDER. S. Kleis* and I.P. Callard, Department of Biology, Boston University, Boston, MA 02215, U.S.A.

Corpus luteum function and progesterone are central to eutherian pregnancy, but the role of progesterone in viviparous nonmammalian animals is not defined. The objectives of this study were to characterize a progesterone receptor in the reproductive tract of *Nerodia* during the reproductive cycle and to correlate quantitative changes in receptor with plasma steroid levels, luteal function and stage of the cycle. Plasma progesterone (P_4) and estradiol-17β (E_2) were measured, and luteal activity estimated by histochemical determination of 3β-hydroxysteroid dehydrogenase (3β-HSD). Progesterone receptor was determined by DNA-cellulose affinity and LH-20 chromatography. E_2 levels were high during follicular growth and vitellogenesis (1700 pg/ml) decreasing prior to ovulation and remaining low (300 pg/ml) during most of pregnancy. Near term, E_2 levels increased sharply (2400 pg/ml), decreasing abruptly postpartum. P_4 also begins to increase during the follicular growth phase, attaining highest levels (10 ng/ml) at mid-term, falling thereafter to postpartum values of 1 ng/ml. The enzyme 3β-HSD is located in follicles during ovarian growth & in the corpus luteum during all of pregnancy. A progesterone receptor (PR) having a KD = 5.6×10^{-10}M and exhibiting low capacity and steroid and tissue specificity was characterized. Cytosolic PR increased initially during pregnancy with progesterone values, but then declined before progesterone values peaked. These data indicate that the P_4 receptor in the snake oviduct has classical characteristics and may be regulated by E_2. The data also support the thesis that progesterone, probably of luteal origin, is physiologically important during pregnancy in this species. (Supported by NSF-81 04144 to IPC)

1048 Influence of time and therapy on the receptor status in human breast cancer. K. Klinga*, M. Kaufmann, B. Runnebaum, and F. Kubli, Universitäts-Frauenklinik, D-6900 Heidelberg, Fed. Rep. Germany

In 43 patients with primary breast cancer and subsequent development of a recidive the estrogen (ER) and progesterone (PR) receptors were determined by use of a standardized charcoal adsorption technique. The mean age of the women was 56 (range 34 to 78) years. The mean disease free interval was 17 (range 3 to 42) months. 23 (53%) of the patients had similar ER concentrations in both lesions. 7 (16%) showed great variability with relatively high ER in one site and borderline concentrations of ER in the other site. 31% of the patients had different ER status in tumor and recidive. PR could be determined in only 23 patients of whom 30% had a change in the receptor status. After surgery of the primary tumor group I (n=9) had no adjuvant therapy at all, group II (n=15) was irradiated, group III (n=9) received a combined chemo- and hormone therapy and group IV (n=10) were treated with cytostatica. In no group, even not in the hormone (tamoxifen) treated group, an uniform influence on the receptor status of the patients could be detected. Furthermore, there was no correlation between the time of occurrence of the recidives and a changing of the receptor status.

1049 RECEPTOR BINDING AND HORMONAL ACTIVITY OF THE CATECHOLS OF DIETHYLSTILBESTROL (DES) AND OTHER ACTIVE METABOLITES. K.S. Korach*, P.J. Sarver, J.A. McLachlan, Lab. Reprod. and Devel. Tox., NIEHS, NIH, Research Triangle Park, NC 27709 USA, J. Liehr, Univ. of Texas, Houston, TX USA

DES is a synthetic estrogen which has been reported to possess carcinogenic properties. The mechanism for this activity is not well understood, but DES has been shown to undergo oxidative metabolism, producing reactive intermediates. We have investigated the receptor binding and estrogenic activity of various catechol stilbene compounds; catechol DES (CD), dicatechol DES (DCD), methoxy catechol DES (MCD) and a unique metabolite of reproductive tract tissue, monomethyl DES (MMD). A reactive intermediate of DES oxidative metabolism, DES-p-quinone (DQ), was also tested. The competitive binding affinity (C_{50}) of the compounds with the mouse uterine cytosol estrogen receptor (ER) gave the following order, DES (0.7), CD (1), DCD (4), MMD (5), MCD (10), DQ (200), and a single component binding curve. At pH 7.2 DQ exhibited a multiple component binding curve with C_{50} values of 5 and 200. Association rate reactions using DQ at 10,50 and 100 fold competitor showed 50,66 and 90% competition similar to DES. These results are not due to DES contamination or formation since at pH 7.2 DQ is oxidized to Z,Z dienestrol which is a poor ligand for ER in both assays. *In vivo* treatment with the DES compounds resulted in nuclear ER translocation of 100% DES, 33% MCD and 14% MMD; CD and DCD had no activity. DES and MMD (20 μg/kg) stimulated uterine DNA synthesis to 800% control. MCD showed 400% at 50 μg/kg dose. Both CD and DCD were ineffective in stimulating the activity at either dose. These findings suggest that reactive DES metabolites formed within target cells can interact and bind to ER and translocate to the nucleus to induce uterine responses.

1050 INDUCTION OF MENSES AT MIDLUTEAL PHASE IN MONKEYS: ANTI-PROGESTERONE RU 486. B. Kreitmann-Gimbal*, O.L. Kreitmann, R.L. Collins and G.D. Hodgen, Pregnancy Research Branch, NIH, Bethesda, MD 20205, USA.

We injected the anti-progesterone, anti-glucocorticoid RU486 at midluteal phase in cycling cynomolgus monkeys. RU486 was administered (5 mg/day, im) on days 17-19 of the menstrual cycle. Menses were induced in monkeys within 2 days of end of treatment given in midluteal phase (determined by midcycle LH surges following E_2 peaks and an expected rise in P_4 level); moreover, the corpus luteum was identified at laparoscopy at day 16. Menses occurred even when P_4 levels in serum were > 1 ng/ml. Anovulatory monkeys, lacking a secretory endometrium, were not induced to menstruate after RU486. Using 4 other monkeys, after the second dose of RU486, total concentrations of steroid receptors for E_2 (E_2R), P_4 (P_4R) and RU486 (RU-R) were measured in endometrium. No change was found in total E_2R ($0.1 < p < 0.05$). There was a statistically significant decrease in total P_4R when measured with ^{3}H-P after 48h of RU486 treatment ($0.01 < p < 0.001$); but, when measured with ^{3}H-RU, total binding to progesterone receptors was not different ($p > 0.5$).

fm/mg DNA ± SE	d 18 normal cycle	d 18 treated cycle
E_2R	1545 ± 202	2813 ± 569
PR (with ^{3}HP)	4035 ± 805	871 ± 260
RU-R		4555 ± 850

We conclude: 1) RU486 induces menses on secretory endometrium but not proliferative tissue; 2) RU486 displaces progesterone from its own receptor and subsequently blocks endometrial progesterone action. These findings demonstrate that RU486 acts upon endometrium as an anti-progesterone binding progesterone receptors, not by its anti-glucocorticoid properties.

1051 PARTIAL PURIFICATION AND PHYSICOCHEMICAL CHARACTERIZATION OF PROGESTERONE RECEPTOR IN BENIGN PROSTATIC HYPERPLASIA (BPH).

S. Ganesan, J.D. Young, and N. Bashirelahi*, University of Maryland, Dental and Medical Schools, Baltimore, Maryland 21201

Although the progesterone receptor has been well characterized in the chick oviduct, there is considerable controversy regarding its structure in the human system. We have characterized a specific progesterone receptor in human benign prostatic hypertrophy (J. Steroid Biochem. 18, 801-809, 1983). We have attempted to partially purify and investigate the physicochemical properties of progesterone receptor in BPH. Maximum precipitation of the receptor occurs at 40% ammonium sulfate. Exposure of cytosol from BPH tissue to phosphocellulose for 2 minutes significantly increased the specific binding of [^{3}H]R5020 as determined by glycerol density gradient centrifugation. Twenty-fold purification was achieved by precipitating the receptor with 40% ammonium sulfate. When BPH cytosol was applied to a column of DEAE-cellulose, the receptor eluted at a salt concentration of 0.18M KCl. Fractions corresponding to the specific receptor were pooled and applied to a phosphocellulose column, the receptor eluted at a salt concentration of 0.1M KCl. These studies so far indicate that the receptor eluted from DEAE-cellulose is homogenous and similar to the B subunit of T47D human breast cancer cells reported by Lessey *et al.*, (Endocrinology 112, 1267-1274, 1983). In conclusion, our preliminary results based on DEAE-cellulose, phosphocellulose chromatography, and analysis of photolinked receptor on denaturing polyacrylamide gel seems to indicate that BPH progesterone receptor consists of a mixture of at least two hormone-binding proteins.

1052 ANDROGEN AND LH/hCG RECEPTORS IN PROTEIN-CALORIE MALNOURISHED RATS.

D.C. Herbert*, P.J. Sheridan, H.G. Klemcke, R.D. Martinez and G.L. Paterick, Department of Cellular and Structural Biology, UTHSCSA, San Antonio, Texas 78284, USA

Protein-calorie malnutrition (PCM) leads to a marked reduction in gonadotrophin and testosterone secretion along with a delay in puberty onset. In light of these findings, we questioned whether PCM induced alterations in androgen (A) and luteinizing hormone (LH) receptor concentrations in several target organs. Twenty day-old male Sprague Dawley rats were fed *ad libitum* a control (C) diet consisting of 27% protein or a low, 8% protein diet for either 30 or 60 days. The hypothalami, pituitary glands, ventral prostates and testes were removed and stored at -70°C for subsequent receptor analysis. On day 50, the concentration of free cytosolic A receptor in the pituitary glands (C vs. PCM rats; 6.2±0.8 vs. 13.0±0.1 fmoles/mg protein) and ventral prostates (10.5±1.7 vs 41.1±9.3) was significantly ($p<0.01$) higher in the PCM rats; no differences were found in binding affinity. Hypothalamic receptor concentrations and K_d were similar in the two animal groups. The results were comparable at 80 days of age. In contrast, there was a significant ($p<0.005$) reduction in testicular LH/hCG receptor concentration in the PCM rats on days 50 (C vs. PCM; 84.8±2.7 vs. 67.9±3.2 fmoles/mg protein) and 80 (98.7±5.0 vs. 66.5±4.2). These data indicate that A and LH receptor concentrations are markedly affected by PCM. The relationship between these findings and the delay in sexual maturation which accompanies PCM will require additional study. Supported by NSF Grant PCM 81188487.

1053 THERMOLABILITY AND DISSOCIABILITY OF METHYLTRIENOLONE-RECEPTOR COMPLEXES WITHIN HUMAN GENITAL SKIN FIBROBLASTS. M. Kaufman* and L. Pinsky, Lady Davis Institute for Medical Research, Centre for Human Genetics, McGill University, Montreal, H3T 1E2, Canada.

Genital skin fibroblast (GSF) monolayers incubated with 3 nM methyltrienolone (M) saturate their basal androgen-receptor (AR) activity within 30 min at a B_{max} of ∿20 fmol/mg protein. GSF incubated for an additional 18 h acquire 2-3 times basal activity (up-regulation). Both basal and up-regulated M-R complexes dissociate homogeneously with a $t\frac{1}{2}(37°)$ = 58 min when chased with 0.6 µM radioinert M. We have studied the thermolability of up-regulated M-R complexes in GSF incubated with 3 nM ^{3}H-M in the presence of 10 µM cycloheximide (to nullify receptor synthesis). Plotted semilogarithmically, the loss of M-R complexes (37-43°C) yielded curves that were progressively curvilinear, yet M-R complexes remaining within GSF after 2 h at 42°C dissociated homogeneously [$t\frac{1}{2}(37°)$ = 58 min]. A mechanism compatible with M-R complexes that dissociate homogeneously but are heterogeneous in regard to thermolability is shown below:

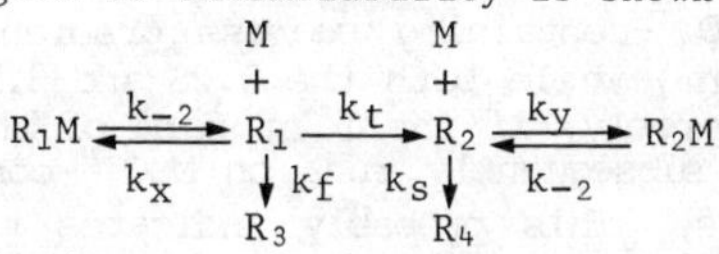

$R_1,R_2:R_3,R_4$ = binding:non-binding forms; $k_x,k_y:k_{-2}$ = association:dissociation [$t\frac{1}{2}(37°)$ = 58 min] constants; $k_f,k_s:k_t$ = thermolability (fast, slow components):transformation constants.

1054 INTERACTION OF THE MONOMERIC GLUCOCORTICOID RECEPTOR WITH A NON-HORMONE-BINDING, CYTOSOLIC MACROMOLECULE. Branka Kovačič-Milivojević* and Wayne V. Vedeckis, Dept. of Biochemistry, LSU Medical Center, New Orleans, LA. 70112, USA.

The untransformed glucocorticoid receptor (GC-R) extracted from mouse AtT-20 cells is an oligomer with a sedimentation coefficient of 9.1S. This moiety can be converted to two transformed (DNA-binding) species, a 5.2S oligomer, and a 3.8-4.4S monomer. The GC-R was transformed by Sephadex G-25 filtration (followed by incubation at 0-4°C for 4 h), applied to a DEAE-cellulose column, and the transformed GC-R step-eluted with 0.12M KCl. This column was subsequently step-eluted with 0.5M KCl. The 0.12M KCl step contained the monomer, which sedimented at 3.8-4.4S on low salt vertical tube rotor sucrose gradients. Addition of the 0.5M KCl step material caused a consistent increase in GC-R sedimentation rate to yield a discrete 6.2-6.8S species. The reaction was rapid, and dependent upon the amount of 0.5M KCl step material added. Partial characterization of this factor revealed that it 1) is macromolecular, 2) does not bind hormone, 3) is heat-stable, and 4) is inactivated by incubation (37°C, 1 h) with 27 U/ml of ribonuclease A ("essentially protease-free"). These results suggest that the GC-R monomer is capable of forming a discrete 6.2-6.8S complex with a cytosolic macromolecular factor, and that this factor may be RNA. Further studies are needed to confirm the chemical nature of this macromolecule, to determine if its interaction with the GC-R monomer is specific, and to see if it is a component of the 9.1S oligomeric, untransformed GC-R complex. Supported by American Cancer Society Grant BC-436.

1055 HPLC SEPARATION OF GLUCOCORTICOID RECEPTOR FORMS EXTRACTED FROM MOUSE AtT-20 CELLS.

Margot C. LaPointe* and Wayne V. Vedeckis, Dept. of Biochemistry, LSU Medical Center, New Orleans, LA, 70112. USA.

Gel-exclusion high performance liquid chromatography has been used, for the first time, to separate forms of the glucocorticoid receptor (GC-R) extracted from mouse AtT-20 cells. Using 200 mM potassium phosphate buffer (pH 7.4) as the eluent, an efficient separation of the untransformed GC-R from the transformed GC-R is attained in 15-20 min. The untransformed GC-R elutes from the columns with a Stokes radius (R_s) of 8.2-9 nm, while GC-R transformed with either heat (25°C, 1 h) or with 0.3M KCl elutes with a R_s of 5.7-6.0 nm. Also, GC-R extracted from the nucleus with either 0.3M KCl or 2 mM sodium tungstate has a R_s of 5.5-6.3 nm. The data are identical either in the presence or absence of 20 mM Na_2MoO_4, suggesting that Na_2MoO_4 is not causing aggregation to produce a larger R_s value than that of the native GC-R.

Sucrose-gradient ultracentrifugation of GC-R produces three forms of the receptor: 9.1S, 5.2S, and 3.8S. The untransformed 9.1S form of the GC-R pooled from a $MoO_4^=$-containing sucrose gradient elutes from HPLC with a R_s of about 9 nm, while both the 5.2S and 3.8S forms elute with a R_s of $\sim$6 nm. Conversely, if the 6 nm form of the receptor is pooled from HPLC, then it subsequently runs on $MoO_4^=$-containing gradients as a 3.5-4.1S species. This probably indicates that the 5.2S, transformed GC-R is unstable and dissociates into the smaller form during HPLC, despite the rapidity of the process. This study was supported by Grant BC-436 from the American Cancer Society.

1056 PROTEIN KINASE ACTIVITY OF PURIFIED RAT HEPATIC GLUCOCORTICOID RECEPTOR.

A.S. Miller*, T.J. Schmidt and G. Litwack, Fels Research Institute, Temple University School of Medicine, Philadelphia, PA 19140.

Highly purified rat hepatic glucocorticoid receptor (G_R) was tested for protein kinase activity. The G_R was purified by a three step procedure which includes elution from an affinity resin. After subsequent filtration through Sephadex G-75, to remove sodium molybdate, purified G_R was incubated with [γ-^{32}P]ATP for 30 min at 25°C. The reaction was terminated by addition of Laemmli "sample buffer" and boiling for 5 min at 100°C. Samples were electrophoresed and gels stained, dried and subjected to autoradiography. The 90 K component of G_R was phosphorylated when incubated in the presence of Ca^{2+}; sodium molybdate, added during incubation, appeared to block incorporation of radioactive phosphate under these conditions. Autophosphorylation of the 90K component was not detected when Mg^{2+} was substituted for Ca^{2+}. Histones (calf thymus Type III) were phosphorylated when incubated with G_R and [γ-^{32}P] ATP in the absence of Ca^{2+}; however, when Ca^{2+} was present during incubation, the 90K component of G_R was preferentially phosphorylated. In the absence of Ca^{2+}, neither exogenous cyclic nucleotides (cAMP or cGMP) or calmodulin promoted autophosphorylation of the 90K component. Preliminary experiments suggest that calcium-dependent autophosphorylation of purified G_R does not occur in the absence of bound hormone. Potential requirement of bound steroid for kinase activity is currently under investigation. These results suggest that the 90K component of G_R can be autophosphorylated in the presence of Ca^{2+} and that the G_R may exhibit protein kinase activity. Research supported by Grants AM-32870 and AM-13531 (NIH).

1057 **EXCESS SERUM MINERALOCORTICOID ACTIVITY IN PATIENTS WITH DEXAMETHASONE-SUPPRESSIBLE HYPERALDOSTERONISM (DSH) ESTIMATED BY THE RAT RENAL RECEPTOR TECHNIQUE.** P.W. Speiser*, K.O. Martin, M.I. New, The New York Hospital-Cornell Medical Center, 525 East 68 Street, New York, N.Y. 10021 U.S.A.

Patients with low renin hypertension may produce an uncharacterized pressor steroid. We have adapted the rat renal slice mineralocorticoid receptor assay (RRA) to assess total mineralocorticoid actitivity in human serum. RIA values of deoxycorticosterone (DOC), corticosterone (B), cortisol (F), and aldosterone were multiplied by the potency of steroid relative to aldosterone in the RRA. The sum of these values, referred to as RIA-aldosterone equivalents, was compared to RRA values in 14 patients with intact adrenal steroidogenesis. Using RU26988 (Roussel-UCLAF) for glucocorticoid receptor blockade, RRA and RIA values correlated closely. These experiments demonstrate that, in normal patients, receptor-binding steroids can be almost totally accounted for by immunoreactive DOC, B, F and aldosterone, while in 3 patients with DSH, RRA was greater than RIA in the basal state ($p < 0.05$). In the 3 patients studied with graded ACTH stimulation, RRA progressively increased in proportion to DOC, B, F and aldosterone. With dexamethasone treatment, RRA values fell markedly. A repeat 360-minute ACTH test while on dexamethasone showed an RRA to RIA ratio comparable to that found with the ACTH test without dexamethasone.

Conclusion: Total mineralocorticoid activity as measured by RRA in DSH patients is greater than measurable immunoreactive DOC, B, F and aldosterone, indicating the presence of an unidentified pressor steroid which is dexamethasone-suppressible and ACTH-stimulable, and appears to be under the same control as other known adrenal steroids.

1058 INTERACTION BETWEEN INSULIN RECEPTORS AND MAJOR HISTOCOMPATIBILITY COMPLEX ANTIGENS. M. Fehlmann*, Y. Le Marchand-Brustel, N. Brossette and E. Van Obberghen, INSERM U 145, Faculty of Medicine, Nice, France.

The possible relationship between insulin receptors and major histocompatibility complex (MHC) antigens was investigated. This study was initiated following the observation that Daudi cells, a human Burkitt lymphoma cell line, express neither Class I MHC antigens nor insulin receptors. Insulin receptors from $H\text{-}2^k$ mouse liver membranes were specifically labeled with a ^{125}I-photoreactive insulin analogue by UV-irradiation. When membranes were solubilized in 1% Nonidet P-40, anti-$H\text{-}2^k$ monoclonal antibodies precipitated approximately 5% of the recoverable labeled insulin receptors, identified by SDS-polyacrylamide gel electrophoresis and autoradiography. No immunoprecipitation was observed with normal serum or with anti-$H\text{-}2^b$ monoclonal antibodies. However, when the detergent concentration was decreased to 0.01%, all recoverable insulin receptors were immunoprecipitated by anti-$H\text{-}2^k$ monoclonal antibodies. Further, preincubation of liver membranes or soleus muscles isolated from $H\text{-}2^k$ mice with anti-$H\text{-}2^k$ monoclonal antibodies (reacting with $H\text{-}2K^k$) reduced insulin binding by 40%. No inhibition was observed with monoclonal antibodies reacting with $H\text{-}2D^k$. Finally, anti-$H\text{-}2^k$ monoclonal antibodies (reacting with $H\text{-}2K^k$) stimulated 2-deoxyglucose uptake in isolated soleus muscles.

In conclusion, the present results demonstrate that insulin receptors are structurally and functionally associated with Class I MHC antigens. This interaction might represent a mechanism for receptor transmodulation that could be involved in the pathogenesis of certain forms of insulin resistance.

1059 INSULIN RECEPTORS IN RAT BRAIN CORTEX SYNAPTOSOMES. KINETIC EVIDENCE FOR A RECEPTOR SUBTYPE IN THE CENTRAL NERVOUS SYSTEM. S. Gammeltoft*, P. Staun-Olsen, B. Ottesen and J. Fahrenkrug, Dept. Clinical Chemistry CL, Rigshospitalet, DK-2100 Copenhagen, Denmark.

The receptor binding kinetics of porcine ^{125}I-monoiodo(A14 Tyr)insulin was studied in purified synaptosomes of rat brain cortex. The binding was rapid and small at 37°C, but the rate decreased and the size increased at lower temperatures. The pH-optimum was 8.0-8.3. At steady state receptor-bound ^{125}I-insulin was inhibited by unlabeled insulin with an apparent K_d of 3 nmol/l. Scatchard analysis revealed a slight binding heterogeneity and a maximal binding capacity of 1 pmol/g wet brain weight. Dissociation kinetics were biexponential with $T_{½}$ of 5 and 180 min, and not influenced by addition of an excess unlabeled insulin. Receptor-bound ^{125}I-insulin was only inhibited by insulin analogues and the binding affinities relative to porcine insulin were: human insulin 100%, rat insulin (I+II) 71%, coypu insulin 47%, multiplication stimulating activity 8%, porcine proinsulin 5%, relaxin < 0.1% and nerve growth factor < 0.1%. No degradation of receptor-bound insulin was observed in the presence of bacitracin although an insulin protease is present in brain. In conclusion, insulin binding kinetics in rat brain cortex synaptosomes are different from those in isolated fat and liver cells regarding insulin specificity and absence of both negative cooperativity and receptor-mediated insulin degradation. It is suggested that an insulin receptor subtype is present in rat brain cortex. The peptide specificity is interpreted that insulin exerts growth-promoting activity in the central nervous system.

1060 **MEASUREMENT OF INSULIN RECEPTORS IN A MITOCHONDRIAL-MICROSOMAL FRACTION PREPARED FROM MILLIGRAM QUANTITIES OF HUMAN FAT, AND ON MONOCYTES PREPARED FROM SMALL VOLUMES OF HUMAN BLOOD.** **B.D. Greenstein*, Department of Pharmacology, St. Thomas's Hospital Medical School, London SE1 7EH, UK.**

A method is described for the measurement of high affinity bound tyrosine A-14 monoiodinated inuslin in a mitochondrial-microsomal fraction prepared from small (50-150 mg) quantities of human adipose tissue, and in a monocyte-enriched fraction prepared from small volumes (20-30 ml) of human blood. Freshly removed fat was weighed and homogenised in ice-cold Tris-HCl buffer, 50 mM, containing sucrose, 0.25 M pH 7.4, and the mitochondrial-microsomal fraction prepared by differential centrifugation. The final pellet was taken up in Tris-HCl, 50 mM, $MgCl_2$, 10 mM, B.S.A. 0.1% (w/v), pH 7.9: 100 mg fat yielded about 5 mg of final pellet. Blood was collected into heparinised vials and a monocyte-enriched fraction was prepared as described by Fotino, Merson and Allen (1971) and was adjusted to 3.5 x 10^6 cells/ml. Insulin receptors were measured in both fractions using the method of Greenstein (1979) and in both preparations the radioactive hormone was bound with low capacity and high affinity (Kd ~ 10^{-10} mol/l) although Scatchard plots obtained were curvilinear. It is suggested that this method is suitable for the routine screening of insulin receptors from fat biopsies and small volumes of blood. This work was supported by Boehringer Ingelheim Ltd.

Fotino, M., Merson, E.J. and Allen, F.H. (1971). Ann.Clin.Lab.Sci.1,131-133.
Greenstein, B.D. (1979). Br.J.Pharmac., 66, 317-322.

1061 MONOVALENT CATIONS STIMULATE THE BINDING OF ANGIOTENSIN II (Ang II) IN NEURONAL CULTURES FROM THE BRAINS OF NORMOTENSIVE (WKY) AND HYPERTENSIVE (SH) RATS. J.B. Feldstein*, C. Sumners, and M.K. Raizada, Dept. of Physiology, Univ. of Florida, Gainesville, FL 32610.

Centrally injected NaCl causes an increase in blood pressure in WKY and SH rats which is mediated by the brain renin-angiotensin system. Neuronal cultures from one day old brains of WKY and SH rats were used to determine the effect of Na^+ and other cations on Ang II receptors in order to understand the mechanism of action of Na^+ at the cellular level. Incubation of neuronal cultures made from WKY rat brains with Na^+ caused a dose dependent increase in the specific binding of ^{125}I-Ang II to its receptors. A 260% increase in the binding was observed with 150 mM NaCl. The increase was rapid (within 30 min) and longer incubations caused no further increase in the binding. Neuronal cultures made from SH rat brains which expressed a higher number of Ang II receptors/neuron compared with WKY, showed a similar Na^+ stimulated increase in the binding. Scatchard analysis revealed that the increase in binding caused by Na^+ appeared to be due to a two-fold increase in the affinity of receptors for Ang II without affecting the total number of receptors. The ability of Ang II to compete for its receptors did not change in the absence or presence of Na^+. Other monovalent cations also caused a dose-dependent increase in ^{125}I-Ang II binding in the order of Li > Na = K = Rb = Cs. These observations indicate that various cations influence the brain renin-angiotensin system by their effect on Ang II receptors and suggest that the stimulatory action of centrally injected NaCl on blood pressure may be mediated by its effects on Ang II receptor affinity in both WKY and SH rats. Supported by an AHA grant.

1062 ACTH RECEPTORS IN RAT ADRENAL GLOMERULOSA CELLS. INTERACTION WITH VASOPRESSIN. N. Gallo-Payet* and E. Escher. Départements de Médecine et de Pharmacologie, CHUS, Sherbrooke, Québec, Canada, J1H 5N4.(spon: D. Bellabarba).
Previous studies have shown that the vasopressin system interacts with the ACTH system to enhance aldosterone secretion in glomerulosa cells. (Payet et al., J. Steroid biochem., 20, 1(1984). The purpose of this work is to assess the role of vasopressin and ACTH at the receptor level, both peptide hormones have not been studied as yet on glomerulosa cells. We have investigated the binding of $[[^{125}I]Tyr^{23}, Phe^{2}, N1^{4}]$ACTH (1-24) in rat adrenocortical glomerulosa and fasciculata cells and membranes. The analogue was iodinated by the iodogen method and separated by HPLC. The iodinated analogue had high specific radioactivity and retained full biological potency. After 30 minutes incubation at 22°C and for a concentration of 2 X 10^{-11}M of ^{125}I-ACTH the specific binding was 6.3% and 3.2%/50.000 glomerulosa and fasciculata cells respectively. In purified membranes, the specific binding after 15 minutes at 4°C was about 60%/mg prot. (11.7 pM/mg prot.) and 28%/ mg prot. (5.6 pM/mg prot.) respectively, for glomerulosa and fasciculata membranes. Scatchard analysis show that the association constants were similar in the two zonae but the number of receptor sites per cell was higher in zona glomerulosa. Also, we have studied the effect of vasopressin on the ACTH binding. The present data demonstrate that zona glomerulosa possess a higher concentration of ACTH receptors than zona fasciculata and that vasopressin interacts with ACTH on aldosterone secretion by postreceptor effects since the binding characteristics of ACTH were not modified by the presence of vasopressin.
N. G-P is a MRC scholar and E.E a CHF scholar; this study was supported by the MRC.

1063 THE HUMAN PROSTATE IS A TARGET ORGAN FOR PROLACTIN. F.K. Habib*, A. Leake and G.D. Chisholm, Dept. of Surgery, Edinburgh University Medical School, Teviot Place, Edinburgh EH8 9AG. Scotland, U.K.

Studies performed in this laboratory have identified the specific prolactin receptor in the human prostate. The receptor protein exhibited a high affinity and low capacity for prolactin. The bulk of the prolactin binding was confined to the microsomal and mitochondrial membrane pellets and appeared to be both time and temperature dependent. Pre-treatment of the membrane pellets with magnesium chloride to dissociate tightly bound endogenous prolactin from its receptors and with dextran coated charcoal to remove possible inhibitors from tissue extracts, resulted in a marked increase in the number of binding sites. The specificity of the prolactin binding sites in the human prostate for the human peptide hormone was confirmed and our measurements revealed that the cross reactivity with the other peptide hormones was minimal. We also investigated the relationship between divalent cations and specific prolactin binding in the two membrane fractions, the data generated indicates that the type of effect achieved was dependent on the metal ion used during the incubation. Clearly, a significant increase in the binding was induced by magnesium and copper ions, whilst zinc, calcium and manganese ions inhibited the binding. In view of the inhibition measured after treatment with ethylenediamine-tetra-acetic acid, one can assume that some divalent cations are essential for optimising the specific binding of prolactin to the human prostate gland. This work was supported by a generous grant from the Medical Research Council.

1064 INSULIN-LIKE GROWTH FACTOR II RECEPTORS ON HUMAN FIBROBLAST MONOLAYERS. R.L. Hintz*, A.V. Thorsson, G. Enberg, and K. Hall, Departments of Pediatrics, Stanford University, Stanford CA, USA and St. Joseph's Hospital, Reykyavik, Iceland, and the Department of Endocrinology, Karolinska Hospital, Stockholm, Sweden

Two major somatomedin peptides have been isolated from human plasma, somatomedin-C/insulin-like growth factor I (SM-C/IGF-I) and insulin-like growth factor-II (IGF-II). Two types of SM/IGF receptors have been defined so far. Type I receptors have a higher affinity for SM-C/IGF-I than IGF-II, and insulin binds to this receptor at high concentrations. Type II receptors have a higher affinity for IGF-II than SM-C/IGF-I, and insulin does not bind to this receptor site. In this study, we have characterized the binding of IGF-II to human monolayer fibroblast cultures, its affinity and specificity. ^{125}-I IGF-II binds to the human fibroblast monolayers with an average specific binding of 12.5%/2000,000 cells. The binding of IGF-I was 25%, and of insulin was 4.5% of the specific IGF-II binding. The IGF-II was bound to a high affinity receptor. Half maximum displacement was seen with 12 ng/ml IGF-II and 45 ng/ml IGF-I. Insulin did not bind to this receptor. The estimated affinity of the IGF-II receptor was 1.2 nM, with a calculated receptor site concentration of 400,000/cell. Unlike SM-C/IGF-I and insulin receptors, no autoregulation of these IGF-II receptors was seen by homologous hormone. On the other hand, serum deprivation led to a 50% increase in IGF-II receptor sites. IGF-II binding to normal human fibroblasts fits the criteria for a type II receptor. There are more IGF-II receptors on these cells than either SM-C or insulin receptors, suggesting an important metabolic role for IGF-II in normal human fibroblasts.

1065 RECEPTOR ANTISERUM BINDS TO PROTEINS OF LH RECEPTOR COMPLEX SEPARATED BY GEL ELECTROPHORESIS. J.L. Luborsky*, A. Lyga and H.R. Behrman, Reproductive Biology Section, Depts. Ob/Gyn and Pharmacology, Yale University School of Medicine, New Haven, CT 06510.

Antisera (A/S) against Triton X-100 solubilized rat LH receptors (RS): specifically immunoprecipitate (Impt) [125]IhCG-RS, are removed by adsorption with original antigen (exposed RS) or with luteal membranes (MEM) (embedded RS) and localize by immunohistochemistry to luteal cell MEM. The A/S do not: displace LH, decrease during downregulation or recognize hCG (BBRC 1979,90; JCB 1982,95). A/S Impt 60-80% of total RS. Various combinations of four A/S were not additive suggesting they recognize similar protein(s). Hence RS complexes lacking proteins recognized by A/S would not be Impt. Bound [125]IhCG was crosslinked with dithiobis (succinimidyl propionate)(DTSP) to luteal membranes, solubilized in SDS + urea, separated by SDS-PAGE (6%), transfered to nitrocellulose filters, incubated with A/S I or nonimmune serum and second antibody coupled to horseradish peroxidase and developed with 4-chloro-1-naphthol. [125]IhCG was localized by autoradiography. Five bands specifically reacted with A/S I with molecular weights X 10[3] of about: 129(A), 114(B), 79(C), 51(D) and 41(E). A,B,D and E reacted strongly and were radioactive. A,B, C,D contained LH RS since radioactivity was absent after DTSP cleavage. E contained hCG alone. A/S I staining of proteins from luteal MEM without hCG was identical. Thus E probably represents multiple proteins. In conclusion A/S I reacts with LH receptors and several smaller proteins that may be part of the LH receptor complex in the absence of SDS. Some of the proteins may be regulatory proteins. (NIH grants HD-14098, HD-10718)

1066 DEMONSTRATION OF LATS BINDING WITH TSH RECEPTOR IN HEN THYROID. Y. Nakajima*, M. Ishida, Y. Ochi[1], Y. Ura[1], T. Miyazaki[2], T. Hachiya[3] and H. Ijichi[3], Inter Med, Nantan Hospital, Yagi, Clin Lab[1]. Shiga Univ. Otsu, and Radiol[2] and Inter Med[3], Kyoto prefect. Univ. of Med, Kyoto. Japan.

LATS is regarded as specific thyroid stimulating IgG for the mammalian species because of no stimulatory action for the nonmammalian (chick and amphibia). TSH receptor antibody (TRAb) in Graves' disease was determined by receptor assay using porcine thyroid and ^{125}I-bTSH (Smith's kit). All of 50 LATS positive cases showed positive TRAb activity, while 70 % of LATS negative cases were positive. No correlation between TRAb activity and LATS activity was observed. Thus, LATS may be one of a heterogenous population of TRAb. In the present study we studied LATS binding with hen thyroid receptor by receptor assay using ^{125}I-bTSH and hen thyroid plasma membrane. TRAb activity was expressed as % inhibition of ^{125}I-bTSH binding by test sera (50 µl). Normal range was ± 17.4 %. LATS negative sera in Graves and sera in Hashimoto's disease showed all normal range. Many LATS positive sera showed negative TRAb activity, but some cases showed positive TRAb (the range; 18-33 %). There was no correlation between TRAb activity and LATS activity. These results suggest that failure of hen thyroid stimulation by LATS may be due to two mechanisms, (1) loss of binding with receptor and (2) the postreceptor defect.

1067 DECREASED NUCLEAR BINDING OF TRIIODOTHYRONINE (T_3) IN CORTISOL-DEFICIENT PATIENTS. Ph. De Nayer*, B. Dozin and J. Crabbé, Hormones and Metabolic Research Unit, ICP and Department of Physiology, University of Louvain, B-1200 Brussels, Belgium.

Increased TSH secretion appears to be a common feature in primary adrenal insufficiency before steroid substitution. "In vitro" thyroid and glucocorticoid hormones exhibit a synergistic effect on the regulation of growth hormone gene expression. We now report that "in vivo" glucocorticoids also influence the interaction of T_3 with its nuclear receptor. This study was conducted in 17 patients: 13 with secondary hypopituitarism, 4 with primary adrenal insufficiency. The binding properties of the lymphocyte nuclear receptors were analyzed in these patients while on or off steroid substitution. In patients deprived from steroids ($\geq$ 48 hrs) the mean affinity constant (Ka, $\bar{X} \pm SD$) was significantly lower ($p < 0.005$) than in normal subjects (3.75 ± 3.8 vs $8.6 \pm 0.46 \times 10^8\ M^{-1}$). Steroid therapy induced within 48 hrs a significant increase of Ka (paired "t" test, $0.01 > p > 0.001$). The value thus obtained ($1.15 \pm 1.3 \times 10^9\ M^{-1}$) was not different from normal. No significant difference was observed in the effects of glucocorticoid substitution on the Ka in secondary and primary failure. The glucocorticoid effect was most striking in 2 adult males with long-standing panhypopituitarism. In summary, the Ka of the nuclear receptors for T_3 is decreased in steroid deficiency, and normalized after steroid substitution. From these results we conclude that steroids may affect the sensitivity to thyroid hormones by acting at the thyroid hormone receptor level.

1068 THYROID HORMONE CYTOSOLIC BINDING PROTEINS ARE PREDOMINANTLY IN NEURONS, IN PRIMARY CELL CULTURE FROM EMBRYONIC RAT BRAIN. J. Francon, F. Chantoux, J. Osty and A.M. Lennon*, Unité 96 INSERM, Bicêtre (France).

Brain cells dissociated from 17 day old embryonic rats and grown in the presence of 10% foetal calf serum in monolayer cell culture contain high affinity cytosolic thyroid hormone binding proteins. The K_A values for triiodothyronine and thyroxine were respectively $1.2\text{-}3.7 \times 10^9\ M^{-1}$ and $3.7\text{-}5 \times 10^8\ M^{-1}$. A second class of lower affinity sites ($\sim$ 10 time lower) was also shown. The highest level of thyroid hormone binding protein was on day 4 in culture (145 fmoles per mg soluble proteins), then remained stable until day 7. During the second week of culture the amount of binding protein decreased for about 10 times. On the contrary no differences in the binding affinities of both sites were observed between day 7 and day 14. The decrease in the level of the binding protein correlates with a diminution in the number of neuronal cells and an over multiplication of the glial cells. Lower amounts of cytosolic binding proteins were found in glial cell cultures virtually free of neurons. We therefore conclude that in our culture conditions high levels of thyroid hormone binding proteins are present only in neurons.

1069 CHARACTERIZATION OF ESTROGEN SULFOTRANSFERASE (EST) IN RL95-2 ENDOMETRIAL CANCER CELLS. David S. Grosso, Department of Obstetrics and Gynecology, Arizona Health Sciences Center, University of Arizona, Tucson, AZ 85724

Although estrogen sulfoconjugation is believed to be important in regulating hormonal sensitivity of the endometrium the study of this system in the human has proved difficult. A cell line, RL95-2, derived from a human endometrial cancer and maintained in continuous *in vitro* culture has been reported to contain estrogen sulfoconjugating activity. This study reports the further characterization of this activity in RL95-2 cells. Sulfurylation was measured using 3H-estrone (E1) as substrate. Enzyme activity was localized in the cytosol and exhibited a pH optimum of pH 8. There was a marked temperature dependence between 24°C and 40°C. Simple kinetic behaior was found at E1 concentrations up to 1μM with a Km of 3.6 nM and a Vmax of 135 fmole/μg DNA/h. The Km for the co-substrate 3'-phosphoadenosine 5'-phosphosulfate was 0.6 μM. Inhibition experiments demonstrated that the enzyme was specific for estrogens. Only estradiol and estriol, in addition to E1, inhibited activity to any significant degree. Dehydroepiandrosterone had only 1% of the inhibitory activity of E1. Other androgens corticoids, progestins, phenols, non-steroidal estrogens and antiestrogens and bile acids had little or no effect on activity. The estrogen sulfoconjugating activity of RL95-2 cells was shown to be that of EST. The high affinity of human EST for estrogens suggests that it may serve as an important regulator of intracellular estrogen levels. The RL95-2 cell line provides a potentially useful model for the study of the role of endometrial estrogen metabolism on tissue sensitivity to circulating hormone and as a source of enzyme for the detailed characterization of human EST.

1070 EVIDENCE FOR A GRANULOSA CELL SITE OF DIHYDROTESTOSTERONE METABOLISM. J. Jarrell* L. Belbeck, McMaster University, Hamilton, Ontario, Canada.

Androgens are important for the regulation of follicular development and atresia. Recent reports have demonstrated the presence of 5α-reductase, which converts testosterone to dihydrotestosterone (DHT), to be localized to the theca and interstitial tissue of the immature rat. It was of interest to determine the location of 3α-hydroxysteroid dehydrogenase which reduces DHT to 5α-androstane-3α,17β-diol (3α-diol). The administration of 6,000 rads over 6 minutes to exteriorized ovaries was done in 30 day old Sprague Dawley Rats. The animals were sacrificed at 45 days with sham-irradiation controls. 3α-HSD was measured by incubating ovarian cytosol with $5x10^{-7}$ M, DHT, $5x10^{-4}$ M NADPH and 0.05 uCi (1,2 ^{3}H)-DHT. Control ovarian and uterine weights were significantly higher than in irradiated rats ($p < 0.01$). Histologically the follicles demonstrated hypertrophical theca and interstitual tissues in irradiated rats. Thecal tissues stained positively for 3β-HSD activity histochemically. Ovarian 3α-HSD activity was significantly higher in sham irradiated rats; 23.44±1.97 nmoles/h/organ, 150.75±5.44 nmoles/h/mg cytosol protein vs irradiated rats, 8.49±0.98 nmoles/h/organ, 86.68±15.20 nmoles/h/mg protein ($p < 0.01$). The findings are consistent with a major site of DHT reduction within follicular granulosa cells. Supported by the MOH of Ontario and Physician's Services Incorporated.

1071 HYDROLYSIS OF ESTRADIOL 17-β-ESTERS IN MOUSE UTERINE HOMOGENATES IS CATALYZED BY ESTERASE-1F TAKEN UP FROM THE PLASMA. S. Kadner, J. Katz, M. Levitz and T. Finlay*. NYU Medical Center, New York, NY 10016.

We recently reported the isolation and purification of a serine esterase from mouse uterine homogenates (hydrolase II) which rapidly increases in immature animals after administration of estradiol (E2). We later showed that hydrolase II activity resulted at least in part from uptake of a plasma enzyme which appeared to be identical to the sexually-dimorphic albumin-esterase called esterase 1F (E1F) by von Deimling et al. Consistent with this we find levels of the plasma esterase are 50% higher in female mice than in males. We now show that all uterine hydrolase II activity occurs as a result of uptake of E1F. Like the uptake of other plasma proteins, uterine uptake of E1F is blocked by prednisolone but not by puromycin. Using immunoprecipitation of ^{35}S-methionine labeled E1F prepared in a cell-free translation system, mRNA specific for E1F was found to be present in mouse liver but not in mouse uterus. Although the natural substrate for E1F (or hydrolase II) is not known, we show that it cleaves lipoidal esters of estradiol. Both uterine homogenates and purified E1F are able to hydrolyze E2-17-valerate. In each case, hydrolysis of the ester is completely blocked by heating or by incubation with DIFP or antibody to E1F. These results suggest that E1F is responsible for the hydrolysis of E2-17 esters in the uterus. It is possible that E1F plays a role in estrogen metabolism or transport.
Supported in part by NIH Grant CA-02071.

1072 EFFECTS OF LONG-ACTING CATECHOLESTROGEN DERIVATIVES ON PITUITARY HORMONE SECRETION IN WOMEN. S. Kishida*, S. Miyabo, T. Sugiyama, M. Kuwabara, T. Hashimoto and Y. Fujii, Fukui Medical School, Fukui 910-11; School of Medicine, Kanazawa University; and Hokuriku University, Kanazawa 920, Japan.

Data on the effects of catecholestrogens (CE), especially of 4-hydroxyestrogens, on human pituitary hormone levels are quite few. Recently we reported that both 4- and 2-hydroxyestradiol (4- and 2-OHE_2) injected as an iv bolus caused a transient suppression of LH and FSH in normal youg women, 4-OHE_2 being more potent than 2-OHE_2. In this experiment, more chronic effects of CE were investigated using depot esters of the steroids. The CE dibenzoates(4- and 2-OHE_2B_2) were synthesized by the method of Emons and extensively purified. At 0800 hr, castrated women, 35 to 49 years of age, were injected subcutaneously with 1 mg 4-OHE_2B_2 or 5 mg 4- or 2-OHE_2B_2 or 1 mg estradiol monobenzoate (E_2B) in aqueous suspension. Serial blood samples were assayed for plasma LH, FSH and PRL by RIA. 1 mg 4-OHE_2B_2 and 5 mg 2-OHE_2B_2 did not change the pituitary hormone levels. 5 mg 4-OHE_2B_2 suppressed LH and FSH to 50-60% of preinjection levels at 20 hrs after injection and the effects persisted for several days. 1 mg E_2B was almost equipotent to 5 mg 4-OHE_2B_2. No positive feedback effects of both steroids were observed. PRL tended to increase over 2-3 days after both treatments, but the superimposition of marked diurnal fluctuations made a definite conclusion difficult.

1073 ANALYSIS OF RADIOLABELLED MEDIA PROTEINS FROM IMMATURE RAT UTERI FOLLOWING ESTRADIOL, PROGESTERONE AND ANTIESTROGEN TREATMENT.
B. Komm* and C. Richard Lyttle, Dept of Obstetrics and Gynecology, University of Pennsylvania, Philadelphia, PA. 19104

Media proteins were analyzed following steroid treatment to study the molecular basis of hormone action. Immature rats were treated for three days with estrogens and antiestrogens alone or in combination with progesterone (P). Uteri were incubated in the presence of ^{35}S-methionine for 6 hours, the media collected, and the proteins were analyzed by SDS-PAGE followed by fluorography. Following treatment the uterine weight increases dramatically with a 4.0-fold increase in the endometrial height. There are two major polypeptides with molecular weights of 87,000 daltons and 66,000 daltons which increased 3.5 fold and 2.4 fold respectively. Treatment with tamoxifen, LY117018, and LY156758 did not demonstrate the uterine weight increase seen following E. This treatment did however cause an increase in endometrial cell height similar to E. Tamoxifen was the most potent stimulus followed by LY117018 and LY156758. Protein analysis shows that the antiestrogens stimulate the synthesis of the same two major proteins as E. Furthermore, the degree of stimulation of the synthesis of these proteins correlates with the changes seen in endometrial cell height, namely Tamoxifen>LY117018>LY156758. When P was given in combination with E there was a slight increase in cell height (1.3X) Similarly, the response in protein synthesis was also diminished (1.2X). The results of combining P with the antiestrogens were similar to P with estradiol. These results indicate that these media proteins may be produced in the endometrium and used as molecular markers.

1074 SEX DIFFERENCES IN RAT LIVER ACID PHOSPHATASE (AP).
J. Downey*, C.E. Bird and A.F. Clark, Depts. of Biochemistry and Medicine, Queen's University, Kingston, Ontario, Canada.

It is well accepted that rat prostate AP is controlled by androgens. While developing techniques for examining prostatic AP we examined liver AP. Adult rat liver AP is located in two principal subcellular sites - cytosol and the mitochondrial/lysosomal fraction. AP in the latter fraction can be solubilized by repeated freezing and thawing. When either fraction is subjected to Sephadex G-75 chromatography, two peaks of AP elute - one close to the void volume (G75I) and one later (G75II). The cytosol G75I AP kinetic parameters with p-nitrophenol phosphate are different for male K_m = 2.3 μM:V_{max} = 19.4 μmoles/h) and females (K_m = 9.2 μM:V_{max} = 69.2 μmoles/h). The K_m for the cytosol G75IAP for castrated male rat livers is 9.2 μM. The kinetic parameters for the other soluble AP (G75II) are the same for the two sexes. There are no sex differences in the optimum pH's and the tartrate or metal ion sensitivities for the four liver AP's. The kinetic differences for cytosol G75IAP could be related to some form of androgenic control of the state of glycosylation. Such is implicated in the androgenic control of prostatic AP characteristics. (Supported by Medical Research Council of Canada).

1075 A GONADOTROPIN-INDUCED PROTEIN FACTOR INHIBITS THE CHOLESTEROL SIDE-CHAIN CLEAVAGE ENZYME SYSTEM IN LEYDIG CELL MITOCHONDRIA.
M-A Hattori, D.R. Aquilano and M.L. Dufau*. ERRB, NICHD, NIH, Bethesda, MD 20205, USA.

The activity of the cholesterol side-chain cleavage (CSCC) system was decreased in Leydig cells (LC) from gonadotropin-treated rats with an early biosynthetic defect in testicular androgen production. This phenomenon was accompanied by the appearance of an inhibiting factor in LC mitochondria. The activity of this factor was investigated using an assay system based in its ability to inhibit the CSCC activity of rat adrenal mitochondria, as measured by [^{14}C]-isocaproic acid formation from labeled cholesterol. Addition of the LC mitochondrial preparation to the adrenal CSCC system caused a marked increase in the Km of this enzyme for NADPH (0.017 mM and 0.111 mM before and after the addition, respectively). This effect was more marked with testicular preparations from hCG-treated rats (Km = 0.37 mM) with no changes in Vmax. The inhibitory factor was of protein nature, was confined to the LC mitochondrion, and was not related to changes in oxidative phosphorylation as indicated by incubations with the respiratory inhibitors rotenone and antimycin A. Acetone-powdered cytosol fractions did not contain inhibitory activity. On gel filtration of detergent-soluble fractions from LC mitochondria the inhibitory activity eluted with a K_{av} of 0.168, giving an apparent Stoke°s radius of 4.8 nm. The inhibitory factor exhibited an isoelectric point of 5.05 ± 0.23 (n=8), was not adsorbed to 2°,5° ADP-Sepharose 4B, and did not oxidize or immobilize NADPH. These results have indicated that a membrane protein of the LC mitochondrion is activated or increased by hCG treatment, and has a competitive inhibitory effect on the CSCC system.

1076 LOW TESTOSTERONE AND LOW FSH IN CRITICALLY ILL MALE PATIENTS.
R. Karl*, D. Engelhardt and S. Braun, Departments of Internal Medicine II and Clinical Chemistry, Klinikum Grosshadern, University of Munich, FRG

Within a scope of a prospective, randomized, clinical trial in preventing acute gastrointestinal bleeding in intensive care unit patients we compared the effect of cimetidine-pirencepine (CP) with the effect of aluminum magnesium hydroxide (A) on serum levels of FSH, LH, prolactin (PRL), testosterone (T), estrone (E1) and estradiol-17β(E2) in male patients. Thirteen patients received 0.4 g C and 10 mg P every 6-8 hrs iv, 12 patients 60-120 ml A per 24 hrs. All hormones were determined before, 48 hrs and 6/7 days after beginning of therapy with CP or A. Statistical analyses showed that the randomization worked well so that changes of hormone levels depending only on C and/or P would be detected. All hormonal levels were measured by RIA's. Statistical analyses were performed with the sign test of Dixon and Mood. E2 showed a statistically significant rise under CP after 48 hrs (p 0.05) but this effect is not definitely specific because in patients treated with A there was also a trend to higher E2 levels. Therapy with CP had no influence on serum levels of FSH, LH, PRL, T or E1 in comparison with A. However, there was a statistically significant fall of FSH and T in intensive care unit male patients irrespectively of a medication with CP or A in part after 48 hrs ($p < 0.01 - < 0.05$) but in any case after 6/7 days ($p < 0.01 - < 0.05$). Therefore, we would create in imitation of the term "low T3-syndrome" the terms "low testosterone syndrome" and "low FSH syndrome" in critically ill male patients without knowing an explanation of this phenomenon.

1077 CHANGES IN PROTEIN METHYLESTERASE DURING SPERM MATURATION. C. Gagnon*[1], D. Harbour[1], E. de Lamirande[1], C.W. Bardin[2] and J.L. Dacheux[3]. [1]Biorégulation cellulaire et moléculaire, CHUL, Québec, Canada and Département de Pharmacologie, Université Laval, Québec, Canada; [2]Population Council, New York, NY; and [3]CNRS, Faculté de Sciences, Tours, France.

Protein-carboxyl methylase (PCM) and protein methylesterase (PME) are the enzymes that reversibly control the extent of protein-carboxyl methylation. Whereas the presence of PCM is well established in spermatozoa, PME has been shown to be present in rabbit spermatozoa but absent in rat spermatozoa. Using a more sensitive assay, we found PME activity in bull and rat spermatozoa and observed drastic changes in specific activity during sperm maturation. In bull, testicular spermatozoa had a PME level of 0.28 pmol/mg protein/20 min. Sperm PME activity increased in caput epididymidis up to 1.29 pmol/mg protein/20 min (segment 3). Then, the level felt progressively to 0.27 in the corpus and to 0.06 pmol/mg protein/20 min in the cauda. Similar results were obtained with rat spermatozoa during epididymal maturation. This drop of sperm PME activity during epididymal transit paralleled the acquisition of motility and is consistent with the hypothesis that a high level of protein methylation is associated with motility.
(Supported by grants from M.R.C. of Canada and N.I.H., U.S.A.)

1078 ISOLATION AND CHARACTERIZATION OF TWO POPULATIONS OF LEYDIG CELLS FROM NEONATAL PIG TESTES. Y. Gauthier*, J.R. Ducharme, R. Collu and W. Gibb. Research Unit on Reproductive and Developmental Biology, Centre de Recherche Pédiatrique, Hôpital Sainte-Justine and Depts. Obs/Gyn & Pediatrics, University of Montreal, Montreal, Quebec, Canada.

Cultures of Leydig cells from neonatal pig testes have been examined by a number of laboratories as a model for mammalian testosterone synthesis. In some studies collagenase dispersed cells have been used directly and in others, including our own, cells have been purified using Percoll gradients. The present study demonstrates that using Percoll gradients two populations of Leydig cells, with different steroidogenic potential, can be isolated from these tissues. After digestion with collagenase the cells were separated by centrifugation on discontinuous Percoll gradients and two bands of cells were recovered, band I at 1.045g/ml and band II at 1.058g/ml. Band I had higher activities of 3β-hydroxysteroid dehydrogenase (3βHSD) (4-fold) and 17β-hydroxysteroid dehydrogenase (17βHSD) (2-fold) when compared with band II. Cells from each were placed in culture for 3-4 days. In each population hCG-stimulated testosterone production increased spontaneously during the culture period. Also, in both populations 3βHSD activity increased during the culture period, being more pronounced in band II than band I. This increase was augmented by hCG treatment. In contrast, 17βHSD activities tended to decrease in both populations. These results indicate that there are at least two populations of Leydig cells in neonatal pig testes as defined by 3βHSD and 17βHSD activities and that a spontaneous increase in T production and 3βHSD activity during culture occurs in both populations. Supported by M.R.C. (Canada) and La Fondation Justine Lacoste-Beaubien.

1079 ANTAGONISTIC ACTION OF ESTROGEN AND URINARY PROTEIN ON TESTICULAR ACTIVITY. P.K. Ghosh* and N.M. Biswas, Dept. of Physiology, University Colleges of Science & Technology, 92, A.P.C. Road, Calcutta 700009, INDIA.

Although estrogen inhibits both alpha-2u-globulin(a urinary protein) synthesis and testicular activities, we have studied the effect of this urinary protein on testicular activities in estrogen-treated rats. Subcutaneous injection of estradiol-17β(50 µg/100 g body wt/day) for 7 days to adult male rats results in inhibition of testicular 17β-hydroxysteroid dehydrogenase(17β-HSD) activity and spermatogenesis while the serum level of gonadotrophins and testosterone are decreased on 22nd day. Administration of urinary protein(1.5 mg/rat/day) for 14 days to estrogen-treated rats causes a stimulation of 17β-HSD activity along with increased concentrations of gonadotrophins and testosterone in the serum while spermatogenesis appears to be normal. The present study concludes that urinary protein antagonises the action of estrogen on both spermatogenesis and testosterone synthesis by inducing gonadotrophin synthesis.

1080 STEROIDOGENESIS IN RAT TESTICULAR MYOID CELL CULTURES. J.B. Hay*, J.P. Mather and C.W. Bardin, Population Council, 1230 York Avenue, New York, NY 10021, USA.

Seminiferous tubules synthesize androgens *de novo* in small quantities and further modify Leydig cell derived androgens needed for spermatogenesis. Cell culture experiments have indicated Sertoli cells as the source of these activities, but other cell lines have not been examined. The steroid metabolizing activities of rat testicular myoid cells (primary cultures and TRM line) are reported. Cells were grown to confluency in Ham's F12, Dulbecco's modified Eagle's medium (1:1) at 37°C in air/CO_2 (95:5,v/v) and incubated in fresh medium for 16h with 3-4 ng of tritiated steroid substrate. Radiosteroids were extracted with ether-ethanol (3:1,v/v), separated by thin layer and paper chromatography and identified by crystallization to constant specific activity. TRM cells converted [^{3}H]testosterone to androstenedione and smaller amounts of androsterone, 5α-androstane-3α, 17β-diol and 5α-dihydrostestosterone. [^{3}H]Androstenedione was metabolized to testosterone, 5α-dihydrotestosterone and 5α-androstane-3α, 17β-diol and some 5α-androstanedione and androsterone. 5-Androstene-3β,17β-diol was the main product of [^{3}H]dehydroepiandrosterone metabolism together with some testosterone and androstenedione. Androgens were not formed in detectable amounts from [^{3}H]progesterone and [^{3}H]17α-hydroxyprogesterone. Primary myoid cell culture metabolized androgens more rapidly than TRM cells with high levels of 3α-hydroxysteroid dehydrogenase. It is concluded that myoid cells contribute to the alteration of steroids entering the seminiferous tubules.

1081 HUMAN SERTOLI CELLS: REGULATION OF TRANSFERRIN SECRETION IN THE ABSENCE OR PRESENCE OF HUMAN PERITUBULAR CELLS.

S.D. Holmes*, L.I. Lipshultz and R.G. Smith, Baylor College of Medicine, Department of Urology, Houston, TX 77030, USA.

Transferrin represents approximately 4% of the total secreted proteins from human Sertoli cells (SC) in culture. The amount of transferrin secreted by the cells is maximal after 4 to 5 days in culture; the time chosen for each media change. The following agents: FSH, insulin, dibutyryl cyclic AMP (DBC) and isobutylmethylxanthine significantly increased transferrin secretion over basal values (1.4 to 3 fold) only when added during the second or third media changes. None of the above compounds enhanced transferrin secretion when added for the first 4 to 5 days in culture. Testosterone and retinol (in the absence or presence of insulin) had no effect. With or without the above stimulators transferrin secretion declines with time in culture. These results suggest that the above agents do not stimulate *per se* but help maintain the secretion of transferrin. Human peritubular (PT) cells when co-cultured with SC significantly elevated the secretion of transferrin. (PT, not detectable; PT+SC, 23.1±2.1; SC, 13.0±3.1 ng transferrin/day/10^6cells). DBC stimulated transferrin secretion when added for the first as well as second media changes when SC were co-cultured with PT cells, (DBC+PT+SC, 80.2±1.2; DBC+SC, 12.9±2.6 ng transferrin/day/10^6cells, first media change). Human fibroblasts or PT cell conditioned medium could not mimic the above effect. These results imply that PT cells play an important role in regulating transferrin secretion and the responsiveness of the SC to stimulation by DBC. Supported by NIH grants AA06167, DA02852 and HD11479.

1082 EXOGENOUS TESTOSTERONE INDUCES CHANGES IN GERM CELL NUMBER IN INTACT RATS.

H. Huang* and E. Nieschlag, Max Planck Clinical Research Unit for Reproductive Medicine, Munster, F.R. Germany and Dept. of Anatomy, UMDNJ, New Jersey Medical School, Newark, New Jersey, U.S.A.

The effect of continuous administration of exogenous testosterone (T) on intratesticular testosterone (ITT) and spermatogenesis was studied in intact rats given subcutaneous implantation of 0.5-50 cm long T filled silastic capsule (TC) for 8 weeks. Serum T was suppressed slightly in rats bearing 1 cm long TC, but was increased by 6-30 folds in rats bearing 10 cm or longer TC implants. Serum FSH was suppressed to 30-60 % of control value. ITT was reduced by 90% in rats receiving 1 or 5 cm long TC implant, but rebound to 80% of the control value when 50 cm long TC was used. Despite the presence of complete spermatogenesis, the number of B spermatogonia and preleptotene spermatocytes was reduced in rats bearing 5 cm or longer TC implants ($P < 0.001$). On the other hand, the number of A_1 spermatogonia increased by 20% uniquely in rats bearing 1 cm long TC implant. The yield of spermiogenesis appeared normal in TC implanted rats except in those with 1 cm TC that the elongated spermatids were reduced in number or were absent. These results demonstrate that complete spermatogenesis can be maintained by as low as 10% of normal ITT level, but a quantitatively normal spermatogenesis cannot be supported by as high as 30 folds of normal serum T levels. Furthermore, the drastic differences in the pattern of germ cell number in the face of comparable ITT and serum FSH states in rats bearing 1 and 5 cm long TC implants demonstrate that these two factors are not the only determinant for the quantitative aspect of spermatogenesis.

1083 IN VITRO DEIODINATION OF L- AND D-T_4 IN RAT, COW AND PIG.

M.Grussendorf*, M.Hüfner, Medizinische Univ. Poliklinik, Heidelberg, FRG

Though extensive in vitro studies on L-T_4 deiodination in rat liver have been performed, little is known about 1. in vitro deiodination of D-T_4 and 2. in vitro conver sion in other animals. Therefore, we have compared 5'-and 5-deiodase activity after incubation of 1 μg L-T4 and D-T4 in liverhomogenate of rat, cow and pig. All experiments were performed under identical conditions at pH 7,5. Because the pH-profiles vary significantly between the species, the results were corrected for the respective pH-optima. The mean values ($\pm$ SD) are shown in Table I (because of the very rapid deiodination of rT3 to T_2' in this system, formation of T_2' was taken as an indicator for 5-deiodination).

	n	LT4-LT3	LT4-LT_2'	DT4-DT3	DT4-DT_2'
rat	20	2,00 $\pm$ 0,62	1,25 $\pm$ 0,75	0,87 $\pm$ 0,20	4,60 $\pm$ 1,84
cow	18	0,87 $\pm$ 0,25	0,44 $\pm$ 0,21	0,63 $\pm$ 0,16	1,10 $\pm$ 0,31
pig	19	0,32 $\pm$ 0,10	1,20 $\pm$ 0,67	0,25 $\pm$ 0,06	0,38 $\pm$ 0,18

Table I: Formation of T_3 and T_2' (pmol/mg prot. x 20 min.) after incubation of 1 μg T_4.

We conclude that there are distinct species differences of D- and L-T4 metabolism and that one should be cautious to transfer results of in vitro experiments to conditions in man.

1084 VARIABILITY OF STIMULATORY EFFECTS OF TSH AND GRAVES' IgG ON CYCLIC-AMP PRODUCTION IN CULTURED HUMAN THYROID CELLS.

M. K. Gupta*, C. Johnson, B. Jacobs, B. B. Barna, C. B. Esselstyn, and O. P. Schumacher. Departments of Immunopathology, General Surgery, and Endocrinology. The Cleveland Clinic Foundation, 9500 Euclid Avenue, Cleveland, OH 44106 USA

Thyroid tissues were obtained from 10 patients undergoing thyroid lobectomy or parathyroid surgery. Cells were cultured in MEM media with 10 - 20% fetal calf serum for a minimum of 10 days. Cultures were tested for cyclic-AMP (c-AMP) production in salt free media by thyroid stimulating hormone (TSH) and by IgG fractions from 7 patients (Graves' disease - 4, self-resolving hyperthyroidism (SRH) - 1 and euthyroid - 2). TSH (20 µU/ml) showed a variable degree of c-AMP production (range, 1.3 x to 10.2 x increase over baseline levels). Further increase in c-AMP was seen by 100 µU/ml of TSH in all cultures except 2. IgG fractions from 4 Graves' patients (all positive by TSH binding inhibition assay) also demonstrated similar variability showing none to 19x increase in c-AMP production or 0 - > 100 µU TSH equivalent activity in different cell cultures. One patient with SRH showed 0 - 2.2x increase or 0 - 14 µU TSH equivalent activity. There seemed to be no relationship between TSH and IgG response. For example, IgG from 1 Graves' patient showed only 10 µU/ml TSH equivalent activity in a cell culture which responded maximally to TSH, while in another cell culture which had low response to TSH the same IgG showed 100 µU/ml TSH equivalent activity. Our data points to the limitation of use of primary thyroid cell cultures in bioassay for a reliable and precise measurement of thyroid stimulating immunoglobulins.

1085 THE EFFECT OF TOTAL FASTING AND KETOGENIC DIET ON SERUM THYROID HORMONE LEVELS IN CHILDREN WITH EPILEPSY. M. Hara*, Y. Fukuyama and H. Demura, Department of Pediatrics and Medicine, Tokyo Women's Medical College, Tokyo, Japan.

To disclose the thyroid hormone changes in the hypoenergetic state of man, eight children with epilepsy, aged 5 years and 8 months in average weighing 19.0$\pm$4.3kg, were observed during a total fasting period of 180 hours and for successive periods of 4:1 ketogenic diet therapy which were carried out for the purpose of antiepileptic treatment. Serum T4, T3, reverse T3(rT3), TSH and prolactin (PRL) levels were measured at frequent intervals. Before fasting, all thyroid hormone levels were normal; T4 6.2$\pm$1.3μg/dl, T3:144,3$\pm$27.9ng/dl, rT3:16.1$\pm$2.7ng/dl). Each, patient demonstrated a transient rise of rT3(rT3:29.6$\pm$13.8ng/dl) and moderate decrease of T3 level (T3:69.4$\pm$28.6ng/dl) by 60 hours of fasting and then marked reduction of all thyroid hormones (T4:2.7$\pm$0.7μg/dl, T3:35.5$\pm$16.7ng/dl, rT3:13.5$\pm$3.2ng/dl) by the end of 180 hours' fasting. Serum T3 was about 20% of its pre-fast level. Both TSH and PRL remained at a low level during the starvation. All thyroid hormones, TSH and PRL were recovered to their pre-fast levels after taking the 4:1 ketogenic diet. These reversible peripheral thyroid hormone changes and the following marked reduction of activity of hypothalamo-pituitary-thyroid axis observed in 180 hours of fasting in young children were thought to be closely related to the rate of caloric deprivation. The biological implication of this phenomenon was speculated as a natural, purposeful reaction of the body to spare energy and body protein under a hypoenergetic state.

1086 CHARACTERIZATION OF CALPAIN AND CALPASTATIN FROM HOG THYROID CYTOSOL. K. Haraguchi*, F. Akasu, T. Endo and T. Onaya, The Third Department of Internal Medicine, University of Yamanashi Medical School, Tamaho, Yamanashi-ken 409-38, Japan

Calcium activated-protease (calpain) and its endogenous inhibitor (calpastatin) have recently been found in many tissues and their various physiological actions such as proteolytic modification of hormone receptors and c-kinases have also been known. Protease activity was assayed using casein as the substrate, and TCA-soluble products released were measured by the method of Lowry. Proteolytic activity of hog thyroid cytosol fraction was found to be 0.045 U (1 U was defined as the amount of the enzyme which produced an increment in A of 1.00 during 30 min). After applying the sample on DEAE-cellulose (DE-52) ion exchange column, the column was eluted with a linear gradient of NaCl (0.0-0.7 M). This procedure resolved the activity into two peaks. One peak was eluted at 0.2 M NaCl and the other at 0.4 M NaCl. Calpastatin was eluted in broad peak of 0.15-0.4 M NaCl. Both activities had broad neutral pH optimum, and were totally dependent on calcium. Half maximum stimulation was obtained by adding 0.5 mM calcium in peak 2. Peak 1 activity was 0.45 U and peak 2 activity was 2.87 U. Both activities were inhibited by leupeptin and E-64 but not by serine protease inhibitors or soybean trypsin inhibitor. Further, they were increased to 6-10 fold by 3.0 mM mercaptoethanol and were reduced by 50 % in the presence of 10^{-5} M monoiodoacetic acid. Therefore, we have demonstrated the existence of calpain and calpastatin in hog thyroid gland although their roles in the thyroid remain to be clarified.

1087 THYROID HORMONE INHIBITION OF BIOSYNTHESIS OF PROTEIN INHIBITORS FOR S-ADENOSYL-L-METHIONINE-MEDIATED METHYLATION OF PHOSPHATIDYLETHANOLAMINE IN RAT LIVER. K. Hashizume*, and M. Kobayashi, Department of Gerontology, Endocrinology and Metabolism, Shinshu University School of Medicine, Matsumoto 390, JAPAN

The methylation pathway of phosphatidylcholine(PC) synthesis has important roles in biological actions of cell membrane. Thyroid hormone is well known to modify the function of plasma membrane in several tissues. We examined the effect of thyroid hormone on S-adenosyl-L-methionine(SAM)-mediated methylation of phosphatidylethanolamine(PE) using thyroidectomized(T_x+saline) or T_4-treated-thyroidectomized(T_x+T_4) rats. When the purified rat liver plasma membranes were used as an enzyme(methyltransferase), two different cytosolic inhibitors for SAM-mediated methylation were separated by gel filtration. The inhibitory activity in T_x+saline rats was higher than that in T_x +T_4 rats. T_4 administration to T_x+saline rats reduced the inhibitory activity. Double reciprocal analysis revealed that T_4 treatment reduces the number of inhibitors. The inhibitory activity of partial purified inhibitors was inactivated by pretreatment with trypsin or by heating at 96°C, but not by pretreatment with RNase. The results indicate that thyroid hormone inhibits the synthesis of protein inhibitors for SAM-mediated methylation of PE and that this inhibition results in a stimulation of methylation pathway of PC synthesis in the plasma membrane.

1088 PERMANENT DEFECTS IN RAT PERIPHERAL AUDITORY FUNCTION FOLLOWING PERINATAL HYPOTHYROIDISM: DETERMINATION OF A CRITICAL PERIOD. R. Hébert*, J.-M. Langlois and J.H. Dussault, Thyroid Research Unit, CHUL, Quebec, G1V 4G2, Canada.

Perinatal thyroid dysfunction in the rat is known to interfere with the development of the central and peripheral auditory systems. The aim of this study was to determine the period during which peripheral auditory function development is most susceptible to hypothyroidism. Rats ($n = 35$) from different litters were treated with propylthiouracil (PTU) for a 10 day period beginning at different ages ranging from 3 days before delivery to 35 days of age. One group of PTU-treated rats also received daily injections of thyroxine (T_4). T_4 replacement doses were calculated from the T_4 production rates in developing rats (Endocrinology 101: 435, 1977). Peripheral auditory function was evaluated by auditory brainstem evoked responses (ABR) performed at 200 days of age. Binaural stimulation consisted of brief 4, 8 and 16 kHz tone-bursts calibrated at 80 dB. The latency (ms) of the first reproducible peak (Wave I) was used as an index of peripheral auditory function. PTU treatment significantly increased ($p < 0.05$) Wave I latency in adult rats when administered from 3 days before birth through 6 days postnatally but was without effect when administered for 10 days starting at 10 days after birth. T_4 replacement during the first 10 postnatal days prevented ($p > 0.1$) Wave I latency abnormalities. Conclusion: In the developing auditory system, the critical period of susceptibility to thyroid hormone deficiency occurs prior to 10 days postnatally (and perhaps as early as 5 days postnatally), before the onset of cochlear activity normally seen at 12 days of age.

1089 POSSIBILITIES FOR THALLIUM 201 IN THYROID ONCOPATHOLOGY. J. Hermans, J.P. De Baets, M. Beauduin, J.F.Gigot and A. Schmitz. Department of Nuclear Medicine, Hôpital de Jolimont, Belgium.

Presented with a diagnosis of a cold thyroid nodule as determined by routine scintigraphy, the clinician must determine if the nodule is cancerous or not. This is a serious problem, since, according to literature, 7-20 % of cold thyroid nodules are malignant.
In 1982 some Japanese authors demonstrated the possibility of using 201Tl in diagnosing the thyroid tumors.
The present investigation of 84 patients who were operated for a thyroid disorder characterized by one or more cold nodules (conventional scintigraphy) enabled us to compare complete descriptions of the thyroid disorders with the results of 201Tl scintigraphies carried out with a gamma-camera using a pinhole collimator. 201Tl uptake by cold nodules was often observed in both benign (benign follicular adenoma) and malignant (carcinoma or lymphoma) tumors of the thyroid.
The reliability, sensitivity and specificity of the method were all above 80 %. Our finding were similar to those of our Japanese colleagues and thus encouraged us to :
1. use this technique as a method of choice when confronted with a cold thyroid nodule and
2. recommend immediate surgery, should the 201Tl scintigraphy prove positive for a cold thyroid nodule.

1090 CASSAVA IS NOT A GOITROGEN IN MICE. J.M. Hershman*, A.E. Pekary, A.W. Reed, M. Adler, L. Turner, F. Balauag, M. Sugawara, J.A. Demetriou, and J.D. Hershman, Wadsworth-UCLA VA Med Ctr, Los Angeles, CA 90073, U.S.A.

Cassava (C) may be a goitrogenic food in man because it contains a cyanogenic glucoside which is detoxified to thiocyanate (SCN) after ingestion. We studied effects of dietary C on the thyroid in Swiss-Webster mice. Mice consumed 8 to 14 g fresh peeled C daily. Mice on C for only 2 days had increased urine and serum SCN levels compared with controls on low iodine diet (LID). After 28 days, the C mice had urine [SCN] 10-fold greater than LID or regular diet (RD) controls; urine [I] was similar to LID mice and only 1/20 that of RD mice. The ratio of SCN/I in urine was 14.9 on C, 4.3 on LID, and 0.07 on RD. The thyroid ^{125}I uptake of C mice was slightly less than LID mice at 4 hr but not at 24 hr, and was higher than uptake in RD mice. The thyroid I trap was studied in vitro in LID and C mice (2 weeks of diet): thyroid/medium I gradient was 18.7+4.3(SD) in LID, 12.7+5.1(n.s.) in C, and only 0.20+0.04 in SCN (1 mM added in vitro) thyroids. Three days of C after 5 weeks of LID reduced serum $PB^{125}I$, serum T_3, and thyroid T_4 and T_3 content. Mice eating C for 7 weeks lost nearly ½ their body weight; thyroid mass was similar to the LID mice when adjusted for body weight; serum T_4 and T_3 levels were reduced compared with the other groups, and serum TSH was not increased. These changes probably result from malnutrition. When C mice were given LID twice weekly to prevent weight loss, thyroid size and TSH did not increase. In summary, cassava may deplete thyroid iodine stores slightly, but the SCN generated by cassava ingestion does not block the thyroid I trap. These results do not support the concept that cassava has a significant goitrogenic potential in humans.

1091 INHERITED LOW-T4 SYNDROME: DEFECTIVE AUTOSOMAL STRUCTURAL GENE FOR THYROXINE-BINDING GLOBULIN. R.L. Himsworth*, Diane Parker, Dorothie Clingan, P.G.H. Byfield. Endocrinology Research Group, Clinical Research Centre, Harrow, Middlesex HA1 3UJ, UK.

An abnormal pattern of thyroid function results has been commonly observed in an Asian community. Affected individuals are euthyroid with a normal TRH test but have low total T4 (51 ± 10 nmol/l) and T3 (1.2 ± 0.3 nmol/l) levels, low T3 resin-uptakes yet normal TBG concentrations (8.4 ± 1.4 mg/l); rT3, free T4 and free T3 measurements are normal. The distribution of ^{125}I-T4 amongst the binding proteins after reverse-flow electrophoresis shows a decreased carriage on TBG (45% versus 75% in normals), consistent with a TBG having reduced avidity for T4. Calculations from Mass Action theory indicate that the observed T4 and free T4 levels could be accounted for by a two-fold decrease in avidity of TBG for T4; this small difference is difficult to demonstrate by equilibrium dialysis methods. A reduced avidity for T4 was confirmed in competitive dialysis, however, as affected TBG accumulated 10% less [^{125}I]-T4 than normal TBG when competing for a common pool of tracer. When T4 contained within peptide linkage, as in thyroglobulin, was used as a ligand TBG from these subjects was 3.5-fold less effective as a binder. The mutant TBG is inherited as a dominant trait with father to son transmission, thus unlike other inherited conditions affecting TBG concentration, this abnormality is not X-chromosome-linked. We propose that the structural gene for TBG is carried on an autosome whilst expression of that gene is controlled from the X-chromosome.

1092 THE INFLUENCE OF THYROID HORMONES ON PLASMA EPINEPHRINE AND NOREPINEPHRINE IN HUMAN. A. Honorat-Moisset*, A. Nadeau and J.H. Dussault, Laboratoires de recherche en Endocrinologie et Métabolisme, CHUL, Québec, G1V 4G2, Canada.

Clinical manifestations suggest that thyroid hormones affect the sympathetic nervous system. To verify the hypothesis that this effect might be mediated by changes in circulating catecholamines, the plasma levels of epinephrine (E) and norepinephrine (NE) were measured by a radioenzymatic method in 17 hyperthyroid, 9 euthyroid and 4 hypothyroid subjects matched for age. The thyroid status (T_4-FT_4-T_3) was determined by specific radioimmunoassays. Statistical analysis was performed by Student's "t" test.

	Hyperthyroid	Euthyroid	Hypothyroid
Age (years)	32.2 ± 3.3 †	35.0 ± 3.4	31.8 ± 1.0
T_4 (ug%)	18.3 ± 1.3	7.2 ± 0.3	2.5 ± 0.9
E (pg/ml)	40 ± 8*	14 ± 4	6 ± 6
NE (pg/ml)	118 ± 2	231 ± 3	400 ± 167**

(† mean ± S.E.M.; *$p < 0.05$ and **$p < 0.01$ vs euthyroid).
There was an excellent positive correlation ($r = 0.475$; $p < .01$) between the T_4 concentration and E whereas the correlation between T_4 and NE was negative ($r = -0.593$; $p < .001$). These results suggest that thyroid hormones influence the circulating levels of epinephrine and norepinephrine in an opposite direction. Further studies are needed to explain this phenomenon.

1093 TSH-BINDING INHIBITING AND T3-STIMULATING ACTIVITY DURING ANTITHYROID THERAPY IN GRAVES' DISEASE. R. Hörmann*, B. Saller, R. Müller, K. Mann and H.J. Karl, Dept. Internal Medicine II, Klinikum Grosshadern, University of Munich, FRG.

The heterogeneity of thyroid autoantibodies in Graves' disease (GD) is well documented by immunological studies using monoclonal technique (Valente, 1982). Some exert only binding, other ones stimulating or blocking activity. We studied T3-stimulating (TSAb) and TSH-binding inhibiting activity (TBII) in serum samples of patients with GD under methimazole treatment to characterize the behaviour of these different antibodies in the follow-up. Sera were obtained from 15 patients with GD before treatment and at 1-2 months intervals over a period of 12 months of methimazole therapy (10-40 mg/day). TSAb activity was determined by an in vitro bioassay according to Atkinson/Kendall-Taylor,1981. Porcine thyroid slices were incubated with sera in a two compartmental system and after dialysing T3 was measured by RIA. TBII were evaluated by radioreceptorassay (TRAK-assay, Henning Berlin) according to Shewring/Smith,1982. All 15 patients were positive for TSAb and TBII before treatment. TSAb activity declined into normal range in 12/15 patients within 1.8± 0.7 months ($\bar{x}\pm$ SD), TBII activity became undetectable in 8/15 patients after 2.8± 2.0 months. After 12 months of therapy TSAb was still positive in 3/15 patients, TBII in 7/15 and both in 3/15. In 8/15 patients the decrease of antibody activities was parallel, but in 4/15 patients a discordant behaviour was observed. In conclusion, TSAb activity decreased more rapidly under methimazole therapy than TBII and TBII persisted in some patients, when TSAb was negative. The dissociation of TSAb and TBII activity is relevant, if Graves' antibodies are used as markers for the activity of GD.

1094 SERUM T3, REVERSE T3 AND THYROID BINDING GLOBULIN (TBG) LEVELS BEFORE AND AFTER MAJOR WEIGHT LOSS IN MORBIDLY OBESE WOMEN. I.M. Hramiak*, J.A.Nisker Department of Medicine, Department of Obstetrics and Gynaecology, University of Western Ontario, London.

Semi-starvation has been shown by some authors to cause a fall in serum T3 levels with a concomitant increase in serum reverse T3 levels. We undertook to study serum T3, reverse T3 and TBG levels in a series of obese women. A group of thirty-six women with a mean weight of 129.5 + 21.3 Kg underwent the operation of gastric plication for obesity. A mean weight loss of 41.6 ± 13.9 Kg occurred over 11.75 ± 4.83 months on a standard gastroplasty diet of 3150 Kilojoules (750 kilocalories). The dietary components were 60% protein, 20% fat and 20% carbohydrate. The patients remained euthyroid throughout the period of observation. The serum T4, T3 and reverse T3 all remained in the normal range with no statistically significant difference between the pre-gastroplasty measurement and the point at which maximum weight loss had occurred. Simple linear regression analysis did not show any correlations between weight loss and serum T4, T3 or reverse T3 levels. The pre-gastroplasty serum TBG levels in these obese women were in the normal range unlike other binding globulins such as Sex Hormone Binding Globulin (SHBG) or Cortisol Binding Globulin (CBG) which were elevated. Furthermore, over the period of weight loss no statistically significant change in the TBG occurred. We conclude that in morbidly obese women, major weight loss is not accompanied by changes in thyroid hormone status or thyroid binding globulin.

1095 THE INNER RING (5-) MONODEIODINATION OF THYROXINE (T_4) TO 3,3',5'-TRIIODOTHYRONINE (REVERSE T_3, rT_3) IN CEREBRAL CORTEX (CC).

T.S. Huang*, A. Beredo, I.J. Chopra, D.H. Solomon, and G.N. Chua Teco, UCLA Center for Health Sciences, Los Angeles, CA 90024

T_4 (0.26uM) was incubated in 0.1M phosphate buffer (pH 7.4) containing 10mM EDTA with rat CC homogenate (~4mg protein) and 400mM dithiothreitol (DTT) for one h at 37C and the rT_3 generated was measured by RIA. There was little or no degradation of rT_3 under these conditions. CC was about 15-50 X more potent than cerebellum in the monodeiodination of T_4 to rT_3. The monodeiodinating activity (MA) in CC increased linearly with incubation period (up to 2 h) and the concentration of protein (up to 8 mg), substrate (up to 1uM) and DTT (up to 400mM); its optimal pH 7.0 and optimal temperature 37C. Its Km and Vmax approximated 0.5uM and 3300 pg/mg protein, respectively. The MA was unaffected by high concentrations of 3',5'-diiodothyronine (3',5'-T_2, up to 2.5uM), propylthiouracil (up to 25uM), methimazole (up to 100uM), sodium salicylate (up to 80uM); 8-anilino-1-napthalene sulfonic acid (ANS, up to 75uM), or ipodate (up to 80uM). Ipodate weakly inhibited the MA when studied using 100mM DTT. T_3 and 3,5-T_2 consistently inhibited T_4 to rT_3 MA in a dose dependent manner; their relative molar potency approximated 100: 12. Conclusions: a) monodeiodination of T_4 to rT_3 is enzymic in nature; b) the known potent inhibitors of the monodeiodination of T_4 to T_3 are poor inhibitors of T_4 to rT_3 MA; c) the monodeiodinations of T_4 to rT_3 and to T_3 in CC are probably catalyzed by separate deiodinases; d) a very active deiodination of T_4 to rT_3 in CC may signify an important physiological role of rT_3 in this tissue; e) Inhibition of rT_3 generation by T_3 and vice vêrsa may be homeostatic.

1096 THE COMPARATIVE VALUE OF ^{131}I WHOLE BODY SCANNING AND PLASMA TG MEASUREMENTS IN THE FOLLOW UP OF PATIENTS WITH DIFFERENTIATED CARCINOMA OF THE THYROID.

M.Hüfner, H.P.Stumpf, M.Grußendorf* and B.Kimmig, Med. Poliklinik u. Strahlenklinik, Universität Heidelberg, 6900 Heidelberg, Hospitalstr. 3, FRG

Out of about 400 patients with differentiated thyroid cancer, treated by total thyrectomy and ^{131}I therapy we have investigated two groups of patients in a retrospective study: 1. Patients who developed recurrency after a disease free intervall of at least 6 months. 2. Patients with persistently elevated plasma Tg levels (> 10 ng/ml) without any evidence for tumor persistence or recurrency (including a negative ^{131}I whole body scan).
Of 27 patients with recurrency in 22 whole body scans with 2 mC ^{131}I were available. 18 of the 22 scans were negative (82%) and only 4 patients (18%) showed a positive uptake of ^{131}I. Plasma TG was measured in all 27 patients and was positive in 21 (78%). In only one patient the diagnosis was established by the whole body scan and in this patient the TG concentration was 200 ng/ml. Secondly, 15 patients were evaluated who showed persistently elevated (> 10 ng/ml) TG levels without other evidence of recurrency. 9 of these patients developed recurrency after a follow up of 4 - 39 months (mean 18 months). Conclusions : 1. After radical ablative primary therapy only a small minority of late recurrencies show a positive ^{131}I uptake. 2. Plasma TG is the most reliable parameter under these conditions. 3. Patients with persistent elevated TG but no other evidence of residual tumor are at high risk to develop recurrency in the follow up.

1097 EFFECTS OF STARVATION ON BASAL AND TRH-STIMULATED SERUM TSH IN NORMAL AND HYPOTHYROID RATS. J.N. Hugues*, E. Enjalbert, J. Epelbaum, E. Modigliani, J. Sebaoun, A.G. Burger ; Avicenne Hospital Bobigny France ; INSERM U 159 Paris France ; Thyroid laboratory Geneva Switzerland.

Starvation decreases serum TSH levels in euthyroid rats. Since thyrotroph secretion is under the negative control of thyroid hormones, we have studied the effects of a 3 day-starvation on basal and TRH-stimulated serum TSH levels in hypothyroid as compared to normal chronically cannulated rats. In both fed and starved adult male wistar rats, a TRH-test (500 ng/100 g B.W.) was performed I.V. at 11.00 and blood was collected before, 10 and 30 minute after TRH injection. 4 groups were tested : rats with a short-term (14 d.) post-thyroidectomy hypothyroidism (group A. n = 6) ; substituted-thyroidectomized rats with a single daily I.p injection of T3 performed at 7.00 for 14 days (group B : 75 ng/100 g B.W. n = 6), (group C 175 ng/100 g B.W. n = 6) normal rats, (group D n = 10). After starvation, basal serum TSH was unchanged in highly hypothyroid groups A-B but was significantly reduced in groups C-D. In hypothyroid rats the TSH response to TRH (Δ TSH max) was significantly higher after starvation (group A : 17,9 $\pm$ 2,6 vs 10,4 $\pm$ 1,9 ng/ml $p<0.01$) ; (B : 28,7 $\pm$ 3,5 vs 16,6 $\pm$ 3,5 ng/ml $p<0.05$) and (C : 45,1 $\pm$ 8 vs 22,8 $\pm$ 2,5 ng/ml $p<0.01$). In contrast in normal rats, starvation did not affect the TSH response to TRH (18,2 $\pm$ 1,3 vs 19,2 $\pm$ 1,8 ng/ml). These results show that starvation is not effective in decreasing basal TSH secretion in hypothyroidism but hormonal replacement restores its effect. They suggest that the greater TSH response to TRH in hypothyroid starved rats could reflect a higher sensitivity to TRH or an increased pool of releasable TSH.

1098 THE HLA ANTIGENS IN KOREAN PATIENTS WITH AUTOIMMUNE THYROID DISEASES. K.B. Huh*, H.C. Lee and S.Y. Lee, Dept. of Internal Medicine, Yonsei University College of Medicine, Seoul, Korea.

HLA-A, -B and -C antigens were determined in 97 patients with Graves' disease and 37 patients with Hashimoto's thyroiditis, with the use of the microcytotoxicity test. HLA-DR antigens were determined in 79 patients with Graves' disease and 33 patients with Hashimoto's thyroiditis. The frequency of HLA-A11 antigen in patients with Graves' disease was significantly increased to 29.9% compared with 15.0% of 100 normal control subjects ($P < 0.025$). HLA-A_2 was significantly increased in patients with Hashimoto's thyroiditis compared with control group ($P < 0.025$). HLA-B_{12} was significantly decreased in patients with Graves' disease compared with control group ($P < 0.05$). There was no increased prevalence of any HLA-B antigens in patients with autoimmune thyroid diseases. Comparing with control group there was no increased frequency of any HLA-C antigens in patient groups. HLA-DRw8 was found in 35.4% of patients with Graves' disease and 42.4% of patients with Hashimoto's thyroiditis and 12.0% of 50 healthy control subjects. These differences in antigen frequencies were statistically significant ($P < 0.01$ and $P < 0.005$). HLA-DR6Y was significantly decreased in patients with Hashimoto's thyroiditis compared with control group ($P < 0.05$). In conclusion, frequencies of HLA-B antigens which are significantly increased in other races are not increased in Korean patients with autoimmune thyroid diseases, but HLA-DRw8 is significantly increased in our patients.

1099 IODOTHYRONINE 5'-DEIODINASE ACTIVITY OF RAT LIVER MICROSOMES: EFFECTS OF METHOD OF PREPARATION AND CHAPS DETERGENT. B.C.W. Hummel*, P. Fung and P.G. Walfish, Department of Medicine and Thyroid Research Laboratory, Harold Tanenbaum Department of Research, Mount Sinai Hospital and University of Toronto, Toronto, Ontario, M5G 1X5, Canada.

As a preliminary to the isolation of 5'-iodothyronine deiodinase (5'-D), we have investigated several different methods for preparing rat liver microsomes (RLM): (a) by differential centrifugation of liver homogenized at pH 7.6 in 0.25 M sucrose/0.1 M Tris-HCl/1 mM EDTA; (b) by precipitation at pH 5.4 followed by centrifugation at 2 x 10^3g/10 min; (c) by chromatography on Sepharose CL4B of a post-mitochondrial supernatant (PMS) of liver homogenized in 0.1 M phosphate buffer pH 7.4; (d) prepared as in (c) but with 0.1 M Tris-HCl buffer, pH 8.0 instead of phosphate; or (e) by centrifugation at 10^5g of the PMS in (c). Using ^{125}I-rT3 (^{125}I-reverse T3) at 370-630 pM in the presence of 6.25 mM DTT, these preparations are found to be active but had different kinetic characteristics. Activity of preparations (a) and (b) showed a linear increase in activity with protein concentration, whereas preparations (c) and (e) showed an increase in activity disproportionately greater than increase in protein concentration, suggesting the presence of limiting qualities of an endogenous activator. Relative specific activities were (a) 100, (b) 309, (c) 209, (e) 109 and (d) 4. Solubilization of 5'-D activity with various concentrations of CHAPS detergent was maximal at 4 mM, with reduced recovery of activity at 6-10 mM. Further studies showed that the extracted 5'-D activity was only weakly inhibited by CHAPS itself, suggesting that at > 4 mM CHAPS an inhibitor of 5'-D may also have been solubilized. These results indicate that (1) the method of RLM preparation can alter 5'-D enzymatic characteristics, and (2) although CHAPS has physical and biochemical properties which make it the detergent of choice for solubilization of 5'-D, the possibility of a CHAPS-induced differential release of 5'-D and its inhibitor at various concentrations should be considered. Supported by MRC (Canada) Grant #MA-8092.

1100 BIOLOGICAL ACTIVITY OF ANTI-TSH RECEPTOR ANTIBODIES AGAINST DETERMINANTS DIFFERENT FROM TSH BINDING SITE IN GRAVES' DISEASE.
Y. Ichikawa*, T. Yoshida, K. Arikawa, T. Shinozawa, S. Kawai, H. Oshima, H. Yamada, H. Tanaka and M. Homma. Department of Medicine, School of Medicine, Keio University, Tokyo 160, Japan.

Present study was performed to determine whether the antibodies against determinants different from TSH binding site may contribute to the pathogenesis of Graves' disease. Methods; ^{125}I-TSH-Triton X-100 solubilized TSH receptor-IgG complex, formed by preincubation for a total of 90 min, was immunoprecipitated by anti-human IgG goat serum. The percentage of radioactivity of washed immunoprecipitate to the total count, minus the mean percentage of normal IgG was considered as specific binding (abbreviated as IP-Ab). TSH displacing activity (TDA), and HTACS were determined according to Smith et al. (1974) and Orgiazzi et al. (1976), respectively. Results; Means of TDA, IP-Ab and HTACS in 41 normal subjects were 100±9.0%, 0±0.33% and 100±13%, while those in 30 untreated Graves' disease were 62.5±21.6% ($p<0.001$ vs. normal), 1.5±1.4% ($p<0.001$) and 140±29(S.D.)% ($p<0.001$), respectively. Positive TDA, IP-Ab and HTACS were found in 83%, 73% and 68% of Graves' patients, while those in 16 Hashimoto's patients were 25%, 25% and 0%, respectively. In untreated Graves' patients, correlation coefficient (r) between IP-Ab and HTACS was 0.64 ($p<0.01$), while r between TDA and HTACS was -0.46 ($p<0.05$). There was no significant correlation betweenIP-Ab and TDA (r=-0.25, N.S.), and all patients but one showed positive IP-Ab and/or TDA. Conclusion; These data suggest that anti-TSH receptor antibodies against determinants different from TSH binding site also contribute to the pathogenesis of Graves' desease.

1101 EFFECT OF THYROID HORMONE ON PEROXYSOMAL FLAVIN ENZYMES.

K. Ichikawa*[a], K. Hashizume[a], T. Yamada[a], and T. Hashimoto[b], [a]Department of Gerontology, Endocrinology and Metabolism, and [b]Department of Biochemistry, Shinshu University School of Medicine, Matsumoto 390, JAPAN

Although the structural modifications of peroxysome, induced by thyroid hormone, has been reported, the effect of thyroid hormone on the function of peroxysome is not known. We have studied the effect of thyroid hormone on the peroxysomal flavin enzymes using thyroidectomized(T_x+saline) or T_4-administered-thyroidectomized rats.

In liver, the activities of L-α-hydroxyacid oxidase A, D-amino acid oxidase, and catalase were reduced by thyroidectomy. The diminished activities of these enzymes were normalized by T_4 administration. The activity of acyl-CoA oxidase, on the contrary, was not affected by thyroidectomy or by T_4 administration. In kidney, the activity of L-α-hydroxyacid oxidase was reduced by thyroidectomy. And the diminished enzyme activity was normalized by T_4 administration. However, activities of D-amino acid oxidase and catalase in kidney were not modified by thyroidectomy or by T_4 administration.

The results indicate that thyroid hormone has roles to stimulate the key enzymes in D-amino acid and in fatty acid metabolism in peroxysome and that these regulation, induced by thyroid hormone, is organ specific.

1102 IMMUNOELECTRON MICROSCOPIC LOCALIZATION OF THYROGLOBULIN IN THE HUMAN THYROID GLAND.

M. Ide* , H. Mori, K. Shimizu and T. Shoji, 2nd Department of Surgery, Nippon Medical School, Tokyo, Japan.

The microidentification of the organelles containing thyroglobulin (TG) in the follicular cells of human thyroid glands was studied by the immunoelectron microscopic method. Fresh human thyroid glands were used for the purification of TG. TG was purified by differential salt fractionation and DEAE-cellulose chromatography. Anti-TG rabbit IgG antibody was obtained by immunization of this purified TG. $F(ab')_2$ fragments of anti-TG rabbit IgG antibody were prepared by pepsin digestion. The specificity of the antibody was tested on an Ouchterlony immunodiffusion plate. Conjugation of the purified $F(ab')_2$ fragments of anti-TG rabbit IgG antibody to horse radish peroxidase was performed in order to use the direct peroxidase labelled antibody method. Under immunohistochemical light microscopy, the lumical colloid and the follicular cells appeared heavily stained. Under immunoelectron microscopy, positive reactions were observed in the rough endoplasmic reticulum, the Golgi apparatus and the apical cell border. To date, no clear direct evidence of the presence of human thyroid cells has ever been reported in immunoelectron microscopic studies. This study indicates that the use of $F(ab')_2$ fragments of anti-TG rabbit IgG antibody is useful for the clear identification of TG in organelles of human thyroid follicular cells.

1103 SPONTANEOUSLY OCCURRING THYROTROPIN BINDING ACTIVITY IN THE PATIENTS WITH GRAVES' DISEASE. M. Iitaka*, and J. Ishii, Saitama Medical School, Saitama, 350-04, Japan.

Thyrotropin(TSH) binding immunoglobulin G(Ig G) with different affinities were detected. One, which showed quite abnormal value(-145) in thyrotropin binding inhibitor immunoglobulin(TBII) assay, had extremely high affinity for TSH. It bound TSH without receptor. This binding was inhibited dose dependently by bovine(b)TSH and human(h)TSH, but b-TSH was about 3 times more potent than h-TSH to inhibit the binding. LH and FSH had little influence on the binding. This activity resided monoclonally in Ig G, λ chain. The chromatographical analysis using Sephacryl S-300 showed that Ig G-TSH complex formed macromolecule with approximate molecular weight of 590,000. The patient has never had an injection of TSH, and this activity remained after the normalization of her thyroid function by subtotal thyroidectomy, which suggests that this Ig G is a spontaneously developed anti-TSH antibody. Another, which had low TSH binding activity, was found in a patient who had low positive TBII value. This binding was also inhibited by b-TSH and h-TSH. There is a hypothesis that TBII may be anti-idiotypic antibody against anti-TSH antibody. However, anti-idiotypic antibody against TBII might also be developed, and it could have TSH binding activity by the structural similarity with TSH receptor. In some rabbits immunized with Ig G containing TBII, TSH binding activity could be detected. This activity was reduced by the absorption with Ig G containing TBII but not by the absorption with normal Ig G. It indicates that anti-TBII antibody has TSH binding activity. These findings could suggest that idiotype-anti-idiotype net work may play an important role in the pathogenesis of Graves' disease. TSH binding Ig G may have a clue for the future studies.

1104 DECREASED THYROID MYOSIN LIGHT CHAIN PHOSPHORYLATION BY THYROTROPIN. M. Ikeda*, M. Ferdows, T.B. Nielsen and J.B. Field, Baylor College of Medicine, Houston, TX 77030, U.S.A.

Thyrotropin (TSH) rapidly induces endocytosis and exocytosis in thyroid. These processes, as in other cells, probably involve contractile proteins and phosphorylation of myosin light chain (MLC). In muscle contraction, MLC phosphorylation regulates interaction between myosin and actin. We examined effects of TSH and other stimulators on MLC phosphorylation in beef thyroid slices and cultured dog thyroid cells prelabelled with 0.2 mCi/ml ^{32}Pi for 45-90 min at 37°. After washing, tissue was incubated for various times with TSH or other stimulators and then the cytoskeletal fraction was prepared using Triton X-100. Myosin was also isolated by immunoprecipitation. The cytoskeleton fraction or immunoprecipitate was subjected to SDS-PAGE followed by autoradiography. In control cells several polypeptides including two of 20K and 19K daltons in cells and 20K daltons in slices, with mobilities similar to phosphorylatable MLC, contained ^{32}P. In 1 min. TSH significantly decreased phosphorylation of only the 20K and 19K polypeptides with a maximal effect at 10 min. TSH decreased MLC phosphorylation at 0.1 mU/ml and maximally at 20 mU/ml. Phosphodiesterase inhibition potentiated the TSH effect. Forskolin and dibutyryl cyclic AMP also decreased MLC phosphorylation. Decreased MLC phosphorylation correlated with cell cyclic AMP suggesting involvement of cyclic AMP. Carbachol had no effect but inhibited the action of TSH. Dephosphorylation of MLC decreases association of myosin with the cytoskeleton. Thus stimulation in thyroid, in contrast to muscle, is associated with decreased phosphorylation of MLC.

1105 PRO-OPIOMELANOCORTIN (POMC)-DERIVED PEPTIDES RELEASED FROM THE PARS INTERMEDIA (PI) OF THE ADENOHYPOPHYSIS: USE OF REVERSED-PHASE LIQUID CHROMATOGRAPHY (RP-HPLC). J. Kraicer, H.P.J. Bennett, B.C. Moor* and J.C.R. Randle, Dept. Physiology, Queen's Univ., Kingston, Ont. K7L 3N6, and Endocrine Lab., Royal Victoria Hosp., Montreal, Quebec H3A 1A1 Canada.

The PI synthesizes POMC, which through post-translational processing, gives rise to a number of structurally related peptides. In order to characterize and quantitate the spectrum of peptides released by this tissue, rat nervosa-intermedias were perifused with medium, followed by medium containing dopamine (DA, 10^{-6}M), and finally, medium alone. The 3 samples were processed by RP-HPLC and the eluted fractions were assayed by αMSH-RIA and BA (bioassay), ACTH-RIA and BA, LPH-RIA and receptor binding assay for morphine-like activity (MLA)). We find a consistent and reproducible profile of basal release, similar to the profile of peptides found in the tissue. The following peaks are found; a) with αMSH-RIA and BA, 7 peptides, the predominant form being N,O-diacetyl αMSH, b) with ACTH-RIA and BA, 10 peptides, the predominant forms being CLIP, both 18-39 and 18-38 (including glycosylated and phosphorylated forms) and ACTH 1-39 c) with LPH-RIA, mainly γ-LPH and d) with MLA, 3 peaks not yet identified. The relative proportions of peptides released do not change with DA. DA results in an approximately equimolar decrease in release of all assayable peptides, implying that DA does not alter post-translational processing of POMC. During the "recovery" period, release of all peptides returns to near pre-DA levels. (Supported by MRC and FRSQ)

1106 COMPARATIVE ASSESSMENT OF ACTH AND LIPOTROPINS DETERMINATIONS IN CUSHING'S SYNDROME. J.M. Kuhn*, D. Seurin, X. Bertagna, J.P. Luton, F. Girard, Service d'Explorations Fonctionnelles, Hopital Trousseau, and Centre de Recherches Endocrinologiques, Hopital Cochin, Paris, France.

In order to evaluate the comparative value of ACTH and Lipotropins (LPH) levels as marker of corticotropic activity, both hormones were simultaneously measured in 131 cases of Cushing's syndrome (CS): 79 Cushing's diseases (CD), 20 adrenal tumors (AT), 32 ectopic ACTH syndromes (ES). Plasma hormones were determined in the same laboratory by specific radioimmunoassays. Basal values (9 a.m.) were :

	ACTH pg/ml		LPH pg/ml	
	mean	range	mean	range
CD	57	<10-200	247	25-800
AT	-	< 15	-	< 20
ES	757	50-10,000	15,000	750-200,000
Controls	-	<10-80	-	<20-160

Both hormones were highly correlated, however in contrast to ACTH, the individual LPH values showed only slight overlap between the 3 different groups of CS.

In 8 CD where ACTH was <10 pg/ml, LPH range between 25-120 pg/ml and LVP test (10 IU IM) induced a rise in ACTH and LPH levels in 6 cases. In the 41 CD who appear cured by transphenoïdal surgery (TS) basal ACTH levels fell from 64 ± 7 pg/ml to 19 ± 4 pg/ml, $p<0.001$ and LPH levels from 250 ± 59 pg/ml to 50 ± 13 pg/ml, $p<0.01$. The follow up (1 to 4 years) showed a progressive return to normal values of basal and post stimulative hormone levels. In the 17 CD not cured by TS the hormone levels did not change. In conclusion : a) basal plasma LPH appear more discriminating than ACTH in etiological investigation of CS; b) both hormone levels provide a good index of follow up in CD treated by TS.

1107 PLASMA CONCENTRATION OF β-ENDORPHIN IN THE PERIOVULATORY PERIOD OF THE MENSTRUAL CYCLE. T. Laatikainen[x], I. Räisänen and K. Salminen, Department I of Obstetrics and Gynecology, Helsinki University Central Hospital, SF-00290 Helsinki 29, Finland.

Administration of an opioid antagonist, naloxone, has earlier been found to increase LH secretion suggesting that endogenous opioids inhibit LH secretion. Thus endorphins may participate in the regulation of the menstrual cycle at the midcycle when there are large changes in the secretion of LH. We followed plasma concentration of β-endorphin in the periovulatory period of the normal menstrual cycle. Follicle development was followed by ultrasound in 5 healthy women in order to estimate the day of ovulation. Plasma samples for β-endorphin assy were taken daily at 13.00 - -15.00 hr. Plasma β-endorphin concentration was determined by radioimmunoassay after purification of plasma β-endorphin by high-performance liquid chromatography using a cation exchange column. This step separated β-endorphin completely from β-lipotropin. The results of β-endorphin determinations were arranged according to the day of ovulation. The mean plasma concentration of β-endorphin was 4.6 ± 0.8 pmol/l 2 days and 4.4 ± 1.4 pmol/l 1 day before, and 5.2 ± 1.2 pmol/l on the day of ovulation, and 8.0 ± 1.3 and 6.5 ± 2.2 pmol/l 1 day and 2 days after the day of ovulation, respectively. Paired comparison of the values on the day before and one day after ovulation showed a significant increase ($p < 0.01$). These results suggest that β-endorphin secretion increases at the time of ovulation. The relationship between this change and that in the serum level of estradiol, progesterone and LH is discussed.

1108 PROPERTIES AND DISTRIBUTION OF γ-ENDORPHIN GENERATING ENDOPEPTIDASE (γ EGE) IN RAT BRAIN AND PERIPHERAL TISSUES. J.L.M. Lebouille*, J.P.H. Burbach, and E.R. De Kloet, Rudolf Magnus Institute for Pharmacology, Vondellaan 6, 3521 GD Utrecht, The Netherlands.

γ-Endorphin (β-endorphin-(1-17), γE) is a biologically active peptide generated from β-endorphin (βE) by γE generating endopeptidase (γEGE). γEGE was quantitated by an assay using as a probe the modified βE fragment Ac-Val-Thr-Leu-Phe-[ε-$^{14}CH_3$]Lys-$NHCH_3$. Initial cleavage site of this fragment is exclusively the Leu-Phe bond when incubated with brain fractions. It is effectively protected against exopeptidases, and is insensitive to cathepsin D. βE inhibited substrate conversion competitively. Thus the fragment is suited to measure specifically γEGE activity. Enzyme activity was inhibited by PMSF, pepstatin and divalent metals. No inhibition occured with EDTA, EGTA and Hg^+, while β-mercaptoethanol and DTT stimulated activity. The pH optimum of γEGE was 8.5. In the brain highest γEGE activity was in the cytosol being 15 to 20 fold higher than in a particulate fraction. Highest cytosolic activity was found in cerebellum and striatum, while lowest activity was found in midbrain, thalamus, hypothalamus and septum. In the particulate fraction highest activity was shown in amygdala, medulla, midbrain and cerebellum, and lowest activity in cortex and hippocampus. γEGE activity differed markedly between rat peripheral tissues. Highest cytosolic activity was found in testis (10 fold higher than brain), while no enzyme activity was detected in plasma. The thyroid gland contained highest particulate activity. In conclusion, γE can be produced by a basic thiol-endopeptidase different from any known one. Its wide distribution suggests that many tissues have the potential to generate γE from βE.

1109 STEROID SPECIFICITY OF GLUCOCORTICOID-INDUCED RESTORATION OF NORMAL WEIGHT GAIN AFTER ADRENALECTOMY IS COMPATIBLE WITH AN ACTION ON BRAIN CORTICOSTEROID RECEPTORS. N. Levin*, C. Cascio, J. Shinsako and M. F. Dallman. Dept. Physiology, University of California, San Francisco, CA 94143 USA.

Although adrenalectomy (ADX) in rats is a rapidly accomplished and fairly minor surgical procedure, we find that ADX decreases the rate of weight gain in growing male rats during the first 48h post-operatively compared to that of sham-operated controls (SHAM). In 7 experiments ADX rats gained between 10 and 50% as much weight as SHAMS during the first 48h (ΔBW, $p \leq 0.05$, each experiment) despite provision of 0.5%NaCl to drink. To test whether lack of corticosterone(B) was responsible for the decreased rate of weight gain, ADX rats were given 20μgB/ml 0.5%NaCl to drink. The intake of B was sufficient to increase B levels in brain to near normal (B in brain(ng/g): SHAM 19.4±4.4, ADX 4.3±0.7, ADX+B 15.6±3.9) and todecrease plasma ACTH 3 min after exposure to ether vapor significantly (ACTH(pg/ml): SHAM 173±13, ADX 1181±111, ADX+B 445±153). In 6 experiments B replacement of ADX rats resulted in weight gains of 66-91% compared to SHAM during the first 48h (ΔBW>ADX, $p \leq 0.05$, each experiment). Dexamethasone (0.5μg/ml0.5% NaCl) inhibited weight gain in both SHAM and ADX rats ($p < 0.05$ vs NaCl). Progesterone (60μg/ml0.5%NaCl) did not affect weight gain of either SHAM or ADX rats (p=NS vs NaCl), whereas deoxycorticosterone (40μg/ml0.5%NaCl) completely restored weight gain of ADX rats to normal without affecting weight gain in SHAM rats. We conclude that: 1. in the absence of B the surgical stress of ADX reduces normal food intake and body weight gain; and, 2. the steroid specificity of the effect suggests that it is mediated by receptors in the central nervous system (see Endocrinol. 113:2043, 1983). (Supported in part by USPHS grant AM28172.)

1110 ELECTRONMICROGRAPHIC LOCALIZATION OF ir-βEP GRANULES IN SUBPOPULATIONS OF RAT GRANULOSA CELLS. A.T.W. Lim*, Z.F. Yen, S.J. Lolait, A. Pyliotis, B.H. Toh and J.W. Funder, Medical Research Centre and Department of Pathology, Prince Henry's Hospital, Melbourne; Monash University Department of Pathology & Immunology, Alfred Hospital, Victoria, Australia 3000.

Previously we have demonstrated and localized immunoreactive β-endorphin (ir-βEP) in the ovary (Nature 303:709, 1983). We here report EM identification of cytoplasmic ir-βEP-positive granules in subpopulations of rat granulosa cells. Adult female S-D rats (250-300g) with 4d cycles were sacrificed at late estrus or diestrus, or immature rats at 20d; ovaries and pituitaries were removed, fixed in periodate-lysine-paraformaldehyde and tissue at -70C sectioned (7-10μm) for staining by the unlabeled antibody (R56:dilution 1/100-1/300) peroxidase-antiperoxidase technique. Two distinct forms of cytoplasmic ir-βEP +ve granules (0.5-0.7μm) scattered randomly within the luteinized granulosa cells were identified. The predominant type were vesicular in late estrus corpora lutea, but much more disperse at diestrus. Smaller ir-βEP +ve granules (0.2-0.3μm), similar to those found in the pituicytes, were seen in corona radiata granulosa cells and in the zona pellucida of pre-antral and small antral follicles of both mature and immature rat ovaries. In contrast, ir-βEP +ve granules were absent in oocytes, membranous granulosa cells, theca and interstitial cells. We conclude that the presence of different ir-βEP +ve granules in subpopulations of granulosa cells supports a paracrine role for βEP or its congeners in follicular development and/or granulosa cell-oocyte interactions. Supported by the National Health & Medical Research Council of Australia, and the Australian Development Assistance Bureau (ZFY).

1111 SECRETION OF PEPTIDE α-AMIDATION ACTIVITY AND CARBOXYPEPTIDASE E BY CORTICOTROPIC TUMOR CELLS. R.Mains* and B.Eipper, Neuroscience Dept., The Johns Hopkins University School of Medicine, Baltimore, MD 21205, U.S.A.

Secretion of the enzyme activities involved in performing two essential COOH-terminal modifications during the biosynthesis of bioactive peptides has been examined. Mouse AtT-20 tumor cells, a model for anterior pituitary corticotropes, were attached to Cytodex beads and perfused at 37° with tissue culture medium containing bovine serum albumin and various secretagogues. Fractions were assayed for ACTH/endorphin-related peptides by immunoassay, for peptide COOH-terminal α-amidation activity using ^{125}I-D-Tyr-Val-Gly, and for peptide carboxypeptidase E activity using ^{3}H-Bz-Phe-Leu-Arg. Four secretagogues caused parallel increases in the secretion rates for hormone, α-amidation activity, and carboxypeptidase E activity: corticotropin releasing factor, isoproterenol (β-adrenergic agonist), cAMP and $BaCl_2$. Stimulated secretion of hormone and both enzyme activities was blocked by physiological levels of glucocorticoids and by 0.2 mM $CoCl_2$. The α-amidation activity was stable for 1 hour at 37° after secretion, and was similar to the secretory granule activity; it was copper and ascorbate-dependent with a pH optimum around 8, an apparent Mr during gel filtration of about 50-60,000, and a Km for D-Tyr-Val-Gly of ~10 μM. Secreted carboxypeptidase E was stable when acidified to pH 5.6 and was similar to the secretory granule-associated enzyme: cobalt-stimulated; guanidinoethylmercaptosuccinate-blocked; pH optimum around 5-6; Km for Bz-Phe-Leu-Arg ~65 μM. The regulation of the tissue levels of hormone and both enzyme activities by chronic exposure to glucocorticoids has been examined. Supported by AM-32948, DA-00266, and The McKnight Foundation.

1112 IN VITRO STIMULATION OF PANCREATIC AMYLASE SECRETION BY ACTH RELATED PEPTIDES. JB Marshall, LP Kapcala, AJ McCullough*, and L. Manning, Department of Medicine, Cleveland Metropolitan General Hospital, Case Western Reserve University, Cleveland, Ohio 44109.

We have identified (RIA) immunoreactive (IR-) ACTH in rat pancreatic extracts. This IR-ACTH appears to be authentic on the basis of typical criteria used to authenticate immunoreactivity. Although previous studies have suggested corticotropin-like intermediate lobe peptide (CLIP = $ACTH_{18-39}$), a natural derivative of $ACTH_{1-39}$, stimulates insulin secretion, effects on pancreatic exocrine function have not been studied. To determine whether CLIP alters pancreatic exocrine function, we studied the effects of CLIP on pancreatic amylase secretion. Increasing concentrations of synthetic CLIP (10^{-9}-10^{-5}M) were incubated with isolated rat pancreatic lobules, and amylase secretion was measured and compared to the effects of recognized amylase secretagogues (secretin, carbachol, cholecystokinin 8 -CCK-8). CLIP produced a dose response stimulation of amylase secretion with the greatest increment (239%) at the highest dose. The stimulated increase in amylase secretion by CLIP was greater than secretin and CCK-8, but similar to carbachol. To investigate further whether the amino terminal portion of $ACTH_{1-39}$ produced any effect on amylase secretion, the response to synthetic $ACTH_{1-18}$ was also studied. Amylase secretion rose with increasing $ACTH_{1-18}$ (10^{-9}M -10^{-5}M), showing the greatest increment (391%) at 10^{-5}M. Conclusions: 1. ACTH related peptides may be potent physiological modulators of pancreatic amylase secretion. 2. Because CLIP ($ACTH_{18-39}$) and $ACTH_{1-18}$ do not share any amino acid homology, these data suggest at least 2 different receptors mediate the stimulation of amylase secretion by ACTH related peptides.

1113 μ, BUT NOT K OR δ OPIATE RECEPTORS MODULATE LUTEINIZING HORMONE AND PROLACTIN RELEASE. A.Martini, F.Petraglia, P.Sacerdote, A.R.Genazzani, A.E.Panerai. Dept.Pharmacology Univ of Milano, and Dept.Obst & Gynaecol. Univ of Modena, Italy.

Pharmacological doses of exogenous or endogenous opiates (B-endorphin, the enkephalins, dynorphin) have been shown to increase LH and decrease PRL secretion. The existence of multiple opiate receptors has been postulated and it is well known that morphine and B-endorphin have higher affinity for the μ receptor, ethylketocyclazocine and Dynorphin for the K receptor and the enkephalins for the δ receptor. However, at the doses usually employed in endocrinological studies, both exogenous and endogenous opiates loose their receptor specificity. In order to better specify the role of the different receptors and endogenous opiates in the regulation of LH and PRL secretion, we employed several opiate antagonists specific for different opiate receptors. We employed graded doses of the following drugs: Naloxone (μ, B-endorphin antagonist), MR 1452 and MR 2266 (K, dynorphin antagonists), ICI 154129 (δ, enkephalins antagonist). The role of different opiate receptors on LH secretion was evaluated in the following animal models: prepuberal female rats, adult male rats; the role of PRL secretion was studied in: lactating rats, stressed female rats, estradiol benzoate-primed ovariectomized rats. The results we obtained indicate that only naloxone is capable of increasing LH and decreases PRL secretion. The other antagonists employed were not effective in modulating LH and PRL secretion although, at the doses we used, affect other behavioral parameters known as K or δ mediated. In conclusion, our results indicate that only the μ receptor is responsible for the opiate modulation of LH and PRL secretion, and that the endogenous opiate most probably involved is B-endorphin.

1114 EFFECT OF γ1-MELANOTROPIN (MSH) ON ALDOSTERONE SECRETION IN ISOLATED RAT GLOMERULOSA CELLS IN VITRO. T. Horiuchi*, K. Tanaka, T. Watabe, M. Hasegawa, K. Nakamura, S. Miyabe, H. Yoshida, T. Kinouchi, A. Kanbegawa and N. Shimizu, First Department of Medicine and Department of Gynecology and Obstetrics, Teikyo University School of Medicine, Tokyo 173 Japan.

The N-terminal fragment (16K fragment) of pro-opiomelanocortin (POMC) has been reported to potentiate ACTH-stimulated aldosterone secretion. To examine the effect of γ1-MSH, which is contained in the 16 K fragment of POMC, on aldosterone secretion, γ1-MSH (10nM-10μM) was incubated with isolated rat adrenal glomerulosa cells (10^5 cells/ml) with or without a Ca ion channel blocker (verapamil, 100nM-100μM) or a calmodulin inhibitor (trifluoperazine, 100nM-100μM) for 2 hrs at 37° C under 95% O_2-5% CO_2. After incubation, the concentrations of aldosterone and cAMP in the medium were determined by radioimmunoassay. γ1-MSH stimulated aldosterone secretion significantly in a dose-responsive manner (127, 239, 371 and 615% of the basal level at 10nM, 100nM, 1μM and 10μM, respectively). Aldosterone secretion stimulated by γ1-MSH was completely suppressed by the addition of either verapamil (100μM) or trifluoperazine (100μM). cAMP in the medium after stimulation with γ1-MSH did not differ significantly from the control level, although a significant rise in cAMP concentration was observed with 1pM to 30pM of ACTH. These results suggest that γ1-MSH may play some physiological role in the regulation of aldosterone secretion. The present data also indicate that stimulation of aldosterone secretion by γ1-MSH is mediated at least in part by Ca ion and that cAMP is probably not involved in this secretory process.

1115 PURIFICATION OF HUMAN ADRENAL ZONA FASCICULATA AND ZONA RETICULARIS CELLS ON LINEAR PERCOLL GRADIENTS. P.J. Hyatt* and K. Bhatt, Biophysical Endocrinology Unit, Dept. of Medical Physics and Institute of Nuclear Medicine, Middlesex Hospital Medical School, Cleveland St.,London W1,U.K.

Collagenase-dispersed adult human adrenal zona fasciculata-reticularis cell preparations containing 49% zona fasciculata (ZF) cells and 51% zona reticularis (ZR) cells were purified by isopycnic centrifugation on linear gradients of Percoll in order to examine the relative steroidogenic potential of the purified ZF and ZR cells. Fractionation of the gradients yielded 6 or 7 cell preparations which had a range of cell purities from 92% $\pm$ 3.5 (mean $\pm$ SEM,n=4) ZR cells at the highest density (1.065g/ml) to 90% $\mp$ 4.2 (mean $\mp$ SEM,n=4) ZF cells at the lowest density (1.024g/ml). Both cell types when incubated produced cortisol,androstenedione, DHA and DHA sulphate, as measured by radioimmunoassay. ZF cells produced relatively greater quantities of cortisol and ZR cells relatively greater quantities of the three androgens measured, both basally and in response to 3 doses of ACTH(10^{-14},10^{-12} and 10^{-8}M). DHA sulphate production was not stimulated by ACTH in ZF cells or in the cells of the two males studied, but was stimulated in the ZR cells of the two females studied, at all three doses of ACTH. In order to examine the relative bias of ZR cells towards androgen production, the ratio of androstenedione + DHA + DHA sulphate/cortisol was examined, and it was found that for basal steroid outputs this ratio was 3 to 25-fold higher for ZR than for ZF cells, indicating the bias of ZR cells towards androgen production. This bias was maintained on stimulation with ACTH. These purified human adrenal cell preparations will be valuable in the future assessment of putative adrenal androgen stimulating factors.

1116 MECHANISM FOR DIVERGENT MINERALOCORTICOID HORMONE (MCH) LEVELS AFTER CONTINUOUS ACTH STIMULATION IN CLASSIC (C) AND NONCLASSIC (NC) TYPES OF 21-HYDROXYLASE DEFICIENCY (21-OHD). C.E. Kater, E.G. Biglieri*, and B. Wajchenberg, Escola Paulista de Medicina, Hospital das Clinicas, São Paulo, Brasil and Medical Service, SF General Hospital, San Francisco, CA USA.

Identification of suspected patients with C or NC type of 21-OHD relies on the often imprecise ACTH-stimulated level of 17α-hydroxyprogesterone. Continuous superphysiologic doses of ACTH produced divergent steroid responses in 9 patients (5-56 yr; 5 C, 4 NC), 6 normal subjects (NS), and 3 women (21-30 yr) with hirsutism and menstrual irregularities (NC subtype). On 20 mEq Na/d, ACTH gel was given every 8 h for 72 h. RIA of plasma cortisol (F), corticosterone (B), 18-hydroxyB (18-OHB), deoxycorticosterone (DOC), 18-hydroxyDOC and aldosterone (A) levels were measured daily at 0800 h. In C F levels in μg/dl (4.9±2.2) were lower than in NC (10.9±3.0, $p<0.05$) and NS (10.7±4.0, $p<0.05$). ACTH produced a subnormal increase to 14.5 by day 3. In NC F rose slower than in NS during the 1st 24 h ($p<0.05$) but reached normal levels at 48 h. B and 18-OHDOC were normal but DOC was elevated (25.3±5.0 ng/dl, $p<0.05$) and all failed to increase with ACTH. A and 18-OHB were elevated in both groups at 29.1±5.9 ($p<0.02$) and 83.8±15.3 ($p<0.01$) ng/dl. Both steroids increased briskly after 24 h of ACTH in all types but did not "turn off" to normal levels in C but did in NC. In the NC ACTH failed to increase DOC, B and 18-OHDOC but F, A and 18-OHB patterns were normal. Paired values of stimulated F and A in NS, C and NC types (n=76) showed negative correlation (r-0.63, $p<0.001$) and suggest a causal effect. ACTH-stimulated A distinguishes C from NC; the unresponsive 17-deoxy pathway of zona fasciculata (DOC, B, 18-OHDOC) is defective in all 21-OHDS.

1117 EVIDENCE OF FAMILIAL TRANSCORTIN DEFICIENCY.

H. Kaufman*, S. Bruhis, A. Roitman, B. Baumann and Z. Laron.
The Endocrinological Laboratory and the Institute of Pediatric and Adolescent Endocrinology, Beilinson Medical Center, Petah-Tikva,Israel.

A screening cortisol test, in a 15 year old boy, with slightly delayed puberty and gynecomastia, revealed very low plasmatic values (0.5-1.5 μg %) and normal urinary values (17 OHCS 6.9-10.8 mgr/24 h; 11 OHCS 25-42 μgr/24 h). These findings and the lack of any other signs of hypothalamo-pituitary-adrenal axis disturbances led us to presume a corticosteroid binding globulin (transcortin) deficiency. Transcortin determinations in six members of the patient's family revealed an undetectable level in the propositus and his sister and about half of the normal values (9.3-13 mgr/L; normal 22.5$\pm$4 mgr/L) in another brother and the two parents (first cousins). The levels of transcortin was normal (21 mgr/L) in only one of the four children. These results suggest a genetically determined transcortin deficiency with an autosomal, codominant or recessive, pattern of inheritance. The free cortisol values in all members of the family were within the normal range. Other estrogen sensitive proteins (SHBG; TBG) were normal. No other evidence of endocrine abnormality was found. The clinical significance is discussed.

1118 DIFFERENCES IN METABOLIC PROPERTIES BETWEEN CORTISOL, PREDNISOLONE AND DEXAMETHASONE IN LIVER AND RENAL DISEASES.

S. Kawai*, Y. Ichikawa, H. Oshima, H. Tanaka, H. Yamada, T. Yoshida, T. Shinozawa, K. Arikawa, and M. Homma, School of Medicine, Keio University, Tokyo 160, Japan.

Since the previous reports about the altered metabolism of various glucocorticoids in liver and renal diseases were inconsistent, this study was undertaken to clarify the metabolism of cortisol, prednisolone and dexamethasone in these diseases by a comparative study. One mg each of these glucocorticoids were given iv simultaneously, after 1 mg of betamethasone was administered on the previous night for suppression of endogenous cortisol. Plasma steroid levels of periodically collected blood samples were assayed by respective RIA after separation by paper chromatography. The results of t1/2 and MCR of cortisol, prednisolone and dexamethasone were as follows: t1/2, 2.1±0.2 (M±SD), 2.5±0.7 and 3.5±1.0 h, MCR, 114±20, 75±25 and 153±45 l/day/m^2 in 16 normal controls; t1/2, 2.8**±0.8, 3.0±0.7 and 5.9**±2.3 h, MCR, 92±35, 61±14 and 98**±43 l/day/m^2 in 20 with chronic liver diseases; t1/2, 2.9**±1.0, 3.7**±1.2 and 2.4**±0.7 h, MCR, 102±42, 47**±22 and 259*± 120 l/day/m^2 in 16 with chronic renal failure, respectively (**P<0.01, *P< 0.02 vs. normal). That is, the metabolism of cortisol was disturbed in both liver and renal diseases, while that of prednisolone was disturbed only in renal diseases. On the other hand, dexamethasone metabolism was disturbed in liver diseases, but was definitely accelerated in renal diseases.

These results suggest that one must pay attention to the kind of glucocorticoids administered for the therapeutic purposes, or for the estimation of hypothalamic-pituitary-adrenocortical axis in patients with chronic liver diseases and chronic renal failure.

1119 INFLUENCE OF INTRAADRENAL PROGESTERONE LEVEL ON IN VITRO PRODUCTION OF CORTISOL IN PIG ADRENAL, L. Kecskés, Central Laboratory, University Medical School, PÉCS, H-7643, Hungary.

Besides the main glucocorticoid, cortisol the human adrenal cortex secretes corticosterone and some steroid intermediates, too, tough in less extent. The homogenates of pig adrenal cortex were used as model to study the relationship between the two glucocorticoids and the steroid intermediates. The in vitro production of cortisol was 1.4-4.4 nM/g/min in oxygen and 0.6-1.4 nM/g/min in air atmosphere. That of corticosterone was 3.4-3.8 nM/g/min and 2.2-4.4nM/g/min respectively. Among the steroid intermediates, progesterone was present in the most significant amount in the samples, its production was 0.08-4.90 nM/g/min in oxygen and 2.8-4.8 nM/g/min in air atmosphere. A negative correlation was observed between the production of cortisol and progesterone. This observation suggests that the intraadrenal elevation of progesterone level during incubation inhibits the cortisol production on the Δ^5-pathway. The corticosterone pathway, however, exerts a shunt effect on the intraadrenal progesterone level. The fall of partial pressure of oxygen decreases the production of cortisol from endogenous substrates during incubation, but hardly touches the shunt effect of corticosterone pathway. The shunt effect of corticosterone pathway has been supported by other investigations. Besides cortisol metabolites, a-tetrahydrocorticosterone was found to be the most prominent steroid in the urine of prepubertal girls during surgical stress.

1120 AUTONOMIC NEUROPATHY IN DIABETICS-AUTONOMIC FUNCTION AND PLASMA CATECHOLAMINE- N.Kikuchi*, M.Nanno, Y.Oki, S.Ohgo, H.Kurahachi and T.Yoshimi, 2nd Div., of Dep. of Int. Med., Hamamatsu University School of Medicine, Hamamatsu, Japan.

In order to evaluate sympathetic function in diabetics quantitatively, we studied the response of plasma norepinephrine(NE) and epinephrine(E) after 10 min of upright posture and 5 min handgrip being upright, and smoking a piece of "Peace" in four age-matched groups. We also studied R-R interval variation of ECG(CV:Coefficient of Variation) as a parameter of parasympathetic function and compared this CV with sympathetic function. Basal NE did not differ in all groups(G). However, NE responses to both standing and handgrip stimuli were markedly reduced not only in 15 diabetics with autonomic disorder(G.4) but also in 15 diabetics with peripheral neuropathy devoid of autonomic disorder(G.3). NE increments in 15 diabetics without complications(G.2) were not so different with those in normal subjects(G.1) Basal E levels did not differ and significant changes were not observed after both stimuli in all groups. After smoking, both NE and E responses were markedly reduced in G.4 and, even in G.3, responses were smaller than those in G.1 and G.2. In diabetics, CV was correlated with NE increments after standing. Also CV was correlated strongly with NE and E increments after smoking. These results suggested: 1) Measuring NE and E after standing, handgrip and smoking is a sensitive, specific and simple method in evaluating sympathetic neuropathy in diabetics. 2) The sympathoadrenomedullary function was already impaired before autonomic disorder appear. 3) There is parallel dysfunction between sympathetic and parasympathetic nervous systems.

1121 11β-HYDROXYSTEROID DEHYDROGENASE: EVIDENCE FOR INDEPENDENT 11-OXIDASE AND 11-REDUCTASE ACTIVITIES. Vijaya Lakshmi* and Carl Monder, The Population Council, 1230 York Avenue, New York, New York 10021.

We are studying the properties of 11β-hydroxysteroid dehydrogenase (11-HSD). The oxidase-reductase (O-R) ratios of rat liver microsomal (mc) enzyme extracted with detergents varied widely and depended on the detergent used. In 3-[(3-cholamidopropyl)dimethylammonio]-1-propanesulfonate (CHAPS), only 11-reductase was detected. Digitonin stimulated oxidase, but not reductase. Zwittergents and Tritons extracted both activities with varying selectivity. O-R ratios were affected by detergent conc's, pH of extraction, ionic strength and temperature. The physical state of the phospholipid matrix affected 11-reductase activity. The transition temp. for mc bound activity determined from Arrhenius plots coincided with the phase transition temp. for mc lipids. Detergent solubilized 11-reductase showed no temp. dependent phase transition. The activation energy of microsomal or solubilized 11-oxidase showed no discontinuities over the entire range of temp. studied. In Triton DF-18, mc 11-oxidase activity increased. Latency was 75% (Latency = 100 $(A_D - A_U)/A_D$, where A_D is activity of mc enzyme in detergent and A_U is unstimulated activity). Triton DF-18 did not alter 11-reductase activity. Lipid dependence of enzyme activity was studied directly by treating mc with phospholipase A_2 and phospholipase C. Losses of 11-reductase activity were 70% and 80%, respectively. Triton DF-18 reactivated phospholipase inactivated reductase. In contrast, both phosphohydrolases stimulated 11-oxidase. We conclude that 11-oxidase and 11-reductase are separate, closely linked components of 11-HSD. Supported by USPH Service grant HD-17043.

1122 A NOVEL APPROACH TO THE BIOLOGICAL SCREENING OF DRUGS AFFECTING ENDOCRINE TISSUES. A. Lambert*, J.C. Ratcliffe and W.R. Robertson, Univ. Manchester, Dept. Chem. Path. Hope Hospital, Salford, M6 8HD, U.K.

Due to the lack of satisfactory in vitro bioassays, the quality of structural or chemical assays for the screening of biopotency of drugs cannot be easily evaluated. We report on the use of dispersed endocrine cells for this purpose. When such cells are maximally and specifically stimulated by the hormone controlling their function, the effect of an agent (eg a drug) which interferes with end-product secretion can be measured. This approach has been studied with trypsin dispersed guinea-pig adrenal cells, cortisol production by which was maximally stimulated by ACTH (>50ng/L). The anti-steroidogenic effect of 8 drugs of differing structure and therapeutic function (aminoglutethimide, metyrapone, trilostane, danazol, epostane, megestrol acetate, stanozolol and etomidate) was tested. Aliquots of the cells were treated for 90 min at 37°C with ACTH (50ng/L) alone or in combination with the drugs, all of which depressed steroid output in a dose-related fashion. The concentration of drug which inhibited cortisol output by 50% was (μmol/l, mean ±S.D.): etomidate 0.097±0.003 (n=4), epostane 0.44±0.04 (n=3), trilostane 1.3±0.3 (n=12), metyrapone 3.5±1.4 (n=6), megestrol acetate 11±3 (n=2), danazol 22±6 (n=6), aminoglutethimide 41±10 (n=5), stanozolol 50±5 (n=2). Thus, etomidate, an anaesthetic, is more potent than the established anti- steroidogenic drugs metyrapone and aminoglutethimide. In conclusion, this bioassay offers a promising new approach to the assessment of biological potency of drugs affecting endocrine tissues.

1123 ADRENOCORTICAL RESPONSE TO ACTH-Z IN THE YOUNG AND ELDERLY MEN.

T. Maki*, K. Kato, K. Muta and H. Ibayashi, Third Department of Internal Medicine, Faculty of Medicine, Kyushu University, Fukuoka 812, Japan

The influence of aging on the steroid secretory capacity of adrenal gland was evaluated by comparing young(20-21 yr, n=5) with elderly (77-86 yr, n=8) healthy male subjects. After the administration of ACTH-Z(1 mg, im) during the treatment of dexamethasone(1 mg, daily), blood samples were taken at time 0,1,2,3,6,12 and 24 h. The mean basal levels of serum pregnenolone(P_5), dehydroepiandrosterone(DHEA), progesterone(P_4), aldosterone(Ald) and cortisol(F) were significantly lower in the elderly men than those in the young men. After the ACTH-Z stimulation, the initial responses for 3 hours of all steroids, such as P_5, 17α-hydroxypregnenolone ($17OHP_5$), DHEA, P_4, 17α-hydroxyprogesterone($17OHP_4$), androstenedione(A), Ald and F, were lower in the elderly men than those in the young men. When the 24-hour secretion rates of steroid hormones were compared by area which indicated the increased area for 24 hours after the ACTH-Z administration, the secretion rate of F showed no significant difference between two groups, but that of DHEA was significantly low in the elderly men. The 24-hour secretion rates of P_5 and P_4 were not impaired, and that of $17OHP_4$ was significantly high in the elderly men. These results indicate that, in elderly men, the adrenocortical sensitivity to ACTH is decreased and the secretory capacity of Δ^5-steroid is impaired, whereas the secretion of Δ^4-steroid is comparable or higher, suggesting the decreased activity of 17,20-lyase in the elderly adrenal gland.

1124 ALTERATION OF GROWTH HORMONE (GH) AND PROLACTIN (PRL) DOPAMINE REGULATION IN AGING.

G. MANCIET*, P. GALLEY, JP EMERIAU, P. ROGER and J. RIVIERE. Service de Médecine Interne-Gériatrie et d'Endocrinologie I - CHU de Bordeaux - 33604 PESSAC - FRANCE

Conflicting results are reported about the age-related alterations of GH and PRL secretion. In order to assess the respective role of age and of illnesses and undernutrition we have studied the response of GH and PRL to different provocative tests in three groups of male subjects : G1 : 5 young controls (age from 24 to 36 y) ; G2 : 15 healthy old men (age from 71 to 89 y) ; G3 : 9 old undernourished patients (age from 70 to 89 y). Basal PRL serum levels and PRL response to TRH are similar in the three groups. PRL decrease after L.DOPA (500 mg per os) was significantly lower in old subjects nadir expressed as percent of the mean basal value : G1 : 43 % ; G2 : 60 % ; G3 : 61 %). GH basal levels are slightly higher in old subjects - TRH elicited a GH surge in 3 subjects of G2 and in five subjects of G3. The main difference occurs in the response to L.DOPA stimulation : the mean peak value is 25,2 $\pm$ 5 ng.ml^{-1*} in G1, 12 $\pm$ 5 ng.ml^{-1*} in G2, but only 2 patients of G3 give a response above 5 ng.ml^{-1*}. It must be noticed that the G3 response to insulinic hypoglycaemia is higher in G3 (53,4 $\pm$ 12 ng.ml^{-1*}) than in G2 (41,9 $\pm$ 9 ng.ml^{-1*}) or in G1 (33,92 $\pm$ 2,5 ng.ml^{-1*}). The present data point out that : 1. the lactotrophs and somatotrophs remain active in old age ; 2. aging is associated with a slight decrease of inhibitory effect of L.DOPA on the lactotrophs ; 3. Dopamine action on GH regulation is altered at the hypothalamic level in old subjects and this latter effect is enhanced by undernutrition.

* mean $\pm$ S.E.M.

1125 CHRONIC EXPOSURE TO VASOPRESSIN IN THE AGING RAT IMPAIRS RENAL RESPONSIVENESS TO VASOPRESSIN. Myron Miller*, VA Medical Center and SUNY Upstate Medical Center, Syracuse, N.Y. 13210, USA.

Two seemingly paradoxical changes in water regulation occur in the aging rat - hypersecretion of vasopressin (ADH) from the neurohypophysial system and progressive decline in renal concentrating capacity. This study tests the hypothesis that chronic exposure of the kidney to increased amounts of ADH impairs renal responsiveness to ADH. Male rats 8-9 months old were injected daily for 28 days with 200 mU vasopressin tannate in oil (PTO) or oil alone. Chronic PTO administration decreased serum Na (144.9 $\pm$ 0.4 vs 146.2 $\pm$ 0.4 mEq/l, $P < 0.025$) and increased plasma ADH concentration (2.8 $\pm$ 0.3 vs 1.2 $\pm$ 0.3 μU/ml, $P < 0.005$). Treatment did not affect basal urine osmolality (Uosm). However, 48 hr of water deprivation increased Uosm by only 593 mOsm in PTO animals in contrast to 875 mOsm in control animals. Similarly, DDAVP injection raised Uosm by 321 mOsm in the PTO group compared to a rise of 519 mOsm in the control rats. Basal cyclic AMP (cAMP) content of kidney medulla slices did not differ in the two groups. Following exposure of the slices to 10^{-6} M DDAVP, cAMP content of medullary tissue from PTO animals did not change while cAMP in control animals rose from 2.56 $\pm$ 0.27 to 4.49 $\pm$ 0.52 p mol/mg ($P < 0.005$). Incubation of renal medullary slices from PTO rats with DDAVP caused no increased release of cAMP into the medium while slices from control animals exhibited an increase from 3.46 $\pm$ 0.54 to 6.63 $\pm$ 1.78 p mol/mg ($P < 0.05$). These impairments of both in vivo and in vitro renal response following chronic exposure to ADH may be a consequence of altered renal membrane receptor function. Chronic ADH hypersecretion in the aging rat appears to be a primary event resulting in decreased water conserving capacity of the kidney.

1126 FUNCTIONAL CLASSIFICATION OF ELDERLY MALE BY SERUM LEVELS OF TESTOSTERONE (T) AND LUTEINIZING HORMONE (LH). K. Muta, T. Maki, K. Kato and H. Ibayashi, Faculty of Medicine, Kyushu University, Fukuoka, Japan.

Age-related changes of serum T and LH are well recognized and we have already reported that serum T shows a gradual decrease from fifties of age and serum LH rises complementally but falls from the eighth decade in male senescence.
To establish an useful index of aging for individual in man, 234 aged subjects (60-101 yrs. old) were devided into 4 groups by the median values of serum T and LH (T; M=403 ng/dl, LH; M'=25.8 mIU/ml, group I (n=50): $T > M$, $LH < M'$, group II (n=40): $T > M$, $LH > M'$, group III (n=34): $T < M$, $LH > M'$, group IV (n=53): $T < M$, $LH < M'$), and hypothalamic-pituitary-gonadal functions (plasma LRH, responses to synthetic LRH and hCG), intelligence score (by the Gikei-kai medical college method) and survival rate of 5 years were compared between these 4 groups.
Group II and III were significantly higher in plasma LRH and the response to synthetic LRH than group IV. Group I showed remarkably higher response to hCG than other 3 groups.
Furthermore, group IV was the lowest in intelligence score and survival rate, and there was statistical significance between group I and IV ($P < 0.05$). These data suggest that the functional classification of elderly males may be possible by the serum levels of T and LH.

1127 Intestinal epithelial tissue hypersensitivity to angiotensin II in thyro-deprived rats. M. Labajos*, M. Morell and R. Alvarez. Dpto. de Fisiología y Bioquímica. Facultad de Medicina. Universidad de Málaga. España.

The effect of angiotensin II at a concentration of 10^{-12} g/ml on intestinal epithelium transport in thyrodeprived rats, previously sensitised to angiotensin II by bilateral adrenal-nephrectomy, was studied. Male Wistar rats were given an iodine deficient diet from the 21st to the 24th day of life in order to facilitate the localisation and extirpation of the thyroid gland. Six days after thyroidectomie the animals received a dose of radiactive iodine to eliminate the possibility of active thyroid tissue remaining. Segments of everted colon from thyrodeprived rats were incubated for an hour in glucosed Krebbs-Ringer solution; firstly without, and then with, angiotensin II in the serosal medium. Net flows were determined for segments of proximal and distal colon. In each case, inhibitions of flow were produced: in proximal colon the values were from 12 $\pm$ 2 to -7 $\pm$ 2 µl/h per 100 mg; and in distal colon, from 11 $\pm$ 2 to -7 $\pm$ 2 µl/h per 100 mg; $p < 0.001$ for both series. A simialr inhibition in the ionic movement of chloride and sodium was produced. This inhibitory effect, similar to the one produced in euthyroid animals by much higher concentrations of angiotensin II (10^{-9} g/ml), may be due to tissue hypersensitivity to angiotensin II resulting from thyroid hormone deprivation; a similar effect at the vascular level has been described in the literature.

1128 OPIATE INVOLVEMENT IN THE RESPONSE OF THE RENIN-ANGIOTENSIN-ALDOSTERONE SYSTEM TO ACUTE SYMPATHETIC STIMULATION IN MAN. K.Lam*, P.Drury, P.Bouloux, A.Grossman and G.M.Besser. Dept. of Endocrinology, St. Bartholomew's Hospital, London and Dept. of Medicine, University of Hong Kong.

It has been suggested that endogenous opiates may be involved in the regulation of systemic blood pressure. We have therefore investigated the effect of naloxone, an opiate antagonist, on the neurohumoral response to acute sympathetic stimulation induced by sustained hand grip. Six normal males (21-28 yrs) on unrestricted sodium diet were studied fasting at 0830h. on 2 occasions at 7-days intervals, with each subject sustaining 30% of his maximal hand grip on a hand dynamometer for 5 min. Either IV naloxone (8 mg bolus) or 20 ml of normal saline was given 5 min.before hand grip in a randomised double-blind cross-over trial. Blood was sampled for cortisol, renin activity, aldosterone (RIA) and catecholamines (HPLC and electrochemical detection). Sustained hand grip induced significant ($p < 0.05$ or less) increases in plasma adrenaline (0.12 $\pm$ 0.02 to 0.24 $\pm$ 0.02 nmol/L; mean $\pm$ S.E.), noradrenaline (0.77 $\pm$ 0.09 to 1.64 $\pm$ 0.27 nmol/L) and renin (0.264 $\pm$ 0.054 to 0.303 $\pm$ 0.064 nmol AI/L/hr.); there was no significant rise in aldosterone and cortisol. In the presence of naloxone, the increments in plasma renin (0.267 $\pm$ 0.062 to 0.457 $\pm$ 0.137 nmol AI/L/hr.) aldosterone (538 $\pm$ 53 to 738 $\pm$ 80 pmol/L) and cortisol (322 $\pm$ 15 to 484 $\pm$ 24 nmol/L) were significantly enhanced; the increment in adrenaline (0.17 $\pm$ 0.03 to 0.50 $\pm$ 0.15 nmol/L) also showed definite but not significant enhancement. The increment in noradrenaline was not affected. These results suggest that endogenous opiates modulate the response of the renin-angiotensin-aldosterone system to acute sympathetic stimulation in man.

1129 RADIOIMMUNOASSAY OF THE SECOND MAIN ALDOSTERONE METABOLITE - 21 DEOXYTETRAHYDROALDOSTERONE.
S. Lewicka*, J. Winter#, V. D. Bokkenheuser#, D. Haack, and P. Vecsei, University of Heidelberg, 6900 Heidelberg, West Germany and St. Luke's Hospital Center, New York, NY 10025 USA#.

A new radioimmunoassay for 21-deoxytetrahydroaldosterone (21-DOTHAldo) was established. 21-DOTHAldo and ^{3}H-21-DOTHAldo synthesized by Eubacterium lentum have a 5 time higher affinity for the tetrahydroaldosterone (THAldo) antibody than does THAldo. Using this system we measured urinary 21-DOTHAldo, THAldo and their glucuronides in patients with essential hypertension (EH), primary aldosteronism (PA), 21-hydroxylase deficiency (CAH), and in 21 controls (C). The excretion in ug/24 h is given below.

	C n=21	EH n=53	PA n=15	CAH n=8
21-DOTHAldo	0.645*±0.112**	1.41±0.323	4.45±1.67	7.35±3.53
21-DOTHAldo gluc.	16.62 ±2.04	30.0±4.445	32.4±6.43	59.7±23.7
THAldo	1.24 ±0.201	3.29±0.548	3.86±1.28	2.95±0.69
THAldo gluc.	29.2 ±1.897	72.1±11.36	105.1±18.5	83.6±15.3

*ug/24 h **mean ± SEM

All patient groups excreted significantly more THAldo and 21-DOTHAldo than did the controls. It is noteworthy that the urinary excretion of 21-DOTHAldo glucuronide is exceptionally high in the CAH. It could reflect a defect in aldosterone synthesis or an altered threshold value for the compound. Urinary 21-DOTHAldo was elevated despite normal THAldo values in some PA patients. These cases may reflect particularly active 21-dehydroxylation by intestinal bacteria.

1130 ROLE OF CORTISOL (F) ON POTASSIUM-MEDIATED ALDOSTERONE SECRETION IN MAN.
J.M.López*,J.A.Rodríguez,D.Mahana and P.Michaud.Dpt. of Endocrinology,School of Medicine, Catholic University of Chile, P.O.Box 114-D, Santiago-Chile.

Six patients with Sheehan's syndrome supplemented with thyroid hormone were given an oral K load with and without F therapy during converting-enzyme inhibition with captopril and fixed electrolyte intake (Na 120, K 50 mEq/d).Daily measurements of urinary aldosterone (UA, μg/d), Porter Silber chromogens (PSC, mg/d) and K (mEq/d) were made for 4 days in Period I (PI) while on chronic F administration (20 mg at 8 AM, 10 mg at 8 PM) and after 4-8 weeks in Period II(PII),having discontinued F 2 days before.K Cl 30 mEq was given orally at 9AM and 9PM on days 3 and 4 of PI and PII.Plasma aldosterone (PA,ng/dl) and K(mEq/l)were measured daily at 9AM and also at 10AM of days 3 and 4 of both periods.Statistical analysis was done by ANOVA for randomized complete block designs.Results are shown as mean ± SE.

Days	PI 1	2	3	4	PII 1	2	3	4
UA	2.1±0.4	1.8±0.3	4.0±1.2	5.8±2.1	3.4±0.9	5.4±1.7	12.4±4.4	14.4±1.9
PSC	8.4±0.7	7.8±0.5	7.9±0.5	8.1±0.5	0.7±0.4	0.5±0.3	0.9±0.4	0.7±0.2
K	43±7	41±4	81±8	92±7	39±7	46±8	71±12	91±9
PA 9AM	2.5±0.5	2.6±0.6	3.1±0.7	4.6±0.6	4.0±0.7	5.1±1.1	8.1±2.5	13.0±1.6
10AM			8.2±2.1	10.5±2.1			22.9±6.5	32.3±2.5
Δ Serum K(9-10AM)			0.6±0.1	0.5±0.1			0.6±0.1	0.4±0.1

F significantly decreased UA and PA($p<0.01$).The stimulatory effect of K on UA($p<0.001$)and PA($p<0.01$)was greater in the absence of F($p<0.02$)in spite of similar serum K increments.A significant effect of the interaction between F and K on UA($p<0.05$)and PA($p<0.01$)was demonstrated.Our results show that F can inhibit basal and K-stimulated aldosterone secretion in man.

1131 GLIPIZIDE REDUCES HIGH PLASMA INACTIVE RENIN LEVELS IN DIABETES MELLITUS.
J.A. Luetscher*, M. Bryer-Ash, G. C-K Liu, C. Lardinois, and G.M. Reaven, Department of Medicine, Stanford University, Stanford, CA 94305, USA.

We have found increased levels of inactive renin, a high-molecular-weight zymogen and putative prorenin, in the plasma of patients with diabetes mellitus, especially but not exclusively in those with nephropathy or retinopathy. 30 Diabetic patients were studied over 1 to 6 months on programs designed to control plasma glucose. 15 Type 2 diabetics received either intensive insulin with monitoring of plasma glucose or insulin supplemented by another oral agent; no consistent change in inactive renin ensued. 15 Type 2 diabetics followed a low-caloric diet to reduce weight (average loss 7 Kg): in 7 of these patients who received glipizide, plasma inactive renin was reduced by 30%, with 6 of 7 patients achieving normal levels (<50 ngAI/ml/h) of inactive renin. Patients not receiving glipizide had an insignificant increase of plasma inactive renin despite equivalent weight reduction and a distinct improvement in glycemia (basal -50 mg/dl vs -87 mg/dl in patients taking glipizide). Camerini-Davalos et al reported (NEJM, 12/22/83) a reduction in muscle capillary basement membrane thickness in patients with chemical diabetes after 16-36 months of glipizide treatment. While other effective methods of controlling hyperglycemia do not consistently reduce inactive renin and have shown limited promise in avoiding diabetic complications, glipizide has shown promising and possibly specific effects on two objective measurements related to early diabetic microangiopathy.

1132 REDUCTION OF ALDOSTERONE STIMULATING FACTOR AND REVERSAL OF IDIOPATHIC HYPERALDOSTERONISM BY LEVODOPA.
C.D. Malchoff*, J.Q. Miller, S. Sen, and R.M. Carey, University of Virginia, Charlottesville, VA, and The Cleveland Clinic Foundation, Cleveland, OH, United States.

Aldosterone secretion is inhibited by dopamine (DA) and stimulated by the anterior pituitary glycoprotein, aldosterone stimulating factor (ASF). Idiopathic hyperaldosteronism (IHA) may be caused by increased ASF. To test the hypothesis that dopamine can reverse the clinical and biochemical manifestations of IHA by decreasing ASF, we used levodopa (LD) to treat a patient with IHA. A 52 year old white man with a Parkinsonism syndrome for 3 years and hypertension for 10 years was found to have IHA by the following evidence: serum K 3.6 meq/l and 24 hour urinary K 82 meq/24h while on a 150 meq Na, 60 meq K diet; plasma renin activity 0.8 ng/ml/hr after furosemide stimulation; plasma aldosterone concentration (PAC) 21 ng/dl before and after saline infusion; PAC increased with upright posture; and bilateral equal uptake of ^{131}I-6 β-iodomethylnorcholesterol on adrenocortical scan. Supine plasma ASF concentration was 150 ng/dl [(N=70±6,mean±SE)] and urinary ASF excretion was 400 ng/24h (N=147±5). During a four hour infusion of DA (4.0 μg/kg/min) PAC decreased from 23 ng/dl to 13 ng/dl. LD was started and gradually increased to 3.0 g/day. Manifestations of IHA resolved: blood pressure, initially 150/100, decreased to 120/70; supplemental K requirements, initially 150 meq/day, decreased to 25 meq/day; supine PAC decreased to 12 ng/dl; supine plasma ASF decreased to 109 ng/dl; urinary ASF excretion decreased to 159 ng/24h. LD reversed the clinical and biochemical manifestations of IHA. The effect of LD may be mediated by its conversion to dopamine, which may act to reduce elevated ASF secretion in IHA.

1133 THE ROLE OF SEROTONERGIC TYPE 2 RECEPTORS IN THE REGULATION OF ALDOSTERONE PRODUCTION. H. Matsuoka*, A. Goto, M. Ishii, and T. Sugimoto. The 2nd Dept. of Intern. Med. University of Tokyo, Tokyo, Japan.

It is well recognized that serotonin(Ser) stimulates aldosterone(Ald) production in adrenal cells. To investigate the roles of Ser-type 1 and type 2 receptors in Ald production, we examined the effects of ketanserin (Ket; a Ser-type 2 selective antagonist) and cyproheptadine(Cyp; a non-selective Ser antagonist) on Ald and cAMP production using rat adrenal collagenase-dispersed capsular cells. Ser ranging in concentration from 10^{-9} to 10^{-6}M significantly increased Ald production from the control value of 24.0 ± 3.3(SE) to the maximal response of 59.5 ± 3.5 ng/10^5 cells in a dose-dependent fashion after 2 hrs of incubation at 37°C. Ket and Cyp showed comparable inhibitory effects on basal Ald production, i.e., Ket and Cyp at a dose of 10^{-7}M decreased Ald production by 28.4 and 26.1 %, respectively. Although 10^{-7}M Ket and Cyp significantly decreased Ald production induced by 10^{-8}M Ser by 26.4 and 26.1 %, respectively, these Ser antagonists did not affect Ald production induced by 10^{-8}M $ACTH^{1-24}$. Ser at a dose of 10^{-6}M increased cAMP production from the control value of 10.6 ± 0.4(SE) to 14.7 ± 1.2 pmole/10^5 cells. Both Ket and Cyp at a dose of 10^{-5}M inhibited basal cAMP production by 16.7 and 11.4 %, respectively. Ket and Cyp which are 10 times as much as Ser on molar basis decreased cAMP production by 26.2 and 20.7 %, respectively. However, these Ser antagonists did not affect cAMP production stimulated by $ACTH^{1-24}$. These results suggest that adrenal Ser type 2 receptors are coupled with adenylate cyclase activity and that these receptors are involved in the regulation of Ald production.

1134 EFFECTS OF Na^+ DEPLETION, BETAMETHASONE AND CAPTOPRIL TREATMENT ON THE RAT ADRENAL ZONA GLOMERULOSA CONTENT OF TRYPSIN-RELEASABLE ALDOSTERONE. McAuley, M.E., Raven, P.W.* and Vinson, G.P. *Department of Biochemistry, St Bartholomew's Hospital Medical College, Charterhouse Square, LONDON, EC1

Rat adrenal zona glomerulosa (ZG) tissue contains sequestered steroid pools from which aldosterone (aldo) and 18-hydroxycorticosterone (18-OH-B) are released by trypsin. To investigate the physiological role of this sequestered steroid, groups of rats were maintained on a Na^+ deplete diet (5 days), or treated with betamethasone (20μg/ml drinking water overnight) or captopril (7.2mg injected/Kg/day for 5 days). Intact ZG preparations from both treated and control animals were incubated for 1hr ± trypsin (1mg /ml) and aldo was measured in the incubation medium. Plasma aldo levels were also measured. Sodium depletion significantly increased plasma aldo while the *in vitro* secretion of aldo under basal conditions was not affected by Na^+ depletion, aldo released by trypsin was increased (266 ± 41 to 776 ± 92ng/adrenal pair) ($p<0.001$, n=6). Both captopril and betamethasone treatment caused a fall in plasma aldo and a decrease in trypsin-releasable aldosterone compared with controls (eg for betamethasone: control 216 ± 22ng, trypsin 263 ± 24ng/adrenal pair ($p>0.1$, n=6) compared with untreated animals: control 208 ± 18ng, trypsin 341 ± 2ng/adrenal pair) ($p<0.001$, n=6). Simultaneous betamethasone (but not captopril) treatment was effective in abolishing the rise in plasma aldo induced by Na^+ depletion, but had no effect on the increased trypsin-releasable aldo from Na^+ deplete tissue. These results suggest that this sequestered steroid plays a role in the physiological responses of the zona glomerulosa to various secretory stimuli.

1135 ROLE OF OXYTOCIN IN MATERNAL BEHAVIOR ONSET IN RATS. S.E.Fahrbach,* J.I. Morrell, and D.W. Pfaff. Laboratory of Neurobiology & Behavior, The Rockefeller University, 1230 York Avenue, New York, NY 10021

Intracerebroventricular (icv) infusion of oxytocin (OXY) facilitates maternal behavior in estrogen-primed virgin rats during the first hr of foster pup contact (Pedersen et al., Sci. 216, '82; Fahrbach et al., Horm. Behav., submitted, '83). This suggests that OXY may have a central nervous system (CNS) role in the onset of maternal behavior at parturition. To test this hypothesis, we used a pregnancy-terminated preparation which yields reliable short-latency maternal behavior. Sprague-Dawley rats (Zivic-Miller) with lateral ventricle cannulae were ovariectomized and hysterectomized (OH) on day 16 of gestation and given a sc injection of estradiol benzoate (EB) or the oil vehicle. The latency to respond to pups of groups receiving EB and 1)icv infusion of antibody to OXY (n=8) 2)icv infusion of an OXY antagonist, $d(CH_2)_5$-ornithine^8-vasotocin (n=6) (Bankowski et al.,Int. J. Peptide Prot. Res. 16, '80) 3)control icv infusions of normal rabbit serum (NRS) or antibody to antidiuretic hormone (ADH) (n=8) was compared with the latency of groups receiving no icv infusion and either EB (n=8) or oil (n=7). Pups were presented 48 hr after surgery; behavioral observations were made for the next 5 hr and periodically for the next 5 days. At the end of the first 5 hr 100% of the EB group were maternal; 87.5% of the NRS/anti-ADH group; 37.5% of the anti-OXY group; 16.7% of the OXY antagonist group; 27.5% of the oil group. We conclude that a temporary reduction in OXY action in the CNS delays the onset of estrogen-dependent maternal behavior.

1136 MOTILIN STIMULATES FEEDING IN FASTED RATS. T.L. Garthwaite,* Medical College of Wisconsin, Wood VA Medical Center, Milwaukee, WI.

Since the isolation of motilin from gut, research has focused on the relationship between it and interdigestive migrating motor complexes (MMCs) in the gastrointestinal tract. Plasma levels of motilin are low in the fed state with peaks of immunoreactivity every 90-120 minutes during fasting in association with MMCs. This apparent interrelationship between plasma motilin levels and feeding prompted an investigation of the effects of motilin on feeding behavior in the rat. Sprague-Dawley rats (200-225 g) were maintained in single wire bottom cages and were fasted for 21 hours beginning at 1600 hours. Groups of fasted rats were injected (i.p.) with varying doses and combinations of synthetic porcine motilin, naloxone, naltrexone, pentagastrin, or vehicle. Following injection, rats were returned to their home cages with a weighed quantity of lab chow, and the chow consumed during the next two hours was quantitated. Motilin injection was associated with a significant increase in food consumed at doses of 2.5, 5, and 10 μg/kg (one-way analysis of variance: $F=14.95$, $p < .001$). Stimulation of feeding was noted at 30, 60, and 120 minutes after injection. Naltrexone (10 mg/kg), naloxone (10 and 0.1 mg/kg), or pentagastrin (5 μg/kg) attenuated the motilin-induced feeding when injected i.p. just prior to the injection of motilin. Similar doses of motilin administered to sated rats were without effect. CONCLUSIONS: 1) These experiments demonstrate a dose-dependent feeding response to peripherally administered motilin in fasted rats; 2) motilin-induced feeding may be mediated through an endogenous opioid pathway.

1137 SODIUM FLUORIDE TREATMENT FOR OSTEOPOROSIS. R.G. Josse*, T.A. Bayley, V.L. Fornasier, J.E. Harrison, T.M. Murray, W. Sturtridge, C.S. Tam and C. Williams, Departments of Medicine and Pathology, University of Toronto, Toronto, Ontario M5S 1A8, Canada.

Sixteen patients with postmenopausal osteoporosis have been followed for 4 years while on sodium fluoride (NaF, 25 mg b.i.d.). Sequential bone mineral measurements of the central third of the skeleton by neutron activation analysis showed variable results with, in 8 cases, significant increases in mineral mass (△ CaBI of 10-21%) and overall, a mean increase of 7.9 ± 2.9% ($p < .05$). Fluorosis on bone histology (increased percentages of formation surfaces with thickened osteoid seams) was associated with a significant mean increase in CaBI of 13.8 ± 2.6%. With fluorosis, bone F retention was 49.3 ± 3.0 mmol/mol Ca. With lower bone F levels, 34.8 ± 4.2 mmol/mol Ca, no histological evidence of fluorosis and no improvement in bone mass was observed (△ CaBI -4.2 ± 5.6%). This lack of bone stimulation by F appears related to inadequate F dose. Fasting serum F levels, however, were comparable in the two groups, with and without fluorosis, 9.2 ± 3.7 and 7.9 ± 2.3 μmol/L respectively, indicating that these serum determinations are unreliable for predicting F response. NaF is the only agent known to produce > 10% increases in osteoporotic bone mass and merits, therefore, further evaluation but further understanding of the optimal F dose, on an individual basis, is required.

1138 HYPOTHALAMIC α-MSH IS NOT UNDER DOPAMINERGIC CONTROL. S. Jégou, J. Guy[π], A. Coquerel, C. Delbende, G. Pelletier[π] and H. Vaudry*.Groupe Recherche Endocrinologie Moléculaire, ERA 891, Fac. Sciences, Univ. Rouen, 76130 Mont-Saint-Aignan, France ; π MRC Group in Molecular Endocrinology, CHUL, Québec GIV 4G2, Canada.

Two neuronal systems containing α-MSH-like molecules have been identified in rat hypothalamus. Since, in the pars intermedia, α-MSH secretion is inhibited by dopamine, we have investigated a possible dopaminergic control of α-MSH-containing neurons. The release of α-MSH-like material by rat hypothalamic slices was studied in vitro using the perifusion technique and a specific radioimmunoassay. The infusion of KCl (50 mM) during 9 min induced a rapid stimulation of α-MSH release (500% over basal level). Removal of calcium from the perifusion medium abolished the potassium-evoked release of α-MSH. Addition of dopamine (10^{-7}M to 10^{-5}M) or its antagonist haloperidol (10^{-5}M) during 24 min did not affect spontaneous and potassium-induced α-MSH release. A possible regulation of hypothalamic α-MSH was also studied in vivo. Intraperitoneal injection of haloperidol (150 μg to 3 mg/kg B.W.) to male rats did not modify α-MSH concentrations in the arcuate nucleus and in the dorsolateral area of the hypothalamus. Reverse phase HPLC analysis revealed that both the dorsal and the ventral parts of the hypothalamus contain two major forms of α-MSH-like immunoreactivity : desacetyl α-MSH and α-MSH. The ratio between these two forms was not altered by haloperidol treatment. These results indicate that, in opposition to the intermediate lobe, hypothalamic α-MSH is not under dopaminergic control. Supported by INSERM Grant n° 81.60.31.

1139 PRODUCTION AND RELEASE OF PRO-OPIOMELANOCORTIN-DERIVED PEPTIDES BY EXTRA-HYPOTHALAMIC BRAIN CELLS. L.P. Kapcala*, T.M. Birk and T.A. Griffin, Dept of Med, Case Western Reserve Univ, Cleve Metro Gen Hosp, Cleveland, Ohio.

Although most studies have suggested brain POMC peptides are synthesized in hypothalamus, others have suggested they may also be produced in the amygdala and cortex. Furthermore, it has been suggested that POMC peptides may be neurotransmitters/neuromodulators in brain, but little is known about their release. To determine whether POMC peptides are produced by extrahypothalamic brain, the production of POMC peptides was assessed by measuring (RIA) the accumulation of immunoreactive (IR-) ACTH and β-endorphin in the media of dissociated fetal rat amygdala and cortical cell cultures incubated for several days, and by comparing the measured quantities to those in cells at plating. To determine whether the release of POMC peptides can be stimulated, IR -ACTH and β-endorphin were measured in amygdala and cortical cells separately incubated with 60mM K^+ with and without Ca^{++}, and with 10^{-9}M corticotropin-releasing factor (CRF). Significant increments ($p < 0.001$) in IR-ACTH/IR-β-endorphin were measured in amygdala (118%/326%) and cortical (171%/446%) cells. Depolarizing concentrations of K^+ with Ca^{++} stimulated increments in release of IR-ACTH/IR-β endorphin by amygdala (111%/105%) and cortical (162%/136%) cells. In addition, CRF stimulated significant increments ($p < 0.025$) in release of IR-ACTH (156%) and IR-β-endorphin (42%) by cortical cells. Conclusions: 1. POMC peptides are produced by extrahypothalamic brain (amygdala/cortex). 2. Release of IR-ACTH/IR-β-endorphin during K^+ stimulated Ca^{++} dependent depolarization suggests these neuropeptides could be neuroregulators in brain. 3. CRF, the potent regulator of POMC peptides in pituitary, may also regulate POMC peptides in brain.

1140 **CALCITONINSTIMULATES 25-HYDROXYVITAMIN D_3-1-HYDROXYLASEINRAT KIDNEY CELLS IN PRIMARY CULTURE.** H. Kawashima*, A. Iida-Klein, and K. Kurokawa, Nephrol. Sect., Med. and Res. Services, VA Wads. Med. Ctr., and Dept. Med. UCLA Sch. Med., Los Angeles, California 90073, U.S.A.

We have previously shown that calcitonin(CT) given in vivo stimulates 25(OH)D_3-1-hydroxylase(1-OHase) in the proximal straight tubules of rat kidney via a mechanism independent of c-AMP. To further define the mechanism of action of CT on 1-OHase, an in vitro system is preferable. Since it takes several hours for CT to stimulate 1-OHase in vivo, it is necessary to maintain these kidney cell functions intact for 6-8 hrs. This has been difficult particulary with rat kidney cells until we established a primary culture system ofrat kidney cells withintact 1-OHase and 25(OH)D_3-24-hydroxylase(24-OHase). Isolated kidney cells were prepared by the method of Turner et al and incubated in a medium of Dulbecco°s MEM and HAM(F12)(1/1) supplemented withinsulin(5 ug/ml) at37C in 95%O_2/5%CO_2. After the culture became confluent, PTH(10U/ml), CT(1U/ml) or 1,25(OH)$_2D_3$ was added to each dish and incubated for 12 hrs. Then ^{3}H-25(OH)D_3 and 25(OH)D_3(10nM) were added to each dish for 5 more hrs incubation. Metabolites of 25(OH)D_3 were identified by chromatography including 3 different HPLC systems. The non-treated cells produced 1,25(OH)$_2D_3$ at a rate of 3 + 0.5 pmol/10^6cells/5hrs. PTH and CT increased the production 2-3-fold and 2-fold, respectively, while 1,25(OH)$_2D_3$ reduced the enzyme activity by 90% and stimulated 24-OHase activity. These results clearly demonstrate that the responsiveness of 1-OHase in our primary culture system of rat kidney cells remains similar to these as shown in vivo, and suggest that the effect of CT is direct.

1141 INDUCTION OF 25-HYDROXYVITAMIN D_3-24-HYDROXYLASE BY 1,25-DIHYDROXYVITAMIN D_3 IN CULTURED KIDNEY (LLC-MK_2) CELLS: EVIDENCE FOR MEDIATION BY A VARIANT FORM OF THE HORMONE RECEPTOR. M. Kelly*, C. Donaldson, M. Haussler and J. Pike, Department of Biochemistry, University of Arizona Health Sciences Center, Tucson, Arizona, USA.

One action of 1,25-dihydroxyvitamin D_3 (1,25$(OH)_2D_3$) is to stimulate 25-hydroxyvitamin D_3-24-hydroxylase (24-OHase) in cells of both renal and extra-renal origin. This actinomycin D-sensitive induction is thought to be mediated by the 1,25$(OH)_2D_3$ receptor, although it has been observed in LLC-MK_2 cells in which high affinity receptor binding is undetectable. We have examined 24-OHase stimulation in both LLC-MK_2 and receptor-rich (5400 molecules/cell) LLC-PK_1 cells. 24-OHase activity was assayed by HPLC separation of lipid extracts of control or 1,25$(OH)_2D_3$ pretreated (12 hr) cells after incubation with 0.5 μM 25(OH)[^{3}H]D_3 for 30 min at 37°C. We observed maximal stimulation of 24-OHase at 1 nM 1,25$(OH)_2D_3$ in receptor-positive LLC-PK_1 while LLC-MK_2 required 100 nM 1,25$(OH)_2D_3$ for optimal induction. This suggested that 24-OHase stimulation in LLC-MK_2 cells might be mediated by a lower affinity variant of the 1,25$(OH)_2D_3$ receptor which escapes detection by classical binding techniques. In fact, DNA-cellulose chromatography of extracts of intact LLC-MK_2 cells incubated with 2, 20 and 100 nM 1,25$(OH)_2$[^{3}H]D_3 indicated the presence of $\geq$600 copies/cell of an atypical receptor molecule which requires $\geq$20 nM 1,25$(OH)_2D_3$ to detect binding. Experiments to immunochemically characterize this potential receptor variant, which may be a good model for hereditary rickets characterized by reduced hormone responsiveness, are currently in progress. (Supported by AM30290 and AM15781).

1142 ON THE ACTION OF 1,25-DIHYDROXYVITAMIN D_3 (1,25-$(OH)_2D_3$) ON RAT SMALL INTESTINE: CHANGES IN TRANSLATABLE MESSENGER RNA SPECIES. M.A. Kessler*, and H.F. DeLuca. Dept. of Biochemistry, Univ. of Wisc. Madison, WI 53706 USA

The active metabolite of vitamin D, 1,25-$(OH)_2D_3$, has been shown to share several characteristics of the classical steroid hormones. These include a high affinity receptor protein, localization in the nuclei of target cells, and induction of specific mRNA species. However, the relation of these molecular events to the physiologic action of vitamin D, stimulation of calcium transport, remains unclear. To define the physical properties of vitamin D-associated gene products and analyze their relationships to the biphasic calcium transport response of rat intestine to 1,25-$(OH)_2D_3$, the time course of changes in translatable mRNA from small intestinal mucosa was studied in vitamin D-deficient rats following an intrajugular dose of 1,25-$(OH)_2D_3$. L-[^{35}S] methionine-labelled translation products were analyzed by high resolution one- and two-dimensional electrophoresis. Dramatic changes were detected in two distinct proteins, M_r 14,000/pI 6.24, and M_r 5,200/pI 4.86. These increased to maxima of 1-2% each of the total *in vitro*-synthesized protein at 12 hours after dosing. This represented a three- and ten-fold increase, respectively, over control values. The time course of these changes suggests that regulation of the levels of the mRNAs coding for these proteins is not involved in the initial (6 hour) peak of 1,25-$(OH)_2D_3$ -stimulated calcium transport in the rat intestine. This study was supported by NIH grant DE 07031.

1143 INCREASE IN ENDORPHIN LEVELS INDUCED BY CALCITONIN ADMINISTRATION.
L. Laurian*, Z. Oberman, E. Horer, E. Graf and R. Chayen, Ichilon Medical Center, Tel Aviv University Medical School, ISRAEL.

The analgesic effect of calcitonin in different bone diseases has been repeatedly reported. Various hypotheses have been put forward regarding the intimate mechanism of this effect. None has been definitely established. We assumed that calcitonin may act centrally by stimulating the endogenous opiate substances. We therefore initiated this study to evaluate the effect of calcitonin on the endorphin levels. We investigated 8 patients with acute painful episodes of osteoporosis. We injected 100 mU salmon calcitonin Sandoz i.v. and estimated the levels of endorphin and cortisol by radioimmunoassay at -15,0,15,30,60,90 and 120 min. The same estimations were done after administration of saline. 6 of the 8 patients showed an average increase of 120% in the endorphin levels at 30 min. and an average increase of 195% in the cortisol levels at 45 min after the calcitonin administration. No changes in endorphin levels were seen throughout the test in the other two patients. No changes in the other two patients. No changes in endorphin levels were seen after saline administration. The cortisol levels decreased mildly throughout the saline test in all the patients. These preliminary results seem to support a stimulative action of calcitonin on endorphin. The investigation is being continued, and will endeavor to ascertain whether the endorphin responseto calcitonin correlates with the basal levels of endorphin. This study was supported by Sandoz.

1144 RELATIONS BETWEEN CIRCADIAN VARIATIONS OF CALCIUM, PHOSPHATE, CT AND PTH IN RAT ; EFFECT OF CALCIUM DEFICIENCY. Lausson S. , Staub J.F. and Milhaud G., LA 163 CNRS, 27 rue Chaligny, 75571 PARIS Cedex 12, France.

Circadian variations of plasma calcium and phosphate are well documented in the rat. We have studied these electrolytes and immunoassayable CT and (1-34) PTH concentrations over 24 h period, in normal and calcium deficient Wistar CF male rats. In normal rat, (40 or 140 days of age), the CT_i level was higher during the dark period. Plasma (1-34) PTH_i fluctuations presented two peaks at transition times between feeding and resting period. The pre and post-prandial CT_i variations didn't seem modified by calcium deficiency as long as plasma calcium level remained nearly normal. A striking finding is that, when plasma calcium was strongly diminished, the hormone rise was limited to the light period. The mean PTH_i level was increased of about 1.5 fold but the pattern of PTH_i fluctuations remained unchanged. In these experimental conditions, calcium paralleled CT_i ($r = .50$, $p < 0.01$) and varied in an opposite way to PTH_i ($r = .55$, $p < 0.01$) over the 24-h day. Thus the predominant effect seems to be an action of plasma calcium changes on hormonal secretions. Studied at each sampling time, only negative correlations ($p < 0.05$) between CT_i versus calcium and CT_i versus phosphate (index of CT control) appeared at 4 h and just before food access, i.e. when calcium level was higher. The present data reinforce the hypothesis reported by Hirsch that feeding schedule is not an essential component for CT secretion in the rat ; results are consistent with the concept that endocrine system and target organs are intrinsically able to generate circadian variations.

1145 Parathyroid Hormone Bioactivity (bioPTH) in Patients with Familial Hypocalciuric Hypercalcaemia (FHH).

N. Loveridge[*1], A. Sangal[2], P.H. Weller[2], and J. Allgrove[3]

[1]Kennedy Institute, London W6 7DW, [2]Dudley Road Hospital, Birmingham B18 7QH and [3]East Birmingham Hospital, Birmingham B9 5ST, U.K.

The aetiology of FHH, an autosomal dominant condition characterized by hypercalcaemia in association with increased renal tubular reabsorption of divalent cations, is unknown. Although the patients are hypercalcaemic, immunoreactive parathyroid hormone (iPTH) levels are usually normal or only slightly elevated but the possibility exists that the biological activity of the PTH secreted is raised. In order to test this hypothesis we have measured bioPTH and iPTH levels in a family in which the father and two sons were hypercalcaemic (>3m moles/L) while the third son and the mother were normocalcaemic. The father and two sons had markedly elevated renal tubular reabsorption of calcium while in the third son this was slightly raised. The mother reabsorbed calcium normally. None of the patients had vitamin D intoxication. iPTH levels were undetectable (<250 pg/ml) and the bioPTH levels, as measured by the cytochemical bioassay, were towards the lower end of the normal range for the father (1.5pg/ml) and two sons (1.5pg/ml and 1.2pg/ml) with FHH. The third son (10pg/ml) and the mother (2.4pg/ml) were also in the normal range for this assay. These results would seem to indicate that the defect in patients with FHH lies in the renal tubule and is not attributable to abnormally increased PTH bioactivity.

1146 ACUTE INHIBITION OF PRL AND GH SECRETION FOLLOWING INTRA-VENTRICULAR INJECTION (IVT) OF CALCITONIN (CT-HUMAN; SIGMA).

H.K.Mangat*[1] and S.M.McCann[2], Dept. of Physiology, UTHSCD, Dallas, Tx-75235, USA and Dept. of Biology, GNDU, Amritsar-143005, India.

Prolactin is under inhibitory control via hypothalamus, however various peptides and proteins can modulate its release. Experiments were performed to determine if CT can effect the release of PRL. Ovariectomized (OVX) rats bearing implanted IVT and jugular cannulae were used. Blood was withdrawn in unanaesthetized OVX, freely-moving animals before and after IVT 0.9% NaCl or 3 or 5 ug of CT. No effect on any pituitary hormone occurred after either IVT or intravenous (IV) saline or CT. With elevated initial PRL by estradiol-priming (E) in OVX rats IVT of both doses of CT caused more effective lowering of PRL. FSH and TSH were not altered by CT. Small and inconsistent declined in LH were seen following IVT CT in either OVX or OVXE-primed rats. A significant lowering of GH occurred in OVX or OVXE primed rats within 60 min. after IVT 5 ug of CT, but none with IV. No effect of CT was there on release of PRL or GH from Hemipituitaries *in vitro*. Consequently, CT has inhibitory action on PRL and GH release via hypothalamic mechanisms. ([1]Ford Foundation Fellow with S.M.McCann 1980-83, [2]Supported by NIH Grants HD-09988, AM-10083, Ford Foundation).

1147 1,25-DIHYDROXYVITAMIN D_3: A NOVEL LYMPHOCYTE ACTIVATION MARKER AND IMMUNOREGULATOR. S. Manolagas*[1], D. Provvedini[1], C. Tsoukas[2], D. Werntz[1], and L. Deftos . [1]University of California, VA Medical Center, and [2]Scripps Research Foundation, La Jolla, California, 92161.

The widespread distribution of receptors for $1,25(OH)_2D_3$ in tissues not regarded to participate in mineral metabolism has made it apparent that this hormone plays a regulatory role for many organ systems. We have examined normal human leukocytes for the presence of receptors for $1,25-(OH)_2D_3$ and the effects of this hormone in immune function. We found that human monocytes possessed a cytoplasmic receptor for $1,25(OH)_2D_3$, while lymphocytes did not. However, upon mitogenic stimulation lymphocytes also became receptor positive. This receptor macromolecule sedimented at 3,3S in sucrose density gradients, and bound ^3H-labelled $1,25(OH)_2D_3$ with specificity and high affinity ($Kd=1-4x10^{-10}M$). The addition of picomolar concentrations of $1,25(OH)_2D_3$ to PHA stimulated lymphocytes suppressed the production of Interleukin 2 (IL2) in the culture supernatant. Fifty percent reduction of IL2 activity occurred at $2-10x10^{-12}M$ of hormone. At this concentration no discernible effects on lymphocyte proliferation were detected. The IL2 suppressive effect was not due to a direct interaction of the hormone with IL2 itself or with the target cells used in the IL2 assay. The order of potency of IL2 suppression by $1,25(OH)_2D_3$ analogs corresponded to the order of their affinity for the specific hormone receptor, suggesting that the IL2 suppression is mediated via the specific receptor of $1,25(OH)_2D_3$ in the activated T cells. The above observations open new avenues of investigation on the interrelationship between the endocrine and the immune system and may have important clinical implications.

1148 UTILITY OF A HUMAN CANCER MODEL FOR DESIGNING NEW TREATMENTS FOR MALIGNANCY ASSOCIATED HYPERCALCEMIA (MAH). S.C. Kukreja*, L.J. Kukla, E.C. Abramson, T.E. Lad, D.H. Shevrin, H. Mishoulam and W.P. McGuire. VA West Side and University of Illinois Medical Centers, Chicago, IL U.S.A.

Tumor tissue from a patient with squamous cell lung cancer and hypercalcemia has been serially transplanted into athymic mice. The animals develop hypercalcemia, hypophosphatemia and elevated urinary cyclic AMP levels in the absence of bone metastases. In this model, we evaluated the effectiveness of cis-Platinum (cis-P) in the treatment of MAH. Cis-P is a cancer chemotherapeutic agent associated with hypomagnesemia and hypocalcemia as side effects. Upon development of hypercalcemia (serum Ca > 11.5 mg/dl), the mice received either normal saline (NS) alone (1.5 ml/day i.p.) or NS + cis-P administered as a single dose of 6 μg/Kg i.p. Serum Ca decreased from 14.3 ± 0.46 (S.E.) to 12.7 ± 0.33 mg/dl in the NS alone group, and from 13.5 ± 0.46 to 10.4 ± 0.48 mg/dl in the NS + cis-P group. Post-treatment serum Ca values were significantly lower in the NS + cis-P group ($p = 0.003$). The decrease in serum Ca was not associated with a corresponding decrease in serum magnesium or reduction in tumor volume. Six patients with lung cancer and hypercalcemia (serum Ca 14.0 to 17.0 mg/dl, mean 15.6) were given cis-P 100 mg/M^2 as a 24 hour infusion. Serum Ca decreased to a level below 11.5 mg/dl in 5 of the 6 patients. Serum magnesium decreased significantly; however, there was no correlation between the hypocalcemic response and the degree of hypomagnesemia. Objective regression of tumor did not occur. Therefore, we conclude that 1) cis-P is an effective treatment for MAH, an effect occuring independent of its hypomagnesemic as well as its anti-tumor effects, 2) the animal model is useful in designing new treatments for MAH of human cancer.

1149 TREATMENT AND BONE IMAGING WITH (3-AMINO-1-HYDROXYPROPYLIDENE)-1,1-BIPHOSPHONATE (APD) IN A PATIENT WITH METASTATIC PARATHYROID CARCINOMA.

K. Mann*, U. Büll, G. Wehmeyer and S. Braun, Dept. Internal Medicine II, Nuclear Medicine, Clinical Chemistry, Grosshadern, University of Munich, Munich, FRG

We report about the treatment of a woman(63y) with metastatic parathyroid carcinoma. In 1979, left side tumor was removed; local relapse was operated in 1981. Hypercalcemia up to 4.5 mmol/l resistant to conventional drug treatment reoccured in 8/83; at this time C-terminal PTH-levels were slightly elevated to 2.7 µg/l. After reducing serum calcium to 3 mmol/l using clodronate(200-500 mg/day i.v.) 7 metastases of the lung were removed.However, high doses of clodronate were necessary, when PTH(up to 40 µg/l) and calcium increased again postoperatively.Giving APD (15-75 mg/day i.v. Henkel, Düsseldorf) calcium fell to 3.5 mmol/l without a dose-relationship. In 11/83 we startet oral medication with APD(600-900 mg/day) keeping calcium in the same range. A routine bone scan was done with Tc-99m DPD and showed only very slight extraosseous accumulation. To experience utilisation, Tc-99m labeled APD(1.98 mCi) was applicated orally. Only 0.05% of the dose was recovered in serum. In 12/83 bone scanning was performed 12 and 140 min after injection of 15 mCi and excellent bone images were documented. In addition, highest intensitiy was found in heart and stomach indicating tissue calcifications. Postmortem, extensive microcalcifications were found in heart and stomach. In conclusion, Tc-99m APD imaged bone and extraosseous calcifications. APD, orally administered, is an effective drug to lower hypercalcemia despite its minimal intestinal absorption. However, tissue calcifications were not hindered. We propose Tc-99m APD scanning concomitantly to ADP treatment to detect early dangerous tissue calcifications.

1150 CORTICOTROPIN RELEASING FACTOR (CRF) LIKE ACTIVITIES IN VARIOUS HUMAN TUMORS.

T.Ihara*, I.Wakabayashi, Y.Tonegawa, M.Hattori, T.Shibasaki[1] and K.Hashimoto[2], Dept Med, Nippon Med Sch, Tokyo 113, [1]Dept Med, Tokyo Women's Med Coll, Tokyo 162 and [2]Dept Med, Okayama Univ, Okayama 700 Japan

Recent studies have described the presence of CRF immunoreactivity (IR-CRF)in endocrine or paracrine cells of gastrointestinal tract. We measured IR-CRF in various human tumors by the RIA developed against ovine CRF(Life Sci 32:1001,1983). The RIA system(^{125}I-Tyr-oCRF,oCRF standards) detected approximately 25% of rat(human)CRF. Control and tumor tissues obtained at autopsy or surgery were homogenized with 1N acetic acid and heated for 10min in boiling water. After centrifugation, the supernatant was used for CRF assay. lR-CRF concentrations in control tissues(ng oCRF/g wt)were:hypothalamus(3)2.17±1.1,thyroid gland(5)ND,lung(5)ND,stomach(4) 0.88±29,pancreas(4)1.90±0.73,adrenal gland(5)1.73±0.36. The figures in various tumors were:medullary carcinoma of the thyroid(2)0.64,1.94,adenocarcinoma of the lung(2)0.42,3.59,small cell carcinoma of the lung (ectopic ACTH syndrome)1.76,adenocarcinoma of the stomach(2)1.12,2.58,adenocarcinoma of the pancreas(1)1.33,pheochromocytoma of the adrenal gland(2)1.21,3.49. Dilution curves of the tissue extracts were paralleled that of synthetic oCRF. When aliquots of tissue extracts were subjected to gel filtration on a Sephadex G-50 column(in 1N acetic acid),lR-CRF resolved into two components:one of which emerged immediately after blue dextran and the other emerged in elution volumes consistent with oCRF.

The results suggest that materials closely related to oCRF are present widely in tissues and tumors outside of the brain.

1151 HIGHLY SPECIFIC AND SENSITIVE MEASUREMENTS OF ASIALO HCG WITH LECTIN-ANTIBODY SANDWICH ASSAYS.

S. Imamura*, E.G. Armstrong, S. Birken and L.A. Cole, Departments of Medicine and Pathology, Columbia University, New York, NY 10032 and Department of Internal Medicine, University of Michigan Medical School, Ann Arbor, Michigan 48109.

Highly specific and sensitive assays have been developed for the measurement of various forms of asialo hCG (ashCG) in urine. These sequential sandwich assays utilize peanut lectin, Arachis hypogea (PNA), to selectively extract ashCG, which is then directly quantified with purified and radiolabeled monoclonal antibodies or rabbit antiserum. PNA is highly specific for the terminal carbohydrate linkage Galβ-(1→3)-GalNAc which is only exposed in hCG when the o-serine linked oligosaccharides of its unique β subunit COOH-terminal peptide (βCTP) region are deficient in sialic acid. AshCG concentrations as low as 0.05 ng/ml can be accurately measured in the presence of excess quantities of hCG or hLH. As many as three different forms of ashCG with intact βCTP regions can be detected, depending upon the binding specificities of the radiolabeled antibody or antiserum used for measurement of lectin bound glycoprotein. R525, a rabbit antiserum to βCTP, detects ashCG, ashCGβ subunit, and free as βCTP. B105, a monoclonal antibody to the hCG β-subunit, detects ashCG and ashCGβ. B107, a monoclonal antibody specific for dimeric hCG, detects only ashCG. Analyses of a sample containing a mixture of these forms of ashCG, using the three antibodies, allow the calculation of the concentration of each component. These assays will be examined for their abilities to detect ashCG in the urines of choriocarcinoma patients, who have been reported to excrete this unusual form of hCG.

1152 AN EM STUDY OF PITUITARY PROLACTIN CELL POPULATIONS IN CARCINOGEN TREATED FEMALE RATS.

P.M.Ingleton* and P.V.Gaitens, Department of Zoology, The University of Sheffield. S10 2TN. U.K.

In the strain of Sprague-Dawley rats used for this study there is only a low incidence of mammary tumours following a single intragastric dose (20mg) of 7,12-dimethylbenz(a)anthracene(DMBA) in 50-60 day old females; 1/8 and 2/14 in two experiments. However,pituitary prolactin(PRL) cells appear to be affected by the treatment,ultimately showing adenomatous changes.PRL cell morphology could be seen to have changed three days after treatment,particularly showing dilated RER cisternae. By eight weeks two populations of PRL cells could be distinguished,one composed of cells with very dilated RER which showed some fragmentation and disorganisation,large Golgi with immature secretory granules and few large pleomorphic hormone storage granules in the cytoplasm. Immunoperoxidase staining with antiserum to rat PRL only showed hormone in the granules,with none in the RER cisternae. These PRL cells had features similar to those of oestrogen treated rats and appeared to be active.Cells of the other major group of PRL cells had dense cytoplasm,abundant RER organised into parallel arrays with narrow lumena and with many free ribosomes. The Golgi of these cells were large,with many immature secretory granules, but also large numbers of mature pleomorphic granules in the peripheral cytoplasm; granule release was frequent and mitosis was only seen in this PRL cell population. The numbers of these cells declined and were very rare eight months after DMBA treatment when other PRL cells showed distinct adenomatous changes.
This study was supported by the Yorkshire Cancer Research Campaign.

1153 INHIBITION OF ESTROGEN BIOSYNTHESIS IN HUMAN TROPHOBLAST TUMORS GROWN IN ATHYMIC NUDE MICE. J.O. Johnston* and C.L. Wright, Merrell Dow Research Institute, Cincinnati, OH 45215, U.S.A.

A human trophoblast choriocarcinoma cell line (JAr), which has the capacity for bioconversion of androgens to estrogens by aromatase, was utilized to evaluate inhibitors of estrogen biosynthesis. In vitro kinetic analyses using JAr cells in culture were used to compare a suicide aromatase inhibitor, 10-(2-propynyl)-estr-4-ene-3,17-dione (MDL 18,962), with inhibitors in clinical use for breast carcinoma. S.c. injections of JAr cells (~2×10^6 cell/site) into nude mice resulted in the development of tumors (~500 mg) in 9-11 days. In tissue culture the clinical agents, aminoglutethimide, a competitive aromatase inhibitor (apparent Ki=830 nM), and Δ^1-testololactone, a competitive and time-dependent inhibitor (apparent Ki=560 nM, $k_{cat}=1.5 \times 10^{-4}$ sec^{-1}) were approximately 1300 times less active in inhibiting aromatase activity in JAr cells in vitro than the suicide inhibitor MDL 18,962, a competitive and time-dependent aromatase inhibitor (apparent Ki=0.6 nM, $k_{cat}=4.4 \times 10^{-4}$ sec^{-1}). MDL 18,962 had a greater affinity for aromatase active-site than the natural substrate, androstenedione (apparent Km=35 nM). Trophoblast tumor aromatase inhibition relative to concurrent vehicle-treated controls for 5-6 mice per treatment group was determined at 6 h after a single subcutaneous injection of each inhibitor. Aminoglutethimide at 100 mg/kg caused 35% inhibition and was inactive at 10 mg/kg. Δ^1-testololactone at 10 mg/kg exhibited 15% inhibition while MDL 18,962 at 10 and 1 mg/kg had 62% and 43% inhibition, respectively. The data indicate that a suicide aromatase inhibitor with a high affinity for the enzyme may offer greater specificity and prolonged pharmacologic action than the current clinically available agents.

1154 THE EFFECT OF CORTISOL ON GROWTH AND AROMATASE ACTIVITY IN FOUR LINES OF CULTURED HUMAN BREAST CARCINOMA CELLS. D.W. Killinger*, L. Kharlip, M. Blackstein, and E. Perel, Department of Medicine and Institute of Medical Sciences, University of Toronto, Toronto, Canada M5R 1A8.

The effects of cortisol on cell growth and aromatase activity were examined in four lines of cultured human breast carcinoma cells (MD, DM, MCF-7, ZR-75). The cells were grown in α-MEM with 15% fetal calf serum. Cell growth was studied over a period of 14 days in medium with and without cortisol (10^{-6}M). Aromatase activity was determined daily starting on day 4 of culture. In both the MD and DM lines, which have previously been shown to possess high aromatase activity, there was no effect of cortisol on the rate of cell division. Aromatase activity in both lines was greatly stimulated by cortisol in the late exponential phase with maximum stimulation occurring as the cells reached confluence (400 to 600%). The growth of MCF-7 cells was inhibited by 40% in the presence of cortisol. Aromatase activity was low under basal conditions and was stimulated by 300% by the addition of cortisol. The growth of ZR-75 cells was inhibited by 50% in medium containing cortisol. Aromatase activity in these cells was also low under basal conditions and there was no detectable stimulation by cortisol. These studies suggest that assessment of aromatase activity in breast carcinoma tissue may be helpful in predicting growth response to hormone manipulation.

1155 REGULATION OF CORTISOL METABOLISM BY LYMPHOCYTES - ISOLATION OF AN ENHANCING FACTOR.

A. Klein*, A.W. - L. Chan and A. Malkin. Sunnybrook Med. Ctr.,University of Toronto, Clinical Biochemistry Dept., Toronto, Canada.

In previous studies, we found that plasma of healthy subjects is characterized by the ability to enhance cortisol metabolism by lymphocytes. This effect was found to be reduced in plasma of carcinoma patients due to lack of enhancing factors or presence of inhibitory factors. This experiment is an attempt to isolate lymphocyte cortisol metabolism enhancing factors (LCMEF). Recently we demonstrated that the factors were sufficiently small to pass through dialysis membranes. In the present study, gel filtration and high pressure liquid chromatography (HPLC) were used in an attempt to isolate and purify these factors. Dialysate of healthy donors' plasma (HDP) and of cancer patients' plasma (CPP) were chromatographed separately on C-10 Sephadex columns. Most of the enhancing effect of the HDP on cortisol metabolism by lymphocytes was found in the region between two conductivity peaks and was related to a factor with a probable molecular weight of 400 D. This enhancing effect was significantly reduced in the same region by the CPP. HPLC carried out with phenyl and NH_2 columns showed that LCMEF - because of its high polarity - is separated on the polar column (NH_2) functioning as normal phase chromatography column. These results show that gel filtration and HPLC could be used for LCMEF isolation. The results obtained with CPP support the assumption that this plasma is lacking LCMEF.

1156 LONG-TERM LHRH-AGONIST TREATMENT OF METASTATIC BREAST CANCER.

J.G.M. Klijn* and F.H. de Jong. Dr Daniel Den Hoed Cancer Center and Erasmus University ROTTERDAM.

In our first study on the endocrine and antitumor effects of chronic intranasal treatment with 3x400/ug of the LHRH-agonist Buserelin = Hoe 766(after 3-7 days 3 mg i.v.or s.c.)in 12 untreated premenopausal pts.with metastatic breast cancer we found an objective tumor response (irresp.of the receptor status)in 4 pts.and stable disease in 4 further ones.The longest duration of response until now is 27+ mths. Because of the observation that with this dose 6 pts.did not show continuous complete suppression of ovarian E^2 secretion(in contrast to Prog.)we have treated 5 menstruating pts.($\bar{x}$-42 yr)using very high doses of 2x1 mg s.c.We decreased the dose gradually during treatment ($\bar{x}$24 wks,range 6-44 w.)to doses between 800 and 1800/ug per day s.c. In all 5 pts. a complete castration was reached within 2-3 wks.with very low mean plasma E_2 levels during long-term treatment i.e.18,31, 25,10 and 12 pmol/l(x=19 pmol/l∾5 pg/ml).All pts. had complaints about flushes.In 4 pts. plasma LH and FSH were clearly suppressed during chronic treatment in relation to pretreatment levels but not to subnormal values. 2 Pts.showed an objective tumor response (9 and 3^+_m) Conclusions: 1) a dose of 3x 400/ug Buserelin i.n.(~25/ug s.c.per day)caused anovulation in all pts. but suppression of follicular maturation in only half of the pts.;however,higher doses s.c.appeared to cause a strong suppression of ovarian E^2 secretion in all pts., 2) medical castration with Buserelin seems as effective (6/17=35% objective response) as surgical castration.

1157 ANTIESTROGEN-BINDING PROTEIN IN NUCLEAR EXTRACT OF HUMAN BREAST CANCER TISSUE. O.L.Kon, Dept of Medicine, Memorial University, Canada, and Dept of Biochemistry, National University of Singapore.

The precise mechanism of antiestrogen action is unclear. A specific antiestrogen binding protein (AEBP) has been identified in many tissues of several animal species including man. The functional role of this protein is unknown particularly as its presence in the nuclear extract of any tissue has not been reported. The present studies demonstrate the existence of AEBP in 0.6M KCl extracts of breast cancer nuclear pellets. In contrast to observations in the rat, differential centrifugation indicates that AEBP in breast cancer does not reside in the microsomal fraction, and KBr density gradient centrifugation demonstrates no association with lipoproteins. Breast cancer nuclear AEBP is present in more than 10-fold higher concentration than cytosolic AEBP. Nuclear and cytosolic AEBP are very similar and share the following characteristics: (1) high affinity binding of [^{3}H]-tamoxifen ($K_d = 10^{-9}$M); (2) little or no binding affinity for steroid hormones; (3) only nonsteroidal antiestrogens (tamoxifen, CI628 nafoxidine, clomiphene, LY117018 and trioxifene) compete for bound [^{3}H]-tamoxifen; (4) large size as judged by gel filtration (agarose 0.5m) and sedimentation analysis; (5) greater thermal stability than the estrogen receptor. DEAE-chromatography also indicates that AEBP is less negatively charged than the estrogen receptor. These characteristics of AEBP from breast cancer tissue are remarkably similar to the AEBP from normal human tissue (myometrium) (J Biol Chem 258:3173, 1983), possibly reflecting a highly conserved structure. Supported by MRC(Canada), NCI(Canada), National University of Singapore and the Shaw Foundation.

1158 CORRELATION BETWEEN CELL GROWTH AND NUCLEAR ANDROGEN RECEPTOR REGULATION IN HUMAN PROSTATIC TUMOR CELL. Y. Koseki* and M.S. Soloway, University of Tennessee Center for the Health Sciences, Memphis, TN 38163, U.S.A.

The effects of dihydrotestosterone (DHT) and 17B-estradiol (E_2) on the growth and the levels and cellular distribution of androgen (AR) and estrogen (ER) receptors in prostatic tumors were examined using human prostatic epithelial cell line DU-145 (metastatic) and 1013L (primary). The cell growth was measured by DNA determination and receptor assay was done by an improved hydroxylapatite (HAP) post-precipitation exchange assay using [^{3}H]methyltrienolone or [^{3}H]estradiol as radioactive ligand.

Dihydrotestosterone alone did not induce the growth of both cell lines and regulated the AR levels differently in each cell line: that increased cytoplasmic AR (ARc) but decreased nuclear AR (ARn) in cell line 1013L and did not change the levels of ARc and ARn in cell line DU-145. On the other hand, DHT (10^{-7}M) along with E_2 (10^{-11}-10^{-9}M) induced the growth of cell line DU-145 only. This combination treatment increased total AR specifically AR_n in cell line DU-145, however that did not change the AR levels in cell line 1013L and the ER levels in both cell lines.

Physiological concentration of E_2 (10^{-10}M, 10^{-11}M) induced the growth of both cell lines, though this induction was not so marked as seen by DHT plus E_2 in growth of cell DU-145, and pharmacological concentration (10^{-8}M) suppressed the growth of cell line DU-145 and did not that of cell line 1013L.

Nuclear AR regulation appeared to be the key mechanism in controlling the growth of human prostatic tumor cell.

1159 LONG TERM FOLOW-UP OF PATIENTS WITH ADVANCED PROSTATIC CARCINOMA TREATED WITH BUSERELIN OR OCHIECTOMY.

M.Koutsilieris*[1], R.Herrera[1] and G.Tolis[1,2], Royal Victoria Hospital[1],Montreal,Quebec,Canada and Hippokrateion Hospital[2] Athens, Greece.

Twenty nine patients with advanced prostatic carcinoma were subjected to orchiectomy or treated medically with an LHRH agonist analogue (Buserelin)(n:20). The evaluation of the patients was done as previously reported by us (P.N.A.S.79:1658,1982) and the response was assessed according to the criteria established by the National Prostatic Cancer Project.

All ten patients with stage C or D_1 entered in ful remission of the disease for up to 3 year follow-up. Among the patients with stage D_2 we documented objective stable in 9 and partial response in 9. Escape from the control of the disease process was primarily evident in the osseous metastases(100%) rather than in the prostate (20%). This occurred within 16 months in 2 of 6 orchiectomised and in 8 of 12 Buserelin treated patients; 2 patients relapsed at 17 and 22 months. Within the 3 years of follow-up we had 8 deaths, all of disease dissemination. At the time of relapse or death plasma testosterone values were in castrate levels and did not differ from those in whom the disease was arrested. The three variables we found of significant predictive value for disease evolution were: a.Histologic grading b.degree of elevation of prostatic acid and bone alkaline phosphatase levels and c.extension of bone metastases. Side effects included impotence and hot flushes; no morbidity was associated with Buserelin. Above data document the value of Buserelin in advanced prostate cancer and suggest that the disease outcome depends on other variables than plasma androgens.

1160 CLONING OF DUNNING PROSTATIC TUMOR mRNAS.

C. Kreis, and J.G. Dodd, A. Hamel, R.J. Matusik*, Department of Molecular Endocrinology, Laval University, Quebec, and Department of Physiology, University of Manitoba, Winnipeg, R3E OW3, Canada.

The purpose of this study was to identify mRNAs that are preferentially or specifically expressed in the androgen dependent rat Dunning R-3327H prostatic tumor. The sequence complexity of the tumor, ventral and dorsal prostate indicates three component classes. However, in the ventral and dorsal prostate the highly abundant class contains 1-3 sequence in contrast to 54 of the tumor. Since the tumor class comprises 34% of the mRNA population, we identified the major proteins by a limited Rot hybrid arrest (12%) and cell free translation. After 2-D gel electrophoresis, we have identified six major proteins. In order to obtain probes to their mRNAs, a cDNA cloned library prepared to tumor mRNAs was screened kinetically to identify preferentially, and differentially to identify specifically expressed genes. Additionally, the colonies were, screened with P^{32}cDNA synthesized to mRNA of regressing tumors (castrated animals) and growing tumors to select androgen dependent genes. By screening 1200 colonies, 5 androgen dependent and 5 androgen independent preferentially expressed genes; and, 2 androgen dependent and 1 androgen independent specifically expressed genes were identified. Furthermore, 3 of the preferentially and 2 of the specifically expressed rat genes show homology to human benign hyperplasic mRNAs. Thus, we have selected probes not only to rat tumor mRNAs but also to express human prostatic genes. Supported by NCI of Canada.

1161 TREATMENT OF ADRENAL ANDROGEN DEFICIENCY IN HYPOPITUITARY ADOLESCENTS. J.C. Job*, and A. Rolland, Faculté Cochin, Paris.

In 17 prepubertal hypopituitary patients (14 M, 3 F) treated with hGH 12-30 IU/kg/yr (m = 20.8) from at least two years, the lack of adrenarche was documented by subnormal plasma DHA and/or DHAS levels at age 14.5 ± 2.1 and bone age 10.4 ± 1.4 yrs. Norethandrolone (N) 0.25 mg/kg/day 2 months/3 was then added, the dose of hGH remaining unchanged. The mean ± SD growth velocity (cm/6 ms) increased from 1.94 ± .77 before N to 3.83 ± 1.02 on the first semester with N (n = 17), 3.57 ± .83 the 2nd (n = 16) and 3.15 ± .70 the 3d (n = 7). Thus height gain rose from 4.47 ± 1.20 to 7.50 ± 1.56 cm for 1 year, and from 6.10 ± 1.18 to 10.12 ± 2.3 cm for 1 1/2 year. Bone age did not advance faster than height age, the ratio BA/HA being 1.02 ± .13 before, 1.00 ± .11 after 1 yr and 1.03 ± .11 after 1 1/2 yr with N. No side-effects were observed. In a control group of 8 hypopituitary dwarfs with similar age conditions and normal adrenarche, association of N to hGH had to be stopped after a short trial since it provoked advance of bone age and/or virilizing side-effects. It is suggested that the management of pituitary deficiency in children would include the follow-up of adrenal androgens, and the prepubertal use of mild androgens when adrenarche is lacking.

1162 CLINICAL AND EXPERIMENTAL STUDIES ON THE ROLE OF GABA IN THE REGULATION OF ACTH SECRETION. M. T. Jones*, B. Gillham, R. Altaher, U. Beckford, +J. Jenkins, +A. Prysor-Jones, ++R. Abraham, ++A. Dornhorst, ++V. Wynn, Department of Gynaecology, St. Thomas's Hospital, London SE1; +Department of Medicine II, St. George's Hospital, London SW17, and ++Alexander Simpson Laboratory for Metabolic Research, St. Mary's Hospital, London W2.

GABA inhibits CRF secretion, induced by 5-HT and acetylcholine from the hypothalamus incubated in vitro, and is implicated in the negative feedback exerted by corticosteroids on CRF release. Sodium valproate (Epilim) has weak GABA-transaminase inhibitory activity but acts mainly by enhancing, postsynaptically, the effectiveness of endogenously released GABA. We initially tested the effect of this drug given over 3-5 weeks on circulating ACTH in six patients suffering from Nelson's syndrome. ACTH levels were significantly ($p < 0.002$) decreased but returned to pretreatment values after withdrawal of treatment. Subsequently, 10 patients were treated with sodium valproate (600-1200 mg/day) for 5-32 weeks, the ACTH levels falling from 2460 ± 1870 to 480 ± 330 ng/l with the return of the ACTH circadian rhythm in two patients. On discontinuing treatment, plasma ACTH levels rose to pretreatment values in 5-12 weeks. Two patients failed to show a second response to treatment. In one patient, a reduction size of a pituitary microadenoma occurred with treatment. 5-10g GABA given orally had no effect on circulating ACTH levels in the control period but caused a profound fall when the patients were on valproate. Neither valproate nor GABA affected ACTH release from tumour tissue incubated in vitro suggesting the effect is primarily at the hypothalamus.

1163 VALUABILITY OF AN ANTI-PLATELET AGGREGATION INHIBITOR(TICLOPIDINE) TO GRAVES' OPHTHALMOPATHY. T. Kakita*, H.Hosojima and S.Morimoto, Department of Medicine, Kanazawa Medical University, Uchinada, Ishikawa, Japan

The treatment of Graves' ophthalmopathy is presently unsatisfactory. We evaluated the new management to these ophthalmopathies. Fifteen patients of Graves' disease treated with PTU or MZI were accompanied with bilateral or unilateral exophthalmus and medicated with ticlopidine. 8 of the patients were cross-overed with predonisolone. In these cases the patients were treated with 30mg/day predonisolone for 3-4 weeks and then medicated with 200-300mg/day ticlopidine. 7 patients were medicated with ticlopidine alone. The improvement of ophthalmopathies were assessed by clinical symptoms and the length of "A" on X-P of orbits CT scanner(c.f. Figure). Predonisolone produced a clinical improvement and a decrease of "A" on CT X-P in 12 of the 13 eyes. "A" of pre-treatment;19.2±2.7mm(mean±SD), post-treatment;16.8±2.9mm(p 0.01). 3 eyes of 2 patients recurred after changing to ticlopidine following predonisolone. "A" of 9 eyes, however, remained 17.0±2.7mm(significant from the pre-treatment "A" values). The effective rate of ticlopidine in 15 patients was 70% clinically and objectively on CT X-P. There were no severe side effect except for hyperemia of one conjectivae. It is difficult to continue the drugs that are previously well known to be effective to Graves' ophthalmopathy for long time because of serious side effects. These result suggust that ticlopidine may be effective in improvement of Graves' ophthalmopathy, while it's mechanism is unknown. This may provide a new perspective regard of the etiology of Graves' ophthalmopathy.

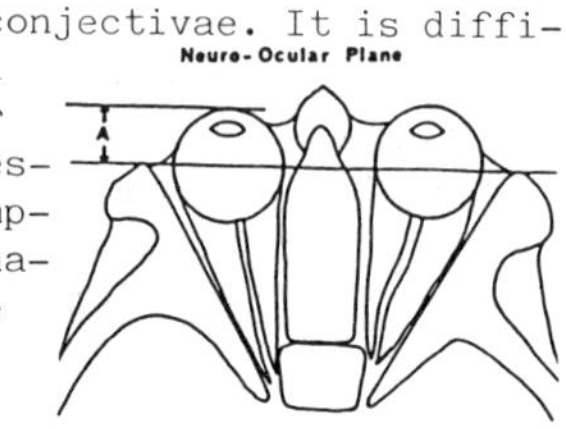

1164 ENDOCRINE ABNORMALITIES FOLLOWING TREATMENT FOR GYNECOLOGICAL MALIGNANCIES. S. Katayama*, K. Shimaoka, M.S. Piver, G. Osman and Y. Tsukada, Saitama Medical School, Saitama, Japan, Roswell Park Memorial Institute and SUNY at Buffalo, New York, U.S.A.

The therapeutic consequences of gynecological malignancies on the endocrine organs were studied in 1265 patients who were diagnosed to have carcinoma of the ovary, and cervix and corpus uteri at Roswell Park Memorial Institute during a 20-year period 1963-1983. Among them, autopsy was performed in 242 cases, which includes ovary 99, cervix 101, and corpus 42. We found 14 cases of adrenal hyperplasia, 17 cases of parathyroid hyperplasia and 10 thyroid adenomas. When these autopsy cases are divided into 150 cases in whom no radiation therapy (RT) or surviving less than 1 yr from RT and 92 cases who survived more than 1 yr after RT, the latter group had significantly higher incidence of adrenal hyperplasia 9 vs 5 ($p < 0.05$) and parathyroid hyperplasia 12 vs 5 ($p < 0.01$). However, thyroid adenoma was found 5 vs 5 and no significant differences. Only 1 of 12 cases with parathyroid hyperplasia in the irradiated group was associated with clinical and biochemical hyperparathyroidism. A higher incidence of chronic thyroiditis was found in the non-irradiated group of ovarian cancer (8/53) as compared to the irradiated patients (1/46). When reanalyzed in relation to chemotherapy all 9 pts had received chemotherapy. This results suggest that irradiation to the pelvic region may increase the incidence of adrenal and parathyroid hyperplasia. Chemotherapy may trigger chronic thyroiditis in the patients with ovarian carcinoma.

1165 ACUTE AND LONG-TERM EFFECT OF CAPTOPRIL (SQ14,225) IN PATIENTS WITH IDIOPATHIC EDEMA.
M. Kawamura*, H. Suzuki, H. Nakane, I. Saito, E. Takeshita, T. Uchida and T. Saruta. Department of Internal Med. and Division of Endocrinology, Laboratory Med., Keio University Hospital, Tokyo, and Department of Internal Med., Urawa City Hospital, Urawa, Japan.

We investigated the acute and long-term effect of captopril, an orally administered angiotensin convering enzyme inhibitor, in patients with idiopathic edema (IE) to study, 1) the role of the renin-angiotensin-aldosterone system in the pathogenesis of this disease and 2) the long-term therapeutic usefulness of this drug. In the acute study, 8 patients with IE and 5 normal controls were studied. The urinary water and sodium excretion during 3hr-recumbency were compared to those during 3hr-standing with or without captopril administration (50 mg/day). The changes in plasma renin activity (PRA), plasma aldosterone (PA) while keeping different postures were also compared between control and patients groups. Compared to 5 normals, patients with IE showed significantly greater reduction in water and sodium excretion and greater increment in PA and PRA in the upright posture. In these patients, captopril significantly restored water and sodium excretion, attenuated the increment of PA and enhanced the rise in PRA in the upright posture. The effects of captopril on these variables were not remarkable in normals. By long-term captopril administration, marked clinical improvement of edema was obtained without remarkable side effect and the dosage of diuretics to control edema state could be minimized or, in some cases, discontinued. These results suggest that an enhanced response of the renin-angiotensin-aldosterone system to standing plays an important role in the pathophysiology of IE and that captopril may be an effective drug for IE in the long-term therapy.

1166 CLINICAL APPLICATION OF PULSATILE GONADOTROPHIN RELEASING HORMONE (GnRH).
E.J.Keogh*, C.Carati, J.Meakin, A.MacKellar, C.Lawson-Smith, S.Laing, S.Banovic, D.Curnow & +C.Matthews. Reproductive Medicine Research Institute, Depts. Clinical Biochemistry and Endocrinology, Queen Elizabeth II Medical Centre, Nedlands, Western Australia, +Dept. Obstetrics and Gynaecology, Queen Elizabeth Hospital, Woodville, South Australia.

Intermittent administration of boluses of GnRH (every 1-2 hours around the clock, 50-200ug per day) has proved effective in the management of cryptorchidism, hypogonadism in men and hypothalamic anovulatory infertility (HAI) in women. GnRH (Ayerst, Australia) was delivered subcutaneously from a battery operated syringe driver (4.5x2x11cm,115gms). One hundred and fourteen cryptorchid boys (1-13 years) received GnRH for 30-100 days. Forty six testes (20/75 unilaterally and 26/78 bilaterally cryptorchid testes) descended and remained in the scrotum. In all but 3 of the remainder, congenital or acquired mechanical barriers to descent were found. Four azoospermic men (28-30 years) received GnRH for 3-18 months. Testicular size, gonadotrophins and testosterone increased and sperm concentration reached 3-120 x $10^6 ml^{-1}$. Three pregnancies resulted in their spouses. Fourteen women (25-35 years) with clomiphene-resistant HAI were treated for 1-9 months. Ten ovulated and 6 conceived. The ovulation and conception rates per month were 60% and 15% respectively. In conclusion, GnRH is effective in various hormonal disorders when frequent, small doses are administered.

1167 A COMPARISON OF ESTROGEN AND ANDROGEN RECEPTOR LEVELS IN PROSTATIC TISSUE FROM PATIENTS WITH NON-METASTATIC AND METASTATIC PROSTATE CANCER AND BENIGN PROSTATIC HYPERPLASIA. R.Y. Kirdani*, L.J. Emrich, E.J. Pontes, R.L. Priore and A.A. Sandberg. Roswell Park Memorial Institute, Buffalo, N.Y.

The utility of receptor levels as markers in prostatic cancer was investigated by determining estrogen (ER, n=72) and androgen (AR, n=33) receptors by a high pressure liquid chromatography (HPLC) method in 72 human prostatic 'large' and 'needle biopsy' specimens obtained at prostatectomy. A total of 27 comparisons were made amongst various groupings of the results. No significant correlation was found between ER and AR values determined in the same tissues, nor was there any significant correlation between ER values measured in needle biopsy specimens taken from a large piece with the corresponding value in the remainder of the large piece. In other analyses, it was found that median values of cytosolic AR in the four cancer stages examined were statistically significant from each other (p=0.01), with AR increasing from stages A through D. Even though ER differences between the four stages were not significant (p=0.13), there was a trend for median ER values to decrease with stages B through D. On the other hand, median BPH values for both ER and AR were found to lie mid-scale compared to the respective cancer stages. Even though it is probable that receptor values cannot be used to distinguish between cancer and BPH in human prostatic tissue, these measurements could be used as a marker of the hormonal status of the tissue. However, more problematic is our finding that receptor values in needle biopsies probably are not representative of the actual values. Even though further refinements of methodology can be achieved, in our opinion, competitive binding techniques may have to be abandoned in favor of an immunologic assay.

1168 USE OF PROTON BEAM IRRADIATION OF THE PITUITARY FOR CUSHING DISEASE TREATMENT. L.E.Kirpatovskaya, E.I.Marova, G.S.Kolesnikova, Yu.V.Morozov*, Institute of Experimental Endocrinology and Hormone Chemistry, the USSR Academy of Medical Sciences, Moscow, USSR.

40 patients with intracellar adenomas or pituitary microadenomas were subjected to proton beam irradiation (PBI). They suffered from light or middle forms of Cushing disease (CD) for less than 3 years. In 12 patients with middle form of CD unilateral adrenalectomy preceded PBI. For PBI of the pituitary plurifield-convergent irradiation method with biplanar rotation of the patient's head was used. PBI was discrete and was carried out from 15-25 fields in the left temporal area. Energy of proton beam was about 200 MEV, maximal single dose in the centre of convergence ranged from 5000 to 11000 RAD; proton beam was roundshaped, 6 to 10 mm in diameter. The results obtained show that PBI is effective in the treatment of light and middle forms of CD. Clinical and biochemical remission was observed in 92% and 89% respectively. PBI of the pituitary may successfully be combined with unilateral adrenalectomy which leads to shortening of remission approach period. During 3 years of observation no relapse, postirradiational side effects or hypopituitarism developed. Along with normalization of ACTH and cortisol secretion plasma GH, FSH, LH and thyrotropin levels also returned to normal values.

1169 THYROID-PITUITARY AXIS IN PATIENTS WITH ANOREXIA NERVOSA

T.Komaki*, S.Sakata, S.Nakamura, K.Kamikubo, N.Kojima and K.Miura. The 3rd Department of Internal Medicine, Gifu University School of Medicine, Gifu 500, Japan.

Serum T3, T4, free T3, free T4, rT3, TBG, and TSH levels were examined in 14 cases of anorexia nervosa and 36 age-matched healthy subjects. In patients with anorexia nervosa, serum T3, T4, free T3, free T4, and TBG levels were 67.9±40.8 ng/dl, 4.8±1.7 µg/dl, 2.1±0.72 pmol/l, 0.82±0.17 ng/dl, and 16.9±3.9 µg/ml (mean±SD), respectively, all of which were significantly lower than those of healthy controls. Serum rT3 levels in patients with anorexia nervosa were 348.7±22.5 pg/ml and were not significantly higher than those of controls. Serum TSH levels in the patients and healthy subjects before TRH administration were 3.3±2.1 µU/ml and 3.9±2.2 µU/ml, respctively. Values of ΣΔTSH, a sum of the increments of TSH after TRH administration, in anorexia nervosa were 63.4±28.7 µU/ml and were higher than those of normal controls (45.5±18.6 µU/ml). Thus low serum thyroid hormone levels and hyperresponsiveness of TSH against TRH administration in anorexia nervosa indicate that they are in mild hypothyroidism.

1170 PROLONGED (24 HOUR) INFUSION OF THE OPIOID ANTAGONIST NALOXONE DOES NOT SIGNIFICANTLY ALTER PLASMA LEVELS OF CORTISOL AND ACTH IN HUMANS.

M.J. Kreek*, B.S. Schneider, J. Ragunath and S. Plevy, The Rockefeller University, NY,NY 10021, USA and the L.I. Jewish-Hillside Medical Center, NY, NY, USA.

Exogenous opioids administered acutely suppress plasma levels of cortisol and ACTH. Reports suggest that acute administration of an opioid antagonist results in elevations of cortisol and ACTH levels. This study was performed to determine the effects of prolonged intravenous infusion of the specific opioid antagonist naloxone on plasma levels of cortisol and ACTH in humans. Thirteen subjects (10F,3M) who were generally healthy except for intestinal hypomotility were studied first while receiving placebo (P) infusion and then while receiving naloxone (N) 29.2mg/24h by steady state infusion, each for 24h on a blinded basis. Bloods were drawn from in-dwelling cannula at time 0,4,8,12 and 24 hours during infusion (9A,1P,4P,8P,9A) and plasma cortisol levels measured by radioimmunoassay. There were no significant differences of plasma levels of cortisol; area under the plasma cortisol level time curve (AUC_{0-24}) also were not significantly different in N vs. P. (N-256±33; P-248±25(SEM)µg/dl/24h.)

Time (N)	Pre (13)		4h (12)		8h (13)		12h (6)		24h (13)	
Treatment	P	N	P	N	P	N	P	N	P	N
µg/dl	14.8	15.2	12.8	15.2	11.5	10.8	5.0	5.6	15.2	14.7
(±SEM)	(0.9)	(1.1)	(1.2)	(2.0)	(1.2)	(1.2)	(1.0)	(1.5)	(1.1)	(1.0)

Plasma levels of ACTH were determined pre- and after 8h of N infusion (10mg in 8h) in 7 similar patients (4F,3M) studied on 12 occasions. Only one ACTH level was elevated (325pg/ml) on N. Mean plasma ACTH levels otherwise were: Pre-infusion-56±14, after 8h of N infusion-62±16(SEM)pg/ml. Specific effects of prolonged naloxone infusion on β-endorphin are being studied.

1171 BLUNTED VENTILATORY DRIVE IN HYPOTHYROIDISM: PREVALENCE, PREDICTION BY SERUM TSH, AND ACUTE REVERSIBILITY WITH THYROID HORMONE THERAPY.

PW Ladenson*, PD Goldenheim, EC Ridgway. Thyroid Unit, Mass. Gen. Hosp. Boston, MA, USA.

To define the prevalence of impaired hypercapnic (CO_2V) and hypoxic (O_2V) ventilatory drive in hypothyroidism, predictive thyroid function parameters, and the potential acute reversibility of these defects, we compared hypothyroid patients (n=37, T4 1.3±0.2 ug/dl*) to euthyroid controls (n=18). Hypothyroid patients were acutely treated with 100 ug T4 or 25-50 ug T3 IV q.d. for 7 days. Ventilatory responses were measured on days 0,3, and 8. There were more abnormal responders to CO_2 (CO_2V <0.95 L/min/mmHg) among the hypothyroid patients than controls (9/27 vs 1/18, p<0.05). Similarly, there were more abnormal responders to hypoxia (O_2V<150 L/min/mmHg) in the hypothyroid group (8/31 vs 0/17, p<0.05). Only 2 hypothyroid patients had abnormal responses to both CO_2 and O_2. For the entire hypothyroid and control groups, however, CO_2V and O_2V were not significantly different (1.27±0.12 vs 1.70±0.25 L/min/mmHg and 227±24 vs 315±41 L/min/mmHg, respectively). TSH levels were higher among the hypothyroid patients with an abnormal O_2 or CO_2 response (141±26 vs 70±14 uU/ml, P<0.05). Among hypothyroid patients with TSH levels >90 uU/ml, 7 of 11 had blunted ventilatory responses. There were no differences in the serum T4 or T3 concentrations of hypothyroid patients with normal vs abnormal responses. Acute treatment of the hypothyroid abnormal responders increased both O_2V(93±12 to 176±31 L/min/mmHg, p<0.01) and CO_2V(0.75+0.06 to 1.18±0.16 L/min/mmHg, p<0.05) by day 8. We conclude: 1) A subset of hypothyroid patients have impaired ventilatory responses to hypercapnea (33%) or hypoxia (28%). 2) Hypothyroid patients with abnormal ventilatory control are distinguished by higher levels of serum TSH. 3) Thyroid hormone therapy acutely enhances ventilatory drive within one week.

1172 **A NEW, QUICK AND VERY EFFECTIVE PREPARATION FOR THYROID SURGERY IN PATIENTS WITH GRAVES' DISEASE.**

E. Lajeunie*, D. Houlbert , D. Julien, P. Tran Ba Huy, R. Caporal and J.M. Segrestaa. Hôpital Lariboisière. Paris. France.

The aim of the present study was to test the efficiency and the tolerance of the combination of dexamethasone (DEX), Carbimazole (C) and potassium iodide (KI) in the preoperative management of hyperthyroidism. 13 patients with Graves' disease in whom subtotal thyroidectomy was considered the most appropriate form of therapy were studied. All patients received for 6 days DEX 2 mg every 6 hours, KI 60 mg every 8 hours and C 15 mg three times daily. Thyroidectomy was performed on day 7. T3, T4 and iFT4 (free thyroxine index) were determined before starting treatment (Day 0) and on successive days (days 1 to 6) before surgery. The mean D0 values ± SEM for T3, T4 and iFT4 were respectively 454 ng/dl ± 41, 20,1 µg/dl ± 2,2 and 25,1 ± 2,7. Normal range : 80-180 ng/dl, 5-14 µg/dl and 4,5-15. The decrease in serum T3 was statistically significant at about 24 hours after beginning treatment (p <0,001) and reached the normal range in all patients on day 4. The changes in T4 and iFT4 were statistically significant 48 hours after beginning treatment (p <0,05) and on day 6 all patients but two were in normal range. At the time of operation all patients were clinically euthyroid. No side effects were observed other than a reversible hypocalcemia. Surgery was carried out in each patient without complications and after 1 year of follow-up observation all patients were biochemically euthyroid. This treatment has proved to be always effective and well tolerated. It has the advantage to reduce the time of preoperative preparation without any inconvinience.

1173 THE EFFECTS OF A LONG-ACTING SOMATOSTATIN ANALOG ON PITUITARY TUMOR GROWTH AND HORMONE SECRETION IN RAT AND MAN. S.W.J. Lamberts*, P. Uitterlinden, J. Zuiderwijk, T. Verleun, M. Neufeld and E. Del Pozo, Dept Medicine, Erasmus University, Rotterdam, The Netherlands and Sandoz, Basel, Switzerland.

SMS 201-999 (SMS) is a potent somatostatin analog, which is in vivo 20 times more active than somatostatin in inhibiting GH secretion and exerts a weaker inhibitory effect on insulin release. In vitro studies with normal cultured rat pituitary cells showed that 10 nM of SMS completely and 1 fM of SMS partially (by 60%) prevented the GRF (10 nM)-induced GH release, while at 10 nM SMS did not affect CRF-stimulated ACTH release. In vivo adm. of SMS (2 and 12 ug/kg/day) for 30 days inhibited the growth of the transplantable PRL/ACTH-secreting rat pituitary tumor 7315a by 40%.SMS (10 nM) also directly inhibited PRL and ACTH release by dispersed 7315a tumor cells by 40% and 16%, resp.In pituitary tumor cell cultures prepared from 4 acromegalic patients, 10 nM of SMS inhibited GH release by 35±4%, while 0.1 nM SMS completely overcame GRF (10 nM)-induced GH secretion.In vivo subc.adm. of 50 ug SMS to 5 acromegalics inhibited GH levels by more than 50% for 10.2±2.1 h (basal GH levels varied between 12 and 47 ng/ml; mean 29 ng/ml). There was a slight transient postprandial increase in blood glucose. SMS 201-995 is a promising drug, because of its high potency and long action after subc.adm. and might be useful in the treatment of acromegaly and for indications in oncology as well.

1174 NON-SUPPRESSIBILITY OF SERUM THYROGLOBULIN TO EXOGENOUS THYROID HORMONE IN THE ASSESSMENT OF THE HYPOFUNCTIONING THYROID NODULE. E. Lechuga* and P.G. Walfish, Dept. of Medicine and Endocrine Division, Mount Sinai Hospital, University of Toronto, Ontario, M5G 1X5, Canada.

In order to assess the risk of underlying neoplasia and/or cancer, patients with hypofunctioning and solid thyroid nodules delineated by radioactive scintiscans and fine-needle biopsy (FNB), respectively, had serial measurements of serum thyroglobulin (Tg) before and after exogenous thyroid hormone feeding with a maximal dose of either L-triiodothyronine (T3) 50-75 ug/day for a 3-4 week period, or 0.1-0.15 mg/day of L-thyroxine for 6-8 weeks. All patients with hypofunctioning nodules were euthyroid and asymptomatic and none had underlying cardiovascular, hepatic or renal disease. The response to thyroid hormone suppression of serum thyroglobulin was compared to the results of FNB cytology performed after obtaining basal Tg as well as to final surgical histology in 40 subjects consisting of 17 with follicular adenoma, 5 Hurthle cell adenoma, 8 thyroid cancers, 7 benign multinodular goiter and 3 benign degenerating colloid nodules. The suppression (mean % decrease from pretreatment level) in serum Tg after thyroid hormone feeding was maximal in patients with degenerating benign colloid goiter and multinodular goiter (63.5% and 40%, respectively). In patients with follicular adenoma, Hurthle cell adenoma and thyroid carcinoma, overall mean Tg suppression was less than 30%. Using a less than 50% suppression response criterion as an index of neoplasia and/or cancer, 25 of 30 (83.4%) were correctly positive and only 5 of 30 (16.6%) were false negative. Suppressibility was not related to nodule size. Although Hurthle cell adenomas were smaller in diameter than follicular adenomas (1.68 vs 3.12 cm) they had the highest basal serum thyroglobulin (98.24 vs. 42.79 pmol/dl). These preliminary results suggest that the % suppressibility of serum thyroglobulin from pretreatment values may provide a non-invasive adjunctive diagnostic aid in the preoperative assessment of hypofunctioning solid nodules which, when combined with FNB, may assist in the detection of thyroid neoplasia and cancer.

1175 MOLECULAR HETEROGENEITY OF VERTEBRATE LUTEINIZING HORMONE-RELEASING HORMONE: STRUCTURAL ANALYSIS OF REPTILE AND TELEOST BRAIN LH-RH.
J.A. King*, R.C. Meinert and R.P. Millar, Department of Chemical Pathology, University of Cape Town Medical School, Observatory 7925, South Africa.

Hypothalamic LH-RHs in birds, reptiles and fish differ structurally from mammalian LH-RH (mLH-RH) in the region Leu^7Arg^8 while amphibian LH-RH is identical to mLH-RH. Isolation and sequence analyses have established the structure of chicken hypothalamic LH-RH (cLH-RH) as Gln^8-LH-RH and salmon brain LH-RH (sLH-RH) as Trp^7,Leu^8-LH-RH. Recent studies utilising region-specific LH-RH antisera and high performance liquid chromatography (HPLC) indicate that reptile (lizard) brain LH-RH and teleost (hake) brain and pituitary LH-RHs are identical to sLH-RH. Immunoreactive (IMR) LH-RH in crude acetic acid extracts and in HPLC-purified extracts was measured with five region-specific antisera generated against mLH-RH and cLH-RH. Comparative antiserum binding studies demonstrated that lizard and hake IMR LH-RHs differ from mLH-RH and cLH-RH at residues 7 and 8, and have similar immunological properties to sLH-RH. In at least four reverse phase HPLC systems specifically designed to yield high resolution of LH-RH analogs (Vydac C-18, Spherisorb ODS, Microbondapak C-18 and Microbondapak Phenyl columns; NH_4Ac/CH_3CN, TFA/CH_3CN, $HFBA/CH_3CN$, $TEAP/CH_3CN$ gradients), lizard and hake IMR LH-RHs were well-separated from mLH-RH and cLH-RH, and consistently co-eluted with the more hydrophobic sLH-RH. In cation exchange HPLC (Partisil PXS SCX column; NH_4Ac/ethanol) lizard and hake IMR LH-RHs co-eluted with sLH-RH, while cLH-RH eluted earlier and mLH-RH later. Isolated and purified hake pituitary IMR LH-RH had identical chromatographic properties to sLH-RH. These studies indicate that the major LH-RH form in lizard brain and hake brain and pituitary is Trp^7, Leu^8-LH-RH.

1176 SEASONAL CHANGES IN SERUM GROWTH HORMONE (GH) LEVELS IN THE GOLDFISH, CARASSIUS AURATUS.
T.A. Marchant* and R.E. Peter, Department of Zoology, University of Alberta, Edmonton, Alberta T6G 2E9, Canada.

Changes in circulating levels of GH in relation to the seasonal somatic growth cycle of the goldfish were studied. Several times throughout the year, the somatic growth rate and mean daily serum GH levels were determined in goldfish held under laboratory conditions simulating natural environmental photoperiods and temperatures. The fastest growth rate occurred in the summer (July) and the slowest growth rates occurred in the winter months; the seasonal changes in growth rates were closely correlated with changes in water temperature. The highest serum GH levels were found in fish sampled in March and June, and the lowest serum GH levels were found in fish sampled in November; there was no evidence for a regular daily cycle in serum GH levels at any time of the year. The changes in serum GH levels appear to be related to seasonal changes in daylength, and it is suggested that changes in the duration of the photophase or scotophase may be the environmental factor by which seasonal changes in circulating GH levels in goldfish are regulated. The data demonstrate a lag period of several weeks between seasonal maxima in mean daily serum GH levels and growth rates. This study was supported by NSERCC.

1177 MITOCHONDRIAL α-GLYCEROPHOSPHATE DEHYDROGENASE ACTIVITY IN LIVER AND BRAIN OF HYPOTHYROID FISH. A.K.Medda*, R.K.Ghosh, S.De and A.K.Ray, Bose Institute, Calcutta-700054, India.

In search of responsiveness of fish liver and brain to thyroid hormone, mitochondrial α-glycerophosphate dehydrogenase(α-GPD) activity was used as a main biochemical index. A significant reduction of α-GPD activity occurred both in liver and brain of Singi fish (Heteropneustes fossilis Bloch) immersed in thiourea-containing medium (1 mg/ml) for 33 days. Goitre was produced during this period. Thiourea treated hypothyroid fish given a single injection of L-triiodothyronine (T_3, 0.5 μg/g) not only restored the α-GPD activity to the normal level, but also raised the activity above the control value on the 3rd day as occurred in case of T_3 injection (0.5 μg/g) in normal fish. Liver appeared to be more responsive than brain to T_3 on the basis of percentage increase in enzyme activity. Mitochondrial protein content of liver and brain, though unaltered in hypothyroid fish, increased after T_3 injection (0.5 μg/g). The total protein and RNA content of liver and brain decreased in hypothyroid fish and increased above the control level after T_3 injection. The results thus show responsiveness of fish liver and brain to thyroid hormone.

1178 TEMPERATURE-DEPENDENT PHOSPHOLIPASE SENSITIVITY OF SMOOTH MUSCLE ADENYLATE CYCLASE. J.F. Krall*, and S.G. Korenman, Dept. of Medicine, UCLA, and VA Medical Center, Sepulveda, CA, USA.

Disrupting the native (membrane) structure of adenylate cyclase (AC) may provide useful insight into the state of the phospholipid bilayer during hormone regulation of cAMP production. Thus, the effect of membrane phospholipid hydrolysis by phospholipase A_2 (A_2) on isoproterenol (ISO)-sensitive AC from the smooth muscle layers of the rat uterus was examined. AC was incubated with porcine pancreatic A_2 at supramaximal concentrations. Membrane phospholipids were hydrolyzed to 62±7 and 51±5 % of control by A_2 treatment at 4 and 16°C respectively. A_2 treatment inactivated AC, subsequently determined by conversion of [^{32}P]-ATP to [^{32}P]-cAMP. A_2 treatment at 4°C decreased basal AC to 65±11 % (mean ± S.D.) and to 39±11 % of control at 16°C in 3 separate preparations. GTP-dependent AC, reflecting the activation step that couples receptor with the AC catalytic subunit, was decreased to 41±12 and 18±5 % of control by treatment with A_2 at 4 and 16°C respectively. ISO-dependent AC was completely abolished by A_2 at either 4 or 16°C. Treatment with snake venom A_2 instead of pancreatic A_2 decreased basal and GTP-dependent AC to 16±3 % of control values at either 4 or 16°C. Conclusions: Since temperature-dependent decreases in phospholipid packing are known to facilitate fatty acid tail hydrolysis by pancreatic but not by venom A_2, receptor coupling may take place in a more fluid membrane environment compared to GTP-dependent activation of the AC catalytic subunit. Therefore, β-adrenergic receptor coupling with AC and the GTP-dependent activation step have distinct and different phospholipid requirements.

1179 PARTICIPATION OF STIMULATORY AND INHIBITORY SUBUNITS IN HORMONAL CONTROL OF ADENYLATE CYCLASE. V.P. Michelangeli, S.A. Livesey and T.J. Martin, University of Melbourne, Department of Medicine, Repatriation General Hospital, Heidelberg, Victoria, Australia.

Current views of hormonal regulation of adenylate cyclase are that stimulatory hormones act solely via the stimulatory (N_s) component of the nucleotide regulatory subunit, whilst inhibitory hormones act solely through its inhibitory (N_i) component. We present evidence to indicate that hormones can produce their net effects by a combined action through both the N_s and N_i subunits. The human breast cancer cell line, T47 D, possesses an adenylate cyclase stimulated by to both calcitonin and PGE_2. The maximal effect on cyclic AMP production is greater with calcitonin than with PGE_2. When maximal concentrations of both hormones were added to cells simultaneously, the amount of cyclic AMP generated was less than that seen with calcitonin alone. When T47 D cells were treated with pertussis toxin (islet activating protein; IAP) which inactivates N_i there was no change in basal or calcitonin-stimulated adenylate cyclase activity. The PGE_2 response was augmented at all dose levels. Moreover, in cells pretreated with IAP, simultaneous addition of PGE_2 and calcitonin resulted in additivity rather than in inhibition of cyclic AMP production. These data are consistent with a model in which calcitonin acts through N_s alone, whereas PGE_2 acts by both N_s and an N_i input. The N_i input is capable of limiting calcitonin effects when the two agonists are used simultaneously. Preliminary data using other cell lines and hormones suggest that this phenomenon can be generally applied to adenylate cyclase control.

1180 CYCLIC AMP DEPENDENT PHOSPHORYLATION OF HIGH MOLECULAR WEIGHT THYROID MEMBRANE PROTEINS. Y. Munari-Silem*, J. Champier, C. Alquier, C. Audebet and B. Rousset, INSERM U.197, Faculté de Médecine A.Carrel, Lyon, France.

Cyclic AMP dependent and independent protein-kinases (PK) are both present in cytosolic and particulate fractions of thyroid tissue.They have been essentially studied using exogenous substrates;little is known about their physiological substrates. In this work we have studied the phosphorylation reactions in thyroid membranes (TM) in order to identify component(s) phosphorylated by TM-PK. TM were purified from fresh pig thyroid fragments forced through a steel sieve in hypotonic medium. The filtrate was centrifuged (95000xg,1h) on 41 % sucrose solution. The interface material used as TM fraction was tested for its PK content by measuring ^{32}P incorporation into histones(H), phosvitin (P) and into intrinsic membrane proteins (IMP). Phosphorylated IMP were analyzed by SDS-polyacrylamide gel electrophoresis and autoradiography. PK activities of TM fraction measured with H(H-PK) and P(P-PK) represented 13 and 1 % of the corresponding total activity in the homogenate; the specific activity of H-PK and P-PK was increased by 28 and 3, respectively. The ^{32}P incorporation into IMP was about 50 % of that obtained with IMP+H. A large number of IMP were phosphorylated. In the absence of cAMP three main bands were observed (MW:115,105 and 42KD); the 42 KD protein was the major product. In the presence of cAMP (10 μM), three additional species of high MW (about 350,270 and 230 KD) were detected. None of these components did correspond to major proteins after Coomassie staining. In conclusion, we found that TM contain selective substrates for cAMP dependent PK ; these substrates are present in low amounts and characterized by their high MW.

1181 IN VIVO AND IN VITRO STUDIES ON THE PRODUCTION OF PLACENTAL PROTEINS (HUMAN CHORIONIC GONADOTROPIN, HUMAN PLACENTAL LACTOGEN AND PREGNANCY SPECIFIC ß1-GLYCOPROTEIN) IN AN ADRENAL CHORIOCARCINOMA. M. Maeyama,* Y. Furuki, M. Munemura and N. Tanaka, Department of Obstetrics and Gynecology, Kumamoto University Medical School, Kumamoto 860, Japan

The ectopic production of placental proteins (human chorionic gonadotropin (hCG), human placental lactogen (hPL) and pregnancy specific ß1-glycoprotein (SP_1)) by an adrenal choriocarcinoma was investigeated experimentally in vivo and in vitro. Using selective adrenal vein catheterization, the concentration of hCG-ß, SP_1 cortisol, and dehydroepiandrosterone were measured. The right adrenal vein blood yielded values of 79 ng/ml, 38 ng/ml, 10.5 ug/ml, and 1.81 ng/ml; the left adrenal vein blood, 65 ng/ml, 34 ng/ml, 10.9 ug/ml, and 4.11 ng/ml; the inferior vena cava blood, 69 ng/ml, 32 ng/ml, 12.1 ug/ml, and 2.19 ng/ml; and the peripheral vein blood, 64 ng/ml, 36 ng/ml, 8.1 ug/ml, and 1.27 ng/ml, respectively. Clinically, the patient was given two courses of double chemotherapy with actinomycin D and methotrexate, followed by hysterectomy and right adrenalectomy. By an immunohistochemical method, the choriocarcinoma tissues were found to react with hCG-, hPL- and SP_1-antibodies. The concentrations of hCG-ß, hPL and SP_1 in the tumor fluid were 1480 ng/ml, 100 ng/ml, and 47 ng/ml, respectively. On incubation of the tumor slices in vitro, the concentration of hCG-ß in the incubation medium increased markedly with increased incubation time: 0 hr, 1.0 ng/ml; 1 hr, 20.2 ng/ml; 2 hr, 24.0 ng/ml; 12 hr, 56.0 ng/ml; and 24 hr, 68 ng/ml.

1182 TOWARDS IMMUNOLOGICAL CONTROL OF FERTILITY·
G.Frajese*, L.Silvestroni, S.Murgiano, A.Magnani, 5th Medical Clinic, University of Rome, 00100 Rome, Italy.
Blood serum of some infertile women contains antibodies which agglutinate spermatozoa. Such condition causes delay in achieving pregnancy, even at low antibody titer. In an attempt to identify and isolate seminal antigens which react specifically with spermagglutinating female antibodies an immunochromatographic system has been developed. In this system the solid phase is represented by purified, total female IgGs, and the mobile phase is represented by seminal glycoproteins. The technique consists in the purification of the glycoproteins by an affinochromatography of vasectomized seminal plasma on Con A-Sepharose followed by an immunoaffinochromatography of the glycoproteins on CNBr-conjugated female IgGs isolated from spermagglutinating blood sera. In this way only specifically reacting glycoproteins are retained in immunocomplexes which are then clivated with NaSCN. The eluted fraction completely absorbed the spermagglutinating activity of female reference sera, while no titre lowering was observed with other seminal proteins or glycoproteins. The SDS-PAGE analysis of the antigen preparation showed the presence of 5 major components which range in apparent molecular weight from 30,000 to 270,000. The same results were obtained in successive experiments using different antibody and seminal batches. The antisera produced with the isolated glycoproteins could produce an efficient contraceptive blockage of the sperm progression into the female genital tract without negative side-effects, as occurs naturally in immune infertility.

1183 ENDOMETRIAL RESPONSES TO THE ANTI-PROGESTERONE STEROID RU 486 IN POST-MENOPAUSAL WOMEN. A. Gravanis*, G. Schaison, J. de Brux, M. George, P.G. Satyaswaroop, E.E. Baulieu and P. Robel, CNRS ER125 and INSERM U 33, Lab. Hormones, 94270 Bicêtre, France ; and Institut de Cytologie Appliquée 75016 Paris, France.

Seventeen post-menopausal women were injected with estradiol benzoate (Eb, 0.625 mg/d) for 15 d. Progesterone (P, 25 mg/d) and/or RU 486 (100 or 200 mg/d), were given to groups of 2-3 patients during the last 6 d of Eb treatment. An endometrial biopsy was performed on the 15th day. Histological examination showed that despite week estrogenic stimulation, either P or RU 486 induced characteristic secretory changes. The affinity of RU 486 for the human progesterone receptor (PR) (Kd = 0.8 nM) was higher than that of P (Kd = 1.2 nM). Both P and RU 486 tended to decrease the concentrations of total and cytosol PR. The largest nuclear "translocation" of PR occured in the patients who received P together with 200 mg RU 486. P and RU 486 also provoked a decrease of endometrial DNA polymerase α and a large increase of estradiol-dehydrogenase (E_2-DH) activities. The latter enzyme was also induced by in vitro 2 d culture of proliferative endometrium with the progestin R 5020 or with RU 486. Nevertheless, RU 486 completely counteracted the induction of E_2-DH produced by P. We concluded that, under the clinical experimental conditions used, RU 486 has not only a clearcut antiprogesterone activity, but also some progesterone-like effects, a result that had not yet been observed in laboratory animals.

1184 ACUTE CHANGES IN MATERNAL NUTRITION ALTER CIRCULATING INSULIN LIKE GROWTH FACTOR (IGF) -I AND -II IN THE OVINE FETUS. P. Gluckman* and J. Butler, Dept. of Paediatrics, University of Auckland, Auckland, New Zealand.

As fetal growth is ultimately determined by the supply of nutritional substrates and in view of evidence suggesting a role for the IGFs in fetal growth, we studied the effect of changes in maternal nutrition upon fetal IGF-I and IGF-II concentrations. 4 pregnant ewes with catheterised fetuses were studied 8 days after surgery (110-135 days gestation). The ewes were fasted for 48 hrs then given 2-4 mg/kg/min glucose (G) iv for 4 hrs then refed. After acid ethanol extraction, fetal plasma IGF-I was measured by immunoassay and IGF-II by rat placental receptor assay. Maternal venous G fell ($p<0.01$) from 52.4$\pm$(SE) 3.2 mg/dl to 29.8$\pm$5.6 mg/dl at the end of the fast, rose to 85.3$\pm$8.9 mg/dl at the end of the G infusion and was 51.7$\pm$13.6 mg/dl after 24 hrs refeeding. Fetal IGF-II was elevated ($p<0.01$, 1728$\pm$317 ng/ml) prior to fasting compared to 11 nonpregnant ewes (701$\pm$111 ng/ml). With 48 hrs fasting, fetal IGF-II fell ($P<0.01$) to 46.8$\pm$9.9% of prefasting values. 4 hrs of maternal G restored ($p<0.05$) IGF-II to 86.2$\pm$9.3% of basal value with no further change on refeeding for 24 hrs (117$\pm$31%). IGF-I was low (21.1+2.4 ng/ml) compared to the adult (30.2$\pm$1.6 ng/ml) and did not alter with fasting. Thus the markedly elevated fetal concentrations of the activity measured by IGF-II receptor assay fall rapidly with maternal starvation and are restored by maternal G administration. In contrast to the postnatal animal, IGF-I was not reduced by starvation. These findings suggest that fetal IGF-II secretion is rapidly modulated by changes in maternal glucose and further suggest a role for IGF-II in the regulation of fetal growth. (Supported by the MRC of NZ.)

1185 RECEPTORS FOR INSULIN-LIKE GROWTH FACTORS (IGFs) IN HUMAN FETAL BRAINS (HFBs). C.G. Goodyer*, L. De Stéphano, H.J. Guyda and B.I. Posner, McGill University, and Y. Lefebvre, Université de Montréal, Montreal, Canada.

We have demonstrated the presence of specific receptors for IGFs in membrane preparations of adult rat anterior pituitary, hypothalami and brains (ENDO, April 1984). We now report that brain tissue from human fetuses of 9.5 - 18 wks fetal age specifically bind (SB) ^{125}I-labelled IGF-II, insulin and IGF-I but not hGH, hPRL, hPL or EGF. Brain tissues from 42 human fetuses were obtained at the time of therapeutic abortion by D&C. 15,000 x g membranes, prepared by differential centrifugation, bound ^{125}I-IGF-II rapidly, reaching maximal SB at 2 h (37°C), 4 h (22°C) or 6 h (4°C). SB increased proportionally with protein and ligand concentration, was reversible (decreasing to 25% of initial total binding by 24 h), and showed a broad pH curve with maximal binding at pH 8.0. SB was unaltered by bacitracin (1 mg/ml), prior washing of the membranes or fetal age. IGF-II, MSA (courtesy of Drs. Nissley and Rechler, NIH) and, to a lesser extent, IGF-I > insulin > proinsulin all displaced ^{125}I-IGF-II, while unrelated peptides had no effect. The predominance of IGF-II binding in HFBs suggests a role for IGF-II in human fetal brain development.

	^{125}I-IGF-II	^{125}I-insulin	^{125}I-IGF-I
HFBs^{+}:	9.8 ± 3.3* (n=39)	4.0 ± 2.5 (n=42)	1.7 ± 0.7 (n=42)

+ Assay conditions: 18-20 h, 4°C, pH 7.5, 400 μg HFB membrane protein.
* %SB: M ± SD (n = number of triplicate observations).

1186 THE NEGATIVE FEEDBACK EFFECT OF CORTISOL (F) ON ACTH RELEASE CAN BE DEMONSTRATED IN FETAL SHEEP YOUNGER THAN 100 DAYS (0.68) GESTATION. B. Hargrave* J. Rose, W. Brooks & L. Winkler. Departments of Physiology/Pharmacology & Obstetrics & Gynecology, Bowman Gray School of Medicine, Winston-Salem, NC

To determine if cortisol (F) can exert negative feedback effects on fetal ACTH release early in gestation we monitored ACTH responses to nitroprusside-induced hypotension in 5 chronically cannulated fetal lambs between 0.65 and 0.72 gestation. Using a paired cross-over design each fetus received in a random sequence a 4 hr intravenous infusion of F (5 ug/min) or saline. Blood pressure was then reduced 25% with nitroprusside. All animals had normal blood gas and pH values. Hypotension increased ACTH in the animals pretreated with saline. The ACTH response to hypotension was inhibited in the group pretreated with F ($p < 0.01$).

Cortisol Treated Group (Fetal Plasma values)

	Control	4 hrs after F infusion	Nipride Started	2.5'	5'	10'
Cortisol (ng/ml)	6±5	34±4		52±6	41±6	40±8
ACTH (pg/ml)	14±8	15±0		17±3	11±3	13±2
Saline Treated Group (Fetal Plasma values)						
Cortisol (ng/ml)	2±1	2±.1		4±3	3±2	4±2
ACTH (pg/ml)	12±5	12±4		17±6	96±23	176±18

In two animals receiving 1 ug/min of F, fetal plasma F levels reached only 12 ng/ml. This also blocked the ACTH response to hypotension.

In contrast to previous reports these data indicate that negative feedback by F can modulate ACTH release in fetuses younger than 100 days gestation. Supported by NIH grant HD11210.

1187 BINDING SITES OF RAT ALPHA$_1$FETOPROTEIN (AFP) : INTERACTION BETWEEN DRUGS AND ESTROGENS.

F. HERVE,[#] K.M. RAJKOWSKI, M.T. MARTIN and N. CITTANOVA.
E.R. N°239 CNRS, UER Biomédicale des Saints-Pères, 45, rue des Saints-Pères 75270 PARIS cedex 06 - FRANCE -

Serum binding proteins, such as albumin or AFP, regulate the action of biological and pharmacological ligands. If competition occurs between the binding of two ligands (a drug and a hormone for example) for the same sites on the protein, there will be an increase in the concentration of the free form of the drug and of the hormone with risks of overdosage and toxicity. Here, we report two sets of results, obtained by equilibrium dialyses, concerning the binding properties of rat AFP : 1) Rat AFP has 0.5 strong affinity binding sites for the drugs warfarin (k=0.8 . $10^6 M^{-1}$), azapropazone (k=0.08 . $10^6 M^{-1}$) and phenylbutazone (k=0.14 . $10^6 M^{-1}$). Charcoal treatment of AFP at neutral pH led to increased affinities (2.5-fold for warfarin, 8-fold for azapropazone and 13-fold for phenylbutazone) without a change in the number of sites, indicating competition for binding at these sites by (an) endogenous ligand(s) which is extractable by charcoal. 2) Rat AFP is known to bind estrogens strongly and competition between the drugs (warfarin, azapropazone and phenylbutazone) and estrogens (estrone, estradiol and ethinyl-estradiol) was studied using charcoal pretreated AFP. The results indicate that estrogens strongly compete for binding with phenylbutazone and azapropazone, but not with warfarin. It may be concluded that :
a) Unlike albumin, warfarin does not occupy the same binding site as phenylbutazone and azapropazone on rat AFP. b) Binding of estrogens could be dramatically perturbated by the presence of drugs administered to the mother during pregnancy.

1188 SOMATOMEDIN (SM) ACTIVITY IN CORD BLOOD OF DIABETIC AND CONTROL SUBJECTS.

W. Hill*, J.L. Kitzmiller, and E. M. Spencer, Lab. of Growth and Development of Children's Hospital, Depts. of OB/GYN and Med., Children's Hospital and UCSF, San Francisco, CA 94118

Somatomedins (SMs) mediate the growth-promoting action of growth hormone. Studies have also implicated SMs as possible regulators of fetal growth. This study investigates the hypothesis that SMs are related to the macrosomia in infants of normal and insulin-dependent diabetic mothers. SM-C/IGF-I was measured by a specific RIA and total SMs by a human placental membrane RRA in 15 diabetic and 29 control subjects at ≥ 36 weeks gestational age. Acid-ethanol extraction was used to separate the SM binding protein. Cord SM-C and total SM levels in appropriate for gestational age (AGA) and large for gestational age (LGA) infants of diabetic mothers (IDM) and infants of control mothers (ICM) are presented in the table:

	SM-C (ng/ml) (mean ± S.D.)		Total SM (ng SM-C equivalents/ml) (mean ± S.D.)	
	IDM (N)	ICM (N)	IDM (N)	ICM (N)
All Infants	(15) 60.8 ± 19.59	(29) 46.4 ± 35.6	(13) 156.1 ± 77.1	(27) 146.1 ± 67.28
AGA	(9) 59.9 ± 19.61	(22) 49.0 ± 20.1	(7) 154.1 ± 49.16	(21) 128.3 ± 52.69
LGA	(6) 62.3 ± 21.34	(7) 84.0 ± 26.9*	(6) 158.3 ±106.58	(6) 208.5 ± 80.18**
Female	(8) 69.2 ± 17.30	(21) 58.1 ± 27.5	(8) 180.2 ± 90.61	(19) 159.2 ± 66.79
Male	(7) 51.3 ± 18.63	(8) 55.8 ± 24.2	(5) 117.4 ± 20.92	(8) 114.9 ± 61.34

*P < .01, LGA vs AGA, ICM   **P < .025, LGA vs AGA, ICM
AGA (10th-90th percentile)   LGA (>90th percentile)

In this study, cord SM-C and total SM levels were significantly higher in LGA than AGA infants of control mothers, but not of diabetic mothers. To further determine the role of SMs in excessive fetal growth, work is in progress to measure SM-A/IGF-II by RIA and to determine SM receptor status in placental and fetal tissues. (Supported by NIAMDDK AM#28098.)

1189 ROLE OF STEROID METABOLISM IN HUMAN FETAL MEMBRANE IN ONSET OF LABOR.

D. Hori*, H. Mori and T. Kigawa, Dept. of Obstetrics & Gynecology, Oita Medical College, Oita, Japan.

To clarify the physiological role of steroids metabolism in the fetal membrane, dispersed cell of decidua (D), chorion (C) and amnion (A) were incubated with pregnenolone (P5) in KRBB, and converted progesterone (P4) was measured by RIA.
C produced P4 in dose-dependent manner by the range of 0-1000 ng/ml of P5; $P4 = (0.8 \times P5 \pm 3.42) \times 10^{-4}$ ($r=0.95$, $p<0.005$). D showed dose-dependency by the range of 100-1000 ng/ml of P5, while A did not show the dose-dependency. P4 production of C in 400 ng/ml of P5 was $(3.25 \pm 0.85) \times 10^{-3}$ pg/cell/hour, which was markedly suppressed by the presence of 400 ng/ml of estradiol (E2), testosterone (T) or dehydroepiandrosterone (DHA) (p 0.005). Such suppressions were not observed in A and D. On the other hand, C of elective cesarean section did not show the suppression of P4 production by E2, T or DHA.
These results suggest that P4 concentration in the neighbouring tissue of the uterine muscle is physiologically regulated by the steroids which are increased towards the parturition, and also suggest that P4 produced in the fetal membrane affects the onset of labor by means of the muscle contractivity.

1190 COMPARISON OF TSH AND T4 ASSAY IN NEONATAL SCREENING FOR CONGENITAL HYPOTHYROIDISM.

H. Inomata*[1)], H. Nakajima[1)] H. Naruse[2)] and M. Irie[3)], 1) Dept. of Pediatr., Univ. of Chiba, Chiba. 2) National Center for Nerv., Ment. and Musc. Disorders, Tokyo. 3) Dept. of Intern. Med., Toho Univ., Tokyo.

In order to compare merits of primary TSH to primary T4 plus supplementary TSH screening, we measured both TSH and T4 in 266,000 samples taken from newborn in Chiba prefecture. Blood was taken from 5 - 7th days old babies generally. However, in case of special centers for premature or high risk babies, blood was taken immediately after a baby was admitted into the centers. Thus, about a thousand samples were taken before 4th day of life. All T4 were measured using the Micromedic Neonatal T4 kit with Concept IV in NCNMMD. TSH in 195,000 samples were measured in NCNMMD using Eiken ICL's TSH-RIA kit and Corning Neonatal TSH-RIA kit, and TSH in 61,000 samples were measured using Daiichi RI's TSH-RIA kit in Toho Univ. 27 cases of premary hypothyroidism were confirmed in Univ. of Chiba and no case of secondary hypothyroidism was detected. In 11 cases out of 27, T4 levels in the first samples were higher than 5 μg/dl, and especially, in 5 cases, the levels of T4 in the first samples were higher than 8 μg/dl. Thus, these five cases might be missed by the premary T4 plus supplementary TSH screening. No patient of hypothyroidism had low T4 and normal TSH in the 1st sample.

1191 STUDY ON PATIENTS WITH CONGENITAL HYPOTHYROIDISM DETECTED BY THE NATIONWIDE NEONATAL THYROID SCREENING PROGRAM IN JAPAN. M. Irie [1]*, H. Nakajima [2] and H. Inomata [2], 1) First Dept. of Med., Toho Univ. School of Med., Tokyo 143, 2) Dept. of Pediatrics, Chiba Univ. School of Med., Chiba, 280, Japan.

This study is a summerized work of the Project Team of the Ministry of Health and Welfare in Japan. In Japan, TSH assay on the filter paper was adopted for the screening method of governmental basis, although T4 is also measured in some screening centers. Nationwide screening started in 1979. By March 1983, 4.473.772 newborns were screened, and 554 cases were reported as congenital hypothyroidism (CH) or its related conditions. Most of these patients were sent to the managing hospitals recommended by the project Team. We report the follow-up study of 506 cases, conducted by means of questionnaire to these hospitals. Among these 506 cases, 400 cases were diagnosed as CH, including 138 male and 262 female patients; 55 as transient hypothyroidism, 56 as the patients with transient hyperthyrotropinemia. The study includes the stastitics on birth year, area distribution, birth month, gestational age, birth weight and height, TSH and T4 concentrations on filter paper, days of screening and the first visit for examination, perinatal symptoms, complications, family history, etiological classification, clinical symptoms and thyroid function at the first visit, initiation day of the treatment, drugs and dose for treatment, clinical course, development and DQ or IQ following treatment, and other related conditions. The physical, mental and neurological development were favorable except the cases complicated with Down's syndrome or de Lange's syndrome.

1192 CHANGES OF SERUM STEROID LEVELS IN PREMATURE INFANTS IN EARLY NEONATAL PERIOD. H. Kato*, M. Hashino, E. Kawamura, T. Kosaki, T. Yanaihara, T. Nakayama and H. Mori. Department of Obstetrics and Gynecology, Showa University School of Medicine, Tokyo, and Teikoku Hormone Mfg. Ltd. Kawasaki, Japan.

Serum steroid hormone levels in five premature infants were measured and compared with those in five normal infants on the 1st, 3rd and 5th day after birth. Conjugated dehydroepiandrosterone(DHA), 16αOH-DHA, pregnenolone(P_5), 20α-dihydro-P_5(20P_5), estradiol(E), free progesterone(P_4), 20α-dihydro-P_4(20P_4) were measured by newly developed method of gas chromatography mas spectrometry using deutreuted steroid as internal standard and cortisol(F) by RIA. All hormone levels decreased in both premature and normal infants as days passed. However, levels of Δ^5-steroids (DHA;2,300, 20P_5;1,431, P_5;1,583 ng/ml on the 1st day) were higher in premature infants than those in normal during the period studied. Significant differences were found in DHA and 20P_5 levels on the 1st and 5th day of life, while no differences for F, P_4, 20P_4 and E levels between premature and normal infants were noticed.

The facts that high serum concentrations of Δ^5-steroid, the main products of fetal adrenal glands, were observed in premature infants, and the levels did not reach to that of normal infants even on the 5th day after birth suggested that the involution of fetal zone of adrenal glands of premature infants was retarded. New information was obtained that the premature infants maintained the secretary function of fetal adrenal steroids in neonatal period.

1193 IMMUNOHISTOCHEMICAL ANALYSIS OF FUNCTIONAL DIFFERENTIATION OF THE HUMAN THYROID GLAND. A.Kawaoi*, M.Tsuneda, N.Nemoto and H.Sato, Department of Pathology, Yamanashi Medical College and 1st Department of Pathology, Nihon University School of Medicine, Yamanashi, 409-38, Japan.

In order to ellucidate the process of differentiation of thyroid function, the immunoperoxidase method was applied to demonstrate triiodothyronine (T3), thyroxine (T4) and thyroglobulin (Tg) in the fetal and neonatal human thyroid tissues, including 18 cases of embryos and fetuses with the crown-rump length from 17 to 275 mm, and 33 cases of newborns with the postnatal age from 0 to 45 days. The thyroid tissues were fixed with either 10 % formalin or zamboni's solution and embedded in paraffin. The serial paraffin sections were cut and immunostained for T3, T4 and Tg respectively. Tg was detected in the immature cords of thyroid tissues of the fetus as early as at 38 to 40 days of developing stage. Later, both T3 and T4 appeared in the fetuses with the gestational ages of 11 to 12 weeks. They increased the stainability as the follicular structure developed, especially at the marginal areas of the thyroid lobules. The immunostaining of the serial sections confirmed the simultaneous localization of T3, T4 and Tg in the most part of the newborn thyroid tissues. Increased stainability of T3, T4 and Tg during the early neonatal stage seemed to correlate with the activated thyroid function at this period.

1194 EVIDENCE AND CHARACTERIZATION OF SPECIFIC HIGH AFFINITY BINDING SITES FOR THE GASTRIC INHIBITORY POLYPEPTIDE (GIP) IN HAMSTER INSULINOMA CELLS. M. Maletti*, B. Amiranoff, J.C. Marie, M. Laburthe and G. Rosselin,
* Fondation de Recherche en Hormonologie, 67 Bd Pasteur, 94260 Fresnes, INSERM U.55, Hôpital Saint-Antoine, 75012 Paris, France.

Gastric Inhibitory Polypeptide (GIP) is a putative candidate for stimulating insulin release from β-cells. In order to demonstrate that GIP can directly act on β-cells, we investigated whether GIP receptors could be detected in the plasma membrane of a transplantable hamster insulinoma, a convenient source of a large amount of β-cell tissue. ^{125}I-GIP purified by HPLC was used as radioactive ligand. Elution of ^{125}I-GIP resulted in two major peaks which possess identical specific binding. High affinity binding sites can be found in membrane preparations from hamster β-cell tumors. Native GIP competitively inhibited the binding of ^{125}I-GIP in the range of 10^{-10}-10^{-6}M and half-maximal inhibition was observed at $1.9 \pm 0.19 \times 10^{-9}$M GIP. The number of high affinity sites was 219 ± 8 fmol/mg protein and the dissociation constant $2.05 \pm 0.1 \times 10^{-9}$M. All peptides tested, structurally related and unrelated to GIP, had only slight effect, if any, on the binding of ^{125}I-GIP. These data are the first evidence for the existence of specific GIP binding sites in mammalian tissues. The presence of those GIP binding sites potentiates the hypothesis suggesting a possible involvement of GIP in the control of insulin release from β-cells.

This work was supported by the Fondation de Recherche en Hormonologie.

1195 INSULIN-RELEASING ACTIVITIES OF SYNTHETIC PHI AND PHM IN PERFUSED ISOLATED RAT PANCREAS. H. Manaka*[1,3], C. Yanaihara[2], K. Nokihara[2], H. Sasaki[3] and N. Yanaihara[1,2], [1]National Institute for Physiological Sciences, Okazaki, Aichi 444, [2]Shizuoka College of Pharmacy, Shizuoka 422, and [3]Yamagata University, School of Medicine, Yamagata 990-23, Japan.

Peptide histidine isoleucine (PHI), peptide histidine methionine isoleucine (PHM, i.e. human PHI) and the related peptides were synthesized by the solution or solid-phase method. Immunoreactive (IR) PHI/PHM was detected in the rat pancreas in concentration of 1.1 ± 0.4 (mean ± SD) fmole/mg wet weight of tissue by a PHI N-terminal specific RIA and 3.2 ± 1.0 by a PHI C-terminal specific RIA versus IR-VIP 1.1 ± 0.4. In the presence of 5 mM glucose, 10^{-7}M PHI and PHM both significantly released insulin in monophasic pattern, while VIP exhibited the same effect at 10^{-8}M. With 16.7 mM glucose, 10^{-9}M PHI and PHM significantly enhanced the biphasic insulin release by the glucose. The integrated insulin release by 16.7 mM glucose during 20 min (242.4 ± 72.9 ng, mean ± SE) was augmented to 614 ± 97.5 ($p < 0.05$) by 10^{-9}M PHI, 543.3 ± 58.0 ($p < 0.05$) by 10^{-9}M PHM and 741.1 ± 167.5 ($p < 0.01$) by 10^{-9}M VIP. And the effects were magnified depending on glucose concentration between 5 and 16.7 mM. Neither PHI(1-15) nor PHI(14-27) showed any insulin-release enhancing effects in the system used. A VIP-PHI hybrid peptide having the N-terminal decapeptide connected to PHI(11-27) also exhibited no effect on insulin release by glucose. The results indicated that in the system employed PHI and PHM, as well as VIP, in 10^{-9}M dose possessed equipotent activities enhancing insulin-release by glucose and that to exert the activities the whole intrinsic molecular structures of PHI and PHM were required.

1196 APPARENT INCREASED SERUM GASTRIN LEVELS ASSOCIATED WITH HYPERLIPEMIA AND NORMAL GASTRIC EMPTYING. J. C. McPherson, III* and J. C. McPherson, Jr., Dept of Clinical Investigation, Eisenhower Army Medical Center, Ft Gordon, GA 30905, Dept of Surgery, Medical College of Georgia, Augusta, GA 30912.

The control of gastric secretion and emptying has been recognized to be under the control of various gastrointestinal hormones. We have shown Triton WR-1339 (TWR), a non-ionic surfactant, to delay gastric emptying, increase gastric secretion and sustain increased levels of gastrin (ENDO ABS #1352, 1982; #827, 1983). This animal model utilized 330-350g male rats, fasted for 48h with water ad libidum, then injected IV with saline, TWR or Pluronic F-127 (F-127), 800mg/kgBW and immediately fed 5ml of tube feeding diet. Additional rats, non-fed, served as controls. Pluronic polyol F-127, a non-ionic surfactant, showed normal gastric emptying, normal gastric secretion and sustained increased levels of gastrin which showed a 7-fold increase over TWR and a 38-fold increase over saline controls in fed rats at 8h. These elevated gastrin levels are associated with cholesterol levels increased 2.5-fold over saline controls and a 2-fold increase over TWR and triglyceride levels increased 28-fold over saline controls and 6.8-fold over TWR. Pluronic F-127 appears to have little if any effect on gastrin release directly since there are no increased levels of serum gastrin during the early time periods when gastrin secretion is stimulated by feeding, in either fed or non-fed animals. In contrast to TWR, where sustained levels of gastrin could be accounted for by prolonged gastric secretion following gastric emptying, Pluronic F-127 appears to maintain even higher levels of circulating serum gastrin following gastric emptying due to an inhibition of gastrin catabolism.

1197 GROWTH HORMONE GENE CLUSTER POLYMORPHISM IN SHORT STATURE. ESTABLISHMENT OF REGISTERY BANK FOR RELPs. Prof. Nemat Hashem, Ain-Shams University Medical Genetics Center, Cairo, Egypt.

Availability of human growth hormone (hGH)cDNA probe and restriction enzymes which identify DNA polymorphisms(RELP)in or near the hGH gene cluster allows definition of any inheritable hGH-linked polymorphism. Since populations of pure homosapien races depict significant quantitative variation of linear skeletal growth(LSG),identifiable hGH gene cluster polymorphism could eventually be traceable to distinct genomic racial variability.The role of such DNA polymorphism in predisposing to genic mutations which impede LSG needs to be explored.Some genetic syndromes which implicate LSG depict specific racial predilictions.Hence establishment of a registry bank for typed hGH DNA RELPs of sampled populations of pure definable races and from short stature(SS) anomalous genetic syndromes from the same population could hasten gene mapping and assignment of linkage gene groups mediating aberrant features associating different SS syndromes.DNA fragments will be collected from inhabitants of different zones of the Nile Valley, Mount-Sinai peninsula, Mediterranean and Red Sea Coasts and from native dwellers of the Egyptian deserts and neighbouring Middle East Countries.Computerized sheets and programs are designed for registry of standared anthropometric features for future correlative analysis of relevant phenotypes with any RELPs at hGH gene clusters or other defined DNA segment polymorphisms collected from dwellers of other continents.

1198 ABSENCE OF A CENTRAL LOCUS FOR THE NALOXONE-MEDIATED SURGE IN TAIL SKIN TEMPERATURE AND LH SECRETION IN THE RAT. M.J. Katovich*, J.W. Simpkins and I-C Song. College of Pharmacy, Univ. of Florida, Gainesville, FL 32610.

We have previously demonstrated that s.c. administration of naloxone (NAL) to morphine (MORP)-dependent rats results in a surge in tail skin temperature (TST) and LH secretion (Life Sci. 32:1957, 1983), which are similar in magnitude, duration and temporal relationship to those observed during a menopausal hot flush. Presently, we attempted to determine the central locus responsible for the NAL-induced increases in TST and LH secretion. Female rats were fitted bilaterally with cannula located in the preoptic area-anterior hypothalamus, olfactory tubercle, medial basal hypothalamus, locus coeruleus, frontal cortex or lateral ventricles. In MORP-dependent rats, TST was monitored every 5 min for 60 min and blood samples were obtained via jugular cannulae at 0, 5, 10, 15, 30 and 60 min following administration of NAL (20µg/2µl, bilaterally). Regardless of the central site of NAL injection, TST was significantly increased 3-5°C and LH secretion was elevated by 40-70ng/ml over control values. Peak surge in both TST and LH secretion occurred in 5 to 15 min with the LH surge preceding that of TST by 5 min. This ubiquitous NAL effect was still present when injection volume was reduced to 0.2µl bilaterally. Additionally, when ^{3}H-NAL was administered to the frontal cortex less than 1% was observed outside the injected site. Collectively, these studies indicate that in MORP-dependent rats, TST and LH surges can be induced by local application of NAL to numerous brain regions and suggest that these responses are subsequent to a locally-induced spreading activation of CNS neuronal activity. (Supported in part by NIH Grant HD18133).

1199 CHLOROQUINE EFFECT ON OVARIAN INTRACELLULAR LH METABOLISM

H. Kawamura*, J. J. Pehrson, and J. L. Vaitukaitis, Department of Medicine, Boston University School of Medicine, Boston, MA. U.S.A.

Chloroquine (CQ) inhibits pseudopregnant ovary lysosomal function, starting 6 hours after a single intraperitoneal injection of 25 mg/kg. That effect persists at least 18 more hours. Since LH appears to be more rapidly metabolized than hCG after internalization within pseudopregnant rat ovaries, studies were undertaken to ascertain whether intracellular metabolism of LH could be significantly altered by inhibiting lysosomal function with CQ. Six hours after treating pseudopregnant rats with CQ, rats were injected intravenously with 1.0 μg hLH (11 I.U.) and groups of animals sacrificed intermittently for the next 5 hours. Serum and ovarian associated LH concentrations were determined by radioimmunoassay. The concentration of free LH/hCG receptor sites in ovarian membrane fractions harvested from control and CQ treated rats was determined by saturation analysis. Serum hLH levels were similar in control and experimental groups. Cytosolic cAMP levels were determined by radioimmunoassay. Although the concentration of free LH/hCG receptor prior to hLH stimulation was significantly greater among CQ treated rats, less circulating hLH bound to the ovarian membrane fraction of CQ treated animals for the first 2 hours after hLH. Cytosolic LH levels were greater among CQ rats for the first hour after hLH stimulation but cytosolic levels were not markedly different between groups thereafter. After hLH stimulation, cytosolic cAMP accumulation was markedly lower among CQ treated rats. The foregoing suggest CQ induced rearrangement of LH/hCG menbrane receptor as well as evidence for both lysosomal and nonlysosomal metabolism of internalized hormone.

1200 IMMUNOLOGICAL EVIDENCE FOR A CONFORMATIONAL CHANGE IN DEGLYCOSYLATED HUMAN CHORIOGONADOTROPIN. H.T. Keutmann*, L. Johnson, I.Z. Beitins and R.J. Ryan, Endocrine Unit and Vincent Research Laboratory, Massachusetts General Hospital, Boston, MA 02114 and Dept. of Cell Biology, Mayo Medical School, Rochester, MN 55905 USA.

Deglycosylated choriogonadotropin (hCG) binds to ovarian membrane receptors but does not activate adenylate cyclase. We detected a reduction in immunoreactivity with antisera to native hCG or hCG-alpha after deglycosylation of hCG by means of hydrogen fluoride (Keutmann, HT, McIlroy, PJ, Kitzmann, K and Ryan, RJ, Biochem. 22:3067, 1983).

In the present study, we probed for conformational changes by use of a region-specific immunoassay to reduced, carboxymethylated (RCXM) alpha subunit. Antiserum 110 recognizes a segment at the N-terminus of the linear sequence, distant from the points of carbohydrate attachment; it normally reacts weakly with native subunit (ID-50=200 ng peptide). After deglycosylation of hCG-alpha, reactivity was enhanced by 6-8 fold, to ID-50 of 30 ng. A similar increase took place after deglycosylation of associated whole hCG. Comparable results were obtained using a second N-terminal antiserum (As 101). Deglycosylation of RCXM subunit itself had no effect on the assay response, so carbohydrate *per se* does not influence the antigenicity or immunoreactivity of these antisera.

These results suggest that after deglycosylation, alpha subunit may assume a more "linear" shape in an area of the primary sequence remote from carbohydrate itself. Altered conformation could thus account, at least in part, for the unique effect of deglycosylation on receptor-cyclase "coupling" in hCG action. Supported by NIH grant #HD-12851.

1201 ISOELECTROFOCUSING (IEF) PROFILES OF BIOACTIVE AND IMMUNOREACTIVE FSH AND LH IN MONKEY PITUITARY PREPARATIONS OF VARYING PURITY. S.A.Khan* and E. Diczfalusy, Reproductive Endocrinology Research Unit, Karolinska Sjukhuset, S-104 01 Stockholm, Sweden.

The suitability of purified monkey FSH (AFP 4348 A:FSH-1 and WP-XV-104C: FSH-2) and LH (WP-XV-20:LH-1 and WP-XV-63-2429:LH-2) preparations to be used as tracer (LH-2) or to replace the expired standard (LER 1909-2) in radioimmunoassays (RIA) was assessed. The preparations were fractionated by IEF on sucrose density gradient (pH range 2.5 to 10.0) and FSH and LH in each fraction was determined by heterologous RIA systems and in vitro bioassays. The ratios of bioactivity (B) to immunoreactivity (I) were: FSH-1: 0.34, FSH-2: 1.5, LH-1: 1.3 and LH-2: 1.5. The FSH/LH ratios of FSH-1 and FSH-2 were 0.38 and 8.3, and the LH/FSH ratios of LH-1 and LH-2 were 1.5 and 114, respectively. Whereas FSH-2 exhibited a high specific activity (S.A) and an IEF profile similar to that of LER 1909-2, the profile of FSH-1 was shifted towards the acidic region and contained an "acidic" LH species absent from all other preparations. LH-1 and LH-2 had high S.A. and exhibited IEF profiles similar to that of the standard; however, LH-1 was heavily contaminated with "alkaline" FSH species, absent from all other preparations, suggesting again artifact formation during purification. It is concluded that neither FSH-1, nor LH-1 are suitable replacements for LER 1909-2, whereas LH-2 and (following the removal of its LH-contamination) FSH-2 are suitable candidates. The IEF profiles of the above preparations will be compared to those of FSH and LH present in unfractionated pituitary glands of normal and gonadectomized monkeys.

1202 THE SEXUAL DEVELOPMENTS OF IDIOPATHIC GROWTH HORMONE DEFICIENCY — THE PROBLEMS OF THE ABSCENCE OF PUBERTY OR THE ACCELERATION OF BONE AGE ON h-GH THERAPY—. S. Kusano*, Y. Shiki, K. Ichimura, S. Amemiya, Y. Nozaki, K. Ohyama and K. Kato, Dep. of Pediatrics, Keio University, Tokyo, 160 Japan.

(PURPOSES and PATIENTS) The children with idiopathic growth hormone deficiency tend to fail to show the onset of puberty, but about one-third of them show the onset of puberty soon after h-GH therapy. And we have recognized that the bone age of the laters rather progress very rapidly. Then we studied the pituitary-testis functions, and the development of puberty of the idiopathic pituitary dwarf male patients (16 patients) with a bone age above 11 6/12 years for mean duration of 3 10/12 years (form 1 year to 6 6/12 years). The specimens of testicular biopsies were also studied. We devided them into 3 groups according to these results.

	number of patients	LH-RH test	testosterone response to HCG loading	basal testosterone
A-group	8	LH: No responses FSH: No responses	No response	very low
B-group	2	LH: low responses FSH: low responses	low response	low
C-group	6	LH: normal responses FSH: normal boderline responses	normal responses	normal

(DISCUSSION and CONCLUSION) In patients with idiopathic growth hormone deficiency, the responses of LH to LH-RH varied from very low to almost normal levels. The patietns with the normal responses of LH showed the onset of puberty during h-GH therapy. The responses of FSH were more or less reduced. From the findings of testicular specimen, their fertility might be disturbed even in the patients with puberty. The patients of group A have been treated with HCG and/or HMG therapy in order to gain puberty. On the other hand, the patients of group C have been placed on the therapy of cyproterone acetate to suppress the rapid progress of their bone age, resulting in the improvement of their stunted final heights.

1203 ASSESSMENT OF PITUITARY ALPHA SUBUNIT mRNA AMOUNTS DURING THE OVINE ESTROUS CYCLE USING cDNA HYBRIDIZATION. T.D. Landefeld*, I. Levitan and J. Kepa, Department of Pharmacology, Reproductive Endocrinology Program, Univ. of Michigan, Ann Arbor, MI 48109.

Changes in the pattern of serum LH during the ovine estrous cycle has been well established, with the highest values being observed during the preovulatory surge. In this study, we have examined the amount of alpha subunit mRNA present during certain times of the cycle to establish the role of alpha synthesis in serum LH concentrations. Five stages of the cycle were examined: Day 12; 24 hrs before estrus; 5, 15 and 25 hrs after the onset of behavioral estrus. These stages were characterized by serum and pituitary LH concentrations, ovarian morphology, and behavioral estrus. Pituitaries were removed and RNA extracted. Amounts of specific mRNA present in cytoplasmic RNA were determined by Northern transfers using 32P-labeled cDNAs of bovine alpha subunit, PRL and GH. In addition, mRNA amounts and activities were assessed in cell-free translation assays. Average serum LH values increased in these groups, reaching peak values of ~200 ng/ml between 5 and 15 hrs after the onset of estrus. Although GH and PRL mRNA amounts did not vary in the groups examined using Northerns and/or cell-free assays, alpha subunit mRNA amounts did differ among groups. Approximately 3X more alpha subunit mRNA was seen in the groups after the onset of estrus than in those groups before the surge and only slightly more alpha mRNA was observed in the estrus minus 24 hr group than in the Day 12 group. These results establish a pattern of alpha mRNA amounts during the estrous cycle of the ewe, specifically near the time of the LH surge. Supported by NIH grants HD12016 and HD11311.

1204 INHIBITION OF LH RELEASE IN RAT ANTERIOR PITUITARY CELL CULTURE BY TESTOSTERONE WITHOUT CONVERSION TO DIHYDROTESTOSTERONE. T. LIANG*, E. J. Brady, A. Cheung, and R. Saperstein, Merck Sharp and Dohme Research Laboratories, Rahway, New Jersey, USA.

Testosterone (T) is converted to 5α-dihydrotestosterone (DHT) in the hypothalamus and the pituitary, but it is not known whether 5α-reduction is required for its feedback inhibition of gonadotropin secretion. We have investigated the effect of 5α-reductase inhibitors on the inhibition of LH release by testosterone in rat anterior pituitary cell cultures. Pituitary cells were incubated in the absence and in the presence of T or DHT (10^{-13}-10^{-6}M) for 17h and then with LHRH (0.5 nM) for an additional 4h. LHRH increased the rate of LH release ~30-fold. The LHRH-induced release of LH was inhibited by T and DHT to a maximum of 50%. DHT (IC_{50} 0.4±0.2 nM) is 6-fold more potent than T (IC_{50} 2.6±1.8 nM). When cells were preincubated with T or DHT in the presence of a 5α-reductase inhibitor (0.2 μM), 17β-N, N-diethylcarbamoyl-4-methyl-4-aza-5α-androstan-3-one (4-MA,JBC2567998,1981) or 17β-N,N-diisopropylcarbamoyl-4-aza-5α-andostan-3-one (DIPA, JBC in press), the inhibition curves of T and DHT were not shifted. ^{3}H-T was incubated with cells for 17 h and the radioactivity was extracted with ethylacetate and chromatographed on TLC. Unmetabolized T accounted for 67.6±2.4% and the metabolites are DHT (13.4±0.5%), androstenedione (16.1±1.3%), and androstanedione (2.9±0.5%). In the presence of 4-MA or DIPA, androstenedione was the only metabolite found. Androstenedione was found to be only 16±4% as potent as T in the inhibition of LHRH-induced release of LH. Thus, both T and DHT inhibit LH secretion and the conversion of T to DHT is not necessary for the inhibition of LH secretion in the pituitary cell culture.

1205 CHARACTERIZATION OF HCG EXPRESSED FROM CLONED cDNA. J. Lustbader*, S. Birken, R. Canfield, A. Beck, E. Cole and N. Hsiung. Department of Medicine, Columbia University College of Physicians and Surgeons, New York, NY 10032 and Integrated Genetics Inc., Framingham, MA 01701.

Human chorionic gonadotropin (hCG) and its subunits expressed in mammalian cells from cloned complementary DNA (cDNA) were studied to obtain information about the processing of expressed recombinant hCG (r-hCG) and to compare r-hCG with purified urinary hCG and the natural hCG forms circulating in pregnancy plasma. Samples of hCG and r-hCG were electrophoresed in two different sodium dodecylsulphate (SDS) gel systems: (1) under reducing conditions using β-mercaptoethanol and (2) on low temperature (5°C) gels where the dimer does not dissociate. Following transfer to nitrocellulose paper the blots were immunochemically developed using the following antisera: anti-reduced carboxymethylated (RCM) hCGα R117, anti-RCM hCGβ R132, anti-native hCGα R111 and anti-native hCGβ R126. R-hCG was purified by classical methods from culture medium and its amino acid composition is similar to purified urinary hCG. Western blot analyses of purified r-hCG following both normal and low temperature SDS gel electrophoresis showed that r-hCG was indistinguishable from hCG by this criteria. It is of equal interest to examine the culture media containing expressed r-hCG since these contain all forms of hCG secreted by the cells containing the specific cDNAs. Western blot analyses of the cell supernates from which the r-hCG was purified showed significant quantities of a variety of higher molecular weight forms of the α subunit and to a lesser extent of the β subunit. In addition, one system produced increased amounts of free β subunit which could recombine with the complementary urinary α subunit.

1206 HUMAN INSULIN-LIKE GROWTH FACTORS I AND II (IGF-I, IGF-II) ARE SYNTHESIZED AS PRECURSORS. M. Jansen*, H.H.M. van Tol, F.M.A. van Schaik, J.L. Van den Brande and J.S. Sussenbach, Depts. of Pediatrics and Physiological Chemistry, State University of Utrecht, the Netherlands.

Recently, we have reported the nucleotide sequence of a human liver cDNA-clone encoding Insulin-like Growth Factor I (IGF-I) as a precursor [1]. By using the BamHI-PstI restriction fragment (500 nucleotides) of this pIGF-I cDNA as a probe, we have been able to select from this cDNA-library another clone showing hybridization with this fragment under moderately stringent washing conditions (1 hr, 1x SSC, 60°C), but not under conditions of increased stringency (½ hr, 0,3x SSC, 60°C). The cDNA-insert of this clone, amounting to approximately 700 nucleotides, encodes the complete amino acid sequence of human IGF-II, flanked by an N-terminal prepeptide region and a carboxyl-terminal extension, indicating that IGF-II, like IGF-I, is synthesized as a precursor protein. The nucleotide sequence of this cDNA-insert will be presented and compared with that of IGF-I and other structurally related peptides.

1) M. Jansen et al., Nature 306: 609-611, 1983.

1207 Cyclic AMP decreases the sensitivity of human fibroblasts to stimulation of aminoisobutyric acid (AIB) uptake by somatomedin C. P. Kaplowitz* and D. Cranin, Dept. of Pediatrics, Medical College of VA, Richmond, VA 23298.

The relationship between cyclic AMP (cAMP) and somatomedin action is controversial. We have examined the effect of agents which elevate intracellular cAMP levels on somatomedin action in human fibroblasts. We have recently reported (J Clin Endo Metab 58:176, 1984) that a 3 hr exposure to somatomedin C (Sm-C) elicits an approximately 2-fold stimulation of the rate of uptake of the amino acid analog AIB into confluent cultures of normal human fibroblasts. The concentration of Sm-C resulting in half-maximal stimulation of AIB uptake (the ED_{50}) ranged in different cell lines from 2 to 10 ng/ml. Addition of theophylline (1 mM) or dibutyryl cAMP (100 μM) resulted in 40-60% and 10-30% inhibitions, respectively, of basal AIB uptake but had no consistent effects on Sm-C stimulated uptake. However, the combination of theophylline and dibutyryl cAMP shifted the Sm-C dose-response curve to the right, increasing the ED_{50} in one experiment from 5.8 to 14 ng/ml. Maximal stimulation of AIB uptake was slightly higher in the treated vs. the control cultures (3.5 vs. 2.8-fold) suggesting that elevation of intracellular cAMP was not toxic to the cells. Similar results were obtained when 8-BrcAMP (100 μM) was substituted for dibutyryl cAMP. Cholera toxin (10 ng/ml) elicited a 20-30% increase in basal AIB uptake and increased the ED_{50} for Sm-C stimulated AIB uptake in a manner similar to theophylline plus the cAMP derivatives. A one hour preincubation with the above agents did not decrease binding of ^{125}I-Sm-C to its receptors. These studies demonstrate that agents which elevate intracellular cAMP levels decrease the sensitivity of human fibroblasts to Sm-C without impairing the ability of cells to respond normally to higher concentrations.

1208 PURIFICATION AND CHARACTERIZATION OF A HUMAN PITUITARY-DERIVED CHONDROCYTE GROWTH FACTOR. S. Kasper*, A.M. Hamel, J. Rowe and H.G. Friesen Dept. of Physiology, University of Manitoba, Winnipeg, Manitoba, Canada R3E 0W3.

In a previous study, we have shown that the human pituitary gland contains, and may secrete, a novel mitogen for chondrocyte proliferation. The chondrocyte growth factor (CGF) is heat and trypsin sensitive, acid labile, and has a MW of 40,000 and an isoelectric point of 7.9. In this study, we report a modification of the purification procedure which results in an improved yield and purification of CGF. In the initial step, the side fraction generated during the purification of hGH was chromatographed on Sephadex G-100. Those fractions which stimulated rabbit fetal chondrocytes in tissue culture were pooled and purified further on hydroxylapatite chromatography and DEAE affigel blue affinity chromatography to yield a 4,000-fold purification of CGF. CGF stimulated cell proliferation in a dose dependent manner down to 0.5 ng/ml with a half maximumal effect of 8 ng/ml. Further studies of the biological effects of CGF have shown that CGF is not only mitogenic for rabbit fetal chondrocytes but also stimulates the growth of primary cultures of fetal rat chondrocytes, adult rabbit and human patellar chondrocytes. Preliminary results also indicate that daily subcutaneous injections of CGF enhances the growth of the Swarm chondrosarcoma transplanted into Sprague Dawley rats. These results suggest that the human pituitary gland contains a novel factor or hormone in addition to growth hormone which may play an important role in cartilage growth and development.

1209 TRANSFORMING GROWTH FACTOR PRODUCTION BY ANTERIOR PITUITARY CELLS

M.S. Kobrin,* J.E. Kudlow, Departments of Clinical Biochemistry and Medicine University of Toronto, Toronto, Ontario, Canada. M5G 1L5

Pituitary glands have been a source of mitogens for fibroblasts and adrenal cells. Culture medium conditioned by normal bovine pituitary cells (CM) contained growth factors which competed with epidermal growth factor (EGF) for binding to the EGF-receptor and stimulated nontransformed rat kidney fibroblasts (NRK) to form colonies in soft agar. Chromatography of the CM on Bio-Gel P-60 in 1 M acetic acid produced three separate peaks of EGF-competing activity in a radioreceptor assay. These peaks had apparent molecular weights of 17,000, 9,000 and 6,000 daltons. The 6,000 M_r peak (Peak 3) contained an EGF-like activity which competed as well as mouse EGF for binding to anti-mouse EGF antibodies, whereas the higher molecular weight peaks (Peaks 1 and 2) had very little EGF-like immuno-activity. Peaks 1 and 2 caused NRK cells to form colonies in soft agar. Peak 3 had no colony-forming activity. Peak 2 contained the majority of colony-forming activity and was further purified by cation exchange chromatography on a Mono S column (Pharmacia) with an ammonium acetate gradient and then by reverse phase high pressure liquid chromatography on a C_{18} column (Pharmacia) with an acetonitrile gradient. This partial characterization of CM suggests the in vitro production of a bovine EGF (Peak 3) and a EGF-like transforming growth factor(s) from normal bovine pituitary cells. This system provides the opportunity to study the secretion of transforming growth factors by normal cells and may indicate they have a role in normal pituitary physiology.

1210 PHOTOAFFINITY LABELLING OF THE ATP BINDING SITE OF THE EGF-DEPENDENT PROTEIN KINASE.

J.E. Kudlow*, Departments of Clinical Biochemistry and Medicine, University of Toronto, Toronto, Ontario, Canada M5G 1L5.

Epidermal growth factor (EGF), after binding to its receptor, activates a tyrosine specific protein kinase which phosphorylates several substrates including the EGF-receptor itself. The effects of a photo-affinity analogue of ATP, arylazido-β-alanyl-ATP, on the EGF-dependent protein kinase in A431 human tumour cell plasma membrane vesicles was investigated. This analogue at 10uM was capable of inactivating the EGF-receptor kinase in a photodependent manner. The photodependent inactivation of the enzyme by the analogue could be partially blocked by 20 mM ATP and more effectively blocked by either 20 mM AMP-PNP or 20 mM GMP-PNP indicating nucleotide-binding site specificity. Arylazido-β-alanyl-[α-^{32}P]ATP was capable of labelling membrane proteins in a photodependent manner. Numerous proteins were labelled, the most prominent of which with a molecular weight of 53,000. Immunoprecipitation of affinity labelled and solubilized membranes with an anti-EGF-receptor monoclonal antibody demonstrated that the 170,000 Mr receptor protein was photoaffinity labelled with the azido-ATP. The 53,000 Mr peptide was not specifically bound by the anti-receptor antibody. The affinity labelling of the receptor was not enhanced by EGF suggesting that EGF-stimulation of the kinase does not result from changes in the affinity of the kinase for ATP. These studies demonstrate that arylazido-β-alanyl-ATP is an effective photoaffinity label for the EGF-kinase and that the EGF-receptor, identified using monoclonal antibodies, contains an ATP binding site providing further confirmation that the EGF-receptor and EGF-dependent protein kinase are domains of the same 170,000 Mr protein.

1211 HUMAN ADIPOCYTE PRECURSORS FROM MASSIVELY OBESE SUBJECTS RELEASE FACTORS MITOGENIC ON CULTURED ADIPOCYTE PRECURSORS. D.C.W. Lau*, C.H. Hollenberg, and D.A.K. Roncari. Departments of Medicine, The University of Calgary and University of Toronto, Calgary, Alberta and Toronto, Ontario, Canada.

In this study, possible paracrine factors in adipose tissue from lean and massively obese subjects were sought. Growth media conditioned by adipocyte precursors derived from lean and massively obese (defined as > 170% of reference weight) persons were tested for their mitogenicity on cultured rat adipocyte precursors. Conditioned medium was collected from omental precursors, initially grown in alpha medium supplemented with 15% fetal bovine serum, at each of the following growth phases: 3 days post-inoculation, 3 days before and at monolayer confluence. Cells were washed with Hanks' balanced salt solution and grown in fresh medium with 1% fetal bovine serum; the conditioned medium was removed 24 h later, filtered, and added to the precursors at 1%-50% (vol/vol). Mitogenicity was quantified by both thymidine incorporation into DNA and direct cell counting. Conditioned media from massively obese precursors stimulated adipocyte precursor replication in a dose-dependent manner, with effects first evident at >5%, with maximal stimulation 8-fold over control ($3.3x10^3$ vs $0.4x10^3$ cpm). Conditioned media from all three growth phases were mitogenic, but those from precursors at monolayer confluence were three times more potent. Corresponding media from lean precursors were much less stimulatory. Thus, adipocyte precursors from massively obese subjects release into the medium factors mitogenic on cultured adipocyte precursors. These principles may act as paracrine or autocrine growth factors contributing to the development of the adipocyte hyperplasia characteristic of massive obesity.

1212 SOMATOSTATIN - RELATED MATERIAL IS NATIVE TO BACTERIA. D. LeRoith*, M. Berelowitz, W. Pickens, L.K. Crosby and J. Shiloach, Div. Endocrinology, Dept. of Medicine, Univ. Cincinnati, Cinti., Ohio.

Recent studies in our laboratory have shown the presence of vertebrate-like hormonal peptides in unicellular eukaryotes including materials resembling insulin, ACTH, somatostatin (SS14) and relaxin (PNAS 77:6184, 1980, PNAS 79:2086, 1982, Endocr 110:1939, 1982, JBC 258:2778, 1983). In extending these studies we have looked for somatostatin-like immunoactivity (SRIF-LI) in the prokaryotes E. coli and B. subtilus. Bacteria were grown in large fermenters using defined medium. Cells were separated from the medium, homogenized and the SRIF-LI extracted in acid-ethanol. Sep-Pak C18 cartridges were used to concentrate the extract and further purification was achieved using Biogel P-6 and HPLC. Between 2-8 pg of SRIF-LI was recovered per G wet weight of cells. Two immunoassays were used; one specific for the N-terminal tetradecapeptide of somatostatin 28 (SS28) molecule and the other specific for SS14 (the C-terminal tetradecapeptide of SS28. On Biogel P-6, two peaks of SRIF-LI were recovered; a large MW peak with a Mr similar to SS28, which demonstrated reactivity in both N- and C- terminal immunoassays, and a second peak with a Mr similar to SS14 which reacted only with the C-terminal assay. Unconditioned medium contained no SRIF-LI while conditioned medium contained 20-40 pg SRIF-LI per liter. These findings suggest that both SS28 and SS14 forms of somatostatin are native to prokaryotes and further support the suggestion that vertebrate peptide hormones have an early evolutionary origin.

1213 A NEW SIMPLE RIA FOR SOMATOMEDIN C BASED ON AN ENTIRELY SYNTHETIC SYSTEM.
A.W. Lindall*, J.W. Orf, W.C. Mahoney, N. Johanson and J.A. Ells. Immuno Nuclear Corporation, 1951 Northwestern Avenue, Stillwater, MN. 55082.

Synthetic peptides to several regions of human somatomedin C were synthesized by solid phase methods and used to generate antibodies. One peptide (residues 53-70) conjugated to Keyhole Limpet hemocyanin and used to immunize rabbits produced antibodies which cross-react with native somatomedin C and allowed the generation of a sensitive RIA. Iodinated (I-125) peptide 53-70 has the additional advantage of not binding to serum binding proteins. Native somatomedin C was isolated from human serum and purified by ion exchange chromatography and reversed-phase high-performance liquid chromatography. Amino acid analysis combined with 22 cycles of automated Edman degradation confirmed the structure of this material as human Insulin-Like Growth Factor I or somatomedin C. This material was subsequently used to calibrate the synthetic system on a mass basis. A method for the extraction and separation of somatomedin C from serum using reversed-phase Sep-Paks® was developed and compared to conventional gel filtration. As an alternative approach, heparin was used to block the binding of somatomedin C to its binding protein, allowing development of a direct assay. This allowed the comparison of an extraction with a non-extraction based method for the assay of somatomedin C. Up to 100% of total somatomedin C in serum can be measured by the non-extraction method, a result that compares well with results obtained with the more involved extraction based method. This new system overcomes many of the problems and simplifies the measurement of somatomedin C in the clinical laboratory.

1214 EFFECT OF GROWTH HORMONE RELEASING FACTOR ON GROWTH HORMONE AND PROLACTIN SECRETION FROM HUMAN PITUITARY ADENOMA CELLS IN CULTURE.
M. Ishibashi* and T. Yamaji Third Department of Internal Medicine, Faculty of Medicine, University of Tokyo, Hongo, Tokyo 113, Japan

To determine the role of growth hormone releasing factor (GRF) in hormone secretion in patients with acromegaly, the effects of GRF as well as hypothalamic hormones including somatostatin (SRIF), TRH, VIP, corticotropin-releasing factor (CRF) and dopamine on growth hormone (GH) and prolactin (PRL) release from cultured pituitary adenoma cells of acromegaly were studied. Human pancreatic GRF(1-44)-NH_2 at concentrations from 10^{-12} to 10^{-8}M significantly increased GH and PRL secretion from adenoma cells from 10 acromegalic patients in a dose-dependent manner. In contrast, no stimulatory effect of GRF on PRL release was observed in adenoma cells obtained from 6 patients with prolactinoma. The magnitude of GH responses to GRF in adenoma cells of acromegaly varied from tissue to tissue and ranged from 107 to 197% of each control incubation. The responsiveness was not related to age, sex and basal GH secretion in individual patients. SRIF (10^{-10}M), on the other hand, uniformly suppressed both GH and PRL secretion in all of the adenoma cells from acromegalic patients and blocked the stimulatory effect by GRF at 10^{-9}M. TRH, VIP and CRF (10^{-7}M) also increased GH secretion in some, though not all, adenoma cells. The responders to CRF and VIP showed a greater GH response to GRF. These results suggest that GRF-stimulated GH release from pituitary adenomas of acromegaly is variable and that PRL-secreting cells associated with pituitary adenomas of acromegaly behaves differently to GRF from those in prolactinomas.

1215 INFLUENCE OF NEONATAL ANDROGEN SECRETION ON PLASMA GH LEVELS, BODY GROWTH AND HEPATIC STEROID METABOLISM IN ADULT MALE RATS.

John-Olov Jansson, Olle Isaksson*, Agneta Mode and Jan-Åke Gustafsson, Dept of Physiology, University of Göteborg, P O Box 33031, S-400 33 Göteborg and Dept of Medical Nutrition, Karolinska Institute, Stockholm, Sweden

The sexually differentiated secretory pattern of rat growth hormone (GH) (higher pulses and lower trough levels in males compared to females) appears to be of importance for the sex difference in body growth (Jansson et al, Acta Endocrinol 99:24,1982). Moreover, the sex differentiated hepatic steroid metabolism seems to be largely determined by the plasma GH trough levels, which are, in turn, influenced by the postpubertal secretion of sex steroids (Mode et al, Endocrinology 111:1692,1982). The aim of the present study was to investigate the role of the neonatal testicular androgen secretion of the male rat in control of these functions.

Blood samples were obtained from the tip of the tail according to an experimental protocol described previously (Mode et al, 1982). Plasma GH was measured by RIA. Longitudinal bone growth, body growth, and the activities of sex differentiated hepatic enzymes were also determined.

Hepatic steroid metabolism was more "feminine", and body growth and plasma GH pulse height were markedly lower in adult male rats after neonatal (day 1) than after prepubertal (day 25) gonadectomy. Neonatal testosterone propionate treatment (0.5 mg s c day 1) reversed these changes.

The results indicate that the neonatal testicular androgen secretion is a determinant for plasma GH pulse height, body growth and hepatic steroid metabolism in the adult male rat.

1216 CLINICAL AND FUNDEMENTAL STUDIES ON ABNORMAL INCREASE OF SERUM GH AFTER TRH INJECTION AND ORAL GLUCOSE TOLERANCE TEST(OGTT) IN CANCER PATIENTS.

K. Kamijo*, T. Kato, K. Kawasaki, A. Saito, M. Suzuki and A. Yachi
1st Dept. of Internal Medicine, Sapporo Medical College,Sapporo 060, Japan

Recently we have demonstrated that TRH injection abnormally stimulated GH release in cancer patients. In order to investigate changes in serum GH levels after TRH, OGTT, LHRH, L-Dopa and bromocriptine(Br) as well as the effect of the operation, weight loss, Br and domperidone(Domp) on paradoxical responses of GH to TRH, GH levels were measured on serum samples obtained from 31 normal subjects and 96 cancer patients by RIA.

TRH injection and OGTT induced significant GH release in cancer patients, whereas there was no significant changes in serum GH after TRH injection in normal subjects, or after saline or LHRH injection in cancer patients. There was no significant correlation of serum GH responses to between TRH and OGTT. Incidence of GH responders to TRH or OGTT are significantly higher in female cancer patients than in males. L-Dopa and Br normally stimulated GH release in cancer patients. Gh responses to TRH are gradually diminished after curative resection of tumors and reappear in postoperative recurrent patients. Weight loss is not significant factor and Br and Domp show suppressive effects on this paradoxical response of GH to TRH.

It is concluded that there is a tumor-dependent hypothalamic-pituitary dysfunction in cancer patients.

1217 **Use of Avian Retroviral-Bovine Growth Hormone Recombinant DNA to Direct Expression of Bovine Growth Hormone by Cultured Fibroblasts.** John J. Kopchick, Richard H. Malavarca, Thomas J. Livelli, and Fred Leung. Merck Sharp and Dohme Research Labs, Rahway, New Jersey 07065 USA

We have constructed a variety of recombinant DNA molecules in which an avian retroviral long terminal repeat (LTR) has been ligated to the bovine growth hormone gene. The retroviral LTR was derived from a plasmid clone of a Schmidt Rupin Strain of Rous Sarcoma Virus while the bovine growth hormone gene was derived from a λ -bacteriophage genomic library. Using a transient eucaryotic expression assay system, the plasmid constructs were screened for their ability to direct expression and secretion of bovine growth hormone. One such recombinant DNA construct was found to be active in the production of bovine growth hormone. Stable mouse fibroblast cell lines have been generated which contain this biologically active plasmid construct integrated into the mouse cell genome. Many of these cell lines express and secrete bovine growth hormone. One of these stable cell lines was found to secrete bovine growth hormone at a rate of 5.0 ug/ml per 10^5 cells per 24 hours. Currently, we are purifying bovine growth hormone derived from this stable mouse cell line.

1218 A PARADOXICAL GROWTH HORMONE RESPONSE TO TRH IN DIABETICS WITH PROLIFERATIVE RETINOPATHY. J.Krassowski*, H.Rogala, W.Jeske, S.Zgliczyński, Clinic of Endocrinology, Medical Ctr. of Postgraduate Education and Clinic of Gastroenterology and Metabolism, Medical Academy, 01-809 Warsaw, Poland.

Since insulin-like growth factor-I/IGF-I/ is elevated in diabetic proliferative retinopathy /PR/ and correlates with GH levels, a disturbance in GH secretion may be an important pathogenetic factor in PR. We studied GH secretion in type I diabetics with PR after stimulation with TRH /Roche/ 0.2 mg iv, bromocriptine /Parlodel,Sandoz/ 2.5 mg orally and L-Dopa /Roche 500 mg orally. Two control groups were also studied: type I diabetics with background retinopathy /BR/ and healthy subjects. TRH induced a marked increase in GH levels in all 9 patients with PR raising GH from the basal value of 7.4 to a peak of 19.6 ng/ml. TRH had no effect on GH release in BR patients and in healthy controls. TRH-induced GH response did not correlate with basal glucose and HbA1 levels. Bromocriptine raised GH levels in BR group and in healthy subjects to 15.3 and 14.6 ng/ml respectively while it was ineffective in PR group. L-Dopa induced a similar GH response in all three groups. These data indicate that dopaminergic control of GH release in diabetics with proliferative retinopathy is disturbed and a paradoxical GH response to TRH is a characteristic feature in these patients.

1219 PLASMA AND PITUITARY CONTENT OF GH, LH AND PROLACTIN IN UREMIC RAT.

B. Lacour, M.T. Bluet-Pajot, J.B. Roullet, T. Drueke and D. Durand*, U. 159 INSERM, 2ter rue d'Alésia, 75014 Paris, and U. 90 INSERM, Hôpital Necker, 149 rue de Sèvres, 75015 Paris (France).

In the rat, thyroid insufficiency was associated with chronic renal failure (CRF) and also with alterations in pituitary functions. In this study, plasma levels and pituitary content of GH, LH and prolactin (PRL) were investigated after four weeks of experimental period, in 8 normal rats fed ad libitum (C), 8 uremic (U) and 8 diet-restricted rats (DR) because CRF was associated with a decrease in food intake. CRF created by electrocoagulation was evaluated by plasma creatinine concentration. U and DR rats had a significantly lesser body weight gain during experimental period than C rats. They had also a marked decrease in pituitary GH content (1239 $\pm$ 98 μg in U, 1374 $\pm$ 109 in DR, and 1834 $\pm$ 189 in C rats, mean $\pm$ SEM) with no change in serum GH concentration. Pituitary LH content was only significantly decreased in U rats as compared to C and DR rats (53 $\pm$ 4.8, 87.5 $\pm$ 10.9, and 90.1 $\pm$ 10.6 μg respectively) with no change in serum LH concentration. Pituitary PRL content was similar to the 3 groups of rats while serum PRL concentration was significantly increased in U rats as compared to C and DR rats (27.2 $\pm$ 6.2 vs 14.7 $\pm$ 1.7 and 12.9 $\pm$ 1.8 ng/ml).
In conclusion, CRF is associated with decreased pituitary LH and GH content. However, the latter perturbation could be due to the malnutrition associated with CRF. Finally the increased serum PRL concentration in U rats was not associated with a modification in pituitary PRL content.

1220 EFFECTS OF GROWTH HORMONE ON FATTY ACID OXIDATION IN LIVER MITOCHONDRIA OF RATS.

V. T. Maddaiah, Dept. of Pediatrics, Nassau County Medical Center, SUNY, Stony Brook, East Meadow, N.Y. 11554.

We have shown that growth hormone (GH) exerts a significant effect on structure-function of liver mitochondria (M) that include fatty acyl and cardiolipin distribution in membranes, activity of respiratory enzymes and also enzymes of urea metabolism. One of the early clinical findings in children during GH therapy has been the increase in plasma free fatty acids. We have now investigated the effects of GH on fatty acid metabolism by measuring the rate of respiration (RR, ng atoms of O_2/min/mg protein) of M using palmitoyl-L-carnitine (PC), with and without malonate, an inhibitor of succinic dehydrogenase, in control,

	Succinate	Succinate + malonate	PC	PC + malonate
Control	194.65±43.81	34.43±11.61	84.71±28.64	70.18±28.44
Hypox	105.42±14.74	26.75± 8.20	56.41±17.70	56.00±21.31
Hypo + GH	142.73±30.23	25.91± 9.63	73.62±14.58	69.96±22.60

hypophysectomized (Hy) and Hy + GH treated (100 ug/rat daily for 7 days) rats (Table). Hy decreased significantly RR with PC and GH administration partially restored it. Malonate caused about 17% inhibition of RR with PC in control but not in Hy. We have measured RR using octanoate and also with K_3 $Fe(CN)_6$ as the electron acceptor. These results suggest that the entry of acetyl CoA into Kreb's cycle may be negligible in Hy rats as the availability of CoA may be limiting.

1221 THE PITUITARY HAS AN INHERENT ABILITY TO SECRETE GROWTH HORMONE IN A PULSATILE FASHION IN THE MALE RAT. C.J. Maltman* and S.H. Shin, Dept. of Physiology, Queen's University, Kingston, Canada, K7L 3N6.

We previously demonstrated that the ectopic pituitary dissociated from hypothalamic control secretes prolactin in a pulsatile manner. In this study, we examined the secretion pattern of rat growth hormone (rGH) from an adenohypophysis grafted under the kidney capsule. Blood samples were taken every 2 minutes via an indwelling right atrial cannula from conscious freely moving rats. The circulating rGH concentration did not remain at a steady level but fluctuated with time in both non-estradiol primed and estradiol primed rats. The fluctuations in plasma rGH concentration were not synchronized with the pulsatile change in prolactin concentration. Grafted rats were injected with a bolus of synthetic hpGRF in order to stimulate a rGH pulse. The declining phase of the pulse was not steady but had discrete small pulses superimposed upon it. Clonidine, an α-adrenergic agonist that stimulates rGH release in the normal rat, neither elevated the height of the pulses nor raised the basal concentration of rGH, indicating that the influence of the hypothalamus did not reach the ectopic adenohypophysis. The results of these studies show that the grafted adenohypophysis, which is not under the direct influence of hypothalamic GRF or somatostatin, has the ability to generate pulsatile changes in the plasma rGH. This ability suggests that the adenohypophysis possesses an inherent communication system to permit synchronized rGH secretion. (Supported by the MRC of Canada)

1222 INHIBITION OF INSULIN SECRETION BY INTRACEREBROVENTRICULAR INJECTION OF PANCREATIC POLYPEPTIDE (PP) IN CONSCIOUS DOGS. A. Inui*, N. Mizuno, H. Morioka, M. Ooya, T. Ogawa and S. Baba, The Second Department of Internal Medicine, Kobe University School of Medicine, Kobe, Japan

We have suggested that endogenous PP might inhibit insulin secretion through the vagal innervation (Excerpta Medica, 1982, pp). Since PP is found not only in pancreas but also in brain or cerebrospinal fluid (Excerpta Medica, 1982 138pp), we have studied the effect of intracerebro-entricular injection of PP on insulin secretion before and after vagotomy. Mongrel dogs were settled with a chronic cannula allowing intraventricular injections in the third or lateral ventricle. Administration of 50-5,000 ng/dog of PP (Porcine PP) caused significant inhibition of insulin secretion by modified sham feeding (sight and smell), intravenous injection of glucose (0.5 g/kg) and CCK-8 (0.07 μg/kg/5min), respectively. The novel finding, however, was shown that the maximal decrease of each insulin response was induced by 50 ng of PP and not in a dose-related fashion. Prior transthoracic bilateral truncal vagotomy abolished the suppressive effect of PP on glucose- and CCK-8-induced insulin secretion. The present data demonstrate that intraventricular PP administration has an inhibitory effect on insulin secretion and that the effect of the peptide is mediated by the vagus nerve. It is suggested that PP might be involved in the central regulatory mechanisms of insulin secretion.

1223 EFFECTS OF GLUCOCORTICOIDS ON TYROSINE HYDROXYLASE ACTIVITY IN HUMAN NEUROBLASTOMA CELL LINES. N. John* and P.S. Timiras, Department of Physiology-Anatomy, University of California, Berkeley, CA, 94720. USA

The inducing effect of glucocorticoids on tyrosine hydroxylase (TH) activity is well known *in vivo* in peripheral and central neurons and has been demonstrated *in vitro* in mouse neuroblastoma. The present study investigated whether a similar effect could be demonstrated in human neuroblastoma. This study utilized two human neuroblastoma cell lines, LA-N-1 and SY-5Y, cultured in basal synthetic growth media (1:1 mixture of Ham's F12 and Dubecco-Vogt Modified Eagles) supplemented with 10% fetal bovine serum. Following treatment with either hydrocortisone or dexamethasone (dosage range 12.7 - 138.0 uM) for a period of 5 - 8 days (media and steroid were changed daily during the treatment period), activity of the rate limiting biosynthetic adrenergic enzyme, TH, was measured. Radiometric results show basal TH activity to be significantly lower in SY-5Y cells than in LA-N-1 cells (.347 $\pm$ .035 nmol/hr/mg protein vs. 8.4 $\pm$ .114 nmol/hr/mg protein) and to be reduced by the administration of the ethanol vehicle (35 nM). Both LA-N-1 and SY-5Y were shown to contain cytoplasmic glucocorticoid receptors and to respond with slightly increased TH activity to steroid treatment. However, compared to mouse neuroblastoma, this inducing effect was significantly lower. Further studies on the molecular level to determine at which point in the hormone-response pathway the glucocorticoid-sensitivity occurs is warranted. This study was supported by NIH Training Grant GM-07379-07.

1224 ISOLATION OF MULTIPLE FORMS OF IMMUNOACTIVE RELAXIN-LIKE POLYPEPTIDES FROM RABBIT PLACENTAS. R. Eldridge*, V. Lee and P. Fields, University of South Alabama College of Medicine, Department of Anatomy, Mobile, Alabama, 36688, USA.

Like the human, relaxin (RXN) can be isolated from the ovary and placenta of the rabbit. Therefore this animal may provide an experimental model for studying the production and release of placental RXN. The first step in determining the feasibility of this model is purification and characterization of the hormone from rabbit tissue. Placentas from rabbits of unknown stages of pregnancy were extracted with 0.7N HCl-acetone (3:5 v/v) containing protease inhibitors. Gel filtration (Sephadex G-50) and ion exchange chromatography (carboxymethyl cellulose) separated a bioactive relaxin-like fraction with a specific activity of 9.4 units/mg as determined by the *in vitro* mouse uterus bioassay. SDS-urea gel electrophoresis of this fraction resulted in protein bands with molecular weights of 30K, 20K, 18K, 12K and 7K. These proteins were electrophoretically transferred to nitrocellulose and stained using peroxidase anti-peroxidase immunochemistry and porcine RXN antiserum (UF 1M). The 20K, 18K, 12K and 7K proteins demonstrated immunoactivity. Sugar moieties were not detected when the gels were stained with either the Alcian blue or Schiff's reagent. Thus like the pig, rat and cow, multiple forms of relaxin-like polypeptides are present in the rabbit. The prohormone form of porcine RXN has been shown to have a molecular weight of 20K. However further studies are necessary to determine whether these immunoactive proteins represent prohormone forms of rabbit RXN. Porcine RXN antiserum was supplied by Dr. M. J. Fields. Supported by NIH #HD-15773 and NSF PCM #8110062.

1225 PURIFICATION AND CHARACTERIZATION OF RAT ATRIAL CARDIONATRINS - POTENTIAL DIURETIC, NATRIURETIC AND VASOACTIVE HORMONES. T.G. Flynn*, M. de Bold and A.J. de Bold, Departments of Biochemistry and Pathology, Queen's University and Hotel Dieu Hospital, Kingston, Ontario, Canada K7L 3N6.

Atrial muscle contains secretory-like storage granules which have histo chemical and morphological features similar to granules that store polypeptide hormones. Extracts of rat atria or of purified granules cause a significant diuresis, natriuresis and hypotensive effect after injection into rats. To determine the chemical nature of the substance(s) responsible for these effects rat atria were homogenized and extracted in a mixture of 1M acetic acid, 1N HCl and 1% NaCl, processed through Sep-Pak cartridges (Waters) and the extracts chromatographed on BioGel P10 followed by reverse phase high pressure liquid chromatography using linear gradients of CH_3CN in either 0.1% TFA or 0.13% HFBA. Four fractions (Cardionatrins I-IV) were identified by these procedures each with significant diuretic and natriuretic activity. Purified Cardionatrion I yielded the sequence S-L-R-R-S-S-C-F-G-G-R-I-D-R-I-G-A-Q-S-G-L-G-C-N-S-F-R-Y with a disulfide bond between C_7 and C_{23}. Predictive secondary and tertiary structure analysis of this peptide shows a compact folded molecule with little ordered secondary structure. Synthetic peptides containing the residues 1-6, 1-12, 1-18 were not biologically active; the disulfide bridge appears necessary for the biological activity of Cardionatrin 1-28. Secretion of cardionatrins by the heart to exert an effect on the kidney suggests a mechanism by which the heart plays an endocrine role in the maintenance of water and salt balance in the body. This study was supported by IDEA Corporation and MRC.

1226 RELEASE OF IMMUNOREACTIVE TRH IN SERUM FREE CULTURES OF RAT HYPOTHALAMIC CELLS. D. Jordan*, M. Veisseire, Y. Germani and R. Mornex, INSERM U.197, Faculté de Médecine Alexis Carrel, 69008 Lyon, France.

Serum free cultures of rat hypothalamic cells were used as a model for studying TRH release in vitro. Cultivation of hypothalamic tissue by mean of the roller-tube technique yields thin histiotypic cultures. Explants con sisted of "punchs" of the paraventricular nuclei area of the anterior hypothalamus of 7 day-old rats. Explants are embedded in a plasma clot on flying coverslips and cultivated the first 4 days in a medium containing 25 % horse serum and then in a serum free medium (BME+insulin 5 µg/ml, transferrin 100 µg/ml, progesterone 20 nM, putrescin 0.1 mM, selenium 30 nM and glucose 30 mM) replaced every 3-4 days. The 16th day of culture experimental procedures were carried out in fresh serum free medium (incubation period:15 min). TRH release in the medium as well as the explant content were measured in a specific TRH-RIA (sensitivity 5 pg). The TRH neurons were visualized by immunocytochemistry using the PAL-PAP method.They appeared as 10-20 µ cells usually grouped by three or four everywhere inside the histio typic explant and also in the escaping individual nerve cells.15.0$\pm$2.6 pg of TRH are released in 15 min from explants containing 63.5$\pm$14.5 pg. An enriched K^+ medium (K^+x10) promotes a significant increase of TRH release,effect prevented by EGTA addition (0.1 mM). The addition of 5HT also induced an increase of medium TRH directly related to 5HT concentration from 10^{-8} to 10^{-4}M. The 10^{-8}M 5HT stimulating effect is prevented by cyproheptadin addition(10^{-6}M).In conclusion, immunocytochemically characterized TRH cells of hypothalamic explant release TRH when cultured in serum free medium.TRH release is increased in enriched K^+ medium and after 5HT addition.

1227 INVOLVEMENT OF HYPOTHALAMIC SOMATOSTATIN (SRIF) AND DOPAMINE (DA) IN THE INHIBITION OF GROWTH HORMONE (GH) AND PROLACTIN (PRL) SECRETION BY GASTRIN RELEASING PEPTIDE (GRP) IN THE RAT. Y. Kabayama*, Y. Kato, A. Shimatsu, N. Matsushita, H. Ohta, T. Inoue, K. Tojo and H. Imura, Second Medical Clinic, Department of Medicine, Kyoto University Faculty of Medicine, Kyoto, Japan.

GRP, a 27 amino acid peptide, has been demonstrated in the rat hypothalamus. However, its possible role in the hypothalamo-pituitary axis remains to be fully elucidated. In the present study, we examined the mode of action of GRP influencing the secretion of GH and PRL in the rat. ICV injection of synthetic porcine GRP (1 μg/rat) almost completely inhibited GH release induced by hpGRF-44-NH_2(hpGRF, 80 ng/100 g BW, iv) in urethane-anesthetized male rats (mean±SE of peak plasma GH: 23.9±7.3 vs 171±32.0 ng/ml, $p<0.05$). Depletion of hypothalamic SRIF by cysteamine pretreatment (30 mg/100 g BW, sc) or by passive immunization with anti-SRIF rabbit serum (0.5 ml, iv) attenuated the inhibitory action of GRP on GH response to hpGRF (ΔGH: 193±66.9 and 268±77.7 vs control 2.9±2.5 ng/ml, $p<0.01$). As previously reported (PSEBM 172:118, 1983), GRP (1 μg/rat, icv) inhibited PRL release induced by a Met^5-enkephalin analog, FK33-824 (10 μg/100 g BW, iv), but did not inhibit elevated plasma PRL levels sustained by a DA antagonist, domperidone (10 μg/100 g BW, iv). In *in vitro* studies with perifused hypothalamic fragments, DA release was increased by GRP (10^{-5}M)(39.5±2.8 vs KRBG control 25.3±5.0 pg/5 min/hypothalamus, $p<0.05$). GRP (10^{-5}M) did not affect GH and PRL release from superfused anterior pituitary cells. These results suggest that hypothalamic SRIF and DA are involved in the inhibitory action of GRP on GH and PRL secretion in the rat, respectively.

1228 PEPTIDE HISTIDINE ISOLEUCINE AMIDE(PHI), BUT NOT VASOACTIVE INTESTINAL POLYPEPTIDE(VIP), MAY BE AN ENDOGENOUS PRL-RELEASING FACTOR IN THE RAT. H. KAJI* K. CHIHARA, H. ABE, N. MINAMITANI, H. KODAMA, T. KITA, Y. KASHIO, Y. OKIMURA AND T. FUJITA Third Div. Dept. of Med. Kobe Univ. Sch. of Med. Kobe 650, Japan

It remains to be controversial whether PHI and VIP are endogenous PRL-releasing factor(PRF). In this studies, first, we examined the effects of PHI and VIP on PRL release in male Wistar rats weighing 300g. The iv injections of pure PHI(0.1, 1 and 10μg)resulted in a significant and dose-related increase of plasma PRL in conscious, freely-moving rats. PHI(10^{-8}-10^{-7}M) stimulated PRL release from rat anterior pituitary tissues perifused *in vitro*. A PRL-releasing potency of PHI was similar with that of VIP both *in vivo* and *in vitro*. Second, we studied the effects of passive immunization with anti-PHI and anti-VIP serum on a sustained elevation of plasma PRL following every 30 min injection of sulpiride(S, 5mg/kg BW). Antiserum was raised in rabbit against pure PHI or synthetic VIP conjugated with bovine thyroglobulin and 1 ml each of them was iv administered 45 min after the first injection of S. The PRL release area for 75 min after the injection of anti-PHI serum(1828±238)was significantly less than those after normal rabbit serum(3891±444) or anti-VIP serum(3671±356). These results strongly suggest that PHI, but not VIP, may be another candidate for hypothalamic PRF. This study was supported by grants from the Japanese Ministry of Education, Science and Culture.

1229 EFFECTS OF HYPOTHALAMIC PERIVENTRICULAR (PV) LESIONS ON SOMATOSTATIN (SRIF) RELEASE FROM PERIFUSED BLOCKS OF PREOPTIC AREA-HYPOTHALAMUS (POA-H). L. W. Kaler*, A. Dyke and V. Critchlow, Reproductive Biology and Behavior, Oregon Regional Primate Research Center, Beaverton, Oregon, U.S.A.

As shown previously, lesions in the hypothalamic PV nucleus reduce median eminence (ME) SRIF content by ≈80% without affecting nonstress plasma growth hormone (GH) levels or the GH response to stress. Our aim was to study the effects of PV lesions on SRIF release during POA-H perifusion. A large deficit in such release would suggest that most SRIF is PV-derived and available in excess for control of GH secretion; no deficit would suggest major extra-PV sources of SRIF. Female rats received anterior or posterior PV lesions; sham-lesioned and intact rats served as controls. At 2, 4, and 16 weeks after surgery, nonstress and stress plasma GH levels were similar in all groups. The rats were killed at 18 weeks and each POA-H was perifused with a Krebs-Ringer-Hepes-Bicarbonate medium saturated with 95% O_2:5% CO_2 (pH 7.4; 37°C) at 0.1 ml/min; effluents were collected at 10 min intervals. The POA-Hs of the PV- and sham-lesioned rats released similar amounts of SRIF (5.9 ± 0.5 pg/ml), and these were higher (P<0.001) than from POA-Hs of intact rats (0.9 ± 0.4 pg/ml). All POA-Hs showed similar increases (P<0.05) in SRIF release after 56 mM K^+. Two rats were chosen randomly from each group to assess ME SRIF content. PV lesions caused 80% depletion; sham lesions did not. These results confirm that most SRIF neurons in the PV nucleus and 80% of ME SRIF content are not essential for apparently normal control of GH secretion under nonstress and stress conditions and indicate that PV or sham lesions in the rostral forebrain enhance *in vitro* SRIF release; this SRIF may stem from neurons located outside of the PV nucleus. Supported by Grants RR00163 and AM32442 from the NIH.

1230 HUMAN GROWTH HORMONE RELEASING FACTOR(1-44)NH_2-LIKE IMMUNOREACTIVITIES IN VARIOUS HUMAN TISSUES AND CEREBROSPINAL FLUID. Y.Kashio*, K.Chihara, H.Abe, T.Kita and T.Fujita. Third Div., Dept. of Med., Kobe Univ. Sch. of Med., Kobe 650 Japan.

A RIA method for human growth hormone releasing factor(1-44)NH_2 (hGRF) was established using the antiserum recognizing the C-terminal portion of hGRF. Minimal detectable value was 1 pg/tube. Various tissues were obtained from 8 patients with non-endocrine diseases at autopsy 2-12 hrs after their death, and extracted with 2 N acetic acid. The cerebrospinal fluid(CSF) was collected by spinal tap from 34 patients with various diseases and lyophilized without extraction. The hGRF-like immunoreactivities(hGRF-LI,pg/mg wet weight) in the median eminence ranged from 228-3300, highest among human tissues, and next rich in the pituitary stalk(85-500) and in the hypothalamus except the median eminence(12-75). Small but detectable amounts of hGRF-LI were contained in the cerebral cortex(0.08-0.46). Contents of hGRF-LI in other tissues were varied among patients; pyrolic antrum nd-0.5, gastric cardia nd-0.6, pancreatic head nd-0.9, pancreatic tail nd-2.4, colon nd-0.6, esophagus nd-0.1, liver nd-0.2, renal cortex nd-0.4, renal medulla nd-0.2, adrenal gland nd-2.1. The hGRF-LI of the CSF were detected in 21 patients ranging from 13.6-61.5 with the mean ± SE value of 31.2 ± 2.9 pg/ml while the remaining 13 patients had the undetectable levels of hGRF-LI. These findings indicate that hGRF-LI are present predominantly in the median eminence of human hypothalamus and sparse in other tissues with a small quantity even if they exist,and also suggest that hGRF-LI were detectable in human CSF. This work was supported by grants from the Japanese Ministry of Health and Welfare.

1231 DUAL ACTION OF GROWTH HORMONE (GH)-RELEASING FACTOR (GRF) ON SPONTANEOUS GH SECRETION IN CONSCIOUS MALE RATS. H. Katakami* and L. A. Frohman, Div. of Endocrinology, Univ. of Cincinnati Coll. of Med., Cincinnati, Ohio

Central nervous system effects of GRF were studied in conscious male rats with indwelling intraatrial and intracerebroventricular (icv) cannulae. Animals were injected iv or icv with 10 ng or 1000 ng hpGRF1-40 and blood samples obtained every 10-20 min from 1000 h to 1400 h. Spontaneous GH secretory pulses occurred from 1120-1300 h in most control animals. The icv injection of 10 ng GRF at 1100 h, immediately before the expected GH pulse, suppressed GH secretion during the 1100-1300 h period (GRF: 22±3 ng/ml vs control: 69±6, $p<0.001$), while the iv injection of 10 ng GRF had no effect (77±11 ng/ml). In contrast, a larger dose of GRF (1000 ng) given icv at 1100 h increased GH secretion with peak values 20 min after injection (GRF: 621±138 ng/ml vs control: 100±24, $p<0.01$). The iv injection of 1000 ng GRF also stimulated GH release with peak values occurring 10 min after injection (307±108 ng/ml, $p<0.01$ vs control). The spontaneous GH secretory pulse following GRF (iv or icv) was suppressed proportionately to the magnitude of the GRF-induced GH secretory response ($r=-0.78$, $p<0.01$). The results suggest that 1) central administration of a low dose of GRF suppresses GH secretion by inhibition of endogenous GRF or stimulation of somatostatin release while a large dose of GRF stimulates GH release by leakage from the CSF to the pituitary, and 2) the magnitude of spontaneous GH surges are influenced by the antecedent (GRF-induced) secretory activity of the somatotrophs.

1232 ELECTROPHYSIOLOGIC MANIFESTATION OF LHRH PULSE GENERATOR ACTIVITY IN THE RHESUS MONKEY: INFLUENCE OF α-ADRENERGIC AND DOPAMINERGIC BLOCKADE. J. M. Kaufman*, J. S. Kesner, R. C. Wilson and E. Knobil, Department of Physiology, University of Texas Medical School, Houston, Texas 77025 USA.

Characteristic, discrete, intermittent increases in neuronal multi-unit activity (MUA), coupled with the initiation of circhoral LH pulses, were recorded from ovariectomized rhesus monkeys bearing chronically implanted electrodes in the region of the arcuate nucleus and tubero-infundibular tract. In 25 experiments in 6 monkeys restrained in primate chairs, hypothalamic MUA was monitored continuously for 4 to 10 h before, and 6 to 15 h after, intravenous injection of α-adrenoceptor blocking or antidopaminergic substances. Blood samples were taken at 10 to 20 min intervals and assayed for LH by RIA. α-receptor blockade with phentolamine (2-5 mg/kg BW), or with the more specific α_1-receptor blockers phenoxybenzamine (1.0 mg/kg BW) and prazosin (0.1 mg/kg BW), resulted in an immediate alteration of the pattern of electrical activity, ranging from a transient reduction in frequency to a prolonged (>12h) arrest of the MUA volleys. These changes were faithfully reflected in the pulsatile pattern of LH secretion. Similar results were obtained with the antidopaminergic drug metoclopramide (0.6 mg/kg BW). The α_2-receptor blocker yohimbine at a dosage of 0.25 to 1.0 mg/kg BW had no distinct effect on pulse generator activity or LH secretion. These observations suggest that, in the rhesus monkey, the frequency of the hypothalamic LHRH pulse generator can be influenced, either directly or indirectly, by noradrenergic and dopaminergic inputs. (Supported by grants from the NICHD and the A.W. Mellon Foundation).

1233 **ESTRADIOL STIMULATES AN INCREASE IN LH-PULSE FREQUENCY IN THE EWE INDEPENDENT OF PRIOR EXPOSURE TO PROGESTERONE.** Alan H. Kaynard* and Fred J. Karsch, Reproductive Endocrinology Program and Dept. of Physiology, The University of Michigan, Ann Arbor, MI, 48109.

An increase in LH-pulse frequency occurs during the follicular phase of the estrous cycle in sheep and is obligatory for ovulation. We recently found that withdrawal of progesterone (P) and maintenance of a basal concentration of estradiol (E) produces a more rapid increase in pulse frequency than does withdrawal of P alone. This raises the question of whether E acts by increasing the rate of removal of P inhibition of frequency or by directly stimulating frequency independent of P withdrawal. This study tested the hypothesis that E can directly stimulate LH-pulse frequency. Five long-term ovariectomized Suffolk ewes were studied in the early breeding season. This time was chosen to avoid the inhibitory effect of estradiol on pulse frequency (only in anestrus) and to precede development of the mid-breeding season castrate frequency (possibly maximal). Each ewe received a Silastic E implant previously shown to produce an early follicular phase serum level of E. LH-pulse frequency was determined (6 min samples) before and 12,24,36,60 and 84 hr after implantation of E. Frequency increased in all ewes as shown by a decrease in inter-pulse interval (IPI). The overall ability of E to decrease mean IPI below control (IPI=41±1 min) was significant ($p<.01$) and was most dramatic at 60 and 84 hr after implantation (IPI=34±1 min; $p<.01$). This increase in LH-pulse frequency is consistent with the hypothesis that, during the follicular phase of the estrous cycle of the ewe, E can stimulate the hypothalamic pulse generator independent of prior exposure to P. NIH HD11311, HD07048

1234 SUBSTANCE P RECEPTORS IN RAT ANTERIOR PITUITARY MEMBRANES.
B. Kerdelhué *, V. Lenoir, P. Hubleau and A. Tartar, Laboratoire des Hormones Polypeptidiques, C.N.R.S., 91190 GIF sur YVETTE, and Faculté de Pharmacie, Université de Lille II, 3, rue du Professeur Laguesse, 59045 LILLE, France.

We have previously demonstrated that Substance P (SP), an undecapeptide structurally unrelated to GnRH, inhibits in a dose-dependant manner the GnRH-induced LH and FSH release from rat anterior pituitary. In the present study, using two different SP receptor ligands, $|^{3}H|$SP and chloramine T $|^{125}$-$|$ (D-Tyr^{0},Nle^{11})SP, we were able to demonstrate SP binding sites in rat anterior pituitary membranes. Binding studies were performed at 0°C in 10 mM Tris-HCl, pH 7.4 in presence of inhibitors (1 mM 1-10 Phenanthroline ; 1 µg/ml α_2-macroglobulin ; 1 mM dithiothreitol, 5 mM EDTA) of SP-degrading enzymes. $|^{125}I|$ SP binding reached maximum after 120 min. This binding was reduced by 90 % when 10 µM unlabelled SP was added. Specific $|^{3}H|$ SP binding exhibited saturation kinetics and plateaued at approximately 6.10^{8}M. Scatchard analysis indicated a single population of binding sites whith a dissociation constant (Kd) of 7.5 ± 2.5 nM and a maximal number of binding sites (B_{max}) of 20 to 40 fmol/mg protein. $|^{125}I|$ SP binding was inhibited by increasing concentrations of unlabelled (D-Tyr^{0}, Nleu^{11}) SP or SP and Scatchard analysis demonstrated a single class of binding sites with a Kd of 13 nM. The binding affinity decreased as amino acids were progressively removed from the N or C terminal part of the molecule. However, the binding was not inhibited by GnRH nor by other neuropeptides. These data demonstrate the presence of a specific receptor for SP in rat anterior pituitary membranes and further support the concept of a specific role for SP in the modulation of gonadotropins release by mechanisms which remain to be elucidated.

1235 STUDIES ON GnRH INDUCED PRIMING AND DESENSITIZATION.

Gy. Kéri[+], K. Nikolics, J. Molnár, I. Teplán, J. Ramachandran
1st Institute of Biochemistry, SOTE 1444. POB. 260. Budapest, Hungary, Hormone Research Lab. UCSF San Francisco Ca 94143 U.S.A.

Preincubation of cultured pituitary cells with various concentrations of GnRH for various time periods caused a biphasic effect on the responsiveness of the cells on subsequent GnRH stimulus. Preincubation of the cells with a submaximal dose of GnRH for a shorter time period caused a significant priming on subsequent GnRH induced LH and FSH release while by increasing the preincubating concentration of GnRH or the preincubation time a concentration and time-dependent desensitization of subsequent GnRH induced LH and FSH release could be observed. The GnRH induced priming and desensitization showed a similar pattern for both LH and FSH release although the ED_{50} values of priming and desensitization slightly differed for LH and FSH release.

Photoaffinity labeling was also applied for studying desensitization. After preincubation of cultured rat pituitary cells with different concentrations of GnRH or a superactive analogue for different periods, the cells were photolabeled with Nitroazidophenylsulfenyl analogue of Orn^8-GnRH. Consequently, LH release induced by covalently bound hormone was measured. These results were in very good correlation with those obtained by consequtive incubations.

1236 ACTIONS OF ARACHIDONIC ACID IN PITUITARY GONADOTROPHS: STIMULATION OF LH RELEASE AND CYCLIC NUCLEOTIDE PRODUCTION.

L. Kiesel*, T. Rabe, B. Runnebaum and K. J. Catt[1], Dept. Obstetrics & Gynecology, Univ. of Heidelberg, 6900 Heidelberg, FRG and [1]Endocrinology and Reproduction Res. Branch, National Institutes of Health, Bethesda, MD 20816, USA.

Recently, we and others have proposed that phospholipids and arachidonic acid (AA) may be involved in the post-receptor mechanism of GnRH action. In the present study, we have investigated various aspects of AA action on LH release and cyclic nucleotide (cAMP and cGMP) production. Enriched gonadotroph fractions were prepared from rat anterior pituitaries by centrifugal elutriation. Cells (3×10^4 /dish) were incubated in 1 ml Medium 199. AA (10^{-7} to 10^{-4} M) stimulated the release of LH dose-dependently in monolayer cell cultures, as well as in superfusion experiments. The effect of AA was maximal at 10^{-4} M and was found to be about 10^4 less potent than GnRH. Other fatty acids (oleic acid, linoleic acid) did not affect LH release up to 10^{-4} M. In addition to exclude toxicity, gonadotrophs were preincubated with AA for 15 min and exposed to GnRH. No change in cell response to GnRH following AA was observed. In superfused gonadotrophs AA enhanced LH release within the first 1-2 minutes and gonadotropin release was stimulated linearly up to 4 h by the fatty acid in monolayer cultures . The production of cAMP and cGMP was enhanced by 2 min incubations of AA up to 80 and 70%, respectively. The levels of cGMP returned to initial values after 5 min, whereas cAMP production decreased slightly between 5 and 30 min and incresed subsequently. In 2 h incubations AA stimulated cAMP production two-fold (maximum at 10^{-5} AA), but cGMP levels remained unchanged. In this report we have shown that AA, which can be released by GnRH, stimulates LH release and its active metabolites may act as mediators of GnRH action in gonadotrophs. (This study was supported by the DFG)

1237 EFFECT OF IN VIVO INTERMITTENT VS CONTINUOUS ADMINISTRATION OF PROGESTERONE LOCALLY INFUSED IN THE RAT MEDIOBASAL HYPOTHALAMUS (MBH) AND LHRH RELEASE AS DETERMINED WITH PUSH-PULL PERFUSION (PPP). K. Kim* and V. D. Ramirez, Dept. of Physiology and Biophysics, University of Illinois, Urbana, IL 61801, USA.

We reported that intermittent infusion of progesterone (P) is highly effective in stimulating *in vitro* LHRH release from hypothalamic fragments from ovariectomized, estradiol-primed (OVX+E) prepuberal rats (Endocrinol. 111:750, 1983). This study attempts to examine the effectiveness of intermittent vs continuous perfusion of P on *in vivo* LHRH release from the MBH from OVX+E adult rat bearing push-pull cannulae. PPP was performed between 10:00-17:00, and perfusates were collected at 10-min intervals. Three groups were studied: 1) control (perfused only with medium), 2) intermittent P perfusion (10 min-on, 20 min-off), and 3) continuous P perfusion. MBH was directly perfused with P (10 ng/ml) following a 3-hr basal collection period. LHRH concentrations were determined by RIA. Cycle detector analysis revealed that intermittent perfusion of the MBH by P was the only effective regimen in stimulating mean LHRH release (pre-P:.72±.08 vs post-P:1.12±.23 pg/10 min) and pulse amplitude (pre-P:1.14±.18 vs post-P:1.99±.53 pg) without changes in spontaneous LHRH pulse frequency (pre-P:48±6 vs post-P:42±5 min). Neither continuous perfusion of P nor control perfusions were effective in changing any of the parameters measured.

The present results suggest that *in vivo* rhythmic secretion of P might be the effective signal activating the rat neural LHRH apparatus.

1238 REGIONAL DISTRIBUTION OF RAT-GROWTH HORMONE RELEASING FACTOR(GRF)-LIKE IMMUNOREACTIVITIES IN RAT HYPOTHALAMUS. T. Kita*, K. Chihara, H. Abe, N. Minamitani, H. Kaji, H. Kodama. and T. Fujita. Third Div., Dept. of Med. Kobe Univ. Sch. of Med., Kobe 650 Japan

The heterologous RIA for rat GH releasing factor (GRF) was established using syntehtic rat GRF(1-43)OH for both standard reference and radioiodination with the antiserum produced against human GRF(1-44)NH_2. The regional distribution of rat GRF-like immunoreactivities(GRF-LI) was examined by this RIA and compared with that of somatostatin-like immunoreactivities (SRIF). Male SD rats were killed by decapitation, brains were removed, frozen, and hypohtalamic nuclei were punched out according to the Palkovits' method. One specimen in the specified hypothalamic area was pooled from 10 rats, sonicated in 2N acetic acid, boiled for 10 min, centrifuged and the supernatant was lyophilized. Both GRF-LI and SRIF-LI contents(ng/mg protein, mean ± SE, n=5) were highest in the median eminence(ME: 32.2 ± 11.4, 109.9 ± 19.9) and next abundant in the arcuate nuclei(ARC: 3.5 ± 0.5, 12.9 ± 1.7). Only small amounts of GRF-LI were contained in the supraoptic (SO: 2.1 ± 0.5), ventromedial(VM: 1.4 ± 0.2), dorsomedial(DM: 1.6 ± 0.2) nuclei and the anterior hypothalamic area(AHA: 1.3 ± 0.5) whereas GRF-LI was not detected in the suprachiasmatic(SC), periventricular(PEV), paraventricular(PV), premammillary ventral(PMV) nuclei and the medial preoptic area(MPOA). Considerable amounts of SRIF-LI were contained in the PEV, VM, SC, PV and AHA in consistent with previous reports. These findings indicate that GRF-LI are localized in the ME and ARC in the rat but their contents are approximately one-tenth of SRIF-LI on a molar basis. This work was by grants from the Japanese Ministry of Health and Welfare.

1239 TWO NEW ANALOGUES OF TRH WITH HIGH BIOLOGICAL ACTIVITY. W. Klingler*, G. Vierke, H. Kalbacher, P. Ball and R. Knuppen, Inst.f. Biochem. Endokr. MH 24 Lübeck and Inst. f. Physiol. Chemie Univ. 74 Tübingen, Fed. Rep. Germ.

During recent years different analogues of TRH with high biological activity have been described. We synthesized two simple analogues of TRH: Pyr-N3-Im-methyl-His-Pro-NH-n-amyl (I) and Pyr-His-Pro-tyramine (II). The TSH-releasing activity of these compounds was tested in comparison with (N3-Im-methyl-His)2-TRH (III) and natural TRH. Since all these peptides were found to produce serum TSH maxima 20 min after i.p. injection potencies and efficiencies were assessed at this point. Potencies were calculated from the regression lines of the TRH dose/TSH serum level relationship, efficiencies were defined as maximal increment of serum TSH irrespective of the peptide dose. Compound I and III showed potencies 5 times, compound II only 0.05 times that of natural TRH. Highest efficiencies, however, were achieved by compound I and II (ΔTSH = 1.7 ng/ml); compound III behaved as natural TRH (ΔTSH = 1.2 ng/ml). From these results and former studies we conclude that the alkylation of the prolin moiety of TRH (compound I and II)seems to enhance the TSH release from the pituitary gland. Moreover, after iodination with I-125, compound II may be suitable for receptor studies with rat pituitaries. We thank Dr. Raiti (NIAMDD-rat hormone distribution program) for providing substances for the rat TSH-RIA.

1240 MAINTENANCE OF SPERMATOGENESIS BY NASAL GNRH-APPLICATION IN PATIENTS WITH KALLMANN'S SYNDROME. D. Klingmüller*, M. Meschi and H.U. Schweikert ,Dept. of Internal Medicine, University of Bonn, D 5300 Bonn, W.-Germany.

Pulsatile substitution with GnRH appears to be the therapy of choice in patients with Kallmann's syndrome (KS), a well defined type of hypogonadotropic hypogonadism. We tried to simplify the treatment and to limit the subcutaneous GnRH therapy to the period absolutely necessary to induce spermatogenesis. Therefore, before GnRH treatment of a 19 year old man with KS we stimulated his testes by hCG administration (2500 IU twice weekly for 390 days). During this treatment testicular volume increased from 1 to 5.5 ml. Thereafter, 5 µg GnRH were administered subcutaneously every 128 minutes by means of a small computerized pump (Zyclomat®) for 12 weeks. During the 90 days of this treatment testicular size increased to normal adult volume (left testis: 15 ml, right testis: 12 ml) and spermatogenesis was induced. Semen analysis showed a total of 0.3×10^6 immobile spermatozoa before GnRH therapy and 59×10^6 with normal motility on day 90 of GnRH therapy. Later on, 200 µg GnRH were administered by nasal spray every 2 hours, 8 times daily. After 6 months of this therapy the spermiogram showed 188×10^6 spermatozoa of normal motility. Similar results could be obtained in a second patient. We conclude: 1. Pulsatile GnRH-application is a new effective therapy of hypogonadotropic hypogonadism. 2. Pretreatment with hCG simplifies the therapy considerably. 3. Spermatogenesis can be maintained by periodic intranasal GnRH application.

1241 IDENTIFICATION OF DOPAMINE RECEPTOR IN THE VARIOUS HUMAN PITUITARY TUMORS.
M.KOGA*, H.NAKAO, M.ARAO, B.SATO, K.NOMA, Y.MORIMOTO, S.KISHIMOTO, S.MORI, and T.UOZUMI, The Third Department of Internal Medicine, Osaka Univ.,Osaka, Department of Neurosurgery of Osaka Adult Center, Osaka, and Department of Neurosurgery, Hiroshima Univ., Hiroshima, Japan.
Since dopamine agonists have been known to affect hormone release as well as tumor growth in some human pituitary tumors, we have studied dopamine receptors in various human pituitary tumors (14 prolactinomas, 12 GH-secreting adenomas and 19 non-functioning adenomas). Plasma membranes fraction of prolactinomas was incubated with [^{3}H]spiperone ± 2 μM nonradioactive fluphenazine at 25°C for 1 h, and membrane bound radioactivity was separated from free by filtration through Whatman GF/C filter. All prolactinomas showed the single class of high affinity binding site. Kd and Bmax were 0.85 ± 0.11 nM and 428 ± 49 fmoles/mg protein, respectively. Compound active upon the D-2 dopamine receptor in the prolactinoma competed with [^{3}H] spiperone for the occupancy of the specific binding site. Guanosine 5'triphospate decreased the affinity of agonist but not antagonist for the specific [^{3}H]spiperone binding sites. Using this procedure, we examined the possibility of the presence of dopamine receptor in other pituitary tumors. In 9 of 12 GH-secreting adenomas, specific [^{3}H]spiperone binding sites were identified. Kd and Bmax of GH-secreting adenomas with measurable binding were 1.65 ± 0.34 nM and 193 ± 37 fmoles/mg protein, respectively. Furthermore, 13 of 19 non-functioning adenomas were also found to contain specific [^{3}H]spiperone binding sites. Kd and Bmax of non-functioning adenomas with measurable binding were 2.22 ± 0.36 nM and 191 ± 27 fmoles/mg protein, respectively. These results suggested that dopaminergic agonists exert their direct effect upon various pituitary tumors via dopamine receptor.

1242 ONTOGENY OF TRH AND HISTIDYL PROLINE DIKETOPIPERAZINE (DKP) IN THE RAT: EVIDENCE THAT DKP MAY ARISE INDEPENDENTLY OF TRH.
P. Lamberton*, R. Lechan, and I.M.D. Jackson, Division of Endocrinology, New England Medical Center, Boston, MA, U.S.A.
His Pro DKP, a cyclized dipeptide, proposed as a metabolite of TRH has been shown to have multiple biologic effects in the CNS, some similar but others opposite to those of TRH. To evaluate the postulated relationship between TRH and DKP the ontogeny of these two peptides in the rat from fetal day 17 to adult was studied (N=4-16 animals per age). Various regions of the CNS as well as whole pancreas were extracted (in 1N HAC and 50% MEOH) and the levels of DKP and TRH determined by specific RIAs. On fetal day 21, large quantities of DKP were present throughout the CNS (e.g. midbrain 527 ± 75, spinal cord 554 ± 91 pg) while these regions contained undetectable or low levels of TRH (<5 and 27 ± 2 pg resp.). Fetal day 21 pancreas contained 211 ± 50 pg DKP and 354 ± 37 pg TRH. In the adult pancreas the content of DKP rose to 20.8 ng ± 3.5 while TRH became undetectable. In the hippocampus where the tissue content of DKP rose from 27 ± 7 pg (day 21 prenatal) to 726 ± 77 pg (adult) TRH was continually undetectable. The molar ratio of DKP:TRH in the hypothalamus at fetal day 21 was 2 but by adult had fallen to 0.3. In the olfactory lobe at fetal day 21 DKP:TRH was 11.6, at postnatal day 7 had risen to 44.3, but then gradually fell to 21.6 (day 10), 2.2 (day 28), and 0.53 (adult). These results indicate that DKP is a neural peptide distributed throughout the CNS as well as in extraneural locations. In various regions of the fetal rat CNS, DKP is present in substantial concentrations although TRH is undetectable. The tissue content of DKP during development shows little relationship to that of TRH suggesting DKP may arise independently of the tripeptide amide.

1243 ATTENUATION BUT NOT ABOLITION OF PITUITARY RESPONSIVENESS DURING CHRONIC TREATMENT WITH AN LHRH AGONIST. B.Laroche*, N.Faure, A.Lemay, G.Robert, R.Plante, M.Thabet, R.Roy and A.T.A. Fazekas, St-François d'Assise Hospital, Laval Hospital, Quebec, G1L 3L5, Canada.

25 patients with prostatic cancer have been treated with the LHRH agonist [D-Ser(TBU)^6-des-Gly-NH$_2$^{10}] LHRH ethylamide (buserelin) for periods up to 21 months. The initial dosage was 500 µg s.c. every 8 hours for 7 days, followed by 400 µg intranasally every 8 hours. Serum testosterone decreased to levels below 1 ng/ml within 3 weeks ($p<0.01$) and remained suppressed (between 0.44 and 0.66) from the 6th week up to the longest time of observation. Basal serum LH decreased from 16 mUI/ml to 10 and 6 mUI/ml after one and 3 months respectively ($p<0.01$) and remained at that level thereafter. Serum FSH decreased by 50% after one month of therapy (from 22mUI/ml to 11 mUI/ml) after one and 3 months ($p<0.01$). However a slight tendancy to rise was observed at 9 and 12 months to levels of 15 mUI/ml ($n=13$, $p<0.05$) and 15 mUI/ml ($n=9$, N.S.) respectively. The 3h-Δ LH (serum levels of LH 3h. after a dose of LHRH-A minus baseline) was already 82% inhibited at the second injection and there was no response after the 4th injection (at 24 h). However, even if the release of LH remains markedly inhibited (over 85%) during the 12 months of suppressive therapy, a small rise in serum LH is seen after each injection of the peptide, suggesting that the pituitary is not completely desensitized but is constantly responding at a much lower level. These data support the reversibility of the pituitary inhibition after LHRH agonist treatment. Temporary interruption of treatment could lead to an escape from that inhibition. However, rapid pituitary recovery would be a positive aspect regarding application of LHRH agonist in male contraception.

1244 EFFECTS OF TESTOSTERONE (T) AND NALOXONE ON LHRH SECRETION *IN VITRO* - RELATIONSHIP WITH HYPOTHALAMIC LHRH CONCENTRATION. Pushpa S. Kalra*, C.L. Leadem and S.P. Kalra, Department of OB/Gyn, College of Medicine, University of Florida, Gainesville, FL 32610, U.S.A.

The effects of *in vivo* T treatment and *in vitro* naloxone infusion on LHRH release *in vitro* and the relationship between LHRH release and hypothalamic (Hyp) LHRH concentration were assessed. The LHRH secretion rates in perifusate from Hyp of intact, castrated and castrated male rats bearing sc T implants (length 5 or 30mm) were compared; Hyp LHRH concentrations of these groups were also determined. Castration depleted Hyp LHRH stores and the LHRH secretion rate was markedly reduced (10.4 ± 0.4 pg/10 min) as compared to that of intact rats (24.0 ± 0.8 pg/10 min). Treatment with 5mm T implants ($\simeq 500$ pg T/ml serum) significantly raised the Hyp LHRH levels but failed to augment release *in vitro* (8.9 ± 0.4 pg/10 min). In contrast, the 30mm T implants ($\simeq 2$ ng T/ml serum) raised Hyp LHRH levels as well as LHRH output (13.6 ± 0.8 pg/10 min). Infusion of naloxone for 30 min during *in vitro* perifusion evoked increases in LHRH release rate which were higher from the Hyp of intact rats as compared to that of castrated rats. These studies show that: (i) T promoted both accumulation and release of LHRH; these two neurosecretory events displayed differential thresholds of response - LHRH accumulation being more sensitive to T than the release response; and (ii) naloxone-evoked LHRH release may be dependent upon the hypothalamic releasable pool of LHRH - lowest pool was found in castrated rats and highest in intact rats. (Supported by NIH HD 11362).

1245 LUTEINIZING HORMONE-RELEASING HORMONE (LHRH) PATHWAYS IN THE SHEEP BRAIN DURING ANESTROUS AND THE MID-LUTEAL PHASE. M.N. Lehman, A.-J. Silverman, J.E. Robinson, and F.J. Karsch, Dept. Anat. & Cell Biol., Univ., New York, NY 10032, and Reprod. Endo. Progr., Univ. Mich., Ann Arbor, MI 48109.

We examined the LHRH neuronal systems of adult intact and ovariectomized (OVX) ewes during anestrous, and estrous cycling ewes during their mid-luteal phase. Animals were perfused with Zamboni's fixative, and coronal vibratome sections (80 um) were processed for LHRH immunocytochemistry using an antiserum provided by Dr. R. Benoit (Salk Institute) and an avidin-biotin-HRP procedure (Vectastain). A majority of LHRH-immunoreactive neurons were found in the medial preoptic area, near the organum vasculosum of the lamina terminalis (OVLT). Clusters of labelled cells were also found in the medial septum and along the ventrolateral surface of the anterior hypothalamus. Few if any cells were seen in the arcuate nucleus. LHRH-immunoreactive fibers could be followed along several routes to dense fiber plexuses in the median eminence and continuing into the neural lobe. In addition, LHRH fibers were seen in the OVLT, the accessory olfactory bulb, the stria terminalis, and the medial amygdala. No differences were seen in the general distribution of LHRH neurons and fibers among the groups examined. However, while LHRH-immunoreactive neurons in the preoptic area of both intact and OVX anestrous ewes were large, multipolar cells with branching dendrites, LHRH cells in the same area of mid-luteal sheep were smaller with fewer immunoreactively-defined dendrites. Whether these differences represent seasonal changes in the morphology of LHRH neurons themselves, or in the manner in which immunoreactive LHRH is synthesized or stored, remains to be determined. (Supported by NIH HD10665, HD11311 and the Whitehall Fdn.)

1246 EVIDENCE THAT THE MATERNAL PITUITARY SUPPRESSES SECRETION OF RELAXIN IN THE PREGNANT RAT. T.G. Golos* and O.D. Sherwood, Dept. of Physiology and Biophysics, University of Illinois, Urbana IL, 61801, USA

The role of the pituitary in regulating relaxin synthesis and secretion by the corpus luteum (CL) during the second half of pregnancy was investigated by hypophysectomizing rats carrying either one conceptus (1C) or a full complement (FC) of conceptuses (≥ 8) on day 13 of pregnancy. Serum and luteal relaxin levels, serum progesterone (P) levels and CL weights in 1C rats were markedly lower during the period from day 14 through day 20 of pregnancy than those in FC rats. Following hypophysectomy of 1C rats (H1C) serum relaxin levels, serum P levels and CL weights increased to values which did not differ significantly from those of FC rats. Additionally, hypophysectomized FC rats (HFC) had higher serum relaxin levels than FC rats. Luteal relaxin content was unaffected by hypophysectomy in spite of increased relaxin secretion and this may indicate that relaxin synthesis also increased following hypophysectomy. Other workers have suggested that placental testosterone (T) may support luteal function during the second half of pregnancy. Serum T levels in 1C rats were markedly lower than those in FC rats but did not increase following hypophysectomy in either H1C or HFC rats. It is concluded that the pituitary has a suppressive effect on relaxin synthesis and secretion as well as on P secretion and CL growth, and that increased luteal function following hypophysectomy is not due to increased placental T secretion. The results of this study are consistent with the hypothesis that relaxin synthesis and secretion, P secretion and CL growth may be regulated through a common mechanism from day 12 to day 20 of pregnancy in the rat.

1247 A POSSIBLE ROLE FOR ESTROGEN IN THE REGULATION OF PLACENTAL ANDROGEN SYNTHESIS DURING RAT PREGNANCY. Jane A. Jackson* and Eugene D. Albrecht, Depts. Ob/Gyn and Physiol., Univ. Maryland School of Medicine, Baltimore, Md. 21201 U.S.A.

Recent studies suggest that the placenta (plac) may be the source of androgen (i.e. androstenedione,Δ^4A) precursor for ovarian estradiol (E2) production during rat pregnancy, but the regulation of it's synthesis is unknown. The present study utilized the antiestrogen enclomiphene (EC) to determine whether estrogen regulates plac synthesis of Δ^4 A. EC in various doses (1,10 or 100 μg) or vehicle alone were injected sc on D9,11 and 13 of gestation. Other rats received an E2 implant on D9 to increase peripheral serum E2 conc by 7.5pg/ml. Plac were obtained on D14 and homogenized in Krebs Ringer buffer (100 mg/ml) and 200 mg was incubated with 2 μCi [7-3H] pregnenolone (P5) and 2.5mM NAD^+ for 2 h at 37°C. [3H] progesterone (P4) and [3H] Δ^4 A were purified by paper chromatography and their formation determined (%dpm [3H]P5→dpm [3H]P4 or Δ^4 A/200mg plac). Mean plac wt was decreased from a control value of 138 mg to 119 mg (P<.05) and 95 mg(P<.001) by 10 μg and 100 μg EC, respectively, while E2 had no effect. EC at 100 μg decreased (P<.01) the mean(±SE) %P5→Δ^4 A from a control value of 53±8(N=8) to 38±8(N=7) and increased (P<.05) the %P5→P4 from a control value of 3.8±1(N=8) to 6.2±2(N=7). Formation of Δ^4A and P4 were not effected by the lower dosages of EC or by E2. The lack of effect of E2 may be due to maximal stimulation by normal E2 conc. EC at 1 and 100 μg decreased serum P4 (ng/ml) from a control value of 72 to 49 (P<.05) and 32(P<.01), respectively, indicating the antiestrogen action of EC. The increase in P4 and decrease in Δ^4 A caused by EC suggests a selective decrease in enzymatic conversion of P4→Δ^4A. Thus, estrogen from the ovary may control it's own production by regulating the synthesis of plac androgen during the second half of rat pregnancy. Whether the action of estrogen is direct or indirect via effects upon P4 is unknown and under further investigation.

1248 EFFECTS OF EPIMESTROL AND CLOMIPHENE ON RECEPTOR LEVELS IN THE RAT UTERUS.

H.J. Kloosterboer*, P.B.A. Loonen and E.W. Bergink, Organon Scientific Development Group, OSS, The Netherlands

Epimestrol, 3-methoxy-17-epiestriol (Stimovul[R]), is used for the induction of ovulation. We studied the effects of epimestrol on the progesterone receptor (Pg-R) and estrogen receptors (E-R, cytosolic, nuclear Types I and II) in the rat uterus and compared them with the effects of clomiphene, a triphenylethylene derivative. The effects of a single low (4,75 nmol/kg) and high (950 nmol/kg) dose (s.c., in oil) of these compounds in ovariectomized rats on receptor levels and uterine weight, 1 and/or 14 days after administration of the compounds, are shown below:

Compound	E-R			Pg-R	Uterine weight
	Cytosol	Nuclear Type I	Nuclear Type II		
Epimestrol (low, 1 d, n=4)	122	295*	117	148*	110
Clomiphene (low, 1 d, n=4)	111	301*	119	170*	107
Epimestrol (high, 1 d, n=4)	125*	109	375*	140*	122*
Clomiphene (high, 1 d, n=4)	76*	112	268*	107	127*
Epimestrol (high, 14 d, n=8)	not determined			150*	104
Clomiphene (high, 14 d, n=8)	not determined			194*	134*

Values are % of untreated control * P < 0,05

Low doses of both compounds show weak estrogenic effects. The high dose of clomiphene shows, in contrast to epimestrol, anti-estrogenic effects. The known long-term effect of clomiphene is confirmed in the 14-day experiment.

1249 THE FERTILITY STATUS IN MALE PATIENTS WITH HYPERTHYROIDISM, BEFORE AND AFTER TREATMENT. G.E.Krassas*, I.Ziannas, G.Koios, Th.Kaltsas and K.Miras, Endocrine clinic, Panagia Hospital, Thessaloniki and Department of Biochemistry, Athens Medical School, Athens, Greece.

Oligospermia has been reported in some male patients with thyrotoxicosis, but the number of reports and patients investigated was small in order to reach definetive conclusions. No data are also available on the effect of treatment on the fertility status of hyperthyroid patients. To evaluate further this problem we studied 23 (aged I8-58) men with thyrotoxicosis. Semen analyses were performed before and 6 months after treatment with antithyroid drugs or radioactive iodine (I-I3I). The results show that I4 patients had sperm counts of less than $40XIO^6$/ml before treatment, while only IO after treatment. In IO out of 23 patients the sperm count increased after treatment. The mean values before treatment was 35.7±5.3 (S.E), while after treatment was 43.3±6.5. However the difference, although about 20%, did not reach statistical significance. When sperm counts were corrected to the normal spermatozoa, with good motility, the mean values was $19.3XIO^6$±3.4, while after treatment was $25.7XIO^6$±7.0. The two groups did not differ statistically. There was no difference between the patients who were treated with carbimazole and those treated with I-I3I. Our results indicate that oligospermia is not a feature of the disease and treatment of hyperthyroidism does not improve the fertility status of the male patients, although "poor" sperm counts with a tendency of improvement with treatment is not an uncommon finding in patients with thyrotoxicosis.

1250 HORMONAL PATTERNS IN FEMALE AND MALE INFERTILITY IN AN AFRICAN POPULATION. S. F. Kuku*, and P. A. Akinyanju, Immunoassay Laboratories, 31, Glover Street, Ebute-Metta, Lagos, Nigeria.

Infertility is a very sensitive medico-social problem in most African communities, especially in women where it is claimed that in 50% pelvic inflammatory disease is responsible. To-date, the aetiological role hormones play in both sexes has received little attention. To study this, sera of patients complaining of infertility sent to our laboratory, an urban reference laboratory, over an 18-month period were analysed by double antibody radioimmunoassay on duplicate samples for luteinising hormone (LH), follicle stimulating hormone (FSH), prolactin and progesterone, in 2047 females in the luteal phase, and LH, FSH, prolactin and testosterone, in 454 oligo /azospermic males. In the females, 1086 (53%) had significant abnormalities in one or more of these hormones. The commonest abnormality was a high prolactin in 543 (26.5%). Low progesterone occurred in 404 (19.7%). Significant elevation also occurred in LH, 316 (15.4%), FSH, 164 (8.0%) and in both LH & FSH, 79 (3.9%). In the males 279 (61.5%) showed abnormalities in one or more of the hormones studied, consisting of high prolactin, 147 (32.4%), LH, 73 (16.1%) FSH, 63 (13.9%), low testosterone, 50 (11.0%) and high LH and FSH, 20 (4.4%). These results show that (a) endocrine abnormalities are not uncommonly associated with male and female infertility in Africans. (b) Hyperprolactinaemia (males and females) and anovulation, both treatable conditions, constitute majority of these abnormalities.

1251 IMMUNOLOGICAL ABNORMALITIES PRECEDE HYPERGLYCEMIA IN MICE TREATED WITH MULTIPLE LOW DOSES OF STREPTOZOTOCIN. H. Itoh*, M. Itoh, K. Sato, M. Funauchi, S. Kisamori, N. Fukuma, Y. Hirooka, and N. Nihei, Hamamatsu University School of Medicine, Hamamatsu, Japan.

Insulitis induced by multiple administrations of subdiabetogenic dose (40 mg/kg BW ip) of streptozotocin (STZ) in mice has been considered as a good model for type 1 diabetes mellitus. However, the precise pathogenesis remains to be elucidated. Immunological functions in STZ-treated mice were compared between multiple-subdiabetogenical and bolus-diabetogenical (200mg /kg BW) injections. Blastogenesis of spleen lymphocytes to PHA and PWM depressed by 40% and 45% respectively ($p<0.001$) were recognized before blood glucose elevation, but blastogenesis of thymocytes to Con A were increased only in multiple-STZ-treated group. Positive islet cell surface antibodies (ICSA) were detected by indirect immunofluorescence method. At the time insulitis appeared later, lymphoblastogenesis (LBG) to PHA still remains suppressed by 25% ($p<0.05$), but the suppression of LBG to PWM was not observed. In bolus group LBG to PHA was depressed by 30% ($p<0.02$), whereas those to PWM and Con A were not different from controls. ICSA was not positive at all. From these results the onset of insulitis might be due to the deterioration of immunological surveilence rather than the destruction of pancreatic B cell per se. Thymus-derived lymphocytes are suggested to play some role in the induction of diabetes accompanied with insulitis.

1252 ABNORMALITIES OF LYMPHOCYTE FUNCTIONS IN INSULIN-DEPENDENT DIABETES MELLITUS: RELATIONS TO GLUCOSE CONTROL, ISLET CELL SURFACE ANTIBODIES (ICSA), AND CIRCULATING IMMUNE COMPLEXES (CIC). M. Itoh*, H. Itoh, M. Hakamata, M. Funauchi, N. Fukuma, S. Kisamori, Y. Hirooka, and N. Nihei, Hamamatsu University School of Medicine, Hamamatsu, Japan.

Several reports indicated the lymphocyte functions were suppressed in poorly-controlled diabetes, but there is no clear evidence about the intrinsic defect in the lymphocytes of diabetic patients. To clarify this point, lymphoblastogenesis (LBG) to phytohemagglutinin (PHA), pokeweed mitogen (PWM), concanavalin A (Con A), monocyte functions determined by the chemiluminescence, and their relations to glucose control, ICSA, and CIC were studied in 13 insulin-dependent diabetes mellitus (IDDM), 32 non-insulin-dependent diabetes mellitus (NIDDM), and 20 normal subjects. LBG's to PHA, PWM, and Con A and monocyte fuctions were suppressed in NIDDM with high FBS and Hb Alc ($p<0.05$). LBG to PHA was suppressed in cases with positive CIC ($p<0.05$) and IDDM with high FBS and Hb Alc ($p<0.01$). The correction of deteriorated glucose metabolism brought normalization of the depressed LBG's to PHA, PWM, and Con A in NIDDM ($p<0.01$), augmentation of LBG's to Con A, and further suppression of LBG's to PWM in IDDM ($p<0.05$). High prevalence of CIC was detected in IDDM with positive ICSA or insulin antibodies, but did not affect responses of LBG. Monocyte functions were more suppressed in IDDM than in NIDDM, but addition of insulin to medium in vitro did not affect LBG nor monocyte functions. In contrast to NIDDM lymphocyte functions in IDDM are suggested to be impaired independent of glycemic control.

1253 REVERSAL OF CYCLOSPORIN PROPHYLAXIS AND PASSIVE TRANSFER OF INSULIN DEPENDENT DIABETES MELLITUS (IDDM) IN THE BB RAT WITH THYMIC OR SPLENIC LYMPHOCYTES. M.A. Jaworski* and L. Honore, Departments of Pediatrics and Pathology, University of Alberta, Edmonton, Alberta, Canada.

To identify the lymphocytes mediating the destruction of beta cells in IDDM, we developed a passive transfer model using the Wistar-derived Bio-Breeding (BB) rat. Spontaneous IDDM occurs between 60-120 days of age in 50% of BB rats from high-risk lines; prophylactic cyclosporin (Cy) therapy instituted at an early age reduces disease incidence to 0%. Sex-matched littermates from high-risk lines were divided into 4 groups. Group I: 40-140 x 10^6 thymic or splenic lymphocytes from acutely diabetic BB rats were incubated for 72 h with 5 ug/ml Concanavalin A (Con A) and injected i.v. into normoglycemic BB rats which were either past the age of developing IDDM, or maintained on continuous Cy therapy (10-20 mg/kg/day p.o.)from 42 days of age until sacrificed. Within 33-50 days of injection, 5/5 recipients developed IDDM, with weight loss and sustained hyperglycemia (mean peak blood glucose 438 mg/dl,range 255-750). Group II: equal numbers of Con A-activated thymic or splenic lymphocytes from nondiabetic donors (from low-risk lines of BB rats) injected into Cy-treated and age-matched littermates induced IDDM in 0/5 recipients; none of the rats developed weight loss or glycosuria. Group III: 0/8 Cy-treated littermates developed IDDM (mean blood glucose 92.5 mg/dl,range 80-107). Group IV: 7/16 (44%) of untreated littermates developed spontaneous IDDM. We conclude that T lymphocytes are required to mediate beta cell destruction in the BB rat and that Cy prophylaxis of autoimmune IDDM is reversible by the administration of mature T lymphocytes. Supported by a grant from the Kroc Foundation.

1254 CYCLOSPORIN (CY A) IMMUNOSUPPRESSION IN TYPE I DIABETES MELLITUS (D.M.): PRELIMINARY RESULTS IN 16 PREPUBERTAL CHILDREN. M. Jenner*, C. Stiller, J. Dupre, P. Keown, A. Laupacis, R. Martell, N. Rodger, B. Wolfe. London Juvenile Diabetes Study Group, University Hospital and War Memorial Children's Hospital, London, Canada.

In a pilot study of pubertal and adult males and females with Type I D.M., greater than 50% were able to sustain euglycemia for up to one year on Cy A as the sole immunosuppressant, treated within 6 weeks from clinical diagnosis. In contrast 16 prepubertal children, 9 females and 7 males (ages 1 8/12 to 9 9/12 years) were treated with Cy A, pure pork insulin and a standard diabetic diet from 18 to 301 days ($\overline{X}$=140 days). Two infants age 1 8/12 and 2 9/12 years at diagnosis received short term prednisone and cyclosporin treatment with no decrease in insulin requirement. Intercurrent viral infections limited the duration of therapy in these very young children. Five children over age 3 years are currently off insulin from 25 to 214 days ($\overline{X}$=136 days). As in the older age group, glucagon stimulated C peptide values greater than 0.6 pmol/ML were predictive of a clinical remission off insulin in most patients. Side effects are clinically minimal to date but include hypertrichosis, gingival hyperplasia, elevated serum creatinine, elevated alkaline phosphatase and small reduction in serum hemoglobin. Linear growth remains normal to date. Temporary remissions off insulin, controlled by diet alone have been achieved in Type I D.M. prepubertal patients over age 3 years under close clinical supervision.

Further clinical studies are required to determine whether these remissions can be sustained and islet B-cell function can be preserved, in the young diabetic without serious detriment from cyclosporin.

1255 INSULIN SENSITIVITY AND METABOLIC CLEARANCE IN MASSIVE OBESITY (MO) AS ASSESSED BY THE GLUCOSE CLAMP METHOD. J. Jimenez*, S. Zuniga-Guajardo, B. Zinman and A. Angel. Department of Medicine, University of Toronto and Institute of Medical Science, University of Toronto, Toronto, Ontario, Canada M5G 1L7.

Insulin resistance is typically found in MO patients (>170% IBW) and explains in part the hyperinsulinemia, glucose intolerance and overt diabetes associated with this metabolic state. In the present study insulin sensitivity was measured by the euglycemic insulin clamp method (40MU/M^2/min) for a 2 hour period. Seven, non-diabetic MO patients (6♀, 1♂) aged 39±3 yrs., 206±4% of IBW were compared to 7 normal controls (C) (6♀, 1♂) aged 25±3 yrs., 92±1.5% IBW. The glucose uptake (M) was significantly reduced 2.17±0.34 in MO vs 7.19±0.57 mg/kg/min in C ($p<0.001$). Similarly, the metabolic clearance rate of glucose (MCRg) was lower 2.23±0.38 in MO and 7.68±0.59 ml/kg.min in C. The plasma insulin levels were not different during the last 60 min in both groups. M/I ratio (glucose metabolized per unit of insulin) was also markedly reduced from 5.45±0.38 in C to 1.44±0.33 mg/kg. min per uU/ml X 100 in MO, ($p<0.001$). These differences between C and MO persisted when calculated in terms of lean body mass rather per kg body weight ($p<0.001$) and thus were not simply due to fat mass. The metabolic clearance rate of insulin (MCRI) calculated on the basis of lean body mass (as estimated by skinfold thickness) were not different in the two groups 8.98±0.36 in C vs 10.97±1.08 ml/kg/min in MO. In summary, non-diabetic MO persons have markedly reduced sensitivity to insulin compared to C even when expressed per unit lean body mass despite similar rates of total body insulin clearance. Thus, abnormalities in insulin sensitivity may occur independent of changes in insulin clearance.

1256 COMBINED TOLAZAMIDE, INSULIN TREATMENT IMPROVES METABOLIC CONTROL IN TYPE I DIABETES MELLITUS (IDDM). U. Kabadi*, VA Medical Center, Des Moines, Iowa

Sulfonylurea agents are known to lower plasma glucose (G) by enhancing the effect of endogenous insulin (INS) in NIDDM. This study was undertaken to assess the efficacy of tolazamide (T), a sulfonylurea drug in facilitating action of exogenous INS in IDDM. 20 male IDDM (25-65 years) with duration of DM, 1½-30 years were studied. IDDM was confirmed by development of ketoacidosis (DKA) within 48 hours on withdrawal of INS. Patients were followed at 2-4 week intervals during the study period. They were continued on their insulin regimen (I) for 12 weeks and then divided into 2 groups according to metabolic control. Group 1: fasting G (FBS) <140 mg/dl, HbA1C <9%; Group 2: FBS >140 mg/dl, HbA1C >9%. T (500 mg, bid) was added to I and continued for 3 months. INS dose was adjusted as needed in Group 1. INS dose, FBS, HbA1C, and number of hypoglycemic episodes (↓S) documented by symptoms and capillary blood G <50 mg/dl are shown below.

Patients	Rx Regimen	INS Dose Units/Day	FBS mg/dl	HbA1C %	↓S
Group 1	I	61± 6	131±11	8.7±0.1	4.0±1.0
(12)	I+T	42± 5†	121±10	8.3±0.1	1.0±0.2†
Group 2	I	60±10	253±13	12.0±0.4	0.5±0.04
(8)	I+T	60±10	126±12†	8.6±0.3†	0.7±0.02

† - Significantly different from I in the same group, $p<0.05$

This study demonstrates that adjuvant therapy with tolazamide lowered insulin dose and number of hypoglycemic episodes, and improved metabolic control in IDDM. It is concluded that sulfonylurea agents may enhance action of exogenous insulin and may help achieve a more uniform metabolic control in IDDM.

1257 SPECIES DIFFERENCE IN EFFECTS OF SUBSTANCE P ON ISLET HORMONE SECRETION — OPPOSITE EFFECTS ON CANINE AND RAT ISOLATED PERFUSED PANCREASES. K. Kawai*, N. Chiba, E. Munekata and K. Yamashita, Institute of Clinical Medicine, University of Tsukuba, Ibaraki-ken, Japan.

Many conflicting results have been reported concerning the effects of substance P (SP) on hormone secretion from pancreatic islet. Since this controversy could arise from the species difference in regulating mechanism of hormone secretion, we compared the effects of SP and its active fragment (SP^{6-11}) on insulin, glucagon and somatostatin secretion from the isolated perfused canine and rat pancreases. In the canine pancreas, 1 nM and 10 nM SP stimulated insulin, glucagon and somatostatin secretion under the perfusate condition with 5.5 mM glucose and 5 mM arginine. In the rat, however, SP inhibited insulin and glucagon secretion under the same condition. Similar differential results were obtained by SP^{6-11} with almost same potency. Whereas the effects of SP^{6-11} continued throughout the infusion period, those of SP were transient, especially in its stimulation of insulin, glucagon and somatostatin secretion from the canine pancreas. To examine the mechanism of the species difference for SP, cAMP concentration in the effluent perfusate was measured in both species. However, no significant change in cAMP concentration was found during the SP infusion.

These experiments provide a direct evidence that the biological peptide oppositely affects the mammalian islet hormone secretion. Thus, it is suggested that each mammalian has a different regulatory mechanism in islet hormone secretion.

1258 AUTONOMIC REGULATION IN EARLY-PHASE OF INSULIN RESPONSE TO GLUCOSE -NON-ISOLATED PANCREATIC PERFUSION SYSTEM IN RATS- H. Kikuoka*, M. Nishi, H. Bessho, G. Matsumoto, K. Nanjo, K. Iwo and K. Miyamura, Division of Endocrinology, Department of Internal Medicine, Wakayama Medical School, Wakayama 640, JAPAN

Autonomic regulation in early-phase of insulin response to glucose was studied in vivo using non-isolated pancreatic perfusion system in rats. This perfusion system was prepared by means of catheterization into the celiac artery and the portal vein without any detachments of the surrounding tissues. The levels of immunoreactive insulin and glucose in the perfusate were measured every one minute during glucose infusion into the femoral vein without direct influence on glucose concentration in the pancreatic perfusion system.

An obvious insulin release from the pancreas before elevation of the glucose level could be demonstrated. Addition of phentolamine or propranolol into the perfusate revealed no effect upon the insulin release preceding the rise of glucose level, although phentolamine addition was followed by gradual elevation of basal insulin out-put. Addition of atropine, on the other hand, significantly depressed the early-phase of insulin response without any effects on basal insulin out-put.

These data suggest that the insulin release triggered by extrapancreatic elevation of blood glucose level was under the regulation of cholinergic vagal nerve. The results implicate the mechanism of rapid insulin response, generally observed in normal but impaired in the diabetic subjects, during intravenous glucose loading.

1259 REDUCED APPEARANCE RATE OF ASIALOGLYCOPROTEIN RECEPTORS IN DIABETIC RATS.
H-J. Kim,* and I. V. Kurup. Metabolic-Endocrine Section, Medical College of Wisconsin, Milwaukee, WI 53226 USA.

Previously we reported that the catabolism of galactose-, or glucose-conjugated plasma albumin, low density lipoprotein (neoglycoproteins) or asialofetuin (ASF) was reduced in diabetic rats. The reduction was due to significantly reduced numbers of the asialoglycoprotein receptors (ASGR) in diabetic liver cells (at 4°C and 37°C 12±2, 42±8.5, mean ± SEM x 10^{-3} binding sites per cell) compared to normal (45±13; 221±32) and insulin treatment reversed the reduction (Clin. Res. 30:780A, 1982). However, the mechanism of the reduced ASGR activity is poorly understood. To assess the kinetics of the ASGR appearance and disappearance, in vivo hepatic clearance of I^{125}-ASF was determined with a portal vein injection technique in ether anesthetized normal and diabetic rats (Pardridge et al J.B.C. 258: 990-994, 1983). The portal injection of 20-1200 µg unlabeled ASF was followed 30s - 30 min later by the portal injection of tracer. Specific extraction of the I^{125}-ASF, which was near zero shortly after a 400 µg loading dose, gradually increased toward normal levels with a t½ of 17.5 min in normal rats (N=40) while the t½ was delayed in diabetes (36 min, N=40). Nonlinear regression analyses of saturation data showed the in vivo kinetics of hepatic clearance of I^{125}-ASF was reduced 50% in diabetics (Km = 0.32±.08 mg/ml; Vmax = 105.9±15 µg/min/g, N=36) compared to normal (Km = 0.29±0.05 mg/ml, Vmax = 201.3±30 µg/min/g, N=36). Extration of extracellular markers, and portal blood flow were not significantly different between two groups. The results suggest that reduced ASGR activities in diabetes are not only due to a reduced receptor number, but also due to reduced recycling or reinsertion of the receptors to cell membrane.

1260 IN VIVO TRANSPORT OF AMINO ACIDS AND GLUCOSE INTO SKELETAL MUSCLE: GLUCOCORTICOID-INSULIN INTERACTIONS. D.J. Koerker* and C.J. Goodner, Univ. of Wash., Seattle, WA. 98195, USA.

Glucocorticoid excess is known to induce insulin resistance and muscle wasting. To examine the effect of glucocorticoids on the insulin mediated transport of glucose and amino acids into 14 separate muscles, rats were treated daily with 1.5 mg/kg dexamethasone (DEX) for one week then compared to a vehicle treated group. The method of Hom et al., (Diabetes, Feb. 1984) for determining transport rate constants was used with (^{3}H)-2deoxyglucose (2DG) and (^{14}C)-methylaminoisobutyric (AIB) used as tracers. Both treatment groups were studied in the basal state and under maximal insulin stimulus (.5U/kg). Calculated rate constants vary 10-15 fold from muscle to muscle and are slightly less for AIB (.001 to .009) than for 2DG (.002 to .03). Insulin increased the rate constants for net uptake of 2DG 3 to 18 fold and for AIB transport 1.5 to 4 fold. DEX treatment had no inhibitory effect on basal 2DG transport rate constants but increased them in 6/14 muscles. In contrast, DEX reduced basal AIB transport in 7/14 muscles. Under maximal insulin stimulus DEX reduced 2DG uptake rates in 6/14 muscles and in AIB transport in 4/14 muscles. These data demonstrate the marked variability between individual muscles for transport of 2DG and AIB. They further suggest that there is a component of post receptor linkage to transport mechanisms which allows enhancement of 2DG transport and impairment of AIB transport in the same tissue at identical insulin concentrations. They also suggest that the dose response curves for insulin stimulated 2DG and AIB transport will be different in individual muscles and between muscles.

1261 GLUCOSE METABOLISM IN EXPERIMENTAL HUMAN HYPERTHYROIDISM. M. LAVILLE*, J.P. Riou, P.F. Bougneres, M. Beylot, P. Serusclat, G. Sautot, F. Berthezene and R. Mornex, INSERM U.197, Faculté Médecine A.Carrel, 69008 Lyon, France.

The relationships between insulin and glucose metabolism in human hyperthyroidism have been studied during an insulin dose response (0.4,1,2,6mU. $kg^{-1}.min^{-1}$) using the euglycemic glucose clamp technique in 5 male volunteers in the control (C) state or during experimentally induced hyperthyroidism (H). T_3 rose from 1.92 ± 0.17 nM in C to 3.66 ± 0.7 nM in H ($p < 0.01$) and resting metabolic rate from 39 ± 0.7 to 48 ± 1 watt/m^2 ($p < 0.001$). Glucose turnover rate (GTR) was measured with ($6\text{-}6\text{-}^2H_2$) glucose as tracer in the basal state and under 0.4 $mU.kg^{-1}.min^{-1}$ insulin. In the basal state hyperthyroidism was characterized by a significant increase in glycemia, in GTR ($mg.kg^{-1}.min^{-1}$: $C=2.3 \pm 0.14$; $H=3.7 \pm 0.1$, $p < 0.01$) and in glucose clearance rate ($ml.kg^{-1}.min^{-1}$: $C=3.3 \pm 0.22$; $H=4.51 \pm 0.22$, $p < 0.05$) without change in insulinemia.

During the insulin dose response study neither the maximal glucose infusion rate ($mg.kg^{-1}.min^{-1}$: $C=15.7 \pm 0.7$; $H=15.8 \pm 0.2$) nor the apparent K 0.5 for insulin effect (mU/l : $C=48 \pm 4$; $H=43 \pm 5$) was affected by hyperthyroidism Hepatic glucose production under 0.4 $mU.kg^{-1}.min^{-1}$ insulin was totally suppressed in C whereas it remained in H (0.96 ± 0.39 $mg.kg^{-1}.min^{-1}$, $p < 0.05$) but the magnitude of the decrease was similar in both state.

In conclusion, glucose metabolism in experimental hyperthyroidism is characterized by 1) an increased GTR, 2) an antagonism between the effect of insulin and hyperthyroidism at the hepatic level, 3) lack of peripheral insulin resistance.

1262 EFFECT OF SUCROSE MEAL ON INSULIN REQUIREMENT IN IDDM AND ITS MODULATION BY ACARBOSE. L. Lecavalier*, L. Germain, P. Hamet and J.L. Chiasson, Clinical Research Institute of Montreal, Montreal, H2W 1R7, Canada.

The purpose of the present study was to evaluate the insulin requirement in response to sucrose meal in IDDM and its modulation by a disaccharidase inhibitor, Acarbose. After an overnight fast, the subjects (n = 5) "were hooked" up to the artificial pancreas (Biostator) to maintain normoglycemia. Each subject was studied during a sucrose meal of 50, 75 and 100 g with and without Acarbose. Blood glucose and insulin requirement were recorded by the Biostator for 120 minutes. After a **50 g sucrose meal** with/without Acarbose, the peak post-prandial (PC) blood glucose was 118/157 mg/dl and the insulin requirement was 4/8 units; the area under the curve for glucose was 2.2/2.6 g/dl and for free plasma insulin 100/163 µU/ml. After a **75 g sucrose meal** with/without Acarbose, the peak PC blood glucose was 134/166 mg/dl and the insulin requirement was 6/10 units; the area under the curve for glucose was 2.3/2.8 g/dl and for free plasma insulin 159/235 µU/ml. After a **100 g sucrose meal** with/without Acarbose the peak PC blood glucose was 130/175 mg/dl and the insulin requirement was 6/13 units; the area under the curve for glucose was 2.5/3.0 g/dl and for free plasma insulin 136/185 µU/ml. Plasma glucagon was not affected by increasing sucrose load with or without Acarbose. Conclusion: In IDDM 1) increasing sucrose load required increasing amount of insulin to maintain comparable normoglycemia, 2) Acarbose decreased the peak blood glucose achieved and the insulin requirement at each sucrose load, and, 3) Acarbose could become a useful adjunct in the treatment of diabetes.

1263 THE EFFECTS OF PHORBOL ESTERS ON RAT GRANULOSA CELL PROGESTERONE AND PROSTAGLANDIN PRODUCTION. Y. Kawai*, M.R. Clark, Repscend Laboratories, Univ. of Miami School of Med, Miami, Florida 33101, USA

TPA (12-0-tetradecanoyl-phorbol-13-acetate) has been shown by others to directly activate a Ca^{2+}- and lipid-dependent protein kinase (protein kinase C). This kinase is postulated to become activated in vivo upon stimulation of phosphatidylinositol (PI) metabolism. We have demonstrated increased PI metabolism by granulosa cells in response to LH and GnRH. Granulosa cells were obtained from immature (28-29 d) rats 48 h after the injection of 20 IU PMSG and incubated for up to 5 h. TPA (25 ng/ml) caused a 2-3 fold increase in prostaglandin E (PGE) accumulation at 5 h. TPA (1-100 ng/ml) did not affect progesterone (P) production. An inactive phorbol ester, PMA, (4B-phorbol 13 α-monoacetate) did not affect PGE or P accumulation at concentrations of 1-100 ng/ml. LH (10 ng/ml) stimulated PGE production more than 4-fold (22.4±1.1 vs 5.0±0.5 pmol/10^6 cells). The effect of TPA on PGE was essentially additive to that of LH, increasing the accumulation to 42.8±8.4. LH (10 ng/ml) also stimulated P production (14.7±0.3 ng/10^6 cells) compared with controls (2.47±0.25). TPA decreased the P response to LH about 25% (10.8±0.4). In addition, [D-Ala^6, des-Gly^{10}]GnRH (GnRHa) (10 ng/ml) stimulated PGE production (18.9±2.4 pmol/10^6 cells) compared with controls (3.1±0.5). The effect of TPA on PGE was similarly essentially additive to that of GnRHa (27.2±3.26). GnRHa slightly increased P production, but TPA did not affect this response. These results suggest that protein kinase C may play an important role in granulosa cell function. Supported by NIH grant HD-17942.

1264 REGULATION OF ORNITHINE DECARBOXYLASE GENE EXPRESSION BY ANDROGENS IN MOUSE KIDNEY. K.K. Kontula*, V.V. Isomaa, C.W. Bardin and O.A. Jänne, The Population Council and The Rockefeller University, New York, New York.

The concentration of ornithine decarboxylase (ODC), the first and one of the rate-controlling enzymes in polyamine biosynthesis, is regulated by androgens in a dual fashion in mouse kidney: via increased de novo synthesis and via prolonged biological half-life of the enzyme protein. To gain more insight into these regulatory mechanisms we have cloned cDNA sequences coding for ODC-mRNA and established nucleic acid hybridization assays for quantitation of this mRNA. Northern blot analyses of mouse kidney poly(A)-RNA indicated the presence of two ODC-mRNA species (2.15 and 2.7 kb) that were both regulated by androgens. In accordance with ODC protein concentration, there was a clear sex difference in the renal ODC-mRNA content with male values being 3- to 5-fold higher than those in females. Androgen administration increased renal ODC-mRNA content within 6 h, with a maximal increase at 24 h after testosterone injection. Prolonged androgen treatment resulted in a 10- to 20-fold increase in ODC-mRNA concentration in castrated male mice, whereas no change in this mRNA content was seen in kidneys of androgen-insensitive (Tfm/Y) animals after a similar treatment. Inhibition of protein synthesis by cycloheximide administration before and during androgen exposure partially inhibited androgen-elicited increase in renal ODC-mRNA concentration. The half-life of ODC-mRNA sequences, as measured after α-amanitin administration to intact male mice, was less than 5 h. Conclusions: (1) Androgens regulate ODC activity in mouse kidney, at least in part, by increasing ODC-mRNA accumulation, (2) Functional androgen receptors are required for this regulation. Grant: NIH HD 13541.

1265 ANTAGONISM OF ANDROGENS TO THE CALCIUM INDUCED CONTRACTION OF THE PREGNANT RAT MYOMETRIUM. C. Kubli-Garfias*, M. Perusquía and H. Ponce-Monter. Unidad de Investigación Biomédica, Centro Médico Nacional del Instituto Mexicano del Seguro Social. México D.F. 03020, MEXICO.

During gestation a variety of androgens exist circulating. Also it is known that testosterone and some of its metabolites produce inhibition of uterine contractility. However, the mechanism of action on the uterus of these steroids has not been explored. Thus, we decide to challenge the effect of some androgens with the Ca^{2+} activation of uterine smooth muscle. Strips of 15 days pregnant Sprague-Dawley rat uterus were bathed in Tris buffer solution in a isolated bath at 37°C, bubbled with O_2. After the recording of the spontaneous activity, the preparation was depolarized with a isotonic K^+ (40 mM), free Ca^{2+} solution, which resulted in a complete relaxation 45 min later. In these conditions the addition of 1 mM of Ca^{2+} to the media produced a tonic contraction. In order to prevent such contraction in a second trial, tissues were incubated 10 min with one of the following steroids (μg/ml): testosterone (17α-hydroxy-4- androsten-3-one, 100), androsterone (3α-hydroxy-5α- androstan-17-one, 20), androstanediol (5α-androstane- 3α,17β-diol, 32) and 5β-dihydrotestosterone (17β-hydroxy-5β-androstan-3-one, 30). A remarkable inhibition of the Ca^{2+} induced contraction was observed as compared with the control (from 49 to 100%). This antagonism of the calcium action in the smooth muscle might explain the relaxant mechanism of the androgens. Likewise, this might be of physiological importance in the regulation of the uterine tonus during pregnancy.

1266 GLUCOCORTICOID RECEPTOR SYSTEM : COMPARATIVE ANALYSIS BETWEEN CYTOSOLS FROM CONTROL AND HYPOTHYROID RATS. A.M. Leseney* and M. Benmiloud Laboratoire de Biochimie Thyroïdienne, Centre Pierre et Marie Curie, Alger, Algérie.

A complex but coherent pattern of a glucocorticoid receptor system arise from recents works. The influence of the metabolic status of the cell on this system remains obscure. We investigated this problem by comparing the receptor systems from liver of control (Te) and hypothyroid (Hy) rats. We show that the physicochemical properties of the native complexes (i.e. complexes protected from transformation and inactivation by molybdate) in both conditions were analogous : KD ≅ 12 μM, pHi = 5.6. However the number of sites per cell is diminished 3 fold in the case of Hy rats ($8.3\ 10^3$) as compared to control rats ($22\ 10^3$). At 22°C, the Hy transformed complexes are less stable than the control used as 100 % (50 % of the binding is lost after 180 min). The dissociation rate of the Hy native complexes is diminished by 30 % as compared to the control. Both transformed and native Hy complexes are more sensitive to the actions of ATP on the system. The dissociation of ^3H dex in the presence of $2\ 10^{-5}M$ progesterone measured at 22°C is greater in the case of Hy complexes (kd = $30\ 10^{-3}\ min^{-1}$) than in the control (kd = $15\ 10^{-3}\ min^{-1}$). These values were related to the degree of hypothyroidism. Our results favor the hypothesis of a diminished concentration or efficacity of the binding factors and reducing equivalent in hypothyroid cytosols. We propose this as a new approach to the analysis of the complex regulations involved in glucocorticoid receptor mechanisms of action. On the other hand, the glucocorticoid receptor system could be used as a probe to test the metabolic modifications observed in hypothyroidism.

1267 HORMONE MEDIATED TRANSLOCATION OF RAT AORTIC AND MYOCARDIAL CYTOPLASMIC ESTROGEN AND ANDROGEN RECEPTORS. Alan L. Lin*, Roberto Gonzalez, Jr., and Sydney A. Shain, Southwest Foundation for Biomedical Research, San Antonio, Texas 78284

We used estradiol-17β (E_2) or testosterone (T) injection of intact male or female AXC rats respectively to examine steroid mediated translocation of cytoplasmic estrogen or androgen receptors. Saturation analysis of nuclear extracts prepared from aorta or myocardium of T injected intact females or E_2 injected intact males consistently showed evidence of limited capacity, high affinity binding of 5α-dihydrotestosterone (5α-DHT) or E_2, respectively. Binding of radiolabeled E_2 or 5α-DHT to aortic or myocardial nuclear estrogen or androgen receptors was effectively inhibited by estrogens or androgens, respectively, whereas progestins and cortisol were ineffective inhibitors. The dissociation constants (K_d) of nuclear E_2 receptors were 1.28 nM (aorta), 0.71 nM (myocardium) and those for nuclear 5α-DHT receptors were 4.46 nM (aorta), 4.32 nM (myocardium). Nuclear extracts prepared from aorta or myocardium of uninjected intact female or male rats failed to have saturable 5α-DHT or E_2 binding. T injection (1.0 mg/rat) of intact females diminished aortic (90%) and myocardial (50%) cytoplasmic androgen receptor content and comparably increased aortic and myocardial nuclear androgen receptor content. E_2 injection (10 μg/rat) of intact male rats caused partial depletion (65%) of both aortic and myocardial cytoplasmic estrogen receptor content and comparably increased aortic and myocardial nuclear estrogen receptor content. The ability of steroid hormones to translocate cardiovascular cytoplasmic estrogen or androgen receptors suggests these receptors are physiologically functional and indicates that steroid hormones may directly influence cardiovascular cell function. (Supported in part by BRSG grant 2 S07 from the DHHS.)

1268 DIRECT STIMULATING EFFECT OF GONADOTROPIN RELEASING HORMONE ON LEYDIG CELL STEROIDOGENESIS IS ASSOCIATED WITH RAPID PHOSPHOLIPID TURNOVER. T. Lin*. Medical Service, William Jennings Bryan Dorn Veterans' Hospital and Department of Medicine, University of South Carolina School of Medicine, Columbia, South Carolina, 29201, U.S.A.

Evidence has been accumulating that direct stimulating effect of gonadotropin releasing hormone (GnRH) on Leydig cell steroidogenesis is calcium dependent and not mediated by cyclic AMP. The present study was designed to investigate the effect of GnRH on phospholipid turnover. Purified Leydig cells were incubated with ^{32}P for 60 min. GnRH analog (GnRHa, des-Gly^{10} (D-Ala^{6})-GnRH) was then added and incubations were carried out for additional periods of time. Phospholipids were extracted and purified by Supelco thin layer chromatography plates. The phospholipids were identified by comparison with authentic standards following autoradiography. Within 30 sec after the addition of GnRHa (10^{-7}M), ^{32}P labeling of triphosphoinositide decreased 15% with a concomitant increase of phosphatidic acid (PA) labeling, 10.0±0.04% (±SE, $p < 0.02$) as compared with respective controls. Phosphatidylinositol (PI) labeling did not change until 2 min after the addition of GnRHa. At 60 min, labeling of PI increased to 258± 13.2% ($p < 0.001$), whereas labeling of PA increased to 292±16% ($p < 0.001$) of respective controls in response to GnRHa (10^{-7}M). The effect of GnRHa on steroidogenesis and ^{32}P incorporation is specific and receptor mediated as it is completely inhibited by GnRH antagonist (DpGlu^{1},D-Phe^{2}, D-Try^{3,6} -GnRH). The addition of nifedipine (1 and 10 ug/ml) inhibited GnRH-stimulated testosterone formation but had no significant effect on ^{32}P incorporation into phospholipids. These studies indicate that GnRH-stimulated steroidogenesis is associated with rapid phospholipid turnover.

1269 ANALYSIS OF MONOMERIC-DIMERIC STATES OF THE ESTROGEN RECEPTOR WITH MONOCLONAL ANTIESTROPHILINS. A.D. Linstedt, N.B. West and R.M. Brenner* Oregon Regional Primate Research Center, Beaverton, Or. 97006, U.S.A.

We used monoclonal antiestrophilins (H222 and H165, provided by Dr. L. Miller, Abbott Labs.) to test the hypothesis that the activated cytosolic (ERc*) and the nuclear (ERn) forms of the ^{3}H-estradiol labeled estrogen receptor from the macaque endometrium are homodimers of the cytosolic (ERc) form. Sedimentation values (S) and molecular weights of receptor-antibody complexes were determined on sucrose density gradients and Sephacryl-300 columns in 0.5M KCl. After incubation with H222(150K), ERc increased from 4S(72K) to 8S(232K) and both ERc* and ERn increased from 5S(134K) to 8S(288K). After incubation with H165(150K), ERc increased to 8S(232K) but ERc* and ERn both increased to 10S(465K). These data suggest that two molecules of H165 can bind to either ERc* or ERn but only one to ERc, and that only one molecule of H222 can bind to any of the receptor forms. We also incubated H165 with aliquots of cytosol that had been heated for various times to induce transformation of ERc to ERc*. We found that the ERc-H165-8S complex disappeared and the ERc*-H165-10S complex appeared at rates appropriate to a dimerization of ERc. We also added either H165, H222 or both to cytosol before the onset of the heat-induced transformation and found that H222, but not H165, would block the formation of ERc* from ERc. These data suggest that ERc is a monomer with one antigenic site for each antibody, that ERc* is a dimer with two available H165 antigenic sites and only one available H222 antigenic site, that after dimerization the H222 site of one (but not both) of the subunits is sterically hindered and that ERn is also a homodimer of ERc. Supported by NIH grants HD-14155 and RR-00163.

1270 CHARACTERISTICS OF INSULIN MEDIATOR FROM RAT SKELETAL MUSCLE AND LIVER . S. L. Macaulay*, J. O. Macaulay, K. L. Kelly and L. Jarett, University of Pennsylvania School of Medicine, Philadelphia, PA USA

Insulin stimulates the production of a substance from plasma membranes that fulfills the role of an intracellular insulin mediator (M). M can be extracted in boiling acid from frozen liver and skeletal muscle of control (C) and insulin-treated (I-T) rats. Larger quantities are extracted from I-T rats. The M is partially purified by ultrafiltration, ethanol extraction and sephadex chromatography and has a MW of 500-2000. The M's were eluted through YM2 filters but retained on YCO5 filters. The M's were insoluble in 100% ethanol. M partially purified from liver and skeletal muscle stimulated pyruvate dehydrogenase (PDH) up to 10 fold, low Km cAMP phosphodiesterase by 30% and inhibited both basal and glucagon-stimulated adenylate cyclase by at least 50%. M extracted from C rats had lesser effects on enzyme activities than did M extracted from I-T rats. The M which stimulated PDH was separable from the M which inhibits adenylate cyclase by Sephadex G-15 chromatography substantiating that there is more than one M. The activity of the M's were stable to boiling in 6N HCl for 24 hrs but were inactivated after 72 hrs. Activity of M's was destroyed by 2.5M NaOH for 1 hr at 24°C, but not by 0.5M NaOH. Protease at mg/ml partially inactivated the M's but lower concentrations (ug/ml) were without effect. These data suggest that the active portion of the M's may not contain simple peptide. These sources of M are being used for further purification and characterization. Supported by NIH, Reynolds Foundation and J.D.F.

1271 INVESTIGATION OF CALMODULIN INVOLVEMENT IN REGULATION OF ADENYLATE CYCLASE ACTIVITY. S. Mac Neil, T. Lakey, D. S. Munro and S. Tomlinson*, Department of Medicine, Clinical Sciences Centre, Northern General Hospital, Sheffield S5 7AU, U.K.

Although calmodulin (CaM)-regulated adenylate cyclase activity was described for brain in 1975, there are comparatively few reports of CaM-regulated adenylate cyclase activity in other tissues. In an investigation of the role of CaM in the regulation of human thyroid (H.T.) and mouse B16 melanoma (B16) adenylate cyclase activity we found agonist-stimulated enzyme activity to be inhibited by CaM antagonists but unresponsive to the addition of exogenous CaM. EGTA-treatment (up to 20 mM) failed to remove endogenous membrane CaM (0.46 μg CaM/mg protein for H.T., 0.72 μg CaM/mg protein for B16) but treatment of membranes with the rare earth, lanthanum (La^{3+}), as described by Schultz and Klumpp (FEMS Microbiology Letters, 1982 13, 303-306) for Tetrahymena membranes, allowed removal of over 90% membrane CaM. Removal of endogenous CaM was associated with a decrease in agonist-stimulated (but not basal) enzyme activity. Similar concentrations of lanthanum were inhibitory to the CaM activation of a CaM-dependent phosphodiesterase enzyme. Preliminary results with La^{3+}-treated membranes now indicate that agonist-stimulated enzyme activity for both H.T. and B16 membranes may be partially restored (to 70% of original response) by the addition of pure calmodulin (6×10^{-7}M). We conclude that for some tissues it is necessary to remove endogenous calmodulin in order to demonstrate direct activation of the enzyme by calmodulin and that La^{3+} is a more useful tool than EGTA in this respect.

1272 ESTRADIOL 17β DEHYDROGENASE ACTIVITY IN MICROVILLI FROM HUMAN PLACENTAL SYNCYTIUM. S. Guller*, A. Gravanis, A. Ross and E. Gurpide. Depts. of Obs. Gyn. & Reprod. Sci. and of Biochem., Mount Sinai School of Medicine, New York, NY 10029, USA.

Microvilli of the syncytiotrophoblast were obtained by mechanical treatment of human term placenta as described by Smith et al (Nature, 252:302, 1974). Purity of these preparations was assessed by electron microscopy. The isolated microvillar vesicles rapidly and completely converted ^3H-E_2 (18 nM) to ^3H-E_1 at 4 or 25 C in the absence of added cofactors. Spectrophotometric measurements of initial velocities of oxidation of E_2 (100 μM) in the presence of excess cofactor (200 μM) indicated that the oxidation proceded more rapidly when NAD^+ rather than $NADP^+$ was used. Reaction rates declined sharply at pH values above 8; this loss of activity was not due to changes in membrane fluidity, which remained unaffected by pH changes at 25 C, as estimated by fluorescence polarization using the diphenylhexatriene probe. Testosterone and 20α-dihydroprogesterone were also substrates of the membrane-bound enzyme. More than 90% of the activity could be solubilized by treatment with 0.3% sodium cholate/2M NaCl for 1 h at 25 C. Other activities found in the microvillar preparation included 3α oxidation of androsterone and 3β oxidation of DHEA. Estradiol 17β dehydrogenase present in syncytial microvilli may influence the relative output of E_1 and E_2 into maternal circulation. The preferred direction of the red-ox reactions occurring under physiologic conditions remains to be determined.

1273 COMPARISON OF PORTAL vs PERIPHERAL HYPERINSULINEMIA ON VLDL-TRIGLYCERIDE KINETICS. T. Kazumi*, M. Vranic, G. Steiner. Depts. Medicine & Physiology, Univ. of Toronto, Toronto, Canada.

The effects of peripherally delivered hyperinsulinemia (HI) on VLDL-triglyceride (TG) kinetics were compared to those of primarily portally delivered HI in rats. HI was produced by delivering crystalline pork insulin (6 U/day) from Alzet minipumps. The pumps were placed subcutaneously (SC) or intraperitoneally (IP). IP pumps produced profound portal HI and less marked peripheral HI. SC pumps produced profound portal HI and equal (greater than IP pumps) peripheral HI. Both HI groups and one control group of rats received 10% sucrose drinking water. All consumed the same amount of sucrose. Another control group received no sucrose. Sucrose supplementation elevated the serum glucose in controls. Although SC-HI lowered the serum glucose, IP-HI did not. Serum TG rose 34% in sucrose supplemented controls, 39% in IP-HI rats and did not change in SC-HI rats. TG production rose 14% with sucrose supplementation alone, 27% with SC-HI and 40% with IP-HI.

Considering the changes in both TG production and concentration together, we conclude that:

1) in SC-HI (i.e. peripheral HI = portal HI), TG removal increases more than does TG production.

2) in IP-HI (i.e. peripheral HI $<$ portal HI), TG production increases more than does TG removal.

1274 RELATIONSHIP OF BODY FAT DISTRIBUTION TO SKELETAL MUSCLE INSULIN RESISTANCE AND GLUCOSE DISPOSAL IN PREMENOPAUSAL WOMEN. A. Kissebah*, J. Evans and A. Pieris, Medical College of Wisconsin, Milwaukee, Wisconsin, USA.

Skeletal muscle sensitivity and responsiveness to insulin and their relationship to overall glucose disposal and insulin binding were determined in 72 premenopausal women of varying body fat topograhy [waist:hips girth ratio(WHR) 0.64-1.02] and obesity level [% ideal body weight 92-230]. As a marker of insulin action, the percentage of total glycogen synthase present in the I form (%GSI) was measured in quadriceps muscle biopsies. The increase in % GSI in response to submaximal steady-state plasma insulin (SSPI) of ∿100 μU/ml achieved by the infusion of somatostatin, insulin and glucose, was significantly lower in obese than in nonobese subjects (8.8 ± 0.9 and $12.5\pm1.2\%$ respectively, $p<0.05$), and was inversely correlated with WHR ($r = -0.51$). The increase in %GSI also correlated inversely with the steady-state plasma glucose (SSPG) concentration ($r = -0.74$), and directly with insulin binding (IB) to circulating monocytes ($r = 0.63$). When obese subjects were separated into 3 weight-matched subgroups on the basis of increasing WHR, significant trends to decreased GSI response, increased SSPG, and decreased IB were found. In 9 women with predominantly upper body obesity, % GSI response to supramaximal SSPI of ∿1000 μU/ml was unimpaired. In 4 subjects, SSPG was normal but was markedly increased in 5 women. Thus in premenopausal women, impaired skeletal muscle insulin sensitivity may contribute to diminished glucose disposal and insulin resistance associated with upper body obesity. This defect may result from a reduction in insulin receptor number. In some upper body obese women, however, a defect in other insulin-sensitive pathways may also be present.

1275 A MONOCLONAL-BASED SOLID PHASE RIA FOR PROGESTERONE. J. W. Orf*, P. A. Schueler, A. W. Lindall, and W. C. Mahoney, Immuno Nuclear Corporation, 1951 Northwestern Avenue, Stillwater, Minnesota 55082.

Hybrid cell lines were generated by fusion of progesterone 11-hemisuccinate-Bovine serum albumin immunized A/J spleen cells and NS-1 myeloma cells in a 4:1 ratio; according to a modification of the method of Oi and Herzenberg, (Cur. Top. in Microbiol. & Immunol. 81: 115 [1978]). The hybrid culture medias were screened with a HPLC purified iodinated (125I) histamine-11-progesterone tracer. The antibody designated BC3-F1 was absorbed to submicron polystyrene beads. The monoclonal antibody solid phase assay reached equilibrium within 20 minutes at room temperature and demonstrated sensitivity at a 50% B/Bo of approximately 40 pg/tube. The affinity constant was 7 x 10^8 L/M. The specificity of this antibody was then checked at 500 ng/ml with the following steroids: 20 alpha-dihydroprogesterone, 17 alpha-hydroxyprogesterone, desoxycorticosterone, pregnenolone, cortisol, and DHEA sulfate. The cross reactivities were: 0.5%, 0.6%, 0.2%, 1.3%, not-detected, 0.1%, respectively. This demonstrates that the use of monoclonal antibodies, with their clonal specificity, is ideal for discrimination of highly similar antigens in complex mixtures.

1276 DYNAMIC STUDIES OF FREE AND OCCUPIED LH RECEPTORS WITH A MONOCLONAL ANTI-LH RECEPTOR ANTIBODY. E.J. Podestá*, M.L. Sánchez, A.R. Solano. Centro de Investigaciones Endocrinológicas, Hospital de Niños "R. Gutiérrez" Gallo 1330, (1425) Buenos Aires. ARGENTINA.

LH receptor (R) internalization was studied by using a monoclonal antibody (aLHR) against the receptor with capacity to act as a Leydig cells stimulator. In order to fluorescence label the R before internalization, Leydig cells (Lc) were incubated with the agonist aLRH at 10°C for 3 hours to produce an aLHR-R complex, followed by an incubation with a fluorescence labelled anti mouse IgG (fIgG) at 34°C, a temperature which allows internalization. 15 minutes at 34°C is sufficient to observe a cytoplasmic fluorescent stain. A marked fluorescence is observed at 60 min, the stain was in the cytoplasm of the cell and no label could be detected in the nucleus. FIgG alone or unrelated monoclonal antibody are without effect.

Being capable to observe internalization of free LHR by using aLHR, we were able to study the behaviour of unnocuppied R on the membrane surface after an initial occupancy of few LHR by LH. Lc were incubated with submaximal dose of LH for 15-45 min at 34°C, washed and incubated for 6 hours at 4°C with aLHR followed by fIgG. ^{125}I-LH studies showed an initial occupancy of 20 % of the receptors and no dissociation occurs at 4°C. The results show that LH interacting with few R produce aggregates, patches, capping and internalization of free R sites. This would explain why the extent of true receptor loss is much greater than the initial occupancy in the period of refractoriness. Cells with free R in state of capping showed to be less sensitive to a second LH stimulation, compatible with the refractoriness without loss of R.

1277 SEROTONINERGIC ELEMENTS PLAY AN IMPORTANT ROLE IN THE ONSET OF THE DIURNAL PLASMA CORTICOSTERONE RHYTHM OF THE RAT.

B. Halász[x], Zs. Bánky and Gy. Nagy, 2nd Department of Anatomy Semmelweis University Medical School, H-1o94 Budapest, Hungary

The information on the involvement of the serotoninergic (5-HT) system in the neural control of the diurnal fluctuations in plasma corticosterone is contradictory. In the present studies an ontogenetic approach was used to study this question. In 16-day-old male rats, ie. before the onset of the corticosterone rhythm (1) a knife cut was made at the meso-diencephalic level interrupting the ascending 5-HT pathways, or (2) 5,7-dihydroxytryptamine (1o ug), which selectively destroys the 5-HT elements was injected into the region of the nucleus raphe dorsalis or the hypothalamic suprachiasmatic nucleus and various weeks later circadian variations in plasma corticosterone (determined by competitive protein binding radioassay) were examined. Both interventions caused a significant delay in the onset of the hormone rhythm. In several cases the rhythm was still not evident 4-5 weeks after intervention no.2. It always existed 7 weeks or later following the injection of the neurotoxin. The data suggest that the 5-HT system is involved in the neural control of the onset of the diurnal corticosterone rhythm.

1278 INSULIN INFUSION NORMALIZES THE ABNORMAL CARDIOVASCULAR FUNCTION AND PLASMA NORADRENALINE AFTER ORAL GLUCOSE IN TYPE 1 DIABETIC PATIENTS. L. Hegedüs*, A. Dejgaard, N.J. Christensen and C. Kühl. Department of Internal Medicine and Endocrinology, Herlev Hospital, and Hvidøre Hospital,Denmark.

We have previously shown that i.v. injection of insulin increased plasma noradrenaline (NA), heart rate and the systolic blood pressure. Furthermore, an oral glucose load increased plasma NA, heart rate and blood pressure significantly in young normal subjects but not in young uncomplicated Type 1 diabetic patients. The aim of this study was to examine if the abnormal regulation of the cardiovascular system and plasma NA observed after oral glucose in insulin-dependent diabetics was normalized by i.v. insulin infusion. Eight insulin-dependent diabetic patients were examined twice after an oral glucose load with and without i.v. infusion of insulin. The latter increased plasma insulin from 0.05 to 0.31 nmol/l. In the control experiment where only glucose was given the heart rate and arterial blood pressure remained unchanged, whereas plasma NA decreased slightly. After oral glucose plus i.v. insulin the heart rate increased 11% ($p<0.01$) and the systolic blood pressure increased 4% ($p<0.01$). The plasma NA averaged 99.8% of basal values during the glucose load alone and 129% after glucose plus insulin ($p<0.05$). Plasma adrenaline did not change. The results obtained in diabetic patients after oral glucose plus insulin are similar to those observed in normal subjects given an oral glucose load. This study indicates that endogenous insulin participates in the regulation of the cardiovascular system and plasma NA during glucose intake.

1279 EFFECT OF ORAL TYROSINE INGESTION ON CIRCULATING CONCENTRATIONS OF PROLACTIN (PRL) AND MONO-AMINE METABOLITES. B. Ishizuka* , M. Maruoka, M. Hayashi, H. Hamada, A. Minegishi, and T. Ishizaki. Dept. of OB-GYN, St. Marianna Univ, Kawasaki, Japan and Division of Clinical Pharmacology, Clinical Research Institute, National Medical Center, Tokyo,Japan

An acute increment in serum PRL levels following oral tyrosine (TS) ingestion has been reported recently <Ishizuka et al JCEM 57(6)>. In an attempt to delineate the neuroendocrine mechanism by which this phenomenon occurs, serial double-blind placebo-controlled studies were performed in fasted normal men. In all studies, blood was drawn at 15-30min intervals between 1100h and 1430h and TS or lactose placebo was given at 1200h. Plasma levels of mono-amine metabolites <(5-HIAA), (DOPAC), (HVA) and (MHPG)> were measured by HPLC with electrochemical detection. In 5 men who ingested 3 different doses of TS (45, 90 and 180mg/kg), serum PRL levels increased significantly in a dose dependent manner (mean basal levels 5.8±1.1ng/ml, mean peak values; 9.2±0.7ng/ml with 45mg/kg, 12.7±1.1ng/ml with 90mg/kg, 13.9±2.2ng/ml with 180mg/kg). Pretreatment with bromocriptine (5mg/day for 1 W) completely abolished the TS-induced PRL rise. In other 5 men, ingestion of TS 90mg/kg decreased mean plasma concentrations of DOPAC significantly at 30min (mean basal levels,2.2±0.2ng/ml). Mean HVA levels were also significantly lowered between 15 and 30min (basal levels 8.1 0.2ng/ml, mean max decrements 31%). Mean MHPG concentrations were significantly lowered between 30 and 60min (basal levels 4.9±0.4ng/ml, mean max decrements 21%), whereas 5-HIAA levels were not changed by TS ingestion. These results suggest that TS ingestion increases pituitary PRL release dose-dependently through temporal changes in the CNS catecholaminergic activitites.

1280 NON-SPECIFIC EFFECTS OF DSP4 ON OPIATE CONTROL OF LH SECRETION. W. Jacobson[1]*, C.J. Gibson[3] and M. Wilkinson[1,2,]**. Dept.[1] Physiol/.Biophys., [2]Obs./Gyn., Dalhousie U., Halifax, and of [3]Pathology, U. W. Ont., London, Canada.

A noradrenergic component is essential in the opiatergic control of LH release. We have used the neurotoxin DSP4, which markedly depletes noradrenaline (NA) without affecting dopamine to further investigate this relationship. Pretreatment of prepubertal female rats or of adult males with 50 mg/kg DSP4 blocked naloxone-induced LH release 2 hrs later. In adult males, the response reappeared in 7 days. Short term (2 hr) exposure of prepubertal females to DSP4 decreased the Bmax of ^{3}H-NAL binding to hypothalamic slices (4215+5 vs 8023+143 cpm/μg protein) without affecting the K_D. In this slice assay, DSP4 has an IC_{50} of 100 nM. There is some recovery of the number of binding sites after 7 days. In an homogenate assay, DSP4 did not affect the Bmax for ^{3}H-NAL binding (control 6020+238 vs DSP4 6208+2283 cpm/μg protein) but the K_D was greatly increased (2.3+0.2 vs 15.4+7.5 nM). The IC_{50} of DSP4 was 5 μM. In adult males, HPLC analysis revealed no change in NA content after 2 hr (i.e. when the NAL response is absent; 1.55+0.21 vs 1.53+0.27 μg/g; control vs 2 hr). At 24 h, NA content decreased to 69% and 73% of control values in prepubertal females and adult males respectively. NA further decreased with time in both males and females, but after 7 days, males showed some recovery. The dissociation between the decrease of hypothalamic NA and the disappearance of the NAL response, and of an effect of DSP4 directly on the opiate receptor, indicate that DSP4 modifies non-catecholaminergic systems. (Supported by MRC and O.M.H.F.; **correspondence).

1281 DEVELOPMENTAL CHANGES IN THE SEROTONERGIC SYSTEM UNDERLIE THE MATURATION OF THE NEUROENDOCRINE RESPONSE TO STRESS IN THE MALE RAT.

C.A. Johnston* and A. Negro-Vilar, Reprod. Neuroendoc. Sect., Lab. Reprod. Devel. Tox., NIEHS, NIH, Research Triangle Park, NC 27709 USA.

Our laboratory has previously (Neuroendocrinol. Lett. 8:79, 1983) shown that infantile rats, while exhibiting an established dopaminergic inhibitory tone over prolactin (PRL) secretion, do not respond to ether stress with the characteristic increase in plasma PRL levels seen during the prepuberal and adult periods. This indicates that infantile rats lack a functional stimulatory mechanism(s) for PRL release. This study analyzes the role of central monoaminergic systems in the maturation and establishment of a full neuroendocrine (rises in PRL, ACTH, β-Endorphin) response to ether stress or to a systemic injection of morphine (MOR). Metabolism of norepinephrine (NE), serotonin (5-HT), and dopamine (DA) in the medial preoptic (MPO) or mediobasal hypothalamic (MBH) regions was evaluated by concurrently measuring the amines and their respective metabolites (MHPG, 5-HIAA, and DOPAC) using HPLC and electrochemical detection. Infantile (14 day old) as well as prepuberal (36 day old) male rats showed an increased NE metabolism in both MPO and MBH 3 min. after ether exposure or 20 min. after MOR injection. Conversely, while prepuberal rats showed increased 5-HT metabolism in MPO and MBH after ether or MOR, infantile rats failed to show an altered metabolism of 5-HT in response to either stimulus. DA metabolism was essentially unaffected. The results suggest that the maturation of a full neuroendocrine response to ether stress or MOR in the rat requires the development of appropriate neuronal circuitry within the serotonergic system.

1282 HUMAN ATRIAL NATRIURETIC POLYPEPTIDES (hANP): PURIFICATION, STRUCTURE AND NATRIURETIC ACTIVITY.

Kenji KANGAWA* AND Hisayuki MATSUO, Department of Biochemistry, Miyazaki Medical College, Kiyotake, Miyazaki 889-16, JAPAN

The present survey for natriuretic factors in human atrial extract was performed by using in vitro assay for the relaxant activity on the contractility of chick rectum. Three distinct components (α-, β- and γ-) of a potent relaxant activity were found in the crude extract. Approximate molecular weights of these components were estimated by gel filtration to be: α-, 3,000; β-, 5,000; γ-, 12,000. As α-component, a 28-amino acid peptide has been isolated in a pure state and found to elicit potent diuretic and natriuretic activities as well as vasorelaxant activity, when injected into assay rats. Accordingly, we proposed a name "α-human atrial natriuretic polypeptide (α-hANP)" for the peptide. The complete amino acid sequence of α-hANP has been determined by microsequencing and confirmed by synthesis. Injection of α-hANP into rat resulted in a rapid increase of Na^+, Cl^- and urine excretions, which reached maximum within 5 min. The responses were essentially completed in 30 min. At the maximum response, α-hANP (0.4 nmole) caused a 20 x fold increase in urine output and a 30 x fold increase in NaCl excretion, comparable to the responses induced by furosemide (ca. 1.0 μmole). A small but reproducible decrease (15-20 mmHg) in blood pressure was also observed during 45 min after injection into rat. These data obviously indicate that α-hANP is one of the substances responsible for the natriuretic effect of the atrial extract.

Furthermore, β-hANP of 5,000 daltons has also been purified and its complete amino acid sequence and activities will also be reported.

1283 FAILURE TO DEMONSTRATE A ROLE FOR CALCIUM ION IN THE ACTION OF PROSTAGLANDIN $F_{2\alpha}$ IN THE RAT CORPUS LUTEUM. M. Lahav*, H. Rennert and D. Barzilai, Endocrinology Institute, Faculty of Medicine, Technion-Israel Institute of Technology, Haifa.

In rat corpora lutea (CL), prostaglandin $F_{2\alpha}$ ($PGF_{2\alpha}$) inhibits the LH-induced cAMP production. We examined the suggestion that calcium ion is a mediator of this effect in CL isolated from PMSG-treated rats (15 i.u. on day 28-30) and incubated in vitro. We reported previously that in functional (10-day-old) CL, the effect of $PGF_{2\alpha}$ (10μM) on cAMP accumulation was intact in calcium-free or verapamil-containing medium, as well as in presence of the calmodulin inhibitor trifluoperazine (3-300 μM). We report now that with another calmodulin inhibitor, pimozide (50 μM), $PGF_{2\alpha}$ inhibited the LH-induced cAMP accumulation by 60% ($p<0.02$), compared to 54% ($p<0.01$) in its absence. N,N-Diethylamino-octyl-3,4,5-trimethoxybenzoate (TMB-8), a putative intracellular calcium antagonist, did not interfere with $PGF_{2\alpha}$ action: with 0, 30 and 150 μM TMB-8, cAMP in LH-treated CL was significantly reduced by $PGF_{2\alpha}$ (by 51, 64 and 58%, respectively). In calcium-free medium with 150 μM TMB-8, $PGF_{2\alpha}$ reduced the LH-induced cAMP accumulation by 58% ($p=0.01$). In 10-day-old CL, LH and LH+$PGF_{2\alpha}$ had no effect on either uptake or efflux of $^{45}Ca^{2+}$; in regressing (14-day-old) CL, calcium uptake and efflux were unaffected by $PGF_{2\alpha}$. Thus, mediation by calcium of $PGF_{2\alpha}$ in rat CL is yet to be demonstrated.

1284 SYNTHETIC PLASTIC SUBSTRATE CAN SUBSTITUTE FOR EXTRACELLULAR MATRIX (ECM) IN THE MAINTENANCE OF BOVINE GRANULOSA CELLS IN VITRO. Richard F. Laherty*, Terre Haute Center for Medical Education, Indiana University School of Medicine, Terre Haute, IN 47809.

It has been shown that bovine granulosa cells can be established and maintained in vitro on extracellular matrix (ECM) (Endocrinology 109:409, (1981). Since the exact chemical composition of ECM has not been determined, and further, varies between batches, its use introduced a degree of uncertainity to experiments. To circumvent this problem, experiments were undertaken to ascertain the effects of a synthetic substrate (Primaria) on bovine granulosa cell growth and function. Bovine granulosa cells were harvested from medium size follicles (<6mm) and plated in 35mm plastic, ECM-coated plastic, or Primaria culture plates. The medium (DME, 10% FCS) was supplemented with fibroblast growth factor (FGF) (100ng/ml/2 days), hFSH (100 mIU/ml), neither, or both. After two weeks in culture, the medium was changed and ^3H-testosterone was added. 25 hr later this medium was aspirated and stored frozen. The granulosa cells were counted. Medium progesterone was measured by RIA, and aromatase activity was determined by quantifying ^3H-H_2O production from ^3H-testosterone. Primaria substrate produced a significant ($p<.01$) increase in final cell number that was comparable to that observed with ECM. FSH stimulated aromatase activity in granulosa cells, no matter which substrate was used, but cells cultured on primaria had higher base (-FSH) aromatase activity. The choice of substrate had no effect upon progesterone production. It was concluded that Primaria plastic can function as a chemically defined substrate in the culture of bovine granulosa cells. (This work was supported by grant #5SO7RR5371, BRSGP, NIH.)

1285 A COMPARISON OF THE ACTIONS OF A GnRH AGONIST, ANTAGONIST AND FOLLICULAR FLUIDS ON GRANULOSA CELL PROGESTERONE SECRETION.

F. Ledwitz-Rigby*, S.H. Petito, T.M. Gross, T.W. Doyle and B.W. Rigby, Dept. of Biological Sciences, Northern Illinois University, DeKalb, IL 60115 U.S.A.

Our data on follicular fluid (FFl) alterations of granulosa cell (GC) steroidogenesis exhibit many similarities to data of others on GnRH actions on GC. We performed the following experiments to determine if GnRH and FFl have identical actions and if a GnRH-like molecule might be responsible for FFl actions on progesterone secretion. GC from small [GC(S)] (1-2mm), medium [GC(M)] (3-5mm) and large [GC(L)] (6-12mm) porcine antral follicles were incubated in monolayer in TC 199 plus 10-50% serum or FFl with or without a GnRH agonist (GNRHa) [des-Gly^{10}, D-Lys^{6}, NαMe, Leu^{7}, Pro-NHEt]-GnRH and/or a GnRH antagonist (GnRH-an) [Ac-D-Phe^{1}, D -p-Cl-Phe^{2}, DTrp3,6]-GnRH. During three day incubations progesterone secretion by GC(S) was stimulated by FFl from large follicles and by $5x10^{-6}$M GnRH-an. FFl and GNRH-an effects were additive. $1x10^{-9}$ to $5x10^{-8}$M GnRHa was partially inhibitory of LH and FFl stimulated progesterone secretion. In experiments with GC(M) and GC(L), basal and LH stimulated progesterone secretion were inhibited by FFl from small follicles (SFFl) and by $5x10^{-9}$ or $5x10^{-8}$GnRHa. In some experiments GnRHa was inhibitory in serum but not in SFFl. $5x10^{-7}$M GnRH-an eliminated the inhibitory action of $5x10^{-9}$M GnRHa but did not decrease the inhibition caused by SFFl. A GnRH-like molecule does not appear to be responsible for SFFl inhibition of progesterone secretion. The possibility remains that a GnRH-antagonist exists in FFl and is involved in FFl's stimulatory action. Dr. A. Hsueh donated the GnRHa and antagonist.

1286 CELLULAR LOCALIZATION OF ZONA PELLUCIDA MATERIAL IN THE HAMSTER OVARY.

M.C. Léveillé*, K.D. Roberts, A.Chapdelaine, S. Chevalier and G. Bleau. Maisonneuve-Rosemont Research Center, Montreal, Canada.

The role of the zona pellucida in the species specificity of fertilization and the possibility of an immunocontraceptive method based on the production of antibodies directed against the zona pellucida (z.p.) have provided renewed interest in the study of this ovum investment. We have prepared doubly labelled antibodies to study the cellular origin of the zona pellucida (z.p.). Fluorescein-labelled anti-rabbit IgG (FITC-IgG) were further labelled with N-[ethyl-2-^{3}H]-ethylmaleimide (^{3}H-NEM). The resulting conjugate (^{3}H-NEM-FITC-IgG) exhibited the same immunoreactivity as the non-derivatized fluorescein labelled antibody as shown using indirect immunofluorescence and immunoradioautography assays on hamster ova. The doubly labelled conjugate was used on sections of fixed hamster ovaries enclosed in paraffin. The sections were first exposed to a rabbit antiserum raised against hamster z.p.; the bound antibodies were then visualized by fluorescence microscopy and radioautography using the doubly labelled antibody. On sections of the ovaries, the fluorescence was detected in the ooplasm and the z.p.. No specific reaction was observed on the granulosa cells. The radioautographic evaluation showed a statistically significant difference between the number of silver grains over the oocytes in incubations with anti-z.p. serum compared to control incubations with normal rabbit serum. This difference was not observed over the granulosa cells. From this study, it is concluded that important immunogenic constituent(s) of the z.p. originate from the oocyte. Supported by MRC and FCAC.

1287 ASYMMETRICAL CHANGES OF OVARIAN LHRH AND LH/hCG RECEPTORS (R) INDUCED BY ELECTRICAL STIMULATION OF THE BRAIN : EVIDENCE FOR A DIRECT NEURAL MODULATION.
B.Marchetti*, M.Cioni and U.Scapagnini, Depts of Pharmacology and Physiology, University of Catania, 95125 Catania, Italy.

Since it has been recently recognized that an efferent neural system from the brain to the ovaries can directly affect ovarian function,the extent of LHRH and LH/hCG-R modulation by neural information in right(r)and left(l) ovary(o)was analysed during the proestrous critical period after unilateral (r)electrical stimulation(UES)of medial preoptic area under pentobarbital anesthesia.Repetitive monophasic pulses(0.1msec;100Hz;100μA)were applied for 30mn at 30-sec intervals,in acutely adrenalectomized rats,some of wich underwent spinal cord transection(SCT,thoraco-lumbar junction).A biphasic pattern of response,opposite for LHRH and LH-R number(with no change in affinity)and asymmetrical for r-and-l ovary followed UES:while LHRH-R concentration was markedly depressed at 15pm in r-o(4.3±0.3 fmol/mg o)compared to l-o(8±0.3 fmol/mg),LH-R number showed a greater increase in r-o(13.7±0.5fml/mg o)than in l-o(9±0.4 fmol/mg).On the other hand,after UES at 17pm,a consistent increase of LHRH-R in r-o(9.5±0.5 fmol/mg)and decrease in l-o(4.5±0.3 fmol/mg)was measured;while a marked drop of LH-R activity greater in r-o(3.2±0.2 fmol/mg)than in l-o(6.2±0.4 fmol/mg)was observed.These effects were abolished by SCT and indicate the existence of a direct neural modulation of ovarian-R activity,possibly mediated via ovarian nerves containing LHRH or other putative transmitters.

1288 EFFECTS OF GRANULOSA CELL ASPIRATION FROM NON-DOMINANT FOLLICLES ON OVARIAN VEIN STEROIDS IN THE PRIMATE.
E.L.Marut*, M.Y.Dawood, & F.S.Khan-Dawood, Depts OB/GYN-Michael Reese Hosp & Med Ctr & U of IL Coll of Med,Chicago,IL

The role of granulosa cells in ovarian steroidogenesis in the primate dominant follicle (DF) has recently been reported (Marut, Huang, & Hodgen, JCEM 57:925, 1983). Aspiration of the DF reduced ovarian vein levels of estradiol, progesterone & androstenedione, but not 17OHprogesterone. This present study asks whether the granulosa cells of non-dominant follicles (NDF) in the late follicular phase of the primate modulate the ovarian vein levels of E_2, P, A & 17OHP. Cycling female cynomolgus monkeys were studied in 5 control & 16 study cycles. Daily peripheral bloods were drawn and assayed for LH, FSH, E_2 & P. Laparotomy was performed between day 9 & 12 of the cycle, when the DF is identifiable grossly. Ovarian vein blood was drawn bilaterally, and again after aspiration of up to 6 NDF on the ovary either sponsoring or lacking the DF. These were assayed for E_2, P, A & 17OHP. For all ovulatory cycles, ovarian vein E_2 & P were greater on the side with the DF, with asymmetry up to 30:1. Asymmetry of A was not as marked, & 17OHP was inconsistent in its concentration gradient. While overall effects of unilateral NDF aspiration were highly variable, the effect of aspiration ipsilateral to the DF diminished ovarian vein E_2 levels in every case, with a mean reduction of 77%. Ovarian vein levels of P,A,17OHP tended to decrease but not uniformly (72% of measurements). Monkeys undergoing NDF aspiration contralateral to the DF, as well as anovulatory monkeys, had no obvious pattern of changing ovarian vein steroid levels. These data suggest that aspiration of NDF, unlike the DF, has an inconsistent effect on ovarian vein steroid levels depending on multiple parameters.

1289 LUTEOLYTIC ACTION OF ANORDRIN IN MONKEYS. R.R. Mehta* and R.T. Chatterton, Jr. Div. of Surg. Oncol., University of Ill. at Chicago, Chicago, IL 60612 and Dept. of Obstet-Gyn, Northwestern Univ. Med. School, Chicago, IL 60611.

Anordrin (2α, 17α-diethynl-A-nor-5α-adrostane-2β, 17β-diol 2, 17 dipropionate), a known post-coital contraceptive agent, was evaluated for its effects on ovarian function. Six adult cynomologus monkeys (Macaca fascicularis) were monitored for at least one complete cycle to establish the occurrence of ovulation prior to anordrin treatment. Plasma, urinary hormonal profiles and vaginal smear cytology were considered as indices of ovulation and luteal function. Three monkeys were given anordrin (two animals 4.0mg/kg b.w., one animal 8.0mg/kg b.w.) on days 9-13 of the menstrual cycle. Blood samples were collected daily from days 10-20 of the cycle. All three animals during control cycles showed typical vaginal smears. Urinary pregnanediol began to rise on day 18-19, peaked on day 20-21 of the cycle, and declined to low levels before next menstruation. Serum progesterone levels also followed a similar pattern. Following the anordrin treatment the number of cornified cells in the vaginal smear reduced significantly. Urinary pregnanediol levels were elevated on days 12-14, peaked on day 14-16, and declined to the baseline levels by day 22 of the cycle. In all three animals urinary pregnanediol levels were significantly lower in the treatment cycles that in the control cycles. Serum progesterone levels began to rise 1-2 days following anordrin treatment but declined to lower levels by day 16-17 of the cycle. All the animals underwent 4-5 months amenorrhea. Our results in the present study suggest that anordrin administration to monkeys during the late follicular phase imparied the ovarian function, leading to luteal insufficiency. Supported by PARFR 309NU/NMH under a co-op agreement from AID (DRE-0546-A-00-1003-00).

1290 REGULATION OF AROMATASE IN RAT OVARIAN GRANULOSA CELLS: EFFECT OF FSH ON THE SYNTHESIS OF NADPH-CYTOCHROME P-450 REDUCTASE. Carole R. Mendelson*, Carolyn Durham, and Evan R. Simpson, Cecil H. and Ida Green Ctr Reprod Biol Sci, Univ Texas Southwestern Med Sch, Dallas, TX, USA.

Aromatase is an enzyme complex that is comprised of a specific form of cytochrome P-450 and a flavoprotein, NADPH-cytochrome P-450 reductase (RED). The objective of this study was to investigate the effect of FSH on the rate of synthesis, cellular concentration and specific activity of RED in rat ovarian granulosa cells in vitro. Granulosa cells from the ovaries of immature, estrogen-primed rats were incubated in the absence or presence of FSH (250 ng/ml) for 72 h. Aromatase activity of cells incubated in the absence of hormone was 4 pmol/mg prot/2h and was increased 75-fold by FSH. RED was immunoisolated from [^{35}S]Met-labeled lysates of granulosa cells, by use of an antibody prepared against porcine liver RED. By analysis of autoradiograms of SDS-polyacrylamide gels we found that a protein of ∿ 80 kDa that co-migrated with purified RED was immunoisolated from cell lysates; the rate of [^{35}S]Met incorporation into this protein was increased 3-fold in FSH-treated cells as compared to controls. By immunoblot analysis we found that the concentration of RED was increased by 1.6-fold in FSH-treated cells compared to controls. RED activity was 10.1 nmol/mg protein/min in membrane fractions from control cells and was increased 1.6-fold by FSH treatment. These findings are indicative that FSH increases the rate of synthesis, specific content and specific activity of RED in ovarian granulosa cells. We suggest that the stimulatory effect of FSH on aromatase activity may be mediated, in part, by an increase in the rate of synthesis of RED.

1291 PREVENTION OF EXPERIMENTAL WATER INTOXICATION WITH THE VASOPRESSIN ANTAGONIST d/CH_2/$_5$Tyr/Et/VAVP IN RAT
F. A. László, Endocrine Unit, First Department of Medicine, University Medical School, Szeged, PB: 469, Hungary.

Treatment of Schwartz-Bartter syndrome is an unsolved problem. A study was made of whether a recently synthetized vasopressin antagonist analogue can be used to treat the syndrome. The essence Schwartz-Bartter syndrome is water intoxication, which was induced in rat with a high subcutaneous dose /2 x 1.5 µg/daily/ of dDAVP, together with the normal water intake /3 x 5 % b.w./. At the same time, some rats received the antidiuretic antagonist vasopressin derivative [1-/β-mercapto-β,β-cyclopentamethylene-propionic acid/,2-O--ethyl-tyrosine-4-valine] arginine vasopressin /3 x 6 µg daily s.c./. In response to dDAVP administration, there was an appreciable water retention, the urinary osmolality and the excreted sodium quantity increased, the serum osmolality and sodium level dropped markedly /serum Na to below 100 mmol/l/, and the water content of the brain rose by 2.8%. The antagonist prevented water retention, enhanced natriuresis and hyponatraemia, and cerebral oedema did not develop. Without water loading, dDAVP alone produced no changes other than the decrease of diuresis. The observations suggest that the vasopressin antagonist might be of use in the future as an effective drug against Schwartz-Bartter syndrome.

1292 ARGININE VASOPRESSIN IN THE RAT AND SHEEP OVARY.
S.J. Lolait*, A.T.W. Lim, J. Abrahams, C.I. Johnston, J.W. Barlow, B.H. Toh and J.W. Funder, Medical Research Centre and Monash Department of Medicine, Prince Henry's Hospital, Melbourne; Ewen Downie Metabolic Unit and Monash Deptment of Pathology & Immunology Alfred Hospital, Prahran, Australia.

There is increasing evidence supporting the production of a variety of neuropeptides by gonadal cells, including immunoreactive arginine vasopressin (ir-AVP) in extracts of human (Wathes et al, Lancet ii, 410, 1982) and bovine ovary (Wathes et al, Endocrinology 113, 693, 1983). In the current study we have used a specific AVP antiserum (Woods & Johnston, Am. J. Physiol. 363, F727, 1982) to show the presence, in extracts of rat and sheep ovaries, of ir-AVP coeluting with standard AVP_{1-9}, and of a high M_r (∿20K) putative precursor form of the peptide consistent with the ovarian production of AVP. Levels of ir-AVP change significantly over the estrous cycle in mature rats, or after administration of estradiol to immature rats. Follicular cell cultures from sheep and rat ovaries, and immunofluorescence studies, suggest that ir-AVP is produced by follicular and luteal cells, that its production is related to the estrous cycle, and that it may thus play an autocrine role in ovarian steroidogenesis. In parallel studies, we have shown by radioimmunoassay and immunofluorescence indistinguishable ovarian levels of ir-AVP in Brattleboro (di/di) and Long-Evans rats. The finding of ir-AVP in the ovary (but not the pituitary) of Brattleboro rats suggests that the gene for the AVP precursor is present in this strain, but is not expressed in the hypothalamus.
Supported by the National Health & Medical Research Council of Australia.

1293 VASOPRESSIN GENE REGULATION IN THE RAT HYPOTHALAMUS.

J. Majzoub*, J. Sokol, J. Habener, Howard Hughes Medical Institute, Massachusetts General Hospital, Harvard Medical School, Boston, MA 02114

Vasopressin (VP), is synthesized in the magnocellular neurons of the hypothalamus (HT), is secreted via axons in the posterior pituitary in response to several stimuli, including systemic dehydration. Although 96 hr of water deprivation results in a 10-fold rise in plasma VP and a 5-fold fall in posterior pituitary VP content, nothing is known about the concommitant VP mRNA regulation in the HT. To study this issue, groups of adult female rats were deprived of water for 12 to 96 hr, followed by rehydration for 8 to 24 hr. After various intervals of dehydration ± rehydration, rats were weighed, sacrificed by decapitation, plasma osmolality was measured, total HT RNA was isolated, and VP mRNA levels were assessed by filter hybridization (Northern) blot analysis using a synthetic oligonucleotide VP probe. During the 96 hr of water deprivation, rats lost 20% of initial body weight, plasma osmolality rose from 275 to 305 mosm/L, and VP mRNA levels rose 10-fold. After 24 hr of rehydration, plasma osmolality fell to 280 mosm/L, body weight increased to 95% of initial weight, but VP mRNA levels remained elevated at 5-fold above the initial value. This persistently high VP mRNA level might indicate a long $T_{1/2}$ for VP mRNA. Alternatively, since posterior pituitary VP content is known to be less than 50% replenished after 24 hr of rehydration, the high VP mRNA levels after 24 hr of rehydration may be related to the diminished posterior-pituitary VP content. This suggests that VP gene expression may be regulated by the intracellular concentration of VP in the magnocellular neurons.

1294 HORMONE RECEPTOR REGULATION OF THE PULSATILE LUTEOLYTIC SECRETION OF PROSTAGLANDIN $F_{2\alpha}$ FROM THE OVINE UTERUS.

J.A. McCracken* and W.C. Okulicz. Worcester Foundation for Experimental Biology, Shrewsbury, MA 01545 USA

During corpus luteum (CL) regression in sheep the uterine luteolytic hormone $PGF_{2\alpha}$ is secreted from the uterus as a series of pulses lasting about 1 h at intervals of 6 h. Our studies indicate that $PGF_{2\alpha}$ synthesis in the endometrium is caused by interaction of oxytocin (OT) with its receptor (rOT), the latter being induced by the action of estradiol (E). During the luteal phase E stimulation of rOT is blocked by progesterone (P), but later, due to a loss of P action, E action returns forming rOT and hence $PGF_{2\alpha}$. Because pulses of oxytocin neurophysin occur synchronously with pulses of $PGF_{2\alpha}$ it seemed that episodes of OT from the brain might fine-tune the secretion of $PGF_{2\alpha}$. Since sheep CL contain $PGF_{2\alpha}$-dischargeable OT we have evidence for the following: With declining P action E causes synthesis of endometrial rOT which coupled with basal levels of OT initiates uterine $PGF_{2\alpha}$. This initial rise of $PGF_{2\alpha}$ causes a discharge of OT from the CL reinforcing the synthesis of $PGF_{2\alpha}$ which now begins luteolysis. Because endometrial rOT are now down-regulated, $PGF_{2\alpha}$ synthesis temporarily subsides. Since rOT are formed by E in 6 h, a similar sequence of events, culminating in an episode of $PGF_{2\alpha}$ secretion, will follow at intervals of 6h. This is consistent with observed endogenous pulse frequency of $PGF_{2\alpha}$ during natural luteolysis and the frequency found essential for the induction of luteolysis with ultra-low pulses of $PGF_{2\alpha}$ (Prostaglandins 26:347,1983). The receptor mediated mechanism proposed for the pulsatile release of $PGF_{2\alpha}$ may also have significance for the pulsatile release of other hormones. (Supported by HD 08129 and HD 06295).

1295 ABLATION OF THE ANTERIOR WALL OF THE THIRD VENTRICLE OF SHEEP DEPRESSES VASOPRESSIN RELEASE. M.J. McKinley,* M. Congiu, D.A. Denton, M. Leventer, R.G. Park, R.S. Weisinger and R.D. Wright, Howard Florey Institute of Experimental Physiology and Medicine, University of Melbourne, Parkville, 3052. Australia.

The aim of this study was to test whether tissue in both the dorsal and ventral parts of the anterior wall of the third ventricle (A3V) is involved in osmotically stimulated vasopressin (AVP) release. Three groups of sheep were studied before and after ablating these brain regions. (1) Sheep with lesions extending dorsally in the midline A3V from the anterior commissure (a.c.) to include the subfornical organ (AD3V-sheep, n=5). (2) Sheep with midline lesions extending dorsally from the optic chiasma up to near the level of the a.c. (AV3V-sheep, n=5). (3) Sheep with total ablation of both dorsal and ventral parts of the A3V (TA3V-sheep, n=3). The supraoptic nuclei were undamaged in all sheep. The increase in plasma [AVP] which results from intracarotid infusion of hypertonic NaCl for 20 min was significantly attenuated in both AD3V- and AV3V-sheep and almost abolished in TA3V-sheep when compared to pre-lesion responses. The pAVP in response to water deprivation for 3 days was also measured pre-lesion and increased from 4±1 to 23±5 pg/ml (mean ± SD). With such dehydration, pAVP reached 32±11 pg/ml in AD3V-sheep, 18±7 pg/ml in AV3V-sheep and 9±2 pg/ml in TA3V-sheep in the post-lesion period. Only the latter value was significantly lower than the pre-lesion level. However plasma osmolality was much higher in dehydrated AV3V-sheep post-lesion compared to pre-lesion, and pAVP may have been inappropriately low. These results indicate that there is tissue in both the dorsal and ventral A3V which is involved in AVP release in response to hypertonicity.

1296 MELATONIN RHYTHM IN SOME IDIOPATHIC HYPOTHALAMIC-HYPOPHYSEAL DISEASES.
Lissoni P.*, Mauri R., Resentini M., Morabito F., °Djemal S. and Fraschini F
Centro Auxologico Italiano di Piancavallo; °Cattedra di Chemioterapia, Facoltà di Medicina, Università di Milano.

In order to evaluate the role of the pineal gland in some idiopathic hypothalamic-hypophyseal diseases, light/dark rhythm of melatonin was studied in 11 patients, of whom 5 were affected by delayed puberty and 6 by isolated or multiple hypophyseal deficiencies, and in 30 healthy subjects of both sexes (15 prepubertal and 15 pubertal). Serum melatonin levels were determined with Wetterberg's RIA method in sample taken at 4 different times of the day (7 a.m., 12a.m., 6p.m., 12p.m.). The results confirmed the existence of a circadian rhythm of melatonin, with a night peak also in man. Male prepubertal subjects showed significantly higher melatonin levels in respect to the pubertal ones. In prepubertal females was higher than in pubertal ones in periovulatory phase and similar to the values found during menstrual bleeding. A functional hyperpinealism condition, with high melatonin levels, was present in patients affected by delayed puberty, and associated with an abnormal rhythm, with a peak of the hormone also at midday. In contrast, a hypopinealism state was observed in the hypopituitarism, with low melatonin levels, and the rhythm was absent in two patients. Concluding, the evaluation of the light/dark rhythm of melatonin can be important in the clinic study of the idiopathic hypothalamic-hypophyseal diseases.

1297 CHANGES IN BRAIN BENZODIAZEPINE RECEPTORS AFTER PINEALECTOMY OR MELATONIN INJECTION TO RATS. P.R.Lowenstein*, R.Rosenstein and D.P.Cardinali, Centro de Estudios Farmacológicos y de Principios Naturales, Serrano 665, 1414 Buenos Aires, Argentina.

The pineal gland has sedative properties on the CNS as shown by the convulsive states arising after pinealectomy (Px) in rats. Melatonin itself acts as an anticonvulsivant and tranquillizer as well as a sleep inducer in several mammalian species. The purpose of this work was to evaluate whether Px-induced hyperexcitability could be related to changes in benzodiazepine (BZP) receptors sites of rat cerebral cortex. BZP receptor activity was assayed by the "in vitro" specific binding of ^{3}H-flunitrazepam (FNZP) to P_2 membrane fractions; dissociation constant (Kd) and number of binding sites (Bmax) were calculated by triplicate in independent experiments for each treatment. Pineal removal depressed Bmax significantly by 17,20 and 40% when assessed 3,7 or 14 days after surgery. No changes in Kd's were detected. The administration of a single injection of melatonin (800 ug/kg) at the 4th h of light (12:12 LD) restored BZP receptor levels in Px rats 3 h later. However melatonin (up to 1600 ug/kg) injected to intact animals either at the 4th or the 10th h of light did not affect FNZP binding to cerebral cortex membranes. Daily injections of melatonin for 5 days increased significantly BZP receptor sites by 27% when injected at morning hours. Addition of melatonin (up to 100 uM) to purified P_2 fractions did not interfere with subsequent binding. These results suggest that the pineal gland modulates through melatonin brain BZP receptor activity. This study was supported by the Consejo Nacional de Investigaciones Científicas y Técnicas, Argentina

1298 ADRENOCORTICOTROPIC REGULATION OF ANGIOTENSIN-I-CONVERTING ENZYME ACTIVITY (ACE) IN RAT ANTERIOR PITUITARY. A.Israel*, M.Niwa and J.M.Saavedra, Laboratory of Clinical Science, NIMH, Bethesda, Md. 20205, USA.

Angiotensin II (AII) acts directly on the anterior pituitary to stimulate ACTH secretion (Spinedi and Negro Vilar, 1983). Bilateral adrenalectomy (ADX) increases AII immunoreactivity in the zona externa of the median eminence (Kilcoyne et al, 1980). ACE and AII receptors are high in anterior pituitary (Guiguere et al, 1982, Chevillard and Saavedra, 1982) These findings suggest a possible interaction between the adrenocortical and angiotensin systems at the pituitary level. In addition, pulmonary ACE decreases in ADX rats, a change reversed by dexamethasone (DEX) treatment (Mendelsohn et al, 1982), and ACTH is a potent noncompetitive inhibitor of lung ACE (Verma et al, 1982). To evaluate the possibility of an interaction between the two systems in the pituitary, we determined the ACE activity of anterior pituitary and median eminence of sham-operated, ADX (10 days after operation) and ADX male rats after DEX replacement (subcutaneous 5 mg pellets implanted for 7 days). All ADX rats were maintained on 0.9% NaCl. Sham operated animals were divided in two groups receiving water or 0.9% NaCl *ad libitum*. There were no differences in ACE activity in the two groups groups of sham operated rats (132± 10 and 110±6 pmol/µg protein/hr). ADX resulted in a marked decrease (-52%) in anterior pituitary ACE activity ($p<0.001$), a change reversed by DEX replacement. There were no changes in median eminence in the three groups of animals. Our findings suggest the possibility of a local control of ACE activity by the adrenocorticotropic system at the anterior pituitary level.

1299 STUDY ON PRIMING EFFECT OF LH-RH TO SUBUNITS OF GONADOTROPIN IN PITUITARY CULTURE. Shun-ichiro Izumi*, Tsunehisa Makino, Masayoshi Arisawa, Takashi Seki, Satoshi Tanimoto, Kazuki Fukuoka, and Rihachi Iizuka, Department of Obstetrics and Gynecology, School of Medicine, Keio University, Tokyo Japan

To clarify the priming effect of leuteinizing hormone-releasing hormone (LH-RH) on gonadotropin synthesis and release of the anterior pituitary gland, the anterior pituitaries of the male rats were cultured in vitro through a LH-RH stimulation and a washing sequence for the analysis of gonadotropins and their subunits. After the first stimulation of gonadotrophs with synthetic LH-RH for 20 minutes and the removal of LH-RH by washing, the alteration of gonadotropin release and its content in the anterior pituitaries were investigated for several hours. The data indicate that the primary stimulation by LH-RH to the gonadotrophs has the late-manifesting effect on the release of gonadotropins, especially LH-beta-subunit, after washing, but that LH-RH, primarily administered, does not change the responsiveness of the pituitary to the secondarily administered LH-RH in terms of the releasing ability. Concerning with the synthesizing ability of the gland, any changes of the tissue contents of these hormones and subunits were not observed, which was attributable to the primary administration of LH-RH. However the ratio of subunit to native hormone was affected to increase only in the pre-treated groups, indicating that LH-RH might have the priming effect only or especially on subunit synthesis.

1300 GROWTH HORMONE VALUES TEN YEARS OR MORE AFTER Y-90 PITUITARY IMPLANTS FOR ACROMEGALY. A. Jadresic*, L. Jimenez and G.F. Joplin, Department of Medicine, Royal Postgraduate Medical School, Hammersmith Hospital, London W12 OHS, England.

Thirty eight acromegalic patients who had not received treatment previously were treated with Y-90 pituitary implants and followed up from 10 to 17 years. 24 were women. Growth hormone (GH) values were determined preoperatively and at 3 months and one year after implant and thereafter at variable intervals. Random GH or mean values during the second hour of a standard oral glucose tolerance test of $\leqslant$ 5mIU/l were obtained in 3 patients (8%) at 3 months and in 7 patients (18%) at one year, but cumulative percentages increased to 24% at 3 years, 29% at 4, 32% at 6, 37% at 8, 53% at 10 and 63% at 12 years to reach 76% at 14 years. Cumulative hypopituitarism after the implant increased from 16% at 3 months to 18% at one year, 21% at 2, 29% at 4, 32% at 7, 37% at 10 and 39% at 14 years. Eight further patients received more than one implant, 4 of these had a full remission at 5, 7, 8 and 11 years from first implant. Hypopituitarism occurred in 3 of them at 4 months, one year and 5 years.
In the whole series of 46 acromegalic patients given one or more Y-90 pituitary implants as the only treatment and followed up for 588 patient-years there has been no instance of relapse.

1301 EFFECT OF HYPERBARIC OXYGEN (HOB) ON PITUITARY HORMONES. M.Janches(*), G. V.Spirito,E.C.Andrada & J.A.Andrada, Instituto de Investigaciones Medicas, University of Buenos Aires,C.P.1427 Buenos Aires,Argentina.

Due to the frequent use of hyperbaric oxygen (HOB) in different conditions as deep diving,astronautic flights,therapeutic applications in several pathological situations,etc.,we asume that it will be important to study its effects on human Physiology. For this purpose we have investigated pituitary secretion under HOB in a group volunteer subjects without endocrine disturbances. The experiment was done on: A) Twelve subjects introduced in a chamber of 3.000 litres,breathing 100% oxygen at 2 atmosphere (ATA) during 1 hour; B) eight subjects introduced in the same chamber breathing compressed air at 1 ATA for 1 hour, and C) seven subjects breathing environmental air. Before (8A.M.) and after the chamber session (10A.M.) blood was drawn for assaying by radio-immuneassay : Prolactin (PRL),Somatotrophin (SH), Gonadotrophins FSH & LH), Thyroxin (T4) and Cortisol. In group C the same scheme was performed.

In 8 of the 12 subjects of group A, PRL raised after HOB (8 A.M. 10.3 ng/ml $\pm$ 2.0, 10 A.M. 18.4 ng/ml $\pm$ 4.1 , $p < 0.02$); under bromoergocriptine this effect disappeared. Group B and C sowed lowering of PRL at 10 A.M. The statistical evaluation between A and C at 11 A.M. exhibited statistical difference ($p < 0.01$). However no differences were detected for the other hormones. The present data demonstrate that HOB may have a stimulatory effect on PRL in normal subjects. Probably this effect is obtained by deppressing prolactin inhibiting factor or stimulating directly pituitary cells.

1302 **HUMAN THYROTROPIC ADENOMA : CELL CULTURE STUDIES OF 2 TUMORS.** P.Jaquet, G.Gunz, J.Hassoun, B.D.Weintràub, Clinique Endocrinologique,Marseille, France and Clinical Endocrinology Branch,NIAMDD, Bethesda, Md, USA.
In patients with a TSH-producing pituitary adenoma, high levels of thyrotropin (TSH) in plasma are generally not modified by thyroid hormones and thyrotropin releasing hormone (TRH). We have studied in vitro the endocrine regulation of TSH in 2 cases of such human tumors obtained after surgery. After dispersion,tumor cells were maintained, in defined serum-free conditions, on extracellular matrix for 4-6 weeks. The ratio of TSHα/TSH released in the culture medium was 4 and 24 according to case. Analysis of tumor TSH by high pressure gel chromatography revealed 3 fractions with apparent M.W of 45K (11%), 28K (70%), 20K (19%).Thyroid hormone (T3) produced a dose dependent inhibition of both TSH and TSHα with half maximal inhibition at 1 or $4x10^{-11}$M according to case.TRH at various concentrations had no effect on TSH or TSHα release. Adenylate cyclase activation by 10^{-11} M choleratoxin elicited an increase of TSH and TSHα (150-190%) according to case. Bromocriptine produced a partial inhibition of TSH and TSHα.Maximal inhibition (37 and 51%) was obtained at 10^{-8} M concentrations and half maximal effect was achieved at 1 to $5x10^{-10}$ M.These data show that 1/ tumor thyrotrophs may be responsive,in vitro, to near physiological concentrations of T3. The in vivo thyroid hormone insensitivity of such tumors might not be the sole pathogenic explanation. 2/ from the partial effect of dopaminergic inhibition it can be inferred that bromocriptine will not be an effective therapeutic agent in most TSH secreting tumors.

1303 NUCLEAR MAGNETIC RESONANCE STUDIES ON METABOLISM OF RAT PITUITARY TUMOURS IN VIVO. J. Jenkins*, R. Prysor-Jones, J. Silverlight, A. Stevens, L. Rodrigues and J. Griffiths, St. George's Medical School, London SW17 UK.

We have previously shown that spontaneously arising rat pituitary tumours are a good model for human prolactinomas. In order to study rapidly changing biochemical events within these pituitary tumours during life, and the effects of agents which may modify their secretion, we have explored new techniques for obtaining nuclear magnetic resonance (NMR) spectra of living tissues in vivo. Pituitary tumours were transplanted into peripheral sites and ^{31}P spectra were obtained using an Oxford Instruments TMR-32-200 instrument and a surface coil. Prominent peaks were observed from phosphocreatine (PCr), inorganic phosphorus (Pi), the 3 phosphates of ATP, and other metabolites including monophosphates and phosphodiesters. In 14 tumours the size of the PCr peak varied considerably, being greatest in the younger smaller tumours and less in large tumours. Repeated examination showed that PCr fell and Pi rose during the course of tumour growth. There was some correlation between prolactin secretion and the ATP/Pi ratio, and as the ratio declined the tumour became more acidic. Intracellular pH (pH_i) is easily measured by NMR, and values ranged from 6.6-7.5 in different tumours. A preliminary investigation of the effects of vaso-intestinal peptide (VIP) on the metabolism of 7 further tumours showed that after i/v injection of VIP there was a consistent fall in pH_i ranging from 0.06-0.77 together with a rise in Pi. Similar changes were not seen with TRH. These initial results promise that NMR will increase knowledge of the intracellular processes concerned with hormone secretion and growth.

1304 MAITOTOXIN AND GROWTH HORMONE RELEASING FACTOR INCREASE ARACHIDONATE RELEASE FROM ANTERIOR PITUITARY CELLS. AM Judd*, K Koike, T Yasumoto, RM MacLeod, University of Virginia, Charlottesville, Virginia, U.S.A.

Secretagogue-induced anterior pituitary (AP) hormone release is generally associated with mobilization of calcium (Ca^{2+}) and may be related to arachidonate (AA) metabolism. We determined whether the calcium channel activator maitotoxin (MTX) affects esterified-AA release from primary AP cultures. These cells were pre-incubated for 90 min with 0.25 μCi/ml ^{3}H-AA (86.6 Ci/mmol) to incorporate ^{3}H-AA into esterified lipids, washed with buffer without ^{3}H-AA, and incubated 30 min with vehicle or MTX. ^{3}H-AA was extracted from the medium with ethyl acetate, applied to silica gel TLC plates, and the dpm in the ^{3}H-AA band determined. MTX significantly ($P<0.01$) increased ^{3}H-AA release from both male (vehicle, 229 ± 10; 5 ng/ml MTX, 4926 ± 35) and female (vehicle, 614 ± 26; 5 ng/ml MTX, 1920 ± 162; 10 ng/ml MTX, 3720 ± 324) rat AP and increased the release of all AP hormones determined. Since growth hormone releasing factor (GRF) appears to mobilize calcium, we determined its effect on AA release from AP. GRF increased AA release from male AP in a concentration dependent manner (vehicle, 577 ± 9; 0.05 nM GRF, 554 ± 31; 1 nM GRF, 662 ± 30^{a}; 100 nM GRF, 750 ± 24^{b}; $^{a}P<0.05$; $^{b}P<0.01$ vs. vehicle) and markedly increased GH release. In conclusion, MTX and GRF increase AA release from AP. Therefore, the mobilization of Ca^{2+} and the release of AA may be related and may be generally important events in the release of AP hormones and specifically in GRF-induced GH release. [Funded by CA-07535 (RMM) and F-32-CA-07137 (AMJ).]

1305 CHARACTERISATION OF DYNORPHIN IN HUMAN PITUITARY TUMOURS. P. Kendall-Taylor*, G. Dawson, A.I. Smith, and D. Mathias. Department of Medicine, Royal Victoria Infirmary, and Neuro-endocrine Unit, Newcastle upon Tyne NE1 4LP. U.K.

Dynorphin A is a potent opioid peptide which has been identified in brain tissue where it exists in several molecular forms, and in posterior pituitary. We investigated the possibility that some pituitary tumours derive from intermediate or posterior pituitary by measuring dynorphin-LI in tumour extracts. The molecular nature of the immunoreactive material has been analysed by HPLC and RIA of fractions. Pituitary tumours were obtained at surgery from 13 patients and normal anterior pituitary tissue from 2 patients. Peptides were extracted by homogenisation in hot 0.1N HCl. The supernatant was submitted to HPLC and peptides eluted with a linear acetonitrile/TFA gradient. Antiserum R3C (a gift from Dr. A. Goldstein) recognised dynorphin A_{1-17} (dyn 1-17) and dyn A1-13 but not smaller fragments of dynorphin. In 3 Cushing's tumours an identical pattern was seen of 2 immunoreactive peaks which co-eluted with synthetic dyn 1-17 and dyn 1-13. Dilution curves for these peaks were parallel to standard curves for dyn 1-17 and dyn 1-13. The range of tissue concentration was: dyn 1-17 1.28 - 2.89 pmol/mg, dyn 1-13 0.64 - 1.6 pmol/mg. Other tumours examined were 7 Cushing's, 1 Nelson's, 2 acromegalic, but no dyn-LI was seen in these or in normal pituitary tissue. Conclusion: in some Cushing's tumours, presumably arising from the neuro-intermediate lobe, there is autonomous production of dyn 1-17 and dyn 1-13.

1306 EVIDENCE FOR THE PRESENCE IN RAT PITUITARY MAMMOTROPHS OF POOLS OF PROLACTIN DIFFERENTLY REGULATED BY DOPAMINE, TRH AND VIP. J. Lafond*, J.R. Ducharme and R. Collu, Res. Unit on Reprod. Develop. Biol., Pediatric Res. Center, Ste-Justine Hospital and U. of Montreal, Montreal, Que., H3T 1C5.

An *in vitro* perifusion system of columns made of enzymatically dispersed rat pituitary cells attached to Cytodex beads was utilized to investigate the control of prolactin (PRL) release by dopamine (DA), TRH and VIP. Cells packed in columns were perifused with Dulbecco's Modified Eagle Medium (DMEM) with or without drugs at a constant rate of 0.2 ml/min. Prior to the experimental period, all columns were perifused for 2 h with DA 10^{-5} M. The experimental period consisted in 1 h of DA infusion preceeded and followed by 2 h of DMEM alone, TRH 10^{-8} M and VIP 10^{-7} M in various combinations. At least 3 perifusions of every combinations were performed. Two distinct peaks of PRL release (1st and 2nd) were thus obtained, separated by 1 h of very low values. Since the total amount of PRL released in the 1st peak varied greatly from column to column under equal experimental conditions, statistical analysis was approched by ANOVA comparing total amount of PRL release in the 2nd peak as % of the 1st peak. With the DMEM-DMEM combination, the 2nd peak (91±3.2%) was not significantly different from the 1st while with DMEM-TRH and DMEM-VIP, the 2nd peaks were significantly increased (201±44% and 166±18% respectively). With TRH-DMEM, TRH-TRH and TRH-VIP, the 2nd peaks were respectively 16±3%, 78±0.3% and 50±9%. With VIP-DMEM, VIP-TRH, VIP-VIP, the 2nd peaks were respectively 54±6%, 62±14% and 47±11%. These results suggest that: 1) TRH and VIP stimulate pools of PRL not released by the suppression of DA inhibition; 2) there is a difference between the mechanisms through which TRH and VIP regulate PRL release.

1307 DATA WITH A NEW GALENICAL FORM OF BROMOCRIPTINE IN SUPPRESSION OF LACTATION. Ioana Lancranjan*[1], R. Rolland[2], and M. L'HERMITE[3],
[1] Clinical Research Department, Sandoz Ltd., Basle, Switzerland.
[2] Academic Hospital St. Radboud, University of Nijmegen, The Netherlands.
[3] University Brugmann Hospital, Bruxelles, Belgium.

A new galenical form of bromocriptine has been developed for the prevention and suppression of puerperal lactation. This is an injectable, retard form which at a dose of 50 mg/dose, injected deep i.m. shows 2 hours after the injection a maximum plasma concentration of bromocriptine of 1.5 ± 0.6 ng/ml, 1.0 ± 0.2 ng/ml one day after, 0.6 ± 0.1 ng/ml 14 days and 0.3 ± 0.1 ng/ml 28 days following the injection. The 24 hour profile of PRL, investigated in 6 male and 4 female, young euthyroid, healthy volunteers by hourly blood collection before, the first day of bromocriptine administration (day 1), 14 and 28 days later showed a suppression of basal and sleep related PRL peak in all volunteers throughout the 28 day study period. Clinical studies were carried out in 300 postpartum women who did not wish to breast feed their children. Prevention of lactation was recorded in 96% of postpartum women and no rebound lactation occured in any of these cases. These excellent clinical results were due to a strong inhibition of PRL secretion (92% decrease from the initial values) which lasted up to 42 days after a single i.m. injection of 50 mg bromocriptine-retard. The very good local and general tolerability (97% of cases) and the excellent acceptance of bromocriptine-retard suggests that this might be the best available treatment of postpartum lactation suppression.

1308 EFFECT OF HYPERPROLACTINEMIA ON LH PULSATION IN MALE RABBITS. J. Larsen* and W.D. Odell, University of Utah School of Medicine, Salt Lake City, Utah, USA.

Intact and 10-14 day castrate (CSTR) adult male rabbits were implanted with internal jugular vein silastic catheters. One to two days later, one group received a priming bolus of 20 μg bovine prolactin (PRL), followed by 50 μg/h PRL infusion for 3.5 h (blood concentration ~ 100 ng/ml). A second group served as controls. Blood was taken Q 3 min for 1 h (after 2 h PRL infusion in PRL animals). All animals were awake and minimally restrained. LH was determined by RIA, and mean LH, LH pulse (P) frequency (freq), amplitude (amp) and duration (dur) were calculated.

	LH mean (ng/ml)	P-freq/h	P-amp (ng/ml)	P-dur (min)
Intact (n=8)	2.57 ± .51	3.24 ± .42	1.65 ± .18	9.8 ± .57
Intact-PRL (n=6)	1.16 ± .4	1.8 ± .3	.96 ± .34	12.4 ± 2.0
CSTR (n=16)	12.98 ± 1.85	2.4 ± .24	8.27 ± .74	19.55 ± 1.82
CSTR-PRL (n=7)	6.26 ± .53	2.52 ± .3	3.2 ± .55	13.2 ± .94

We conclude that: a) castration results in increased LH P-amp (p<.01), increased mean LH (p<.01) and increased LH P-dur (p<.01); b) in castrate animals, PRL decreases mean LH values (p<.01), as well as LH P-amp (p<.01) and P-dur (p<.01); and c) in intact animals, PRL decreases P-freq (p<.05), as well as decreasing mean LH (p<.05).

1309 METABOLIC ACTION OF PROLACTIN (PRL) IN THE RAT PROSTATE: AN ACTION WHICH IS INDEPENDENT OF THE ANDROGEN ACTION.

C. Lee*, C. Smith, D. Assimos and J.T. Grayhack, Northwestern University Medical School, Chicago, Illinois, U.S.A.

Hyperprolactinaemia is known to cause a delay in castration-induced regression in the lateral prostate of rats. Since it is possible that a small amount of endogenous androgen present in the prostate at the time of castrationacts synergistically with the elevated PRL to cause this delay in prostate regression, the present study was conducted to explore if this action of PRL was mediated through the action of androgen. Two female pituitaries were grafted under the renal capsule of adult Sprague-Dawley rats. Seven days later, bilateral orchiectomy and unilateral nephrectomy were performed. In half of the rats, the kidney bearing the grafts was removed and, in the other half, the contralateral kidney was removed. Rats bearing the grafts had a higher level of serum PRL (93±7ng/ml) than in rats without the grafts (26±3ng/ml). The rate of protein degradation in the lateral prostate, as judged by the amount of radioactivity remaining in the protein fraction following a single pulse of ^{3}H-leucine, was significantly slower in graft-bearing animals than in those without the grafts. However, the rate of protein synthesis, as judged by both the in vitro and the in vivo incorporation of ^{3}H-leucine into the prostatic protein, was not different between the two groups of animals. Nor was the total content of cathepsin D in the prostate different. These results indicate that the effect of PRL on protein metabolism in the rat prostate is not consistent with the parameters known as the androgen effect. Therefore, we conclude that the action of PRL is not mediated through the action of androgen. (Supproted by NIH grant HD 11611)

1310 FETAL EXPOSURE TO SPIRONOLACTONE LEADS TO HYPOPROLACTINEMIA IN THE ADULT MALE RAT.

T. Lemarchand-Béraud*, V. Jaussan, MG. Zürich, F. Gomez, Division d'Endocrinologie et Biochimie Clinique, CHUV, 1011 Lausanne, Switzerland.

The endocrine effects of fetal exposure to Spironolactone (SP), an aldosterone antagonist with weak antiandrogen and gestagen properties, were studied in the male offspring of rats that had been treated daily from gestation day 14 to 20 with 20 mg SP or the solvant vehicle (controls, C). Compared to C rats, at 70-80 days of age SP rats showed no alterations in their external genitalia but the weights of the ventral prostate (VP) and seminal vesicles (SV) were decreased. Basal and GnRH-induced LH, FSH, testosterone and 5αDHT were similar to C, but plasma and pituitary PRL were reduced (SP 6.8 ± 1.0 vs C 15.8 ± 2.8 ng/ml and 6.1 ± 1.2 vs 11.6 ± 1.8 µg/pituitary; mean ± SEM). The suggested partial peripheral androgen resistance underlying the low weights of VP and SV in the presence of normal androgen did not appear to be due to modifications of androgen receptors since cytosolic and nuclear androgen receptors in VP were normal. The decreased growth of the sex accessory organs may be attributed to the low PRL secretion in view of the known trophic effect of PRL on these organs. Similar results were observed in rats exposed in utero to Cyproterone acetate (an antiandrogen and gestagen) but not in rats exposed to Norethisterone (gestagen only) suggestive that the effect of SP on PRL is due to its antiandrogenic properties. In conclusion in utero exposure to SP is associated with a normal testicular function in the adult offspring in spite of hypoprolactinemia.

1311 POSSIBLE ROLE OF THE TESTIS IN THE INHIBITORY EFFECT OF THE ADRENAL ON PROLACTIN SECRETION IN THE MALE RAT. A. Lopez-Calderon and J.A.F. Tresguerres*, Chair Exptl. Endocrinology. Dept. Physiology. Fac. Medicina, Univ. Complutense, Madrid-3, SPAIN.

Adrenalectomy in the intact rat is associated with an increase in prolactin (PRL) levels (105 ± 15 ng/ml ± s.e.m. vs 74 ± 12 ng/ml ± s.e.m. in the fourth day), whereas chronic treatment with 1-24 ACTH (3 IU/100 g b.w.) or dexamethasone (DXM) (50 µg/100 g b.w.) shows a marked reduction of PRL plasma values reaching nearly the 12% of the control values in both cases ($P < 0.001$). The testis seems to be involved in this action since adrenalectomy or ACTH administration are not able to modify plasma PRL values 7 days after castration. In the long term castrated rat (62 days after) DXM exerts a marked reduction of plasma PRL levels in the sham operated rat whereas a significantly lower decrease can be found in orquidectomized animals. In order to study the possible role of gonadal steroids on this effect, castrated or sham operated rats chronically treated with ACTH or DXM where submitted to a challenge with 50 µg of estradiol benzoate (EB), plasma PRL response was studied 24 and 48 h. later. ACTH treatment completly blocks and DXM significantly reduces PRL response to EB in castrated and sham operated rat. These results suggest that glucocorticoids may antagonice the stimulatory action of gonadal steroids on PRL secretion. This work has been possible through the grant nº 4290 of the CAICYT. PRL has been supplied by the NIAMDD.

1312 PROLACTIN SECRETION BY INDIVIDUAL LACTOTROPES: A POPULATION ANALYSIS. E.H. Luque*, M. Munoz de Toro and J.D. Neill. Dept. of Physiology and Biophysics, Univ. of Alabama in Birmingham, AL 35294 USA

Prolactin (Prl) secretion from individual lactotropes can be microscopically visualized and measured using a reverse hemolytic plaque assay (Endocrinology 112: 1135, 1983). In the present study, we investigated whether rat lactotropes can be grouped into sub-populations (Prl secretion/lactotrope) under basal, inhibited, or stimulated conditions. In proestrus, ovariectomized (ovx.), and estrogen(E)-treated ovx. animals, ∿ 55% of the adenohypophyseal cells secreted prolactin; however, mean Prl secretion/lactotrope, as measured by extent of hemolysis (plaque size) in ovx. animals was about half that in proestrus or E-treated ovx. animals. The frequency distribution of amount of Prl secreted/lactotrope in proestrus rats was unimodal. Maximally inhibitory doses of dopamine (DA) (10^{-5}M) and bromocryptine (Br) (10^{-7}M), as determined from complete dose response curves, reduced Prl secretion/lactotrope to ∿ 20-25% and the number of secretory cells to ∿ 70% as compared to control proestrus levels. TRH increased Prl secretion/lactotrope to 125-150% of control levels without affecting the number of secretory cells. TRH (10^{-7}M) partially reversed the inhibitory effect of Br (10^{-7}M) and DA (10^{-5}M). The frequency distribution remained unimodal after DA or Br, TRH, and TRH/Br -- Prl secretion/lactotrope being shifted to smaller numbers and to larger numbers, respectively. Based on responsiveness to inhibitory and stimulatory secretagogues, lactotropes appear to be composed of a single population.

1313 THE TEMPORAL PATTERN OF HUMAN PROLACTIN RELEASE IS GENETICALLY DETERMINED.
M. L'Hermite*, E. Van Cauter, M. Baleriaux, J. Mendlewicz and P. Linkowski, School of Medicine, Free University of Brussels, Belgium.

The 24-h profile of plasma PRL was obtained at 15-min intervals in 8 pairs of male monozygotic twins, aged 16-28. All were studied in the same laboratory following the same protocol, including similar bedtimes, mealtimes and periods of adaptation to the environment. Sleep was polygraphically monitored. The same data were used to form 8 pairs of age-matched non-twin profiles by random selection. PRL levels were measured by radioimmunoassay using AFP reagents of the NPA, NIH. A best-fit curve, based on the periodogram method, was computed for each profile. This method allows for the estimation of the timing and magnitude of the nocturnal PRL elevation independently of episodic variations. Each 24-h PRL profile was quantitatively characterized by the mean level during the wake period, mean level during sleep, ratio of sleep mean to wake mean and level and timing of the nocturnal acrophase. The similarity of each of these parameters was determined from the coefficients of variation (CV) within each pair of profiles. For the 8 non-twin pairs of PRL profiles, the CV were: wake mean: 14.9 ± 17.2%, sleep mean: 25.8 ± 13.7%, sleep/wake ratio: 21.0 ± 12.2%, level of nocturnal acrophase: 26.7 ± 13.2%. The corresponding values for the 8 twin pairs were significantly lower: 4.4 ± 4.1% (p=.03), 12.1 ± 12.6% (p=.02), 10.9 ± 14.4% (p=.03) and 11.5 ± 8.2% (p=.01). There was no significant difference in the reproducibility of the timing of the nocturnal acrophase. These results indicate that the temporal organization of spontaneous PRL release has a genetic component.

1314 EFFECT OF BROMOCRIPTINE(BE) AND TRH ON PLASMA CATECHOLAMINES(CA) IN NORMAL SUBJECTS AND PRL-SECRETING TUMOR PATIENTS.
A. Mancini*, M. Barontini, I. Armando, G. Levin, J. Razumny and I. Molocznik. CEDIE Hospital de Niños. Medicina Nuclear-Endocrinología, Hospital Español, Av. Belgrano 2975-(1209) Buenos Aires, Argentina.

The effect of placebo or chronic BE(5mg/day/5 days) on plasma epinephrine (E), norepinephrine(NE), dopamine (DA), PRL and LH was studied in 4 normal (C) and 6 PRL secreting tumor women (P). Blood was sampled each 15 min. during 210 min. No significant differences were found between C and P when studied on placebo in E, NE, DA and LH levels. During the study period plasma CA levels showed clear fluctuations (25% above the $\bar{X}$ 210 min. concentration) in either C or P. BE induced: 1) a decrease in PRL (placebo C 12±3; P 122±51 ng/ml) which was similar in both groups (C 67%; P 70%). 2) a decrease in NE in all C (placebo 277±47; BE 163±14 pg/ml, $p<0.05$) and half of the P. The effect of TRH(200 μg) either in subjects on placebo or BEC was also studied. TRH was injected after the 210 min. sample and 2 additional samples were drawn. Under placebo TRH induced in C a 6 fold increase in PRL, while it only increased in 1 P(p=0.048). Under BE, TRH induced PRL increments in all C and 3 P. TRH induced no consistent changes in E, NE, DA and LH neither under placebo nor under BE. This study shows that chronic BE induces in normals a decrease in plasma NE, as it was shown in acute studies. No consistent response was found in tumoral patients.

1315 ABNORMAL PITUITARY FUNCTION IN PATIENTS WITH SEVERE CYCLICAL MASTALGIA AND NODULAR BREASTS. R.E. MANSEL,* S. KUMAR, M. SCANLON, UNIVERSITY DEPARTMENTS OF SURGERY AND MEDICINE, WELSH NATIONAL SCHOOL OF MEDICINE, CARDIFF CF4 4XN UK.

We have tested the hypothalamic control of pituitary hormones in patients with severe cyclical mastalgia with lumpy breasts (CM), non cyclical mastalgia (NCM) and controls (C) in two separate groups. Gp.1 by TRH/LH-RH (Numbers CM=17, NCM=7, C=11) and Gp. 2 by Domperidone (CM=12, C=11) i.v. bolus injections. All subjects were premenopausal with no endocrine problem or intake of exogenous hormones. All cases were tested in luteal phase, between 9am to 1pm and sera were batch assayed by automated radioimmunoassay. Non parametric and parametric analysis on log transformed data were performed. Samples were serially collected from an indwelling cannula and estimated for Prolactin, TSH, LH and FSH. The basal samples were also assayed for free and total T3 and T4, Progesterone and Oestradiol 17β and these did not differ significantly in patients and controls and remained within normal limits. Peak TSH responses to TRH and dopamine blockade were not different in any of the groups suggesting a normal thyroid status. The peak Prolactin responses to both TRH and Domperidone were significantly greater (Gp.1 $p<.05$; Gp.2 $p<.002$) in CM as compared to NCM and controls (Gp.1 CM=3792±920; NCM=1297±239; C=1587±325 and Gp.2 CM=8138±768; C=4028±581 mU/L±1SE). LH and FSH peak responses to LH-RH were also significantly greater in CM patients (LH: CM=39±5; C=22±5 U/L±1SE and FSH: CM=11±1; C=7±1 mU/L±1SE, $p<.05$). Altered endogenous dopaminergic activity or relative hyperoestrogenism could account for these responses although one could not exclude hypothalamic disturbance. This study provides a putative hormonal basis for cyclical mastalgia.

1316 IN VITRO PRODUCTION OF PROSTACYCLIN METABOLITE ($6KPGF_{1\alpha}$) BY UTERINE (UT) AND OMENTAL (SYS) ARTERIES FROM EARLY AND LATE POSTPARTUM EWES: EFFECT OF ANGIOTENSIN II (AII) AND SARALASIN(S). Ronald R. Magness*, Kwabena Osei-Boaten, Murray D. Mitchell, Charles R. Rosenfeld, Depts. Peds, Ob-Gyn, and Biochem., Southwestern Med. Sch., Dallas, Texas.

Ovine and human pregnancy are associated with reduced systemic pressor responses to AII. Furthermore, in pregnant ewes the uterine vasculature is less responsive than systemic vasculature to AII-induced vasoconstriction. To determine if this refractoriness might be due to alterations in vessel production of prostacyclin, we obtained ovine UT and SYS artery segments (∿30mg) from ewes on postpartum days 1-4 (early; n=10) or >7 days (late; n=7), and incubated them for 1hr in 4ml of oxygenated (95:5%=O_2:CO_2) Krebs-Hengseleit (37°C; pH=7.43) alone, with aspirin, or with 4 doses of AII ($5x10^{-9}$ to $5x10^{-6}$M). Aspirin inhibited $6KPGF_{1\alpha}$ formation in both UT and SYS vessels*. Control early-UT and -SYS arteries produced more $6KPGF_{1\alpha}$ than late vessels (165±34 [$\bar{X}$±SE] pg/mg·hr and 79±22 versus 13±7* and 27±7*, respectively). Although $6KPGF_{1\alpha}$ synthesis by early-UT arteries was greater than SYS vessels*, this was not seen with late vessels. AII led to increased $6KPGF_{1\alpha}$ synthesis only in early-UT arteries; however, there was no dose response, $6KPGF_{1\alpha}$ increasing to a mean of 255±24. The addition of S inhibited $6KPGF_{1\alpha}$ production at all 4 doses of AII studied* (e.g., $6KPGF_{1\alpha}$ was 261±61 without S and 173±35 with S at $5x10^{-6}$M AII). During pregnancy, systemic vascular refractoriness to AII and reduced sensitivity of the uterine as compared to systemic vasculature may be mediated by vessel production of prostacyclin. *$p<.05$.

1317 CORTICOTROPIN-RELEASING FACTOR (CRF) STIMULATES NOT ONLY PLASMA CORTICOSTERONE BUT ALSO ALDOSTERONE AND 18-HYDROXYCORTICOSTERONE IN THE RAT.

C. Maser-Gluth*, A. Toygar and P. Vecsei. Dept. of Pharmacology, University Heidelberg, FRG.

The reaction of aldosterone and 18-hydroxycorticosterone to corticotropin-releasing factor (CRF) has been studied in the rat. 8 µg of ovine CRF was injected intravenously in nembutal anaesthetized rats and the animals were decapitated between noon and 1.p.m. to eliminate circadian variations.CRF caused a significant increase in aldosterone and in 18-hydroxycorticosterone 0.5h after injection ($p<0.01$). This was accompanied by an expected rise in corticosterone and ACTH. 2h after CRF administration ACTH and corticosteroid levels were still elevated. However, after 6h, a dissociation between corticosterone, 18-hydroxycorticosterone and aldosterone was seen. The aldosterone concentration remained moderately but significantly higher (10.8 ± 2.9 ng/dl) than the corresponding control (4.3 ± 1.3 ng/dl), while the 18-hydroxycorticosterone and corticosterone levels were decreased (43.7 ± 4.0 ng/dl vs. 104.4 ± 23.0 ng/dl for 18-hydroxycorticosterone, and 2.5 ± 0.7 µg/dl vs. 12.6 ± 9.1 µg/dl for corticosterone).

The present data clearly demonstrate the aldosterone and 18-hydroxycorticosterone stimulating effect of CRF. The dissociation between corticosterone, 18-hydroxycorticosterone and aldosterone is unusual since under numerous experimental and pathological conditions both steroids show parallel changes. The reason for the lowering of corticosterone and 18-hydroxycorticosterone levels observed 6h after CRF administration is yet unclear since the ACTH concentration remained unaltered. It is apparently mediated through an ACTH independent mechanism.

1318 LATE PUBERTAL DEVELOPMENT: THE ROLE OF OPIOID TONUS.

M. Giusti*, G. Mazzocchi, L. Granziera, D. Bessarione, M. Contessini, W. Tarditi, D. Mignone and G. Giordano.
Department of Endocrinology, University of Genoa, I-16132 Genoa, Italy.

Opiate peptides have been shown to decrease LH release in man while naloxone, a specific blocker drug of opioid receptors, has an opposite effect. In this study we have evaluated the effect of continuous infusion of naloxone on LH,FSH,Testosterone (T) and Prolactin (PRL) secretion in a group of 9 sexually immature children aged 11.3-16.5 yrs. Saline solution (0.9%) on the 4th day of hospital life, and naloxone-HCl (0.05 Kg/BW hour) on the 5th day were infused by means of a portable pump. Blood samples were collected hourly with a continuous sampling technique. Lights were turned off between 22:00-07:00 hour, sleep was monitored visually by trained medical personnel. LH,FSH,PRL and T were assayed by RIA. The analysis of the data was performed by using the paired "t" test. The sleep period was superimposable during the 2 nights. During the saline infusion: a sleep related surge of LH titers was present in 5; a nocturnal increase of T levels was found in 3 patients, while a sleep-wake rhythm of PRL secretion was observed in all children. During naloxone administration: no variations in PRL and T secretory patterns but an increase of LH titers in 5 patients, were observed. No correlation between LH response to naloxone and cronological or bone age and between LH and T rates was found. These data seem to esclude a role of the opioid tonus in the physiopathology of delayed puberty with hypogonadotropinism, and indicate that the blockade of opioid receptors can cause a LH secretory response even in some subjects with variable degrees of delayed pubertal development and androgenic priming.

1319 APPLICATION OF A SIMPLE RECEPTOR ASSAY TO STUDY ANDROGEN ACTION IN THE ANDROGEN INSENSITIVITY SYNDROME. I.A. Hughes* and B.A.J. Evans, Department of Child Health, Welsh National School of Medicine, Cardiff CF4 4XN, U.K.

A simple, reproducible dispersed cell assay was used to study androgen-receptor binding in genital skin fibroblasts established from patients with the phenotype of: (a) complete androgen insensitivity syndrome (CAIS, n=6) (b) partial androgen insensitivity syndrome (PAIS, n=11) and (c) a mixed group of micropenis/hypospadias (M/H, n=10). Normal values were determined in cell lines established from 19 circumcised children. Parameters of binding routinely measured included: (1) receptor concentration (Bmax) and binding affinity (Kd) determined at 37°C using [^{3}H]-DHT (2) thermolability of binding at 40°C defined as a change in specific binding outside a range of 84-110% of binding at 37°C and (3) augmentation of specific binding after preincubation with 3nM [^{3}H]-DHT for 20 hr, expressed as a ratio of basal binding; a normal response was an augmented: basal ratio more than 1.4:1. Bmax and Kd in normals was 804 $\pm$ 172 x 10^{-18}moles/ug DNA (mean $\pm$ SD) and 0.92 $\pm$ 0.32 x 10^{-10}M respectively. CAIS (33%), PAIS (82%) and M/H (100%) patients were receptor positive; all had a normal Kd. In 2 patients (1 CAIS, 1 PAIS) the receptor was thermolabile (62% and 38% respectively). Augmentation did not occur in 29% of PAIS studied, whereas 2 receptor positive CAIS patients with a markedly elevated Bmax did augment further following androgen preincubation. The dispersed cell assay provides a useful initial functional classification of patients with AIS, and serves as a possible in vitro bioassay to predict in vivo responsiveness to exogenous androgens given after birth or endogenously produced at puberty.

1320 DIRECT EVIDENCE FOR ACTIVATION OF THE CNS-PITUITARY MECHANISM FOR LH SECRETION AT PUBERTY IN THE MALE RAT. A.E. Karpas*, A.M. Matsumoto, and W.J. Bremner, Endocrinology, VA Med Ctr; Dept. Med., Univ. Wash., Seattle, WA 98108.

The mechanism underlying the pubertal rise in testosterone (T) levels at 45-60 days of age (D) in male rats is controversial since little change occurs in LH levels at this time. We determined whether experimental maintenance of stable, early pubertal T levels in these animals as they passed through the normal age of puberty would allow demonstration of a major increase in serum LH levels. At 15D, 160 male rats were divided into three groups. 80 rats were castrated and implanted with silastic capsules containing T (CASTR+T), 40 rats were left intact and implanted with empty capsules (INTACT), and 40 rats were castrated and implanted with empty capsules (CASTR). At 29,36,40,43,47,51,54 and 58D, blood was drawn from 5-8 animals in each group for measurement of LH and T by RIA. Only CASTR+T rats whose T was <1.6 ng/ml were considered (upper range for intact early pubertal controls). In these rats, T level was 0.9±0.03 ($\bar{x}$±SEM) with no significant difference among age groups (ANOVA); LH levels were suppressed (<100 ng/ml RP-1) until 47D when they rose to 212±42 (p<0.05) and reached 653±95 by 58D. In INTACT rats, T levels remained <1.6 until 54D and rose to 3.2±0.1 by 58D; LH levels (80±7) did not differ among age groups. In CASTR rats, LH reached adult castrate levels (765±105) by 29D while T levels remained <0.2 throughout the study. **Conclusions:** Constant, early pubertal levels of T are able to suppress LH levels in CASTR rats until the normal age of puberty (45-60D), at which time LH levels increase markedly. These results provide direct evidence for activation of the CNS-pituitary mechanism for LH secretion at puberty in the male rat. The CASTR+T rat is a good model for studying the CNS-pituitary changes underlying normal puberty.

1321 MOLECULAR CLONING OF A cDNA FOR THE CHICKEN PROGESTERONE RECEPTOR B ANTIGEN, M. Kulomaa*, T. Schulz, D. Headon, N. Weigel, M. Baez, and B. W. O'Malley, Baylor College of Medicine, Dept. of Cell Biology, Houston, TX. 77030 USA; D. Edwards, and W. McGuire, University Texas Health Science Center, Dept. of Medicine, San Antonio, TX. 78284 USA.

A cDNA library generated from size-selected poly(A)$^+$-RNA isolated from oviducts of estrogen-stimulated chicks was screened by a high-affinity monoclonal antibody (αPR^B; 9G10) raised against the B subunit (M_r=108K) of the hen oviduct progesterone receptor (PR^B). Positive clones were used to hybrid select mRNA, which was translated in a rabbit reticulocyte lysate system. One clone, pPRB-1, specifically yielded a translation product of 108K which could be precipitated with αPR^B. The immunoprecipitated $[^{35}S]PR^B$ co-migrated with authentic PR^B when analyzed for size and isoelectric point on 2-D gels. Moreover, comparison of peptides produced by partial digestion of PR^B and $[^{35}S]PR^B$ showed similar patterns. Using a $[^{32}P]$-labelled cDNA insert from pPRB-1 as a probe, additional cDNA clones for PR^B have been isolated. Furthermore, a mRNA of sufficient length to encode PR^B was identified by Northern analysis of oviduct total RNA. Finally, the concentration of the mRNA was greatly reduced in the oviduct of estrogen withdrawn chick when compared to that of hormonally stimulated chick. This corroborates earlier studies showing that cellular levels of PR^B in the oviduct are regulated by estrogen.

1322 STEROID RECEPTORS IN OVARIAN TUMORS OF HUMAN SUBJECTS. H. Kusanishi*, T. Tamaya and H. Okada, Dept. of OB/GYN, Kyoto Pref. Univ. Med., Kyoto 602, Japan.

Steroids have the bilogical effects on the normal ovaries and even the therapeutic effects on the malignant ovarian tumors in human subjects. Therefore receptors for estrogens(ER), progestogen(PR) and androgen(AR) were investigated in ovarian tumors. Steroid receptors, especially in ovarian cancer cytosol, were sedimented to 8S and 5S and had a dissociation constant(Kd) of (18.7±7.5)nM (n=20) for ER, (8.4±2.2)nM (n=10) for PR and (7.8±2.4)nM (n=6) for AR in ovarian malignant tumors. Ovarian benign and malignant tumors contained various steroid receptors, where cytosol ER was detected in 79%(n=43). It is speculated that estrogen action may be present in ovarian tumors. Mucinous cystadenocarcinoma and endometrioid adenocarcinoma contained cytosol ER and PR with high quantity and frequency. Cytosol PR and AR were not detected in most cases of serous cystadenocarcinoma and undifferentiated adenocarcinoma. After the operation and chemotherapy, the stage II and III cases with ER presence and PR absence in cytosol showed longer term of remission than those with the presence of both ER and PR. The latter cases may be responsive to endocrine therapy. In nuclear KCl extract and KCl-resistant fractions of given cases, steroid receptors were detected. These findings suggest that each steroid demonstrate the effect on nuclear mechanism. The morphometric analysis showed that the level of ER and PR was not related to the nuclear configuration constant. The results indicate that histological grade was not related to steroid receptor level, possibly due to the histological complexity of malignant ovarian tumors.

1323 HIGH AFFINITY BINDING SITES FOR TRIPHENYLETHYLENE ANTIESTROGENS IN THE CHICKEN.

C.B. Lazier*, P.R. Murphy, C. Butts, A. Gillis, K. Lonergan. Department of Biochemistry, Dalhousie University, Halifax, Nova Scotia, Canada B3H 4H7.

In addition to interaction with the estrogen receptor (ER) in estrogen target tissues, the antiestrogens (AE) bind with high affinity and distinctive specificity to estrogen non-competable AE binding sites (AEBS) in a number of tissues and in serum. We have examined the tissue and intracellular distribution and ligand specificity of the AEBS using competitive binding analysis with [^{3}H]-tamoxifen (TAM). Highest concentrations (20-40 pmol/g tissue) of AEBS are present in cytosol and microsome fractions of liver from male and female immature chickens and in oviduct of estrogen-treated birds. In addition, salt extracts of purified nuclei (NSE) from these tissues contain about 3 pmol/g of a single class of high-affinity (Kd 2-4 nM) AEBS. The concentration of the liver NSE AEBS is not altered on estrogen treatment even though the level of ER increases 10X. The relative binding affinities of various AE for these sites are as follows: nafoxidine (126%) > TAM (100%) >> N-desmethylTAM (15%) = CI628 > 4-OH-TAM (8%) = LY156758. Estradiol and 7 other steroids do not compete. Assay of the NSE AEBS is significantly enhanced by pretreatment of the tissue preparations with dextran-charcoal. Ether extracts of cockerel serum, whole nuclei or NSE from liver or oviduct contain a potent competitive inhibitor of [^{3}H]-TAM binding to the NSE AEBS. Sequential purification in 3 TLC systems separates the inhibitor from common estrogens. The purified material binds AEBS but not ER. These data suggest that the nuclear AEBS may be occupied in vivo by an endogenous ligand. Supported by the MRC and NCI, Canada.

1324 REGULATED EXPRESSION OF A METALLOTHIONEIN-SOMATOSTATIN FUSION GENE IN A HAMSTER KIDNEY CELL LINE.

M Low*, P Dee, R Goodman, R Palmiter, and J Habener, Department of Medicine, New England Medical Center, and Division of Molecular Endocrinology, Massachusetts General Hospital, Boston, MA, Department of Biochemistry, University of Washington, Seattle, WA.

To test the hypothesis that the proteolytic processing of pre-prosomatostatin (pre-proSS) to somatostatin 14 (SS14) and SS28 is specific to brain/gut cells that normally secrete SS we investigated the biosynthesis of SS in a cell line that does not normally produce peptide hormones. A DNA fragment containing the entire coding sequence for rat pre-proSS, previously cloned from a cDNA library of a medullary thyroid carcinoma, was ligated into a plasmid containing the metallothionein (MT) promoter. By inserting the SS cDNA next to the MT promoter SS production is controlled by ambient heavy metal levels. Baby hamster kidney (BHK) fibroblasts were cotransfected by calcium phosphate precipitation with this MT-SS fusion gene and a neomycin resistance gene. BHK cells containing integrated rat SS genes were selected by their resistance to a neomycin analog. Immunoreactive SS (IR-SS) was quantitated by RIA of acetic acid cell extracts and acidified media. Cells containing the fusion genes synthesized and exported nanogram amounts of IR-SS that chromatographed in positions compatible with the intact prohormone, SS14, SS28, and a predominant 7 K intermediate form. Incubation with 100 uM zinc sulphate caused a four to ten fold increase in IR-SS content of cells and media demonstrating that the SS gene expression was positively regulated by the MT promoter. We conclude that the enzymes responsible for processing of pre-proSS are not specific to neuroendocrine and gut secretory cells.

1325 PROGESTIN RECEPTORS IN THE BRAIN AND PITUITARY OF A PROGESTERONE "RESISTANT" PRIMATE N.J. MacLusky, G.P. Chrousos, D. Brandon, D.M. Renquist, D.L. Loriaux, M.B. Lipsett and F. Naftolin Dept. of OB/GYN, Yale University Medical School, New Haven, CT 06510 and Developmental Endocrinology Branch, NICHD, NIH, Bethesda, MD 20205
Female squirrel (SQ) monkeys (Saimiri sciureus) have higher circulating progesterone levels and lower progesterone sensitivity than 'Old World' monkeys such as the cynomolgus macaque (CYNO; Macaca Fascicularis). Previous studies have shown that the estrogen-inducibility of uterine cytoplasmic progestin receptors (PRCs) is lower in SQs than CYNOs (Chrousos et al, JCEM 55:364, 1982). The present study was performed to determine whether a similar difference exists in the hypothalamus-preoptic area (HPOA) and pituitary (PIT). SQ and CYNO monkeys were ovariectomized two weeks prior to use, treated with estradiol i.m. in sesame oil (10 µg./kg BW/day) for 2 days, then killed. Uterine, HPOA and PIT PRCs were labelled with [3H] R5020 and measured by Sephadex LH-20 gel filtration, as previously described (MacLusky et al., Endo 106:185, 1980). High-affinity, progestin-specific [3H] R5020 binding was detected in all tissues, from both species. There were no significant differences between SQ and CYNO tissues in the apparent equilibrium dissociation constants for [3H] R5020 binding (approx. 0.3 nM). Differences in PRC levels (fmoles/mg cytosol protein) were observed in the uterus (SQ 880±210, N=3; CYNO 3550±303, N=3) and PIT (SQ 106±24, N=5; CYNO 202±20, N=4); but not the HPOA (SQ 8.7±1.4, N=4); CYNO 10.1±1.8, N=4). These results confirm that the estrogen-inducibility of PRCs is lower in SQ than in CYNO monkeys; but suggest that this difference may not extend equally to central and peripheral progesterone target tissues. (Supported by NS19610 and HD13587)

1326 IDENTIFICATION AND HISTOCHEMICAL LOCALIZATION OF ^{3}H-21-DEHYDRO ORG2058 AFFINITY LABELED HUMAN PROGESTERONE RECEPTOR.
B.Manz*, T.Beck, A.Heubner, H.-J.Grill and K.Pollow. Abt. f. Experimentelle Endokrinologie, Universität Mainz, F.R.G.

Two independent lines of evidence are used to identify the 21-dehydro Org2058 labeled receptor in crude uterine cytosol. Fast protein liquid chromatography (FPLC) on Mono Q (ion exchange) and Mono P (chromatofocusing) columns concurrently identify only one specifically labeled protein. Native R5020, Org2058, progesterone or affinity labeled receptors elute at superimposable positions at both, sodium chlorid (Mono Q) or pH (Mono P) gradients.
Anti-Org2058 antibodies were obtained in rabbits by use of the 21-CMO-BSA-conjugate of 21-dehydro Org2058. The antibodies are able to recognize the affinity labeled receptor in crude cytosol and the resulting complexes are retained on protein A-sepharose columns. When progesterone receptor positive tissue slices are affinity labeled, specifically bound 21-dehydro Org2058 can be demonstrated with a modified peroxidase-antiperoxidase-(PAP-)method.

1327 POST-CASTRATION INTERVAL DOES NOT INFLUENCE ANDROGEN RECEPTOR LEVELS IN VARIOUS TISSUES OF THE MALE RHESUS MONKEY (M. mulatta). L.C. Krey* and R.M. Sapolsky. The Rockefeller University. New York, New York.USA.

In male monkeys testosterone is the primary testicular product responsible for the negative feedback control of gonadotropin release. However, long-term (6+weeks) castrates fail to respond to this steroid with a suppression of LH/FSH secretion. To examine the neuroendocrine bases for this deficit, we used ^{3}H-methyltrienolone (^{3}H-1881) to quantify androgen receptors in the hypothalamus+preoptic area (HPOA), anterior pituitary and other tissues from short-term (2day, n=3) and long-term (6-8weeks, n=3) castrate monkeys. Tissues were homogenized in a 10 mM Tris buffer (pH7.4) containing 1.5mM EDTA, 25mM sodium molybdate, 1mM dithiothreitol and 10%(v/v) glycerol. Cytosolic extracts (108,000xg) were incubated with 0.05-10nM ^{3}H-1881 (plus a 200-fold molar excess of triamcinolone acetonide) in the absence or presence of a 500-fold molar excess of 5α-dihydrotestosterone. Macromolecular-bound ^{3}H-1881 was separated on Sephadex LH-20 columns. Scatchard analyses of the specific binding data revealed the presence of a saturable, one-component binding site with affinity characteristics ($K_D \sim 10^{-10}$M) similar to those reported for androgen receptors in other species. Mean receptor levels (fmoles ^{3}H-1881/mg cytosolic protein) were highest in the seminal vesicle (65) and prostate (65) and lower in the pituitary gland (26), HPOA (20), liver (23) and heart (9). Significantly, receptor levels in the long-term castrates were comparable to or greater than those in the short-term castrates. Thus, these animals possess the physiologic potential to process a testosterone "signal" in both reproductive tract and neuroendocrine tissues. (Supported by a grant from the Rockefeller Foundation)

1328 BLOCKADE OF ANDROGEN ACTION BY ANANDRON, A PURE AND LONG ACTING ANTIANDROGEN. Moguilewsky, M.*, Coussedière, D., Pottier, J., Philibert, D., Raynaud, J.P. Centre de Recherches Roussel Uclaf 93230 Romainville, France.

Anandron (RU 23908) is a non steroidal pure antiandrogen. At 10 mg/kg, it antagonizes the androgen activity of testosterone propionate (TP) (50 μg/rat) in the castrated (CX) male rat. In vitro, anandron interacts weakly and transiently with the cytosolic androgen receptor (AR) since its relative binding affinity is 4.5, 1.1 and 0.4% of that of testosterone respectively after 30 min, 2 h and 24 h of incubation at 0°C. In vivo, anandron interacts with the prostatic AR as early as 15 min and up to 24 h after an oral administration of 10 mg/kg to CX rats, as indicated by the absence of free binding sites after 1 h incubation at 0°C with (^{3}H)RU 1881 in cytosols prepared from the prostates of treated rats. However anandron was rapidly exchanged in vitro by prolonging the time of incubation with (^{3}H)RU 1881, indicating that AR is still present in the cytosol and that no nuclear translocation has occured. When administered concomitently with TP (50 μg /rat), anandron impedes the binding of testosterone to AR and blocks the TP-induced cytosolic AR depletion and nuclear translocation, up to 24 h after the treatment. Thus, there is a sharp contrast between the rapid dissociation of anandron from the cytosolic AR in vitro and its in vivo sustained interaction with AR even in the presence of androgens. This difference might be explained by the unusual pharmacokinetic profile of plasma anandron. Following oral administration (10 mg/kg) to male rats, bioavailabitity is complete and the plasma concentration of anandron plateaus (5 μg/ml) for up to 6 h; thereafter, elimination is slow (half-life of about 7 h). The sustained plasma level of unchanged compound, also observed after an i.v.injection, might explain the antiandrogen activity of anandron in spite of its very low affinity for AR. Thus in vivo, the persistant large supply of anandron will achieve a constant blockade of androgen action by preventing the "activation" of the cytoplasmic AR.

1329 INTERACTION OF ANDROGEN RECEPTORS WITH RNA AND DNA.

E.Mulder*, A.A.Vrij, A.O.Brinkmann and H.J.van der Molen,
Dept.of Biochemistry, Erasmus Univ.Rotterdam, The Netherlands

Androgen receptors were isolated from prostates of castrated and non-castrated rats and partially purified by chromatography on 2',5'-ADP-Sepharose. The receptors were labelled with ^{3}H-5α-dihydrotestosterone; for the receptor from non-castrated rats an incubation period of three days at 4°C was necessary for optimal exchange. The partially purified receptor preparations were free of DNAse activity. From the castrated rats a receptor was isolated with sedimentation value and Stokes radius of approximately 4S and 2.8 nm. For a smaller form of the receptor obtained from the intact rats these values were 3S and 2.3 nm respectively. Some potent inhibitors of proteolysis added during isolation, did not have any significant effect on the form of the receptor. Both forms could be bound by ADP-Sepharose, but only the 4S-form showed a high affinity for DNA-Sepharose and ds DNA. In contrast both the 4S and 3S receptor forms interacted with equal affinity with prostate RNA. Certain polyribonucleotides were strongly bound by both forms of the receptor (e.g.poly UG) and competed more effectively for the receptor binding site than prostate RNA. These observations provide evidence that for DNA binding a different or additional part of the receptor molecule is required than for RNA and polyribonucleotide binding.

1330 STUDY OF GLUCOCORTICOID RECEPTOR IN MUSCLE ATROPHY.

Y. Miyachi*, K. Tanaka and H. Ideshita, Department of Internal Medicine and Nuclear Medicine, Shizuoka General Hospital, Shizuoka, Japan.

Exposure of muscle in vivo to glucocorticoids(G) results in a significant depression of protein synthesis and of muscle volume, however, the role of intramuscular G receptor(Grc) in the development of atrophy remains still unknown. In the present investigation we studied the levels and physico-chemical characteristics of Grc in the atrophied rat gastrocunemius muscle induced by unilateral sciatic nerve cutting and also in the atrophied muscle in patients with neurogenic myopathy. The atrophied muscles were homogenized in Tris-HCl buffer, centrifuged at 104,000G for 1 hour and the supernatant was used for the analysis of Grc. The binding capacity of Grc in the atrophied gastrocunemius muscles increased gradually without changes in Kd values after sciatic nerve cutting, and at 28days it was 0.076 ± 0.005pmoles/mg protein, three times that of the control muscle. Since the muscle volume decreased gradually, the total contents of Grc were slightly higher in the atrophied muscle. The molecular weight of Grc in the control and atrophied muscles, analyzed by Sephacryl S-300 gel chromatography, was found to be approximately 80,000daltons. Grc in the atrophied muscle degradated rapidly in vitro at 20 and 37C compared with that in the control muscle, suggesting the increase of Grc in the atrophied muscle is not the inhibition of Grc degradation. The addition of sodium molibdate(10mM) protected partly the degradation of Grc in the atrophied muscle. The very similar findings were observed in the Grc of the atrophied muscle in patients with neurogenic myopathy. These results suggest that the known catabolic effects of G on muscle may relate the increase in Grc with enhanced G actions.

1331 DIFFERENT LOCALIZATIONS OF MINERALO- AND GLUCOCORTICOID RECEPTORS IN RAT HIPPOCAMPUS. M. Moguilewsky*, C. Gueniau, D. Lecaque and M.M. Bouton, Centre de Recherches Roussel-Uclaf, F93230 Romainville, France.

Aldosterone (A), corticosterone (B) and dexamethasone (DM) bind to at least 2 sites in the rat hippocampus. Autoradiographic studies revealed ^{3}H-B and ^{3}H-A neuronal labeling (pyramidal neurons of CA_1 and CA_2 areas), while they suggested that the lower ^{3}H-DM labeling could be confined to glial cells. We studied the influence of a 30 min forebrain ischemia (Pulsinelli) (which leads to a total degradation of the pyramidal neurons after 3 days followed by an appearance of glial cells 14 days after in the CA_1 area of the dorsal hippocampus), on ^{3}H-B, ^{3}H-A and ^{3}H-DM binding sites concentration and specificity in the hippocampus. In sham-operated rats CA_1 area, only ^{3}H-B and ^{3}H-A specific binding sites were detectable (200 and 80 fmoles/mg protein respectively) while no high affinity ^{3}H-DM binding sites could be detected. Three days and 14 days after ischemia, a total loss of ^{3}H-A and a partial loss (60%) of ^{3}H-B binding sites were recorded concomitently with the neuronal destruction. No ^{3}H-DM binding sites still could be detected even when glial cells appeared (14 days). The specificities of the ^{3}H-B and ^{3}H-A receptor in this CA_1 area, were strictly similar and of the "mineralocorticoid" type (B $>$ A=cortisol $>$ DM $>$ spironolactone and no displacement by RU 38486,a potent antiglucocorticoid, nor by RU 26988, a pure glucocorticoid). In the other hippocampal regions, ^{3}H-DM bound not only to a similar mineralocorticoid receptor but also to a classic "glucocorticoid" receptor (RU 38486 $\geq$ DM=RU 26988=B $>$ cortisol $\gg$ A). These results confirm the neuronal localization (pyramidal neurons) of ^{3}H-B and ^{3}H-A binding sites in the CA_1 area of the rat hippocampus (same mineralocorticoid specific receptor?) and the absence of ^{3}H-DM binding (glucocorticoid receptor) in these neurons.

1332 CHICK ERYTHROCYTE GLUCOCORTICOID RECEPTOR.
T. Murakami* and N. Ohsawa, The Third Department of Internal Medicine, Faculty of Medicine, University of Tokyo, 7-3-1 Hongo, Bunkyo-ku, Tokyo, Japan.

Human circulating red cell does not have glucocorticoid receptor probably due to the lack of nucleus. We have characterized the glucocorticoid receptor in chick erythrocytes which have nuclei. The Scatchard plot analysis of (^{3}H)-dexamethasone (Dex) binding to chick erythrocytes showed a single class of binding sites at 20°C. The apparent K_d of (^{3}H)-Dex binding to erythrocytes was 0.31 nM after 1 hour incubation and decreased to 0.12 nM after 8 hours incubation at 20°C. The maximum binding capacity was 5.1 fmol/10^7 cells. This value was approximately 1/10 of the value for goat mononuclear leukocytes (MNL)(1). Cells were incubated at 20°C in 5.0 nM (^{3}H)-Dex for the kinetic studies of (^{3}H)-Dex binding. The association rate constant (k_1) was $11.8 \times 10^6 M^{-1} min^{-1}$. A 1000 fold chase of unlabeled Dex was added to study the subsequent dissociation of bound (^{3}H)-Dex. The dissociation of (^{3}H)-Dex from erythrocytes consists of two components. The rate constants were $-16 \times 10^{-3} min^{-1}$ (k_{-1}) for the rapid component and $-1.2 \times 10^{-3} min^{-1}$ (k'_{-1}) for the slow component. These values were very similar to those reported for goat MNL (1). The value of k'_{-1}/k_1 was 0.10 nM. This value approximates to the K_d after 8 hours incubation. The apparent K_d of (^{3}H)-Dex binding to cytosol receptor was 0.6 nM. Steroid binding specificity was similar to that reported for goat MNL. These data demonstrate that chick erythrocyte has a high affinity glucocorticoid receptor.

(1) Murakami et al., Endocrinology 104: 505, 1979.

1333 DEMONSTRATION OF A GENETIC DEFECT IN THE INSULIN RECEPTOR KINASE OF CULTURED FIBROBLASTS IN TYPE A SYNDROME OF INSULIN RESISTANCE.

F. Grigorescu*, G.L. King and C.R. Kahn, Joslin Diabetes Center, Boston, MA.

The Type A syndrome of insulin resistance and acanthosis nigricans is characterized by a major impairment of insulin action at the cellular level. Recently we have shown that this may be accompanied by an abnormality of phosphorylation of insulin receptors on circulating erythrocytes. To define a possible genetic defect of the insulin-receptor kinase, we have examined binding and phosphorylation of the insulin receptor using fibroblasts cultured from a patient with this syndrome. ^{125}I-insulin binding to fibroblasts was decreased by 70% when compared to normal. This decrease in binding persisted up to 10 passages of these cells. IGF-I and MSA (IGF-II) binding were normal, as was cellular growth and insulin stimulated thymidine incorporation into DNA. The kinase properties of the receptor were measured in the Triton-extracted receptor either by direct immunoprecipitation with anti-receptor antibody or in a receptor partially purified by wheat germ agglutinin affinity chromatography. When normal receptor was incubated with [^{32}P-γ] ATP, Mn^{2+} and various concentrations of insulin, a 3-5-fold stimulation of phosphorylation of the β-subunit of the receptor could be identified by gel electrophoresis and autoradiography. With receptors from the patient, phosphorylation was decreased by 70-80% over the entire dose-response curve. This was consistent with the insulin binding defect and was persistent during serial passage. We conclude that the Type A syndrome of insulin resistance is due to a genetic defect in the insulin receptor which is reflected in its binding and kinase properties.

1334 INSULIN RECEPTORS: REDOX STATE AND SUBUNIT LABELING; EFFECT OF COLLAGENASE TREATMENT.

F. Haynes* and C. Yip, Dept. of Physiology and Banting and Best Dept. Med. Res. Univ. Toronto, TORONTO, Ont. Canada, M5G IL6.

Receptors for insulin are comprised of glycoprotein subunits linked by disulfide bonds. Light-sensitive derivatives of insulin identified these receptors as Mr 380 kDa proteins. Endogenously, disulfide bonds between subunits are differentially reduced such that the 380 kDa species were resolved into three forms of 380, 300 and 230 kDa, during gel electrophoresis, through the loss of non-covalently attached subunits. Sulfhydryl alkylating agents converted the 300 and 230 forms to the 380 kDa species while dithiothreitol converted the 380 form to the 300 and 230 kDa species. In hepatic tissue subunits of Mr 110, 100, 80 and 40 kDa were identified which, upon reduction, changed to 130, 115, 90 and 40 kDa respectively indicating the presence of internal disulfide bonds. Collagenase treatment of PM from adipose, hepatic, placental, muscle and kidney tissue altered the electrophoretic mobility of the receptor from 380 to 300 kDa. In hepatic PM, this treatment also decreased the amount of 110 kDa subunit detected, but, increased the labeling of the 115 kDa subunit. A 115 kDa subunit was also labeled in placental and brain PM. The 115 kDa subunit in brain PM was insensitive to neuraminidase. Compared to hepatic tissue, the receptor in adipose tissue existed in a more oxidised state, and upon reduction yielded subunits of 130, 90, 85 and 40 kDa. Consequently, insulin receptors demonstrate tissue specific differences in redox state and subunit labeling. These findings may relate to the differences in insulin binding and action in these tissues.

* Commonwealth Scholarship Awardee. Study supported by, MRC and Best Fdn.

1335 INSULIN-LIKE ACTIVITY OF BOUND WHEAT GERM LECTIN ON CELLS WITH FEW OR NO SURFACE INSULIN RECEPTORS.

C. Hofmann*, P. Bruns, and P. Hessel, Dept. of Surg. and Biochem., Loyola University Stritch School of Medicine, Maywood, IL and Research Service, VA Hospital, Hines, IL USA

In Madin-Darby canine kidney (MDCK) cells, specific plasma membrane binding of ^{125}I-insulin was undetectable. Correspondingly, neither insulin-stimulated incorporation of [^{14}C]glucose into glycogen, nor insulin-induced uptake of radiolabeled α-aminoisobutyrate ([^{3}H]AIB) could be demonstrated. When MDCK cells were preincubated with serum containing antibodies to the insulin receptor and subsequently incubated with ^{125}I-protein A, no insulin receptors were radiolabeled. Comparable studies in control hepatoma cells (H4) showed that these cells bound insulin, responded with increased glycogen synthesis and amino acid uptake, and possessed immunologically recognizable insulin receptors. In MDCK cells, the lectin wheat germ agglutinin (WGA, 30μg/ml) induced the insulin-like response of stimulated [^{3}H]AIB uptake (166%, control= 100%). Furthermore, when these cells were preincubated for 30 minutes with WGA (30μg/ml), rinsed to remove unbound lectin, and further incubated 4 hours, induction of stimulated [^{3}H]AIB uptake still occurred. Such stimulation was completely reversed by simultaneous incubation of cells with N-acetyl-D-glucosamine (10mM) and WGA, but was also depleted when the saccharide was added following the initial incubation with WGA. Thus, while MDCK cells appeared to have few or no cell surface insulin receptors, binding of the lectin WGA produced an insulin-like effect which could be terminated by dissociation of the bound lectin.

1336 MONENSIN AS RECYCLING INHIBITOR ENHANCES DOWN REGULATION OF hGH RECEPTOR.

N. Hizuka*, K. Takano, S. Hasegawa, S. Saito, N. Honda and K. Shizume Dept. of Medicine, Tokyo Women's Medical College, Tokyo 162, JAPAN

Polypeptide hormone binds to cell surface receptor and is subsequently internalized by the cell as function of time and temperature. The receptor is also internalized with hormone, and the internalized receptor might be degraded or recycled to cell surface. It has been hypothesized that the recycling of receptor is involved in the process of receptor down regulation. To test the hypothesis, we have investigated the effect of monensin as recycling inhibitor on hGH receptor of cultured human lymphocytes (IM-9 cells). When the IM-9 cells were incubated with 125I-hGH at 37°C, in which condition hGH was rapidly internalized in the presence or absence of monensin, monensin (0.1 - 10 μM) increased the cell-associated 125I-hGH. In addition, monensin decreased dissociation of 125I-hGH from the cell and the degradation of 125I-hGH at 37°C. At 15°C, however, monensin had no effect. When the cells were preincubated with unlabeled hGH (5 ng/ml) at 37°C for 3 hours, the 125I-hGH binding to the cells was decreased to 68.0 ± 0.9 % of control binding preincubated without hGH (i.e. down regulation of hGH receptor was occured). Presence of 10 μM monensin in the preincubation media enhanced the down regulation of hGH receptor, i.e. the 125I-hGH binding to the cells was decreased to 55.4 ± 2.4 % of control (p<0.01). These data support the concept that the recycling of receptor is involved in down regulation of receptor.

1337 CHANGES IN THYROTROPIN DISPLACING IMMUNOGLOBULINS(TDI) IN SERA OF PATIENTS WITH GRAVES' DISEASE DURING LONG TERM TREATMENT WITH THIONAMIDE DRUGS: DETERMINATIONS BY RADIORECEPTOR ASSAY. T.Iiri*, H.Uchimura, N.Akimoto, T.Mitsuhashi, K.Kubota, N.Kuzuya, Y.Imai, H.Ikeda, F.Matsuzaki, and L.F.Kumagai, The Third Department of Internal Medicine, Faculty of Medicine University of Tokyo, Hongo, Tokyo, Japan.

TDI's are presumed to be closely related to the pathogenesis of Graves' disease. Recently a radioreceptor assay kit for TDI using solubilized porcine TSH receptors has become available for routine clinical use (Japan Travenol,Inc.). The present study was aimed to evaluate its usefulness in determining TDI's as markers during treatment and follow-up of Graves' patients. TDI's were measured in sera of 288 patiens with Graves' disease who were followed 0-25 years (21 untreated; 237 under therapy; 30 in remission assessed by T_3 suppressibility). Assays were performed by using 50μl of serum. Nonspecific binding by sera was a little higher than by using IgG, albeit negligible. All untreated patients showed positive TDI. Frequency of positive patients decreased yearly with treatment. 20% remained positive after 6 years treatment. TDI's were positive in 13 of 16 patients (81%) treated longer than 13 years; drug therapy could not be stopped because of recurrence. TDI's were strongly positive in 2 of 30 patients in remission; one for 16 years, the other for 5 years. These results suggest that most TDI positive patients are very likely to relapse after stopping drug therapy. TDI activity detected by the kit can be useful in following Graves´disease patients during therapy with thionamide drugs, and can be easily performed.

1338 PITUITARY GONADOLIBERIN (GnRH) RECEPTOR: PURIFICATION, CHARACTERIZATION, RAISING OF ANTIBODIES. M.T. Jansem de Almeida Catanho, A. Bérault, M.Théoleyre and M. Jutisz*, Laboratoire des Hormones Polypeptidiques, CNRS, 91190 Gif-sur-Yvette,France.

The GnRH receptor contained in plasma membranes from bovine pituitary glands was solubilized in Triton X-100. The binding properties of the soluble material were shown to be the same as those of the membrane-included receptor. Chromatography of this preparation on a Concanavalin A-Sepharose column resulted in 33-fold purification. A second affinity chromatography on a column of a GnRH agonist immobilized on Sepharose, yielded, after 4 successive recyclings, a 14,000-fold purification over the membrane preparation with an overall yield close to 40 %. The binding capacity of an iodinated GnRH analog, used for radioreceptor assay, increased from 16 fmoles/mg of protein in the crude material to 225 pmoles/mg in the purified preparation. The product appeared almost homogeneous in HPLC chromatography and in other chromatography systems and its apparent molecular mass, as determined by electrophoretic analysis, was about 60,000 Da. Using a purified receptor preparation, antibodies were raised in rabbits and purified by affinity chromatography. Purified antibodies inhibit the binding of GnRH to its receptor sites and stimulate cultured rat anterior pituitary cells with releasing of LH. With these antibodies a radioimmunoassay (RIA) of GnRH receptor was developed. The present data demonstrate that the GnRH receptor from the pituitary gland can be solubilized and purified. It appears to be a glycoprotein with a molecular weight of about 60,000 . Antibodies raised against the receptor allowed us to develop a RIA of the receptor.

1339 [^{3}H]-AVP BINDING SITES IN BEEF KIDNEY MEDULLA AND CORTEX. M.H. Jawadi* and L.S. Ho, Univ. Kans. Sch. Med-W and VAMC, Wichita, Kansas, 67214

Previous studies of renal binding sites were performed in rodents and pigs with use of [^{125}-I]-AVP or with [^{3}H]-Lysine vasopressin (LVP). [125-I]-AVP has little or no demonstrable renal biological activity, whereas LVP is not a native hormone in rodents and most other mammals. With the availability of [^{3}H]-AVP, AVP binding sites, its characteristics and distribution in the various portions of kidneys were investigated. Partially purified membranes (PPM) were prepared from medulla (ME) or cortex (CO) of beef kidneys. [^{3}H]-AVP binding assay was performed in triplicate in the presence of [^{3}H]-AVP (.2-20nM). The specific binding ranged 50-75% of the total binding. The max. binding was obtained at 25°C in about 60 min. Scatchard analysis showed number of binding sites for medulla and cortex to be 160 and 80 fm/mg respectively, and Kd was 3.2 nM for both preparations.

COMPETITIVE BINDING OF NON-LABELED PEPTIDES AND [^{3}H]-AVP TO MEMB. PREP. (50% INHIBITION, nM)

	AVP	VDAVP[1]	dPVAVP[2]	LVP	MAVP[3]	Oxytocin
ME PPM	3.0	6.5	30	130	800	1300
CO PPM	3.0	6.5	30	100	300	520

[1]=[4-valine, 8-D-arginine]-vasopressin [2]=[-deaminopenicillamine, 4-valine]-arginine vasopressin [3]=[1-(β-mercapto-β, β-cyclopentamethylene propionic acid), 2-(O-methyl) tyrosine]-arginine vasopressin

We conclude that a.) AVP binding sites are found not only in the medulla but also in the cortex. b.) Of the tested analogues only VDAVP and dPVAVP have been reported to have a more potent antidiutetic effect, however; they showed less affinity than that of AVP to the renal binding sites.

1340 DOWN-REGULATION OF PROLACTIN RECEPTORS (PRLR) IN CULTURED MAMMARY TUMOR CELLS BY AN INHIBITOR OF PROSTAGLANDIN (PG) SYNTHESIS. P. Reichel*, L.A. Cohen, R. Karmali and D.P. Rose. Division of Nutrition and Endocrinology, Naylor Dana Institute, Valhalla, NY 10595, USA.

The objective of this study was to assess the effects of the PG synthetase inhibitor flurbiprofen on the growth and PRLR binding capacity of cultured neoplastic cells derived from dimethylbenz(a)anthracene (RBA) and N-nitrosomethylurea (NMU)-induced mammary adenocarcinomas. These were seeded in T-75 flasks and incubated at 37°C in Eagles medium plus 10% fetal bovine serum. One day later, flurbiprofen was added at 100 and 10 μg/ml in fresh growth medium, and the cells incubated for 72 hr. Control cells received vehicle only (0.1% ethanol). Growth medium was then removed for PG assay. A 1,500 x g membrane fraction prepared from the cells was used for the PRLR assay. PGs were extracted from the medium with diethylether and measured by radioimmunoassay. Flurbiprofen was toxic at 100 μg/ml. At 10 μg/ml, growth was inhibited by 33% (NMU) and 27% (RBA) of controls. Flurbiprofen (10 μg) significantly depressed the biosynthesis and release of PGs. Medium PGE_1 and $PGF_{2\alpha}$ were markedly reduced in both cell lines. PGE_2 was decreased in the NMU but not in the RBA cells. PRLRs were also decreased significantly in cells treated with 10 μg flurbiprofen, total specific PRL binding decreasing from 117,780 (cpm/mg protein) to 50,360 in NMU cells, and from 30,690 to 3,000 in RBA cells. The above observations suggest that inhibition of mammary tumor cell growth by inhibitors of PG synthesis may be mediated via alterations in PRL binding capacity.

1341 CHARACTERIZATION OF THE LH/hCG RECEPTOR IN LUTEINIZED RAT OVARIES.
P. C. Roche and R. J. Ryan*, Dept. of Cell Biology, Mayo Medical School, Rochester, MN 55905

The LH/hCG receptor is a membrane protein which can be extracted by certain nonionic detergents, but the lability of solubilized receptor has hampered its purification and characterization. By including 20-30% glycerin in solubilization buffers, we have been able to obtain stable, soluble LH/hCG receptor from luteinized rat ovaries. Soluble receptor retains 85% of hCG binding activity after storage for 2 weeks at 10°C. Stabilization of soluble receptor has allowed further biochemical characterization. 75-85% of ovarian receptors are solubilized by 1% Triton X-100 at 0°C after 30 min extraction. Only 30-50% are solubilized by 1% Lubrol PX. Soluble receptor in low ionic strength buffer binds to immobilized Blue B dye and quantitatively elutes with 1.0 M KCl. Adsorption to Concanavalin A cannot be achieved in the presence of 0.1% detergent. The major peak of hCG binding activity elutes from Sephacryl S-300 (equilibrated with 0.1% detergent) with an apparent M_r = 350,000. hCG-receptor complexes also elute with the same M_r. Free receptor adsorbs to DEAE-cellulose (pH 7.4) and to hCG-Sepharose, but a functional receptor cannot be eluted from either media. Covalent coupling of ^{125}I-hCG to receptor followed by SDS-PAGE and autoradiography produces radiolabelled bands of M_r = 210,000 (major) + 180,000 (minor). Reducing agents do not alter band migration. Further purification and characterization studies of the LH/hCG receptor are in progress. (Supported by HD 9140, HD 7108 and the Mayo Foundation).

1342 DIRECT ASSESSMENT OF β-ADRENERGIC RECEPTORS IN INTACT ADIPOCYTES: A REEVALUATION WITH THE HYDROPHILIC β-ANTAGONIST ^{3}H-CGP 12177.
Y. Giudicelli*, D. Lacasa and B. Agli. Dep^t of Biochemistry, C.H.U. Paris-Ouest, 78303 Poissy, France.

Although the β-adrenergic receptors of the fat cells have been well characterized on membrane preparation, studies on intact adipocytes are scarce and have generally yielded non-specific binding, B_{max} and agonist-K_D values far higher than those obtained in membrane preparations. Since these discrepancies seem to be due to the lipophilic nature of the ligands used, we have attempted to characterize the β-adrenergic receptors on intact rat adipocytes using the hydrophilic β-adrenergic antagonist ^{3}H-CGP 12177. While non specific binding of this ligand was low (less than 40 % of total binding at saturation), its specific binding reached equilibrium within 30 min at 37°C, was reversible, of high affinity (K_D = 2 ± 0.4 nM), saturable and stereospecifically displaceable by β-antagonists and agonists with an order of potency typical of binding to β_1-receptors. While competitions by β-antagonists resulted in sigmoidal curves, competition with agonists resulted in shallow curves consistent with the existence of two affinity states of the binding sites for agonists. The number of binding sites also varied with the cell size (34 500 ± 6 500 sites in a 60 μm diameter cell vs 116 800 ± 14 500 sites in a 85 μm diameter cell, $0.001 < P < 0.01$). Finally, as the ability of β-agonists to promote cyclic AMP production in the adipocytes closely correlated with the ability of catecholamines to displace ^{3}H-CGP 12177 specifically bound to the cell, it is concluded that ^{3}H-CGP 12177 is a valuable tool for detailled studies on the molecular mechanisms involved in the β-adrenergic regulation of fat cell metabolism.

Supported by the INSERM (Grant CRL 824005).

1343 **BINDING OF APOLIPOPROTEIN AI AND AII AFTER RECOMBINATION WITH PHOSPHOLIPID VESICLES TO THE HIGH DENSITY LIPOPROTEIN RECEPTORS OF LUTEINIZED RAT OVARY.**

Jaulang Hwang* and K. M. J. Menon, The University of Michigan, Ann Arbor, Michigan 48109

To determine which apolipoprotein is recognized by HDL receptor, ApoAI and ApoAII purified from HDL were reconstituted into dimyristoyl phosphotidyl choline (DMPC) vesicles and their abilities to bind to luteinized rat ovarian membranes were examined. Both ^{125}I-ApoAI·DMPC and ^{125}I-ApoAII·DMPC were shown to bind to ovarian membranes with K_d = 2.87 μg/ml and 5.70 μg/ml, respectively. The binding of ApoAI·DMPC was inhibited by ApoAII·DMPC and vice versa, suggesting that ApoAI·DMPC and ApoAII·DMPC bind to the same receptor. The binding site for ^{125}I-ApoAI·DMPC and ^{125}I-ApoAII·DMPC was also shown to be the HDL receptor, since the binding of these ligands was inhibited by intact HDL. In addition, the binding of both ^{125}I-ApoAI·DMPC and ^{125}I-ApoAII·DMPC was inhibited by unlabeled apolipoprotein alone (ApoAI and ApoAII) but not by DMPC vesicles, suggesting that the binding ability of the reconstituted lipoprotein is conferred by the apolipoprotein moiety rather than the liposome vesicles. We have shown that HDL receptor concentration in rat ovary was induced by in vivo hCG treatment (Hwang and Menon, J. Biol. Chem. 258, 8020, 1983). If the binding site for ^{125}I-ApoAI·DMPC and ^{125}I-ApoAII·DMPC is the HDL receptor, then the number of binding sites for these ligands should also increase by hCG treatment. As expected, the binding sites were induced by hCG. These results further support our conclusions that the HDL receptor of luteinized rat ovary specifically recognizes both ApoAI and ApoAII and its concentration is hormonally regulated. (Supported by NIH-HD06656).

1344 TWENTY MINUTES MEASUREMENT OF ESTRADIOL & ESTRIOL BY HIGH PERFORMANCE LIQUID CHROMATOGRAPHY (HPLC) AND ITS EVALUATION AS COMPARED TO RADIO-IMMUNOASSAY (RIA).

Zenjiro Kondo*, Tsunehisa Makino, Nobuhiro Uchida, Shinichi Yoshimura, Toshiki Kawabe+, Masao Fushimi+, Toshiyuki Dohji+, Fumio Kamiyama+ and Rihachi Iizuka, Department of Obstetrics and Gynecology, School of Medicine, Keio University, Tokyo, Japan, Medical Division, Sekisui Chemical Co., Ltd.+

Measurement of Estradiol(E2) and Estriol (E3) within 20 minutes by high performance liquid chromatography (HPLC) was achieved in this study and the values was compared with those of Radioimmunoassay (RIA). A totally computerized HPLC method was developed for measurement of unconjugated E2 and E3 in the sera of pregnant women. The serum samples were injected directly into the apparatus and transfered to a pretreatment column, where estrogens were absorbed while hydrophilic components such as proteins and carbohydrates were excluded. The estrogens then passed into another separation column containing a new type of polymer gel. The mobile phase consisted of an acetonitrile/water mixture, and separation was achieved by a reversed phase mechanism. The eluent was monitored for fluorescence. All these procedures were monitored and controlled by in-housed microcomputer. The sera samples from 61 normal pregnant women at 20 to 41 weeks of pregnancy were concomitantly assayed by HPLC and RIA.
The correlation of values with HPLC and RIA is; E3:Y=0.875 X - 0.172, the coefficient of correlation is 0.899, E2:Y=0.972 X + 6.791, the coefficient of correlation is 0.841 (Y=RIA values, X=HPLC value). The quick measurement of E2 & E3 by HPLC can be a useful method to evaluate the feto-placental function.

1345 PROGESTERONE MAY NOT DIRECTLY INDUCE GENE REGULATION IN ESTROGEN WITHDRAWN CHICK OVIDUCTS. B. Littlefield, J. Hora, B. Gosse, K. Rasmussen, N. Jiang, and T. Spelsberg*, Departments of Cell Biology-Biochemistry and Laboratory Medicine, Mayo Clinic, Rochester, MN 55905.

Many studies on the progesterone regulation of specific genes have utilized the oviducts of estrogen withdrawn chicks. However, data in this laboratory indicate that the progesterone receptors in this physiological state of the chick are inactivated, i.e., incapable of binding to nuclear acceptor sites. Considering this information and the reports that glucocorticoids (Glu) and other steroids can also induce the transcription of the same specific genes in these animals, the idea arose that progesterone may be metabolized to a Glu and other steroids which in turn regulate the expression of these genes. $[^3H]$Progesterone ($[^3H]$P) was injected (S.C.) into 10-day estrogen withdrawn chicks and the blood and oviduct cytosol and nuclei isolated at various periods post injection. Extracted radiolabeled steroids were analyzed by high pressure liquid chromatography using reverse phase and radioimmune analyses. At 1/2 hour, a marked (~50%) metabolism of the parent $[^3H]$P was measured with the appearance of Glu, estrogens and androgens in the serum. Interestingly, the only nuclear localized radiolabeled steroid was a Glu-like steroid. These data support that in the withdrawn chicks, $[^3H]$P is rapidly metabolized to other active steroids including glucocorticoids and that the latter may regulate and the secretory protein genes. Studies are underway to determine whether $[^3H]$R5020 (a synthetic progestin) can bind the oviduct Glu receptor and whether it can enhance ovalbumin mRNA levels in the oviducts of these chicks. Supported by NIH grants HD9140 and HD16705 from the NICHHD and the Mayo Foundation.

1346 TAMOXIFEN INHIBITS PROTEIN SYNTHESIS IN STROMAL CELLS FROM PROSTATES OF PATIENTS WITH BPH. J. Liu*, J. Albert and J. Geller. Mercy Hospital and Medical Center, San Diego, California 92103

Growth of the stroma of the human prostate may be regulated by estrogen since there are reports that estrogen concentrations are highest in the nuclei of prostate stromal cells. To test this hypothesis, we studied the effect of <u>in vivo</u> administration of tamoxifen, a non-steroidal anti-estrogen, on human prostate stromal protein synthesis <u>in vitro</u>. This was done by measuring ^{3}H-proline incorporation <u>in vitro</u> in the stromal cells separated enzymatically with 0.5% collagenase and trypsin from prostate tissue removed at surgery. Treated patients (10 cases) were given 20 mg. of tamoxifen b.i.d. for ten days prior to surgery. The blood level for tamoxifen at the time of surgery ranged from 200-500 picomoles/ml in all tamoxifen-treated patients. Control tissues were obtained from patients (11 cases) who were untreated. The results indicated that tamoxifen inhibited protein synthesis in stromal cells of treated patients compared with control (mean 37,809 counts/minute/mg protein, 119,927 counts/minute/mg protein, respectively, $p < 0.02$). These results support the concept that estrogen regulates, at least in part, stromal protein synthesis and suggests a role for estrogen in the pathophysiology of BPH.

This study is supported by NIH Grant No. AG 02776-01A1.

1347 ESTROGEN SYNTHETASE ACTIVITY IN HUMAN TERM PLACENTAL CELLS IN MONOLAYER CULTURE. J. Lobo* and F. Bellino, Dept. of Biol. Sci., SUNY/Buffalo, Buffalo, NY 14260 USA

Trophoblast cells of human placenta are known to produce both steroid and polypeptide hormones during pregnancy. hCG, hPL and progesterone secretions from placental cultures have been investigated; reports on estrogen secretion are limited. This study examines the estrogen synthesizing capacity of human placental cells in monolayer culture. Placental cells, isolated using trypsin (Hall et al.,1977), washed by centrifugation and treated with NH_4Cl, were plated in medium 199 + 10% fetal bovine serum with medium changed daily. Estrogen synthetase (aromatase) activity was assessed by ^3H_2O released from $(1\beta-^3H,4-^{14}C)$androstenedione (0.7 nmol). The aromatase activity (pmol/min/mg prot. ± SE) in placental tissue before trypsinization (21.3±0.4,n=6) decreased to 0.63±0.04,n=15 in freshly released cells. Aromatase activity of the attached cells in monolayer culture increased linearly to about 14.8±1.1,n=13 at 72-96 h after plating and then declined. Cells exposed to 1mM $(Bu)_2$cAMP plus 1mM theophylline (combination called dbT) for 72 h showed decreased aromatase activity ($p < 0.05$). The viability of these cells was demonstrated by the increasing hCG secretion into the medium throughout 96 h of culture, with dbT-grown cells secreting about three times the amount from control cells. The morphological changes of these cells in culture are striking. Freshly isolated, primarily mononuclear cells (25.1±2.1 µm,n=4) grew to large multinucleated cells by 72 h (347.1±2.1 µm,n=4) suggesting differentiation of these cells from cytotrophoblast to syncytiotrophoblast in culture. Supported by grant HD 16593 from the U.S.D.H.H.S.-Nat. Inst. of Health.

1348 MODULATING EFFECTS OF NEFAs ON THE INTERACTIONS BETWEEN SEXUAL STEROID AND HUMAN SEX BINDING PROTEIN (SBP). Martin, M.E., Vranckx, R., * Benassayag, C., Nunez, E.A. - U. 224, INSERM - ERA 881, CNRS - Faculté de Médecine Xavier Bichat - 16, rue Henri Huchard - 75018 PARIS.

Several lines of researchs suggest that NEFAs could play an important role in the mechanisms of hormonal action. Notably our recent studies have shown that the NEFAs modify the estrophilic properties of some seric or tissular proteins. It has been previously demonstrated that in the rat, the unsaturated NEFAs inhibit the estrogen binding to the uterine receptors of immature rat as well as to the seric murine AFP. In human, the unsaturated NEFAs potentialize the estrogen binding to cytosoluble uterine proteins. The aim of this work is to investigate the effects of physiological levels of NEFAs on the interactions between purified human SBP which specifically binds the sexual steroid hormones in the serum. SBP has been purified from pooled pregnancy human sera through a 3 step procedure (ammonium sulfate fractionation, phenylsepharose and cortisol 21-hemisuccinate HMD-AcA 44 gel chromatographies). The influence of NEFAs on the binding of dihydrotestosterone, testosterone, estradiol to purified SBP has been studied by three methods : polyacrylamide gel electrophoresis, cross immunoautoradiography and equilibrium dialysis. Whatever the method used, physiological levels (0,1 mM) of saturated NEFAs increase by 1,5 to 2 fold the binding of the three steroids to the SBP. Conversely, unsaturated NEFAs such as the oleic (18:1) or docosahexaenoic (22:6) acids highly inhibit the binding to the protein. This inhibition is dose dependant and inversely correlated with the association constant of each steroid for the SBP. In human, our data clearly point out the opposite effect of the NEFAs on either seric or tissue binding proteins.

1349 11-KETOTESTOSTERONE (11-T; ANDROST-4-ENE-17-ß-OL-3,11-DIONE) IN HUMAN AND TROUT PLASMA. H.K. Kley, R. Schlaghecke and H.L. Krüskemper*.
2. Medizinische Klinik C, University of Düsseldorf, West-Germany

The physiological role of 11-keto- and 11-hydroxyandrogens is still unknown in man. To determine 11-T a highly specific RIA was established using antisera to 11-T-3-BSA and (1,2-^{3}H)11-T as marker. At 8 a.m. plasma levels of 11-T were 0.64 ± 0.22 ng/ml (n: 25) without sex differences. No oscillation was found when blood was drawn in 20 min intervals. Diurnal variation was considerable exhibiting a decrease of 55% from 8 a.m. to 11 p.m. When stimulating testicular synthesis by HCG (3times 5000 U i.m.) plasma 11-T remained unaffected, suggesting adrenal origine of 11-T. After dexamethasone (3 mg orally at 11 p.m.) 11-T decreased to 0.12 ± 0.05 ng/ml. However, in contrast to cortisol, ACTH stimulation decreased 11-T by 30% after 1 h. When adrenal stimulation was performed over a period of 8 h decrease was even 60%. As compared to male trouts (50.6 ± 14.2 ng/ml) levels of 11-T were low in man. Both T and 11-T were bound by human (97.8 ± 0.2 and 89.9 ± 1.1%) and trout plasma (98.6 ± 0.2 and 90.5 ± 2.2%). Conclusions: 11-T can be measured in human and trout plasma. The physiological role of 11-T is unknown in man. 11-T appears to originate from the adrenal cortex though ACTH stimulation decreased 11-T levels considerably. 11-T is bound less than T in human and trout plasma.

1350 ANDROGEN CONVERSION TO ESTROGENS IS LOW IN IDIOPATHIC HEMOCHROMATOSIS (IHC); COMPARISON WITH ALCOHOLIC LIVER CIRRHOSIS (AC). H.K. Kley*, W. Stremmel, C. Niederau, R. Hehrmann, E. Keck and H.L. Krüskemper, Medizinische Klinik C, University of Düsseldorf, West-Germany.

Gynecomastia is found in AC but not in IHC. Therefore, we studied whether differences are present in sexual hormones, in the production rates (PR) of testosterone (T) and androstenedione (A), and in conversion ratios (CR) of T and A to estrone (E1) and estradiol (E2) in 12 age-matched male patients with IHC and AC. Severity of impotence both in IHC and AC was correlated to more than 60% decreased plasma T. However, patients with IHC showed basal E1 levels of 29.8 ± 3.1 pg/ml and significantly lower E2 levels (17.7 ± 6.3 pg/ml) as compared to controls (E1: 32.5 ± 5.6; E2: 28.5 ± 8.5 pg/ml) and to AC (67.8 ± 20.8 and 36.0 ± 4.7 pg/ml). Despite decreased T and E2 levels in IHC LH was low and insufficiently stimulated by LHRH. When studying sexual hormones after ACTH and HCG application plasma E1 and E2 were significantly reduced in IHC and increased in AC. PR of T was reduced by about 60% in both IHC and AC, whereas PR of A was increased in AC. CR from androgens to estrogens were more than doubled in AC; In IHC, however, they were found to be in the range of the controls. Conclusions: In IHC hypogonadism is mainly due to pituitary hypofunction. In contrast to AC, in IHC E1 levels are normal, and plasma E2 is even reduced. Lack of gynecomastia in IHC can be explained by decreased formation of estrogens. Therefore, T might be used for substitution therapy in IHC.

1351 COMPENSATORY RISE OF SERUM TESTOSTERONE DEFIES THE ANTIANDROGENIC EFFECT OF FLUTAMIDE (FL) IN YOUNG HEALTHY MEN - A DOUBLE BLIND CROSSOVER STUDY.
U.A. Knuth*, R. Hano and E. Nieschlag, Max Planck Clinical Research Unit for Reproductive Medicine, Steinfurter Str. 107, D4400 Münster, FR Germany

The antiandrogens FL and cyproterone acetate (CPA) differ in their activity as FL lacks the gestagenic property of CPA. Although well established in rats, the endocrine implications of this difference have not been fully assessed in men since most data derive from uncontrolled studies in prostatic carcinoma patients. In a split double blind crossover study two groups (2x10) of volunteers received 250 mg FL t.i.d or 50 mg CPA b.i.d. for two weeks followed or preceeded randomly (interval: 4 weeks) by 14 days of placebo. Serum T (nmol/l), E_2 (pmol/l), LH and FSH (µg/l WHO-HRP) were measured on days 1, 5, 8 and 14. Corresponding results (mean±SEM) were compared between placebo and drug period. During FL treatment serum T increased gradually up to day 14 (17.4±1.4 vs 26.9±1.5, $p < .01$). CPA had the opposite effect on T (14.6±1.8 vs 3.3±0.6, $p < .01$). E_2 concentrations paralleled this development (FL: 114±12 vs 177±20; CPA: 95±13 vs 35±6). Serum LH increased during 14 days of FL (63±6 vs 88±7, $p < .01$), indicating an interruption of the negative feedback by blocking hypothalamic androgen receptors. A simultaneous inhibition of gonadotropin secretion seen at the end of CPA administration (LH: 58±7 vs 29±4; FSH: 2.3±0.3 vs 1.5±0.1) did not occur under FL. FSH, however, was not affected by FL. Only two out of ten volunteers treated with FL complained of loss of libido, whereas this expected side effect occurred in 8 men receiving CPA ($p < 0.002$). The data suggest that rising serum T levels attenuate the antiandrogenic effect of FL.

1352 RAT TESTIS GONADOTROPIN AND PRL RECEPTORS (R), STEROIDOGENESIS, AND THEIR RESPONSE TO hCG-STIMULATION AFTER BLOCKADE OF GnRH-R WITH A POTENT GnRH ANTAGONIST.
I.T. Huhtaniemi[1,*] and K.J. Catt[2]. Dept. of Clin. Chem.[1], and Dept. of Immunol. and Bacteriol.[1], Univ. of Helsinki, Finland, and Endocr. Reprod. Res. Branch[2], NICHD, NIH, Bethesda, MD, USA.

Adult male rats (n=24) were injected with a potent GnRH antagonist (N-Ac-D-p-Cl-$Phe^{1,2}$,D-Trp^3,D-Lys^6,D-Ala^{10}-GnRH; Ant.); 1 mg/kg BW s.c. at 0, 12 and 24 h. Half of the rats received an injection of hCG (600 IU/kg s.c.) at 12 h. All animals were killed at 36 h, and subjectee to R and hormone measurements. Ant. blocked >95% of the available pituitary and testicular GnRH-R, decreased testicular Prl-R by 60% ($p<0.01$), but had no effect on LH- and FSH-R. Ant. decreased serum and testicular testosterone (T) by 90%, and testicular in vitro capacity to produce T by 50% ($p<0.01$). No decrease was observed in production rates of cAMP and progesterone (P). hCG alone abolished testicular LH-R, decreased Prl-R by 55% ($p<0.01$), and GnRH-R by 65% ($p<0.01$). Desensitization of cAMP and T production, and increase in P/T ratio was seen after hCG. hCG + Ant. treatment resulted in R-, cAMP and steroid responses indistinguishable from those after hCG alone. The main conclusions are: (1) Ant.-induced hypogonadotropism decreases testicular Prl-R and T production, (2) Testicular GnRH- and Prl-R are subject to heterologous down-regulation by hCG, and (3) Inhibition of the putative GnRH mediated regulation of testis by Ant. blockade of the GnRH-R does not change testicular response to hCG. Hence, the present observations still leave the physiological role of testicular GnRH-R open.

1353 TRIETHYLENEMELAMINE (TEM) EFFECTS ON DOG SPERMATOGENESIS.
W. L. Hunt* and R. H. Foote, Departments of Animal Science and Biological Sciences, Cornell University, Ithaca, NY.

After 5 wks of standardization during which semen was collected 3x/wk by digital manipulation from 20 sexually mature Beagle males, dogs were grouped according to sperm output and randomly assigned to 4 groups--control, biopsy, and a single injection of 0.2 mg TEM/kg or 0.4 mg TEM/kg. After treatment semen collections continued for 20 wks. Testicular biopsies were performed on one randomly selected testis at the end of wks 1, 5 and 9 in all but controls. Unilateral castration of the biopsied testis and one testis of the controls was performed at end of wk 16. Remaining testes were removed from all dogs at the end of wk 20. Sperm output (10^6/wk/dog) during standardization averaged 851, 901, 1007 and 873, respectively, for the 4 groups. Three dogs in the 0.4 mg TEM group died. TEM caused a progressive decline for 16 wks in sperm output in the 0.2 mg TEM group (>65%) and the 0.4 mg TEM group (>89%) with no effect on sperm motility. Compared to controls TEM dogs exhibited progressive denudation of spermatogenic cells throughout 20 wks. Cellular destruction, disorganization and sloughing occurred mildly, moderately and extensively within the seminiferous tubules of wks 1, 5 and 9 biopsies, respectively. Reductions in sperm output coincided with low cell counts. Active regeneration of spermatogenic cells was not observed in TEM treated dogs during the 20 wks.

1354 GONADOTROPIN AND ISOPROTERENOL STIMULATED ADENYLATE CYCLASE ACTIVITIES IN RAT TESTICULAR TISSUE DURING CRYPTORCHIDISM.
T.Jahnsen*[1], B.Karpe[2], A.Erichsen[1], H.Attramadal[1], M.Ritzen[3], E.Haug[4] and V.Hansson[1].
1. Institute of Pathology, Rikshospitalet, Oslo, Norway. 2. Department of Pediatric Surgery, St.Gøran Hospital, 11281 Stockholm, Sweden. 3. Pediatric Endocrinology Unit, Karolinska Hospital, 10401 Stockholm, Sweden. 4. Aker Hospital, Oslo, Norway.
During unilateral cryptorchidism in adult rats there is a selective decrease in the adenylate cyclase responses to gonadotropin stimulation in the abdominal testis. This is associated with a parallel decrease in specific FSH and LH binding. There is no reduction in the response of testicular adenylate cyclase to PGE_1 or fluoride stimulation, indicating that both the GTP binding protein (N-component) and the catalytic subunit of the adenylate cyclase complex are intact. Furthermore, we have shown that cryptorchidism is associated with an increased responsiveness of isoproterenol sensitive adenylate cyclase in testicular membrane particles from abdominal testes. Maximal isoproterenol responses are seen 3-4 weeks after the rats are made cryptorchid. Following orchidopexy there is a gradual normalization of the isoproterenol response and two to three months after orchidopexy the isoproterenol response in the rat testis had decreased to normal control values. Thus, experimental cryptorchidism in rats is associated with a decreased responsiveness of gonadotropin sensitive adenylate cyclase activity, but an increased responsiveness of isoproterenol sensitive adenylate cyclase activity in testicular membrane particles from abdominal testes.

1355 IDENTIFICATION OF VASOPRESSIN-LIKE SUBSTANCES IN THE RAT TESTIS. Barry G. Kasson*, Rina Meidan, and Aaron J.W. Hsueh, Dept. of Reprod. Medicine, Univ. of Calif., San Diego, La Jolla, CA 92093 U.S.A.

A direct inhibitory effect of vasopressin on hCG-induced androgen production by cultured testicular cells has been previously reported by our laboratory (Nature 293:650, 1981). Pituitary arginine vasopressin (AVP) is unlikely to affect testis function since its circulating concentration is very low. The present studies were conducted to determine whether an endogenous vasopressin-like ligand is present in the testis. An acid extract (0.2N HCl) of homogenized testicular tissue displaced ^{125}I-AVP binding to AVP antiserum in a manner parallel to that of synthetic AVP. When this extract was further purified by acetone and ether extractions, competitive displacement of ^{3}H-AVP from specific receptors in an enriched interstitial cell preparation could also be demonstrated. Parallel competition curves for synthetic AVP and the tissue extract suggest the testicular substances may be endogenous ligands for testis AVP receptors. Gel filtration chromatography of acid extracts on Biogel P2 or Sephadex G-25 resulted in two peaks of vasopressin immunoreactivity. One peak co-chromatographed with authentic AVP. However, the major portion (95%) of the immunoreactivity was of higher molecular weight and eluted prior to either synthetic AVP or oxytocin. Since the testicular concentration of the observed vasopressin-like substance is very high ($\sim$10ng/testis), our data suggest the presence, by radioimmunoassay and radioreceptor assay, of endogenous substances which may function as intratesticular modulators of steroidogenesis.

1356 SYNTHESIS OF ANDROGEN BINDING PROTEIN (mABP) IN SERTOLI CELL-ENRICHED CULTURES FROM CYNOMOLGUS MONKEYS. Hugh S. Keeping*, Stephen J. Winters and Philip Troen, Department of Medicine, Montefiore Hospital, University of Pittsburgh, Pittsburgh PA 15213 USA

The male human and subhuman primate produces two extracellular androgen binding proteins: serum testosterone-estradiol binding globulin (TeBG) and testicular ABP. We have studied the in vitro synthesis of mABP using Sertoli cells obtained from prepubertal monkeys. Sertoli cell-enriched cultures were derived from testis by sequential trypsin and collagenase dispersion. The cells were maintained in a serum-free, chemically defined, hormone supplemented media containing 0.5 µg/ml hFSH. After 9 days of culture, the methionine concentration of the media was reduced 10-fold, ^{35}S-methionine (10 µCi/ml) was added and the cells were incubated for an additional 16 hr. The media was concentrated 5-fold and loaded onto an androgen affinity column consisting of 17α-epoxypropyl-dihydrotestosterone (DHT) bound covalently to Thiopropyl Sepharose-6B, provided by Ray et al. (Endocrinology (Suppl.) 112, 244, Abst. 653, 1983). The affinity beads were washed with column buffer until trace amounts of radioactivity were detected in the eluant, then buffer containing 10 mM DHT was added to the column to displace ABP bound to the immobilized androgen. The eluted radiolabeled protein was analyzed by polyacrylamide gel electrophoresis under denaturing conditions and then processed for fluorography. Two bands corresponding to apparent molecular weights (M.W.) of 48,000 and 46,000 were found, with the lower M.W. band being more intense. The ratio of these subunits differs from those reported for mTeBG. In conclusion, Sertoli cells from a species which produces TeBG are able to synthesize and secrete ABP in culture.

1357 TESTICULAR RESPONSE TO HCG DURING AND AFTER ACUTE LH SUPPRESSION BY DIHYDROTESTOSTERONE (DHT).

J.M. Kuhn, J. Mahoudeau*, P. Leymarie, M.H. Laudat, J.P. Luton and L.M. Wolf, C.H.U., 14000 Caen, and Hopital de Boisguillaume, 76000 Rouen, France.

Testicular hormone response to HCG seems to be related to the previous gonadotropin status. Since DHT has been shown to acutely decrease plasma LH, we have evaluated the response to HCG in 8 healthy men before, during and 1 week after percutaneous administration of DHT (250mg daily for 3 weeks). Morning (8-9am) plasma levels of testosterone (T), estradiol (E2), 17OH-progesterone (17OHP) and DHT were measured by RIA before HCG, and daily for 3 days after HCG (5000 IU). The results (m±SD) are below:

	Before DHT		During DHT		After DHT	
	base	HCG peak	base	HCG peak	base	HCG peak
T ng/ml	6.5±1.9	12.5±3.4	2.6±1.5	10.1±2.6	4.5±2.2	16.0±3.5
E2 pg/ml	28±7	88±23	30±19	57±20	17±4	62±33
17OHP ng/ml	1.3±0.2	3.2±0.9	0.8±0.3	1.9±0.4	0.8±0.3	2.4±0.7
DHT ng/ml	0.8±0.3	0.9±0.2	3.4±1.4	3.4±0.9	2.5±1.5	2.0±0.8

Although the T peaks prior to DHT and under DHT were not different, the increase in plasma T was slower under DHT. The peaks of E2 and 17OHP were markedly decreased under DHT. We conclude that acute LH suppression by DHT results in 3 reversible changes: 1. a decreased basal T; 2. a slower T increase after HCG; 3. a striking decrease of E2 and 17OHP. These data are in agreement with the dissociated responses of T and E2 found in hypogonadotropic males.

1358 CLINICAL AND PATHOLOGICAL CHARACTERISTICS OF ACUTE EXACERBATION OF HASHIMOTO'S THYROIDITIS.

T.ISHIHARA*, N.WASEDA, K.IKEKUBO and T.MORI DEPARTMENT of INTERNAL MEDICINE, KOBE GENERAL HOSPITAL, JAPAN.

Acute exacerbation of Hashimoto's thyroiditis is a rare occurance, and its clinical and pathological details have never been well documented. In a 76 y.o. female, 12 episodes of acute exacerbation, which were manifested by a high fever with a chill, pain and tenderness on a multinodularly enlarged thyroid and general malaise, were observed over a period of 4 months. Finally, a total thyroidectomy was performed and she became free from the episodes. Laboratory findings revealed accelarated ESR, high IgG and Tcell ratio, and positive CRP,RA and ANF. T_4,T_3,T_3U,fT_4 and TSH were within normal range, anti-Tg was negative, and anti-M was weakly positive. Thyroid 99mTc O_4-uptake was lower, and scintigraphy showed heterogeneous RI accumulations. Ultrasonogram showed localized hypoechoic region coincidental with the inflammatory lesion. Clinical worsening was associated with elevations of ESR, CRP and serum Tg, but not of circulating hormone levels. Four needle biopsies were performed. Together with typical findings of Hashimoto's thyroiditis, the specimen obtained immediately after the episodes particularly, had characteristic features of loosely arranged fibrosis indicative of edema. These findings rapidly disappeared within 1 or 2 days with intrathyroidal steroid administration. Only steroid medication gave her transient relief, but none of plasmapheresis, D-penicillamine, or various antibiotics were effective. Acute exacerbation of Hashimoto's thyroiditis is considered to be not related directly to humoral factors but mostly composed of intrathyroidal localized edematous inflammation.

1359 THYROID STIMULATING IMMUNOGLOBULIN ASSESSED BY FOLLICLE-FORMING CELLS OF PORCINE THYROID GLAND. O.Isozaki*, T.Tsushima, M.Saji, K.Sato and K.Shizume, Department of Internal Medicine,Tokyo Women's Medical College,Tokyo,Japan.

Monolayer cultured thyrocytes have been often used to assess thyroid stimulating immunoglobulin (TSI) of Graves' disease. But thyrocytes are arranged with their specific structure and polarity in thyroid gland. Therefore, we have compared the response of thyrocytes in monolayer and in follicles to Graves' IgG. porcine thyrocytes were prepared with Dispase, cultured in Ham's F-12 medium with 0.5 % fetal calf serum in dishes pre-coated with agarose and allowed to form follicles. On the 3rd day,follicles were shifted to Hanks' solution and exposed to Graves' IgG (10mg/ml). After 120 min medium and cells were extracted and cAMP was meassured by RIA. IgG of 35 out of 38 untreated patients (92.1 %) caused significantly greater response (more than 160 % of basal) than normal IgG. In monolayer cultured cells from the same thyroid gland, the response was always less than that in follicles and only 50 % of IgG from untreated patients caused significant cAMP production. With IgG of treated patients who had been euthyroid for more than one year, the increase of cAMP in follicles correlated significantly with 20 min uptake of ^{131}I after T3 suppression test ($r=0.58$, $p < 0.001$). The ^{131}I uptake also correlated with thyrotropin displacing activity (TDA) assayed by TSH-RRA ($r=0.48$, $p<0.02$). TSI correlated significantly better with the ^{131}I uptake than TDA did. There was a positive correlation between TSI and serum thyroglobulin values in these euthyroid patients ($r=0.85$, $p<0.001$).

Thus thyrocytes in follicles were more sensitive to TSI compared to cells in monolayer and proved to be useful for TSI determination.

1360 PERIPHERAL T LYMPHOCYTE SUBSETS AT POSTPARTUM AGGRAVATION OF AUTOIMMUNE THYROID DISEASES. Y. Iwatani*, N. Amino, H. Mori, H. Tamaki, M. Aozasa, M. Mori, O. Tanizawa, Y. Kumahara and K. Miyai, Department of Laboratory Medicine, and Obstetrics and Gynecology, Osaka University Medical School, Osaka 553, Japan.

In order to elucidate the mechanisms of postpartum aggravation of autoimmune thyroid diseases, we examined serially peripheral T lymphocyte subsets in the postpartum period. T lymphocyte subsets were measured by FACS analysis with monoclonal antibodies (Leu series). At 2-6 months postpartum, the percentages of total T cells (E rosette or Leu 1 positive), suppressor T cells (Leu 2a) and helper T cells (Leu 3a) decreased and that of B cells (EAC rosette) increased transiently in both Graves' disease (postpartum relapse (4 cases), euthyroid (3), destructive thyrotoxicosis (3)) and Hashimoto's disease (destructive thyrotoxicosis (2), euthyroid (1)). Changes of these lymphocyte subsets were more obvious in the patients who had marked postpartum thyroid dysfunction. However, there was no definite change of the helper T/suppressor T cell ratio in any group of Graves' disease or Hashimoto's disease, and the treatment of methimazol had no effect on the ratio. The Leu 2a antigen density on suppressor T cells decreased at postpartum relapse of Graves' thyrotoxicosis. These data indicate that there are transient decreases of total T cells, suppressor T cells and helper T cells and a increase of B cells, but no definite change of the helper T/suppressor T cell ratio at postpartum aggravation of autoimmune thyroid diseases. B cell increase, rather than the unbalance of helper T/suppressor T cell ratio, may induce postpartum aggravation of autoimmune thyroid diseases.

1361 FACTORS WHICH INFLUENCE THE IODINE CONTENT OF SERUM THYROGLOBULIN(Tg).

M. Izumi*, S. Morita, S. Yamashita, S. Ohtakara, S. Okamoto, T. Miyamoto°, N.Mochinaga°, S. Nagataki, The First Department of Internal Medicine, The Second Department of Surgery°, Nagasaki University, Nagasaki 852, Japan

The purpose of the present study was (1) to compare the iodine content of serum and intrathyroidal Tg in normal subjects and in patients with thyroid nodules and (2) to investigate changes in iodine content of Tg in serum obtained before and sequentially after the operation of these patients. Tg in serum and supernatant of homogenate of thyroid tissue was precipitated by ammonium sulfate. The precipitate was resolved and dialyzed against phosphate buffer. These solutions were fractionated by isopycnic centrifugation in 34.5% RbCl and Tg concentration of each fraction was measured by radioimmunoassay. Serum Tg of normal subjects migrated significantly faster than that of patients with thyroid nodules. There was no significant difference between migrations of serum Tg of patients with thyroid carcinoma and adenoma. Serum Tg migrated significantly slower than intrathyroidal Tg in both normal subjects and patients with thyroid nodules. After operations of patients with parathyroid adenoma (normal thyroids), levels of serum Tg increased extremely because of destruction of normal thyroid tissue and serum Tg immediately after operation migrated to the same fraction of intrathyroidal Tg. The migration of serum Tg became slower thereafter and finally reached to that before operation within 48 hours, although the serum Tg concentrations were 10 times more than the preoperative levels. It is suggested that iodine content of serum Tg is influenced by both (1) iodine content of intrathyroidal Tg and (2) removal of iodine of serum Tg during circulation.

1362 FAMILIAL INCREASE IN NUCLEAR T3 RECEPTORS WITH HYPERRESPONSIVENESS TO THYROID HORMONES.

C. Jaffiol*, L. Baldet, J. Bismuth, J. Torresani and C. Papachristou. Dept. of Endocrinology, Hopital St Eloi, 34059 Montpellier Cédex and Lab. of Medical Biochemistry 13385 Marseille Cédex, France.

We have described previously a new syndrome of 'pseudo-hyperthyroidism' with increased nuclear T3 receptors (1).We now have evidence of a familial disturbance.Two brothers were investigated.Patient A complained of severe paroxysmal tachycardia without goitre or exophthalmos.Repeated investigation excluded cardiac or adrenergic disease and although thyroid hormones were normal, the TSH response to TRH was blunted. The paroxysmal tachycardia remitted on carbimazole (CBZ) treatment but relapsed on withdrawal of CBZ. T4 fell but the patient remained clinically euthyroid on CBZ. Patient B complained of intermittent bouts of tachycardia and was euthyroïd. The brothers' father was deceased but had complained throughout life of intermittent palpitation. Nuclear T3 receptors were measured for both brothers in lymphocytes separated on a Ficoll-Hypaque gradient, and incubated with increasing concentrations of labelled T3. Nuclei were isolated by washing in Triton X 100. The apparent affinity constants for T3 were normal (A: ka = 1.42×10^{10} M^{-1}, B: ka = 1.85×10^{10} M^{-1} ; N = $1.84 \pm 0.19 \times 10^{10}$ M^{-1}).The concentration of binding sites was increased in both patients (A : 9.85 fmol/100 µg DNA ; B: 5.6 fmol/100 µg DNA ; N: 3.7 fmol/100 µg DNA).These data suggest that the increment in nuclear T3 receptors may be inherited, and may explain the increase in responsiveness of peripheral tissues to thyroid hormones and the onset of thyrotoxic symptoms in the presence of normal thyroid function.

(1) Jaffiol et al 12 ETA meeting Brussels 1982. Abstr. No.60

1363 INHIBITION OF T4-5'-DEIODINASE ACTIVITY DECREASES HEPATIC UPTAKE OF rT3 IN THE PERFUSED RAT LIVER. A. S. Jennings*, Endocrine Section, University of Pennsylvania, Philadelphia, PA 19104, USA.

Many drugs and nonthyroidal illnesses decrease extrathyroidal production of T3 from T4 and decrease the metabolic clearance of rT3. Studies using liver homogenates have attributed these changes to decreased T4-5'-deiodinase activity; however, we have shown in the perfused liver that decreased hepatic T3 production can result from decreased T4 uptake (fasting) as well as decreased T4-5'-deiodinase activity (PTU, diabetes, hypothyroidism). To investigate the metabolism of rT3 in similar situations, rat livers were perfused at 37°C with Krebs-Ringer bicarbonate buffer containing albumin (3g/dl), RBCs, and rT3 and the disappearance of rT3 from the medium was monitered by RIA. Perfusate rT3 levels decreased exponentially with a T 1/2 of approximately 4 minutes. When livers were perfused with 125-I-rT3, there was a similar rapid release of 125-I into the perfusate, indicating rapid deiodination of rT3. There was no change in the rate of metabolism of rT3 over a concentration range of 35 to 800 ng/dl, demonstrating a large capacity for deiodination. When rT3 and PTU (a T4-5'-deiodinase inhibitor) were perfused simultaneously, rT3 uptake was significantly decreased. These data suggest that the uptake and deiodination of rT3 by the liver are tightly coupled events, whereas the uptake and subsequent deiodination of T4 to T3 appear to be separately regulated.

1364 TISSUE-SPECIFIC CHROMATIN STRUCTURE OF A TRIIODOTHYRONINE (T_3) RESPONSIVE GENE. DB Jump* and JH Oppenheimer, Division of Endocrinology, Department of Medicine, University of Minnesota, Minneapolis, MN 55455 U.S.A.

Whereas $mRNA_{S14}$ (Spot 14; 18,000 Mr; 4.9 pI) is expressed both in liver and spleen, regulation by T_3 occurs only in liver. Accordingly, we have examined the organization of the Spot 14 gene in chromatin to determine whether structural differences may account for the tissue specific Spot 14 regulation. DNAse I hypersensitive sites around the Spot 14 gene were examined by mildly digesting nuclei with DNAse I. The DNA was subsequently isolated, digested with Eco RI, electrophoretically separated and transfered to nitrocellulose. Eco RI (E) cuts the Spot 14 gene in the intervening (open bar) and flanking sequences (line) to give a 14.7 Kb 5′-fragment and a 4.7 Kb 3′-fragment thus enabling us to examine potential cleavage sites beyond the 5′ and 3′ boundaries of the Spot 14 gene. The ^{32}P-cDNA(E_7) recognizes only the 3′-fragment, whereas the ^{32}P-cDNA(F_5) recognizes both 3′ and 5′-fragments. Using differential hybridization we found 9 hypersensitive sites in liver (↑) and 5 hypersensitive sites associated with the Spot 14 gene in spleen (↓).

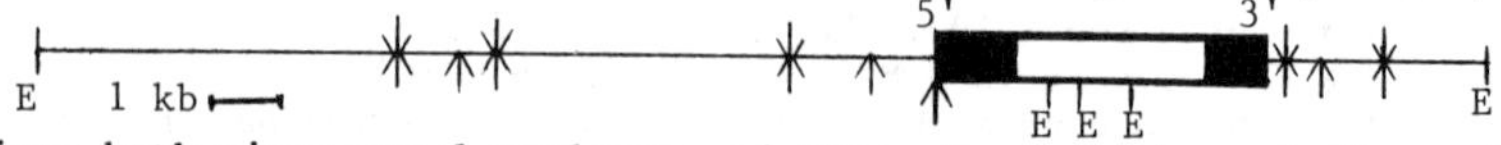

Since both micrococcal nuclease and DNAse I recognize similar sites in liver nuclei the 5′ and 3′-hypersensitive sites appear to be freely accessible to DNA-protein interaction. Unique loci found in liver but not spleen may contain specific signals leading to the tissue specific regulation of the Spot 14 gene.

1365 THYROID HORMONE BINDING TO HUMAN ALBUMIN: EFFECTS OF OTHER LIGANDS

K. Kamikubo*, T. Komaki, S. Nakamura, S. Sakata, K. Yasuda and K. Miura Department of Internal Medicine, Gifu University School of Medicine, Gifu 500, Japan.

Effects of several ligands on thyroid hormone binding to human serum albumin (HSA) were studied by utilizing ^{125}I-labeled thyroid hormones and HSA-Sepharose. Association constant and number of the primary binding site for T4 were 6.1×10^5 M^{-1} and 1/mole, respectively. Those of the secondary T4 binding sites were 0.5×10^5 M^{-1} and 5/mole. Association constant and number of the primary binding site for T3 were 2.4×10^5 M^{-1} and 1/mole, respectively. 8-Anilino-1-nephthalenesulfonate (ANS) non-competitively inhibited the T4 binding to the primary site. The ANS inhibition of T4 binding was evident even at low [ANS]/[HSA] ratios ([ANS]/[HSA]>1). T4 had virtually no inhibitory effect on ANS binding to HSA as measured by the fluorescence intensity of ANS. These results indicate that ANS allosterically inhibits the primary T4 binding. Covalent modification of ^{34}Cys with either N-ethylmaleimide or p-chloromercuriphenylsulfonate failed to affect the T4 binding. These results suggest that T4 primarily binds to a site distinct from but near to the ANS binding site, which is located on the domain 1 of HSA. It is likely that ^{34}Cys on the domain 1 is not involved in the primary T4 binding. Bilirubin and long chain fatty acids at high concentrations ([bilirubin]/[HSA] > 10,[fatty acid]/[HSA] > 50) inhibited the T4 binding to HSA. Steroid hormones (hydrocortisone, DHEA) showed no effect on the T4 binding. These results suggest that these natural ligands little affect the thyroid hormone binding to HSA in physiological conditions.

1366 A NEW CASE OF HYPERTHYROIDISM WITH ELEVATED SERUMβ-TSH AND TSH-AUTOANTIBODY(AT).

K.Kamoi*,S.Ishikawa,O.Arai,H.Sato,M.Yokoyama, R.Tanaka, N.Mituma and R.Yamada, Nagaoka Red Cross Hospital,Niigata University, Aichi Medical College, Shinshu University,Niigata,940,Japan.

Hyperthyroidism(HT) with elevated serum(s) TSH and β-TSH is rare. We report a case in which the HT might be related to the elevated sTSH and β-TSH by the AT. A 27 year old man with a history of hypertension with hypersweating and palpitation. Height 170 cm, BW 54.5 kg, BP 150/90 mmHg, puls rate 130/m. His struma was soft and diffuse. His exophthalamos was not found. I^{131} uptake(24h) 61.5%, BMR+ 42%. TGHA(-), MCHA(-), LATS(-), TSI-71.3%. Elevated sT3, T4, FT4, TSH and β-TSH were 569.6 ng/dl(85-200), 21.6 ug/dl(5-12), 10↑ ng/dl(0.8-2.2), 77.8 uU/ml(2-10) and 3.9 ng/ml(<0.5), respectively, but sα-TSH(0.5 ng/ml) and TRH(6 pg/ml) were normal level. S-TSH value (77.8) by double antibody RIA method was reduced in 3.0 uU/ml by single antibody method. AT to TSH of the IgG(r>k) class which bound human TSH alone was demonstrated using specific RIA and radioimmunoelectrophoretic method. ST3, T4, β-TSH and TSH were not responded to the given TRH, insulin, l-DOPA or T3. However, oral given dexamethasone(4 mg/day x4) suppressed these elevated levels. After the given steroid, these parameters were gradually decreased and now he is euthyroid without elevation of sTSH, β-TSH and the AT. The sT4 level was correlated with sTSH level ($TSH=10^{2.4}$ $T4^{1.8}$, r=0.92) and the sTSH level was also correlated with the AT level ($TSH=10^{0.7}AT^{0.09}$,r=1.0). Moreover, the sβ-TSH level was correlated with sTSH level(β-TSH=0.05TSH+0.1, r=0.97). These results indicated that the thyrotoxicosis might be related to the AT production. This case is unique among repored cases of HT.

1367 STUDY ON THE INCIDENCE OF PATIENTS WITH THYROID DYSFUNCTION IN ADULT, SCREENED BY MESURING TSH AND T4 ON FILTER PAPER. S. Kantoh[1]*, T. Hyodo[1], K. Tsuboi[1], N. Hoshiko[2], T. Masuda[3] and M. Irie[1], 1) First Dept. of Med., Toho Univ. School of Med., Tokyo 143, 2) Nippon Telegr. & Teleph. Public Coop., Tokyo Health Administr. Center, 3) Kanto Teishin Hosp., Tokyo, Japan.

We have collected blood of 11.463(male 9.069, female 2.394) adult normal workers and school students on filter paper, on the occasion of their annual physical examination, and measured TSH and T4 by radioimmunoassay. Either TSH or T4 or both showed abnormal values in 94 cases. For these subjects, serum TSH, Total T4 and T3, Free T4, TBG, antimicrosomal and antithyroglobulin antibody were estimated. From these results, diagnosis was made as follows: hyperthyroidism 4, primary hypothyroidism 14(including 4 subclinical hypothyroidism who showed elevated TSH and normal T4 values) and TBG abnormality 13(increase 2, decrease and deficiency 11). The incidence by this method was; hyperthyroidism 0.35(male 0.33, female 0.45)/1000, primary hypothyroidism 1.22(male 0.99, female 2.08)/1000, TBG increase 0.17(male 0.11, female 0.42)/1000, TBG decrease and deficiency 0.96(male 1.3, female 0)/1000. In 49 subjects among these 94 cases, the subjects with positive antimicrosomal antibody were present in 6 cases (12.3 %), and subjects with positive antithyroglobulin were present in 4 cases (8.2 %). Most of these patients with thyroid dysfunction were not diagnosed before this screening test. The fact that the incidence of hypothyroidism was higher than hyperthyroidism was apparent in this study. We plan to cover the subjects with all age distribution in future.

1368 T CELL SUBSETS IN GRAVES' DISEASE. A. Kapoor* and R. Dattwyler, Division of Endocrinology and Allergy-Immunology, Department of Medicine, SUNY at Stony Brook and NVAMC, New York, USA.

Graves' Disease is generally considered to be a form of organ-specific autoimmune disease. Previous studies of peripheral blood lymphocytes in patients with this disorder utilizing indirect fluorescent microscopy have yielded conflicting results. We sought to improve the accuracy of these results by utilizing a fluorescent activated cell sorter, analyzing 10,000 cells per parameter, not just 200 as in the other studies. Four patients with newly diagnosed, active, untreated Graves' Disease as well as age and sex matched controls were studied using monoclonal antibodies against Helper Cells (T4), Suppressor/Cytoxic Cells (T8), Total T Cells (T11), and Natural Killer Cells (Leu 7). 20cc of Heparinized venous blood was obtained from each patient and the mononuclear cells were isolated using a standard Ficoll-Hypaque gradient. The cells were incubated with the appropriate monoclonal antibody washed and then incubated with goat antimouse Ig conjugated with FITC. The labelled cells were analyzed on a Coulter Epics V cell sorter. No significant difference in total T cells, helper cells, suppressor/cytoxic cells, NK cells or helper/suppressor ratios as compared to the normal controls were found. We, therefore, conclude that Graves' Disease is not accompanied by alterations of peripheral T-cell subsets. This does not exclude an abnormality of the functional status of peripheral T-cells, however.

1369 A HIGHLY SENSITIVE METHOD OF BIOTIN-AVIDIN SOLID-PHASE EIA DETECTS THYROGLOBULIN ANTIBODY SYNTHESIS IN VITRO.

M. Kawagoe*, W. Hirose, M. Hara A. Kitani, T. Hirose and H. Nakamura, 1st Dept. Int. Med. National Defense Medical College, Tokorozawa, Saitama 359, Japan.

To estimate in vitro thyroglobulin(TG) antibody(Ab) synthesis by the peripheral blood lymphocytes(PBL) of Hashimoto thyroiditis, we improved EIA method by introducing Biotin-Avidin(B-A) system. PBL from 8 Hashimoto patients and 6 normals were cultured with TG and/or staphylococcus aureus cowan I(SAC) for 5 days and in fresh medium for another 2 days. TG-Ab in the culture supernatants was assayed by B-A EIA. Immunoplate was coated with bovine TG, and sample, biotinylated anti-human Ig, Avidin D-horse-radish peroxidase and o-PD were applied in this order. The sensitivity of B-A EIA was 5 times greater than that of tanned red cell hemagglutination. Hashimoto's PBL were classified into 3 groups upon their respose to TG and /or SAC. Group I(3 cases): TG-Ab production was increased by TG but suppressed by SAC. In these cases B cells had been stimulated with TG already in vivo and could not respond to SAC, and might be suppressed through a immunological feedback regulation. All these cases were in hypothyroid state and had elevated TSH and CPK. Group II(3): The response to TG was negative and to SAC was positive. However the response to SAC and TG was increased. Group III(2): They responded to neither TG nor SAC. Only 2 cases out of Group II and III had the episode of hypothyroidism. Therefore, the patterns of PBL respose to TG and/or SAC in vitro detected by B-A EIA could be a valuable immunological indicator of Hashimoto thyroiditis.

1370 IMMUNOHISTOCHEMICAL STUDY OF IODINATED PROTEINS IN THE NORMAL HUMAN THYROID GLAND.

R. Kawano*, N. Mishima, A. Ikeda , T. Harada**
Department of Anatomy, **Division of Endocrine Surgery, Department of Surgery, Kawasaki Medical School, Kurashiki 701-01, Japan.

Thyroid albumin is defined as an iodinated albumin isolated from normal and pathological thyroid gland. However, the nature of this protein remains controversy. The aim of this study is to explore the origin and characteristics of the thyroid albumin extracted from normal human thyroid gland.

Amino-acid analysis revealed a difference of the basic amino-acid composition between the thyroid albumin and the serum albumin. Immunodiffusion study of each fraction extracted by flat-bed isoelectric focusing was also performed to confirm their pI range; the thyroid albumin ranged from 4.70 to 5.21 and the serum albumin ranged from 4.85 to 6.16.

Double diffusion agar gel method was carried out to elucidate the relationship between thyroid albumin and T_3. The thyroid albumin reacted with anti-human albumin and $-T_3$ serum, but not with anti-thyrogloburin serum. However, there was no presipitin reaction of the T_3-free sample, prepared by charcoal absoaption, with anti-T_3 serum.

In the foregoing study, it seems likely that the thyroid albumin is the tissue specific protein which might participate in transportation of the thyroid hormone, liberated from thyrogloburin or iodine oxidated in the follicular cells.

1371 EFFECTS OF DOPAMINE ANTAGONISTS ON THYROTROPIN AND PROLACTIN SECRETION -EVIDENCE FOR DISSIMILAR MODIFICATION- M. Kikuoka*, H. Kikuoka#, E. Suzuki, Y. Momotani, H. Bessho#, G. Matsumoto#, K. Nanjo#, K. Iwo#, K. Miyamura# and Y. Higashi, Dept. of Neuropsyciatry, #Div. of Endocrinology, Dept. of Internal Medicine, Wakayama Medical School, Wakayama 640, JAPAN

Dopamine, a well-known inhibitor of prolactin (PRL) release, has also regulatory effects on thyrotropin (TSH) in the various thyroid diseases. The aim of this study is to describe the discrepant effects of various dopamine antagonists upon TSH and PRL secretion in euthyroid subjects and to clarify the dissimilarity between dopaminergic control of PRL and TSH secretion. Nineteen normal male volunteers, aged 20 to 40 years, were studied. One of three dopamine antagonists, 20 mg of metoclopramide (MCP), 25 mg of chlorpromazine (CPZ) and 100 mg of sulpiride (SLP), was diluted with 200 ml of xylitol and infused over 30 minutes. Blood samples drawn at directed time were subjected to radioimmunoassay for PRL and TSH.

Administration of MCP or CPZ was followed by significant rise in TSH from basal level. SLP could not show any significant rises in TSH. Maximal TSH increment induced by CPZ was highest and significantly higher than that induced by SLP. On the contrary, PRL responses to SLP were maximal and those to CPZ were minimal. Additionally, the significant rises of TSH provoked by CPZ and MCP were long after discontinuance of infusion in spite of their prompt effects upon PRL.

These data suggest that, although TSH secretion as well as PRL is under the dopaminergic control, the neuroregulatory "pathway" to TSH secretion is different from that to PRL secretion.

1372 CONSISTENT DECREASE IN CIRCULATING THYROID-STIMULATING IMMUNOGLOBULINS DURING ANTITHYROID DRUG THERAPY. R. Kleinmann*, West Virginia University Medical Center, Charleston Division, Charleston, WV, USA.

The effect of antithyroid drug (ATD) therapy on circulating thyroid adenylate cyclase-stimulating immunoglobulins (TSI) and the clinical significance of TSI measurements during ATD therapy were evaluated. Sera from 15 patients with untreated Graves' disease were assayed for TSI, as were serial samples during ATD therapy in the 10 patients so treated. Immunoglobulins (Ig) extracted from sera were incubated with human thyroid cell membrane homogenates and {32P}ATP. A TSI index was defined as the amount of {32P} cAMP generated in the presence of sample Ig, expressed as the percent above that generated in the presence of Ig from pooled normal sera. The mean TSI index of 33 determinations in 10 normal subjects was 2.9 (SE 1.1); the highest value in a normal subject was 11.6. One untreated Graves' serum was negative for TSI (TSI index 5.6); the other 14 were positive (range 17.4-255.3, mean 68.2). The TSI index decreased during each of 10 courses of propylthiouracil or methimazole. The mean TSI index was 73.5 before treatment and 42.4 after a mean of 12 wks of treatment ($p<0.005$ by paired *t* test). In 4 patients the TSI index became normal during ATD therapy and ATD's were discontinued: 2 had a marked rise in TSI index and a relapse of thyrotoxicosis within 20 wks; 1 had a prolonged remission (>1 yr) and 1 was lost to follow up. In conclusion, (1) there is a consistent decrease in circulating TSI during ATD therapy, and (2) disappearance of circulating TSI during ATD therapy does not predict a long term remission. (The meticulous technical assistance of Amy Vaughan is gratefully acknowledged. This work was supported by NIH grant AM-30586).

1373 INTRACTABLE GRAVES' DISEASE DETERMINED BY CIRCULATING THYROGLOBULIN(Tg) CONCENTRATION.

I. Kobayashi*, H. Ishihara, M. Murakami, M. Takahashi, H. Shimizu, Y. Shimomura, K. Ohshima, M. Mori, N. Kamio, T. Kondo and S. Kobayashi, Division of Endocrinology, First Department of Internal Medicine, Gunma University and Isesaki City Hospital, Maebashi 371, Japan.

There is no reliable parameter indicating intractable Graves' disease resistant to antithyroid drug therapy. We attempted to determine whether measurement of circulating thyroglobulin(Tg) reflected thyroid activity in such patients. One hundred patients with Graves' disease had been treated propylthiouracil or methimazole for periods ranging from 1 to 10 years. Serum T_4, T_3 and TSH were measured by RIA. Tg autoantibody-negative sera were used. The positive suppression group in the conventional T_3 suppression test was defined as the post T_3 uptake(24-h) less than 35 %. Serum Tg determined by RIA from the positive group was 47.8±7.6 ng/dl, while that from the negative group was 118.7±30.8 ng/dl($p < 0.01$). On the other hand, serum Tg in all 20 patients with long term antithyroid drug therapy($\geq$ 5 years) remained high throughout the study(203.8±36.3 ng/dl), similar to the level of untreated Graves' disease(210.1±35.2 ng/dl). In contrast, circulating thyrotropin-receptor antibody(TRAb, Smith's kit) was detected in 60 % of the patients in intractable cases.

Conclusion: Determination of circulating Tg appeared to be of practical value in predicting the outcome of medical treatment. Sustained high levels of circulating Tg may be a more sensitive marker for the intractable Graves' disease than TRAb activity.

1374 THYROID HORMONE MODULATION OF PHOSPHATIDYLINOSITOL-SPECIFIC PHOSPHOLIPASE C ACTIVITY IN RAT LIVER: POSSIBLE ROLE OF Ca^{2+}.

M. Kobayashi* and K. Hashizume, Department of Gerontology, Endocrinology and Metabolism, Shinshu University School of Medicine, Matsumoto 390, JAPAN

When mammalian tissues are exposed to peptide hormone or chemical transmitters enhancement of phosphatidylinositol turnover is observed. It is well known that thyroid hormone induces a modification of peptide hormone- or catecholamine-sensitive reactions in several tissues. In this study, we examined the effect of thyroid hormone on the phosphatidylinositol-specific phospholipase C(PIPC) activity in rat liver.

Young male rats were thyroidectomized and 14 days after operation, saline(T_x+saline) or T_4(10 μg)(T_x+T_4) was administered. Thyroidectomy increased the activity of PIPC in liver. T_4 administration to T_x+saline rats reduced the activity of PIPC. The inhibition of the enzyme induced by T_4 was noncompetitive type. The diminished enzyme activity obtained from T_4-treated animals recovered by treatment of the enzyme with 1 mM EGTA in vitro. The enzyme activity derived from T_x+saline rats was not affected by EGTA treatment. Furthermore, the higher concentrations of Ca^{2+} strongly inhibited the enzyme activity obtained from T_x+saline rats. These results suggest that thyroid hormone induces an inactivation of PIPC activity through the mobilization of large amount of Ca^{2+} in intracellular space.

1375 BROMOCRIPTINE AS TREATMENT FOR THYROID HORMONE RESISTANCE.
J. Köbberling*, H. Dirks and G. Hintze, Dept. of Medicine University of Göttingen, D 3400 Göttingen, Germany (FRG)

Resistance to thyroid hormones is characterized by persistently elevated levels of total and free T_4, high TSH and recurrent goitre. Some patients with a predominant resistance of pituitary receptors are mildly hyperthyroid. They cannot be treated with T_4 without deterioration of hyperthyroidism. Patient 1: 29-year-old male, thyroidectomy at the age of 13, referred to the clinic with mild signs and symptoms of hyperthyroidism and with recurrent goitre (about 200 ml); TSH 8.7 µU/ml, T_4 14.5 µg/dl, T_3 233 ng/dl. Similar biochemical abnormalities were found in his father, uncle, son and nice. Patient 2: 55-year-old female, thyroidectomy at the age of 29, referred to the clinic with recurrent goitre (about 260 ml); TSH 12.4 µU/l, T_4 16.1 µg/dl, T_3 444 ng/dl. A pituitary tumor, antibodies to T_3 or T_4 and abnormalities of binding proteins were excluded. Medication of thyroxin had to be discontinued due to severe side effects. Both patients were treated with 7.5 g bromocriptine per day for periods up to 2 years without any side effects. TSH and thyroid hormone levels were reduced to normal or nearly normal. No further enlargement of the thyroid volume was observed. Symptoms of tracheal compression improved or disappeared. Thus, bromocriptine seems to be an adequate treatment for patients with thyroid hormone resistance especially for those with signs or symptoms of hyperthyroidism.

1376 MAPPING OF LIGAND BINDING SITE CHARACTERISTICS OF IODOTHYRONINE DEIODINASE (ITH-D). J. Köhrle*, M. Auf'mkolk, R.-D. Hesch; Division Clinical Endocrinology, Medical University, D-3000 Hannover 61, Postf.610180, W. Germany.

Analysis of structure-activity relationships of more than 30 inhibitory ITH-analogs competing with the substrates L-T4 and rT3 in an in vitro ITH-D assay (ID-50%:10^{-8}-10^{-4}M) let us develop characteristics of the substrate (ligand) binding site of the enzyme. Optimal inhibitory potency was achieved for analogs with 1. a negatively charged side chain if it requires minimal conformational space; 2.bulky substituents in 3- and/or 5-position which diminish rotational freedom between the two aromatic rings; 3. phenolic ring substituents capable of forming hydrogen bonds, increasing the acidity of the phenolic OH-group(s), carrying negative charge, or which are able to interact by charge-transfer reactions similar to iodine. 4. Neither iodine in 3', 5'-position nor a 4'-OH-group are absolutely required for inhibition. 5. "Conformationally blocked analogs" are potent inhibitors,too. 6. Some of the analogs compete with L-T4 or rT3 not as "inhibitors", but serve as substrates of the ITH-D themselves, provided iodine is present as substituent. ITH-D does not catalyze debromination or dehalogenation as shown by HPLC- and RIA-methods for product analysis. We conclude a marked similarity of the ITH-(analog) ligand binding sites between rat liver type I ITH-D and the thyroxin binding prealbumin (TBPA), but to a less extent also with TBG and the nuclear T3-receptor. The conservation of the ITH ligand binding site of ITH binding and metabolizing proteins and their high affinity for iodinated aromates suggest a common ancestor protein in the evolution and this may help in the further characterization of these functionally different cellular, membrane and serum proteins. Ackn.: ITH-analogs were kindly obtained by Drs.Cahnmann, NIH; Cody, Buffalo; Emmett,SK&F England; Rokos, Henning Berlin.

1377 CLINICAL AND LABORATORY OBSERVATIONS IN HYPOTHYROID PATIENTS HAVING TSH-BINDING INHIBITOR IMMUNOGLOBULINS. J. Konishi*, Y. Iida, K. Kasagi, T. Misaki, T. Nakashima, K. Endo, '. Mori, Y. Nohara, N. Matsuura, and K. Torizuka, Departments of Nuclear Medicine and Internal Medicine, Kyoto University School of Medicine, Kyoto, 606 and Department of Pediatrics, Hokkaido University School of Medicine, Sapporo, 060, Japan.

Since 1978, we have experienced 11 hypothyroid patients who have potent TSH-binding inhibitor immunoglobulins (TBII) in their sera. In the present study clinical features and laboratory findings of these patients including 3 cases previously reported were analyzed. The patients, 1 male and 10 females, ranged in their onset of hypothyroidism from 15 to 49 y.o. All of them were nongoitrous and were myxedematous at the time of diagnosis with markedly elevated serum TSH levels. In a screening of 43 patients with primary mydexema, the incidence of cases with potent TBII (>50 % inhibition of ^{125}I-TSH binding) was 12 %. ^{99m}Tc or ^{125}I thyroid uptake in these patients were significantly lower than that in TBII-negative patients with primary myxedema. All except one were positive for antimicrosomal antibodies. Transient hypothyroidism was observed in all 5 babies born to 4 mothers after the onset of the disease. IgG preparations from these patients did not stimulate cAMP accumulation in cultured human thyroid cells and rather inhibited the cAMP increase induced by bTSH. Above clinical and laboratory findings are compatible with the blocking nature of their TBII and support the concept that TBII play a pathogenic role in a group of patients with primary myxedema. Further, the study revealed the usefulness of TBII measurement for the prediction of neonatal hypothyroidism.

1378 INTERFERENCE OF ANTITHYROGLOBULIN AUTOANTIBODIES IN RADIOIMMUNOASSAY OF T-4, T-3 AND rT-3. J. Kosowicz and M. Gembicki*, Department of Endocrinology, Medical Academy, Poznan, Poland.

Laboratory animals immunized with human thyroglobulin /Tg/ develop antibodies which usually bind also thyroid hormones. The aim of our studies was to find whether sera of patients with Tg-autoantibodies show a similar binding of T-4 T-3 and rT-3. In sera of 50 patients with anti-Tg antibodies and sera of 60 control subjects without antibodies the binding of 125-I-T-4, 125-I-T-3 and 125-I-rT-3 was studied by 13% polyethyleneglycol precipitation, binding onto Protein A Sepharose minicolumns and immunosorbents of T-4, T-3 and rT-3 agarose. Our results revealed that in anti-Tg positive sera the binding of labelled T-4, T-3 and rT-3 is 3 to 15% higher than in control sera and in 64%, 52% and 57% of anti-Tg positive sera respectively, which change the results of thyroid hormone assays. The present data demonstrate that high titre anti-Tg autoantibodies show interference in radioimmunoassay of T-4, T-3 and rT-3, hence proper evaluation of thyroid function requires determinations of these antibodies.

1379 "GIGANTOMASTIA"-AN UNUSUAL PRESENTING FEATURE OF PRIMARY HYPOTHYROIDISM.

L.G. Krishnan*, A. Kapoor, and Z. Rosenwaks, Divisions of Endocrinology and Reproductive Endocrinology, Departments of Medicine and Obstetrics and Gynecology. SUNY at Stony Brook, New York, 11794, USA.

Gigantomastia is a rapid and massive hypertrophy of one or both breasts in a female. It is a very rare occurrence usually developing around puberty, postpartum, and menopause. It has, so far, not been linked to any demonstrable hormonal abnormalities. We report a 75 year old caucasian female, who presented with bilateral, massive and progressive breast enlargement of four years duration. Physical examination was unremarkable except for emphysema and gigantomastia. She had no palpable breast masses or nipple discharge. The abnormal serum chemistries included: cholesterol 335 mg/dl, SGOT 113 IU/L, SGPT 67 IU/L, GGTP 122 IU/L, CPK 1534 IU/L, LDH 483 IU/L. Serum T4 (R.I.A.) of less than 3 micrograms/dl (nl: 5.5-11.5), T3 RU 25.5% (23-32%) and TSH greater than 50 MU/L. Her other endocrine data including serum prolactin, DHEA-S, Progesterone, Androstenedione, B-HCG and total plasma and urinary (24 hour) estrogens were normal. The Maturation Index on the PAP smear was 100% parabasal cells. The CT scan of the adrenal gland and an ovarian sonogram were normal. The patient was then treated with gradually increasing doses of L-thyroxine till euthyroid. Thereafter her serum chemistries returned to normal. There was immediate cessation and partial regression of her breast enlargement. Primary hypothyroidism has been known to cause gynecomastia in men. However, this is the first case report of hypothyroidism stimulating massive breast enlargement in a female.

1380 SPECIFIC LOSS OF ABILITY TO α-AMIDATE NEWLY SYNTHESIZED α-MELANOTROPIN(αMSH) IN PRIMARY RAT INTERMEDIATE PITUITARY CULTURES.

V. May*, Neuroscience Dept.,The Johns Hopkins Univ. Med. Sch.,Balt., MD 21205 USA

Alpha-amidation is important in conferring optimal biological activity to many neuroendocrine peptides. An enzyme capable of forming α-amidated product from its glycine extended precursor has been identified in rat intermediate pituitary and shown to require ascorbate, copper and molecular oxygen (Eipper et al., PNAS 80:5144, 1983). Rat intermediate pituitary cells in primary culture exhibit time-dependent loss of αMSH amidation leading to synthesis of ACTH(1-14)OH-related molecules (Eipper et al., JBC 258:7292, 1983). To define the specific factors involved in maintaining α-amidation, a complete serum-free medium (CSFM) was developed. Enzymatically dispersed intermediate pituitary cells were cultured in CSFM containing DMEM:F-12 (1:1), bovine serum albumin, insulin, transferrin, putrescine, T3, $CuSO_4$, ceruloplasmin and trace elements. Tryptic digests of αMSH-related molecules, biosynthetically labeled with [^{3}H]Trp for 3h in pulse-chase experiments, were analyzed by RP-HPLC. Total production of αMSH-sized molecules did not decline in culture. Approximately 85% of the newly synthesized αMSH material was amidated in freshly isolated cells, 20% after 24h and 6% after 72h. Addition of 1 mM ascorbate to the culture medium during the 2h chase period of 72h cultures raised the amidation level to 20%; inclusion of ascorbate during the entire pulse-chase period increased the production of amidated αMSH to 40%. Other factors regulating amidating activity in cultured cells are being investigated. Supported by DA-00266 and ES-07094.

1381 ENDOTOXIN-INDUCED PROLACTIN AND β-ENDORPHIN RELEASE IN THE RAT: EFFECTS OF NALOXONE AND INDOMETHACIN.

M.F. Mazurek*, N.W. Kasting and J.B. Martin, Dept. of Neurology, Massachusetts General Hospital, Boston, MA 02114, USA.

We have shown that endotoxin administered intravenously to the rat results in a prompt rise of plasma prolactin (PRL) and plasma β-endorphin (β-END). We now report that the PRL release is inhibited in a dose-dependent manner by pretreatment with either naloxone or indomethacin, while the β-END release is unaffected. Experiments were performed on freely-behaving male rats. Endotoxin was administered i.v. to all animals at 11:00. Blood was sampled every 30 minutes for 4 hours. Mean baseline PRL values in all groups were <2 ng/ml. In animals receiving endotoxin alone (N=9), PRL rose to 21.0 ± 4.7 ng/ml within 60 minutes. Pretreatment with i.v. naloxone 1 mg/kg (n=6) attenuated this response (peak PRL 6.3 ± 1.1 ng/ml) while naloxone 5 mg/kg (N=5) further suppressed it (peak PRL 2.9 ± 1.5 ng/ml). Pretreatment with s.c. indomethacin 1 mg/kg (n=5) also inhibited the PRL response to endotoxin (peak PRL 4.0 ± 1.5 ng/ml), while indomethacin 5 mg/kg (N=6) abolished it (peak PRL 1.0 ± 0.3 ng/ml). With none of these treatments was there a corresponding inhibition of the plasma β-endorphin (β-END) response to endotoxin. Baseline β-END levels were <85 pg/ml for all groups. Peak β-END levels were: endotoxin alone 1276 ± 56 pg/ml; naloxone 1 mg/kg pretreatment 1350 ± 93 pg/ml; naloxone 5 mg/kg pretreatment 1095 + 85; indomethacin 1 mg/kg pretreatment, 1218 ± 25 pg/ml; indomethacin 5 mg/kg pretreatment 919 ± 165 pg/ml. These results show that both naloxone and indomethacin produce dose-dependent inhibition of endotoxin-induced PRL release without affecting plasma β-endorphin release. Supported by AM26252.

1382 PRO-OPIOMELANOCORTIN (POMC) MODULATION BY CORTICOSTEROID TREATMENT FOR HUMAN SEPTIC SHOCK.

Lorraine McLoughlin*, S.F. Evans, R.L. Patience, C.J. Hinds and Lesley H. Rees, Departments of Chemical Endocrinology, Anaesthetics and Intensive Care, St. Bartholomew's Hospital, London, EC1A 7BE, U.K.

Sephadex G50 chromatography has been utilised to observe the neuroendocrine changes associated with the administration of corticosteroids for the stabilisation of severe shock conditions. Blood samples were obtained at time 0, 1h and 2h after a bolus injection of methyl prednisolone 30mg/kg. Following chromatography the fractions were assayed for ACTH, β-endorphin and γ-MSH immunoreactive content. At time 0' elevated levels were noted of ACTH, 1-76 POMC, β-LPH and β-endorphin, which were subsequently suppressed over the 2h period, with a converse rise in larger molecular weight precursor peptides, and smaller immunoreactive fragments. A feature of the endorphin chromatography was the apparent heterogeneity of β-LPH. HPLC with a Propan-1-ol/0.13%HFBA/H_2O system on an Altex C_3 column, was used to investigate this and supportive evidence was obtained, showing the early fractions to have the elution properties of β-LPH at 23 min, and the second peak to elute at 16 min. The chemical nature of this latter peak awaits elucidation. HPLC analysis of the endorphin fractions using an acetonitrile/H_2O gradient in 0.1% TFA demonstrated at least 3 major forms. The major peak co-elutes with synthetic 1-31 β-endorphin standard at 10 min. The second of these has the elution characteristics of β-LPH at 15 min, and the third that of acetylated 1-27 β-endorphin, the standard of which does not cross-react in the C-terminal β-endorphin assay (<3%).

1383 GONADOTROPIN REGULATION OF PRO-OPIOMELANOCORTIN (POMC) mRNA IN GRANULOSA CELLS. M.H. Melner*+, Y. Luo+, R.D. Koos+, M.R. Clark+, J.L. Roberts**, and D. Puett+, +REPSCEND and the Depts. of Biochemistry and Ob/Gyn, Univ. of Miami Sch. Med., Miami, FL 33101, USA and **Dept. of Biochemistry, Columbia Univ., New York, NY 10032, USA.

Recent evidence has demonstrated the presence of β-endorphin and adrenocorticotropin immuno-reactivities in the sheep ovary and follicular fluid. The objectives of this study were: (1) to determine whether this localization reflects synthesis of the POMC precursor in granulosa cells versus an accumulation of the processed peptides and (2) to investigate whether POMC expression is under gonadotropin regulation. Granulosa cells were harvested from intact, immature, diethylstilbestrol-primed rats. Cells were plated at a density of 3.4×10^6 cells per 5 ml of serum-free DMEM:Ham's F-12 (1:1) medium in 35 mm culture dishes pre-coated with rat tail collagen. The cells were cultured under standard conditions or in the presence of highly purified ovine FSH (Papkoff FSH 211B; 10 ng/ml). After 48 hr of FSH treatment, additional cultures received ovine LH (100 ng/ml) for 24 hr. POMC mRNA was detected by dot-blot hybridization on nitrocellulose using a cDNA for the rat pituitary POMC sequence inserted into PBR 322 plasmid as a probe. The probe was nick-translated to a specific activity of 2.2×10^6 cpm/μg. Positive hybridization was detected in both control and gonadotropin-treated cells. A marked increase in POMC mRNA levels relative to controls was evident throughout much of the 72 hr culture period beginning as early as 1 hr after FSH treatment. Treatment with LH plus FSH appeared to reduce POMC mRNA relative to FSH alone. These studies are the first demonstration of POMC gene expression in granulosa cells and suggest that this expression is under gonadotropin control. Supported by NIH: AM33973.

1384 TWO STIMULI OF IN VIVO IMMUNOREACTIVE ACTH PRODUCTION BY HUMAN LYMPHOCYTES: W. J. Meyer*, E. M. Smith, G. E. Richards, A. Cavallo, A. C. Morrill and J. E. Blalock, Departments of Pediatrics and Microbiology, University of Texas Medical Branch, Galveston, Texas, USA.

Lymphocytes from 21 children (16 with normal pituitary ACTH production [NORMAL] and 5 with ACTH deficiency [ACTH DEF]) were examined for *in vivo* ACTH production by immunofluorescence (IF) with antibody to ACTH (1-13 amide). Children underwent 3 study periods: control, insulin induced hypoglycemia, and typhoid vaccine (an interferon-α inducer). Plasma cortisol and lymphocyte ACTH IF were measured at 0, 1, 2, 4, 6, 8 and 10 hours after each 9AM stimulus. All patients demonstrated positive baseline ACTH IF. NORMAL had an increase in the number of ACTH IF-positive cells at 5PM (6 hr) on the control day (20 ± 4% to 37 ± 8%, $p<.02$), a rise at 1 hr after insulin (25 ± 5% to 44 ± 6%, $p<.01$) and no change with typhoid. ACTH DEF had no change on the control day or after insulin and a significant rise at 5PM (6 hr) on typhoid day (24 ± 14% to 57 ± 7%, $p<.05$). *In vitro*, lymphocytes incubated with ACTH do not increase in IF positivity. Insulin, and/or hypoglycemia, do not increase lymphocyte immunoreactive ACTH production, but typhoid vaccine does (<10 to 75%). Synthetic porcine corticotropin releasing factor (CRF) also caused a significant increase from 10 to 40% IF-positive cells. We conclude that human lymphocyte production of immunoreactive ACTH is increased by at least 2 stimuli: 1) a central factor made by the hypothalamic pituitary axis, (possibly CRF), accounting for the *in vivo* rise 1 hr after insulin in NORMAL and *in vitro* with CRF, and 2) an interferon inducer (e.g., typhoid vaccine) accounting for the typhoid induced rise *in vivo* in ACTH DEF and *in vitro* with typhoid vaccine.

1385 CHRONIC HALOPERIDOL SELECTIVELY ALTERS THE MOLECULAR FORMS OF β-ENDORPHIN IN THE INTERMEDIATE LOBE OF THE RAT PITUITARY. W.R. Millington*, M.C. Chappell, T.L. O'Donohue and G.P. Mueller, Dept. of Physiology, Uniformed Services University and Exper. Ther. Br., NINCDS, NIH, Bethesda, MD USA

β-endorphin (β-END) is post-translationally processed in the intermediate lobe (IL) through N-terminal acetylation and C-terminal cleavage to multiple molecular forms which differ markedly in their bioactivities. We found that chronic haloperidol (HAL) administration, which has been shown to accelerate IL β-END synthesis, differentially alters the concentration of each molecular form of β-END in the IL. HAL treatment (2mg/kg; 21 days) increased the IL content of total immunoreactive β-END (iβ-END) two-fold without affecting anterior lobe or plasma concentrations of iβ-END by 24h after the last injection. Cation exchange chromatography (SP Sephadex) revealed that the predominant forms of IL β-END, specifically, N-Ac-β-END 1-26, 1-27 and 1-31, constituted 29%, 48% and 10% of total iβ-END, respectively. HAL dramatically increased the amount of N-Ac-β-END-1-27 in the IL (accounting for 67% of the HAL-induced increase in total iβ-END) and substantially lowered N-Ac-β-END-1-26 (from 29% to 10% of total iβ-END). Consistent with the increase in total N-Ac-β-END, the activity of opiomelanotropin acetyltransferase (OMAT), the enzyme which acetylates β-END peptides, was similarly increased two-fold by HAL treatment. These data indicate that treatment conditions which accelerate β-END synthesis both increase the activity of OMAT, an enzyme importantly involved in the post-translational processing of β-END, and alter the pattern of β-END peptides contained in and released from the IL.

1386 EFFECTS OF NALOXONE ON CATECHOLAMINE SECRETION IN CULTURED BOVINE ADRENOMEDULLARY CHROMAFFIN CELLS AND HUMAN PHEOCHROMOCYTOMA CELLS. N. Morii*, K. Nakao, T. Yoshimasa, M. Suda, M. Sakamoto, Y. Ikeda, I. Tanaka, S. Oki, K. Kumakura, S. Matsukura and H. Imura, 2nd Div., Dept. of Med. and Div. of Clin. Nutrition (S.M.), Kyoto Univ. Sch. of Med., Sakyo-ku, Kyoto 606 and Life Science Institute (K.K.), Sophia Univ., Tokyo, Japan.

Recently we reported the existence of a high amount of opioid peptides in the adrenal medulla and some human pheochromocytomas (Yoshimasa et al. JCI 69, 643, 1982). In order to elucidate a pathophysiological role of endogenous opioid peptides in the adrenal medulla and pheochromocytoma, effects of naloxone on catecholamine (CA) secretion were studied in cultured bovine adrenomedullary chromaffin cells and human pheochromocytoma cells. In bovine chromaffin cells, a low dose of naloxone ($\leqq 10^{-6}$M) did not affect either basal CA secretion or acetylcholine (ACh) stimulated CA secretion. Addition of a high dose of naloxone (10^{-4}M) also did not affect basal CA secretion, but showed 46% inhibition of CA secretion stimulated by 10^{-4}M ACh. In human pheochromocytoma cells, a low dose of naloxone (10^{-6}M) had no significant effects on basal nor ACh stimulated CA secretion. A high dose of naloxone (10^{-4}M) exerted an increase of basal CA secretion which was comparable to the response to ED_{30} of ACh. However, the presence of a high dose of naloxone caused 75% inhibition of CA secretion stimulated by 10^{-4}M ACh. Since a high dose of naloxone acts not only as an opioid antagonist but as an agonist, further studies as to whether or not the effects of naloxone on CA secretion is mediated via endogenous opioid peptides are ongoing in our laboratory.

1387 A BENZODIAZEPINE RECEPTOR MECHANISM REGULATES THE RELEASE OF PITUITARY β-END IN RATS. G.P. Mueller*, S. Maiewski, K.M. Hargreaves, and R.A. Dionne. Dept. Physiol., USUHS, and NAB, NIDR, NIH, Bethesda, MD, USA

Our recent studies in humans have revealed that benzodiazepine-sensitive anxiety covaries with the release of pituitary immunoreactive β-END (iβ-END). This raises the possibility that an interaction exists between pituitary iβ-END, benzodiazepine receptor mechanisms and the perception of anxiety. To further examine this question we have evaluated the effects of three classes of benzodiazepine receptor acting drugs on the release of pituitary iβ-END in rats. Neither the "active agonist", diazepam, nor the "inactive antagonist", RO 15-1788, altered basal secretion of pituitary iβ-END over time. By contrast, the "active antagonist", ethyl β-carboline-3-carboxylate (βCCE), which causes anxiety, evoked dose-related (up to 30 mg/kg, ip) increases in plasma iβ-END which were maximal (four-fold) by 10 min. This response was attenuated by pretreatment with either diazepam (2.5 mg/kg) or RO 15-1788 (10 mg/kg) but not by morphine (5 mg/kg). CGS 8216, another benzodiazepine receptor antagonist, also evoked dose-related (.2 to 5 mg/kg) increases in circulating iβ-END (maximal by 15 min); the iβ-END response to CGS 8216 was attenuated by pretreatment with RO 15-1788. Gel filtration chromatography revealed that the majority of circulating iβ-END following βCCE treatment resembled beta-lipotropin in molecular size, a marker for pars distalis secretion. This finding, taken together with the observation that dexamethasone pretreatment completely prevented the βCCE plasma iβ-END response, suggests that a benzodiazepine receptor mechanism regulates hypothalamic corticotropin releasing factor and, thereby, pars distalis iβ-END.

1388 INCREASED SECRETORY ACTIVITY OF ACTH AND MSH CELLS IN THE PITUITARY OF RATS BY OVINE AND BOVINE CRF. D.V. Naik*, R.M.G. Nair+, and T.Fairwell++, *Dept. of Anatomy, Kuwait Univ., Kuwait, +VA Medical Center, Charleston, SC, and ++Molecular Disease Branch, NHLBI, Bethesda, MD, USA.

Pars intermedia (PI) and its rostral zone in the pituitary contain both ACTH and MSH cells innervated by nerve fibers, whereas pars distalis (PD) contains only ACTH cells. To study the comparative regulatory activities of ovine and bovine CRF on both ACTH and MSH cells, 200 ng of synthetic ovine or bovine CRF was infused in the lateral ventricle of 15 male rats. The animals were sacrificed 5 and 15 minutes after infusion, and their PI and PD were studied by electron microscopy. Five minutes after infusion, ACTH and MSH cells showed very high level of activity. ACTH cells showed an abundance of granules towards the periphery, with granule extrusion in the pericapillary and intercellular spaces. MSH cells were loaded with enlarged granules, many of which were released in the intercellular spaces. In both ACTH and MSH cells, the endoplasmic reticulum, Golgi apparatus and the Golgi cisternae showed hyperactivity with an abundance of pleomorphic granules in the region of the Golgi complex. Fifteen minutes after the infusion, hyperactivity had tapered off in both ACTH and MSH cells. ACTH cells were on their way to recovery, while most of the MSH cells still showed exhaustion. Our results indicate that ovine and bovine CRF activates increased synthesis and release of ACTH and MSH granules in both the ACTH and MSH cells of the pituitary. The peptides were found specific to these two types of cell populations. Supported by Kuwait University Grant and by the Veterans Administration.

1389 THE LASTING EFFECT OF ACTH ON STEROIDOGENESIS IN GUINEA PIG ADRENOCORTICAL CELLS : EVIDENCE FOR STIMULATION OF PRE- AND POST-PREGNENOLONE PATHWAYS OF CORTISOL SYNTHESIS. F. Lambert ☆, J. Lammerant and J. Kolanowski, Dept. Physiol., Medical School, Namur (Belgium).

Aside from its well-known acute effect on the overall adrenocortical steroidogenesis, ACTH may also exert a prolonged stimulatory influence on cortisol (F) synthesis. In the present study, this lasting effect of ACTH was evaluated on adrenocortical cells harvested from control (C) and ACTH-treated guinea pigs (A; 50 μg $ACTH_{1-24}$, s.c. twice, 24 h before the experiment) . The maximal production of F in response to ACTH was increased from 342 ± 36 ng (C) to 663 ± 38 ng (A). In the presence of trilostane, added to block the conversion of pregnenolone (P) into F, the maximal production of endogenous P and 17-hydroxypregnenolone (17OHP) in response to ACTH was increased in A group (450 ± 36 ng P and 86 ± 11 ng 17OHP *vs* 269 ± 36 ng P and 44 ± 9 ng 17OHP in C). In addition, the conversion of 5 μg of exogenous P into F was significantly greater in A (2193 ± 139 ng) than in C (1277 ± 124 ng) while 11-deoxycortisol (S) accumulation was decreased in A which suggests an enhanced 11 β hydroxylase activity. Moreover, the maximal capacity to convert exogenous P into F was also increased in cells from ACTH-treated animals (3423 ± 211 ng F formed from 5 μg S *vs* 2074 ± 185 ng in C). Thus, ACTH exerts a prolonged stimulatory effect both on the capacity of adrenocortical cells to produce pregnenolone, which quantitatively account for the increase in steroidogenic potency of these cells, and on the conversion of this common precursor of steroidogenesis into cortisol.

1390 PROENKEPHALIN- AND ENKEPHALIN-LIKE IMMUNOREACTIVITIES IN THE ADRENAL GLAND AND BRAIN OF THE FROG. F. Leboulenger*, Y. Charnay[π], P.M. Dubois[π], G. Pelletier[&], J. Rossier[§], and H. Vaudry, Lab. Endocrinol., Fac. Sciences Rouen, 76130 Mt-St-Aignan, France; [π] Lab. Histol. Embryol., Fac. Medicine Lyon-Sud, 69600 Oullins, France; [&] MRC Group in Molecular Endocrinol., CHUL, Quebec; § Lab. Physiol. Nerveuse, CNRS, 91190 Gif-sur-Yvette, France.

We have recently raised antibodies against synenkephalin, the N-terminal 77-amino-acid residues from bovine adrenal proenkephalin, which does not contain any enkephalin sequence. These antibodies have now been used to elucidate the localization of proenkephalin in the adrenal gland and brain of the frog. In the adrenal gland, immunofluorescence studies on adjacent sections showed that synenkephalin-like immunoreactivity (LI) was present, together with Met- and Leu-enkephalin-, and vasoactive intestinal peptide (VIP)-LI, in all cells which stained for tyrosine hydroxylase (chromaffin cells). At the electron microscope level, we have observed the coexistence of both VIP-, Met- and Leu-enkephalin-, and dopamine β-hydroxylase-LI in 200-400 nm dense-core secretory granules of frog chromaffin cells. Immunocytochemical localization of synenkephalin in these secretory granules is in progress. In the frog brain proenkephalin- and enkephalin-LI had the same distribution. Cell bodies were restricted to the infundibulum and the central tectum whereas fibres were largely distributed (infundibulum, preoptic area, cerebral cortex, lateral funiculus of the rhombencephalon...). No proenkephalin- or enkephalin-LI could be detected in any part of the hypophysis. These results demonstrate that, in frog as in mammals, Met- and Leu-enkephalins derive from a pro-hormone and they indicate that the structure of proenkephalin is highly preserved in all vertebrate species.

1391 ADRENAL STEROID RESPONSES TO ACTH STIMULATION IN YOUNG NORMAL AND HIRSUITE FEMALE HUMANS. Peter A. Lee*, Maria D. Urban, Roberto Lanes, Departments of Pediatrics, University of Pittsburgh, Pittsburgh, PA; Wright State University, Dayton, OH: North Shore University Hospital, Manhasset, NY, USA

Ten normal 15 hirsuite females aged 15-30 had steroid levels determined before and 30 minutes after 100 units of ACTH (Cortrosyn). Plasma levels of 17-hydroxypregnenalone (17 Preg), 17-hydroxyprogesterone (17 Prog), progesterone (Prog), desoxycortisol (Cmpd S), dehydroepiandrosterone (DHA), DHA sulfate (DHAS), and androstenedione (Δ4) were determined by radioimmunoassay after column chromatography separation.

Normal Females - Follicular Phase

	17-Preg (ng/dl)	17-Prog (ng/dl)	Prog (ng/dl)	Cmpd S (ng/dl)	DHA (ng/dl)	DHAS (ng/dl)	Δ4 (ng/dl)
				Basal Levels			
$\bar{x}$	171	58	29	57	353	1503	169
SD	86	31	15	39	113	794	67
Range	(37-305)	(37-104)	(09-38)	(19-136)	(174-515)	(546-2878)	(101-289)
				Incremental Rise (30 Minutes)			
$\bar{x}$	294	85	40	67	746	207	60
SD	202	42	19	36	419	249	40
Range	(25-599)	(09-145)	(16-69)	(04-143)	(42-1316)	(01-337)	(20-84)

Thirteen of 15 patients had abnormal hormonal rises; 12 had elevated baselines including the 2 without increased increments. 3 had abnormal Cmpd S levels (± abnormal values proximally in the metabolic pathway); 3 abnormal 17 Prog ± proximal steroids; and 5 abnormal 17 Preg and androgen levels. The remaining 4 had only elevated androgen levels.

1392 CHARACTERIZATION OF HMG-CoA REDUCTASE IN A VIRILIZING HUMAN ADRENAL CARCINOMA. J.G. Lehoux*, S. Bélisle and D. Bellabarba. Faculty of Medicine, Sherbrooke University, Sherbrooke, Quebec, Canada, J1H 5N4.

3-Hydroxy-3-methyl glutaryl coenzyme A (HMG-CoA) reductase is a key regulatory enzyme of cholesterol synthesis. We have characterized this enzyme in a tissue producing an excess of steroids, namely a human virilizing adrenal carcinoma. Tissue was homogenized in an Imidazole buffer containing 1mM PMSF, 0.1mM leupeptine and 5.5mM DTT. The HMG-CoA reductase activity assay was performed on microsomal preparations preincubated at 37°C for 30 min., followed by incubation in the presence of (^{14}C)-HMG-CoA and a NADPH generating system. The authenticity of (^{14}C) mevalonate formed was verified by silica gel chromatography as the free acid, and as its lactone-, and amide derivatives. HMG-CoA cleavage activity was also assayed and found to be less than 4% under conditions used. HMG-CoA reductase activity was maximal in the presence of 5mM EDTA, 5.5mM DTT, 250mM NaCl and at pH 7.2. Km_s for the substrates (S)-HMG-CoA and $NADP^+$ were 5µM and 80µM respectively. Maximal reductase activity was 994 ± 74 pmol/mg prot/min (mean ± SE, N=10). This activity was decreased 32% when NaF was present in the homogeneisation and incubation media. NaF also prevented the activation of the reductase by liver phosphorylase phosphatase. In the absence of NaF the preincubation alone increased the reductase activity 1.7 ± .16 fold (mean ± SE, N=10). Two fractions, one inhibiting, the other enhancing the reductase activity were also partially isolated from the tumor. The high level of HMG-CoA reductase activity suggests that the tumor had acquired a high capacity for *de novo* cholesterol synthesis; presumably a requirement for its high steroid production. Supported by a grant from MRC (Canada).

1393 REPEATED SMALL HEMORRHAGE (HEM) POTENTIATES ADRENAL CORTISOL AND CATECHOLAMINE RESPONSES IN AWAKE DOGS. M.P. Lilly*, W.C. Engeland, and D.S. Gann, Brown Univ/RI Hospital, Providence, RI 02902 USA

Potentiated adrenal responses to the second of 2 hems 24h apart are seen in the pentobarbital anesthetized(PA) dog(Endo 111:1917,1982; Endo 112:681, 1983). However, PA may affect baseline and posthem responses of hemodynamic and hormonal parameters in the dog. Therefore, we studied this effect in awake trained dogs with chronic adrenal venous catheters.Dogs were bled 8.7 to 21.8% I-131 blood volume(BV) over 3m, and peripheral and adrenal blood was sampled. Blood was reinfused 1h later, and the dogs were fed. Experiments(exp) were repeated 24h later.Catecholamines and steroids were assayed by HPLC, ACTH by RIA. Secretory rates of epinephrine, norepinephrine and cortisol were calculated(E,NE,F).Maximal F(MaxF)was determined after injection of 100mU ACTH following each exp. Dogs with large hem(18.9+2.1%BV;n=9) showed a greater E and NE response to hem on day2($P<0.05$). Dogs with small hem(11.6+2.3%BV; n=8) showed no difference on the 2 days. Dogs whose day 1F after hem was submaximal(15.9+3.1%BV;n=7)showed a greater F response to hem on day2($p<0.005$). This increased F response to hem was accompanied by increased responses in ACTH presentation rate(APR)($p<0.025$) and by increased adrenal sensitivity to ACTH(slope F vs logAPR)($p<0.025$).No potentiation was seen if post hem F reached MaxF and MaxF did not change on the 2 days. No hemodynamic differences were seen on the 2days in any group.These data confirm and extend our results in the PA dog. Whereas potentiation was seen in both E and NE responses to a 2nd 10%hem in PA dogs,larger hem(20%) was needed to elicit this effect in awake dogs. In contrast, PA does not alter the expression of potentiated F responses. However,cortisol potentiation may be limited to repeated submaximal stimuli. Thus, potentiated adrenal cortical and medullary responses to repeated hem occur in both awake and PA dogs,yet important differences in the threshold and manifestation of this effect are seen. This work was supported by NIH grants AM26831 & GM27946.

1394 90 MINUTE OSCILLATION IN CORTICOSTERONE SECRETION RATE IN CONSCIOUS, NORMAL DOGS. L.L. Loring, L.A. Benton and F.E. Yates*, Crump Institute for Medical Engineering, UCLA, Los Angeles, CA 90024, U.S.A.

Cortisol secretion rate (FSR) and adrenal blood flow oscillate with periods of 3 and 90 min in conscious, unrestrained dogs; blood flow oscillates also at 6 min (L. A. Benton, L. L. Loring, and F. E. Yates: The Physiologist 26: A-19, 1983). To test whether or not corticosterone secretion rate (BSR) shows similar rhythms, we collected 1146 spontaneous adrenal blood samples from 7 dogs in 17 experiments. We obtained samples every 15 or 20 sec, for 25 min; 5 min, for 240 min; or 10 min, for 480 min. Corticosterone concentration was determined by a double-antibody radioimmunoassay developed in our laboratory. Mean BSR in these normal, resting dogs was 0.5 ug/min, although the moment-to-moment range was 0.0-18.8 ug/min. After a 1 U i.v. bolus of ACTH (supramaximal stimulus to corticosteroid secretion) BSR increased to peak (range 0.3-14.7 ug/min) in 15 min. Maximum BSR lagged maximum blood flow, however, by 10 min. Data (before ACTH) from individual experiments were analyzed for periodic behavior by spectral analysis. We could have detected oscillations with periods of 1.25-10 min (15 or 20 sec sampling) or 25-160 min (5 or 10 min sampling). We did not detect oscillation in BSR at 3 min, previously found in FSR and adrenal blood flow, or at 6 min, previously found in blood flow but not FSR. In 4/8 cases, however, BSR oscillated at approximately 90 min. Conclusion: These results are additional evidence that 90 min is the period of a major organizing rhythm in the conscious, normal dog. Supported by NIH Grant GM 23732.

1395 LATE ONSET CONGENITAL ADRENAL HYPERPLASIA(CAH) IN WOMEN WITH POLYCYSTIC OVARY SYNDROME(PCO). A.A.LUCIANO*, R.N. Turksoy, F.K. Chapler, and B.M. Sherman, Depts. of Ob-Gyn and Med., U. of Iowa and Tufts University, Boston, Massachusetts 02111.

Late onset CAH has been reported to occur in 2-20% of hirsute women. Since the clinical presentation of CAH is indistinguishable from that of PCO, its diagnosis must be based on the abnormal response of 17-hydroxyprogesterone (17-OHP) to ACTH stimulation. To further define the incidence of CAH and to better characterize its endocrine profile, we evaluated 60 PCO patients with extensive baseline and perturbation studies, using gonadotropin releasing hormone, dexamethasone suppression and ACTH stimulation (Cortrosyn 0.25 mg I.V.). CAH was diagnosed in 4 patients by an exaggerated 17OHP response to ACTH, as shown below. Urinary free cortisol (F) were lower and baseline DHEA-S levels were higher in CAH patients (p<.05).

		F ug%	17-OHP ng%	DHEA-S ug%	A-Dione ng%	Test. ng%
Basal	PCO	12.3±2	112±12	303±21	603±32	87±5
	CAH	9.9±1	678±200**	508±30**	659±39	142±11**
After ACTH	PCO	22.4±4	190±10	250±29	550±40	101±12
	CAH	16.7±3	5990±300**	479±27**	732±52	122±14

Conclusions: 1) In our population of patients with symptom complex of PCO, the incidence of CAH is 6.7%; 2) Mean urinary F levels are significantly lower in CAH patients; 3) The basal levels of at least one of the adrenal steroids were sufficiently elevated in each of the four patients with CAH to strongly suggest its diagnosis and to allow for selective utilization of the ACTH stimulation test to render this test cost effective in PCO patients at risk. **p<.05

1396 CLONING OF cDNA ENCODING BOVINE $P450_{scc}$ (20,22 DESMOLASE). K.J. Matteson, B.C. Chung, and W.L. Miller*, Dept. of Pediatrics, University of California, San Francisco, CA., 94143

The first, rate-limiting, and hormonally regulated step in the conversion of cholesterol to all steroid hormones is cholesterol side chain cleavage (SCC) by 20,22 desmolase. This enzyme is a single 49,000 dalton mitochondrial cytochrome P450, termed $P450_{scc}$ which is synthesized as a 54,500 dalton precursor. We prepared polyadenylated messenger RNA (mRNA) from demedulated bovine adrenals and used this mRNA as template for the synthesis of double-stranded (DS) complementary DNA (cDNA), and cloned DS cDNA larger than 1kb in the Pst I site of pBR322 by the dC.DG "tailing" procedure, yielding >10,000 clones. Pools of 4 to 10 clones together with a previously prepared bovine growth hormone cDNA clone were assayed by hybrid-selected translation using a rabbit-anti-bovine $P450_{scc}$ antiserum (M.R. Waterman, Dallax, TX.) and rabbit-anti-ovine growth hormone antiserum as an internal control. Although cell-free translation of bovine adrenocortical mRNA followed by immunoprecipitation with anti-bovine $P450_{scc}$ suggested about 1.0 to 1.5% of bovine adrenal mRNA encodes $P450_{scc}$, we screened over 700 clones before finding a pool of 4 clones which specifically selected $P450_{scc}$ mRNA. The cloned DNA from the positive clone in this pool should provide the amino acid sequence of a $P450_{scc}$ and should be useful for studying the hormonal regulation of this enzyme. This work was supported by NIH grant HD16047.

1397 EFFECT OF SOMATOSTATIN ON THE GROWTH AND STEROIDOGENIC CAPACITY OF THE RAT ADRENAL CORTEX. G.Mazzocchi, P.Rebuffat and G.G.Nussdorfer*, Department of Anatomy, University of Padua, 35100 Padua, Italy.

Some lines of evidence indicate that somatostatin exerts an inhibitory effect on rat zona glomerulosa cells cultured in vitro (Aguilera et al., Nature 292:262,1981). The effects of somatostatin are now investigated in vivo, using hypophysectomized rats administered maintenance doses of ACTH (4 IU/kg). Stereology demonstrated that 5 daily subcutaneous injections of somatostatin (100 μg/kg) induce a noticeable decrease (about 40%) in the volume of zona glomerulosa cells. The decrease in the volume of zona fasciculata cells was much less conspicuous (about 18%), but still significant. The atrophy of adrenocortical cells was principally due to a dramatic decrease in the volume of smooth endoplasmic reticulum and mitochondria, the two cytoplasmic organelles containing the enzymes of steroid synthesis. Radioimmunoassay showed that somatostatin chronic administration provokes a significant fall in both plasma and intracellular concentrations of aldosterone (30% and 52%, respectively). Plasma corticosterone concentration did not display any significant change, while intracellular corticosterone level was noticeably lowered (about 35%). These findings suggest that somatostatin plays a major role in the control of rat zona glomerulosa growth and steroidogenic capacity. However, a slight inhibitory action of this polypeptide on the zona fasciculata cannot be excluded.

1398 RADICAL OVARIAN RESECTION ACCELERATES ONSET OF ACYCLICITY AND PERSISTENT VAGINAL CORNIFICATION (PVC) BUT ONLY TRANSIENTLY DISRUPTS THE REPRODUCTIVE HYPOTHALAMIC-PITUITARY AXIS (HPA) IN C57BL/6J MICE. J. Nelson* & L. Felicio Centre for the Study of Reproduction & Department of Ob/Gyn, McGill Univ., Montreal, Quebec, H3A 1A1, Canada.

Aging of the female reproductive HPA in laboratory rodents is attributable in part to exposure during adulthood to ovarian secretions. Although estradiol (E2) is implicated, neither the duration nor pattern of hormonal exposure required to disrupt HPA function is known. This study was designed to determine whether ovarian secretions during PVC, the predominant post-cyclic phase (low but relatively steady plasma E2), are more detrimental to the HPA than those associated with regular cyclicity (E2 levels are elevated but fluctuating). To examine these two hormonal states independent of age, cessation of cyclicity and subsequent onset of PVC were advanced by resecting 90% of the ovarian tissue from 4-mo-old mice. At 13 mos., mice were acutely ovariectomized and given 4-mo-old ovarian grafts under the renal capsule to assess the potential of the HPA to support estrous cycles. At that age, median duration of exposure to PVC in resected mice was 2.5 mo. compared to 1 mo. in shams ($P<0.001$, Mann-Whitney U-test (MWUT)). During the first month after grafting, resected mice had only half the cycles of shams ($P<0.005$, MWUT). However, total cycles experienced by the two groups during months 2 and 3 after grafting were indistinguishable. These results suggest that the ovarian secretions associated with PVC are more detrimental to the HPA than those of regular cyclicity, but that the deleterious effects of PVC are only transient at this age. Supported by MRC of Canada; JN is a MRC Scholar.

1399 IODINE KINETIC ANALYSIS (IKA) IN THE ERDERLY. W.Nicolau, Y.Grandjean-Thomsen, Y.L.Long, P.A.Costa and E.C.Carvalho Fº., Unity of Endocrinology - São Paulo University - CP 8091 - São Paulo, Brazil.

IKA was performed in 7 normal (5 females and 2 males) subjects older than 70y. (71 to 89y). Serum thyroxine (8.76±1.59ug%), T_3 (148±27.1ng%), TSH (3.5±1.4uUI/ml) and 24h^{131}I uptake (25.1±4.4) were in the normal range. Three compartimental model was utilized. After I.V. ^{131}I administration serial determinations were made for the thyroid (T) isotope content and PB^{131}I. To the extent possible all parameters were measured at 2,4,8h and daily intervals until equilibrium (Eq.) was reached, observed by the assimptotism of PB^{131}I curve. In Eq. T. iodine Pool (Qg), T. iodine secretion release rate (Kgb), T. secretion (H) and actual T. ^{131}I T1/2 (T.T1/2) were calculated. For this purpose we utilized the equilibrium and theoretical maximum T.uptake, PB^{131}I (PB^{131}I/T_4I) specific activity and the slope of the T. uptake curve. Our data show: 1) A lower than habitual Qg (5,152±3,820ug), 4 out 7 presenting less than 5,000ug, 2) a high Kgb (0.0266±0.0089d^{-1}), 3) a low T.T1/2 (28.8±11.8d) and 4) H not different (138±47ug.d^{-1}) from that reported as normal for younger adults, although three of them presented somehow high values (163, 187 and 196 ug.d^{-1}). These findings are in concordance with fibrosis, celular infiltration and folicular alterations encountered in advancing age allowing to a diminished Qg and high turnover of glandular iodine. It is also possible to speculate about the high Kgb and H presentend by some elderly, that could represent non hormonal spillage of thyroidal iodine.

1400 AGE-RELATED CHANGES IN SERUM PREGNENOLONE AND ITS SULFATE CONCENTRATIONS AND THE RESPONSES TO ACTH IN MEN. K.Ono*, K.Kato, T.Maki, R.Takayanagi, and H.Ibayashi, Third Department of Internal Medicine, Kyushu University, Fukuoka 812, Japan.

In order to determine the basis for the decline of serum adrenal androgens in aged men, serum concentrations of pregnenolone(P_5) and its sulfate(P_5-S) were measured by simultaneous RIA in 74 healthy men(20-89 y.o.), before and after the administration of dexamethasone(1 mg), and at 0, 1, 2, 3, 6, 12, 24 hours after the i.m. injection of ACTH-Z(1 mg) with premedication of dexamethasone(1 mg). P_5-S hydrolyzed with HCl by the method of T.Aso, et al. was separated by sephadex LH-20 column chromatography. The basal serum P_5 and P_5-S levels showed a gradual decline from 20 years of age. After the administration of dexamethasone, serum P_5 and P_5-S were suppressed to 27.7±8.1 % (M±SE) and 30.3±1.9% of the corresponding baseline value, respectively, in the young, and to 63.6±7.8% and 55.3±7.6%, respectively, in the aged. The increments of serum P_5 and P_5-S after ACTH-Z were significantly lower in the aged than in the young. These results indicate that in men serum P_5 and P_5-S are mainly of adrenal origin and decline with advancing age, and suggest that the decrease in serum adrenal androgens in aged men is due to the delayed steroidogenic response to ACTH and in part to an impairment in P_5 biosynthesis in the adrenal cortex.

1401 DOES PROLACTIN (PRL) CONTRIBUTE TO THE REPRODUCTIVE DYSFUNCTION SEEN IN THE AGED PROLONGED DIESTROUS (PD) RAT? A. Ratner* and B. C. Wiggins, Dept. Physiology, Univ. New Mexico Sch. Medicine, Albuquerque, NM, USA

Prolactin (PRL) levels increase during aging and it has been suggested that this may contribute to the reproductive dysfunction seen in the aged female rat. To test this hypothesis, we examined the effect of pimozide (a dopamine antagonist) treatment in young cycling rats to see if we could induce some of the naturally-occurring effects of aging. Rats were given 0.1 or 0.5 mg pimozide/kg every 48 hours for a total of 4 weeks. Both treatments produced in most animals a leukocytic vaginal smear pattern throughout the treatment period. Some rats had pseudopregnancies of shorter duration, ranging from 17 to 21 days. At the termination of the treatment period, basal serum PRL values were increased some 5-fold in rats which had received 0.5 mg pimozide/kg. PRL levels were not altered in the group which received the lower dose of pimozide. However, while not changing basal PRL levels, this dose of pimozide did produce a nocturnal PRL surge similar to that which we found in 13-14 month old prolonged diestrous (PD) rats. Interestingly, these 13-14 month rats did not have increased basal PRL levels. When examining older PD rats (24-25 months), we found that they had increased basal PRL levels, but did not exhibit nocturnal PRL surges. Our results suggest that a change in the PRL secretory pattern may contribute to the dysfunction seen in aged PD rats and that this may, in part, be due to a dopaminergic deficit.

1402 DIAGNOSIS OF LOW RENIN STATES BY CONVERTING ENZYME INHIBITION. R. Mongeon*, R. Goldstone, E. Carlson and W. Hsueh, Section of Endocrinology, LAC/USC Medical Center, Los Angeles, California.

Basal levels of plasma renin may be normal in hyporeninemic hypoaldosteronism and primary aldosteronism so that physiologic stimulation is required to uncover a renin deficiency. Sodium restriction often requires hospitalization. Another method, IV furosemide, may not be sufficient stimulus in renal insufficiency. Since removal of angiotensin II negative feedback is a potent stimulus to renin release, we tested the ability of converting enzyme inhibition (CEI) to diagnose low renin states. The 4 hr ambulatory plasma renin concentration in response to A) 20mEq/day Na diet for 5 days, B) intravenous furosemide, 60mg, and C) captopril, 50mg, was tested in I) 8 renal insufficient hyperkalemic patients, creatinine clearance (C_{cr}), 36±5cc/min, II) 4 eukalemic patients, C_{cr} 30±2cc/min, III) 4 patients with nonsuppressible aldosteronism and normal C_{cr}, IV) age-matched normals. Patients were on 100-200mEq/day sodium intake for B and C. Baseline supine values were I) 2.7±0.8 (mean±SE), II) 6.2±1.5, III) 1.0±0.6, IV) 3.4±1.0ng/ml/hr. The increases times baseline were:

	A	B	C
I	1.5±0.3*	1.6±0.1*	2.1±0.6*
II	2.5±1.0	1.8±0.9*	4.7±1.2
III	1.2±0.3*	1.8±0.7*	1.8±0.7*
IV	5.0±1.0	4.8±1.4	7.3±2.0

(* p <0.01 compared with IV)

We conclude that CEI is a better method than furosemide to stimulate renin release particularly in patients with chronic renal insufficiency. Thus, CEI may be more reliable in the diagnosis of low renin states.

1403 A NEW MEDICAL THERAPY FOR PRIMARY ALDOSTERONISM: CALCIUM CHANNEL BLOCKADE.

J.L. Nadler*, A. Nimalasuriya, R. Horton and W. Hsueh, Section of Endocrinology, Dept. of Medicine, LAC/USC Medical Center, Los Angeles, Ca.

Evidence suggests that calcium (Ca) plays an important role in mineralocorticoid production and that Ca channel blockade in normal subjects inhibits angiotensin II (AII) induced aldosterone release. The role of Ca in aldosterone synthesis in primary aldosteronism (PA) is not known. To determine the potential therapeutic effect of Ca blockade in PA, 8 supine patients (4 adenoma, 4 hyperplasia) documented by endocrine testing and/or surgery were given nifedipine (N, 20mg sublingual). Their response was compared to 6 normal controls (C) on a 25mEq Na diet. N reduced mean Bp in C (87±3 SE mmHg to 77±2, $p < 0.01$). Active renin (AR) increased (2.5 times baseline) with a reciprocal decrease in acid activated inactive renin (IR). Plasma aldosterone (A) decreased by 3 hours (16±4ng/dl to 9±4). In all PA patients, N lowered systolic (S) and diastolic (D) Bp for 4-6 hours (158±6 to 128±4 S; 104±3 to 84±4 D, $p < 0.01$). AR and IR were low and not altered by N. Plasma cortisol and potassium did not change. However, N reduced A to normal levels in all PA patients within 2 hours (20±4 to 6±2, $p < 0.01$) including the 4 subjects with adenomas (23±4 to 11±3, $p < 0.05$). We conclude that Ca channel blockade: 1) in C stimulates AR with a reciprocal fall in IR. 2) In PA, reduces Bp to normal for up to 6 hours after a single dose. 3) Acutely lowers plasma aldosterone to normal in subjects with adrenal hyperplasia and adenoma. This suggests that Ca both mediates AII stimulated aldosterone synthesis and plays a direct role in aldosterone secretion in PA. The marked hormonal and clinical response suggests that Ca blockers may provide a new medical therapy for PA.

1404 HIGH LEVEL OF PLASMA INACTIVE RENIN IN BARTTER'S SYNDROME.

H. Nagai*, M. Matsunaga(1), K. Ogawa, T. Kuwahara, K. Kanatsu(2), C.H. Pak, A. Hara(3), T. Tamura(1), T. Kono(4) and C. Kawai.

III and II(4) Dept. Int. Med., and Coll. Med. Tech., Kyoto Univ., Kyoto, Dept. Int. Med., Hyogo Hosp.(2), Hyogo, and I Dept. Int.Med., Fukui Med. School(3), Fukui, Japan.

In 10 cases of Bartter's syndrome, plasma active and inactive renin(AR and IR) were measured by two different methods. First, plasma renin activity (PRA), and total renin activity(TRA) after activating IR with trypsin, were measured by radioimmunoassay(RIA) of angiotensin I(AI) generated from endogenous substrate. And secondly, plasma active renin concentration(ARC) and total renin concentration(TRC) were measured by RIA of AI generated in the presence of an excess of exogenous substrate. The difference between TRA and PRA, and between TRC and ARC were designated as inactive renin activity(IRA) and inactive renin concentration(IRC), respectively. Small amounts of IRA were found only in 2 cases and no IRA in 8 cases. However, the existence of large amounts of IR in Bartter's syndrome was revealed by the IRC determination. This suggests that the shortage of endogenous renin substrate, consumed by the markedly increased AR, may have interfered with the detection of IRA in Bartter's syndrome, though the IR is markedly increased as well.

1405 IMMUNOHISTOCHEMICAL LOCALIZATION OF RENIN IN HUMAN ENDOCRINE TISSUES. K. Naruse*, M. Murakoshi, Y. Osamura, M. Naruse, H. Demura, T. Inagami and K. Shizume. Tokyo Women's Medical College, Tokyo 162, Japan, Tokai University School of Medicine, Isehara 259-11, Japan, and Vanderbilt University School of Medicine, Nashville, TN 37232, USA.

We have previously reported the presence of renin activity which is sensitive to anti-renin antibody in various extrarenal tissues. However, the localization of renin in the human tissues has not been elucidated except for in the brain. We investigated the location of renin in various human endocrine tissues by immunohistochemical techniques. Antiserum against purified human renal renin was produced in rabbits. Endocrine tissues obtained from autopsy cases were fixed in the Bouin's fixative, dehydrated and embedded in paraffin. Sections were cut and stained with anti-human renin antisera by the enzyme-labeled antibody method using diaminobenzidine. In the pituitary, renin was localized within oval cells scattered throughout anterior lobe but not in the posterior lobe. In the adrenal, renin was localized in the zona glomeruloza and in the inner layer of the zona reticularis. Furthermore, renin was stained in the Leydig cells of the testis and in the follicular epithelial cells of the thyroid gland and the prostate. Control staining with normal rabbit serum or anti-human renin antisera absorbed with purified kidney renin did not show positive staining. The present results show a specific localization of renin in human endocrine tissues and indicate an important role for the tissue renin in the regulation of endocrine functions.

1406 BIOCHEMICAL PROPERTIES AND REGULATORY MECHANISM OF RAT ADRENAL RENIN. M. Naruse*, M. Nakamaru, K. Naruse, Y. Yamori, H. Demura, K. Shizume and T. Inagami. Vanderbilt University School of Medicine, Nashville, TN 37232, USA, Tokyo Women's Medical College, Tokyo 162, Japan, and Shimane Medical College, Izumo 693, Japan.

We have previously reported the presence of renin in the rat adrenal gland. The purpose of this study was to investigate biochemical properties and the regulatory mechanism of the adrenal renin. Adrenals were obtained from male Sprague-Dawley rats after nephrectomy and perfusion with saline. Renin activity in the extracts was determined by RIA of angiotensin I generated at pH 7.0 with nephrectomized rat plasma. The difference before and after preincubation with anti-renin antibody was defined as specific renin activity. Various biochemical properties were investigated. Furthermore, the effects of the following treatments on the adrenal renin level were investigated: low salt diet (LS), high potassium diet (HK), DOCA-Salt treatment (DS), Captopril treatment (CPT), ACTH treatment (ACTH), hypophysectomy (Hypox) and adrenal denervation (DN). Active renin was shown to have an affinity to pepstatin-Sepharose and concanavalin A-Sepharose, a molecular weight of 40,000, isoelectric points of 5.30 and 5.06, and neutral optimal pH. Furthermore, trypsin-activatable inactive renin was separated from active renin by pepstatin-Sepharose. Adrenal renin activity per mg of protein increased by LS, HK, CPT and DN. In contrast, it decreased by DS and did not change by ACTH and Hypox. These results indicate adrenal renin has similar biochemical properties as kidney renin and has close relation to electrolyte balance and adrenal innervation. Supported by NIH grants HL-24112 and HL-14192.

1407 ALDOSTERONE SECRETION IS REGULATED BY A NOVEL SERUM FACTOR STIMULATED BY METOCLOPRAMIDE.
G.Norbiato*,M.Bevilacqua,R.Meroni,D.Scorza,R.Dagani,G.Frigeni and E.Malacco,Endocrine Unit and Internal Medicine Department,Ospedale L. Sacco (Vialba),Via GB Grassi 74 - 20157 Milano ITALY

Metoclopramide stimulates aldosterone secretion in man independently of aldosterone regulating mechanisms (renin,ACTH,potassium).Metoclopramide does not increase aldosterone *in vitro*.To examine the possibility of a humoral mediator of metoclopramide we evaluated the effect of serum of 10 normal subjects injected with the drug on aldosterone production by collagenase dispersed calf adrenal zona glomerulosa cells.Serum collected from 5 to 30 min after the injection stimulated aldosterone production (*P<05).The effect disappeared at 40min, when plasma aldosterone was still elevated in the subjects.The stimulatory action was not abolished by Sar^1Ala^8angiotensin II;it was not related to ACTH since serum did not stimulate cortisol.The maximal aldosterone response *in vivo* was correlated to that observed *in vitro* (r^2=0.69,P<.01).Metoclopramide elicites the appearance *in vivo* in man of a novel,potent aldosterone stimulating factor.

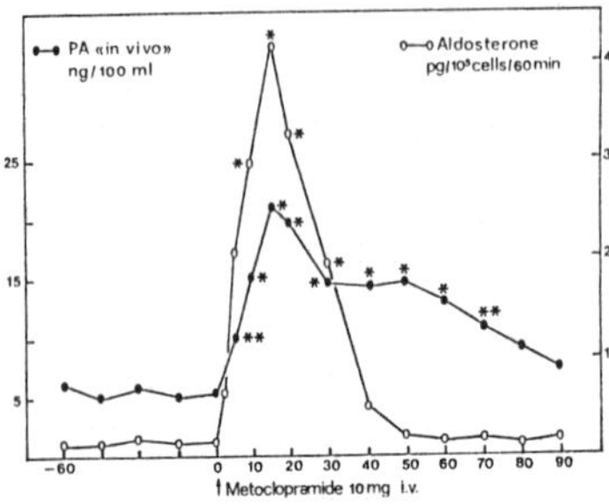

1408 STIMULATING EFFECT OF METOCLOPRAMIDE (MCP) ON ALDOSTERONE SECRETION IN VITRO.
M.NOZAKI* and S.MURAKAWA, 3rd Depertment of Internal Medicine, Kyorin University School of Medicine, Mitaka, Tokyo, Japan.

In vitro effect of MCP on aldosterone scretion is still controversial. We have compaired the effect of MCP on aldosterone secretion using rat adrenal glomerulosa cells isolated by tripsin treatment in two different procedures, superfusion and incubation. For superfusion experiments about 10^6 cells were packed with Cytodex into a teflon column and were perfused with Krebs Ringer bicarbonate buffer containing tripsin inhibitor at a rate of 0.8 ml/min and the perfusate was collected every five minutes to determine the aldosterone concentration. MCP increased aldosterone output dose relatedly like as Angiotensin II (AII), and this effect of MCP was not influenced by addition of dopamine or cyproheptadine. Trifluoperadine (TFP) decreased aldosterone response to MCP and AII. On the other hand, isolated cells were incubated at the concentration of 10^5 cells per ml with Krebs Ringer bicarbonate buffer for 120 min. A portion of the buffer was taken serially at 15 min.,30 min.,60 min. and 120 min., and aldosterone was assayed by RIA. MCP increased aldosterone secretion only at 15 min.,thereafter no significant differences were observed compaired to the control. Stimulating effect of MCP at 15 min. was suppressed by adding TFP. These results suggest that MCP stimulates aldosterone secretion directly probably mediated through calmodulin.

1409 DIRECT MICROASSAY FOR PLASMA ALDOSTERONE. J. Nussberger*, B. Waeber, H.R. Brunner , J.F. Burris, W. Vetter. Division of Nephrology and Hypertension, Centre Hospitalier Universitaire, Lausanne, Switzerland.

A direct radioimmunoassay for aldosterone in unextracted plasma was developed using a highly sensitive and specific antiserum and ^{125}I-labeled aldosterone. Plasma or standard (10 or 25 µl) was added to 75 µl buffer and mixed with 500 µl antiserum containing ^{125}I-aldosterone (2000 cpm). After incubation (4°C, 48 h) free aldosterone was separated from antibody-bound hormone by adsorption to dextran coated charcoal. The method was compared to the previously used assay based on methylene chloride extraction and column chromatography and to a micromethod utilizing methylene chloride extraction alone. Unlike previously described methods, the new assay requires neither binding protein digestion or inhibition nor the addition of aldosterone-free plasma to the standard curves. Concentrations of 2 pg/ml of aldosterone can be measured in 25 µl of plasma. The within-assay coefficient of variation ranged between 4.0 and 5.3% over a six-fold range of aldosterone concentrations and the between-assay coefficient of variation between 8.0 and 9.4% over a two-fold range. The correlation coefficients among the 3 methods varied between 0.97 and 0.99, the results being virtually identical between the new direct and the standard chromatography method. Normal values on unrestricted salt intake were 68 $\pm$ 28 pg/ml (n = 30, mean $\pm$ SD) in seated humans. In conclusion, this is an extremely simple, truly direct microradioimmunoassay for plasma aldosterone, which is accurate over a wide range of plasma concentrations, is exquisitely sensitive and provides results identical to those obtained with established methods.

1410 PSYCHOLOGICAL AND ENDOCRINE REACTIVITY IN HYPOTHALAMIC AMENORRHEA (HA) AND POLYCYSTIC OVARY SYNDROME (PCOS). D. Goldstein*, S. Goldstein, J. Sachchidananda and F.I. Reyes, Dept. OB-GYN and Psychiatry, SUNY, Downstate Medical Center and Hillside-Jewish Hospital, Brooklyn, N.Y. 11203, U.S.A

Experimental studies indicate that stressful situations can disrupt the hypothalamic-pituitary-gonadal axis (HPG) function, and clinical observations suggest a causal relationship between psychological stress and HA and PCOS. However, the reason(s) and mechanism(s) why HPG function is affected by stress in some persons and not in others remains unknown. In order to prove if this difference results from the individual reactivity and perception of the stressor, this study explored under controlled conditions the psychological and endocrine reactivity to mental stressors of normal (EU) and amenorrheic women. EU (n=6) and HA (n=5) volunteers had, as demonstrated by the STAI-2 evaluation a higher basal anxiety trait level than the PCOS group (n=6). At that time of the stressor test (serial subtraction, digit span tests), the HA group showed a higher level of anxiety (STAI-1 score), and responded with higher anxiety scores to the stress applications than the EU and PCOS volunteers. The latter group showed not only the lowest basal scoring, but also the lesser stress-reactivity. Basal serum F, GH and PRL levels tended to be high, but within the normal range in all volunteers. Definite hormone change responses occurred following the application of stress challenges in all groups. These results suggest that individual psychological, but not endocrine reactivity to mental stress may be related to the development or maintenance of HPG dysfunction in HA and PCOS. (Part.supported by grant MO1 RR-318, GCRCP, NIH).

1411 TSH RESPONSE TO TRH(TSH/TRH) IN PATIENTS WITH NEUROTIC DEPRESSION (ND).

Gutman R*;Zambrano D.;Mileo R.;Goldberg V.;Canovi A.;Scherle J.;Ricón L.
Endocrinology and Psycopathology Services-Htal.Italiano-Bs.As.-Argentina.

Among other neuroendocrine abnormalities,a low TSH/TRH has been claimed to be useful as a diagnostic aid of Endogenous Major Depressive Disorder (ED). We studied 20 drug free patients(26-60 y.o.,18 fem.)classified as ND (WHO classification 300.4)by psychiatric interviews.Severity of depression was rated by Hamilton and Raskin Covi scales and a self appraisal scale.Serum TSH(uU/ml),Prolactin(PRL ng/ml),HGH (ng/ml) and ACTH (pg/ml)were measured before (B) and 20 and 30 minutes(')after 200 ug i.v. TRH. Six out of the 20 patients showed blunted TSH responses as indicated by significantly lower values of Σ B,20' and 30' TSH: X $\pm$ SEM 12.0 $\pm$ 1.23(range-r-:8.65-16.9)as compared to either the remaining 14 patients: 38.6 $\pm$ 2.58 (r:25.2-63.9; $p<0.001$) or 20 normal controls: 33.87 $\pm$ 2.25 (r:21.9-58.8; $p<0.001$). No significant or consistent abnormalities were observed in the patterns of the other measured pituitary hormones: peak values after TRH: PRL 48.6 $\pm$ 6.2; HGH: 4.02 $\pm$ 1.2 and ACTH: 25.15 $\pm$ 5.78. Fifteen patients were blindly rerated for depression and retested biochemicallyafter 6 weeks on 1 to 4 mg of alprazolam daily plus weekly psychiatric interviews. Although all patients experienced one of various degrees of clinical improvement,no significant changes were seen after treatment in the individual TSH/TRH responses of either the six patients with blunted responses before treatment (14.05 $\pm$ 1.57, r:8.2-20.0) or in the remaining 9 reexamined patients who originally showed a normal TSH response (37.7 $\pm$ 4.1; r: 19.3-56.5).
Our results indicate that the TSH/TRH test may not be a useful diagnostic tool of ED.Persistence of a low TSH response after clinical improvement suggests that this finding may be a trait dependent rather than a state dependent neuroendocrine abnormality in a sub group of ND patients.

1412 LONG KNOWN ALDOSTERONE DERIVATE A PHYSIOLOGICAL PRODUCT ?

K. Lichtwald*, H. Bauer, U. Soltek and P. Vecsei. Dept. of Pharmacology, University Heidelberg, Im Neuenheimer Feld 366, 6900 Heidelberg, FRG.

Recently we described the formation of 11,18;18,21-diepoxyaldosterone (DEALDO), the intramolecular acetal of aldosterone under acidic conditions generally applied for aldosterone estimation in urine samples. However, we claimed that a material with analog paper chromatographic behaviour (Bush B5: Rf=0.85; BHMW: Rf=0.75) could be extracted with dichlormethane from crude unprocessed urine. DEALDO was synthesized as was the tritium labelled compound. The antiserum used was the immune response to an aldosterone-21-hemisuccinate-BSA complex and showed 32% crossreaction compared to aldosterone. DEALDO like material was estimated after paperchromatography in Bush B5. From 35 chromatograms prepared for estimation of urinary free aldosterone the last portions (Rf$\geq$0.6) were gathered and eluted with 100 ml dichloromethane. Rechromatography of the residue revealed an average value of 0.06 µg/24h for DEALDO-cochromatographing material. Ten randomly selected urines were individually estimated for the same material. ^{3}H-DEALDO (3500 CPM) was added to 10 ml urine for loss correction. Extraction was performed with 5 ml of dichloromethane, chromatography as mentioned. The mean value was 0.43 µg/24h (range 0.29-0.62). The concentration range is somewhat similar as the free fraction of aldosterone is. It will be clarified in future by selected ion monitoring if the estimated material is identical with DEALDO. Implication for diagnosis of aldosteronism has to be studied.

1413 THE EFFECT OF GASTRIN-RELEASING PEPTIDE (GRP) ON GROWTH HORMONE SECRETION IN THE RAT. S. Kentroti* and S.M. McCann, Univ of Texas Health Sci Center, Dept of Physiology, Dallas, TX 75235,

Several investigators have reported GRP-like immunostaining in several regions of the rat brain. The objective of this study was to determine the possible regulatory effect of this peptide on growth hormone (GH) release. The 27-residue porcine GRP was administered intraventricularly (2 µl, 3rd ventricle, 3V) to ovariectomized female rats. A significant (p<.001) decrease in basal GH release, as evidenced by decreased plasma GH levels, was observed within 10 min lasting 90 min after 3V injection of 2 µg GRP. In addition all GH pulses were abolished during this time period. In subsequent experiments the GRP-induced blockade of GH release was challenged after 20 min with human pancreatic growth hormone-releasing factor (hpGRF)(0.2 µg/gm, i.v.). GRP abolished the response to hpGRF observed in the control animals. Plasma LH was determined as well and there was little effect of GRP on plasma LH or the response to LHRH (0.1 ng/gm, i.v.). The inhibitory effect of GRP on GH release was further tested on overnight cultured pituitary cells. The cells were pre-incubated with GRP at concentrations of 10^{-6}, 10^{-7} or 10^{-8} M for 20 min after which 4×10^{-10} M hpGRF was added and the cells were incubated for 2 hours. The cells displayed a dose-dependent inhibition of GH release which was greatest at a GRP concentration of 10^{-6} M. The minimal effective dose was 10^{-7} M. The results of this investigation suggest that GRP serves a role as an inhibitory neuromodulator of GH release by a direct action on the somatotrophs. Supported by NIH grant 32928.

1414 ROLES OF OPIOID PEPTIDES IN THE ESTROGEN ACTIVATION OF SEXUAL RECEPTIVITY. K. Kubo* and M. Torii, Department of Physiology, Institute of Constitutional Medicine, Kumamoto University, Kumamoto 862, Japan

We have recently demonstrated that β-endorphin acts to modify the estrogen feedback effects on LH release and behavioral receptivity. Thus, in order to discriminate the β-endorphin action from the actions of enkephalins, and to clarify a role of β-endorphin neuronal system in the estrogen activation of sexual receptivity, the effects of intra-third ventricular injections of β-endorphin, Met-enkephalin, Leu-enkephalin, naloxone, and anti-β-endorphin antiserum on lordosis response were studied in the ovariectomized rats. The rats were primed with estradiol benzoate (EB) and progesterone with an interval of 43 h. After 48 h of EB-priming, lordosis behavior in response to male mounts was tested. Each drug was injected either at the time of EB priming or 1 h before the behavioral test. Results are summarized in the table (↑ facilitation, ↓ inhibition, - no change of lordosis response).

Time of injection	β-End 1 µg	β-End 10 µg	Met-Enk 1 µg	Met-Enk 10 µg	Leu-Enk 1 µg	Leu-Enk 10 µg	Naloxone 1 µg	Anti-β-End Antiserum
EB-priming	↑	↑	↓	↑	↓	↓	↓	↓
1 h before the test	-	↓	↑	↑	-	-	↓	-

Present results indicate that: a) Functional differences among opioid peptides are obvious. b) β-endorphin neuronal system contributes primarily to the development of estrogen activation of behavioral receptivity. c) In the course of estrogen actions in the CNS, a role of each opioid system has altered. d) Met-enkephalin neuronal system is involved mainly in the control of behavioral expression.

1415 EVIDENCE FOR C-24 AND C-23 OXIDATION OF 25-HYDROXYVITAMIN D_3 IN ESTABLISHED KIDNEY CELL LINES. S. Marion*, M. Kelly, C. Donaldson and M. Haussler, Department of Biochemistry, University of Arizona Health Sciences Center, Tucson, Arizona, USA.

The metabolism of both 25-hydroxyvitamin D_3 (25(OH)D_3) and 1,25-dihydroxyvitamin D_3 (1,25(OH)$_2D_3$) has been studied by several groups using kidney and intestinal mucosa homogenates and perfused kidneys, and has been found to proceed primarily via a C-24 oxidation pathway. We have investigated these same enzymatic reactions using cultured kidney cells from established lines. LLC-PK_1 or LLC-MK_2 cells were incubated with 0.5 μM 25(OH)[26,27-^{3}H]D_3 for 30 min and a lipid extract submitted to HPLC employing a Zorbax-SIL column eluted with 10% isopropanol in hexane. Five peaks were collected between the 25(OH)[^{3}H]D_3 substrate and the major product, 24,25(OH)$_2$[^{3}H]D_3; each yielded a single peak upon rechromatography in 6% isopropanol in hexane. Each peak was then subjected to three different HPLC systems--hexane:isopropanol:methanol (94:5:1) on a Zorbax-CN column; dichloromethane:isopropanol (98:2) or methanol:chloroform:hexane (1:2:22) on a Zorbax-SIL column. Based upon comparison of the migration of the unknown peaks with published results, we have tentatively identified four metabolites, all of which are enhanced by pretreatment of the cells with 1,25(OH)$_2D_3$: 25(OH)-24-oxoD_3; 25(OH)-23-oxoD_3; 23,25(OH)$_2$-24-oxoD_3; and 23,25(OH)$_2D_3$. These data demonstrate the capacity of intact cells to metabolize 25(OH)D_3 by both the C-24 and C-23 oxidation routes, although C-24 oxidation predominates. The LLC-PK_1 and LLC-MK_2 cell lines should be valuable models for characterizing the significance of these new routes of vitamin D metabolism. (Supported by AM30290 and AM15781).

1416 DEMONSTRATION AND CHARACTERIZATION OF CALCITRIOL RECEPTORS IN BASAL CELLS OF EPIDERMIS OF NEONATAL MICE. J. Merke*, D. Schwittay, G. Fürstenberger, F. Marks and E. Ritz, Departm. Medicine (Univ. Hdbg) and Cancer Research Center, Heidelberg, FRG.

Skin plays a key role in photosynthesis of 7-dehydrocholesterol, but little is known on actions of calcitriol on skin. To demonstrate and characterize epidermal calcitriol receptors, epidermis of neonatal and adult mice was studied *ex vivo*. Trypsination flotation procedure of Yuspa (1974) ; receptors as described (Merke, Eur.J.Biochem.130:303 (1983)). Nuclear and cytosolic receptors for calcitriol were found in neonatal and adult mouse epidermis. Binding was specific and reversible. K_D was 1.6 x 10^{-10} M for cytosolic and nuclear fractions, binding capacity was 54 fmol/mg protein in cytosol and 108 in nuclear fractions resp.. Half max. displacement of ^{3}Hcalcitriol occured with 80-fold molar excess of calcidiol and 200x 1a(OH)D_3. As studied with sucrose dens. gradients binding occured via 3.5-S macromolecule (distinct from 6-S binding protein for calcidiol). Binding sensitive to proteases, not nucleases and sensitive to SH reag. (N-ethylmaleimide) in unoccupied, less in calcitriol occupied form (suggesting SH groups in binding site). Different cytosolic receptor recovery in high vs. low ionic strength media suggested partially unoccupied nuclear receptors. After keratinocyte separation by percoll centrifugation, receptors were located in basal, but not suprabasal cells. The technique is promising for application in humans.

1417 EFFECTS OF FORSKOLIN AND W-7 ON PARATHYROID HORMONE RELEASE. H. Niki*, A. Niki, T. Koide, T. Tsuzuki and M. Yamaguchi, Dept. of Medicine and Dept. of Pharmacology, Aichigakuin University, Nagoya, 464 Japan.

Exocytosis is generally considered to be induced by an increase in cytosolic calcium (Ca) concentration. Unlike the majority of exocytotic systems, parathyroid hormone (PTH) release is inhibited by elevated extra- as well as intracellular Ca concentrations, and cyclic AMP (cAMP) appears to be the intracellular messenger. Forskolin was recently discovered to act directly on the catalytic subunit of adenylate cyclase and non-specifically increase intracellular cAMP. A new calmodulin inhibitor, W-7, is known to be highly specific and easily penetrate cell membranes. Using these two agents, we have studied on the role of cAMP and calmodulin in PTH release. Parathyroid glands were isolated from male Wistar rats. Batches of two glands were incubated at 37°C for 2 hrs in Krebs-Ringer bicarbonate buffer containing 5 mg/ml bovine serum albumin and variable $CaCl_2$, with or without test substances. PTH in the media and cAMP in the glands were measured by radioimmunoassay. Significantly higher PTH release and cAMP accumulation were observed in low (1 mM) Ca than in normal (2.5 mM) Ca media. Forskolin (1-100 μM) increased cAMP in a dose-dependent manner, independent of concomitant Ca concentrations, but did not affected on PTH release at any Ca concentration. W-7 at 50 μM, a nearly maximal effective concentration to inhibit calmodulin, failed to modify PTH release or cAMP level. These results suggest that non-specifically elevated cAMP or calmodulin in parathyroid cells is not involved in PTH release.

1418 HUMAN PARATHYROID HORMONE (hPTH) 1—38: ENHANCED BINDING AFFINITY AND ADENYLATE CYCLASE ACTIVATION COMPARED TO BOVINE PTH 1—84 AND HUMAN PTH 1—34 ANALOGUE SEQUENCES. S. Nussbaum* and M. Rosenblatt, Endocrine Unit, Massachusetts General Hospital and Harvard Medical School, Boston, MA 02114, USA.

Previous structure-activity studies of parathyroid hormone in multiple in vivo and in vitro bioassay systems have shown that full biological activity of the 84 amino acid secreted peptide is present in the amino terminal 34 residues. The 25—34 sequence of PTH represents the principal binding domain for parathyroid hormone. Conformational predictive models indicate that the region 28—37 has potential for beta sheet conformation, thereby favoring receptor interaction. Therefore, we studied the biological activity of synthetic hPTH 1—38 in a radio-receptor binding assay and in stimulation of adenylate cyclase in canine renal membranes. HPTH 1—38 bound to renal membranes with an apparent K_B of 3.5×10^{-10}M whereas bPTH-(1—84), hPTH-(1—34), and [Nle^8,Nle^{18},Tyr^{34}]bPTH-(1—34)amide, an analogue of enhanced bioactivity, bound 50-fold less avidly than hPTH 1—38. There was an approximately 3-fold enhanced stimulation of adenylate cyclase when hPTH 1—38 was compared to bPTH 1—84 and [Nle^8,Nle^{18},Tyr^{34}]bPTH-(1—34)-amide. Our studies suggest that the enhanced biological activity of hPTH 1—38 may, in part, reflect greater receptor binding favored by a shift toward beta sheet secondary structure. Further structure-activity studies of PTH analogues with carboxyl-terminal amino acid extension to position 38 may lead to the development of more potent parathyroid hormone inhibitors.

1419 DEMONSTRATION OF BIG-CALCITONIN IN MEDULLARY THYROID CARCINOMA.
Y. Ochi*, Y. Ura, M. Ishida[1], Y. Nakajima[1], T. Miyazaki[2], T. Hachiya[3], H. Ijichi[3] and K. Kuma[4], Clin Lab. Shiga Univ. Otsu, Inter Med, Nantan Hosp[1], Yagi, Radiol[2] and Inter Med[3], Kyoto prefect. Univ of Med, Kyoto, and Kuma Hosp[4], Kobe. Japan.

Measurement of calcitonin(CT) and CEA is useful for diagnosis of medullary thyroid carcinoma(MTC). In the present study we examined the size heterogeneity of CT in MTC by RIA. Many cases showed the increase of serum CT of more than 1,000 pg/ml (normal range: $<$ 100), and also the simultaneous increase of both CEA and NCA levels. However, ferritin and α_1-acid glycoprotein were increased in a few cases. CA 19-9 was almost normal range. There was slightly positive correlation between CT level and CEA level. When sera with extremely high CT levels ($>$ 280 ng/ml) were gel-filtrated by Sephadex G-200 (or G-100), the high MW CT (big-CT, MW is about 20,000-100,000) besides the low MW CT (MW is about 3,500) was found. The similarly high MW CT was also found by the gel-filtration of the extract from tumor tissue of MTC. When the authentic ^{125}I-CT preparations in RIA kit of both Eiken and Daiichi Lab were gel-filtrated, the small peak (MW is about 40,000) besides the main peak (MW is 3,500) was found. These evidence indicate that the increase of CT, CEA and NCA is specific for MTC than other tumor markers, and that the increased CT in serum is usually associated with the increase of big-CT which may be pro-CT. The increase of big-CT in MCT may be general phenomenon.

1420 CLINICAL SIGNIFICANCE OF OSTEOCALCIN IN HEMODIALYZED PATIENTS - EFFECT OF ACTIVE VITAMIN D TREATMENT ON OSTEOCALCIN IN HEMODIALYZED PATIENTS -
Y. Ohnishi*, T. Miki, H. Morii, Y. Nishizawa, K. Iba, K. Kikunami#, Y. Matsushita#, and T. Inoue#, The Second Department of Internal Medicine, Osaka City University and #Inoue Hospital, Osaka 545 Japan.

Osteocalcin (OC) is vitamin K-dependent protein in the bone. The immunologically identical protein was found in the serum. Its serum level was reported to be high in hemodialyzed patients, but its clinical significance is not well known. We investigated clinical significance of OC and of vitamin D effect on serum OC level in patients under regular hemodialysis. Fifteen patients were administered 1α-(OH)D3 (VD) for 13.6±5.1 months (mean ±SD), and serum OC, PTH and Ca were measured before and after treatment. Serum Ca increased significantly from 3.83±0.32 mEq/L to 4.24±0.46 mEq/L ($p<0.01$) after treatment. OC level was independent of the duration of hemodialysis. Mean OC level prior to VD treatment was 25.9±21.5 ng/ml, and it was significantly increased to 46.9±44.4 ng/ml ($p<0.05$) with VD treatment. Positive correlations between OC ana PTH both before treatment ($r=0.57$, $p<0.05$) and after treatment ($r=0.74$, $p<0.01$) were found. The change of OC level correlated with that of PTH level ($r=0.71$, $p<0.01$). Although positive correlations ($r=0.46$; pre-VD, $r=0.45$; post-VD treatment) were found between alkaline phosphatase (AP) and PTH, they were lower than those of OC and PTH. These results suggest that OC is a better indicator than AP, because of frequent complication of liver damage in hemodialyzed patients. As active vitamin D reportedly increases synthesis of OC, significant increase of serum OC in this study may be induced by VD. Natural course is not a possible explanation for the increase, because no significant positive correlation was found between OC and the duration of hemodialysis.

1421 EFFECTS OF MAGNESIUM ON PARATHYROID HORMONE(PTH) RELEASE FROM MAGNESIUM DEPLETED PARATHYROID CELLS AND ADENYLATE CYCLASE ACTIVITY IN LOW MAGNESIUM RED BLOOD CELLS IN A PATIENT.

Y.Okamoto*, E.Shimizu, M.Moriyama, K.Ota, J.Maeda and L.M. Sherwood. Division of Gerontology, Department of Medicine, Wakayama Medical College, Department of Laboratory Medicine, Wakayama Medical College, Japan and Albert Einstein School of Medicine, New York.

Effect of magnesium(Mg) is well known to make an inhibition of parathyroid hormone(PTH) secretion in higher or in lower Mg medium, mediated via adenylate cyclase activation. A patient is presented and diagnosed as low Mg induced hypoparathyroidism. Our attempt is focussed on the study of PTH secretion via membranous adenylate cyclase activity in low Mg content of red blood cells in a patient. PTH secretion from Mg depleted parathyroid cells was higher responsive, by the addition of 1.0mM Mg in incubation medium and also the activation of membranous adenylate cyclase activity was more accentuated in low Mg content of red blood cells in a patient than those of normal Mg content, by the addition of Mg and the supplement of Mg in a patient was able to detect serum PTH. The assay of red blood cell membranous adenylate cyclase activity is suggested to be representative of the status of PTH secretion from parathyroid glands in patients.

1422 A SPECIFIC CLONED cDNA TO STUDY THE CONTROL OF 9 000 MW CHOLECALCIN (9K CaBP) BIOSYNTHESIS BY 1,25-DIHYDROXYVITAMIN D_3.

C. Perret, C. Desplan, A. Bréhier and M. Thomasset*, INSERM U120 44 Chemin de Ronde Vésinet France

Rat intestinal cholecalcin, a vitamin D-dependent 9K CaBP is an intracellular protein mainly located in the duodenum. The cDNA to cholecalcin mRNA was cloned in pBR322 (J Biol Chem 258, 2763, 1983). Nucleotide sequence analysis of the longest cDNA insert (375bp) permitted the assignement of 207 nucleotides of the coding region and 104 nucleotides of the entire 3'-noncoding region of the cholecalcin mRNA (J Biol Chem 258, 13502, 1983). We now report the use of this cloned cDNA to characterize cholecalcin mRNA and study the control of the expression of the 9K CaBP gene.

Cholecalcin mRNA and cell free translation products of cDNA-hybridized mRNA isolated from duodenum, kidney and cerebellum in vitamin D-replete rats and in vitamin D-deficient rats after $1,25(OH)_2D_3$ dosing were analyzed. CaBP mRNA was measured by dot-blot hybridization and CaBP assayed by radioimmunoassay. Only the duodenum contains a cDNA hybridizing mRNA. The specific cloned cDNA does not hybridize with the 28K cholecalcin mRNA from cerebellum and kidney, paralleling the lack of cross-reactivity between 9K and large CaBP antibodies. Nothern hybridization analysis shows a major 500-1000 base mRNA. The hybridized mRNA translated in a cell free system directs only the synthesis of rat intestinal cholecalcin. CaBP mRNA was present all along the intestine and abundant in duodenum and cecum.

The control of cholecalcin mRNA synthesis by $1,25(OH)_2D_3$ was clearly demonstrated in rat duodenum and cecum and occured with apparent time lag suggesting that the primary response to the hormone is at the transcriptional level.

1423 HYPOCALCEMIA IS MODERATE IN A KINDRED WITH AUTOSOMAL DOMINANT HYPOPARATHYROIDISM, SINCE SERUM 1,25(OH)$_2$-VITAMIN D LEVELS ARE NORMAL. W.E. Nolten*, R. Chesney, S. Dabbagh, J. Lutz, J. Lemann, E. Slatopolsky and H. DeLuca, Depts. of Medicine, Pediatrics, Nursing and Biochemistry, Univ. of Wisconsin, Madison, WI, 53792, USA; Depts. of Medicine, Medical College of Wisconsin, Milwaukee, WI and Washington Univ., St. Louis, MO.

Autosomal dominant hypoparathyroidism was found in 9 members of a kindred over 3 generations. Mean serum calcium (Ca) was 7.8±SD 0.5 mg/dl, mean Ca^{++} was reduced to 3.48±0.18 mg/dl; iPTH was low in 7 subjects. All patients were asymptomatic. Intravenous parathyroid extract (300 U) resulted in 3 patients in a brisk rise in urinary cAMP, typical of the response in hypoparathyroidism. Infusion of EDTA (50 mg) in one subject caused a fall in Ca^{++} from 3.44 to 2.76 mg/dl, but iPTH remained undetectable. Vit. D metabolites were measured in 5 patients and showed normal concentrations of 25(OH)D_2, 25(OH)D_3 and 1,25(OH)$_2$D. Mean 1,25(OH)$_2$D in these hypocalcemic patients was 39±8 pg/ml (nl = 20-70), significantly higher than the value of 16±4 pg/ml measured in 13 sporadic hypoparathyroid patients; p<.001. Treatment with vitamin D_2 (50,000 to 150,000 IU/day) or 1,25(OH)$_2$D (1 to 2 μg/day) did not normalize hypocalcemia in 3 patients. These results suggest that familial hypoparathyroidism may often present with mild hypocalcemia, possibly because serum 1,25(OH)$_2$D values are higher than in other forms of hypoparathyroidism. The stimulus for 1,25(OH)$_2$D synthesis in familial hypoparathyroidism remains unknown. It may be assumed that the higher values of 1,25(OH)$_2$D support greater intestinal Ca absorption resulting in higher serum calcium levels.

1424 CALMODULIN BINDING PROTEIN IN RAT TESTIS: CHARACTERIZATION AND THE EFFECTS OF SURGICAL CRYPTORCHIDISM. T. Ono*, Y. Koide, Y. Arai and K. Yamashita, Institutes of Applied Biochemistry and Clinical Medicine, University of Tsukuba, Ibaraki, Japan.

Calcium ion (Ca^{2+}) regulates a variety of cellular functions through its interaction with calmodulin and calmodulin binding proteins. Although testis contains high amount of calmodulin, its physiological role has not been clarified. Therefore we investigated the properties of calmodulin binding proteins in rat testis and the effects of surgical cryptorchidism on calmodulin and calmodulin binding protein contents. The application of heat-treated supernatant of rat testis on DEAE-cellulose column yielded two fractions of phosphodiesterase inhibitor activity, i.e. unadsorbed fraction (Fr.I) and adsorbed fraction (Fr.II) eluted with 0.2 M NaCl. Fraction II was purified to 860 fold with calmodulin-Sepharose 4B chromatography. This inhibitor formed a complex with calmodulin only in the presence of Ca^{2+}, and was revealed to be an acidic monomer protein stable to heat and acid with molecular weight of 32,000. Fraction I was separated into three fractions with CM-cellulose and calmodulin-Sepharose chromatography. They also formed a complex with calmodulin in the presence of Ca^{2+}. Seminiferous tubules contained higher amount of calmodulin and calmodulin binding protein of Fraction II than interstitial cells. Surgical cryptorchidism caused a significant decrease in the content of calmodulin (50% of control) by the 5th day, and of calmodulin binding protein (14% of control) by the 3rd day. The results suggest that rat testis contains several types of calmodulin binding proteins, and that calmodulin and calmodulin binding protein are involved in the regulation of spermatogenesis.

1425 STUDIES OF A CORTISOL-BINDING MACROMOLECULE IN HUMAN BREAST CANCER.

*M. Krelenbaum and A.G. Fazekas, Dept. of Surgery, McGill University, The Mont-General Hospital, Montreal, Quebec, H3G 1A4, Canada.

In an attempt to better characterize endocrine sensitivity of human breast tumors, over 3000 specimens were investigated for the presence of cortisol receptors. High levels of binding (>1000 fmole/g tissue) were found in over 90% of cases. This can be largely attributed to a binding protein which resembles plasma trancortin. It sediments at 4S (M.Wt. ~60,000) has a K_d in the range of 10^{-8}M and does not bind synthetic fluorinated corticosteroids. It is distingquishable from the larger (8S), higher affinity (Kd=10^{-9}M) receptor which is present in 25% of breast tumors and binds dexamethasone. The cortisol binder showed differences in elution pattern from plasma transcortin on DEAE-A50-Sephadex columns. This binder has not been detected in the nuclei, suggesting that it may have a different role from that of the classical glucocorticoid receptor. The possibility that the binder is synthesized by the cancer cell is currently being investigated by studying the incorporation of ^{14}C-labelled amino acids into the cortisol binder by tissue slices and tissue explants. It is suggested that the intensive binding of cortisol by the tumor relative to the adjacent normal tissue (tumor/breast ratio as high as 25) might be used for early detection of breast cancer by a gamma-emitting cortisol tracer.

1426 UNOCCUPIED ANDROGEN RECEPTORS ARE BIOLOGICALLY ACTIVE IN RAT PITUITARY GONADOTROPHS,

F. Labrie* and J. Simard, MRC Group in Molecular Endocrinology, CHUL, Québec G1V 4G2, Canada.

Androgens exert a specific inhibitory effect on LHRH-induced LH release in rat anterior pituitary cells in culture (Endocrinology 98, 1528, 1976). This parameter can thus be used as a highly precise and sensitive in vitro bioassay for agonistic and antagonistic androgenic compounds. Following 4 days of preincubation of the pituitary cells in the absence of steroids, 0.3 nM LHRH causes an approximately 4-fold stimulation of LH release during a 3-h incubation period. While preincubation of the cells for 48h with 10 μM Anandron (5,5-dimethyl-3[4-nitro-3-(trifluoromethyl)-phenyl]-2,4-imidazolidinedione) has only a small (20%, $p < 0.05$) stimulatory effect on spontaneous LH release, it causes a 2-to 3-fold stimulation (over control) of 0.3 nM LHRH-induced LH release. The potent stimulatory effect of the pure antiandrogen is exerted at an ED_{50} value of ~ 10 μM. The present data have major implications for the treatment of androgen-sensitive diseases, especially cancer, since they indicate that unoccupied androgen receptors are highly active even in the absence of androgens. The logical implication is that removal of the source of endogenous and/or exogenous androgens is not sufficient for the treatment of androgen-dependent diseases, and that blockade of the androgen receptor with a pure antiandrogen is required for full blockade of androgen receptor action.

1427 A PERMANENT GONADOTROPE CELL LINE FROM RAT PITUITARY ADENOMA. E. H. Leiter*, W. G. Beamer, H. G. Bedigian, and M. T. Davisson, The Jackson Laboratory, Bar Harbor, ME 04609. USA

A pituitary adenoma from a 1100 day-old ACI/Mai_f female rat was enzymatically dissociated and maintained as cell aggregates in shaking culture for 6 days. These aggregates, when plated into stationary culture flasks, produced epithelial cell outgrowths. Fibroblasts were eliminated by serum deprivation, and a well-differentiated epithelial cell line, designated RC-4B/C, was established from one culture which had been maintained in culture medium supplemented with 2.5 ng/ml epidermal growth factor. The cell line has been maintained in vitro for 6 years; population doubling time has gone from 33 hr (year 3) to 28 hr (year 5). Cells were diploid (2n = 42) at year 3; modal chromosome number had shifted slightly (to 45) by year 5. During the 5th year, an endogenous rat type C virus was spontaneously expressed. The cells were uniform in appearance, and classified as gonadotropes both on ultrastructural appearance of their numerous secretory granules and on their ability to secrete in response to 1 μg/ml gonadotropin release hormone. Chromatographic analysis of labeled cell proteins showed FSH-like molecules with bioactivity (expansion of mouse oocyte-cumulus cell complexes), but not immunoreactivity with rabbit antiserum against normal rat FSH. Thus, the adenoma-derived gonadotropes appeared to produce an abnormal form of FSH. This study was supported by NIH.

1428 BINDING OF INSULIN AND EPIDERMAL GROWTH FACTOR (EGF) TO RAT LIVER CELLS DECREASES SHARPLY DURING THE CHEMICAL HEPATOCARCINOGENESIS. A.Lev-Ran*, B.I.Carr, Z.Josefsberg, C.Tomkinson, G.Barseghian, and D.Hwang. City of Hope National Medical Center, Duarte, California 91010, USA.

We studied the binding of insulin and EGF (both known hepatic mitogens) to microsomal and Golgi receptors of liver cells of male F344 rats fed 0.02% 2-acetylaminofluorene (AAF). Specific binding was expressed as per cent per 0.5 mg protein for microsomes and per 0.1 mg protein for Golgi. The binding to Golgi receptors in control rats and in rats fed AAF for 2,4,8, 21,34,46, and 85 days was: for insulin 10.0;5.9;3.4;2.3;1.5;1.6;4.0 and 2.7% and for EGF 15.3;9.4;3.4;1.4;0.8;1.0;1.8 and 1.6% (significant drop in both after 2 days). The decrease in binding started later and was less pronounced in microsomes: for insulin 19.1;21.0;18.0;15.7;14.2;13.9;10.8; and 10.7% (significant after 46 days) and for EGF 26.3;22.3;17.4;19.5; 16.1;9.6;7.5 and 8.4% (significant after 4 days). Animals given AAF for 3 months and then returned to a basal diet for 2 months showed only partial restoration of EGF binding and no restoration of insulin binding. The competition curves showed a decrease in apparent number of receptors and no changes in their affinity. In vitro neither AAF nor its metabolites hydroxy- and acetoxy-AAF influenced the binding of insulin or EGF. Thus, decreased binding to intracellular receptors is a very early effect of AAF and probably is not toxic in character. Preliminary results showed that human liver microsomes specifically bind insulin and EGF but the binding of EGF is much weaker than in rats. In one case of hepatoma the binding of EGF was very low but that of insulin was normal.

1429 CATECHOL FORMATION FROM FLUORO- AND BROMO-SUBSTITUTED ESTRADIOLS IN HAMSTER LIVER MICROSOMES: EVIDENCE FOR DEFLUORINATION. J.J. Li*, J.K. Klicka, R.H. Purdy, and S.A. Li. Med. Res. Labs., V.A. Med. Center and Univ. of Minnesota Med. Sch., Minneapolis, MN 55417, and Dept. of Organic Chemistry, Southwest Med. Fdn. for Biomedical Res., San Antonio, TX 78284.

Since halogen-substituted estrogens have been used as probes to assess the significance of 2- and 4-hydroxylation in estrogen carcinogenesis in the hamster, we have examined the usefulness of this approach. Hamster liver microsomes were incubated with 2-, 4-fluoro-, or 2,4-difluoroestradiols and analogous bromo-substituted estradiols to determine the extent of 2- and 4-hydroxylation with these substrates. Estrogen-2/-4 hydroxylase activity was evaluated by radioenzymatic assay and the [^{3}H]-labeled products identified by HPLC. The fluoroestradiols exhibited significantly greater catechol estrogen formation than their corresponding bromoestradiols. Using 17β-estradiol as substrate, 95.5% of the product formed was 2-hydroxylated and 3% 4-hydroxylated. With 2-halogen estradiols, 2-fluoroestradiol exhibited more than twice the ability to form catechol estrogens than the corresponding 2-bromoestradiol. HPLC analyses indicated at least a 6-fold greater ability to form 2-hydroxylated compounds with 2-fluoroestradiol(35.5%) compared to 2-bromoestradiol(5.7%). Interestingly, 2-hydroxylation using 4-fluoroestradiol exceeded that of 17β-estradiol. Strikingly, 2,4-difluoroestradiol showed a substantial ability to form 2-hydroxy products compared to insignificant amounts formed from 2,4-dibromoestradiol. These data clearly provide evidence for defluorination of such substituted estrogens, particularly in the C-2 position and seriously question the use of fluoroestrogens in assessing either the hormonal or carcinogenic activity of the parent hormone(NCI Grants CA 22008,24629, and NIEHS Grant 1K07 ES 00094).

1430 MODULATION OF NATURAL KILLER ACTIVITY BY THE PINEAL GLAND
P.Lissoni,O.Marelli,R.Mauri,P.Franco,M.Resentini and F.Fraschini,Chair of Chemotherapy,Faculty of Medicine,University of Milan,Italy.

Some data seem to suggest that the pineal gland can inhibit the growth of some tumors,and this is a consequence,at least in part,of the anti-mitotic action of melatonin and other pineal factors;instead,the influence of the pineal gland on the immunity has not yet been established. In order to study the relationship between the pineal gland and the lymphocytic subgroups, we have evaluated the effect of melatonin on NK activity,that is involved in inhibiting the tumor growth. We studied 5 healthy volunteer young subjects of both sexes;melatonin was given at a dose of 10 mg(dissolved in 95% ethanol)i.v.infusion in 100 ml of saline solution for 30 min at 3 p.m. on December. Venous blood samples were drawn at 0,2,4 and 6 hours after melatonin infusion. NK activity was determined using a standard ^{51}Cr release assay with radiolabeled K 562 cells. NK activity response to melatonin showed a two-phase trend,with an increase after 2 hours and a marked decrease at 6 hours. This behaviour,difficult to interpretate,could depend upon a variety of endocrine effects induced by melatonin. We may conclude that the pineal gland can modulate natural killer cells activity in man;however,more data and further studies,with different doses of melatonin and during different periods of the day,are required to establish if melatonin can be used to stimulate the immunological system in the treatment of the neoplastic diseases.

1431 APPLICABILITY OF SALIVARY STEROID MEASUREMENTS FOR THE DIAGNOSIS OF PROSTATE CANCER. M. Luisi*, G.F. Argenio, D. Barletta, M. Gasperi, G. Gravina and F. Franchi, Endocrine Research Unit of the C.N.R., Pisa University School of Medicine, 56100 PISA, Italy.

Conflicting data are reported on circulating steroids in prostate cancer. Since saliva has recently offered the possibility to determine biologically available steroids, we have measured mean (± SD) morning salivary (pmol/l) and plasma (nmol/l) levels of testosterone (T), dihydrotestosterone (DHT) and estrone (E_1) in 14 men (59-74 yrs) with prostate cancer and in controls (n = 11; 58-72 yrs). Salivary T (510±118) and DHT (140±39) in patients were significantly higher (P <0.001) than in controls (T = 293±92 DHT = 77±20), while plasma T (18.4±4.9) and DHT (1.18±0.15) did not differ from normals (T = 19.6±5.2; DHT = 1.23±0.14). E_1 in patients was elevated both in saliva (59±15 vs. 25±8; P <0.001) and in plasma (241±62 vs. 147±35 P <0.001). We tentatively conclude that the higher steroid levels in saliva, reflecting the biologically active molecule, may be of aid in the diagnosis of the neoplasia and may affect the course of the disease also in terms of prognosis and response to endocrine therapy. Moreover, our data provide further evidence that measurement of steroids in saliva appears to be more sensitive than plasma to pathophysiological conditions and consequently useful in evaluating various endocrine functions in health and disease. This study was supported by the C.N.R. (Roma).

1432 OCCURRENCE AND CHARACTERIZATION OF PROLACTIN-RECEPTORS (PRL-R) IN HUMAN PATHOLOGIC BREAST. M. L'Hermite-Balériaux*, S. Casteels, G. Noël°, C. Loriaux, A. Vokaer and M. L'Hermite, Lab. de Gynécologie (ULB and FRESERH), Hôpital Brugmann; and °Cliniques St-Luc, U.C.L.; Bruxelles, Belgium.

The significance of PRL-R within mammary tumors is presently well documented in several animal species, while their characterization and clinical implications in the human remain to be established. We investigated 90 cases of human breast tumoral tissue, using different methodological approaches for membranes preparation : a) as classically used for animal PRL-R (according to Shiu); b) as for E-R and Pg-R determination; c) without removing the mitochondrial fraction (according to Peyrat et al.). The membrane preparations (± 400 µg protein) were incubated with I_{125} oPRL, in presence (N Sp B) or absence (Sp B : specific binding) of an excess oPRL. When (Sp B minus N Sp B) was ≥ 0.8 %, the tumor was considered PRL-R +. The occurrence of PRL-R + cases varied according to the procedure used : a) 8 out of 22 (36 %); b) 7 out of 47 (14 %); c) 4 out of 21 (19 %), with an overall rate of 23 %. It appears thus that the standard procedure used for E-R and Pg-R assays is not optimal to evidence the presence of PRL-R. In 3 cases of carcinoma (including one male patient) from which enough material was available for Scatchard analysis, the K_d ranged from 2.09 to 8.54 10^{-10} mol/l and the N from 2.79 to 20.0 fmol/mg protein. The characteristics of the PRL-R detected in human breast carcinoma are thus comparable to those reported for animals; this finding, at the light of animal data, reinforces thus the requirement to further establish the clinical relevance of PRL-R in human pathologic breast.

1433 IS DIETHYLSTILBESTROL (DES) MORE THROMBOGENIC THAN OTHER ESTROGENS?
J.J. Mandoki*, N. Mendoza-Patiño, E. Zavala, G. Silva, C. Rubio-Póo, and C. Lemini. Departamento de Farmacología, Facultad de Medicina, Escuela Nacional de Estudios Profesionales Zaragoza, Universidad Nacional Autónoma de México, 04510 México, D.F., México.

The effects of DES on blood clotting time were studied in male CD1 mice. A single intraperitoneal injection of a large dose (2 mg/100 g), produced a biphasic effect; an initial increase of blood clotting time observed 6 hours after the injection, was followed by a smaller, and more prolonged decrease below control values. The biphasic effect was similar to those produced by the administration of estrone (E1), estradiol-17β (E2), or mixed conjugated equine estrogens (MCEE). The same dose of DES, and a dose 10 times larger, administered daily for three days, reduced blood clotting time on the fourth day by 25 %. This effect contrasts with the lengthening of blood clotting time observed after similar treatments with E1, E2, and MCEE (Mandoki et al., Proc. West. Pharmacol. Soc. 26: 45-48, 1983). These observations, and the marked clinical thrombogenicity of DES in patients with prostatic cancer, suggest that DES administered repeatedly, is more thrombogenic than E1, E2, and MCEE, and that DES should be replaced by other estrogens in the treatment of prostatic cancer. Treatment with large doses of MCEE (10 mg/day), shown by Stamler et al., (1963) to reduce the risk of thrombogenesis, should be the first choice, as the smaller doses of MCEE used in the Coronary Drug Project (1970, 1973) increase somewhat the risk of thrombogenesis. By eliminating the increased risk of thrombogenesis, estrogen therapy could be initiated at earlier stages of the disease, increasing thereby greatly its benefits.

1434 ISOELECTRIC HETEROGENEITY OF HCG IN TROPHOBLASTIC TUMORS.
K. Mann and G. Spöttl*, Dept. Internal Medicine II, Grosshadern, University of Munich, FRG

Molecular heterogeneity of purified, urinary hCG has been well documented. However, it is widely unknown wether tumor-specific variants exist in serum- and urine-samples of patients with trophoblastic diseases. We studied IEF-pattern of untreated serum samples from 16 patients with non-seminoma germ cell tumors of the testis (NSGCT), 2 with hydatidiform moles and 1 with choriocarcinoma as well as in dialysed urinary samples of 3 patients. Sera and urine of 6 pregnant women and hCG CR 119 (NIAMDD) served as controls. IEF was carried out on polyacrylamide flat bed gels with a linear gradient from 3-7 and in a second run from 3-5. Gels were sectioned into 47 slices (5mm), extracted wit 1 ml PBS containing 1% BSA. HCG was determined by RIA and IRMA using poly- and monoclonal anti-hCG-ß antibodies. HCG CR 119 was resolved into 6 components from pH 4.1 to 5.3, whereus hCG in sera of pregnant women focused as 7 components from 4.1 to 5.8. These 7 components were also observed in serum samples of 16 patients with testicular cancer and in moles and choriocarcinoma. However, in 15/16 patients with NSGCT more neutral pI components were absent or reduced and the isoelectric profile shifted to the acid components. In serum samples of all patients 1 to 4 acid variants (pI 3.2-3.9) were found and recovered in urine. Fraction, which did not bind to Con A-sepharose focused mainly at pH 3.7 and 3.9, whereus the Con A reactive fractions had pattern similar to hCG in pregnancy. In conclusion, acid isoelectric variants of hCG were found in patients with trophoblastic diseases, which are not found in normal pregnancy. Con A nonreactivity indicates altered carbohydrate moiety.

1435 ROLE OF POLYAMINES IN MEDIATING THE EFFECTS OF PROLACTIN AND GROWTH HORMONE ON THE GROWTH OF EXPERIMENTAL BREAST CANCER. A. Manni* and C. Wright, Dept. of Medicine, Div. of Endocrinology, The M.S. Hershey Medical Center, The Pennsylvania State University, Hershey, PA 17033

We have observed that the integrity of the polyamine pathway is essential for the full expression of the stimulatory effect of estradiol on the growth of the hormone-responsive N-nitrosomethyl-urea (NMU)-induced rat mammary tumor cultured in vitro in soft agar (Manni and Wright, Clin. Res., 1984, in press). This study was designed to evaluate whether the polyamines putrescine, spermidine and spermine are also involved in mediating the effects of ovine prolactin (oPRL) and ovine growth hormone (oGH) on the growth of this tumor in vitro using the soft agar clonogenic assay. Single cell suspensions of NMU-mammary tumors were plated under serum-free media conditions. The number of stem-cell derived colonies (aggregates >50 cells) formed on day 6 after plating was the parameter used to assess mitogenesis. Under these conditions, physiologic concentrations of oPRL (20, 50, 200 ng/ml) and oGH (1, 10, 50, 100 ng/ml) were found to stimulate colony formation in a dose-dependent fashion. Such effect was blocked by α-difluoromethylornithine (DFMO)(1 mM), an inhibitor of ornithine decarboxylase, the rate-limiting enzyme of polyamine biosynthesis. Exogenous administration of putrescine (2.5 mM), spermidine (0.1 mM), and spermine (0.1 mM) reversed the inhibitory effect of DFMO and restored the action of oPRL and oGH. Our results suggest that in this system the polyamine pathway plays an essential role in mediating the effects of both steroid and peptide hormones on the growth of experimental breast cancer.

1436 METABOLIC CLEARANCE RATE OF Op'DDD IN 2 CASES TREATED FOR CUSHING DISEASE. S. Leiba,* R. Weinstein, B. Shindel, E. Stern and H. Kaufman, Department of Endocrinology, Beilinson Medical Center, Petah Tikva, Israel, 49 100.

A patient with Cushing disease who became pregnant while receiving Op'DDD (mitotane (Lysodren)) and who underwent abortion because of the known teratoxicity of this type of compound, wished to have a child and therefore posed the problem of metabolic clearance rate of this drug. Biopsy of adipose tissue performed one month after discontinuation of the drug showed it to be the storage site of considerable quantities of the drug. Determination of serum levels at various intervals after discontinuation of treatment in this patient as well as in another patient with a similar history of drug ingestion showed that it took more than one year until the blood level approached that found in the control group. These findings indicate: 1) that the adrenals remain under the influence of this drug for a long period of time after its withdrawal, 2) that pregnancy should be avoided for approximately one and a half years after discontinuation of treatment, 3) that since there is an undesirable accumulation of the drug in the adipose tissue, smaller doses may be sufficient to control the disease.

1437 CRYOSCOPIC THERMOGRAPHY (CT): PART VI. DIFFERENTIATION OF SUBACUTE THYROIDITS (SAT) FROM GRAVES' DISEASE (G). F.K. Leung, The American Institute Of Medical Research, Wilmington, Delaware.

Previous experiences in CT have demostrated that it is useful to diagnose G (Clin. Res. 30:2, 273A, 1982) and thyroid cysts (Clin. Res. 30:4, 720A, 1982). The present study involved 35 normals, 56 newly diagnosed G and 6 SAT. Normal thermograms revealed cold areas overlying the thyroid cartilage and trachea, which are outlined by warm areas over the communicating branch of the anterior jugular vein. All G patients have at least one of the following abnormal thermographic findings: 1) hypervascularity 2) warm spots over the thyroid gland, or 3) intense heat over the anatomical veinous system of the neck. Although both groups of SAT and G have elevated thyroid function tests, 5 SAT have normal thermograms which were easily distinquishable from G thermograms. Three had flourescent scans showing diffusely decreased iodine content. One SAT showed asymmetrical pattern, thermally cold lobe had decreased iodine content. CT is a simple technique to differentiate SAT from G hyperthyroidism. The whole procedure takes only a few minutes. The differences between SAT and G thermograms appeared clear-cut in this study.

1438 EFFECT OF GROWTH HORMONE THERAPY ON PLASMA CHOLESTEROL IN GROWTH HORMONE DEFICIENT CHILDREN. J.H. Levine*, A. Thienemann, H. Wohltmann, and M.L. Virella, Medical University of South Carolina, Charleston, S.C.

Plasma cholesterol (TC) and that fraction bound to high density lipoprotein (HDLC), is altered in adult men with hypopituitarism, and can be modified by thyroid and androgen therapies. Since the HDLC/TC ratio seems to be a predictor of coronary artery disease, we measured plasma lipids in growth hormone (GH) deficient male children before and at 3 month intervals after starting GH therapy. Six boys aged 56-204 months had partial or complete hypopituitarism. All were below the 3rd percentile for height, had bone ages delayed at least 3 years, and were receiving L-thyroxine; two received glucocorticoids. Before GH, the patients' triglycerides were similar to those reported by Berenson et al. for both age-matched and surface area-matched boys. Mean TC for the GH deficient boys was 207 mg/dl $\pm$ 42; m $\pm$ SD (range 153-263) compared to 170 $\pm$ 6 for controls ($p > .05$). Mean HDLC was 39 $\pm$ 6 mg/dl compared to 68 $\pm$ 22 for controls ($p < .001$). The HDLC/TC ratio of the GH deficient boys was 0.19 $\pm$ .04 (range .15-.25) vs a control ratio of 0.47 $\pm$ .03 (range .45-.51) ($p < .001$). Five boys received GH for at least 2 years. Mean growth rate was 7.2 cm/yr (range 2.7-12.8). No change in triglycerides or TC was observed but HDLC increased to 50 $\pm$ 5 ($p < .01$). The HDLC/TC ratio rose from 0.19 to 0.28 $\pm$ .04 ($p < .01$), but was still below control levels. Conclusions: Although plasma cholesterol levels are normal, HDLC levels are decreased in GH-deficient boys, producing a reduced HDLC/TC ratio. GH treatment is associated with an improvement, but not a normalization, of this ratio.

1439 INAPPROPRIATE TSH SYNDROME (ITSHS) WITH CARDIAC ARRHYTHMIA. E.S. Lightner*, Dept. of Peds., Univ. of Arizona, Tucson, AZ; J. Magner and B. Weintraub, National Institute of Health, Bethesda, MD., USA.

Cardiac arrhythmias are rare in juvenile thyrotoxicosis; we report a patient with ITSHS who developed a life-threatening arrhythmia during surgery. A six year-old male with goiter and symptoms of thyrotoxicosis (T4 24 μg, T3RU 45%, TSH 3.5 μU/ml) was treated with PTU. Both goiter and symptoms increased. Repeat thyroid studies were T4 2.6 μg, T3 580 ng/ml, TSH 240 μU/ml, I-131 uptake was 61.2 and 46.6% at 2 and 24 hrs. Pituitary CT was normal. T4 (.15 mg) was added to the PTU. T4 and T3 increased to 10.4 μg and 626 ng; TSH decreased to 30 μU/ml. Therapy was stopped; 60 days later a TRF test was done, the PRL response was normal.

	T4 μg	T3 ng	TSH μU	α TSH ng/ml	β TSH ng/ml
BASELINE	29.7	576	2.9	0.8	0.5
30'	29.0	524	18.0	2.7	0.6
60'	29.1	600	14.4	2.1	0.4
120'	26.5	726	5.2	1.3	0.4

The data are consistent with ITSHS, not due to a pituitary tumor, but of resistance to thyroid hormone action at the level of the pituitary gland. Cytomel(25 μg) was given bid, then tid. Initially, subjective but no laboratory improvement occurred. After six months of Cytomel, repeat TRF test showed a basal TSH of <1.5 μU, a maximum level of 3.9 μU/ml. During surgery, bigeminal rhythm, then ventricular tachycardia occurred-but resolved spontaneously with termination of surgery. Perhaps these patients are candidates for propranolol to reduce the risk of cardiac arrhythmias, especially during surgery.

1440 MEDICAL TREATMENT OF CUSHING'S DISEASE (CD) AND NELSON'S SYNDROME (NS). P.Loli*, M.Berselli and M.Tagliaferri Division of Endocrinology, Ospedale Niguarda Cà Granda, 20162 Milano, Italy

The value of chronic treatment with bromocriptine (Br) or sodium valproate (Sv) was assessed in 12 patients with CD and in 2 with NS. Eleven patients with CD and 1 with NS received Br 7.5-20 mg/day for 4-19 months;2 patients with CD and 1 with NS received Sv 600 mg/day for 1-5 months. Clinical as well as hormonal parameters (24 h excretion of 17OHCS, plasma ACTH and cortisol levels) were taken into account in evaluating the effects of treatment. Since even in cases of ACTH secreting pituitary macroadenomas neurosurgery often fails in eradicating the tumor, a possible tumor shrinking effect of treatment was investigated by CT scan in 3 patients with CD and 2 with NS who had evidence of macroadenoma. Only 2 patients with CD, treated with Br showed a definite but transient clinical and biochemical improvement. The responses to metyrapone, low-dose dexamethasone, insulin-induced hypoglycemia were unaffected by either treatment. In none of the patients with NS were plasma ACTH levels or skin pigmentation affected by drug administration. Tumor size was unchanged after 3-6 months of treatment in 5 patients with large adenomas. We conclude that Br and Sv are of limited value in controlling ACTH hypersecretion in patients with CD and NS; moreover we cannot confirm preliminary observations of other Authors showing that these drugs can reduce the size of ACTH secreting tumors.

1441 GH-STIMULATION WITH GROWTH HORMONE RELEASING FACTOR (hpGRF$^{1-44}$) IN ACROMEGALY BEFORE AND AFTER TRANSSPHENOIDAL OPERATION

M. Losa+, G.K. Stalla, O.A. Müller, R.Hartl and K. von Werder
Medizin. Klinik Innenstadt, Univ. of Munich, 8 München 2, FRG

100 µg of human pancreatic growth hormone releasing factor (hpGRF$^{1-44}$) was given as an i.v. bolus to 18 active acromegalics (11 males, 7 females). In 7 patients the GRF-test was repeated 6 weeks after ts-op. All patients were also subjected to standard diagnostic tests with TRH, Gn-RH, insulin hypoglycemia and oral glucose.
Out of 18 patients 9 had not been treated before, 7 had been operated, 4 were also irradiated. All had active acromegaly at time of investigation. GH-levels ranged from 3.5 to 440 ng/ml. After GRF administration GH rose by more than 100 % over baseline in 14, whereas 3 previously treated patients showed only a minimal rise after GRF. There was no correlation between the GH response to GRF and the other diagnostic tests. One girl with gigantism and a metastasizing GRF-oma (GRF-levels: 40-50 ng/ml; normal < 1 ng/ml) had also no GH response to GRF. After ts-op 5 out of 7 patients had GH levels below 10 ng/ml with a normal maximal rise after GRF to 11.6 ± 3.0 ng/ml ± SE. The GRF-oma patient had no GH response to GRF after ts-op and one postop. active acromegalic had basal and GRF-stimulated GH-levels reduced by the same magnitude.
These findings show that GH secretion can be stimulated by GRF in the majority of acromegalics. Lack of GH response in untreated acromagalics may indicate an ectopic GRF source. Previous treatment may also lead to blunting of the GH-response in active acromegaly. A normal GH response after ts-op may serve as an indicator for normal postop. pituitary function.
Supported by DFG (We 439/4-1)

1442 IMPROVEMENT OF MICROSURGERY IN ACROMEGALY BY IMMEDIATE INTRA- AND POSTOPERATIVE GROWTH HORMONE RADIOIMMUNOASSAY (GH-RIA).

D.K. Lüdecke *, H.C. Müchler and H.-D. Herrmann, Department of Neurosurgery, University-Clinic, 2000 Hamburg 20, Germany.

Measurements of perioperative plasma GH profiles were carried out since 1980 regularly the day after transnasal microsurgery In case of persistent GH excess (10 out of 50) a second transnasal operation was performed within 5-11 days (6 out of 10). Follow-ups of at least two years confirmed the effectiveness of this regimen. The normalization rate in macroadenomas could be increased from 59 to 85% when compared with an evaluation of 224 primary operations using the criteria of basal GH (normal= < 4,5 ug/l). Short half life of tumor GH (about 15 minutes) and reproducability of GH decrease after complete tumor removal now led us to a trial of intraoperative GH measurements. Reliable results of GH plasma levels were obtained within 90 minutes by a modification of a commercial GH-RIA-Kit (RIA-mat(R)HGH, Byk Mallinckrodt). Thus, in 6 out of 8 patients normalization could be proved before closure of the transnasal access. In the other two patients additional tumor could be detected and removed. Complete normalization, however, was achieved only after a second transnasal operation after 7 days in one patient. The other was referred to radiation treatment. We conclude that close GH monitoring helps to improve microsurgical results in acromegaly.
Supported by Deutsche Forschungsgemeinschaft, SFB 34.

1443 AUTOIMMUNE THYROIDITIS ASSOCIATED WITH MELASMA IN NON-PREGNANT WOMEN

R. Lutfi, M. Fridmanis, A. Misiunas, D. Pafume, E. González, J. Villemur, M. Mazzini and H. Niepomniszcze*, Complejo Médico Policial "Churruca-Visca". Buenos Aires, Argentina.

We have recently demonstrated that in non-pregnant women attended for melasma (a localized hyperpigmentation over the forehead, upper lips, cheeks and chin) there is a high incidence of thyroid alterations, being autoimmune thyroiditis the most frequent. Among 62 women with melasma (aged 24-52 yr), 19 cases (30.6 %) had positive titers of circulating thyroid microsomal antibodies (MCHA). Six of them were euthyroid and without goiter, with basal serum TSH: 3.4 ± 1.0 μU/ml; and 15.8 ± 1.8 μU/ml after i.v. stimulation with 200 μg TRH. MCHA titers were 1:100 in two cases and 1:400 in the rest. The remaining 13 patients, whose MCHA titers ranged from 1:100 to 1: 102400, were: a) Diffuse goiter and euthyroidism: 6 patients, basal TSH: 3.2 ± 1.1 μU/ml; TSH post TRH: 11.7 ± 1.2 μU/ml. b) Diffuse goiter and subclinical hypothyroidism: 5 patients, basal TSH: 9.0 ± 4.6 μU/ml; TSH post TRH: 47.8 ± 11.4 μU/ml. c) Subclinical hypothyroidism without goiter: 2 patients, basal TSH: 6.5 and 10 μU/ml; TSH post TRH: 45 and 31 μU/ml, respectively. The incidence of goiter in the general population is less than 5 %, and the expectation of autoimmune thyroiditis with goiter and/or subclinical hypothyroidism is even lesser. It is concluded that there is a true association between autoimmune thyroiditis and melasma in approximately one third of the women affected by this hypermelanosis. However, the thyroid compromise appears to be rather mild.

1444 GROWTH HORMONE-RELEASING HORMONE TEST IN PATIENTS WITH HYPOTHALAMIC DISEASE, CUSHING'S SYNDROME, AND ACROMEGALY.

N. Lytras,* A. Grossman, J.A.H. Wass, °D.H. Coy, Lesley H. Rees and G.M. Besser, Department of Endocrinology, St. Bartholomew's Hospital, London, UK, and °Department of Medicine, Tulane University, New Orleans, Lo, USA.

Growth hormone-releasing hormone-(1-40) and -(1-29)NH_2 are equipotent releasers of serum GH in normal subjects. We have therefore administered both peptides to patients with various pituitary-hypothalamic diseases to assess whether some have an endogenous defect in GHRH synthesis or release. Sixteen adult patients with growth hormone deficiency (age range 21 - 50y) were studied, 8 had craniopharyngiomas, 2 large pituitary tumours, 1 germinoma, 1 suprasellar arachnoid cyst, 3 idiopathic hypopituitarism, 1 neurosarcoidosis. Each was administered either GHRH-(1-40) 200μg (2p) or GHRH-(1-29)NH_2 200μg (14p) as a bolus, and serum GH was measured over 2h. A rise in serum GH (>10mU/l) was seen in 5 patients (3 craniopharyngiomas, 1 germinoma, 1 prolactinoma), indicating a functional defect in endogenous GHRH release. Fifteen patients with acromegaly were also administered GHRH-(1-29)NH_2 200μg as an intravenous bolus. A rise in serum GH was seen in 14 patients, ranging from 8% to 1600% of basal values. The non-responder had a metastatic carcinoid tumour associated with high levels of circulating endogenous GHRH-like immunoreactivity (25,000pg/ml; normal range < 60pg/ml). There was no correlation between serum GH responsiveness to exogenous GHRH and basal GH, previous radiotherapy, or bromocriptine responsiveness. Finally, 4 patients with Cushing's syndrome received GHRH-(1-29)NH_2 200μg; there was no serum GH response to GHRH, suggesting that high levels of corticosteroids suppress the capacity of the somatotroph to synthesize or release GH.

1445 A TIME-RESOLVED IMMUNOFLUOROMETRIC ASSAY (IFMA) FOR SEX HORMONE BINDING GLOBULIN. O. Mäentausta*, N.J.Bolton and G.L. Hammond, *Farmos Diagnostica, SF-90460 Oulunsalo, Finland and Dept. OB-GYN, University of Western Ontario, London, Canada.

The steroid binding activity of human sex hormone binding globulin (SHBG) deteriorates when the protein is isolated in pure form and limits the use of pure SHBG standards or labeled SHBG in immunoassays. This may be overcome by using labeled antibodies in immunometric assays and has largely been achieved by labeling with ^{125}I. However, this isotope has a short shelf-life, is hazardous, and presents disposal problems. We have therefore developed an assay based on time-resolved fluorometry in which a Europium labeled monoclonal SHBG antibody (Eu-MAb) is used as the tracer. The assay protocol involves addition of standards (dilutions of human pregnancy serum of known SHBG content, 0.1 ml) or dilutions (0.1 ml, 1:200) of serum samples to microtiter cuvettes passively coated with polyvalent rabbit anti-SHBG antiserum (RAb). The standards range from 6.25 to 100 fmol/cuvette. Eu-MAb (0.15 ml) is added to each well and incubated for 1 h at 20° C. The reaction mixtures are then aspirated and the wells washed (3 x 0.3 ml Tris buffer, pH 7.6) before addition of an organic "enhancing solution" (0.25 ml) prior (15 min) to counting for 1 sec only. The standards ranged from 4,000 to 25,000 cps with a background of 1,200 cps. Intra-assay precision (CV %) of serum controls was $<$ 6 %. Serum concentrations of SHBG determined by the IFMA agreed with binding capacity measurements (r = 0.85) and immunoradiometric assay values (r = 0.81). The unlimited shelf-life of the Eu-MAb and the rapidity and sensitivity of the IFMA reflect its potential as an important clinical endocrinological test.

1446 IS LOW INSULIN RESPONDER PREDIABETES? H. Makimura*, K. Kitada, K. Ishii, M. Kimura, M. Hasegawa and A. Matsuoka, Dept. of Clin. Pathology and Clin. Laboratory, Hyogo College of Medicine, Nishinomiya, Japan.

Using a glucose monitoring device, 75g O-GTT had performed in 30 healthy subfects with a normal insulin response and 21 "apparently" healthy subfects with a low insulin response to investigate the difference in the response of insulin secretion between two groups. Blood glucose and plasma IRI levels were determined every 2 minutes and 6 minutes respectively for 3 hours. In the normal responders the sum of plasma IRI levels was 1.8-fold higher than that in the low responders, while there was no difference in the sum of blood glucose levels between two groups. Further, between the sum of blood glucose levels and the sum of plasma IRI levels no significant correlation was observed. However, in the normal responders the peak appearance time of plasma IRI was significantly delayed (7.9±1.9 min M±SE) as compared with that of blood glucose, while in the low responders the former was closely corresponded (0.4±0.9 min) to the latter which was not different from that in the normal responders. The difference in the ratio of increased rate of plasma insulin to that of blood glucose until 30 minutes after the glucose load was not statistically significant between two groups. Plasma levels of TG, NEFA and ketone bodies in low responders were not higher than those in normal insulin seems to be released at the minimum effective amount at the optimal time to show the maximum effects. It is therefore not reasonable to consider that low insulin responder is equal to prediabetes, though some prediabetics may be low insulin responder.

1447 AUTONOMOUS THYROID ADENOMAS IN CHILDHOOD AND ADOLESCENCE. Arline L. A. Martin and Malcolm M. Martin.* Georgetown University School of Medicine, Washington, D.C., USA.

Autonomous solitary thyroid nodules are rare in childhood; prior to 1980 there were only 5 documented cases. A recent review of 7 adolescents with solitary hyperfunctioning thyroid nodules reported elevation of serum T-3 and blunted TRH responses indicative of subtle hyperthyroidism. We have seen 9 patients with autonomous hyperfunctioning thyroid nodules in the past 5 years. All were teenage girls except one 26-year-old female and one 4-year-old boy. The only presenting complaint was a mass in the neck in 8 of the 9 patients. The patients appeared euthyroid though one of the 9 was found on laboratory evaluation to be hyperthyroid with elevated T-4, Free T-4 and T-3, and suppressed TSH. In the remaining 8 all thyroid parameters were normal except T-3 which was elevated in 2 patients. Thyroid antibodies were absent in all subjects. Thyroid scans revealed hot nodules in 4 and hot/cold nodules in 5 with suppression of I-131 uptake in the extranodular thyroid. The nodules were not T-3 suppressible and TRH responses were absent except in the 4-year-old boy when first seen. Sonograms showed cystic areas in 6/6 cases. Seven of the patients chose surgery including the 3 with elevated T-3 which became normal post-op in 2. The 1 with hyperthyroidism became hypothyroid post-op due to fibrosis and follicular atrophy in the remaining thyroid gland. Pathology showed benign follicular cystadenoma in all cases. In the past routine ablation of non-toxic autonomously functioning thyroid adenoma was the customary treatment. However, observation with sonography appears safe and appropriate for smaller lesions.

1448 UNILATERAL ADRENAL MEDULLARY HYPERPLASIA, A CAUSE OF EPISODIC HYPERTENSION RESEMBLING PHEOCHROMOCYTOMA. S.P. MARYNICK*, Depts. of Internal Medicine & Pathology, Baylor University Medical Center, Dallas, Texas 75246 U.S.A.

Intermittent hypertension associated with tachycardia, sweating and pallor or flushing is characteristic of episodically secreting pheochromocytoma. In two patients with the above symptoms evaluation for pheochromocytoma was unrevealing as urinary VMA and metanephrine, plasma catecholamines and adrenal computed tomography were normal. When these patients developed symptoms of hypertension and tachycardia there was an elevation of plasma epinephrine on selective venous sampling with unilateral elevation of epinephrine from an adrenal vein (data in table). On laparotomy both patients were found to have unilateral adrenal enlargement with the enlarged gland demonstrating adrenal medullary hyperplasia both grossly and microscopically. Both patients are asymptomatic regarding episodes of hypertension associated with sweating and tachycardia following unilateral surgical adrenalectomy for 24 and 12 months respectively. Cortisol levels have remained normal in both patients.

	Norepinephrine				Epinephrine			
	Adrenal Vein		Vena Cava		Adrenal Vein		Vena Cava	
	Right	Left	Inferior	Superior	Right	Left	Inferior	Superior
Pt.#1:	120	3,730	509	545	5	14,192	154	251
Pt.#2:	580	2,383	147	439	3,363	26,488	77	104

It is concluded that adrenal medullary hyperplasia may present clinically in a manner similar to episodically secreting pheochromocytoma and is benefited by surgical therapy.

1449 CHARACTERIZATION OF GOITROUS PATIENTS WITH NORMAL T4 AND T3 AND BLUNTED TSH RESPONSE TO TRH.

R. Matte*, J.M. Boutin, P. D'Amour, F. Gilbert, R. Bélanger, J. Havrankova, R. Chartrand, M. Zakarija and J.M. McKenzie, Un. of Montreal and Miami.

The nature of the thyroid disorder presented by patients with goiter, normal T4 and T3 but blunted TSH response to TRH has not yet been clarified. In this study we compare different thyroid function tests in 16 of these patients with those of 14 controls and 10 hyperthyroid patients. Basal total T4, free T4, total T3 and iodine uptake were similar to controls but significantly ($p<.001$) lower than in hyperthyroid patients. In contrast, basal TSH, ΔTSH after TRH stimulation, and decrease of T4 during T3 suppression test were similar to hyperthyroid patients but significantly ($p<.001$) lower than in controls. TSI were measured in 8 patients with blunted TSH response and were positive in only one, while TSI were clearly positive in five and of borderline value in two of 8 hyperthyroid patients. Iodine uptake was measured before and 18 hours after IM injection of 10 units of TSH in all patients. Patients with blunted TSH response to TRH had a percent increase of uptake of $216 \pm 52\%$ post TSH while this increase was $94 \pm 12\%$ in controls ($p<.05$) and $6 \pm 6\%$ in hyperthyroid patients ($p<.001$). The percent increase in uptake was at least 25% in all patients with TSI lower than 0.6 pmole/cAMP/mg and less than 5% in all but one patient with higher values of TSI. Our results do not support claims that the presence of TSI is responsible for the thyroid autonomy in patients with normal T4 and T3 and blunted TSH response to TRH. Moreover increase in iodine uptake after TSH stimulation allows a clear distinction of these patients from controls and hyperthyroid patients.

1450 STRUCTURE/ACTIVITY RELATIONS OF LH-RH in VERTEBRATES: REQUIREMENTS FOR AMINO ACID RESIDUES IN POSITIONS SEVEN AND EIGHT.

R. Millar*, J. King, R. Roeske, W. Day, J. Rivier and P. Licht, *Department of Chemical Pathology, University of Cape Town, Observatory 7925, South Africa; Department of Biochemistry, Indiana University; Peptide Biology Laboratory, The Salk Institute; and Department of Zoology, University of California.

Hypothalamic LH-RH from birds, reptiles and fish differs structurally from mammalian hypothalamic LH-RH at amino acid residue Arg^8 or at residues Leu^7 and Arg^8. To establish the functional significance of these structural differences, analogs with substitutions for Leu^7 and Arg^8 were synthesised, and their biological activity and receptor binding was compared. LH release from ovine pituitary cells in culture was markedly decreased by any neutral amino acid substitution for Arg^8. Acidic amino acid substitutions had lowest LH-releasing activity. Some activity was retained with basic amino acid substitutions (e.g. Lys^8-LH-RH had 10%). The K_ds of binding of all the analogs to rat pituitary receptors closely paralleled the biological activity. Neutral amino acid-substituted analogs had high activity in stimulating LH release from dispersed chicken pituitary cells, as did mammalian LH-RH. Analogs Phe^8- and Trp^8-LH-RH and salmon LH-RH (Trp^7, Leu^8-LH-RH) were more active in the chicken system than chicken LH-RH (Gln^8-LH-RH). Mammalian, chicken and salmon LH-RH had equal biological activity in a teleost fish. In the amphibian (bullfrog), in which the endogenous hypothalamic LH-RH has the same structure as mammalian LH-RH, chicken LH-RH had full gonadotropin-releasing activity. These findings indicate that the mammalian pituitary receptor has high "fidelity" for the amino acid in position eight of LH-RH while the receptor in birds, fish and amphibians is "promiscuous".

1451 SEASONAL EFFECTS OF CORTICOSTERONE INJECTION OR STRESSFUL STIMULI ON LHRH CONCENTRATION IN MICRODISSECTED HYPOTHALAMIC AREAS OF MALE NEWTS. Frank L. Moore* and R. T. Zoeller, Zoology Dept., Oregon State Univ., Corvallis, OR, 97331, USA.

Stressful stimuli can stimulate corticosterone (CS) secretion and disrupt reproductive functions in newts (Taricha granulosa, Amphibia). To test the hypothesis that CS inhibits LHRH release during stress-induced inhibition of reproduction, LHRH was measured in specific brain areas. When male newts were stressed (confined for 1 hr), concentrations of irLHRH were significantly higher in the preoptic area (POA), infundibulum (IF), and rostral hypothalamus (RH) of stressed males compared to controls. When male newts were injected with CS, concentrations of irLHRH were significantly higher in the POA, IF, and RH of the CS-injected males compared to controls. Stressed and CS-injected males had lower plasma testosterone concentrations than the controls. These data, from February experiments, support the hypothesis that corticosterone inhibits LHRH release during stress-induced inhibition of reproduction. In a June experiment, which is after the breeding season, neither plasma testosterone concentrations nor hypothalamic concentrations of irLHRH were influenced by stress or CS injection, as observed in February. Thus the sensitivity of LHRH release to corticosteroids appears to change seasonally. Supported by NSF and NICHD (PCM 83-16001,1 K04 HD00407).

1452 STEROID SULFATASE ACTIVITIES AND LIPID CONTENT IN LIVER MICROSOMES OF NON-PREGNANT AND PREGNANT FEMALE GUINEA-PIGS. M. Nicollier*, S. Roblin, O. Prost, M. Moutaouakkil and G.L. Adessi, INSERM U198, Rte de Dôle, 25000, Besançon, France.

In a previous study, we have reported an increase of estrone sulfatase activity in the liver of female guinea-pigs during pregnancy. As membrane-bound steroid sulfatases could be phospholipid dependent enzymes (McNaugh and France.J.Ster.Biochem. 13,363-373,1980), the steroid sulfatase activities and the lipid content of liver microsomes have been compared in non-pregnant and pregnant guinea-pigs. Estrone and DHEA-sulfatase activities were significantly increased($P<0.05$) in liver microsomes of pregnant guinea-pigs compared to mature females. Cholesterol: 2.6% $\pm$ 0.2 v.s 1.7% $\pm$ 0.3 (in percentage of total lipids $\pm$ SD),and sphingomyelin: 2.3% $\pm$ 0.5 v.s 1.5% $\pm$ 0.3, were significantly higher ($P<0.05$) in the liver microsomes of pregnant guinea-pigs than in mature females. Cholesterol/phospholipids ratio increases from 0.089 $\pm$ 0.022 in mature females to 0.140 $\pm$ 0.024 in pregnant females. Cholesteryl sulfate which represents 0.2% of total lipids does not vary between the two groups of animals. These results show a variation in lipid content of liver microsomes in pregnant guinea-pigs and corroborate the fundamental role of lipids on the activity of membrane bound steroid sulfatases.

1453 EFFECT OF ATRIAL NATRIURETIC FACTOR (ANF) IN GENETICALLY HYPERTENSIVE RATS. S.C. Pang*, M.C. Hoang, J. Tremblay, M. Cantin, R. Garcia, J. Genest and P. Hamet, Clinical Research Institute of Montreal, Quebec, H2W 1R7, Canada.

The natriuretic and vasorelaxant effects of ANF are well known; the concomitant, 10-fold increase of urinary cGMP suggests that these effects are related to or may even be resulted from elevated level of the cyclic nucleotide. The present study was designed to analyze the differential effect of ANF on arterial blood pressure, and urinary sodium content and cGMP level in a genetically hypertensive rat model. Female hypertensive SHR and SHRSP, and normotensive WKY were anesthetized; femoral vessels and urinary bladder were catheterized for ANF infusion, arterial pressure recording, and urine collection. The collected urine was analyzed for sodium and cGMP content. ANF decreased systolic blood pressure by 31(15%), 33(16%) and 8(8%) mmHg, and increased diuresis (15, 12 and 5 times the basal level) and natriuresis (22, 20 and 7 times the basal level) in SHRSP, SHR and WKY, respectively. However, a 10-20 fold increase in total urinary cGMP level by ANF was not significantly different among the 3 groups. Results of the present study demonstrate that the blood pressure-lowering, diuretic and natriuretic effects of ANF were more pronounced in hypertensive than in normotensive rats. These data also suggest that although the production of cGMP is similar in the three strains of rat, the cGMP effector system may be abnormal which lead to the observed differences in arterial pressure and natriuresis in this animal model. Supported by the MRC and CHF.

1454 CALMODULIN (CM) AND CALCIUM DEPENDENCE OF PITUITARY ADENYLATE CYCLASE (AC) ACTIVITY. Glenn T. Peake* and J. Alvin Smoake, Univ. of New Mexico and New Mexico Tech. Albuquerque 87131 and Socorro, New Mexico, USA.

We sought here to determine whether pituitary AC required CM for activation and to ascertain which component of the AC system was regulated by CM. AC activity was measured in isolated pituitary plasma membranes. Mg^{++} and Ca^{++} from .05 to 10 mM each increased AC activity up to 10 and 50 fold respectively. However, in the presence of free Mg^{++} (up to 3 mM in excess of ATP substrate), Ca^{++} had biphasic effect on the enzyme. Above 0.1 mM Ca^{++}, there was a progressive decline in AC activity from 50 pmoles/mg/min cAMP formed to reach a nadir of 11 pmoles/mg/min at 1.0 mM C^{++} and then a rise in activity at 5 and 10 mM Ca^{++} to reach a peak of 85 pmoles/mg/min. Thus, this regulation of the enzyme occurred over the physiologic range of calcium concentration. EGTA (2.5 mM) reduced enzyme activity from 12.9$\pm$1 pmoles/min. to 7.6$\pm$2 and 1.0 mM TFP reduced it to 1.51$\pm$0.2. Forskolin, guanidoimidodiphosphate and NaF all of which increased AC activity presumably by activating the guanine nucleotide binding subunit (GNs), were blocked by TFP. However, 10 mM Ca^{++} increased AC from 17.8$\pm$0.6 pmoles/10 min. 20 275$\pm$18 and the addition of TFP did not decrease enzyme activity. CM presence in the membranes was further established by demonstrating that EGTA and TFP blocked phosphodiesterase (PDE) activity in the isolated membranes and that heated membranes could be used as a source of CM to activate a CM deficient PDE. We conclude that CM is a necessary component of the pituitary AC system and that it is necessary for the (GNs) activation of the catalytic subunit. High concentrations of Ca^{++} appear to directly stimulate the catalytic subunit.

1455 DESENSITIZATION OF β-ADRENERGIC RESPONSIVENESS OF HAMSTER BROWN ADIPOCYTES DURING VOLUNTARY OVEREATING. Richard J. Schimmel, Department of Physiology, Rutgers Medical School, Piscataway, N.J. 08854.

Thermogenesis in brown adipose tissue (BAT) is activated during hyperphagia and the stimulus appears to be increased sympathetic activity. Catecholamines elicit heat production in BAT by stimulation of adenylate cyclase resulting in an increase in cyclic AMP (cAMP) levels which in turn activates lipolysis. The resultant production of FFA increases mitochondrial respiration. In many cells, chronic hormone exposure leads to a state of diminished responsiveness to the same hormone. The present study investigates brown fat cells from hyperphagic hamsters to determine if the sympathetic stimulation of BAT during hyperphagia modifies cell responsiveness to catecholamines. Hyperphagia was induced by including several palatable foods in the diet (cafeteria-diet). cAMP accumulation in brown fat cells of hyperphagic hamsters was increased by isoproterenol to a smaller extent than in cells from chow fed animals. Addition of forskolin, however, partially restored the responsiveness of cells from hyperphagic hamsters. Isoproterenol-stimulated adenylate cyclase activity was also lower in brown fat cells from hyperphagic hamsters. In contrast, when glycerol production was measured as an index of lipolysis, cells from hyperphagic hamsters were more responsive to isoproterenol than were cells from chow fed animals. These data are consistent with decreased coupling between β-adrenergic receptors and adenylate cyclase in brown fat cells of hyperphagic hamsters and suggest that regulatory factors exist to preserve optimum rates of lipolysis.

1456 STUDY ON THE OXYTOCIN-LIKE SUBSTANCE IN THE HUMAN PLACENTA.
Kazumi Nakazawa*, Tsunehisa Makino, Akihiko Nakayama, Ichigen Haginiwa, Kazumi Ui, and Rihachi Iizuka, Department of Obstetrics and Gynecology, School of Medicine, Keio University, Tokyo, Japan

Oxytocin(OT)-like substance was extracted with acetic acid from fresh human placenta of various periods of gestation. The extracts were studied for (1) quantitative measurement of immunoreactive OT by radioimmunoassay, (2) molecular characterization by gel-filtration and ion- exchange chromatography, (3) bioactivity on the rat uterine muscle, (4) immunohistochemical localization. The results are as follows; 1), 2), 3), 4), 5), 6). These findings suggest that OT-like substance might play some role in the mechanism of initiation of labor.

1) The placental tissue content of immunoreactive OT increases from 12.7ng/placenta at first trimester to 4.1μg at second trimester, 12.5μg at third trimester, respectively.
2) The mean immunoreactive OT concentration of 1gm of the placental tissue is 1.6 ng/gm at first trimester then significantly increases to 22.0ng/gm at second trimester maintaining the level till third trimester.
3) The dilution curve of placental tissue nearly parallels with that of synthetic OT in RIA dose response curve.
4) The elution curve of placental tissue through CMC column chromatography shows similar pattern with that of synthetic OT.
5) The placental tissue extract causes the similar contraction to that of synthetic OT, however the uterine contraction was diminished when this placental extract was incubated with the anti OT serum.
6) In immunohistochemical study with anti rabbit OT serum, OT- like substance was detected in the synsytiotrophoblastic layer.

1457 THE ANTI-PROGESTIN AND ANTI-GLUCOCORTICOID ACTIVITIES OF 11ß-SUBSTITUTED STEROIDS CAN BE SEPARATED. D.A.Henderson*, G.Neef, C.Bengtson and M.Töpert. Research Laboratories of Schering AG, Müllerstrasse 170-178, D-1000 Berlin 65.

We have established culture systems which allow the demonstration of anti-progestin and antiglucocorticoid effects in vitro. Initial characterisation used RU 38486 (11ß-(4-N,N'-dimethylaminophenyl)17ß-hydroxy-17α-propynyl4,9 (10)estradiene-3-one), a compound known to have both anti-progestational and anti-glucocorticoid properties. Organ cultures of post partum rat uterus produce collagenase which can be measured from the concentration of hydroxyproline in soluble peptides in the culture medium or using 3H-collagen as substrate. Repression of collagenase activity by progestin or glucocorticoid is reversible by RU 38486. This system displays progestin control independent of estrogens. In our second test system, the glucocorticoid inhibition of growth of S49.1 mouse lymphoma cells is followed by measuring DNA synthesis (3H-TdR incorporation). This system is not significantly affected by progestins and the inhibitory effect of cortisol can be completely reversed by RU 38486. Using these two models, we can therefore distinguish the two anti-hormonal effects. Results will be presented which indicate the possibility of separating anti-progestational and anti-glucocorticoid activity by appropriate modification of the 11ß-phenyl substituted steroid. Thus it may be possible to develop a progesterone antagonist free from other anti-hormonal activities.

1458 A FERTILE WOMAN WITH XO SEX CHROMOSOME CONSTITUTION.

E.Kehyayan*[1], R.Fortuna[2], M.G.Tibiletti[3], L.Dalprà[3].

1-Ospedale Regina Elena, Milano. 2-Laboratorio di Citogenetica I.C.P., Milano. 3- III Clinica Ostetrica e Ginecologica, Università di Milano.

The occurrence of a successful pregnancy in patients with 45,X karyotype is a very rare event. A review of the literature indicates that no more than 40 cases had been described, and most of these were mosaics with a 46,XX or 47,XXX cell line in addition to the 45,X cells. We present a fertile 45,X patient showing a typical Turner's phenotype having given births to two normal children. The correlation between femal fertility and X chromosome abnormalities with particular emphasis to X monosomy is discussed. The woman was refered to our hospital at the age of 10 years because of her short stature. Lymphocytes chromosome analysis by conventional staining technique shoved a 45,X karyotype. Hormonal substitutive therapy was refused by the patient. From 13 years of age she had sporadic menstrual cycles. The cytogenetic study was repeated on both lymphocytes and fibroblasts by means of QFQ and RBA banding techniques. An homogeneous 45,X cell population was found in the analyzed tissues.

1459 EFFECTS OF MATERNAL ETOH CONSUMTION ON LIPID SYSTHESIS IN NEONATAL RATS. T. Kepic*, A. Snyder, S.Singh. Chicago Medical School and VA Medical Center, North Chicago, IL 60064.

Because of the major role nutrition and hormones play in fetal development, we studied the effects of chronic maternal ethanol (EtOH) consumption on neonatal lipid synthesis. Timed pregnant Sprague-Dawley rats were assigned to three groups: one group (EF) received liquid diet with EtOH, 5% w/v; control diet was by pair feeding (PF) or ad libitum (AF); liver (LI), lung (LU) and placenta (PL) from cesarean-delivered term fetuses were used for wet weights and for a modified Jungas fatty acid synthesis analysis. Pooled plasma was used for corticosterone (F) analysis by RIA. Weight gain was reduced in both EF and PF dams ($p<0.001$). There was a significant decrease ($p<0.001$) in LU and a significant increase ($P<0.001$) in PL relative weights in the EF pups as compared to the PF and AF pups. Prepared tissue for total rate of lipid synthesis (TRLS) (umole/min/gm BW) in the LI showed no significant difference (NSD) in the EF pups as compared to the PF and AF pups. There was a significant increase ($p<0.01$) in the TRLS in the LU of the EF pups (0.770 ± 0.278) as compared to PF (0.423 ± 0.25) and to AF pups (0.596 ± 0.260). There was NSD in the PL TRLS. Moreover, plasma F levels showed a significant decrease in the maternal EF group (16.68 ± 1.25 ug/dl) as compared to the PF (51.24 ± 8.40) and AF (37.30 ± 1.0) dams. There was NSD in the plasma F levels in the Ef pups as compared to the PF and AF groups. This study was supported by the North Chicago Veterans Administration.

1460 GLYCEROL PHOSPHATE DEHYDROGENASE LEVELS AND FUNCTIONAL GLUCOCORTICOID RECEPTORS IN DEVELOPING RAT BRAIN. E. Kitraki, F. Stylianopoulou,* and M. N. Alexis† Dept. of Histology-Embryology, Univ. of Athens Medical Sch., and †Natl. Hellenic Res. Found., 48 Vas. Constantinou Ave., Athens 501/1 Greece.

Glycerol phosphate dehydrogenase (GPDH) activity was measured in developing brain cytosol from intact and adrenalectomized rats. In adult rats, adrenalectomy caused a decrease in GPDH activity of approximately 30%, when measured two weeks following operation. This decrease was reversed by glucocorticoid replacement effected by means of corticosterone tablet implantation. In intact rats GPDH activity could be detected throughout postnatal development in both cortex and limbic system areas. By 40 days of age, enzyme activity in limbic system area was almost twice as much as in cortex. Adrenalectomy did not affect GPDH activity during development in either brain area, until day 40, at which time adrenal control of brain GPDH activity was analogous to that seen in the adult rat. Day 40 coincides with the time when adult enzyme activity has been attained in the intact rats, in both brain areas studied. Parallel studies of brain cytosolic glucocorticoid receptors revealed that receptor binding could be detected as early as the 17th day of gestation, and that adult receptor levels were attained by the age of two weeks. Rat brain glucocorticoid receptor functionality, as judged by the capability for in vitro activation, and in vitro and in vivo nuclear translocation, was observed throughout development. Our results show that no direct correlation exists between brain glucocorticoid receptor changes in concentration or properties and control of GPDH activity by glucocorticoids.

1461 FETAL LEYDIG CELL CULTURE-AN IN VITRO SYSTEM FOR THE STUDY OF GnRH ACTION.
G. F. Knox*, M.L. Castellon, K. J. Catt and M. L. Dufau. Mol. Endo. Section, ERRB, NICHD, NIH, Bethesda, MD 20205, U.S.A.

We have recently demonstrated that inhibitory actions of GnRH agonists (GnRHa) on steroidogenesis accompany the expression of GnRH receptors in short-term cultures of 20.5 day fetal rat testes (Dufau et. al., J. Biol. Chem., 1984). The present studies were performed to define the characteristics of this inhibition and to develop long-term fetal Leydig cell cultures. Collagenase-dispersed Leydig cells were cultured for 80 days with preservation of LH receptors and steroidogenic functions. After 4 days of exposure of cultures to daily additions of oLH, 8-Br-cAMP, forskolin, or cholera toxin, in the presence or absence of GnRHa, testosterone (T) and pregnenolone (P) were measured in the incubation media. T production was maximally stimulated during incubation of cultures with 8-Br-cAMP, CT and forskolin, to the levels attained in cultures exposed to oLH. In cultures maximally stimulated by LH or cAMP-elevating agents, addition of GnRHa caused marked (60 to 80%) inhibition of T production. However, P accumulation in LH-stimulated cultures (measured in the presence of cyanoketone and spironolactone) was not reduced by GnRHa. These studies indicate that a major component of the steroid inhibitory effect of GnRHa occurs beyond cAMP production. The lack of reduction of P formation indicates that a late biosynthetic lesion (distal to P) is largely responsible for the decrease in androgen production. The fetal Leydig cell can be maintained in long-term culture with preservation of receptor-activated steroidogenic responses, and provides a valuable model for studies of GnRH action in the testis.

1462 CORD BLOOD THYRONINES IN NEWBORNS FROM IODINE DEFICIENT ENVIRONMENTS: NEW INSIGHTS INTO THE PATHOGENESIS OF "NERVOUS CRETINISM"

N. Kochupillai, M.M. Godbole*, C.S. Pandav and M.G. Karmarkar, Department of Endocrinology, A.I.I.M.S., New Delhi, India.

As the independent feto-placental unit metabolise thyroxine differently and as thyronine profile is important to the developing brain, we studied cord blood thyronines in two different parts of India with severe (Gonda) and mild (Delhi) environmental iodine deficiency. 130 and 160 cord sera from Gonda and Delhi respectively were analysed for T_4, T_3, r-T_3 and TSH by sensitive and specific RIAs. The cord sera from Gonda had significantly higher T_3 and TSH levels and significantly lower T_4 & r-T_3 levels. Five newborns from Gonda were hypthyroid. An ongoing Neonatal Screening programme in these two areas show 4% incidence of neonatal hypothyroidism in Gonda while among thousand newborns screened from Delhi only one could be detected to be hypothyroid. 9% of the normal newborns from Gonda had cord blood T_3 levels above 110 ng/dl. Interpretation of these data in the context of modern knowledge in developmental neurobiology may explain the pathogenesis of neurological defects associated with severe environmental iodine deficiency. The work was supported by DST, Govt. of India.

1463 PLASMA LEVELS OF SOMATOSTATIN-LIKE IMMUNOREACTIVITY (SLI) IN NEWBORNS AND INFANTS. T. Koshimizu*, K. Ohtsuka and Y. Ohyama, Department of Pediatrics, Kitasato University School of Medicine, Sagamihara, Japan.

Plasma SLI was measured together with plasma gastrin at 2 - 3 h after suckling in 98 healthy newborns and infants. As an animal model study, the concentrations of SLI and gastrin in the cardiac and hepatic portal plasma were also measured in neonatal rabbits during the first 40 days of life. Plasma SLI was determined by RIA after extraction with acetone-petroleum ether. No significant difference was found by age in gel filtration patterns of the extracts of these plasma samples. The plasma levels of SLI increased progressively with age during the neonatal period. The mean level of plasma SLI was higher in infants aged 1 - 3 months than in newborns and tended to decrease in infants aged 6 - 9 months after weaning. The mean levels of plasma SLI were significantly higher in newborns and infants less than 9 months old than in older children aged 8 - 12 years (mixed cord plasma: 18.5±7.5, newborns aged 1-5 days: 29.0±17.2, infants aged 1 - 3 mos: 45.5±25.8, infants aged 6 - 9 mos: 31.6±7.9, older children: 10.2±4.6 pg/ml). The mean concentrations of SLI in the cardiac and portal plasma also increased progressively with age in rabbits less than 15 days old and decreased after weaning, while the mean portal levels were 4 - 8 times higher than the mean cardiac plasma levels. These changes of plasma SLI with age were found to be well correlated with those of plasma gastrin in both humans and rabbits. These findings suggest that high concentrations of somatostain are present in the portal and peripheral circulations in immature suckling animals and that this peptide plays an important role as a hormone in nutrient homeostasis in newborns and infants.

1464 CHANGES OF MATERNAL PLASMA LEVELS OF 11-DEOXYCORTISOL PRECEDING ONSET OF HUMAN LABOR. Y. Kuwabara*, M. Mizuno and S. Sakamoto, Dept. of Ob-Gyn, Faculty of Medicine, Univ. of Tokyo, 7-3-1 Hongo, Bunkyo-ku, Tokyo, Japan.

In humans, because of the difficulties to monitor the activity of corticosteroidogenesis of the fetal adrenal cortex, it is not known whether fetal cortisol triggers the start of labor. In this work it is shown that maternal plasma levels of 11-deoxycortisol (S) might be the good index of fetal adrenal corticosteroidogenesis and the changes of maternal levels toward labor were investigated. Plasma S was determined using the specific RIA. Sixty nine normal pregnant women and 17 women with abnormal pregnancies were chosen for analysis. Furthermore, samples in 13 normal cases were obtained serially every two days for the last three weeks before labor. Concentrations in maternal plasma increased with progression of pregnancy and reached a peak at 39 weeks. The levels decreased very rapidly in the postpartum period. In cases of intrauterine fetal death and anencephalic pregnancies, the values were apparently lower than normal. In cases of bilaterally adrenalectomized women, the maternal plasma levels were almost normal. The maternal levels were high in cases of twin pregnancies. Therefore it is assumed that the fetus, especially, fetal adrenal cortex is the source of the increased S in maternal plasma during late pregnancy. During the last three weeks maternal S levels increased continuously and reached the highest value about 10 days before the onset of labor. Because of this definite pattern of the maternal plasma S levels, it is strongly suggested that the maturation of fetal adrenal function is a prerequisite for the initiation of human partrition.

1465 THE INFLUENCE OF NEONATAL HYPERTHYROIDISM ON SOMATIC GROWTH, SERUM T4 AND SUBMANDIBULAR GLAND (SMG)- AND SERUM NGF CONCENTRATIONS IN ONE MONTH OLD MICE.

J. Lakshmanan*, U. Beri, J. Alm, T. Macaso, H. Kim and D.A. Fisher. Harbor-UCLA Medical Center, UCLA School of Medicine, Torrance, CA 90509

Newborn female Swiss-Webster mouse pups were randomly divided into control (vehicle injected) and L-thyroxine (T4) treated (0.4 μg/g BW/day) groups. Pups were injected with vehicle or T4 from birth through day 6. T4 treatment accelerated eyelid opening and incisor eruption but impaired somatic growth. Retardation in body weight gain was evident from day 9; linear growth retardation (nose to rump length) was observed from day 15. In addition T4 treatment abolished the normal ontogenic peak serum T4 and T3 levels seen on day 15. Normal values were restored by day 21. Somatic growth and SMG- and serum-NGF concentrations in control and treated mice at one month were as follows:

Treatment	Body Weight (g)	Length (cm)	SMG-NGF (ng/mg protein)	Serum-NGF (ng/ml)
Vehicle	21.8±0.47	8.99±0.11	24.2±7.60	1.72±0.04
Thyroxine	16.48±0.48*	7.87±0.10	1.4±0.38*	2.09±0.14**

*p<0.001 **p<0.05

SMG-NGF and serum-NGF concentrations were significantly reduced at 30 days. Conclusion: Neonatal hyperthyroidism a) accelerates maturation; b) impairs growth; c) alters the normal ontogenesis of circulating T4 and T3 levels; d) impairs normal ontogenic maturation of SMG-NGF concentration and e) increases serum NGF levels.

1466 DEHYDROEPIANDROSTERONE METABOLISM IN TESTICULAR TISSUE FROM HUMAN EMBRYOS EXPOSED OR UNEXPOSED TO A COMBINATION OF ETHINYL ESTRADIOL AND NORETHINDRONE ACETATE.

G. Laudahn*, M. Pulkkinen and H.U. Schweikert, Schering AG, Berlin, W.-Germany, Dept. of Obstetrics and Gynecology, The University of Turku, Finland, Dept. of Internal Medicine, The University of Bonn, W.-Germany.

It has been postulated that hypospadias - a common congenital birth defect - might be caused by the maternal ingestion of progestins and/or estrogens during the critical period of male phenotypic sexual differentiation. It has been suggested that these steroids inhibit the activity of the 3β-hydroxysteroiddehydrogenase Δ^5-isomerase (3β-HSD), an enzyme of critical importance for the fetal testicular synthesis of testosterone. To test this hypothesis 3β-HSD-activity was assessed in testicular tissue (mean weight 2.6 mg) obtained from 4 embryos (10-16 weeks of gestation) whose mothers ingested 20 mg norethindrone acetate and 40 mg ethinyl estradiol 24 hours before legal abortion. 4 embryos (10-17 weeks of gestation) unexposed to these steroids served as the controls. Small tissue fragments (mean weight 2.6 mg) were incubated with ^{3}H-dehydroepiandrosterone and the metabolites formed were separated by thin layer chromatography. Results: 1. Due to the minute size of the tissues used for incubations morphological analysis of each sample was feasable thus allowing to prove both origin and integrity of the tissue examined after incubation. 2. Androstenedione and testosterone formation was demonstrated in substantial amounts in all samples. 3. Compared to the controls 3β-HSD was not decreased in testicular tissue of embryos exposed to synthetic steroids. Thus, it seems reasonable to conclude that the tested synthetic steroids do not affect genital development by the inhibition of 3β-HSD as proposed previously.

1467 DIHYDROTESTOSTERONE MODULATES ESTRADIOL PRODUCTION IN HUMAN TERM PLACENTAL EXPLANTS. W.Y. Ling*, W. Wrixon and T. Acorn, Departments of Obstetrics/ Gynecology & Physiology/Biophysics, Dalhousie University, Halifax, Canada.

Estradiol (E2) regulates many important physiologic processes in late pregnancy. The effect of dihydrotestosterone (DHT) on the conversion of E2 from ^{3}H-esterone-3-sulfate (^{3}H-E1S), and on the interconversion of ^{3}H-labeled E2 and E1 were studied. Explants from normal term placentas were cultured for 0.5-24 h in media supplemented with either ^{3}H-E1S, ^{3}H-E1 or ^{3}H-E2 and with or without added test agents. Using ether-extraction, column chromatography and recrystallization techniques, the formation of labeled E2 and E1 was quantitated. With 0.25 μM (equivalent of late pregnancy plasma level) ^{3}H-E1S as substrate, DHT (0.05-5 μM) caused a significant dose and time related increase of ^{3}H-E2 (e.g. 1.6X, 3.3X, 6.5X at 0.05, 0.5 and 5 μM after 1 H). The presence of 50 μM hydroxyflutamide (an antiandrogen) did not influence the DHT effect. At equimolar substrate concentration (0.1 μM), the interconversion of ^{3}H-E1 and ^{3}H-E2 showed that DHT exerted a dose and time dependent action in favor of E2 formation. These results indicate that (a) DHT may increase placental E2 production from circulating E1S, and this action is probably not mediated via androgen receptors; (b) DHT influences placental estradiol-17β-hydroxydehydrogenase (17EDH) activity towards E2. Since placental 17EDH controls the ultimate placental synthesis of the bioactive E2, DHT may regulate its overall E2 production, (c) This androgenic effect may have important implications in other normal or pathological estrogen sensitive tissues (breast, endometrium) that synthesize both estrogens and DHT.

1468 EFFECTS OF ACUTE METABOLIC ACIDOSIS ON ARGININE VASOPRESSIN (AVP) AND CATECHOLAMINE (C) RELEASE IN THE OVINE FETUS. Tom Lowe*, Daniel J. Faucher, Abbot R. Laptook, John C. Porter and Charles R. Rosenfeld, Depts Peds and OB-Gyn, Southwestern Medical School, Dallas, TX., U.S.A.

In fetal sheep, acute asphyxia, i.e, hypoxia, hypercapnia, and acidosis, results in 75-and >20-fold rises in plasma AVP and C, respectively. Hypoxia alone results in only a 5-fold rise in AVP; the effects of either acidosis or hypercapnia alone on AVP release are unknown. To study the effect of acidosis on AVP and C release and interaction, we induced acute metabolic acidosis in 8 fetal sheep (n=10, 137±1.4 [$\bar{x}$±SE] days gestation), infusing NH_4Cl,.03-.07mEq/min·kg for 120min, and monitoring mean arterial pressure (MAP), heart rate (HR), PaO_2, pHa, and $PaCO_2$, and plasma AVP, dopamine (DA), norepinephrine (NE) and epinephrine (E) before, at 20min intervals during, and every 30 min for 6h after NH_4Cl. MAP, PaO_2 and $PaCO_2$ were unchanged; pHa fell from 7.38±.01 to 6.99±.07* at 120min of NH_4Cl, returning to 7.36±.02 at 24h. HR rose ∿25%* after NH_4Cl. Plasma AVP rose gradually during NH_4Cl from 2.85±.23 to 5.26±1.1μU/ml* at 120min, returning to control levels 60min after NH_4Cl although pHa remained <7.10*. AVP rose as a function of falling pHa during NH_4Cl, r=-.67, p<.0001 (n=37). Although D and NE levels rose, they were not significant; however, E rose from 79±28 to 279±123pg/ml* after 120min of NH_4Cl. Neither the rise in AVP nor fall in pHa correlated significantly with changes in C. In contrast to an asphyxial insult in fetal sheep, marked metabolic acidosis alone results in only mild rises in AVP and E secretion and a tendency for increased D and NE release. Since correlations between secretion of these neurohormones are not obvious, their interaction in fetal stress responses remains unclear. *p<0.05.

1469 PHORBOL ESTER INHIBITS STIMULATION OF H^+ SECRETION BY ISOLATED RABBIT GASTRIC GLANDS. N. Raphael* and T.E. Machen, Dept. of Physiology-Anatomy, Univ. of Calif., Berkeley, CA 94720, USA.

Whereas stimulation of H^+ secretion by histamine is mediated by rapid increases in intracellular cAMP, muscarinic agonists and gastrin are thought to utilize Ca^{2+} as second messenger. These latter secretagogues have been linked to activation of Ca^{2+}, phospholipid dependent protein kinase (C-kinase) in other systems. Because phorbol esters activate C-kinase, we tested the effects of 12-O-tetradecanoylphorbol-13-acetate (TPA) on the H^+secretory response in gastric glands using the accumulation of the weak base, [^{14}C]-aminopyrine (AP), as an index of H^+ secretion. TPA (10^{-10} to 10^{-6} M) had no effect on resting AP uptake ($AP_r = 25.3 \pm 3.6$) but inhibited secretagogue stimulated AP_r between 20-100%. TPA caused a noncompetitive shift in the dose-response to histamine. At the maximally stimulatory dose of histamine (10^{-4} M), 10^{-7} M TPA reduced AP_r from 81.9 ± 5.1 to 56.8 ± 8.8 and also caused a 63% inhibition of the response to a maximally stimulatory dose of dibutyryl cAMP (10^{-3} M). These data suggest that: (1) TPA causes a rapid inhibition of H^+ secretion by oxyntic cells; (2) this effect occurs distal to the generation of cAMP; (3) there may be an antagonistic role for C-kinase; and (4) muscarinic agonists and gastrin do not share a common mechanism of action with phorbol esters during normal oxyntic cell activation. Supported by NIH AM19520.

1470 ROLE OF EXTRACELLULAR SODIUM IN PANCREATIC INSULIN RELEASE. P. Ronner* and A. Scarpa, Department of Biochemistry and Biophysics, University of Pennsylvania, School of Medicine, Philadelphia, PA 19104, USA.

The splenic Brockmann body of channel catfish (Ictalurus punctatus) was perfused in vitro. When sodium in the perfusion medium was replaced isotonically with either choline chloride or tris(hydroxymethyl)-aminomethane chloride, glucose-induced (15mM) insulin and somatostatin release were abolished. Tetrodotoxin (2-10μM), a highly specific inhibitor of voltage-dependent sodium channels, had no effect on glucose-induced hormone release in the presence of normal extracellular sodium, although this same concentration of tetrodotoxin was effective in completely blocking veratridine-induced (150μM) hormone release. In addition, neither arginine-induced (2mM glucose present) nor potassium-induced insulin and glucagon release were inhibited in the absence of extracellular sodium. Thus, these results demonstrate that the terminal events of insulin release do not appear to involve a voltage-dependent sodium channel or an influx of sodium across the plasma membrane; rather, a step in the sequence leading to B-cell glucose recognition may be affected in the absence of extracellular sodium. Thus, the inhibition of glucose-induced insulin release may provide a valuable tool in determining the stimulus recognition site for insulin secretion. Since hormone release from the catfish Brockmann body closely resembles hormone release from perfused mammalian pancreata, similar mechanisms can be expected to operate in mammalian B-cells as well. (Supported by NIH grant AM-27546 and by a grant from the R.J. Reynolds Fund.)

1471 FORSKOLIN INHIBITS THE EXPRESSION OF SUCRASE-ISOMALTASE IN THE ENTEROCYTE-LIKE HUMAN COLON CARCINOMA CELL LINE Caco-2 IN CULTURE.

M. Rousset*, M. Laburthe, M. Pinto, N. Triadou, N. Boige, C. Rouyer-Fessard, E. Dussaulx, G. Chevalier, J.L. Brun and A. Zweibaum, INSERM-CNRS, PARIS, FRANCE.

The human colon carcinoma cell line Caco-2 exhibits in culture a typical enterocytic differentiation characterized by : brush border on the apical surface and high activities of Sucrase-Isomaltase (SI) (Pinto et al., Biol. Cell., 1983, 47, 323-330). The activity of SI, tested in both the cell homogenate (H) and the brush border fraction (BB), is growth related with low activities in the exponential phase (0.4 mU/mg of prot. in H and 5 in BB), and, when confluency is reached (day 7) a regular increase up to 40 mU/mg of prot. in H and 300 in BB at day 20. The addition of Forskolin (FK) to the culture medium results in an important and permanent increase of cyclic AMP accumulation (30 fold at FK 10^{-5}M). Chronic exposure of cultured cells to FK 10^{-5}M always results in an inhibition of the expression of SI : 1) addition of FK from the beginning of the culture results in an almost complete absence of increase of SI activity in both H and BB after confluency (3 mU/mg of prot. in H and 20 in BB at day 20). 2) Addition of FK from day 13, i.e. when SI is increasing in untreated cells, results in an arrest of this increase in both H and BB. The inhibition of expression of SI was confirmed by both immunofluorescence with anti SI antibodies and immunoblotting. Several other effects of FK are observed : morphological modifications of cell junctions and important modifications of glucose metabolism (2 fold increase of glucose consumption and lactic acid production, 3 fold decrease of glycogen accumulation). These results suggest that Caco-2 cells are an ideal model to study the role of cyclic AMP on the regulation of the expression of Sucrase-Isomaltase.

1472 HEREDITARY PREWEANLING ANOREXIA IN MICE.

L. J. Maltais*, P. W. Lane and W. G. Beamer, The Jacskon Laboratory, Bar Harbor, ME 04609, USA

A recessive lethal mutation, anorexia (anx), that causes starvation in preweanling mice has been located on Chromosome 2. The mutant mice are recognized by a lack of thrifty appearance throughout the preweanling period. Abnormal behavior including headweaving, body tremors, uncoordinated gait and hyperactivity observed in mutants beginning at 18 days could be approximated by manipulation of serotonin activity in normal littermates. Death occurs at 22 days. Although anorexic mice ingest significantly less milk, the temporal pattern of stomach content mass was identical with their control littermates. Anorexic mice are also characterized by spleens that are small in size and pale in color, livers that are histologically lacey in appearance and devoid of fat and glycogen, and brains that are enlarged and have a reduction in size of the ventricular system. Hematocrits, hemaglobin, total RBC and mean cell volume are normal. Deficient dietary and serum zinc associated with anorexia and immunodeficiency could not be demonstrated. Hypothermia is evidenced at 20 days though there is a tendency for lower body temperatures during the preweanling period. The data indicate that these mutant mice fail to ingest the quantity of food to sustain life and are therefore characterized as anorexic. Although the site of the anx gene action is still not known, the reduction in the size of the brain ventricular system may be contributing to the alteration of the sucking response in anx/anx mice. This animal provides opportunities to study the neurobiology of suckling in the neonate. This study was supported by NIH.

1473 THE EFFECT OF pH ON THE DISTRIBUTION OF IMMUNOREACTIVITY OF OVINE LUTROPIN (oLH) SUBMITTED TO HIGH PRESSURE LIQUID CHROMATOGRAPHY (HPLC).

A Madej* and P. Hallin, Dept. of Clin. Chem., Swedish University of Agricultural Sciences, S-750 07 Uppsala, Sweden, Dept. of Zoophysiology, Uppsala University, S-751 22 Uppsala, Sweden.

Recently it was demonstrated a marked difference in the immunoreactivity between fractions obtained by reverse-phase HPLC fractionation of LH standards at pH 3.3 [1,2]. In the present study oLH (NIH-LH-S18) was submitted (each time approx. 1 mg) to the same chromatographic system, except that the pH of the buffers were adjusted to 4.3 and 5.3. As a control served the fractionation at pH 3.3. All eluted fractions were tested by means of radioimmunoassay for LH. It was found that regardless of pH, the material corresponding to the first peak occurred at 31.5-32.1 min. after injection and contained no LH immunoreactivity. The absorbance at 280 nm for this peak tends to decrease as pH increases. The fractions which form the second peak (retention time 34.7 min.) comprised LH immunoreactivity almost equal to native LH. This peak was never recorded at pH 3.3, although slight LH immunoreactivity in fractions collected at similar retention time was found. Retention time for the third peak observed at all applied pHs was 38.6-39.3 min. In conclusion, the increase of pH from 3.3 to 5.3 changed the distribution of LH immunoreactivity and chromatographic pattern after reverse-phase HPLC fractionation of oLH.

1. P. Hallin and A. Madej (1983). Acta Endocrinol. (Copenhagen) Suppl. 256,232
2. P. Hallin, A. Madej and L.-E. Edqvist. Submitted for publication.

1474 PROGESTERONE-MEDIATED INHIBITION OF CHORIONIC GONADOTROPIN ß-mRNA IN TROPHOBLASTIC TISSUES CULTURED IN VITRO.

T. Maruo*, H. Matsuo, T. Otani, M. Hoshina and M. Mochizuki, Department of Obstetrics & Gynecology, Kobe University School of Medicine, Kobe 650, Japan

In order to elucidate the inhibitory regulation of hCG synthesis, the dynamics of synthesis and secretion of hCG were investigated by culturing explants of trophoblastic tissues from early placneta and choriocarcinoma in the presence and absence of pregesterone, and then were compared to that of hPL. The dynamics of mRNAs encoding hCG (α, ß) and hPL were assessed by grain counts in the tissue sections hybridized in situ with labeled cDNA probes corresponding to these mRNAs. In control culture of early placenta, hCG, hCG α and hPL in the medium showed marked increases compared to the initial tissue levels, whereas hCG, hCG α and immunoreactive hCGß in the tissue explants remained constant. Progesterone suppressed the secretion of hCG and hCGα by placental tissue after 48 hours culture in a dose-response manner and simultaneously decreased the tissue level of immunoreactive hCGß. However, neither hPL secretion nor hPL tissue level were decreased by progesterone. The in situ hybridization revealed that grain counts for hCGß-mRNA in the sections prepared from placenta cultured with progesterone were markedly decreased compared to those prepared without progesterone, whereas grain counts for hPL-mRNA remained unchanged. In culture of explants from choriocarcinoma, no inhibition of synthesis and secretion of hCG by progesterone was found. From these results it will be concluded that progesterone inhibits hCG synthesis through the inhibition of hCGß-mRNA accumulation and that regulation of hCG synthesis in choriocarcinoma is different from that in normal placenta.

1475 GONADOTROPINS AND TESTOSTERONE IN PATIENTS AFTER MONOLATERAL SPERMATIC CORD TORSION. I.Mastrogiacomo*, R. Zanchetta, L. De Besi, W. Gomiero and P.Graziotti, Institute of Semeiotica Medica, Medical School, University of Padua, Padua, Italy.

Seminal alterations are often found in patients that had suffered spermatic cord torsion. The pathogenesis of such testicular damage is still unknown. We considered the gonadotropins, testosterone and their correlation with the seminal alterations in 65 patients (mean of age 17±3.5 years, M±SD) that had spermatic cord torsion. Thirty-eight patients had the spermatic cord torsion before puberty. Seven patients were orchidectomized at the time of the acute episode because the severity of the necrosis; in 28 patients the testis became atrophic while the other 30 patients still showed a normal testis. As controls we studied the gonadotropins and testosterone in 12 healthy men. The patients with normal testis showed a normal seminal analysis while the patients with an atrophic testis showed a significant ($p < 0.01$) decrease of number of spermatozoa/ml (29.500.000 ± 27.5 x 10^6). The values of testosterone were normal while a significant increase of FSH (10.7 ± 4.3 mIU/ml; $p < 0.005$), a significant alteration of the LH/FSH ratio (1.1 ± 0.6; $p < 0.01$), and an inverse correlation of the LH/testosterone ratio in patients with testicular atrophy and in orchidectomized patients were found. On the contrary, no correlation exists between high values of FSH and seminal alterations. Therefore, the increase of FSH and the slight hypogonadism may be due to a compensating phenomenon. Indeed in orchidectomized patients we found an increase of FSH with normal seminal analysis.

1476 PHYSIOLOGICAL EPISODIC LH SECRETION IN MEN WITH NORMAL AND ABNORMAL SEMEN ANALYSIS. C.D. Matthews*, J.C.Peek, J.M. Crocker and C. Kirby. Dept. of Obstetrics & Gynaecology, University of Adelaide, The Queen Elizabeth Hospital, Woodville, South Australia.

An attempt has been made to recognise temporal or other defects in episodic gonadotrophin secretion in men with varying states of reproductive incompetence. A series of 35 men have been investigated by multiple venous blood sampling (10 minutely for 5-7 hours) in order to investigate the problems associated with the recognition of endogenous pulses of LH, to further elucidate the physiology of the endogenous pulse generator and to clarify which subjects might benefit from pulsed GnRH. Peaks were defined by using 3 coefficients of variation of the assays. The subjects demonstrated a range in the number of peaks identified (0-3) over the sampling period. The number of peaks was correlated with mean (LH) ($r = 0.44$ $p < 0.05$). Peak height (maximum (LH) minus base line (LH) was also correlated with mean (LH) ($r = 0.77$, $p << 0.001$). These relationships suggest that the pulsatile component of LH secretion largely determines the overall (LH). For 11 men with 2 or more pulses recognisable, the time between peaks of LH was 117±34 (x±sd) min. Although mean testosterone (T) was correlated with mean (LH) ($r = 0.52$, $p < 0.05$) when (LH) <10 IU/L, there was no obvious temporal relationship between patterns of LH and T secretion (FSH) showed less fluctuation than (LH). Men with both normal and abnormal semen analyses showed a range in frequency and amplitude of LH peaks. At the present time the identification of those men who might benefit from therapy rests on the further understanding of the dynamic relationship between gonadotrophins and the testes.

1477 CROSSLINKING OF RAT FOLLICLE STIMULATING HORMONE TO ITS RECEPTOR IN RAT OVARY AND TESTES. O. Moctezuma*, A. Ulloa-Aguirre and F. Larrea, Department of Reproductive Biology, National Institute of Nutrition, México City.

Follicle stimulating hormone (FSH) is believed to mediate a variety of events ocurring in both testis and ovaries through its binding to specific membrane receptors. In the present study we describe the crosslinking (CL) of (^{125}I)-FSH to testicular and ovarian membrane preparations to be used as a specific probe for studing FSH-receptor structure.The bifunctional CL reagents disuccinimidyl suberate (DSS) and dithiobis (succinimidyl propionate) (DTSP) were used as CL agents. Rat FSH as iodinated by the lactoperoxidase method was specifically bound to ovarian and testicular membranes with a Kd of 1.3×10^{-9}M and 1.22×10^{-9}M respectively. CL of (^{125}I)-FSH to its receptors was performed by adding either DSS or DTSP after the equilibrium of FSH and receptor was obtained. Following incubation in the presence of CL-agents the non-dissociated FSH was evaluated by the addition of 2 vol of 4M $MgCl_2$. In all instances DTSP was more efficient than DSS to specifically CL rat FSH to its receptor in both tissues. The efficiency (% of initially bound (^{125}I)-FSH) of DTSP to covalently bind FSH to testes and ovary was; 64% and 62 % respectively whereas DSS resulted in only 35% and 45% efficiency for testes and ovary respectively. Our results are consistent with the presence of covalently bound FSH to specific receptors in membrane preparations from rat testis and ovaries.

1478 PRESERVATION OF HUMAN CHORIONIC GONADOTROPIN (HCG) AND PLACENTAL LACTOGEN (hPL) SECRETION FOLLOWING LONG-TERM CULTURE OF NORMAL HUMAN PLACENTAL CELLS. D.W.Morrish*, O.Siy, Department of Medicine, University of Alberta, Edmonton, Alberta, T6G 2G3, Canada.

To study long-term regulation of placental hCG and hPL secretion, we have developed a monolayer culture system that preserves the morphology and functional integrity of normal placental cells. Minced term placenta was incubated at 37°C in 0.25% trypsin-500 U DNAse I in Ringer-bicarbonate buffer for four 10 min periods. Dispersed cells were cultured in 60 mm Petri dishes in 3 ml Dulbecco's modified Eagle medium containing 10% fetal calf serum, 20 mM HEPES, 100 U/ml penicillin, 100 ug/ml streptomycin Light microscopic morphology of cells was similar at day 0 and day 50 of culture. No fibroblast overgrowth occurred. Representative values of hCG and hPL secretion (ng/ml; mean$\pm$SD) were:

DAY	2	4	6	9	13	50
hCG	6.8±0.9	8.9±1.6	2.4±0.5	2.2±0.3	2.7±0.5	0.065±0.026
hPL	2468±391	114±27	47 ±6	118 ±18	50 ±14	2.5 ±0.7

Medium collected at 49-96 h of dibutyryl cAMP (1 mM)-theophylline (1 mM) stimulation on day 13 of culture showed: control = 0.17±0.06 ng/ml, stimulated = 0.73±0.06 ng/ml ($p<0.005$). The same treatment on day 50 showed a similar magnitude of stimulation: control = 0.039±0.01 ng/ml, stimulated = 0.39±0.01 ng/ml ($p<0.05$). These data demonstrate that normal functioning human placental cells can be maintained in long-term culture and may provide a model for study of the regulation of hCG and hPL secretion.

1479 EFFECT OF PROGESTERONE METABOLITES ON GONADOTROPIN SECRETION IN PMSG-PRIMED LIGHT-BLOCKED RATS. L.L. Murphy and V.B. Mahesh*, Department of Endocrinology, Medical College of Georgia, Augusta, Georgia 30912.

In previous work from our laboratory it was demonstrated that the injection of 5α-dihydroprogesterone (5α-DHP) to estrogen-primed immature ovariectomized rats or to adult cycling rats ovariectomized on the morning of proestrous resulted in the selective release of follicle stimulating hormone (FSH). On the other hand, injection of 3α-hydroxy-5α-pregnane-20-one (3α,5α-tetrahydroprogesterone; 3α,5α-THP) to estrogen-primed ovariectomized immature rats resulted in selective release of luteinizing hormone (LH). Because the selective effect of progesterone metabolites on gonadotropin release appeared novel, these effects were investigated in another animal model. The model was the immature rat maintained in constant light (LL) since 22 d of age and injected with 8 IU of pregnant mare serum gonadotropin at 28 d of age. Control rats exposed to 14 h L/10 h D (LD) exhibited surges of LH and FSH at 6 p.m. on the second day after PMSG. In LL rats, the PMSG-induced surges of LH and FSH were delayed until 10 a.m. on Day 3 after PMSG and gonadotropin surge levels were greatly attenuated compared to LD controls. An injection of 5α-DHP (0.4 mg/kg) at 9:30 a.m. on Day 2 after PMSG, significantly stimulated FSH release at 10 a.m. on Day 3 in LL rats but had no effect on LH. Treatment with 3α,5α-THP (0.4 mg/kg) enhanced the secretion of LH at 10 a.m. on Day 3 but did not alter FSH. These results extend earlier findings in the immature ovariectomized estrogen-primed rat and suggest that the 5α-reduced metabolites of progesterone may have a significant role in the regulation of FSH and LH secretion. Supported by grant # HD 16688.

1480 UNIQUE CARBOHYDRATE STRUCTURE OF HUMAN CHORIONIC GONADOTROPIN PRODUCED BY CHORIOCARCINOMA. *R.Nishimura*[1]*, *T.Mizuochi*[2], *T.Hamamoto*[1], *T.Utsunomiya*[1], *T.Taniguchi*[2], *A.Kobata*[2] and *M.Mochizuki*[1], [1]*Department of Obstetrics and Gynecology, Kobe University School of Medicine, 5-1 Kusunoki-cho 7 chome, Chuo-ku, Kobe 650, Japan and* [2]*Department of Biochemistry, the Institute of Medical Science, the University of Tokyo, Tokyo, Japan.*

The structure of the asparagine-linked sugar chains of human chorionic gonadotropin (hCG) were investigated comparatively between normal pregnancy, hydatidiform mole and choriocarcinoma. The identical methods were employed for the extraction and purification of hCG from urine of all cases. The sugar chains were quantitatively liberated as radioactive oligosaccharides from polypeptide portion by hydrazinolysis followed by N-acetylation and NaB^3H_4 reduction. The structures of these sugar chians were determined by the combination of sequential glycosidase digestion, periodate oxidation and methylation analysis. Although hCGs from various sources contained four asparagine-linked sugar chains in one molecule, only the structure of hCG from choriocarcinoma was prominently different from the others. hCG from choriocarcinoma contained unusual biantennary complex-type sugar chains in addition to regular tri-, bi- and monoantennary sugar chains as indicated below. These sugar chains had two outer chains linked at C-2 and C-4 position of the same α-mannosyl core. The occurence of Galβ1→4GlcNAcβ1→4 group and the increase of fucosylated sugar chains were characteristic features of hCG from choriocarcinoma.

```
±(Galβ1→4GlcNAcβ1→2)Manα1↘                        ±(Fucα1↘
                          6                                6)
±(Galβ1→4GlcNAcβ1↘        3 Manβ1→4GlcNAcβ1→4GlcNAc
                  4)               ↗
 Galβ1→4GlcNAcβ1→2  Manα1
```

1481 SHORT PHOTOPERIOD EFFECTS ON KIDNEY GROWTH IN SYRIAN GOLDEN HAMSTERS Joy L. Logan*, Bryant Benson, and Stanley M. Lee, Departments of Internal Medicine and Anatomy, University of Arizona, Tucson, Arizona, U.S.A.

Although photoperiod is known to regulate body growth and reproductive function in a variety of animals, little is known about the effects of varying photoperiods on kidney growth. Male Syrian golden hamsters weighing 90-100 g were acclimatized in long photoperiod (LP; L/D=14/10 hrs) for two weeks when half were transferred to short photoperiod (SP; L/D=10/14 hrs). After 2, 5 and 8 weeks in SP, groups of 6 underwent left nephrectomy (Nx) or sham operation (S-Nx). LP hamsters were similarly treated. All animals were sacrificed two weeks after surgery. At 10 weeks the SP S-Nx animals showed a significant increase in body weight (BW). Kidney weight (KW), expressed per 100 g BW, was significantly depressed in S-Nx animals at seven weeks (LP = 0.71 ± 0.02 vs SP = 0.65 ± 0.01; $P < 0.01$) and ten weeks (LP = 0.69 ± 0.01 vs SP = 0.60 ± 0.02; $P < 0.001$). After Nx, KW/100g BW was significantly depressed in animals kept in SP for ten weeks (LP = 0.49 ± 0.01 vs SP = 0.43 ± 0.01; $P < 0.001$) but absolute increase in KW was not different. SP caused a significant increase in percent body fat in 7 week S-Nx animals ($P < 0.05$). When corrected for lean BW (carcass wt - wt of fat) the observed significant difference between KW in these animals was negated. Kidney growth in hamsters may be a function of lean BW. Age related kidney growth is retarded by short photoperiod, but compensatory renal hypertrophy remains unaffected.

1482 USE OF AFFINITY CHROMATOGRAPHY TO PURIFY ENDOGENOUS OVARIAN GROWTH FACTOR. A. Makris*, Z. Petro, M. Klagsbrun, and K.J. Ryan, Laboratory of Human Reproduction and Reproductive Biology, Harvard Medical School and Dept. of Surgery, Children's Hospital Medical Center, Boston, MA, 02115 USA.

Endogenous ovarian growth factor (EOGF) stimulates the growth of cultured granulosa and BALB 3T3 cells[1]. Previous purification schemes for EOGF from ovarian tissue have yielded a partially purified preparation (300X) from cytosol extract and a less than 0.1% yield[2]. More recent results using affinity chromatography of the active fraction, obtained after Bio-Rex 70 cation exchange chromatography of whole ovary cytosol, results in a 12,400X increase in purity of EOGF and an increased yield of 3% of the original activity. The protein fraction is applied to a heparin-sepharose column and elutes from the column at 1.5M NaCl. Half maximal activity, measured by ^{3}H-DNA synthesis in cultured quiescent cells, is seen at a protein concentration of 10 ng/ml. SDS-PAGE analysis indicates a protein band with a molecular weight of about 18,000, which is compatible with earlier HPLC data. Present evidence indicates that a further 10 fold increase in specific activity is needed for EOGF to be purified to homogeneity. Affinity chromatography is indicated to be a significant step of the purification of EOGF. Supported by NIH Grant 1 RO1 HD 14709-01A1

1. Makris et al., Biology of Reproduction 29:1135 (1983).
2. Makris et al., Abstr. 65th Annual Endocrine Soc., San Antonio, TX 1983.

1483 PRODUCTION OF SOMATOMEDIN (SM) BINDING PROTEIN BY ADULT RAT HEPATOCYTES IN PRIMARY CULTURE. Janet L. Martin*, Carolyn D. Scott and Robert C. Baxter, Department of Medicine, University of Sydney and Department of Endocrinology, Royal Prince Alfred Hospital, Sydney, NSW Australia

In conjunction with a study of SM-C production by primary cultures of adult rat hepatocytes, the release of SM binding protein (SMBP) by these cells has been measured. SMBP was separated from endogenous SM by high-pressure gel permeation chromatography at pH 2.7, with quantitative recovery. Binding activity was measured by incubating samples with ^{125}I-SM-C (125pg) for 2h at 20°C, and separating bound from free tracer using charcoal. Proportionality with added protein was seen up to at least 25% binding. The predominant binding species had a mol. wt. of 40,000 and a pI of 6.9, and bound to concanavalin-A. The affinity of SMBP for SM-C, determined by Scatchard analysis, was 4×10^{10}L/mol (n=6). Expressed as pmol SM-C binding sites/mg cell protein/24h, cells from normal rats released SMBP at a rate of 1.72±0.24 (SD,n=6), increased by 200ng/ml bovine GH to 2.27±0.34 (p=0.01). Cycloheximide (15μg/ml) decreased SMBP production to 0.13±0.06, while dexamethasone (3μM) increased the rate to 2.65±0.33 (p<0.005). A reduction in SMBP of over 90% was seen in cells from hypophysectomized rats. From a comparison with SM-C data we conclude that production of rat liver SMBP, a neutral glycoprotein, is under similar hormonal control to SM-C. Supported by NH&MRC Australia.

1484 THE SIGNIFICANCE OF THE MEASUREMENT OF PLASMA TRANSFERRIN AS A GROWTH FACTOR. M.Matsubara*, K.Nakagawa, K.Akikawa and M.Kubo, Second Department of Medicine, Hokkaido University School of Medicine, Sapporo, 060 Japan.

We previously reported the significance of total iron binding capacity (TIBC) values in various endocrine diseases. In the present study we investigated the significance of the measurement of plasma transferrin(pTf, by the immunodiffusion technique) as a growth factor in patients with these diseases before and after treatment. The pTf levels in healthy subjects were 256±9(mean±SE)mg/dl for men and 271±11 for women. In patients with active acromegaly, they elevated to 350±8(n=10), while lowered to 179±22(n=6) in patients with hypopituitarism. They were normalized after treatment. The pTf levels in 8 patients with anorexia nervosa were low(231±13), and the negative correlation was observed between the extent of deficit from the ideal body weight and pTf (r=-0.77). In 22 patients with hyperthyroidism, the pTf tended to decrease and correlated negatively with the serum T_3 levels(r=-0.61) within this group. The pTf in 11 patients with Cushing's syndrome was also slightly lower(236±11), but that in hyperprolactinemia was normal. The value was elevated in the pregnancy, especially in the late stage. A significant correlation was observed between the somatomedin-C(SM-C, by the RIA kit of Nichols Ins.) and pTf levels in these subjects(r=+0.73). The measurement of pTf which changed with the endocrinological condition and correlated with the SM-C was useful for the evaluation of growth factors in endocrine diseases. However, these values should be assessed carefully in cases with specific Tf abnormalities.

1485 PURIFICATION OF A HUMORAL FACTOR WITH GROWTH-PROMOTING ACTIVITY TOWARDS PROSTATIC EPITHELIAL CELLS. G. Mc Kercher*, S. Chevalier, G. Bleau, K.D. Roberts and A. Chapdelaine. Maisonneuve-Rosemont Res. Center and U. of Montreal, Quebec, Canada. H1T 2M4.

The presence of a humoral non-steroidal factor in dog serum results in the proliferation of cultured canine prostatic epithelial cells. Its properties upon ultrafiltration and gel filtration, as well as the decrease in activity observed following treatment with amino- and carboxy-peptidases allowed us to conclude that the humoral growth-promoting factor is a low molecular weight peptide. Further purification includes the following steps: a 90% ethanol precipitation of serum with the growth factor remaining in the supernatant; chromatography on a C-18 column for the separation of hydrophobic compounds from the growth factor, the latter remaining in the aqueous phase; a Bio Gel P-2 column resulting in the recovery of the growth factor at a molecular weight of approximately 1200; following anion exchange chromatography at pH 10, growth factor activity is retained on the column and eluted between pH 6 and 5. As a further step, a cation exchanger at pH 3.5 retains the growth factor and elution is obtained between pH 6 and 8. HPLC in different hydrophobic systems with C-18 resins results in no retention of the growth factor. A final purification of at least 4000-fold with a recovery of approximately 10% was achieved. Parallel studies with human urine, seminal plasma and prostatic tissue resulted in the detection of a growth factor with similar chromatographic and growth-promoting properties in each of these samples. The role of these growth-promoting factors in HBP and prostatic cancer awaits further purification and sequence determination. (Supported by MRC, FRSQ and FCAC).

1486 EPIDERMAL GROWTH FACTOR (EGF) RECEPTORS IN THE RAT UTERUS. V.R. Mukku* and G.M. Stancel, Department of Pharmacology, The University of Texas Medical School at Houston, Houston, Texas 77025.

Estrogen treatment stimulates growth of the immature rodent uterus in vivo, but such hormone stimulated growth is diminished under certain circumstances without a decrease in estrogen receptor levels, e.g., in hypothyroidism (Endocrinology 103: 1164, 1978). One possible explanation of such observations is that other factors function in concert with estrogens to stimulate the growth of estrogen responsive tissues. To explore this possibility we have begun a study to identify receptors for other hormones and growth factors in normal uterine tissue, and report here the presence of EGF receptors in the immature rat uterus. Uterine membranes contain high affinity (K_d approximately 1 nM), saturable binding sites for ^{125}I-EGF. The binding of labelled EGF is specific since it is abolished by excess unlabelled EGF but not by excess unlabelled insulin, fibroblast growth factor or multiplication stimulating activity. Incubation of ^{125}I-EGF with uterine membranes, followed by chemical crosslinking with discuccinimidyl suberate and detergent extraction reveals a single species of specifically bound EGF (MW = 170,000) visualized by autoradiography of SDS gels after electrophoresis of the extracts. In detergent solubilized preparations EGF also stimulates the phosphorylation of a single major species with an identical MW (170,000) as seen by autoradiography of SDS gels. These results indicate that the rat uterus contains high affinity EGF binding sites with the properties expected of EGF receptors, including an EGF stimulated kinase activity. (This work was supported in part by NIH grant HD-08615.)

1487 PURIFICATION AND CHARACTERIZATION OF OVINE PITUITARY-DERIVED RENOTROPIN.
K. Nomura*, H. Demura and K. Shizume, Dept. of Medicine, Tokyo Women's Medical College, Tokyo, 162, Japan.

Ovine pituitary-derived renotropin, shown to be distinct from other pituitary hormones (K. Nomura et al., Proc. Natl. Acad. Sci. USA, 79:6675, 1982), was further purified by a series of chromatographic steps including CM-cellulose, Concanavalin A, G-100 and HPLC with reverse phase column (TMS-250, Toyosoda). Bioassay was done as follows: Kidney slices from castrated hypophysectomized rats injected with a sample 8 h before sacrifice were incubated in a Krebs Ringer Bicarbonate buffer containing [3H] thymidine, then [3H] thymidine incorporation into renal DNA was measured as a indicator of renotropic activity. The most highly purified fraction, obtained at a yield of 3.9 g from 1 kg of lyophilized ovine pituitary powder, was found to be homogeneous judged by symmetrical elution profiles at G-100 and HPLC (a linear gradient of acetonitrile), and also by the presence of only two staining bands at SDS-PAGE. Its molecular weight was estimated at 38000 by G-100 and 35000 by SDS-PAGE analysis, which showed renotropin was composed of two subunits (19000 and 16000 each). It appeared to be a glycoprotein because it was absorbed by Concanavalin A and absorbed renotropin was eluted by methylmannoside. A single injection (400 μg) of renotropin enhanced [3H] thymidine incorporation 2-2.5 times. Our data demonstrates that ovine pituitary-derived renotropin could be highly purified and demonstrated its physicochemical properties.

1488 PLANT GROWTH HORMONES ACTIVATE MAMMALIAN GUANYLATE CYCLASE ACTIVITY.
D.L. Pack, J.L. Hudson, J.L. Pipkin, Jr., and D.L. Vesely*, National Center for Toxicological Research, Jefferson, Arkansas, and Division of Endocrinology & Metabolism, University of Arkansas for Medical Science, Little Rock, Arkansas, U.S.A.

Plant growth hormones are known to increase RNA and protein synthesis in plants. *In vivo* injections of plant growth hormones increase the growth of animals as well as plants. Since cyclic GMP also increases RNA and protein synthesis, the present investigation was designed to study the effect of various representatives of all classes of plant growth stimulating hormones on the rat guanylate cyclase-cyclic GMP system. Thus, auxins (indole-3-acetic acid; indole-3-butyric acid; B-naphthoxyacetic acid; 2,4,5,-trichlorophenoxy acetic acid and p-chlorophenoxy acetic acid); gibberellins (gibberellic acid) and cytokinins (N_6 benzyl adenine) all increased rat lung, colon, liver and renal cortex guanylate cyclase activity 2- to 4-fold at the 1 nM concentration. Dose response curves revealed that maximal stimulation of guanylate cyclase by these plant growth hormones was at 1 nM; there was no augmented guanylate cyclase activity at 0.01 nM. The activation of guanylate cyclase by the auxins and cytokinins required the presence of manganese ion, while activation by gibberellic acid did not.

Conclusions: 1) Auxins, gibberellins, and cytokinins all activate the guanylate cyclase-cyclic GMP system. 2) Manganese was important as a cofactor for auxins and cytokinins, but not for gibberellic acid, enhancement of guanylate cyclase. These data suggest that guanylate cyclase may play a role in the mechanism of action of plant growth hormones at the cellular level.

1489 INFLUENCE OF RANITIDINE AND PIMOZIDE ON THE SLEEP INDUCED GROWTH HORMONE (GH) SECRETION. G. Mayer*, J. Köbberling, W. Hund, Dept. of Medicine, University of Göttingen, D 3400 Göttingen, Germany (FRG)

The mechanisms regulating sleep induced GH secretion are still not fully elucidated. Besides many others histamine and dopamine receptors are assumed to be involved. We investigated the influence of ranitidine, an H_2 receptor blocker, and of pimozide, a dopamine receptor blocker, on sleep induced GH secretion in 10 healthy male volunteers well adapted to our sleep laboratory. EEG and EOG registration was continously performed. Cubital vein blood was withdrawn from an adjacent room in 15 min. intervals for GH determination (RIA). The integrated hormone secretion between onset of deep sleep and the end of peak secretion was calculated. Besides a basal test each proband was retested after treatment with ranitidine (2x150mg/day p.o. for 8 weeks) or pimozide (16mg or 4mg p.o. in 5 probands each). All probands showed a marked sleep induced GH secretion. Ranitidine caused a significant reduction to 44.6% compared to control tests ($p<0.05$). Pimozide in the high dose caused a clear GH reduction to 18.7% but with the smaller dose the difference was not significant. There war no change in the mode of sleep cycle during treatment with ranitidine or pimozide. Our data suggest that mechanisms acting via H_2 receptors and probably also via dopamine receptors are involved in the control of sleep induced GH secretion.

1490 GROWTH HORMONE EXCRETION IN NORMAL AND DIABETIC HUMAN URINE. E.Mikuni*, K.Hayashi, S.Yamada, and K.Miyamura, Wakayama Rosai Hospital, Nat'l Osaka South Hospital, and Wakayama Medical School, Wakayama 640 and Kawachi-Nagano, JAPAN.

Urinary growth hormone (GH) was measured by radioimmunoassay(RIA) and radioreceptor assay(RRA) (VI International Congress Endocrinology, #250). Sample were obtained from 18 normal volunteers and 15 diabetics without albuminuria (DM). We also performed serial studies on five patients with diabetic ketoacidosis (DM coma) untill their recovery.

The 24 hrs urinary excretion of GH were 38.5 ± 18.0 ng in normal subjects, 45.4 ± 16.8 ng in DM, and 2000 - 3000ng in DM coma at the start of treatment (GH excretion in DM coma were more elevated than those in acromegalics). GH value estimated by RIA was well consistent with that by RRA. In diabetics with nephropathy, there was some discrepancy in urinary GH values between RIA and RRA, and the GH-like material did not always consist of monomeric form on gel filtration. In DM coma, urinary excretion of β_2-microglobulin was 500-fold. Clearance of GH was about 6-fold, that of β_2-microglobulin was about 150-fold, and creatinine clearance was 0.2-fold in DM coma at the start of treatment. GH and β_2-microglobulin fell progressively towards the normal range. At the time of discharge, all had normal levels of plasma creatinine and urea. Urinary GH in DM coma and pituitary GH showed assay parallelism by RIA and RRA. Gel filtration patterns of GH in ketotic urine consisted of mainly monomeric form (22K).

Urinary GH usually reflects integrated plasma GH in normal subjects and diabetics without nephropathy. In DM coma, the renal tubular dysfunction should be considered in addition to high plasma GH levels.

1491 THE MECHANISM BY WHICH α_2-ADRENERGIC BLOCKADE SUPPRESSES GH SECRETION IN CONSCIOUS MALE RABBITS; AN ENHANCED SOMATOSTATIN RELEASE WITH A CONCOMITANT INHIBITION OF GRF. N.Minamitani*,K.Chihara,H.Kaji,H.Kodama,T.Kita, and T.Fujita. Third Div. Dept. of Med. Kobe Univ. Sch. of Med. Kobe, 650, Japan

It remains to be clarified how central α-adrenergic mechanism regulates the hypothalamic Growth Hormone(GH) Releasing Factor(GRF) and somatostatin (SS), thereby affecting the GH secretion, though we have reported that central α-adrenergic mechanism plays an important role in the regulation of GH secretion in conscious male rabbits as well as other species. In this study we investigated the effects of α_1-,α_2-and D_2-blockers on spontaneous GH secretion and plasma GH response to iv administered human GRF(1-44)-NH_2(hGRF) in freely-moving male animals. In saline-injected control animals, episodic GH release was observed during a 6h period(1030-1630) and iv injections of 2µg hGRF caused a further increase in plasma GH. Yohimbine(Y),2.5mgx3/kg iv ,α_2-blocker, inhibited hGRF-induced GH rises as well as spontaneous GH episodes, whereas neither prazosin(P),2mgx3/kg,α_1-blocker, nor sulpiride(S), 5mgx3/kg iv,D_2-blocker, did. The highly oscillated GH release observed in rabbits treated with anti-SS-γ-globulin(ASG) was abolished by simultaneous injection with Y. However, treatment with ASG disinhibited a suppression by Y of hGRF-induced GH release. These results suggest the followings ; 1) Central α_2-adrenergic mechanisms play a more important role in the regulation of rabbit GH secretion than do α_1-adrenergic mechanisms. A2-blockade results in suppression of the release of hypothalamic GRF and an enhanced release of SS, thereby suppressing the GH secretion. 2) D_2-dopaminergic mechanisms appear to play a minor role in regulating GH secretion. This study was supported by the grants of the Ministry of Health and Welfare, the Ministry of Education and Foundation of Growth Science, Japan, 1982.

1492 CHARACTERISTICS OF THE SOMATOTROPIC GROWTH HORMONE BINDING. Moore, W.V.*, Kover, K. and Hung, C.H., Department of Pediatrics, University of Kansas Medical Center, Kansas City, Kansas 66103 USA

Growth hormones and prolactins form a closely related family of hormones with lactogenic and somatotropic activities. Human growth hormone binds to receptors on female rat liver plasma membranes with the following characteristics: (1 pH optimum of binding at pH 5.5-6, (2 stable binding by 120-180 min of incubation, (3 partial displacement of bound hGH by hGH, (4 dissociation of bound hGH in the presence of disulfide reducers, (5 enhancement of binding by monovalent and divalent cations, (6 relatively low nonspecific binding, (7 competition of binding with lactogenic hormones, especially oPrl. We have studied the characteristics of somatotropic growth hormone binding to homologous liver plasma membranes. This includes bGH, oGH, rGH and hGH. The characteristics of binding of these hormones to homologous membranes include the following: (1 no optimum pH of binding in the absence of divalent cations with an optimum pH of binding at pH 5-6 in the presence of divalent cations, (2 stable binding by 60-120 min incubation, (3 partial displacement of bound GH by unlabeled GH, (4 no dissociation of bound GH in the presence of disulfide reducers, (5 a requirement of divalent cation for binding with no enhancement of binding by monovalent cations, (6 relatively high nonspecific binding, (7 no competition for binding with lactogenic hormones. The somatotropic growth hormone-receptor interaction exhibits unique and distinguishing characteristics of binding. This comparison suggests that differences between lactogenic and somatotropic hormone-receptor interactions resides in the receptor and not the hormone.

1493 GH DEFICIENT CHILDREN WITH INSULIN DEPENDENT DIABETES MELLITUS. LONG TERM TREATMENT WITH HGH AND INSULIN. O. Mori*, T. Yazawa and M. Ogawa, Department of Pediatrics, School of Medicine, Nagoya University, Nagoya, Japan.

The pathological conditions of both growth hormone and insulin deficiency in children are not only extremely rare, but also of significant interest in studying the interaction between GH and glucose metabolism. Two brothers visited our clinic with the chief complaint of short stature. Both of them were diagnosed isolated GH deficiency and insulin deficient diabetes mellitus. The typical Houssay's phenomenon was observed. Insulin treatment could not be initiated to correct their hyperglycemia, because of recurrent hypoglycemia and insulin hypersensitivity. Diabetic ketoacidosis was not encountered even without insulin therapy. HGH therapy was adopted when the boys were 9 and 7 years old, respectively. HGH administration caused exaggerated hyperglycemia and ketosis instead of disappearance of Houssay's phenomenon. Therefore, insulin therapy was required to control the diabetic status. It was necessary to change the insulin dosage day by day, because the diabetogenic effect of HGH was observed for about 24 hours. The average insulin dosage for one week have to be increased to attain the usual requirement in IDDM after 4 years of HGH administration. Height velocities in both cases were remarkably increased during 5 years HGH therapy. Control of diabetes was fairly good without any serious side effects. In conclusion, long-term HGH and insulin therapy for 5 years in two brothers with GH deficiency and insulin dependent diabetes mellitus were effective, and both showed clinical improvement.

1494 GROWTH HORMONE /GH/ AND PROLACTIN /PRL/ SYNTHESIS AND RELEASE IN RATS WITH HYPOTHALAMIC CUT OR LESION. I. Nagy†, I. Kakucska, Gy. Horváth, M. Kurcz and G.B. Makara, Heim Pál Pediatric Hospital, Institute of Experimental Medicine of Hungarian Academy of Sciences, CHINOIN Pharmaceutical Works Co., Budapest, Hungary.

Anterior pituitaries from rats bearing an anterolateral cut /ALC/ around the medial basal hypothalamus /MBH/ or MBH lesion were incubated with ^{3}H-leucine, the newly synthetized GH and PRL separated with polyacrylamide gel electrophoresis, quantitated and compared to radioimmunoassayable hormone data. GH synthesis and release failed to change one day after ALC but was decreased one week and one month after operation. A lesion of the MBH was followed by a marked decrease in GH content and release, and the share of the GH in protein synthesis was decreased. Combined thyroxin and dexamethasone treatment of ALC rats restored GH synthesis and release to that of the sham-operated controls. The marked decrease in *in vitro* GH release and synthesis following ALC may be - at least in part - secondary to decreased thyroid and adrenocortical hormone secretion. Synthesis and release of the newly synthetized PRL was markedly stimulated by MBH lesion but not by ALC one month after the surgery. The share of radioactive PRL in protein synthesis was increased.

1495 EFFECT OF DEXAMETHSONE ON GH RESPONSE TO GH-RELEASING FACTOR(GHRF) IN ACROMEGALY IN VIVO AND IN VITRO. K. Nakagawa*, K. Akikawa, M. Matsubara, M. Kubo and Y. Ito, Second Department of Medicine, Hokkaido University School of Medicine, Sapporo, 060 Japan.

Glucocorticoids have been considered to be a potent inhibitor to the secretion of GH to various stimuli in vivo. Recently, however, the potentiation of GH response to GHRF by glucocorticoids in vitro has been demonstrated. To examine this discrepancy, the effect of dexamethasone (D) on GH response to GHRF in vivo in patients with acromegaly as well as in vitro in the GH-secreting pituitary tumor cells obtained from these same patients. One hundred μg of human pancreatic GHRF(1-44 amide) was injected intravenously in 5 patients with active acromegaly before and after the oral administration of 9 mg/day of D for 2 days. Before D, plasma GH levels(RIA) ranged from 4.8 to 18.5 ng/ml in basal state and increased to 27.9 to 86.5 ng/ml;the peak/basal ratios were 6.54 ± 2.93 (mean ± SE). After D, the basal GH levels were -56 to +17 % of those before the treatment. The peak levels were lower in all cases(19.0 to 39.3 ng/ml) but the ratios of the peak levels to the basal were not changed(6.57 ± 3.17). Plasma somatomedin-C levels(RIA) decreased in all cases by 12 to 50 % and blood glucose levels increased by 18 to 31 % after D. On the other hand, 2-day treatment with 5×10^{-8} M of D added to the monolayer culture of dispersed pituitary adenoma cells from 2 of these patients augmented the release of GH by 10^{-10} to 10^{-9} M of GHRF. These results indicate that the potentiating action of 2-day treatment of D in vitro is overwhelmed in vivo by some extra-pituitary action of glucocorticoids also in patients with acromegaly.

1496 EFFECTS OF INTRACELLULAR GLUCOPENIA ON PULSATILE GROWTH HORMONE (GH) SECRETION: MEDIATION BY GH-RELEASING FACTOR (GRF) AND SOMATOSTATIN (SRIF). J.C.Painson*, N.Ling and G.S.Tannenbaum, McGill University-Montreal Children's Hospital Research Institute, Montreal, Quebec, H3H 1P3, Canada.

We examined the effects of 2-deoxy-D-glucose (2DG)-induced cellular glucoprivation on GH secretory dynamics in freely-moving rats bearing chronic intraventricular and intracardiac venous cannulae. Intravenous (iv) administration of 2DG (400 mg/kg) caused a striking suppression in amplitude and duration of spontaneous GH surges, and plasma GH levels remained significantly depressed for 6h (mean 6-h GH level:28.7±13.2 vs 146.6±12.2 ng/ml in normal saline controls; P<0.001) in the presence of pronounced hyperglycemia (308.7±13.2 vs 144.5±4.0 mg/dl; P<0.001). Intraventricular administration of 50-100 fold lower doses of 2DG also markedly attenuated GH pulse amplitude and raised plasma glucose levels, however, these low doses were without effect when injected systemically, suggesting a central site of action. To elucidate the mechanism(s) mediating the 2DG-induced GH suppression response, we assessed the involvement of the 2 hypothalamic GH regulatory peptides SRIF and GRF. Passive immunization with a specific SRIF antiserum failed to restore the amplitude of GH peaks, although basal GH levels were elevated and the mean 6-h plasma GH level (77.9±10.5 ng/ml) was significantly (P<0.001) greater than that of 2DG-normal sheep serum controls (18.8±3.0 ng/ml). In contrast, administration of 3 iv bolus injections of human pancreas GRF-44 (10 μg/0.3 ml) at 90 min intervals, resulted in a rapid release of GH to values as high as 1200 ng/ml (vs 76 ng /ml in 2DG controls). We conclude 1) that central glucopenia is a potent inhibitor of pulsatile GH release, and 2) that this response is mediated by the interaction of the 2 hypothalamic peptides GRF and SRIF.

1497 DIFFERENTAL EFFECTS OF METHAMPHETAMINE AND CHOLECYSTOKININ ON THE RAT HYPOTHALAMIC NUCLEI.

T. Kaneyuki*, T. Morimasa, M. Ikeda and T. Shohmori, * Okayama Prefectural Junior College, Okayama, Japan and Department of Clinical Neurochemistry, Institute for Neurobiology, Okayama University Medical School, Okayama, Japan.

Cholecystokinin (CCK) has an anorectic action. Whether this effect becomes manifest via a peripheral mechanism or centrally is in dispute. We studied the effect of CCK on monoamine metabolites in the brain from rats pretreated with oral methamphetamine for one week. Rats were killed by decapitation 30min after intraventricular (i.v.; 100ng/10ul) or intraperitoneal (i.p.; 30ug) CCK-8-Sulfate. The brains were removed and ventromedial hypothalamic area (VMH) and lateral hypothalamic area (LH) dissected. Monoamine metabolites in tissue were measured using HPLC-ECD. The i.v. CCK caused no variation in blood sugar and insulin, brain DOPAC, 5-HIAA and HVA levels. The i.p. CCK increased the already lowered blood insulin with methamphetamine drinking to the control level. The methamphetamine-induced 5-HIAA increase in LH was lowered to the control level by the i.p. CCK. The methamphetamine-induced DOPAC increase in LH remained at higher level even after the i.p. CCK. HVA level in LH was not changed by methamphethamine but decreased by the additional i.p. CCK. Methamphetamine induced no variation of amine metabolites in VMH but only HVA level was decreased with the additional i.p. CCK. The present data suggest that peripheral CCk antagonizes the central action of methamphetamine in some ways.

1498 THE SEXUALLY DIMORPHIC NUCLEUS OF THE PREOPTIC AREA (SDN-POA): LACK OF A DEVELOPMENTAL INFLUENCE OF THE THYROID AXIS.

L.P. Karaviti*, R.A. Gorski, and J. Shryne. Department of Anatomy and Laboratory of Neuroendocrinology, UCLA School of Medicine, Los Angeles, CA 90024, USA.

The SDN-POA is a model of the influence of gonadal hormones on the differentiation and development of the rat hypothalamus. Since thyroxin (T4) is also known to influence neural development, the present studies were designed to examine the possible role of T4 on the development of this nucleus. Three studies were performed. In the first, pregnant females received daily injections of propylthiouracil (PTU); 4mg, or saline from day 11 until parturition. When born, the rat pups exposed prenatally to PTU received daily injections of PTU 0.5mg. Pups born of mothers treated with saline either continued to receive saline or T4 3μg/day postnatally. In the second study, PTU or saline treatment continued until sacrifice at day 16. The animals were perfused with neutral formalin and brains processed histologically for analysis of SDN-POA volume. In both studies two way ANOVA demonstrated that treatment with either PTU or T4 failed to modify absolute volume of the SDN-POA at the ages analyzed, whereas the expected sex difference in SDN-POA volume remained. In the third study, additional animals were independently treated with PTU, T4, or saline, as described above, and serum T4 measured at sacrifice on postnatal day 8 or 16. Animals treated with PTU were hypothyroid (T4<0.1μg/dl) and those treated with T4, hyperthyroid (T4>20μg/dl). These data suggest that during the developmental period analyzed, SDN-POA volume is not affected by alterations in T4 levels. This lack of an effect of T4, a known neurotrophic factor, on SDN-POA volume supports the view that development of this nucleus may be specifically dependent on steroids. (HD-01182)

1499 RELAXIN AND COLLAGEN METABOLISM IN THE RAT UTERUS. E.H. Frieden* and W.C. Adams, Kent State University, Kent, OH 44242.

We have previously demonstrated that the uterotrophic effects of relaxin are correlated with increased incorporation of several amino acids into uterine protein in vitro. Our data also indicate that collagen appears to be especially sensitive to the anabolic effect of relaxin, since incorporation of ^{3}H-proline into uterine collagen of immature, ovariectomized, estrogen-primed rats was nearly doubled as compared to its incorporation into soluble protein (Federa. Proc., 42, 1873(1983)).

Both the mass and collagen content of the rat uterus decrease to 10% of their parturient values within 4 days post-partum; this phenomenon provides an opportunity to study collagen turnover in a rapidly involuting uterus. Unilaterally pregnant rats were given porcine relaxin (0.1 mg) every 12 hours, beginning at parturition and continuing until day 4. Both gravid and non-gravid uteri were removed at intervals and examined for changes in size and Hyp as a measure of collagen content. In other experiments, rats were ovariectomized at parturition and given estrogen and relaxin, alone or in combination, during the post-partum period.

In intact animals, both gravid and non-gravid uteri involute more slowly when relaxin is given. In non-gravid uteri, weights and collagen contents averaged 40% larger than controls after four days. Although the effects of relaxin in ovariectomized animals were borderline, relaxin clearly potentiated estrogen inhibition of involution in these animals. Our results indicate that collagenolysis in the post-parturient rat uterus is sensitive to the action of relaxin. Relaxin may therefore be a significant factor in alterations in uterine collagen during gestation in the rat.

1500 PURIFICATION OF INHIBIN FROM PORCINE FOLLICULAR FLUID. M. Godbout* and F. Labrie, MRC Group in Molecular Endocrinology, CHUL, Québec G1V 4G2, Canada.

Much evidence suggests that not only LHRH and sex steroids but also an inhibitory substance of ovarian and testicular origin called "Inhibin" is involved in the control of LH and FSH secretion by a direct action at the pituitary level. Changes of spontaneous or LHRH-induced FSH release in rat anterior pituitary cells in primary culture were used as assay of inhibin activity and results were expressed in terms of specific activity, one unit (U) being defined as the amount of inhibin inducing half-maximal inhibition of FSH release. Following treatment of porcine follicular fluid (PFF) with dextran-coated-charcoal (PFFc.t.), salting out with ammonium sulfate (20-40%), adsorption on CM-AFFI Gel Blue and Concanavalin-A-Sepharose columns and, finally, preparative polyacrylamide gel electrophoresis (PAGE) (gradient 3-12%), the material was electroeluted. Analysis of the purified material was performed on 10-20% SDS-PAGE (pH 8.3) and by EIF (pH 3.5-9.5). The fraction which possesses highest Inhibin activity (12,000-14,000 U/mg) migrates on 10-20% SDS-PAGE at an apparent molecular weight of 140,000 daltons and electrofocuses on IEF at pH 5.5 and 5.6 as two single bands. The fraction of Inhibin is at least 80% pure according to the above-mentioned criteria and is biologically active at ED_{50} values of 60-70 ng/ml as compared to 5,000 ng/ml for the starting material, thus representing a purification factor of approximately 75. Assuming a M.W. of 140,000 daltons, the purified material inhibits FSH secretion at an estimated ED_{50} value of $5 \times 10^{-10}M$, a concentration similar to the action of other hormones acting on the pituitary gland.

1501 REVERSAL OF β-ENDORPHIN (βE)-INDUCED BLOCKADE OF PREOVULATORY LH RELEASE AND OVULATION WITH PROSTAGLANDIN E_2 (PGE_2) IN RATS.
C.A. Leadem and S.P. Kalra*, Department of OB-Gyn, College of Medicine, University of Florida, Gainesville, FL 32610 U.S.A.

These studies examined the effects of intraventricular (Ivt) administration of βE on preovulatory LH release, ovulation and the mechanism that may be involved in opioid action. Female rats were implanted with permanent cannulae in the third ventricle and were allowed to recover 4-day estrous cyclicity. Intrajugular cannulae were placed on diestrus II. The following day on proestrus, rats received Ivt either saline (2 μl) or βE (10 μg/2 μl) at 1300, 1430 and 1600 h. In addition, at 1600 and 1700 h they were injected Ivt with either vehicle (CSF or saline) or one of the following compounds: epinephrine (15 μg), norepinephrine (15 μg) or PGE_2 (6 μg). Blood samples for LH measurements were taken at 0, 10, 30 and 60 min after these additional injections. βE blocked the preovulatory LH surge and ovulation. Administration of opiate receptor antagonist naltrexone (10 mg/kg) reversed these effects. Catecholamines stimulated LH release in the βE-treated rats, but this was insufficient to induce ovulation. On the other hand, PGE_2 reversed the βE blockade of LH surge and normal ovulation occurred in these rats. These studies show that blockade of ovulation and LH surge may not be due to adverse effects of βE on the intraneural secretory events in the LHRH neurons, but that βE may decrease the influx of neurogenic stimuli responsible for activation of preovulatory LHRH secretion during the critical period on proestrus. (Supported by NIH HD 08634 and 14006).

1502 REGIONAL DISTRIBUTION OF HUMAN PANCREATIC GROWTH HORMONE-RELEASING FACTOR-LIKE IMMUNOREACTIVITY IN HUMAN HYPOTHALAMUS BY RADIOIMMUNOASSAY.
John W. Leidy, Jr* and Richard J. Robbins, Div of Endocrinology, Univ of Colorado Hlth Sci Ctr, B151, Denver, CO 80262, USA.

Human pancreatic growth hormone releasing factor (hpGRF-44) is a potent stimulator of growth hormone release; however, its relationships to native human hypothalamic growth hormone-releasing factor (GRF) remains uncertain. We have developed specific antisera to synthetic hpGRF-44 in rabbits and have examined extracts of human brain tissue for the presence of hpGRF-44-like immunoreactivity (iGRF). Antisera were produced using hpGRF-44 with methylated BSA and complete Freund's adjuvant. One antiserum (1972) was further characterized and a radioimmunoassay established. Characteristics of antiserum 1972 included a titer of 1/40,000, a sensitivity of 30pg per tube and a high specificity for hpGRF. There was no cross reactivity with the glucagon-secretin family (including PHI-27, VIP, GIP), hypothalamic releasing factors (LHRH, TRH, SRIF), and anterior pituitary hormones. The distribution of iGRF was determined in acetic acid extracts of human hypothalamus. The majority of iGRF was found in the pituitary stalk with smaller amounts in the ventral and infundibular regions. No iGRF was present in cortex and thalamus. Dilutions of hypothalamic iGRF demonstrated parallel displacement curves with synthetic hpGRF-44. We conclude that 1) the distribution of iGRF in the human hypothalamus is similar to the predicted distribution of native GRF, 2) there is close immunologic structure between human hypothalamic iGRF and hpGRF-44. The results provide further evidence that hpGRF-44 is structurally similar to native hypothalamic GRF. These studies were supported by PHS grants AM 07445 and AM 30451.

1503 REVERSIBLE HYPOESTROGENISM INDUCED BY REPETITIVE LHRH AGONIST ADMINISTRATION IN THE TREATMENT OF ENDOMETRIOSIS. A.Lemay,* R.Maheux, N.Faure, C.Jean and A.T.A.Fazekas, Endocr. of Reprod. St-François d'Assise Hospital, Quebec Canada.

Ten women having endometriosis (stage I to IV) as evaluated by laparoscopy received 200 ug of [D-Ser(TBU)^6-des-Gly-NH$_2$^{10}) LHRH ethylamide (buserelin HOE 766) by s.c. injections every 12 hrs for 5 days beginning on day 3 to 6 of the cycle. 400 ug of the LHRH agonist was then administered intranasally every 8 hours for 25 to 31 weeks. The pituitary response was already refractory after the second injection, serum FSH levels returning to basal values on the second day of treatment. Serum LH levels progressively decreased to normal within 4 weeks. Serum estradiol decreased below early follicular phase levels within 7 to 30 days and continued to decrease to castrate levels. Light to moderate estrogen withdrawal bleeding was followed by amenorrhea with occasional bleeding or spotting in 4 women. Abdominal pain and dyspareunia disappeared or were ameliorated after 2 months of treatment. At the end of treatment, laparoscopy showed resorption of endometrial implants. The endometrial biopsy revealed inactive endometrium or weak proliferation. Ovulation returned within 45 days and 2 out of 4 sexually active women became pregnant during cycle 3 and 5. Dysmenorrhea was relieved and abdominal pain continued to be improved in all but one patient during a 6 month follow-up period. The treatment was well accepted in spite of the expected hot flushes and vaginal dryness. Biosafety evaluation during and after treatment did not reveal any abnormalities. Reversible down-regulation of pituitary-ovarian function by repetitive LHRH agonist administration can be a worthwhile approach to medical treatment of endometriosis.

1504 EFFECTS OF DOPAMINE (DA), MORPHINE AND VIP ON HYPOTHALAMIC SOMATOSTATIN RELEASE IN VITRO. A.M.J. Lengyel*°, A. Grossman, Lesley H. Rees+, and G.M. Besser, Departments of Endocrinology and Chemical Endocrinology+, St. Bartholomew's Hospital, London, EC1A 7BE, UK.

Several neurotransmitters and peptides influence GH secretion. In the rat, VIP and morphine increase serum GH, while the effect of DA is disputed. The site of action of these substances is unclear. Therefore we studied the effect of DA, VIP and morphine on SMS release from rat hypothalamic fragments in vitro. Hypothalamic fragments from male rats were incubated in Earle's medium. After 60 min preincubation medium from two 20 min incubations was collected and SMS levels measured by RIA. DA 10^{-8} to 10^{-4}M induced a progressive increase in basal SMS levels (r=0.41;p<0.01). K^+30mM-induced SMS release was also increased by increasing doses of DA (r=0.54; p<0.01). Metoclopramide (MCP) 10^{-5}M blocked the DA (10^{-6}M) induced increase in SMS release (control (C) = 130±17; DA=200±25; DA + MCP: 81±19pg/ml). At high concentrations of VIP (10^{-6}M) SMS release was stimulated (C:131±15pg/ml; VIP 10^{-6}M: 196+31), while at low concentrations SMS release fell (VIP 10^{-10}M: 86±10; 10^{-9}: 99±10pg/ml). No effect was obtained on K^+30mM SMS release. Basal SMS was negatively correlated with morphine concentrations (r=0.63; p<0.01) while no significant correlation was found with K^+30mM depolarization. Conclusion: 1) DA inhibits GH release in the rat through an increase in SMS release, 2) VIP has a dual effect on hypothalamic SMS release, decreasing at low concentrations and increasing at high concentrations, 3) morphine decreases SMS release, accounting, at least in part, for the increased GH secretion after morphine in vivo.

°Supported by FAPESP (80/1522-5), Brazil.

1505 HETEROGENEITY AMONG CORTICOTROPES OF THE RAT ANTERIOR PITUITARY. D.A. Leong*, D.N. Orth, and M.O. Thorner, Department of Internal Medicine, University of Virginia Medical Center, Charlottesville, VA 22908, and Vanderbilt University Hospital, Nashville, Tennessee, USA.

We describe ACTH release from individual corticotropes using the reverse hemolytic plaque assay technique introduced by Neill and Frawley (Endocrinology 112:1135,1983). Complement mediated antibody-directed lysis of erythrocytes is exploited in such a way that ACTH release from single corticotropes triggers the lysis of a surrounding monolayer of ACTH-sensitive erythrocytes. A cell releasing ACTH is distinguished within a mixed population of cells as a single cell surrounded by a zone of hemolysed erythrocytes. Dispersed anterior pituitary cells were mixed with ACTH-sensitized erythrocytes, separated into batches, and exposed to different concentrations of ovine CRF (0.3, 1.0, 10.0 nM) for different periods of time (1.5, 3.0, 4.5 hours). A representative study of 3 separate experiments is expressed as the % of ACTH plaque forming cells (mean area of plaque) in the table below:

CRF concentration	1.5 h	3.0 h	4.5 h
10.0 nM	6.5 (767)	7.5 (738)	8.6 (1610)
1.0 nM	5.2 (366)	5.8 (583)	5.6 (497)
0.3 nM	2.1 (216)	4.7 (423)	4.8 (292)
0.0 nM	2.2 (149)	1.9 (151)	2.0 (131)

These data suggest that CRF has the potential to stimulate ACTH release, in a dose-dependent fashion, by regulating the amount of ACTH released and the number of active corticotropes.

1506 POTENT INTERACTION BETWEEN THYROTROPIN RELEASING HORMONE (TRH) AND HUMAN PANCREATIC GROWTH HORMONE-RELEASING FACTOR (hpGRF) IN STIMULATING CHICKEN GROWTH HORMONE (cGH) IN VIVO

F. C. LEUNG*, J. E. TAYLOR, and C. A. BALL
Department of Animal Physiology, MSDRL, Rahway, NJ 07065

HpGRF and TRH were reported to be potent releasers of cGH in vitro and to stimulate cGH release in an additive manner when they were added together in the culture medium (Endocrinology, 1983, 113:1913). The purpose of this study was to determine the interaction of hpGRF and TRH on cGH release in vivo. Four-week old cockerels (~1 kg) were injected with hpGRF (1.0 μg/bird), TRH (0.1 μg/bird), or hpGRF (1.0 μg/bird) in combination with TRH (0.1 μg/bird). Blood was taken 5 min post-injection and serum cGH was determined using a homologous RIA for cGH. The results showed that hpGRF and TRH were potent stimulators of cGH release, 5 and 6 fold, respectively, over the control birds, and hpGRF and TRH administered in combination gave a synergistic stimulation of cGH release (>20 fold). In separate experiments, pretreatment of birds with αMT (250 mg/kg) blocked the stimulatory effect of TRH, but not that of hpGRF, on cGH release. The present data demonstrated that hpGRF and TRH are each potent stimulators of cGH release and when they are administered together a synergistic effect on cGH release is obtained. Our results also indicate that hpGRF acts at the pituitary level which TRH acts on both the hypothalamus and pituitary in causing the release of cGH.

1507 DIFFERENCES BETWEEN SPECIES IN THE SENSITIVITY TO THE ANTIPITUITARY AND ANTIOVULATORY EFFECTS OF A POTENT LHRH ANTAGONIST. P. Limonta*, S. Pavlou, K. Sundaram and R.B. Thau, The Population Council, New York, N.Y. 10021

The effects of the potent LHRH antagonist [Ac-D-NAL(2)^1,4F-D-Phe^2,D-Trp^3,D-Arg^6]-LHRH (A), on ovulation in mature rats and rabbits and on plasma LH levels in ovariectomized rats and rabbits were investigated. Dose-response studies show that 1 µg (4 µg/kg) A was sufficient to inhibit ovulation completely in cycling rats (N=9 to 11 per group), while 500 µg (135 µg/kg) were required to inhibit mating induced ovulation in 8 of 11 rabbits. Two of the three rabbits which ovulated in spite of the A treatment and subsequently became pregnant, had delayed LH surges, reaching maximal LH levels at 4 h as compared to 2 h for mated controls. The mean LH peak (ng AFP-559-B/ml) of the 3 rabbits (6.0 ± 1.4, mean ± SE) was significantly ($p < 0.0005$) lower than that of controls (18.4 ± 3.3, N=12). These results suggest that rabbits are less sensitive to the inhibitory action of A than rats. Pituitary release of LH, as measured by plasma LH levels following A treatment (100 µg/kg) in ovariectomized rabbits and rats, also showed lower sensitivity of the rabbit pituitary. Plasma LH levels in rabbits reached their lowest values less rapidly as compared to rats (2 versus 1 h) and began to recover sooner (by 4 versus 24 h). In rats A was also effective at a lower dose (10 µg/kg). The differences between rats and rabbits may be due to differences in receptor binding. The affinity of A to pituitary receptors was 5 fold higher in rats as compared to rabbits. Conclusion: significant differences between rats and rabbits were found with respect to the antipituitary and antiovulatory effects of a potent LHRH antagonist.

1508 RELEASE OF oCRF-LIKE IMMUNOREACTIVITY FROM OVINE MEDIAN EMINENCE IN VITRO: EFFECT OF VASOPRESSIN. E.A. Linton* and P.J. Lowry, Protein Hormone and Recombinant DNA Laboratory, St Bartholomew's Centre for Clinical Research, Dominion House, 59-60 Bartholomew Close, London EC1.

Investigations on neuropeptide and neurotransmitter regulation of CRF have produced conflicting data, possibly caused by difficulty in measuring CRF directly. Following the characterization of ovine-CRF (oCRF), a 41 residue peptide with potent ACTH-releasing ability, and the availability of a radioimmunoassay for its measurement, we have studied the effect of various substances on the release of oCRF-like immunoreactivity from ovine median eminence in vitro. 8-10 ovine median eminences were hand-dissected into approximately 1mm longitudinal sections, suspended in a 2ml plastic column in a total volume of 500µl, and perfused at a rate of 0.25ml/min with Earle's Balanced Salt solution. 8-min pulses of stimulants were applied and responses measured by oCRF radioimmunoassay in 4-min fractions of the column effluent. Basal oCRF levels (500-800pg/ml) represented less than 0.1% of the total extractable oCRF-like immunoreactivity. 70mM $[K^+]$ elicited a rapid increase in oCRF release (by 159% above background) which was Ca-dependant. Arginine-vasopressin at 10^{-8}, 10^{-6} and 10^{-4} M also stimulated oCRF release, by 58, 77 and 153% above background respectively. No significant effect of dopamine on oCRF release was obtained. These results suggest that vasopressin plays a complex role in ACTH secretion, causing the release of oCRF from the hypothalamus, in addition to its known intrinsic ACTH-releasing activity. This in vitro method may be useful in investigating the action of other neuromodulators on oCRF release.

1509 SOMATOSTATIN (SRIF) INHIBITS CORTICOTROPIN RELEASING FACTOR (CRF) INDUCED ACTIVATION OF ADENYLATE CYCLASE (AC) AND cAMP-DEPENDENT PROTEIN KINASE (PK) IN AtT20 CELLS. Y. Litvin*, M. Leiser, N. Fleischer and J. Erlichman. Dept. of Medicine, Albert Einstein College of Medicine. Bronx, N.Y. U.S.A.

We have studied the effects of SRIF on CRF and forskolin stimulated cAMP formation and PK activation in intact AtT20 cells, and the effects of SRIF on the AC in isolated membranes from these cells. In the presence of 0.5mM methylisobutylxanthine (MIX), CRF (100nM) and forskolin (10uM) stimulated cAMP accumulation in intact cells by 15- and 80-fold respectively. The degree of activation of cAMP-dependent PK isoenzymes was assessed by employing specific antisera directed against their regulatory subunits. When cells were incubated with 0.5mM MIX and 100nM CRF for 5 min., 100% of PK I and 50% of PK II were activated. When cells were incubated under the same conditions in the presence of 1uM SRIF cAMP levels were reduced by 90% and cAMP induced activation of PKs I and II was reduced to 60% and 20% respectively. In the presence of MIX forskolin activated both PKs completely. Low concentrations of forskolin (100nM) in the absence of MIX resulted in a partial activation of PK I (43%) and PK II (10%). In the presence of SRIF (1uM) activation of PKs I and II was reduced to 10% and 3% respectively. Using isolated membranes 100nM CRF stimulated AC activity 4- to 5-fold. SRIF inhibited CRF stimulated AC in a dose dependent manner, however, AC activity was still 2-fold above basal at 10uM SRIF. Forskolin (10uM) stimulated AC activity 15-fold but was only slightly (15%) inhibited by SRIF. Minimal effects of SRIF on basal AC activity were seen. These studies show that SRIF inhibits hormone sensitive AC and thereby blocks hormone induced cAMP formation and PK activation in intact AtT20 cells.

1510 HYPERSENSITIVITY TO HUMAN PANCREATIC GROWTH HORMONE-RELEASING FACTOR (hpGRF-40) OF PITUITARIES DISCONNECTED FROM THE CENTRAL NERVOUS SYSTEM. V. Locatelli, S.G. Cella, S. Loche°, C. Pintor° and E.E. Müller*. Dept. of Pharmacol. Univ. Milan and °Dept. Pediatrics Univ. Cagliari, Italy.

hpGRF can be profitably exploited to study pituitary GH function of subjects with growth disorders due to an organic or functional alteration of the CNS. The aim of our study was to investigate in the rat the effect of a short-lasting hypothalamo-pituitary disconnection on the GH responsiveness to hpGRF. Adult S.D. female rats were either sham-operated (sham-op) or underwent complete ablation of the mediobasal hypothalamus (HA) by a stirrup shaped knife. One and three wks following surgery sham-op and HA rats were anesthetized with urethane and injected intrajugularly with saline or hpGRF-40 (20,100 and 500 ng/rat). In sham-op rats hpGRF-40 stimulated GH release only at the dose of 500ng (from 14±2.5 to 193±62 ng/ml at 5 min), while in 1wk-HA rats it elicited a GH response already apparent at 20ng, clear-cut at 100 ng and striking at 500 ng (from 32±4 to 1023±120 ng/ml at 5 min). In 3wk-HA rats the GH response to hpGRF-40 was similar to that evoked in sham-op rats, being significant only at the dose of 500 ng (from 15±1.5 to 161±29 ng/ml at 5 min). GH pituitary concentrations were as follows: sham-op rats 92±11 µg/mg, 1wk-HA rats 38±2 µg/mg; 3 wk-HA rats 17±2 µg/mg.

These data indicate that, despite a clear-cut reduction in the GH secretory pool, pituitaries shortly disconnected from the CNS show an enhanced (1wk) or preserved (3wks) GH responsiveness to hpGRF-40, thus implying development of somatotroph hypersensitivity to the neurohormone.

1511 REGRESSION OF LEIOMYOMATA UTERI FOLLOWING HYPOESTROGENISM INDUCED BY REPETITIVE LHRH AGONIST TREATMENT. R.Maheux, C.Guilloteau, A.Lemay and AT.A. FAZEKAS. Department of Obstetrics and Gynecology, Division of Reproductive Endocrinology, St-François d'Assise Hospital, Quebec City, Canada.

11 patients aged between 31 and 51, harboring leiomyomata uteri positively identified by gynecologic exam, ultrasonographic exam and/or by laparoscopy were treated with [D-Ser (TBU)^6-des-Gly-NH_2^{10}] LHRH ethylamide (buserelin, HOE 766) 200 µg s.c. T I D x 7 days thereafter 500 µg s.c. die for a total treatment period of 6 months. Initial volume of the myomas was between 14.5 and 720 cc. Significant reduction of the myomas up to 90% has been observed in 10 out of the 11 patients. The regression has been observed principally during the first two months of treatment followed by a much slower regression rate during the rest of the treatment period. Serum estradiol and gonadotropin levels were significantly suppressed and reached menopausal levels after the first month of treatment. 5 out of 11 patients presented an episode of bleeding after the first month of treatment; none thereafter. Significant hot flushes were the only side effect noted. Uterine myomas are the most common tumors of the female pelvic organs and the first indication of abdominal hysterectomy. Based on preliminary evidence, therapy with LHRH agonist results in important regression of uterine myomas and may be an acceptable medical alternative to surgical treatment for woman harboring myomata uteri.

1512 EFFECT OF LONG-TERM LESION OF THE HYPOTHALAMIC PARAVENTRICULAR NUCLEUS (NPV) ON PITUITARY-ADRENAL FUNCTION AND IMMUNOREACTIVE CRF-41 IN THE STALK-MEDIAN EMINENCE OF RATS. G.B. Makara*, E. Stark and G. Kapocs, Inst. of Exp. Med., Hung. Acad. Sci., Budapest 1450, Pf. 67., Hungary

Plasma corticosterone response to ether - venesection stress was impaired by one week but not 6 weeks after PVN lesioning. On the 6th week after PVN lesioning plasma ACTH was increased markedly in response to ether-laparotomy stress or adrenalectomy (performed 8 days previously), although the levels attained were lower than in the controls. oCRF-41 immunoreactive material in the SME was 577 fmol/SME in the controls and less than 35 fmol/SME in the rats with PVN lesion. Six weeks after PVN lesioning the in vitro ACTH release in response to synthetic oCRF-41 was slightly enhanced when compared to the sham-operated controls.

The data show that several weeks after lesioning the PVN region a marked recovery of the pituitary-adrenal system occurs without reappearence of oCRF-41 immunoreactive material in the SME. Inhibition of the plasma ACTH responses can be seen at a time when the plasma corticosterone response is restored. We suggest that besides hypothalamic CRF-41 other hypothalamic factors may also have a significant role in the control of the pituitary-adrenal system.

1513 THE DISTRIBUTION OF GROWTH HORMONE RELEASING FACTOR (GRF) IN THE HUMAN HYPOTHALAMUS.

P.E. Marshall, J.B. Martin*, W.J. Millard, S.M. Sagar, D.M.D. Landis. Department of Neurology, Mass. Gen. Hosp., Boston, MA 02114

In the human hypothalamus the distribution of GRF has been studied with immunocytochemical techniques using an antiserum directed against human pancreatic GRF 1-40 (supplied by W. Vale). Human postmortem tissue was usually fixed in formalin. Numerous immunoreactive perikarya were visualized in the ventral medial hypothalamus (VMH) where their distribution overlapped with, but was not defined by, the boundaries of the VMN and tuberal (arcuate) nucleus. Additional cells were concentrated in the perifornical region, and sparsely in the periventricular zone (PVZ). Cell somata most frequently were bipolar (22x12um). A varicose axon arose either from the cell body or proximal dendrite; dendrites branched infrequently. The median eminence, supplied by fibers from the lateral margins of the stalk, contained the highest concentration of axon terminals. They were seen throughout the external zone and associated with portal capillaries. Fibers were generally associated with areas containing GRF cell bodies. However, they were also densely distributed in the suprachiasmatic anterior hypothalamus, PVZ and mediodorsal hypothalamus. Sparse fibers were found in the lateral hypothalamus and midline thalamus. Terminal axons were identified in the VMH and similar arborizations were seen within areas of fiber distribution. The widespread distribution of fibers suggests that GRF may have a hypothalamic function in addition to its recognized role in the tuberoinfundibular system. Supported by NIH grants AM26252 and NS16367.

1514 THE EFFECTS OF GLUCOSE AND FREE FATTY ACIDS ON GROWTH HORMONE-RELEASING FACTOR-MEDIATED GH SECRETION IN MAN.

A. Masuda*, T. Shibasaki, T. Imaki, M. Nakahara, T. Tsushima, H. Demura, K. Shizume and N. Ling[1]. Department of Medicine, Tokyo Women's Medical College, 10 Ichigaya-Kawada-cho, Shinjuku-ku, Tokyo 162, Japan, [1]Laboratories for Neuroendocrinology, The Salk Institute for Biological Studies, La Jolla, California 92037, U.S.A.

The effects of glucose and free fatty acids (FFA) on growth hormone-releasing factor (GRF)-mediated GH secretion were examined in normal young males. In two paired experiments the six subjects drank a 75-g glucose solution or an equal volume of water 30 minutes before receiving intravenously 100 µg of hpGRF-44. Thirty minutes after hpGRF-44 administration mean plasma GH level reached the peak concentration in both experiments. However, the GH response was significantly diminished in the experiment where the subjects had received glucose (plasma GH: 8.12 ± 1.12 ng/ml) versus the one where they had drank only water (23.70 ± 8.46). The effect of FFA on GRF-mediated GH secretion was examined. Six subjects were intravenously infused 250 ml of lipid-heparin solution or an equal volume of saline during 150 minutes. Thirty minutes after infusion started, 100 µg of hpGRF-44 were injected intravenously. Thirty minutes after hpGRF-44 administration, mean plasma GH level reached the peak concentration in both groups. However, the GH response was significantly diminished in the subjects who were given FFA (plasma GH: 8.4 ± 1.7 ng/ml) compared with the control (28.9 ± 7.1). These data suggest that acute hyperglycemia and elevation of plasma FFA attenuate the GH secretion induced by hpGRF-44.

1515 EFFECTS OF CONTINUOUSLY ADMINISTERED LHRH AGONIST ON THE PITUITARY-GONADAL AXIS IN MACAQUE MONKEYS. G.I. McRae*, L.M. Sanders and B.H. Vickery, Syntex Research, Palo Alto, California, USA.

Nafarelin acetate, a highly potent LHRH agonist was microencapsulated into microspheres of poly(d,l lactic-co-glycolic acid), PLGA, at a level of 1% using a phase separation process, to give a formulation affording controlled release over a prolonged period of time. Intramuscular injection of a suspension of these microspheres(3mg nafarelin) into female monkeys caused suppression of basal levels of LH and FSH for the 36 days in which the agonist was measurable in the blood. Gonadotropin levels then rose and a normal menstrual cycle followed. In contrast, when nafarelin is administered daily by injection, although ovulation is also prevented, basal levels of gonadotropins are unchanged, pituitary responsivity persists and only the preovulatory gonadotropin surge fails to materialize. In male monkeys the discrepancy between continuous and daily dosing is even more marked. Plasma testosterone declined to castrate levels in 2 of 3 animals by 3 weeks after intramuscular injection of PLGA containing 3.7mg of nafarelin whereas daily injection of agonist persistently evoked testosterone elevations. The qualitative differences in response to continuous versus daily treatment suggests that such formulations may be the treatment of choice for gonadal hormone dependent syndromes such as endometriosis and prostate cancer.

1516 IMMUNOCYTOCHEMICAL LOCALIZATION OF GROWTH HORMONE RELEASING FACTOR (GHRF) IN THE RAT BRAIN. I. Merchenthaler*, A. Arimura, C.R. Thomas and S. Vigh. Laboratories for Molecular Neuroendocrinology and Diabetes, Tulane University, Hebert Research Center, Belle Chasse, LA 70037 (I.M., A.A., C.R.T.) and Dept. of Medicine, Tulane Univ., New Orleans, LA 70112 (S.V.), USA.

Immunoreactive GHRF was present in perikarya, neuronal processes and terminals in the rat brain by using both the anti-human pancreatic (SV#97) and the anti-rat hypothalamic (#565) antisera. Colchicine dramatically increased the number of GHRF-immunopositive perikarya as well as the intensity of their staining. Medium sized, bi-or multipolar GHRF-containing neurons were observed in the following areas of the brain: perifornical regions of the anterior and lateral hypothalamus, arcuate nucleus, medial and lateral borders of the ventromedial nucleus, paraventricular and dorsomedial hypothalamic nuclei, and the lateral basal hypothalamus. Antiserum #565 stained perikarya in the hypothalamus in a fashion as that seen with antiserum SV#97, and occasionally immunopositive cells in the amygdala. Fibers from the perifornical, paraventricular and dorsomedial cells formed a fan-like projection to the external layer of the median eminence (ME), where a dense accumulation of GHRF-immunoreactive terminals was observed. Fibers from the arcuate nucleus reached the ME above the pathway coming from the perifornical cells. Fibers from the perikarya in the lateral basal hypothalamus joined the pathway arising in the perifornical region, close to the base of the hypothalamus. The localization of GHRF in the ME reinforces the view that this peptide plays a physiological role in the control of the release of GH from the anterior pituitary.
Supported in part by NIH Grant AM09094.

1517 EFFECTS AND EVOLUTION OF hpGRF IN SOMATOTROPES OF RAT PITUITARY GLAND. AN IMMUNOCYTOLOGICAL APPROACH. P. Mesguich, F.J. Hemming, G. Morel and P.M. Dubois*, CNRS-ERA 981, Univ. of LYON, OULLINS, France.

Secretion of GH is increased by injection of synthetic human pancreatic Growth hormone-Releasing Factor (hpGRF) (Guillemin et al. Science, 1982). To study its effects on ultrastructure and its evolution in somatotropes 1) a semi-quantitative immunoelectron microscopic method (Morel and Dubois, Neuroendocrinology, 1982) and 2) conventional immunoelectron microscopy were performed on pituitaries of rats I.V. injected with 1 µg hpGRF, sacrified at various times (from 30 sec to 120 h after injection). Somatotropes were identified with an anti-hGH serum. Injected hpGRF was localized with an anti-hpGRF (451-6, a gift from Dr. P. Brazeau) which does not cross react with rat GRF. As early as 30 sec after injection, immunoreactive hpGRF was localized both in the cytoplasm and in the secretory granules, while it was only observed in the nucleus after 2 min. It rose rapidly to a peak at 15 min, and then dropped gradually to a plateau lasting from 60 min to the 2nd day. Forty-eight hours after injection, no immunoreactive GRF could be observed. The main ultrastructural modifications were swelling of the Golgi apparatus, appearance of microfilaments and especially of granular extrusions. These data suggest that exogenous GRF was rapidly internalized in somatotropes and gradually eliminated after provoking exocytosis of granules.

1518 α- AND β-ADRENERGIC REGULATION OF GROWTH HORMONE SECRETION: EVIDENCE FOR GROWTH HORMONE-RELEASING FACTOR (GRF) MEDIATION. N. Miki*, M. Ono and K. Shizume, Department of Medicine, Tokyo Women's Medical College, Tokyo 162, Japan

We have recently found that α- and β-adrenoreceptors exert the opposite effects on growth hormone (GH) secretion. The present studies were performed to examine which factor, GH-releasing factor (GRF) or somatostatin (SRIF), is involved in the adrenergic regulation of GH secretion in the conscious rat. Adult male rats weighing 250-300 g were implanted with chronic cannulae into lateral ventricle of the brain and/or right atrium. When rats were passively immunized with antiserum to rat hypothalamic GRF (rGRF), it completely inhibited the episodic GH secretion over 6 hrs and abolished GH release induced by intravevous injection of clonidine (125 µg /kg BW), an α-adrenergic agent, indicating that α-adrenergic mechanism stimulates GH release via endogenous rGRF. This GRF-mediated GH release by clonidine was totally suppressed by intraventricular injection of β-adrenergic agent, dl-isoproterenol (0.5 µM) or dobutamine (0.1 µM). Activation of central β-adrenoreceptor also significantly inhibited GH release by FK 33-824 (100 µg/kg BW), an enkephalin analogue, which we have recently found to act on GRF. However, this GH inhibitory effect of β-adrenergic agonist, was not reversed under passive immunization with anti-SRIF serum. In contrast, either isoproterenol or dobutamine failed to suppress GH response to a synthetic rGRF (1 µg/kg BW), which was grately enhanced when rats were pretreated with anti-SRIF serum prior to β-agonist administration. These results suggest that rGRF mediating the GH stimulatory role of α-adrenoreceptor may also be involved in GH inhibitory β-adrenergic mechanism.

1519 GLUTAMIC ACID DECARBOXYLASE (GAD) CONTAINING AXONS INNERVATE ARCUATE NEURONS CONTAINING WHORL BODIES AND/OR NEMATOSOMES. C. Leranth, H. Sakamoto, N.J. MacLusky and F. Naftolin. Dept. of OB/GYN, Yale Medical School, New Haven, CT. 06510.

The hypothalamic arcuate nucleus (AN) of the rat contains high concentrations of gamma aminobutyric acid (GABA) and its synthesizing enzyme, (GAD). The activity of GAD is regulated by sex steroids. Morphologically, AN contains neurons with whorl bodies (WB) and nematosomes (NS), the numbers of which are also controlled by gonadal steroids. In this study, we attempted to see whether these estrogen sensitive cells with WB and/or NS receive GAD input and, if so, whether the GAD axons are intrinsic or extrinsic. Female rats (200-250 gm) were treated for 3 weeks as follows: Group I. Ovariectomized (OVX); Group II. OVX 1 week; estradiol valerate (EV; 2.0 mg. S.C.); Group III. OVX and injected with 1.5 mg EV 3 weeks prior to sacrifice. AN were immunocytochemically stained for GAD using the PAP technique. In group I, frequent WB were observed in the AN. Group II showed coexistence of WB and NS in neurons, but the frequency of the former was much less than in group I. Group III was characterized by large numbers of NS but no WB. These data confirm that WB and/or NS are controlled by gonadal status and steroids. In all 3 groups, GAD immunopositive axons form symmetric (inhibitory) synapses through the AN, some of them establishing axo-somatic connections with neurons containing WB/NS. These terminals remained after complete AN deafferentiation, suggesting that they are intrinsic to the AN. Supported by NIH HD13587 and the Andrew Mellon Foundation.

1520 AN ACTIVE SODIUM TRANSPORT INHIBITOR (ASTI) RELEASED BY CULTURED RAT HYPOTHALAMIC CELLS. K. Morgan*, SM. Foord, G. Spurlock, BM. Charalambous, C. Dieguez, MF. Scanlon and MA Mir. Department of Medicine, Welsh National School of Medicine, Heath Park, Cardiff, CF4 4XN, U.K.

Investigations showing the hypothalamus contains an inhibitor of Na^+-K^+-ATPase have been criticised because these extracts contained high concentrations of interfering substances. To overcome these problems we cultured fetal rat hypothalamic cells in monolayer and capillary perfusion systems. We used media alone and the media from cortical cells as controls. Erythrocyte sodium transport and ^{3}H-ouabain binding were used as assays for inhibitory activity. Hypothalamic media reduced the total sodium efflux rate constant from 0.487±0.014 to 0.408±0.013 ($P<0.001$) and the 'active' ouabain-sensitive constant from 0.305±0.015 to 0.240±0.016 ($P<0.01$); it also showed a dose-dependent displacement of ^{3}H-ouabain binding to erythrocytes. Both controls had no effect in either assay. Twelve peptides (DKP, ACTH 1-24, TRH, SS14, GNRH, CRF, Neurotensin, Oxytocin, DDAVP, GRF, αMSH and Substance P) failed to reduce sodium transport. Exposure of hypothalamic cells to 60 mM K^+ in the presence of 2.5 mM Ca^{2+} significantly increased the release of ASTI in the monolayer ($P<0.025$) and capillary perfusion systems ($P<0.001$). Gel filtration of hypothalamic media on Sephadex G-25 resulted in elution of inhibitory activity in the past-salt fraction. This material caused 30% displacement of ^{3}H-ouabain binding to intact erythrocytes and inhibited canine kidney Na^+-K^+-ATPase by 19% ($P<0.025$). These studies demonstrate that fetal rat hypothalamic cells contain and release a low molecular weight factor which inhibits Na^+-K^+-ATPase.

1521 PROSTAGLANDINS (PGs) ARE INVOLVED THROUGHOUT THE DECIDUAL CELL REACTION (DCR).

T.G. Kennedy*, MRC Group in Reproductive Biology, University of Western Ontario, London, Ont. N6A 5A5 Canada.

The results of studies in which PG production was inhibited for a limited time by the sc administration of indomethacin (IM) have suggested that PGs are involved in the growth and differentiation of decidual cells. In the present experiments, IM (0.5 mM in phosphate buffered saline containing gelatin) was infused into the uterine lumen from Alzet osmotic minipumps to reduce uterine PG production during the DCR. Mature ovariectomized rats, treated with a regimen of estradiol and progesterone to sensitize the uteri for the DCR, were used. To determine the effect of mode of administration of IM on the DCR, rats received a single sc injection of IM (2 mg ≃ 3 h before pump insertion) or its vehicle, and intrauterine infusion of IM or its vehicle, in a 2x2 factorial experiment. The effects of the IM treatments on the DCR, as assessed 5 days later by uterine weights, were statistically additive; geometric mean weights of infused uterine horns were 949 mg for controls, 619 mg for intrauterine IM, 556 mg for sc IM and 304 mg for intrauterine plus sc IM. PGE and PGF concentrations 24 and 48 h after the insertion of the pumps were lower in the IM-infused horns, suggesting that the infusion of IM reduced uterine PG production. PGE2 and $PGF2_{\alpha}$ (1 μg/h), alone or combined, infused in 0.5 mM IM into the uterine lumen of rats treated sc with IM, overrode the inhibitory effects of IM (geometric means: vehicle, 210 mg; PGE_2, 1242 mg; $PGF_{2\alpha}$, 811 mg; PGE_2 + $PGF_{2\alpha}$, 1020 mg). These data suggest that PGs are required during the growth and differentiation of decidual cells from endometrial stromal cells. (Supported by the MRC)

1522 BIOSYNTHESIS OF PROSTAGLANDINS IN ENDOMETRIUM OF PREGNANT MOUSE AROUND IMPLANTATION.

K. Kinoshita*, K. Satoh, O. Ishiwara, O. Tsutsumi, M. Nakayama, M. Mizuno and S. Sakamoto, Dept. of Ob. and Gyn. Faculty of Medicine, Univ. of Tokyo, Hongo, Bunkyo, Tokyo, Japan

In an attempt to elucidate the role of prostaglandins (PGs) in blastocyst implantation, biosynthesis of PGs by endometrium of pregnant mouse around the days of implantation and the invivo effect of indomethacin with PGs on implantation were studied. The endometrium obtained from Day 1 to 7 of pregnant mouse was incubated in medium 199 (pH 7.4) with 10% FCS containing C^{14}-arachidonic acid (10.2 nmol, 0.5 μCi) at 37°C for 24 hours and PGs generated in endometrium were analysed. One group of pregnant mice was treated with both 300 μg of indomethacin and 150 μg of PGE_2 on two days of Day 3 and 4. (Day 1 = first day of vaginal plaque) The PGs formed by endometrium were mainly PGE_2, 6 keto PGF_1 and PGF_2 and the production of PGE_2 increased from Day 1 (7.5×10^{-2} nmol/mg prot) to Day 4 (16.3×10^{-2} nmol /mg prot), the day previous to implantation, followed by decrease of the formation of PGs thereafter. The number of implanted blastocysts was 2 ± 1 (n=3) in the mouse treated with indomethacin on Day 3 and 4, but it was 11 ± 2 (n=3) in the mouse trated with both indomethacin and PGE_2, being equivalent to the control group untreated. These data suggested that PGE_2 formed in endometrium on Day 4 of pregnant mouse was very likely to be one of the compounds necessary for implantation.

1523 MALE INFERTILITY AS A RESULT OF DEFICIENCIES IN ACROSOMAL ENZYMES.

J. Langlais*, A. Chapdelaine, G. Bleau and K.D. Roberts. Maisonneuve-Rosemont Research Center and University of Montreal (Quebec), Canada.

The presence of a normal acrosome is essential for fertilization. Several cases of male infertility as a result of acrosomal defects have been evaluated in our clinic. Of special interest, two cases of round-headed spermatozoa have been investigated. This rare type of teratospermia is associated with a lack of the acrosome and patients with this defect are reputed to be infertile. In each case, artificial insemination with donor semen resulted in pregnancies. Semen analysis showed a normal sperm count with low motility. Scanning and transmission electron microscopy revealed a spherical shape in all of the spermatozoa. A complete lack of acrosomal matrix was also observed. In some instances, intracellular membrane remnants were found. The complete absence of acrosomal contents was corroborated biochemically by the failure to detect any appreciable amounts of acrosin by spectrophotometric analysis. Some evidence for the presence of proteolytic activity was observed by digestion of casein-agar gels. Moreover, phospholipase A_2 activity was extremely low in both cases (assay based on sperm phospholipase A_2-induced hemolysis). These results were compared with the zona-free hamster ova penetration assay. In both cases, no penetration of the vitelli was observed, an observation which is in good agreement with the low levels of phospholipase A_2 and the absence of the acrosome, both of which are implicated in the fertilization process.

(Supported by the MRC, FRSQ, FCAC).

1524 INTRANASAL LH-RH CHRONIC AND PULSATILE ADMINISTRATION IN NORMOGONADOTROPIC IDIOPATHIC OLIGOSPERMIA.

O. Levalle*, N. Aparicio, R.Fiszbein, N. Pacenza, A. Guitelman. Servicio de Endocrinología. Hosp. Alvarez. Aranguren 2701, Bs. As. Argentine.

The aim of this study was to evaluate the therapeutical response of infertile men with idiopathic normogonadotropic oligoasthenospermia (INO) to a chronic treatment with LH-RH intranasally administered. Fourteen men with long lasting infertility ($>$3 years) considered with INO based on at least 3 previous spermograms($<$ 20.0x10^6 sperm/ml; $<$30% forwardly progressive spermatozoa), normal LH, FSH, prolactine and testosterone (T) levels and absence of other abnormalities were incorporated. All of them were treated with LH-RH nasal spray 6 shots per day during 90 days (200 ug per shot). Control spermograms were performed monthly during treatment. Eight patients performed spermograms up to 90 days after treatment. Before and at the end of treatment it was studied the LH and FSH response to LH-RH administration.

The LH response was significant and sustained after the initial shots. No decay of this response was observed after treatment (area under curve ($\bar{x}$ $\pm$ SE): LH Pre 46.9$\pm$10.8; post 41.9$\pm$4.5 and FSH Pre 23.9$\pm$4.1; post 22.3$\pm$2.4 mUI.h/ml). T levels before and after treatment were similar ($\bar{x}\pm$SE)(3.3 $\pm$0.4 and 3.4$\pm$0.3 ng/ml respectively). Five patients (35.7%) experienced a normalization of sperm count and motility at the end or after LH-RH treatment. Other 4 patients experienced significant improvements without achieving normalization. In 6 patients the response was nil. Pregnancy was achieved by 3 patients. LH-RH by intranasal application could be a useful alternative for patients with INO. Pituitary exhaustion was not evident in these patients after 3 months of treatment.

1525 PREGNANCY ESTABLISHMENT AND MAINTENANCE IN THE ABSENCE OF OVARIAN FUNCTION.
P. Lutjen*, A. Trounson, J. Leeton, J. Findlay+ and C. Wood, Dept. Obstetrics/Gynaecology, Monash University, Queen Victoria Medical Centre and MRC Prince Henry's Hospital+, Melbourne, Australia, 3000.

A cyclic regimen of oestradiol-17β(E2) and progesterone (P4) designed to mimic endogenous steroid production throughout the normal ovulatory cycle has been used in women with premature ovarian failure. This sequential steroid replacement produces histological changes in the uterine endometrium and results in plasma oestradiol and progesterone levels consistent with a normal ovulatory cycle. Utilizing techniques of in vitro fertilization and embryo transfer, a donated oocyte fertilized by the recipient's husband was transferred to one of these women on the 16th day of her third treatment cycle. Pregnancy was confirmed 10 days post-transfer by normal changes in human chorionic gonadotrophin. The dose of oestradiol valerate and progesterone was altered to maintain the patient's peripheral plasma levels of E2 and P4 within the normal range for pregnancy. Oestrogen and progesterone therapy were withdrawn at 12 and 19 weeks of gestation, respectively. Minimal changes were observed in plasma 17α-hydroxyprogesterone around the time of embryo transfer. The absence of a functional corpus luteum and primordial follicles at delivery and HLA-typing of the infant confirmed that the baby originated from the donated oocyte and that the pregnancy had been maintained by exogenous hormones. These results show that embryo donation and steroid replacement can be used successfully for the treatment of human infertility due to primary ovarian failure.

1526 HLA ANTIGENS IN KOREAN PATIENTS WITH JUVENILE-ONSET INSULIN-DEPENDENT DIABETES MELLITUS.
H.C. Lee*, K.B. Huh and S.Y. Lee, Department of Internal Medicine, Yonsei University College of Medicine, Seoul, Korea

Specific allelic associations vary among ethnic groups. We studied the distribution of HLA-A, -B, -C and -DR antigens in 33 Korean patients with insulin-dependent diabetes mellitus (IDDM) and compared the frequencies with those in the control population (HLA-A, -B and -C, 86 and -DR, 68 cases). HLA typing for the A,B,C and DR antigens was performed by the standard microcytotoxicity test. The incidence of HLA-Bw54 was significantly increased ($P < 0.005$, relative risk 6.5) in the IDDM group (24.2%) as compared with controls (4.7%). There was no difference in the incidence of Bw22 in IDDM patients (24.2%) and the controls (11.6%). HLA-A26 was significantly decreased in patients with IDDM ($P < 0.05$). The remaining HLA-A, -B and -C alleles did not demonstrate significant differences in the frequencies between the patient and control populations. Although the data suggest the increasing tendencies in the frequencies of HLA-DR3 (15.1 versus 5.9%) and -DR4 (57.6 versus 36.8%) in the patient population, these differences were not statistically significant. DR2 was decreased in the diabetics (9.1%) as compared with controls (26.5%) without statistical significance. It is concluded that the pattern of HLA and diabetes association in Korean diabetics might appear to be different from that in most other racial groups. There is, however, a need to further study larger numbers of diabetics and control population so that a clearer picture may emerge.

1527 CARBOHYDRATE METABOLISM IN GLUCAGONIMMUNIZED RABBITS.

V. Maier*, A. Haas, D. Grube[1)], A. Greischel and E.F. Pfeiffer.
Center of Internal Medicine, University of Ulm and Dept. of Anatomy, University of Hannover[1)], Germany.

Pancreatic glucagon is a poor antigen. In order to raise antibodies rabbits have to be immunized for at least 8 months. In glucagon immunized rabbits the pancreas and carbohydrate metabolism was investigated:
a) By immunocytochemistry and electron microscopy glucagon-, insulin- and somatostatin-producing cells were investigated ("PAP"-method). In the islets of immunized animals the number of A-cells was increased from 24 % to 66 %. The number of B-cells was diminished from 70 % to only 28 %. A-cells showed ultrastructural features of increased cellular activities.
b) Although the number of B-cells is dramatically reduced tolerance tests do not yet show a diabetic state. There is a tendency to increased hypoglycemia after a glibenclamide load.
Conclusions: Antibodies (titer 1 : 4000) circulating in longtime immunized rabbits appear to neutralize endogenous glucagon. The increased cellular activities in the A-cells support the hypothesis of an autocrine regulation. If immunization is continued the ratio of B-/A-cells might be shifted more and offer a new model of diabetic animals.
Supported by Deutsche Forschungsgemeinschaft, Bonn - Bad Godesberg, SFB 87/G 3.

1528 INTRANASAL AEROSOLIZED INSULIN: COMPARISON OF THE PHARMACOKINETICS AND BIOACTIVITY WITH INTRAVENOUS INSULIN IN NORMAL AND DIABETIC SUBJECTS.

J.E. Manson*, G. Griffing, R. Salzman, E. Stoltz, J. Armstrong, A. McCall, N.B. Ruderman, and J.C. Melby, Evans Memorial Department of Clinical Research and the Department of Medicine, University Hospital and Boston University School of Medicine, Boston, Massachusetts 02118.

Aerosolized insulin can be absorbed across the nasal mucosa and lower plasma glucose levels in man. To examine the pharmacodynamics and relative bioactivity of intranasal insulin (INI), fasting normals (n=4) and type I diabetics (n=8) received either placebo or INI (0.1, 0.5, 1.0, or 1.5 U/kg) or intravenous insulin (IVI)(0.01, 0.05, 0.1, or 0.15 U/kg). Plasma insulin (I) and glucose (G) were measured over several hours. All normals responded to 0.5 U/kg and diabetics to 1.0 U/kg INI; smaller doses produced a less consistent effect. As shown in the table, approximately 10 times more INI than IVI had to be given to produce a similar decrement in G. In normals, plasma G returned toward baseline within 60-120 minutes following both IVI and INI; in contrast, in diabetics plasma G was still depressed after four hours. These data indicate that nasal insulin is rapidly absorbed and can improve glucose regulation in Type I diabetics. They suggest that investigation of INI's therapeutic efficacy is warranted.

		0	30	60	120	240	Insulin $T_{\frac{1}{2}}$ (min)	IVI:INI Dose Ratio
Normal	INI (1.0 U/kg)	84	43	46	68	ND	8	1:12
	IVI (0.1 U/kg)	82	23	57	77	ND	5	
Diabetic	INI (1.0 U/kg)	247	198	141	122	121	25	1:9
	IVI (0.1 U/kg)	212	120	106	127	128	11	

1529 GLUCAGON AND OTHER COUNTERREGULATORY HORMONE RESPONSES TO INSULIN-INDUCED HYPOGLYCEMIA IN TOTALLY PANCREATECTOMIZED PATIENTS. T. Matsuyama*, H.Horie, M. Namba, K. Nonaka, S. Tarui, A. Yamatodani and H. Wada, The Second Department of Internal Medicine and The Second Department of Pharmacology, Osaka University Medical School, Osaka 553, Japan.

Totally pancreatectomized patients (Px) easily fall into severe hypoglycemia during insulin therapy. We measured plasma levels of glucagon, epinephrine (E), norepinephrine (NE), cortisol and growth hormone (GH) during insulin-induced hypoglycemia to clarify the role of hormonal responses in recovery from hypoglycemia in Px. Six normal subjects and four Px (well controlled by multiple insulin injection or continuous subcutaneous insulin infusion) were given 0.15~0.2 U/kg of iv Actrapid insulin after overnight fast. Blood samples were obtained at every 10 min for 90 min. Plasma glucose fell from 88.7±2.0 to 29.7±5.0 mg/dl at 30 min and returned to 67.7±6.2 mg/dl at 90 min in normal subjects. In Px, glucose fell from 79.5±5.8 to 18.2±4.9 mg/dl at 40 min and did not rise until glucose or glucagon was given. Glucagon, measured by specific radioimmunoassay for C-terminal of glucagon, rose 29.2±6.7 to 83.7±12.2 pg/ml at 40 min in normal subjects, whereas glucagon, probably of gastric origin in Px, did not change significantly from 30.5±2.9 pg/ml. E and NE, determined by a novel, sensitive catecholamine analyzing system, rose both in normal subjects (E: 43±8 to 732±102 pg/ml, NE: 186±52 to 338±43 pg/ml at 40 min) and in Px (E: 27±3 to 899±289 pg/ml, NE: 229±43 to 744±313 pg/ml at 70 min). Cortisol and GH also rose in normal subjects and Px. So, we can conclude that not catecholamine but glucagon response is essential to recover from hypoglycemia.

1530 DIRECT EFFECT OF INSULIN ON THE ABUNDANCE OF TYROSINE AMINOTRANSFERASE (TAT) MESSENGER RNA IN RAT HEPATOMA CELLS IN CULTURE. J.L. Messina*, J. Larner and J. Hamlin, University of Virginia School of Medicine, Charlottesville, Virginia, USA, 22908.

Tyrosine aminotransferase, a liver specific enzyme, accounts for 0.03% of the total hepatic cytosolic protein content. Insulin stimulated the synthesis of TAT in liver as well as in cultured H4IIEC3 hepatoma cells, a clonal derivative of Reuber H35 cells. Insulin stimulation of TAT synthesis is associated with an increase in the TAT-mRNA as measured by in vitro translation of total poly(A)$^+$RNA. However, insulin also increases the overall efficiency of translation. The purpose of the present study was to explore the direct effects of insulin on the amount of hybridizable TAT-mRNA using a cDNA for TAT. H4IIEC3 cells were grown to subconfluence, were exposed to insulin for varying times, and total RNA was purified by centrifugation through cesium chloride after disruption with guanidine isothiocyanate. Total RNA was electrophoresed on agarose-formaldehyde gels and transfered to nitrocellulose. Specific hybridization of ^{32}P-labelled TAT-cDNA to the RNA samples was measured by autoradiography. Insulin (5 x 10^{-9} M) added directly to the monolayer cultures increased TAT-mRNA by 2-5 fold after 1 hr at 37°. This effect was maximal at 1-2 hr after insulin addition and was followed by a gradual decrease in the amount of TAT-mRNA by 6 hr. The effect was dose-dependent, with small increases observed at 1 x 10^{-12}M insulin. Increasing concentrations of insulin did not change the time-course of the accumulation of TAT-mRNA suggesting a rate limiting step in the induction of TAT-mRNA. Our data indicate that insulin has a rapid and direct effect on the amount of TAT-mRNA and suggests that insulin alone can stimulate transcription of the TAT gene.

1531 HIGH PREVALENCE OF AUTOIMMUNE THYROID DISEASE IN INSULIN-DEPENDENT DIABETES MELLITUS WITH PERSISTING ISLET CELL ANTIBODY S. Miyake*, K. Toyama, Y. Yamaguchi, A. Takahashi, Y. Ueda, N. Kuriya, Y. Ikeda and S. Nagataki The First Department of Internal Medicine, Nagasaki University, Nagasaki 852, Japan

It is well known that islet cell antibody (ICA) is transient in most patients with insulin-dependent diabetes mellitus(IDDM), but ICA generally persists for many years in patients with polyendocrine disease. In the present study, the incidence of autoimmune disease was investigated in IDDM who had ICA for more than 1 year after the onset of diabetes. ICA was determined by our method using peroxidase-labeled protein A. In brief, fresh frozen sections of human pancreas and serum samples were incubated and treated with peroxidase-labeled Protein A. Treated sections were then reacted with diaminobenzidine. Anti-thyroid microsomal(TMA) and anti-thyroglobulin(TA) antibodies were determined using commercial kits (Fuji zoki Ltd.). Among 10 patients with IDDM, in whom ICA was detected for more than 1 year, 8 patients had TMA and 5 of them had clinical hyperthyroidism and one had chronic thyroiditis. None of them showed positive TA. One had been diagnosed as having hyperthyroidism prior to the onset of IDDM and the remaining 4 acquired hyperthyroidism at the time of onset of IDDM or within the second years after IDDM was diagnosed. Among 6 patients with autoimmune thyroid disease, 4 developed IDDM after 25 years old. In 27 ICA negative patients with IDDM, none showed abnormal thyroid function during follow up period. although 4 of them had TMA. These results indicate that persistence of ICA is associated with high prevalence of clinical autoimmune thyroid disease.

1532 DECREASED CAMP RESPONSE TO GLUCAGON IN NON-OBESE TYPE II DIABETIC PATIENTS WITH MACROANGIOPATHY. H.Miyakoshi*,I.Miyamoto,K.Ohsawa,Y.Nishimura,A.Sanada,T.Yamamoto,Y.Noto and N.Hattori. First Department of Internal Medicine, Faculty of Medicine,Kanazawa University,Kanazawa,Ishikawa,Japan.

Although it is well known that cAMP inhibits replication of many different cell lines and cGMP has opposite actions to cAMP,it is not clear whether these cyclic nucleotides have any clinical significance in the progress of atherosclerosis.To elucidate the interrelationships between plasma cyclic nucleotides levels and diabetic macroangiopathy,cyclic nucleotides responses to glucagon were investigated in 16 non-obese type II diabetic patients(6 patients with macroangiopathy-M+,10 patients without macroangiopathy-M-) and 10 normal controls.Macroangiopathy was regarded as positive when one of the following findings were detected; 1)aortic wall calcification on chest X-ray film,2)ischemic ST-T changes on ECG,3)impalpable pedal artery.After an overnight fast,glucagon(100μg) was injected intravenously and venous samples were obtained at 0,5,10 and 15 minutes for cAMP,cGMP, blood glucose,IRI and IRG(only basal) estimations.Basal levels of cyclic nucleotides were similar among M+,M- and control groups.CGMP showed no response after glucagon injection in the 3 groups.However, cAMP response to glucagon was significantly lower at 5 minutes in diabetic patients than in controls.Interestingly,the response of cAMP to glucagon was significantly lower at 5 and 15 minutes in M+ than in M-.There were no significant differences between M+ and M- in age,%obesity,degree of diabetic microangiopathy,renal function,blood glucose,IRI and IRG levels.These results suggest that decreased cAMP response to glucagon may have some clinical significance in the progress of diabetic macroangiopathy.

1533 POSSIBLE RACIAL DIFFERENCES IN IMMUNOLOGICAL CHARACTERISTICS OF INSULIN DEPENDENT DIABETES MELLITUS AMONG ASIAN POPULATIONS.

M. Miyano*, K. Nanjo, R. Sowa, K. Okai, Y. Nomura, T. Sanke, M. Kondo, K. Miyamura, R. Miyashita, K. Kashii[1], A. Kawa[2], M. Nakazawa[3], R. Fernando[4] and A. Vichayanrat[5], Dept. of Medicine and Paediatrics, Wakayama Medical School, Wakayama 640[1], Kyorin University, Tokyo 181[2], Nakazawa DM Clinic, Kagoshima 890, Japan[3], Mary Johnston Hospital, Manila 734, Philippines[4] and Dept. of Medicine, Mahidol University, Bangkok 7, Thailand[5].

To clarify possible racial differences in immunological characteristics of insulin dependent diabetes mellitus (IDDM) among Asian populations, the incidences of islet cell surface antibodies (ICSA) and anti-thyroid microsomal antibodies (ATMA) were examined in 119 IDDM patients (73 Japanese, 20 Thai and 26 Filipino) and 189 healthy controls (90 Japanese, 45 Thai and 54 Filipino).

The incidences of ICSA and ATMA in the patients were significantly higher than those in the respective controls. In Japanese patients the duration dependent decrease of the incidences was observed, while this was not the case in Thai and Filipino patients. Thus the incidences of ICSA and ATMA in Thai and Filipino patients with a longer duration were significantly higher than those in Japanese patients with a longer duration.

These results indicate that 1) autoimmunity found in IDDM is not specific for islet antigens, and 2) in Japanese the autoimmunity is transient, while in Thai and Filipino the autoimmunity is persistent. The latter findings strongly suggest that there exist racial differences in immunological characteristics of IDDM among Asian populations.

1534 VALIDATION OF MEASUREMENT OF NONSTEADY POST-HEPATIC INSULIN APPEARANCE IN THE DOG: A NEW NONINVASIVE METHOD FOR DETERMINATION OF HEPATIC INSULIN EXTRACTION. T. Morishima*, C. Bradshaw, and J. Radziuk. Depts. of Medicine and Physiology, University of Western Ontario, London, Ont and Dept. of Biochemistry, University of Geneva, Geneva.

The rate of post-hepatic insulin appearance (Ra) was determined using a constant infusion of B1-[H^3-Phe]-insulin and two-compartment analysis. To verify the calculations, unlabelled insulin was infused into 4 overnight-fasted dogs at continuously variable rates up to 250 mU/min. Somatostatin (0.6 ug/kg-min) was infused to suppress endogenous insulin production. Normoglycemia was maintained with a glucose infusion. Plasma levels of immunoreactive (IRI) and H^3-insulin were measured after initial purification on a C-18 column. IRI varied between 5 and 930 uU/ml. Over this range the fractional disappearance rate of insulin (k) changed from basal (0.198 ± 0.040 min^{-1}) to a minimum of 54.5% below basal. The regression line for $\bar{k}$ as % of basal was 94.8-0.0625xIRI, under these nonsteady state conditions. The system is therefore highly nonlinear. To asses the matching of the calculated Ra to the rate of insulin infusion, the absolute value of the area between the curves was determined as a fraction of the area under the infusion curve and was $10.5 \pm 2.2\%$. Our previous work (Diabetes 32: 41A,1983) showed that prehepatic insulin secretion could be calculated to the same degree of accuracy using C-peptide levels and mathematical deconvolution. CONCLUSIONS: Both post and prehepatic insulin secretion can be calculated within a 10% error. Subtraction yields a continuous noninvasive determination of the first-pass hepatic uptake of insulin. (Supported by MRC Canada)

1535 PARTIAL REVERSAL OF THE DECREASED HEPATIC mRNA FOR α_{2u} GLOBULIN IN DIABETIC RATS WITH THYROXINE. C.V.R. Murty, W.F. Demyan, B. Chatterjee and A. K. Roy*, Oakland University, Rochester, MI 48063, U.S.A.

Experimental diabetes causes about 90% reduction in the hepatic concentration of the mRNA for α_{2u} globulin within the total hepatic mRNA population (Roy et al., J.B.C. 255, 11614, 1980). Hypoinsulinemic diabetes results in both decreased level of circulating T_3 and the hepatic T_3 receptor (Gonzalez et al., Endo. 107, 2099, 1980). In order to elucidate the contributory role of thyroxine in the diminution of hepatic mRNA for α_{2u} globulin, we have examined the possible stimulatory role of this hormone in α_{2u} globulin synthesis in streptozotocin diabetic rats. Hepatic concentration of α_{2u} globulin was determined by RIA, α_{2u} globulin mRNA was quantitated both by *in vitro* translation assay and by molecular hybridization with a cloned cDNA probe. The rates of synthesis of α_{2u} globulin and its mRNA were performed by pulse labeling and by nuclear run off experiments, respectively. Results show that thyroxine (1.5 μg/100 g, daily for 8 days) can increase the rate of synthesis of hepatic α_{2u} globulin by about 8 fold over the diabetic control. Thyroxine mediated increase of α_{2u} globulin synthesis in the diabetic rat also correlated with corresponding increases in the hepatic concentration of α_{2u} globulin mRNA and its rate of synthesis as judged from the results of nuclear run off experiments. Despite this stimulatory effect, thyroxine was only 33% as effective as insulin in reversing the hepatic concentration of α2u mRNA in the diabetic rat. These results, therefore, underscore the complex interacting influence of various hormones in the multihormonal regulation of α2u globulin. Supported by grants from NIH (AKR) and ADA (BC).

1536 ERYTHROCYTE SODIUM,POTASSIUM PUMP IN DIABETIC PATIENTS AND EFFECT OF INSULIN ON Na^+,K^+-ATPase. S.Nagamatsu*[1] S.Murakawa[1] N.Inoue[2] Y.Hayashi[2] and H. Matsui[2] 3rd Dept.of Internal Medicine[1] and Dept.of Biochemistry[2] Kyorin University School of Medicine, Shinkawa, Mitaka, Tokyo Japan

It has been reported that the metabolic abnormalities in diabetes affect the erythrocyte deformability and membrane fluidity. While recent studies have characterized the changes of Na^+,K^+-ATPase on erythrocyte in obesity and thyroid disease, little work has been done concerning the enzyme in diabetes. Therefore we have measured the number of Na pump(=Na^+,K^+-ATPase) on erythrocyte by ^3H-ouabain binding and the activity of pump by ouabain inhibitable ^{42}K or ^{43}K uptake and the turnover rate has been calculated. Furthermore we have studied the effect of insulin on Na^+,K^+-ATPase in both membrane preparations and intact cells. The maximal ouabain binding(Bmax) was 335 ± 47(n=17) site/cell in control and 342 ± 120(n=14) in diabetics. There were not significant differencese between two groups, though, large variation was observed in diabetics. The maximal velocity of K^+ influx(Vmax) in diabetics was slightly higher(197 ± 53 nmol/hr/10^9cell,n=9) compaired with Vmax in control(159 ± 17,n=10; $p<0.05$), but the turnover rate was not significantly different between control(2445 ± 480 /min,n=10) and diabetics(3040 ± 955,n=9). Addition of insulin 10^{-7}M *in vitro* to the erythrocytes from control and diabetic groups revealed no effect on the number of ouabain binding and K^+ uptake. Insulin had no effect on both Na^+,K^+-ATPase in erythrocyte ghosts and the purified one from canine kidneys. The present data suggests that insulin has no direct effects on human erythrocyte Na^+,K^+-ATPase.

1537 GELSOLIN, A Ca^{2+}-SENSITIVE ACTIN-BINDING PROTEIN IN A HAMSTER INSULIN-SECRETING CELL LINE. T Yap Nelson* and A E Boyd III, Department of Medicine, Baylor College of Medicine, Houston, Texas, USA.

A transient, Ca^{2+}-dependent solation of the actin cytoskeletal network is postulated to be necessary for the recruitment of insulin-containing granules to the plasma membrane. Gelsolin is a 90 kDa protein which binds to the rapidly growing, barbed end of actin filaments and controls the rate of actin polymerization in vitro. The objective of this study was to isolate this protein from an insulin-secreting (HIT) cell line and compare the immunologic properties and peptide maps with gelsolin obtained from rabbit macrophages and human platelets. DNase I-Sepharose retains HIT cell actin-binding proteins in 1mM $CaCl_2$; the 90 kDa protein is eluted with 5 mM EGTA. The remaining actin-binding proteins are then eluted using a buffer containing SDS. The Coomassie-stained gel of EGTA peak fractions showed two major protein bands with M_r = 90 and 42 kDa, suggesting that a 90 kDa protein-actin complex was eluted from the DNase I-Sepharose column. Specific antibodies to human platelet and rabbit macrophage gelsolins (antibodies and gelsolin preparations were generous gifts of Drs J Bryan and H Yin) identified the 90 kDa bands in the EGTA eluate, but did not cross-react with other actin-binding proteins in the SDS fraction. Tryptic peptide maps of radioiodinated HIT 90 kDa protein, human platelet and rabbit macrophage gelsolins were compared and the autoradiographic maps of the 3 proteins are indistinguishable. The HIT cell, platelet and macrophage gelsolins share antigenic determinants as well as considerable homology in primary sequence and must be closely related if not identical. Thus, gelsolin is found in HIT cells as well as macrophages and platelets and may link a transient increase in Ca^{2+} cellular levels with actin polymerization.

1538 MOLECULAR CLONING OF TRIIODOTHYRONINE RESPONSIVE RAT LIVER mRNAs AND STUDY OF THEIR NONCOORDINATE REGULATION. M.A. Magnuson* and V.M. Nikodem, NIADDK, NIH, Bethesda, MD, USA 20205.

In order to study the factor(s) responsible for the pre-translational regulation of rat liver mRNAs by the thyroid hormones we have sought cDNA clones for these T_3 regulated genes. A cDNA library was constructed with poly(A)$^+$ RNA obtained from animals treated with T_3 and fed a high carbohydrate diet. This library was screened by differential hybridization with probes made from hypothyroid and hyperthyroid liver RNA. Eight different clones were obtained and studied further. The corresponding mRNA size for each clone was determined by Northern blotting. The response of hypothyroid animals to a receptor saturating dose of T_3 (200 µg/100 g BW) for times from 0 to 48 hours and steady state levels for animals at different thyroidal and dietary states was examined by hybridization assay. We found delays in induction from less than 4 to greater than 24 hours and in levels of induction from several to about 30 fold. There was no necessary correlation in the level of induction by T_3 and in that by a high carbohydrate diet. Unique responses for various thyroidal and dietary states were found for each clone. Two cDNAs corresponding to mRNAs of 2300 and 1300 nucleotides were determined by hybrid-selected translation to code for proteins of 46 and 27 kD, respectively. We conclude that the marked differences in the kinetics of induction of the various clones by T_3 and the unique responses with regards to the estimated nuclear occupancy suggests different factors are involved in the regulation of separate liver mRNAs by T_3.

1539 EFFECTS OF PROGESTINS ON 5α-REDUCTASE (5αR) ACTIVITY OF PUBIC SKIN FIBROBLASTS (PSF). E. Melanitou*, M.C. Portois, I. Mowszowicz. The Population Council, New York, New York and Department of Biochemistry, Pitre'-Salpetriere, Paris, France.

Androgen induced 5αR activity in PSF, can be inhibited by cyproterone acetate (CPA). However, CPA alone is also capable of inducing 5αR acitivity. This prompted us to study the effects of other progestins on 5αR activity of PSF. Steroids were added to cultures containing 5% fetal calf serum (FCS) and 5αR activity was measured 72 h later by incubating intact cell monolayers with ^{3}H-testosterone and chromatography of the metabolites. CPA or medroxyprogesterone acetate (MPA) (10^{-7} M) stimulated 5αR to the same extent as dihydrotestosterone (DHT) at the same dose. However maximal response was obtained with MPA or CPA at a concentration of 2×10^{-9} M, while DHT required 10^{-7} M for peak stimulation. By contrast, progesterone (P) or promegestone (R5020) had no effect. The fact that the effect of CPA, MPA was suppressed by actinomycine D (1 ug/ml, 19h) suggests that the action of these steroids is mediated by RNA synthesis. To further elucidate the mechanism of this induction, we studied the effect of CPA and MPA on 3 cell strains of PSF derived from patients with the complete form of the testicular feminisation syndrome (TF) and lacking androgen receptor (AR). Both CPA and MPA were capable of stimulating 5αR in these cells, indicating that this effect was not mediated by the AR. We conclude from these studies that some progestins are capable of stimulating 5αR in PSF by a mechanism independent of AR.

1540 LHRH AND PROSTAGLANDIN $F_{2\alpha}$ BUT NOT PGE_2 STIMULATE PHOSPHATIDIC ACID-PHOSPHATIDYLINOSITOL TURNOVER IN RAT OVARIAN CELLS. T. Minegishi*, J. Sun and P.C.K. Leung, Dept. of Ob/Gyn. and of Physiology, University of British Columbia, Vancouver, Canada.

We have demonstrated previously that LHRH and $PGF_{2\alpha}$ causes acute alterations in phospholipid turnover in the rat corpus luteum. In the present study, granulosa cells and luteal cells were prepared from immature female rats treated with 4 IU PMSG or with PMSG and hCG, respectively. After 3 days in culture, the cells were incubated for 20 min in the presence of ^{32}P orthophosphate (200 μCi/ml). In both granulosa and luteal cells, addition of 1 μM LHRH stimulated ($p<0.01$) the incorporation of radioactivity into phosphatidic acid (PA) and phosphatidylinositol (PI) but not phosphatidylcholine (PC), phosphatidylethanolamine (PE) or phosphatidylserine (PS). During a 10 or 20 min incubation period, addition of 1 μM $PGF_{2\alpha}$ to either cell culture also caused specific increases in ^{32}P labeling of PA and PI ($p<0.05$), although $PGF_{2\alpha}$ was slightly less effective than LHRH in granulosa cells. In contrast, 1 μM PGE_2, LH or FSH (1 μg/ml) failed to affect ^{32}P incorporation into the various phospholipid fractions in either cell type ($p>0.05$). The time-course of the stimulation of PA-PI turnover by $PGF_{2\alpha}$ was remarkably similar to that of LHRH. Addition of 2 mM dibutyryl cAMP or 5 mM 8-bromo-cAMP to luteal cells markedly attenuated the LHRH or $PGF_{2\alpha}$-induced PA-PI labeling. These data further support the hypothesis that LHRH and $PGF_{2\alpha}$ (but perhaps not PGE_2) share a common mechanism in ovarian cells involving acidic phospholipid metabolism. (Supported by the BCHCRF and the MRC of Canada)

1541 QUANTITATIVE AND QUALITATIVE ANALYSYS OF RAT LIVER MALIC ENZYME IN ALTERED THYROID STATES. T. Mitsuhashi*, K. Kubota, N. Kuzuya, H. Ikeda and H. Uchimura, Third Department of Internal Medicine, University of Tokyo, Hongo, Tokyo, Japan.

It is recognized that T_3 affects the quantity of rat liver malic enzyme(ME), but little is known about its qualitative effects. This study was done to see whether T_3 exerts a qualitative change in ME. Adult male Wistar rats were used in 3 groups: intact; thyroidex on low I diets ; thyroidex + T_3(100μg/d/100 g BWt) 7d. Liver homogenates were centrifuged 100,000 xg and photometric and specific RI assays for ME were done and remainder of supernatants was salted out ($(NH_4)_2SO_4$). Precipitates were purified with affinity chromatography, gel filtration and ion exchange chromatography. ME properties in the 3 groups were determined by mol wt, electrophoresis, kinetic and immunological studies. ME activity measured by photometric assays and ME concentrations determined by specific RIA were significantly lower in hypothyroid and markedly increased in hyperthyroid rats compared to normals. No differences were found in enzyme specific activities or kinetic activities among the 3 groups. Isoelectric focusing(IEF) patterns of ME in all groups were generally similar; however, zymograms of ME demonstrated some differences in microheterogeneity among the groups. Mol wt of ME was found to be 242 K by light scattering photometry and 61 K by SDS-PAGE, and again, no differences were noted in the 3 groups. In conclusion, no major qualitative differences in liver ME were observed in hypothyroid, normal and hyperthyroid rats and some differences in microheterogeneity among the groups were noted with IEF.

1542 ACTIONS OF ANDROGENS AND FOLLICLE-STIMULATING HORMONE ON PROGESTERONE METABOLISM BY RAT GRANULOSA CELLS IN VITRO. Y.S. Moon*, A. Duleba and H. Takahashi, Department of Obstetrics and Gynaecology, University of British Columbia, Vancouver, B.C. V6H 3V5, Canada.

The present study was designed to investigate the mechanisms underlying the stimulatory effect of FSH and androgens on progesterone accumulation by rat granulosa cells. The cells (2.5×10^5 cells/ml) were cultured for 24 h with or without testosterone (T, 0.5 μM), 5α-dihydrotestosterone (DHT, 0.5 μM) and/or follicle-stimulating hormone (FSH, 1 μg/ml). Subsequently, the cells were washed and reincubated for 3 h with [4-^{14}C] progesterone (0.5 nmol/ml, 56 mCi/mmol). Androgens significantly decreased the utilization of radiolabeled progesterone by 18-31% both in the presence and absence of FSH. FSH alone did not alter progesterone utilization nor modulate the androgen stimulated effect. The major metabolites of progesterone were 20α-hydroxy-4-pregnen-3-one, 3α-hydroxy-5α-pregnan-20-one, and 5α-pregnane-3α,20α-diol. The conversion to 20α-hydroxy-4-pregnen-3-one was decreased by 18 to 54% with androgens and/or FSH. The conversion to 3α-hydroxy-5α-pregnan-20-one was increased by 24 to 69% with both androgens and FSH. The conversion to 5α-pregnane-3α,20α-diol was increased 51% by FSH and decreased 29% by T. Androgens and FSH or DHT alone had no effect on 5α-pregnane-3α,20α-diol accumulation. The present results indicate that androgens and FSH modulate progesterone metabolism by decreasing 20α-hydroxysteroid dehydrogenase and by increasing 5α-reductase activities.
This study was supported by the MRC and the BCHCRF.

1543 DEXAMETHASONE INHIBITION OF NON-INSULIN STIMULATED GLUCOSE TRANSPORT IN 3T3-L1 FIBROBLASTS.

D. K. Murray* and D. H. Nelson, Departments of Anatomy and Medicine, University of Utah, Salt Lake City, Utah, USA.

Dexamethasone is well known to inhibit insulin stimulation of glucose transport (GT). Studies were undertaken to determine whether GT stimulated by cholesterol, or other factors, is also inhibited by dexamethasone. 3T3-L1 fibroblasts were incubated with or without insulin or the exogenous lipids, cholesterol (Chol), phosphatidylcholine (PC), or phosphatidylethanolamine (PE) in concentrations of 1 mg/ml for four hours. The cells were washed, and GT was then determined using (^{14}C)2-deoxy-glucose. Chol or PC treatment increased GT significantly over control values ($P<0.01$), but PE did not. Insulin (IN) stimulation of GT with or without the above lipids was significantly different from controls ($P<0.001$), but not from the lipids alone. Treatment of the cells with Dex (10^{-7}M) increased sphingomyelin (Sph) and Chol membrane content ($P<0.05$) and also inhibited IN stimulated GT in these cells ($P<0.01$). Dex blocked Chol stimulated GT (which was 96% over controls) completely if the cells were preincubated for 24 hours with the hormone ($P<0.001$). These studies confirm the finding that lipids added to the cell membrane can directly influence GT. Dex inhibition of the effect is further evidence that membrane lipids are involved in the regulation of GT. The action of Dex to increase plasma membrane Sph and Chol and also to alter the effects of exogenously added lipids on GT, suggests that corticosteroids have the capacity to reorder membrane lipids to produce an effect on GT.

1544 HORMONAL REGULATION OF DNA POLYMERASE β IN ENDOCRINE ORGANS.

A. Nagasaka* S. Yoshida°, A. Nakai, T. Aono, T. Ohyama, H. Nakagawa and K. Iwase. Fujita-Gakuen Univ. School of Med. and Inst. for Deveropmental Res. Aichi Pref. Colony, Toyoake, Aichi 470-11, Japan.

We have shown that the activity of DNA polymerase β in rat adrenal gland was regulated by the level of ACTH (Endocrinology 111, 1345, 1982).

Here we extended our work to the thyroid and testis of hypophysectomized (hypox) rats. Crude extracts from thyroid glands and testes from hypox rats were assayed for DNA polymerase α, β and γ with poly(dA)·oligo$(dT)_{12-18}$, activated DNA and poly(rA)·oligo$(dT)_{12-18}$ as template-primers, respectively.

1 and 2 W after hypox, the activity of DNA polymerase β in rat testes decreased to 1/3 and 1/7 (per μg DNA) of the control in parallel with the decrease of serum testosterone. Furthermore, apparent molecular size of testicular DNA polymerase β increased by hypox; from 3.3 S to 4.5 S. These changes were similar to those observed with adrenal gland. On the other hand, the level of β-enzyme in the thyroid was affected by hypox only slightly, but the changes in its molecular size was also observed. These changes in either the activity level or the molecular weight were reversed by injections of LH and FSH or TSH. In contrast, DNA polymerase α and γ activities were relatively resistant to hypox.

These results suggest that DNA polymerase β in endocrine organs is generally regulated by pituitary hormones. It can be speculated that DNA polymerase β might play some role in the cell differentiation in endocrine organs.

1545 POST-TRANSCRIPTIONAL REGULATION OF A THYROID HORMONE RESPONSIVE GENE IN RAT LIVER.

P. Narayan and H.C. Towle*, Department of Biochemistry, University of Minnesota, Minneapolis, MN 55455.

Administration of triiodothyronine (T3) to a hypothyroid rat results in a rapid and dramatic increase in the level of hepatic mRNA coding for Spot 14 - a polypeptide with a Mr of 17000 and a pI of 4.9. To investigate the site of regulation by T3, the levels of nuclear precursor for Spot 14 mRNA following treatment of hypothyroid rats with T3 were measured. The nuclear precursor for Spot 14 mRNA was found to be present in increased amounts as early as 10 minutes following acute hormone administration, suggesting this gene may be regulated directly by the receptor-hormone interaction. This increase preceded the earliest detectable rise in mature mRNA. A 12- to 15-fold increase in the levels of both the nuclear precursor and cellular mRNA for Spot 14 was found in chronically treated hyperthyroid rats, compared to the hypothyroid controls. Thus, regulation of production of Spot 14 mRNA was due to some step leading to increased accumulation of the nuclear precursor and not to alterations in the rates of splicing, transport or cytoplasmic mRNA stability. Nuclear 'run off' experiments were performed to estimate relative rates of Spot 14 gene transcription. Following acute injection of T3, a transient increase of approximately 2-fold was found within 30 minutes. However, no further increases in the transcription rate occurred at later times following injection or in chronically hyperthyroid animals. Thus, increases in the transcription rate can only account for a small portion of the rise in Spot 14 mRNA levels. These data suggest that the regulation by T3 of this gene occurs by altering the nuclear stability of the mRNA precursor.

1546 CHARACTERIZATION OF A COMMON 43K PROTEIN INDUCED BY GLUCOCORTICOIDS IN MAMMALIAN CELLS AND TISSUE.

N. Nichols*, K. Tracy, M. McNally and J. Funder, Medical Research Centre, Prince Henry's Hospital, Melbourne, Australia 3004.

We have studied adrenal steroid effects on newly synthesized proteins in a variety of mammalian cells and tissues by high resolution 2-D gel electrophoresis and autoradiography. After treatment with steroids in vivo (20 µg/d for 5d post-adrenalectomy) or in vitro (10^{-7} M for 24h in the absence of fetal calf serum) and ^{35}S-methionine pulsing, we found a similar protein (M_r ∿43K, pI ∿6.5) to be invariantly (112/112) increased by dexamethasone in three rat tissues and eight human, bovine, and rat cell lines. The protein was constitutively synthesized in all tissues; densitometry showed a ∿2-fold induction by dexamethasone in all systems. Glucocorticoid-specific, but not sex steroids increased 43K synthesis. Preliminary characterization of 43K in human skin fibroblasts showed an effect on synthesis as early as 2h after steroid treatment with a maximal effect by 4h. Following 4h treatment and pulse, 43K was induced in all sub-cellular fractions; the highest specific activity of incorporation (∿3X) was found in the 20,000xg supernatant. Neither constitutive nor steroid-induced 43K was secreted into media after 4 or 24h exposure to steroid. The protein bound neither to concanavalin A nor lentil lectin; 2-D gel analysis of ^{32}P-labeled proteins showed that 43K is not a phosphoprotein in the presence of absence of dexamethasone. The nature of this ubiquitous glucocorticoid-induced 43K protein, and its possible physiological roles, remain to be established.

Supported by the National Health & Medical Research Council of Australia.

1547 EVIDENCE THAT GLUCOSE INDUCTION OF MALIC ENZYME mRNA IS MEDIATED BY A PRODUCT OF PYRUVATE OXIDATION. CN Mariash* and JH Oppenheimer, Division of Endocrinology and Metabolism, Department of Medicine, University of Minnesota, Minneapolis, MN 55455, USA

We have previously proposed that the induction of the mRNA for malic enzyme (ME) is mediated by a product of glucose metabolism. In order to identify the proximate stimulus, we have tested the possibility that induction is specifically related to pyruvate oxidation. To this end we compared the effect of glucose to chlorinated hydrocarbons known to stimulate pyruvate dehydrogenase (PDH); dichloroacetic acid (DCA), trichloroacetic acid (TCA), and 2-chloropropionic acid (CPA). In 6 day cultured hepatocytes we measured the level of ME activity and the activity of PDH by quantitating the generation of $^{14}CO_2$ from 1-^{14}C pyruvate. An excellent rank correlation was observed between ME formation and PDH activity. DCA was the most potent and CPA the least potent of the PDH activators. In addition, we determined the mRNA activity profile by 2D-gel electrophoresis of reticulocyte lysate translated products directed by mRNA obtained from cultured hepatocytes. A striking overlap in responses between DCA and glucose stimulation was apparent. Four out of 7 glucose stimulated changes were reproduced by DCA. Moreover, the mRNA for ME (Spot 2) was proportional to ME activity. Lastly, *in vivo* administration of DCA resulted in hepatic mRNA activity profiles similar to those produced by sucrose *in vivo* and by glucose and PDH activators *in vitro*. We conclude that pyruvate oxidation may generate the putative intermediate involved in the induction of ME mRNA and that DCA strikingly mimics the response of glucose at the genomic level.

1548 LIPOGENIC EFFECTS OF HYPOTHALAMIC EXTRACTS OBTAINED DURING SPONTANEOUS WEIGHT GAIN AND WEIGHT LOSS. R.B. Melnyk*and J.M. Martin, Research Institute, The Hospital for Sick Children, Toronto, M5G 1X8, Canada.

Partially purified hypothalamic extracts enhance lipogenesis in adipocytes. Material from fasted rats is more potent than that from fed donors. To determine whether hypothalamic concentrations of the active material vary with spontaneous changes in food intake and body weight, we studied dormice (*Glis glis*), hibernators showing two-month weight cycles when kept in 12 h light cycles and 23°C. Lab chow and water were available *ad lib*. 24-h fasted High (HF) and Low Food Intake (LF) animals were decapitated when they achieved intakes ⩾20 or ⩽ 5 g/day for 2-4 consecutive days, respectively. Noncycling (NC) dormice with relatively stable weights were also studied. The hypothalamus was homogenized and extracted at 4° with 0.1 M acetic acid. After filtration (Whatman #4) and centrifugation, the lyophilized supernatant was chromatographed using reverse phase HPLC (μ-Bondapack C-18 column, 25 min. linear gradient [25-100% MeOH + 0.1% TFA]). D-[2-^{3}H(N)] glucose incorporation into total lipid was measured in rat adipocytes incubated for 2 h at 37° in 2 ml KRBA-2% (pH 7.4) with 0.5 mM glucose (0.25 μCi/μmol), plus test fractions. In all three groups (HF, LF and NC), lipogenesis was characteristically enhanced by material eluting with the void volume (15, 23 and 27% relative maximal insulin stimulation, respectively). Lipogenic activity tended to be inversely correlated with food intake, suggesting a dissociation between insulin-mediated and hypothalamic effects on fat cell metabolism, but increased hypothalamic concentrations of the active principle could reflect reduced turnover during weight loss, since pancreatic insulin levels are also higher at this time. Supported by MRC (Canada).

1549 ARE CONVENTIONAL ISOTOPIC METHODS FOR DETERMINATION OF IN VIVO KETONE BODY KINETICS VALID?

J. Miles*, W. Schwenk, J. Gerich and M. Haymond, Mayo Clinic and Foundation, Rochester, MN, USA 55905.

Isotope dilution studies of ketone body (KB) [acetoacetate (AcAc), plus β-hydroxybutyrate (βOHB)] turnover in vivo are ordinarily performed with a single ^{14}C KB tracer using so-called "total KB specific activity" (TKBSA). The present study was conducted to evaluate the validity of conventional isotopic methods, using a stable isotopic tracer and a dual isotope model. KB kinetics were traced with simultaneous constant infusions of ^{14}C βOHB and ^{13}C AcAc in 7 conscious postabsorptive dogs. After baseline arterial blood sampling, unlabelled Na AcAc (10 $\mu mol \cdot kg^{-1} \cdot min^{-1}$) or Na D-(-)-βOHB (7.5 $\mu mol \cdot kg^{-1} \cdot min^{-1}$) was infused for 2 hrs. TKB turnover was calculated by TKBSA, TKB moles percent enrichment (MPE), and by an open two-pool model. During Na AcAc infusion, ^{14}C TKBSA underestimated exogenous inflow by ~60% ($p < 0.01$), and TKB MPE provided a ~15% overestimate; TKB flux was ~97% exogenous inflow using the dual isotope model, however. In contrast, during Na D-βOHB infusion ^{14}C TKBSA underestimated exogenous inflow ~15%, ^{13}C TKB MPE provided an overestimate of >150% ($p < 0.01$), and the dual isotope model predicted ~90% of exogenous inflow. Plasma FFA did not change during the studies. Rates of KB interconversion increased ~15-fold during both infusions. Conclusions: When KB kinetics were determined with a single isotope, significant errors in estimates of inflow occurred. A dual isotope model predicted exogenous inflow of both AcAc and βOHB nearly quantitatively (~95%). Furthermore, the dual isotope technique can estimate rates of whole body KB interconversion. Thus, the dual isotope technique appears to be superior to single isotope methods for examining KB metabolism in vivo.

1550 CHARACTERIZATION OF MONOCLONAL ANTIBODIES TO HUMAN GROWTH HORMONE (hGH)

Y. Sato,* T. Tsushima, N. Emoto and K. Shizume, Department of Internal Medicine, Tokyo Women's Medical College, Tokyo 162, Japan

Monoclonal antibodies (MoAb) to hGH were prepared and studied for their immunological properties. BALB/c mice were immunized with hGH and spleen cells were fused with mouse myeloma cells (SP 2/0) with 50 % polyethylene glycol. The cells were cultured in HAT selection medium. Cloning was performed by the limiting dilution technique. Three MoAb belonging to IgG_1 subclass were obtained. These antibodies recognized different parts of hGH molecule, judged by crossreaction of digested, chemically modified hGH, fragments of hGH (gifts of U.J.Lewis) or hPL. Binding of ^{125}I-hGH to each MoAb was quite rapid, reaching to maximum within 10 min, while equilibrium required more than 24 h in the case of polyclonal antibodies (PoAb) which were derived from sera of immunized mice. Dissociation of MoAb-bound ^{125}I-hGH was also much faster than that of PoAb-bound ^{125}I-hGH. RIA for hGH using either of MoAbs was insensitive, and half maximal displacement of ^{125}I-hGH was attained at 30-50 ng/ml hGH. When mixtures of two or three MoAb were used, sensitivity of RIA increased significantly and half maximal displacement occurred at 15 and 5 ng/ml, respectively. Although delayed addition of ^{125}I-hGH increased sensitivity of RIA with PoAb, it was totally ineffective in RIA with single MoAb. The effect of delayed addition of tracer appeared again if two or three MoAbs were combined. These results strongly suggest that binding of ^{125}I-hGH to MoAb is reversible, whereas binding to PoAb is much less reversible. This may account for difference in sensitivity of RIA using MoAb and PoAb.

1551 MONOCLONAL ANTIBODY PRODUCTION/HYBRIDOMA METABOLISM DEPENDS ON THE METHOD OF CULTURE. S.S. Seaver*, J.L. Rudolph, and J.E. Gabriels, Millipore Corporation, 80 Ashby Road, Bedford, MA. 01730. USA.

Hybridoma cells are increasingly being used to produce monoclonal antibodies. Yet little is known about their metabolism or how culture methods affect production. We have monitored cell growth, viability and antibody, glucose, lactic acid, glutamine and alanine levels using two different culture methods-stationary and stirred-in two different cell lines: SP 2/0-Ag-14 myeloma-based hybridoma and P3-NS1-Ag-4-1 myeloma-based hybridoma. In stationary culture antibody levels plateaued while cell viability was still $>90\%$, 2-3 days after cells stopped dividing. Glucose utilization and lactic acid production was greatest (1-2 mg/10^6 cells/day) during cell proliferation. Little glucose was consumed once cells stopped dividing. Glutamine levels decreased continuously and were not correlated with cell proliferation. When glutamine levels decreased to <0.5mM, cell viability started to decrease. Alanine, the only other amino acid that was affected markedly, increased when cell viability was high ($>90\%$). Nutrient usage, metabolite production and cell proliferation were similar in stirred cultures. However, in the SP 2/0 hybridoma antibody levels plateaued as soon as proliferation ceased at 1/10 the level of that found in stationary culture. In the NS-1 hybridoma maximum antibody levels, 50-75% of that measured in stationary culture, were obtained 6-8 days after cells had stopped dividing, as cell viability decreased to $<50\%$. Thus the amount and timing of antibody secretion are affected by the way hybridoma cells are cultured.

1552 DOPAMINE (DA) RECEPTOR BLOCKER, PIMOZIDE, BLOCKS THE STIMULATORY EFFECT OF CHOLECYSTOKININ (CCK)-8-S IMPLANTED IN THE MEDIAL PREOPTIC AREA (MPO) ON LH SECRETION IN THE RAT. F. Kimura*, R. Hashimoto and N. Mitsugi, Department of Physiology, Yokohama City University School of Medicine, 2-33 Urafune-cho, Minami-ku, Yokohama 232, Japan.

We have shown that implantation of CCK-8-S or DA into the MPO in the ovariectomized estrogen-primed rat induced an increase of LH secretion. Since immunohistochemical and behavioral-physiological investigations have suggested a possible functional interaction of CCK-8-S and DA in the brain, this study was done to examine if there is certain interaction between CCK-8-S and DA concerning the regulation of anterior pituitary hormone secretion. The effects of CCK-8-S or DA implanted into the MPO through the chronically implanted guide cannula on the serum LH concentration in the ovariectomized estradiol(20 μg, sc)-primed rat was compared between the pimozide(1 mg/Kg body weight, ip, at 12.00 h on the day of experiment)-treated and pimozide-untreated conditions. An inner cannula with CCK-8-S or DA at the tip, as well as an empty cannula as the control, was implanted into the MPO at 12.00 h, and blood samples were obtained sequentially after-wards. In the pimozide-untreated group, the mean serum LH concentration at 16.00 or 18.00 h was higher in rats implanted with CCK-8-S or DA than that in control rats, whereas in the pimozide-treated group, neither CCK-8-S nor DA could induce a significant increase in the serum LH concentrations. It was apparent that both the CCK-8-S and DA effect on LH secretion are blocked by pretreatment of DA receptor blocker, pimozide, and was thus indicated that DA receptors are required to be intact for CCK-8-S manifesting its action concerning the stimulation of LH secretion.

1553 ALTERATIONS OF HORMONAL RESPONSES FOLLOWING LITHIUM TREATMENT IN THE RAT.
J.I. Koenig*, H.Y. Meltzer and G.A. Gudelsky, Dept. of Psychiatry, Univ. of Chicago and ILL. State Psychiatric Inst., Chicago, ILL. 60637 USA

Lithium(Li), a monovalent cation, has been used for the treatment of manic depression. One action of Li is thought to involve an enhancement of serotonergic(5HT) function in the CNS. The present study addresses the issue of whether Li alters the neuroendocrine effects of 5HT agents. Adult male rats were fed rat chow containing 0.23% Li_2CO_3 for seven days. Plasma PRL, corticosterone(B) and beta-endorphin(B-E) were determined by RIA after the administration of the 5HT agonist, 5-methoxy-N,N-dimethyltryptamine(5MeODMT), or the solvent vehicle. The inclusion of Li in the diet for seven days caused a marked decrease in plasma PRL concentrations and an increase in plasma B levels, whereas B-E levels were unaltered. The effect of 5MeODMT to increase plasma PRL concentrations was significantly potentiated in rats maintained on the Li diet. The PRL- releasing effects of quipazine and 5-HTP were also significantly greater in Li-treated rats. Plasma concentrations of B-E were increased following the administration of 5MeODMT and, like the PRL response, the plasma B-E response to 5MeODMT was potentiated by Li treatment. Unlike the PRL and B-E responses, the incremental elevation of plasma B concentrations induced by 5MeODMT was similar in control and Li-treated rats. Thus, Li administration alters the concentration of both PRL and B by an, as yet, undefined mechanism. The ability of Li to potentiate the PRL-, B- and B-E-releasing activity of several 5HT agonists is suggestive of an effect of Li to enhance the sensitivity of 5HT receptors in the neuroendocrine axis.

1554 CIRCADIAN CHANGES IN CONCENTRATIONS OF DOPAMINE (DA) AND NOREPINEPHRINE (NE) IN RAT MEDIAN EMINENCE (ME), INTERMEDIATE (IL) AND POSTERIOR (PL) PITUITARY LOBES.
M. Koulu*, N. Bjelogrlic, J.M. Saavedra and M. Linnoila, CPB, NIMH, Bethesda, MD, USA.

There are marked diurnal variations in the secretion of several pituitary hormones. The important role of monoamines in neuroendocrine regulation of pituitary function prompted us to study how DA and NE concentrations in tuberoinfundibular and -hypophyseal DA systems and in the corresponding NE-terminals change during the 24 h cycle. Male Sprague-Dawley rats, housed in regular LD-cycle (lights on 7 am to 7 pm), were killed at 7 time points throughout the 24 h cycle. DA and NE concentrations were analyzed by HPLC using electrochemical detection. In ME, DA concentrations were highest at 1 pm, and decreased gradually to a nadir at 1 am (593±61 pmol/mg protein, vs. 329±50; $p<0.05$; mean±SEM). In IL and PL DA levels were similarly lowest at 1 am (60±4 and 33±2, resp.). Peak daytime values were obtained at 8 am (115±12 for IL; $p<0.01$; 55±4 for PL; $p<0.05$). The NE levels of ME followed the same time pattern as DA: a decrease from 251±14 to 140±19 ($p<0.001$). In PL NE levels decreased during the dark period from 21±2 at 8 pm to 14±1 at 1 am ($p<0.05$), while NE levels in IL remained unchanged. These marked circadian changes in DA and NE concentrations in ME, IL and PL may be related to circadian rhythms in pituitary hormones, such as PRL.

1555 INCREASED ADRENAL DOPAMINE SYNTHESIS ACCOMPANIES THE RISE IN BLOOD PRESSURE OF SPONTANEOUSLY HYPERTENSIVE RATS. O. Kuchel*, K. Racz, and N.T. Buu, MRC Group in Hypertension, Clinical Research Institute, University of Montreal, Montreal, Quebec, H2W 1R7, Canada.

Dopamine (DA) is known to affect blood pressure (BP) but the rate of endogenous DA synthesis in hypertension is unknown. We studied the relationship between BP and adrenal DA synthesis in Wistar-Kyoto (WKY) and spontaneously hypertensive rats (SHR) after labelling the catecholamine (CA) pool with ^{3}H-tyrosine. Rats of ages 4,8 and 14 weeks received iv pulse injections of ^{3}H-tyrosine (700 µCi/kg) and were killed at various time intervals thereafter. Specific activities and half-lives of adrenal CA were estimated using reverse phase HPLC for separating individual CA.

Age	WISTAR-KYOTO RATS 4 weeks	8 weeks	14 weeks	SHR 4 weeks	8 weeks	14 weeks
systolic BP (mmHg)	106±3	113±3	106±2	109±3	147±5*	189±9*
adrenal DA content (nmol/pair)	1.0±0.1	1.2±0.1	1.3±0.1	1.0±0.1	1.6±0.1*	1.8±0.1*
T 1/2 of adrenal DA (min)**	96±9	86±9	67±8	86±9	68±4*	46±2*

Values are means ± SE from groups of 5-12 rats; *p < 0.05 between SHR and WKY groups of the same age; ** apparent half-lives calculated from disappearance of ^{3}H-labelling between 15 and 75 min.

There was a shorter half-life of ^{3}H-DA and a higher DA content in 8 and 14 week old SHR while the norepinephrine and epinephrine content and labelling were similar in SHR and WKY at each age. The selectively increased DA synthesis in adrenals of hypertensive SHR, in conjunction with an increased urinary free DA excretion (51 ± 12 vs 20 ± 0.5 nmol/24h in WKY rats) suggests that increased adrenal DA (but not NE and E) release is involved in the sequence of events associated with hypertension in SHR.

1556 IS PLASMA ACTH LEVEL INFLUENCED BY CIRCULATING CATECHOLAMINES IN RATS UNDER STRESS? R. Kvetňanský*, F.J.H. Tilders+, J. Čulman, M. Dobrakovová, M. Vigaš and P.G. Smelik+, Institute of Experimental Endocrinology CPS, Slovak Academy of Sciences, 833 06 Bratislava, Czechoslovakia and +Department of Pharmacology, Free University, 1007 MC Amsterdam, The Netherlands.

Literary data show that plasma catecholamines along with CRF and other factors participate in the regulation of ACTH release. Is this finding valid also for rats under stress? During 5-10 min exposure of rats to immobilization stress (IMO) there is a 7-12-fold increase of plasma ACTH and a 6-12-fold increase of plasma corticosterone (B) levels. In thus immobilized animals, plasma epinephrine (EPI) and norepinephrine (NE) levels show even more pronounced increases. IMO applied to rats with removed adrenal medullas which were also sympathectomized (6-week administration of guanethidine; 30 mg kg^{-1} i.p. every day) resulted in virtually the same rise in plasma ACTH and B levels as recorded in intact animals, and that despite complete blockade of plasma EPI and NE increase. In adrenalectomized plus sympathectomized rats with already increased basic plasma ACTH (about 20-times) there was a further significant IMO-induced rise of plasma ACTH in spite of the fact that plasma EPI and NE conc. were practically negligible. The present data suggest that in rats exposed to immobilization stress an activation of the peripheral sympathetic-adrenomedullary system is not significantly involved in the regulation of ACTH release.

1557 NOREPINEPHRINE (NE)-INDUCED SUPPRESSION OF LH PULSE FREQUENCY IN OVARIECTOMIZED RATS DURING PUSH-PULL PERFUSION OF THE MEDIAL PREOPTIC AREA. R.E. Leipheimer* and R.V. Gallo, Physiology Section, Biological Sciences Group, and Department of Biobehavioral Sciences, University of Connecticut, Storrs, CT. USA

A previous study in this laboratory demonstrated that intraventricular infusion of 0.3 or 1.8 µg NE/h suppressed pulsatile LH release solely by decreasing LH pulse frequency (Gallo, Neuroendocrinology, In press). The present study utilized the technique of push-pull perfusion to determine whether the medial preoptic area (MPOA) was a site mediating this inhibitory effect. Ovariectomized rats were bled continuously at a rate of 50 µl whole blood/7 min for 2h prior to perfusion, and during a 2-3h period of perfusion of the MPOA (20 µl/min) with artificial CSF, or 2 or 20 pg NE/min. In another group of rats LH levels were only determined during a 2-3h period of MPOA perfusion with CSF. Pulsatile LH release was not affected by push-pull perfusion with CSF when a comparison was made to pre-perfusion LH values in the same rats. Moreover, LH levels obtained from rats only bled during MPOA perfusion with CSF were not different from LH values in the pre-perfusion periods in the other groups. However push-pull perfusion of the MPOA with 2 or 20 pg NE/min decreased mean LH levels by causing a 35-45% reduction in pulse frequency. As in the previous intraventricular infusion study, no decrease occurred in LH pulse amplitude. These studies demonstrate that NE acting at the level of the MPOA can suppress pulsatile LH release solely by decreasing LH pulse frequency. Supported by NIH HD17728.

1558 IS 21-DEOXYCORTISOL (21-DF) PRODUCED BY THE OVARY? A. Milewicz*, G. Tupikowska, J. Szymczak, M. Grabinski and P. Vecsei. (Intro M.A. Kirschner) Dept. of Endocrinology, Wroclaw, Poland and Pharmacology Institute -Steroid Laboratory, Heidelberg, FRG.

Using a new specific RIA we explored 21-DF responses to HCG in 11 normal women, 7 with idiopathic hirsutism (IH) and 15 with polycystic ovary syndrome (PCO). HCG was given I.M. daily x 2 days, with plasma assayed in basal state, after 24 and 48 hours. Values for 21-DF are compared with simultaneously measured plasma 17-hydroxyprogesterone (17-OHP).

		21-DF (ng/dl)	
	Basal ± S.E.	HCG Day = 1	HCG = 2
Normal women	8.3 ± 0.47	8.0 ± 0.41	8.8 ± 0.59
IH	7.9 ± 0.58	8.3 ± 0.3	7.7 ± 0.2
PCO	18.2± 1.4	23.1± 2.2	30.1± 4.1
		17-OHP (ng/dl)	
	Basal	HCG Day = 1	HCG Day = 2
Normal women	175 ± 17	292 ± 20*	478 ± 20*
IH	135 ± 16	323 ± 43*	455 ± 41*
PCO	117 ± 28	233 ± 49*	388 ± 45*

*Significant from basal at P .05

These data show significant elevations of 17-OHP in normal, IH and PCO patients after HCG, as expected. To our surprise, we found a 2-fold increase in serum 21-DF after 2 days of HCG in women with PCO. Each of the 15 PCO patients exhibited significant increments of 21-DF over basal levels, in contrast to control in IH patients.

Since HCG has not been observed to normally stimulate adrenal steroidogenesis, these data suggest that 21-DF may not be a unique adrenal hormone.

1559 REDUCTIONS IN PLASMA OESTRADIOL (E2) DURING DIOESTRUS-2 AND EARLY PROESTRUS DELAY OVULATION IN THE RAT. C.M. Milne*, R.L. Hasmall, S. Watson and M.C. Middleton, Central Toxicology Laboratory, Imperial Chemical Industries PLC, Alderley Park, Macclesfield, Cheshire, UK.

We are studying the effect of a substituted triazole, known to inhibit sterol biosynthesis in fungi, on female reproductive processes in rats. Ovulation was delayed by a mechanism involving inhibition of the preovulatory peaks of LH, FSH and progesterone. The underlying reasons for inhibition of gonadotrophin secretion are uncertain. The proestrus peak of E2, known to be an important controlling factor in gonadotrophin secretion, was unaffected by the triazole (dosed 1200h, dioestrus-2). However, during late dioestrus-2 and early proestrus (6-24 hours after dosing with the triazole) plasma E2 levels were significantly reduced. Exogenous E2, administered during the first 12 hours after dosing, attenuated the inhibitory effects of the triazole on ovulation. The observed reductions in E2 levels may involve inhibition of aromatase activity. In vivo, reductions in plasma E2 at the time of maximal aromatase activity (late proestrus) are an indication of aromatase inhibition. In this respect the triazole (dosed 1000h on proestrus) was equipotent with aminoglutethimide, a compound with known aromatase inhibitory activity. Thus, the triazole delayed ovulation by reducing circulating E2 levels during late dioestrus-2 and early proestrus. This may prevent adequate E2 priming of the pituitary and inhibit the subsequent gonadotrophin surges. However, the triazole also has antiuterotrophic activity and it is possible that antioestrogenic actions at the level of the hypothalamus/pituitary may contribute to inhibition of gonadotrophin secretion.

1560 PARTIAL ISOLATION OF GONADOTROPIN_RELEASING HORMONE (GnRH) LIKE SUBSTANCE FROM THE PORCINE OVARY. H. Minaguchi*, J. Mori and T. Uemura, Department of Obstetrics and Gynecology, Yokohama City University,School of Medicine Yokohama, 232, Japan.

It has been recently reported that both in the ovary and testis of several species there exists Gonadotropin-Releasing Hormone (GnRH) like substance, which may act directly on the gonad to regulate its function. Present study was undertaken to extract and isolate the substance from the porcine ovary. Porcine ovaries were homogenized in ether:chloroform:acetic acid:H_2O(810:90:5:95) or 0.02N acetic acid. Supernate from 3000xg spin was freeze-dried. The extract was defatted with ether and incubated overnight with dry charcol. Removal of steroids from the extract was confirmed by RIA. In rat pituitary monolayer culture system, 41.8 millifragments of the extract induced a significant increase of LH in the medium. The dose response curves of LH and FSH were observed to various amounts of native LHRH and the crude extract. However, the extract was not immunoreactive to LHRH antiserum in RIA. In RRA, 2.6 millifragments significantly inhibited the binding of radioactive ligand (^{125}I-[D-Ser(Tbu)^{6}des-Gly-NH_2^{10}]LHRH ethylamide) to rat pituitary membrane preparation. Parallel dose response was also present between LHRH and the extract. When the extract was dialyzed with Spectrapore no. 3 membrane tubing (mol wt cutoff, 3500) against distilled water, the retentate showed both biological and binding activities. Gel filtration of the retentate by Sephadex G-75 demonstrated that the activities were located in one zone. The results indicate that GnRH like substance, which is chemically and immunologically different from native LHRH, exists in the porcine ovary.

1561 EXISTENCE OF SOMATOSTATIN-LIKE IMMUNOREACTIVITY IN PORCINE OVARIES AND ITS ROLE IN GERMINAL VESICLE BREAKDOWN.

T.Mori[1]*, Y. Ohno[2], M. Irahara[2], E. Hoshi[3] and H. Saito[3], Department of Gynecology and Obstetrics, Faculty of Medicine, Kyoto University, Kyoto , Department of Obstetrics and Gynecology and Laboratory Medicine , University of Tokushima School of Medicine, Tokushima, Japan.

The present study was undertaken to clarify the existence and characteristics of somatostatin (SRIF) in the porcine ovaries and its histological effects on germinal vesicle breakdown (GVB). Measurements of SRIF by RIA in porcine ovarian tissues after removal of follicular fluid revealed the existence of immunoreactive (IR)-SRIF at the concentration of 2.2 $\pm$ 0.6 ng/g wet weight tissue (mean $\pm$ SD). On gel chromatographe analyse of ovarian extracts, one major and two minor components with IR-SRIF have been detected. The major component was co-eluted with SRIF-14 (59.5% of total IR-SRIF). The two other components seemed to have almost the same molecular weight to SRIF-28 (25.1%) and to preprosomatostatin (15.4%). In _in vitro_ studies using cultured porcine oocytes, when seven different concentrations of synthetic SRIF-14 ranging from 1 pg to 1 ug/ml were added to culture medium, % of oocytes with GVB of total cultured oocytes (% GVB) gradually decreased with increasing concentrations of SRIF reaching to maximum inhibition rate of 59.6% of control at 1 ug/ml. The inhibitory effects of SRIF was blocked following neutralization with rabbit anti-SRIF serum added to the medium. These findings suggest that (1) SRIF with molecular heterogenity exists in porcine ovaries and (2) SRIF plays a physiological role as an oocyte maturation inhibitor.

1562 ENDOCRINE STUDIES ON OVARIAN ANDROBLASTOMAS (SERTOLI-LEYDIG TUMORS).

M. Munemura*, S. Inoue, R. Himeno, J. Mizumoto, Y. Sakoda and M. Maeyama, Department of Obstetrics and Gynecology, Kumamoto University Medical School, Kumamoto 860, Japan.

Endocrine studies were made on 4 women with ovarian Sertoli-Leydig cell tumors of varying degree of differentiation. Clinically, all 4 patients showed evidence of increased androgen production, manifested by either hirsutism or virilization. The calculated ratios of steroid hormones between the affected ovarian venous values and peripheral values for testosterone (T), androstenedione (A), and dehydroepiandrosterone (DHEA) in 3 patients, were 1.4-18.6, 4.2-24.4 and 3.7-10.0, respectively. The peripheral levels of the hormones before salpingo-oophorectomy in all the patients were T, 0.97-45.0 ng/ml; A, 2.92-114.0 ng/ml; and DHEA, 13.0-20.9 ng/ml. In the 3 juvenile patients, elevated basal levels of LH and normal or subnormal levels of FAH (high LH:FSH ratio) were found. In a 12-year-old patient with 1900 g of tumor composed predominantly of Stertoli cells with lipid storage, the peripheral serum levels of T and estradiol (E_2) were 114 ng/ml and 1890 pg/ml, respectively. The present data suggest that: 1) androblastomas have a biosynthetic capacity for androgen, estrogen, or both in which both the Δ^5 and Δ^4 pathway are involved, and 2) little correlation exists between the endocrine function and cellular composition of the tumor or their degree of differentiation.

1563 Ovarian steroids in postmenopausal women with endometrial cancer.
M. Nagamani*, E.V. Hannigan, E. Dillard and D.V. Tung, Department of Obstetrics and Gynecology, UTMB, Galveston, Texas, USA.

The purpose of the present study is to evaluate the endocrine function of the ovary in postmenopausal women with endometrial cancer to see whether there is an increase in the secretion of ovarian steroids in women with cancer. Levels of testosterone (T), androstenedione (A), estradiol (E2) and estrone (E1) were measured by specific radioimmunoassays in the peripheral and ovarian vein samples obtained at the time of hysterectomy from 16 postmenopausal women with endometrial cancer and 9 women without cancer. Patients and the controls were matched for age and years since menopause. In the normal controls, there was a significant difference between ovarian and peripheral vein concentrations of testosterone. (623 ± 108 pg/ml vs 156 ± 21 pg/ml, $P < 0.001$). Ovarian vein levels of A, E1 and E2 were not significantly different from the levels in the peripheral blood. In women with endometrial cancer, a significantly higher ovarian than peripheral vein concentrations were found for all the hormones measured. T(3847 ± 1184 pg/ml vs 204 ± 42 pg/ml, $P < 0.01$), A(5225 ± 1743 pg/ml vs 1249 ± 183 pg/ml, $P < 0.05$), E2(50 ± 11 pg/ml vs 22 ± 3 pg/ml, $P < 0.05$) and E1(80 ± 12 pg/ml vs 32 ± 3 pg/ml, $P < 0.05$). In conclusion, (1) the ovaries of postmenopausal patients with endometrial cancer secrete significantly more T and A than normal controls resulting in increased prehormone availability for extraglandular E1 formation. (2) they secrete minimal amounts of E2 and E1 (3) this increase in ovarian steroid secretion might play a role in the pathogenesis of endometrial cancer.

1564 AUTORADIOGRAPHIC STUDIES ON THE DISTRIBUTION OF GONADOTROPIN-RELEASING HORMONE RECEPTOR (GnRH-R) IN THE OVARY.
T.NAMIKI*, T.UEMURA, H.MINAGUCHI, Department of Obstetrics and Gynecology, Yokohama City University, School of Medicine, Yokohama, 232, Japan.

Gonadotropin-releasing hormone receptor (GnRH-R) has been recently demonstrated in the ovary. Autoradiographic studies are undertaken to clarify its distribution and regulatory mechanism in immature rats during sexual maturation. 3×10^5 cpm/g/BW of ^{125}I-D-Ser(Tbu)^6 des-Gly^{10}-NH$_2$ LHRH ethylamide (GnRHa) (SA:800-1000uCi/mg) were injected intravenously with or without 1000 fold excess of cold GnRHa. One hour after the injection, rats were sacrificed, perfused with 0.9% NaCl and 3% glutalaldehyde, and post-fixed with PAF. The sections were processed for autoradiography and grains were counted. Uptake (cpm/mg wet wt.) of ^{125}I-GnRHa to the ovary increased gradually by age to reach a peak at 21 days and declined prepubertally. Autoradiographic studies demonstrated GnRH-R in all components of granulosa cells, theca cells and interstitial tissue. Quantitative analysis of grain distribution indicated that GnRH bound predominantly to the interstitial tissue before 21 days of age. However, after 28 days of age, GnRH mainly bound to granulosa cells and GnRH binding to theca and interstitial tissue was relatively decreasd, which corresponded with prepubertal decrease in GnRH uptake by the ovary. In large follicles, the distribution of GnRH was heterogeneous and localized in special cells of granulosa. PMSG treatment in young immature rats induced these prepubertal changes. Small number of silver grains was found in luteal tissue. These results indicate that GnRH distribution changes in the ovarian component by follicular development during sexual maturation.

1565 STIMULATION OF RELAXIN SECRETION IN RHESUS MONKEYS DURING PROLONGED EXPOSURE TO HCG: A FUNCTION OF AGE OF THE CORPUS LUTEUM.
J. Ottobre*, R. Stouffer and W. Nixon, Dept. of Physiology, Univ. of Arizona, Tucson, AZ 85724, and Developmental Endocrinology Branch, NICHD, NIH, Bethesda, MD, USA 20205.

Endogenous chorionic gonadotropin (CG) in early pregnancy or exogenous human (h) CG during the luteal phase of the menstrual cycle induces relaxin (RLX) secretion in women and monkeys. To determine if this induction by CG is influenced by the age of the corpus luteum, female rhesus monkeys received a 10-day regimen of hCG (Ayerst APL) beginning in the early (n=4), mid (n=6) or late (n=4) luteal phase of the cycle (5.3 ± 0.3, 8.3 ± 0.5, and 12.0 ± 0.4 days post-LH surge, respectively; $\bar{x} \pm SE$). Increasing doses of hCG were injected im twice each day to mimic the pattern and circulating levels of macaque CG in early pregnancy. Femoral venous blood was collected daily and serum LH, hCG, progesterone (P) and RLX-like activity were measured by RIA. RLX was not detectable during hCG treatment that began in the early luteal phase; however levels near the limit of detection were observed in one monkey after termination of treatment (192 ± 10 pg/ml). In contrast, circulating RLX appeared in 7 of 10 animals 5.0 ± 0.7 days after onset of hCG treatment at mid or late luteal phase. Although mean RLX levels were similar in these groups (315 ± 51 vs 247 ± 48 pg/ml), peak levels occurred later in monkeys treated at mid than at late luteal phase (13.0 ± 0.0 vs 6.0 ± 0.6 days after onset of hCG treatment, $p<0.001$). Whereas CG treatment rapidly enhanced circulating P levels, serum RLX often peaked just prior to menses after P concentrations declined to ≤ 2 ng/ml. Thus, 1) the young, developing corpus luteum of the menstrual cycle did not respond to CG with initiation of RLX secretion, and 2) peak RLX release by the corpus luteum during prolonged CG exposure was associated with luteolysis. NIH HD12333

1566 CLINICAL AND LABORATORY FEATURES OF PATIENTS WITH PRIMARY POLYDIPSIA.
Arnold M. Moses*, VA Medical Center and Dept. of Medicine, SUNY, Upstate Medical Center, Syracuse, NY 13210, USA.

Urine volume ranged from 4.1 to 6.4 l/24 hr in 7 patients (5 females, 2 males) with primary polydipsia (PP). Five patients had no evident organic process, while 2 had hypothalamic disease. The 2 latter patients markedly improved when treated with dDAVP. Six types of laboratory observations revealed that: (1) 5U AVP doubled urine osmolality (Uosm) over a 4 hour period when the patients were hydrated ad libitum, (2) osmotic threshold values were normal or low, (3) Uosm was normal or increased in relation to plasma osmolality (Posm) during dehydration, (4) 5U AVP did not increase Uosm when injected at the plateau in Uosm during dehydration, (5) urine AVP was generally below normal in relation to Posm during dehydration, (6) Uosm was normal in relation to urine AVP. PP can be differentiated from central and congenital nephrogenic diabetes insipidus (DI) by using the above 6 tests as follows:

	(1)	(2)	(3)	(4)	(5)	(6)
PP vs central DI	−	+	+	+	−	+
PP vs nephrogenic DI	+	+	+	+	+	+

In summary, primary polydipsia can be readily differentiated from central and congenital nephrogenic DI. The kidneys of patients with PP are less resistant to AVP than the kidneys of patients with central DI. Some patients with PP can be effectively treated with dDAVP.

1567 OXYTOCIN RELEASE FOLLOWING INTRA-ATRIAL OR INTRA-VENTRICULAR INFUSION OF HYPEROSMOLAR SOLUTION OF VARIOUS SOLUTES IN THE RAT. H. Negoro, T. Higuchi, K. Honda and T. Fukuoka, Dept. of Physiology, Fukui Medical School, Matsuoka, Fukui, 910-11 Japan.

It has been established that vasopressin release is stimulated by solutes to which cell membranes are impermeable and not affected by those to which cell membranes are permeable. Oxytocin was also reported to be released in response to hypertonic NaCl. This study was carried out to investigate characteristics and location of osmoreceptors for oxytocin release. A cannula was inserted into the right atrium of male rats. In some animals a stainless steel cannula was implanted in the third cerebral ventricle in addition to the atrial cannula. Each rat was infused at 1 µl/sec via the atrial cannula with Locke solution to which 1.2 osmol/l of either NaCl, mannitol or urea was added or with Locke solution alone. Plasma oxytocin concentration determined by radioimmunoassay showed a significant increase in response to NaCl and mannitol but was not affected by urea in spite of a significant increase in plasma osmolality. Artificial cerebrospinal fluid (CSF) made hypertonic by addition of NaCl, mannitol or urea was administered into the third ventricle in the other group of rats. Plasma oxytocin also increased significantly following the infusion of the CSF containing NaCl or mannitol but was not affected by the CSF containing urea or the CSF alone. These data suggest that the osmoreceptor mechanism controlling oxytocin release is analogous to that for vasopressin release and that the osmoreceptors are located in a region of brain accesible from both outside and inside of blood brain barrier.

1568 PROCESSING OF PROVASOPRESSIN: IDENTIFICATION OF A CARBOXYPEPTIDASE ASSOCIATED WITH NEUROSECRETORY GRANULES. W.G. North*, Department of Physiology, Dartmouth Medical School 03756

Processing of provasopressin to form hormone (AVP), neurophysin and glycopeptide(s) appears to take place within the neurosecretory granules (NSG) of hypothalamic neurons during movement from perikarya to storage sites in the neural lobe. The published sequences for provasopressins and our isolation of glycosylated proneurophysins as possible intermediates during processing has suggested the following scheme for the generation of active hormone:

(a) ProAVP —(ProAVPase1)→ AVPdodecapeptide + proneurophysin

(b) AVPdodecapeptide —(ProAVPase2)→ AVPdecapeptide + Lys + Arg

(c) AVPdecapeptide —(ProAVPase3)→ AVP (active nonapeptide) + glyoxylic acid

Step (b) in this scheme requires the presence of a carboxypeptidase-like activity to form vasopressin (Gly^{10}) decapeptide. We now report partial charactierization of such an activity contained in NSG isolated from rat neural lobes by sucrose-gradient ultracentrifugation. The enzyme(s) converts the dipeptide N-CBZ-Phe-LeuOH to N-CBZ-PheOH. The pH optimal for this conversion is 4.5 with little activity below pH 3 and above pH 6. The amount of this activity in NSG was 203 nmole dipeptide/nmole AVP for the 2 h period of incubations at pH 5.0.

1569 NEUROHYPOPHYSIAL HORMONES IN THE ADRENAL GLAND. S.S. Nussey*, V.T.Y. Ang and J.S. Jenkins, St. George's Hospital Medical School, London, SW17, U.K.

Using highly specific radioimmunoassays (RIA) we have previously reported the presence of immunoreactive oxytocin and vasopressin in the adrenal medulla of rat, cow and man in concentrations far greater than those in plasma. The purpose of the present studies was to determine the source of these hormones. Immunocytochemical staining of rat, human and bovine adrenal tissue showed patchy staining of medullary cells for both oxytocin and vasopressin. Ultracentrifugation of adrenal homogenates followed by RIA showed that the peptides were present in the chromaffin granule fraction. The possibility that the paraventricular nucleus of the hypothalamus was the ultimate source of the neurohypophysial hormones found in the adrenal was studied. Four rats were subjected to stereotactic lesions of the paraventricular nuclei but when the adrenal concentrations of oxytocin and vasopressin were compared in these animals with sham-operated rats no difference was observed. To determine whether there was direct synthesis of peptides, slices of bovine adrenal were incubated in Krebs Ringer-bicarbonate-glucose in the presence of ^{35}S-cysteine. The slices were homogenized, extracted with acid and subjected to Sephadex chromatography, thin layer chromatography and finally high-pressure liquid chromatography. Significant radioactivity was obtained in the eluates corresponding with retention times of oxytocin and vasopressin. There is therefore evidence that these "neurohypophysial" hormones can be synthesised outside the hypothalamic nuclei, and thereby providing further impetus to investigate the functional role of vasopressin and oxytocin in the adrenal gland.

1570 INTERACTION OF DIPHENYLHYDANTOIN AND NALOXONE ON VASOPRESSIN SECRETION IN NORMAL RATS. Y. Oiso*, and A. Tomita, First Department of Internal Medicine, Nagoya University School of Medicine, 65 Tsurumaicho, Showaku, Nagoya 466 Japan.

Diphenylhydantoin(DPH) has various pharmacological effects besides its anticonvulsant action. DPH has been used for treatment of syndrome of inappropriate secretion of ADH(SIADH) because of its inhibitory effect on vasopressin(VP) secretion. However, the effect of DPH in normal osmoregulation has not been well elucidated. We investigated the effect of DPH on VP secretion in intact rats and also examined its interaction with endogenous opioid which has been proposed as an inhibitor of VP secretion. Conscious male Sprague-Dawley rats were treated with hypertonic saline(600 mOsm/kg : i.p.). Subsequently, the animals received DPH(25 mg/kg : i.v.) and/or naloxone(10 mg/kg : s.c.). Trunk blood was collected for measurement of plasma VP(p-VP) and plasma osmolality(p-OSM) 30 min after the administration of drugs. When DPH was given without naloxone, no significant difference was observed in p-VP(3.2 ± 0.5 pg/ml : M ± SD) and p-OSM compared with control(p-VP : 2.7 ± 1.1 pg/ml). However, combined administration of DPH and naloxone elevated p-VP(5.1 ± 0.9 pg/ml : $p<0.02$) without influencing p-OSM. Naloxone alone did not affect both p-VP(2.8 ± 0.1 pg/ml) and p-OSM. These data indicate that the effect of DPH on VP secretion is different in normal rats and in cases of SIADH with impaired osmoregulation. These findings also suggest that DPH may modify the opioid-dependent process of VP secretion.

1571 ALLOXAN-INDUCED DIABETES CHANGES PINEAL INDOLES IN RATS AT MID-LIGHT AND MID-DARK. S.F. Pang* and F. Tang, Department of Physiology, University of Hong Kong, Hong Kong.

The effects of alloxan treatment on the pineal levels of N-acetylserotonin and melatonin, and serum levels of melatonin were studied. Male rats (250 g) were kept under 12:12 light:dark cycle with lights on at 0600 hr. Food and water were given ad libitum. Alloxan (170 mg/kg.) or vehicle was injected subcutaneously and the rats were checked weekly for the presence of glucose in the urine. Only rats with positive results were considered diabetic and used as experimental animals. Four weeks after alloxan injection, the rats were sacrificed at mid-light (1200 h) and mid-dark (2400 h). Pineal indoles and serum melatonin were extracted by methanol or dichloromethane and determined by radioimmunoassay. Our results demonstrated that the pineal levels of N-acetylserotonin in the diabetic rats were significantly higher ($P<0.05$) than those of the control rats at mid-light and mid-dark. On the other hand, pineal and serum levels of melatonin in the control animals were significantly higher ($P<0.05$) than those of the experimental animals in the two time points studied. Thus, alloxan-induced diabetes may decrease pineal melatonin synthesis at the level of hydroxy-indole-O-methyl-transferase, leading to a decrease in melatonin secretion.

1572 EPISODIC SECRETION OF MELATONIN IN PRE- AND POST-PUBERTAL GIRLS AND BOYS. R. Penny*, University of Southern California School of Medicine and LAC-USC Medical Center, Dept of Pediatrics, Los Angeles, CA, U.S.A.

The concentration of melatonin was determined in serum samples obtained at 15 minute intervals during a 4-hour period from seven normal girls, 9.5-16.5 years of age, and eight normal boys, 9.0-16.8 years of age. All samples were obtained between 08:00 and 13:00 hours. An episodic pattern of melatonin secretion was found in all subjects. There was no significant ($p >0.1$) difference between girls and boys as to mean $\pm$ SD number of episodes (3.1 ± 0.4 vs 3.4 ± 0.5 per 4 hours), absolute melatonin increase (49 ± 6.7 vs 50.4 ± 4.1 pg/ml) or "apparent melatonin half-life" (20.3 ± 0.8 vs 20.8 ± 1.0 minutes). Mean absolute increase during secretory episodes correlated ($r= 0.843$, $p <0.005$) with the mean melatonin concentration per 4 hours, and a significant ($p <0.05$) inverse correlation ($r= -0.508$) was found between the mean percent increment of the melatonin secretory episode and the mean "apparent melatonin half-life". A significant correlation between melatonin secretion and previously reported (JCEM 45:307, 1977) episodic luteinizing hormone secretion was not found. In girls and boys, mean melatonin concentration increased with advancing puberty. The increase in melatonin concentration was due to an increase in the amplitude of secretory episodes. These data are consistent with an influence of gonadal function on melatonin secretion but do not support a role for melatonin in the onset of normal puberty in man.

1573 AUTONOMOUS PROLACTIN SECRETION INDUCED BY PRIMARY HYPOTHYROIDISM.

Baruch Landau*, Itzhak Rosenberg and Bella Shindel, Department of Endocrinology, Beilinson Medical Center, Petah Tikva, and Tel Aviv University Medical School, Israel

Three female patients who presented with galactorrhea and elevated prolactin levels were found to be suffering from primary hypothyroidism. Treatment with thyroid extract re-established the euthyroid state and normalized the previously high levels of thyroid stimulating hormone. The high levels of prolactin were not affected by prolonged thyroid treatment. Dynamic studies of prolactin secretion indicated that in these three patients the lactotroph cells were functioning autonomically. This clinical course suggests that the process of hyperplasia of the pituitary can develop into an autonomic adenoma.

1574 PURIFICATION, IMMUNOCYTOCHEMICAL LOCALIZATION AND PRIMARY STRUCTURE OF A NOVEL POLYPEPTIDE FROM HUMAN PITUITARIES.

R. Leduc*, S. Benjannet, N.G. Seidah, C. Lazure, T. Antakly and M. Chrétien, Clinical Research Institute of Montreal, Montreal, Quebec, Canada, H2W 1R7.

The pituitary gland contains many biologically active polypeptides. In the human, hormones present in the anterior lobe include: prolactin, gonadotropin, thyrotropin, growth hormone and POMC, the precursor form of ACTH/β-end. The posterior lobe, innervated by neurons originating in the hypothalamus, contains oxytocin, vasopressin, neurophysins, C-terminal of pro-pressophysin and dynorphin. We report the characterization of a new polypeptide from whole human pituitary extracts isolated during our ongoing growth hormone purifications. It has a molecular weight of about 10,000 daltons estimated on gel permeation HPLC, which means a protein in the range of 80-90 amino acids. The quantities having been purified to date are minimal (1-4 nanomoles) so it was necessary to digest the polypeptide into fragments so as to obtain maximal information on its primary structure. After having identified 79 residues, a computer data-bank search using a mutation data matrix and comparison with over 340,000 segments revealed no homologies with existing sequences. We are therefore dealing with a substance that could be classified as a protein belonging to a new family. Using an antibody produced against a fragment following a pair of basic residues, immunocytochemical staining revealed the presence of material in the pars intermedia of rat pituitary gland. No staining was observed in the anterior or posterior lobes which is interesting since only POMC secreting cells have been characterized in the intermediate lobe to date.

1575 EFFECTS OF STEROIDS ON INHIBITION OF GONADOTROPIN SECRETION BY INHIBIN

V.W.K. Lee*, N. Colvin, J. McMaster, H. Quigg and H.G. Burger
Medical Research Centre, Prince Henry's Hospital, Melbourne, Australia 3004

The inhibition of follicle-stimulating hormone (FSH) release and content in cultured pituitary cells have been used as reliable endpoints for inhibin (INB) bioassay. We have examined the effects of steroids on responses to increasing doses of INB standard (RTFS) in isolated pituitary cells from immature female rats. Following treatment with 0.5% tryspin the cells were dispersed in Dulbecco Modified Eagle's Medium containing 10% foetal calf-serum. Cell incubations were performed for 48h using varying doses of RTFS $\pm 10^{-6}$M progesterone (P), testosterone (T), androstenedione (A), or estradiol (E) or with combination of all steroids. FSH in the media and in 0.1% triton treated cell lysates were assayed by RIA. Total FSH (cells plus medium) and release (medium alone) were increased by P (2.0 fold) and androgens (T or A, 1.4 fold). Despite elevated FSH release the inhibition slopes of RTFS were similar to those with RTFS alone or in the presence of E (Range of slopes: 29.4-37.4; indices of precision (λ): 0.04-0.09). The sensitivities of the inhibition curves were, however, decreased in the presence of P and androgens; 1.8 and 1.4-fold greater doses of RTFS respectively were required to cause 40% FSH inhibition. Similar trends in results were obtained when total FSH levels were used as the index but the inhibition curves were less precise and sensitive (Range of slopes: 16.8-21.4; λ: 0.10-0.14). The present data demonstrate that INB acts directly and independently of steroids in the suppression of FSH release from pituitary cells and that P or androgens may decrease the suppressive action of INB at the pituitary cell. This study was supported by the NH&MRC of Australia.

1576 EFFECTS OF HUMAN PANCREATIC GH RELEASING FACTOR-44 (hpGRF-44) ON PLASMA GH LEVELS IN ACROMEGALY.

A.Liuzzi*, P.G.Chiodini, G.Oppizzi, G.Verde and D. Dallabonzana, Division of Endocrinology, Ospedale Niguarda Cà Granda, 20162 Milan, Italy.

One hundred mcg of hpGRF-44 have been injected to 34 acromegalics and the observed GH changes have been compared with those obtained after bromocriptine (Br, 2.5 mg) and TRH (200 mcg). hpGRF-44 significantly increased GH levels in the whole group (bas 29 $\pm$ 9.8 ng/ml; mean $\pm$ SE; peak 108 $\pm$ 24 ng/ml; $p < 0.01$) but the individual percent GH changes were highly variable (9-3611%) and inversely correlated ($r = 0.34$; $p < 0.05$) to those induced by Br but not by TRH nor with basal GH, PRL, somatomedin C levels. When dividing the patients according to their responsiveness to TRH or Br, the GH releasing effect of hpGRF-44 was not different between TRH responders (GH increase by 100% over the baseline) and nonresponders, but it was significantly lower ($F = 2.31$; $p < 0.01$) in Br responders (GH decrease by 50% below baseline) than in nonresponders. We conclude that: 1) the weak GH response to hpGRF-44 of Br responders may be interpreted with the presence of tumoral somatotrophs with receptorial properties of the lactotropes and thus less sensitive to a specific stimulus for GH secretion ("mammosomatotropic" cells), 2) the marked GH increase after hpGRF-44 of Br nonresponders would suggest the prevalence of pure somatotrophs in the tumor, 3) the lack of correlation between the effects on GH of TRH and hpGRF-44 could be explained on considering that the TRH induced GH release, found also in pathological conditions other than acromegaly, is a less specific marker than the Br induced GH inhibition for the presence of "mammosomatotropic" cells. (Supported by CNR, Special Project "Control of Neoplastic Growth", grant no. 820033496).

1577 DIETHYLSTILBESTROL (DES) REDUCES TUMOR SIZE AND INHIBITS GROWTH OF MtTW15 RAT PITUITARY TUMOR WHILE MODIFYING EXPRESSION OF PROLACTIN AND GROWTH HORMONE BY TUMOR CELLS. R. V. Lloyd*, T. Landefeld, and I. Masler, University of Michigan Medical Center, Ann Arbor Michigan 48109

Silastic tubing implants of DES (20 mg) placed in Wistar/Furth rats with palpable (1 cm^3) transplantable prolactin (PRL) and growth hormone (GH) secreting MtTW15 tumors reduced tumor size and inhibited tumor growth. After 3 weeks of treatment, DES-treatment significantly reduced tumor weight (control:27.8 ± 4.9 g; treated:0.594 ± 0.251 g) and plasma PRL levels (control:63.8 ± 20.0 ug/ml; treated 1.22 ± 0.334 ug/ml). Mitotic counts showed 2.8 mitoses/10^4 tumor cells in controls and 0.8 mitoses/10^4 tumor cells in DES-treated rats. When DES was removed after 3 weeks, the tumors resumed growth. Immunohistochemical studies showed that tumors from controls had 62.5% PRL and 18.6% GH cells (n=6) while DES-treated rats had 10.2% PRL and 57.1% GH cells (n=6). The pituitaries of controls weighed 7.6 ± 0.57 mg and had 26.3% PRL cells and 23.6% GH cells, while the pituitaries of DES-treated rats weighed 23.5 ± 2.0 mg and had 65.0% PRL cells. In situ hybridization studies with a cloned ^{3}H-DNA complimentary to rat pituitary PRL mRNA (rPRL cDNA probe gift of R. Maurer) showed more labeling in M+TW15 tumors from controls compared to normal rat pituitaries. Further studies are being performed to characterize the PRL and GH mRNA in DES-treated and control tumors. These results indicate that DES inhibits growth of MtTW15 tumors by inhibiting mitotic activity, reduces tumor size, and also modifies the expression of immunoreactive PRL and GH by the tumor cells. (Supported by Am Cancer Soc No. IN-40W and BMRG RRO 5383).

1578 MAITOTOXIN STIMULATES CALCIUM FLUX IN GH_3 AND NORMAL PITUITARY CELLS. IS Login*, AM Judd, G Schettini, K Koike, T Yasumoto, MJ Cronin, RM MacLeod, University of Virginia, Charlottesville, Virginia, U.S.A. and Tohoku University, Sendai, Japan.

Maitotoxin (MTX) stimulates pituitary hormone release and $^{45}Ca^{2+}$ uptake (Koike et al., Soc. Neurosc., 711, 1983). To define the $^{45}Ca^{2+}$ flux response, GH_3 or normal anterior pituitary cells were exposed to $^{45}Ca^{2+}$ and MTX, as well as other agents, and cellular $^{45}Ca^{2+}$ flux measured after washing and vacuum filtration. In GH_3 cells 10 ng/ml MTX stimulated calcium uptake from 31 ± 4 to 181 ± 10 pmol $Ca^{2+}/10^6$ cells within 1 min; at isotopic equilibrium MTX induced a net $^{45}Ca^{2+}$ influx within 10 sec. $^{45}Ca^{2+}$ uptake due to MTX and 50 mM K^+ was blocked by the calcium antagonists, reserpine (Casteels et al., J. Physiol. 340: 403, 1983) and D-600. MTX-stimulated $^{45}Ca^{2+}$ uptake was dose dependent between 0.4 and 10 ng/ml. In normal cells 10 ng/ml MTX and 50 mM K^+ each increased uptake at 1 and 5 min and the effect was blocked by reserpine. Calcium uptake induced by the ionophore A23187 was not blocked by a calcium antagonist. Therefore, MTX, like K^+, rapidly increases net calcium influx into these cell types. The action is dose related and blocked by calcium channel antagonists. We conclude that unlike A23187, which has ionophoretic properties, MTX appears to activate physiological calcium channels. K07 NS00454 (ISL), K04 NS00601 (MJC), F05 TWO 3767 (GS), F-32-CA-07137 (AMJ), CA-07535 (RMM).

1579 PITUITARY SECRETORY GRANULES CONTAIN GLUTATHIONE AND DIVALENT CATIONS.
M.Y. Lorenson, L.S. Jacobs*, University of Rochester, Rochester, New York.

We have recently shown that most thiols, including reduced glutathione (GSH), stimulate prolactin and growth hormone release from isolated pituitary secretory granules and can cause granule dissolution (Endocrinology 110:1164,1982). In contrast, divalent cations profoundly inhibit hormone release from granules (J. Biol. Chem. 258:8618,1983). Thiols and divalent cations also exert powerful influences on the structure of storage PRL so as to enhance (thiols) or inhibit (cations) its ability to be measured by immunoassay (Endocrinology 112:1880,1983). Because of these observations, we have examined pituitaries for their content of divalent cations and GSH; atomic absorption spectrophotometric and fluorometric methods were used, respectively. Calcium, magnesium, and zinc were readily detectable in homogenates of bovine (b), porcine (p), and rat (r) pituitaries with values (μg/gm wet wt) of:

	(b)	(p)	(r)
calcium	226 ± 25	166 ± 25	290 ± 19
magnesium	162 ± 8	211 ± 19	121 ± 8
zinc	19.7 ± 0.7	19.9 ± 1.3	11.1 ± 0.6

The zinc concentration in bovine secretory granules was about 1.1 mM, more than 10 times that required to inhibit hormone release and assayability. GSH in pituitary homogenates was 1.3 (b) and 1.5 ± 0.2 (r) μg/mg protein; these values were similar to those measured in rat liver (1.8 ± 0.3 μg/mg). The GSH in rat cytosol was 3.9 μg/mg and that in secretory granules was 0.92 ± 0.17 μg/mg, yielding an intragranular concentration of about 3mM. Thus, pituitary secretory granules contain compounds which are capable of altering hormonal structure, functionality, and release. The regulation of these effects *in vitro* and *in vivo* remains to be studied.

1580 PITUITARY ADENOMAS: PATTERNS OF HPRL AND HGH SECRETION AS REVEALED BY HIGH RESOLUTION IMMUNO-CYTO-CHEMISTRY. N.D. Maestracci*, M. Bendayan and J. Hardy, Depts. of Medicine, Anatomy and Neurosurgery and the Notre-Dame Hospital, University of Montreal, Montreal, Quebec.

Seven human pituitary adenomas obtained by transsphenoidal surgery were investigated for the intracellular localization of PRL and GH, using the protein A-gold immunocytochemical technique. Among the seven cases, two were prolactinomas, two were GH secreting adenomas and three were mixed PRL and GH secreting adenomas. When PRL or GH were revealed, immunoreactivity was found in the cellular compartments involved in protein secretion, RER, Golgi apparatus and secretory granules of corresponding secreting cells. An increasing gradient in the intensity of labeling was observed from the RER to the Golgi and the granules which may correspond to the increasing concentration of the proteins occurring along their secretory pathway. Table : Comparative Density of Labeling

		anti hPRL protein A gold	anti hGH protein A gold
RER		19.14 ± 2.45	16.40 ± 1.50
Golgi		46.99 ± 3.89	22.98 ± 2.06
Secretory Granules	Immature	361.33 ± 43.96	134.97 ± 19.53
	Mature	583.17 ± 30.35	291.09 ± 9.84
Nucleus		3.81 ± 0.48	3.19 ± 0.45
Mitochondria		7.69 ± 0.78	3.50 ± 0.73

The distribution of immunoreactivity demonstrates that in the different adenomas studied, secreting cells: 1) have retained their differentiation; 2) may retain some specificity; 3) exhibit the same pattern of secretory events both for PRL and GH peptides.

1581 HISTIDYL-PROLINE DIKETOPIPERAZINE (HDP) FAILS TO SUPPRESS PROLACTIN SECRETION FROM HUMAN PITUITARY ADENOMAS IN VITRO. S. Marcovitz*, C. G. Goodyer, and J. Hardy. McGill University, Montreal, Quebec, Canada.

Human pituitary tissue from 4 PRL-secreting tumors and 1 mixed GH/PRL adenoma was obtained at transsphenoidal adenomectomy and maintained for 4 weeks in explant culture on stainless steel grids in Ham's F-10 medium with 10% fetal bovine serum and antibiotics. At 2-day intervals after day 5 in culture the tissues were subjected to 2 consecutive 3h incubations, the first in control medium (C) and the second (E) in either medium containing the test substances TRH or HDP (both at 10-6M - 10-9M) or control medium. The various agents were tested in random sequence on a total of 6-12 grids of each tumor. PRL was measured in the media by RIA. Results were expressed as log of the ratio E/C for paired data on each grid. The significance of differences between treatment groups and controls was calculated by ANOVA and Duncan's multiple range test. In 3 of the tumors (2 PRL and 1 GH/PRL), response to TRH was blunted (25-50% rise) in vivo and significant at 10-6M - 10-7M in vitro, while 2 PRL tumors showed no signficant response to TRH either in vivo or in vitro. HDP had no significant effect on PRL secretion in vitro from any of these 5 tumors. These results are at variance with the report of Melmed et.al. (Clin. Endo. 16:97, 1982) of an inhibitory effect of HDP on PRL secretion from human adenomas in culture. This would suggest that human pituitary tumors have variable responses to HDP.

1582 BIPHASIC TIME COURSE OF ESTRADIOL ON PROLACTIN PRODUCTION IN CELLS GROWN IN A COLLAGEN MATRIX. A. Martinez-Campos* and P.S. Dannies, Dept. of Pharmacology, Yale School of Medicine, New Haven, Conn. USA

Collagen has been used to improve growth, function and survival of primary cultures of cells from different tissues. We examined responses of PRL cells surrounded by this extracellular matrix. Dispersed anterior pituitary glands from male rats were seeded in a 1:1 mixture of DMEM and Ham's F10 medium supplemented with 15% gelding serum (which has low E_2 levels), in medium alone or a gel made of medium and rat tail collagen. Cells in the gel responded normally to bromocriptine; 30 nM caused a 2-fold or greater decrease in PRL in the medium on top of the gel. The response to 10^{-11} to 10^{-7} M E_2 was unexpected. E_2 stimulated PRL production 3 to 6 d after plating. At later times (9-18 d), E_2 decreased PRL production about 50% from cells in collagen, but still stimulated PRL production 2- to 5-fold in cells on plastic or on a thin layer of collagen. In one experiment, we quantitated PRL cells by immunostaining and found E_2 increased the number of PRL cells in collagen 75% above controls after 18 d, while PRL production decreased 50%, indicating the decrease is not caused by a toxic effect on PRL cells. We see cells with long processes in collagen that stain for A_2B_5, a possible neuronal marker. We are investigating whether these cells have other neuronal markers and whether E_2 decreases PRL by inducing these or other cells to produce inhibitory factors.

1583 LONG-LASTING PRL INHIBITING PROPERTIES OF AF1,A NEW ERGOLINE DERIVED COMPO=UND:IN VITRO STUDIES. A.Menegus,M.Boscaro,S.Mazzari°,F.Mantero*,Istituto di Semeiotica Medica,Università di Padova,Padova and°Fidia Research Laborato=ries,Abano Terme,Italy.

Almost all dopaminergic drugs of clinical use in long-term treatment of hyperprolactinemia have a short lenght of action and require multiple daily doses. Thus the availability of a new ergoline derived compound,AF1,provided with marked tropism for neuronal membrane,prompted us to evaluate the degree and duration of its PRL-inhibiting properties in a in vitro perfusion system of rat pituitary cells. PRL and ACTH were measured by RIA(NIAMDD antisera). Dopamine(DA)5.10^{-6}M infusion markedly suppressed PRL secretion but when DA was removed from the perfusion medium,PRL secretion rapidly(within 3.5 minutes)increased. Perfusion with Bromocriptine(B)(10^{-7}-10^{-5}M)inhibited PRL secretion with=in 30 min.;after its withdrawal,when only saline was added to the perfusion medium,PRL secretion slowly increased but did not reach maximal levels until more than 2 hours after withdrawal of B. AF1 10^{-6}M infusion decreased PRL secretion within 15 min.; however,this inhibitory effect was lower than that obtained with B and higher concentrations(10^{-5}M)failed to show any greater PRL inhibition. However,when only saline was infused a further progressive decrease of PRL secretion up to 4.5 hrs. after AF1 infusion was demonstrated. AF1 fai=led to inhibit both basal and Adrenalin- or LVP-induced ACTH secretion. These preliminary data demonstrate that AF1 inhibits PRL secretion from isolated rat anterior pituitary cells through a direct action and that this inhibiting effect is markedly long-lasting.

1584 MOLECULAR SIZE HETEROGENEITY OF HUMAN LACTOGENIC HORMONES (PRL, GH, hPL) AS SEEN BY IMMUNOPEROXIDASE ELECTROPHORESIS. S. Meuris*, M. Svoboda, J. Christophe and C. Robyn, Human Reproduction Research Unit and Dept. of Biochemistry and Nutrition, Medical School, U.L.B., 1000-Brussels, Belgium.

Size and charge heterogeneity of human lactogenic hormones, prolactin (hPRL), growth hormone (hGH) and placental lactogen (hPL) have been widely studied. The findings of molecular variants of hGH (Lewis, U.J. et al., B.B.R.C. 92:511,1980) and hPRL (Meuris, S. et al., FEBS L. 154:111, 1983) led us to reassess the molecular size (Mr) heterogeneity of lactogenic hormones under reducing conditions by immunoperoxidase electrophoresis with rabbit sera raised against hGH, hPL and rat, ovine and hPRL.

Two major monomeric immunoreactive variants of hGH with Mr 20000 and 22000 were found in all crude homogenates of human pituitaries (n=5).

Only one band with Mr 24000 was detected with the anti-hPL serum in crude homogenates of human placenta (n=5) and in amniotic fluid (n=5).

Two immunoreactive hPRL forms with Mr 17000 and 25000 were only found in 5 highly purified preparations of human pituitary PRL. In addition to these two forms, an other immunoreactive PRL with Mr 29000 was also found in crude homogenates of human pituitaries (n=5), of prolactinomas (n=5) and in amniotic fluid (n=5). By densitometry, the Mr 29000 PRL form represented 20-30% of the total immunoreactive hPRL recorded.

We conclude that different molecular heterogeneity and thus distinct cellular processing routes exist for each of the three lactogenic hormones. Moreover, the presence in the amniotic fluid of the Mr 29000 hPRL form, beside the known Mr 25000 hPRL, suggests that it can be a secretory product.

1585 PROLACTIN DIFFERENTIALLY ALTERS CARDIOVASCULAR REACTIVITY TO NOREPINEPHRINE AND ANGIOTENSIN IN THE RAT. D. Mills*, and R. Ward, Dept. of Health Studies, Univ. of Waterloo, Waterloo, ONT., N2L 3G1, Canada.

Low doses of ovine prolactin (oPRL) increase vascular pressor responses to norepinephrine (NOR) and angiotensin (ANG) in isolated preparations, and high doses inhibit the responses. This may contribute to the bell-shaped response curve of blood pressure (BP) to oPRL in vivo. This study examined effects of chronic oPRL infusion (via 7 day osmotic pump implanted ip. day 1) at 0, 0.15, 0.30, 0.60, 1.20, 2.40, and 4.80 µg/hr on resting BP (on days 1 and 7). Acute BP responses to i.a. NOR (4.3 µg) and ANG (0.125 µg) were also measured on day 7. oPRL infusion did not significantly change resting BP over the 7 days. However, oPRL tended to increase the BP response to NOR at 0.15 and 0.30 µg/hr, and significantly raised it at 0.60 and 4.80 µg/hr ($p<0.01$) vs. controls. Reactivity to NOR at 1.20 and 2.40 µg/hr was identical to controls. Body weight increases during the study were also greater in groups receiving 0.15, 0.30, 0.60, and 4.80 µg oPRL/hr ($p<0.05$), than in controls. BP reactivity to ANG tended to decrease at all higher oPRL doses, significantly at 0.30 and 1.20 µg/hr ($p<0.01$). These data suggest that 1) oPRL enhances vascular reactivity to NOR at low and high, but not moderate rates of infusion, 2) oPRL may induce fluid retention, resulting in body weight gain at these same rates of infusion, 3) oPRL depresses vascular reactivity to ANG at moderate and high infusion rates, and 4) the vascular effects of oPRL may not be evident under resting conditions. These data support a role for PRL in cardiovascular regulation during conditions of altered sympathetic activity. Supported by Ont. Heart Fund.

1586 DIETHYLSTILBESTROL INDUCTION OF PROLACTIN-SECRETING PITUITARY TUMORS: RESPONSE OF TUBEROINFUNDIBULAR DOPAMINERGIC NEURONS. W. W. Morgan*, A. Bartke, M. S. Smith and R. W. Steger, Depts. of Anatomy and Ob/Gyn, The Univ. of Tex. Health Sci. Ctr. at San Antonio, TX 78284 and Dept. of Physiology, Univ. Pittsburgh School of Med., Pittsburgh, PA 15261.

Response of the tuberoinfundibular dopaminergic neurons (TIDA) to elevated circulating prolactin (PRL) was examined after different intervals of diethylstilbesterol (DES) treatment or after DES removal. Fisher 344 male rats received Silastic capsules containing 8-9 mg DES or empty capsules for 3, 7, 14 or 30 days and had the capsules removed 22 days before sacrifice. In one group the DES-containing capsules were retained until killing. All rats received NSD-1015, a dihydroxyphenylalanine (DOPA) decarboxylase inhibitor, and the subsequent accumulation of DOPA provided a measure of dopamine (DA) synthesis. Anterior pituitary weights and plasma PRL levels were elevated in those rats treated for 30 days or continuously with DES. DA synthesis was elevated in the median eminence (ME) of rats treated with DES for 14 or 30 days but was not different from control in continuously DES-treated rats despite markedly elevated PRL. The results show that the TIDA respond to DES induced hyperprolactinemia but only after DES removal. Enhanced TIDA function may be a factor in the ensuing involution of the pituitary tumor while the suppression of TIDA function by DES may be a factor in the initial proliferation of the PRL secreting cells. (Supported by HD12671: RCDA DA 00083 to WWM.)

1587 MECHANISM OF INDUCTION OF OVULATION BY BROMOCRIPTINE IN EUPROLACTINEMIC ANOVURATORY WOMEN-ROLE OF OCCULTED HYPERPROLACTINEMIA IN ANOVULATION.
H.Mori*,K.AISAKA,R.Matsuoka and T.Kigawa,Dept.OB.GYN.,Oita Medical College ,Oita,Japan

It has been well documented that ovulation was induced by the treatment with bromocriptine in euprolactinemic-amenorrheic women.Present study has been performed to clarify the underlying mechanism.16 women with euprolactinemic anovulation had been treated with 5 mg of bromocriptine daily. Their prolactin secreting capacities were tested by 500 ug of TRH injection.Besides,the measurment of serum prolactin levels were performed in every 2 hours for 24 hours in 8 cases to examine their circadian prolactin secretion.

7 ovulated cases were observed out of 16 cases. In ovulated cases,the maximal response of serum prolactin to TRH was 138.0±34.7,which was higher than 66.6±25.3 in anovulated cases(ng/ml,M±S.D.,$P<0.005$).The circadian study revealed as following:prolactin level in ovulated cases at 24:00H was 48.7±10.0,at 2:00H 67.4± 28.2 and at 4:00H 47.4±17.5,which were higher than those of 15.6±10.1,22.5±12.3 and 16.2±3.8 in anovulated cases,respectively(ng/ml,M±S.D.,$P<0.05$).

These results conclude that the underlying mechanism of effectiveness of bromocriptine on euprolactinemic anovulation bases on the increased prolactin secreting capacity and hyperprolactinemic state during night,which should be called as the occulted hyperprolactinemia.

1588 "PROLACTIN STRESS TEST (PST)": A SIMPLE TOOL TO RULE OUT NON-PATHOLOGICAL HYPERPROLACTINEMIA.
O. Muneyyirci*, D. Goldstein, E. Kirpan, E. Modell and F.I. Reyes, Dept. OB-GYN, SUNY, Downstate Medical Center, Brooklyn, N.Y. 11203, U.S.A.

Prolactin (PRL), like cortisol (F) and growth hormone (GH) secretion, may increase in response to venipuncture or catheterization, as a result of anticipating anxiety or distress during the procedure. This may lead to a false diagnosis of pathological hyperprolactinemia. In order to exclude this possibility, we studied oligo- or amenorrheic patients, who had shown initially high serum PRL levels on 2 or more occassions, by serial blood samplings (q 15'x5) for PRL, F and GH determination under resting conditions (PST). Six patients out of 31 were found to have stress-venipunctured related hyperprolactinemia (SVH). Three of them still showed high PRL levels at the beginning of the PST, but concentrations fell within normal limits at 30-60'; the other 3 showed normal values throughout the test. Consistently high serum PRL levels were found in all the other patients. A pituitary adenoma was demonstrated in 6 of them (2 macros) by CT-scan; while the other showed no sellar or parasellar radiological abnormalities. Initial serum F levels tended to be high normal in all patients, but more so in patients with SVH (2 borderline elevated), but levels declined thereafter. A similar, but less conspicuous picture was also seen in GH levels. These results demonstrate that the PST is a helpful tool to rule out pathological hyperprolactinemia in anxiety-prone patients.

1589 REGULATION OF PRL AND LH SECRETION BY THE POSTERIOR PITUITARY IN THE NON-ANESTHETIZED RAT. Ichiro Murai*, and Nira Ben-Jonathan, Department of Physiology, Indiana University Medical School, Indianapolis, IN 46223 USA
Using urethane anesthetized rats, we previously reported (Endocrinology 110:1861, 1982) that the posterior pituitary modulates PRL and LH release. This study was designed to evaluate posterior lobe contribution to the control of hormone secretion in conscious rats, and examine the profile of PRL and LH release for a prolonged time after posterior lobectomy (LOBEX). LOBEX or sham surgery were performed under brevital anesthesia on the morning of estrus. Blood (0.4 ml) was collected at 1 h intervals for 6 h, and at 0900h, 1300h and 1700h for 4 days. Within 1 h after LOBEX, plasma PRL and LH elevated 2 fold. Throughout the collection period, PRL was 3-4 times above control, whereas LH reduced to near control levels by 6 h. During the next 3 days, plasma PRL levels were 5-6 times above control, and reduced by 50% on the fourth day. In contrast, plasma LH remained low and unaltered. None of the LOBEX rats showed estrous vaginal cyclicity for at least 6 days; 65% resumed normal cyclicity after 6-9 days, and the rest after 10-16 days.
Conclusions: 1. The sustained marked rise of plasma PRL after LOBEX indicates a significant contribution by the posterior lobe, probably via a dopaminergic (DA) mechanism, to the regulation of PRL release in cycling rats. 2. The pattern of plasma PRL after LOBEX differs from that during pseudopregnancy, and the resumption of cyclicity after 6-9 days may result from compensatory activation of hypothalamic DA. 3. The posterior lobe also participates in the control of LH secretion; the lowering of plasma LH following LOBEX may be caused by hyperprolactinemia.
Supported by NIH grants NS 13234, HD 14348 and RCDA NS 219.

1590 NEURAL STRUCTURES MEDIATING THE SUCKLING INDUCED PROLACTIN RELEASE. Gy, Nagy[x], K. Köves and B. Halász, 2nd Department of Anatomy, Semmelweis University Med. Sch. H-194 Budapest, Hungary

Location of the pathways in the rat hypothalamus mediating the suckling-induced prolactin (PRL) release were investigated. Unilateral and bilateral anterior and posterior hypothalamic deafferentations were made or 5,7-dihydroxytryptamine (5,7-DHT) was injected into the dorsal raphe nuclei (DRN) 5-11 days after delivery. Basal and suckling-induced PRL levels were determined by RIA in freely-moving lactating rats bearing indwelling cannula in the jugular vein. Bilateral anterior cut behind the optic chiasm and bilateral posterior cut interrupting the anterior or posterior connections of the hypothalamus respectively reduced the basal PRL levels and completely prevented the suckling-induced PRL release. A similar unilateral anterior cut also interfered with the PRL response. Unilateral posterior cut was ineffective. Injection of 5,7-DHT into the DRN reduced both the basal level of PRL and the suckling-induced hormone release. Data suggest that the pathways mediating the suckling-induced PRL release enter the hypothalamus from caudal and from rostral. The ascending fibers passing on one side of the hypothalamus are sufficient for the mediation while the pathways on one side entering the hypothalamus from rostral are insufficient. The ascending pathway contains serotonergic fibers.

1591 STIMULATION OF PROSTAGLANDIN ENDOPEROXIDE SYNTHASE ACTIVITY BY A SUBSTANCE IN HUMAN AMNIOTIC FLUID.
Murray D. Mitchell*, Douglas A. Craig, Sheikh A. Saeed and Daniel M. Strickland, Departments of Biochem. and OB-Gyn, The Cecil H. and Ida Green Center for Reproductive Biology Sciences, The University of Texas Southwestern Medical School, Dallas, TX.

The objective of this study was to characterize a substance in human amniotic fluid (HAF) that is stimulatory of prostaglandin (PG) biosynthesis by a microsomal-enriched preparation of bovine seminal vesicles. By use of gel exclusion chromatography and anisotropic ultrafiltration it was demonstrated that the stimulatory substance has a molecular weight of less than 500. Stimulation of PG biosynthesis by this substance is time- and concentration-dependent; maximal stimulation of 1.2-1.8-fold being observed by 20 min in the presence of 1 ml-equivalent of stimulant fraction. Stimulatory activity is demonstrable both in the presence of reduced glutathione (1.3 mM) and L-tryptophan (20 mM) either separately or combined and in the presence of exogenous arachidonic acid (5-120 μM). In the absence of added cofactors the stimulatory substance increases the rate of biosynthesis of PGE_2 and $PGF_{2\alpha}$ to an equal extent. The amount of stimulatory substance added is correlated positively with increased oxygen consumption by the PG synthase preparation. The stimulatory substance is stable to heating at 100°C for 10 min but is inactivated substantially (<20% of original activity) by treatment with pronase. We conclude that HAF contains a substance of low molecular weight, which is proteinaceous in character, that acts to stimulate prostaglandin endoperoxide synthase activity.

1592 EFFECT OF CHRONIC GLUCO- OR MINERALOCORTICOIDS ADMINISTRATION ON PROSTAGLANDIN GENERATION IN RAT MESENTERIC ARTERY.
I.Miyamori*, S.Yasuhara, H.Koshida and R.Takeda, The Second Department of Internal Medicine, School of Medicine, Kanazawa University, Kanazawa 920, Japan.

In order to elucidate the interplay between steroid hormones and known vascular prostaglandins(PGs), we studied the effects of chronic administration of glucocorticoids and mineralocorticoids on rat mesenteric artery PGs generation. Male Wistar rats weighing 150-180g were randomly divided into three groups. In each group of rat, either 12.5 mg/Kg of DOCA or 0.1 mg/Kg of Dexamethasone(Dx) or veicle alone was given subcutaneously and fed for three weeks on normal chow with free access to water. From each group of rats, mesenteric artery preparation was obtained at weekly interval and perfused with oxygenated Krebs-Ringer solution. Perfusion pressure was continuously monitored and perfusate was collected at every 30 sec after the perfusion system was fully equilibrated. Prostaglandin E_2 and 6-oxo-$PGF_{1\alpha}$ in the perfusate were measured by radioimmunoassay. In DOCA group 6-oxo-$PGF_{1\alpha}$ output was 1.28±0.36 ng/min and in Dx group 0.76±0.24 ng/min on one week which remained within the same range on the third week. These values were significantly lower than controls (2.28±0.92 ng/min, $P < 0.01$). PGE_2 showed a similar response. Substantial suppression of vascular PGs generation in Dx group may partly explain for

1593 TREATMENT OF FAMILIAL MALE PRECOCIOUS PUBERTY WITH SPIRONOLACTONE. Daniel Kenigsberg*, Ora Pescovitz, Florence Comite, Karen Hench, D. Lynn Loriaux Gordon B. Cutler, Jr., DEB, NICHD, NIH, Bethesda, Md. 20205

Five male children aged 4-8 years with familial precocious puberty (FPP) were treated with spironolactone, an antiandrogen and testicular cytochrome P-450 inhibitor, in doses of 1.5 mg/kg/day to 5.7 mg/kg/day for 3-6 months. All patients had low basal and peak levels of LH and FSH and a prepubertal response to LHRH. Testosterone levels were in the normal adult male range. Four of 5 subjects had not responded to LHRH analog treatment and the fifth had no prior therapy. All patients had a positive family history of precocious puberty and a negative evaluation for CNS, gonadal, adrenal, or HCG-producing neoplasms and for congenital adrenal hyperplasia. Spironolactone treatment decreased plasma testosterone from 322 ± 29 to 200 ± 31 (SE) ng/dl ($p < 0.05$, paired t-test). Free testosterone, measured in 3 patients, underwent a parallel decrease (2.6 ± 0.5 to 1.4 ± 0.3 ng/dl). Acne, a prominent complaint in 2 patients, improved markedly and the frequency of spontaneous erections decreased. In 3 patients reexamined after 6 months of treatment, pubertal stage did not advance. Testicular volume did not change significantly (7.6 ± 1.3 to 6.0 ± 0.5 ml). Linear growth rate did not change (8.8 ± 1.7 to 10.5 ± 3.5 cm/y). Bone age advancement was not slowed. One patient developed Tanner stage 2 gynecomastia. These preliminary results suggest that spironolactone causes a moderate decrease in plasma testosterone in FPP, has a beneficial effect on acne and spontaneous erections, and may retard pubertal progression. Linear growth rate and bone age advancement, however, have not benefited to date.

1594 SEQUENTIAL STUDY OF GONADOTROPIN (GT) SECRETION IN THALASSEMIC PATIENTS WITH DELAYED PUBERTY. M.Langer*, S.Alagna, PA.Cossu, GB.Cuccuru, G.Granieri, A.Masala, PP.Rovasio, and A.Stangoni. Service of Endocrinology of the University and Immunohematology and Transfusional Unit, USL 1, Sassari, Italy.

Delay or lack of sexual maturation is frequent in thalassemic patients and is attributed to GT deficiency due to iron overload. To evaluate whether GT secretion may improve or deteriorates with time and whether it might be of any prognostic value we determined at 2 years interval serum FSH and LH and their responses to GnRH (50µg iv) in 12 patients with β-thalassemia major, 5 M. aged 15-19 and 7 F. aged 15-20, all in Tanner's puberty stage 1. Mean FSH (5.3±2.2 mU/ml) and LH(4.8±2.5) were lower but not significantly, than in 8 sex and age matched controls (7.5±3.1 and 7.0±3.6). Peak values after GnRH (FSH: 10.7±5.7; LH: 18.1±11.9) were lower than in controls(15.9±7.8 and 33.5±18.0; $P<0.05$). Individually the LH response to GnRH was prepubertal(3.7–10.2, mean 6.6±2.8) in 6 pts. pubertal in the other (13–37 mean 23.9±8.9). Two years later the mean basal and stimulated levels were not significantly different; however, individually peak LH values increased markedly in 3 pts. 2 of whom developed puberty stage 2, decreased in 3 and remained about unchanged in 6; the clinical puberty stage in these 9 patients remained unchanged. Sexual immaturity in thalassemic patients is not always associated with permanent GT deficiency; gonadotropic function may improve with age and they may reach late puberty. Conversely a deterioration may be due to hemosiderosis and implies a bad prognosis for sexual maturation.

1595 FORMATION OF 5β- AND 5α-C_{19}-STEROIDS IN IMMATURE HAMSTER TESTES...PATHWAYS, LOCALIZATION AND HORMONAL REGULATION.

K. Matsumoto* and B. Sato, Departments of Pathology and Internal Medicine, Osaka University Medical School, Kita-ku, Osaka, Japan.

Whole testes, separated seminiferous tubules and interstitial tissues from golden hamsters at 8-60 days of age, 28-day-old testes irradiated with X-rays at 23 days of age (lack of germ cells) and 28-day-old testes from hypophysectomized hamsters injected with NIH-LH-S_{19} or NIAMD-oFSH-13 for 5 days were used. Tissue homogenates were incubated with radioactive androstenedione, progesterone and/or 5β- or 5α-pregnanedione and steroid metabolism were estimated. The major C_{19}-steroids formed by immature testes from progesterone were 5β- and 5α-products such as androsterone, etiocholanolone and 5β- and 5α-androstane-3α, 17β-diol, though the major steroids formed by neonatal and adult testes were testosterone and androstenedione. The 5β-C_{19}-steroids were formed from progesterone through androstenedione and testosterone, but the 5α-C_{19}-steroids were formed predominantly via 5α-C_{21}-steroids in immature testes. In immature testes, the high 5β-reductase activity, which was regulated by FSH, was found in cytosol of the seminiferous tubules, especially in non-germ cells, while the high 5α-reductase activity which was stimulated by LH in the presence of FSH, was present in microsomes of the interstitial tissue. The results indicate that 5β-reduction of testosterone takes place in cytosol of Sertoli cells under the influence of FSH, while the formation of 5α-C_{19}-steroids via 5α-C_{21}-steroids occurs in microsomes of interstitial cells under the influence of LH and FSH in immature hamster testes.

1596 17β Estradiol (E_2R) and Progesterone (PR) receptor sites before and after parturition in placenta at term.

O Martin* (SPON: V Cortés-Gallegos) and V Cortés-Gallegos. División Fisiología Gonadal, Unidad de Investigación Biomédica, Centro Médico Nacional IMSS. Apartado postal 73-032 México City México.

It is accepted that E_2R and PR sites of endometrium and myometrium are themselves regulated throughout the menstrual cycle and pregnancy. The placental synthesis of both steroids is significant at the end of pregnancy. Placental tissue was obtained by Cesarean Section with and without labour and after parturition, our findings (n=6) show an increase in the population of E_2R sites in the citosol with a consistent nuclear translocation which might be correlated with the labour work, reaching the maximum after parturition (8515 Fmol/mg DNA). However the nuclear PR sites decrease from 9525 to 735 Fmol/mg DNA including also the citosolic and total sites. These data agree with the compartamentalization through the menstrual cycle and partially with the decidual endometrial behavior. The possible molecular role of the 17β estradiol is its association required for the E_2R in the placenta and might induced the oxytocin receptor sites in the myometrium with the subsequent parturition.

1597 POSSIBLE MECHANISMS FOR THE DIFFERENCES BETWEEN IN VITRO AND IN VIVO ESTROGENICITY OF α-ZEARALANOL (P-1496) IN RAT LIVER. C. Mastri*, T.C. Sloop and G.W. Lucier, NIEHS, P.O. Box 12233, RTP, NC 27709.

We have shown recently that α-zearalanol (P-1496) binds to the estrogen receptor (ER) of rat liver, in vitro, with the same affinity as estradiol-17β(E_2). However, in vivo, P-1496 is much less potent than E_2. In the present study we investigated possible mechanisms underlying these differences. Interactions of DNA with cytosolic components prelabeled with P-1496 or E_2 were examined by DNA-cellulose chromatography. In the female, elution of DNA-bound radioactivity with KCl resulted in two main peaks (0.23 and 0.28M KCl) for both P-1496 or E_2. In the male, three main peaks of radioactivity were obtained (0.20, 0.23 and 0.28M KCl) with either P-1496 or E_2. However, quantitative differences between the two compounds were observed in both sexes. The time course of ER translocation into the nucleus was examined in vivo after a single injection of either P-1496 or E_2. With both compounds, two peaks of nuclear ER levels were observed at approximately 30 minutes and 4.5 hours after injection. We also examined the binding of P-1496 to cytosolic components. Saturation experiments with [^{3}H]-P-1496 after incubation with radioinert E_2(2μM) indicated the presence of a binding site specific to P-1496 (Kd~8nM) and distinct from the antiestrogen site. This component was found in both males and females, did not translocate P-1496 to the nucleus, and did not bind to DNA-cellulose. Our studies show similarities between P-1496 and E_2 with respect to nuclear translocation of ER. However, some differences are observed in the binding to DNA-cellulose and to cytosolic components of rat liver.

1598 MONOCLONAL ANTIBODIES TO CHICK PROGESTERONE RECEPTOR SUBUNIT A. A. P. McHale*, W.T. Schrader and B.W. O'Malley, Department. of Cell Biology, Baylor College of Medicine, Houston, TX 77030, USA.

Subunit A (M_r=79K) of chick oviduct progesterone receptor is structurally similar to its companion B subunit (M_r=108K). We purified subunit A from laying hen oviducts and produced antibodies to it by injection of BALB/C mice, detected using an ELISA assay. Monoclonal hybridoma lines were obtained by fusing splenocytes with mouse myeloma cells (P3 x 63Ag 8V) and screening by ELISA. Stable cloned lines were grown as ascites tumors in pristane-primed BALB/C mice. Two antibodies have been obtained. Antibody $4B_4$ (class IgM) was unable to bind to denatured subunit A in dot or Western immunoblot assays. The antibody was coupled to CNBr-activated Sepharose, and used successfully to purify receptor A under non-denaturing conditions. Elution (pH 2.5) and immediate neutralization yielded a single receptor protein band (pI-5.8; M_r=79K) which retains DNA sequence preference for the ovalbumin gene 5' flanking DNA receptor site. Yield was 70%. This antibody recognizes only receptor complexed in vivo with progesterone and not receptor labeled in vitro with [^{3}H]progesterone. The second antibody $4A_1$ (class IgG_1) reacts with denatured subunit A protein in immunoblot assays but not with the native protein. Proteolytic mapping studies place the epitope on the protein within a 27K receptor fragment containing the hormone site but not the DNA site. Both antibodies are specific for receptor A subunit, and do not recognize either companion B subunit, other steroid receptors nor unrelated chicken proteins.

1599 CROSSLINKING AND DENSITY SHIFT EXPERIMENTS TO STUDY THE SUBUNIT NATURE OF THE 5S NUCLEAR ESTROGEN RECEPTOR COMPLEX IN MCF-7 BREAST CANCER CELLS.

M. A. Miller*, A. Mullick, and B. S. Katzenellenbogen, Department of Physiology and Biophysics, University of Illinois, Urbana, Illinois 61801.

We have used chemical crosslinking and density shift experiments to study the subunit nature of the 5S nuclear estrogen receptor (ERn). Salt-extracted ERn prepared from MCF-7 cells labeled with ^{3}H-estradiol or ^{3}H-antiestrogen were treated with 2-iminothiolane. The crosslinked receptor complexes sediment as 5S species on 3M urea-containing sucrose gradients while non-crosslinked species are 4S. SDS-PAGE analyses of crosslinked ERn covalently labeled with ^{3}H-tamoxifen aziridine reveal a species of Mr 120,000-130,000 while the non-crosslinked or the crosslinked but mercaptan cleaved receptor is 62,000. In turnover studies, cells exposed for different time periods to dense (^{2}H, ^{13}C, ^{15}N) amino acids were labeled with ^{3}H-estradiol or ^{3}H-antiestrogen (trans-hydroxytamoxifen or CI628M), and salt-extracted ERn were separated on sucrose gradients under conditions that maintain the 5S form of the receptor. The normal density 5S form shifted to a broader and finally to a more dense, sharply sedimenting species (complete by 8 h). The time-course of this shift is the same as that seen for the 4S urea-disaggregated nuclear receptor form, suggesting that the 5S nuclear receptor is composed of 2 species which turnover at the same rate. We conclude that the nuclear 5S receptor complex consists of two similar sized units both of which turnover with similar half-lives. These data are consistent with the hypothesis that the 5S nuclear receptor is a homodimer. (Supported by NIH CA18119 and CA31870).

1600 CROSS-REACTIVITY OF CHICK OVIDUCT ESTROGEN RECEPTOR (ER) WITH MONOCLONAL ANTIBODIES RAISED AGAINST CALF UTERUS ER ; STUDIES IN CHROMATIN.

She Wei Ming, Bruno Moncharmont, Marie-Claire Lebeau, Nelly Massol and Etienne-Emile Baulieu. Lab Hormones, 94270 Bicêtre, France.

Monoclonal antibodies raised against ER purified from calf uterus cytosol interact with chick oviduct ER. Four antibodies (out of a library of five (Moncharmont et al., 1982, Biochemistry 21, 6916)) were able to recognize the oviduct ER in both its cytosol and its nuclear or chromatin associated forms. The antibody showing the best affinity (JS 34/32) was used to purify chick oviduct cytosol ER and to isolate ER-bearing chromatin fractions. In soluble chromatin, prepared by micrococcal nuclease digestion of hen oviduct nuclei (Massol et al., 1978, Nucl. Acids Res. 5, 723 ; Lebeau et al., 1982, Biochem. J. 204, 653), the ER peak which originally sedimented in sucrose gradients at 13-14S, was shifted to 18-19S after interaction with these antibodies. This allowed to easily separate chromatin-associated RE from the bulk of mono- and di-nucleosomes. The nature of the DNA sequences and proteins associated with the ER in the 18-19S peak was investigated.

1601 CONVERSION OF ESTROGEN RECEPTOR (ER) FROM A STATE WITH FAST INTO A STATE WITH SLOW ESTRADIOL (E_2) DISSOCIATION DOES NOT REQUIRE 4S TO 5S TRANSFORMATION. R. E. Müller*, A.M. Traish, T. Hirota and H.H.Wotiz.
Boston University School of Medicine, 80 E. Concord St., Boston, MA 02118

Calf uterine $R(^3H)E_2$ formed at 0°C (low affinity state, fast E_2 dissociation with $T_{1/2}$ = 6 min) was immobilized on hydroxylapatite (HAP) without (8S oligomer) or with (4S monomer) 0.4M KCl and heated (28°C) in the presence of unlabeled DES. In contrast to $R(^3H)E_2$ free in cytosol, the heat-promoted conversion of HAP-bound 8S and 4S $R(^3H)E_2$ into a higher affinity state (E_2 diss. $T_{1/2}$=90min) was not accompanied by receptor transformation, since the HAP eluate (0.4M phosphate) contained only the 4S monomer; upon reheating or desalting (0°C) of this eluate 4S to 5S transformation occurred. $R(^3H)E_2$ bound to HAP in 0.4M KCl (4S), heated (28°C) and eluted from HAP as 4S, remained in the slow dissociating high affinity state. Addition of pyridoxal 5'-phosphate (PLP) to slow dissociating high affinity 5S $R(^3H)E_2$ (heat-transformed 5S cytosol) induced rapid $(^3H)E_2$ dissociation although $R(^3H)E_2$ remained unaltered as 5S dimer. This effect was reversed by addition of lysine. The 4S monomer exists in two conformational states; upon E_2 binding to the low affinity state a temperature accelerated conformational change of the estrogen binding site results in stronger R interaction with E_2 and slower E_2 dissociation. Concomitant with this conformational change, but independent from it, is the heat-accelerated alteration of the dimerization domain of the 4S subunit; thus, when RE_2 is free in solution, 4S to 5S transformation accompanies RE_2 conversion from the lower into the higher affinity state.

1602 PATTERN OF CHANGES IN ANDROGEN RECEPTOR LEVEL AND FUNCTIONALITY IN RESPONSE TO ACUTE TESTOSTERONE STIMULATION. T.G. Muldoon* and W.I.P. Mainwaring, Dept. of Endocrinology, Med. Coll. of Georgia, Augusta, GA 30912, USA, and Dept. of Biochemistry, Univ. of Leeds, Leeds, England.

This study was based on our seemingly-unrelated observations that (a) two functionally-distinct forms of androgen receptor (AR) exist in rat ventral prostate (VP) cytosol and (b) a temporally biphasic pattern of protein synthesis is induced in VP cells in response to androgen. We have measured cytoplasmic and nuclear VP AR, as well as association rate kinetics and the rate of approach to equilibrium of androgen-receptor interactions at intervals from 12 h to 7 days following Silastic implantation of testosterone into 7-day-castrate adult male rats. Cytosol AR levels initially fell in concert with rising nuclear AR titer in a typical receptor translocation fashion, reaching a nuclear peak within 24 h. Subsequently, nuclear AR concentration fell to castrate levels by 3 days, while cytosol AR remained low. Between days 3 and 4, a second rise in nuclear AR occurred, this time unaccompanied by any change in cytosol AR; this nuclear surge subsided within a subsequent 24-h period. The pattern of nuclear AR fluctuation was closely coincident with the biphasic protein synthesis response. The cytoplasmic receptors gradually changed from high- to lower-avidity binders of androgen during the course of the first nuclear receptor rise, and then reverted to the higher-avidity form just prior to the second peak of nuclear binding. The results suggest a relationship among receptor-mediated cell responsiveness, nuclear AR level, and patterns of differential protein synthesis in the response of the VP to androgen.
(Supported by a Burroughs Wellcome Travel Award to TGM.)

1603 REGULATORY EFFECTS OF GLUCOCORTICOIDS ON THE DUNNING PROSTATE R3327H-G8-A1 CELL LINE. Abhijit Nag*, Allan J. Syms, James S. Norris and Roy G. Smith, Baylor College of Medicine, Dept. of Urology, Houston TX and (JSN) Dept. Med., Univ. of Arkansas School of Med. Sci., Little Rock, AR.

The R3327H-G8-A1 cell line derived from rat prostate adenocarcinoma contains receptors for both androgen and glucocorticoids. While the growth of these cells in culture are stimulated by androgens, and receptor augmentation is promoted by androgens (1.7 fold in 6h) the potent glucocorticoids triamcinolone acetonide (TA) and dexamethasone dramatically inhibit both these androgenic effects; aldosterone, estradiol and progesterone are ineffective. The glucocorticoid effect on receptor augmentation and cell proliferation is maintained for at least 96h whereas nuclear residency and total concentration of glucocorticoid receptors is maximal only during the first 30 min. One could therefore speculate that if TA induces synthesis of a repressor molecule(s) that the repressor should have a long half-life. Incorporation of ^{35}S-methionine into proteins synthesized in the presence of TA was analyzed by SDS gel electrophoresis and autoradiography. While the synthesis of a 54K protein was elevated, two proteins of molecular weight, 41K and 66K, were repressed. It is postulated that glucocorticoids regulate the function of these prostate derived tumor cells by inhibiting the synthesis of regulatory proteins such as the androgen receptor and that the temporal relationship with glucocorticoid mediated events is possibly associated with de novo synthesis of a protein repressor(s).

Supported by NIH Grant #CA36264

1604 ANDROGEN RECEPTOR IN RAT SUBMANDIBULAR GLAND. M. OTA*, N. SATO, T. NEMOTO, Y. NEMOTO and S. KYAKUMOTO, Department of Biochemistry, Iwate Medical University School of Dentistry, Morioka, 020 Japan

The characteristics of cytosol androgen receptor in the submandibular gland, androgen-dependent organ, of intact female rats and castrated male rats was investigated using ^{3}H-methyltrienolone (R1881). The Scatchard analysis revealed that R1881 binds to a single class of sites of the receptor in both sexes and that the Kd and the number of binding sites were 3.6 nM and 66 fmol/mg protein in males, and 2.5 nM and 159 fmol/mg protein in females, respectively. The competitive experiments showed that ^{3}H-R1881 was displaced by 5α-dihydrotestosterone=testosterone > cortisol > estradiol in both sexes in the presence of a 100-fold excess. Androgen cytosol and nuclear exchange assays were performed in the submandibular gland. The cytosol exchange activity in male rats was lower than that in female rats, whereas, the nuclear exchange activity in males was 2-fold higher than that in females. A linear glycerol (15-30%) gradient density centrifugation at low salt ionic strength exerted that ^{3}H-R1881 receptor complex sediments at 8 S in both sexes. This 8 S receptor complex converts to 4 S by warming at 20° C for 30 min, indicating that the activation occurred. This activated ^{3}H-R1881 receptor complex was shown to bind DNA using DNA-cellulose resin in both sexes. These findings suggest that, similar to receptors in other androgen target organs, a receptor, which binds androgen specifically with high affinity and low capacity, exsists in the cytosol of the submandibular gland of male and female rats, and that the R1881-receptor complex interacts with DNA following the activation.

1605 THERMOLABILE AND ACTIVATION-LABILE GLUCOCORTICOID RECEPTOR OF CULTURED SKIN FIBROBLAST IN THE PATIENT OF GLUCOCORTICOID RESISTANCE SYNDROME. H.Nawata*, K.Sekiya, K.Higuchi, T.Yanase, K.Kato and H.Ibayashi, Third Department of Internal Medicine, Kyushu University, Fukuoka, 812 Japan.

To clarify the end-organ resistance to cortisol in man, glucocorticoid receptor(GR) of cultured fibroblasts was characterized, which were obtained by skin biopsy from patient FK who had high plasma cortisol and ACTH concentration, increased urinary free cortisol, 17-OHCS and 17-KS excretions, resistance to adrenal suppression by dexamethasone(Dex.), hyperresponse of plasma ACTH by CRF, LVP and metyrapone, no suppression of plasma ACTH by FK-33824 and absence of any symptoms and signs of Cushing's syndrome, and was compared with those of healthy controls and the patients with typical clinical symptoms of Cushing's disease. GR of the patient FK was found to have increased dissociation constant using whole cell assay and decreased binding capacity using cytosol assay, compared with those of healthy controls and Cushing's disease. Cytoplasmic GR of the patient FK was more thermolabile than controls. [^{3}H]Dex.-GR complex activated by temperature of the patient FK showed reduced affinity to DNA and lower peak eluted at the position of stable activated complex on DEAE cellulose column chromatography compared with controls. The incroporation of [^{3}H]thymidine into DNA of cultured fibroblasts was less inhibited by Dex. in the patient FK. The present study demonstrated that GR of the patient FK was thermolabile and activation-labile to form stable activated [^{3}H]Dex.-GR complex translocated into nucleus. This abnormal GR status explains the mechanism of glucocorticoid resistance of the patient FK.

1606 CHARACTERIZATION OF THE PARTIALLY PURIFIED UNBOUND GLUCOCORTICOID RECEPTOR OF RAT LIVER. K.NOMA*, S. KASAYAMA, Y.NISHIZAWA, B.SATO, S.KISHIMOTO, and K. MATSUMOTO, The Third Department of Internal Medicine and The Second Department of Pathology, Osaka University Hospital, Fukushima-ku, Osaka, 553, Japan

Rat liver glucocorticoid receptor(GR) in the crude cytosol is different from other targets with respect to the steroid specificity and the stability. In order to characterize the GR itself by excluding the effects of other cytosol factors, we have partially purified the unbound GR in the presence of molybdate(Mo) and dithiothreitol(DTT). The rat liver cytosol was prepared in 10mM Tris HCl,pH 7.4- 20mM Mo. The unbound GR elutes from DEAE cellulose at 0.15M KCl and purified about 10 folds in 30% yields by addition of DTT(to 10mM). The dexamethasone(Dex) labelled GR elutes at 0.25M KCl in the non-activated form and at 0.15M KCl in the activated form. The unbound GR elutes in the similar position to the activated bound GR.However, this purified unbound GR cannot bind the rat liver nuclei and by ^{3}H-Dex postlabelling elutes at 0.25M KCl. In low salt conditions, the sedimentation coeff. is measured as 9.5-10S by sucrose density gradient and its Stokes Radius,66A by Cellulofine gel filtration. These parameters are consistent with those of the nonactivated occupied GR in the crude cytosol in the presence of Mo. The rat liver cytosol GR is more stable than other targets(thymus, spleen) and DTT effect is not significant. Dex binding in the 0.15M KCl elute becomes very labile and by addition of DTT increases 3 times. In the crude cytosol, progesterone(P) and deoxycorticosterone(DOC) have little inhibitory effects in the competitive study for ^{3}H-Dex binding, while by partial purification 50% binding inhibitory conc. of P &DOC are 3-5x10^{-6}& 5-9x10^{-8}M respectively as thymus, spleen and brain cytosol.

1607 COMPARISON OF THE EFFECTS OF CHAOTROPIC (NaSCN) AND NON-CHAOTROPIC (KCl AND NaCl) SALTS ON THE GLUCOCORTICOID RECEPTOR.

L. Olinger and C.A. Barnett* Dept. Biology, San Diego State Univ., San Diego, CA 92182-0057, USA.

We (Biochemistry 19:5446, 1980) have previously noted that factors which stimulate the rate of activation of glucocorticoid receptor (GR) complexes (heat, salt, dilution, various chemical treatments) also stimulate the rate of inactivation of unoccupied GR suggesting that both processes may involve similar biochemical mechanisms. Recently Kalimi and Hubbard (Biochim. Biophys. Acta 719:488, 1982) suggested that the chaotropic salt NaSCN represents an exception to this generalization and reported that NaSCN alters GR properties in ways which are distinct from that of other salts such as KCl or NaCl. Specifically Kalimi and Hubbard reported that (1) NaSCN inhibits heat induced activation of the GR complex (25C) and (2) that stimulation of inactivation of the unoccupied GR by NaSCN was molybdate insensitive. In contrast we find that NaSCN stimulates the rate of activation of the GR complex at both 0C and 15C and has no effect on activation or DNA-cellulose binding at 25C (30 min). The stimulation of activation of the GR complex by NaSCN is blocked by molybdate. In addition we find that molybdate stabilizes the unoccupied receptor against both KCl and NaSCN stimulated inactivation at 25C. Although the dose response curves are different, NaSCN being more potent, we find no evidence to suggest that the effects of chaotropic salts on the GR are qualitatively different than other salts such as KCl or NaCl.

1608 BIOCHEMICAL NATURE OF INSULIN RECEPTOR ISOLATED FROM TWO CULTURED HUMAN HEPATOMA CELL LINES HEP3B & HA22T.

Ming-Ya Huang[1], Chung-Ming Chang[1], Lo-Tung Ho[2] & Chen-Kung Chou*[1,3]
Dept. of Medical Research[1], Internal Medicine[2], Veterans General Hospital. Shih-Pei, Taipei.
Inst. of Biological Chemistry[3], Academia Sinica. Taipei, Taiwan.

Specific insulin binding of two cultured human hepatoma cell lines HA22T and Hep3B were examined. The Kd for high affinity insulin receptors of both HA22T and Hep3B are about 4nM and 1nM respectively. On the other hand, both cell line carries similar number of receptor ($4X10^4$/cell). We further examined the protein kinase activity associated with insulin receptor. Receptors were solubilized with 1% Triton x-100 and then purified by WGA-agarose chromatography. Both receptor preparations show insulin activated protein kinase activity. Besides the major phosphorylated protein band with molecular weight 94K dalton which is the β subunit of insulin receptor, HA22T also carries another phosphorylated band with molecular weight about 50K. Insulin concentration for half maximum activation of both receptor kinase activity is between 10^{-8} to 10^{-9} M which close to the Kd of insulin receptor measured on intact hepatoma cell. HA22T and Hep3B provide us a good model system to examine biochemical nature of human hepatic insulin receptor and its relationship to the mechanism of insulin actions.

1609 ^{125}I-INSULIN INTERNALIZATION INTO RAT LIVER ENDOSOMES. EVIDENCE FOR DIFFERENT PATHWAYS. M.N. Khan*, S. Savoie, J.J.M. Bergeron and B.I. Posner, McGill University, Montreal, Canada, H3A 2B2.

Colchicine inhibits the early uptake of ^{125}I-insulin (^{125}I-IN) (J.Cell.Biol. 93: 560) while chloroquine augments ^{125}I-IN accumulation into Golgi fractions (J.Biol.Chem.257:5789). In this study we compare the effect of chloroquine and colchicine on the pattern and extent of ^{125}I-IN uptake into endosomes, isolated from lysosomal (L) and microsomal (P) fractions of rat liver. Endosomes were prepared by fractionating P and L fractions on discontinuous sucrose gradients. From the L fraction the endosomes ('unique' vesicles) were recovered at 0.60/0.86M (L_3) and 0.86/1.0M (L_4) sucrose interfaces and corresponding Golgi-enriched endosomes (P_3 and P_4) were obtained from the P fraction. The time course of ^{125}I-IN uptake peaked earlier (2 min) in P_3 and P_4 than in L_3 and L_4 (5 min). Radioautography of all endosomes demonstrated radiolabeled hormone in lipoprotein-containing vesicles. Chloroquine treatment augmented (4 - 11 fold) internalized ^{125}I-IN in both P_3/P_4 and L_3/L_4 fractions. The time of peak uptake in P_3/P_4 remained unaltered while in L_3/L_4 it shifted to 10 min postinjection. Colchicine inhibited (>2-fold) ^{125}I-IN uptake into P_3/P_4 at 2 min post-injection, while increasing uptake into L_3/L_4 (~2-fold). Whereas clearance of ^{125}I-IN from P_3/P_4 was comparable to control that from L_3/L_4 was considerably slowed. These data provide evidence for the existence in rat liver of two endosome vesicle populations participating independently in the internalization of insulin.

1610 BIOCHEMICAL ANALYSIS OF RECEPTORS FOR INSULIN AND IGFS ON CELLS FROM MICRO- AND MACROVESSELS. G.L. King*, I. Jialal, M. Crettaz, C.R. Kahn and A. Moses Joslin Diabetes Center and Beth Israel Hospital, Boston, Massachusetts

We have shown that retinal capillary endothelial cells and pericytes are more responsive to the effects of insulin and IGFs than aortic endothelial and smooth muscle cells. To determine the cause for this difference, the receptors of insulin, IGF-I and MSA (a rat IGF-II) on these cells were studied biochemically by covalently cross-linking the ^{125}I-peptides to their receptors using DSS followed by PAGE and autoradiography. The α- or binding subunit of the insulin receptor in all cells was found to have Mr = 145,000 under reduced conditions. Labeling of this band was inhibited by 10^{-9}M of insulin, anti-insulin receptor antibodies and 10^{-8}M of IGF-I, but not by MSA. The β-subunit of the insulin receptor in endothelial cells was identified by its ability to be autophosphorylated when stimulated by insulin and found to have Mr = 99,000. Both α and β subunits are 4-10,000 larger than in other cells. Labeling of IGF-I receptors revealed a Mr = 145,000, similar to insulin receptor, except that IGF-I was 100 fold more potent than insulin in competing with ^{125}I-IGF-I for binding. ^{125}I-MSA (IGF-II) receptors in all cells had a Mr = 260,000 and 210,000 under reduced and non-reduced conditions, respectively. IGF-I competed weakly with ^{125}I-MSA, whereas insulin was ineffective. ^{125}I-MSA also bound to the IGF-I receptor with Mr = 145,000. In summary, receptors for insulin, IGF-I and MSA on cells from micro- and macrovessels, are biochemically similar to those in other cells. Interestingly, the subunits of insulin receptor seem larger than those of other cell types suggesting differences in the insulin receptor or its biological role in endothelial cells.

1611 NATIVE AND SYNTHETIC ESTROGENS AUGMENT GONADOTROPIN-STIMULATED LH RECEPTOR CONTENT IN CULTURED RAT GRANULOSA CELLS. B. Kessel*, A.J.W. Hsueh, Dept. Reprod. Med., Univ. Calif., San Diego, La Jolla CA 92093

Both follicle-stimulating hormone (FSH) and low concentrations of luteinizing hormone (LH) stimulate LH receptor formation in rat granulosa cells in vivo. We have shown that estrogens enhance gonadotropin-stimulated aromatase activity in cultured granulosa cells. The effect of estrogens on gonadotropin-stimulated LH receptor induction was studied in vitro using granulosa cells from immature hypophysectomized, estrogen-primed rats. Granulosa cells were cultured for 3 days with increasing (3-25 ng/ml) concentrations of FSH with or without 17β-estradiol or diethylstilbestrol. Both estrogens enhanced FSH-stimulated LH receptors by decreasing (1.6-3.2-fold) the ED_{50} of FSH. Some granulosa cells were also primed with FSH for 2 days to induce LH receptors, and were further cultured for an additional 3 days in the presence of rat LH (30 ng/ml) with or without varying concentrations of estrogens. Four native estrogens tested enhanced LH-stimulated LH receptor formation by 3-6-fold with relative potencies of 17β-estradiol = estrone > 17α-estradiol > estriol. Several synthetic estrogens were also effective, with relative potencies of hexestrol > moxestrol > ethynyl estradiol >>> mestranol. The effects of the native and synthetic estrogens to enhance gonadotropin-stimulated LH receptors are in keeping with their reported binding affinities to estrogen receptors in other target tissues, suggesting mediation through ovarian estrogen receptors. Thus, local estrogens in ovarian follicles may enhance LH receptor formation and increase granulosa cell responsiveness to the LH surge, with subsequent ovulation and adequate corpus luteum formation.

1612 THYROTROPIN DISPLACING IMMUNOGLOBULINS (TDI) IN GRAVES' DISEASE PATIENTS TREATED 10 YEARS EARLIER: IN RELAPSE OR IN REMISSION. N. Kuzuya*, Y. Hirota, T. Mitsuhashi, K. Kubota, H. Ikeda, H. Tamai, K. Kuma, K. Itoh, and H. Uchimura, Third Department of Internal Medicine, University of Tokyo Tokyo, Department of Psychosomatic Medicine(Y.H. and H.T.), Kyushu University, Fukuoka, Kuma Hospital(K.K.), Kobe, and Itoh Hospital(K.I.), Tokyo, Japan.

The natural course of Graves' disease is complex; some patients have prolonged remissions after drug therapy, whereas, others require much longer therapy because of relapses. Thyrotropin displacing immunoglobulins (TDI) have been detected in sera of Graves' disease patients and are thought to be related to it's pathogenesis. TDI is measured by an ^{125}I-TSH radioreceptor assay. In the present study, sera from 46 patients whose initial diagnosis of Graves' disease was established more than 10 yrs earlier were examined for TDI. Patients were divided into 2 groups: A. 13 who were being treated with antithyroid drugs for greater than 10 yrs because of relapses, and B. 33 in remission for 5 yrs without therapy. Serum thyroid hormone levels were within the normal range in both groups at the time of study. IgG's were separated from sera by using Protein A - Sepharose and TDI activity was measured using human thyroid membranes and expressed as TDI indices. In group A, 10 of 13 patients (77%) had positive TDI indices, but none of 33 patients in group B had TDI activity. These data indicate TDI is present in the large majority of patients who have frequent relapses after drug therapy and is normal or absent in patients in prolonged remission. TDI appears to be closely related to the clinical activity of Graves' disease.

1613 BINDING AND INTERNALIZATION OF EPIDERMAL GROWTH FACTOR (EGF) IN HUMAN TERM PLACENTAL CELLS IN CULTURE: RELATIONSHIP TO BIOLOGICAL RESPONSE. W.H. Lai*, H.J. Guyda and J.J.M. Bergeron, Departments of Pediatrics & Anatomy (JJMB), McGill University, Montreal, Canada.

The relationship between ^{125}I-EGF internalization and biologic response in primary cultures of human syncytiotrophoblast has been assessed by quantitative electron microscope radioautography. Continuous labeling of cultures with ^{125}I-EGF (0.20 nM, 150 µCi/µg) at 37 C revealed a progressive increase in intracellular EGF with 5% of total label in intracellular organelles at 2 min and 88% by 60 min. Detailed analysis showed a progressive transfer of ^{125}I-EGF from microvillar processes to the base of microvilli followed by uptake into vesicular and polymorphic endosomes as well as multivesicular bodies. Since incubations were carried out with subsaturating doses of EGF with minor degradation of EGF, the results suggest a temporal transfer of occupied and unoccupied EGF receptors into intracellular compartments. Chloroquine (CHL, 100 µM), cholchicine (COL, 100 µM) and bacitracin (BAC, 1 mg/ml) augmented EGF specific binding from 45% in control cultures to 60%, 60% and 65% respectively, with a majority of the ligand (72-83%) being observed in endosomal structures and multivesicular bodies after 60 min of incubation. EGF-stimulated uptake of ^{14}C-3-0-methyl glucose at 30 min was increased by CHL ($p < 0.001$), COL ($p < 0.05$) and BAC ($p < 0.05$). No significant effect of the same inhibitors was observed on ^{14}C-α-amino isobutyric acid uptake. In summary, EGF induced the internalization of occupied and possibly unoccupied EGF receptors. Agents interfering with EGF degradation resulted in greater receptor occupancy especially at intracellular sites. The results are consistent with some EGF actions being exerted at the loci of endosomes and/or multivesicular bodies.

1614 IN VITRO RADIOAUTOGRAPHIC LOCALIZATION OF SOMATOSTATIN-14 (S14) AND SOMATOSTATIN-28 (S28) RECEPTORS IN THE RAT BRAIN. P. Leroux* and G. Pelletier, MRC Group in Molecular Endocrinology, CHUL, Québec, G1V 4G2, Canada.

The localization of somatostatin receptors in the rat brain was studied by "in vitro" radioautography using the agonists [^{125}I]-[Tyr^{0}-DTrp^{8}]S14 (supplied by Dr. D.H. Coy) and [I^{125}]-[Leu^{8}-DTrp^{22}-Tyr^{25}]S28 (supplied by Dr. J. Rivier) as tracers. The binding of either radiolabel was similarly distributed and could be prevented by concomittant incubation with either 10^{-6}M S14 or S28. High density binding occurred principally in the deep layer of the cortex, the hippocampus, the locus coeruleus and the medial and lateral nucleus of amygdala. Moderate and low binding was found in definite regions, particularly the caudate-putamen nucleus. Treatment with cysteamine (300 mg/kg B.W.), which caused a somatostatin depletion, was required to observe labeling in the dorsal hypothalamus. These results indicate a good correlation between the localization of somatostatin receptors and that of immunoreactive somatostatin, except for hypothalamus. The saturability and specificity of the binding was also studied in the same conditions by counting performed on scrapped off serial sections. The scatchard analysis of saturation curves with each tracer gave one site interaction kinetics with K_D value of 0.42 ± 0.09 nM and 0.32 ± 0.04 nM for S14 and S28 iodinated analogs respectively. The competition potencies of the agonists themselves with the binding of both tracers was 10-fold higher than those of the native hormones with a DE_{50} in the nanomolar range. The common localization of S14- and S28-analog binding and the biochemical characteristics of this binding strongly suggest that there is one type of high affinity somatostatin receptor able to bind either S28 or S14.

1615 EVIDENCE FOR THE PRESENCE OF DISULFIDE LINKED NON-IDENTICAL SUBUNITS IN THE LH-hCG RECEPTOR. B.B. Saxena,*, B. Dattareyamurthy, H. Ota, P. Rathnam, Cornell University Medical College, New York, New York 10021

An aliquot of 25 mg of LH-hCG receptor purified from bovine corpora (J. Biol. Chem. 258:3140, 1983) was dissociated into its subunits by reduction with 50mM dithiotreitol (DTT) in the presence of 2% sodium dodecyl sulfate (SDS) and alkytaled with 100mM N-ethylmaleimide (NEM). The subunits were fractionated by gel permeation chromatography on the columns of sepharose 6B, Ultrogel (AcA-34 and AcA-44). The final isolation of the subunits was achieved on a column of sephadex G-75. The total yield of the purified subunits of Mr. of 85K and 38K was approximately 6 mg and 4 mg respectively. Each subunit migrated as a single protein band in SDS-polyacrylamide disc gel electrophoresis indicating high degree of homogeneity. The amino acid analysis of the subunits showed differences. A non-equilibrium double antibody radioimmunoassay system using LH-hCG receptor labeled with ^{125}I by chloramine-T method was developed to determine the immunoreactivity of the LH-hCG receptor and its subunits. The immunological non-identity of the subunits was indicated from the observations that LH-hCG-receptor monomer of an approximate Mr. of 120K-140K showed 80% specific binding with an antisera raised against LH-hCG receptor, however the subunits of 85K and 38K showed only 20% and 10% specific binding. On the other hand when the subunits were assayed together, little specific binding was observed, whereas when the subunits and the monomer of 120K-140K were mixed, a 70% restoration of the immunoreactivity was observed. The LH-hCG receptor monomer of an Mr. of 120K-140K specifically bound ^{125}I-hCG. The subunits also bound ^{125}I-hCG but the bound ^{125}I-hCG could not be displaced with excess cold hCG. On the other hand, NEM-treated subunits failed to bind ^{125}I-hCG suggesting that a disulfide exchange may be involved in hormone receptor binding. These results suggest that the monomer of LH-hCG receptor has a Mr. of 120K-140K and consists of two non-identical disulfide linked subunits of 85K and 38K. Support-NIH CA 13908, Mellon Foundation, N.Y.

1616 SECRETION OF AN INHIBITOR OF FSH BINDING TO RECEPTOR BY THE BACTERIA SERRATIA. P.M. Sluss* and L.E. Reichert, Jr., Department of Biochemistry, Albany Medical College, Albany, New York 12208.

Bacterial growth in contaminated porcine follicular fluid (PFF) was associated with increased concentrations of a large molecular weight (M_r > 6000) inhibitor of ^{125}I-hFSH binding to calf testis membranes (FSH-BI) (Biol. Reprod., 29:335, 1983). To identify the bacteria and determine if the inhibitor was a secretory product, bacteria were isolated by culture on agar plates and pure strains tested for generation of FSH-BI when grown in sterile PFF. Only one of 39 pure bacterial colonies generated the M_r > 6000 FSH-BI. The bacteria were tentatively identified as *Serratia liquifaciens* and subsequently shown to also secrete FSH-BI when grown in synthetic media. Six strains of *Serratia*, obtained from the American Type Culture Collection, also secreted FSH-BI. FSH-BI secreted by *Serratia liquifaciens* was inactivated by heat ($T_{1/2}$ = 30 min at 60°C) or exposure to pH 2 (2 hours at 25°C). FSH-BI was insoluble in ether, 75% acetone or 40% ammonium sulfate. Protease activity, using a casein substrate, was undetected in doses which effectively (50%) inhibited ^{125}I-hFSH binding. Preincubation of FSH-BI with either membranes or ^{125}I-hFSH ("non-equilibrium assays") was utilized to study the mechanism of binding inhibition. Our results suggest that FSH-BI was due to effects on membranes rather than on the radioligand. These data demonstrate that *Serratia liquifaciens* secrete a substance of M_r > 6000 which interacts with testis membranes to inhibit receptor binding of ^{125}I-hFSH. Furthermore, the FSH-BI appears to be secreted constituitively by all (7) strains of *Serratia* tested.

1617 ECDYSTEROID RECEPTORS IN TISSUES OF THE BLOWFLY. G. Käuser and P. Karlson*, Physiol.-Chem. Institut, Universität Marburg, 3550 Marburg GFR

Ecdysteroids control a number of important growth and differentiation processes. A major target tissue is the epidermis. In order to understand the mode of action of ecdysteroids, we studied the ecdysteroid binding proteins ("receptors") of the epidermis of blowfly larvae in comparison to the corresponding protein(s) of other blowfly tissues. Cytosolic extracts were prepared and incubated with tritiated ponasterone A (ponA) which is a 25-deoxy analogue of the moulting hormone. The amount of protein-bound label was determined by gel filtration and corrected for unspecific binding measured by incubation in the presence of an excess of unlabelled ponA. Saturable binding of tritiated ponA could be detected in fat body, epidermis, and brain. Binding of ponA (in relation to protein concentration) was highest in cytosol of the epidermis which was used for further analysis. By Scatchard plots K_d values for ponA between 10^{-8} and 10^{-9} M were measured. The K_d of 20-hydroxyecdysone (20-HO-E) (determined with tritiated 20-HO-E) was one order of magnitude higher. Tritiated ponA bound could be displaced not only by unlabelled ponA, but also by higher concentrations of 20-HO-E and even higher concentrations of ecdysone. Surprisingly the insecticide azadirachtin was able to displace tritiated ponA bound to cytosolic proteins from larval tissues (brain and epidermis). However, no interaction with specific ponA binding proteins extracted from pupal tissues could be detected. Whether this is due to differences between larval and pupal receptors remains to be tested.

1618 COMPARISON OF PROPERTIES OF EPIDERMAL GROWTH FACTOR (EGF) BINDING SITES IN THE INTRACELLULAR ORGANELLES AND MICROVILLUS PLASMA MEMBRANES (MPM) FROM TERM HUMAN PLACENTA. N. Ramani*, B. Stadig, Ch. V. Rao, P. Woost and G. Schultz, University of Louisville, Louisville, KY 40292, USA

The MPM as well as intracellular organelles of term human placenta contain EGF binding sites. The present studies investigated the properties of the intracellular organelle sites and compared them to the MPM sites. The specificity and macromolecular nature of intracellular organelle sites were similar to MPM sites. Kinetics of ^{125}I-EGF binding to rough endoplasmic reticulum (RER) and lysosomes (LY) were different from MPM. Scatchard plots of ^{125}I-EGF specific binding to the intracellular organelles and MPM were curvilinear which was due to negative cooperativity. The Kds in all the organelles were similar, i.e. 0.05-.01 nM. The total number of sites were, MPM-8220 fmol/mg protein > smooth ER-5800 > LY-4320 > RER-3147 > Golgi (G) 2243. While ^{125}I-EGF dissociation rates in 50 X dilution media were similar in all the organelles, the rates in the presence of excess unlabeled EGF were slower in RER and LY compared to MPM. The optimal pH for binding to all the organelles except LY was 7.0. For LY it was 6.0. LY sites were more susceptible to thermal inactivation at 55°, RER sites were more susceptible to dinitrofluorobenzene and smooth ER sites were less susceptible to acetic anhydride and p-chloromercuribenzoate pretreatment compared to MPM sites. Two major proteins of ~140 K and 160K daltons were labeled after incubation with ^{125}I-EGF. The 160 K protein was labeled predominantly in MPM, smooth ER and G, whereas 140 K protein labeled predominantly in LY and both proteins were equally labeled in RER. Small amounts of other labeled proteins (< 140 K & >160 K) were also found in all the organelles.

1619 FREQUENT SUPPRESSION OF ANDROGEN LEVELS BY DEXAMETHASONE WITH RESUMPTION OF REGULAR OVULATION IN POLYCYSTIC OVARY SYNDROME. T.J. McKenna* and T. Loughlin, Dept. of Endocrinology, St. Vincent's Hosp., Dublin, Ireland.

We have assessed androgen, oestrogen and gonadotrophin status in 15 women with polycystic ovary syndrome (PCO) and amenorrhoea before and after 3 months treatment with dexamethasone, 0.5 mg taken at night only. Plasma testosterone (TEST), androstenedione (A4), the TEST/sex hormone binding globulin (SHBG) ratio, oestrone levels and the LH response to LH-RH were all significantly elevated in PCO: SHBG levels were significantly suppressed. The TEST increment following endogenous adrenal stimulation using metyrapone was significantly elevated in PCO: normal women, 1.02 ± 0.53 (mean ± SD), and PCO 1.55 ± 0.7 nmol/l, $p<0.02$. Following the administration of dexamethasone TEST, TEST/SHBG and A4 were significantly suppressed. Oestrone levels fell from 293 ± 136 to 238 ± 113 pmol/l. Ten patients resumed regular ovulation. When the steroidal pattern of response to dexamethasone was assessed in the group of responders and non-responders separately it was noted that in the responders TEST levels fell from 1.93 ± 0.72 to 1.24 ± 0.48 nmol/l, TEST/SHBG fell from 11.14 ± 8.4 to 5.08 ± 2.2 nmol/l and A4 levels fell from 10.07 ± 3.38 to 6.7 ± 2.3 nmol/l, $p<0.05$. In the non-responders there was no significant change in the hormonal values. In our PCO patients there is a large subgroup with an exaggerated androgen response to adrenal stimulation and when androgen levels are suppressed with dexamethasone ovulatory menstrual cycles resume. These findings support the theory that PCO frequently arises due to increased adrenal androgen secretion and suppression of plasma androgens with glucocorticoids predicts a satisfactory therepeutic response.

1620 DIFFERENTIAL ISOTOPE EFFECTS IN THE C-19 HYDROXYLATIVE STEPS OF AROMATIZATION. S. Miyairi and J. Fishman*, The Rockefeller University, New York, NY 10021 USA.

Two sequential hydroxylations at C-19 methyl of androgens are the primary and necessary steps in estrogen biosynthesis. Deuterium substitution at C-19 results in a substantial isotope effect for aromatization as a whole (Can. J. Chem. 59:2809, 1981). We sought information on the nature of this isotope effect and whether it reflected one or both of the C-19 hydroxylations. High specific activity [$19C^3H_3$]-androstenedione was synthesized (Biochem. Biophys. Res. Commun. 117:392, 1983) and converted to [$19C^3H_2$]-19-hydroxyandrostenedione by placental enzymes. Both of these ^3H labeled substrates were incubated together with the corresponding [$4^{14}C$]-labeled substances with human placental microsomes. The formation of ^3H_2O and ^3HCOOH was monitored and the $^3H/^{14}C$ of incubation products and recovered substrates was determined. The results revealed that a) at saturation the isotope effect at the first C-19 hydroxylation has a magnitude KH/KT of 3.2, b) there is no isotope effect in the second hydroxylation irrespective whether the [$19C^3H_3$] or [$19C^3H_2OH$] substrate is employed. Kinetic analysis furthermore showed that the isotope effect is concentrated in the Vmax component of the reaction. This data implies that the two hydroxylations at C-19 have different mechanisms and that separate catalytic sites for the two purposes may be involved. This work was supported by grant CA22795 from the National Cancer Institute.

1621 DEHYDROEPIANDROSTERONE SULFATE (DHEA-S) BLOCKS THE PROGESTERONE (4P) RISE INDUCED BY LOW DENSITY LIPOPROTEIN (LDL) IN CULTURED HUMAN CHORIOCARCINOMA JEG-3 CELLS. J. Moise*, J. Ilekis, A. Scommegna and R. Benveniste, Div. Reproductive Endocrinology & Infertility, Dept. OBGYN, Michael Reese Hosp. Med. Cntr., University of Chicago, Chicago, IL 60616, USA.

The JEG-3 cell retains several secretory characteristics of the normal trophoblast and was presently used to study the regulation of 4P secretion. The focus was on LDL (a cholesterol ester carrier) and DHEA-S, two physiological precursors of the distinct pathways leading to 4P and estradiol (E2), respectively. We report: (i) JEG-3 cells in serum-free Dulbecco's modified Eagles medium (DMEM) form De Novo cholesterol leading to a basal 4P secretion of about 20 ng/ mg cell protein/ 24 hr; (ii) in DMEM alone, the cells do not secrete E2 nor other DHEA-E2 intermediates. Addition of DHEA-S to DMEM (5 to 5 x 10^3 ng/ml) results in a dose-related secretion of DHEA, androstenedione, testosterone, estrone, and E2 with a DHEA-S rate of conversion of about 65%; (iii) the effect of DHEA-S in enhancinq the activity of the E2 pathway takes place without significant effect on basal 4P secretion; (iv) LDL isolated from man sera and added to DMEM (.03 to 1 mg LDL protein/ ml) induces a dose-related increase in 4P secretion up to about 400% of basal levels; (v) addition of DHEA-S (5 to 5 x 10^3 ng/ ml) to DMEM + LDL induces a dose-related inhibition of the LDL stimulatory effect on 4P secretion and a return of 4P to basal levels. Conclusion. Our results suggest that (i) the JEG-3 cell retains the main steroidogenic properties of the normal trophoblast, and (ii) DHEA-S inhibits LDL contribution to 4P secretion, a mechanism which may be relevant to the understanding of parturition when a rise of DHEA-S is associated with a drop of 4P.

1622 ESTRADIOL (E2) ACTION ON PITUITARY LUTEINIZING HORMONE (LH) SECRETION IS ATTENUATED BY SERUM PROTEIN BINDING. George W. Moll, Jr., M.D., Ph.D.* and Robert L. Rosenfield, M.D., Dept. Ped., Univ. of Chicago, Chicago, Il. 60637.

We directly tested the influence of protein binding upon the E2 inhibitory effect on LH responsiveness to LH releasing hormone (LHRH) in perifused rat pituitaries. An initial LHRH pulse (#1) was given in protein-free medium. Medium was then changed to continue perifusion ±E2 ±1gm/dl albumin. LHRH pulse#2 was given 1 hr after the change of medium. LH secretion ratios (LH response to LHRH#2/LH response to LHRH#1 in each study) were compared.

E2(pg/ml)	Albumin	LH Secretion Ratio[a]	p Value[b]	n
0	−	1.14 ± 0.06		8
11.0	−	0.78 ± 0.02	<.01	3
11.0	+	1.91 ± 0.18	<.05	3
272.0	−	0.49 ± 0.03	<.001	3
272.0	+	0.71 ± 0.03	<.05	3

[a]Mean±SEM. [b]LH secretion ratio in Table vs that without E2 or albumin.

These data show that at 11 pg/ml E2, half-maximal inhibition of LH secretion occurs in the absence of albumin. In the presence of 1 gm/dl albumin (free E2 conc. 2 pg/ml), the inhibitory effect of E2 is blocked (the LH secretion ratio resembles that seen with albumin alone). At 272 pg/ml E2, maximal inhibition of LH secretion occurs in the absence of albumin. The presence of 1 gm/dl albumin (free E2 conc. 46 pg/ml) attenuates the E2 effect to the extent expected for this amount of bioavailable E2 with a superimposed modest enhancement of LH secretion by albumin.

We conclude that this inhibitory effect of E2 upon LH responsiveness to LHRH is dependent upon the free E2 concentration and that albumin attenuates this effect to the degree that it binds E2.

1623 PLASMA ANDROGENS IN FEMALES WITH HIRSUTISM AND ANDROGENETIC ALOPECIA.

J. Montalto*, A. Callan, P. Smith, J.F. Connelly, H. Davies and S. Lewis.
Department of Clinical Biochemistry, Royal Children's Hospital, Melbourne, Australia.

Plasma androgen studies were performed on adult female patients with hirsutism (17-51 yrs)and androgenetic alopecia (18-46 yrs)and these resul--ts compared with those from normal adult females. Androgens estimated included 5∝androstane 3∝17βDIOL sulphate (3∝DIOL-S)by radioimmunoassay (RIA) after solvolysis and LH 20 chromatography; testosterone (T), Δ4--androstenedione (Δ)and dehydroepiandrosterone sulphate (DHEA-S)by specif--ic RIA; dihydrotestosterone (DHT)by RIA after removal of T by permangan--ate oxidation. The following results (mean ± S.E.M.) were obtained:-

STEROID	NORMALS (N)	HIRSUTE (N)	ALOPECIA (N)	SYMBOLS
DHEAS (umol/l)	4.7±0.3 (25)	4.6±0.4 (30)	4.6±0.6 (16)	* p< 0.05
Δ (nmol/l)	4.0±0.3 (20)	5.7±0.5** (17)	5.8±0.8* (17)	** p< 0.005
T (nmol/l)	1.4±0.4 (17)	2.6±0.2** (30)	2.4±0.3* (17)	(N) =numbers
DHT (nmol/l)	0.6±0.07 (20)	0.6±0.06 (23)	0.5±0.05 (12)	tested.
3∝DIOL-S (nmol/l)	38 ±3.6 (22)	72 ±8.4** (29)	56 ±7.0* (17)	

Within the hirsute group, 23 patients had elevated T levels, and of these 17 had an elevated 3∝DIOL-S; in only 1 patient was an elevated 3∝DIOL-S associated with a normal T level. In the alopecia group, 10 patients had an elevated T level and of these 8 had an elevated 3∝DIOL-S. No patient with alopecia and elevated 3∝DIOL-S showed a normal T level. The findings of elevated 3∝DIOL-S together with elevated T and normal DHT levels in bo--th groups of patients suggests that 3∝DIOL-S may be of physico-patholo-gical importance providing information on androgen metabolism occurring within the liver and/or peripheral target cells.

1624 TRANSIENT ALTERATION OF GONADAL FUNCTION IN SPONTANEOUSLY HYPERTENSIVE RAT.

Pavel Komanicky*, Christopher Longcope and James C. Melby. Departments of Medicine, Texas Tech University School of Medicine, Amarillo, TX 79106, University of Massachusetts School of Medicine, Worcester, MA 01605 and Boston University School of Medicine, Boston MA 02118, U.S.A.

The mechanisms of the development of hypertension in the spontaneously hypertensive rat (SHR) have not been fully elucidated. In this study we examined male SHR and their respective Wistar-Kyoto (WKY) control rats from the pre-hypertensive (age 4 weeks) through the stage of well established hypertension (age 20 weeks). We measured systolic blood pressure, body weight and testes weight; and, by radioimmunoassay, plasma levels of estrone (E_1), estradiol (E_2), testosterone (T), 5α-dihydrotestosterone (DHT), Δ^4-androstenedione (A), dehydroepiandrosterone (DHEA) and dehydroepiandrosterone-sulfate (DHEA-S) at predetermined time intervals of 4, 8, 12, 16 and 20 weeks of age. The SHR became hypertensive by week 8 and remained so thereafter as compared to WKY controls. Body weight (BW) was significantly lower ($P<0.05$) in SHR at week 4 and higher at weeks 16 and 20. Testes weight in μg/g BW, was significantly lower in SHR at weeks 4 and 16. At week 4 plasma levels of T and DHT were significantly lower and the ratios E_1/DHT, E_1/A, E_2/DHT and T/DHT higher in SHR than in controls. However, at week 8 plasma levels of E_2, DHEA-S and ratio E_2/DHT became significantly lower in SHR. At weeks 12 and 16 only plasma ratio E_2/DHEA was lower in SHR, whereas at week 20 hormone levels were similar in both groups. Thus, in the pre-hypertensive stage SHR exhibit hypogonadism with a relative excess of estrogens. Subsequently, with progression of hypertension and age, the abnormality gradually disappears. Sex hormones may play an important role in the etiology of hypertension in SHR.

1625 PROPERTIES OF 5α-REDUCTASE FOR TESTOSTERONE, THE ABILITY OF ANDROGEN RECEPTOR AND TESTOSTERONE AND 5α-DIHYDROTESTOSTERONE CONCENTRATIONS IN RAT SUBMANDIBULAR GLAND. Shinri Koshika*, Yoshiyuki Nakayama, Mayumi Tarui, Shuichi Takemura and Masahiko Hosaka!, Department of Biochemistry, Kanagawa Dental College, Yokosuka, Japan, !Department of Urology, Yokohama City University School of Medicine, Yokohama, Japan.

To evaluate the significance of androgen in the submandibular gland, the property of 5α-reductase for testosterone, the ability of androgen receptor and intra-submandibular testosterone and 5α-dihydrotestosterone concentrations were studied using rat submandibular gland. Testosterone-4-^{14}C and the microsome obtained from the submandibular gland were used for the elucidation of 5α-reductase properties. The binding capacities of cytosol receptor to methyltrienolone(R1881) and 5α-dihydrotestosterone were determined. Testosterone and 5α-dihydrotestosterone concentrations were measured by a specific radioimmunoassay. Apparent Michaelis constant(Km) value of 5α-reductase for testosterone was 1.02×10^{-6}M in the female . On the other hand, two kinds of Km values as 1.12×10^{-6}M and 1.10×10^{-5}M were determined in the male . The androgen-receptor complexes in the cytosol fractions were sedimented at 4S and 8S in both male and female. Intra-submandibular testosterone and 5α-dihydrotestosterone concentrations showed marked increse from 4 weeks of age. Subsequently, the concentration of 5α-dihydrotestosterone became dominant with the advance in age. There was no sexual difference in the androgen concentration. Getting together, it was conclued that rat submandibular gland was proved as an androgen target organ by biochemical procedures. Furthermore, a definite sexual difference was shown in the properties of 5α-reductase.

1626 VARIATION WITH AGE IN THE LEVELS OF SEX STEROID BINDING PLASMA PROTEIN AS DETERMINED BY RADIOIMMUNOASSAY. Y. Maruyama*, N. Aoki, Y. Suzuki**, H. Shinohara** and T. Yamamoto, Departments of Internal Medicine and Biochemistry**, Kinki University School of Medicine, Sayama, Osaka 589, Japan.

Human sex steroid binding plasma protein (SBP) was isolated from pooled plasma by affinity chromatography on testosterone-17α ethynylcarboxyaminoethyl Sepharose 4B followed by hydroxyapatite column chromatography. This procedure produced a purified SBP preparation, concentrated 6,000 fold over pooled plasma with an overall recovery of 3%. Purified SBP showed a single band in polyacrylamide gel electrophoresis and had a dissociation constant of 5.7 nM for dihydrotestosterone and a binding site per 95,000 daltons. Using the SBP preparation, specific antiserum was obtained in a rabbit and radioimmunoassay for SBP was constructed basing on a double antibody method utilizing anti-rabbit IgG in goat (MILES) as second antibody. In this assay, no cross reactivity was observed with transferin, alubmin, testosterone, estradiol and dihydrotestosterone. The intraassay variation coefficient was 6.0 and interassay coefficient of variation was 9.1. With this assay, SBP was determined in sera of 138 normal men and 169 nonpregnant women, ranging in age from 11 to 87 years. The results indicate (i) that SBP levels in both sexes increased gradually with age up to mid-eighties, (ii) that the average levels in the eighties were approximately twice those in the twenties, (iii) that SBP levels in women were about twice as high as those in men of corresponding age, and (iv) that the mean values of overall results in men and women were 2.1 and 4.4 μg/ml respectively.

1627 FURTHER INVESTIGATION INTO THE APPARENT LOSS OF PROGESTERONE BINDING TO MICROSOMAL CYTOCHROME P450 DURING HCG-INDUCED DESENSITIZATION OF THE RAT TESTIS.

N.Kühn-Velten[+] and W.Staib, Institut f. Physiologische Chemie II, Universität, Moorenstrasse 5, D-4000 Düsseldorf, Germany.

It is well known that injection of a single dose of hCG results in an apparent diminution of several steroidogenic enzyme activities in rat testis microsomes, especially of the cytochrome P450-dependent 17a-hydroxylase/C-17,20-lyase complex. Kinetic studies have revealed that the Vmax is reduced whereas the Km values are probably not affected. This pattern may be explained by either a real loss of enzyme protein or by formation of an enzyme complex with a non-competitive inhibitor during hCG action. In order to investigate this problem, microsomes were prepared from testes of control rats or of rats injected with 100 IU hCG 48 hours prior to the experiment s.c. After hCG administration, apparent maximal progesterone binding (spectral differences A390-420nm) is reduced from 76 to 9 pmol/mg protein. Cytochrome P450 content (CO-induced A450-490nm) is reduced from 83 to 18 pmol/mg protein. Heme content (pyridine hemochromogen; dithionite-induced A558-575nm) is reduced from 106 to 52 pmol/mg protein. The maximal spectral shift (A420-390nm) induced by metyrapone (which does not bind directly to the substrate binding site of microsomal cytochrome P450) is reduced from 0.0032 to 0.0006/mg protein. Finally, oxidation and destabilization of a possible complex of reduced cytochrome P450 with an inhibitor by potassium hexacyanoferrate(III) does not restore progesterone binding ability of cytochrome P450 in testes of hCG-treated animals. These results allow the conclusion that real loss or irreversible conformational change rather than complexation of testicular cytochrome P450 result from hCG administration.

1628 MAINTENANCE OF SPERMATOGENESIS IN HYPOPHYSECTOMIZED MONKEYS WITH TESTOSTERONE (T).

G.R. Marshall*, F. Jockenhövel, D.K. Lüdecke, and E. Nieschlag, Max Planck Clinical Research Unit for Reproductive Medicine, Steinfurter Straße 107, D-4400 Münster, F.R. Germany.

As part of a series of studies on the regulation of spermatogenesis in primates, 5 adult monkeys (M. fascicularis) received twenty 5 cm long T-filled Silastic capsules at the time of hypophysectomy. Completeness of hypophysectomy was confirmed by lack of LH response to GnRH stimulation. In an untreated hypophysectomized monkey serum LH and T levels were undetectable by 7 days and the testicular volume declined rapidly, reaching a nadir of 30 % of the presurgical volume by 5 weeks postsurgery. The seminiferous tubules contained only Sertoli cells and spermatogonia. Leydig cells could not be seen. The T-filled capsules elevated serum T levels from 22 $\pm$ 6 nmol/l (mean $\pm$ sd) to constant levels averaging 149 $\pm$ 11 nmol/l. By the 8th week of treatment, testicular volumes were still 75 % of presurgical values and the seminiferous tubules contained typical spermatogenic cellular associations. Sperm counts remained unchanged during treatment. When the capsules were removed after 14 weeks, testicular volumes were around 60 %. Biopsies showed seminiferous tubules having typical cellular assocations but about 15 % of the tubules had only a few germ cells. Leydig cells were not seen. After removal of the capsules, the testicular volumes and serum T levels declined precipitously. It is concluded that testosterone alone can maintain spermatogenesis in a nonhuman primate.

1629 INVOLVEMENT OF LYSOSOMAL ENZYMES IN TESTICULAR FUNCTIONS AS ALTERED BY PITUITARY HOMOGRAFTS. P.P. Mathur* and S. Chattopadhyay, Department of Zoology, Kurukshetra University, Kurukshetra 132 119 and Dept. of Physiology, B.H.U., Varanasi India.

Pituitary glands grafted under the kidney capsule provide a continuous supply of prolactin due to the absence of hypothalamic inhibitory factor. Increase in the level of prolactin in the rat may affect availability of hormone for reproductive function. Single pituitaries were transplanted under the kidney capsule of male rats. After six weeks of the transplant, the recepient rats were sacrificed and trophic activity of testosterone and intratesticular functions were assessed. The weights of ventral prostate and seminal vesicles, full and empty, showed significant increase from the control, 53%, 18% and 6%, respectively. The activity of beta glucuronidase in kidney, an androgen inducible enzyme, also increased in comparison with the control 3.1 and 2.6 units, respectively. Testicular ascorbic acid content increased significantly from the control values. Incorporation of ^{32}P in the nucleic acid fraction showed an increase. The increased rate of testosterone production and an alteration in spermatogenesis was associated with increased activity of acid phosphatase and decreased activity of beta glucuronidase. The active mediation of lysosomal enzymes in testicular function modified by prolactin was indicated.

1630 METHYLTRANSFERASE INHIBITION REDUCES LEYDIG CELL STEROIDOGENESIS. W.H. Moger*, Departments of Physiology & Biophysics and of Obstetrics & Gynacology, Dalhousie University, Halifax, Canada, B3H 4H7.

Stimulation of Leydig cell steroidogenesis is associated with an increase in phospholipid methyltransferase activity (Nieto and Catt, Endocrinology 113:758, 1983). In this study the effects of methyltransferase inhibition with 3-deazaadenosine (DZA) and homocysteine thiolactone (HTL) are reported. Collagenase dispersed murine testicular interstitial cells were preincubated for 1 hr with DZA and HTL and then incubated for 2 hr with the inhibitors and luteinizing hormone (LH), dibutyryl cyclic AMP (dbcAMP) or pregnenolone (preg). DZA (10-1000 μM) caused a dose-dependent inhibition of LH (100 ng/ml) stimulated androgen production when 100 μM HTL was also present. Maximum inhibition was 50% (51 ± 4 vs 102 ± 8 ng/10^6 cells/2 h). The inhibitory effect of DZA-HTL on LH and dbcAMP stimulated androgen production was similar; the maximum rate of androgen production was significantly inhibited (LH; 50%:dbcAMP; 33%) while the EC_{50} was only slightly reduced (LH; 3.4 ± 1.9 ng/ml vs 6.6 ± 3.7 ng/ml:dbcAMP 291 ± 1 vs 544 ± 4 μM). Andorgen production from preg (0.1-3 μM) as exogenous substrate was unaffected by DZA-HTL treatment. It is concluded that LH induced phospholipid methylation may be necessary for LH to maximally stimulate Leydig cell steroidogenesis.

Supported by the MRC of Canada.

1631 ENDOCRINOLOGY OF A TRANSPLANTABLE LEYDIG CELL TUMOR AND RESPONSE TO A CYTOXIC. Ian D. Morris, Department of Pharmacology, University of Manchester, Manchester M13 9PT, U.K.

Leydig cell tumors may provide an in vivo as well as in vitro model for characterization of the physiology and pharmacology of the Leydig cell. Ethylene dimethanesulphonate (EDS) will reversibly destroy the Leydig cell. Tumors were grown s.c. in Fisher rats treated after 3-4 w. with EDS 100 mg/kg i.p. At this time the tumor weighed about 8g, serum testosterone (T) had increased 20-fold, and prostate and seminal vesicles (SV) were enlarged. Testes, epididymides and spermatogenesis appeared normal, gonadotropins were undetectable. hCG binding was 50% lower in the tumor than in testes. After EDS tumor size decreased by 80% at 6d, however growth resumed and at 20d the experiment was terminated (6d in untreated rats). Serum T fell by 6d but was still elevated, at 20d T was 100 ng/ml. No changes were seen in prostate yet SV weight reflected T changes. In contrast to the profound and prolonged testicular and epididymal regression normally seen after EDS, the testes in tumor bearing rats were unchanged except for a small decrease after 2d, epididymal weight was increased and spermatogenesis unchanged. Testicular hCG binding fell to a nadir after 6d compared to 2d in normal rats. Tumor hCG binding was variable, levels fell but the changes were not significant. In conclusion Leydig cell tumor regression was not prolonged as predicted which may reflect the rapid cellular proliferation of a fundamental cellular change. Testes in tumor bearing rats were partially protected from the cytoxic probably by the elevated serum androgen.

1632 HORMONE BINDING AND RESPONSIVENESS IN TESTICULAR CELLS. Patricia L. Morris* and Jennie P. Mather. The Population Council, New York, NY 10021.

To further investigate the sensitivity of testicular cells to tropic factors,we compared several cell lines with primary cultures of immature rat testis. Binding characteristics for gonadotropin (hCG) and epidermal growth factor (EGF) were determined. Responsiveness was analyzed as a function of steroid production (progestin(P) or androgen(A)),and, cell growth *in vitro*. Leydig cells were characterized by LH-induced P or A response and hCG binding capacity (fmoles per 10^6 cells or not detectable, ND). hCG sensitive (P): MA-10 (40fmoles);hCG insensitive (A):TM_3, I10A, R2C, LC-540(ND).Growth and assay in serum-free media with Insulin and Transferrin (2F) did not alter hCG binding. Growth in 2F revealed that EGF is mitogenic for the Sertoli cell line(TM_4) but not the Leydig cell lines. A comparison of EGF binding revealed capacity differences among the cell lines viz. Sertoli (TM_4:40fmoles),Leydig (TM_3,R2C,MA-10:120fmoles and LC-540:30fmoles) endothelial(TR-1:40fmoles) and peritubular myoid (TR-M:35fmoles per 10^6cell) Ligand binding analysis showed differences in the time course of EGF binding among the cell lines. Further studies of surface binding vs. internalization revealed differences in EGF handling from data published for fibroblasts. Growth in 2F with various doses of EGF markedly reduced binding sites for all cell lines within 24 h. Primary Leydig cells were cultured in 2F with a rapid and complete loss of hCG binding activity. On day 4 of culture, levels of EGF binding were different (Sertoli:10fmoles;Leydig:130fmoles/10^6cells). Primary myoid cells (7.5% serum)had levels of 50fmoles/10^6cells. EGF pre-incubation decreased EGF binding in primary Sertoli and Leydig cultures. Comparisons of these parameters will allow the study of the effects of single factors on testicular function.

1633 SUBTOTAL THYROIDECTOMY CAUSES ALTERATIONS IN ACTIVITIES OF THREE THYROID LYSOSOMAL ENZYMES: CATHEPSIN D, β-GLUCURONIDASE AND ARYL SULFATASE A.

P.P. Krupp*, J.R. Starling, J. Golstein and P. Nève, Dept. of Anatomy & Neurobiology, Univ. of Vermont College of Medicine; VA Hospital and Univ. of Wisconsin, Madison; Institut de Recherche Interdisciplinaire (LMN), Free University of Brussels; and Laboratory of Experimental Medicine, Montigny-Le-Tilleul, Belgium.

Subtotal thyroidectomy causes an increase in endogenous secretion of TSH by cells in the anterior pituitary. This results in chronic stimulation of residual thyroid tissue. There is a subsequent increase in synthetic and secretory activity of individual thyroid cells. This study focuses on alterations in lysosomal enzymes which occur during a 6 week period of chronic endogenous stimulation following subtotal thyroidectomy. In order to verify a condition of chronic stimulation serum TSH and T_4 were measured in all experimental and control animals. The specific activities of cathepsin D, β-glucuronidase and aryl sulfatase A were elevated at both 3 and 6 weeks following subtotal thyroidectomy when compared to enzyme activities in age and sex matched sham operated animals. The amount of cathepsin D and aryl sulfatase A activity in the S_2 fraction was also significantly elevated at these times. In addition, the activities of all 3 lysosomal enzymes increase during the period from 3 to 6 weeks following subtotal thyroidectomy. This increase is consistent with an increase in physiological secretory activity of individual thyroid cells under the stimulation of increased circulating TSH. This work was supported in part by Grant #PHS5429-32, Fonds de la Recherche Scientifique Medicale (Contract 3.4518.80), and VA Hospital Research Funds.

1634 EVIDENCE THAT CALMODULIN MAY REGULATE RELEASE OF INTRATHYROIDAL FREE T_4 IN MICE: DEMONSTRATION BY CALMODULIN INHIBITORS.

K. Kubota*, T. Mitsuhashi, N. Kuzuya, H. Ikeda and H. Uchimura, The Third Department of Internal Medicine, Faculty of Medicine, University of Tokyo, Hongo, Tokyo 113, Japan.

The mechanism of thyroid hormone release from the follicular cell is not well defined. We have previously demonstrated that intrathyroidal free hormones play a physiological role in their secretion in TSH-stimulated mice. The present study was aimed to examine if calmodulin regulates the release of the thyroid hormone in mice. Thyroid lobes of male DDY mice were excised en bloc, preincubated in KRB buffer (0.1% glucose, 0.2% BSA) for 30 min at 37°C in 95% O_2-5% CO_2, and incubated with or without test materials for additional 3 hours. Then, lobes were homogenized in 0.03 M Tris buffer pH 8.5 (0.02 M methimazole) and intrathyroidal free T_4 (FT_4) was extracted directly with methanol-ammonia. T_4 in the incubation media (released T_4; RT_4) and in the extracts (FT_4) were measured by RIA. In some mice, thyroid lobes were homogenized in 0.125 M borate buffer pH 8.4 (1 mM EGTA) and calmodulin in the homogenates was measured by RIA after heat treatment. FT_4 was increased by TSH in dose-related manner as well as RT_4. When thyroids were incubated with 1 mU/ml TSH, thyroidal calmodulin was significantly increased. When lobes were incubated with W-7 or W-5, a specific calmodulin inhibitor and its control, in the presence of 1 mU/ml TSH, these agents inhibited increase in RT_4 at the concentrations of 100 μM W-7 and 200 μM W-5 or more and that in FT_4 at 500 μM W-7. FT_4 was not affected by 500 μM W-5. Very similar results were obtained by substituting dibutyryl cAMP for TSH. These results indicate that calmodulin may regulate the release of FT_4, probably at the site after adenylate cyclase-cAMP system.

1635 LEAN BODY MASS IN HYPOCALORIC FEEDING WITH AND WITHOUT SUPPLEMENTAL THYROID HORMONE. J. C. LaRocque*, K. Lyons, J. Thomas, J. T. O'Brian, U.S. Naval Hospital, and the Uniformed Services University of the Health Sciences, Bethesda, Maryland, 20814, USA.

During starvation or hypocaloric feeding, serum T3 declines, and the TSH response to TRH is suppressed. A beneficial effect of these changes may be relative protection from loss of lean body mass while fasting. To examine this hypothesis, potassium-40, which is a naturally occurring isotope of potassium virtually confined to lean body mass, was measured in five female obese subjects during three two week periods of near fasting (400 cal/day): during an unsupplemented fast; during a fast supplemented with 30mcg/day of T3; and during a fast supplemented with 100mcg/day of T4. Net potassium-40 emissions were measured in a whole body counting chamber, using a five inch thick, sixteen inch diameter sodium iodide scintillation detector, with subjects in supine, Z-chair configuration. During the unsupplemented fast, the net average K-40 counts were reduced 2.9 ± 1.2 % from baseline (p=ns). During the T3 fast, K-40 counts were reduced 4.9 ± 1.7% ($p<.05$), while during the T4 fast, K-40 counts were reduced only 2.2 ± 2.1 % (p=ns). Changes in serum T3 during the fasts were similar to those reported previously: a slight rise during T3 administration; a decline during the unsupplemented fast; and no change during the T4 fast. These data suggest that supplementation with T3 during hypocaloric feeding causes a significant loss of total body potassium, and hence lean body mass. Such a loss of lean body mass during the T3 fast is analogous to that observed clinically in hyperthyroidism, and supports the concept of the protective role of the fall in T3 during starvation.

1636 THE LYSOSOMAL METABOLIC PATHWAYS IN THE THYROID GLAND STUDIED BY MEANS OF ANALYTICAL MICROSCOPY. E. Larras-Regard*, F. Escaig, S. Halpern, L. Neveu, Laboratoire Biologie Vertébrés, 91405 Orsay; Département de Biophysique, 94000 Créteil; Laboratoire Labcatal, 92120 Montrouge, France.

In the thyroid cell iodine metabolism is present in lysosomes but the ability of these organelles to concentrate mineral elements is questionable. Thyroid cells from aged mice containing numerous dense bodies are helpful for this work. In addition to the presence of halogen that of Al and Au has been studied after intraperitoneal injections of these metals in salt form, by means of secondary ion mass spectroscopy (SIMS) and electron probe microanalysis (EPMA). On SIMS pictures from controlled and treated mice, iodine is distributed in follicular lumens and is locally concentrated in epithelial cells, inside organelles of various size and shape. In treated mice the distribution of Al and/or Au deposits is limited to small spots in some epithelial cells. The EPMA study performed on ultrathin sections shows that organelles where iodine is found correspond to lysosomes. The punctual concentration of halogen is correlated to the electron density of the lysosome rather than to its size. Once injected, Al and/or Au detected form small size dense bodies or dark granules and crystals contained in larger lysosomes. High punctual concentrations of P are always assiociated with the presence of Al and/or Au. Iodine is never apparent in P and metal rich lysosomes. These results indicate that in thyroid cells lysosomes have a double function regarding hormonal metabolism as well as storage of mineral elements. The absence of both iodine and Al (or Au) in a given lysosome suggests that these two fundamental functions occur in two different types of lysosomes.

1637 LITHIUM THERAPY INDUCES AUTOIMMUNE THYROID DISEASE. J.H. Lazarus* M. Ludgate, A.M. McGregor, R. Hassman, F.M. Creagh, J.C. Kingswood, Department of Medicine, University Hospital of Wales, Heath Park, Cardiff, CF4 4XN, Wales.

Patients receiving lithium therapy develop goitre due to a direct thyroidal action of lithium in blocking thyroid hormone release. There is a higher prevalence of thyroid autoantibodies in these patients compared with age and sex matched controls and some become hypothyroid. To examine whether lithium could cause thyroid auto-immunity and to study its effect on established thyroid disease we have therefore evaluated thyroid function prospectively in 37 psychiatric patients receiving lithium carbonate for manic depressive psychosis over 16 months. The development of positive titres to thyroglobulin and microsomal antibodies (measured by ELISA) or a significant change in existing levels of antibody was observed in 35% of subjects. There was no relationship between thyroid function or antibody level and serum lithium or clinical response. We have also examined the effect of lithium on an animal model of thyroiditis produced in the August strain rat by injection of Freund's adjuvant and thyroglobulin. The data obtained show that lithium can increase or decrease thyroid antibody levels depending on the duration of disease in the animal. We conclude that lithium can trigger the development of auto-immune thyroid disease in man and affects the progression of the established disease in animals and man.

1638 BEHAVIOUR OF HUMAN GRAVE'S DISEASE THYROID TISSUE IN NUDE MOUSE. J.Leclère*, M.C.Béné, A.Duprez, G.Faure, J.L.Thomas, J.M.Vignaud and C. Burlet, Faculté de Médecine de Nancy, 54500 Vandoeuvre les Nancy, France.

Thyroid in Grave's disease seems to contain the main elements of the autoimmune reaction, including secreting plasma-cells. Thus, this thyrotoxic tissue could be hyperfunctional in an autonomic way. In order to test this hypothesis, eight diffuse toxic thyroids were transplanted to athymic nu/nu inbred mice (2 to 4 mice for each thyroid). Transplants were removed after 10, 20 or 30 days, and their quality controlled by histology and historadiography after intra-peritoneal injection of 131 I before removal. The initial thyroid tissue and the transplants were studied by immunological methods including the assessment of B lymphocytes, plasma cells, T human lymphocytes and subsets (OKT3, OKT4, OKT8), NK cells (Leu 7) macrophages, IgG, IgA, IgM, C1q, C3 and C9 deposits, HLA antigens (ß2 microglobulin and D|DR). In transplants, were also studied T murine lymphocytes, mouse specific Ia antigens and mouse immunoglobulin deposits. The initial thyroids showed the immunological patterns previously described in Grave's disease : presence of most cells involved in immune reactions (except macrophages), Ig and complement fractions deposits on vesicles'basement membranes. All these elements disappeared in transplants as well as the hyperfunctional state. Conversely, three toxic nodules remained hyperfunctional. It is concluded that in Grave's disease, thyroid is not autonomized, and probably needs an immunological environment to remain hyperfunctional.

1639 EVIDENCE THAT THYROID PHOSPHOLIPIDS FUNCTION AS IODIDE SCAVENGERS DURING HORMONE SECRETION. S. Levasseur, M. Kostelec, and G. Burke*, Dept. of Medicine, Cook County Hospital, Chicago, Illinois 60612.

Work by Rabinowitz' group (Biochem. Biophys. Res. Commun. 68, 1161, 1976; Biochem. J. 168, 155, 1977) has suggested that thyroid phospholipids (PL) may function as iodide scavengers during hormone secretion, although we are unaware of any reports which test this interesting hypothesis directly. In the present study, we prelabeled mice thyroids in vivo with ^{131}I. After injecting mice with either thyrotropin (TSH, 25 mU; 3 h) or long-acting thyroid stimulator (LATS) - positive sera (0.5 ml; 20 h), thyroids were removed, extracted and resolved using thin-layer chromatography into 3 PL fractions: phosphatidylserine and phosphatidylinositol (PS+PI), phosphatidylcholine (PC), and phosphatidylethanolamine (PE). An incorporation index was calculated as follows: [cpm in specific PL fractions)/(cpm in aqueous + total PL fractions)/mg wet weight] x 10^5; blood ^{131}I index = [(cpm at 3 hr (TSH) or 20 h (LATS)/(cpm at 0 h) x 100. The data below are $\bar{x}$ ± SD from 3 separate determinations (2 mice per determination).

Treatment	PI+PS	PC	PE	Blood ^{131}I Index
BSA	0.20±0.08	0.18±0.03	0.30±0.09	92±2
TSH	0.69±0.36	0.58±0.03	0.60±0.28	229±18
BSA	0.17±0.07	0.23±0.03	0.60±0.11	88±15
LATS	4.26±1.33	6.57±1.29	4.94±1.19	1656±593

These data provide convincing evidence that PL function as iodide scavengers during hormone secretion in thyroid. (Supported by USPHS AM 17561).

1640 THYROID STIMULATING ANTIBODY (TSAb) AND T LYMPHOCYTE (L) SUBSET CHANGES IN PATIENTS WITH GRAVES'DISEASE TREATED BY CARBIMAZOLE (C). A.M. Madec, J. Orgiazzi*, A. Stefanutti, N. Genetet+, B. Genetet+, R. Fauchet+, M. Gueguen+and H.Allannic+, INSERM U.197, Lyon and G.U.R.I.F.A,Rennes,France.

Groups of patients with Graves' disease treated with C only were studied either before (t0;N=50), after 6 (t6;N=53) or 18 months of treatment (t18; N=24) and at relapse (N=15) or in remission,i.e. euthyroid 2 years after drug discontinuance (N=23). Overall, 124 patients were studied, 37 of whom at two or more time-points. TSAb was determined in whole serum by a cAMP-human thyrocyte culture stimulation assay and expressed in ul-equivalent of a TSAb standard/ml. Peripheral T L counts (HTLA and E EAT rosette) and subsets (OKT4, OKT8) and HLA A,B and DR antigens were also determined. Before treatment, TSAb was present, ranging from 5 to 150 ul-eq/ml, in 90 % of the patients and decreased, as expected, during treatment to become undetectable in 22/53 and 15/24 at t6 and t18, respectively. On the average T8 L number and T4/T8 ratio, markedly abnormal at t0, did not normalize during treatment. There was no individual correlation between TSAb and T8 or T4/T8 values at any time-point. Moreover, longitudinal studies between t0 and t6 in 20, and t6 and t18 in 7 patients, showed independent variations of TSAb and L counts. At relapse, TSAb was present in 13/15 and T4/T8 was supranormal in 8/15 ; however,in the 23 patients in remission, although TSAb was absent in 21, T4/T8 remained elevated in 8. Finally, when patients subgrouped according to B8 and/or DR3 antigens were compared, no significant differences in the above parameters were observed. In conclusion, changes in TSAb levels, even during C treatment, reflect only partially, at most, abnormalities of the immune system in Graves' disease.

1641 HETEROGENEITY OF T4 AND rT3 5'-MONODEIODINASES IN RAT PITUITARY AND LIVER.

M. Maeda*, F. Tsukahara, M. Obayashi and T. Nomoto, Dept. of Pharmacology, Tokyo Women's Medical College, Kawada-cho, Shinjuku, Tokyo, 162, Japan.

The finding of at least 2 different types of 5'-monodeiodinases(MD) in the pituitary has been reported by Visser et al,and Maeda and Ingbar.The former have suggested that pituitary rT3-5'MD in euthyroid or T3-treated rats is similar to hepatic 5'MD. The present studies were undertaken to determine the heterogeneity of the 5'-MDs in pituitary and liver as well as their properties or factors influencing their activity. Two groups of rats were studied: thyroidectomized(Tx) and Tx plus T3(1.5ug/100gBW) given s.c. as a single injection and sacrificed 24h later. Both groups were investigated under the following conditions: starvation(72h); streptozotocin-induced diabetes; and dexamethasone administration(0.5mg/100gBW)s.c.x3days. Metabolism of 125I-T4 and 125I-rT3 was studied in paired homogenates of pituitary and liver from the same rats in the presence of 10mM dithiothreitol. Metabolites were analyzed by paper chromatography, results beinq related to tissue protein content. Hepatic T4-5'MD activity was significantly inhibited following starvation, dexamethasone or with diabetes in both Tx and Tx+T3 rats, but pituitary T4-5'MD was unaffected; pituitary rT3-5'MD was also unaffected in both Tx and Tx+T3 rats under the same conditions. This latter finding indicates that pituitary rT3-5'MD in T3-treated rats is different from hepatic T4-5'MD because otherwise an inhibition of activity would have been expected. In conclusion, the data indicate that pituitary rT3-5'MD in T3-treated animals is different from hepatic T4-5'MD or is influenced differently under various conditions, suggesting a greater heterogeneity of 5'-monodeiodinases in various tissues.

Quebec, Canada G1V 4G2

1642 GROWTH PROMOTING ACTIVITY AND PLASMINOGEN ACTIVATOR ACTIVITY IN OVINE THYROID CELLS IN PRIMARY CULTURE.

W.W. Mak, L.K. Bachrach, M.C. Eggo and G.N. Burrow, Banting & Best Dept. of Medical Research and Dept. of Medicine, University of Toronto, Toronto, Canada. M6G 1L7

We have recently identified high levels of plasminogen activator (PA) activity in ovine thyroid cells in culture, which was stimulated by TSH in a dose-dependent manner. At day 4, the addition of 500 uU/ml TSH resulted in an increase in PA activity from 24.5 $\pm$ 3.6 Ploug Unit/ml to 82.5 $\pm$ 10.5 PU/ml. These levels of PA activity are higher than those in normal cells (0.1 to 0.5 PU/ml) and comparable to those in transformed cells (10-50 PU/ml). The addition of plasminogen to the culture medium containing PA resulted in the formation of the protease, plasmin, which stimulated 3H-thymidine incorporation 2 to 5-fold in human foreskin fibroblasts. The addition of conditioned medium obtained from thyroid cell cultures both in the presence and absence of TSH stimulated 3H-thymidine incorporation 3 to 4-fold in the fibroblast culture. This growth-promoting activity was present even when the conditioned medium was treated with bovine pancreatic trypsin inhibitor and aprotinin, which inhibit PA and other serine protease activities. The stimulatory effects of the conditioned medium and epidermal growth factor were additive. These data suggest that ovine thyroid cells are capable of producing growth-promoting agents which appear to differ from EGF or factors modulated by PA.

1643 FREE THYROID HORMONES IN AUTONOMOUS THYROID ADENOMA (A.T.A.) R. Maoui *, F. Bakiri, N. Abdelmoumene, M. Benmiloud. Service d'Endocrinologie, Centre Pierre et Marie Curie, Alger - Algérie.

We have studied the thyroid function in 66 patients with a solitary hot nodule from an endemic area. They were clinically and biologically euthyroid (total T_4 and total T_3 within the normal range). TRH I.V. test was positive in 28 % (group A), negative in 67 % (group B) and equivocal in 5 % (group C). On ^{131}I scanning the extra nodular tissue was totally suppressed in 63 % (group I) and partially inhibited in 37 % (group II). As compared to a control group (T) : 1) Total T_4 was not significantly different while total T_3 was higher ($p < 0.02$) in all the groups. 2) FT_3 and FT_4 were higher ($p < 0.001$). FT_3 and FT_4 were significantly increased in group B as compared to group A (p 0.001) and in group II as compared to group I ($p < 0.001$). There was a negative correlation between ΔTSH and FT_3 ($r = -0.5$ $p < 0.001$) among all groups. 3) 23 untreated patients were followed for a period of 3-9 months : variations in TRH response and serum concentration of hormones were noted in 16 cases ; the 7 others became thyrotoxic, their initial FT_3 was significantly higher (mean = 6.30 ± 1.66 $p < 0.005$) than in the remaining patients (3.99 ± 1.14). The inhibition of extra nodular thyroid tissue and the responsiveness to TRH are related to a relative increase of FT_3, especially its unbound fraction. This inhibition exists in presence of varying secretion of the thyroid gland. The high incidence of overt hyperthyroidism is probably due to the conjunction of thyroid autonomy with iodine deficiency. FT_3 appears to be the most selective criterion for the prognosis of development of toxic adenoma.

1644 EVIDENCE THAT NORMAL CONCENTRATIONS OF ENDOGENOUS PLASMA THYROID HORMONE INDUCE PROTEIN INHIBITORS OF TSH SECRETION TO PRESERVE A EUTHYROID STATE. S. Maruta* and M.A. Greer, Section of Endocrinology, Oregon Health Sciences University, Portland OR 97201, USA.

High doses of both T_3 and T_4 induce a protein which inhibits TRH-induced TSH secretion. However, the role of this phenomenon in the homeostatic maintenance of euthyroidism *in vivo* has not been documented. The present study was designed to investigate this possibility in adult male rats with chronic atrial catheters. All doses were per 100 g BW. TRH (1 μg) was injected iv every 15 min for 2 h and blood was sampled every 15 min for 3 h. In some groups, 80 μg Actinomycin-D (ActD) was injected 4 h before the first TRH injection at 0 h. In euthyroid rats not given ActD, 1 μg T_4 at -4 h significantly inhibited TRH-induced TSH secretion ($P < 0.05$) but had no effect if given at 0 h ($P > 0.1$). 10 μg T_4 at 0 h suppressed TSH secretion after 45 min ($P < 0.05$). In euthyroid rats, TRH-induced TSH secretion was significantly higher in ActD than in control groups ($P < 0.05$). 1 μg T_4 at -4 h significantly diminished the ActD-enhanced TSH response but 1 or 10 μg T_4 at 0 h had no effect. In hypothyroid rats, ActD pretreatment had no effect on TRH-induced TSH secretion. Conclusions: Synthesis of a protein inhibitor of TRH-induced TSH secretion is under tonic stimulation by euthyroid concentrations of circulating thyroid hormone. Production of the inhibitor is proportional to the plasma concentration of thyroid hormone. Variations in the pituitary concentration of inhibitor may be more important than those of TRH in the feedback regulation of pituitary-thyroid homeostasis.

1645 GAMMA HEAVY CHAIN DISEASE ASSOCIATED WITH PRIMARY PLASMACYTOMA OF THE THYROID.

Sunao Matsubayashi, M.D.*[1)], Shuji Fukata, M.D.[1)], Hajime TAMAI, M.D.[1)], Fumio Matsuzuka, M.D.[2)], Kanji Kuma, M.D.[2)], Toshimitsu Suzuki, M.D.[3)], Shigenobu Nagataki, M.D.[4)]
1)The Dept. of Psychosomatic Medicine, Faculty of Medicine, Kyushu University, Fukuoka; 2)Kuma Hospital, Kobe; 3)The Dept. of 1st Pathology, School of Medicine, Niigata University, Niigata; 4)The Dept. of 1st Internal Medicine, Nagasaki University School of Medicine, Nagasaki, Japan.

We encountered a 65-years-old man with gamma heavy chain disease associated with primary plasmacytoma of the thyroid. Serum electrophoresis revealed an abnormal fast gamma band that cross-reacted with anti-IgG(Fcγ) on immunoelectrophoresis. Intracytoplasmic monoclonal immunoglobulin, IgG(Fcγ), was demonstrated in tissue sections using an indirect immunofluorescence method. After the operation, the abnormal fast gamma band of patient's serum rapidly decreased and disappeared. As of this writing, the patient is alive 7 months after the operation.

1646 ATROPHIC AUTOIMMUNE THYROIDITIS (PRIMARY MYXEDEMA) IN CHILDHOOD.

N.Matsuura*[1)], H. Fujita[1)], K. Fujieda[1)], Y. Nohara[1)], Y. Iida[2)], K.Endo[2)], J. Konishi[2)], Department of Pediatrics, Hokkaido University School of Medicine[1)] and Department of Nuclear Medicine, Kyoto University School of Medicine[2)], Japan

The pathogenesis of atrophic autoimmune thyroiditis is still obscure. In order to elucidate the pathogenesis of AAT in childhood, clinical features, laboratory findings and TSH receptor antibodies were analyzed in 13 children c̄ AAT and in 33 children c̄ goitrous autoimmune (Hashimoto) thyroiditis (GAT). Short height, gain in weight and clinical features of hypothyroiditis were more marked in AAT. None of children c̄ AAT had papable thyroid glands. Much lower T_4, T_3 c̄ elevated TSH and higher cholesterol values were observed in AAT. Degree of T_gHA and McHA titers was not significantly different. Mean 24 hr I^{123}-uptake (%) was 4.2±23, whereas in GAT, it was 47.3±17.4. Mean age of onset (yr) in AAT and GAT was 8.1±1.7 and 11.0±2.0, respectively. TBII were undetectable in both AAT and GAT. In addition, immunoglobulins from children c̄ AAT did not block TSH induced cAMP increase while immunoglobulins from adult primary myxedema often block it. From these findings, it was suggested that 1) pathogenesis of AAT is different from that of GAT; 2) the two types of thyroiditis do not simply represent different facets of the same disease etiology; 3) TBII and blocking type immunoglobulins for cAMP stimulation are not responsible for thyroid dysfunction and atrophy in childhood AAT; 4) pathogenesis of AAT is heterogenous.

1647 RECENT CHANGES IN THE AETIOLOGY OF HYPERTHYROIDISM. J.McConnon* and A.Macdonald, Department of Medicine and Trinity College, University of Toronto and Peel Memorial Hospital, Brampton.

421 hyperthyroid patients were seen in one consulting endocrine practice in a community hospital in Southern Ontario between 1972 and 1982. 339(80.5%) had Graves disease, 19 (4.7%) had hyperthyroidism due to De Quervains thyroiditis and 47 (11.6%) had transient hyperthyroidism. The remaining 16 (3.8%) consisted of all other causes of hyperthyroidism. 98% of all hyperthyroid subjects had a radioactive iodine uptake performed. Only 2 cases of transient hyperthyroidism were seen between 1972-1974. In 1981-82 it had become the second commonest cause after Graves disease and constituted 14% of the total seen. Least square regression between time and the proportion of cases of transient hyperthyroidism over the total cases showed a significant increase. (p 0.05). There was no significant change in the incidence of Graves disease. Subjects with transient hyperthyroidism had an average age of 33 years compared to 39.5 years for Graves disease and 44 years for De Quervains thyroiditis. Two-thirds of the subjects with transient hyperthyroidism had significant titres of thyroid antibodies and it occurred within six months of delivery in 45% of women under 40. This would suggest the possibility of an autoimmune cause. This study was funded by The Physicians of Ontario through the Physicians Services Incorporated Foundation.

1648 THE EFFECT OF CARBIMAZOLE ON THYROID AUTOANTIBODY SYNTHESIS BY THYROID LYMPHOCYTES. S.M. McLachlan,* C. Pegg, E.T. Young, F. Clark and B. Rees Smith. University of Newcastle upon Tyne, University of Nottingham and Welsh National School of Medicine, Cardiff.

Thyroid autoantibody synthesis by cultures of thyroid lymphocytes and lymphocytes extracted from lymph nodes in the region of the thyroid has been studied in patients treated preoperatively with carbimazole or propranolol. In the case of thyroid lymphocytes from 6 carbimazole treated patients, only small amounts of IgG (1.9 ± 1.3μg/10^7 cells) were secreted and thyroid microsomal or thyroglobulin autoantibody production (measured by ELISA) was undetectable. However, lymphocytes extracted from the lymph nodes of all 6 patients secreted relatively large amounts of IgG (69 ± 19μg) and cultures from 4/6 patients synthesised detectable levels of thyroid autoantibody. In contrast to carbimazole treated patients, thyroid lymphocytes from 6 patients treated pre-operatively with propranolol synthesised relatively large amounts of IgG (50 ± 17μg) and cultures from 3/6 patients contained detectable levels of thyroid autoantibodies. Lymph node lymphocytes from the propranolol treated patients produced similar amounts of IgG (42 ± 17μg) and autoantibodies to the carbimazole treated patients. In addition to differences in IgG and autoantibody synthesis, thyroid lymphocytes from propranolol treated Graves' patients had an increased ability to survive in culture (38 ± 13% recovery of the original numbers seeded compared with 1 ± 0% in lymphocytes from thyroid tissue of patients taking carbimazole). Lymph node lymphocytes, however, had similar capacities for survival in culture whether isolated from propranolol or carbimazole treated individuals (18 ± 6% compared with 30 ± 8%). Therefore carbimazole appears to have a marked effect on thyroid but not lymph node lymphocytes.

1649 TSH RECEPTOR ANTIBODIES IN LARGE MULTINODULAR UNTREATED ENDEMIC GOITER: EFFECT OF IODIZED OIL PROPHYLAXIS.
G. Medeiros-Neto*, M. Knobel, H. Cavaliere & N. Lima, Thyroid Laboratory, Hospital das Clinicas, Univ São Paulo Med School, C. Postal 8091, São Paulo, Brazil.

We have studied the effect of IgG concentrates from sera of 36 patients with large multinodular goiters, living in an area of chronic iodine deficiency (I<40μg) on the inhibition of binding of labeled TSH to detergent solubilised TSH receptors. Sera was also obtained 6-12 months after a IM injection of I-oil. At baseline studies serum T4 (8.2±2.5μg/dl) and T3 (170±53ng/dl) were within the normal range but basal TSH levels (6.5±2.4μU/ml) and serum Tg (47.5±36.5ng/ml) were significantly higher than in normal controls ($p < .01$). TSH-receptor antibody activity (TBII index) indicated that 12 patients had a positive value, greater than 15% inhibition of TSH binding (range: 15.2-51.0). Four subjects had a TBII index > 25%. After I-oil there was a significanty higher mean value of serum T4 (13.8±2.8μg/dl). T3 (196±59ng/dl), a lower TSH (2.1±1.9μU/ml) and Tg (27.9±25ng/ml). Similarly there was a significant reduction in TBII index in all patients ($p<.01$, Mann-Whitney test) and a marked reduction in goiter size. In four patients, after I-oil, it was observed clinical and laboratory evidence of thyrotoxicosis (Jod-Basedow). A positive and significant correlation ($r=.51$, $p<.05$) was found between serum T3 and the TBII index. No correlation was found between the TBII index, serum T4, TSH or Tg concentrations. We concluded that TSH-receptor antibody activity may be elevated in 25% of patients with large multinodular endemic goiter and this abnormality seems to be corrected by I-oil prophylaxis.

1650 IN VIVO DEMONSTRATION OF DIIODOTYROSINE (DIT) FORMATION BY T4 ETHER-LINK CLEAVAGE AND EFFECTS OF MONONITROTYROSINE AND AMINOTRIAZOLE.
H. Meinhold*, R. Buchholz, Thyroid Res. Group, Dept. Nuclear Medicine and Endocrine Dept., Klinikum Steglitz, Free University Berlin, Berlin, F.R. Germany.

Recent observations suggesting that the formation of DIT by ether-link cleavage (ELC) of T4 may be an extrathyroidal pathway of T4 metabolism need confirmation by direct in vivo investigations. This report describes in vivo studies on ELC of T4 and the effects of mononitrotyrosine (MNT) and 3-amino-1,2,4-triazole (AT) on this pathway in thyroidectomized rats substituted with synthetic T4 (16 μg/d for 1 week). Metabolic clearance rates of ^{131}I-DIT and ^{125}I-T4 were determined without and with additional MNT treatment (50 μmol/d for 1 week). Serum concentrations of DIT, T4, T3 and rT3 were measured by RIA. Results in $\bar{T}$ rats under T4 substitution without additional treatment were as follows: Serum levels (nmol/l) DIT 0.243 ± 0.130 (SD), T4 173 ± 34. MCR (ml/h·100 g) DIT 19.0, T4 0.65. T4-to-DIT conversion ratio (percentage of circulating T4 degraded to DIT) 4.1%. Administration of MNT, a substance known as iodotyrosine deiodinase inhibitor, resulted in a decreased MCR of DIT (9.9 ml/h·100 g) and caused a strong reduction of both serum levels (< 0.020 nmol/l) of DIT and T4-to-DIT conversion ratio (< 0.2%). Treatment with the catalase inhibitor AT in amounts up to 40 μmol/d for 1 week did not significantly influence serum DIT levels derived from T4. Our data confirm the in vivo generation of extrathyroidal DIT from T4. The inhibitory effect of MNT on this process requires further studies for confirmation and elucitation of its mechanism.

1651 MODULATING INFLUENCE OF D,L-PROPRANOLOL ON T_3-INDUCED SKELETAL MUSCLE PROTEIN DEGRADATION. J.L. MILLER*, F. ISMAIL, J.K. WALIGORA and W. GEVERS, University of Cape Town School of Medicine, Cape Town, South Africa.

Thyrotoxicosis induces higher β-adrenoreceptor density on some target tissues. Clinical and electromyographic studies have shown improvement in muscle power of patients with thyrotoxic skeletal myopathy treated with β-adrenoreceptor blocking agents alone. We have studied the effects of D,L-propranolol on T_3-induced enhanced in situ proteolysis of white muscle fibres of the extensor digitorum longus group of young Long Evans rats. In situ proteolytic rates were measured by estimation of tyrosine liberated from the muscle into the incubation medium. In situ proteolysis was significantly enhanced in T_3-treated animals (30μg/day for 7 days) when compared to controls (0.79±0.04 vs 0.45±0.02). This effect of T_3 was significantly reduced by simultaneous treatment of animals with propranolol (0.01, 0.1 or 2mg per day) (0.79±0.04 vs 0.58±0.02); propranolol treatment alone yielded similar results to controls. This effect of propranolol was duplicated by Atenolol, a β-adrenoreceptor blocker devoid of membrane-stabilizing effect. We conclude that propranolol significantly reduces the T_3-induced increment of in situ proteolysis of white muscle fibres and suggests a role for the adrenergic system in the genesis of thyrotoxic skeletal myopathy.

1652 IMMUNOHISTOLOGIC CHARACTERIZATION OF THYROID-INFILTRATING LYMPHOCYTES IN AUTOIMMUNE THYROID DISEASES. T. Misaki*, J. Konishi, T. Nakashima, K. Kasagi, K. Endo, K. Torizuka and K. Kuma#, Department of Nuclear Medicine, Kyoto University School of Medicine, Sakyo-ku, Kyoto 606 and Kuma Hospital#, Chuo-ku, Kobe 650, Japan.

To clarify pathogeneic mechanisms involved, subsets of thyroid-infiltrating lymphocytes were identified by their surface markers in frozen tissues of Hashimoto's thyroiditis and Graves' disease. T cell antigens and a natural killer cell-associated antigen were located with murine monoclonal antibodies (OKT3, Leu-3a and OKT8, and Leu-7, respectively) in a 3 step immunoperoxidase staining (IP). For B cells, anti-immunoglobulin D (IgD) antisera was employed in a 2 step IP. In Hashimoto's thyroiditis, density of lymphocytes infiltrating between thyroid epithelial linings was about ten times as much as that of Graves' disease. In both diseases, most of these cells were phenotypically OKT3 positive T cells (OKT3+), with numerical superiority of OKT8+ (suppressor/cytotoxic) subset over Leu-3a+ (helper/inducer) population. Some Leu-7+ were also found, but surface IgD positive mature B cells (IgD+) were almost absent in these sites. In contrast, IgD+ were densely populated in primary lymphoid follicles and mantle zones of secondary follicles. In these areas, numerous Leu-3a+, less frequent OKT8+ and small number of Leu-7+ were found. In germinal centers, some Leu-3a+ and Leu-7+ were scattered, but IgD+ and OKT8+ were rarely seen. Thus, the arrangement of lymphocytes in lymphoid follicles of these thyroid tissues appeared similar to that of peripheral lymphoid organs such as lymphnodes and tonsils.

1653 INCIDENCE AND PROPERTIES OF LABELED TSH BINDING GLOBULIN (LTBG). T. Mori*, T. Akamizu, H. Ishii and H. Imura, 2nd Div. of Internal Med., Kyoto Univ. School of Med., Kyoto, Japan.

Through Thyrotropin Binding Inhibitor Immunoglobulin (TBII) assay, we found 3 Graves' patients with anti-TSH antibody of very high affinity. This prompted us to study individual Labeled TSH Binding Globulin (LTBG) in TBII assay. Among 379 determinations, elevated LTBG were observed in 40 cases. 34 of them were Graves' disease including 16 untreated and active. Elevated LTBG were often associated with high TBII activities and 12 of them had TBII levels exceeding 60 %. Further, 35 sequential studies in one patient with malignant exophthalmos revealed a close correlation between LTBG and TBII. IgG concentration also showed significant correlation with LTBG but in less degree. Using 19 Graves' Immunoglobulin (Ig), LTBG with 125-I b TSH and those with 125-I h TSH were compared. Both LTBG showed a good correlation in 14 Ig, however, there were 3 Ig dominant in b TSH binding and 2 in h TSH, respectively. Addition of corresponding nonlabeled TSH resulted in specifical reduction of LTBG in these 5 cases, but none of others showed any significant changes. Further, addition of non-radioactive iodinated b TSH picked up 2 other Ig showing reduction in LTBG. LTBG seemed to have thyroid related antibody like properties, and some of them were found to be specific for b-, h TSH, or iodinated b TSH. Further studies are necessary to clarify LTBG non specific for these TSH preparations.

1654 MEASUREMENT OF ANTI-THYROID MEMBRANE ANTIBODY S. Morita*, M. Izumi, S. Yamashita, S. Okamoto, S. Noguchi° and S. Nagataki, The First Department of Internal Medicine, Nagasaki University, Nagasaki 852. Japan. ° Noguchi Thyroid Clinic and Hospital FND. Beppu. Japan.

We have developed a new method to detect antibodies against thyroid membrane in serum as well as in medium of lymphocyte culture. Graves' thyroids obtained at operation were homogenized and centrifuged at 800g. The supernatant was further centrifuged at 10000g. The membrane proteins of the pellet were solubilized with 1% Lubrol and centrifuged at 100000g. The supernatant was used as the thyroid membrane antigen. Falcon microplate was coated with the thyroid membrane antigen. After washing the plate, 40μl of human IgG samples were added and incubated for 60min at room temperature. After washing the well 6 times with 1% BSA, 40μl of ^{125}I anti-human IgG antibody, $F(ab')_2$, was added and incubated for 60min. The radioactivity of the well was measured to detect anti-human thyroid membrane antibody which was expressed as the ratio of the well to the total radioactivity. When 10μg/ml of serum IgG was employed, the ratios of the well to the total radioactivity were less than 2% in all normal subjects, while values in patients with Graves' disease ranged from 1% to 20%, and 70% of Graves' patients showed values greater than 2%. Even when 1μg/ml of IgG was employed, the difference of values between Graves' patients and normal subjects was significant. Anti-thyroid membrane antibodies in culture medium of peripheral lymphocyte obtained from a Graves' patient and transformed by EB virus, could be detected by this new method. This new method is simple and sensitive and is especially useful for detecting monoclonal antibodies of lymphocyte culture.

1655 CORRELATION BETWEEN CLINICAL FEATURES AND TUMOR CONTENTS OF PROENKEPHALIN A DERIVED OPIOID PEPTIDES IN HUMAN PHEOCHROMOCYTOMA. K. Nakao*, T. Yoshimasa, M. Sakamoto, M. Suda, N. Morii, Y. Ikeda, I. Tanaka, S. Oki, S. Matsukura, and H. Imura, 2nd Div., Dept. of Med. and Div. of Clin. Nutrition (S.M.), Kyoto Univ. Sch. of Med., Sakyo-ku, Kyoto 606, Japan.

We observed a marked difference in methionine-enkephalin (Met-Enk) and leucine-enkephalin (Leu-Enk) contents between two adrenal pheochromocytomas and two extraadrenal pheochromocytomas (Yoshimasa et al. JCI, 69, 643, 1982) and concomitant secretion of these opioid peptides and catecholamines from the tumors (Yoshimasa et al. JCEM, 57, 706, 1983). In order to elucidate pathophysiological roles of proenkephalin A derived opioid peptides in human pheochromocytomas, we have correlated clinical features with tumor contents of proenkephalin A derived opioid peptides in 18 cases of pheochromocytomas. Nine of 18 cases had adrenaline-producing pheochromocytomas (A type) and the remaining 9 cases had noradrenaline-producing pheochromocytomas (NA type). Nine cases showed paroxysmal hypertension, whereas 8 cases exhibited sustained hypertension. Twelve tumors were adrenal and six tumors were extraadrenal. The tumor contents of proenkephalin A derived opioid peptides were measured by RIAs for Met-Enk, Leu-Enk, Met-Enk-Arg^6-Phe^7 and Met-Enk-Arg^6-Gly^7-Leu^8. The tumor contents of these opioid peptides were much higher in A type than in NA type. A significantly high amount of opioid peptides were detected in the tumors from the patients with paroxysmal hypertension and in the adrenal tumors.

These results suggest the pathophysiological significance of proenkephalin A derived opioid peptides in human pheochromocytomas.

1656 CONCOMITANT SECRETION OF THE PRO-OPIOCORTIN N-TERMINAL FRAGMENT (N-POC) WITH CORTICOTROPIN (ACTH) AND β_h-ENDORPHIN (β_h-EP) IN CULTURED HUMAN CORTICOTROPINOMAS AS DETECTED BY A SPECIFIC RADIOIMMUNOASSAY (RIA). M. Nixon*, M. Westphal, J. Ramachandran and C. B. Wilson, Hormone Research Laboratory, Laboratory of Molecular Endocrinology, and Department of Neurological Surgery, University of California, San Francisco, CA 94143.

Peptides derived from the POC precursor are thought to be secreted in concert by the corticotroph. In this study we developed an RIA for N-POC to determine whether human pituitary tumors secrete N-POC in parallel with ACTH and β-EP. Human N-POC 1-49 was synthesized by solid phase methods. Antisera were raised in rabbits against N-POC 1-49 conjugated to BSA. An RIA was developed using [^{125}I]-iodinated Bolton-Hunter modified synthetic N-POC 1-49 as the radioligand. The RIA sensitivity was 50 fmoles and the ED_{50} was 200 fmoles. No cross-reactivity was detected for other pituitary peptides, isolated salmon N-POC 1-76 or synthetic N-POC 1-28. Human corticotropinomas were obtained at transsphenoidal surgery for Cushing's Disease. Dispersed cells were cultured on extracellular matrix derived from corneal endothelia. Conditioned cell culture media were assayed by RIA for N-POC immunoreactivity (IR). In five cases arginine vasopressin and corticotropin-releasing factor caused an increase in secretion of N-POC IR, up to 5-fold, and cortisol suppressed secretion by approximately 35%, when tested. In all cases the secretion of N-POC IR followed the pattern of secretion of ACTH and β-EP. It appears that the secretion of POC-derived peptides by human tumor cells _in vitro_ is similar to that described for other species _in vivo_ and _in vitro_. This work was supported by CA-16417 (NCI), GM-2907 (NIH) and Deutsche Forschungsgemeinschaft (MW).

1657 REGULATION OF IMMUNOREACTIVE β-ENDORPHIN(ir-β-END) LEVELS IN RAT HYPOTHALAMIC NUCLEI BY DOPAMINERGIC COMPOUNDS. A. Nohtomi* and M. Itoh, Department of Neuropsychiatry, Fuculty of Medicine, Kyushu University, Fukuoka, 812, Japan.

Effects of dopamine receptor antagonists on the levels of ir-β-END in rat hypothalamic nuclei were investigated. Rats were treated with sulpiride(1.25, 5 or 20 mg/kg) or domperidone(2.5 mg/kg) intraperitoneally and killed by microwave irradiation 2 hr after the injection. The hypothalamic nuclei were dissected according to the method of Palkovits(1973) and the levels of ir-β-END were measured using RIA for β-END. Single injection of sulpiride significantly and dose-dependently decreased the levels of ir-β-END in nucleus paraventricularis(PA, 66% of control), nucleus arcuatus(ARC, 66% of control) and median eminence(ME, 58% of control). On the other hand, repeated injections of sulpiride for 2 weeks significantly and dose-dependently increased the levels of ir-β-END in nucleus periventricularis(PE, 154% of control), ARC(166% of control) and ME(202% of control). These findings suggest that sulpiride may affect the release and/or biosynthesis of β-END in these hypothalamic nuclei via dopamine receptor. In addition, single injection of domperidone significantly decreased the levels of ir-β-END in ARC(61% of control) and ME(72% of control). The present results suggest that both sulpiride (a centrally active dopamine receptor antagonist) and domperidone (a dopamine receptor antagonist with reportedly preferential actions outside of the blood-brain barrier) can affect the release and/or biosynthesis of the peptide in certain hypothalamic nuclei.

1658 ACTH-LIKE IMMUNOREACTIVITY AFTER RP-HPLC IN NORMAL AND ABNORMAL ACTH SECRETION. G.Opocher*, M.Boscaro, T.Luzzi, D.D'Agostino and F.Mantero, Institute of Semeiotica Medica, University of Padova, Italy

The specific measurement of ACTH and ACTH-related peptides is complicated by the lack of specific antisera and cross-reactivity for different peptides. Recently reverse phase high performance liquid chromatography(RP-HPLC) has been used for high resolutive separation of these peptides. In order to elucidate the immunochromatographic profile of ACTH in normal and abnormal ACTH secretion we have set up a RP-HPLC system for ACTH and other small peptides which allows a complete separation of ßMSH,αMSH,1-24 ACTH,γMSH, 1-39 ACTH and ß-Endorphin. After Sep-Pak extraction, glycine-HCl-treated plasma samples have been processed by RP-HPLC: in eluted fractions ACTH-like immunoreactivity was detected by RIA(West's antiserum NIH). Results: in normal plasma (n=5) two distinct ACTH-like peaks with retention times respectively corresponding to 1-39 ACTH and between α and γ MSH were detected. In the cases of abnormal ACTH secretion (Cushing d. n=2,Nelson s. n=2, ectopic production n=1) the immunochromatographic profiles revealed the presence of a third peak with a retention time similar to γMSH. Conclusions: these procedures demonstrate the presence in normal plasma of a ACTH-like compound probably smaller than 1-39 ACTH. In pituitary or ectopic tumors another ACTH-like peptide co-eluted with MSH is present. The chemical nature of these componds remains to be clarified.

1659 HAEMORRAGIC STRESS IN CONSCIOUS SHEEP ELEVATES PLASMA BUT NOT CEREBROSPINAL FLUID BETA-ENDORPHIN. P.C. Owens*, R. Smith, D. Green and J. Falconer, Faculty of Medicine, University of Newcastle, Newcastle, N.S.W. Australia.

Endogenous opiates appear to be involved in stress-induced analgesia but it is not known whether they act on peripheral tissues or within the central nervous system. (CNS) The effect of haemorragic stress on β-endorphin (β-EP) in cerebrospinal fluid and plasma was examined in six conscious sheep which were chronically catheterized (cisterna magna, carotid artery, jugular vein). Cerebrospinal fluid (CSF) and venous plasma were obtained before and after arterial haemorrage (n = 8) and during sham experiments (n = 4). Cortisol and β-EP were measured by radioimmunoassay (RIA). The ovine β-EP RIA has a sensitivity of 2.5 fmol/ml and ovine β-lipotropin (β-LPH) has 37% molar crossreactivity. Samples extracted prior to β-EP assay, had β-EP and β-LPH recoveries of 83% and 28% respectively. Concentrations of immunoreactive (ir) β-EP did not change significantly in control experiments and were higher ($p<0.001$) in plasma (30.9 ± 2.6 fmol/ml, x ± SEM) than in CSF (6.0 ± 0.8). Cortisol and ir β-EP concentrations in plasma increased within 45 min after haemorrage, and returned to baseline by 1.5h (β-EP) and 2.25h (cortisol). The changes in plasma cortisol and plasma ir β-EP were significant ($P<0.01$) using analysis of variance. No significant changes in CSF ir β-EP were observed. Chromatography of extracted plasma revealed a major peak co-eluting with βo-EP and a minor peak with βo-LPH. This study suggests that if β-EP mediates pain suppression induced by haemorragic stress, its actions are not via the CSF but may be at a peripheral site. Supported by the NH & MRC of Australia.

1660 VASOPRESSIN AND PROSTAGLANDIN E_2 AFTER CHANGES IN THE HYPOTHALAMIC STIMULATION OF ACTH AND ß-ENDORPHIN RELEASE. W. Knepel*, M. Vlaskovska, D. Nutto and D.K. Meyer, Department of Pharmacology, University of Freiburg i. Br., Hermann-Herder-Str. 5, D-7800 Freiburg i. Br., Federal Republic of Germany.

Vasopressin can be released from the rat medial basal hypothalamus (MBH) in vitro (Knepel and Reimann, Brain Res. 238, 484, 1982). Vasopressin-induced release of ACTH and ß-endorphin-like immunoreactivity (ß-EI) from anterior pituitary quarters in vitro is modulated by locally formed prostaglandin (PG) E_2 (to be published). This study was to examine whether long-term activation (by adrenalectomy) or reduction of the hypothalamic stimulation of the pituitary corticotrophs (by lesions of the paraventricular nuclei, PVN) may influence the above mentioned events in subsequent in vitro experiments. 1) Electrically induced vasopressin release in vitro from the MBH of adrenalectomized rats or of PVN-lesioned rats was enhanced about 7-fold or almost abolished, respectively, when compared to controls. 2) The vasopressin (10 nM)-induced ß-EI release from anterior pituitary quarters was changed neither by adrenalectomy nor by PVN lesions. By contrast, the vasopressin-induced PG E_2 release was enhanced to about 300 % of controls after adrenalectomy but decreased after PVN lesions. The observed variations suggest that hypothalamic vasopressin and pituitary PG E_2 are related to mechanisms controlling ACTH and ß-endorphin release. Supported by the DFG.

1661 ROLE OF DIFFERENT OPIATE RECEPTORS AND OF HISTAMINE IN THE RELEASE OF ACTH IN RATS.

A.Pfeiffer* and D.G.Pfeiffer. Medizinische Klinik II, Universitaet Muenchen, Klinikum Grosshadern D-8000 Muenchen 70, Germany-West and Developmental Endocrinology Branch, NICHHD, Bethesda, MD 20205.

Opiates are known to release ACTH in rats possibly through modulation of CRF. However, the opiate antagonist naloxone also releases ACTH after injection of high doses. To investigate which type of opiate receptors participates in these actions, we injected selective mu- and kappa-opiate agonists intracerebroventricularly (icv.) into handled rats which were implanted with intracardial catheters to permit withdrawal of blood samples from undisturbed animals. The selective mu-opioid agonist (D-Ala,MePhe^4,Gly^5-ol)enkephalin (DAGO) and the benzomorphan kappa-opioid agonist MRZ both increased ACTH after icv. injection of 1-10 nmol by 3-14-fold over baseline levels 30-60 min after injection. The preferential mu-opiate antagonist naloxone (5 mg i.v.) and saline (i.v. or icv.) did not affect ACTH levels significantly while the benzomorphan mu- and kappa-opiate antagonist MR 2266 (2 mg/kg) increased ACTH levels briefly but significantly after 10 min. MR 2266 (2mg/kg) significantly antagonized the 7-fold increase in ACTH by MRZ (250 µg/kg). The histamine antagonist diphenhydramine 3 mg/kg did not affect ACTH release when given alone but significantly lowered the effect of MRZ (250 µg) on ACTH. These data show that: i) ACTH is released by mu- and kappa opiate agonists ii) endogenous kappa-opiate agonists may inhibit release of ACTH through a separate pathway iii) histamine may mediate the action of exogenous kappa-agonists.

1662 ONTOGENY OF ENDORPHIN AND MSH-SIZED PEPTIDES DURING RAT PITUITARY DEVELOPMENT.

J.E. Pintar*, D.T. Krieger and A.S. Liotta, Dept.Anat.&Cell Bio. Columbia P & S, NY 10032, Div. Endo, Mt. Sinai Med. School, NY 10029.

We have analyzed extracts of embryonic day 15 (e15)-postnatal day 6 (p6) rat pituitary glands for acetylated (AC), non-acetylated (NAC) and trimmed forms of B-endorphin (B-EP) and melanocyte stimulating hormone (MSH) using specific antisera to assay fractions isolated by successive use of gel filtration, ion exchange chromatography, and HPLC. Only B-EP(1-31) and desacetyl-a-MSH are present in extracts of whole e15-e17 rat pituitary glands. Authentic a-MSH, AC-B-EP(1-31) and AC and NAC B-EP (1-26) and B-EP(1-27) are not detected prior to day e18. Since AC and trimmed B-EP forms are present only in adult intermediate lobe, e21 and p6 anterior and neurointermediate (NI) lobes were separated before extraction. At e21, acetylated and shortened B-EP forms are present only in the NI lobe; AC-B-EP(1-31) is the predominant form and >90% B-EP(1-26) and B-EP(1-27) are acetylated; however, even at p6, the relative abundance of AC B-EP(1-26) and AC-B-EP(1-27) is still lower than that found in adult intermediate lobe. At e21, >90% a-MSH in extracts of NI is acetylated, while only 25% is di-AC; desacetyl-a MSH is present in the anterior lobe both at this stage and at p6.

These results demonstrate a temporal dissociation during development between production, AC, and trimming of B-EP and production and AC of a-MSH. Ontogeny of these modifications parallels the biosynthetic pathway established in adult intermediate lobe. Since AC and NAC peptides have different biological activities, these observations should provide a basis for assessing the role of these peptides in development.

Supported by HD-18952 (JP) and NB-02893-15 (DTK).

1663 RADIOIMMUNOASSAY OF β-ENDORPHINS AND β-LIPOTROPINS. A.Reuter*
Y. Vrindts-Gevaert, J. Joris , M. Chretien and P. Franchimont,
IRE Fleurus, Service de Radioimmunologie, CHU, Liège and
Université of Montreal.

It is well known that β lipotropin and ACTH are derived from a common precursor molecule containing 265 A.A. called pre-pro-opiomelanocortin. β Endorphin in turn is derived from β lipotropin (β LPH) by cleavage into β endorphin and γ LPH. Very sensitive antisera were obtained with a detection limit of 2 pg/tube for β endorphin and 10 pg/tube for β LPH. Endorphin was labeled with chloramine T at specific activity (S.A.) of 100 mCi/mg and β LPH with lactoperoxidase at S.A. of 150 mCi/mg. Cross reaction were investigated with α MSH, β MSH, α , β , γ , δ endorphins, met and leu enkephalins, prolactin and ACTH. This study shows that the β endorphin antiserum is specific for the COOH terminal fragment and partly for the whole configuration of β endorphin. The ratio between β LPH and β endorphin immunoreactivity is 1/6 with anti β endorphin serum. The LPH antiserum is specific for NH_2 terminal fragment of the molecule and thus displayed no cross reaction with β endorphin. Plasma concentrations are validated by molecular sieving on ACA 54.

1664 REGULATION OF CHOLESTEROL METABOLISM IN RAT ADRENAL GLANDS. K. Mikami*,
T. Nishikawa, Y. Saito, Y. Tamura and S. Yoshida, The 2nd Department of
Internal Medicine, School of Medicine, Chiba Univ., Chiba 280, Japan.

We have compared the regulation of acyl-CoA synthetase with that of cholesterol ester hydrolase in order to investigate the regulation of cholesterol metabolism in the rat adrenal. The mechanism in adrenal glands of regulation of acyl-CoA synthetase producing acyl-CoA which is used as a substrate for acyl-CoA/cholesterol acyltransferase has not been reported yet. A significant increase in acyl-CoA synthetase activity and decrease in cholesterol ester hydrolase activities were observed in 24-h hypophysectomized rats. Acute injection of ACTH, however, reversed these changes, whereas dexamethasone administration had no effect. When 4-aminopyrazolo [3,4-d] pyrimidine was given to rats, adrenal cholesterol ester content and the acyl-CoA synthetase activity declined and activities of the cholesterol ester hydrolases were increased in association with the rise of plasma ACTH concentration. When dexamethasone, which suppresses ACTH secretion, was simultaneously administered with 4-aminopyrazolo [3,4-d] pyrimidine no changes except for a decrease in plasma cholesterol level occurred. In hyperlipidemic rats the acyl-CoA synthetase activity increased when a high cholesterol diet was given and the plasma cholesterol level was increased. These results suggest that acyl-CoA synthetase is under the influence of ACTH and also the plasma cholesterol concentration, and that cholesterol ester hydrolases are mainly regulated by ACTH.

1665 THE ADRENAL STEROIDOGENESIS IN WOMEN WITH POLYCYSTIC OVARY DISEASE (PCOD)

A. Milewicz*, P. Vecsei, G.Tupikowska,M.Grabinski,J.Szymaczak,Dept. of Endo crinology,Wroclaw,Poland, Dept. of Pharmacology,Heidelberg, FRG.

The site of androgen synthesis was determined in 21 women with polycystic ovary disease (PCOD) using radiographic studies,catheterization of ovarian and adrenal veins, and/or inferior vena cava samplings. Gradients of testosterone,androstenedione and dehydroepiandrosterone sulfate (DHEA-S) were determined by comparing the levels in adrenal and ovarian veins with those found in anticubital veins.In six patients, the adrenals were predominant site of androgen synthesis (Group I).In five patients, both the ovaries and the adrenals participated equally in androgen production (Group II).Group III (10 women) presented the predominant androgens appeared to come from ovarian secretion. The plasma dehydroepiandrosterone,DHEAS,androstenedione (A), testosterone,17-hydroxyprogesterone and cortisol levels were determined before and 12h after i.m. ACTH(2 times 25IU.Cortrophin-Z-Organon).

	DHEA ng/dl		DHEAS μg/dl		Androstenedione ng/dl	
	basal	ACTH	basal	ACTH	basal	ACTH
Gr.I	1660.6 ±297.8	1186.4 ±248.2 *	347.1 ±47.2	493.6 ±128.3 *	440.6 ±160.4	469.8 ±137.9 *
Gr.II	580.2 ±194.2	980.4 ±197.6	260.8 ±66.8	357.2 ±177.6	341.4 ±64.0	422.6 ±133.6
Gr.III	468.4 ±169.5	668.4 ±187.6	210.3 ±37.8	339.8 ±143.2	326.4 ±37.7	554.6 ±152.9

In Group I significant increase of DHEA and DHEA-S but not A were observed, that can be suggested secundary partial 3-beta-ol-steroid dehydrogenase and delata 4,5isomerase deficiency in some patients with PCOD.No correlation was found between morphology and hormonal disturbances.

1666 DIRECT EFFECTS OF GLUCOSE, INSULIN AND GLUCAGON ON RAT ADRENAL CATECHOLAMINE SECRETION. T. Mitchell*, A. Gustafson and R. Kalkhoff, Medical College of Wisconsin, Milwaukee, Wisconsin, 53226, USA.

Insulin-induced hypoglycemia elevates plasma catecholamines (CATS) in part via autonomic cholinergic stimulation of the adrenal medulla. However, little is known about possible direct effects of glucose, insulin and glucagon on adrenal CAT secretion. 60 studies were performed on isolated, denervated adrenal glands of fasted female rats perfused in situ through the aorta with albumin-KHB buffer, 0.2 ml/min. After 30 min at 200 mg/dl glucose, mean basal secretion (± S.E.M.) of epinephrine (E) and norepinephrine (NE) was 2395±452 and 998±195 pg/ml/min, respectively, (n = 14). Subsequent reduction of medium glucose to 100 or 50 mg/dl suppressed secretory rates more than 50% which were restored to original rates with 200 mg/dl glucose. Insulin (100, 500, 1000 μU/ml) also suppressed basal E and NE release 32-89% ($P < 0.025$). Acetylcholine (ACh) dose response curves revealed maximal stimulation of E and NE to 4- and 2-fold above baseline, respectively, at 10^{-4} M. Similar effects were observed with glucagon, 500-1000 pg/ml. Neither glucose (50-300 mg/dl) nor insulin (100-1000 μU/ml) influenced the ACh or glucagon effect. 20 min pulses of glucagon in the presence or absence of insulin blocked subsequent ACh-stimulated CAT secretion. We conclude that while low glucose or high insulin concentrations suppress basal CAT secretion, they do not impair ACh or glucagon action on CAT release. This suggests that cholinergic stimulation of the adrenal medulla in response to insulin-induced hypoglycemia overrides direct negative effects of low glucose or high insulin concentrations on CAT secretion.

1667 EFFECT OF ANGIOTENSIN II (A-II) ON THE ACTH-INDUCED CYCLIC AMP PRODUCTION BY BOVINE ADRENAL CELLS IN CULTURE. A.M. Morera*, M.A. Chauvin, G. Andoka and J.M. Saez, INSERM U. 162, Hôpital Debrousse, 29 Rue Soeur Bouvier, 69322 Lyon Cedex 05, France.

The modulating action of A-II on cyclic AMP by calf adrenal cells in primary culture, were studied. A-II alone, even at high concentrations (10^{-7} M) had no effect on cAMP production by either freshly isolated or cultured adrenal cells. Likewise, A-II did not modify cyclic AMP production induced by ACTH in freshly isolated cells, but after two days of culture A-II enhanced significantly the ACTH effect on cAMP production. Both, the cAMP response to ACTH-(1–24) (10^{-8} M) and the potentiating action of A-II increase progressively from day 2 to day 9 of culture. On day 4, the effect of A-II on ACTH-(1–24)-induced cAMP production was dose-dependent. Half maximal and maximal responses were obtained with 10^{-9} M and 10^{-7} M of A-II respectively. Moreover A-II (10^{-7} M) lowered about 10 fold the ACTH ED-50 value and increased 1.5 to 2 fold the maximal cAMP response. The specificity of this effect of A-II was inferred by the fact that an A-II antagonist ($Sar_1 Ala_8$ A II) completely inhibited the potentiating effect of 10^{-7} M A II on ACTH-induced cAMP production but did not affect the production of cAMP induced by ACTH alone. A II also potentiated the effect of forskolin and cholera toxin on cAMP production by cultured adrenal cells. These studies confirm that A II alone has no effect on cAMP production by adrenal cells and demonstrate for the first time, that this hormone potentiates the action of several effectors on cAMP production, by cultured bovine adrenal cells.

1668 ASCORBIC ACID AND CATECHOLAMINE SECRETION FROM DIGITONIN TREATED CHROMAFFIN CELLS. K. Morita, M. A. Levine*, and H. B. Pollard, N.I.A.D.D.K., N.I.H., Bethesda, Maryland U.S.A. 20205

Ascorbic acid and catecholamines have been found to be concomitantly secreted from cultured bovine chromaffin cells but to originate from different intracellular compartments. We have now treated chromaffin cells with digitonin to further differentiate the origin of secreted ascorbate and catecholamines. In the presence of 20 uM free calcium, catecholamine secretion was 30% of total at 30 minutes, while in the absence of calcium catecholamine secretion was 5%. As expected, secretion of dopamine beta hydroxylase was nearly half of catecholamine secretion. We then predicted that if secreted ascorbate had a cytoplasmic origin, in the presence of digitonin most of the ascorbate would simply leak out of the cells. Indeed, in [^{14}C] ascorbate preloaded cells treated with digitonin, more than 80% of the labelled ascorbate was secreted, regardless of the presence of calcium. As a control for cytosolic localization, we used dimethylepinephrine, a permanently charged epinephrine analog which is transported into chromaffin cells but not into chromaffin granules. In cells preloaded with [^{3}H] dimethylepinephrine and treated with digitonin, more than 80% of free dimethylepinephrine was secreted, identical to ascorbic acid secretion under the same conditions. We conclude that ascorbic acid appears to be secreted from a cytoplasmic compartment in digitonin treated chromaffin cells, in striking contrast to catecholamine secretion. Furthermore, since the calcium dependence of ascorbic acid secretion is lost in digitonin treated cells, the site responsible for calcium dependent ascorbate secretion may be directly located on the plasma membrane.

1669 THE IN VIVO EFFECTS OF PROLACTIN (PRL) ON RAT ADRENAL STEROIDOGENIC ENZYME ACTIVITIES.

A.K. Munabi, M.L. Sienkiewicz, V. Mericq, M. Koppelman, F. Cassorla, D.L. Loriaux and B.D. Albertson*. DEB, NICHD, NIH, Bethesda, MD 20205

We examined the effect of PRL on adrenal microsomal 3β-hydroxysteroid dehydrogenase (3β-HSD), 21-hydroxylase (21-OH), 17-hydroxylase (17-OH) and mitochondrial 11-hydroxylase (11-OH) activities in hyperprolactinemic rats and controls. Hypophysectomized, ACTH replaced Fisher rats were made hyperprolactinemic by isografting 3 pituitaries under the kidney capsule. Controls received skeletal muscle isografts. All rats were sacrificed by decapitation 7 days later and serum PRL was measured in each. The adrenals were resected, pooled according to PRL levels, and mitochondrial and microsomal fractions were prepared from each pool. Specific activities of 3β-HSD, 21-OH, 17-OH and 11-OH were measured using as substrates ^{14}C-dehydroepiandrosterone, 17-hydroxyprogesterone, progesterone and deoxycorticosterone, respectively. The results are shown below:

		PRL†	3βHSD§	21-OH§	17-OH§	11-OHλ
Female	↑ PRL	217±18*	15.0±0.3*	5681±80*	41±3	6.0±1.0*
	control	17±8	13.0±0.5	4714±57	31±3	2.0±0.4
Males	↑ PRL	241±22*	7.0±0.2*	1701±34*	19±3	3.0±0.6*
	control	11±4	8.0±0.2	1950±47	28±4	6.0±0.8

*p<0.05 †=ng/ml, §picomol/mg protein/min, λ=nanomol/mg protein/min

3β-HSD, 21-OH and 11-OH activities increased in female hyperprolactinemic rats compared to controls, whereas they decreased in males. There was no significant change in 17-OH in either experiment. We conclude that PRL increases the activity of the enzymes of the glucocorticoid pathway in female rats and inhibits them in male rats.

1670 ROLE OF ADRENAL FUNCTION IN HYPERANDROGENIC ANOVULATORY WOMEN.

O. Narita*, T. Masahashi, M. Asai, MC. Wu, M. Osawa, N. Suganuma, A. Takada, and Y. Tomoda, Department of Obstetrics and Gynecology, Nagoya University School of Medicine, Nagoya, Japan.

Twenty five patients with hyperandrogenic anovulation were studied in order to determine a possible etiologic cause of hyperandrogenism. Adrenal steroid responses to adrenocorticotropic hormone stimulations were evaluated and the results were compared to those in six normally menstruating and non-hirsute women. In the patients' group, it was suggested that there was a possibility of the reduced enzymatic activity of 21-hydroxylase in four patients, 11β-hydroxylase in one patient, 3β-ol-dehydrogenase in two patients. In one of four patients with 21-hydroxylase deficiency, polycystic ovary was proved histologically. The patients' group exhibited significantly elevated serum luteinizing hormone and low or normal follicle-stimulating hormone concentrations. In conclusion, a subtle imcomplete form of enzymatic deficienty may exist in hyperandrogenic anovulatory women with androgen excess inappropriate gonadotropin secretion.

1671 EFFECT OF CYTOCHALASIN B, A SPECIFIC MICROFILAMENTS DISRUPTING AGENT, ON ADRENAL STEROIDOGENESIS IN FROG. P. Netchitailo*, I. Perroteau, I. Lihrmann and H. Vaudry. GREM, ERA CNRS 891, Lab. Endocrinol., Fac. Sci., 76130 Mont-Saint-Aignan, France.

If cytoskeleton implication in transport and exocytosis process of peptidics hormones is well known, investigations concerning the role of microfilaments in adrenal steroidogenesis have led to conflicting results. Both stimulatory and inhibitory actions on adrenal secretions have been shown. We have investigated the actions of cytochalasin B, an antimicrofilament agent, on frog interrenal fragments to determine in vitro, a possible intervention of the cytoskeleton in steroidogenesis. Interrenal dices were perifused for 12 hours and both corticosterone and aldosterone were radioimmunoassayed in the effluent perifusate. Micromolar concentration of cytochalasin B was responsible for an inhibition of corticosteroid production. The effect of cytochalasin B was reversible and dose-dependant from 1 to 100 μM. Addition of cytochalasin B (50 μM) led to a 95% and 92% decrease of the corticosterone and aldosterone release, respectively. Corticosteroid biosynthesis returned to normal levels within 100 min after withdrawal of the drug. In addition, we showed that cytochalasin B (50 μM) inhibited totally the stimulatory effect of angiotensin II (10^{-7}M), PGE_1 (8.8 10^{-8}M) and VIP (10^{-5}M) and induced to a 80% decrease of the stimulation of steroidogenesis by ACTH (10^{-9}M) and dbc AMP (4 mM). Since the mechanism of action of angiotensin and prostaglandin on the one hand, and ACTH, dbc AMP and VIP on the other are totally different, our results indicate that, microfilaments must represent a common later step in the response of frog adrenocortical cells to all corticotropic peptides.

1672 ADRENAL REGULATION OF CORTICOSTEROID-BINDING GLOBULIN (CBG). L. K. Nieman*, G. P. Chrousos, H. M. Schulte, D. L. Loriaux and B. C. Nisula. Developmental Endocrinology Branch, NICHD, NIH, Bethesda, MD 20205, USA

The role of the adrenal gland in regulating the concentration of CBG is controversial. To address this issue, we measured CBG during acute and chronic alterations in adrenal function. Blood was drawn before and 90 min after ovine-corticotropin releasing factor (CRF) was given to 11 healthy volunteers (Control) and 12 hypercortisolemic patients (CS), 4 with ectopic ACTH secretion (EA) and 8 with Cushing's disease (CD). Five (4CD, 1EA) were retested 1-6 months after after curative surgery (CS-postop). CBG was determined using a solid phase Con A-Sepharose assay; similar results were obtained with or without removal of steroids with dextran-coated charcoal. Total cortisol (TF) was measured by RIA and free cortisol (FF) was calculated with a computer program. Results are shown below as mean ±SE:

	CBG (ug/dl)		TF (ug/dl)		FF (ug/dl)	
Group	Basal	90 min	Basal	90 min	Basal	90 min
Control	17.2±0.9	14.3±0.6	2.9±0.6	12.2±0.6	0.1±0.3	1.1±0.1
CD	12.2±1.4	10.9±0.9	21.5±2.6	39.7±6.0	4.2±0.7	10.9±2.2
EA	12.2±2.1	13.1±2.1	31.7±3.2	33.5±3.2	7.5±0.1	7.9±0.9
CS-postop	18.5±3.3	14.2±2.0	3.4±2.0	6.0±1.8	0.02±02	0.3±.14

Basal CBG was significantly decreased in CD (P<.01) and EA (P<.05) as compared to Control, while the CS-postop group was not different from Control. After CRF, FF increased in Control (P<.01), CD (P<.01) and CS-postop (P<.05) and CBG decreased in Control (P<.01), CD (P=.08) and CS-postop (P<.05). In EA, CRF did not alter either FF or CBG. We conclude: Both acute and chronic changes in adrenal function modulate the principle glucocorticoid transport protein in a manner that amplifies glucocorticoid action.

1673 DOPAMINERGIC NEURONS IN THE MEDIOBASAL HYPOTHALAMUS OF OLD RATS: EVIDENCE FOR REDUCED AFFINITY OF TYROSINE HYDROXYLASE FOR COFACTOR AND SUBSTRATE.

M.J. Reymond*, J. Arita, C.A. Dudley, R.L. Moss and J.C. Porter, Depts Ob-Gyn/Physiol, Univ of Texas Health Sci Ctr at Dallas, Dallas, TX, USA.

The hypersecretion of PRL observed in old female rats was previously shown to be associated with a decreased secretion of hypothalamic dopamine (DA) into hypophysial portal blood and a reduced synthesis of DA in tuberoinfundibular neurons of the hypothalamus. The effect of aging was studied on the activity of tyrosine hydroxylase (TH) and on the number of TH-containing perikarya in the hypothalamus of female rats. The activity of TH in the mediobasal hypothalamus (MBH) of old (20-24 months) rats was significantly ($P < 0.025$) less than in young (3-4 months) rats. The Km of TH for the cofactor 6-methyl-5,6,7,8-tetrahydropterine as well as for the substrate tyrosine was markedly greater in old rats than in young rats (0.485 ± 0.015 vs. 0.230 ± 0.010 mM, and 0.086 ± 0.003 vs. 0.047 ± 0.001 mM, respectively). Vmax was slightly ($P < 0.05$) reduced in old animals. Contiguous coronal sections of the brain of an old and a young rat were immunocytochemically stained for TH, and the TH-positive perikarya in the hypothalamus were counted. In the arcuate region, 2868 TH-positive perikarya were detected in the young brain and 2760 in the old brain. In the circumventricular region, 6793 and 6632 TH-positive perikarya were present in the young and old brain, respectively. It is concluded that the reduced TH activity in the MBH of old rats is not a consequence of a reduction in the number of TH-containing perikarya in the arcuate or circumventricular regions of the hypothalamus but is due to a reduction in the affinity of TH for its cofactor and substrate.

1674 EFFECT OF AGING ON SERUM T3, T4 AND TSH LEVELS IN HEALTHY SUBJECTS.

S.Sakata, S.Nakamura, K.Kamikubo, N.Kojima, T.Komaki and K.Miura. The 3rd Department of Internal Medicine , Gifu University School of Medicine, Gifu, 500, Japan

Serum T3, T4 and TSH levels were measured in healthy adult subjects (220 males and 176 females) aged 20～80 years who were carefully selected on the basis of their medical histories and various blood chemistries including a 50 g oral glucose tolerance test. In males, serum T3, T4 and TSH concentrations in the third decade were 134.8 ± 25.8 ng/dl, 9.6 ± 2.1 μg/dl and 3.9 ± 2.2 μU/ml (mean ± SD), respectively. These values were not significantly different up to the eighth decade, except for T3 values of seventh decade (154 ± 19.1 ng/dl) being higher than that of third decade. In females, serum T3, T4 and TSH concentrations in the third decade were 149.3 ± 23.5 ng/dl, 9.0 ± 2.0 ug/dl and 4.0 ± 1.1 μU/ml, respectively. These values were not significantly different up to the eighth decade except for TSH levels of fifth decade (4.8 ± 1.0 μU/ml), sixth decade (5.7 ± 1.4 μU/ml) and seventh decade (5.8 ± 1.6 μU/ml) being higher than that of third decade. Thus in carefully screened healthy subjects aging per se had no effect on serum T3 and T4 levels. Decreased levels of serum T3 and T4 in the aged previously reported by other workers could be due to the presence of non-thyroidal illnesses affecting thyroidal functions.

1675 EFFECT OF AGE AND SEX ON TSH AND PROLACTIN RESPONSE TO THYROTROPIN IN THE ELDERLY. J.L. SCHLIENGER, C. JACQUES, C. SIMON*, F. KUNTZMANN, Service de Médecine Interne, Hôpital de Hautepierre et Service de Médecine Interne-Gériatrie, CHU STRASBOURG 67098 (FRANCE).

Since there is disagreement about the TSH response to TRH in old age and since a hypothalamo-pituitary dysfunction has been postulated in the elderly, we have studied the thyroid function and the responsiveness of TSH and prolactin (PRL) to TRH in euthyroid healthy geriatric inpatients. Basal plasma levels of total and free thyroxine (T4), triiodothyronine (T3), reverse T3 (rT3), TSH and PRL and the response of TSH and PRL to an i.v. bolus injection of 250 µg TRH were determined in 26 control subjects aged from 50 to 65 years (15 menopaused females,11 males) and in 56 patients (32 females and 24 males) shared out in three groups according to the age (70-79,80-89, 90 or more). In the elderly patients there is a decrease in T3 ($p<0.01$) and an increase in rT3 levels ($p<0.02$) ; T4, free T4, basal TSH and PRL levels were comparable to the controls. The mean TSH and PRL responses to TRH were reduced in patients ($p<0.01$) but there was no age effect within the elderly patients. A significant effect of sex was apparent only in patients. The mean TSH response was reduced in males (2.8 ± 0.3 vs 4.9 ± 0.7 µU/ml, $p<0.01$) as well as the mean PRL response (11.2 ± 2.6 vs 23.3 ± 3.1 ng/ml, $p<0.001$). No correlation may be found between TSH response and age, thyroid hormones or PRL responses in patients. No response of TSH was noted in 8 out of the patients.

In the elderly 1) there is a reduction in the TSH and the PRL response to TRH more pronounced in males 2) absence of TSH response to TRH does not in itself indicate the presence of hyperthyroidism 3) a simultaneously blunted TSH and PRL response may be in favour of a central dysfunction.

1676 THE EFFECT OF HUMAN MENOPAUSAL GONADOTROPINS ON OVARIAN FOLLICULAR SELECTION IN WOMEN.

J. SHALEV, T. SAADON, B. LUNENFELD, S. MASHIACH, D.M. SERR, J. BLANKSTEIN.
Departments of OB/GYN and the Institute of Endocrinology, Sheba Medical Center, Tel-Hashomer, Israel.

In order to answer the question whether human menopausal gonadotropins(HMG) can override the normal mechanism of ovarian follicular selection, we administered HMG to 10 infertile women using the different schemes: HMG was administered on day 2 of the menstrual cycle, before the existence of the dominant follicle as documented by ultrasound. In the second group HMG was administered from day 9 of the menstrual cycle. Following the first treatment cycle, the treatment schemes were changed in a way that those who received the treatment on day 2 received it on day 9 and vice-versa (cross-over design). All women were followed by serial ultrasound examinations and by frequent determinations of urinary and blood levels of estrogens.

It was found in those women in whom the treatment was started earlier had significantly more follicles (8.2 ± 1.9 follicles on day 2 and 4.4 ± 1.7 follicles on day 9, $P < 0.001$); moreover the number of the mature follicles was also significantly higher when treatment was started on day 2 (2.4 ± 1.2) mature follicles vs. 1.1 ± 1.1, ($P < 0.05$) when treatment was started on day 9. Since it has been shown in primates (Dizerga and Hodgen J.C.E.M. 1980) that selection of the follicle destined to ovulate had already occurred a week before ovulation, it can be concluded that HMG therapy can override the natural selection process in women, especially if it is administered prior to the selection of the dominant follicle.

1677 DEMONSTRATION OF RENIN-ANGIOTENSIN IN PURIFIED RAT LEYDIG CELLS.

K. Pandey*, M. Melner, K. Misono and T. Inagami, Department of Biochemistry, School of Medicine, Vanderbilt University, Nashville, TN. 37232, USA.

Recent findings suggest that Leydig cells may be an important source of peptide hormones whose roles in male reproductive system are as yet unknown. More recently, specific localization of renin in Leydig cells of rat testes has been demonstrated by histochemical methods. The apparent biological role of renin is related to its capacity to generate angiotensin. In an attempt to study the existence of a renin-angiotensin system in the testis we have utilized purified rat Leydig cells. Testes were excised from adult male rats, decapsulated and dissociated with 0.4 mg/ml collagenase treatment. Leydig cell population I and II were purified by discontinuous Metrizamide gradient centrifugation. The lysates of Leydig cell populations I and II exhibited renin activity of 332.96 ± 25.26 pg angiotensin I (AI)/h/10^6 cells and 163.55 ± 19.86 pg AI/h/10^6 cells, respectively. Both cell populations I and II contained inactive (latent) renin which was activated with dithiothreitol by 4-fold and 8-fold, respectively. Active and latent renin both showed strong affinity to an anti-rat renin IgG-Sepharose column indicating that the activity is due to specific renin. Furthermore, Leydig cell lysate contained angiotensin I, angiotensin II and angiotensin III which were determined by high pressure liquid chromatography and specific radioimmunoassays. These findings together indicate the existence of an intracellular renin-angiotensin system in testicular cells. The physiological function of renin-angiotensin in testis remains to be established. Supported by NIH grants HL-07323, HL-14192 and HL-24112.

1678 IDENTITY OF APPARENT MOLECULAR WEIGHT BETWEEN RAT TESTICULAR AND KIDNEY RENINS.

M. Parmentier*, T. Inagami and R. Pochet, Lab. Histology, School of Medicine ULB, 2, rue Evers, Brussels, Belgium. Dept Biochemistry, Vanderbilt University, Nashville, USA.

Renin-like activity or immunoreactivity have been described in various extrarenal organs such as brain, pituitary, blood vessels, uterus, adrenal, and submaxillary gland. For many of those localizations, the identity of renin-like subtances with true renin has not been proven. Using very specific antisera against pure rat renin, and a very sensitive immunohistochemical method we have described the presence of a renin immunoreactivity in the Leydig cells of the adult rat. This renin-like substance appeared to be under gonadotropin dependence. Renin enzymatic activity has been confirmed by biochemical studies on whole testis and Leydig cells cultures. Kidney and testicular homogenates have been submitted to SDS PAGE and the proteins have been transferred to nitrocellulose sheets by the Western Blotting method. The immunodetection of renin-like substances revealed the presence of two bands of 63000 and 60000 daltons in rat kidney. Two major bands of 63000 and 58000 and a minor one of 60000 daltons was found for rat testis, strongly suggesting that both organs do contain two identical forms or renin.

1679 ANGIOTENSIN II RECEPTOR REGULATION DURING ALTERED SODIUM INTAKE IN PRIMATES.
M. P. Platia*, K. J. Catt, G. D. Hodgen and G. Aguilera, NICHD, ERRB and PRB, NIH, Bethesda, MD, U.S.A.

In the rat, angiotensin II (AII) receptors of the adrenal glomerulosa and smooth muscle undergo reciprocal forms of regulation that parallel the changes in AII sensitivity during changes in sodium intake. However, the relative role of AII receptor regulation during sodium-induced changes in AII sensitivity in primates is not clear. In the monkey (Macacca fascicularis) we analyzed the changes in AII receptors after 4 to 6 days of high vs low sodium diet in adrenal and bladder membrane-rich particles. Consistent with the decreased pressor response to AII, smooth muscle AII receptors were lower in sodium-restricted monkeys (93±6 fmol/mg) than in sodium loaded monkeys (171±8 fmol/mg). However, in contrast to the rat, regulation of zona glomerulosa AII receptors in monkey adrenal was similar to that in smooth muscle, decreasing with sodium restriction and increasing with sodium loading (344±64 and 660±68 fmol/mg, respectively). Altered sodium intake caused no change in AII receptor affinity in either smooth muscle or adrenal particles. In spite of the decrease in adrenal AII receptors, 18-hydroxylase activity was markedly elevated in adrenal mitochondria from sodium-restricted monkeys (74±8 fmol/mg/min) compared with sodium-loaded animals (28±11 fmol/mg/min). Increased adrenal sensitivity to AII despite a fall in adrenal AII receptors indicates that full activation of steroidogenesis by AII can be maintained with partial receptor occupancy, and that post-receptor events including increased 18-hydroxylase activity are important determinants of the aldosterone response to AII during sodium restriction.

1680 EFFECT OF INSULIN TREATMENT ON RENIN AND ALDOSTERONE IN THE DIABETIC RAT.
J.H. Pratt*, C.A. Parkinson, M.H. Weinberger, and W.C. Duckworth. Indiana University School of Medicine, and the VA Hospital, Indianapolis, IN, USA.

Insulin deficiency can lead to decreases in renin secretion and aldosterone production (AP). We examined effects of alloxan-induced diabetes on the renin-aldosterone system in rats, and compared effects of 3 weeks of insulin treatment of diabetes (DM-Ins) with no treatment of diabetes (DM-unTx). At the end of this period, plasma renin activity (PRA) was 18.1+3.1 (SEM) in a control group (CTL), 5.6+1.3 in DM-unTx, and 22.8+3.7 ng/ml/3 hr in DM-Ins. The decrease in PRA in DM-unTx ($p<0.001$ when compared to either DM-Ins or CTL) was not anticipated since these rats were volume contracted (as evidenced by an increase in BUN with normal creatinine), a result of a marked osmotic diuresis in DM-unTx (10-fold greater than DM-Ins). In an additional set of animals, adrenals were removed and the capsular portion (zona glomerulosa) isolated and perifused to assess *in vitro* AP. Basal and potassium stimulated (4.0 mM/L increase in potassium for 60 min) AP (ng/min/mg protein) is tabulated below:

	n	basal	10 min	30 min	60 min
CTL	4	0.7+0.1	0.8+0.1	2.4+0.2	2.0+0.2
DM-unTx	6	0.6+0.1	0.7+0.1	1.8+0.4	1.6+0.3
DM-Ins	10	1.5+0.3	2.0+0.4	3.6+0.5	3.2+0.6

Basal as well as stimulated AP was greater in DM-Ins than in either DM-unTx or CTL ($p<0.05$). In conclusion, insulin treatment restored PRA to normal in diabetic rats. AP also increased after insulin therapy, a result of insulin having increased PRA in diabetic rats, but also insulin may have had a direct trophic influence on the zona glomerulosa.

1681 MECHANISM OF THE BLOOD PRESSURE RESPONSE TO INTRAVERTEBRAL ANGIOTENSIN II.

E.W.Quillen, Jr.* and I.A.Reid, UCSF, San Francisco, CA 94143, USA.

Intravertebral (ivb) infusion of angiotensin II (AII) increases mean arterial pressure (MAP) in dogs but the contribution of cardiac output (CO) and peripheral resistance (TPR) to this increase is not clear. Therefore, CO and its distribution were studied with microspheres in 4 conscious dogs with chronic femoral arterial and venous, left atrial, and vertebral artery catheters. 0.66ng/kg/min AII ivb increased CO from 2390±191 to 3684±363 ml/min($p<.05$), MAP from 102.6±1.9 to 112.0±3.3 mmHg($p<.05$) and heart rate (HR) from 96.3±5.5 to 103.5±7.1 bpm($p<.05$). Compartmental resistances (R_C), expressed as fractional changes from control, were decreased in the kidneys(.78), spleen(.71), digestive tract(.82), skin(.81), heart(.78), brain(.84), skeletal muscle(.77) and bone(.84). No changes were observed with 0.66ng/kg/min AII iv. 2.0ng/kg/min AII ivb caused greater increases in MAP (99.5±2.1 to 115.0±3.5 mmHg, $p<.05$) and HR (92.8±6.3 to 104.3±6.8 bpm, $p<.05$) but the increase in CO (3284±364 to 3511±320 ml/min) was smaller. R_C were increased in the kidneys(1.24), digestive tract(1.18), skin(1.05), heart(1.04), brain(1.04) and skeletal muscle(1.28) but decreased in the spleen(.89) and bone(.87). In contrast to ivb AII, 5.0ng/kg/min AII iv increased R_C in the above vascular beds except muscle and bone over a range of 1.10 to 2.28X and CO fell from from 3630±215 to 3111±102 ($p<.05$) while MAP rose from 101.6±4.4 to 123.3±3.8 ($p<.05$) without a change in HR. The data show that with a low dose of ivb AII, the increase in MAP is due to an increase in CO concomitant with a decrease in TPR while at a higher dose, the increase results both from increased CO and TPR. Whether the increase in resistance at higher AII levels is due to sympathetic stimulation or direct vasoconstriction from recirculated AII remains to be determined. Supported by NIH AM07265 and HL29714.

1682 DOPAMINE-3-SULFATE INHIBITS ALDOSTERONE SECRETION IN MONOLAYER BOVINE ADRENAL CELL CULTURE.

K. Racz*, N.T. Buu, O. Kuchel and A. De Léan, Clinical Research Institute, Montreal, Quebec, H2W 1R7, Canada.

Dopamine (DA) has been demonstrated to inhibit aldosterone (Aldo) secretion in bovine adrenal cells *in vitro*. Since circulating DA is present cverwhelmingly in the sulfoconjugated form and free DA, DA sulfate and the sulfoconjugating enzyme, phenolsulfotransferase, can be found in the bovine adrenal cortex, we examined whether the DA sulfates could also inhibit Aldo secretion by cultured bovine adrenal cells, and we then compared their action with that of free DA. Cocultured subcapsular and medullary cells from bovine adrenal glands responded to 10 nM Angiotensin II (A II) stimulation by a 10-12 fold increase in Aldo output (1. ± 0.2 to 11.3 ± 1.2 pmol/1.5 X 10^6 cells/3h). This stimulatory effect was partially inhibited by the addition of free DA and DA-3-sulfate but not by DA-4-sulfate. Both free DA and DA-3-sulfate produced their maximum inhibitory effect at a concentration of 100 μM, with a decrease in Aldo secretion of 61% (free DA) and 44% (DA-3-sulfate). The inhibition curves for DA and DA-3-sulfate indicated a slightly different potency for each substance: on equimolar basis DA-3-sulfate was about 2.5 times less potent than free DA. The inhibitory effect of DA-3-sulfate on the A II-stimulated Aldo secretion cannot be explained by liberation of free DA since less than 1% free DA was detected after the incubation of the cells with sulfoconjugated DA. Comparison of bovine adrenocortical concentrations of free and sulfoconjugated DA with those added to the *in vitro* cell culture system indicates that DA-3-sulfate may complement the dopaminergic inhibition of aldosterone secretion at the adrenal level.

1683 RELATIONSHIPS BETWEEN GLUCOSE-INDUCED (GI) PARADOXICAL ELEVATION OF SERUM POTASSIUM (SK) IN THE UPRIGHT POSTURE (UP) AND HORMONAL CHANGES DURING CAPTOPRIL (CAP) TREATMENT. J.P. Radó*, Gy. Gercsák, and É. Pató, Department of Medicine, Emil Weil Hospital, Budapest, Hungary.

The study was undertaken to explore the influence of CAP on the interrelationship between changes in SK and hormone levels (plasma aldosterone /PA/ and insulin /IRI/) in the course of glucose tolerance test (GTT). In 16 drug-resistant hypertensive patients who responded to CAP by a decrease of mean BP from 130±4 mmHg to 114±5 mmHg ($p<0{,}001$) four GTT-s were performed one in the recumbent and one in the UP both before and after CAP (2,2 mg/Kg BW/100 ml GFR). In 8 patients (Group 1) GI elevation of SK was found in the UP under CAP ($p<0{,}01$), while in Group 2 a normal hypokalemic response to glucose was obtained ($p<0{,}01$). PA and IRI were measured by commercial RIA kits. In the pre(glucose)loading PA both CAP and UP caused a significant change ($p<0{,}001$) and an interaction was found only in Group 1 by analysis of variance. In the whole patient material the relationship between SK and PA (% decrease in response to CAP) is expressed by $\Sigma\Delta SK = -0{,}023\ PA - 0{,}7$; $r = -0{,}6$; $p< 0{,}05$. Significant depression of IRI was found only in UP at 180 min of GTT uninfluenced by CAP and at 90 min during CAP ($p<0{,}05$). $\Sigma\Delta SK = -6{,}22\Sigma\Delta IRI + 0{,}88$; $r = -0{,}54$; $p<0{,}05$. Conclusion: interaction between influences of CAP and UP on PA combined with an IRI depressing effect of both may provide a plausible explanation for the observed postural GI SK elevation.

1684 COMPARISON OF THE STIMULATORY EFFECTS OF ACTH AND ANGIOTENSIN II ON ALDOSTERONE AND CORTICOSTEROID LEVELS IN CONSCIOUS DOGS. H. Raff*, J. Shinsako, C.E. Wade, L.C. Keil, and M.F. Dallman. Dept. of Physiol. UC San Francisco, CA 94143, Letterman Army Hosp., San Francisco, CA 94129, and NASA- Ames Research Center, Moffett Field, CA 94035.

This study examined the relative potencies of ACTH and angiotensin II (AII) as stimuli to mineralocorticoid and glucocorticoid secretion *in vivo*. We performed 60 min iv infusions of saline (control), 0.5 and 1 ng/kg/min 1-24 ACTH, and 2.5 and 5 ng/kg/min AII in 5 normovolemic, sodium-replete, conscious dogs. These infusion rates produce elevations of ACTH and AII within the physiological range. Plasma concentrations of ACTH, aldosterone (ALDO), and corticosteroids (CORT) were measured by RIA. Control ACTH after saline infusion was 70±6 pg/ml. Control ALDO and CORT were 7±1 ng/dl and 1.5±0.7 ug/dl respectively. After 60 min of 0.5 and 1 ng/kg/min ACTH, ALDO increased to 15±3 and 23±1 ng/dl respectively. After 60 min of 2.5 and 5 ng/kg/min AII, ALDO increased to 25±6 and 38±6 ng/dl respectively. After 60 min of 0.5 and 1 ng/kg/min ACTH, CORT increased to 7.5±0.4 and 11.1±1.3 ug/dl respectively. CORT responses to AII were small (+1.3 ug/dl) and not dose related. We conclude that (1) 1 ng/kg/min ACTH and 2.5 ng/kg/min AII produce equivalent ALDO responses (2) both ALDO and CORT responses to ACTH infusions were dose related (3) by comparing measured ACTH and calculated AII concentrations on a molar basis, ACTH is more potent than AII as an acute stimulus to ALDO and (4) AII has little direct effect on CORT levels. This study was supported by NASA-Univ. Interchange NCA2-OR 665-201, AM28172, and AM06704.

1685 ETHOSECRETOGRAM - PHASE RELATION OF BEHAVIOR TO PLASMA CORTICOSTERONE IN FREELY MOVING RATS.

T. Hiroshige* and I. Shiraishi, Department of Physiology, Hokkaido University School of Medicine, Sapporo, 060 Japan.

An ethosecretogram, which illustrates phase relation between animal's behavior and plasma hormone levels, was constructed in conscious rats. A catheter was introduced into the right atrium in male rats 2 days before blood sampling. Plasma corticosterone levels were monitored individually through the catheter every 5 min over a period of several hours under freely moving conditions on an Animex which records spontaneous locomotor activity. The results showed that the bursts of locomotor activity were temporally correlated with those of plasma corticosterone level, the peak of the former preceding the hormone peak by 15 min. As to the type of locomotor activity, feeding and grooming were significantly correlated with the subsequent hormone elevation, whereas drinking was not. In separate series of experiments, effects of feeding and drinking on plasma corticosterone levels were examined in conscious rats which had been fasted or water-deprived for 24 or 48 h. In each combination, feeding induced a more pronounced elevation of hormone level than drinking, although locomotor activity counts *per se* increased more sharply in the latter. It is concluded that in the ethosecretogram specific types of locomotor activity such as feeding and grooming induce a phase-locked elevation of plasma corticosterone in freely moving rats.

(This work was supported in part by a grant to T.H. from the Ministry of Education, Science and Culture of Japan, no. 57440028).

1686 KAPPA-SELECTIVE OPIOIDERGIC PATHWAYS AND MEMORY.

D. Jefferys*, J.H. Boublik and J.W. Funder, Medical Research Centre, Prince Henry's Hospital, Melbourne, Australia 3004.

Adrenalectomized (adrx) and intact rats show indistinguishable levels of immobility during an initial 15-minute swimming test. In a 5-minute re-test 24 hours later, however, adrx rats show reduced immobility (∿30%; intact ∿70%). This effect is reversed by the administration on test, but not re-test, of glucocorticoids (dexamethasone (DM) 6µg; corticosterone 6mg) or D-ala^{2}-met^{5}-enkephalinamide (DAMEA; 5µg) but not 6mg deoxycorticosterone (Jefferys et al., Eur. J. Pharmacol. 92:99, 1983). Naloxone (20µg-2mg), but not quaternary analogs progressively reduced immobility in intact animals, and equivalently antagonized DM and DAMEA reversal of the effects of adrenalectomy. In specificity studies, ketocyclazocine (7.5µg), and dynorphin 1-17 (23µg) reversed the effects of adrenalectomy, whereas D-ala^{2}-D-leu^{5}-enkephalin (50µg), dynorphin 1-8 (10µg), morphine sulphate (67µg) and MR2266 (200µg), a mixed opiate agonist/antagonist, were inactive; MR2266 (200µg) antagonized the reversing effect of ketocyclazocine (7.5µg). From these studies we conclude (i) that the incorporation of information post-stress involves at least two opioidergic pathways, (ii) that the integrity of at least one of these is essential for incorporation to occur, (iii) that at least one of these pathways appears kappa-selective, suggesting a possible physiological role for dynorphin(s) in memory.

Supported by the National Health & Medical Research Council of Australia.

1687 JUVENILE HYP MICE MALABSORB CALCIUM FROM ISOLATED DUODENAL SEGMENTS IN VIVO DESPITE NORMAL ABSORPTION IN ADULT MICE AND NURSING PUPS: A ROLE FOR THE INTESTINE IN HYPOPHOSPHATEMIC BONE DISEASE. R.A. Meyer, Jr.*, P.R. Delzer, and M.H. Meyer, Marquette University, Milwaukee, WI 53233 USA

Four week old male X-linked hypophosphatemic (Hyp) mice malabsorb calcium from their intestines while adult Hyp mice absorb calcium normally. In this study Hyp mice of varying ages were tested for malabsorption to determine the extent of this defect and whether heterozygous female Hyp mice were also affected. ^{45}Ca was put into the lumen of 2 cm segments of the duodenum in 150 mM NaCl + 2 mM $CaCl_2$ vehicle. Both normal and Hyp male and female (Hyp/+) mice were used, n = 10/group. Absorption was measured at the time needed for normal mice to absorb 50% of the ^{45}Ca, which was 2, 4, 8, and 20 minutes for mice at 2, 4, 7, and 10 weeks of age respectively. At this time 2 and 10 week old Hyp mice of both sexes had plasma ^{45}Ca and % absorption from the duodenum not significantly different from normal. However, the 4 and 7 week old Hyp mice of both sexes had plasma ^{45}Ca at 50 $\pm$ 12% of normal and reduced absorption at 62 $\pm$ 6% of normal. In 4 and 7 week old Hyp mice half-way through the collection period plasma ^{45}Ca was also depressed to 35 $\pm$ 10% of normal. In conclusion, rapidly growing Hyp mice malabsorb calcium from their intestine, and this defect occurs equally in hemizygous males and heterozygous females. Nursing Hyp pups at 2 weeks of age and adult mice at 10 weeks of age and older absorb calcium normally. This defect correlates with low intestinal vitamin D-dependent calcium-binding protein and a failure of bone growth. We suggest that intestinal malabsorption is a significant factor exacerbating the bone disease.

1688 STEROID AND OPIOID MODULATION OF PROLACTIN SECRETION. P. Limonta, R. Maggi, F. Piva and L. Martini*, Department of Endocrinology, Via A. del Sarto, 21, 20129 Milano, Italy.

Sex steroids modulate the secretion of anterior pituitary hormones and interfere with the activity of several brain neurotransmitters. In addition to their feedback effects, sex steroids also exert "organizational" effects during the perinatal period. To evaluate the role of the neonatal steroid environment on the opiatergic control of prolactin secretion, naloxone (an opioid antagonist) has been acutely administered to normal male and female rats as well as to female rats androgenized immediately after birth (1.25 mg testosterone propionate) and to male rats orchidectomized on day 2 of life. Naloxone (2.5 mg/kg) was injected s.c. to the four groups of rats on days 16, 26 and 60 of life. Saline injected animals served as controls. The animals were killed 20' later and serum prolactin was assayed by RIA. On days 16, 26 and 60 of life prolactin was decreased by naloxone in normal males and in neonatally androgenized females, but not in normal females and in neonatally orchidectomized males. It is concluded that: 1) the central opioid systems controlling prolactin secretion are different in males and in females; 2) the differentation of these systems seems to be due to the endocrine environment existing at time of birth. (Supported by CNR through the Project "Preventive and Rehabilitative Medicine").

1689 DECREASED BRAIN CONCENTRATIONS OF CORTICOTROPIN RELEASING FACTOR AND ARGININE VASOPRESSIN IN SPONTANEOUSLY HYPERTENSIVE RATS COMPARED TO NORMOTENSIVE RATS. K. Murakami*, K. Hashimoto, K. Fujino, M. Niimi and Z. Ota, Third Department of Internal Medicine, Okayama University Medical School, Okayama 700, Japan

Fisher et al. (Regulatory Peptides, 5:153, 1983) reported that an intraventricular administration of corticotropin releasing factor (CRF) increased blood pressure by stimulating the noradrenergic sympathetic nervous flow. In this study here, we examined the CRF and arginine vasopressin (AVP) concentrations in spontaneously hypertensive rats (SHR) and normotensive Wistar Kyoto rats (WKY). The test animals were decapitated, and the brain were immediately removed. The major brain regions were dissected out and weighed. The tissue was extracted by acid acetone (80% acetone-20% 0.5 N HCl)-petroleum ether extraction. CRF was measured by radioimmunoassay in which rat CRF was used for tracer labelling and reference preparation. In both SHR and WKY the hypothalamus showed the highest levels of CRF and AVP. CRF and AVP immunoreactivities were also detected in the thalamus, cerebral cortex, cerebellum, pons, midbrain and medulla oblongata. CRF immunoreactivity was lower in the hypothalamus, thalamus, medulla oblongata and midbrain of SHR, and AVP immunoreactivity was lower in the hypothalamus and thamalus compared with WKY. These results in SHR suggest that CRF and AVP might be involved in hypertension of SHR, but exact roles remain to be clarified.

1690 CALCEMIC HORMONE EFFECTS ON INOSITOL LIPID METABOLISM IN LIMB BONES AND CALVARIA. Mark S. Rappaport* and Paula H. Stern, Northwestern University, Chicago, IL 60611, USA.

Numerous hormones and neurotransmitters affect turnover of phosphatidylinositol (PI) and other acidic phospholipids in target tissues. These phospholipids may be involved in intracellular events in hormone action. Parathyroid hormone (PTH) has been reported to increase ^{32}P incorporation into rat bone total phospholipid and to stimulate PI turnover and increase total acidic phospholipids in renal tubules. We have examined hormonal effects on inositol lipid metabolism in relation to bone resorption in two *in vitro* culture systems. Neonatal mouse calvaria were treated with .1 U/ml PTH, 10 ng/ml calcitonin (CT), or 10^{-9} M 1,25(OH)$_2$vitaminD$_3$ for 24 h. Bones were then labeled 30 min with 2μCi/ml ^3H-inositol, extracted in chloroform-methanol, and lipids separated by TLC. PI labeling was increased 39% by PTH and 16% by 1,25(OH)$_2$vitaminD$_3$. In contrast, CT decreased PI labeling 22%. After simultaneous PTH and CT treatment, labeling was not different from control. These differences could not be explained by changes in free inositol pool size. Bone resorption, assessed as medium Ca^{2+} following 24 h culture, was increased 15% by PTH and 9% by 1,25(OH)$_2$vitaminD$_3$, and inhibited 16% by CT and 13% by CT plus PTH. In other studies, fetal rat limb bones were incubated with 10^{-7} M PTH and ^3H-inositol for 2 h. PTH increased PI labeling 31%. The early occurrence of changes in PI metabolism and their correlation with resorptive events suggests that hormonally mediated changes in PI metabolism may have an integral role in the calcemic actions of these hormones. Supported by NIH grant AM11262 (PHS) and PMAF fellowship (MSR).

1691 ACTIVITY OF GUANINE NUCLEOTIDE REGULATORY PROTEIN IN THE ERYTHROCYTE MEMBRANE AND ITS CORRELATION WITH CLINICAL FINDINGS IN PATIENTS WITH TYPE I PSEUDOHYPOPARATHYROIDISM. T. Saito* and S. Ishikawa, Division of Endocrinology and Metabolism, Jichi Medical School, Tochigi 329-04, Japan.

Patients with Type I pseudohypoparathyroidism (PHP-I) have findings that stem from the failure of hormonal actions mediated through cAMP. The significance of deficiency in guanine nucleotide regulatory protein (N-protein) in the cell membrane which couples hormone receptors and catalytic units of adenylate cyclase in the development of clinical symptoms of PHP-I was examined in Japanese patients. The activity of N-protein in the erythrocyte membrane was assayed by the reconstitution method of Lubrol extract of N-protein with plasma membrane of S49 cyc^- mouse lymphoma cells, which lacks N-protein. The activity of N-protein expressed as adenylate cyclase [% of pooled standard, mean ± SE (n)] was 78.9±6.1 (18) in the patients, which was significantly ($p<0.01$) lower than that in normal subjects, 99.5±2.4 (30). The N-protein activities (Y:%) in the patients were in significant correlations with three clinical parameters examined (X): with body height in standard deviation score from the mean of the normal population at the corresponding age, Y=89.4+10.4X ($r=0.616$, $p<0.01$); with urinary excretion of cAMP (nmol/mg creatinine), Y=56.3+72.0X ($r=0.501$, $p<0.05$), and with TSH levels in plasma (μU/ml), Y=129-3X ($r=0.639$, $p<0.01$). The decrease in cAMP production due to N-protein deficiency in the cell membrane may be involved in the development of the clinical symptoms of PHP-I including short stature, decrease in urinary excretion of cAMP and latent or manifest primary hypothyroidism associated with TSH elevation in plasma.

1692 CYTOCHEMICAL BIOASSAY OF HUMAN PARATHYROID HORMONE FRAGMENTS. K. Sakaguchi[1]*, M. Fukase[2], T. Fujita[2], T. Kimura[3], S. Sakakibara[3], S. Katsuragi[4], K. Morita[4] and T. Noda[4], North Hyogo Med. Orthoped. Center[1], Third Div. Dept. of Med. Kobe Univ. Sch. of Med.[2], Peptide Institute[3] and Toyo Jozo Research Institute[4], Japan

In view of the absolute requirement of two N-terminal amino acids for the development of biological activity of parathyroid hormone (PTH), Nle^8, Nle^{18}, Tyr^{34} bPTH(3-34)NH_2 and Tyr^{34} bPTH(7-34)NH_2 were synthesized as inhibitors of PTH action without agonist action in vivo. The cytochemical bioassay using guinea pig kidney sections to measure glucose-6-phosphate dehydrogenase activity in the distal convoluted tubule as the index of PTH action which was shown to be the most sensitive and specific mehtod to detect PTH activity in vitro was therefore applied to test the biological activity of bPTH(1-84), hPTH(1-84), hPTH(3-34), Tyr^{34} hPTH(7-34)NH_2 and Tyr^{34} hPTH(13-34)NH_2 and other synthetic PTH fragments. At the concentration range between 10^{-16}-10^{-13}M, hPTH(3-34), Tyr^{34} hPTH(7-34)NH_2 and Tyr^{34} hPTH(13-34)NH_2 were as active as bPTH(1-84) and hPTH(1-84) on molar basis as complete agonists. When added to bPTH(1-84) and hPTH(1-84), all these fragments were not only devoid of inhibitory actions on PTH, but also were additive in their agonist actions. Unlike the reported absence of agonistic actions in vivo of synthetic PTH inhibitors, hPTH(3-34) and Tyr^{34} hPTH (7-34)NH_2 showed no inhibitory actions on PTH and proved to be complete agonists in cytochemical bioassay. Such discrepancy between results obtained by different methods of assay might indicate the multiplicity and complexity of PTH action, indicating a need for multiple assays to draw an overall picture of the action of each fragment.

1693 PROBLEMS IN THE ESTIMATION OF NEPHROGENOUS CYCLIC AMP K. Sato*, F. Kakezono, S. Okamoto, N. Yokoyama, S. Morita, S. Yamashita, T. Tanabe, S. Ohtakara, M. Izumi, and S. Nagataki, The First Department of Internal Medicine, Nagasaki University, Nagasaki 852 Japan.

It has been known for some time that parathyroid hormone stimulate the production of cyclic AMP by the kidney and we have undertaken a study to calculate nephrogenous cyclic AMP (NcAMP) by the usual methods. We found some problems in this because plasma cAMP (PcAMP) is unstable and quickly degrades even with the additional EDTA. We have shown this instability by measuring cAMP in plasma at various times after the sampling. A sample of blood was taken into an ice-cooled tube containing 10 mM EDTA solution, and was immediately centrifuged at 4°C. Plasma aliquotes were put into several tubes. One tube was frozen immediately in dry-ice acetone, while the other tubes were incubated in ice or at room temperature, and then were frozen at various times ranging from 15 min. to 6 hours after the sampling. The concentration of PcAMP decreased significantly with time, especially during the first 3 hours in which PcAMP decreased by 20 to 30%. Addition of 100mM EDTA could not prevent this decline. Therefore, if the plasma sample is not frozen promptly the PcAMP result will be lower than it should be. In order to assess the accuracy of the calculation of NcAMP we took hypoparathyroid patients and measured PcAMP by taking a sample of blood, separating it, freezing it within 15 minutes and then doing assay after quick thawing. In the cases, calculated NcAMP was negative. Also it is not known whether filtered cAMP is reabsorbed in the kidney, but careful estimation and therefore very careful interpretation is necessary for NcAMP.

1694 RENAL 25-HYDROXYVITAMIN D_3 -1α-HYDROXYLASE ACTIVITY IN PATIENTS WITH RENAL DISEASE. K. Satomura*, Y. Seino, K. Yamaoka, Yos. Tanaka, M. Ishida, H. Yabuuchi, Yoko Tanaka[1] and H. F. DeLuca[1]. Department of Pediatrics, Osaka University Hospital, Osaka 553, Japan. Department of Biochemistry, University of Wisconsin-Madison, U.S.A.[1]

It is important to measure $25OHD_3$-1α-hydroxylase (1α-hydroxylase) in understanding the pathogenesis of diseases involving disturbance in the vitamin D endocrine system. We have already reported a micro detemination of renal 1α-hydroxylase activity in renal biopsy specimens. In this study, we have measured the renal 1α-hydroxylase activities in thirteen patients with renal disease. The 1α-hydroxylase activity of seven patients with asymptomatic proteinuria and/or hematuria ranged between 25.1 and 117.0 pg/mg tissue/20 min. Since these patients did not show any impaired mineral metabolism or pathological changes in the tubules, we presume that these results indicate the normal range in man. The 1α-hydroxylase activities of two patients treated with prednisolone (15 mg/day) showed 86.1 and 46.1 pg/mg tissue/20 min. The 1α-hydroxylase activity seemed not to be reduced after the administration of prednisolone. The 1α-hydroxylase activity showed 55.2 and 85.3 pg/mg tissue/20 min two patients with mild renal insufficiency and 10.5 and 7.1 pg/mg tissue/20 min in two patients with severe renal insufficiency. The 1α -hydroxylase activities, therefore, not to be reduced in mild renal insufficiency but it is reduced in severe renal insufficiency. The new method for measurement of renal 1α-hydroxylase activity would seem to be useful in the clinical studies on vitamin D endocrine system.

1695 GENETIC TRANSMISSION OF PARATHYROID HORMONE (PTH) GENE VARIANTS IN MAN.
J. Schmidtke* and D.N. Cooper, Institut für Humangenetik der Universität, Nikolausberger Weg 5a, D-3400 Göttingen, FRG.

Restriction fragment length polymorphisms (RFLP's) in and around cloned DNA sequences are a useful tool in the diagnosis of human inherited disease, in that they may serve as markers for linked mutations giving rise to genetic disease. Impaired PTH (parathyroid hormone) gene expression is one possible cause of primary hypoparathyroidism in man. We have looked for and identified RFLP's in the region of the human PTH gene by a combination of Southern blotting of genomic DNA and molecular hybridisation using a cloned human PTH genomic fragment and a cDNA clone as probes. We present here our data on the genetic transmission of three such RFLP's detected with the restriction enzymes Pst I, Taq I, and Xba I. The results are consistent with Mendelian segregation of the allelic variants. It will now be possible to use these RFLP's to search for primary gene defects.

1696 CALCIUM REGULATION OF CALCITONIN mRNA.
Segond, N.*, Jullienne, A., Taboulet, J., Milhaud, G. and Moukhtar, M.S., U113 INSERM, 27 rue Chaligny, 75571 Paris cedex 12, France.

Calcium raises the relative abundance of calcitonin (Ct) mRNA as early as 2 minutes after its administration in rats. This could be due to an increase in transcription rate, or to post transcriptional modifications of Ct mRNA. We report here the effect of actinomycin D on the levels of Ct mRNA in rats subjected to acute hypercalcemia. Ct mRNA was quantified by its ability to direct the synthesis of preprocalcitonin in a cell free system, or by hybridization to a ^{32}P cDNA probe specific for Ct mRNA. Actinomycin D injected 5 hours before Ca administration provoked a moderate decrease in basal Ca levels, but did not inhibit the rise in plasma levels of Ca or Ct (measured by a specific radioimmunoassay). Incorporation of ^{3}H adenine in liver and thyroid was diminished. Ct mRNA extracted from the thyroids of rats, treated or not with the antibiotic, directed the synthesis of the same quantities of preprocalcitonin (estimated by integrating autoradiographies of polyacrylamide gel electrophoresis of specific immunoprecipitates). In control rats, 2 minutes after calcium injection, an 8 fold increase in preprocalcitonin synthesised was observed. In the actinomycin D pretreated animals this rise was not observed. Quantification of Ct mRNA levels by hybridization assay showed no change in mRNA levels. Therefore the increase in translatable Ct mRNA level after Ca stimulation is probably due to post transcriptional modifications involving or not the expression of other genes.

1697 Differential Diagnosis of Hypoparathyroid Disorders During Childhood.
Y. Seino*[1)], Y. Tsuchiya[2)], N. Matsuura[3)], A. Okuno[4)] and T. Iijima[5)]
Department of Pediatrics, Osaka University School of Medicine, Osaka 553[1)], Tokyo Metropolitan Children's Hospital, Tokyo 204[2)], Hokkaido University School of Medicine, Hokkaido 060[3)], Asahikawa Medical School, Hokkaido 078-11[4)] and Yamasa Shoyu Co., Ltd., Chiba 288, Japan[5)].

Changes in the plasma and urinary adenosine 3',5'-monophosphate (cyclic AMP) levels on infusion of parathyroid hormone were studied in 18 normal children, 11 children with idiopathic hypoparathyroidism, 14 children with pseudohypoparathyroidism type I, 3 children with pseudohypoparathyroidism type II, and 1 child with pseudopseudohypoparathyroidism. In normal children the plasma concentration of cyclic AMP ranged from 12.4 to 44.0 pmol/ml under basal conditions, and increased to a peak of about 12-times of the basal 10 minutes after infusion of parathyroid hormone.

Infusion of parathyroid hormone caused no increase in plasma cyclic AMP in patients with pseudohypoparathyroidism, but caused increase 31-times in untreated patients with idiopathic hypoparathyroidism and 16-times in such patients under treatment.

The measurement of plasma cyclic AMP before and 10 minutes after infusion of parathyroid hormone is concluded to be a simple and effective method for differential diagnosis of hypoparathyroid disorders.

1698 MAITOTOXIN, A Ca^{2+} CHANNEL ACTIVATOR, STIMULATES PITUITARY cAMP GENERATION AND PROLACTIN SECRETION: INHIBITION BY DOPAMINE.
G Schettini*, K Koike, IS Login, MJ Cronin, EL Hewlett, AM Judd, T Yasumoto, RM MacLeod, University of Virginia, Charlottesville, Virginia, U.S.A.

Maitotoxin (MTX) stimulates prolactin (PRL) release and Ca^{2+} uptake from both normal and clonal anterior pituitary (AP) cells. In AP primary culture MTX (1-50 ng/ml) induced a dose dependent stimulation of cyclic AMP (cAMP) accumulation and PRL release. In the presence and absence of 0.2 mM IBMX, 50 ng/ml MTX stimulated cAMP accumulation within 1 min ($P < 0.05$), reached a maximum at 10 min, and returned to or below the baseline after 30 min. Enhanced PRL release was achieved by 50 ng/ml MTX within 1 min (with IBMX) and 3 min (without IBMX) and was sustained for 30 min. The cAMP accumulation induced by 5 ng/ml MTX, but not 10 ng/ml, was reduced by coincubation with 1 or 10 µM dopamine (DA) ($P < 0.01$). PRL release induced by either 5 or 10 ng/ml MTX was reduced by DA ($P < 0.01$). Bromocriptine (0.01, 0.1, and 1 µM) also inhibited the enhanced cAMP accumulation and PRL release produced by 10 ng/ml MTX ($P < 0.01$). Finally, a preincubation of hemi-AP glands for 10 min with 100 ng/ml MTX activated adenylate cyclase from 32 ± 0.9 to 46.5 ± 3.1 pmol cAMP/mg protein/min ($P < 0.01$). The addition of 10 µM DA to the pituitary membrane preparation reduced both basal and MTX-stimulated adenylate cyclase activity ($P < 0.01$). In conclusion, it is likely that the activation of Ca^{2+} flux induced by MTX stimulates both PRL release and cAMP accumulation; these latter effects are attenuated by DA. Although we cannot exclude an effect of DA on Ca^{2+} flux, the present results suggest a direct inhibitory action of DA on adenylate cyclase activity in membranes previously activated by MTX *in vitro*.

1699 EFFECT OF ETHANOL ON CALCIUM UPTAKE AND INSULIN RELEASE FROM RAT ISLETS.

R. Sethi*, G. Pullen, A. Snyder, F. Ellyin and S. Singh. Veterans Administration Medical Center, North Chicago, Illinois 60064, USA.

Evidence suggests that ethanol inhibits glucose mediated insulin release from pancreatic islets. Studies were undertaken to correlate effects of ethanol on Ca^{45} uptake and insulin release from rat islets. Incubations were carried out with 16.7 mM glucose for 30 min. Ethanol (ETOH) concentrations of 600 mg%, 300 mg%, and 100 mg% significantly inhibited Ca^{45} uptake by islets from 4.32 $\pm$ 0.12 pmoles/islet (control) to 2.68 $\pm$ 0.20, 2.84 $\pm$ 0.16, and 3.7 $\pm$ 0.18 pmoles/islet respectively ($p<0.05$), and insulin release from 191.3 $\pm$ 11.3 μU/10 islets (control) to 107.7 $\pm$ 13.6, 81 $\pm$ 6.2, and 107 $\pm$ 6.3 μU/10 islets respectively ($p<0.05$). Experiments were performed with A23187 (20 μM), high extracellular calcium (7.5 mM), and acetylcholine (ACH) (20 μM), with and without 600 mg% ETOH, to determine if the inhibition of insulin release can be reversed by increasing Ca^{++} influx. A23187 increased insulin release from islets to 330 μU/10 islets. In the presence of ETOH, insulin release was 175 $\pm$ 9.9 μU/10 islets ($p<0.05$). Incubations with high Ca^{++} and ACH increased insulin release to 354.3 $\pm$ 26.5 and 233 $\pm$ 14.6 μU/10 islets while, in the presence of ETOH, insulin release was 190.7 $\pm$ 16.3 and 181.6 $\pm$ 12.0 μU/10 islets respectively. A23187, high Ca^{++} and ACH increased Ca^{45} uptake in ETOH groups to values not significantly different from those without ETOH. Thus, membrane inhibition of calcium uptake by ETOH may not be the primary site of action for inhibition of insulin release.

Supported by the Veterans Administration.

1700 DEHYDROEPIANDROSTERONE INHIBITS THE GROWTH OF THE DUNNING R-3327 RAT PROSTATIC ADENOCARCINOMA.

J. R. Matias*, C. P. De Feo III, V. Malloy, and N. Orentreich. New York University Medical Center and The Animal Sciences Laboratory, Orentreich Foundation for the Advancement of Science, 910 Fifth Avenue, New York, New York, USA 10021.

Dehydroepiandrosterone (DHEA) has been demonstrated to inhibit the onset of various spontaneous and chemically induced tumors in laboratory animals. However, little is known about its influence on the growth of transplantable tumors. The present study was undertaken to evaluate the effect of DHEA on the growth rate of the androgen dependent, transplantable R-3327 prostatic cancer of the Copenhagen rat. DHEA at a dose of 10 mg/kg of body weight was injected subcutaneously on alternate days in adult male rats implanted with 2 mm^3 of the tumor. In comparison to the vehicle injected controls, the rate of tumor growth was slower in rats treated with DHEA. At 130 days after tumor implantation, the mean tumor volume in the DHEA treated and control groups were 29.9 cm^3 and 10.5 cm^3, respectively ($P< 0.001$). Rats injected with DHEA for 4 weeks prior to tumor inoculation showed the same tumor take as the control rats. Significant differences in the rate of food consumption and body weight were not observed between the control and experimental animals. The data demonstrate that prostatic cancer may be included among the types of tumors inhibited by treatment with DHEA.

1701 ANIMAL MODEL FOR HYPERCALCEMIA OF MALIGNANCY: ADENOCARCINOMA DERIVED FROM APOCRINE GLANDS OF ANAL SAC IN DOGS (CA).

D.J. Meuten, C.C. Capen*, G.V. Segre, E.F. Voelkel, L. Levine, A.H. Tashjian, Jr., L.A. Nagode, and G.J. Kociba, Dept. Vet. Pathobiol., The Ohio State University, Columbus; Dept. Med., Mass. Gen. Hosp.; and Lab. Toxicol., Harvard School Public Health, Boston, MA, USA.

Hypercalcemia associated with malignancy was investigated in 36 aged (mean: 10 yr.), female (92%) dogs with a naturally occurring CA and persistently elevated blood calcium (15.7 ± 0.56 mg/dl). All tumors had histologic features of malignancy and 96% metastasized to regional lymph nodes. Bone metastases were found in only one dog. Lamellar arrays of endoplasmic reticulum, prominent Golgi apparatuses, and small (150-400 nm) secretory granules with a dense core were present in the neoplastic cells. Plasma iPTH (pg/ml) in dogs with CA (168 ± 40) was not significantly different from normocalcemic tumor-controls (264 ± 46) and clinically normal (322 ± 33) dogs. iPTH was not detected in tumor tissue. Parathyroids were atrophic and composed of inactive chief cells. Surgical removal of the CA resulted in normocalcemia within 24-48 hr. and a marked (2- to 20-fold) increase in plasma iPTH. Regrowth of the CA was associated with a recurrence of hypercalcemia. Histomorphometric evaluation of lumbar vertebrae revealed significantly decreased trabecular bone volume, increased total resorptive surface, and increased osteoclast/mm bone surface compared to age-matched controls. The plasma 13,14-dihydro-15-keto prostaglandin E_2 was not significantly different from control groups. Serum 1,25-$(OH)_2D$ levels (pg/ml) of 23 ± 5 in dogs with CA were inappropriately high for the degree of hypercalcemia and were similar to normocalcemic tumor-controls (16 ± 4) and clinically normal (26 ± 5) dogs. Supported by State of Ohio Canine Research Funds.

1702 GROWTH RATE AND CELLULAR EVENTS REGULATED BY ANABOLIC STEROID HORMONES IN S-180 SARCOMAS IN VIVO AND IN VITRO.

H. Michna*[1], C. Stang-Voss[2], Institute of Anatomy [1], Medical University of Lübeck, Institute of Experimental Morphology[2], DSHS Cologne, FRG

The aim of this study is to characterize the implications of catabolic effects of anabolic steroid hormones on fibroblasts (Michna 1983) with their possible therapeutic effects on malign tumors of mesenchymal origin. Since such in vivo experiments do not exhibit whether a pharmacologically induced effect acts directly or whether cells of the reticulo-endothelial system mediate, it is expedient to provide information of effects in tissue culture on sarcomas. **In vitro** the absolute cell number, cell density, mitotic index and the number of cells without cytoplasmic processes were estimated after treatment with DIANABOL® (1,2 μ/ml medium). **In vivo** the time dependent effect of 3 mg DIANABOL®/kg body weight /week was studied on female mice (SPF-NMRI). With stereological methods the tumor volume and the portion of necrosis were quantified. By means of electron microscopy the cellular reaction pattern of the sarcoma cells was characterized in vivo and in vitro. We present evidence that anabolic steroids, which mediate protein synthesis via activation of cAMP, are involved in the release of catabolic reaction patterns of sarcomas. Although the results indicate a cytotoxic influence of the anabolic steroid on S-180 sarcoma cells in vitro, which in vivo may lead to dramatic effects on sarcoma growth rate, it is not possible to decide whether enhanced necrosis of bigger sarcomas after 4 weeks compared to controls indeed is due to a direct catabolic effect of the hormone or whether an inadequate capillary supply of the bigger sarcomas have to be taken into account.

1703 CHARACTERISATION OF THE PERITONEAL MACROPHAGE RESPONSE TO ANABOLIC STEROIDS IN CANCER BEARING MICE: A COMBINED BIOCHEMICAL, IMMUNOLOGICAL AND MORPHOLOGICAL STUDY.

H. Michna[I], H. Twilfer[I] and C. Stang-Voss[2]* Institute of Anatomy[I], Medical University of Lübeck, Institute of Experimental Morphology[2], DSHS Cologne, FRG

Compelling demonstrations have shown that anabolic steroids may stimulate the activity of the monocyte-macrophage system, which might be due to the existence of the appropriate steroid receptor machinery in these cells. Therefore it is of special clinical interest to investigate in which way anabolic steroid hormones may modulate the potencies of macrophages during immune response to cancer. Peritoneal macrophages from sarcoma 180-bearing mice treated with a synthetic anabolic steroid (3 mg DIANABOL®/kg body weight/week) were studied in vitro. In a short term study (1 week) and in a long term study (3 or 4 weeks) the changes in macrophage number of the peritoneal exudates, the macrophage migration and the chemotactic activity as well as the phagocytic and cytotixic activities were determined. DIANABOL®treatment enhanced the chemotactic activity markedly at an early stage and slightly at an advanced stage of tumor growth but chemotaxis did not reach the level of untreated controls of the advanced stage. Furthermore, with continued tumor growth the phagocytic activity of macrophages is potently and their natural cytocoxicity slightly enhanced, accompagnied by an increased total number of macrophages. These findings are correlated with the ultrastructure, the biochemical activity of lysosomal enzymes and the production of o_2^-.

1704 THE BISPHOSPHONATE APD HAS AN INHIBITORY EFFECT ON TUMOUR CELL MULTIPLICATION. H.W.Minne*, L. Gozariu, L. Lumpp, P.A. Lohse, R. Ziegler, Dept. Int. Med. VI, Univ. Heidelberg, West Germany, Dept. Endocrinol, Univ. Cluj, Rumania

Bisphosphonates inhibit bone resorption and thus influence paraneoplastic hypercalcemia in man and in the rat with the transplantable hypercalcemic Walker carcinosarcoma 256. In the latter, the bisphosphonate APD does not only lower serum calcium but also decreases elevated iPTH. The question was, whether this followed changes in PTH metabolism or a direct effect of APD on the malignant tumour itself. We therefore studied the effect of APD on the in vitro growth of the Walker tumour and of two additional human tumours (mammary cancer, malignant lymphoma). The tumour cells were cultured in vitro in the absence or presence of various doses (1 - 250 μMol/l) over a two or more weeks period. Cell counts served as parameter of cell multiplication, trypan blue exclusion test verified the vitality of the counted cells. We found, that increasing doses of APD inhibited tumour cell multiplication dose related. Removal of APD from the culture medium led to recovery of tumour cells. Increase in medium calcium potentiated this "cytostatic" APD-effect. We have to conclude, that the effect of APD on paraneoplastic hypercalcemia may have an additional reason: it does not only inhibit bone resorption but also inhibits tumour cell multiplication. This study was supported by the DFG, SFB 136

1705 ANALYSIS AND CHARACTERISTICS OF EPIDERMAL GROWTH FACTOR (EGF) RECEPTORS IN HUMAN BREAST CANCER. V.R. Mukku, J.L. Wittliff* and G.M. Stancel, Dept. of Pharmacology, Univ. Texas Med. Sch. at Houston, Houston, TX. 77025, and the Dept. of Biochemistry and James Graham Brown Cancer Center, Univ. of Louisville Health Science Ctr., Louisville, KY. 40292.

While measurements of sex steroid receptor levels and characteristics have improved the ability to predict the response of breast cancer patients to endocrine therapy, it is not yet possible to predict with certainty the response to this or other treatment modalities. Since this suggests other factors may be involved in regulating tumor growth, we initiated a study of receptors for other growth factors in human breast cancer. Membranes prepared from breast tumors contain high affinity ($K_d \simeq 1$ nM) binding sites for EGF. The binding of ^{125}I-EGF is blocked by excess unlabelled EGF, but not insulin, fibroblast growth factor or multiplication stimulating activity. In detergent solubilized preparations EGF stimulates the phosphorylation of two major proteins (MW = 170,000 and 150,000) observed by autoradiography of SDS polyacrylamide gels. Following ^{125}I-EGF binding to membranes, chemical crosslinking with disuccinimidyl suberate, detergent extraction and analysis by autoradiography of SDS gels, two bands of identical MW are observed. Analysis of 12 individual tumor samples revealed variable specific binding of EGF, ranging from undetectable levels to 18 fmol/100 μg protein. These results indicate that individual human mammary tumors contain varying levels EGF binding sites with the properties expected of EGF receptors, including an EGF stimulated kinase activity. (Supported by USPHS Grants HD-08615 and CA-19657.)

1706 EFFECTS OF LY117018 (LY) ON MCF 7 BREAST CANCER CELL GROWTH IN VITRO. RELATIONSHIP TO AFFINITY FOR ESTROGEN RECEPTOR(ER) AND ANTIESTROGEN BINDING SITE(AEBS). L.C. Murphy* and R.L. Sutherland. Ludwig Institute for Cancer Research (Sydney Branch) University of Sydney, N.S.W. Australia. 2006.

The nonsteroidal antiestrogen Tamoxifen (Tam) exerts 3 effects on the growth of MCF 7 human breast cancer cells in vitro: an E_2-reversible growth inhibition, an E_2-irreversible growth inhibition and a cytotoxic effect. Previous studies with Tam-related derivatives indicated that potency with regard to the first effect was correlated with affinity for ER and maximal potency with regard to the two latter effects occurred in those triphenylethylene derivatives which had a basic ether sidechain and a high affinity for AEBS. To extend further these structure-activity studies we investigated the effects of LY, a benzothiophene derivative with a basic sidechain, high affinity for ER (E_2=100%, LY=41%, Tam=2%) and low affinity for AEBS (Tam=100%, LY=2%), on the growth of MCF 7 cells in vitro. Drugs were added to exponentially growing cells and after 4 population doublings of control cultures, cell number and cell cycle kinetic parameters were estimated. At concentrations where Tam produced E_2-reversible effects (< 10μM), LY was a more potent growth inhibitor than Tam, but was less potent than Tam at concentrations (> 10μM) where the effects of Tam were E_2-irreversible LY showed no cytotoxicity at those doses where Tam had potent cytotoxicity. These data extend and confirm our previous observations which are consistent with E_2-reversible growth inhibition being mediated through ER while indiccating that other factors are likely to be involved in the mechanism of action of E_2-irreversible growth inhibition and cytotoxicity in vitro.

1707 PREINCUBATION WITH ESTROGEN INCREASES LACTOGENIC RECEPTOR CONCENTRATION IN CULTURED HUMAN BREAST CANCER CELLS. L.J. Murphy* and L. Lazarus. Garvan Institute of Medical Research, St. Vincent's Hospital, Sydney, 2010, Australia.

Recent studies in this laboratory have demonstrated a correlation between estrogen and lactogenic receptor concentration in a series of cultured breast cancer cell lines. To further investigate the relationship between estrogen and lactogenic receptors in this system we examined the effect of pre-incubation with β-estradiol (E2) on 125I-hGH binding to T47-D and MCF-7 cell monolayers. Confluent monolayers were incubated for varying time periods with 0-1μM of E2. A dose-dependent increase in specific 125I-hGH binding to both MCF-7 and T47-D cells was seen, with significant stimulation at E2 concentrations of 5 and 10nM ($p<0.025$) respectively. The maximal effect of E2 was seen in the presence of serum-free medium or in medium containing up to 1% charcoal-stripped FCS. Maximal increase in 125I-hGH binding to T47-D monolayers (144.6±6.1% of control, N=13) required 1μM E2 while similar enhancement of 125I-hGH binding to MCF-7 cells occurred at 100nM. A significant increase in specific 125I-hGH binding was observed with pre-incubations as short as 6h. The effect of E2 on specific binding of 125I-hGH was maximal after a 24h preincubation and persisted at submaximal levels for up to 72h. Tamoxifen (1μM) did not diminish the E2 response. Scatchard analysis of binding data for T47-D cell monolayers preincubated with or without 1μM E2 demonstrated an increase in lactogenic receptor number without any significant change in receptor affinity. These data demonstrate that E2 increases lactogenic receptor concentration in cultured breast cancer cells and suggest that estrogens may regulate lactogenic receptors in breast cancer tissue in vivo.

1708 SUPPRESSION OF ADRENAL ANDROGENS BY AMINOGLUTETHIMIDE IN PATIENTS WITH ADVANCED BREAST CANCER. By Robin Murray & Paula Pitt*, Cancer Inst. MELB.

Aminoglutethimide (A/G) is now an established treatment in advanced breast cancer (B/c). There is a profound fall in plasma oestrogens with this drug but secretion of adrenal androgens is relatively well preserved[1]. This study was to determine whether while basal levels of androgens might be maintained there was a significant fall over the day. 22 patients with actively progressing B/c had 2 hourly blood samples for 8 hours prior to & after receiving 250mg, 500mg and 750mg per day of A/G+37.5mg of cortisone acetate per day. DHEA-SO4 and testosterone (T) were measured by RIA. Results are expressed as mean ±SD. Prior to commencement of A/G there was no change in DHEA-SO4 between 8am(9±0.1umol/1) and 4pm while T fell from 1.3±.08 at 8am to 1.0±0.03umol/1 at 4pm - ($p>0.05$). Following 250mg of A/G again there was no fall in DHEA-SO4 while T fell progressively from 1.2±0.1 to 0.5±0.04nmol/1 ($p<0.05$). After 3 days on 250mg bd of A/G basal levels of DHEA-SO4 (0.35±.05umol/1) were significantly less ($p<0.05$) than pretreatment, but again there was no fall over an 8 hour period after 250mg of A/G. In contrast, basal T levels were not suppressed (1.0±.16) but again fell significantly after 250mg of A/G to 0.5±.16nmol/1. Results were similar after a further 3 days on 250mg of A/G tds. These findings suggest that A/G causes a slow but significant fall in plasma DHEA-SO4 and that T falls sharply after A/G only to rebound to near pretreatment levels overnight. Mean T levels through the day are lower in patients on A/G and this may be a factor influencing response to treatment.

REFERENCES

SAMOJLIK E, VELDHUIS J, WELLS S, SANTEN R. J. Clin Invest. 1980 65:602-612

1709 ESTROGEN STIMULATED CELLULAR ACCUMULATION AND SHEDDING OF A HIGH MOLECULAR WEIGHT (>500 k daltons) GLYCOPROTEIN IN MCF7 and ZR-75 BREAST CANCER CELLS.
M. L. Nicholson*, K. D. Pierotti, D. M. Hess, B. D. Manning, M. A. Harvey, K. L. Travis, L. M. Stundtner and P. M. Chen, Biomedical Research Group, Sullivan Park, Corning Glass Works, Corning, N.Y. 14831

Mouse monoclonal antibodies produced in our laboratory were found to react with a cell surface antigen that is present on normal and malignant breast epithelial cells. One of these antibodies, 21DD5, reacts with a family of high molecular weight glycoproteins whose accumulation and shedding are augmented by treatment with 10^{-8} M (17β) estradiol. MCF7 and ZR-75 cells, depleted of hormones by a 5 day exposure to media containing 10% fetal calf serum treated with dextran-coated charcoal, were exposed to estradiol for 2 or more days. Both cells and media were assayed on 5-16% SDS-PAGE gels following Western blot transfer to nitrocellulose and subsequent radioimmunoassay. The amount of cell lysate or media in each lane was relative to the amount of protein in the cells. Within 2 days there was a stimulation of this antigen in both cell lines. The initial stimulation in the estrogen treated MCF7 cells was followed by a decrease below the level in the control cells. This could be accounted for, however, by increased shedding of this antigen into the media. ZR-75 cells that were exposed to estrogen maintained an increased level of the antigen in the cells but shed relatively less of it into the media. However, these cells no longer shed the antigen at all if the last 3 days of a 5 day exposure to the hormone was done in serum-free media. It would appear, therefore, that estrogen stimulates the production of this antigen and that both estrogen and some element contained in serum augment its release from the cell.

1710 SELF-PRIMING EFFECT OF LH/hCG UPON THE BIPHASIC TESTICULAR RESPONSE TO hCG.
J.P. Méndez*, V. Diaz-Sánchez, G. Pérez-Palacios and A. Ulloa-Aguirre. Inst. Nal. de la Nutrición, México 14000, D. F.

The present study was conducted to investigate if the early (2-6h) testicular response to a single dose of exogenous hCG depends on previous exposure to luteinizing hormone activity. Four different groups of subjects were studied: Normal adult men (n = 5; group A) and pubertal children Tanner Stage 1 (bone age $\geq$ 10 years) to 4 (n=16; group B); patients with complete androgen insensitivity (n = 2; group C) and patients with hypogonadotrophic eunuchoidism (n = 4; group D). Each subject received an im injection of hCG (40 IU/kg) at day 1 and blood samples were drawn before and 1-8, 24, 48 and 72 h after injection. At 96 h, a second dose of hCG was given (80 IU/kg) and blood samples were obtained at the same time sequence as the first hCG administration. Plasma testosterone (T) was measured by RIA after celite chromatography. The first administration of hCG evoked a biphasic response of T in groups A to C, with an early peak at 2-8 h and a second peak at 48 - 72 h. In group D, the early response did not occur and the late peak was attenuated and delayed (96 h). After the second hCG dose, all groups exhibited a biphasic T response. This study demonstrates that previous exposure to luteinizing hormone activity is an obligatory prerequisite for the hCG-mediated biphasic testicular response; this self-priming effect of LH/hCG is essential only for the occurrence of the early response. In contrast to previous reports, this study demonstrates that as early as immediately before puberty a single dose of exogenous hCG induces a biphasic testicular response. (Supported by grants from WHO, Geneva, Switzerland and CONACYT, Mexico).

1711 IS BREAST-FEEDING IN MOTHERS WITH GRAVES' DISEASE COMPATIBLE WITH PROPYLTHIOURACIL THERAPY?

N. Momotani*, R. Yamashita, K. Ito, and M. Shimizu, Ito Hospital, and Department of Pediatrics, School of Medicine, Keio University, Tokyo, Japan.

Although the advantages of breast-feeding are well known, lactation has been discouraged when mothers are receiving thionamides because these agents have been thought to be excreted in milk. There have been studies reporting that PTU reaches breast milk in an insignificant dose for suckling infants; however, they have had little information enough to substantiate the result. To examine whether there is any effect on suckling infants of PTU ingested by mothers, free T4 and TSH were measured in 9 infants by RIA and PTU in 3 of these infants by high speed liquid chromatography. Mothers were under treatment with 100 to 300mg of PTU daily for Graves' disease and the infants had been continuously breast-fed after birth. The infants' age varied from 1 to 7 months when examined. Neonatal Graves' disease was ruled out by either measuring TSH-binding inhibiting immunoglobulin at birth or considering the months of age at examination. Free T4 levels of mothers on the day when their infants were examined were slightly higher than normal in two mothers and within the normal range in the others. The free T4 values of the infants ranged from 1.0 to 1.9 ng/100 ml; the TSH values ranged from 1.0 to 4.0 uU/ml. These were all normal. There was no dose dependency of PTU on these values. PTU could not be detected in any of the sera from infants investigated. Conclusion: Infants of mothers with Graves' disease who are receiving PTU may be breast-fed without any adverse effect on thyroid status.

1712 THYROID HORMONE SECRETION AND METABOLISM IN MYASTHENIA GRAVIS

K.Murakami*, K.Sahashi, T.Mitsuma, and A.Takahashi in IVth Department of Internal Medicine, Y.Ishizuki in Ishizuki Thyroid Institute. Nagakute, Aichi, Japan.

Thyroid hormone secretion and metabolism were studied in myasthenia gravis. 24 cases of myasthenia gravis were divided into 3 groups according to Osserman's classification, namely type I(4),type IIa(16) and typeIIb(4). Plasma total and free thyroxine(T4,FT4), 3,3'5triiodothyronine(T3,FT3), 3,3'5'triiodothyronine(rT3), 3,3'diiodothyronine(3,3'T2), thyroxine binding immunoglobulin(TBG), thyrotropine(TSH) and TSH binding inhibiting immunoglobulin(TBII) were determined by radioimmunoassay. Anti-thyroglobulin antibody(TGHA) and anti-microsomal antibody (MCHA) were measured by commercial kits. T3,FT4 levels increased significantly in myasthenia gravis and tended to increase T4 and FT3,but not significantly. T3,FT3,3,3'T2 and rT3 levels tended to increase in type I,comparering with the control. In type IIa,T4 showed the tendency to increase. FT4,TBG and TSH tended to increase in type IIb. TBII was positive in 8 cases out of 24 cases,in which no cases were observed after thymectomy. MCHA was positive 8 cases out of 24 cases and TGHA was positive in 3 cases. The present findings suggest that the abnormality of secretion,metabolism and immunological abnormality in thyroid may exist.

1713 MASS SCREENING PROGRAM FOR THYROID DISORDERS IN EARLY PREGNANCY.

M. Murata*(1), K. Sawada(1), M. Kanbara(1), K. Okada(2), N. Momotani(3), K. Ito(3), M. Matsumoto(4), (1)Tokyo Women's Medical College, The 2nd Hospital, (2)Tokyo Branch of Japan Association for Maternal Welfare, (3)Ito hospital, (4)Tokyo Association of Health Service, Tokyo, Japan.

A screening program for thyroid abnormalities in pregnants has been performed since November 1980. At the initial medical consultation of pregnants blood samples were obtained on filter paper and these were sent to the screening center (Tokyo Association of Health Service) for measuring TSH, T4, free T4 (FT4), TBG and antithyroid antibodies (Microsome Test and Thyroid Test, Fuji Zoki, Tokyo, Japan). Free thyroxine index was calculated by Shishiba's equation. TSH and FT4 are thought to be most sensitive indicators for hypothyroidism (hypox) and hyperthyroidism (hyperx) respectively. By the end of August 1983, 21,830 pregnants were screened. Among them 150 cases suspected to have thyroid abnormalities. Among these, 103 cases agreed to be performed endocrinological examination in detail. The results are that hypox 9 cases, hyperx 22 cases, goiter 23 cases, other abnormalies 14 cases and 35 normal cases. If all of the suspected pregnants were further endocrinologically examined and the frequency of each thyroid disease was not changed, incidence of hypox would be 1 per 1665 pregnants (1/1665), that of hyperx would be 1/680 and that of goiter would be 1/650. All of the pregnants with thyroid disorders who were found by the screening had no clear clinical signs and symptoms and two thirds of hyperx and all of hypox need treatments. These facts mean this screening has practical significance.

1714 OESTRONE SULPHATE IN PLASMA IN MEN WITH CHRONIC ALCOHOLISM AND FATTY LIVER.

O. Myking* and A. Aakvaag, Hormone Laboratory, University of Bergen, Norway

Oestrone sulphate (E_1S) - derives from nonglandular conversion of plasma oestrone (E_1) and oestradiol (E_2), presumed to take place primarily in the liver. Decreased plasma E_1S and increased E_1 and E_2 have been found in men with liver cirrhosis and fatty liver. In the present study the plasma concentrations of E_1S in 20 men with chronic alcoholism and fatty liver were related to plasma E_1, E_2, testosterone (T), sex hormone-binding globulin (SHBG), the appearent free testosterone (AFT), dehydroepiandrosterone sulphate (DHEAS) and the clinical findings of feminization and hypogonadism. For each patient there was a healthy control subject matched for age and weight. The plasma concentrations (mean ± SD) in the alcoholics and the controls were; E_1: 286 ± 99* - 198 ± 48 pM, E_2: 61.2 ± 18.1* - 44.6 ± 9.3 pM, E_1S: 627 ± 175* - 957 ± 188 pM, T: 16.5 ± 1.9 - 16.6 ± 2.7 nM, SHBG: 57.4 ± 13.1* - 45.9 ± 9.6 nM, AFT: 200 ± 28* - 221 ± 21 nM and DHEAS: 5.1 ± 2.8* - 7.5 ± 1.4 uM (* significant at the level of $2p < 0.01$). No correlation was seen between SHBG and T, and between E_2 and T in the patients in contrast to the findings in the controls. In both groups a significant correlation existed between SHBG and E_2. Eight of the 20 patients showed symptoms and/or signs of hypogonadism. The patients with hypogonadism did not differ from the remaining patients regarding the parameters of endocrine function measured. The ratio E_1S/E_1, however, was in every case lower than in the matched control and tended to be even lower in the patients with hypogonadism, suggesting a more marked deterioration of the liver function in these patients.

1715 CLINICAL AND LABORATORY INVESTIGATION OF A VIRILIZED WOMAN WITH PLACENTAL-SITE TROPHOBLASTIC TUMOR (PSTT).

S B Nagelberg* and S W Rosen, Clinical Endocrinology Branch, NIADDK, Bethesda, Maryland, USA.

The novel association of virilization and PSTT, an uncommon form of gestational trophoblastic disease, is described in a 32-year-old woman. Chemotherapy lowered serum concentrations of chorionic gonadotropin (CG) (8.7 to 2.1 ng/ml), pregnancy-specific β_1-glycoprotein (SP_1) (32 to 3.9 ng/ml), and testosterone (T) (400 to 74 ng/dl). Subsequent hysterectomy revealed a 2 cm tumor nodule within the myometrium, and one week postop serum concentrations of CG (0.5), SP_1 (1.3), and T (20.7) had all returned to normal. Catheterization of the ovarian veins before chemotherapy demonstrated 50-fold elevation of T concentrations, whereas 17β-estradiol (E_2) concentrations were only two-fold higher than normal. Direct sampling of the uterine veins during hysterectomy documented T and E_2 production, presumably by the PSTT. Wedge biopsy of the ovaries disclosed minimal histologic changes compatible with CG stimulation. Immunoperoxidase staining of tumor sections demonstrated CG and placental lactogen, even though the latter was barely detectable in the peripheral circulation (1.6 ng/ml). We conclude that 1) despite the lowering of serum placental protein concentrations by chemotherapy, hysterectomy was necessary to eradicate this patient's PSTT, 2) although the trophoblast in PSTT may contribute to sex steroid production, CG-stimulated ovarian production of T was the dominant endocrine alteration in this patient, and 3) the failure of the PSTT to produce large amounts of estrogen, in contrast to normal pregnancy and hydatidiform mole, resulted in marked androgen/estrogen imbalance, high circulating levels of free T, and virilization. These physiologic perturbations were reversed by removal of the gonadotropic stimulus.

1716 THYROID HORMONE AUTOANTIBODIES (THAA) IN A FAMILY.

S.Nakamura*, S.Sakata, K.Kamikubo, T.Komaki, N.Kojima, K.Yasuda, and K.Miura, The 3rd Department of Internal Medicine Gifu University School of Medicine, Gifu 500, Japan.

Two sisters (case 1 : 13 years old, case 2 : 10 years old) were admitted to our hospital because of short stature. They were clinically hypothyroid and serum TSH levels were high in both cases. A diagnosis of Hashimoto's thyroiditis in each case was made by open biopsy of the thyroid gland.
In case 2, in contrast to low level of serum T4 (0.9 µg/dl), serum T3 was extremely high (375 - 1660 ng/dl), suggesting the presence of THAA in serum. Further studies demonstrated that case 1 and case 2 had both anti-T4 (both cases : IgG, κ type) and anti-T3 (case 1 : IgG, κ ; case 2 : IgG, $\kappa+\lambda$) autoantibodies in their sera. Treatment with L-T4 was started and their heights and weights increased. After the 1 year treatment, bindings of ^{125}I-T3 and ^{125}I-T4 to serum γ-globulin were decreased. Acid-charcoal treatment of sera which we had shown to eliminate the interferences of endogeneous and/or therapeutic thyroid hormones with these bindings, however, demonstrated still high bindings of labelled thyroid hormones to serum γ-globulin in both cases. The presence of anti-T4 autoantibodies (IgG, $\kappa+\lambda$) was also detected when serum from another sister (case 3 : 5 years old) was treated with the acid-charcoal.

1717 SECONDARY HYPOGONADISM IN IMPOTENT MEN. H.R. Nankin, T. Lin, J. Osterman, D. Markuck, D. Powell, J. Carnes, E.P. Murono, and K. Krzyzaniak. Medical Research, and Surgical Services, Wm.Jennings Bryan Dorn Veterans' Hospital, and Departments of Medicine, Surgery and Psychology, University of South Carolina, Columbia, South Carolina.

In an earlier report we noted that 35% of 118 men with secondary impotence of six months or longer had low mean testosterone levels (<350 ng/dl). Since the average age in the group was 56 years (range 30-73 years), and since Leydig cell responsiveness progressively decreases with aging, we expected to find LH elevations in sera from the men with low testosterone concentrations.

Using an LH radioimmunoassay, we analyzed serum samples from 44 impotent low testosterone (Low T) men. Results were compared to values obtained in 18 normal men, ages 20 to 85 years of age. The results for Low T men were:

Serum LH (compared to normals)	Number Low T Men	Percent
Less than the mean	19	43.2
High normal	16	36.4
Borderline elev.	5	11.4
Elevated	4	9.0

Thus, most of these Low T men have LH values that are inappropriately low.

In conclusion, 35% of secondarily impotent men have low testosterone concentrations in serum, and less than 10% of this group have significant elevations of serum LH. These data suggest that many of these men have altered hypothalamic or pituitary function of an undefined etiology.

1718 SUCCESSFUL TREATMENT OF CUSHING'S SYNDROME WITH THE GLUCOCORTICOID ANTAGONIST RU 38486. L K Nieman, G P Chrousos, I Spitz, B C Nisula, G B Cutler*, G R Merriam, C W Bardin, D L Loriaux, NICHD, Bethesda, MD, USA and Population Council, New York, NY, USA.

RU 38486 (RU) is a 19-nor steroid competitive antagonist of cortisol at the receptor level. We report here the successful treatment of a 25 year old man who presented with severe depression and signs and symptoms of Cushing's syndrome (CS) due to ectopic ACTH secretion. This syndrome persisted despite partial resection of an ACTH-positive carcinoid tumor and therapy with metyrapone. He was treated for 2 months with oral RU in increasing doses of 5, 10, 15 and 20 mg/kg/day. We monitored treatment efficacy by clinical status and several glucocorticoid-sensitive parameters that included fasting blood sugar (FBS), blood sugar at 120 min after oral glucose (BS-120), peak TSH increment after TRF (ΔTSH), and the concentration of CBG, TeBG and free testosterone (T). All normalized despite continued hypercortisolism; UFCs were 100-10,000 μg/d.

	RU Dose mg/kg/d	FBS mg/dl	BS-120 mg/dl	ΔTSH μU/ml	CBG μg/dl	TeBG μg/dl	Free T ng/dl
patient	0	140	269	4.3	7.4	0.06	3.5
	10	88	157	0.6	15.5	0.35	21.3
	15	76	147	>6.0	10.6	0.68	29.5
	20	76	110	>6.0	16.8	1.02	17.4
normal	0	<105	<140	>6.0	14-20	0.2-1.0	5-30

The somatic signs of CS (buffalo hump, central obesity, moon fascies) improved, the depression resolved, and libido returned. No side effects or toxicity were seen. We conclude that in this patient RU 38486 was a safe, well-tolerated, and effective medical treatment for hypercortisolism.

1719 GYNECOMASTIA IN A HOSPITALIZED MALE POPULATION. C.B. Niewoehner* and F.Q. Nuttall, Endocrine Section, VA Medical Center, Minneapolis, Minnesota, 55417, USA.

Two hundred fourteen hospitalized adult males ages 27-92 (mean age 63.5 years) were examined for the prevalence of palpable gynecomastia. No subject had mastodynia. The presence of gynecomastia was correlated with age, body mass index, disease states and medications. The overall prevalence was 65%. In all but 11 subjects gynecomastia was bilateral. The prevalence was greatest in the 50-69 year old age group (72%). It was lower in the 70-89 year old (47%, $p < .01$) and the 30-49 year old (54%, $p < .05$) groups. The prevalence of gynecomastia increased strikingly with increasing body mass index (BMI). More than 80% of those with BMI ≥ 25.0 kg/m^2 had gynecomastia. (Mean BMI for all subjects 24.7 kg/m^2.) The diameter of breast tissue also increased with increasing BMI ($r = 0.52$, $p < .001$). The decreased prevalence of gynecomastia after the seventh decade could be explained by the lower BMI (23.1 kg/m^2) in this group ($p < .05$). The youngest group did not have a lower BMI; an independent age factor appears to be present. [These results plus a previous study by one of us (FQN, J. Clin. Endocrinol. Metab. 48:338, 1979) indicate an increasing prevalence of gynecomastia with age from the 3rd to the 8th decades.] Because of the high overall prevalence of gynecomastia and the overriding effect of a high BMI, independent effects of diseases or medications could not be determined. We conclude that palpable bilateral gynecomastia is present in many older males, is correlated with the amount of body fat, and does not require further evaluation unless symptomatic or of recent onset.

1720 ROLE OF CIRCULATING IMMUNECOMPLEX IN PATHOGENESIS OF GRAVES' DISEASE. N. Nihei*, M.Funauchi, N. Fukuma, S. Kisamori, M. Itoh and Y. Hirooka, Third Internal Medicine, Hamamatsu University School of Medicine, Hamamatsu, Shizuoka-ken, 431-31, Japan.

Existence of circulating immunecomplex (CIC) in Graves' disease(GD) has been reported by several investigators, but the pathogenetic role of CIC is not well documentedyet. In order to clarify the role of CIC in GD, relationship between CIC and TBII or clinical symptoms in GD was observed.Forty patients with GD and fifteen healthy volunteers were randomized for this study. Determination of CIC was performed by three different methods as polyethyleneglycol precipitation method(PEG), C_{1q} binding assay(C1q) and Protein A binding assay(PA). TBII was measured by Smith's method. In GD, CIC levels by three methods distributed from normal rang to abnormally high level. Incidence of abnormally high level of CIC was 17.7% by PEG, 30.2% by C_{1q} and 52.5% by PA in GD. This incidence increased in the cases with small goiter size, exophthalmos or pretibial myxoedema. CIC levels by all three methods showed negative correlation with TBII($p<0.01$) and that by C_{1q} showed negative correlation with serum thyroxine level ($p<0.01$). These data suggested that CIC may have a role to inhibit the stimulatory activity of TBII to thyroid gland in GD.

1721 EFFICACY OF INTRENASAL OR INTRAVAGINAL LHRH AGONIST IN THE TREATMENT OF ENDOMETRIOSIS.

N. Nishi*, T. Koyama, K. Ichimiya, M. Saito and S. Isshiki, Dept. of Obstet. & Gynecol. and Dept. of Central Pharmacy, Tokyo Medical & Dental University, Tokyo, Japan.

Cases with endometriosis were treated with LHRH agonist, D-Leu^{6}-LHRH ethylamide(TAP,144), by way of either intranasal drop or vaginal suppository. 15 cases were treated with suppository, contained 50ug of peptide, from day 5 through the last day of the menstrual cycle. 35 cases were treated by nasal drop, 50ug once daily, started on day 5 for 14 days. All cases, other than 3, manifested remarkable relief of pain, dysmenorrhea as well as hypermenorrhea. Anemias were also improved. Serum levels of E_2 and P were depressed during nasal administration. On the other hand, follicular FSH and E_2 levels were raised to mean values of 42±38miu/ml and 360±160ug/ml respectively in cases with vaginal suppository. P levels were also raised to 15,8± 3.2ng/ml in the same group.

1722 FUNCTIONAL DEVELOPEMENT OF CHILD ADRENAL CORTEX.

Y.Nozaki*, T.Shinozuka, K.Ohyama, K.Kato, S.Kusano, K.Ichimura and S.Amemiya, Dept. of ped., Yamanashi Medical College, Yamanashi, 409-38 Japan.

Fetal pattern of steroidogenesis was known to continue to early life of infancy, however, there was little information after that period. Our study was performed to assess the functional aspects of steroidogenesis by measuring plasma levels of steroids. Plasma steroids were evaluated at basal levels(B-levels) and the levels after ACTH stimulation (A-levels) in the group under 2Y/O(Y-group, n=10) and in the group over 10Y/O(O-group, n=8). In normal children, results of mean plasma levels of B-levels and A-levels in Y-group and O-group were 26.5, 166.7, 8.76, 38.5mcg/ml for compound F, 1.36, 11.6, 0.44, 5.8ng/ml for compound S, 7.67, 40.8, 2.32, 35.1ng/ml for compound B, 0.35, 1.75, 0.102, 0.96ng/ml for DOC, 1.31, 11.6, 1.07, 3.56ng/ml for 17OHP(17α-hydroxyprogesterone),and 2.64, 9.0, 0.1,0.5ng/ml for 21DOF(21-deoxycortisol), respectively. Plasma bioactive metyrapone (reduced metyrapone+metyrapone) levels over 6mcg/ml induced the maximum suppression of the indices of $\frac{S}{S+F}$x10^2 and $\frac{DOC}{DOC+B}$x10^2. Plasma bioactive metyrapone levels at 50% suppressive levels of $\frac{S}{S+F}$x10^2 and $\frac{DOC}{DOC+B}$x10^2 were 0.38, 0.2mcg/ml in Y-group(n=10) and 0.56, 0.15mcg/ml in O-group(n=9), respectively. High plasma levels of 21 DOF and 17OHP, and high index of $\frac{21DOF}{21DOF+F}$x10^2 were noted in Y-group. This could be due to the decreased activities of 21-hydroxylase. On the other hand, high plasma levels of S and DOC were detected in Y-group, but the indices of $\frac{S}{S+F}$x10^2 and $\frac{DOC}{DOC+B}$x10^2 were not significantly higher in them. This finding may suggest lower metabolic clearance in Y-group. From the data of exogenous enzyme blocker, 11β hydroxylase activity of glucocorticoid pathway was more sensitive in Y-group, but that of the mineralcorticoid pathway was less sensitive, there were opposite in O-group. This showed the heterogeneity of the maturation even about the same enzyme.

1723 GENETIC CONTROL OF THE PRODUCTION OF ANTI-HUMAN THYROGLOBULIN AND ANTI-THYROID HORMONE ANTIBODIES IN MICE IMMUNIZED WITH HUMAN THYROGLOBULIN. K.Okuda, S.Sakata, Y.Aihara, S.Nakamura, T.Komaki, O.Tarutani and K.Miura. Dep.of Bacteriology, Yokohama City Univ. Sch. of Med, Yokohama. Dep. of Int. Med. Gifu Univ. Sch. of Med. Gifu. Inst. for Endocrinology, Gunma Univ. Maehashi, Japan.

Various strains of mice with different H-2 and Igh allotype were immunized with human thyroglobulin (HTg) and genetic control of the production of anti-HTg and anti-thyroid hormone antibodies was examined. Among the mice of independent haplotypes, high responders against HTg were $H\text{-}2^a$, $H\text{-}2^d$, $H\text{-}2^q$ and $H\text{-}2^k$, while low responders were $H\text{-}2^b$ and $H\text{-}2^s$. Using various recombinant strains of mice, it was concluded that the Ir-gene for the production of anti-HTg antibodies is located in the I-A subregion of H-2. Anti-HTg antisera obtained from different strains of mice were examined for the presence of anti-thyroid hormone antibodies. The Ir-gene which controls the production of anti-T4 antibodies by immunization with HTg was identified in the I-A subregion. The presence of Ir-gene(s) outside the H-2 is also suggested. Concerning the production of anti-T3 antibodies , only 3 strains were high responders and therefore we were unable to identify the Ir-gene(s) for them. These results indicate the presence of Ir-gene which controls the immune response in mice against HTg and thyroid hormones.

1724 HETEROLOGOUS APPLICATION OF CANINE PROLACTIN RIA TO SERA FROM WOLVES, SEALS, AND TIGERS. E.K.Peterson[1]*, U.S.Seal[2], J.A.Parsons[1]. [1]Department of Anatomy, University of Minnesota, Minneapolis, Mn. USA. [2]VA Medical Center, Research Services, Minneapolis, Mn. USA.

We have been studying the effect of PRL on reproduction in animals other then rodents and ungulates, in particular the large carnivores. Since a canine PRL RIA was available (NIADDK), we have investigated the heterologous application of this assay for evaluation of immunoreactive PRL in other large carnivores. Anterior pituitary (AP) extracts from dogs, wolves, and tigers showed parallel displacement curves to canine PRL standards. Immunoreactive PRL was elevated following IV TRH in dogs, wolves, seals, and tigers (dog 0 min=9ng/ml, 10 min=40ng/ml; wolf 0 min=7ng/ml, 10 min=54ng/ml; seal 0 min=20ng/ml, 20 min=70ng/ml; tiger 0 min=6ng/ml, 10 min=60ng/ml). Wolves evaluated for seasonal baseline variation of PRL immunoreactivity showed high serum levels (60ng/ml) during summer and low levels (1-5ng/ml) during winter (45 degrees N. Latitude). Wolf pup studies showed a similar increase in immunoreactive PRL until midsummer (1ng/ml at 1 month of age, 20ng/ml at 5 months of age). Assuming the cross reacting component in AP and sera from carnivores is PRL our data shows that the NIADDK canine PRL RIA can be used to evaluate immunoreactive PRL in wolves, tigers,and seals. The data further show that these carnivores respond to TRH and that seasonal variation of PRL is probably present in these animals. This study supported in part by NIH grant AM26962 (JAP) and in part by VA research funds (USS).

1725 SLEEP DISORDERS AND CEREBRAL MONOAMINE (CMA) LEVELS CHANGES IN TETANY.
S. Poenaru*, S. Rouhani, H. Aymard, A. Opriou, and J. Regnard, Laboratoire de Neuroendocrinologie, Département de Physiologie, UER Biomédicale, 45, rue des Saints-Pères F-75270 Paris cedex 06, France.

In this study, electropolygraphic records (EPG) were obtained during afternoon sleep from 100 patients with positive electromyographic test of tetany due to hypomagnesemia and from 60 normal subjects. The results were compared with EPG vigilance states of 36 Mg^{++} -deficient Wistar rats (MDR) (18 of which were treated with a magnesium complex (Bio-Mag^R) (TR)) and in 14 normal rats (NR). Tissue levels of CMA and their metabolits were measured in all 3 groups of rats. The same disorders of sleep : decrease of N-REM sleep percentage and rarity of REM sleep, were present in patients and untreated animals. In the MDR a significant increased of brain dopamine (DA : 2023 $\pm$ 223.73 ng/g ; $p < 0,001$) and a brain 5-hydroxindol 3-acetic acid (5-HIAA : 668.3 $\pm$ 54.99 ng/g ; $p < 0.01$) was observed as compared to the NR (DA : 961.08 $\pm$ 75.33 ng/g ; 5-HIAA : 474.62 $\pm$ 18.76 ng/g). In the TR the sleep stages %, the DA and 5-HIAA levels returned to normal. These data give the evidence of sleep disorders associated with disturbances in CMA levels in tetany due to Mg^{++} deficiency and of their reversibility after treatment by magnesium.

1726 Analysis of the Steroid Receptor in a Eukaryotic Microorganism.
R. M. Riehl* and D. O. Toft, Dept. of Cell Biology, Mayo Clinic, Rochester, MN, USA.

Sexual reproduction in fungi of the *Achlya* genus is unique because it is controlled by two steroid hormones. Antheridiol is the steroid constitutively produced by females that induces the development and differentiation of male sex organs. We have previously reported the detection of a high affinity (Kd = 0.7 nM) binding protein in the cytosol of *A. ambisexualis* male cells that is specific for antheridiol and a tritium-labeled analog. Current studies have revealed that, in the presence of sodium molybdate, this macromolecule has a sedimentation coefficient of 8.1S in sucrose gradients of low ionic strength, a Stokes' radius of 56.6 A (Sephacryl S-300 columns), a molecular weight of 192,000 g/mole, a frictional ratio of 1.5, and an axial ratio of 8.9. The binding protein can be eluted with 0.24 M KCl as a single peak from DEAE-Sephadex A-25 columns. When sucrose gradients are prepared containing 1 M KCl without molybdate, a shift in sedimentation coefficient from 8.1S to 3.6S occurs. These results indicate that this steroid binding protein from a primitive eukaryotic microbe has *in vitro* biochemical properties that are similar to those of other known steroid receptors in higher organisms and that these properties may have been evolutionarily conserved. This work was supported by NIH grant AM 25625.

1727 ISOLATION OF A FORSKOLIN-RESISTANT MUTANT FROM Y1 ADRENOCORTICAL TUMOR CELLS. B.P. Schimmer* and J. Tsao. Banting and Best Department of Medical Research, University of Toronto, Toronto, Ontario, Canada M5G 1L6

Forskolin increases adenylate cyclase activity in many tissues. In order to determine the mechanism of forskolin action and to determine if this mechanism is shared by hormones and other agonists of the adenylate cyclase system, we have isolated and partially characterized a spontaneous forskolin-resistant mutant from Y1 adrenal cells. The addition of forskolin (10 μM) to parental Y1 cells causes most of the population to round up and detach. This response is typically elicited by agonists which raise the intracellular level of cyclic AMP in Y1 cells. One colony resistant to this action of forskolin emerged from cells grown in the presence of 10 μM forskolin. In this mutant, resistance to forskolin was stable, resulted from a defect in cyclic AMP accumulation rather than cyclic AMP action, and was associated with a reduced ability of forskolin to stimulate adenylate cyclase activity in cell homogenates. Whereas corticotropin (ACTH) stimulated adenylate cyclase activity over 20-fold in cell homogenates from the Y1 adrenal parent, ACTH had only marginal effects on the adenylate cyclase system of the mutant clone. These results suggest that the resistance to forskolin resulted from a mutation in the adenylate cyclase system at a locus common to the actions of forskolin and ACTH. (Supportd by MRC, Canada).

1728 Immunological Quantitation Of Regulatory Subunits Of cAMP Dependent Proteinkinases Type I And II In Human Mammary Tumors. H.Schröder*, J.Kaufmann, G.Trams. Institut für Physiologische Chemie, Universitätskrankenhaus Hamburg, D-2000 Hamburg 20, F.R.G.

In contrast to estrogen-receptor (ER)-free human mammary carcinomas, the ER containing tumors display a slower proliferation and a higher differentiation grade (1,2). The pattern of cAMP dependent proteinkinase isoenzyme I and II contents is assumed to be a function of the proliferation and differentiation status of tissues (3). These enzymes can rapidly be quantitated by immunotitration of their regulatory subunits RI and RII with the aid of specific antibodies in a test including Protein A-Sepharose as a precipitating agent (4). 24 human ER-containing mammary tumors and 13 tumors without ER have been investigated for their relative and absolute amounts of RI and RII. The results were referred to DNA content of the tumors. No correlation was found between ER and absolute RI or RII contents. Instead, a significant negative correlation between ER and the relative amount of RI per total high affinity cAMP binding capacity (RI+RII) was discovered. A respective positive correlation holds for ER and RII. In conclusion, the correlation of high RI:RII-ratios and low ER (signifying low differentiation and rapid growth) in human mammary tumors corroborate the hypothesis mentioned in (3). (1)Maynard,P.V. et al (1978),Br.J.Cancer 38,745. (2)Silvestrini,R. et al (1974),Cancer 34,1252. (3)Miyazaki,K. et al (1980),Eur. J.Biochem. 104,543. (4)Weber,W. et al (1981),Biochem.Biophys.Res.Comm. 99, 475. I am indebted to Prof.Helmuth Hilz, Hamburg. The study was supported by the DFG.

1729 REGULATION OF PROTEIN KINASE 380 CATALYZED PHOSPHORYLATION OF EUKARYOTIC INITIAL FACTOR 2α BY CYCLIC AMP-DEPENDENT PROTEIN KINASE. R.K. Sharma*, S. Nishimatsu and Y. Kuroda, Department of Biochemistry, University of Tennessee Center for the Health Sciences, Memphis, TN 38163.

Protein kinase 380 (PK 380) is a novel adrenocortical cyclic nucleotide-independent protein kinase that catalyzes the phosphorylation of a serine residue(s) of the α subunit of the eukaryotic initation factor eIF-2 (Kuroda Y., Merrick, W.C., and Sharma, R.K., 1982, Arch. Biochem. Biophys. 213, 271-275). When PK 380 was further purified by either chromatofocusing (pH 4.4 peak) or by phosphocellulose chromatography, the PK 380-dependent eIF-2α kinase activity was lost. The activity could be restored by the addition of the catalytic subunit (C subunit) of cyclic AMP-dependent protein kinase which could be blocked in turn by the heat-stable inhibitor. The regulatory subunit of cyclic AMP-dependent protein kinase also inhibited the C subunit increment of the PK 380 activity; the activity was restored, however, by cyclic AMP. Together, these results indicate that PK 380-catalyzed phosphorylation of eIF-2α is regulated by the C subunit, raising the possibility that in adrenal cortex certain cyclic AMP-mediated events are indirectly regulated by PK 380. (Supported by grants NCI CA-16091 and NSF PCM-800873)

1730 INTRASPLENIC TESTICULAR TUMOR INDUCED BY LONG-TERM LH STIMULATION: HORMONE RECEPTORS AND STEROIDOGENIC ACTIVITY M. Nozawa*, I. Otsu, J. Kurokawa, M. Hattori and K. Wakabayashi, Dept. of Surgery, Josai Dental University and Institute of Endocrinology, Gunma University, Sakado, Saitama, Japan.

Heterotopic infantile testicular graft into the spleen of castrated male rat (Group A) caused the development of testicular tumor which was mainly composed of Leydig cell-derived cells having 3β-ol dehydrogenase activity. On the other hand, if the recipient rats had been operated to form porta-caval shunt (Group B), the implanted testes either shrunk or disappeared. In Group A, the recipients showed significantly higher levels of serum LH and FSH than intact rats and those in group B. Testosterone levels in the portal blood in Group A were much higher than those in the peripheral blood. The tumors over one year old showed an increased cyclic AMP production in response to ovine LH (NIAMOD-oLH-24). ED50 (oLH) was 0.1 nM and the maximum cAMP production was 154 pmol/10^6 cells ([oLH]=1 nM) in the presence of phosphodiesterase inhibitor (MIX) and 106 pmol/10^6 cell in the absence of MIX. They specifically bound LH with an association constant $Ka=1.35\times10^{10}M^{-1}$ and Maximum Binding=50.0 fmol/mg protein which were not competitively inhibited by prolactin, GH, TSH or FSH. However, the binding of FSH to the tumors was not observed. These results seem to indicate that the hepatic inactivation of testosterone causes an enhanced secretion of LH from the pituitary, and the long-term stimulation of the implanted testis in the spleen by LH induced the formation of a neoplasm which has LH receptor and produces testosterone in response to the hormone.

1731 COMPENSATORY HYPERTROPHY OF THE UTERUS IN THE RAT. BIOLOGICAL COMPENSATION OF THE DECREASE IN THE NUMBER OF PROGENIES.
M. Kurcz*, Cs. Kiss and I. Nagy, Res. Lab. Clin. Biochemistry, CHINOIN, Centr. Lab. Heim Pál Hosp., and Dept. Obstr. Gynec. Róbert Károly Hospital, Budapest Hungary.

CFY female rats were used with the same age,weight and regular sexual cycle. One of the uterine horns was removed on the first day of estrus or diestrus. The same number of animals was sham-operated. The operation did not disturb the normal cycle. Ten animals were sacrificed on days 8-10,16-20, and 40 after operation i.e. in the same phase on 2nd, 4th and loth cycle. The contralateral uterine horn was removed or both of horns of sham-operated rats, and ovaries, adrenals, thyroid and pituitary gland. The weight of organs was weighted and the dry weight of uterus,too. It was found,that-after 8 days-the weight of intact horn increased, and on the 16-20 and 40 days were significantly heavier, then the half of total uterus weight of control animals. In another experiments unilateral hysterectomy was done on 120 females. After 40days they were mated, together with control females. No difference was found in the pregnancy rates. However, the number of progenies of mothers with one uterine horn was more, than the number of progenies of control rats calculated for one horn of uterus. Till now left described in the literature the possibility of compensatory hypertrophy of uterus and s.c."biological compensation mechanism", counteracting the decrease of the number of progenies.

1732 INHIBITORY EFFECT OF GOSSYPOL ON MAINTENANCE OF IMPLANTATION AND PREGNANCY IN RATS.
Y. C. Lin*, T. Fukaya and Y. Rikihisa, VA-MD Regional College of Veterinary Medicine, VPI&SU, Blacksburg, VA 24061, USA.

In rats exhibiting 3 consecutive 4-day cycles, i.m. administration of gossypol acetic acid (GP) in 10% EtOH at 25 mg/kg/daily from day of proestrus induced an irregularity of the cyclic pattern for as long as treatment is continued. The normal estrous cycle resumed 5-7 days after GP treatment was stopped. On the day of sperm-positive vaginal smear (day-0 of pregnancy) other rats were given similar dosages of GP for 8 consecutive days. At laparotomy on day-8 of pregnancy, the no. of implantation sites (IS) in control, 12.5 and 25 mg/kg/daily treated rats were 14±3, 11±4, and 8±4, respectively; the no. of pups born at term were 11±2, 9±2 and 0, respectively. Progesterone (P) and estradiol (E2) values averaged 18.70±0.95 and 0.12±0.01 in treated, vs 35.80±2.35 and 0.17±0.01 ng/ml, in controls respectively. In rats given GP at 25 mg/kg on day-2 of diestrus and mated on day of proestrus, zero IS were found on day-8 of pregnancy. When supplements of combined P (2 mg) and E2 (0.2 ug) s.c. in 100 μl sesame oil/rat/daily a normal no. (14±4) of IS were found on day-8. With continued steroid treatments some pregnancies went to term. Our results suggest that: 1) GP exerts its inhibitory effect on ovarian steroid synthesis causing the cyclic irregularities in normally cycling rats and disturbs normal implantation in pregnant rats. 2) Blocking of ovulation or mating behavior will not occur if GP treatment is given on day-2 of diestrus and day of proestrus. 3) Failure of treated rats to continue pregnancy to term without exogenous steroids implies dysfunction of the CL or placenta during the latter portion of pregnancy. Supported by NIH Grants HD 17627 and HD 16883.

1733 IN VIVO ADRENOCORTICOTROPIN (1-24)-INDUCED ACCUMULATION OF cAMP BY OVINE FETAL ADRENAL CELLS IS INHIBITED BY CONCOMITANT INFUSION OF METOPIRONE.
S.J. Lye* and J.R.G. Challis. MRC Group in Reprod. Biol., St. Joseph's Hospital Research Institute, Univ.West.Ontario, London, Canada, N6A 4V2

Activation of the ovine fetal adrenal (FA) gland following pulse ACTH (P-ACTH) administration is associated with an increase in plasma cortisol (F) levels. We have investigated whether F may play a role in this adrenal activation process. The ability of FA cells to accumulate cAMP in response to ACTH in vitro was compared in fetuses (d132 gestation) that had received infusions (100h) in utero of 1) saline (0.5ml for 15min/2h) (n=4); 2)P-ACTH (66.6ng/min for 15min/2h (n=3); 3) P-ACTH+metopirone (MET; an inhibitor of F production, 31.3mg/h; n=4); 4) P-ACTH+MET+F (2.4mg/24h (n=3) or 24mg/24h (n=4) for 100h). Control fetuses showed no increase in plasma F and no accumulation of cAMP by their FA cells in response to ACTH in vitro. Plasma F rose from 2.21±0.47ng/ml at 0h to 35.7±11.6ng/ml at 96h in fetuses receiving P-ACTH in vivo. This was associated with a significant ($P<0.05$) ACTH-induced accumulation of cAMP by FA cells in vitro (mean increment Δ=48pmol). MET blocked the rise in plasma F, accumulation of cAMP by FA cells and the increase in adrenal weight normally consequent upon P-ACTH treatment.P-ACTH treatment resulted in an increase in cortisol binding capacity (CBC) of fetal plasma. This effect was also blocked by MET but exogenous F at both doses overcame the MET block on CBC. However, systemic F did not reverse the effect of MET on P-ACTH-induced increases in cAMP accumulation and fetal adrenal weight. These data suggest that ACTH increases the capacity of FA cells to accumulate cAMP in vitro and that local cortisol may mediate this effect. Supported by MRC Canada.

1734 BLOCKADE OF NEONATAL ACTIVATION OF PITUITARY-TESTICULAR AXIS WITH CONTINUOUS GNRH AGONIST TREATMENT IN MALE RHESUS MONKEYS.
D.R. Mann, M. Davis-DaSilva, K. Wallen, and D.C. Collins*, Morehouse School of Medicine, Yerkes Regional Primate Research Center, and Emory University School of Medicine/VA Medical Center, Atlanta, GA 30310, USA.

Five male infant monkeys were treated continuously with a GnRH agonist (Ag; Wyeth Labs; Wy-40972; 10 µg/day) beginning at 10-13 days of age for 112 days using osmotic minipumps. Five additional animals served as controls; two received sham implants. No differences were observed between controls with and without implants. Three wk of Ag treatment reduced serum LH (bioassay) to undetectable values where they remained throughout treatment. Mean levels of serum testosterone ± SE (T) fell from 1.5 ± 0.5 ng/ml (before treatment) to 0.38 ± 0.09 ng/ml after three wk of Ag treatment. Serum T did not exceed 0.60 ng/ml in Ag treated animals after that time. In contrast, serum LH (mean range, 0.53-1.36 µg/ml) and T (1.6-6.0 ng/ml) were elevated over the first two postnatal mo in control infants, but then declined to values that were indistinguishable from Ag treated infants by four mo of age. Serum LH and T responses to five µg GnRH/kg BW were abolished with seven wk of Ag treatment. Age-matched controls exhibited a five-fold increase in serum LH and a four-fold rise in serum T in response to GnRH. At four wk posttreatment, Ag treated and control infants showed similar serum LH and T responses to GnRH. Our data suggest that continuous Ag treatment desensitizes the pituitary to GnRH and abolishes activation of the pituitary-testicular axis in the infant male rhesus monkey. Supported by Wyeth Laboratories and NIH Grants RR-08006 and RR-00165.

1735 REGULATION OF HEPATIC GLYCOGEN METABOLISM IN PRENATAL RATS.

R. Margolis, Dept. of Anatomy, Howard Univ., Washington, D.C.

The last stage of gestation in the rat is characterized by large scale synthesis and accumulation of hepatic glycogen, which is then mobilized as free glucose within the first day after birth. Recently, a role for hepatic smooth ER-associated synthase phosphatase (SP) and phosphorylase phosphatase (PP) activities in regulation of activation of glycogen synthase catalyzed glycogenesis and inactivation of glycogen phosphorylase catalyzed glycogenolysis has been demonstrated for adult rats (Margolis and Curnow, Endoc.113:2113,1983). In this present study glycogen first appeared on day 18 of gestation (22 day term), increasing slowly to day 20. A large burst of glycogenic activity occurred from days 20 to 21. This was marked by increased ER-SP and ER-PP activities and corresponding activation of synthase and inactivation of phosphorylase. This period was also marked by large increases in the amount of SER, particularly in areas of the hepatocyte cytoplasm where new glycogen deposits were present. Following birth massive glycogenolysis occurred, accompanied by decreased ER-SP and ER-PP activities and concomitantly decreased activation of synthase and increased activation of phosphorylase. These data are consistent with a role for the SER and associated enzymes in regulation of hepatic glycogen metabolism in prenatal rat liver. Supported by grants from the JDF, the Kroc Foundation, and the ADA, Wash.,D.C. Affiliate.

1736 COMPARATIVE STUDY OF T4 CONCENTRATION IN DETECTED HYPOTHYROID INFANTS WITH APLASTIC AND ECTOPIC THYROID GLAND.

J. Morissette* and J.H. Dussault, The Quebec Network for Genetic Medicine, CHUL, Ste-Foy, P.Q., Canada.

In order to evaluate the compensatory mechanism involved in the thyrotropin (TSH) stimulation of the residual tissue in ectopic thyroid gland, data was pooled from different hypothyroid mass screening Program (Quebec, New England, Tokyo, Osaka, Brussels, Toulouse, Heidelberg, Lille). The thyroxine (T_4) concentration for the first week of life was obtained from filter paper spot specimen, whereas the others were obtained from serum specimen. The following table shows the mean T_4 and the standard error of the mean for hypothyroid infants with aplastic (A) and ectopic (E) gland.

T_4 ± S.E.M. (mg/dl)

Age in week	1	2	3	4
Hypo				
A	3.4 ± 0.85	1.9 ± 0.35	1.8 ± 0.22	1.6 ± 0.20
(n)	(6)	(36)	(61)	(73)
E	3.4 ± 0.6	4.5 ± 0.52	5.0 ± 0.51	4.3 ± 0.46
(n)	(9)	(31)	(48)	(46)

These results indicate that the compensation phenomena does not occur before two weeks of life. Thus the assumption that hypothyroid infants with ectopic thyroid gland are missed by primary T_4 screening program because of the compensation mechanism is rejected.

1737 IN VITRO HORMONE SECRETION BY THE SUPERFUSED HUMAN PLACENTA. G.H.Mulder*, H. van Kessel and N.F.Th. Arts, Dept. Obst./Gyn. Free University Hospital, de Boelelaan 1117, 1081 HV Amsterdam, the Netherlands.

In spite of much effort from both the research lab and the clinic, the search for better indicators to evaluate fetal well-being and placental function continues. Physical data, obtained during pregnancy (ultrasound, FHR) or after birth (placenta weight, morphology) have aided immensely in separating pathology from the 'normal' state, but virtually nothing is known about biochemical parameters, i.e. the regulation of the production of hormones that play a role in fetal growth and development. In order to delineate the placental contribution to the endocrine milieu of the fetus, we have set out to investigate its in vitro hormone production.To that end we have developed a system utilizing superfusion of fresh placental fragments obtained from normal, term pregnancies.By collecting fractions (10 min) of medium effluent from four identical samples ($1\frac{1}{2}$ g each)taken from a pool of tissue fragments from one placenta,we can simultaneously monitor the dynamic hormone response to three different, carefully timed signals in comparison to the spontaneous hormone secretion rate. Thus far we have limited ourselves to assaying one steroid (progesterone) and several protein hormones (HCG,HPL,PRL,ACTH,SP-1). The number of signals we can present to the tissue is virtually unlimited, but we have started with 'obstetrical'(β-mimetics,oxytocin) and 'pharmacological' agents (CAMP,DA,norepi). The results thus far point toward a substantial degree of autonomy of in vitro placental hormone secretion.Nevertheless we will present data showing clear and strong effects of various substances on placental hormone secretion.Comparing results from various tissues (diabetes,growth retardation)should yield information on the hormonal derangement.

1738 NEONATAL THYROID SCREENING BY ENZYME IMMUNOASSAY MEASURING TSH IN DRIED BLOOD SPOTS. H.Naruse*[1]), N.Takasugi [2]), N.Kunita [3]), O.Maeda [4]) and H.Shirane [5]). [1])National Center for Nerv., Ment. & Musc. Disorders, Tokyo. [2])Sapporo City Inst. of Public Health, Sapporo. [3])Osaka Prefectural Public Health Inst., Osaka. [4])Kyoto City Inst of Public Health, Kyoto. [5])Central Inst. of Fuji Revio Co. Ltd., Tokyo.

For the purpose of avoiding many problems caused by a use of radioisotope and of obtaining a better non-isotopic method which can measure TSH in dried blood, an enzyme immunoassay method was developed by Naruse et al. in 1979 and the method was adopted in a routine neonatal screening for primary hypothyroidism. The method is a competitive EIA and is using a double antibody solid phase method with a special bead. Fluorometry was introduced into a step determining the enzyme activity in order to obtain the better sensitivity. TSH-β-galactosidase and TSH-horse raddish peroxidase conjugates were produced and both were equally usable, but the former was used in the routine screening. The method is more sensitive than usual RIA kits for TSH in dried blood, and can measure TSH in one of 3 mm disc of dried blood spot exactly. Four screening laboratories adopted the method. Three of them compared the results obtained by the EIA method with that by RIA, and all laboratories tested the intra- and interassay CV% casefully, and the results were all satisfactory. About 157,330 newborn samples were tested by the EIA method and 28 patient were detected. During an initial stage of this study, it was revealed that some sample contained "unknown" compounds which produced enhanced fluorescent intensity, and revisions were achieved to overcome this problem.

1739 ATYPICAL UTERINE RESPONSE TO ESTROGEN IN MICE TREATED PRENATALLY WITH DIETHYLSTILBESTROL (DES).

R.R. Newbold, D.B. Maier, K.S. Korach, J.A. McLachlan*, Lab. Reprod. and Devel. Tox., NIEHS, NIH, Research Triangle Park, NC 27709 USA

Developmentally estrogenized animals express permanent alterations in genital tract differentiation, including neoplasia. The mechanisms underlying these changes are not known, but probably involve alterations in the tissue response to hormones later in life. Thus, mice were treated on days 9-16 of gestation with DES (100 μg/kg/day). In the period just before puberty (days 21-24) prenatally DES treated mice respond to estrogen stimulation with uterine weight increases approximately 50% of controls. Uterine luminal fluid (ULF) volume and protein content are also depressed; ULF protein profiles are altered as determined by two-dimensional gel electrophoresis. Additionally, uterine estrogen receptor levels in DES mice are only half those of control mice in the peripubertal period. Prior to estrogen stimulation no difference in uterine luminal epithelial mitosis is observed between control and treated mice. Following 3 days of estrogen treatment, the uterine epithelia of DES treated mice has a mitotic rate approximately half of controls. There is extensive squamous metaplasia; mitosis in these squamous cells is low compared to the columnar cells. Ovariectomy on day 17 prevents the appearance of uterine squamous metaplasia, but treatment of ovariectomized mice with estrogen for 3 days results in 100% induction of squamous metaplasia which persists in the absence of further estrogen treatment. Thus, prenatally induced alterations in patterns of cell differentiation profoundly influence later hormone responses in the genital tract.

1740 HIGH LEVELS OF α-MSH IMMUNOACTIVITY IN FETAL PLASMA: EVIDENCE FOR TONIC DOPAMINE INHIBITION.

C. Newman*, S. Wardlaw, R. Stark, S. Daniel, and A. Frantz, Depts. of Medicine and Pediatrics, Columbia University College of Physicians and Surgeons, New York, New York.

α-MSH is present in high concentrations in the intermediate lobe of the fetal pituitary, and has been implicated as a regulator of fetal adrenal steroidogenesis and fetal growth. However, there are few data regarding α-MSH levels in fetal plasma or the control of fetal α-MSH secretion. In this study, chronic arterial and venous catheters were implanted into 4 pregnant ewes and their fetuses in utero, and serial experiments were performed 1 week later (121 - 138 days gestation). Plasma was extracted with talc, and α-MSH measured by a specific RIA using an antibody with no cross-reactivity with ACTH. In 12 simultaneously drawn basal samples, mean fetal plasma α-MSH was 33.1 ± 2.4 (SEM) pg/ml, and mean maternal α-MSH 8.6 ± 1.2 pg/ml. In 6 studies, injection of metoclopramide (MCP) .25 mg/kg into the fetal jugular vein stimulated α-MSH secretion into fetal plasma from 33.9 ± 2.8 pg/ml to 139 ± 28 and 130 ± 19 pg/ml 15 and 30' after MCP. Simultaneous maternal plasma α-MSH did not change. In 6 newborn sheep (2 hrs -10 days), mean plasma α-MSH rose from 45.2 ± 13 pg/ml to a peak of 211 ± 38 pg/ml 15' after MCP .25 mg/kg IV. In 3 adult ewes, MCP 5 mg IV stimulated plasma α-MSH from 9.4 ± 2.0 pg/ml to a 30' peak of 19.5 ± 4.5 pg/ml. These data demonstrate that fetal and newborn sheep contain significantly higher plasma α-MSH immunoactivity than adult ewes, and that in these animals, α-MSH secretion is subject to inhibitory control by dopamine.

1741 A MODEL FOR FETAL DEVELOPMENT IN SPONTANEOUS GESTATIONAL DIABETES: THE db/+MOUSE. H.C. Nielsen*, C.P. Fawcett, J. Warshaw. Depts. Pediatrics and Physiology, Southwestern Med. Sch., Dallas, Tx., USA.

The development of maternal glucose intolerance during pregnancy in the heterozygous diabetes (db/+) mouse has recently been described (Kaufmann et al, AJOG 141:479,1981). Newborn mice of these pregnancies weighed more than controls. We hypothesized that the maternal glucose intolerance would cause endocrine and biochemical changes in the fetus. We measured blood glucose, pancreatic insulin and glucagon content, and lung glycogen content in fetuses of db/+ mice and of normal Swiss Webster mice (SW) at 18 days gestation (day 19=term). After maternal sacrifice, fetal blood was obtained and fetal pancreases and lungs rapidly removed and frozen on dry ice. Blood glucose was measured by micro-glucose oxidase assay. Pancreases were lyophilized and extracted with acid alcohol. Insulin and glucagon were measured by radioimmunoassay (glucagon antibody courtesy of Dr. R. Unger, Dallas, Tx). Lungs were homogenized and glycogen content measured as the formation of NADPH from glucose-6-phosphate. Fetal blood glucose in db/+ and SW mice were not different. Pancreatic insulin content was significantly decreased in db/+ fetuses (db/+: 12.3±4.6 mU/mg wgt; SW: 20.8±8.4 mU/mg wgt; p<.0001). Pancreatic glucagon content was unchanged (db/+: 61.6±32.8 ng/mg wgt; SW: 55.4±11.5 ng/mg wgt). Lung glycogen was significantly elevated (db/+: 643±92.8 µg/mg prot; SW: 262±57.8 µg/mg prot; p<.0001). All values are mean ± SD. These findings suggest a state of increased fetal glucose utilization, depleting insulin stores and prolonging fetal glycogen formation or storage. We propose that this model will be useful to study fetal development as affected by the spontaneous development of maternal glucose intolerance.

1742 THYROTROPIN RELEASING HORMONE EXTRACTION AND METABOLISM BY THE FETAL SIDE OF THE GUINEA PIG PLACENTA. T. Nogimori*, R. Matys, C.F. Wu, S. Alex and C.H. Emerson, Division of Endocrinology and Metabolism, University of Massachusetts Medical School, Worcester, MA, USA.

Studies in the fetus suggest that extrahypothalamic TRH could be more important than hypothalamic TRH for fetal thyrotroph function. This would be less likely if there are major losses of fetal TRH through the placenta. To evaluate this, the extraction and metabolism of TRH by the intact guinea pig placenta was examined. Under anesthesia the fetus was removed and perfused through an umbilical artery with ^3H-H_2O in Krebs Heinselait buffer (KHB). Placental effluent fractions (PF) were collected from the umbilical vein and analyzed by specific RIAs for TRH and deamido TRH (TRH-OH). TRH was not detected in PF when KHB alone was perfused but was detected after addition of TRH to the KHB. TRH levels stabilized during the last hr of the 90 min perfusions. The fractional extraction (FE) of TRH was 22% of the FE ^3H-H_2O. It was similar at all 6 collection periods in each perfusion regardless of whether 10, 1.0, or 0.01 µg TRH/ min was perfused (FE-TRH, Mean ± SE of all collection times at 10 µg TRH/min = 23 ± 2, 6 ± 1 and 18 ± 6; at 1.0 µg TRH/min = 7 ± 2, 15 ± 3, and 10 ± 4; at 0.01 µg TRH/min = 5 ± 1, 15 ± 1 and 7 ± 2). A portion of the TRH extracted by the placenta was converted to TRH-OH and fetal-maternal transfer of TRH was also detected. Conclusions: Fetal TRH can be converted to deamido-TRH in the placenta and is also transferred to the maternal circulation. However, a large percentage of fetal TRH perfusing the placenta returns to the fetus. This finding is surprising in view of current concepts that the placenta is relatively permeable to TRH.

1743 Effect of brain-gut peptides on glucose output from isolated perfused rat liver.

H. Sasaki*, K. Yamatani, N. Sato and M. Hara, Third Dept. of Internal Med., Yamagata Univ. Yamagata, Japan

To investigate if the hyperglycemic brain-gut peptides act directly on the liver, glucose output and cyclic AMP output from the isolated perfused rat liver was examined. The liver was obtained from male Wistar rats weighing 250g fed ad lib according to Sugano's method and perfused non-cyclically with hemoglobin free Krebs-Henselite bicarbonate buffer gassed continuously with a humidified mixture of 95% O_2 and 5% CO_2. Glucose output from the liver increased soon after adrenalin administration, but later and persistently by glucagon. Glucose output was increased at as low as physiological concentration of glucagon, 10^{-11}M, together with an increase of cyclic AMP, but it was increased with 10 times higher than physiological concentration of adrenalin, 10^{-8}M, without any changes of cyclic AMP output. Glucagon and adrenalin were additive in glucose output but not in cyclic AMP output. Secretin raised cyclic AMP output without changes of glucose output. Secretin and adrenalin were not additive in glucose production but inhibitory in cyclic AMP production. Neither neurotensin, bombesin, CCK nor caerulein increased both glucose output and cyclic AMP output. These results indicated that 1) glucagon and adrenalin induced glucose output from the liver through different mechanism. 2) Adrenalin may act on the liver directly in the case of exaggerated secretion. 3) Secretin increases cyclic AMP in the liver and may exert other effect on the liver than glucogenolysis. 4) Neurotensin, bombesin, CCK and caerulein do not act on the liver directly.

1744 PORCINE PROSOMATOSTATIN: ISOLATION OF THE PEPTIDE AND PARTIAL AMINO ACID SEQUENCE. W.E. Schmidt*, J.M. Conlon, V. Mutt and W. Creutzfeldt
Div. of Gastroenterology/Metabolism, Dept. of Medicine, Univ. of Goettingen, W. Germany and Dept. of Biochem. II, Medical Nobel Inst., Karolinska-Inst., Stockholm, Sweden.

The m-RNA of preprosomatostatin of different species (human, rat, anglerfish, catfish) has been cloned and sequenced. It has been postulated that the cleavage of the N-terminal signal peptide occurs at position -79 and -78 (gly-ala), but so far no sequence data are available for the primary structure of the somatostatin precursor. Here we report the isolation of the prosomatostatin peptide from a porcine gut extract using conventional gel filtration and ion exchange chromatography. Final purification was obtained by high pressure liquid chromatography (HPLC) on a reversed phase C-18 column. The purification procedure was monitored by radioimmunoassay with an antiserum directed towards the central residues of somatostatin-14. Porcine prosomatostatin was cleaved by trypsin and staphylococcus aureus V8 protease and the enzymatic digests were separated by HPLC. Using automated liquid phase sequencing and manual DABITC-Edman degradation, the sequence of the 31 amino acids at the N-terminus of porcine prosomatostatin were elucidated as:

A P S D P R L R Q F L Q K S L A A A A G K Q E L A K Y F L A E ...

Conclusion: The signal peptide is removed from porcine preprosomatostatin at the alanine residue corresponding to position -78 of human preprosomatostatin. The N-terminal 31 amino acids of porcine prosomatostatin are identical with the corresponding sequence in human preprosomatostatin. Supported by DFG, Stiftung Volkswagenwerk and Smith Kline Dauelsberg Foundation.

1745 TWO MESSENGER RNAs ENCODE POLYPEPTIDES RELATED TO GASTRIN-RELEASING PEPTIDE IN A HUMAN PULMONARY CARCINOID TUMOR. E.R. Spindel*, W.W. Chin, A.B. Oser, J.S. Moon, J. Price, L.H. Rees, G.M. Besser and J.F. Habener. Laboratory of Molecular Endocrinology, Massachusetts General Hospital and Howard Hughes Medical Institute Laboratories, Boston, MA and St. Bartholomew's Hospital, London, England.

Gastrin-releasing peptide (GRP) is a 27-amino acid-peptide related to amphibian bombesin and is a member of a large family of mammalian bombesin related peptides. In order to define the structures of the members of this family we have prepared and cloned a cDNA library from mRNA derived from a pulmonary carcinoid tumor rich in bombesin immunoreactivity. Synthetic, mixed deoxynucleotide probes complementary to two different portions of amphibian bombesin were used to select 13 bacterial colonies which contained hybridizing cDNA inserts. Sequence analysis of one such clone containing a 450 base insert demonstrated that it encoded a human GRP with marked homology to porcine, avian and canine GRP. Northern blot hybridization analysis of the tumor mRNA using [^{32}P]-labeled cDNA revealed two mRNAs of approximately 800 and 850 base pairs in length. Restriction enzyme mapping of the other cDNAs revealed that all were closely related in structure. Southern blot analysis of human genomic DNA revealed only single hybridizing bands suggesting that a single gene may code for human GRP. Thus the presence of 2 mRNAs encoding GRP precursor proteins in the face of a single GRP gene suggests alternate processing of the RNA transcript. Sequence analysis of the remaining cDNAs is now in progress to determine the exact difference between the two mRNAs.

1746 ONCOGENE (myc-gene) EXPRESSION IN PRE- AND POSTIMPLANTATION RAT EMBRYOS. S. Sarkar, V. Maharajan*, M. Sanyal and W. Summers. Depts. of Obstetrics and Gynecology, Human Genetics, and Therapeutic Radiology, Yale University School of Medicine, New Haven, CT 06510

It is known that proto-oncogenes are present but not expressed in normal vertebrate cells, but such genes (e.g., myc gene) are expressed in malignant cells. In this study, a 35-S labeled v-myc probe was prepared by nick translating v-myc DNA sequences and utilized for in situ cytohybridization with RNA of pre- and postimplantation embryos of different developmental stages. The cytohybridization procedures permitted detection of specific DNA-RNA hybrids in glutaraldehyde fixed embryos and embryonic tissue sections by autoradiography with exposure for 3-4 days. Under the conditions of hybridization, embryos of both preimplantation (1-and 2-cell) and postimplantation (pregnancy days 9 and 11) stages showed the presence of RNA transcripts homologous to myc genes. In 1-and 2-cell embryos, myc gene probe hybridized more intensely, indicated by numerous silver grains. The intensity of hybridization was relatively reduced in the postimplantation embryonic tissues. In contrast, control experiments with adult rat liver, spleen and uterine tissues exhibited only a few silver grains following hybridization with the myc gene probe. Therefore, these preliminary observations suggest the possibility that there is expression of genes homologous to myc-gene during early embryonic development. It is not known whether the factors which control the expression of oncogenes in embryonic tissues are similar to those operating in malignant cells. (Supported by NIH grant HD14587)

1747 CARBOHYDRATE COMPOSITIONS OF THE HUMAN PITUITARY GLYCOPROTEIN HORMONE SUBUNITS (ISOLATED BY HIGH PERFORMANCE LIQUID CHROMATOGRAPHY) INDICATE DIFFERENTIAL OLIGOSACCHARIDE PROCESSING. T.F. Parsons* and J.G. Pierce, Dept. of Biological Chemistry, UCLA School of Medicine, Los Angeles, CA 90024

The carbohydrates of the human pituitary glycoprotein hormones LH, TSH and FSH are N-linked to asparagine residues, and contain 3 Man, 2 GlcNAc and Fuc typical of complex type oligosaccharide cores. The contents of NeuAc, Gal, GlcNAc, GalNAc and sulfate are different, indicating differential processing of the oligosaccharides. LHα, LHβ, TSHα and TSHβ contain one residue of GalNAc and one residue of sulfate per oligosaccharide, and are resistant to enzymatic deglycosylation. We have previously shown that the carbohydrates of bovine LH and TSH contain terminal O-sulfated GalNAc and O-sulfated GlcNAc residues which result in the resistance to enzymatic deglycosylation (Parsons, T.F. and Pierce, J.G. (1980) Proc. Natl. Acad. Sci. USA 77, 7089-7093). We propose that the oligosaccharides of human LHα, LHβ, TSHα and TSHβ contain one residue of O-sulfated GalNAc. FSHα and FSHβ, however, are susceptible to enzymatic deglycosylation and do not contain sulfate. FSHβ, in contrast to the other subunits, does not contain GalNAc. The role of differential processing in the biosynthesis and secretion of the glycoprotein hormones remains to be determined. A single method of reverse phase high performance liquid chromatography was used to separate the subunits. This rapid and easy method is applicable for the separation of subunits from as little as 10 μg or as much as 100 mg of hormone. Separation is achieved by chromatography on a Vydac 218TP1010 column with a linear (60 min) gradient of 0.1 M sodium phosphate pH 6.8 to a solvent containing 50% acetonitrile and 50% 0.1 M sodium phosphate pH 6.8. (Supported by USPHS Grant AM 18005.)

1748 IN VITRO TRANSLATION OF PORCINE AND HUMAN PITUITARY GONADOTROPIN mRNAs. O. Pascal and J. André[+] Biochimie Endocrinienne, UER Lyon Nord, INSERM-U.34 Hôpital Debrousse. 29 rue Soeur Bouvier. 69322 Lyon Cedex 05. France.

We published results suggesting that porcine α and β-LH subunits are encoded by distinct mRNAs (BBRC, 1984). The aim of the present work was to bring further evidences supporting this conclusion and to determine whether a human pituitary gonadotropin adenoma contains high concentrations of corresponding mRNAs. RNAs were extracted from the anterior pituitary (AP) of castrated male pigs, from a pituitary adenoma removed from a 27 year old man with isolated high serum FSH concentration (23 IU/l) and from Macaca fascicularis AP. Poly A rich RNAs were translated in wheat germ extracts in the presence of ^{35}S-cysteine-methionine. We show that in the translation products (TP) of pig RNAs that the 14 K proteins precipitated by antisera directed against denatured α or β-p-LH subunits are clearly different from each other according to their behavior on electrofocusing in non equilibrium conditions and the finger-prints of their trypsin digests. These results are new evidences in favor of distinct mRNAs coding for α and β-p-LH subunits. The electrophoretic pattern of human adenoma RNAs TP shows a prominent band of ≃ 18 K which is under current immunological characterization and which corresponds to that of ovine and rat pre-β-FSH. Proteins of molecular weight similar to the pre-α-subunit (≃ 14 K), pre-PRL (≃ 25 K) and pre-GH (≃ 23 K) were present in limited amounts compared to those found in the TP of RNAs extracted from normal AP of pig and M. fascicularis. These results suggest this human adenoma is enriched in β-FSH mRNA. Thanks are due to J. Trouillas and B. Claustrat for providing adenoma and hormone RIAs. This study was supported by the INSERM and the UER Lyon Nord.

1749 EVIDENCE FOR A STIMULATORY BETA-ADRENERGIC COMPONENT IN THE RELEASE OF LH IN THE RAT.

S.L. Petrovic*, J.C. Bedran de Castro and S.M. McCann. Dept of Physiology, Univ of Texas Hlth Sci Center, Dallas, TX 75235

Single injections of a powerful beta-adrnergic blocker, FM-24 (30 mg/kg, i.p.) to acutely orchidectomized rats resulted in a complete (>90%) blockade of visceral beta-receptors (recovery T/2, >= 12 hrs), and of brain beta-receptors (recovery T/2, >= 6 hrs). In blood collected at 30 min intervals from conscious, freely moving rats 0-6 hrs after the injection (18-24 hrs after castration), a 45% mean decrease (n = 6, p<0.005) in LH levels was noted in comparison to diluent-injected controls (n=5), while in collections 18-24 hrs after orchidectomy and 16-22 hrs after FM-24 there was a 35% mean decrease (n=4, p<0.01). The anterior pituitary content of LH rose significantly by 29% (n=7, p<0.025) at 24 hrs after FM-24 (48 hrs after castration), and by 51% (n=8, p<0.01) two days after the injection compared to castrated controls (n=7). These results indicate that a sizable component of LH release in vivo might be controlled by beta-adrenergic mechanisms, possibly via a direct action on the gonadotrophs since β agonists are inhibitory at the hypothalamic level. The data are consistent with our recent finding of parallelism in the post-orchidectomy increase of anterior pituitary beta-receptors and the levels of plasma gonadotropins (Petrovic, McDonald, Snyder and McCann, Life Sci., submitted). Supported by HD 09988.

1750 THE EFFECT OF DOPAMINE AGONISTS ON CIRCULATING GONADOTROPHIN LEVELS IN PATIENTS WITH POLYCYSTIC OVARY SYNDROME

G.Prelević*, M.Vircburger, D.Mijalković, Lj.Perić, A.Popović, Belgrade University, School of Medicine, City Clinic Hospital, Raja Sekulića 172, 11000 Belgrade, Yugoslavia

Data about the modulatory role of dopamine on gonadotrophin secretion in humans are still controversial. The aim of this study was to determine whether the administration of dopamine agonists modulates gonadotropin secretion in PCO patients. Either L.dopa (500mg) or bromoergocryptine (2,5mg) were administered orally on the 4th day of menstrual cycle to 16 patients with PCO and 9 normal healthy women. Blood samples were taken at 30 min intervals during the first two hours after the administration of the drug and at 2 hourly intervals during the following 8 hours of the test. Changes in plasma LH and FSH levels were expressed as percent change of the mean basal level. LH and FSH concentrations were determined by RIA. Both dopamin e agonists induces significant reduction in plasma LH but not FSH levels in PCO patients. A significantly greater supression of LH levels occurs in PCO patients after bromocriptine administration(50,92% v.s.21,33% in the controls).The greatest decline in LH levels is estimated 2 hours after the administration of both dopamine agonists. A significant rebound in LH release is observed 7-8 hours after L-dopa administration, and the magnitude of rebound is greater in PCO patients when compared with the controls. No rebound in LH release occurs during the 10 hours after bromocryptine.

1751 SECRETION OF BIOLOGICALLY INACTIVE LH BY A GONADOTROPIN-PRODUCING PITUITARY ADENOMA. H.E. Scaglia*, I. Molocznik, A.M. Brizzio, C. Zylbersztein, G.E. Bur and E. Pardal, Reference Center of Radioimmunoassay, CRRIE, La Plata, and Costa Buero Institute, Buenos Aires, Argentina.

We have studied a 62-yr-old man with a pituitary adenoma and gonadal failure and elevated LH and FSH levels whose LH did not have biological activity and eluted normally on gel filtration. In basal conditions, LH, FSH and Testosterone (T) circulating levels determined in multiple blood samples were (Media $\pm$ SD): 44.0 $\pm$ 6.5 mIU/ml, 48.4 $\pm$ 7.5 mIU/ml and 0.4 $\pm$ 0.03 ng/ml, respectively. A normal gonadotropin response was induced by LH-RH administration. Neither gonadotropin levels nor gonadotropin response to LH-RH were significantly modified by T propionate (100 mg/day/5 days). A 3 mm pituitary adenoma and a portion of non tumoral pituitary were removed. Cell citoplasms loaded with secretory granules were seen at electronmicroscopy. Following transsphenoidal adenomectomy LH and FSH decreased to 20 mIU /ml. Tumor LH and FSH concentrations were 2200 and 2800 U/mg tissue while in the non tumoral tissue they were 3500 and 3800 U/mg tissue, respectively. LH was partially purified from both tissues. LH biological activity could not be detected in the tumoral or the non tumoral tissue in in vitro (T production in rat isolated Leydig cells) or in vivo (testicular response in prepubertal rats) conditions. Results show that the tumor and the pituitary of this patient produce gonadotropins not inhibited by T and under LH-RH control without LH biological activity and suggest: 1) the biosynthesis of gonadotropins with structural alterations might be induced by the lack of androgens and 2) the hyperplasia might be due to the sustained LH-RH stimulus.

1752 MODE OF ACTION OF CLOMIPHENE CITRATE ON THE LHRH-STIMULATED RELEASE OF LH AND FSH BY THE RAT PITUITARY GLAND. G.A. Schuiling* and T.R. Koiter, Department of Obstetrics and Gynaecology, University of Groningen, 59 Oostersingel, 9713 EZ Groningen, THE NETHERLANDS.

The action of the ovulation-inducing drug clomiphene citrate on the LHRH-stimulated release of LH and FSH (LHRH was infused for 21 h at the rate of 1000 ng/h), was studied in 2-weeks ovariëctomized rats pretreated with either oestradiol benzoate (OB; 3 µg s.c.) for 3 days, with LHRH (250 ng/h, delivered for 6 days by Alzet osmotic minipumps) or with LHRH plus OB. In rats not pretreated with LHRH OB enhanced the LHRH-stimulated release of both LH and FSH (positive effect of oestrogen), but clomiphene enhanced only the secretion of LH. In rats pretreated with LHRH OB strongly suppressed the stimulated release of LH and FSH (negative effect of oestrogen), but clomiphene enhanced this release. Clomiphene also prevented OB to cause the negative oestrogen effect. The present results suggest:

1. the negative oestrogen effect on the pituitary gland develops when, at the moment of OB administration, the pituitary gland is exposed to significant amounts of LHRH; 2. the positive effect of oestrogen on the pituitary gland develops only in the absence of (significant amounts of) LHRH; 3. clomiphene is not only a (weak) oestrogen, able to exert the positive oestrogen effect on the pituitary gland, but, rather, a partial oestrogen, unable to cause the negative oestrogen effect.

1753 *MONOCLONAL ANTIBODIES (MCA) FOR PROBING THE EPITOPES OF HUMAN CHORIONIC GONADOTROPIN (HCG) AND FOR MEASURING HOLO-HCG AND/OR ITS FREE SUBUNITS.* *S.Schwarz*, P.Berger, & G.Wick, University of Innsbruck, School of Medicine, Institute of General & Exper. Pathology, Innsbruck, Austria/Europe*

Monoclonal antibodies (MCA) against HCG were raised, characterized as to their main specificity (α-subunit (sbt), or β-sbt or intact(holo)HCG (=conformational, "c") directed) and as to affinity by direct binding assay using ^{125}iodine-tracers and subsequent SCATCHARD-plot evaluation. Then, by combining in a chess-board-type fashion 21 different MCA that were coated to tube with 8 different iodinated MCA in a consecutive incubation sandwich assay design, the antigenic surface of the HCG molecule was probed: 4 α-, 3 β- and only one single c-epitope were distinguished. - On this basis, a selected number of MCA could be combined for generating 3 different species of 2-site ImmunoRadioMetric Assays (IRMA) that specifically recognize either holo-HCG alone or holo-HCG + free α-sbt or holo-HCG + free β-sbt. The coexistence of these 3 molecular entities of HCG could thus clearly be demonstrated in patients with trophoblastic tumors as well as in choriocarcinoma cell line (BeWo and JAr) supernatants and -cytosols. Most obviously, there was a striking dis-balance in the production and secretion of holo-HCG and its free subunits.

Supported by the Austrian Cancer Research Fund, 1982/83.

1754 CENTRAL EPINEPHRINE ACTIVITY DURING THE RAT ESTRUS CYCLE. R. Sheaves, R. Laynes and P. MacKinnon*, Department of Human Anatomy, Oxford University, England, OX1 3QX.

Central epinephrine (E) neurons have been implicated in the control of the estrogen-stimulated gonadotropin surge in rats. Concentrations and turnover of E in the medial preoptic area (mPOA), the medio-basal hypothalamus (MBH) and the perifornical area (PFA) have been measured in groups of 4-day cycling rats at various times of the estrous cycle. After decapitation, brains were removed and sectioned (250u) in a cryostat (-12°C). The relevant tissue was removed by needle punch (0.85 mm i.d.) with the aid of a dissecting microscope. Concentrations of E were measured by radioenzymatic assay, turnover being assessed 2h after administration of a centrally active E synthesis inhibitor, SKF 64139. During the 'critical period' at the start of the preovulatory gonadotropin surge (1500-1700h) E activity, as reflected by increases in its concentration and turnover, was increased (P 0.05). Such changes were not found in these areas at metestrus or diestrus or in the PFA at any time. This pattern of central E activity at the sites of synthesis (mPOA) and release (MBH) of the GnRH neuron appears to be closely related to the preovulatory output of gonadotropins. An additional finding was of much larger increases (P 0.01) in concentration and turnover in the MBH on proestrous evening (2100-2300h) and the estrus afternoon (1500-1700h). That these events may also be related to the neural control of gonadotropin (FSH and/or prolactin) output across the periovulatory period cannot be ignored. (MRC Grant G8215236N)

1755 LACK OF GROWTH HORMONE DEPENDENT SOMATOMEDIN LIKE ACTIVITY IN FETAL SHEEP.

M.J. Parkes*, D.J. Hill and G.S. Dawes, Nuffield Institute for Medical Research, Oxford University and Department of Paediatrics, Sheffield University.

The role of somatomedins in fetal growth is not known, and previous incompleted studies disagree as to the existence of growth hormone dependent somatomedins in fetal sheep. Somatomedin like activity was therefore measured in the plasma of intact and hypophysectomised fetal sheep, and during chronic intravenous infusion of ovine Growth Hormone or ovine prolactin into hypophysectomised fetuses. Hormone levels were measured by radio immunoassay, and plasma somatomedin like activity by the pig costal cartilage bioassay. Fetal hypophysectomy did not consistently lower plasma somatomedin like activity, either when compared to the levels in other intact fetuses, or in the same fetus before hypophysectomy. Neither growth hormone nor prolactin infusion into hypophysectomised fetuses, to give the same or three times the levels in intact fetuses, changed the plasma somatomedin like activity. Yet the growth hormone preparation was biologically active both in hypophysectomised rats and fetal sheep. The results demonstrate that the factors in fetal plasma which stimulate the incorporation of ^{35}Sulphate into cartilage, are not growth hormone dependent.

1756 NEONATAL MOUSE URINARY EPIDERMAL GROWTH HORMONE CONCENTRATION: ONTOGENY, AND RESPONSES TO THYROXINE, GH AND TESTOSTERONE.

J. Perheentupa *, J. Lakshmanan, A. Grueters, T. Macaso, and D.A. Fisher, Harbor-UCLA Medical Center, UCLA School of Medicine, Torrance, California, U.S.A.

Using a specific and sensitive RIA we quantified urinary concentrations of epidermal growth factor (U-EGF) in neonatal mice from birth through day 18. We observed 3 developmental phases. First, U-EGF remained unchanged from day 0 (mean 1.75 ng/mg Urea-N) to day 6 (3.7 ng/mg). Second, there was a rapid increase to a plateau of 40-48 ng/mg on days 12-15. Third, there was a new increase (day 18, 86 ng/mg). Sephadex G50 column chromatography revealed a single peak of EGF-immunoreactive material, similar in molecular size to standard mouse submandibular gland (SMG) EGF. We studied modifications of the above ontogeny induced by thyroxine (T4, 0.4 µg/g BW/day for 6 days), bovine GH (bGH, 6 µg/g BW/day for 8 days), or testosterone propionate (TP, 0.4 µg/g BW/48 h for 4 doses). In addition to U-EGF we also measured SMG-EGF (pg/mg protein). Group means were (C, controls; *, $p < 0.05$; ***, $p < 0.001$):

	Exp. 1			Exp. 2			Exp. 3		
	C		T4	C		bGH	C		TP
U-EGF, ng/mg	86.6	***	618	20.1	*	30.7	11.8		12.3
SMG-EGF, ng/mg	120		114	629		251	132	***	61
Body weight, g	4.0		4.1	4.7		5.0	4.7	*	5.4

Summary: There is a progressive 50-fold increase in U-EGF during the first 18 days of life. During the first week this increase can be accelerated by T4 or GH but not TP. These effects are independent of changes in SMG-EGF.

1757 TRANSFORMING GROWTH FACTORS IN HUMAN MILK: ISOLATION AND PARTIAL CHEMICAL AND BIOLOGICAL CHARACTERIZATION.

P.E. Petrides*, M. Hosang, E.M. Shooter and P. Böhlen, Dept. of Neurobiology, Stanford University School of Medicine, Stanford, CA. 94305, and Laboratories for Neuroendocrinology, The Salk Institute, 10010 North Torrey Pines Road, La Jolla, CA. 92037.

Using a purification scheme entirely based upon reverse phase liquid chromatography we have isolated from human milk and partially characterized three polypeptides that can compete with murine epidermal growth factor (mEGF) for human placental membrane receptor sites. These peptides have molecular weights of about 6000 and differ from human epidermal growth factor/urogastrone as well as from each other in their amino acid compositions. None of them interacts with rabbit anti-mEGF antibodies. They show different affinities for the placental membrane EGF-receptor (K_i of 1, 2.5 and 7 ng resp.). All three peptides stimulate the anchorage dependent proliferation of human neonatal skin fibroblasts in culture as well as the anchorage independent growth of rat kidney fibroblasts in semisolid media. Based on these properties they can be classified as type α transforming growth factors (αTGFs). Whereas their potencies for the stimulation of anchorage dependent growth (half maximal stimulation at 1 ng/ml) and anchorage independent growth (half maximal stimulation at 2.5 ng/ml) are similar, one of the three has a higher intrinsic α-TGF activity than the others. These results provide evidence for the existence of a family of EGF related polypeptides in humans which are involved in the regulation of cell proliferation.

1758 INSULIN-LIKE GROWTH FACTOR I (IGF I): REGULATION BY PLATELET DERIVED GROWTH FACTOR (PDGF), EPIDERMAL GROWTH FACTOR (EGF) AND FIBROBLAST GROWTH FACTOR (FGF).

B. Pfeifle*, H. Ditschuneit, University of Ulm, Internal Medicine II, Ulm, FRG.

Serum contains a number of mitogens, which regulate growth of cells. We examined the binding of ^{125}I-insulin-like growth factor I (IGF I) to cultivated smooth muscle cells of the rat aorta in the presence of platelet-derived growth factor (PDGF), epidermal growth factor (EGF) or fibroblast growth factor (FGF)(10-1000 ng/ml) using 0.1 M HEPES buffer pH 7.4 with 0.2% HSA and an incubation time of 90 min at 20°C. ^{125}I-IGF binding was not displaced by PDGF, EGF or FGF. Preincubation of the cell layers in medium with 1 μg/ml PDGF for 0.5 - 4 hr led to an increase of the ^{125}I-IGF binding after 2 hr. This was followed by a decrease in binding after 4 hr. When the cells were preincubated with 1-100 ng/ml PDGF a dose-dependent decrease in ^{125}I-IGF binding was observed. Preincubation of the cells with 100 ng/ml FGF led to an increase of the ^{125}I-IGF binding after 30 min. Preincubation with 100 ng/ml EGF caused no change in the ^{125}I-IGF binding. In medium with 1% fetal calf serum (FCS) PDGF, EGF, IGF and FGF (10-1000 ng/ml) stimulated DNA synthesis in a dose-dependent mode. In medium without FCS IGF, FGF and PDGF produced only a low stimulation of DNA synthesis. EGF had a similar activity than in the presence of 1% FCS. Incubation of the cells with PDGF and IGF in medium without FCS led to an increase of the DNA synthesis, whereas FGF and IGF caused no additional increase of DNA synthesis. EGF activity was not potentiated by IGF.
This study was supported by the DFG.

1759 ALTERED SOMATOMEDINS AND SOMATOMEDIN INHIBITORS IN EXPERIMENTAL DIABETES.
LS Phillips,* AC Fusco, TG Unterman, and S Goldstein, Depts. of Medicine, Northwestern and Emory Univ. Med. Sch.,Chicago, IL and Atlanta, GA, USA.

Diabetes is associated with poor growth despite elevated GH. Skeletal GH effects are mediated by somatomedins (SM); in diabetes, SM by RIA are normal yet SM activity by bioassay (reflecting SM and SM inhibitors) is low. We asked if this discrepancy could reflect discordant changes in circulating SM and SM inhibitors.

Graded severity of diabetes was induced in rats by injection of streptozotocin (STZ) at 37, 73, 146, and 293 mg/kg; after 2 days, metabolic derangement varied from nl BOHB with slight ↑ glucose and Δ wgt -1 g to BOHB 11 mM, glucose 450 mg/dl, and Δ wgt -32 g. After fractionation of serum on Sephacryl S-300 pH 7.0, SM and SM inhibitors were measured by hypox rat cartilage bioassay. SM (K_d 0.25-0.50) were unchanged from control levels despite BOHB 2, glucose 500, and Δ wgt -11 g at 73 mg/kg STZ and fell only at higher STZ doses. In contrast, SM inhibitors (K_d 0.62-0.88) began to rise at the lowest STZ dose and increased with higher STZ. SM correlated weakly with BOHB only ($r=-0.49$, $p<0.05$), while SM inhibitors correlated significantly with all indices, paricularly BOHB ($r=0.78$, $p<0.0001$).

Summary: SM inhibitors rise early and progressively with increasing severity of STZ-induced diabetes, correlating strongly with BOHB; SM do not fall until BOHB is >2 mM. The early rise in inhibitors but late fall in SM could explain low SM activity (and poor growth) despite normal SM by RIA; inhibitor measurement may provide an index of growth potential in human diabetes. In addition, the correlation of SM inhibitors with BOHB may indicate that inhibitor regulation is linked to ketogenesis.

1760 ISOLATION OF SOMATOMEDIN BINDING PROTEIN FROM HUMAN AMNIOTIC FLUID AND DEVELOPMENT OF A RADIOIMMUNOASSAY FOR ITS DETERMINATION. G. Povoa, G. Enberg and K. Hall*, Department of Endocrinology, Karolinska Institutet, S-104 01 Stockholm, Sweden.

From human amniotic fluid a somatomedin binding protein has been isolated with high yield. The binding protein was identified through its competition with human placenta membrane for labelled SMA/IGF-1. The purification scheme consists of three steps; precipitation with ammoniumsulphate, hydrophobic chromatography on phenylsepharose and anionexchange chromatography (Mono Q column FPLC) eluted with a liniear NaCl gradient. SDS PAGE disclosed one band with a molecular size of 36000 daltons, which correspond to results from gelchromatography. The pI of the binding protein determined by chromatofocusing was 4.3. The amino acid composition of the protein has been determined but not the sequence. Both SMA/IGF-1 and IGF-2 binds to the protein with high affinity and can be displaced by pure IGF-2. The protein does not bind to placenta membranes.

A radioimmunoassay (RIA) has been developed this somatomedin binding protein with antibodies raised in rabbits. Separation of bound and free was achieved with second antibody technique. In this RIA amniotic fluid and human serum showed displacement curves parallel with the pure protein curve. In serum from new borns considerable higher levels were found than in adults. Determination of serum fraction after gelchromatography disclosed that not only the small molecular form of binding protein in serum but also the larger GH regulated form crossreact in the RIA.

1761 CHARACTERIZATION OF INSULIN-LIKE GROWTH FACTOR (IGF) RECEPTOR DYNAMICS IN CULTURED RAT CHONDROCYTES BY PHOTOAFFINITY LABELING.
D. Reismann*, C. Emler, M. Sanazaro and D. Schalch. University of Wisconsin Hospital, Madison, WI, USA.

We have used the technique of photoaffinity labeling to identify two separate IGF receptors (types I and II) on rat chondrocytes (RC), known target cells of IGF activity. ^{125}I-labeled IGF-I and IGF-II, reacted with N-succinimidyl-6-(4'-azido-2'-nitrophenyl)-amino hexanoate to produce photosensitive cross-linking derivatives, were incubated with monolayer cultures of RC and subjected to polyacrylamide electrophoresis and autoradiography. The type I IGF receptor complex consists of specific bands of Mr 350,000 and 305,000 under nonreducing, and Mr 200,000, 130,000 and 86,000 under reducing conditions. The type II receptor complex consists of a single specific band of Mr 230,000 under nonreducing, and Mr 275,000 under reducing conditions. Densitometric analysis of these bands indicates that RC possess considerably more type II than type I IGF receptors and that the type I receptor hormone complex is more trypsin sensitive than the type II. Excess equimolar amounts of unlabeled IGF-I and IGF-II displaced the ^{125}I-labeled ligands from both type I and II receptors, while insulin only partially displaced them from type I receptor sites. Incubating RC in the presence of 200 μM chloroquine indicates that the type I receptor (Mr 130,000 subunit) may be degraded by the lysosomal pathway to a greater extent than the type II. We conclude: 1) cultured RC possess both types I and II IGF receptors, with a clear prevalence of the latter, 2) data derived under nonreducing and reducing conditions suggest that the type I receptor is a disulfide-linked heterotetramer while the type II receptor is a monomer containing at least one internal disulfide bridge, and 3) types I and II receptors differ both in their degradative pathways and trypsin sensitivity.

1762 DIFFERENT OLIGOMERIC FORMS OF EPIDERMAL GROWTH FACTOR RECEPTORS FROM RAT LIVER AND HUMAN A-431 CELLS.
Richard A. Rubin* and H. Shelton Earp, Cancer Research Center and Department of Medicine, University of North Carolina at Chapel Hill, Chapel Hill, N.C. 27514.

The oligomeric structure of the epidermal growth factor (EGF) receptor was investigated. Rat liver membranes solubilized with Triton X-100, and fractions purified from this prep by wheat germ agglutinin (WGA)-agarose, were phosphorylated in the presence of EGF and [γ-^{32}P]ATP. Some samples were reduced with β-mercaptoethanol (BME) prior to analysis by SDS/polyacrylamide gel electrophoresis and autoradiography. In unreduced samples, EGF caused several-fold stimulation of phosphorylation of proteins of M_r 170,000 (p170), 210,000 (p210) and 340,000 (p340). p170 corresponds to the hepatic EGF receptor; more than 50% of the EGF-stimulated ^{32}P incorporation was into forms larger than p170. In reduced samples, EGF-stimulated phosphoproteins of M_r 170,000 and 50,000 (p50) were observed. All these phosphoproteins were predominantly labeled on tyrosine residues. Electrophoretic isolation and chemical reduction of p340 with BME yielded p170, while p210 yielded p170 and p50. EGF receptor purified by EGF-Affigel affinity chromatography showed the same pattern of bands, but EGF had little or no effect on their phosphorylation in this prep. In human A431 carcinoma cell membranes, only p170 and a small amount of p340 were seen. Thus, the hepatic EGF receptor exists both as a separate 170,000 dalton subunit as well as two disulfide-linked forms: a p170 dimer, and p170 linked to a discrete, 50,000-dalton EGF-stimulated tyrosine residue phosphoprotein. The 50,000-dalton component, and its dimer with p170, were absent from A-431 cells. Supported by NIH grant AM31683.

1763 THE BRATTLEBORO RAT : DECREASED HEPATIC GROWTH HORMONE (GH) RECEPTORS AND LOW PLASMA SOMATOMEDIN ACTIVITY. F. Picard , B. Wolf, J-N. Hugues, D. Durand, J. Charrier, P. Czernichow and*M-C. Postel-Vinay, INSERM U.30, Hôpital des Enfants-Malades, 75015 Paris, France.

Growth failure, without clear reduction of GH secretion has been observed among the Brattleboro strain rats with hereditary diabetes insipidus (DI). Body weight was significantly lower in 3 month-old DI male rats than in Long Evans (LE) rats of the same age. GH pituitary content was not different in DI and control rats (519 ± 66 µg and 569 ± 36 µg per anterior pituitary gland, respectively. Pulsatile GH release and mean 6-h GH plasma levels did not appear significantly different in chronically cannulated DI and control animals. Plasma somatomedin bioactivity was significantly lower in DI male and female rats (0.63 ± 0.07 U/ml) than in LE rats (0.87 ± 0.05 U/ml). Microsomal membrane fractions were prepared from the livers of 3 month-old DI and LE male rats. 5'nucleotidase activity was not different in microsomal membranes of DI and LE rats. ^{125}I-bGH (bovine GH) binding, expressed as the percentage of total radioactivity per mg of membrane protein, was 13.9 ± 1.1 for DI male rats and 20.2 ± 1.1 for LE rats. The specific binding of ^{125}I-insulin was 1.5 times higher in liver microsomal membranes of DI rats than in membranes of LE rats. Since the receptors of bGH and insulin were oppositely affected, a non specific effect of the DI state on peptide hormone liver receptors is unlikely. The low level of GH binding and the subsequent low plasma somatomedin activity explain, at least in part, the growth retardation of the Brattleboro rats.

1764 BASAL GROWTH HORMONE LEVELS IN PATIENTS DURING THE FIRST 48 HOURS OF ACUTE MYOCARDIAL INFARCTION. V. K. Piziak, M.D.*, Scott & White Clinic, Temple, Texas, and T. Bratcher, Ph.D., Baylor University, Waco, Texas.

The effect of acute myocardial infarction (AMI) on unstimulated serum growth hormone (HGH) is controversial. This study was conducted to determine whether a significant difference exists between basal HGH levels of patients with AMI and a similar control population with chest pain in whom AMI was excluded. Risk factors for AMI and the degree of cornary artery disease were equivalent in both groups. AMI was diagnosed by electro-cardiographic changes, history, and elevation of CPK-MB fraction.

The AMI group was divided into three subgroups: stable, complicated, and Streptokinase treated patients. The results are summarized in the accompanying table.

Mean HGH levels were significantly higher in patients with myocardial infarction, stable, complicated, or Streptokinase treated, than in the control population. The p values compared to the control group are noted in the table. In addition, the group treated with Streptokinase had a significantly higher mean basal HGH level than the stable AMI population (p<.05).

	Controls	AMI Stable	AMI Complicated	AMI Streptokinase Therapy
Number of patients	13	16	4	6
Mean HGH (ng/ml) over 48 hrs.	1.4	1.99	2.5	2.5
		p<.01	p<.0005	p<.0005

1765 SPECIFIC AND LONG-ACTING SUPPRESSION OF GH SECRETION BY THE SOMATOSTATIN ANALOGUE SMS 201-995 IN ACROMEGALY. G. Plewe*, J. Beyer, U. Krause, M. Neufeld and E. del Pozo, Dept. of Endocrinology, University of Mainz, Germany and Dept. of Exp. Therapeutics, Sandoz Ltd., Basle, Switzerland.

Due to its short half-life (2-3 min) natural somatostatin is not suitable for the treatment of acromegaly. The somatostatin analogue SMS 201-995 (SMS), which possesses a half-life of 113 min after s.c. injection in humans, has been found to exert a prolonged inhibitory action on GH secretion and a short-lasting suppression of insulin. In the present study the effect of single dose SMS on the release of GH, insulin, glucagon, TSH, T3, cortisol, LH, FSH and PRL was investigated in 6 subjects with active acromegaly. Injection of 50 µg s.c. led to a rapid fall in serum GH in all 6 cases (30 ± 12 to 1.4 ± 4 (SE) ng/ml), returning to pre-administration levels 9 hours post-injection. Plasma glucagon was lowered to 60% of the initial concentration for 6 hours. A distinct rise in insulin was observed after a standard meal (10 Kcal/kg b.w.) following SMS administration, but the peak was lower in comparison to a similar control period (36 ± 11 vs. 88 ± 17 uU/ml) and glucose levels were accordingly higher (116 vs. 130 mg%). Serum TSH, T3, cortisol, LH, FSH and PRL were not altered by SMS. It can be concluded that SMS may represent a new option in the medical management of acromegaly as an alternative to bromocriptine or as combined therapy with dopamine agonists.

1766 GH,PRL AND CORTISOL SECRETION DURING GLUCOSE AND FFA CHANGES IN THE RHESUS MONKEY. H.-J. Quabbe*, B. Bratzke, T. Walz, S. Bunge, Dept. of Endocrinology, Klinikum Steglitz/FUB, 1 Berlin 45, W-Germany.

In man, plasma glucose and free fatty acids (FFA) modulate the secretion of GH. To establish a primate model for studies on the central mediation of these effects, male adult rhesus monkeys received (1) insulin-hypoglycemia (IHG), (2) glucose infusion (GLU), (3) FFA suppression by nicotinic acid infusion (NA), (4) lipid infusion (LIP). Blood was sampled for 3 hr (IHG) or 6 hr via chronic jugular catheters from freely moving animals. IHG (n=8/20 for animals/tests): Glucose fell < 2.2 mmol/l. GH and cortisol rose significantly (4.7 → 17.4 ng/ml at 30 min and 115.0 → 253.5 µg/l at 90 min). A PRL rise was not significant (4.9 → 10.3 ng/ml). GLU (n =7/18): Glucose rose to 10 mmol/l. GH was moderately suppressed (max. 5.3 ng/ml vs approx. 9 ng/ml in spontaneous GH surges of untreated animals at same clock time (1)). PRL and cortisol were essentially unaffected. NA (n= 6/15): FFA were suppressed to 130 µEq/l (basal: 314 µEq/l). GH rose significantly (2.1 → 17.9 ng/ml at 5 hr). PRL was unaffected. A cortisol rise was not significant (132 → 170.9 ng/ml). LIP (n=10/23): FFA rose to 2500 µEq/l. GH was entirely suppressed (max. 2.6 ng/ml). PRL and cortisol were essentially unaffected. Conclusions: The GH reaction to glucose and FFA changes in the rhesus monkey is identical to that in man (increase during substrate lack, suppression during substrate excess). In contrast to man, PRL is unaffected by IHG. As in man, cortisol rises during IHG and is unaffected by glucose excess and FFA changes. The rhesus monkey may serve as a model for metabolic influences on human GH secretion. (1) Quabbe et al. Endocrinology 109: 513, 1981. Supported by Deutsche Forschungsgemeinschaft.

1767 EVALUATION OF TREATED ACROMEGALIC PATIENTS WITH NORMAL GROWTH HORMONE LEVELS DURING ORAL GLUCOSE LOAD. M. Rieu*, J.M. Kuhn, H. Bricaire and J.P. Luton. Centre de Recherches Endocrinologiques, Hôpital Cochin, 27 rue du Faubourg Saint Jacques - 75674 Paris cédex 14, France.

Activity in acromegalics was evaluated in 21 treated patients with plasma GH levels ⩽ 5 ng/ml at 60 min. of an oral glucose tolerance test (OGTT). Serum Insulin-like growth factor (IGF) levels, measured by a competitive binding assay, were above the normal mean + 3 S.D. in 10, normal in 8 and low in 3 patients. Urinary calcium excretion (CaU), measured 24 hourly, was above the normal mean + 3 S.D. in 9 of the 10 patients whose IGF levels were high, whereas only one of the 11 patients with normal or low IGF levels was hypercalciuric. After TRH injection, a paradoxical rise in GH levels (above the normal mean + 3 S.D. at 15, 30 or 60 min. of the test) was observed in 5 of the 10 patients whose IGF levels were high, whereas all patients with normal or low IGF levels showed no GH response to TRH. GH levels ⩾ 10 ng/ml occurred during Ornithine (ORN) test in 6 of the 18 patients with normal or high IGF levels : the remaining 12 patients showing no GH rise during ORN included 2 cases in which IGF levels were high and GH rose following TRH and 2 cases in which IGF levels were normal and GH were ⩾ 10 ng/ml during Insulin-induced hypoglycemia, thus excluding a GH deficiency. These results show that acromegaly is not cured in certain treated patients with normal GH levels during OGTT. In order to assess the disease activity in these patients, it seems that IGF and CaU determinations are valuable parameters, in contrast to GH response to ORN. Also GH response to TRH has a relative value.

1768 EXOGENOUS GROWTH HORMONE (GH) INHIBITS GROWTH HORMONE RELEASING FACTOR ($GRF-44-NH_2$)-INDUCED GH SECRETION IN NORMAL MEN: FURTHER EVIDENCE FOR GH AUTOREGULATION. S.M. Rosenthal*, J.A. Hulse, S.L. Kaplan, M.M. Grumbach, Department of Pediatrics, University of California San Francisco, CA, USA

Previous studies from this laboratory (J Clin Invest 50:940, 1971) and by others in humans, monkeys, and rats support the concept that GH can regulate its own secretion through an autofeedback mechanism. Such studies demonstrated that exogenous GH either blunted the GH response to provocative stimuli or blunted pulsatile GH secretion. The anatomic locus or loci for this mechanism have not been determined, but are presumed to be either at the hypothalamic or pituitary level, or both. To investigate further the site of GH autofeedback in vivo, we administered GRF (1 μg/kg IV bolus, obtained from R. Guillemin and N. Ling) before and after 5 days of placebo (1 ml normal saline IM q 12 h), and before and 12 h after 5 days of biosynthetic methionyl GH (5 U IM q 12 h, provided by Genentech, Inc.) in 4 normal men (32-34 yr). Twelve hours after the last GH injection, plasma GH levels ranged from 2.3-3.2 ng/ml. The GRF-induced plasma GH response, determined both by peak increment over time 0 and by integrated area, was significantly inhibited after GH treatment (2.3-11.2 ng/ml before and 0-1.3 ng/ml after treatment; 122-699 area units (ng·min/ml) before and 0-11 area units after treatment; $p<0.05$, Mann-Whitney test), but was not affected by placebo. Fasting blood glucose levels were unchanged following GH treatment. These results demonstrate that exogenous GH inhibits GRF-induced GH secretion. This impaired pituitary response to GRF may be mediated indirectly by stimulation of somatomedin and/or somatostatin, or by a direct effect of GH itself; these data suggest that the autofeedback effect of GH is not solely a consequence of the inhibition of hypothalamic GRF.

1769 DIMINISHED RESPONSE OF GROWTH HORMONE (GH) TO SYNTHETIC HUMAN PANCREATIC GROWTH HORMONE-RELEASING FACTOR (hpGRF) IN PATIENTS WITH PITUITARY-DEPENDENT CUSHING'S SYNDROME. G.W. Rothman*, S.H. Roman, D.T. Krieger, and M.O. Thorner, Mount Sinai Medical Center, New York, NY, and University of Virginia School of Medicine, Charlottesville, VA, USA.

Previous studies have shown diminished release of GH in response to insulin-induced hypoglycemia in patients with both Cushing's syndrome and hypercortisolemia due to long-term,high-dose glucocorticoid therapy.In an effort to clarify the mechanisms for this inhibitory effect of glucocorticoids,we administered hpGRF, 1 μg/kg as an intravenous bolus,to 3 patients with pituitary-dependent Cushing's syndrome,diagnosed by standard criteria. In normal young men(n=10),the mean$\pm$SE ΔGH after such a dose of hpGRF is 32.0$\pm$6.9 ng/ml,with maximum levels attained at an average of 49.5 min post hpGRF. In the patients,baseline GH levels were 1.0, 2.1, and 0.5 ng/ml. Maximum values after hpGRF were 2.3, 4.6, and 9.3 ng/ml,respectively. The peak value in the third patient was reached 90 min after hpGRF. In this patient,the highest GH level after placebo was 3.2 ng/ml. In a control patient receiving at least 30 mg of prednisone daily for over 2 months there was no response to hpGRF; maximum GH level was 1.6 ng/ml. The preliminary results of this small series suggest that glucocorticoids--whether endogenous or exogenous--diminish the response of GH to hpGRF. Further studies are currently underway to elucidate the mechanism for this suppressive effect of hypercortisolemia. Possible mechanisms include (1) a direct inhibition at the pituitary level of GH release, or (2) decreased GRF production or release by the hypothalamus, leading to "unprimed" somatotropes which are unresponsive to this dose of exogenous GRF.

1770 GROWTH HORMONE (GH) RESPONSE TO SYSTEMIC THYROTROPIN-RELEASING HORMONE (TRH) AND GH-RELEASING FACTOR (GRF) ADMINISTRATION IN RATS: EFFECT OF HYPOTHYROIDISM AND THYROID HORMONE REPLACEMENT. P.C. Ruestow*, D.E. Kramer and M. Szabo, Michael Reese Hospital and the University of Chicago, Chicago, IL 60616, USA

Whereas TRH exerts a direct stimulatory effect on GH release in cultured adenohypophyseal cells of chronically hypothyroid but not euthyroid rats, the GH response to GRF is unaffected by thyroid status. We have now explored the influence of thyroid status *in vivo*. Hypothyroidism was induced by surgical thyroidectomy followed by 131-I injection. Thyroid hormone replacement was by daily ip injection of T_4 (20 μg/kg). Secretagogues were injected into the carotid artery of urethane-anesthetized rats; blood samples were collected at 0, 2, 5, 10, and 20 min. In euthyroid rats, 1 μg/kg TRH caused a small, transient stimulation of plasma GH. The plasma GH response to 5 μg/kg GRF was significantly greater and more prolonged. Chronic hypothyroidism (9 weeks) suppressed basal plasma GH, abolished the GH response to both TRH and GRF and markedly depleted intrapituitary GH. T_4 replacement partially restored intrapituitary GH and significantly enhanced the GH response to TRH but not to GRF to above that of euthyroid rats. The stimulatory effect of T_4 replacement on the GH response to TRH was maximal at 2 days. Longer replacement progressively suppressed the response to below that of euthyroid rats. The minimal duration of hypothyroidism required to sensitize the somatotroph to TRH was 6 weeks, with 8 or more weeks being optimal. We conclude that chronic hypothyroidism selectively sensitizes the somatotroph to TRH and that short-term thyroid hormone replacement is needed to replete a readily releasable pool of GH and allow the expression of an enhanced GH secretory response to TRH.

1771 INTRACISTERNALLY INJECTED TRH INDUCES STIMULATION OF GASTRIC SECRETION. ROLE OF BRAIN CATECHOLAMINES. D. Lesiège*, R. Collu, Y. Taché, Pediatric Research Center, hospital Ste Justine, Québec, H3T 1C5, Canada.

Intracisternal (ic) administration of Thyrotropin-Releasing Hormone (TRH) elicited a dose-dependent stimulation of gastric acid secretion which is vagal dependent (Nature 287; 149, 1980). Studies were carried out, in pylorus-ligated rats, to further elucidate neural pathways through which TRH (5 µg, ic) exerts its gastric stimulatory action. Pharmacologic manipulations designed to block dopaminergic, serotoninergic, GABAergic or peripheral catecholaminergic receptors using respectively haloperidol (25 µg, ic), combined treatment with 5,6-dihydroxytryptamine (50 µg, ic) and p-chlorophenylalanine (316 mg/Kg, ip), bicuculline (1 mg/Kg, sc) or guanethidine (40 mg/Kg, ip, 5 days a week, during 5 weeks) in adrenalectomized rats, did not modify the increase in gastric output induced by intracisternal TRH. Spinal cord transection or hypophysectomy did not alter this effect either. Depletion of brain catecholamines by the combined treatment with 6-OH-dopamine (400 µg, twice in 48 h) and α-methyl tyrosine (250 mg/Kg, ip, 18 and 4 h before experiment) totally abolished the secretagogue action of intracisternally administered TRH. These results indicate that TRH action on gastric secretion requires the integrity of brain catecholamine pathways.

1772 INTRA-HYPOTHALAMIC 5,7-DHT AND N. RAPHE TRANSPLANT EFFECTS ON SEXUAL BEHAVIOR: CORRELATION WITH SEROTONIN LEVELS IN THE HYPOTHALAMUS V. Luine*, K. Renner, M. Frankfurt and E. Azmitia, Rockefeller University, New York, N.Y. 10021 and New York University, New York, N.Y. 10003.

Placement of 5,7-dihydroxytryptamine (5,7-DHT) into the hypothalamus of female rats results in selective loss of 5HT containing neurons and a facilitation of female sexual behavior (Brain Res. 264 : 344, 1983). The present studies have utilized HPLC techniques to measure 5HT and monoamine levels in hypothalamic nuclei from 1 to 10 weeks after 5,7-DHT. Results show that loss of 5HT in the ventromedial nucleus is correlated with presence of facilitated female sexual behavior. Facilitated behavior declines between 8 and 10 weeks after 5,7-DHT and the decline is associated with a restoration of 5HT in the ventromedial nucleus. Transplantation of fetal brain tissue rich in n. raphe cells into the hypothalamus of 5,7-DHT treated females resulted in a more rapid decline in facilitated behavior. Five weeks after 5,7-DHT treatment, females receiving transplants no longer exhibited facilitated sexual behavior. Implants of cortical tissue did not affect behavioral recovery. Measurement of monoamines showed a more rapid restoration of ventromedial hypothalamic 5HT in females receiving raphe transplants.

Results support the hypothesis that serotonergic innnervation of the ventromedial nucleus exerts tonic inhibiton on gonadal hormone induction of female sexual behavior. They also suggest that fetal n. raphe transplants can exert functional regulation over a complex, innate behavior. (Supported by NIH Grant HD12011 and NSF Grant BN579064-74).

1773 A CASE OF THE PITUITARY TUMOR WHICH COMBINED HYPERTHYROIDISM AND ACROMEGALY - TSH AND GH PRODUCING TUMOR -

A. Ishihara*, H. Nasu, M. Hieda, T. Sasho, Y. Shiokawa, H. Nogami[1], H. Ishikawa[1] and R. Ariwa[2] Dept. of Internal Medicine, Juntendo University, [1]Dept. of Anatomy, Jikei University and [2]Tokyo Metropolitan Okubo Municipal Hospital.

We have experienced a very rare case of the pituitary tumor which combined hyperthyroidism and acromegaly. The tumor was removed by Hardy's method. Microscopic and electron microscopic study of the tumor by Peroxidase Anti-Peroxidase method revealed the same cell produced Growth Hormone and Thyroid Stimulating Hormone. The case: 29 years old male complained of weightloss, fatigue, sweat, palpitation, visual disturbance and enlargement of foot. This findings diffuse goiter and hand tremor were recognized. Laboratory data of his basal values were as followed: Sugar; 81 mg/dl, IRI; 26 μU/ml, GH; 23 ng/ml, T_3; 3.6 ng/ml, T_4; 19 μg/dl, TSH; 13 μU/ml, PRL; 4.1 ng/ml and ACTH; 12 pg/ml. The findings of X ray and CT Scan of the sella turcica revealed the pituitary tumor. The tumor was removed by Hardy's method. After the operation he recovered visual sight, TSH and GH level decreased. Tumor was sliced and fixed with 1% GLA and 1% OSO_4, embed with Epon. Two ultra thin specimen facing each other were immunological stained by two different antibodies, one was stained by anti hGH and the other was stained by anti-r THSß. As for microscopic study, some cells showed positive for both antibodies, but most of cells reacted for either one of them. By electron microscope, there were no distinct structural difference among cells which reacted for both antibodies, and there were irregular cells which has few small secretary granula.

1774 STRUCTURE-ACTIVITY RELATIONSHIPS OF SEX STEROID ANALOGS DETERMINED IN VITRO IN A THYROID HORMONE-RESPONSIVE MEMBRANE Ca^{2+}-ATPase MODEL.

W.D. Lawrence*, Y. Osawa, P.J. Davis and S.D. Blas. V.A. Medical Center, SUNY at Buffalo School of Medicine and Medical Foundation of Buffalo, Buffalo, New York.

Ca^{2+}-ATPase activity of rabbit mature red blood cell membranes is stimulated in vitro by L-thyroxine (T_4, 10^{-10}M)(Endocrinology 110:297, 1982). In immature red cells (reticulocytes), nature of the T_4 response of Ca^{2+}-ATPase in vitro is sex-dependent: female retic enzyme is stimulated by T_4 (+0.129 ± 0.025 μmoles P_i/mg membrane protein/90 min vs. control, P <0.01), whereas male enzyme is inhibited by T_4 (-0.126 ± 0.026, P <0.01). In vitro incubations showed that testosterone (T, 5 x 10^{-11}M) converted female retic response to male (inhibition of Ca^{2+}-ATPase) and that 17β-estradiol (E, 5 x 10^{-11}M) converted male retic response to female (stimulation of enzyme by T_4). With this in vitro T/E retic model we analyzed structure-activity relationships of sex steroid analogs (5 x 10^{-11}M):

Female retic membranes	% T effect	Male retic membranes	% E effect
17-Epitestosterone	30	Estrone	128
17α-Methyltestosterone	22	Estriol	-19
5α-Androstan-17β-ol-3-one	28	2-Hydroxyestrone	19
5β-Androstan-17β-ol-3-one	102	DES	34
5α-Androstan-3α-ol-17-one	24		
5β-Androstan-3α-ol-17-one	112		
19-Nortestosterone	22		

In summary, T and E analogs have direct membrane effects in the rabbit retic. Critical to unusual pattern of T effect are 5β and Δ^4-3-ketone non-planar ring conformations. Equally important are side group constituents at C-17, C-19. E analog activities are similar to those in other systems.

1775 DOSE-RESPONSE CHARACTERISTICS OF VARIOUS PEPTIDES WITH GROWTH HORMONE (GH)-RELEASING ACTIVITY IN THE UNANESTHESIZED MALE RAT. W.J. Millard, G.F. McCormick*, T.M. Badger, C.Y. Bowers, J.B. Martin. Departments of Neurology and Gynecology, Massachusetts General Hospital, Vincent Research Laboratories, Boston, MA 02114.

We have recently shown that human pancreatic growth hormone-releasing factor 1-44 (hpGRF-44) and growth hormone-releasing peptide (GHRP), a synthetic cyclic hexapeptide, elicited linear increases in GH secretion in vitro using a pituitary perifusion system. In the present study we investigated the dose-response characteristics of hpGRF-40, hpGRF-44, rat hypothalamic GRF-43 (rhGRF-43), and GHRP in vivo. To assure stability in basal GH secretion, eliminate spontaneous GH pulses, and minimize interference of endogenous somatostatin, unanesthesized, chronically-cannulated male rats were pretreated with diethyldithiocarbamate (400 mg/kg) and anti-somatostatin serum. GRF doses from 10 ng/kg to 5 ug/kg were given iv in random order at 1.5 hour intervals. GHRP was administered in doses of 100 ng/kg to 50 ug/kg. The plot of $\log_{10}$ dose vs peak area was linear for all releasing factors. The maximum peak height was reached at the 500 ng/kg dose for hpGRF-40, hpGRF-44, and rhGRF-43, with larger doses only broadening the peak. The minimum dose of GHRP needed to stimulate GH secretion was a hundred-fold higher than the other releasing factors. The GRF activity was comparable to that previously reported for animals pretreated with monclonal anti-GRF and anti-somatostatin serum. This model appears useful for investigating the pituitary actions of GRF in vivo. Supported by NIH grants AM 26252 and HD 17364.

1776 STRUCTURAL DETERMINATION OF THE SECOND GONADOTROPIN-RELEASING HORMONE IN CHICKEN HYPOTHALAMUS (CHICKEN GnRH-II). K. Miyamoto*, Y. Hasegawa, M. Igarashi, Department of Obstetrics and Gynecology, Gunma University, School of Medicine, Maebashi, Gunma 371, Japan, and K. Kangawa, and H. Matsuo, Department of Biochemistry, Miyazaki Medical College, Kiyotake, Miyazaki 889-16, Japan

A new peptide having gonadotropin-releasing activity distinct from the known luteinizing hormone-releasing hormones (LH-RH's) has been identified in a chicken hypothalamic extract. The existence of $[Gln^8]$-LH-RH in avian hypothalamus has independently been reported by our group and by King and Millar. The new molecular species of gonadotropin-releasing activity, named chicken gonadotropin-releasing hormone II (chicken GnRH-II), has recently been isolated in a yield of 7 μg starting from 10,000 chicken hypothalami. Structural analyses have been performed on the peptide fragments derived from chymotryptic and thermolytic digests of chicken GnRH-II by amino acid analyses as well as terminal analyses. The full sequence of chicken GnRH-II has been determined to be; pGlu-His-Trp-Ser-His-Gly-Trp-Tyr-Pro-Gly-NH_2.

A synthetic decapeptide with the above sequence was verified to be chromatographically identical to natural chicken GnRH-II. For further structural confirmation, chymotryptic and thermolytic peptides from synthetic and natural chicken GnRH-II were also identified. Thus, the structure of chicken GnRH-II has been definitely established. The gonadtropin-releasing potency of chicken GnRH-II was about 32% of that of mammalian LH-RH and 8 times more potent than chicken LH-RH.

1777 TRH CHANGES HETEROGENEOUS COMPONENTS OF GLYCOSYLATED TSH, BUT NOT ITS QUANTITIES, WITHIN THE RAT ANTERIOR PITUITARIES. M. Mori*, M. Murakami, H. Ishihara, Y. Shimomura, I. Kobayashi, S. Kobayashi and K. Wakabayashi, Division of Endocrinology, First Department of Medicine, Institute of Endocrinology, Gunma University, School of Medicine, Maebashi 371, Japan

Information on the role of TRH in TSH biosynthesis associated with glycosylation is still limited. We explored effects of TRH on heterogeneity of glycosylated TSH during de novo biosynthesis in rat anterior pituitaries (APs). Contents of cold TSH measured by RIA and radioactivities of ^{3}H-Glucosamine (Glc)-relating TSH determined by using an anti-TSH serum in APs and media were increased progressively with the incubation time (1, 3 and 6 h). In media, these values were greater in the presence of 10 ng/ml TRH than in its absence, whereas TRH did not cause any change in radioactivities of Glc incorporated into TSH in APs. Amounts of cold TSH and of Glc-relating TSH were increased in media in the dose-dependent manner of TRH (0, 1, 10 and 100 ng/ml), but these values were not changed in APs. Analysis of extracts from APs on isoelectric focusing showed that APs were composed of four component peaks (isoelectric point (pI) 2.5, 5.3, 7.8 and 8.7) of Glc incorporated into TSH, and addition of TRH caused an appearance of new components (pI 6.5 and 7.2) associated with a slightly decreased amounts of pI 5.3-peak. These observations indicate that TRH did not elicit an accumulation of glycosylated TSH, but changed its heterogeneous components within APs, which were assumed to be glycosylated forms ready to be secreted under the increasing TSH biosynthesis induced by TRH.

1778 IMMUNOCYTOCHEMICAL LOCALIZATION OF CORTICOTROPIN-RELEASING FACTOR (CRF) AND GROWTH HORMONE-RELEASING FACTOR (GRF) IN THE HUMAN HYPOTHALAMUS. T. MOURI, O. MURAKAMI*, A. SASAKI, K. YOSHINAGA, N. ANDO, N. SASANAO, T. SUDA and Y. TAKEI, 2nd Dept. of Int. Med., 2nd Dept. of Pathol., Tohoku Univ. Sch. Med., Sendai, Dept. of Int. Med., Tokyo Women's Medical College, Tokyo and Dept. of Pathol. Lab. Med., Emory Univ. Sch. Med., Atlanta, GA.

CRF and GRF immunoreactivity in the human hypothalamic cells was demonstrated by immunocytochemical technique. Brain tissues of coronal section including the hypothalamus were obtained at autopsy, fixed with 10% formalin and made into paraffin sections. The peroxidase-antiperoxidase methods were performed using anti-ovine CRF(1-41), anti-rat CRF(1-41) and anti-human pancreas GRF(1-44) antiserum. In 6 out of 18 cases without steroid treatment, the CRF immunoreactivity was confirmed in the parvocellular cells of the paraventricular nucleus (PVN), but not in the magnocellular cells. In the supraoptic nucleus (SON), no reactivity was detected. Immunoreactive CRF nerve fibers were found in the perivascular space in the pituitary stalk. On the other hand, GRF immunoreactivity was confirmed in the nerve cells of the infundibular nucleus (IFN), but not in PVN nor SON. This study indicates that, in human, CRF regulating ACTH secretion is produced in the parvocellular perikarya in PVN and GRF regulating GH secretion is produced in the perikarya in IFN.

1779 THE EFFECTS OF CORTICOTROPIN-RELEASING FACTOR ON CARDIOVASCULAR SYSTEM IN MAN. M. Nakahara*, T. Shibasaki, A. Masuda, T. Imaki, T. Takemiya, F. Kurimoto[1)], H. Sakurai[1)], H. Demura, K. Shizume and N. Ling[2)]. Department of Medicine, Tokyo Women's Medical College, Tokyo 162, Japan, [1)]Mitsubishi Yuka Laboratory of Medical Science Company, Tokyo, [2)]Laboratories for Neuroendocrinology, The Salk Institute, La Jolla, CA 92037, U.S.A.

In order to investigate the effects of corticotropin-releasing factor (CRF) on cardiovascular system, blood pressure, heart rate and finger plethysmogram were recorded and concentrations of plasma catecholamines and ADH were measured in six healthy young males who were intravenously given 500 µg synthetic ovine CRF. Four of six subjects felt cold sensation on hands within 2 min after CRF injection, which lasted 15 min. Transient decline in brachial arterial blood pressure was observed within the first 15 min in three volunteers. The amplitude of a forefinger plethysmogram was suddenly decreased by about 60 % of basal value within 60 seconds after CRF injection and gradually recovered at 15-30 min. This change in finger plethysmogram was dose-dependent. Furthermore, the fall of skin temperature by more than 3 C in hand fingers was found in thermogram. Plasma catecholamines increased at 15-30 min after CRF injection but each value stayed almost in normal ranges. Plasma ADH increased at 10-30 min after CRF injection, especially in subjects who showed severe degree of hypotention. These results indicated that cold sensation on fingers was due to constiriction of small arteries in fingers. Since the decreases of amplitude in finger plethysmogram were observed in all the subjects regardless of degree of changes in blood pressure, CRF might act directly on small peripheral arteries.

1780 GONADOTROPIN RELEASING HORMONE STIMULATES PHOSPHATIDYLINOSITOL TURNOVER IN CULTURED PITUITARY CELLS. Z. Naor, J. Molcho and H. Zakut, Department of Hormone Research, The Weizmann Institute of Science, Rehovot 76100, Israel

This report describes the effect of gonadotropin-releasing hormone (GnRH) on phospholipid (PL) metabolism in cultured rat pituitary cells. The cells were incubated with $[^{32}P]Pi$ to label endogenous PL (10-60 min) and then stimulated with GnRH for up to 60 min. Cellular PL were separated by two-dimensional thin layer chromatography and the radioactivity was determined. Phosphatidylinositol (PI), a minor constituent of cellular PL, was the major labeled PL accounting for 45% of the total radioactivity. On the other hand, the major cellular PL, namely phosphatidylcholine (PC) was labeled only to a maximum of 32% of the total radioactivity. The remaining labeling was distributed among phosphatidylethanolamine (4.2%), cardiolipin (3.4%), phosphatidic acid (PA, 2.5%), and phosphatidylserine (1.8%). GnRH increased ^{32}P labeling of PA and PI significantly at 1 and 5 min of incubation respectively (2 fold). Labeling of other PL was not affected by GnRH treatment. The half-maximal stimulating dose (ED_{50}) for PI labeling and LH release was 0.75 and 0.5 nM respectively and the stimulatory effect was blocked by the potent GnRH antagonist [D-pGlu^{1},pclPhe^{2},D- Trp^{3,6}]GnRH. GnRH stimulated PA and PI labeling could not be demonstrated after 1 and 45 min of incubation respectively or when the prelabeling was conducted for 60 min rather than 10 min. These results suggest heterogeneous compartmentalization of gonadotroph PA and PI pools and indicate that increased PI-PA turnover might be a transducing signal in the early events that follow gonadotroph GnRH-receptor activation.

1781 INVOLVEMENT OF HYPOTHALAMIC VASOACTIVE INTESTINAL POLYPEPTIDE (VIP) IN PROLACTIN (PRL) SECRETION BY SEROTONIN IN THE RAT.
H. Ohta*, Y. Kato, A. Shimatsu, K. Tojo, Y. Kabayama, T. Inoue, N. Yanaihara and H. Imura, Second Medical Clinic, Department of Medicine, Kyoto University Faculty of Medicine, Kyoto, and Bioorganic Chemistry, Shizuoka College of Pharmacy, Shizuoka, Japan.

It is well known that PRL secretion is stimulated by serotonergic agents such as serotonin (5HT) and a precursor, 5HTP. We have reported that both 5HT and 5HTP raises plasma VIP levels in the hypophysial portal blood and that 5HT stimulates VIP release from the hypothalamus in vitro. Since VIP can stimulates PRL release by acting directly at the pituitary, PRL release induced by the serotonergic mechanisms may be mediated by hypothalamic VIP. In the present study, we further examined by the passive immunization method the role of hypothalamic VIP in 5HT-induced PRL secretion in urethane-anesthetized male rats. Three anti-VIP were generated in rabbits against VIP-PVP mixture (R501, R502) and VIP-bovine thyroglobulin conjugate (KRV-1). Kd and Bmax were 4.9×10^{-12}M and 0.8nmol/ml (R501), 7.7×10^{-12}M and 0.9nmol/ml (R502), and 2.4×10^{-10}M and 7.2nmol/ml (KRV-1), respectively. Normal rabbit serum was used in controls. PRL release induced by 1-5HTP (5mg/100g BW iv) was blunted by anti-VIP (KRV-1 0.5ml/rat iv)(peak plasma PRL; 208±38ng/ml vs 454±72ng/ml, $p<0.05$). 5HT (10μg/rat icv)-induced PRL release was also blunted by anti-VIP (R501, 10μl/rat icv)(24±7 vs 85±10ng/ml, $p<0.05$). When anti-VIP (R502) was infused into a single hypophysial portal vessel at a rate of 2μl/min, 5HT (10μg/rat icv)-induced PRL release was blunted (55±16 vs 119±20ng/ml, $p<0.05$). These findings indicate that PRL secretion induced by serotonergic stimulation may be mediated by hypothalamic VIP release into the hypophysial portal blood in the rat.

1782 ROLE OF GROWTH HORMONE-RELEASING FACTOR (GRF) ON GROWTH HORMONE RELEASE BY IMMUNONEUTRALIZATION OF ENDOGENOUS SOMATOSTATIN IN THE RAT.
M. Ono*, N. Miki and K. Shizume, Dept. of Medicine, Tokyo Women's Medical College, Tokyo 162, Japan.

The method of passive immunization with anti-somatostatin (SRIF) serum has widely been used to study the role of endogenous SRIF in growth hormone (GH) secretion. Anti-SRIF serum (ASS) administration in vivo has been reported to produce a rapid and transient elevation of plasma GH in rats. The present studies were performed to examine whether GH-releasing factor (GRF) is involved in GH release by ASS. The experiments were done under urethane anesthesia using adult male rats implanted with chronic right atrial cannulae. An anti-rat GRF serum (AGRF) was raised in rabbit by injecting a synthetic rat GRF coupled to bovine thyroglobulin by glutaraldehyde. This antiserum could bind 30 % of ^{125}I-rat GRF at final dilution of 1:120000, and immunoneutralized 5 μg synthetic rat GRF to stimulate GH release in vivo at a dose of 1 ml/rat. Intravenous injection of goat ASS (1 ml) produced a rapid increase in plasma GH with a peak value of 321.7 ± 75.7 ng/ml at 15 min post-injection. Passive immunization with AGRF (1 ml) inhibited plasma GH response to ASS by 67 % ($p< 0.01$). However, the peak GH value of AGRF treated rats was significantly higher than that of control given normal rabbit and goat sera ($p< 0.001$). In the next study, effects of various amounts of AGRF on GH release by ASS were examined. AGRF suppressed ASS-induced GH release in a dose-related fashion with a maximum (~70 %) inhibition being observed after administering 0.25 to 1.0 ml of AGRF. These results indicate that GH release by immunoneutralization of endogenous SRIF is mediated largely via endogenous GRF in the rat.

1783 ULTRASHORT-LOOP POSITIVE FEEDBACK OF CORTICOTROPIN-RELEASING FACTOR (CRF) TO ENHANCE ACTH RELEASE IN STRESS.

N. Ono*, J. Bedran-De Castro, and S.M. McCann, Univ of Texas Hlth Sci Ctr, Physiology Dept, Dallas, Texas 75235.

In our previous experiments we have shown that intraventricular (3rd ventricular, 3V) injection of ovine (o)CRF in freely moving, ovariectomized rats evoked a significant, dose-related increase in plasma ACTH, with a minimal effective dose of 50 ng. The higher doses of oCRF were associated with a decline in plasma GH and LH suggesting a hypothalamic action to inhibit the release of these hormones. The stimulation of ACTH release was thought to be via a pituitary action after uptake via portal vessels. To determine if CRF might have any action to alter its own release in stress, the dose of oCRF was reduced and it was injected into the 3V of freely moving, ovariectomized animals 5 min prior to application of ether stress. No significant change in plasma ACTH occurred following administration of oCRF in doses of 500 pg or less. The amplitude of the increase in ACTH following application of ether stress at 2 and 5 min was enhanced by the prior injection of oCRF at doses of 500, 150, or 50 pg. The enhancement was statistically significant at 2 ($p<.025$) and 5 ($p<.05$) min after injection of the 150 pg dose. The results suggest that CRF may have a positive ultrashort-loop feedback action to enhance stress-induced ACTH release. (Supported by PHS grants AM 10073 and HD 09988).

1784 RESPONSES TO CORTICOTROPIN-RELEASING HORMONE (CRH) IN CUSHING'S AND NELSON'S SYNDROMES.

D. Orth*, G. DeCherney, C. DeBold, W. Sheldon, R. Jackson; A. Atkinson, D. Hadden, L. Kennedy; M. Chretien, F. Gilbert; D. Krieger, S. Roman, G. Rothman; and D. Cook. Vanderbilt Med. Ctr., Nashville, TN, USA; Royal Victoria Hosp., Belfast, N. Ireland; Clinical Res. Inst., Montreal, P.Q., Canada; Mt. Sinai Med. Ctr., New York, NY, USA; Oregon Health Sci. Univ., Portland, OR, USA.

We measured basal plasma ACTH (pg/ml) and cortisol (F) (µg/dl) levels and increments (Δ) at -15, 0, 5, 10, 15, 30, 60, 90 and 120 min after iv oCRH (J. Rivier, W. Vale) 1 µg/kg body wt in patients with active or treated Cushing's syndrome or with Nelson's syndrome. All ACTH and most F RIAs were performed on unextracted EDTA-plasma at VMC. Results [range (mean ± SEM)] in active disease were:

Etiology	n	Basal ACTH	ΔACTH	Basal F	ΔF
Pituitary	21	9-280(44±12)	3-430(106±26)	7-30(16±1.2)	3-35(17±2.3)
Adrenal	2	< 10, < 10	0,0	6.2, 32	1.1, 3.0
Ectopic	2	210, 185	10,-35	24,45	3.0, -7.1
Nelson's	5	1.2-29K(7.7±5.4K)	4.4-36K(32±26K)	2.7-6.6	-1.5-0.7

Variable responses in pituitary Cushing's did not correlate with basal F ($r=0.3990$, $p>0.05$), but lowering F with metyrapone increased ΔACTH 3- and 13-fold in 2 patients preop and giving only 10 mg F 8 h before oCRH blocked ACTH response postop. Nelson's ΔACTH was great, but % rise was normal. Four pituitary Cushing's cured by irradiation had normal response by 1 yr; 3 not cured hyperresponded. Eight pituitary Cushing's cured by microadenomectomy had normal response by 1 yr, 1 had a hypo- and 1 a hyperresponse, and 2 of 3 requiring steroids 0.3-5 yr postop had normal ΔACTH. CRH may be useful in diagnosis of Cushing's etiology and in evaluating hypothalamic-pituitary functional abnormalities after treatment.

1785 UTILIZATION OF THE SYNTHETIC SUBSTRATE LEUCINE-P-NITROANILIDE TO INVESTIGATE A POSSIBLE PHYSIOLOGICAL ROLE OF LHRH INACTIVATING ACTIVITY; VALIDATION BY HPLC AND SEPHADEX ISOELECTRIC FOCUSING. J.O'Conner* and C. Lapp, Department of Endocrinology, Medical College of Georgia, Augusta, GA 30912.

LHRH inactivation in the hypothalamus and pituitary is of interest as a potential site of modulation of ovulation. The present studies monitored LHRH inactivating activity through the estrous cycle with particular attention to the proestrous LH surge. Hypothalami and pituitaries from cycled rats were homogenized in 0.05 M Tris-HCl (pH 7.4), centrifuged 10,000 x g 1 h and the supernatant used as enzyme source. The activity was monitored utilizing the synthetic peptidase substrate leucine-p-nitroanilide (Leu-p-NA) which was validated by several methods. Initially, kinetic studies utilizing this crude supernatant indicated that LHRH would inhibit degradation of the synthetic substrate when both were present in the 37-280 µM range. In subsequent experiments, inactivating activity toward LHRH (as indicated by the formation of peptide fragments detectable on PAGE and HPLC) and the synthetic substrate co-fractionated on the basis of molecular sieving (Sephadex G-200), isoelectric point (Sephadex IEF) and charge/size (PAGE). The proestrous LH surge was accompanied by the highest hypothalamic and blood levels of LHRH seen during the cycle. Immediately previous to and accompanying the surge, inactivating activity in the hypothalamus and pituitary evidenced a significant decrease. Simultaneously, E_2 was elevated and P_4 was decreased. As the LH surge terminated, hypothalamic and blood LHRH levels decreased, hypothalamic and pituitary enzyme activity resumed, while E_2 levels decreased and P_4 levels increased. The results suggest facilitation of the surge by an inverse relationship between LHRH levels and inactivating activity, possibly modulated by gonadal steroids. Supported by NIH HD16433.

1786 **GLUCOCORTICOIDS INHIBIT SOMATOSTATIN PRODUCTION AND LOWER SRIH mRNA LEVELS IN CULTURED HUMAN C-CELLS.** W.N. Palmer*, R.F. Gagel, K. Leonhart, and S.S. Leong, The Baylor College of Medicine and the Veterans Administration Medical Center, Houston, TX 77211 and Roswell Park Memorial Institute, Buffalo, NY 14263, USA.

Somatostatin (SRIH) production by normal rat and rabbit C-cells has been demonstrated, but evidence for its production by normal human C-cells has been lacking. The TT cells, a model of the human C-cell derived from a malignant tumor, produce large amounts of calcitonin. We have now, in addition, demonstrated production of large amounts of SRIH by these cells using four techniques. First, immunoreactive SRIH (iSRIH) was demonstrated in cells (2-12 ng/million cells) and growth medium (3-10 ng/million cells/48 hours) by a specific radioimmunoassay. Second, gel filtration of cell extracts, under denaturing conditions, revealed two peaks of iSRIH with the smaller-sized peak eluting in a position similar to that of somatostatin-14. Third, messenger RNA (mRNA) from TT cells, but not from a variety of other cell lines, hybridized to a specific bovine SRIH complementary DNA probe (provided by L. Chan and G. Saunders). Fourth, translation of mRNA isolated from TT cells in a reticulocyte lysate system, followed by immunoprecipitation with anti-SRIH and gel electrophoresis, showed a single protein band with a MW of 13.7K. Treatment of the TT cells with dexamethasone resulted in a dose- and time-related decrease (10-50% of basal) in cell and medium iSRIH and SRIH mRNA content; cell growth was also inhibited. A maximal effect on cell growth and SRIH production (corrected for cell number) was observed at a dexamethasone concentration of 10^{-7} M with a half-maximal effect between 10^{-8} and 10^{-9} M; the effect was maximal by four days of treatment. These results demonstrate SRIH production by a continuous line of human C-cells which can be regulated by glucocorticoids.

1787 HUMAN PANCREATIC GROWTH HORMONE RELEASING FACTOR (hpGRF) IN TELEOST BRAIN AND PITUITARY: MULTIPLE MOLECULAR FORMS AND TWO DISTINCT NEURONAL SYSTEMS

JX Pan*, R Lechan, HD Lin, S Reichlin and IMD Jackson, Division of Endocrinology, Tufts-New England Medical Center, Boston, MA 02111

To determine whether hpGRF was present in teleost brain, we assayed 1N HAc codfish brain extracts and studied the immunohistochemical distribution in the hypothalamic-pituitary complex using 2 antisera, one directed against the C-terminus of hpGRF$_{1-44}$NH$_2$ (raised in this laboratory), the other recognizing the mid portion of hpGRF$_{1-40}$OH (gift of Drs. W Vale and J Rivier). On Sephadex G-25, 3 peaks of teleost (t) GRF$_{1-44}$NH$_2$ were identified, a large (A), an intermediate (B) and a small (C). Peak B behaves similar to synthetic hpGRF$_{1-44}$NH$_2$ on exclusion chromatography (Sephadex G-50, Biogel P-10) and C$_{18}$ u-Bondapak HPLC (CH_3CN/HFBA) while peaks A and C do not. Only peak B is reactive with anti-GRF$_{1-40}$OH. All three peaks were at least as active in releasing GH from a rat pituitary monolayer culture as synthetic hpGRF $_{1-44}$NH$_2$. Topographically distinct, peptide specific neuronal systems were immunostained. The one directed against hpGRF$_{1-44}$NH$_2$ stained cell bodies in the rostral pars distalis exclusively with cytoplasmic processes adjacent to capillaries. The other immunoreactive with hpGRF$_{1-40}$OH revealed parvocellular and magnocellular neuronal cell bodies in the preoptic area of the hypothalamus and gave rise to axons which projected toward the median eminence. Axons entered the pituitary gland and were concentrated primarily in pars nervosa tissue. Axons also entered the proximal pars distalis but not the rostral pars distalis or intermediate lobe. These findings document in fish brain-pituitary 2 distinct neuronal GRF systems, a GRF with similarities to hpGRF$_{1-44}$NH$_2$, and at least 2 additional molecular forms of GRF, and possibly a third.

1788 Corticotropin-Releasing Factor (CRF) Action Involves Cyclic AMP-Dependent Protein Phosphorylation.

R. Pasmantier*, N. Fleischer and U.K. Schubart, Albert Einstein College of Medicine, Bronx, New York

The available evidence suggests that corticotropin-releasing factor (CRF) stimulates ACTH release from the pituitary via a mechanism involving cAMP. In order to identify cAMP-stimulated phosphoproteins that may mediate this effect of CRF, phosphoproteins of AtT-20 mouse pituitary tumor cells were analyzed in $^{32}PO_4$-labeled cells exposed to CRF or other secretagogues. The cellular phosphoproteins were resolved by two-dimensional electrophoresis, visualized by autoradiography and analyzed by computer-assisted densitometry. ACTH release and cAMP formation were measured in parallel incubations. At 30 nM CRF, a concentration at which ACTH release was maximally stimulated (three-fold) and cAMP levels were raised two-fold, two closely migrating 16,000 dalton peptides (isoelectric pH 5.6 and 5.3, respectively) showed ^{32}P-labeling that was 160% and 140% respectively greater than in control cells. When the phosphodiesterase inhibitor isobutyl methylxanthine (0.5 mM) was added with CRF, there was an additional 20-fold rise in cAMP while ACTH release and phosphorylation of the two 16,000 dalton peptides showed only minor additional increases. The effects of CRF on ACTH release, cAMP generation and protein phosphorylation were mimicked by other agents known to raise cellular cAMP levels including isoproterenol (10 μM), 8-bromo-cAMP (2.5 mM) and forskolin (0.1 mM). In contrast, 40 mM K^+-induced ACTH release was not accompanied by changes in cAMP or in the phosphorylation of the two 16,000 dalton peptides. The data suggest that the mechanism of CRF-induced ACTH release involves cAMP-dependent protein phosphorylation.

1789 CYSTEAMINE (CSH) INDUCES A LOSS OF SOMATOSTATIN-28 (S-28) WHEN MEASURED AS $S\text{-}28_{(15-28)}$ LIKE IMMUNOREACTIVITY (LI) BUT NOT WHEN ASSESSED AS $S\text{-}28_{(1-14)}$ LI:EVIDENCE THAT THE DISULPHIDE BOND IS IMPORTANT FOR CSH ACTION.

Y.C. Patel* and I. Pierzchala, Fraser Labs, McGill University, Royal Victoria Hospital, Montreal, Quebec H3A 1A1.

It has been proposed previously that CSH "depletes" tissue somatostatin -14 (S-14) but not S-28 when both molecules are assayed by specific RIAs (Bakhit, Reg. Peptides 6:169,1983). Since S-28 can be monitored both as $S\text{-}28_{(1-14)}$ LI and as $S\text{-}28_{(15-28)}$ LI, we have compared the effects of CSH on the concentrations of the two immunoreactivities in a tissue rich in S-28, the jejunum (JEJ). Acetic acid extracts of JEJ were prepared from rats 4 h after a single s.c. injection of saline or CSH (300 mg/kg). $S\text{-}28_{(1-14)}$ LI was measured by RIA using antibody R22 directed towards the 1-14 region of S-28 which recognizes S-28 but not S-14 or $S\text{-}28_{(1-12)}$. $S\text{-}28_{(15-28)}$ LI was measured by antibody R149 directed towards the ring segment of S-28 which detects S-28 and S-14 equally. JEJ $S\text{-}28_{(15-28)}$ LI was reduced from 0.8 ± 0.05 to 0.21 ± 0.03 pmol/mg protein ($P < 0.01$). By Sephadex G-50 chromatography (in 6 M urea) 55-60% of $S\text{-}28_{(15-28)}$ LI coeluted with synthetic S-28 (Mr=3.1K) and 30% with S-14 (Mr=1.6K), the relative proportions of the two forms remaining unchanged following CSH. By contrast, JEJ S-28 monitored as $S\text{-}28_{(1-14)}$ LI was unaltered after CSH (1.5 ± 0.07 pmol/mg vs 1.3 ± 0.06). On G-50 columns > 65% of $S\text{-}28_{(1-14)}$ LI before and after CSH consisted of a peak of Mr=3.1K the remainder being a higher m.w. form. These data suggest that CSH acts on the 15-28 segment of the S-28 molecule and renders it non-immunoreactive probably through disruption of the disulphide bond. This mechanism probably also accounts for CSH-induced S-14 loss.

1790 MEASUREMENT AND CHARACTERISATION OF GH-RELEASING FACTOR IN HUMAN PLASMA.

Elizabeth S. Penny*, Erica Penman, A.M. Sopwith, Janet Price, J.A.H. Wass, N. Lytras, G.M. Besser and Lesley H. Rees, Departments of Chemical Endocrinology and Endocrinology, St. Bartholomew's Hospital, London, U.K.

Two human pancreatic tumour growth hormone-releasing factors (hpGRF-40 and hpGRF-44) have recently been isolated and their sequences determined. However to our knowledge there are no reports of the characterisation of GRF in human plasma. Therefore we have recently developed a specific RIA for GRF in human plasma. hpGRF-40 (Bachem) was used for both standard and tracer. It was iodinated using chloramine-T and purified on ODS silica with a 1-propanol/1%TFA gradient. The antiserum was raised using synthetic hpGRF-40 (a gift of Dr. David Coy) and is directed against the central region of the molecule, cross-reacting on an approximately equimolar basis with hpGRF-40 and hpGRF-44. Plasma samples were extracted onto Vycor glass prior to RIA. Immunoreactive GRF (IRGRF), measured at 9am after an overnight fast in 37 normal subjects ranged from <10-60pg/ml (mean=21pg/ml). A 32 year old woman with a carcinoid tumour of the lung and widespread metastases, who became clinically acromegalic after the primary tumour had been resected, had a plasma IRGRF level of 25,000pg/ml. Her growth hormone level at this time was 42mU/l, and plasma immunoreactive somatostatin was normal. To further characterise the IRGRF, G50 gel filtration chromatography of plasma from this patient was carried out under acid dissociating conditions. A single peak of immunoreactivity was seen coeluting with hpGRF-40. In conclusion, we report for the first time: 1) measurement of IRGRF in normal human plasma, 2) characterisation of IRGRF in plasma from a patient with a GRF secreting tumour.

1791 GROWTH HORMONE-RELEASING FACTOR (GRF) THERAPY OF GROWTH HORMONE DEFICIENCY: MEASUREMENT OF ANTIBODIES TO GRF BY ENZYME-LINKED IMMUNOSORBANT (ELISA) TECHNIQUES. O.H. Pescovitz, W.E. Nixon, M.C. Gelato, M. Pescovitz, D.L. Loriaux, and G.R. Merriam*. DEB, NICHD, NIH, Bethesda, Md. USA 20205.

We have recently shown that repeated administration of GRF can accelerate linear growth in growth hormone deficient (GHD) children. GRF and its analogs may thus become useful therapeutic agents. It is possible, however, that chronic GRF treatment might induce neutralizing antibodies, which would limit its effectiveness and could potentially reduce growth if used in non-GHD children. To screen for this possibility, we developed an ELISA binding assay for anti-GRF antibodies. Plasma samples were obtained from 11 adult normal volunteers and 8 GHD patients prior to and 3wks-10 months following single or multiple iv or subcutaneous doses of GRF 1-44NH_2 (GRF-44). GRF-44 was adsorbed to microtiter plates and incubated with serial dilutions of patient plasma. Sera from rabbits and mice which had been immunized with a GRF-BSA conjugate in complete Freund's adjuvant were used as positive controls. Species-specific peroxidase-conjugated second antibodies were used in the presence of orthophenyldiamine substrate to detect GRF-binding antibodies colorimetrically. Sera from immunized mice and rabbits had binding titers up to 1:12,800. No increased binding, however, was detected in any post-injection human samples, though there was some low-titer (<1:32) nonspecific binding present both prior to and after GRF administration. We conclude that ELISA techniques are a convenient and rapid means of screening for GRF antibodies; and that no subject developed such antibodies. This suggests that GRF-44, like other releasing factors, is of low immunogenicity and may be safe for chronic therapeutic trials.

1792 HUMAN CHORIONIC GONADOTROPIN (HCG) STIMULATES GONADOTROPIN-RELEASING HORMONE (GnRH) SECRETION IN PERIFUSED RAT HYPOTHALAMI. D.G.Pfeiffer*, O.F.X.Almeida, G.R.Merriam and D.L.Loriaux, Developmental Endocrinology Branch, NICHD, Bethesda, MD 20205, U.S.A.

It has been shown recently that, while basal Gonadotropin-Releasing Hormone (GnRH) secretion does not differ during the rat estrous cycle, the GnRH response of perifused hypothalami to stimulation with KCl is differential and greatest in proestrus. Since differential response to stimulation may be caused by hormonal changes such as changes in steroids or gonadotropins, we have studied the effects of estradiol (E_2) and Human Chorionoc Gonadotropin (HCG) on the secretion of GnRH by the perifused rat hypothalamus. The effects of E_2 on GnRH secretion were tested in hypothalami obtained from ovariectomized (ovx) or hypophysectomized (hpx) Sprague-Dawley rats. After 2hrs of preincubation, different doses of E_2 (ranging from 10^{-8} to $3x10^{-3}$M) in ethanol were injected into the perifusion chamber. For reasons of solubility the ethanol concentration had to be increased (to 2.5%)in the higher dose ranges. No effect of E_2 was observed at lower doses; only some of the hypothalami treated with very high doses showed a varying increase in GnRH. This increase was caused by the vehicle (ethanol) rather than the E_2 and we were able to show a dose dependent release of GnRH by ethanol. Effects of HCG on GnRH secretion were tested by injecting different doses of the highly purified material (batch CR-121) into perifusion chambers containing hypothalami from either ovx, hpx or hpx and with Human Menopausal Gonadotropin (HMG) primed animals. After HCG significant increases in GnRH secretion were observed in hpx (3 fold) and in shortterm (2-7d) ovx animals (10 fold). No HCG effects were found in longterm ovx (3 weeks) and in hpx, HMG primed animals. Thus, HCG but not E_2can stimulate GnRH secretion by the perifused rat hypothalamus.

1793 ACTION SITES OF ESTROGEN IN THE ANTERIOR HYPOTHALAMUS OF FEMALE RATS.

H. Morishita*, S. Kuroiwa and T. Mori, Department of Obstetrics and Gynecology, School of Medicine, The University of Tokushima, Tokushima, Japan.

In cycling rats exposed to a controlled lighting schedule of 12 h of light daily from 22:00 to 10:00, the concentration of estradiol (E) in the anterior hypothalamus at 5:00-6:00 on the day of proestrus was significantly higher than those at 0:00-1:00 on the days of diestrus 1 and estrus, and was about two-fold higher than serum E concentration which reached to a peak at 5:00-6:00 on the same day. The concentration of cytosol E receptor in the anterior hypothalamus at 5:00-6:00 on the day of proestrus was significantly lower than those at 0:00-1:00 on the days of diestrus 1 and estrus. Autoradiographically, the uptake of tritiated E by nuclei of neurons in the nucleus (n.) preopticus pars suprachiasmatica (POSC), n. preopticus periventricularis (POP), and anterior part of n. anterior hypothalami (AAH) was significantly higher at 1:00 on the day of diestrus 1 than at 6:00 on the day of proestrus and at 1:00 on the day of estrus. These results suggest that the POSC, POP and AAH may be the target sites in the anterior hypothalamus of E for its feedback action.

1794 FAMILIAL HYPERINSULINEMIA ASSOCIATED WITH STRUCTURALLY ABNORMAL INSULIN "INSULIN WAKAYAMA".

K. Nanjo*, T. Sanke, M. Kondo, M. Miyano, K. Okai, R. Sowa, K. Sakamoto, Y. Moriyama, K. Miyamura[1], A. Rubenstein, H. Tager and D. Steiner[2], Dept. of Medicine, Wakayama Medical School, Wakayama 640, Japan[1] and Dept. of Medicine and Biochemistry, The University of Chicago, Chicago, Illinois 60637, U. S. A.[2]

The first case of structurally abnormal-insulinemia was found by Given et al. in U. S. A. (1980). We identified an additional and unrelated patient with the same clinical syndrome.

The patient was a 59 year-old, non-obese female with diabetic glucose intolerance and marked fasting hyperinsulinemia (IRI 87 μU/ml, CPR 1.8 ng/ml). Her hepatic and renal functions were normal. Levels of circulating insulin-antagonistic hormones were within normal limits. Her serum did not contain insulin antibodies. She showed normal tolerance to exogenously administered insulin. Almost her serum IRI was recovered in the same position as authentic insulin by gel filtration. Four of five members in her family (Sister, Brother, Son and Grandson) have also hyperinsulinemia with normal levels of CPR and plasma glucose. The specific binding and the Kd at the high affinity site of her erythrocyte insulin receptors were similar in degree to those in healthy controls. The hydrophilicity of her insulin by HPLC method was different from that of the first case. The difference between two cases was also revealed by leucocyte DNA analysis.

The insulin from this patient was named "Insulin Wakayama". The discrepancy between abnormally high levels of serum IRI and normal levels of serum CPR is considered as one of the most important characteristics in such cases with structurally abnormal insulin.

1795 THE EFFECT OF RELAXIN AND INSULIN ON PLASMINOGEN ACTIVATOR SECRETION BY HUMAN FETAL MEMBRANE CELLS *IN VITRO*, E.S.C. Koay, G.D. Bryant-Greenwood* and F.C. Greenwood, Departments of Biochemistry and Anatomy, University of Hawaii, Honolulu, Hawaii 96822, USA.

We recently demonstrated that relaxin (Rlx) increases the secretion of two collagenolytic enzymes, plasminogen activator (PA) and collagenase (C) from dispersed human fetal membrane cells *in vitro*. Rapid time and temperature dependent binding of ^{125}I-Rlx to these cells has also been demonstrated. However, competitive binding studies showed that porcine insulin (INS) prevented ^{125}I-Rlx binding to these cells with a dose-inhibition curve parallel to that of porcine Rlx and with a molar potency relative to Rlx of some 40 %. INS was then shown to stimulate PA secretion by these cells either through the INS or Rlx receptor. To determine whether the PA responses to Rlx and INS are mediated by their respective receptors, dose-response studies have been carried out at physiological concentrations of both hormones. The dose-response effect of Rlx on PA secretion at 20 h of culture with 10, 50, 100, 500 and 1000 ng Rlx/ml gave 1.30 ± 0.05, 3.54 ± 1.77, 7.55 ± 3.84, 13.92 ± 2.43 and 25.48 ± 5.05 PA units/ 2 x 10^5 cells respectively. INS on the other hand at 100, 500 and 2000 ng INS/ml gave 1.57 ± 0.59, 2.87 ± 1.01 and 5.09 ± 0.97 PA units/ 2 x 10^5 cells. PA levels in controls were 0.94 ± 0.30 PA units/2 x 10^5 cells. Thus the effect of Rlx and INS on PA secretion by the human fetal membrane cells *in vitro* appears to be mediated through a Rlx receptor. This study was supported by NIH grant 06633.

1796 IMMUNOHISTOCHEMICAL LOCALIZATION OF RELAXIN IN THE HUMAN. E.S.C. Koay, C.A. Bagnell*, L.H. Larkin and G.D. Bryant-Greenwood. Departments of Biochemistry and Anatomy, University of Hawaii, Honolulu, HI, 96822 and Department of Anatomy, University of Florida, Gainesville, FL, 32610, USA.

The primary source of relaxin (Rlx) in the human is the corpus luteum of pregnancy. From isolation studies, it has been demonstrated that Rlx is also present in the placental basal plate and decidua, but the cells producing the hormone were not identified. It has recently been reported that the syncytiotrophoblast is its site of origin (Yki-Jarvinen *et al*, JCEM 57:451 1983). We have repeated this with four different antisera to purified porcine Rlx using their methodology on tissues from 14 elective Cesarean section deliveries. Five micron sections of these tissues were pretreated to remove endogenous peroxidase activity and then processed using the biotin-avidin immunoperoxidase technique. Identically processed sections of human corpus luteum of pregnancy and uterine endometrium from pregnant guinea pigs served as positive controls. Specificity of the reaction was demonstrated by substitution with either normal rabbit serum or anti-Rlx after absorption with pure Rlx. The cells that showed positive staining were the decidual cells of maternal origin in the decidua and placental basal plate. In contrast the syncytiotrophoblast at its periphery stained less and those within the chorionic villi failed to stain. We conclude that the maternal decidual cells are the major site of Rlx production, supporting our isolation studies of Rlx within the human fetal-placental unit. Supported by NIH grants HD06633 and HD08552.

1797 THE USE OF PENTOXIFYLLINE IN THE TREATMENT OF MILD ASTHENOZOOSPERMIA. M. Manenti*, M. Varengo, R. Giannella, R. Quadri, P. Carpano Maglioli, G. Bellomo and D. Fonzo, Patologia Medica E. Istituto di Medicina Interna, via Genova 3, 10126 Torino.Italy.

Xanthines derivatives are known to enhance quality and duration of sperm motility by reducing phosphodiesterase levels and consequently by increasing cAMP concentrations. Pentoxifylline has the greatest hydrosolubility and the loger lasting activity. The aim of our study has been the evaluation of the increase of sperm forward motility in mild asthenozoospermic patients during treatment with pentoxifylline per os 1200 mg/die (400 mg x 3) within a period of three to nine months. The investigation has been carried in 24 patients aged between 25 and 40 with at least two years of barren marriage, sperm count higher than 20 millions ml and forward motility higher than 20% at the second hour. Pituitary- testicular axis abnormalities, genito-urinary infections, varicocele and antisperm antibodies have been excluded. Mild to sharp improvement in sperm forward motility has been observed in 15 (62.5%) out of 24 patients treated. The wives of four patients (16.6%) became pregnant during the therapy with pentoxifylline.

1798 TREATMENT OF HYPOGONADOTROPHIC HYPOGONADISM IN MEN BY PULSATILE LUTEINISING HORMONE-RELEASING HORMONE (LHRH) INFUSION. D. Morris*, R. Adeneyi Jones, P. Sonksen and H.S Jacobs, Depts of Endocrinology, Middlesex Hospital, London, W1 and St Thomas' Hospital, London,SE1, U.K.

We have investigated the effect of chronic subcutaneous infusion of luteinising hormone-releasing hormone (LHRH) on gonadotrophin (Gn) secretion and testicular function in a group of 17 men with hypogonadotrophic hypogonadism (HH)(Mean age±SEM=30.4±2.1 years). 10 had idiopathic and seven secondary HH, which in 5 resulted from pituitary surgery. LHRH (mean±SEM 14.8±0.8 μg per pulse, range 2.5-20μg) was infused every 90 minutes by miniature pumps for between 1 and 18 months. 3 of the men with primary HH and four of those with secondary HH responded with increased secretion of LH, FSH and testosterone (mean serum testosterone±SEM after 3 months therapy 13.5±1.3nmol/l). Spermatogenesis increased in all these patients and 3 pregnancies have resulted. 7 patients with idiopathic HH produced an initial increase in Gn secretion, but the testosterone response was inadequate in 2 and absent in 5. The latter group demonstrated a progressive decline in LHRH sensitivity. 2 men with post-surgical HH failed to produce any increase in Gn secretion and 1 patient with secondary HH became allergic to LHRH. The initial Gn response to 100μg bolus LHRH injection did not predict the result of therapy. Chronic pulsatile LHRH infusion has a useful clinical role in the treatment of some men with HH.

1799 AMENORRHEA ASSOCIATED WITH WEIGHT LOSS.

Y. Nakamura*, T.Kobayashi, T.Ichinose and R.Iizuka, OB and GY, Keio Univ. School of Med. Tokyo, Japan.

Cessation of the normal menstrual cycle caused by rapid weight loss was defined as amenorrhea associated with weight loss.

All patients devloped secondary amenorrhea in a setting of weight loss. Over 80% of these patients (243 cases) were under 20 years of age.

More than half of the patients with amenorrhea associated with weight loss engaged in intentional food restriction for cosmetic reasons.

LH-RH test revealed that at the onset basal levels of serum LH were low and LH responses were impaired, while both basal and stimulated levels of FSH were comparable to normal. With an improvement of amenorrhea, the basal and stimulated levels of LH were found to rise to normal while FSH responses exceeded the normal response. Regardless of the rate of wight loss, both basal and LH responses were significantly lower than normal, while those of FSH were within normal or higher than normal. There was no significant correlation between rate of weight loss and responsiveness to LH-RH. The recovery rate of body weight in improved cases tended to be more rapid than that observed in unimproved patients.

Induction of ovulation with clomiphene was seccesful in 95% of 40 patients with Ist grade amenorrhea, while 96% of 54 patients with IInd grade amenorrhea failed to ovulate. Eighty per cent of 19 patients with IInd grade amenorrhea ovulated and 4 patients conceived by gonadotropin therapy.

1800 INSULIN DEGRADING ENZYME (IDE) FROM HUMAN (H) ERYTHROCYTES (E) AND MYOCYTES (M) HAVE A COMPARABLE MICHAELIS-MENTEN CONSTANT (K_m).

S.G.Nerurkar and K.K. Gambhir*, Molecular Endocrinol. Lab., Dept. of Med., Howard University, Washington, D.C. 20060 , USA.

Previously we have reported intracellular localization of IDE in HE. IDE has been shown to possess a K_m value of 163 nM in HM, 14-170 nM in rat M, 130 nM in rat adipocytes and 100 nM in rat hepatocytes. Now we report K_m for partially purified IDE from HE.

Insulin (I) degradation was determined at 37°C and pH 7.4 by trichloroacetic acid precipitation technique using ^{125}I - I (100 pg/ml) as a tracer mixed with 0-5000 ng/ml unlabeled I.

K_m was determined by Lineweaver-Burk (LB) as well as Eadie-Hofstee (EH) kinetics.

Expt.#	K_m (nM) (LB plot)	r	K_m (nM) (EH plot)	r
1	123.3	0.99	118.4	0.95
2	245.7	0.99	179.3	0.88
3	51.9	0.97	85.1	0.85
4	190.6	0.97	149.8	0.84
5	200.2	0.97	73.2*	0.56
Average	162.3		133.2	

*This value was not included in determination of the average K_m.

These results show that IDE in HE has a K_m comparable to the same in M from both human and rat. The physiological significance of these studies is unclear at present. However, IDE in HE may play a role in I metabolism and internalization. These studeis were partially supported by Latham Trust Fund.

1801 VAGAL REGULATION OF PANCREATIC HORMONES SECRETION BY ELECTRICAL STIMULATION IN VITRO. S. Nishi*, Y. Seino, M. Morimoto and H. Imura. Second Division, Department of Internal Medicine, Kyoto University School of Medicine, Kyoto 606, Japan.

Electrical stimulation of the vagus nerve has been shown to elicit both insulin and glucagon release in vivo. However, phenomena caused by in vivo vagal stimulation, such as changes in pancreatic blood flow and glucose level, make it difficult to ascertain the direct neural effect on pancreatic endocrine function. Therefore, we have established a new in vitro modification of the isolated rat perfusion procedure to investigate the direct effect of vagal stimulation on pancreatic hormone secretion. The vagus nerves were cut just beneath the diaphragm, leaving them attached to the isolated perfused rat pancreas. The distal end of the subdiaphragmatic vagus nerves was then stimulated with square wave impulses (2-10Hz, 1mS duration, 10V) for a 5 min period. Electrical stimulation of the vagus nerve produced a significant rise in both insulin and glucagon in proportion to the pulse frequency. Somatostatin release was unaffected by vagal stimulation in the presence of 5.5 mM glucose. When 10^{-5}M atropine sulfate was infused, both the insulin and glucagon response to vagal stimulation was partially suppressed, whereas somatostatin release was significantly enhanced. Furthermore, in the presence of 10^{-4} hexamethonium bromide, vagal stimulation failed to affect the insulin, glucagon, or somatostatin secretions. These findings suggest that not only a cholinergic but also a noncholinergic, probably peptidergic, neuron may be involved in vagal regulation of pancreatic hormones secretion and that these neurons may be under the control of preganglionic vagal fibers via nicotinic receptors.

1802 INSULIN SECRETION AND PROTEIN PHOSPHORYLATION. J M Oberwetter*, A E Boyd III, Departments of Cell Biology and Medicine, Baylor College of Medicine, Houston, Texas, USA.

An SV40 transformed beta-cell line (HIT cells) is being used as a model system to investigate the role of protein phosphorylation in insulin secretion. These cells rapidly secrete insulin in response to: glucose, glucose with IBMX, glucagon, amino acids, sulfonylureas and 40 mM K^+. Insulin secretion requires the presence of extracellular Ca^{2+} and is inhibited by verapamil, a Ca^{2+} channel blocker. At 5μM the calmodulin-binding drug, W13, inhibits insulin secretion in a reversible manner, whereas the less active analog, W12, has no effect, demonstrating a requirement for calmodulin in insulin secretion. In smooth muscle cells calmodulin activates the myosin light chain kinase which phosphorylates the Mr 20,000 myosin light chain, promoting an interaction with actin, generating tension. To test if this reaction might provide the motile force for insulin secretion in vivo, phosphorylation patterns of stimulated and control cells were quantitated using 2D gel electrophoresis and autoradiography. Five proteins of Mr = 16K, 20K, 24K, 67K and 68K are rapidly and specifically phosphorylated (1-5 min.) in association with insulin secretion brought about by depolarization of the cell membrane with 40 mM K^+. The Mr 20K phosphoprotein has a pI similar to that of the myosin light chain of smooth muscle. In conclusion, the reversible inhibition of insulin secretion by Ca^{2+} depletion, verapamil and a calmodulin antagonist, and the identification of a 20K protein which is phosphorylated in association with insulin secretion, are consistent with the hypothesis that Ca^{2+} and calmodulin regulate insulin release by activating the myosin light chain kinase.

1803 INDIRECT EFFECT OF DEXAMETHASONE ON GLUCOSE UPTAKE BY SKELETAL MUSCLE IN OBESE(ob/ob) MICE. K. Ohshima*, N. Shargil, T. M. Chan and G. A. Bray, Department of Medicine and the Institute of Toxicology, University of Southern California, School of Medicine, Los Angeles, CA 90033, U.S.A.

In previous studies from this laboratory, we have demonstrated that adrenalectomy reverses the defect in glucose uptake and insulin response by skeletal muscle in obese(ob/ob) mice. The present experiment has tested the possibility that hypercorticism could act directly to skeletal muscle to produce insulin resistance. Uptake of 2-deoxyglucose(2DG) with (1 mU/ml) or without(0 mU/ml) insulin(INS) was examined using the perfused hindquarter preparation. Ob/ob mice were adrenalectomized(ADX) at 4 weeks age. Dexamethasone(DEX)(5 mg/kg) was administered for following 9 days before 2DG uptake measurement. 2DG-6-phosphate(2DGP) accumulation in DEX treated ob/ob mice was significantly lower than vehicle treated group in both INS doses(in 1 mU/ml INS, 53±11 vs. 152±14; in 0 mU/ml INS, 40±2 vs. 68±9 n mole/15 min./g tissue). In the other experiment, the hindquarter of ADX ob/ob mice was perfused for 5 hours in physiological condition with(0.1 μg/ml) or without DEX followed by 2DG uptake measurement. Unlike the *in vivo* DEX treatment, there was no significant difference between DEX perfused group and vehicle perfused group(in 1 mU/ml INS, 102±8 vs. 81±9; im 0 mU/ml INS, 55±5 vs. 64±4 n mole/15 min./g tissue).
Conclusion: These results suggest that hypercorticism acts indirectly on skeletal muscle to produce insulin resistance in ob/ob mice.

1804 ENDOCRINE PANCREATIC FUNCTION IN POLYTRANSFUSED PATIENTS WITH HOMOZYGOUS β-THALASSAEMIA. C. Phenekos*, J. Lazarides, A. Karamerou and C. Politou, Endocrine Unit and Dracopoulion Blood Transfusion Center, Red Cross Hospital, Ampelokipi, Athens, Greece.

The functional status of the endocrine pancreas, as expressed by the secretion patterns of insulin and glucagon, was studied in 10 patients of both sexes aged 12-20 years suffering from homozygous β-thalassaemia without family history of Diabetes Mellitus (D.M.) and lacking any clinical or even biochemical evidence of the disease (Normal Oral Glucose Tolerance Test - OGTT). The patients had been regularly transfused and treated for the resulting iron overload with continuous subcutaneous infusion of Desferrioxamine. 10 normal subjects matched for sex and age and with no family history of D.M were used as controls. It was found that although the OGTT was normal in all patients studied the rise in their blood glucose was significantly higher ($p<0.01$) at 30, 90 and 120 min and the insulin response to hyperglycaemia was significantly smaller ($p<0,01$) at 30, 60 and 90 min compared to controls. Basal glucagon levels and the rise at 30, 60 and 90 min following stimulation with arginine infusion were lower in the patients than in the controls ($p<0,05$). No correlation was found between the serum ferritin levels or iron excretion and the degree of the secretory abnormality observed. It is concluded that even before the development of overt clinical or even biochemical findings of D.M in polytransfused patients with homozygous β-thalassaemia, there may be an initial abnormality of both insulin and glucagon secretion presumably due to iron deposition in both α and β-cells.

1805 CHLORPROPAMIDE INHIBITS GLUCONEOGENESIS IN HEPATOCYTES ISOLATED FROM FASTED RATS. T. Pillsworth, Jr. and S. Goldstein*, Dept. Pharmacology, Uniformed Services University of the Health Sciences, Bethesda, MD., 20814, USA.

It has been suggested that the ability of the hypoglycemic sulfonylureas to lower blood glucose is a result of alterations in hepatic carbohydrate metabolism. We therefore investigated the direct effects of chlorpropamide on gluconeogenesis in suspensions of isolated rat hepatocytes. Hepatocytes were isolated from 24 hour-fasted rats, pre-incubated for 20 min in the absence of substrates, and then incubated for 60 min with glucose, 10 mM; lactate, 5 mM; [^{14}C(U)]-lactate, 0.1 uCi/ml; glutamine, 5 mM; and Minimal Essential Media amino acid mixture. Conversion of [^{14}C]-lactate to [^{14}C]-glucose was determined by ion exchange chromatography and concentrations of gluconeogenic intermediates were measured using NAD^+ and NADH-coupled assays. Chlorpropamide (0.7-2.0 mM) decreased the conversion of lactate to glucose by 19-48% ($p < .05$) in a concentration-dependent manner. The non-hypoglycemic sulfonylurea analog HOE 17,710 was ineffective in decreasing the conversion of lactate to glucose. Decreased gluconeogenesis could be related to an inhibition of the conversion of malate to phospho(enol)pyruvate (PEP). Malate was elevated by 43% and PEP was decreased by 37% in cells incubated with 2.0 mM chlorpropamide compared to control incubations. The concentrations of 2-phosphoglycerate and 3-phosphoglycerate were also decreased in these cells. These data demonstrate that the hypoglycemic sulfonylurea, chlorpropamide can directly inhibit basal gluconeogenic rates in isolated rat hepatocytes which may in part explain their ability to lower blood glucose upon chronic administration.

1806 TERATOGENESIS IN RAT EMBRYOS UNDER HYPERGLYCEMIC CULTURE CONDITIONS: ULTRASTRUCTURAL ANALYSIS OF THE YOLK SAC AND NEURONAL TISSUE. E. Pinter*, A. Reece, C. Leranth, M. Sanyal, J. Hobbins, F. Naftolin and M. Mahoney, Dept. of Ob/Gyn, Yale University School of Medicine, New Haven, CT 06510

Organogenesis is a critical stage during embryonic development when embryos are highly susceptible to anomalous development. Rat conceptuses of pregnancy day 10 (Witschi stage 13, neurula) during organogenesis were cultured in male rat serum with and without added D- or L-glucose (750 mg/dl) for 45 or 93 hr under standard conditions. In the D-glucose exposed group, gross examination revealed decreased conceptus size with paler appearing yolk sac and neural tube defects (NTD) which occurred in 1/2 of all embryos. The same concentration of L-glucose in culture medium had relatively no effect upon the embryos compared to controls. Ultrastructural examination of affected or unaffected conceptuses treated with D-glucose demonstrated fewer yolk sac capillaries and blood cells. The visceral endoderm layer of these yolk sacs showed a marked reduction in endoplasmic reticulum and mitochondria. In embryos with NTD in contrast to controls, mitotic cells were located away from the luminal surface. The neural tubes also had advanced neuropile formation, and their cell cytoplasm contained dense granules. Embryos exposed to L-glucose were slightly decreased in size, but had normal cellular ultrastructures. These findings demonstrate the teratogenic effects of D-glucose, and suggest that the primary effect may be on the yolk sac, including blood forming elements, with a subsequent indirect effect on the neural tissue. (Supported by NIH HD14587, Andrew W. Mellon and Friedman Foundations)

1807 THE METABOLIC CLEARANCE OF INSULIN FROM THE CIRCULATION. THE EXISTENCE OF PLASMA DEGRADATION PRODUCTS OF INSULIN. J. Radziuk*, T. Morishima, S. Pye, C. Bradshaw, R.E. Offord. Dept. of Medicine, Royal Victoria Hospital and McGill Nutrition Centre, Montreal, Que. and Dept. of Biochemistry, University of Geneva, Geneva.

In ten 18hr-fasted dogs, the steady-state metabolic clearance of insulin (MCR) at various insulin concentrations was determined by simultaneous stepped infusions, of unlabelled insulin and a constant infusion of H^3-(B1-Phe)-insulin. Somatostatin was used to suppress endogenous insulin secretion. Glucose was given to maintain normoglycemia. H^3-insulin was determined in plasma samples after purification 1) on a C-18 column 2) with a SepPak (C-18) and by gel filtration. Immunoreactive insulin (IRI) was determined in plasma and after extraction on a C-18 column. It was found that 1) the basal MCR of insulin was 39.9+3.4 ml/kg-min and decreased with increasing IRI levels. The % change in MCR was 11.6ln (IRI)+30.6 2) A difference in H^3-insulin after the two extraction methods suggested the presence of partially degraded plasma insulin. Degradation was saturable since the % H^3 products decreased with IRI (=50.2 -9.8 log (IRI)). The % difference in IRI after the two methods of extraction varied as 29.7-5.0 log (IRI) showing some crossreactivity of these products with insulin. The time course of the development of these products was examined in a series of studies where H^3-insulin was infused at a primed constant rate. The difference between H^3 counts after gel filtration and HPLC increased from 5.8+2.3% at 1 min to 23.7+0.5% at 15 min. Thus insulin is cleared at a saturable rate and yields plasma degradation products, similar in size to insulin. (Supported by MRC Canada).

1808 COMPARISON OF REGIONAL CONCENTRATION AND IMMUNOCYTOCHEMICAL LOCALIZATION OF ISLET HORMONES IN NORMAL, DIABETIC AND ADRENALECTOMIZED DOGS. K.S. Rastogi*, S. Efendic and M. Vranic, Dept of Physiology, Univ. of Toronto, Toronto, Canada and Dept of Endocrinology, Karolinska Sjkhuset, Stokholm, Sweden.

We observed that not only in diabetes but also in adrenalectomized dogs, there is hyperglucagonemia and hypoinsulinemia. Therefore, we compared distribution of islet hormones in 5 normal, alloxan diabetic and adrenalectomized dogs. In normal dogs, single and double staining immunocytochemical method showed that, in contrast to some other species, A(glucagon) and D(somatostatin)cells are randomly distributed while B (insulin) cells are found in central region. Insulin conc. and content was high in the tail (T=175+27μg/gm) and body (B=168+27) and lower in the head (H=84+20). In diabetic dog only minimum amounts were seen (2.2+0.9, 1.3+0.6 and 1.1+0.4). Glucagon conc. were 18.5+1.3(T), 10.3+1.8(B), 0.6+0.3(H)μg/gm and were unaffected by diabetes. However, since the number of islets decreased by 50%, glucagon conc. per islet was substantially increased. Somatostatin was 0.69+0.3(T), 0.28+0.1(B) and 0.26+0.04(H)μg/gm. In diabetes, its conc. increased in H and B by 4x(0.96+0.32) and 2x(0.56+0.15). In adrenalectomized dogs, insulin conc. decreased by 16% (T=147+35) and 30% (B=118+28), glucagon increased 78% (B=18.4+3.9) and somatostatin was greatly augumented 5x(H=1.56+0.42), 5x(B=1.46+0.3). Thus hormones of adrenal gland are important for the control of islet function. Adrenalectomy, caused a small reduction in insulin and a marked increase in somatostatin and glucagon. These changes were much larger than in diabetes.

1809 ENCAPSULATED RAT INSULINOMA CELLS REVERSE HYPERGLYCEMIA IN DIABETIC MICE (STREPTOZOTOCIN INDUCED). A. Ricker*, H. Mori, A. Powers, A. Jarvis and G.S. Eisenbarth, Joslin Diabetes Center and Damon Biotech, Boston and Needham, Massachusetts, U.S.A.

Rat insulinoma (RINm5F) cells grown in tissue culture were encapsulated using poly-L-lysine, alginate polymeric capsules with and without polyvinyl amine and then injected intraperitoneally in varying doses [0.25×10^5 - 1.25×10^5 cells (250,000 cells/cc capsule)] to Balb/c mice made diabetic with streptozotocin (220 mg/kg). Unencapsulated cells in equivalent amounts were injected in a parallel experiment. 1) Plasma glucose returned to normal or hypoglycemic range in all mice receiving encapsulated cells (mean nadir glucose: 85 ± 24 mg%; nadir glucose range: 30-175 mg%) while there was only transient lowering of plasma glucose (mean nadir glucose: 412 ± 39 mg%; nadir glucose range: 296-464 mg%) in those animals receiving equivalent unencapsulated cells. 2) There was a dose response; those animals receiving the largest number of cells (1.25×10^5 cells) became hypoglycemic, others euglycemic. Reversal of diabetes lasted for up to 49 days from the time of injection of capsules. In contrast to intraperitoneal injection, subcutaneous injection of incapsulated RINm5F cells did not reverse hyperglycemia. The continuous RINm5F cell line provides an unlimited source of insulin producing cells to study encapsulation parameter for islet cell transplantation. Encapsulated cells can maintain insulin secretion indefinitely *in vitro* and are protected from normal rejection phenomena for up to 7 weeks *in vivo*.

1810 ISLET CELL ANTIBODIES IN ONE POPULATION AND IN CHILDHOOD DIABETICS IN JAPAN. T. Sakurami, K. Notsu*, J. Endo, A. Yaita, T. Nakamura, N. Nabeya, S. Kuno and S. Note, Department of Internal Medicine, Shimane Medical University, Izumo 693, Japan.

In 1981, we studied islet cell antibodies (ICA) in one population in Japan. Six cases out of 1,125 adults (0.5%) were positive for ICA. These six cases suffered from neither type I nor type II diabetes at that time. We examined these cases in oral glucose torelance tests in 1982. In CPR levels, all cases had low; however, only one case showed a diabetic pattern in plasma glucose levels. Serum samples in this population had been obtained once a year from 1979 and we studied ICA, complement-fixing (CF) ICA and other autoantibodies in each serum sample in these cases. One case, showing a diabetic pattern, have been positive for both ICA and antithyroid antibodies in 1980, 1981, 1982 and 1983. Another one had both ICA and antinuclear antibodies in 1981 and 1982. None of them, however, had CF-ICA. Identical tests for ICA were performed on 149 childhood diabetics with insulin treatment and 473 normal children. The incidence of ICA in type I diabetics was 26.2% and was the highest in cases within a year from the onset. However, the incidence of ICA in Japanese was low. Two cases out of 473 children were positive for ICA and ANA. However, none of two children or six adults suffer from insulin-dependent diabetes until now.

1811 EFFECTS OF CALCIUM ANTAGONISTS ON REACTIVE HYPOGLYCEMIA.
T. Sanke*, M. Kondo, Y. Moriyama, E. Satogami, K. Nanjo, and K. Miyamura, Department of Medicine, Wakayama Medical School, Wakayama, 640, Japan.

Clinical usefulness of calcium antagonist (Ca-AT) was studied in three patients with reactive hypoglycemia including one with idiopathic reactive hypoglycemia and two with postgastrectomic hypoglycemia. All patients had hyperresponse of plasma insulin (IRI) after oral glucose ingestion.

Ca-AT (diltiazem-HCl 90mg/day or nifedipine 30mg/day) was administered orally for about two months. Oral glucose tolerance test (OGTT) was performed at each of (A) before treatment with Ca-AT, (B) two months after the start of treatment, and (C) a month after discontinuation of the treatment. Intravenous glucose tolerance test (IVGTT) was also carried out in a patient with postgastrectomic hypoglycemia at (A) and (B), respectively.

In all cases, postprandial hypoglycemic symptom disappeared completely after about a month treatment. Hyperresponse of plasma IRI after oral glucose load observed at (A) and (C) was markedly reduced at (B). Plasma IRI response and glucose disappearance rate (K value) were also reduced at (B) compared with (A).

In addition, IVGTT was performed in seven patients with hypertension who were treated with Ca-AT at (A) and (B), respectively. In these patients group, plasma IRI response and K value were reduced at (B) compared with (A).

These results indicate that Ca-AT is useful as therapeutic agent for the treatment of reactive hypoglycemia associated with hyperinsulinemia, and suggest that as one of main mechanisms of action of Ca-AT it acted directly on pancreatic B-cell to inhibit glucose-induced insulin release.

1812 ESTROGEN-INDUCED MESSENGER RNAs OR SECRETARY PROTEINS IN RAT UTERUS AND THEIR RESPONSES TO A LARGE DOSE OF ESTROGEN. Y. Nishizawa*, B. Sato, K. Noma, S. Kishimoto and K. Matsumoto. The Third Dept. of Internal Medicine and The Second Dept. of Pathology, Osaka University Hospital, Fukushima-ku, Osaka 553, Japan.

Although the rat uteri have been the subject of numerous inventigations in elucidating estrogen (E) action mechanisms, more information about E effects on mRNAs and protein synthesis seems to be needed. Messenger RNAs was prepared from rat uteri and their cell-free translational products were separated on gel electrophoresis. Administration of estradiol (E_2) and diethylstilbestrol to ovariectomized rats was found to induce four mRNAs coding the proteins with the molecular weight of 26,500, 32,000, 38,000 and 53,000. We have then tried to identify the proteins coded by these mRNAs. Incubation of uterine tissues with [^{35}S] methionine failed to demonstrate E-induced proteins. The addition of tunicamycin in the medium, however, succeeded in the demonstration that E_2 induced secretary proteins with the molecular weights similar to those produced by E-induced mRNAs. The effects of daily injection of a large dose (0.1 µg/g body weight) of E_2 on the induction of these E-induced mRNAs were next asked. This treatment caused marked elevation of these mRNAs on day 3 and then their rapid disappearance on day 7, although E_2 was persistently injected. In addition, it should be mentioned that progesterone receptor, a most widely used E marker, remained at the high level on day 7. These data suggest that 1) E-induced mRNAs identified in this study, which probably code secretary proteins, can be used as a useful marker for E action; 2) a pharmacological dose of E_2 first induces new mRNAs and subsequently antagonizes their induction. This study was supported by grants-in-aid from the Ministry of Education, Tokyo, Japan.

1813 **THE ROLE OF NON-ESTERIFIED FATTY ACIDS (NEFAs) IN THE MECHANISMS OF ESTROGEN ACTIONS.**
*Nunez, E.A., Benassayag, C., Vallette, G., Hassid, J., Martin, M.E., Vranckx, R. - U. 224, INSERM - ERA 881, CNRS - Faculté de Médecine Xavier Bichat - Laboratoire de Biochimie - 16, rue Henri Huchard 75018 PARIS.

Many works mainly performed in the rat have recently cleared up that AFP seems to regulate some estrogen actions. These effects are different from those of albumin. The exact mechanisms by which AFP is working are not yet elucidated. However the fact that unsaturated NEFAs are competitors of the estrogen binding by murine AFPs, opens new perspectives. Furthermore the AFPs of the other species studied are not estrophilic but they bind NEFAs with high affinity.
These facts prompted us to investigate the role of different fatty acids on the binding of estrogens by the rat and human uterine cytosoluble proteins. We have shown that physiological concentrations of unsaturated NEFAs inhibit the binding of estradiol to the rat uterine cytosoluble proteins. By contrast, using a human uterine preparation, we observe an important potentialization of the estradiol binding when adding the unsaturated NEFAs. In these conditions, it can be envisaged that the NEFAs binding properties of AFP and/or albumin can modulate the estrogen actions during normal or neoplasic development.
Furthermore we have recently demonstrated that the binding of sexual steroids by the human sex binding protein (SBP) can be influenced by the NEFAs.
In view of these results, we present two models of the putative role of NEFAs and some binding proteins (AFP, albumin, SBP) on the mechanisms of the estrogen actions.

1814 ANDROGEN RECEPTOR BINDING TO THE C3(1) SUBUNIT GENE OF RAT PROSTATEIN.
S.T. Perry,*D.H. Viskochil, K. Fong, D.W. Stafford, E.M. Wilson, and F.S. French. Cancer Research Center and The Laboratories for Reproductive Biology, University of North Caorlina, Chapel Hill, North Carolina, 27514.

We have used cloned C3(1) prostatein gene fragments to investigate androgen receptor binding to sequences in and around this androgen-dependent gene. Cytosol from the Dunning tumor, R3327H, was labeled with [^{3}H]-dihydrotestosterone and partially purified by column chromatography on phosphocellulose. C3(1) prostatein gene fragments, subcloned into the Eco R1 site of pBR322, were isolated by agarose gel electrophoresis and treated with S1 nuclease to generate blunt ends. Androgen receptor binding to specific C3(1) gene fragments was analyzed in a competition assay. The fragments were added to receptor pre-bound to blunt-ended calf thymus DNA-cellulose, and the amount of receptor displaced was determined. A 300 base pair (bp) fragment, comprising the 5' end of the first exon and adjacent upstream DNA, competes for receptor 3-fold better than does equimolar amounts of calf thymus DNA of equivalent size. The 300 bp fragment displaces 50% of receptor bound to calf thymus DNA-cellulose with 0.25 equivalents of DNA. A region of even higher affinity (5-fold greater than calf thymus DNA) is found within a 500 bp fragment in the first intron. This fragment displaces 50% of receptor at concentrations of 0.15 equivalents of DNA. Receptor binding to other regions of the C3(1) gene are of lower affinity, similar to that of calf thymus DNA. These findings suggest that the androgen receptor binds selectively to nucleotide sequences near the start site of transcription and sequences within the C3(1) gene.
Supported by grants NCI CA07551-01 and CA32458-02.

1815 INHIBITION BY PROGESTINS OF THE CALCIUM ACTIVATED MYOMETRIAL CONTRACTIONS.
M. Perusquía*, H. Ponce-Monter and C. Kubli-Garfias. Unidad de Investigación Biomédica, Centro Médico Nacional del Instituto Mexicano del Seguro Social. México D.F. 03020, MEXICO.

Modulation of uterine contractility depends strongly of hormonal influences. Thus, 5β-reduced progesterone metabolites have shown an important relaxant effect on the myometrium. Since progesterone acts by blocking the Ca^{++} influx it is possible that its metabolites share this property. Therefore, we decide to study the effect of some progestins on the Ca^{++} induced contractions of uterine smooth muscle. Rings of Sprague-Dawley rat uterus in diestrous were bathed in Tris buffer solution in a isolated bath at 37°C, bubbled with O_2. After the recording of the spontaneous activity, the preparation was depolarized with a isotonic K (40 mM), free Ca^{++} solution which resulted in a complete relaxation 45 min later. In these conditions the addition of 1 mM of Ca^{++} to the media produced a tonic contraction. In order to prevent such contraction in a second trial tissues were incubated 10 min with one of the following steroids (μM): progesterone (4-pregnen-3,20-dione, 25), 5α-pregnanedione (5α-pregnane-3,20 dione, 25), pregnanolone (3β-hydroxy-5β-pregnan-20-one, 7) and epipregnanolone (3α-hydroxy-5β-pregnan-20-one, 16). Under the progestins effect a decreased contracture was observed ranging from 45 to 68% regarding with the control. The exception was 5α-pregnanedione which was ineffective. By the results it can be concluded that natural progestins (Δ4 and 5β-reduced) are able of counteract the Ca^{++} influx produced by the K^+ depolarization in the myometrial cell. Therefore, the relaxant effect observed with these steroids might be by blocking the Ca^{++} muscle activation mechanism.

1816 LONG-TERM TREATMENT WITH CATECHOLAMINES (CA) MAY LEAD TO ENHANCEMENT OF OTHER ENDOGENOUS CA.
S.Porta*,I.Rinner,S.Supanz,B.Rangetiner,U.Ertl,A.Sadjak
Institute of Functional Pathology,University of Graz,Austria.

Four groups of male Sprague Dawley rats were treated with either Adrenaline (A),Noradrenaline (NA),Isoprenaline (ISO) or placebo,given by a long term controlled release system. The system consits of a coated Eudragit tablet,implanted in the neck fold of the animals. A number of animals out of each group was carefully sacrificed 6, 12 or 20 hours after tablet implantation.Tablets were removed to determine residual CA concentration and blood samples were collected for estimation of blood glucose and plasma CA levels.CA output of the tablets was linear (HP 9845 B computer) and in the range of μgs/min.A treatment enhanced A plasma levels but did not affect NA plasma levels.NA treatment enhanced NA plasma levels and also considerably increased A concentration. ISO treatment enhanced ISO levels as well as A and NA plasma concentrations.Increase of A during NA and ISO treatment is probably due to changes in glucose availability, reflected by changing blood sugar levels.ISO is known to facilitate NA release from a variety of tissues.We conclude, that during long term tests with NA and ISO also a considerable elevation of endogenous CA is to be expected.

1817 IS CORTICOSTEROID NEGATIVE FEEDBACK MEDIATED BY PROSTAGLANDINS (PG)?
E. Redei*, B.J. Branch and A.N. Taylor, BRI Lab. of Neuroendocrinology, UCLA and West L.A./Brentwood VA Medical Center, Los Angeles, CA 90024, USA.

PGE is known to stimulate CRF and ACTH through cyclic AMP and corticosterone (B) has been shown to inhibit PG biosynthesis. Thus it was of interest to determine whether B feedback inhibition of ACTH secretion involves PG. We perfused rat medial basal hypothalamic (MBH), anterior pituitary (AP) and adrenal gland (AG) fragments. Two-min fractions were collected from AP and AG and ACTH and B were measured by RIA. Backflow (feedback) to MBH and AP was established with 1/3 of the perfusate from AG. Without feedback, 50 nmol acetylcholine (Ach) produced 300% increases of ACTH at 6 and 15 min and 150% and 100% increases of B at 15 and 33 min, respectively. Feedback from AG caused 43% and 40% inhibition of Ach-induced ACTH increases at 6 and 15 min, respectively. Perfused MBH and AP responses to Ach (1, 5, 10 and 50 nmol) were dose-related with equal ACTH increases at 6 and 15 min. Ach (1 nmol) plus B (50 nmol) caused 50% inhibition of the 15-min increase only. Ach (1 nmol) plus PG biosynthesis inhibitors (PGBI, aspirin or indomethacin, 50 nmol) produced 50% inhibition of both Ach-induced increases while PGBI alone produced no change in ACTH. In contrast, at the AP, PGBI increased basal ACTH secretion. PGE_2 (5 and 10 nmol) by itself caused dose-related but unequal ACTH increases. These data suggest that B negative feedback may involve PG biosynthesis inhibition at the hypothalamus, while the mechanism for B's action on the pituitary appears to be more complex. (Supported by NIH-HD 07228 and VA Medical Research Service.)

1818 INHIBITION BY DEXAMETHASONE OF AMINO ACID TRANSPORT IN PLASMA MEMBRANE VESICLES OBTAINED FROM RAT HEPATOMA CELLS. S. B. Reichberg *, New York Medical College, Valhalla, NY 10595 and The Brookdale Hospital Medical Center, Brooklyn, NY 11212, U.S.A.

Exposure of rat hepatoma tissue culture (HTC) cells to the glucocorticoid dexamethasone (dex.), results in marked inhibition of three major plasma membrane amino acid transport systems and in a drastic decrease of hexose uptake rates. To determine whether dex. produces these effects by alterating the plasma membrane itself, and to procure a cell-free experimental system in which to study biochemical changes of the plasma membrane produced by dex., a method was perfected to prepare and purify from HTC cells, plasma membrane vesicles capable of active transport.

Cells were disrupted by nitrogen cavitation followed by differential centrifugation. The resulting concentration of plasma membrane vesicles was enriched 3.8 times on average compared with the starting cell extract, as determined by increases in specific activities of alkaline phosphodiesterase I and 5' nucleotidase. The amounts of mitochondrial, endoplasmic reticulum and lysosomal membranes was estimated by the activities of succinate dehydrogenase, cytochrome c reductase and β-glucuronidase.

Amino acid transport was measured by the uptake of ^{14}C-2-aminoisobutyric acid (AIB). This model amino acid was taken up against a concentration gradient, intravesicular content reaching a maximum 1-2 min after the start of incubation. AIB uptake was consistently decreased in vesicles obtained from cells previously exposed to dex. for 30 hours, as compared with vesicles obtained from control cultures (Supported by grants from the Juvenile Diabetes Foundation and N.I.H. No. AM 31638)

1819 CHRONICALLY ENHANCED ADRENALINE (A) PLASMA LEVELS ACCELERATE A INACTIVATION.

I.Rinner*,S.Porta,G.Egger,B.Rangetiner,A.Sadjak
Institute of Funktional Pathology,University of Graz,Austria

Long term application of A by subcutaneously implantable tablets with different A content leads to a linear A output of 1.8 μg/min qnd 3.9 μg/min up to 2o hours.Radioenzymatic measurement of A plasma levels 6, 12 and 20 hours after tablet implantation showed a discontinuous pattern.Since A synthesis and secretion are not regulated by a negative feed-back regulation (Porta et al.),other systems must be involved in the alteration of the A plasma levels.In vitro investigation of the catecholamine-metabolizing enzymes in the rat liver showed,that MAO,but not COMT activity was elevated after continuous A administration.This was cross-checked by histochemical detection of MAO activity.Although COMT is the first A metabolizing enzyme,the rise of MAO activity is not due to the elevation of the O-methylated product,Metanephrine,which is also a substrat to MAO.This was proved by a 12 hours lasting in vivo pretreatment with 4.2 μg/min Metanephrine, whereafter no stimulation of MAO activity could be observed. Treatment with the two different A doses lead after 6 hours to different A levels,but to similar low MAO activities.After 20 hours treatment comparable low A levels coincide with with different MAO activities.This may account for a time-consuming,dose-dependent de novo synthesis rather than for further activation of pre-exsisting enzyme.

1820 INSULIN-LIKE GROWTH FACTOR I (IGF-I) STIMULATES TYROSINE KINASE ACTIVITY IN PURIFIED RECEPTORS FROM A RAT LIVER CELL LINE (BRL 3A2).

N. Sasaki*, Y. Zick, S.P. Nissley and M.M. Rechler. NIADDK and NCI, National Institutes of Health, Bethesda, MD 20205 USA.

Type I IGF receptors are structurally and immunologically similar to insulin receptors. Recently, it has been reported that IGF-I stimulates phosphorylation of tyrosine residues on the Mr~90K β-subunit of Type I IGF receptors. We now demonstrate that IGF-I stimulates tyrosine kinase activity towards exogenous tyrosine-containing substrates. Microsomal membranes were prepared from BRL 3A2 cells, solubilized and the receptors purified on wheat germ agarose. These preparations contain abundant Type I and Type II IGF receptors but few insulin receptors. Purified receptors were incubated with peptide, [γ-^{32}P]ATP and the synthetic substrate poly (glu,tyr) 4:1. IGF-I stimulated ^{32}P incorporation into substrate by 4-10 fold (ED_{50} ~5 nM). IGF-II and insulin were active at 5-fold higher concentrations. Insulin-stimulated phosphorylation was not decreased after depletion of insulin receptors with anti-insulin receptor IgG. These results suggest that the 3 peptides act via the Type I IGF receptor. Casein, poly (ala,glu,lys,tyr) 6:2:5:1 and poly (glu,ala,tyr) 6:3:1 also were effective substrates for the IGF-I-dependent tyrosine kinase, whereas poly (glu,tyr) 1:1 and poly (lys,tyr) 1:1 were not phosphorylated. In the absence of substrate, 100 and 1000 ng/ml of IGF-I or insulin stimulated phosphorylation of a Mr~98K protein (reduced), presumably the β-subunit of the Type I IGF receptor, that exists in a Mr >300K complex before disulfide reduction. CONCLUSION: We propose that the β-subunit of the Type I IGF receptor possesses IGF-I-dependent tyrosine kinase activity.

1821 ACROMEGALIC HYPERTRIGLYCERIDEMIA: A NEW GROUP OF HYPERLIPOPROTEINEMIA SECONDARY TO A DISORDER IN ENDOCRINE FUNCTION.

T. Murase*, N. Yamada, H. Itakura, M. Kawakami, F. Matsuzaki and F. Takaku, The Third Deparment of Internal Medicine, University of Tokyo, Hongo, Tokyo, Japan

We have suggested previously that acromegaly is frequently accompanied with hypertriglyceridemia (hyperTGmia) and this may be, at least in part, a consequence of defective TG removal due to the decreased lipoprotein lipase (LPL) activity (Metabolism 29:666,1980). In the present communication, we have further attempted to characterize plasma lipoprotein abnormalities. Of 16 patients with active acromegaly, 9 patients had type IV hyperlipoproteinemia (HL), 2 patients type IIb HL and 2 patients type V HL. Only 3 patients were normolipidemic. Plasma HDL-cholesterol levels were low (31±8 mg/dl) and the levels of apoA-1, a major constituent of HDL, were decreased as well (64±15 mg/dl). Plasma apoA-II tended to be low, whereas both apoC-II and apoE were normal. Ultracentrifugation analysis of plasma lipoproteins revealed increases of VLDL and IDL, indicating that TG-rich lipoprotein removal might be impaired. As shown in previous report, postheparin plasma LPL activity was significantly decreased. Although half of the patients (8 of 16 cases) had diabetes, patients without diabetes also had hyperTGmia with low LPL activity. This indicates that acromegaly itself may be a factor causing hyperTGmia and, as suggested earlier (Life Sci. 28:199,1981), probably the excess of growth hormone causes the decrease in adipose tissue LPL activity, resulting in the defective removal of circulating plasma TG. We propose here that acromegalic hyperTGmia is a new group of hyperlipoproteinemia secondary to a disorder in endocrine function.

1822 METABOLIC FATE OF NORETHISTERONE ACETATE (NETA) IN RHESUS MONKEY (MACACA MULATTA).

K. Murugesan*, U. Verma, K.R. Laumas and A. Farooq, Department of Reproductive Biology, All India Institute of Medical Sciences, NEW DELHI-110029, India.

The pharmacokinetics of NETA in monkeys has been carried out to elucidate its fate under constant infusion conditions. Three doses of NETA, 640 µg, 320 µg and 100 µg were infused at a constant rate for 4 hours. The plasma level of norethindrone (NET) was measured by a specific radioimmunoassay. The plasma level of NET at steady state conditions were highest in case of 640 µg dose and lowest at 100 µg NETA/4 hr. studies. However, the levels were not absolutely proportional to the dose infused. The plasma metabolites of NETA revealed the formation of NET and tetrahydro NET in the ether extractable free fractions. The analysis of conjugated metabolites revealed two important events (1) NETA is conjugated to glucuronides of NETA at the earliest and also converted to NET and (2) the unconjugated NET is reduced to tetrahydro NET. *In vitro* studies reveal that the conversion of NETA to NET can occur in the blood plasma and erythrocytes. However, NETA was metabolised to tetrahydro NET in the tissue compartments. 5α-dihydro norethisterone is one of the metabolites identified in plasma apart from NET and tetrahydro NET. Thus the metabolism of NETA to NET and the contribution of tissues and blood is significant in the biodegradation of NETA in this species.

1823 INSULIN RESISTANCE IN PRIMARY HYPERPARATHYROIDISM: DECREASED INSULIN RECEPTOR NUMBER AND DIMINISHED PERIPHERAL INSULIN SENSITIVITY. R.Prager*, G. Schernthaner, J.Kovarik, H.Graf. 2nd Dept.of Internal Medicine and Ludwig Boltzmann-Institute of Clinical Endocrinology,University of Vienna,Austria.

To evaluate the contribution of peripheral insulin sensitivity on impaired carbohydrate metabolism in primary hyperparathyroidism (pHPT) insulin receptor binding to monocytes and erythrocytes was compared between 10 patients (pat) with pHPT and 20 controls (C). Furthermore, in 9 pat with pHPT glucose tolerance, insulin secretion and peripheral insulin sensitivity were quantitated by means of the hyperglycemic clamp technique in comparison to C. In 3 pat hyperglycemic clamp studies were repeated 8 to 12 weeks after parathyroidectomy.

Insulin binding to monocytes and erythrocytes was significantly lower in pat with pHPT in comparison to C($p<0,01$). This was mainly due to a decrease of absolute receptor number. The amount of glucose metabolised (M, mg/kg b.w.min) was significantly lower in pat with pHPT compared to C ($6,7 \pm 3,3$ vs. $10,0 \pm 3,3$, $p<0,01$). The ß-cell response (insulin secretion:I) to hyperglycemia was almost identical between C ($59,8 \pm 36,1$ mU/L) and pHPT-pat ($64,3 \pm 34,0$ mU/L). Tissue sensitivity to insulin (M/I ratio, mg/kg b.w.min per mU/L x 100) was significantly lower in pHPT-pat compared to C($9,2 \pm 2,3$ vs.$17,9 \pm 2,0$, $p<0,01$). After parathyroidectomy glucose tolerance (M) and insulin sensitivity (M/I-ratio) were significantly improved but not completely normalized.

The present data demonstrate that decreased insulin receptor binding and peripheral insulin resistance are the major causes for disturbed carbohydrate metabolism in pHPT, whereas the ß-cell response is essentially normal.

1824 IMMUNOLOGICAL DIAGNOSIS OF MEDULLARY CARCINOMA OF THE THYROID USING MONOCLONAL ANTIBODY A2B5. K. Shimizu*, M. Ishio, H. Nozaki, M. Ide, K. Akimaru, H. Kanauchi, T. Shoji and K. Itoh, 2nd Department of Surgery, Nippon Medical School, Tokyo, Japan

Although medullary carcinoma of the thyroid gland (MCT) has characteristic biochemical (high level of serum calcitonin and CEA) and pathological (amyloid deposition) futures among the thyroid nodules, one sometimes comes across the diagnostic problems because of its macroscopic appearance compared with other thyroid malignant tumors, occasional lack of amyloid deposition and anaplastic findings. Therefore, the exploitation of specific marker for this tumor will be a great help for making a diagnosis. The antigen of our monoclonal antibody A2B5 is a GQ ganglioside of neurons and binds to the membrane receptors of APUD cells and their tumors. It is known that MCT is one of the APUD tumors. We have studied 103 cases of various thyroid nodules including 3 MCTs and 20 carcinomas from other organs with the indirect immunofluorescent method using A2B5. All MCT showed strong positive reaction, while other thyroid tumors and 20 carcinomas from other organs (non-APUD tumors) resulted in negative outcomes except for one follicular adenoma and one follicular carcinoma of thyroid which were weakly positive. As the next step, protein A affinity purified radiolabeled A2B5 was applied for in vitro pre-experiment of radioimmunodetection of MCT using permanent cloned rat MCT cell line (CRL 1607). Radiolabeled A2B5 bound well to CRL 1607 and its binding was blocked by unlabeled A2B5. It will be concluded that A2B5 is a specific marker for MCT and useful tool for not only post-operative but pre-operative diagnosis of this tumor.

1825 MONOCLONAL HUMAN ISLET CELL ANTIBODIES: ENDOCRINE CELL CROSS REACTIVITY.

S. Srikanta*, A. Ricker, A. Rabizadeh and G.S. Eisenbarth, Joslin Diabetes Center and Brigham and Women's Hospital, Boston, Massachusetts, U.S.A.

Monoclonal human islet cell antibodies generated using human islets, human insulinoma cells and neuronal cells were tested for reactivity with unfixed endocrine tissues, isolated endocrine cells or cell lines (indirect immunofluorescence). With the exception of H-22 (which reacts only with pancreatic islets) all other McAbs cross react with endocrine cells in differing patterns. A: H-1, 4, 9 and 14 react with pancreatic islets (PI), anterior pituitary (APC), thyroid follicular (TFC), melanoma (MC) and glioblastoma (GC) cells; B: H-7 reacts with islets and gastric parietal cells (GPC); C: H-19 reacts with islets and pituitary cells, and D: anti-ganglioside McAbs A2B5 and 3G5 react with islets, thyroid calcitonin (TCC) and adrenal medullary (AMC) cells. Variable patterns of cross reactivity of the anti-islet McAbs, a) indicate considerable diversity of the islet cell antigens, b) may imply common function or development origin, and c) may have possible significance in the variable pattern of co-occurence of multiple autoimmune disorders. Common cross reactivity pattern (H-1, 4, 9 and 14) was associated with recognition of an identical antigen (100K cell surface protein by immunoprecipitation and affinity chromatography).

McAb	PI	APC	TFC	TCC	ACC	AMC	TLC	MC	GC	GPC	TEC
H-1,4,9,14	+	+	+		-	-	-	+	+	-	-
H-7	+	-	-		-	-	-	-	-	+	-
H-19	+	+	-		-	-	-	-	-	-	-
A2B5	+	-		+	-	+	-	-	-	-	+
3G5	+	+*			-	+	-	-	-	-	-

ACC: adrenal cortical cells; TLC: testicular Leydig cells; TEC: thymic endocrine cells; *: subset of cells.

1826 EVIDENCE FOR THE INVOLVEMENT OF ENDOGENOUS OPIOID PEPTIDES (EOP) IN THE TONIC RELEASE OF TSH IN THE RAT.

W.J. Litto* and J. Rabii, Dept. Biol. Sci., Rutgers U., Piscataway, NJ 08854, USA.

There is evidence for involvement of EOP in regulation of TSH release. Controversy exists, however, in regard to the role of EOP in tonic release of this hormone. This is in part due to a reported lack of effect of opioid antagonists on basal TSH levels. Thus, we undertook a detailed examination of effects of the opioid antagonist naloxone (NAL), administered by different routes, on TSH release under basal conditions and in response to stress. Intravenous (IV), intraperitoneal (IP), and subcutaneous (SC) injection of 1.0 and 10.0 mg/kg NAL produced a significant elevation in plasma TSH at 30 and 60 min. The elevation of TSH at 30 and 60 min. after the IP and IV administration of NAL was dose related. Infusion of 1.0 and 10.0 μg NAL into the third cerebral ventricle produced a significant increase in plasma TSH at 30 and 60 min. Immobilization stress for 10 min. produced a significant decline in plasma TSH levels, 30 minutes after termination of the stress stimulus. This inhibition was abolished in animals pretreated with IV injection of 1.0 or 10.0 mg/kg NAL. These results provide strong evidence in support of a role for EOP in maintenance of basal levels of TSH in the rat. They also suggest an involvement of EOP in stress-induced inhibition of TSH release. Supported by the Busch Memorial Fund and NIH Grant DA02227.

1827 CAPSAICIN SENSORY DENERVATION ABOLISHES PERIPHERAL CHOLECYSTOKININ INDUCED SATIETY IN THE RAT. D. MacLean,* Dept. of Medicine, Bowman Gray School of Medicine of Wake Forest University, Winston-Salem, NC 27103.

Cholecystokinin (CCK), when injected ip produces short-term satiety in the rat. This effect is blocked by vagotomy or section of vagal sensory rootlets. Capsaicin is an excitatory neurotoxin that when injected neonatally permanently damages unmyelineated sensory neurons in the rat. Neonatal rats were injected with 50mg/kg capsaicin (CapRx), or vehicle (VehRx). CapRx survivors were predominantly female. Treated rats were insensitive to intraocular capsaicin; in an age-matched group of similarly CapRx, vagal content and transport of substance P was reduced 90% vs. VehRx controls. Weights of surviving female CapRx were identical to VehRx litter mates (256±18 vs. 261±18g, $\bar{x}$±SD). In VehRx, CCK-8 (8ug/kg ip) reduced ½ h food intake by 50% ($p<.02$) vs. only 10% in CapRx (NS; and $p<.05$ between groups). Saline ip did not reduce food intake in either group. Both groups ate significantly but equally more during the 8 hours following sc insulin, 16 u/kg. Subsequent bilateral lesioning of the ventromedial hypothalamus (VMH) resulted in a significant and equal degree of obesity in both groups. Conclusions are: 1) neonatal capsaicin administration permanently destroys sensory fibers mediating peripheral CCK-satiety. Compensatory mechanisms do not occur. Substance P is one possible neurotransmitter mediating this phenomenon. 2) Centrally induced feeding responses (insulin and VMH lesioning) are not altered by the absence of the peripheral CCK-satiety reflex arc. Long-term weight regulation is likewise unaffected. This model may be useful for further studying the interactions between peripheral and centrally mediated mechanisms of appetite regulation.

1828 CHOLINERGIC MUSCARINIC RECEPTORS MEDIATE APOMORPHINE-INDUCED GROWTH HORMONE SECRETION IN MAN. F. Massara*, D. Tangolo, S. Goffi, E. Ghigo, G.M. Molinatti. Clinica Medica B, Università di Torino, C.so Polonia 14, 10126 Italy.

Recently pirenzepine (Pire), a specific blocker of muscarinic receptor, has been shown to be able to inhibit the glucagon- and arginine-induced GH secretion, indicating that these receptors participate in the regulation of human GH secretion. To verify whether these receptors are involved also in the mediation of GH response to dopaminergic stimulation, the effect of pretreatment with Pire on apomorphine (Apo)-induced GH secretion has been studied in 6 normal volunteers. Each subject received in two separate occasions, Apo alone (12 µg/kg b.w. sc) and Apo preceded by Pire (0.6 mg/kg b.w. iv 5 min before Apo). Plasma GH was determined (CEA-IRE-Sorin Kit RIA) every 15 min for 90 min before and after Apo. The GH increase induced by Apo (peak at 30-45 min: mean ± SEM 23.3 ± 4.9 ng/ml; sum of the increases over the baselines: 83.4 ± 15.8 ng/ml) was completely or strongly inhibited by Pire in all subjects (peak: 2.7 ± 1.1, sum: 5.9 ± 2.7 ng/ml $p<0.001$). In conclusion the GH response to activation of dopaminergic pathways seems to be mediated by cholinergic muscarinic receptors. Since Pire does not cross the BBB, it may be supposed that interaction between the dopaminergic and cholinergic pathways occurs in the median eminence and/or hypophysis. Cholinergic mediation seems to be one of the terminal steps in the mechanisms controlling the GH release.

1829 CONTRASTING EFFECTS OF FLUOXETINE ON THE E_2 INDUCED LH SURGE IN OVARIECTOMIZED RATS. D. Meyer* and D. Eadens, University of Louisville, Louisville, Kentucky, 40292, USA

The role of serotonin in modulating the E_2 induced LH surge in ovariectomized rats depends on the timing and regional changes in serotonergic neurotransmission. To examine the role of serotonin in phasic LH secretion adult female rats, 2 weeks post ovariectomy, were given silastic capsule E_2 implants. An indwelling cannula was stereotaxically implanted in the anterior hypothalamus and the jugular vein cannulated for chronic blood sampling. In this system E_2 stimulated a late light increase in LH, and when PCPA, a serotonin synthesis blocker, was given i.p., the LH surge was decreased. However, a 10 μg dose of Fluoxetine, a serotonin reuptake blocker, infused into the anterior hypothalamus further decreased the plasma LH level in these PCPA treated rats when given 1 hour prior to the expected LH surge. In these same rats 24 hours later a decrease in LH was again found during the late light period when compared to previously treated (PCPA 125 mg/kg) controls. When Fluoxetine (75μg) was given i.c. in this model system there was a small decrease in LH but within 24 hours a significant increase in LH was found when compared to controls. These results suggest that the effect of in vivo Fluoxetine on phasic LH secretion is dependent on the site and timing of injection, and may ultimately involve stimulation of feedback inhibition of serotonin synthesis.
This study was supported by NICHD to D.M.

1830 ENDOGENOUS OPIATES DO NOT REQUIRE NORADRENERGIC PATHWAYS TO INFLUENCE LH SECRETION. M.A. Miller*, D.K. Clifton, and R.A. Steiner, Depts. of Ob/Gyn, PBIO, Psych., Univ. Wash., Seattle, WA., USA 98195

The ability of endogenous opiate pathways (EOP) to influence LH secretion may depend upon a functional noradrenergic (NE) system, since pretreatment with the α-blocker, phenoxybenzamine (PBZ), blocks the LH increase occurring in response to naloxone (NAL). We hypothesized that if EOP required an interacting NE system to influence LH secretion, then rats that have ascending NE tract lesions would not respond to NAL. To test this hypothesis we challenged NE-lesioned and sham-lesioned rats with NAL. Young, adult male, Sprague-Dawley rats received either a NE-lesion (cut) or a sham-lesion (sham-cut) and six weeks later were challenged with NAL (2mg/kg, iv). NAL significantly increased LH levels in both the cut (n=7) and sham-cut (n=8) groups. Failure of NE lesions to block the LH response to NAL was not due to the presence of active residual NE fibers, because pretreatment with PBZ (20mg/kg, iv) failed to block the NAL response in NE-lesioned animals (n=8), whereas it did so in the sham-lesioned animals (n=7). Mean LH response, (ng/ml), from baseline for each group is tabulated below:

	Cut	Sham-Cut
NAL	(a) 0.52 ± .12	(b) 0.38 ± .07
PBZ-NAL	(c) 0.53 ± .24	(d)-0.01 ± .01

(a) vs (b): not significant
(b) vs (d): $p < 0.001$
(c) vs (d): $p < 0.05$
(a) vs (c): not significant

Conclusion: EOP can influence LH secretion independently of the NE system.

1831 RELATIONSHIP OF PINEAL SEROTONIN-N-ACETYL TRANSFERASE (SNAT) LEVELS TO SUPRACHIASMATIC NUCLEUS (SCN) BINDING OF α-BUNGAROTOXIN (α-BTX) IN THE RAT. M.M. Miller* and R.B. Billiar, Department of Reproductive Biology, Case Western Reserve University, Cleveland, Ohio 44106, USA.

α-BTX, a nicotinic cholinergic antagonist, binds to the rat hypothalamic SCN in male and female rats and castrated males but not to the SCN of ovariectomized rats. Nicotinic cholinergic neurotransmission has been suggested to mediate the SCN light entrainment and inhibition of circadian pineal melatonin biosynthesis, of which SNAT is the rate-limiting step. We studied the nocturnal increase in pineal SNAT activity and its reversal by light and observed that the levels in intact and ovariectomized females were similar during the dark (695±70 pmol/min/gland vs 590±68) or after 20' of lights on (107±5 vs 105±8). Carbachol injected at midnight into the lateral ventricles of orbitally enucleated rats simulated the lights-on effect in both intact and ovariectomized rats. However, purified α-BTX (fractions 2.2 or 3.3) injected into either the 3rd ventricle or bilaterally adjacent to the SCN had no effect on either the night-time increase or lights-on inhibition of pineal SNAT in either intact female or male rats or ovariectomized rats. While gonadal steroids appear to affect the binding of α-BTX to nicotinic cholinergic receptors in the SCN, this hormone-receptor interaction probably does not affect the modulation of pineal activity by the SCN.

1832 PARTICIPATION OF 2-HYDROXYESTRONE IN THE INITIATION OF PREOVULATORY LH SURGE IN RATS. S.K. Panda*, D. Cecchini and S.C. Chattoraj, Dept. of Obstetrics and Gynecology, Boston University School of Medicine, Boston, Massachusetts 02118 U.S.A.

Since 2-hydroxyestrone(2-OHE$_1$) is the major metabolite of estradiol-17β(E$_2$) and high level of E$_2$ is one of the causes for initiating LH surge, we have studied the correlation between the plasma level of 2-OHE$_1$ and LH in the rats at the day of proestrus. Adult female Sprague Dawley rats were taken for experiments and estrous cycle were monitered by vaginal smears taken in the morning. From each group, 6 rats were sacrificed at 3 h intervals on the day of proestrus from 900 h through 2400 h. Plasma LH and 2-OHE$_1$ levels were analyzed by radioimmunoassay. The 2-OHE$_1$ levels were 7 and 3 pg/ml at 900 h and 1200 h respectively while it was 9-12 pg/ml in the afternoon and reached 18 pg/ml at 2400 h. The plasma level of LH was high at 1200 h and peaked at 1500-1800 h and came to basal level by 2400 h. From the present observation it is concluded that low level of plasma 2-OHE$_1$ may be the one of the important factors for initiating the LH surge.

1833 EFFECTS OF FOLLICULAR ATRESIA ON THE IN VITRO UPTAKE OF C^{14}-ACETATE BY THE GRANULOSA CELLS OF THE RAT OVARY. R.K. Parshad* and S.S. Gurava, Department of Zoology, Punjab Agricultural University, Ludhiana 141004, India.

The granulosa cells in the preovulatory follicles get luteinized under influence of LH surge with the deprivation of which they become atretic. During either state they show accumulation of lipids. In order to elucidate the functional differences between the granulosa cells of normal and atretic preovulatory follicles, we have studied the in vitro uptake of C^{14}-acetate by both the types of granulosa cells. Rate of C^{14}-acetate uptake per hour is significantly more in the granulosa cells of atretic than those of the normal follicles. Addition of follicular fluid and human chorionic gonadotropin (HCG) separately and simultaneously significantly increase the uptake of C^{14}-acetate by the granulosa cells of normal follicles, but had no effect on those of atretic follicles. The atretic follicles were obtained from rats deprived of preovulatory gonadotropin surge with pentobarbitone administration. These studies, thus indicate that the granulosa cells of atretic follicles which were deprived of LH surge in vivo fail to respond to follicular fluid and HCG in vitro possibly because of the loss of gonadotropin receptor sites.

1834 LIPOPROTEIN UTILIZATION IN RAT LUTEAL CELLS DURING GONADOTROPIN-INDUCED REFRACTORY STATES. K.G. Rajendran* and K.M.J. Menon, Dept. Ob. Gyn., Univ. Michigan Med. Sch., Ann Arbor, MI 48109, U.S.A.

The loss of in vitro responsiveness of ovaries isolated from PMSG/hCG primed rats to exogenous gonadotropins for progesterone production could possibly be related to depletion of endogenous steroid substrate in the ovary. Ovaries from pseudopregnant rats desensitized in vivo with 50 IU of hCG showed 50 % depletion of cellular cholesteryl ester content within 30 min with concomitant increase in progesterone secretion. This treatment resulted in a loss of gonadotropin response of the isolated ovarian cells as early as 1 h after the injection, but exogenous Low Density Lipoprotein (LDL) and High Density Lipoprotein (HDL) were capable of stimulating progesterone production upto 4 h of hormone injection. There was no significant incorporation of tritium from [^{3}H]cholesteryl linoleate-LDL ([^{3}H]CL-LDL) into progesterone by the cells from the hormone-injected group, though the uptake of [^{3}H]CL-LDL was 3-fold higher than that seen in the control animals. When subcellular fractions from hCG desensitized rats preincubated with [^{3}H]CL-LDL were examined, it was found that receptor-bound LDL is internalized as efficiently as in the control cells but its degradation and utilization for steroid synthesis are impaired. These results suggest that i) steroidogenesis can be stimulated upto 4 h following hCG injection but not afterwords, ii) during the refractory period, the ovaries from hCG injected rats were capable of binding and internalizing exogenously supplied cholesterol-carrying lipoproteins and that iii) LDL internalization is intact but its degradation into steroids was impaired in desensitized ovaries. Supported by NIH Grant HD-06656

1835 BIOLOGICAL PROPERTIES OF CHEMICALLY DEGLYCOSYLATED HUMAN ASIALOCHORIOGONADOTROPIN IN GRANULOSA CELLS.

T. Ranta*, H-C. Chen, Y. Shimohigashi, A. J. Baukal, M. Knecht and K. J. Catt, ERRB, NICHD, NIH, Bethesda, MD. U.S.A.

The ability of chemically deglycosylated human asialochoriogonadotropin (AHF-hCG) to modify the actions of FSH and LH was studied in granulosa cells from DES-implanted immature rats. When added to 48 h FSH-treated granulosa cells, AHF-hCG bound to LH receptors with approximately 2-fold higher binding affinity than that of native hCG, and about 14-fold higher affinity than that of ovine LH. AHF-hCG acted as a partial LH agonist since it slightly increased cAMP production, and stimulated progesterone (P) production to the same extent as LH. However, it inhibited LH-stimulated cAMP formation by 70%, but not P production, consistent with its action as an LH antagonist at the level of adenylate cyclase. When added with FSH to freshly prepared granulosa cells, AHF-hCG inhibited FSH-stimulated P production by 50% and increased cGMP formation 2-fold during 48 h of culture, but only slightly reduced cAMP formation. Such a decrease in P production suggests that spare FSH receptors are not present during granulosa cell differentiation. In contrast, native hCG did not alter FSH-induced cAMP or P production, but reduced cGMP production in response to FSH or choleragen. Whereas native hCG displayed only 0.1% cross-reaction in the FSH receptor assay, AHF-hCG bound to FSH receptors of ovarian homogenates from DES-treated rats with about 5% of the binding affinity of ovine FSH. These results indicate that removal of the sugar moieties of hCG increases its binding affinity for both LH and FSH receptors, with a relatively greater increase in FSH receptor affinity, and confers the ability to modify target cell responses to both gonadotropins.

1836 LH STIMULATES PLASMINOGEN ACTIVATOR (PA) IN RAT PREOVULATORY FOLLICLES

R. Reich, R. Miskin and A. Tsafriri*, Departments of Hormone Research and Biochemistry, The Weizmann Institute of Science, Rehovot 76100, Israel

Production of PA by granulosa cells (GC) and its stimulation by gonadotropins led to the suggestion that PA is involved in ovulation. However, while only LH may be regarded as the physiological ovulation-inducing hormone in the rat, FSH was found to be much more potent than LH in enhancing GC PA production. Assuming that the entire follicular wall, rather than isolated GC, is the tissue involved in follicular rupture, we have compared the potency of LH and FSH in stimulating PA activity by rat preovulatory follicles in culture. LH (NIH-LH-S21) was 5-fold more potent than FSH (NIH-FSH-S14), and purified ovine LH and FSH, generously provided by Dr. Sairam, were equally potent in enhancing follicular PA activity. Furthermore, injection into the ovarian bursa of proestrous rats of ε-caproic acid (CA) and benzamidine (0.05-0.25 mmole), inhibitors of serine proteases, resulted in a dose dependent inhibition of ovulation without causing changes discernible by histological examination. Administration of the inhibitors prior to hCG up to 2 h after it inhibited ovulation (>60%) but had limited effect after 3 h (<20% inhibition). CA not only inhibited ovulation but also reduced breakdown of *in vivo* labeled ovarian collagen as measured by labeled hydroxyproline from ovarian acid hydrolyzates separated by HPLC. The extent of inhibition of ovulation and of collagenolysis correlated with the dose of CA employed. In conclusion, LH is as potent as FSH in stimulating follicular PA activity and the involvement of serine proteases, most probably plasmin, in preovulatory breakdown of collagen and ovulation was corroborated. Supported by the Rockefeller Found.

1837 ISOLATION OF INHIBIN FROM BOVINE FOLLICULAR FLUID (bFF). D.M. Robertson*, L.M. Foulds, L. Leversha, F.J. Morgan, M.T. W. Hearn, H. Burger and D.M. de Kretser, Department of Anatomy, Monash University, Medical Research Centre, Prince Henry's Hospital, and St. Vincent's School of Medical Research, Melbourne, Victoria, Australia.

In order to obtain a purified preparation of ovarian inhibin, bFF free of cystic fluid was collected on ice in the presence of protease inhibitors. Neat bFF was fractionated by gel filtration on Sephacryl S200 using ammonium acetate pH7.0 as eluting buffer and the void volume fraction (mol. wt.>10^5) chromatographed on Sephadex G100 under acidic elution conditions. The inhibin fraction was then fractionated on reversed phase HPLC and preparative polyacrylamide gel electrophoresis. The purification procedure was monitored by an *in vitro* bioassay based on the graded suppression of FSH content in cultured rat pituitary cells using a bFF preparation as standard, and a parallel line bioassay design. Evidence of sample cytotoxicity in the bioassay was monitored by cell morphology, evidence of non-parallelism with the standard, a ^{51}Cr release procedure and effects on other pituitary hormones. The final product, based on biological activity, was about 1000 fold purified with recoveries ranging from 1-5%. On SDS polyacrylamide gel electrophoresis, this preparation consisted of two bands within the 55,000-62,000 molecular weight range of which the major band (~ 55,000) is biologically active. The purified preparation suppressed FSH but not LH, TSH or PRL in the *in vitro* bioassay. The results represent a significant purification of a large molecular weight material with markedly enhanced inhibin bioactivity. This study was supported by N.H. & M.R.C. of Australia.

1838 IDENTIFICATION OF AN OVARIAN MEMBRANE PROTEASE THAT MAY MEDIATE HORMONAL STIMULATION OF ADENYLATE CYCLASE. P. C. Roche* and R. J. Ryan, Dept. Cell Biology, Mayo Medical School, Rochester, MN 55905

Adenylate cyclase (AC) can be stimulated by serine proteases and inhibited by low-molecular-weight protease inhibitors (LMPI). This suggests the involvement of a membrane serine protease(s) in hormonal stimulation of AC. The membrane enriched 2000 xg pellet from luteinized rat ovaries contains numerous proteases of varying molecular weights. These proteases can be resolved and visualized in casein-containing SDS-polyacrylamide gels as previously described (BBA 745:82,1983). None of these enzymes are inhibited by LMPI's that block hCG stimulation of AC. In gelatin-containing gels, however, we have identified a previously undetected membrane protease of M_r = 54,000 which may be involved in cyclase activation. This enzyme is selectively inhibited by LMPI's at concentrations that also block hormonal stimulation of AC. 2.5% SDS will efficiently solubilize and reversibly inhibit this protease but Triton X-100 will not. Although it migrates with an M_r = 54,000 by SDS-PAGE, the protease gel filters on Sephacryl S-200 in nonionic detergent (Lubrol PX) with an apparent M_r = 150,000. This protease will not bind to Concanavalin A but is retarded on an arginine-Sepharose column. The gelatinase activity of the enzyme appears optimum between pH 5 and 7. Further purification is being undertaken and studies are in progress to determine if this membrane protease displays hormonally responsive activity. (Supported by HD 9140, HD 7108 and the Mayo Foundation).

1839 FURTHER STUDIES ON OVINE SMALL LUTEAL (SL) AND LARGE LUTEAL (LL) CELLS.
R.J. Rodgers*, J.D. O'Shea and J.K. Findlay, Veterinary Preclinical Sciences, University of Melbourne, and Medical Research Centre, Prince Henry's Hospital, Melbourne, Australia.

We have shown that both SL and LL cells produce progesterone (P) *in vitro*, but only the SL cells respond to LH by increased P production (J. Reprod. Fert. 69, 113, 1983). Here we report the effects of various agents and hormones on P production (see Table, n = 5 per treatment, paired t-tests), and an investigation into potential interactions between SL and LL cells in P production.

AGENT	% OF CONTROL		AGENT	% OF CONTROL	
	SMALL	LARGE		SMALL	LARGE
Ca Ionophore (0.1μM)	101.9	103.0	LH-RH (1μg/ml)	87.7	111.2
Verapamil (100μM)	20.4**	31.8*	Oestradiol (250ng/ml)	86.5	105.1
Colchicine (10μM)	83.8*	73.0*	GTP analogue (100μM)	94.6	105.1
Cytochalasin B(5μg/ml)	80.8*	84.0*	Isoprenaline (10μM)	115.2	145.9*
			Oxytocin (50miu/ml)	111.8	92.7

*P<0.05 **P<0.01 compared with control.

The results suggest that P production *in vitro* by both cell types is dependent on calcium fluxes, microtubules and microfilaments, and that isoprenaline can stimulate P production by LL cells. P production by SL and LL cells after recombination of SL and LL cells in ratios similar to those found *in vivo* was the same as the sum of P production by equivalent numbers of SL and LL cells incubated separately, thus providing no evidence of synergism between SL and LL cells in P production.

1840 ENDOGENOUS DOPAMINE IS INVOLVED IN THE CONTROL OF VASOPRESSIN RELEASE AS AN INHIBITORY FACTOR. Y.Oki*, S.Ohgo, N.Kikuchi, M.Nanno, H.Kurahachi and T.Yoshimi, 2nd Div.,Dep.of Int. Med., Hamamatsu University School of Med., Hamamatsu, Japan.

In order to investigate the role for central dopaminergic system in the control of vasopressin (VP) release, two series of studies were done. (I) The changes of plasma VP concentrations and dopamine (DA) concentrations in the neurohypophysis (NH) were studied in rats when deprived of water or injected with hypertonic (4.5%) saline (HS) intraperitoneally (25 ml/kg of BW). Water deprivation for 24 h caused significant increases in both plasma VP and NH DA, and for 48 - 72 h caused further increases in them. 30 min after injection HS caused marked increases in both plasma VP and NH DA, and 120 min after the injection plasma VP and NH DA were depressed as compared to those at 30 min though still above the control values. Increases in plasma VP and NH DA did not dissociate in time under all the conditions examined. (II) The effects of DA on VP release from rat hypothalamo-neurohypophyseal complex (HNC) were studied in vitro. HNC prepared by the method of Sladek et al. was perifused at 37°C with Krebs-Ringer-Bicarbonate buffer containing 0.5% BSA and 0.2% glucose under 95% O_2 and 5% CO_2 at a speed of 1 ml/fraction/2.5 min. Using this perifusion system, 3 - 5 fold increase of VP release were demonstrated by increase of NaCl by 20 mM and marked increase of VP release by increase of KCl by 50 mM in the medium. Increase in VP release in response to increase in NaCl (by 20 mM) were abolished by addition of DA to the medium to 10^{-7}M. These results would suggest that central DA has an important role, probably inhibitory, in the control of VP release.

1841 IDENTIFICATION OF FIVE DIFFERENT CELL TYPES IN THE PREOPTICO NEUROSECRETORY SYSTEM OF THE SEA BASS, DICENTRARCHUS LABRAX (TELEOSTEI). F. Ollevier*, W. Verdonck, M. Cambre, E. Kühn and F. Vandesande, Catholic University of Leuven, Zoological Institute, Naamsestraat 59, B-3000 Leuven, Belgium.

An immunocytochemical investigation of the hypothalamo-hypophysial axis of the sea bass, Dicentrarchus labrax, reveals the presence of at least 5 different cell types in the nucleus preopticus (NPO). Using the single and double unlabeled antibody peroxidase anti-peroxidase method in the NPO specifically staining cell bodies are found with anti-CRF, -somatostatin, -enkephalin, -arginine vasotocin and -isotocin. The absence of a portal system between the hypothalamus and the hypophysis makes it possible to follow fibres from these perikarya into the neurohypophysis. In the anterior part of the neurohypophysis CRF positive fibres are found, terminating close to the basal lamina that lines the rostral pars distalis. SRIF-like containing fibres are present in the neurohypophysis penetrating the proximal pars distalis. In the distal part of the neurohypophysis not only enkephalin, arginine vasotocin and isotocin positive fibres are found but also numerous CRF positive fibres. In order to relate the terminals of the specific neuronal fibres with some cell types of the hypophysis, ACTH-, α-MSH-, LH-, STH-, and TSH-cell types of the hypophysis are immunologically stained and determined.

1842 CHARACTERIZATION OF SPECIFIC VASOPRESSIN BINDING IN A RAT AORTA MEMBRANE PREPARATION. A. Frances Pearlmutter*, Mary Szkrybalo, and Gary Pettibone, Department of Biochemistry, Medical College of Ohio, Toledo, OH 43699 USA

Arginine vasopressin (AVP) has been shown to have a direct pressor effect on the smooth muscle of the vasculature. As part of our continuing efforts to elucidate the role of vasopressin and vasopressin receptors in the maintenance and elevation of blood pressure levels, we have identified and characterized specific binding sites for AVP in the rat aorta. Rat aortas were removed immediately after decapitation and placed in Krebs-Ringer solution, pH 7.3. After tissue homogenization, the 1000 x g pellet was discarded and membranes that centrifuged between 1 and 100 K were used for binding studies. With 5 mM Mg^{2+} in Tris-maleate buffer at pH 7.6, Scatchard analysis with ^{3}H-AVP of high specific activity showed a Kd of 1.7 nM, well within the physiological range. With 5 mM Co^{2+}, Ni^{2+}, and Mn^{2+}, the Kd was lower, 10 nM. The Rmax for all of the metal ions varied between 0.2 and 0.6 nM/mg protein. Time course studies showed that equilibrium for specific binding was reached at about 30 min with 90% of the total specific binding occuring within the first 3 min. Temperature studies indicated that at 10 C and 20 C, maximum binding was reached within 30 min with no further dissociation for the next 60 min. At 37 C, the ^{3}H-AVP was rapidly degraded in the presence of the membranes. Structure-function studies to determine the specificity of the binding have shown that AVP is more potent than either deamino AVP or d$(CH_2)_5$Tyr(OMe)AVP in displacing ^{3}H-AVP from specific binding sites. We conclude that we are measuring physiologically relevant binding sites in rat aorta and that these binding sites may be those involved in the pressor effects of AVP. This work was supported by a grant from the Northwest Ohio Heart Association.

1843 OXYTOCIN RECEPTORS IN SHEEP AND RAT MYOMETRIUM: HIGH OR LOW AFFINITY BINDING SITES?

V. Pliška*, J. Heiniger, A. Müller-Lhotsky and B.A. Ekberg, Institut für Tierproduktion, Eidg. Technische Hochschule, CH-8092 Zürich, Switzerland and FERRING AB, S-20062 Malmö, Sweden.

High K_{diss}-values for oxytocin in rat myometrium plasma membranes as reported by Soloff & Schwartz (J. Biol. Chem. *249*, 1376) and Crankshaw et al. (Eur. J. Biochem. *86*, 341) markedly contrast with low pA_2 values for inhibitors structurally similar to oxytocin. We have therefore reinvestigated the oxytocin binding to sheep and rat myometrium using short-time monolayer cultures (0 to 12 days) of myometrium cells. Experiments carried out with tritiated oxytocin (26 Ci/mmol) and suspensions of vital cells indicate populations of binding sites with following approx. K_{diss}'s: 10^{-9} (minor population), 5×10^{-8} and $>10^{-4}$ mol/l. Binding on all the sites is displaceable by cold oxytocin; however, a saturation of the latter population has not been achieved at concs of up to 5×10^{-4}M. Binding sites with $K_{diss}\simeq5\times10^{-8}$ seem to be identical with oxytocin receptors: 1) pA_2 values for most of the substances acting as competitive inhibitors of oxytocin range from 6 to 8 (K_{diss}: 10^{-6} to 10^{-8}); 2) computation of K_{diss} for oxytocin from side chain contributions to pA_2 (Pliška, Experientia *34*, 1190) yields a value close to 10^{-7}; and finally, 3) a similar value can be obtained from titration of oxytocin receptor in rat uterus by irreversible inhibitors (Pliška & Marbach, Eur. J. Pharmacol. *49*, 213).

Supported by Swiss National Science Foundation, Grant 3.705-80.

1844 PSYCHOGENIC POLYDIPSIA AND HYPONATREMIA: EVIDENCE FOR A RESET OSMOSTAT.

V. Ragavan*, J. Verbalis, M. Wood, P. Randels, G. French and A. Robinson. VA Medical Center, Coatesville, PA and U. of Pittsburgh, Pittsburgh, PA, USA

Psychogenic polydipsia is found in up to 3-4% of psychiatric patients and in a subset of these patients, hyponatremia can lead to seizures, coma and death. Osmoregulation of vasopressin (AVP) secretion was studied in 6 institutionalized psychiatric patients with polydipsia of 5-20L/day and hyponatremia ($p[NA^+]\leq120$mEq/L). All patients had documented chronic schizophrenia and no evidence of drug induced SIADH. All patients received 1. Hypertonic saline infusion (3% NaCl of 0.25 ccs/kg/min given IV over 60' after an initial water load of 1.2L PO). 2. Standard Miller-Moses dehydration tests with either pitressin (PIT) (5Units SQ) or urea (30g PO) given at peak Uosm. During each test, $p[NA^+]$, Uosm and volume, Posm and plasma AVP (pAVP) level by RIA were measured. In 3 of 6 subjects, we observed 1. Uosm was suppressed to <100mOsm/kg despite inappropriately low mean $p[NA^+]$ of 119±3(S.E.M.)mEq/L following water load. 2. After hypertonic saline, increases in pAVP were seen at a mean $p[NA^+]$ of 126±2mEq/L with peak pAVP levels of 4.4±1.3μU/ml occurring at mean $p[NA^+]$ of 134±2mEq/L. 3. Oral urea significantly stimulated pAVP levels. Before PIT pAVP (μU/ml) was 3.6±0.9 and 4 h later 3.0±0.4 (N.S.) whereas after urea, pAVP rose from 2.9±0.4 to 4.2±0.5 (P<0.02). Because a significant fraction of our patients excreted maximally dilute urine following water loading with an inappropriately low threshold for AVP secretion, we conclude that many patients with polydipsia and hyponatremia have a reset osmostat for AVP secretion. Additionally, in these patients, AVP secreting neurones seem to be stimulated abnormally by urea. A reset osmostat in these patients may explain the presence of stable hyponatremia despite continued polydipsia.

1845 THE GONADAL ATROPHY INDUCED BY SHORT PHOTOPERIOD IS TEMPERATURE DEPENDENT IN THE GOLDEN HAMSTER. P.Pévet (1,2) and B.Vivien-Roels (1). (1), Lab.Zool. exp.Embryol.,Strasbourg,France, (2), The Netherlands Inst.Brain Res.,Amsterdam, The Netherlands.

In their natural habitat, hamsters are submitted,in autumn, to a decrease of photoperiod and also to a decrease of environmental temperature. The aim of this study was to examine the effects of temperature on the phenomenon of gonadal atrophy induced by short photoperiod (SP).

All the adult male hamsters, used in this study, were always kept under long photoperiod (LP) at 22°C before the experiment. They were then divided into groups of 5 animals and kept either under LP (14L/10D) or SP (10L/14D) at temperatures of respectively 5,15,22 or 25°C. Groups were sacrificed after 3,5,8,10 and 18 weeks (w). Gonadal activity was determined by testicular weight (T.W.) and plasmatic testosterone concentrations (Test.).

Under LP, independently of the temperature, animals remained sexually active (T.W.≈ 1300mg,Test.3-5ng/ml). After 8w under SP the gonads of all animals kept at 5,15 or 22°C were atrophied (T.W.≈ 150mg, Test.< 1ng/ml) while those of animals kept at 25°C weighed yet 300mg. The gonadal atrophy in these animals was not achieved after 10w but was complete after 18w. After 5w the gonadal atrophy was complete in hamsters kept at 5 and 15°C while the gonads of those kept at 22 and 25°C were active. After 3w, a complete gonadal atrophy was only observed in animals kept at 5°C. In those kept at 15°C only a small inhibition was evident (T.W.≈ 800mg).

This experiment demonstrates that the rate at which the SP induces gonadal atrophy in the hamster is dependent of the environmental temperature. Studies are now in progress to determine if the pineal is implicated in this synergic effect of the temperature and the SP on the gonadal axis.

1846 BLIND, ANOSMIC FEMALE RATS DO NOT HAVE DAILY LH SURGES. David R. Pieper*, Mark R. Mortiere, Peter R. Shipley and Yue-Kuang Tang, University of Detroit, Department of Biology and Health Sciences, Detroit, MI 48221 USA.

Previous Studies have shown that female hamsters on short photoperiod become acyclic, possibly due to daily LH surges, and that these effects are eliminated if the animals are pinealectomized PX) before being placed on the short photoperiod. Pre-pubertally blinded (BL) and olfactory bulbectomized (BX) female rats also have irregular estrous cycles, and this effect is also eliminated by PX (Endo Rev 1:109,1983). The main question addressed by the present study was whether the BL+BX rats also have daily LH surges. Twenty-five day old female Sprague-Dawley rats were divided into 5 groups: LD 14:10 Sham (Control); BL+BX; BL+BX+PX; LD 6:18 Sham and LD 6:18 BX. Ten weeks following surgery, all animals were sampled (0.5 ml) every 5 hrs for 2 days from an indwelling atrial catheter. Daily vaginal smears indicated that the BL+BX group were in estrus much less frequently than Controls (15.8 ± 1.8 vs 27.3 ± 1.5 percent of days cornified cells,>10 rats/group smeared for more than 23 days each) and in general had longer, irregular cycles. the other 3 groups all had smear patterns similar to Controls. All 5 groups had LH surges on the day of proestrus (>200 ng/ml maximum value) but no group had LH surges on 2 sequential days or an LH surge on any day of diestrus. These results indicate that (1) BL+BX female rats do become acyclic but do not have daily LH surges (2) BX female rats maintained on short photoperiod neither become acyclic, nor have daily LH surges and (3) the acyclicity of BL+BX rats is not analogous to the acyclicity of female hamsters on short photoperiod. Supported by NSF grant PCM 81-21327.

1847 INHIBITORY FEEDBACK CONTROL EXERTED BY CORTISOL AND ANDROGENS ON THE PITUITARY CELL IS REVERSIBLE. N.D. Maestracci and H. Beauregard*, Depts. of Medicine and Notre-Dame Hospital, University of Montreal, Montreal, Quebec.

Little is known about the inhibitory control exerted by cortisol and androgens on the normal human pituitary cell. A pituitary gland was obtained during the autopsy of a 55 years old cushinoid woman who died of a highly secreting adenocarcinoma of the adrenal (cortisoluria > 600 μg/24 hrs, total androgens > 2227 mg%). After its removal, the hypophysis was processed for monolayer cell culture and maintained 12 days on extracellular matrix and a variety of measurements were made. We studied the in vitro basal secretion of gonadotrophic and corticotrophic hormones and their regulation by their respective hypothalamic releasing factors. 1) R.I.A. assays were performed for all hormones every 24 hours. The total amount of pituitary hormonal secretion is as follows on day 5: PRL 32624 ng, GH 26 904 ng, LH 262 mIU, FSH 232 mIU, α subunits 137 ng, ACTH 250 pg, hNT 14808 ng. 2) In vitro incubation with physiological concentration of GnRH induced a response of all subunits LH, FSH and α (7x, 4x and 6x respectively). 3) The molar ratio of α to LH and/or FSH is < 1 and remains normal during stimulation by GnRH. 4) The corticotropin and its precursor both increased after CRF and/or vasopressine stimulation. These results indicate that monolayer cell culture is a suitable method to maintain an acquired phenotype of pituitary cells and a reliable one for dynamic test. In this case we have demonstrated that eventhough pituitary hormones were under tremendous long lasting suppressing effect, the cells retain their receptors to hypothalamic factors and also their capacity of secretion.

1848 SIMULTANEOUS BILATERAL SELECTIVE SAMPLING FOR 5 PITUITARY HORMONES IN PROLACTINOMA. J. Mahoudeau, J. Théron, P. Leymarie*, H. Herrou, G. Muller and G. Travert, C.H.U., 14000 Caen, France.

9 patients with surgically demonstrated prolactinoma were studied by prolactin (PRL) assays in blood collected from both inferior petrosal sinuses (IPS) during a phlebography procedure. This study was performed between 1977 and 1980, when CT-scan was not yet precise enough and surgical indications still frequent. Plasma levels of PRL (ng/ml $\pm$ SD) in peripheral vein, dominant side of IPS (IPSmax) and opposite side (IPSmin) were, respectively: 137 $\pm$ 192, 581 $\pm$ 871, and 209 $\pm$ 249. The PRL gradient (IPSmax/peripheral) was 4.60 $\pm$ 2.42 (range 2.33 - 9.44). The venous drainage of pituitary PRL was asymmetrical (IPSmax/IPSmin > 1.1) in all patients. During the surgical operation, performed after the study, the adenoma was found to be lateralized in 8/9 cases. Blood PRL level in IPS was highest on the side of the tumor in only 5 cases, and on the opposite side in 3 cases. In 5 patients, 4 other hormones were measured in the same blood samples; the mean gradient (IPSmax/peripheral) of these hormones was: LH, 1.17; FSH, 1.18; TSH, 1.83; GH, 3.70. All 5 hormones were more concentrated on the same side in all patients, including 4 patients with a lateralized tumor and one case with a median tumor. In no case, the side of PRL drainage was the opposite of that of other hormones. Although it was suggested from 3 cases (JCEM 57: 1070, 1983) that selective sampling could show the side of lateralized ACTH-secreting adenoma, we conclude that this technique fails to indicate the side of a PRL-secreting tumor.

1849 TREATMENT OF HYPERPROLACTINAEMIA, ACROMEGALY AND CUSHING´S DISEASE WITH DOPAMINE AGONISTS LISURIDE AND TERGURIDE /TRANS-DIHYDROLISURIDE/.

J. Marek*, J.Šrámková and K.Řežábek, 3rd Dept.of Medicine, Charles University, and Research Institute for Pharmacy and Biochemistry, Prague, Czechoslovakia.

Reports on long-term treatment with lisuride /LD/ and on outcomes of pregnancies enabled by this therapy are scarce. 57 patients with prolactinomas /PMA/, 21 with acromegaly and 6 with Cushing´s disease were treated with LD in doses 0.075-6 mg/day up to 7 years. The therapy enabled conception in all 19 women with PMA desiring pregnancy. In 15 patients with large invasive PMA, incompletly removed by surgery, LD normalised prolactin /PRL/ levels and prevented regrowth of the tumours. In 5 men LD restored plasma testosterone and normal sexual function. In 32 patients with PMA LD increased somatomedin /SM/ levels measured by chick embryo bioassay. In acromegaly complete normalisation was achieved in 2 patients, partial improvement in 5. In 9 acromegalics SM levels fell to normal despite elevated GH levels. A significant fall in urinary free noradrenaline was found in 9 patients during the treatment. Terguride /1-6 mg/day/ was given to 21 patients /15 with PMA, 6 with acromegaly/ for 6-24 months; 8 of them did not tolerate LD previously. Effects on PRL and GH were similar as of LD, however less side effects, especially no decrease of blood pressure, were observed.

1850 IS THERE AN INFLUENCE OF A CALCIUM-ANTAGONIST (VERAPAMIL) ON THE REGULATION OF THE PRL, TSH, LH, FSH RELEASE ?

C. Mazzi*, G. Re Sartò, L.Mattaini, Endocrinology Department, St Anthony Hospital, 21013 Gallarate, Italy.

Verapamil (Isoptin, Knoll) has been administered orally, daily dose 120mg, for eight days, to nine females,aged 57 to 74 yrs, hospitalized for chronic atrial fibrillation. Blood samples were taken for estimations (RIA) of PRL, TSH, LH, FSH. At the end of verapamil treatment, no modification have been registered in basal PRL (before: 9.5 ± 1.5; after: 9.4 ± 1.6 ng/ml) and in basal TSH (before: 1.4 ± 0.2; after: 1.7 ± 0.2 mcU/ml) and in their replies to 200 mcg i.v. TRH (PRL peak: before: 36.6 ± 4.1; after:42.3 ± 5.0 ng/ml - TSH peak: before: 6.4 ± 1.5; after: 6.1 ± 1.2 mcU/ml). Also no significant changes have been registered in basal LH (before: 58.2 ± 9.3; after: 55.4 ± 10.1 mUI/ml) and in basal FSH (before: 70.3 ± 9.0; after: 74.4 ± 11.0 mUI/ml) and in their replies to 100 mcg i.v. LHRH (LH peak: before: 125.7 ± 20.1; after: 127.0 ± 18.8 mUI/ml - FSH peak: before: 99.1 ± 19.6; after: 92.0 ± 13.1 mUI/ml). These data have been shown that verapamil had no effect on baseline hormone levels and on their responses to Releasing Hormones. But remain to be established long term endocrine effects on the calcium-antagonists. More informations are requised on the precise intracellular actions of the calcium-antagonists before they can be used to study the role of calcium in hormone release in vivo.

1851 PITUITARY ADENOMAS IN OLD SPRAGUE-DAWLEY RATS. D.J. McComb*, K. Kovacs, J. Beri and F. Zak, Dept. of Pathology, St. Michael's Hospital, University of Toronto, Toronto, Ont., M5B 1W8 Canada; Dept. of Toxicological Pathology Ciba-Geigy Ltd., Basel, CH-4002, Switzerland.

Spontaneous pituitary adenomas occur in man and a variety of animal species. In our study, 27 male and 39 female Sprague-Dawley rats over 24 months of age, control material in a long-term toxicology study, were killed and pituitaries removed and processed for light and electron microscopic investigation, including immunocytochemistry at the light and electron microscopic level. Adenomas were found in 70% of male and 78% of female rats. Prolactin (PRL)-containing adenomas were most common (47.2%) while immunonegative adenomas (16.3%), luteinizing hormone (LH)-containing adenomas (14.2%), PRL/growth hormone (GH)-containing adenomas (10.9%), thyroid-stimulating hormone (TSH)-containing adenomas (3.6%), adrenocorticotropic hormone (ACTH)-containing adenomas (3.6%), GH-containing adenomas (1.8%) were also identified. Unexpected combinations were observed in 3 tumors: a GH/LH-containing adenoma, a PRL/ACTH-containing adenoma and a PRL/LH/TSH-containing adenoma were noted. One ACTH-containing intermediate lobe adenoma and one metastatic plasmacytoma were diagnosed. Ultrastructural investigation revealed that the tumors also exist in different morphologic forms, as do those occurring in human patients. These results indicate that all known cell types of the rat adenohypophysis can give rise to adenomas. Spontaneous adenomas in rat should prove useful models of the human disease. (This work was supported, in part, by a grant from the St. Michael's Hospital Research Society)

1852 HUMAN GROWTH HORMONE EXPRESSION BY HUMAN-RAT SOMATOTROPH CELL HYBRIDS. S. Melmed*, S. Slanina and M. Leung, Dept. of Medicine, Cedars-Sinai Medical Center-UCLA School of Medicine, Los Angeles, CA 90048.

Interspecific somatic cell hybrids were isolated after fusion of human acromegaly tumor cells (oubain-sensitive) with GH_3 rat pituitary tumor cells (aminopterin-sensitive). After fusion with PEG, hybrids were grown in double selection medium containing hypoxanthine, aminopterin and thymidine (HAT) and oubain (10 uM). This was lethal to both parental cells and only true interspecific hybrids survived. Hybrids were cloned and cells secreting human GH (hGH), rat GH (rGH) and rat PRL (rPRL) were subcultured. Levels of hGH ranged from 10-2400 ng/flask/24 h after subculture and were sustained for 4-6 weeks. hGH co-eluted with ^{125}I-hGH standard on Sephadex G-75. Cytoplasmic mRNA specific for hGH was detected by nitrocellulose hybridization of cell extracts with a ^{32}P-cDNA probe for hGH. Hybrid nature of the cells was confirmed by the mixed human-rat karyotype and expression of both human and rat forms of lactic dehydrogenase isozymes. hGH secretion declined despite the presence of chromosome 17 (containing the structural gene for hGH) in over 50% of metaphase spreads, suggesting either a translocation of 17, or loss of other regulatory genes. Treatment of hybrids cells with hydrocortisone (HCT 100 nM) stimulated hybrid cell proliferation by 60%, whereas GH_3 parental cell growth was inhibited by HCT. HCT stimulated both hGH and rGH secretion 2-3 fold respectively and suppressed rPRL. Conclusion: Interspecific hybrids displayed both concordant hormonal expression of hGH and rGH, as well as regulation of both these genes by HCT. hGH expression is induced by HCT in phenotypic pituitary hybrid cells.

1853 EFFECT OF ACTINOMYCIN D AND CYCLOHEXIMIDE ON ESTRADIOL MODULATED PITUITARY GnRH BINDING CAPACITY.

M. Menon, H. Peegel*, V. Katta and K.M.J. Menon, Dept. of Ob./Gyn, University of Michigan, Ann Arbor, MI 48109 USA.

This study was designed to investigate the mechanism by which 17-β estradiol (E_2) potentiates the action of GnRH on the pituitary *in vitro*. Immature female rat pituitary cells were cultured in media with adsorbed sera. Cultures exposed to E_2 exhibited a dose (10^{-10} to 10^{-6} M) and time (0-48 h) dependent augmentation of LH release in response to a 4 h GnRH (10 nM) challenge when compared to controls. After 48 h E_2 pretreatment, the amount of LH released was increased from 6401 ± 537 (control) to 9541± 350 ng/ml. A similar stimulatory effect was observed when binding studies were performed utilizing ^{125}I-labeled [D-Ala^6] GnRH ethylamide. Cultures incubated with E_2 at different concentrations and for various lengths of time showed a significant increase in GnRH binding capacity when compared to controls . GnRH binding increased from 1.6 ± 0.04 to 3.0 ± 0.08 fmol/ 10^7 cells after 48 h exposure to 10^{-9} E_2. To determine whether the increase in GnRH receptor activity was sensitive to transcription and translation inhibitors, pituitary cells were incubated for 48 h with E_2 in the presence of Actinomycin D or cycloheximide. It was observed that 5 μM Actinomycin D and 20 μM cycloheximide treatment directly reduced the binding of GnRH by 32% and 40%, respectively. In contrast, control cultures did not exhibit a significant decrease in GnRH binding capacity under these conditions. These results suggest that 1) the E_2 potentiation of LH release *in vitro* in response to GnRH is mediated by an increase in GnRH receptors and 2) there may be E_2 initiated sequence of transcription/translation events leading to the increase in GnRH receptor number. (Supported by NIH Grant HD07729).

1854 PITUITARY ADENOMAS STUDIED WITH POSITRON EMISSION TOMOGRAPHY WITH ^{11}C-METHIONINE AND ^{11}C-BROMOCRIPTINE.

C Muhr*, P O Lundberg, G Antoni, K Bergström, P Hartvig, H Lundqvist, B Långström, C G Stålnacke, Department of Neurology, University Hospital and other institutions, Uppsala University, Uppsala, Sweden

Recent years´ research in neuroendocrinology has been intensive and led to new concepts and underlined the necessity of further differentiation of pituitary adenomas. Positron emission tomography offers unique possibility to perform *in vivo* regional dynamic autoradiography. Nine patients, 5 females and 4 males, age range 26-80 years, with a pituitary adenoma were studied with the PET-technique using ^{11}C-methionine, ^{11}C-bromocriptine and ^{68}Ga-EDTA. The labelled substance was administered intravenously in a dose of 35-180 MBq. Results: The different adenomas showed an interesting variation of the uptake and dynamics of the labelled substances. The ^{11}C-methionine uptake was in all tumors higher than in normal brain tissue,usually2-3 times higher with a variation among the tumors and in 6 tumors higher and in 3 tumors relatively lower uptake. The ^{11}C-bromocriptine uptake was higher in 5 patients and relatively lower in 4 patients. The dynamic uptake of ^{11}C-bromocriptine when subtracted and corrected for the blood concentration showed in some patients with time falling concentration, in other patients a more stable uptake was noticed which was interpreted as some form of entrapment of bromocriptine within the tumor tissue. There is so far no method to evaluate tumor activity in pituitary adenomas and of great interest is to find out if the uptake of ^{11}C-methionine correlates to tumor activity and if the uptake and dynamic of ^{11}C-bromocriptine in the adenoma correlates to the effect of treatment with this drug.

1855 GAMMA AMINOBUTYRIC ACID IS NOT A PROLACTIN RELEASE INHIBITING FACTOR (PIF).
M.C. Obonsawin*, S.H. Shin and L. Bates, Dept. of Physiology, Queen's University, Kingston, Canada, K7L 3N6.

The major PIF is thought to be dopamine. However, there is evidence that a dopamine-free fraction of the hypothalamus can exert an inhibitory influence on prolactin (PRL) secretion. One of the major candidates for this agent is gamma aminobutyric acid (GABA). We first examined GABA's effect on PRL release *in vitro*. Confirming previous work, we found that, in a primary monolayer cell culture system, GABA inhibits PRL release in a dose-related manner. We then examined the physiological role of GABA in the regulation of PRL release *in vivo*, with conscious, freely moving male rats bearing indwelling atrial cannulae. All drugs were administered and blood samples collected via this cannula. In the first experiment, we removed all dopaminergic influence on PRL secretion by prior administration of a dopamine receptor blocker, pimozide (3 mg/kg). GABA (0.1 g/kg and 1.0 g/kg) had no significant effect on plasma PRL in either normal or estradiol primed rats. In the second experiment, we removed all dopaminergic influence on PRL secretion using hypophysectomized rats that had an ectopic pituitary grafted to the renal capsule. Again, no consistent inhibiting effect of GABA (0.1 g/kg or 1.0 g/kg) on PRL secretion was seen. To see if GABA exerted a tonic inhibition on PRL secretion, we administered bicuculline (300 ug/kg), a GABA receptor blocker, in pimozide treated rats. There was no significant increase in plasma PRL concentration. We conclude that, although the pituitary contains receptors for GABA, and GABA may have a pharmacological effect on PRL secretion, it has no physiological role as a PIF. This study was supported by the MRC of Canada.

1856 MECHANISMS OF PROLACTIN MODULATION OF LH ACTION ON THE LEYDIG CELLS OF RATS AND MICE.
W.D. Odell* and J. Larsen, University of Utah School of Medicine, Salt Lake City, Utah, USA.

In *in vivo* studies in the rabbit (Laborde & Odell, 1983), prolactin (PRL) decreased LH stimulation of testosterone (T) secretion and prevented the postcastration rise in LH and FSH. To clarify the mechanisms of PRL effects on the testes, an *in vitro* Leydig cell bioassay for T secretion (Dufau *et al*., 1974) was employed. Using testes from both rats and mice, dose-response curves for human LH (hLH) were established. Then, using a constant submaximal dose of hLH, dose-response curves of PRL were determined. PRL exhibited a biphasic response, inhibiting LH-stimulated T secretion at doses between 0.1 and 10 ng/ml, and stimulating T secretion at high doses of 100 to 1000 ng/ml. Doses of PRL that inhibited T secretion also inhibited progesterone and 17 OHP secretion. In the presence of constant inhibiting doses of PRL, the LH-stimulated T dose-response curves were shifted rightward (decreased sensitivity to LH) and the maximal response was decreased. LH receptor numbers, estimated from Woolf plots, were not changed by prolactin. We conclude that: a) prolactin exerts a biphasic effect on LH stimulation of T secretion; b) the mechanism of inhibition is a postreceptor action and results in inhibition of steroid synthesis at an early step; and c) conflicting data in the literature on whether prolactin stimulates or inhibits T secretion may be explained by differences in doses of prolactin studied.

1857 CYSTEAMINE DOES NOT CHANGE RATIO OF RAT PROLACTIN ISOFORMS. W.S. Oetting* and A.M. Walker. Div. of Biomedical Sciences, University of California, Riverside, CA. 92521.

Prolactin (PRL) is known to exist in multiple forms which differ from each other in their net charge, immunoreactivity and biological activity (Nyberg et.al., 1980, BBA 625:255). Recently, cysteamine (CYS) has been reported to alter the immunoreactivity of rat PRL without affecting its release or degradation (Zawalich and Dannies, 1983, Endo. 112:162A). In this study we explored the possibility that CYS may be affecting the formation of one or more of the PRL isoforms without altering the total amount of PRL being produced within the cell. Dispersed anterior pituitary cells derived from female Sprague-Dawley rats were cultured for 44 hours, washed and incubated for 60 min in 0.5 mM CYS, washed again and then labeled with (3H)-proline (50 µCi/ml for 6 h) in the presence of 0.5 mM CYS and 0.1% gelatin. Control cells underwent the same treatment but were not exposed to CYS. At the end of the 6 h labeling period both media and extracted cellular proteins were subjected to two-dimensional PAGE (denaturing conditions, pH 4 to 6.5) and the resultant protein pattern visualized by fluorography. Multiple forms of PRL were found in both the media and cell extracts but no differences were found in the ratios of these multiple forms when CYS-treated cells were compared to control cells. This was found to be true for both PRL released into the media and for the intracellular PRL. In addition, the relative amounts of newly synthesized intracellular PRL do not appear to be significantly altered by CYS treatment when compared to other proteins in the two-dimensional pattern. We conclude that cysteamine's effect on the immunoreactivity of PRL is not achieved by an alteration in the isoforms being produced. NIH grants AM 28534, RR 05816 and AM 07310.

1858 LACK OF ROLE OF INSULIN IN POSTPRANDIAL PROLACTIN SECRETION. G. Pepper*, S. B. Reichberg, T.W. AvRuskin, D.T. Krieger, S.Ram. The Brookdale Hospital Medical Center, Mt.Sinai Hospital Medical Center, New York,USA 11212

Protein-rich meals increase blood prolactin concentrations in human subjects, an effect suggested to result from elevation of blood amino acid levels (Ishizuka,B. et al J. Clin. Endocrin. Metab. 1983,57:1111). Since amino acids are potent stimuli for insulin secretion, this effect on prolactin could be mediated by increased concentrations of insulin. To determine the influence of endogenously secreted insulin on plasma concentrations of prolactin, we orally administered glucose and fructose, carbohydrates which stimulate insulin secretion to different degrees, to healthy volunteers. On three separate occasions, four males and two females were given either 100g glucose or 100g fructose dissolved in 200ml of water, or 200ml of water alone. Samples for measurement of insulin, glucose, and prolactin were obtained by an indwelling cathether at -15, 0,30,60,120,180 min. Neither carbohydrate had a statistically significant effect on prolactin concentration compared with water (1.27±0.5, 1.17±0.5, 0.94±0.4 ug x ml^{-1} x min ±SD, 0-180 min. integrated prolactin concentration for water, glucose, fructose respectively), despite a marked difference in serum insulin levels (9.92±5.3 vs. 2.58±0.8 mU x ml^{-1} x min. ±SD, 0-180 min. integrated serum insulin concentrations, glucose vs. fructose respectively). This data would indicate that endogenous insulin levels do not influence the regulation of postprandial prolactin secretion. (Supported in part by N.I.H. grant Am 31638 and the HANID foundation).

1859 QUANTITATION OF THE PROLACTIN CELL POPULATION IN THE MALE RAT PITUITARY: YOUNG ADULT, AGED AND TUMOROUS. Carol Phelps*, Department of Anatomy, University of Rochester School of Medicine and Dentistry, Rochester, N.Y. 14642, U.S.A.

Although prolactin (PRL) secretory patterns and regulation are frequently studied in laboratory animals of both genders, quantitation of the lactotroph population has been confined exclusively to the female. In order to provide this information for the male rat, the respective distribution and number of PRL cells were determined immunocytochemically in horizontal sections of embedded whole anterior pituitaries and in replicate preparations of individual glands enzymatically dissociated and maintained 4 days in vitro. Hormone was comparably localized using 2 primary rabbit antibodies ("W3", courtesy of W.C. Hymer, and NIAMDD anti-rat PRL-RC-1) and peroxidase-labeled second antibody. As has been previously noted, PRL cells in sectioned glands were distributed homogeneously; the total population appeared larger than has been estimated. This observation was confirmed by counts made among cultured cells, where PRL cells accounted for 22.0 ± 1.7% of the total among young (49 - 154 days old) males, compared with 30.4 ± 0.7% in diestrous female littermates. Aged (32 m.o.) male rats (n=4) showed 28.9 ± 2.4% of dispersed cells to be PRL-positive. That percentage increased to 42.3 ± 3.3% in a spontaneous tumor-bearing gland in an aged male; a similar increase in number was noted in sections of pituitaries bearing steroid-induced tumors in males, and is comparable to numbers previously reported for such induced tumors in female rats. Preliminary computerized analysis (Joyce Loebl/Nikon Magiscan) revealed a heterogeneity of staining intensity and size among PRL-positive cells. Supported by USPHS Grant HD 18243.

1860 DIFFERENT AGONISTS REGULATE PROLACTIN PRODUCTION BY DISTINCT MECHANISMS IN GH_4C_1 PITUITARY CELLS. J.S. Ramsdell* and A.H. Tashjian, Jr., Laboratory of Toxicology, Harvard School of Public Health, Boston, MA 02115, U.S.A.

Prolactin production (PRL-P) is stimulated by several physiological and pharmacological agents. To distinguish mechanisms which enhance PRL-P, we have examined the actions of 3 secretagogues on the GH_4C_1 strain of rat pituitary cells grown in serum supplemented Hams F10 medium ($F10^+$). PRL-P was stimulated by maximal doses of thyrotropin-releasing hormone (TRH), 12-0-tetredecanoyl phorbol 13-acetate (TPA) or epidermal growth factor (EGF) to 148, 330, or 280% of control levels, respectively, over 72 h (n=2). Treatment with any combination of maximal doses of TRH, TPA or EGF yielded fully additive increments in PRL-P (values = ± 10% of summed individual treatments). We next investigated their abilities to stimulate PRL-P and alter free cytosolic calcium ($[Ca]_i$) in Earle's MEM supplemented with 10% Bauers serum substitute (MEM-SS), with extracellular calcium ($[Ca]_e$) varied from 10 to 660μM (measured by atomic absorption). Cultures were grown 6 days in $F10^+$, washed and preincubated 24 h in MEM-SS with various $[Ca]_e$ prior to a 24-h incubation with secretagogue. In the absence of secretagogue, increasing $[Ca]_e$ from 10 to 660μM increased PRL-P from 1.1 to 4.1μg/ml/24 h (n=2) and $[Ca]_i$ from 93 to 425nM (measured by Quin 2 fluorescence). TRH caused an acute increase in $[Ca]_i$ at all $[Ca]_e$ tested. All 3 agents stimulated PRL-P at 10μM $[Ca]_e$; however, the stimulation by TPA was less than by TRH or EGF. At 74μM $[Ca]_e$, TRH, TPA and EGF caused similar increases in PRL-P (4.7, 4.5 and 5.0μg/ml/24 h, n=2) yet no increase in $[Ca]_i$ was observed 24 h after incubation with any secretagogue. At $[Ca]_e$>74μM, only EGF caused a further increase in PRL-P. We conclude that TRH, TPA and EGF have distinct actions on PRL-P with differing dependencies on $[Ca]_e$ and $[Ca]_i$.

1861 PROLACTIN RESPONSE (PR) TO HYPOGLYCEMIA (H) AND TRH IN GROWTH HORMONE DEFICIENT (GHD) AND NON GHD (NGHD) CHILDREN. R. Rapaport*, N.H. Ertel, C. Delfaus, C.T. Chien and A. Sheffet, Children's Hospital of N.J., VA-MC, E. Orange, UMDNJ-New Jersey Medical School, Newark, N.J., U.S.A.

Reports of PR to H have yielded conflicting results in adults and are rare in children. We compared the PR to H, induced by a standard Insulin Tolerance Test (ITT) (0.1 u Ins/kg IV) with that produced by a known stimulus of PR-TRH (7 µg/kg IV). 6 GHD children, ages 6-13 (2♀), and 8 NGHD children, ages 7-16 (1♀), all prepubertal (Tanner Stage I-II), underwent both stimuli. All developed H (blood glucose <40 mg/dl) on ITT.

	GHD n=6		P	NGHD n=8		P
Mean Prolactin(ng/ml)	ITT	TRH	ITT vs TRH	ITT	TRH	ITT vs TRH
Base	9.7	9.3	NS	5.1	8.3	P<.05
Peak	17.4	28.2	<.05	7.0	24.3	P<.002
P Base vs Peak (paired t test)	N.S.	<0.005		N.S.	<0.002	

In neither group of patients did ITT result in a significant rise in prolactin over baseline; however, both baseline and peak PR to ITT were higher in the GHD group vs NGHD (P<.05). The mean increments in prolactin were not different between the groups. TRH resulted in expected rises in prolactin equally (N.S. difference) in both groups. The PR to ITT showed no significant correlation with GH response in the NGHD children. PR to ITT in neither group was correlated with baseline prolactin, nor with PR to TRH. We conclude that maximum PR to H was not significant, though higher in GHD children, and not correlated with GH responses or PR to other stimuli. Therefore, ITT does not seem to be a good test of prolactin dynamics in children. TRH evoked equally good PR in both patient groups studied.

1862 NEUROENDOCRINE RESPONSES IN UNDISTURBED LACTATING RATS DURING MULTIPLE SUCCESSIVE SUCKLING EPISODES. P. RISKIND*, W. MILLARD, J. SOUKUP, AND J.B. MARTIN , DEPT. OF NEUROLOGY, MASS GENERAL HOSP, AND COMPUTER SCIENCE FAC, HARVARD SCHOOL OF PUBLIC HEALTH, BOSTON, MA

We have investigated plasma levels of anterior pituitary hormones during suckling in undisturbed rats without artificially separating pups and mother. This model was intended to approximate natural conditions of suckling in the rat. Rats were implanted with Silastic atrial catheters on days 14-17 of pregnancy, and transferred with their pups to special isolation/blood sampling cages on day two postpartum. On days 5-7 rats were sampled every 10 min from 8 am to 1 pm or from 1 pm to 6 pm (lights on from 9 am to 9 pm). Plasma was assayed by RIA for levels of prolactin (PRL), beta endorphin-like-immunoreactivity (β-END-LI), thyrotropin (TSH), and growth hormone (GH). Attachment of pups to the teat was observed through a viewing window. The relationships of hormone levels and behavioral observations were analysed by computer-assisted linear regression. Rises and levels of plasma PRL were tightly correlated with simultaneous values of plasma β-END-LI, and to a lesser extent, with plasma TSH. Interestingly, high PRL and β-END-LI levels were positively correlated with separation of the mother from her pups. These results suggest that: a) under "natural" conditions suckling may result in simultaneous elevations of plasma PRL and β-END-LI, as well as TSH; b) suckling episodes may be "paced" with peak hormone levels coinciding with cessation of a suckling episode. Supported by grants 1R23 AM 3277-01,1 RO1 AM 26252, and HD 17364.

1863 SERUM PROLACTIN AND IMMUNOCYTOCHEMICAL STAINING FOR PROLACTIN IN PITUITARY MACROADENOMAS. R. Ross*, A. Grossman, Lesley H. Rees, I. Doniach and G.M. Besser, Depts. of Endocrinology, Chemical Endocrinology and Histopathology, St. Bartholomew's Hospital, London, EC1A 7BE, U.K.

Hyperprolactinaemia associated with pituitary macroadenomas results either from prolactin (PRL) secretion from the tumour or interference with delivery of PRL-inhibiting hypothalamic factor(s) to the normal pituitary. It is important to know the relationship between raised serum PRL and the presence or absence of a PRL secreting tumour. We report pre-treatment serum PRL and PRL immunostaining (PRL.IS) in pituitary tumours from 38 patients. Only one patient had a PRL.IS+ve tumour and normal serum PRL. There

PRL IMMUNOSTAINING IN TUMOURS		N	SERUM PRL mU/l (normal < 360 mU/l) MEDIAN	RANGE
NEGATIVE		22	650	150-2700
POSITIVE	<10% cells	5	2400	270-2600
	10-50%	3	3360	2900-3800
	>50%	8	4400	2500-759000
	Total	16	3500	270-759000

was a difference ($P<0.001$) between the serum PRL of patients with PRL.IS+ve and PRL.IS-ve tumours. The serum PRL in patients with PRL.IS+ve tumours correlated with the proportion of PRL.IS+ve cells ($r_s=0.85$, $P<0.01$). Conclusion: In our patients a serum PRL>2700 mU/l was associated with PRL. IS+ve tumours. All PRL.IS-ve tumours had serum PRL<2700 mU/l. It is possible but unusual to have a normal serum PRL and PRL.IS+ve cells; 16 out of 31 tumours from hyperprolactinaemic patients did not immunostain for PRL.

1864 METHERGOLINE IN STERILE WOMEN WITH NORMOPROLACTINEMIA-AMENORRHEA. V. Ruíz-Velasco *. Centro para el Estudio de la Fertilidad. México City. C.P.11560.MEXICO.

Twelve sterile women with secondary amenorrhea were studied. All of them had less than 35 years old; a normal hormonal profile (FSH, LH, PRL, T_4); normal hematic and biochemical tests, and had no treatment since at least four months.

They were treated in a double blind way, six with Metergoline and six with placebo. The treatment was done by 4 months and only was stopped in cases of pregnancy. Clinical and laboratory test controls were done each month and at the end of the study, repeating all the tests done before treatment, adding P in the second half of the cicle and BBT.

The results were succesfully. Two pregnancies, four normal ovulation and return of bleeding in five women (one left the study for drug intolerance) were obtained in the six patients treated with Metergoline. This study open a new treatment for the sterile woman with anovulation or amenorrhea with normal PRL.

At present we are treating sterile anovulatory women or with Lutheal fase defect with normal PRL, with metergoline or Bromocriptine.

1865 CHARACTERIZATION OF PROSTAGLANDIN-9-KETO-REDUCTASE ACTIVITY IN UTERINE DECIDUA VERA. Stefan Niesert*, Murray D. Mitchell, Paul C. MacDonald, and M. Linette Casey, Cecil H. and Ida Green Ctr. for Reprod. Biol. Sci., Univ. of Texas Southwestern Medical School., Dallas, TX 75235. U.S.A.

There is evidence in support of the view that PGE_2 of amnion origin acts to initiate and maintain labor in women. During labor, the levels of PGE_2 in amniotic fluid rise strikingly; PGE_2 is the near exclusive prostanoid of amnion. Moreover, PGE_2 is much more active as a contractile agent in myometrium than is $PGF_{2\alpha}$. Yet, it is the levels of $PGF_{2\alpha}$ metabolites (and not PGE_2 metabolites) that increase strikingly in blood of women in labor. To address this apparent paradox, we evaluated the possibility that PGE_2 is converted to $PGF_{2\alpha}$ by 9-keto-reductase in decidua of pregnant women. In endometrial stromal cells in culture, a model system for decidua, we found that PGE_2 is converted to $PGF_{2\alpha}$ (as measured by RIA) in the presence of indomethacin (2 μM). Because of the importance of this reaction in regulating the tissue concentrations of PGE_2, we characterized the activity of 9-keto-reductase in cytosolic fractions of decidua vera tissue of pregnant women. In the presence of NADPH, $[^{14}C]PGE_2$ was converted to $[^{14}C]PGF_{2\alpha}$ and radiolabeled metabolites thereof. The formation of $PGF_{2\alpha}$ and metabolites was linear with time from 2 to 15 min; the apparent K_m of 9-keto-reductase for PGE_2 was 14 μM. The specific activity of the enzyme in cytosolic fractions of decidua varies widely up to 1 nmol/min/mg protein. We suggest that the reaction catalyzed by this enzyme may account for the striking rise in $PGF_{2\alpha}$ metabolites during labor when, apparently, the parent PG that facilitates parturition is PGE_2 of amnion origin.

1866 DIETARY RIBOFLAVIN DEFICIENCY INCREASES PGE_2 AND $PGF_{2\alpha}$ BIOSYNTHESIS IN RAT RENAL MEDULLA AND PAPILLA IN VITRO. N. Pelliccione, R. Karmali, R. Rivlin*, and J. Pinto, Memorial Sloan-Kettering Cancer Center and Cornell University Medical College, New York, New York 10021, U.S.A.

Prompted by previous reports that riboflavin deficiency increases the proportion of linoleic acid and decreases that of arachidonic acid, a prostaglandin (PG) precursor, in tissue and plasma phospholipids, we studied the effects of riboflavin deficiency on activity in vitro of prostaglandin synthetase in rat kidney homogenates. For 2-5 months weanling rats were fed a diet deficient in riboflavin or equal amounts of a diet identical in composition except for the addition of riboflavin. In further experiments each group of rats was treated for 10 days with either a prostaglandin inhibitor (flurbiprofen) or buffer. Following sacrifice by decapitation, PG biosynthesis in vitro was measured by RIA following extraction with diethyl ether both in the absence and presence of glutathione, and again in the absence and presence of glutathione plus flurbiprofen. Dietary riboflavin deficiency increased both PGE_2 and $PGF_{2\alpha}$ biosynthesis in vitro in rat renal medulla and papilla. When both control and riboflavin deficient rats were treated with flurbiprofen for a 10 day period, PGE_2 biosynthesis in vitro was markedly inhibited. This inhibition of PGE_2 biosynthesis was partially overcome by addition of reduced glutathione in vitro. The addition of glutathione plus flurbiprofen in vitro prevented the restoration of PGE_2 biosynthesis by glutathione. The rate of prostaglandin biosynthesis in kidney homogenates from riboflavin deficient rats remained higher than that of pair-fed controls with each experimental manipulation. These data suggest a role for riboflavin in regulating renal prostaglandin biosynthesis.

1867 ACTION OF SEROTONINERGIC SYSTEM ON THE POSITIVE FEED-BACK EFFECT OF OVARIAN STEROIDS ON LH SECRETION IN PREPUBERTAL RATS. J.A.Moguilevsky*, M.R.Faigón, P.Scacchi and B.Szwarcfarb. Instituto de Fisiología.Facultad de Medicina.Universidad de Buenos Aires.Paraguay 2155.Buenos Aires.Argentina

The positive feed-back effect of ovarian steroids on LH secretion maturates between 22-24 days of age in the female rat and this mechanism is an important event involved in the onset of puberty.The effect of 5-hydroxytryptophan (5-HTP),a serotonin (5-HT) precursor, and p-chloroamphetamine (PCA) a 5-HT neurotoxin,selective for serotoninergic neurons, that depletes 5 HT levels in brain,on the LH release response to estrogen-progesterone (E-P) were studied in prepubertal rats of different ages.E-P decreased LH levels at 16,18 and 20 days of age increasing the concentration of tne pituitary hormone in rats of 26 days old.Destruction of serotoninergic system advances the onset of the positive feed-back mechanism, since the rats pretreated with PCA showed at 20 days of age LH release by E-P administration while in the controls of the same age the ovarian hormones decreased LH concentration.On the other hand in rats of 26 days of age in which the LH release response to E-P is present, this response is significantly reduced by the administration of 5-HTP and increased by the pretreatment with PCA.These results indicate the serotoninergic system has an inhibitory action on the positive feed-back effect of ovarian steroids on LH secretion in prepubertal female rats and this effect is probably connected with the participation of 5-HT neurons in the onset of puberty.

1868 REDUCED FOOD INTAKE ALTERS THE TIMECOURSE OF POST-CASTRATION RESPONSE AND ESTROGEN FEEDBACK IN THE PREPUBERTAL FEMALE RAT. B.E. Piacsek*, Dept. of Biology, Marquette University, Milwaukee, WI 53233, U.S.A.

Female rats(Holtzman) were maintained after weaning on either ad libitum(control=C) or 60% of normal(reduced=R) food intake. Lights were on 500 to 1900 hrs and temperature was 22±1°C. At 31 days of age, animals were ovariectomized (OX) and the following studies were conducted. In Exp.I, rats were sacrificed at 4, 12, 24, 72 and 120 hrs after OX. In Exp.II, rats were allowed to recover for one week after OX, at which time they received a single injection of 0.5 ug 17β Estradiol benzoate per 100 g body weight. Rats were sacrificed at 1, 2, 4, 8 and 24 hrs after injection. Sera from both experiments were assayed for follicle stimulating hormone (FSH) and luteinizing hormone (LH). Results of Exp.I indicate an identical timecourse for the post-castration rise of FSH in both groups. The rise of LH secretion in C rats showed two peaks. The first was observed between 12 and 24 hrs, while the second and larger rise occured between 72 and 120 hrs. In R rats, the first peak did not occur until 48 hrs after OX, while the second was observed between 72 and 120 hrs, but was significantly lower than in C rats. In Exp.II, the response of FSH secretion was again similar in C and R rats, but the pattern of LH secretion was significantly altered in R rats. In C rats, LH values reached a nadir (41% decrease) by 1 hr, remained low through 4 hrs and rose sharply (189%) by 24 hrs. In R rats, the nadir was not reached until 8 hrs, but values remained at this suppressed level through 24 hrs. These results suggest that the delayed puberty observed in R rats may be due in part to a slower response of the LH releasing mechanism to changes in circulating estrogen titers. Support. PHS Gr. HD 14555

1869 TREATMENT (RX) OF PRECOCIOUS PUBERTY WITH THE SYNTHETIC GnRH AGONIST BUSERELIN (HOE 766). C. Rouwé*, S. Drop M. Jansen, and B. Otten. Departments of Pediatrics, University of Groningen, Rotterdam, Utrecht, Nijmegen, the Netherlands.

20 girls and 3 boys (age range 2-8 yrs.) with precocious puberty (PP) were treated with HOE 766, administered subcutaneously for a period of up to 8 mo.. Cyproterone acetate (CPA) (100-150 $mg/m^2/d$), previously given in 11/23 patients, was tapered during the first 4 wks. of Rx. In 18 pat. HOE 766 was given in a dosage of 10 µg/kg b.i.d. s.c. for 1 wk. and once a day for the ensuing 6-20 wks. After the initial induction, basal LH serum values ranged from 3-10 lU/l. The LH/ FSH response to LH-RH (100 µg i.v.) was blunted. After the first week, basal serum estradiol (E_2) values (before HOE 766 Rx: 40-300 pmol/l) in creased to >1000 pmol/l. After 6-20 wks. E_2 values ranged 50-150 pmol/l in 13/15 girls. The sexual signs did not regress and menses persisted. Therefore, 20 µg/kg b.i.d. HOE 766 was given for 1 wk, followed by the same dose once a day (evening). Another 5 pat. were started on this protocol. Basal LH values were 4-6 lU/l, E_2 concentrations fell to <40 pmol/l, pubertal signs regressed and menses stopped. The 3 boys required several adjustments of the dose (up to 20 µg/kg b.i.d.) in order to reach testosterone serum values <1 nmol/l.The s.c. administration was well tolerated; no side effects. Especially in the CPA treated patients, activity and behavior improved. We conclude that daily s.c. HOE 766 Rx is effective in suppressing gonadal function in children with pp. Careful monitoring of anthropometric and hormonal data and individualization of the dosage are necessary for long-term gonadal suppression and will lead to an improvement of final height prediction.

1870 NON-COOPERATIVE BINDING OF ESTROGEN RECEPTOR (ER) TO ESTRADIOL (E_2) IN INTACT CELLS IN VIVO AND IN VITRO. EFFECTS OF ESTRIOL (E_3) ON RE_2 ACTIVATION AND TRANSFORMATION.

R.E. Müller, A.M. Traish and H.H. Wotiz*.
Boston Univ. School of Medicine, 80 E. Concord St., Boston, MA 02118 USA

Mature ovariectomized rats were treated for 16 days with E_2, E_3 or mixtures of these two. Steroids were delivered through implanted Alzet pumps at a constant hourly rate (E_2: 0.04µg; E_3: 0.4 µg and 0.04 µg: E_2 and E_3: 0.04 µg + 0.4 µg). The effects on uterine growth, induction of progesterone R synthesis, and activation (nuclear binding) of ER demonstrate that E_3 acted as a full agonist and did not inhibit E_2 action. Incubation of uteri at 37°C with 1 or 10nM $(^3H)E_2$ gave different degrees of receptor saturation; subcellular localization of $R(^3H)E_2$ complexes, however, was constant (80% nuclear, 20% cytosolic). The presence of 0-8 nM nonradioactive E_3 did not alter the subcellular distribution of $R(^3H)E_2$ complexes, suggesting that E_3 at these concentrations does not inhibit activation of $R(^3H)E_2$. Similarly, 4S to 5S transformation of $R(^3H)E_2$ in intact uteri was not inhibited by estriol. Equilibrium binding of $(^3H)E_2$ to uterine cell suspensions at physiological temperature (37°C) was noncooperative; nonradioactive E_3 did not alter the affinity of the ER for $(^3H)E_2$. Dixon plot analysis of $(^3H)E_2$ binding to intact uterine cells at 37°C in the presence of estriol suggests that the latter is a purely competitive inhibitor of $(^3H)E_2$ binding.

1871 STUDIES OF THE ESTROGEN RECEPTOR (ER) BY ASSAY OF FREE (F) RATHER THAN BOUND (B) LIGAND (L) CONCENTRATIONS. James Murai and Pentti K. Siiteri*, Ph.D., Reproductive Endocrinology Center, Dept. OB/GYN, University of California, San Francisco, San Francisco, CA 94143
We have compared the dextran coated charcoal (DCC) method with the isodialysis (ISO) method for measurement of FL in studies of estradiol (E_2) binding to the cytoplasmic rat uterine ER. Scatchard plots were prepared by calculating FL (DCC) or BL (ISO) and values of K_D were obtained by nonlinear least squares regression analysis. At 4° the value of K_D by ISO (.02 + .01 nM, n=10) was approximately 100 fold lower than that measured with DCC (2.04 + .71 nM, n=5) in low salt. In 0.4M KCl K_D was 0.06 nM. The values for maximal binding (B max) were not different. The value of K_D (ISO) slowly increases irreversibly when DCC treated cytosol is warmed at temperatures between 22 - 37°; 4°C=0.02 nM; 22°C=0.06 nM; 37°C=0.45 nM. Sedimentation constants also changed from 8S to 4S(22°) or aggregates (37°). These results indicate that 1) affinity constants obtained by calculation of FL may be unreliable, and 2) separate classes of binding sites for E_2 may represent transitional forms of the native receptor following exchange assays.

1872 ESTROGENICITY OF COUMESTROL IN THE MOUSE: FLUORESCENCE DETECTION OF INTERACTION WITH ESTROGEN RECEPTORS. Katherine Nelson*, Edward J. Pavlik, John R. van Nagell, Jr., Michael B. Hanson, Elvis S. Donaldson, and Robert C. Flanigan, University of Kentucky College of Medicine, Lexington, Kentucky 40536.

The estrogenicity of coumestrol, a fluorescent phytoestrogen, has been examined in murine uteri. Coumestrol competed with $^3H-E_2$ for binding to cytoplasmic estrogen receptors (ER), translocated cytoplasmic ER to the nucleus, and induced progesterone receptors. Using size exclusion HPLC (SEHPLC), the interaction of coumestrol with ER was examined directly by monitoring the fluorescence associated with macromolecules having ER properties. These analyses were made possible by the addition of dimethylformamide (7.5%) to the elution buffer, so that ER recoveries were improved without interfering with receptor binding. It was possible to detect fluorescent coumestrol at ∿ 0.5 nM. All determinations were performed with preparations in which ER activity was 3-10 nM. Exposure of cytosol to coumestrol (50 nM) resulted in the elution of increased fluorescent activity in the regions where ER eluted during SEHPLC. This fluorescence was reduced when DES, E_2, hexestrol, or tamoxifen were present as competitors (2 uM), but was unaffected by testosterone or progesterone. DES reduced fluorescence below endogenous levels and thereby displayed a fluorescence quench property which was not observed with other ligands. Using hepatic and renal ER preparations, the injected receptor activity was observed to be the major limiting factor in detecting the interaction of coumestrol with ER. These observations are relevant to attempts to visualize ER in tumor cells and demonstrate that fluorescent ligands can satisfy accepted criteria for direct documentation of receptor interaction.

1873 ENDOMETRIAL ESTROGEN AND PROGESTERONE RECEPTORS IN WOMEN BEARING AN INTRAUTERINE DEVICE.

E.M. Niu*, G.S. Cai and Z.H. Tang, The International Peace Maternity and Child Health Hospital of the China Welfare Institute, Shanghai, The People's Republic of China.

Our objective was to determine whether variations of endometrial cytosolic estrogen receptor (ER) and/or progesterone receptor (PR) levels could contribute to the contraceptive efficacy of intrauterine devices (IUDs). The contents of ER and PR in endometrial biopsies from 93 women bearing hormone-free IUDs were assayed using various concentrations of [^{3}H]estradiol and [^{3}H]R5020 and dextran-coated charcoal. Endometrial specimens from 116 women with normal menstrual cycles served as controls. The mean IUD bearing time was 5.3 years. ER and PR contents ranged from 7-640 and 6-2508 fmol/mg protein for the IUD group and 1-364 and 11-3051 fmol/mg protein for controls, respectively. The mean values of ER in both proliferative and secretory phases for the IUD group were higher than in controls ($p<0.001$ and $p<0.01$); PR values were lower, but not significantly. Cyclic variations of PR content were not altered by IUD use, but the peak of ER content was shifted to the early proliferative phase, followed by a gradual decline. Our findings indicate that alterations of endometrial function reflected in the binding of estrogens and progestins to their receptors may be initiated by local mechanical stimulation by an IUD.

1874 A SERUM COMPONENT IN RAT AND HUMAN FEMALE SERA REDUCES THE RELATIVE BINDING AFFINITY OF DIETHYLSTILBESTEROL (DES) TO NUCLEAR ESTROGEN RECEPTOR.

W.C. Okulicz* and Lorna D. Johnson. Worcester Foundation for Experimental Biology, Shrewsbury, MA 01545, and New England Regional Primate Research Center, Southboro, MA 01772 (USA).

A recent study has reported that the relative binding affinity (RBA) of DES was greater for nuclear estrogen receptor (Re) than for cytosol Re (Hendry and Leavitt, J. Steroid Biochem. 17:479, 1982). Since serum binding proteins can alter the relative potency of estrogens and cytosol preparations are susceptible to serum contamination, this study sought to determine if serum could account for the above discrepancy. High salt (0.5 M KCl) extract of rat uterine nuclei was incubated with tritiated estradiol (E_2) (0.75 nM) and different concentrations (0.04 nM-4μM) of unlabeled competitor with or without charcoal stripped sera (1/20, v/v). The molar concentration of competitor required to reduce specific ^3H-E_2 binding by 50% (IC_{50}) was used to calculate RBA (E_2=100). Addition of 4μM testosterone to human sera was shown to block binding of ^3H-E_2 to SBGH. In the absence of serum, DES was a more potent competitor (RBA= 245±36; IC_{50}=2.1±.2x10^{-10}M) than E_2 (IC_{50}= 5.2±.7x10^{-10}M). Human female serum lowered the RBA of DES to 52±7 (IC_{50}= 10±2x10^{-10}M) without affecting the IC_{50} of E_2 (5.0±.x10^{-10}M). Similarly, rat serum lowered the RBA of DES to 43±1 (IC_{50}=12.5x10^{-10}M) and the IC_{50} of E_2 remained unchanged (5.4±.5 x 10^{-10}M). Ammonium sulfate fractionation and affinity chromatography (Affi-Gel Blue) of ^3H-DES bound to rat or human sera suggested a role for serum albumin as a DES binder. These data demonstrate that a component in human and rat sera can reduce the RBA of DES to nuclear Re and suggest that this component could modulate DES action. (Supported by HD 06295).

1875 ISOLATION OF ISOFORMS OF THE A-SUBUNIT OF THE PROGESTERONE RECEPTOR.

L. O'Connor*, A.P. McHale, W.T. Schrader, B.W. O'Malley, Department of Cell Biology, Baylor College of Medicine, Houston, TX 77030. USA.

We have described two subunits of the chicken oviduct progesterone receptor. The A subunit (Mr=79K) contains a high affinity DNA binding sites while the B subunit (Mr=108,000) binds weakly to DNA but does bind to chromatin. QAE Sephadex chromatography has been employed to resolve 3 isoforms of the A subunit isolated from chick oviduct. The PI's have been shown by 2-D gel electrophoresis to have values of 5.7, 5.8, and 5.9. All isoforms have molecular weight of 79,000, demonstrated by covalent labelling with $[^3H]$R5020. Peptide maps of the purified isoforms are identical, showing a closely related primary structure. All 3 forms bind preferentially to OV1.7, a 1.7 kilobase DNA fragment flanking the 5' end of the chicken ovalbumin gene. Only 2 isoforms bind $[^3H]$progesterone *in vitro*. The third form is occupied by endogenous progesterone when isolated from mature egg-laying hens, but does not bind $[^3H]$progesterone *in vitro*. This isoform is the only subunit A protein which reacts with monoclonal antibodies raised against subunit A purified from laying hen oviducts. The antigenic isoform is present in excess over the *in vitro* hormone binding forms. Thus, progesterone receptor A subunit exists in at least three chromatographically distinct states, exhibiting functional as well as biochemical differences.

1876 THREE TYPES OF HEREDITARY PARTIAL ANDROGEN RESISTANCE CLASSIFIED ACCORDING TO A MODEL OF NORMAL ANDROGEN-RECEPTOR (A-R) COMPLEX TRANSFORMATION.

L. Pinsky* and M. Kaufman, MRC Group in Medical Genetics, Lady Davis Institute for Medical Research, Montreal, H3T 1E2, Canada.

Genital skin fibroblasts incubated with 3 nM 5α-dihydrotestosterone (DHT) or methyltrienolone (M) saturate their basal A-R activity at a B_{max} ∿20 fmol/mg protein within 0.5 h and at an app K_d ∿0.2 nM within 2 h. At 0.5 h they have higher, more variable values of K_d (0.3-1.8 nM). When incubated with 3 nM DHT or M for 0.5-2 h, they have a rate constant of dissociation ($k_{37°}$; by chase) of 0.006 min^{-1} (DHT) and 0.012 min^{-1} (M), and if incubation is prolonged DHT increases basal A-R activity by 35% in 20 h while M does so by 100% in 24 h («up-regulation»). These data fit a model whereby time and initial ligand concentration codetermine the transformation of initial, low-affinity A-R complexes to serial states of higher-affinity, the highest-affinity state being necessary but not sufficient as a signal for up-regulation.

Normal: A-R ⟶ A=R ⟶ A≡R ⟶ [A≡R] = up-reg$^+$

Mutants:

Class 1 DHT-R / M-R -/->

Class 2 DHT-R / M-R -/-> DHT=R / M=R -/-> DHT≡R / M≡R -/->

Class 3 DHT-R ⟶ DHT=R -/-> DHT≡R -/->
M-R ⟶ M=R ⟶ M≡R ⟶ [M≡R] = up-reg$^+$

Affinities:
A-R < A=R < A≡R

1877 PARTIAL PURIFICATION AND CHARACTERIZATION OF ANDROGEN RECEPTORS IN HUMAN PROSTATIC TISSUES. F. Radwan*, M. Elhilali, M. Carmel, and J.G. Lehoux. Fac. of Medicine, Sherbrooke University, Sherbrooke, Qué., Canada, J1H 5N4.

We have studied the transformation of androgenic receptors in human hyperplastic prostate. Tissues obtained after surgery were kept in liquid nitrogen until used. The 105,000 xg cytosol was prepared by homogenization and differential centrifugation in a 20 mM Tris HCl buffer pH 7.4 containing 1.5mM EDTA, 20mM sodium molybdate and 25mM monothioglycerol. Endogenous steroids were adsorbed on charcoal (10 min.). The cytosol was incubated with (^{3}H)-** R1881 5nM for 3 h at 4°C or for 2 h at 4°C followed by 1 h at 25°C in the presence or absence of 5uM nonradioactive R1881 for non specific binding determination; 5uM triamcinolone acetonide was also added. After incubation, preparations were chromatographed on phosphocellulose. Elution was done with a buffer containing 0.6M KCl. Without heating, 60-65% of the complex was specifically retained by the column. With heating the binding to phosphocellulose increased by 20-25%. In another series of experiments the cytosolic extract was chromatographed on phosphocellulose prior to incubation. Two fractions were obtained: one excluded and one retained by the column which was eluted with 0.6M KCl. The excluded, retained and reconstituted fractions were incubated separately in the presence of (^{3}H)-R1881 for 18 h at 4°C. The excluded fraction lost its capacity to bind the hormone whereas the retained fraction could still weakly bind (^{3}H)-R1881. The recombined fraction regained the property to bind up to 90% of the hormone and was retained on phosphocellulose. We believe that during fractionation on phosphocellulose, receptors could have been separated from endogenous activation factor(s).(** R1881, methyltrienolone). Supported by the NCI (Canada).

1878 PRELIMINARY INVESTIGATIONS OF A NEW RADIOLIGAND, [^{3}H]-MIBOLERONE, FOR USE IN ANDROGEN RECEPTOR RESEARCH. Valarie A. Randall* & W.I.P. Mainwaring. Department of Biochemistry, University of Leeds, Leeds, U.K.

A new ligand for androgen receptors, [^{3}H]-mibolerone, or 7α, 17α-dimethyl-19-nortestosterone, has recently been produced by Amersham International. At present, the synthetic steroid, methyltrienolone, or R1881, is almost universally used in work on human tissues to avoid the simultaneous measurement of plasma sex hormone binding globulin (SHBG), which occurs with the natural ligand, 5α-dihydrotestosterone (5α-DHT). However, [^{3}H]-R1881 is photolabile and unstable. On sucrose density gradients (5-20%) of rat prostate cytosol only a single peak of binding in the 8-9 S region, saturable with 200 x excess unlabelled 5α-DHT, was obtained with [^{3}H]-mibolerone and [^{3}H]-R1881; with [^{3}H]-5α-DHT virtually unsaturable 4S binding was also detected. Saturation analysis using the dextran-coated charcoal method (0.1-10 nM; ± 200 x unlabelled 5α-DHT) showed a plateau of specific binding at c. 1 nM : KD = 0.93 nM by Scatchard plot. Using the controlled pore glass bead assay (Sigma CPG pore 500, mesh 120-200) all three steroids (5 nM ± 1μM unlabelled 5α-DHT) gave similar specific binding with rat prostate cytosol, but only [^{3}H]-5α-DHT showed any binding to human plasma. Background counts using [^{3}H]-R1881 were higher than with [^{3}H]-mibolerone, probably due to its greater instability. Studies using human benign hypertrophic prostate are in progress. In conclusion, since [^{3}H]-mibolerone binds to the androgen receptor in rat prostate (rodents have no SHBG), but not to human SHBG, it should prove an invaluable aid in androgen receptor research.

1879 REGULATION OF GLUCOCORTICOID RECEPTOR BY GLUCOCORTICOID IN HUMAN PERIPHERAL LYMPHOCYTES. H. Oshima*, Y. Ichikawa, S. Kawai, H. Tanaka, K. Arikawa, T. Shinozawa, T. Yoshida, H. Yamada and M. Homma Department of Medicine, School of Medicine, Keio University, Tokyo 160, Japan.

The regulation of glucocorticoid receptor in man is not well known. We have studied the effect of glucocorticoid on its own receptor in human peripheral lymphocytes. The receptor number in lymphocytes was measured by a whole cell binding assay with [^{3}H]dexamethasone at 25C for 2h incubation. Nuclear receptor was determined by lysing cells in hypotonic $MgCl_2$(1.5mM) after incubation. The receptor content in intact lymphocytes of 20 patients with collagen diseases taking prednisolone(mean;25mg/day) was 7.74±2.20 fmol/10^6cells(M±SD), which was significantly reduced as compared to those of 10 patients with collagen diseases taking no glucocorticoid and 21 healthy controls(11.47±3.02;$p<0.01$, 10.85±2.50;$p<0.01$), respectively. The number of nuclear receptor in patients treated with prednisolone also significantly decreased when compared with controls(3.61±1.37 vs 6.21±1.70, $p<0.01$). The receptor number in intact cells and that in nuclei of patients were both negatively correlated with the daily dosage of prednisolone. There were no significant differences in the dissociation constants of intact cells and nuclei among the three groups(6-8nM). When lymphocytes were incubated *in vitro* with 10^{-7}M prednisolone at 37C, the receptor number in intact cells and that in nuclei did not change after 1 and 24h, but showed 33 and 36% decreases, respectively, after 48h incubation as compared to the control. This depletion was not observed with estradiol and testosterone. These results suggest that glucocorticoid down-regulates its own receptor in intact cells and in nuclei of human peripheral lymphocytes.

1880 EFFECTS OF ADRENAL STEROIDS ON α-LACTALBUMIN PRODUCTION IN THE RAT MAMMARY GLAND. S.J. Quirk*, M.J. Fullerton, J.E. Gannell and J.W. Funder, Medical Research Centre, Prince Henry's Hospital, Melbourne, Australia 3004.

In the mouse mammary gland, the non-physiological ligand cortisol was reported to have a biphasic effect on the production of the specific milk protein, α-lactalbumin (Ona & Oka 1980 Cell 19:474). Both Type I receptors (affinity corticosterone (B) = aldosterone >> dexamethasone (DM)) and Type II (classical DM-binding) receptors have been identified in rat mammary gland during pregnancy and lactation (Quirk et al, 1983 Endocrinology 113:1812). Using RU26988, a synthetic steroid highly specific for Type II receptors, and the physiological ligand B, we have examined the pattern of adrenal steroid control of rat α-lactalbumin production by mammary gland explants from mid-pregnant rats. Explants were cultured in medium with insulin (5μg/ml), prolactin (1μg/ml) and steroid for 48h; medium was renewed at 24h. Tissue and medium α-lactalbumin was estimated by RIA at 48h. With RU26988 (1-300nM) α-lactalbumin production was maximal (3-4 x baseline) at ∿3nM i.e. $\sim K_d$ for Type II receptors. Thereafter values progressively declined to baseline at 300nM RU26988. B (3-300nM) increased α-lactalbumin production in a dose-related fashion to 3-4 x baseline, an effect progressively blocked by spirolactone (0.1-10μM). We conclude that (i) given the specificity of RU26988, effects on α-lactalbumin via classical glucocorticoid receptors are truly biphasic (ii) the physiological glucocorticoid B appears to act at least in part via Type I, spirolactone-sensitive, receptors in the mammary gland.
Supported by the National Health & Medical Research Council of Australia.

1881 RU486 INHIBITS PERIPHERAL EFFECTS OF EXOGENOUS GLUCOCORTICOIDS IN MAN.
M.Rieu, X.Bertagna*, C.Basin, M.Hucher, B.Varet, M.A.Dugue, and J.P.Luton, Centre de Recherches Endocrinologiques, Cochin, Paris 75014; Institut Roussel-Uclaf, Paris 75007, France.

In order to further evaluate the antiglucocorticoid action of RU486 (RU) we examined its ability to antagonize the effects of acutely administered glucocorticoids. In a first study, 7 healthy males received placebo (P), 1 mg dexamethasone (D), or D + RU (400mg) at 0700h and blood leukocytes were counted at 1300h and expressed as percent of basal (0700h); for eosinophils P: 106.9 $\pm$ 16.2 (mean $\pm$ SE), D: 9.3 $\pm$ 4.5, D + RU: 57.3 $\pm$ 26.5; for lymphocytes P: 112.3 $\pm$ 13.3, D: 56.3 $\pm$ 3.7, D + RU: 93.0 $\pm$ 7.8; for neutrophils, P: 140 $\pm$ 17,8, D: 195 $\pm$ 28.2, D + RU: 125 $\pm$ 16.8. For all 3 parameters D induced changes were significant ($p < 0.02$) compared to P and significantly antagonized by RU ($p < 0.02$) being then not different from P. Six healthy males underwent an oral glucose tolerance test (OGTT) at 0900h after P, cortisone acetate (E) alone (50mg at 0100h and 0700h) or E + RU (400mg at midnight). Blood samples were taken every 30 min for 3 hours for glucose and insulin determinations. The mean levels (mean $\pm$ SE) over the OGTT were: for glucose (mmol/l) P: 5.2 $\pm$ 0.1, E: 5.9 $\pm$ 0.2, E + RU: 6.0 $\pm$ 0.2; for insulin (μU/ml), P: 30 $\pm$ 3 E: 44 $\pm$ 4, E + RU: 34 $\pm$ 3. For both parameters, the E induced changes were significant ($p < 0.05$ and $p < 0.01$, respectively) compared to P, but only the insulin change was significantly ($p < 0.01$) antagonized by RU being then not different from P. In conclusion RU antagonizes the peripheral effects of pharmacological doses of glucocorticoids: this action may not appear after the administration of RU alone because of the compensatory cortisol rise.

1882 KINASE ACTIVITY OF GOLGI MEMBRANE INSULIN (INS) RECEPTORS FROM SALINE AND INS-INJECTED RATS. Kenneth M. Lerea* and James N. Livingston, University of Rochester Medical School, Rochester, NY 14642.

The ability of liver plasma membrane (PM) and Golgi membrane (GM) INS receptors from saline - and INS-injected rats to autophosphorylate was examined. INS receptors from PM and GM were purified by lectin chromatography and subjected to phosphorylation studies. Receptors isolated from saline-injected animals demonstrated an INS dependent autophosphorylation on tyrosine residues in a 90K subunit from GM and 90K and 84K subunits from PM. The concentration of INS that produces half maximal stimulation in both membrane systems is 1nM, which is similar to the high affinity Kd value for INS binding to both PM and GM. A major difference was observed however in the magnitude of phosphorylation that exists between GM and PM receptors. Golgi receptors demonstrated 3-4 times more phosphorylation per fmol of INS binding activity than receptors from PM. INS binding studies with liver membranes isolated from INS injected rats (1μg/gm body wt.) reveals a 50% decrease in receptor numbers in PM compared to the number of receptors in PM isolated from saline-treated rats. Conversely, following INS injection the overall receptor number in the GM increased by a factor of 2. Using equivalent INS binding activities, the Golgi receptors from INS-injected rats phosphorylated to the same magnitude as Golgi receptors isolated from saline-treated animals. Overall, this suggests that INS receptors of GM are tyrosine kinases with a greater kinase activity per INS binding than the receptors at the PM. INS injection causes an increase in the number of receptors in the Golgi and thus directs activated receptor kinases to the Golgi apparatus.

1883 KINETICS OF ZINC-FREE INSULIN BINDING TO ISOLATED RAT FAT CELLS AT 15°C.
E.W. Lipkin*, D.C. Teller and C. de Haën, Dept. of Medicine, Univ. of Washington, Seattle, WA 98195, U.S.A.

A description of Tyr A14 ^{125}I-labeled insulin binding to fat cells was sought that can reconcile kinetic and equilibrium data quantitatively. A temperature of 15°C was chosen because under these conditions receptor internalization can still occur, but fusion of lysosomes with endosomes is abolished. Binding equilibrium was measured after 4 h of incubation. In addition, binding association and dissociation experiments were performed, including dissociation experiments of labeled insulin in the presence and absence of large concentrations of cold Zn-free insulin. Various models for insulin binding were fitted to the data using the method of maximum likelihood. In kinetic experiments the differential equations were fitted. The fits of the various models were evaluated by the Akaike Information Criterion. This and other criteria identified the following model as best describing the kinetic and equilibrium situation:

$$I + R' \underset{k_{23}}{\overset{k_{32}}{\rightleftharpoons}} I + R \underset{k_{21}}{\overset{k_{12}}{\rightleftharpoons}} IR \underset{k_{32}}{\overset{k_{23}}{\rightleftharpoons}} IR' ,$$

where I is insulin, R is the receptor mediating biological activity and R' is the same receptor in an altered state or cellular localization. We actually suggest that R' constitutes an intracellular localization. In this model equilibrium is given by a simple binding isotherm with $K = k_{21}/k_{12} = 5x10^{-9}M$. The kinetic rate constants are: $k_{12} = 4.3x10^{5}$ l $mol^{-1}s^{-1}$, $k_{21} = 2.3x10^{-3}$ s^{-1}, $k_{23} = 2.3x10^{-4}$ s^{-1}, $k_{32} = 2.8x10^{-4}$ s^{-1}. The total number of receptors is 150,000 receptors/cell. This study was supported by NIH grants AM02456, AM00682, GM13401 and the American Diabetes Association.

1884 THE EFFECT OF OBESITY AND AGE ON INSULIN RECEPTOR STATUS OF LEAN AND OBESE HYPERGLYCAEMIC MICE.
J. M. Lord and T. W. Atkins*, Dept. of Biological Sciences, Univ. Aston in Birmingham, Birmingham, B4 7ET, England, U.K.

Both obesity and aging may be associated with carbohydrate intolerance and reduced insulin sensitivity. To confirm this insulin receptor binding to hepatocytes and soleus muscle and soleus muscle insulin stimulated ^{14}C-glycogen synthesis have been determined over the complete life span of lean (3-60 weeks) and obese mice (3-40 weeks). Obese mouse hepatocyte high affinity receptor number was significantly reduced at 10 and 20 weeks and empty sites affinity ($\bar{K}e$) was significantly reduced at 40 weeks compared to age matched lean mice. Obese mouse hepatocyte receptor number increased again at 40 weeks. Lean mouse hepatocyte low affinity receptor number gradually decreased with age reaching a nadir at 60 weeks. Receptor affinity was not affected. Obese mouse soleus muscle insulin binding was significantly lower at 10, 20 and 40 weeks compared to lean, the latter remained constant over 3-40 weeks but was significantly reduced at 60 weeks. Obese mouse soleus muscle insulin stimulated ^{14}C-glycogen synthesis was significantly reduced between 5-40 weeks compared to lean with a dramatic fall at 40 weeks. The age related development of insulin resistance in obese mice suggests a postreceptor defect(s) of insulin action as the primary cause. The age related decline in lean mouse receptor binding was probably caused by increased down regulation.

1885 SELF-REGULATION OF VASOPRESSIN RECEPTORS IN THE PITUITARY GLAND. B.Lutz-Bucher and B.Koch*, Laboratoire de Physiologie, ULP, 67000 Strasbourg, France.

Vasopressin (AVP) participates in the regulation of ACTH secretion, because the peptide bears intrinsic CRF-like activity and potentiates the effect of CRF on the pituitary. We have determined binding properties of putative receptors for [^{3}H]AVP in pituitary membranes and examined a possible self-regulation of sites. None of the various neuropeptides tested competed for binding and especially not CRF. The receptor (one population of sites with a K_D=0.4-0.6 nM) recognized AVP and analogs according to the following order: AVP=vasotocin > oxytocin ≥ d(CH2)5Tyr,Val4-AVP > dDAVP > dPAVP. GTP failed to affect binding. Concentration of receptor was inversely related to levels of endogeneous AVP: B max decreased from 99.0 to 28.0 and 12.5 fmol/mg protein in glands from control, AVP-treated (10 IU/day/7days) or adrenalectomized (2weeks) rats, respectively. Dexamethasone injections (40 µg/day) reversed the effect of adrenalectomy. Mere occupation of sites by endogeneous AVP was precluded by the observation that i.v. injection of high doses of AVP (100ng/100g b.w.) to Brattleboro rats (genetically deficient in AVP, i.e. with unoccupied receptors) reduced binding of tracer less than 20% vs. control. The present data demonstrate the presence of highly specific AVP receptors in the pituitary, clearly different from those for CRF, whose concentration appeared to be down-regulated by the neuropeptide.

1886 ARGININE VASOPRESSIN (AVP) BINDING SITES IN THE RAT TESTIS. Rina Meidan* and Aaron J.W. Hsueh, Dept. of Reproductive Medicine, University of California, San Diego, La Jolla, CA 92093 U.S.A.

We have shown previously that AVP directly modulates testicular steroidogenesis *in vitro* (Nature 293:650, 1981). AVP binding to interstitial cells of the rat testis was studied using ^{3}H-AVP. Binding equilibrium was reached by 60 min at 4°C. Scatchard plot analysis revealed the existence of one class of high affinity, low capacity binding sites (Kd=1.2±0.3nM, Bmax=8.5 fmol/10^6 cells). The rates of association and dissociation were calculated to be 0.024 nM^{-1} min^{-1} and 0.09 min^{-1}, respectively. Naturally occurring neurohypophysial hormones as well as synthetic analogs exhibited parallel displacement curves, indicating binding to the same binding sites. The order of potency for these peptides was found to be: AVP = lysine vasopressin = arginine vasotocin (IC_{50} ∿5x10^{-10}M) > oxytocin = valitocin = mesotocin (IC_{50} ∿5x10^{-7}M). Two potent vasopressor antagonists [d(CH_2)$_5$Tyr(Me)AVP] and [dPTyr(Me)AVP] competed with ^{3}H-AVP binding with a higher affinity than native AVP (IC_{50} ∿ 10^{-11}M). In addition, a specific antidiuretic agonist, dDAVP, also competed for receptor binding, suggesting that the testis may contain both V_1 and V_2 receptor subtypes. AVP binding sites could also be demonstrated in rat liver, kidney, testis and anterior pituitary (10.7, 4.9, 2.6 and 1.7 fmoles/mg protein), whereas adrenal, prostate and cerebellum were devoid of AVP binding sites. Thus, we have demonstrated the presence of high affinity, stereospecific receptors for the neurohypophysial hormones in the interstitial compartment of the rat testis. These receptors may mediate the direct action of these peptides on testicular steroidogenesis.

1887 ULTRASTRUCTURAL RADIOAUTOGRAPHIC LOCALIZATION OF SOMATOSTATIN-28 (S28) IN THE RAT PITUITARY GLAND.

G. Morel*, P. Leroux and G. Pelletier, MRC Group in Molecular Endocrinology, CHUL, Quebec G1V 4G2, Canada.

In order to identify the cell type(s) containing S28 receptors in the rat pituitary gland and to evaluate the possible internalization of the peptide, radioautography was performed at different time intervals after intravenous injections of the iodinated agonist of S28, [Leu^{8}-$DTrp^{22}$-Tyr^{25}]S28 (supplied by Dr. J. Rivier). The highest specific uptake of label occurred at the 5 min time interval. As previously shown by immunocytochemical localization of endogenous somatostatin-like immunoreactivity (Morel et al., Neuroendocrinology 36, 291, 1983), three cell types were consistently labeled: somatotrophs, mammotrophs and thyrotrophs. In somatotrophs, the time course study demonstrated that, two min after injection, most silver grains were associated with the plasma membrane. Five and fifteen minutes after injection, label was found in both the plasma membrane and cytoplasmic organelles, especially the Golgi apparatus, secretory granules and lysosomes. At the longest time interval (60 min), labeling was mostly associated with the cytoplasmic organelles and also with the nucleus. The binding of label was prevented by concomittant injection of an excess of unlabeled peptide, an indication of the specificity of the reaction. These results indicate that S28 receptors are present only in those cell types in which somatostatin is known to regulate secretory functions. The present data also show a rapid internalization of the radiolabeled peptide, with ultimate migration to the nucleus.

1888 IGF-II AND INSULIN STIMULATE PROLIFERATION OF H-35 CELLS THROUGH THE INSULIN RECEPTOR RATHER THAN THE IGF-II RECEPTOR.

C. Mottola* and M. P. Czech, Department of Biochemistry, University of Massachusetts Medical School, Worcester, MA 01605.

Insulin-like growth factor II (IGF-II) specifically binds with high affinity to a receptor associated with the plasma membrane of several cell types, however, the role of this receptor in the cellular physiology is still unclear. IGF-II (optimal concentration 10 M) and insulin (optimal concentration 10 M) induce proliferation in rat H-35 cells. By affinity crosslinking, the plasma membrane of these cells appears to be very rich in IGF-II receptor and to contain insulin receptor but no IGF-II receptor. In order to investigate the participation of the receptor for IGF-II in mediating the cellular growth stimulation due to this peptide, we employed an antibody directed against IGF-II receptor. This antibody, elicited in rabbit with purified rat placenta IGF-II receptor inhibits the binding of IGF-II to its receptor in rat and in mouse (with lower affinity), but not in human; it does not inhibit the binding of any hormone either to the insulin or the IGF-I receptor in all the species tested. Concentrations of antibody that inhibit about 70 to 80% the binding to H-35 of IGF-II in the range of 1 to 20nM do not shift the dose-response relationship of ^{3}H-thymidine uptake stimulation by IGF-II in these cells. At 20nM IGF-II the incorporation of labeled nucleoside is twice the control value in the presnece or absence of anti-receptor immunoglobulin. The insulin-induced proliferation is similarly unaffected by anti-IGF-II receptor immunoglobulin. The antibody itself does not mimic hormone action on cell growth, while a specific human anti-insulin receptor antibody (B-9) increases ^{3}H-thymidine uptake to the same extent as insulin.

1889 POLYAMINE-GONADOTROPIN RECEPTOR INTERACTION IN TESTIS: EFFECTS ON THE BINDING EVENT. T.A. Swift* and J.A. Dias, Department of Biochemistry, Albany Medical College, Albany, NY 12208.

The effect of the polyamine spermine on the interaction of radioiodinated human Follicle Stimulating Hormone (^{125}I-hFSH) with membrane bound FSH receptors was studied utilizing membranes (31,000 x g) derived from immature bovine testis. All experiments were performed at 34°C utilizing 0.05 M Tris buffer made 0.1 M with sucrose and 20 mM with $MgCl_2$ (pH 7.5). The dissociation of the preformed hormone receptor complex in the presence of spermine was examined by incubation of membranes (10 mg) for 1 h with ^{125}I-hFSH (5 ng), washing, and subsequent incubation in the presence of various concentrations (5-40 mM) of the polyamine. Membrane bound radioactivity, representing the preformed hormone receptor complexes, decreased up to 38% over a 3 h period when compared to controls in which spermine was absent. Pretreatment of calf testis membranes with spermine (5-40 mM) for 1 h followed by incubation with ^{125}I-hFSH in the continued presence of polyamine resulted in a dose-related inhibition of ^{125}I-hFSH binding (13-84%). However, if membranes were washed prior to the addition of ^{125}I-hFSH, a polyamine dose dependent increase (20-94%) in specifically bound ^{125}I-hFSH was observed. Thus, spermine may act to stabilize the membrane bound receptor at 34°C. Alternatively, spermine may unmask unoccupied cryptic receptor sites or cause the dissociation of endogenously bound hormone. FSH increases the rate of synthesis of the polycationic polyamines. These data demonstrate that spermine affects the longevity of the interaction of FSH with its receptor.

Supported by NIH-HD-16675.

1890 BINDING SITES FOR GROWTH HORMONE AND PROLACTIN IN PURIFIED PLASMA MEMBRANES FROM PREGNANT RABBIT LIVER. C.F. Webb*, M. Wallis and H.F. Cadman, Biochemistry Laboratory, School of Biological Sciences, University of Sussex, Falmer, Brighton BN1 9QG, U.K.

The liver of pregnant rabbit has been found to be particularly rich in growth hormone (GH) receptors and may be a target tissue for somatogenic hormones. This seems particularly likely in view of observations that many anabolic effects of GH are mediated by the somatomedins, a major production site of which is the liver. Binding of ^{125}I-labelled human GH (hGH) to plasma membranes from this source and to membranes solubilised with 0.5% Triton X-100 is time and temperature dependent, binding being slower at 4°C than at 25°C. Binding is also dependent on divalent cations, Ca^{2+} being more effective than Mg^{2+}, and on receptor concentration, a maximum of 52% specific binding being obtained. Some non-primate somatogenic hormones (e.g. bovine GH) and some lactogenic hormones (e.g. ovine prolactin) displaced labelled hGH from receptors, but those from various other species were rather ineffective. Receptors purified by affinity chromatography on hGH linked to Sepharose 4B, and eluted with 5M $MgCl_2$, had high specific binding (35%) and contained a major component of molecular weight of 68,000. The results suggest that there are few specifically somatogenic or lactogenic receptors in these plasma membranes and that the complex nature of the binding is a property of the receptors associated with plasma membranes and not a consequence of heterogeneity of the membranes, since these results are very similar to those obtained using microsomal membranes.

1891 EPIDERMAL GROWTH FACTOR (EGF) BINDING SITES IN BASOLATERAL PLASMA MEMBRANES (BPM) ARE DIFFERENT FROM MICROVILLUS PLASMA MEMBRANES (MPM) SITES IN TERM HUMAN PLACENTA. Ch. V. Rao*, N. Ramani, B. Stadig, P. Woost and G. Schultz University of Louisville, Louisville, KY 40292, USA

The EGF binding sites were shown to be present in MPM which are exposed to maternal circulation and in BPM which are in close proximity to fetal circulation. The present studies were undertaken to investigate whether the properties of EGF binding sites in MPM and BPM differed. The EGF binding specificity, pH optima, the protein functional group requirements and sensitivity to enzymes were similar in MPM and BPM. The ^{125}I-EGF binding to MPM reached a near maximum by 5 min (38°) or 10 min (22°), whereas 60 min were required for maximal binding to BPM at 22° and 38°. The Scatchard plots of ^{125}I-EGF specific binding to MPM and BPM were curvilinear which was due to negative cooperativity. The Kds calculated from the initial slopes were similar for MPM and BPM (0.07-0.12 nM) but the total number of available sites calculated from the X-axis intercepts of low slope lines were greater in MPM (8220 fmol/mg protein) compared to BPM (4880). While ^{125}I-EGF dissociation rates in 50 X dilution media were similar in MPM and BPM, the rates in the presence of excess unlabeled EGF were greater for MPM than for BPM. The BPM sites were relatively insensitive to thermal inactivation of 37° or 45°. Two major proteins of ~140 K and 160 K daltons in MPM and BPM were radiolabeled following incubation with ^{125}I-EGF. The 160 K protein was predominantly labeled in MPM, whereas the 140 K protein was labeled predominantly in BPM. In addition, several other proteins were labeled to a lesser extent in MPM (80K, 115K, 180K) and BPM (80K, 115K, 180K, 190K, 200K, 220K).

1892 EVIDENCE FOR THE PARTICIPATION OF DISULFIDE BONDS IN THE ALPHA-1 BINDING SITE OF NEOCORTICAL TISSUE. **T.A. Reader *, R. Brière and L. Grondin** , Centre de recherche en sciences neurologiques, Faculté de Médecine, Université de Montréal, Montréal, Québec H3C 3J7, Canada.

The tritiated alpha-1 antagonist Prazosin ([3H]-PRZ) binds specifically and with high affinity to postsynaptic adrenoceptors in membrane preparations obtained from rat cerebral neocortex and can be extremely useful in the molecular characterization of the cortical alpha-1 receptor site. Since receptors are of protein nature, we examined the role of disulfide (-SS-) bridges in fixation of [3H]-PRZ. For this purpose the -SS- bridges were reduced with DL-1, 4-dithiothreitol alone, or in combination with the alkylating agent N-Methylmaleimide (NMM). After DTT, which reduces disulfides quantitatively and maintains monothiols in the reduced state, specific binding was significantly decreased, thus suggesing that a possible requisite for [3H]-PRZ binding is the integrity of -SS- groups. After treatments with both DTT and NMM, the decreases in specific binding were comparable to those produced by DTT alone. Interestingly, NMM alone had a more prodound effect than DTT or DTT+NMM. Since the results with DTT indicate intact -SS- bonds as a requisite for specific binding, it is here proposed that the alpha-1 ligand has to "break" or reduce these bridges in order to bind. Alternatively, NMM may affect in some other way the -SS- bridges, and alters the confomational state (and the binding properties) of the alpha-1 adrenoceptor protein. [Supported by the MRC (MA-6967), the Quebec Heart Foundation and the Savoy Foundation for Epilepsy].

1893 UTEROTROPIC ACTIVITY OF THE MAJOR CONJUGATES OF ESTRADIOL IDENTIFIED IN BOVINE LIVER. J. Overpeck*, J. Williams, S. Colson, M. Applestine and J. Hohmann, Division of Drug Biology, FDA, Washington, D.C. 20204 USA

The conjugates of estradiol-17B(E-17B) found in the livers of steers treated with the estrogen have been profiled by others. A major component of the conjugate pool was identified as 17a-estradiol-17B-D-glucopyranoside, a compound of unknown uterotropic activity. The uterotropic activities of the glucuronide conjugates have been historically regarded as weak, but this assumption has prevailed based on data obtained by s.c. injection. The uterotropic activities of two free & four conjugated metabolites were estimated using the immature rat uterine weight assay. The 3-monoglucuronide and the 3,17-diglucuronide of E_2-17B were surprisingly active when given orally being about 1/2 as potent as E_2-17B. The 17-monoglucuronide was somewhat weaker. E_2-17a and the E_2-17a-glucopyranoside have 1/20th and 1/60th the oral activity of E_2-17B. When given s.c. the glucuronides were weakly uterotropic (less than 1% of E_2-17B). The E_2-17a-glucopyranoside is less than 1/1000 as active as E_2-17B when given s.c. Over the last several years this laboratory has been asked to test a variety of materials, i.e., pharmaceuticals and food samples, where estrogenic contamination was suspected. The surprisingly high activities of orally given glucuronides are an indication of the extent of intestinal hydrolysis and absorption and is an indication of their contribution to the uterotropic activity of the entire estrogenic pool.

1894 URINARY CATECHOLESTROGENS IN NORMAL MENSTRUATING AND PREGNANT WOMEN. E.D. Plotka*, R.E. Burrill, M.J. Heindel and D.A. Tewksbury, Marshfield Medical Foundation and Marshfield Clinic, Marshfield, WI 54449, USA.

Total catecholestrogens, mainly 2-hydroxyestrone and 2-hydroxyestradiol, were measured by radioimmunoassay (RIA) in 151 grab samples of urine from 5 menstruating women and 183 samples from 20 pregnant women in the second and third trimester of pregnancy. During the mid-follicular phase of the menstrual cycle, levels averaged 11.5 ± 0.9 (mean ± S.E., expressed as nanograms of 2-hydroxyestrone per milligram of creatinine; ng/mg C) whereas during the mid-luteal phase, levels averaged 19.4 ± 1.4 ($P<0.001$). During pregnancy, levels averaged 267 ± 44 (N=54) for the second trimester and 338 ± 52 (N=128) for the third trimester (t=1.05 with 18 df, NS). Normal values ranged from 61 to 1011 ng/mg C during the last month of pregnancy. The women appeared to fall into one of three groups based on catecholestrogen excretion: (1) average levels less than 200 ng/mg C with less than 2 individual values 200 or over; (2) average levels between 200 and 600 ng/mg C and no more than two individual values out of this range; and (3) more than two individual measurements greater than 600 ng/mg C. Monthly averages in each of these groups were significantly different starting 180 days prior to parturition and remained different throughout the remainder of pregnancy. Three women who had or became hypertensive during pregnancy, had levels of catecholestrogens that fell into Group 3. Levels in these women were significantly higher ($P<0.05$) in the third trimester than the average in normotensive women.
(Supported in part by grants from the Marshfield Clinic and Medical Foundation and NIH No. HL23707.)

1895 INHIBITION BY AMINOGLUTETHIMIDE OF AROMATIZATION OF TESTOSTERONE AND 19-HYDROXYTESTOSTERONE.

A. Purohit & R.E. Oakey*, Division of Steroid Endocrinology, School of Medicine, Leeds, England.

Aminoglutethimide (AG) a known inhibitor of steroid hydroxylations inhibits aromatization of $C_{19}\Delta^4$-3-oxosteroids which involves sequential hydroxylations at C-19, C-19 and C-2β. To study the site of inhibition, we measured, by RIA, the yield of oestrone (the only oestrogen formed) when testosterone or 19-hydroxytestosterone (6.9 pmol) was incubated with washed placental microsomes, NADPH, O_2 and AG (0 - 50 μmol/l). Conversion of both substrates 79% and 65%, respectively, was diminished by 50% in the presence of AG (14 and 4 μmol/l, respectively) whose effect therefore was not restricted to the first hydroxylation of the series.

We thank Ciba-Geigy for a supply of aminoglutethimide.

1896 THE SYNTHETIC PROGESTIN ^{3}H-ORG 2058: ITS LOCALIZATION IN THE BRAIN AND OTHER TISSUES OF FEMALE MONKEYS. Howard D. Rees* and Richard P. Michael, Department of Psychiatry, Emory University School of Medicine, and Georgia Mental Health Institute, Atlanta, GA 30322, U.S.A.

Progesterone acts on the primate brain to inhibit gonadotropin release and it also depresses primate sexual behavior. To help identify possible target neurons for progesterone, two female *Macaca fascicularis* (body wt. 2.5 kg) were ovariectomized and given daily injections of 20 μg estradiol benzoate sc for 1 week. After tranquilization, they were given 1 mCi of ^{3}H-ORG 2058 (Amersham; 54 Ci/mmol) iv and killed 1 h later. A sample of uterus chromatographed by HPLC revealed that 97% of the nuclear radioactivity was in the form of ORG 2058. Thaw-mount autoradiograms from one animal revealed intense accumulation of radioactivity in the nuclei of many neurons in the medial basal hypothalamus, particularly in the ventromedial nucleus (n.), arcuate n., ventral premammillary n., and periventricular n. Neuronal labeling was also observed frequently in the medial preoptic n., and occasionally in the anterior hypothalamic area, paraventricular n., and organum vasculosum of the lamina terminalis. No labeled cells were found in the septal area-bed n., amygdala, hippocampus, brain stem, or spinal cord. In the pituitary, intense labeling was observed in many cells of the pars distalis, but not in the pars intermedia or pars nervosa. The brain of the second animal is currently being processed. We conclude that the distribution of progestin target cells in the primate brain is both more restricted than that in the rodent brain, and more restricted than the distribution of estrogen and androgen target cells in the primate brain. Supported by USPHS Grant MH 33766.

1897 PROLAME, A NEW AMINO-ESTROGEN WITH MARKED ANTICOAGULANT EFFECT. C. Rubio-Póo*, C. Lemini, J.M. Fernández-González, A. de la Peña, F. Cruz, N. Mendoza-Patiño, and J.J. Mandoki. Departamento de Farmacología, Facultad de Medicina, Escuela Nacional de Estudios Profesionales Zaragoza, and Instituto de Química, Universidad Nacional Autónoma de México, 04510 México, D.F., México.

Estrogens with pronounced anticoagulant effects may be useful in the treatment of prostatic cancer, without increasing the risk of thrombo-embolic accidents, and in the prevention of coronary thrombosis. Prodiame, a di-amino-estrogen has been shown to have a marked anticoagulant effect (Rubio et al., 1983), but produces convulsions at large doses. Prolame (N-|3-hydroxy-estra-1:3:5(10)-triene-17β|-1,3-propanolamine), a mono-amino-estrogen, was prepared, and its anticoagulant and estrogenic effects were studied. Male and ovariectomized CD1 mice, and Wistar male rats were used. 25 μL of blood were drawn from the tip of the tail into a glass microhematocrit tube, and were made to flow continuously by gravity between two marks 45 mm apart, until the flow ceased (end point). Vaginal cornification was the estrogenic effect observed. Dose-related increases in blood clotting were detected 24 hours after a single subcutaneous injection, and in the rat, a considerable effect could be observed even after 96 hours. At 24 hours, the maximal observed increases in blood clotting time were 45 % in male mice, 113 % in ovariectomized mice, and 71 % in male rats. Vaginal cornification lasted considerably less with prolame than with equivalent doses of estradiol-17β. Prolame did not increase motor activity, and appears to be a promising agent for the treatment of prostatic cancer, and the prevention of coronary thrombosis.

1898 SEX HORMONES AND ANDROGENS PLASMA ACTIVITY IN UREMIC MALE PATIENTS ON HEMODIALYSIS. I.Mastrogiacomo*, L.De Besi, P.Zucchetta, E.Serafini, I.Karbowiak, S.Lorenzi", P.Dean', D.Armanini. Institute of Semeiotica Medica, University of Padova- Dialysis Units Hosp. of "Venezia,'Verona. Italy.

Uremia causes a male primary hypogonadism whose features are not fully known. In 161 uremic male patients on chronic periodic hemodialysis and in 83 helthy sex and age-matched subjects the following hormones were assessed by RIA methods: testosterone (T), androstenedione (A), estrone (E_1), estradiol (E_2) and DHEA-S. Moreover in 44 patients the total androgen plasma activity was determined by a radioreceptor assay employing castrated swiss mice kidney cytosol, incubated with tracer amount of 3H-RU 1881. Data obtained confirm the existence of a hypogonadism with significantly lower (vs. controls) T levels (289 ± 125 vs. 467 ± 190 ng/100 ml;$p < 0.001$) and lower androgens activity (1.29 ± 0.36 vs. 1.70 ± 0.73 nMEq RU 1881;$p < 0.02$). Significantly diminished were DHEA-S (1.4 ± 1.4 vs. 2.8 ± 2 mcg/ml;$p < 0.001$) and E_2 (11.8 ± 3 vs. 30.6 ± 16.5 pg/ml;$p < 0.001$), whereas A (0.83 ± 0.27 vs. 0.55 ± 0.1 ng/ml;$p < 0.001$) and E_1 (64.3 ± 31.7 vs. 41.5 ± 20 pg/ml;$p < 0.001$) were increased. Also increased and positively correlated between each other were the A/T and E_1/E_2 ratios. Total androgens activity was positively correlated with T ($r=0.36$ $p < 0.05$) and negatively with A/T ratio ($r=-0.43$ $p < 0.01$). In conclusion uremic damage seems to impair the conversion of A to T and of E_1 to E_2, that is the activity of the 17-dehydrogenase. Adrenal androgens production (DHEA-S) is also lessened. Though the levels of A are increased, the total androgens plasma activity is reduced as compared to control subiects. The increase of the A/T ratio seems to be the best index of the hypogonadism, which affects uremic male patients.

1899 CULTURED HAIR FOLLICLE CELLS HAVE LOW 5 α-REDUCTASE ACTIVITY.

Thierry Maudelonde, MD*, Robert L. Rosenfield, MD and Elaine Fuchs, PhD, Departments of Pediatrics, Medicine and Biochemistry, University of Chicago, Pritzker School of Medicine, Chicago Illinois, 60637 (USA).

Because certain hairs are androgen targets, and because the pattern of androgen metabolism by target cells is an important determinant of androgen action, we have determined the pattern of testosterone (T) and dihydrotestosterone (DHT) metabolism in cultured, occipital hair follicle cells.

Anagen hairs (H) were plucked from the scalp vertex of 4 normal volunteers. Epithelial cells (E) and fibroblasts (F) were obtained from 4-5 circumcised neonatal foreskins. H and E trypsinized in EDTA were grown in primary co-culture with 3T3 cells in DMEM containing 20% FCS, insulin, EGF, T3, cortisol, and cholera toxin. After 1-3 subcultures without 3T3 cells, followed by 24 hours in DMEM alone, incubations with 4 nM 1,2 ^{3}H-T and 1,2 ^{3}H-DHT were carried out. Metabolites were isolated by TLC.

Initial velocities, normalized as % substrate/ng DNA/min ($\bar{x} \pm$ SEM):

	5 α-reductase	17 β-HSD	3 α-KS-reductase	3 β-KS-reductase
H	4.59 ± 2.84	8.45 ± 4.39	1.35 ± .40	0.22 ± 0.08
E	1.53 ± .072	12.33 ± 3.95	7.73 ± 3.07	0.47 ± 0.27
F	191.8 ± 92.77	91.60 ± 28.78	14.80 ± 6.62	0.22 ± 0.22

Hair cell 5 α-reductase activity is 5% that of fibroblasts. The pattern of T and DHT metabolism in hair cells resembles that of foreskin epithelium, with metabolism predominantly via the 17 β-hydroxysteroid dehydrogenase (17 β-HSD) pathway at similar rates.

Since T predominates in the plasma and is not metabolized efficiently by hair cells, these data suggest that T is the predominant androgen within hair cells.

1900 DISSOCIATED PRL AND TSH RESPONSE TO TRH IN KLINEFELTER'S SYNDROME

Modena G*, Foresta C., Lo Giudice C., Patarnello T., Manente P. and Scandellari C.
Divisione Medica 2^, Ospedale di Castelfranco Veneto-Treviso
Cattedra di Patologia Medica III^ Università di Padova-Italy

In twenty-five patients with Klinefelter's syndrome (KS) plasma PRL and TSH levels have been measured after stimulation with exogenous TRH (200 mcg i.v.). According to the literature, in our KS we have found a PRL response to TRH significantly higher ($p<0.01$) than in controls. Mean TSH response in KS was not significantly different from that of normal subiects; not only, but in eleven of them (44%) TSH response resulted clearly impaired. Furthermore the statistical analysis showed an inverse correlation between the peack of TSH and the peack of PRL after TRH ($r=-0,45$, $p<0.05$). Our data show the presence of a dissociated PRL and TSH response to TRH in KS, contrary to what is found in other forms of primitive hypogonadism, where both hormones responde exaggerately to TRH.

This response strongly suggests that KS is associated with alterated dopaminergic control. In those patients the hypotalamic dopaminergic system may affect inversely hypophiseal secretion of PRL and TSH, and a reduced central dopaminergic activity may contribute to better underline this alterated mechanism.

1901 INDUCTION OF ORNITHINE DECARBOXYLASE BY GONADOTROPINS IN MOUSE TESTIS INVOLVES INCREASED mRNA ACCUMULATION. A.M. Nakhla*, K.K. Kontula, C.W. Bardin and O.A. Jänne, The Population Council and The Rockefeller University, New York, NY 10021

Both LH and FSH have been shown to increase activity of ornithine decarboxylase (ODC) in rodent testis. The mechanisms by which gonadotropins influence ODC activity are not fully understood although indirect evidence suggests synthesis of new enzyme molecules. In the present work we have studied the *in vivo* effect of LH and FSH on mouse testicular ODC activity, enzyme protein concentration and accumulation of ODC-mRNA. Male NCS mice were given a single i.p. injection of bovine LH (10-250 U/kg bw) or ovine FSH (2 mg/kg) in physiological saline and killed at different time intervals. ODC activity was measured by using L-[1-^{14}C] ornithine as substrate and its concentration by a specific RIA. Relative ODC-mRNA concentration was determined by Northern blot analysis of testicular poly(A)-RNA using cloned cDNA for ODC-mRNA (pODC16) as the hybridization probe. Administration of LH resulted in dose-dependent (10-250 U/kg) 74-275% increase in ODC activity with maximal stimulation occuring at 4 h after LH administration and then rapidly subsided. The response to LH was similar in hypophysectomized and intact males. FSH also stimulated the enzyme activity by 4 h after hormone administration. Elevated ODC activity after gonadotropin treatment was accompanied by 2- 3-fold increased ODC-mRNA concentration in testes. Conclusions: 1) a single injection of LH or FSH stimulates ODC activity in mouse testis in a time- and dose-dependent manner; 2) this study provides the first evidence that increased ODC-mRNA accumulation is involved in the induction of ODC by peptide or glycoprotein hormones.

1902 EVIDENCE THAT β-ENDORPHIN INHIBITS SERTOLI CELL PROLIFERATION IN FETAL RATS Joanne M. Orth*, Department of Anatomy, Temple University School of Medicine, Philadelphia, PA 19140.

It has been suggested recently that fetal Leydig cells produce β-endorphin. This peptide may act locally in the testis, since injection of the remaining testis of hemi-castrate pups with naloxone, an opiate blocker, produced enhanced compensatory hypertrophy (Gerendai et al, Androl.15:398, 1983). Since we recently showed that increased Sertoli cell proliferation plays a central role in the response of the testis to hemi-castration (Orth et al, Biol. Reprod. in press), the aim of the present work was to determine whether blocking opiate receptors in the testis affects Sertoli cell division. Testes were removed from fetal rats on day 20 and placed in organ culture with or without naloxone (1 μg/ml). ^{3}H-thymidine was added at the start of culture. After 24hrs, testes were fixed and processed for LM autoradiography by routine techniques. The % of Sertoli cells labeled was determined by sampling 1500 or more cells in each testis by methods already described. In control (n=3) and treated (n=4) testes, 25.3±1.6% and 36.4±1.5% of the Sertoli cells incorporated label, respectively. This represents an increase (p .01) of 35% in the portion of the Sertoli cell population preparing to divide in testes exposed to naloxone. These preliminary findings suggest that β -endorphin, perhaps from Leydig cells, may play a role in modulating proliferation of fetal Sertoli cells. Recent data from this laboratory indicate that FSH from the fetal pituitary stimulates Sertoli cell division in rat fetuses (Orth, J.Cell Biol.97:18a, 1983). Therefore, ongoing studies are aimed at exploring the possible relationship between these two factors in controlling expansion of the Sertoli cell population during perinatal life. (Supported by NIH Grant #HD15563)

1903 EFFECTS OF FSH ON ACIDIC NUCLEAR PROTEIN SYNTHESIS IN CULTURED PIG SERTOLI CELLS. M.H. Perrard* and A. Dazord, INSERM U. 162, Hôpital Debrousse, 69322 Lyon Cedex 05, France.

Using a primary culture of immature porcine Sertoli cells, we have studied the effect of FSH on the nuclear protein synthesis. Sertoli cells were cultured in a chemically defined medium and treated with porcine FSH (50 ng/ml) for several times (4, 8, 25 and 64 hours). About 65 spots (pHi lower than 8) were identified by a two-dimensional polyacrylamide gel electrophoresis. After 25 hours of FSH treatment, we observed an increase of five proteins, a slight decrease of two and the disappearance of one. For the short times of FSH treatment (4 and 8 hours) no effect of FSH on nuclear protein synthesis was observed. After 64 hours of FSH treatment, the synthesis of all nuclear proteins appeared to be decreased. The data show that FSH affects the synthesis of pig Sertoli cells nuclear proteins. We are probably dealing with acidic proteins since we have only looked to the proteins whose pHi is lower than 8. Since non-histone proteins are involved in gene expression and in the control of transcription, our results suggest that FSH could act at the gene expression level, via modification of nuclear acid protein synthesis.

1904 LOCALIZATION OF AROMATASE IN SEMINIFEROUS TUBULES OF THE GROUND SQUIRREL, CITELLUS LATERALIS. J. Pudney*, J.A. Canick, J. Knapp, and G.V. Callard. Dept. of Biol., Boston Univ., Boston, MA, 02215, and Dept. of Pathol., Women & Infants Hosp., Brown Univ., Providence, RI 02908.

In the rat, aromatase has been detected in immature Sertoli cells and in mature and immature Leydig cells. We have investigated the intratesticular site of aromatase in another rodent species, the ground squirrel, using both mature and immature animals. Expt. I. The testes of mature animals were manually dissected into seminiferous tubules and interstitial components. Both fractions were homogenized and aromatase activity determined by incubation with ^3H androstenedione ($\Delta 4$) plus NADPH. Product estrone (E_1) and estradiol (E_2) were separated by TLC and purified by phenolic partition, methylation, and recrystallization. Results are expressed as fmol E_1 + E_2 produced/min/mg prot: Whole testis=0.50; Interstitium= non detectable; tubules=0.60. Expt. II. Immature animals (3 per group) were injected sc with either ovine LH (ovine LH#23, 100μg/inj) or saline twice daily for four days. The testes were decapsulated and microsomes prepared. Aromatase activity was determined as above using either ^3H $\Delta 4$ or ^3H 19-hydroxy$\Delta 4$, Results are expressed in units given above: S=19-hydroxy$\Delta 4$, saline=3.72, LH=3.60; S=$\Delta 4$, saline=6.05; LH=6.61. LH had no effect on aromatase. Morphologically, Leydig cells were hypertrophied, correlating with increased titers of circulating testosterone (LH=2.0ng/ml, saline <0.2ng/ml) and stimulation of sex accessory glands. These data support results from the first experiment indicating that aromatase is localized in the seminiferous tubules in the ground squirrel.

1905 EFFECTS OF TESTICULAR DENERVATION ON THE TESTIS FUNCTION OF MATURE AND PRE PUBERAL MALE RAT. A.A.M.Rosa*, A.L.V.Favaretto**, T.L.L.Carvalho**, A.L. Ferreira**, J.Antunes-Rodrigues**. *Depto. de Morfologia e Fisiologia Animal, F.C.A.V. - Unesp, 14870, Jaboticabal, SP, Brasil. **Depto. de Fisiologia, F.M.R.P. - USP, 14100, Ribeirão Preto, SP, Brasil.

The functional role of testicular innervation has been discussed. Does it have activity on the gametogenic and secretory function of the testis? In order to study this possibilities adult (200 g body weight) and immature (90 g body weight) male rats were submitted to a local application of 10% phenol. The animals were studied 30 days later to determine: 1) Testicular histology, 2) Plasma levels of LH, FSH and testosterone (T) and 3) T secretion, 30 and 60 minutes after hCG administration (2,5 UI/100g). Similar results were obtained in adult and immature rats, although the results were more evident when the phenolization were done in the immature rats. 1) Besides the normal histological aspects of the seminiferous tubules, phenolized (P) animals show an enhancement of the VII and VIII stages of the spermatogenetic cycle, refleting an accumulation of mature spermatozoa the gonad. 2) In this same sense, they also present higher plasma levels of LH and T and diminished plasma levels of FSH, 3) In response to hCG, P male rats show 100% higher T concentration than the control. The present data demonstrate that testicular innervation has a role in modulating testicular fuction in adult and immature male rat. This study was supported by FINEP.

1906 EFFECT OF VITAMIN A ACID ON THE TESTIS OF THE EGYPTIAN TOAD. I.A. Sadek* and I. Sabry, Zoology Department, Faculty of Science, Alexandria University, Alexandria, Egypt.

Sterility is a common side effect in men treated with chemotherapeutic drugs. On the other hand, the therapeutic effects of vitamin A in the prevention of neoplasms is well documented. The Egyptian toad, Bufo regularis, was chosen for the present study as a new model to show the effect of 13-cis-retinoic acid (RA) on spermatogenesis. Male toads were treated orally with high doses of RA (0.25 mg/50 g body weight, 3 times/week) for 6 weeks. This aromatic retinoid clearly induces a reduction of the germinal epithelium and stops spermatogenesis. These histological changes in the testes were reversible within 6 weeks after withdrawal of the drug. The exact mechanism of vitamin A action in the process of spermatogenesis remains to be clarified.

1907 DIFFERENTIAL BINDING RATES OF T3 & T4 TO DIPALMITOYL PHOSPHATIDYLCHOLINE VESICLES.

E. G. Movius*, M. A. Phyillaier, CEB, NIADDK, NIH, Bethesda, MD, USA 20205.

The entry of T3 & T4 into cells has been postulated to occur via passive diffusion, active transport, and receptor-mediated endocytosis. Regardless of the mechanism, the first step of transport probably involves binding to the cell membrane. We have previously noted a perturbation of pyrene fluorescence by T3 & T4 in dipalmitoyl phosphatidylcholine (DPPC) vesicles (Endocrine Society, Abstracts 1983, #482), and have employed this perturbation to measure the kinetics of binding of T3 & T4 to DPPC bilayer membranes. Unilamellar vesicles of DPPC (0.5 mg/ml) with pyrene (10 µm) were prepared by sonication in 50 mM sodium phosphate buffer, pH 7.0. Pyrene fluorescence at 390 nm was monitored continuously while T3 or T4 (50 µm) was rapidly mixed with the vesicles. A progressive quenching of fluorescence was observed due to the binding of T3 or T4 to the outer vesicle leaflet. Using nonlinear least squares a half-time (T1/2) of binding was calculated. At 35° C. (gel phase) the T1/2's for T3 & T4 were 54.5±1.4 and 36.1±2.8 sec. ($p<.01$), and at 45° C. (liquid-crystal phase) the T1/2's were 9.7±1.7 and 12.8±4.8 sec. ($p>.05$) respectively. From these studies we conclude that both T3 & T4 bind to phospholipid membranes very rapidly when the lipid is in the liquid-crystal phase. The faster binding rate of T4 in the gel phase may be due to its greater lipophilicity compared to T3.

1908 THYROID STATE MODULATES THE GLUCOREGULATORY RESPONSE TO GLUCAGON

M.J. Müller*, P.Hunzinger**, U. Paschen** and H.J. Seitz**,*Abt. Klinische Endokrinologie, Med.Hochschule Hannover and **Institut f. Physiol. Chemie Universitäts-Krankenhaus Eppendorf, Hamburg, West Germany

Plasma glucagon is frequently enhanced in hyperthyroidism, thus probably contributing to thyroid hormone induced increase in glucose production. Therefore, the effect of different thyroid states on glucagon stimulated glucose production was investigated in (i) 24 h starved conscious mini-pigs and (ii) in isolated perfused rat livers.For details of the methods see (1, 2). In euthyroid pigs, arginine stimulated glucagon secretion caused a transient rise in blood glucose (+12%,$p< 0.05$) and in tracer determined glucose production (+36%,$p< 0.01$).The effect was reduced in hypothyroid pigs,but blunted in experimental hyperthyroidism.Correspondingly,infusing glucagon (3ng/kgxmin) in euthyroid pig transiently increased blood glucose (+25%,$p< 0.01$)and glucose production (+25%,$p< 0.05$),whereas in hypothyroidism the effect was reduced and hyperthyroid pigs did not response at all.-In the isolated perfused liver,glucagon (10^{-11}-10^{-7}M)ordBcAMP(10^{-6}-10^{-3}M)were less effective in hypo- than in euthyroid livers in stimulating gluconeogenesis (from alanine)and deactivating pyruvate kinase;this was normalized by inhibiting phosphodiesterase.In hyperthyroid livers gluconeogenesis was increased,which was not further stimulated by glucagon or dBcAMP.

It is concluded that the glucoregulatory response to glucagon is blunted in hyperthyroidism;in hypothyroidism the response is reduced,probably due to alterations in tissue cAMP turnover.

(1) M.J. Müller, U. Paschen, H.J. Seitz, Am. J. Physiol. 244, E 236 (1983)
(2) M.J. Müller, H.J. Seitz, Biochim.Biophys. Acta 756,360 (1983).

1909 COMPARATIVE STUDIES OF T_3 SUPPRESSIBILITY DETERMINED BY SERUM T_4, FREE-T_4 AND THYROGLOBULIN(Tg).

M. Murakami*, I. Kobayashi, M. Mori, K. Ohshima, N. Kamio, Y. Shimomura, T. Kondo and S. Kobayashi, Division of Endocrinology, First Department of Internal Medicine, Gunma University and Isesaki City Hospital, Maebashi 371, Japan.

Thyroid suppression test has been widely used to predict the outcome of medical treatment with antithyroid drug therapy for Graves' disease. We attempted to determine a new T_3 suppression test compared with the conventional method. Studies were conducted with 50 patients with Graves' disease who were regarded as euthyroid during a maintenance dose of antithyroid drug, since their serum T_4, T_3 and Free-T_4 were within normal ranges. Each patient was given 75 μg T_3 daily for 8 days and measured 24-h thyroid ^{131}I uptake after T_3 administration(post T_3 uptake). The positive suppression was defined as the post T_3 uptake lower than 35 %. Serum T_4, Free-T_4 and Tg were determined by RIA before and after T_3 administration. Serum T_4 and Free-T_4 after T_3 administration(% of the initial value) were significantly lower in the positive suppression group(27 cases, T4 68.4±2.5 %; Free-T4 62.1±3.2 %) than in the negative suppression group(23 cases, T_4 91.2±6.5 %; Free-T_4 108.6±7.2 %). Serum Tg level from the positive group was 52.5±6.3 %, while that of the negative group was 71.5± 6.3 %.
Conclusion: We propose a simple and stable T_3 suppression test; when serum T_4 or Free-T_4 after T_3 administration was 70 % or less of the initial value, it suggests the positive suppression. In addition, greater suppressibility by T_3 of circulating Tg in the positive suppression group was demonstrated.

1910 SYNTHESIS OF BIOACTIVE THYROXINE-BINDING GLOBULIN (TBG) FROM HUMAN LIVER mRNA.

Y. Murata*, S. Refetoff, G. Vassart and H. Seo, Depts. of Medicine and Pediatrics, Univ. of Chicago, IL USA; IRIBHN, Free Univ. of Brussels, Belgium; and Research Inst. of Env. Medicine, Univ. of Nagoya, Japan.

TBG is a glycoprotein of hepatic origin which transports thyroid hormone in serum. Synthesis, as a monomer with pH-dependent microheterogeneity, is controlled by the X-chromosome. RNA was extracted from 3 human livers (HL) and from a human hepatoma cell line (Hep G2) and the mRNA was selected by oligo-dT. Translation of mRNA was carried out in rabbit reticulocyte lysate (RRL) and in the Xenopus laevis oocyte (XLO). The product of translation was analyzed for TBG immunoreactivity (precipitation with anti-TBG sera,(specific for either tertiary or primary structure of TBG), TBG bioactivity [specific thyroxine (T4)-binding] and by dodecylsulfate polyacrylamide electrophoresis (SDS-PAGE). mRNA derived from HL and Hep G2 directed the synthesis of a protein precipitable with anti-TBG serum and displaceable with purified TBG. It migrated as a single band on SDS-PAGE of 45K (when translated in RRL) and 61K (when translated in XLO). Pre-TBG constituted about 0.005% of the total product of HL mRNA translation in the nuclease treated RRL. Only XLO injected with either HL or Hep G2 mRNA contained a protein which bound specifically T4. Approximately 0.8 fmole of TBG was synthesized in 24h by 10 XLO injected each with 50 ng HL mRNA. It is concluded that HL contains active TBG mRNA which yields non-glycosylated pre-TBG and glycosylated, bioreactive TBG when translated in the RRL and XLO systems, respectively. Further analysis of these translation products of mRNA from individual HL will determine whether the microheterogeneity of TBG is of genetic origin. Supported by USPHS Grant AM-15070.

1911 LOCALIZATION OF THYROXINE 5'-MONODEIODINASE ACTIVITY IN THE RENAL PROXIMAL TUBULES IN RABBITS. N. Murayama*,[1] K. Yoshida,[2] T. Sakurada,[2] S. Torikai,[3] Y. Asano[1] and K. Yoshinaga[2] Div. of Nephrology, Dept. of Cardiology[1] and Dept. of Pharmacology,[3] Jichi Med. Sch. Tochigi and Dept. of Internal Med. Tohoku Univ. Sch. of Med.[2] Sendai, Japan

We have recently reported (Endocrinol Jap. 30:211, 1983) that the potency of T_4 5'-monodeiodinase activity in dog renal tissues was in the decreasing order of cortical tubule, cortical homogenate, glomerulus and inner medullar tubule. In order to determine the localization of T_4 5'-monodeiodinase activity in rabbit nephron segments, the formation of T_3 from T_4 was measured in the presence of 5mM dithiothreitol in kidney homogenate (0.5 mg protein) and in isolated nephron segments (10 ~ 40 μg protein) obtained by the micro-dissection method. In order of decreasing activity, homogenates of rabbit renal cortex, outer medulla and inner medulla were capable of converting T_4 to T_3. In the isolated nephron segments of the rabbit cortex, the mean net T_3 production from T_4 in the proximal convoluted and proximal straight tubules (PCT and PST) was 23.7 ± 8.8 (mean ± SE, n=9) and 20.1 ± 4.6 pg T_3/μg prot/200 ng T_4/h, respectively. On the other hand, the activities were not detected in the segments including the cortical thick ascending limb of Henle's loop (CAL), the distal convoluted tubule (DCT), the connecting tubule (CNT), and the cortical collecting tubule (CCT). These results indicate that both PCT and PST are the sites of T_3 production from T_4 in the rabbit kidney.

SEGMENT LOCATION ALONG MICRODISSECTED RABBIT NEPHRON

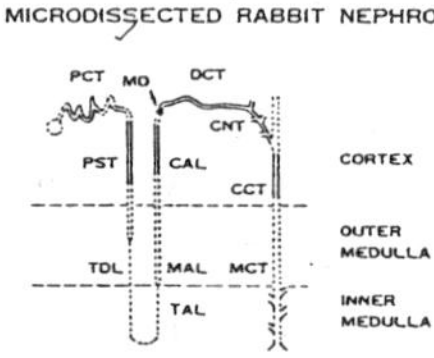

1912 S-100 PROTEIN IN THE TISSUE OF VARIOUS THYROID DISORDERS. A. Nakai*, A. Nagasaka, K. Iwase, H. Hidaka°, H. Umekawa°, S. Ohkubo°, T. Aono, T. Ohyama, H. Nakagawa, K. Miura, K. Kawase and H. Isaji, Fujita-Gakuen Univ. and °Mie Univ. School of Med., Toyoake, Aichi 470-11, Japan.

The S-100 protein first isolated by Moore as a soluble, highly acidic and nervous tissue-specific protein has been detected in various peripheral non-nervous tissues, but the potential physiological significance still remains obscure. We examined the presence of S-100 protein and evaluated its biological significance in various thyroid disorders. The human thyroid specimens, obtained surgically, were homogenized and fractionated. The content of S-100 protein in the soluble fraction was measured by a sandwich enzyme immunoassay system using antibodies labeled with -D-galactosidase. Immunohistochemical analysis was performed immunoperoxidase staining. The S-100 protein was detectable in the soluble fraction of thyroid tissues. The concentration of S-100 protein in the tissue of thyroid cancer was 3-5 times higher than that contained in the tissue of normal thyroid and thyroid adenoma. In the tissue of cancer of stomach and the other digestive organs, the increase of S-100 protein concentration was not remarkable. The calmodulin content increased in thyroid cancer but the increment was low in comparison to the S-100 protein. Our results confirmed the presence of S-100 protein in the thyroid tissue. In contrast to the remarkable decrease in the protein content observed in T lymphocytes from patients with acute T lymphocytic leukemia, S-100 protein content increased in the well differentiated thyroid cancer. This suggests that S-100 protein may be linked to cell maturation.

1913 EFFECT OF TYROPANOATE ON THYROID HORMONE RELEASE FROM THE LIVER BY ISOLATED RAT LIVER PERFUSION. M. Nakazono*, Y. Fujioka, H. Yashiro, T. Irie, H. Kikuchi and K. Takebe, The Third Department of Internal Medicine, School of Medicine, Hirosaki University, Hirosaki, Japan.

It was demonstrated that tyropanoate (Ty) caused thyroxine (T4) release from the liver by the in vivo experiment in man (Felicetta,JV et al, 1980). We observed whether Ty caused thyroid hormone release from the isolated rat liver in the perfusion experiment with the Miller-type apparatus. The isolated rat liver was perfused by 180 ml of bovine serum albumin, 10 mM glucose and 3.1 gHb/dl of bovine red blood cell, with adding 20 mcg of T4 15 min after preperfusion and 300 mg/kgBW of Ty 45 min after T4-addition (Ty-group). We collected 1 ml of the perfusate at intervals of 15 min for 180 min. The increase of T4 level in the perfusate was no significant difference between Ty-group and a group without Ty-addition (Normal group), nor as the volume of T4 distribution in the liver. However, the increment of triiodothyronine (T3) in the perfusate was 9.38 ng/g (of liver) for 15 min after Ty-addition, in comparison with 0.64 ng/g in Normal group ($p < 0.001$). Moreover, the increments of T3 in the perfusate after Ty-addition were proportional to the increases in quantity of Ty. The volume of T3 distribution in the liver in Ty-group was decreased more than that in Normal group ($p<0.001$). These results suggest that tyropanoate causes T3 release from the liver although the compound is known to inhibit the conversion of T4 to T3. This study implies a mechanism for altering hepatic content of thyroid hormones, that could be the site of physiologic regulation or of disease. And the isolated rat liver perfusion system may be useful for the study of the mechanism.

1914 CURRENT TRACER METHODS FOR MEASURING DIALYZABLE FREE T_4 UNDERESTIMATE FREE T_4 IN THE LOW T_4 SYNDROME
*Nelson, J.C., Weiss, R.M., White Memorial Medical Center, Los Angeles, California 90033 USA

We have developed a new T_4 RIA for the direct measurement of Free T_4 (FT_4) in equilibrium dialysates and compared the measurement of FT_4 by direct RIA to measurement by a conventional tracer dialysis method (TD). FT_4 by RIA was lower than FT_4 by TD but the discrepancy between the two methods (Δ) varied with the type of serum studied and the extent of serum dilution used for dialysis.

Progressive dilution of the serum sample caused a progressive fall in FT_4. This fall was more rapid in LT_4S than in NS and the LT_4S FT_4 levels were greater than, equal to, or less than NS FT_4 levels depending on dilution of serum used for dialysis.

The Δ between RIA and TD was greater with less dilute sera and less with more dilute sera. The Δ was strikingly less for LT_4S than for NS. Since the Δ between RIA and TD might be explained by $^{125}I^-$ contamination of dialysate tracer T_4 the chemical identity of dialysate radioactivity was studied by acetonitrile gradient HPLC. Dialysates of normal sera contained a 2.7 to 3.2 fold greater contamination of tracer with $^{125}I^-$ than dialysates of LT_4S compatible with decreased T_4 deiodination by LT_4S.

Conclusions: (1) Serum dilution reduces FT_4 to a greater extent in LT_4S than in NS (2) Dialysate tracer T_4 contamination with I^- is less in LT_4S than in NS (3) The measurement FT_4 by current tracer methods using diluted serum samples underestimates FT_4 concentrations in LT_4S.

1915 DIURNAL RHYTHMICITY IN PERIPHERAL T4 TO T3 CONVERSION IN MAN.
A. Nimalasuriya*, C. A. Spencer, and J.T. Nicoloff. USC School of Medicine, Los Angeles, CA.

To determine if a diurnal variation in T4 to T3 or rT3 conversion occurs in man, serum TSH, T4, T3 and rT3 values were measured by RIA at 4-hour intervals during a 3-day control period (C) and the last 3 days of a 6-day fast (F) in 12 healthy, mildly obese (131% of ideal weight) females. To negate the effects of hemoconcentration and to selectively show T3 or rT3 production variations, T3/T4 and rT3/T4 ratios were used. Results: TSH showed a distinct nocturnal (2200-0200) peak (121% rise) which occurred before (4), during (2) and after (6) a less prominent (28% rise) T3/T4 peak. The Mean daytime (D), (0800-2000) T3/T4 value of 14.88±0.78 was less than the nighttime (N), (2000-0800) value of 16.37±1.01 ($p < 0.004$). No correlation of the magnitude of TSH and T3/T4 was noted ($p > 0.6$). During the fast, diurnal TSH pattern was maintained while T3/T4 was completely lost (D-7.79±0.49, N-7.58±0.40, p = NS). T3/T4 ratio began to fall within 1 day of fasting and leveled after 3 days at 62% of control value. In contrast, a rise in rT3/T4 ratio did not occur until 2 days after the onset of fasting. No diurnal rhythmicity of rT3/T4 was seen during either C or F period. Conclusions: 1) Diurnal variations in T3 but not rT3 production occur in man, 2) altered T3 production is not secondary to TSH but to changes in peripheral T4 to T3 conversion, 3) a sensitive regulation of T4 to T3 conversion system exists which responds to some unknown dietary signal(s), and 4) as is seen during the first 3 days of fasting, serum T3 values can be regulated independently of changes in rT3 thus indicating independent 5' deiodinase systems.

1916 ANTITHYROID ANTIBODIES AND SERUM THYROTROPIN IN JAPANESE POPULATION.
K. Notsu*, T. Sakurami, M. Hirata, F. Oseko, J. Endo and S. Note, Department of Internal Medicine, Shimane Medical University, Izumo 693, Japan.

Since 1979, we have studied antithyroid antibodies (ATA) in one population in Japan. In the 1981 survey, 15 patients with overt thyroid disorders and 111 cases with asymptomatic autoimmune thyroiditis (AAT) were detected in 1242 participants. The incidence of AAT in Japanese population was much the same in European survey and age-specific prevalence of AAT gradually increased in those over 40. The mean serum TSH level in AAT (3.9 uU/ml) was significantly higher than in controls (2.3 uU/ml) matched according to sex and age. Furthermore, there was a significant correlation between the serum TSH levels and the titers of ANA (r=0.35, p 0.01). In four years observation, from 1979 to 1982, 17 cases out of 459 men (3.7%) and 40 cases out of 600 women (6.7%) had been positive for ATA. Furthermore, 13 patients became positive for ATA in this four years survey. In 15 cases, being over 6 uU/ml in serum TSH levels, out of these 70 patients, TRH tests were performed and all cases showed exaggerated rise in TSH. Serum T4 levels in 5 cases with high TSH levels (10 uU/ml) was significantly lower than those in 10 cases with normal TSH levels; however, none of cases with AAT had overt hypothyroidism in four years observation.

1917 EFFECTS OF FINE-NEEDLE ASPIRATION BIOPSY (FNAB) OF THYROID NODULES ON SERUM LEVELS OF THYROGLOBULIN (TG) AND CALCITONIN (Ct). K.Oeff* and A.Franke, Department of Nuclear Medicine, Klinikum Steglitz, Free University of Berlin, D-1000 Berlin 45, F.R.G.

Serum levels of Ct and TG were measured by radioimmunoassay in 139 patients subjected to FNAB of thyroid nodules. A significant, but short-lived increase in the serum levels of Ct 10 min after FNAB was observed. The means ± SD of the concentrations of Ct were 12.2 ± 8.4 pmol/l before and 16.1 ± 8.8 pmol/l after FNAB ($p<0.001$). Means ± SD of serum levels of TG were 67.9 ± 57.9 µg/l before and 132.1 ± 130.8 µg/l 10 min after FNAB ($p<0.001$). Fluids obtained from cystic lesions in 29 patients revealed a higher concentration of Ct (mean ± SD 23.3 ± 9.6 pmol/l) as compared to the serum concentration (mean ± SD 16.1 ± 8.0 pmol/l) in the same patients ($p<0.001$). The average concentration of TG in the cyst fluids of 48 patients was 4000 µg/l (range 51.3 up to 32400 µg/l). The possible mechanism of destruction-induced release of TG and Ct as well as of concentration of Ct and TG in the cyst fluids are discussed with respect to molecular heterogeneity, appearance and disappearance rates of both substances.

1918 SCINTIGRAPHIC IMAGING OF MEDULLARY THYROID CARCINOMA WITH A NEW TUMOR SEEKING AGENT, TECHNETIUM(V)-99m DIMERCAPTOSUCCINIC ACID. H. Ohta*, K. Endo, A. Yokoyama and K. Torizuka, Tamatsu Hospital, Tamatsu-cho Nishi-ku Kobe, Japan and Kyoto University Nuclear Medicine, Sakyo-ku. Kyoto. Japan.

Recently, a very promising tumor seeking agent a Tc(V)-99m dimercaptosuccinic acid (Tc(V)-DMS), has been developed. Tc(V)-DMS was labelled under pH 8 and low $SnCl_2$ concentrations. An equilibrium between a stable form and a dissociated form of anion TcO_4^{3-}, structually analogous to PO_4^{3-}, was postulated from in vitro and in vivo studies. Structual similarity of Tc(V)-DMS (TcO_4^{3-}) with PO_4^{3-} led us to the scintigraphic studies in patients with medullary thyroid carcinoma (MTC), which is known to secret calcitomin and, in some cases accumulate Tc-99m phosphate compoound. Studies were performedin 5 patients with confirmed MTC (3 untreated and 2 treated). Scintigrams were made 60-120 min after i.v. administration of 10 mCi Tc(V)-DMS using a conventional gamma camera. All patients showed intense accumulation of Tc(V)-DMS in the tumor of MTC and its cervical or lung metastasis, and in one case, postoperatively serum calcitonin level continued still high and non-palpable residual tumors of the neck were clearly revealed. Different from Tl-201 chloride or Tc-99m pertechnetate, there was no significant uptake of Tc(V)-DMS in the normal thyroid glands, salivary glands and stomach. In other thyroid malignancies, including 15 patients with papillary or fallicular adenocarcinoma or one patient with thyroid lymphoma or one patient with undifferentiated carcinoma, no significant uptake of Tc(V)-DMS was observed. Although the exact mechanism of Tc(V)-DMS accumulation remains to be elucidated, this accumulation may be specific and Tc(V)-DMS scintigram may be useful in the diagnosis and follow up of MTC.

1919 IMMUNOPRECIPITATION OF TSH-TSH RECEPTOR COMPLEXES. A. Parkes, B. Rees Smith, P. Buckland, C. Rickards, F. Creagh, R. Howells, Endocrine Immunology Unit, Welsh National School of Medicine, Cardiff. U.K.

The possibility that TSH receptor antibodies found in Graves' sera can bind to the receptor at the same time as TSH has been investigated. TSH receptors in guinea pig fat cell membranes were used to avoid interactions involving microsomal and thyroglobulin antibodies. The receptors were solubilised using 1.0 % Lubrol and complexed (in the dark) to 125-I-labelled TSH conjugated to the photo-active cross-linking reagent N-hydroxysuccini - midyl-4-azido benzoate. Covalent cross-linking between hormone and receptor was effected by exposure to U.V. light and the cross-linked complexes separated from aggregates and free TSH by gel filtration. The effectiveness of cross-linking was evident from the inability of unlabelled TSH, Graves' sera, 2M NaCl or 0.1 % SDS to dissociate the complexes. Sera from normal donors, Hashimoto and Graves' patients, were incubated with the cross-linked TSH-TSH receptor complexes and any binding of the patients' IgG to the complexes assessed by addition of anti IgG. In the presence of normal sera ($n = 14$) and Hashimoto sera ($n = 13$) 0.86 ± 0.46 % (mean ± SD) and 0.88 ± 0.59 % respectively of the complex was precipitated. In the case of Graves' sera ($n = 24$) the mean precipitation was slightly higher at 1.7 ± 1.4 %, but not significantly so ($p > 0.05$). 19 of the Graves' sera readily inhibited the binding of labelled TSH to free TSH receptors and low levels of this activity were also detectable in 3 of the Hashimoto sera. Our studies indicate therefore that although Graves' sera contain antibodies which bind to the TSH receptor in such a way as to inhibit TSH binding, they do not appear to contain significant levels of antibodies which can bind to the receptor at the same time as TSH. This suggests that the receptor anti - - bodies are principally directed at a site closely related to the TSH binding site and that a very limited number of autoantigenic sites are involved in the interaction between the TSH receptor and the immune system in Graves' disease.

1920 IS IODINATION THE STOP SIGNAL FOR THE TSH MESSAGE ?

M. Pavlovic-Hournac* and S. Tawadrause - Unité Thyroide, INSERM 78, rue du Général Leclerc - 94270 BICETRE (France).

Protein iodination, which takes place at the apical plasma membranes of thyroid cells, is controlled by TSH via cAMP formation and cAMP-dependent protein kinase activation. The molecular mechanism of this control is, however, not yet well understood. In order to elucidate their role, the correlation between protein kinase and peroxidase activities were studied in purified thyroidal plasma membrane preparations. These preparations contain regularly protein kinase activity, and only occasionally the peroxidase activity, which is in accord with data reported by other authors. In the preparations in which the peroxidase activity was present, the protein kinase activity was significantly inhibited during the process of iodination. In the absence of peroxidase the protein kinases were not affected.

The inhibition of the protein kinase activity is proportionnal to the level of iodination. It was found that peroxidase acts both, on the inhibition of kinase dissociation by cAMP and on the inactivation of the catalytic subunits of already dissociated enzymes.

These results seem indicate that peroxidase and protein kinases cannot be active simultaneously, which suggests that TSH regulation of protein iodination via cAMP does not involve the control of the peroxidase activity itself. This regulation may concern the steps preceding the activation of the peroxidase. However, once triggered, the iodination inhibits the protein kinase activity. It could be speculated therefore, that iodination may represent the stop signal for the TSH message.

1921 AMIODARONE INHIBITS T_4 TO T_3 CONVERSION AND LOWERS αGPD IN RAT LIVER. A.E. Pekary*, A.W. Reed, L. Turner, and J.M. Hershman, VA Wadsworth Medical Center and UCLA Department of Medicine, Los Angeles, Calif.

Amiodarone (A) has been found to decrease serum T_3 by blocking peripheral T_4 5'-deiodinase. This reduction in T_3 levels may contribute to the effectiveness of this drug in moderating cardiac arrhythmias. To further characterize the effect of A on thyroid hormone metabolism and biological action, 125 g male Sprague-Dawley rats were thyroidectomized and then fed 500 μg T_4 or 50 μg T_3 and 500 mg A/kg of powdered diet for 6 to 8 weeks. Hepatic levels of α-glycerophosphate dehydrogenase (αGPD) and malic enzyme (ME) were used as an index of thyroid hormone action at the cellular level. Conversion of T_4 to T_3 was measured in homogenates of liver from T_3-treated rats, mean ± SD.

	(n)	Body wt(g)	TSH(μU/ml)	T_3(ng/dl)	T_4(μg/dl)	αGPD	ME	rT_3(ng/dl)
T_4	(8)	374±37	566±183	28 ± 10	6.2 ±1.8	7.0±1.4	15±8	5.5 ± 2.8
T_4+A	(10)	320±57	625±104	13 ± 4	4.5 ±1.5	4.6±2.3	7±6	7.3 ± 3.2
p		<.05	N.S.	<.001	N.S.	<.05	<.05	N.S.
								$T_4 \rightarrow T_3$
T_3	(9)	494±42	29±80	23 ± 6	0.5 ±0.2	14 ± 7	13±7	2.8 ± 0.6
T_3+A	(10)	486±48	64±74	18 ± 7	0.5 ±0.2	16 ± 4	19±7	1.7 ± 0.9
p		N.S.	N.S.	N.S.	N.S.	N.S.	N.S.	<.01

A usually reduced hepatic αGPD with statistical significance but its effect on ME was less consistent.

Conclusions: A inhibits hepatic T_4 to T_3 conversion resulting in a decreased availability of T_3 in the circulation and at the cellular level, thus reducing hepatic αGPD.

1922 ACCUMULATION OF ANTI-THYROGLOBULIN (Tg) ANTIBODY BY NORMAL THYROID CELLS OF MONOLAYER CULTURE S. Ohtakara*, M. Izumi, H. Hirayu, S. Morita, S. Yamashita, S. Okamoto, S. Nagataki, The First Department of Internal Medicine, Nagasaki University, Nagasaki, Japan

We have previously reported that ^{125}I anti-Tg antibody was accumulated by thyroid carcinoma and adenoma, but not normal thyroid tissue. Similar results were obtained in thyroid tissues transplanted into nude mice. In order to elucidate the difference of the accumulation of ^{125}I anti-Tg antibody between normal tissue and carcinoma or adenoma, the present study was undertaken to investigate whether ^{125}I anti-Tg antibody can be accumulated by normal human thyroid cells of monolayer culture. Normal thyroid tissues were obtained at operation of thyroid adenoma or carcinoma. One ml of 1×10^6 thyroid cells/ml containing 10mIU/ml TSH was cultured in the well of 1.6cm diameter for 6 days changing culture medium every other day. On the last day of culture, after ^{125}I anti-Tg antibody was incubated with the cells for 30min, monolayers were digested with trypsin and the radioactivity of the digestion medium was measured. ^{125}I anti-Tg antibody was clearly accumulated by normal human thyroid cells compared with fiboblasts and this accumulated ^{125}I anti-Tg antibody was significantly displaced by cold Tg and anti-Tg antibody, but not by normal human IgG. When ^{125}I normal human IgG was incubated with both normal human thyroid cells and fiboblasts, ^{125}I normal human IgG was not accumulated significantly by both the cells. These results of the difference between thyroid tissues in vivo and thyroid cells in culture suggest that in order to accumulate ^{125}I anti-Tg antibody, it is essential that Tg is secreted through cell membranes exposed to ^{125}I anti-Tg antibody.

1923 THYROID FUNCTION ASSESSMENT WITH TECHNITIUM- 99m NECK-THIGH RATIO AND THYROID UPTAKE RATIO. A.E. Ohwovoriole*, O.T. Ogunleye and D. Campbell, Departments of Medicine and Radiation Biology and Radiotherapy, Lagos University Teaching Hospital, P.M.B. 12003, Lagos, Nigeria.

Conventional methods of thyroid function assessment include plasma thyroid hormone quantitation and thyroidal radioactive iodine uptake (RAIU). Hormone analysis remains the most reliable method but time required, iodination facilities and production of antibodies are some of the drawbacks. RAIU also has several well known limitations. Technitium uptake has been suggested as an alternative or additional index of thyroid function. This is the report of a study that compared the results of thyroid function using technitium uptake studies and those obtained by hormone analysis and RAIU. The 10'/2' thyroid technitium uptake ratio correlated poorly with the free thyroxine index and failed to distinguish between euthyroidism and hyperthyroidism. The 15min neck-thigh ratio of technitium uptake correlated significantly with the results of the conventional methods and distinguished fairly clearly between hyperthyroidism and euthyroidism. Both the 10'/2' ratio and the 15min neck-thigh ratio were poor discriminants of hypothyroidism. The results of the study suggest that the 15min neck-thigh ratio of technitium uptake in agreement with previous reports, is useful in the thyroid function assessment in the work-up of suspected hyperthyroidism. The method is cheap, fast, safer and more convenient to the patient and deserves clinical application.

1924 AN ENHANCEMENT OF CONCANAVALIN A-INDUCED SUPPRESSOR CELL ACTIVITY BY ANTITHYROID DRUGS(MMI & PTU). N. Okabe*, R. Mori, K. Inoue, K. Okamura, A. Shiroozu, H. Nishitani, M. Yoshinari, T. Tokuyama, K. Sato, H. Ikenoue, T. Nakashima and T. Omae. Department of Virology(N.O. & R.M.) and The Second Department of Internal Medicine, School of Medicine, Kyushu University, Fukuoka 812, and National Sanatorium, Miyazaki-Higashi Hospital (K.I. & H.N.), Miyazaki 880, Japan.

It has been postulated that a primary immunological alteration plays a major role in Graves' disease. There is a hypothesis that defects of suppressor T lymphocytes play a crucial role in the pathogenesis of Graves' disease. A decrease in suppressor cell function in patients with Graves' disease was demonstrated using functional assays for concanavalin A(Con A)-induced suppressor cell activity. However, the abnormalities in suppressor activity was reported to disappear in Graves' patients who became euthyroid on antithyroid drugs.

In the present study, therefore, we attempted to demonstrate whether antithyroid drugs(methimazole:MMI & propylthiouracil: PTU) are capable of enhancing the suppressor cell activity *in vitro* and obtained data that both MMI and PTU had enhancing effects on Con A-induced suppressor activity. In the light of these data, an enhancement in suppressor activity by MMI and PTU may contribute, in part, to a remission of Graves' disease.

1925 HIGH RESOLUTION TWO-DIMENSIONAL ELECTROPHORESIS OF HUMAN THYROGLOBULIN
S. Okamoto*, N.C. Kendrick°, M. Izumi, N. Yokoyama, S. Morita, S.Yamashita, S. Ohtakara, T. Tanabe, and S. Nagataki, The First Department of Internal Medicine, Nagasaki University, Nagasaki 852 Japan, °Kendrick Lab. Madison, Wis. 53713, U.S.A.

Previous Studies in our laboratory have shown the physical properties of thyroglobulin (Tg) in various disease states. Two-dimensional polyacrylamide gel electrophoresis (2-D.E.) is known to be a powerful tool for the analysis of proteins, but its application for Tg is very difficult because 19S Tg is too large a molecule to put into this system. We therefore had to cleave Tg with urea before electrophoresis. Also some modifications were made to the normal O'Farrell 2-D.E. system. The samples were obtained at operation and Tg was purified as previously reported. The samples were then subjected to cleavage with 9.0 molar urea for 14 hours. Modification of the density of acrylamide isoelectric focusing (IEF) tube gel was necessary, because of difficulties to get Tg to enter the gel. Also the fragility of the SDS slab gels used to resolve high molecular weight proteins made them impossible to silver stain and the Tg samples themselves did not stain well. Once these problems had been resolved the procedures became quite easy to use. In this study, three samples of normal thyroid tissue were used. The results are as follows: the Tg from the normal thyroid produced two streaked bands. The molecular weight was about 300,000. Two-dimensional electrophoresis of human thyroglobulin might be useful for the discrimination of the Tg from thyroid tissue in neoplastic and non-neoplastic disease states from normal tissue.

1926 THE RESPONSES OF CIRCULATING CATECHOLAMINES AND THE THYROID AXIS OF NORMAL SUBJECTS TO ACUTE COLD EXPOSURE. B P O'Malley*, N Cook, A Richardson, D B Barnett and F D Rosenthal. University of Leicester, UK

It has been suggested that in cold exposed rats the elevated plasma noradrenaline (NA) levels might contribute to the observed rise in circulating T3 levels via increased peripheral conversion, but TSH levels were not reported (Storm et al, 1981, Acta Endocrinologica, 97, 91). We have investigated the responses of body temperature, circulating catecholamines, TSH and thyroid hormones during 30 minutes of acute cold exposure (4^oC) and a subsequent 90 minutes at room temperature in 8 normal volunteers. Serum TSH levels were measured by a sensitive RIA method (0.3µU/ml), serum T4 and T3 levels by RIA kits and plasma catechols by a HPLC technique. In response to acute cold exposure, mean rectal temperature in the 8 subjects initially rose from 37.15 ± 0.08^oC to 37.31 ± 0.07^oC ($P < 0.01$) during the first 30 minutes, but subsequently fell to 36.76 ± 0.09^oC over the next 90 minutes ($P < 0.005$). During the 2 hour study period, mean serum TSH levels rose from 1.98 ± 0.22µU/ml to 3.25 ± 0.42µU/ml ($P < 0.0005$), and mean plasma NA levels also rose from 2.59 ± 0.41pmol/ml to 5.98 ± 0.76pmol/ml ($P < 0.001$). However, over the same period plasma adrenaline levels were undetectable. Mean serum T4 and T3 levels were also elevated following acute cold exposure, rising from 62.63 ± 5.3nmols/l to 88.5 ± 7.1nmols/l (T4) ($P < 0.01$) and 1.03 ± 0.13nmols/l to 1.37 ± 0.12nmols/l (T3) ($P < 0.001$). There was no significant change in the T4/T3 ratio at any stage of the study. There was a significant positive correlation between the levels of plasma NA and serum TSH levels ($r = 0.71$; $P < 0.01$). Thus on acute cold exposure, a rapid elevation of circulating NA levels accompanied a brisk rise in serum TSH levels, suggesting a possible causal role for NA in the latter.

1927 THE INHIBITORY EFFECTS OF CALMODULIN ANTAGONISTS ON TSH-STIMULATED THYROID HORMONE RELEASE BY MOUSE THYROID LOBES. T. Onaya*, K. Takazawa and T. Endo, The Third Department of Internal Medicine, University of Yamanashi Medical School, Tamaho, Yamanashi-ken 409-38, Japan.

Calcium ions have been shown to play an essential role in the release of various hormones from a wide variety of endocrine organs. More recently, in vitro evidence suggests that a calcium-binding protein, calmodulin, is also involved in the release of insulin from pancreatic islets. So, we studied the effects of several kinds of calmodulin antagonists on TSH-stimulated thyroid hormone release in vitro. Mouse thyroid lobes (one thyro-tracheal unit/tube) were incubated in Krebs-Ringer bicarbonate buffer at 37 C for 4 hours. Free thyroxine (fT_4) released in the incubation medium was measured by radioimmunoassay. TSH (5 mU/ml) and dibutyryl cyclic AMP (DBC) (200 µg/ml) caused two to four-fold increases in thyroidal release of fT_4. The stimulatory effects of TSH on fT_4 release were inhibited by trifluoperazine and prenylamine lactate in a dose-related manner at concentrations from 5×10^{-5}M to 2.5×10^{-4}M. More specific calmodulin antagonists, W-7 and W-13, were also shown to inhibit TSH stimulation of fT_4 release at the concentration of 5×10^{-5}M. In contrast, TSH stimulation of fT_4 release was not depressed by non-specific antagonists, W-5 and W-12, at the same concentration as 5×10^{-5}M. Further, W-13 also markedly inhibited DBC-stimulated fT_4 release at the concentration of 5×10^{-5}M. These results suggest that calmodulin play an important role in TSH-stimulated thyroid hormone release and further that this mechanism exists at the site subsequent to the generation of cyclic AMP.

1928 ANDROGENS AS POSSIBLE ENHANCERS OF THYROID TUMOR INCIDENCE IN RADIATED RATS. R. Oslapas*, C. Hofmann, K. Ernst and E. Paloyan, Dept. of Surg. and Biochem., Loyola Univ. Stritch School of Med., Maywood, IL 60153 and Research Service, Hines VA Hospital, Hines, IL 60141, USA

We have reported that radiation treated male rats had a higher incidence of thyroid tumors than females, and that castration of males prior to radiation treatment markedly reduced this incidence (Surg. 92:839, 1982). Since elevated TSH is a reported requisite for development of radiation-associated thyroid tumors, we examined effects of testosterone (T) on serum TSH levels. In a short term experiment, 20 castrated male Long-Evans rats were s.c. implanted with continuous delivery T pellets (17.5, 175 & 525mg) and were bled weekly for 10 weeks. Serum TSH levels in castrate animals were elevated in the presence of the highest T replacement dose. In another experiment, 15 each of intact, castrate, and castrate male rats treated with T, were radiated with $Na^{131}I$ at 8 weeks and bled at age 6 months. Serum TSH levels were highest in radiated castrated males with T implants (1347±148ng/ml), followed by intact males (1182±157ng/ml) and castrates without T implants (576±65ng/ml). In a long term experiment, a total of 50 each of intact, castrate male, and intact female rats were radiated as above, and thyroid tumor incidence at 24 months was recorded. TSH levels failed to correlate with thyroid tumor incidence, since intact radiated males with 58% tumor incidence had a mean TSH level of 1141±292ng/ ml, whereas female rats with 28% incidence had 2123±387ng/ml TSH. Thus, an indirect effect of T on early stimulation of TSH may be at least partly responsible for higher incidence of radiation-induced thyroid tumors in male rats.

1929 LOW T_3 AND HIGH REVERSE T_3 SERUM CONCENTRATIONS IN SUNCUS MURINUS: AN EXPERIMENTAL MODEL FOR LOW T_3 SYNDROME. Y. Ozawa*, Y. Shishiba, S. Oda and T. Shimizu. Division of Endocrinology, Toranomon Hospital, Tokyo 105 and University of Nagoya, Nagoya 464, Japan.

We had a chance to examine the serum concentrations of thyroid hormones of suncus murinus (house musk shrew), and found that this animal has low T_3 and high rT_3 serum concentrations compared to rat (T_4: 2.82$\pm$1.29 vs 4.00$\pm$1.43 μg/100ml, T_3: 8.2$\pm$2.6 vs 62.6$\pm$22.2 ng/100ml, rT_3: 178.9$\pm$16.6 vs 36.3$\pm$11.3 ng/100ml). We further compared in vitro T_4 outer ring monodeiodinating activities of the liver and kidney of this animal to those of rat. T_3 generation by the incubation of liver and kidney homogenates (30 mg of protein) with T_4 (0.5 μg) for 15 min at 37°C was 0.74$\pm$0.30 ng and non-detectable in suncus murinus, and 6.61$\pm$0.65 and 4.65$\pm$0.69 ng in rat, respectively. Thus, this animal showed low T_3 and high rT_3 serum levels due to the low activities of T_4 outer ring monodeiodination. In this animal and rat, we studied the effects of T_3 by measuring the activities of total ATPase, Na, K-ATPase, α-glycerophosphate dehydrogenase, and malic enzyme in the liver before and after the administration of T_3 (200 μg/100g body weight, sc, every 24 h for 3 days). The responses of those enzyme activities to T_3 were +39%, NS, +12% and +20%, respectively, in suncus murinus, and +50%, +134%, +33% and +250%, respectively, in rat. Those results showed that this low T_3 animal had low response to T_3. In conclusion, above results indicated that suncus murinus presented low T_3 syndrome in terms of 1) serum thyroid hormone profile, 2) mode of deiodinating pathway and 3) enzyme response to exogenous T_3.

1930 PLASMA BETA-ENDORPHIN ACTIVITY DURING THE OXYTOCIN STRESS TEST
P.Riss+, Ch.Bieglmayer, A.Reinthaller, R. Rudelstorfer
2nd Department of Obstetrics and Gynecology, University Hospital, Spitalgasse 23, A-1090 Vienna, Austria

Beta-endorphin activity is increased in maternal plasma during labor, with the highest values seen at the time of delivery. However, it is not clear whether the painful stress of labor or the contractions per se are responsible for the elevation of maternal endorphin peptides. We therefore studied maternal plasma beta-endorphin like immunoreactivity in 20 pregnant women at term with normal or complicated pregnancies (placental insufficiency, postdatism). Blood samples were drawn before, during, and after the oxytocin stress test. Beta-Endorphin activity was determined without prior extraction by means of a radioimmunoassay (New England Nuclear).
Maternal plasma endorphin activity rose significantly during the oxytocin stress test; when oxytocin was discontinued, maternal plasma levels fell again (difference not significant). In view of the presumed inhibitory effect of oxytocin on endorphin release (Genazzani, personal communication) our results would indicate that it is the pain of labor rather than the blood levels of oxytocin which are responsible for the rise in maternal endorphin activity.

1931 MORPHINE INHIBITS THE PITUITARY-ADRENAL RESPONSE TO CORTICOTROPIN RELEASING FACTOR(CRF). R. Rittmaster*, G. Cutler, D. Sobel, M. Koppelman, D. Loriaux and G. Chrousos, Developmental Endocrinology Branch, NICHD,NIH, Bethesda,Md

β-Endorphin suppresses basal plasma ACTH and cortisol concentrations in normal volunteers (JCEM 57:592). This study was designed to determine the locus of negative feedback of opiates on ACTH secretion. Six normal volunteers were given CRF (1 μg/kg) iv at 2000 on each of 2 days. Thirty min before CRF, they received 10 mg of sc morphine sulfate (MS) or placebo. Plasma ACTH and cortisol were measured by radioimmunoassay at 0, 5, 15, 30, 45, 60, 90 and 120 min after CRF administration. MS suppressed plasma ACTH for the first 30 min and cortisol for the first 60 min after CRF.

Plasma ACTH (mean ± SE, pg/ml) after CRF (*P<0.05, paired t test)

Time (min)	0	5	15*	30*	45	60
Placebo	8±2	15±4	26±8	27±7	18±2	22±5
MS	8±2	11±1	10±1	12±2	17±5	20±4

In vitro, rat pituitary cells, dispersed and perifused in columns (Am J Physiol 240:E591), received 2 pulses of 10 nM CRF, 60 min apart. From 30 min before until 30 min after each pulse, the columns were perifused with media containing 1 μg/ml MS or media alone. There was no difference in any aspect of the ACTH peaks in the 2 groups (mean area under curve = 6173±299 for MS and 6074±288 for controls, n=6). Also, in rat pituitary cell monolayer culture (Neuroendocrinol. 36:49), MS, up to 10 μg/ml, had no effect on the amount of ACTH secreted into the media during 3 h incubations with 5nM CRF. We conclude that MS blunts the early response of the pituitary gland to CRF *in vivo*. Based on the lack of an effect of MS on rat pituitary cells *in vitro*, we postulate that morphine given *in vivo* inhibits the pituitary ACTH response to CRF indirectly through a suprapituitary factor(s).

1932 DOPAMINE MEDIATION OF KCl INDUCED INHIBITION OF β ENDORPHIN SECRETION FROM RAT NEUROINTERMEDIATE LOBE.

D.C. Roeger and S.J. Judd*, Departments of Medicine and Clinical Biochemistry, Flinders Medical Centre, Bedford Park, South Australia, 5042.

In vivo studies have shown that Dopamine (DA) inhibits the secretion of β endorphin (βE) from the neurointermediate lobe (NIL) of the rat. Our earlier work indicated that KCl also inhibits rβE secretion in vitro and this prompted investigation into the possibility that KCl inhibition of rβE may be mediated by DA released from tuberohypophysial (THDA) nerve terminals. NILs were dissected from adult male Porton rats and were perfused in groups of 4 with Krebs Ringer bicarbonate (KRB) or KRB containing test substances. Aliquots were collected each minute for 60 - 80 min and were assayed for rβE and DA. DA concentration ([DA]) was measured in NIL tissue at the conclusion of the perfusion. Repeated application of KCl (50 mM over 5 min) produced a consistent (52.4±3.9 %; $p < 0.01$) inhibition of rβE and an increase in perfusate DA of 63 % ($p < 0.05$) and in NIL [DA] from 11.5±0.6 to 17.9±0.8 ng/mg protein ($p < 0.001$). The influence of THDA neurons on NIL was inhibited by 1) prior perfusion of d-butaclamol (10^{-6}M), 2) by pretreatment of rats with 6-hydroxydopamine (6-OHDA), given 30 hours prior to decapitation or 3) by mechanical dispersion of NIL tissue. There was an increase in secretion of rβE after each of these treatments: after d-butaclamol the mean increase (± SEM) was 304±41 % ($p < 0.001$), after 6-OHDA was 142±4 % ($p < 0.001$), and after mechanical dispersion was 247±79 % ($p < 0.001$). We conclude 1) KCl stimulates the release of endogenous DA from THDA nerve terminals in perfused, intact, rat NILs and 2) the inhibition of rβE is dependent on intact connection between THDA neurons and NIL cells. Supp. by Flinders University Research Budget.

1933 PARTIAL PURIFICATION AND CHARACTERIZATION OF THYMORPHIN (TM) 1 AND 2.
A. Rule*, P. Bailey, D. Carr, and H. Miller, Boston College, Chestnut Hill, MA 02167; Massachusetts General Hospital, Boston, MA 02114; and Michigan State University, East Lansing MI 48917, USA.

Anterior pituitary and thymus glands arise from the pharyngeal gut during embryogenesis; pituitary beta-endorphin (B-EP) binds both brain and lymphocyte receptors. We have isolated two previously undescribed thymic factors TM-1 and TM-2 of neonatal calf origin which bind and activate pre T-lymphocytes in vivo and in vitro and have homology with B-EP. Neonatal calf thymus glands obtained using sterile technique were purified by homogenization, centrifugation, acetone extraction, molecular weight and hydrophobic column chromatography, isoelectric focussing and disc gel electrophoresis. Purity of TM-1 and 2 was shown, respectively, by one band on SDS-disc gel. Both TM-1 and 2 induce the theta and Ly-1 differentiation antigens on bone marrow lymphocytes obtained from normal mice or splenic lymphocytes obtained from nude (athymic) mice; reconstitute the immune response in lethally irradiated, thymectomized mice; enhance antibody production to sheep RBC's as demonstrated by plaque forming cells 2-10 times background; and significantly enhance antibody titers in thymectomized adult mice. Both TM-1 and 2 display immunologic identity with B-EP in Ouchterlony gel using antiserum to the carboxy terminus region of B-EP. Both are highly active in B-EP RIA using another antiserum directed at different carboxy terminus sites. Increasing TM purity is directly related to quantitative rises in immunoactive B-EP and biologic (helper) activity, These data suggest a functional role for TM-1 and 2 in thymic-pituitary-adrenal regulation of the immune response.

1934 LARGE MOLECULAR WEIGHT ADRENOCORTICOTROPIN RELATED SUBSTANCES IN A PATIENT WITH ADRENOLEUKOMYELONEUROPATHY (ALMN).
E. Saito* and M. Kinoshita, The Fourth Department of Medicine, School of Medicine, Toho University, Tokyo 153, Japan.

Very high adrenocorticotropin (ACTH) immunoactivity was measured by direct radioimmunoassay in the plasma of a patient with typical adrenoleukomyeloneuropath (ALMN), who showed the normal response to rapid ACTH test. Treatment of 8 mg of dexamethasone at 2100 h did not suppress plasma ACTH level on the next morning. Interestingly, ALMN patients with normal response to rapid ACTH test and very high plasma ACTH levels have occasionally been seen in the literature. Possible artifacts in the radioimmunoassay technique were carefully examined, but ACTH immunoactivity in the patient's plasma does not seem to be the result of artifacts for reasons as following; (1) The slope of dose-response curve of ACTH immunoactivity in the patient's plasma was identical with that of standard ACTH. (2) When ACTH immunoactivity was measured in tubes containing both the patient's plasma and standard ACTH, the total activity was measured in an additive fashion. (3) The addition of trypsin inhibitor did not modify the level of ACTH immunoactivity. (4) Pretreatment of standard ACTH with the patient's plasma did not affect its immunoactivity. (5) Pretreatment of [^{125}I]iodo-ACTH with the patient's plasma did not change its elution profile through Sephadex G50 columns. When the patient's plasma was passed through Sephadex G75 SF column, most of ACTH immunoactivity was eluted in a single peak corresponding to the molecular weight of 55,000 dalton. The present paper strongly suggest the presence of large molecular weight ACTH related substances in the plasma of, at least, some patients with ALMN.

1935 PROENKEPHALIN A DERIVED OPIOID PEPTIDES IN HUMAN GUT. M. Sakamoto*, K. Nakao, T. Yoshimasa, M. Suda, N. Morii, Y. Ikeda, I. Tanaka, S. Oki, K. Takasu, S. Shimbo and H. Imura, 2nd Div. Dept. of Med. Kyoto Univ. Sch. of Med. and Kyoto City Hosp. (K.T., S.S.), Kyoto 606, Japan.

Proenkephalin A contains four copies of methionine-enkephalin (Met-Enk) and one copy each of leucine-enkephalin (Leu-Enk), methionine-enkephalin-Arg^6-Phe^7 (Met-Enk-Arg-Phe) and methionine-enkephalin-Arg^6-Gly^7-Leu^8 (Met-Enk-Arg-Gly-Leu). We previously demonstrated the existence of Met-Enk, Leu-Enk, Met-Enk-Arg-Phe and Met-Enk-Arg-Gly-Leu in the human stomach in a molar ratio similar to a ratio of these peptides contained in proenkephalin A (Sakamoto et al. JCEM 56, 202, 1983.) To elucidate the distribution and tissue localization of these proenkephalin A derived opioid peptides in the human gut, we have examined extracts from various parts of the human gastrointestinal tract. HPLC coupled with the RIAs for these four peptides showed the existence of Met-Enk, Leu-Enk, Met-Enk-Arg-Phe and Met-Enk-Arg-Gly-Leu in the esophagus, stomach, duodenum, jejunum, ileum and colon. The molar ratio of these four opioid peptides in each tissue was similar to the ratio of these peptides contained in proenkephalin A. Gel filtration showed that immunoreactivities of these peptides emerged at the elution position of each synthetic peptide without any detectable high molecular weight forms. In addition, most each of Met-Enk, Leu-Enk, Met-Enk-Arg-Phe and Met-Enk-Arg-Gly-Leu were detected in the muscular layer. These results indicate the wide distribution of Met-Enk, Leu-Enk, Met-Enk-Arg-Phe and Met-Enk-Arg-Gly-Leu in the muscular layer of the human gut and suggest that these peptides are derived from proenkephalin A and that its processing is almost completed in the human gastrointestinal tract.

1936 THE N-TERMINAL FRAGMENT (NTF) OF PRO-OPIOMELANOCORTIN (POMC) -STRUCTURAL AND BIOSYNTHETIC STUDIES - M.A. Seger* and H.P.J. Bennett, Endocrine Laboratory, Royal Victoria Hospital, Montreal, Quebec, Canada, H3A 1A1.

The major forms of NTF have been purified from mouse and rat pituitary neurointermediate lobes (NILs) by reversed-phase HPLC. They have been found to be NTF_{1-74}, NTF_{1-49} and $Lys^1\gamma_3MSH$ (i.e. NTF_{50-74}). The yields of each form indicate that 30-50% of NTF_{1-74} is processed to form NTF_{1-49} and $Lys^1\ \gamma_3MSH$. NTF_{1-74} was found in multiple forms, all of which contained glucosamine (up to 3 moles per mole peptide). This represents N-glycosylation at Asn 65. About 50% of NTF_{1-74} contained galactosamine (up to 1 mole per mole peptide). This represents O-glycosylation at Thr^{45}. NTF_{1-49} contained no amino-sugars. $Lys^1\gamma_3MSH$ contained only glucosamine (up to 3 moles per mole of peptide). We have used pulse/chase biosynthetic experiments to show that the partial conversion of NTF_{1-74} to NTF_{1-49} and $Lys^1\gamma_3MSH$ takes place between 2 and 4 hours after the initial synthesis of POMC. This suggests that the conversion is taking place within the secretory granule fraction. We have incorporated ^3H-galactose into both N-and O-glycosylation sites of NTF_{1-74} and into the single N-glycosylation site within $Lys^1\gamma_3MSH$. As expected we failed to incorporate ^3H-galactose into NTF_{1-49}. The observed absence of the O-glycosylation of NTF_{1-49} suggests that the carbohydrate group is removed during the formation of this peptide from NTF_{1-74}. Alternatively the O-glycosylation site at Thr_{45} may mask the cleavage site at $Arg_{49}Lys_{50}$ and this could be an important mechanism in the control of NTF_{1-49} and $Lys^1\gamma_3MSH$ biosynthesis by the intermediate lobe of the pituitary.
This study was supported by the MRC and FRSQ.

1937 SECRETION OF PEPTIDES DERIVED FROM PRO-OPIOMELANOCORTIN IN PATIENTS WITH CUSHING'S DISEASE AND ADDISON'S DISEASE. K. Sekiya*, H. Nawata, K. Kato, H. Ibayashi, T. Motomatsu & H. Takahashi, Third Department of Internal Medicine, Faculty of Medicine, Kyushu University, Fukuoka 812, Japan. Medical Institute of Bioregulation, Kyushu University, Oita 874, Japan.

To evaluate the secretion patterns of pro-opiomelanocortin (POMC)-derived peptides from pituitary, plasma ACTH, β-LPH, β-endorphin (β-Ep) and N-terminal (N-t) were measured at every 3 hour and after ovine CRF stimulation in 22 normal subjects, 17 patients with Cushing's disease (C-d.) and 12 patients with Addison's disease (A-d.). In normal subjects, mean basal ACTH level (09:00) was 81.0 ± 14.6 (SE) pg/ml and molar ratios of β-LPH, β-Ep and N-t to ACTH in plasma were 1.15 ± 0.18, 0.3 ± 0.05 and 1.24 ± 0.37, respectively. In C-d., ACTH level was 96.1 ± 9.1 pg/ml and its molar ratios of β-LPH, β-Ep and N-t to ACTH were 1.95 ± 0.37, 0.65 ± 0.1 and 1.73 ± 0.35, respectively. The molar ratio of β-LPH/ACTH was less than 1 in three patients of C-d. whose pituitary adenomas located at the inter-mediate lobe and was more than 1 in other three patients of C-d. whose pituitary adenomas located at the anterior lobe. In A-d., ACTH level was 525.6 ± 117.8 pg/ml and its molar ratios of β-LPH, β-Ep and N-t to ACTH were 4.0 ± 0.48, 0.43 ± 0.08, 1.26 ± 0.19, respectively. In C-d., these peptides did not show diurnal rhythm, while in A-d. and normal subjects the diurnal rhythm was observed and the molar ratio of β-LPH/ACTH showed significant diurnal variations. After CRF stimulation, all the peptides studied were secreted in the same molar ratio to that in the basal conditions in normal subjects, C-d. and A-d.

1938 IN VIVO DEMONSTRATION OF EXOCRINE PANCREAS AS A TARGET TISSUE FOR CORTICOTROPIN (ACTH). R. Sikstrom*, C. Linard, M. Cantin, N. Seidah and M. Chrétien, Clinical Research Institute of Montreal, H2W 1R7, Canada.

An in vivo morphological method previously used to show binding of peptide hormones (J. Histochem. Cytochem., 1980 28:824) was adapted to screen tissues for ACTH binding sites. ^{125}I-ACTH (160 × 10^6 CPM/0.1ml) was injected, in the absence (experimental) or presence (control) of 50μg of unlabeled ACTH, into the jugular vein of an anesthetized 80g rat. 3.5 minutes later whole body intracardiac perfusion was performed successively with lactated Ringer's buffer and glutaraldehyde (2.5% in 0.05M Phosphate buffer pH 7.4) and followed by conventional processing of the pancreata for quantitative radioautography. To verify the authenticity of the injected hormone to bind to ACTH receptors the adrenals from these rats were also processed. Adrenal tissue from experimental animals showed a high retention of ^{125}I-label (7300 CPM/mg) which was largely displaced in the control (803 CPM/mg) suggesting that true ACTH receptors were binding the injected hormone specifically. The pancreas overall also showed high radioactivity (4550 CPM/mg) in the experimental compared to the value (791 CPM/mg) in the control. When the experimental pancreas tissue was processed for radioautography a high density of silver grains (10.7 grains/frame) was found overlying acinar cells while the islets of Langerhans showed much lower levels (1.2 grains/frame) comparable to the control (2.0 grains/frame). We conclude that the exocrine pancreas has a high density of binding sites and probably represents a previously unreported target tissue for ACTH action. This study was supported by the MRC and NIH.

1939 INTRACELLULAR MODULATION OF CHOLESTEROL METABOLISM BY APOPROTEINS IN RAT ADRENAL GLANDS.

T. Nishikawa*, K. Mikami, Y. Saito, Y. Tamura and S. Yoshida, The 2nd Department of Internal Medicine, School of Medicine, Chiba University, Chiba 280, Japan.

It is well known that lipoproteins are used for adrenal steroid biosynthesis, although the function of apoproteins is still unknown. We therefore examined the effect of apoproteins on cholesterol esterase (CEase) and cholesterol lyase in the rat adrenal in order to clarify the intracellular regulation of cholesterol metabolism. A substrate containing only cholesteryl oleate and apo-HDL increased CEase activity. CEase activity was also increased by a substrate containing apo-HDL plus cholesteryl oleate and phosphatidylcholine more than by a substrate containing cholesteryl oleate plus apo-LDL or BSA and phosphatidylcholine, suggesting that apo-HDL as part of the substrate for CEase may play a crucial role in regulation of CEase. However, substrate mixtures containing cholesterol plus apo-HDL or apo-LDL produced great enhancement in cholesterol lyase activity, indicating that both apo-HDL and apo-LDL may modify the substrate state for the cholesterol lyase reaction. The present study has demonstrated that plasma lipoproteins not only provide cholesterol for adrenal steroidogenesis, but also that the intracellular apoproteins may regulate both CEase and cholesterol lyase. Thus, lipoproteins and apoproteins have two functions dealing with steroidogenesis: (1) carrier of cholesterol as a substrate for steroidogenesis and (2) regulator of cholesterol metabolism in adrenals.

1940 THE ACTIVITY OF ENZYMES INVOLVED IN STEROIDOGENESIS AND CHOLESTEROL METABOLISM IN THE OUTER AND INNER ZONES OF THE GUINEA PIG ADRENAL CORTEX.

T. Nishikawa* and C. A. Strott, NIH, Bethesda, MD 20205, U.S.A. and Chiba University School of Medicine, Chiba City 280, Japan.

We have used the guinea pig as an animal model to examine the steroidogenic activity of the zona reticularis. The guinea pig adrenal cortex is composed of a brown inner zone (reticularis) and a yellow outer zone (fasciculata/glomerulosa). We have previously reported that steroid production for the zona reticularis is low and that there is little or no response to ACTH or cAMP. In order to investigate this finding in more detail, we have examined the activity of various enzymes involved in steroidogenesis as well as cholesterol metabolism. The activity of 3β-hydroxysteroid dehydrogenase (3βHSD) (disappearance of NAD) was significantly lower in the inner zone while the activity of 17-hydroxylase (^3H_2O formation from [17α-^{3}H]-pregnenolone) was essentially the same for the two zones. The activity of 11-β hydroxylase (cortisol formation from 11-desoxycortisol) was significantly higher in the inner zone. Optimum activity for cholesterol ester hydrolase (CEHase) was found at pH 4.5 and 7.5 in the outer zone, while there was no apparent activity at pH 7.5 in the inner zone, suggesting that a defect in neutral CEHase exists in the inner zone. In addition, basal activities of ACAT and acyl CoA synthetase were significantly lower in the inner zone. In conclusion, these results suggest that the low steroid production and poor response to ACTH and cAMP by the zona reticularis in this animal model may be due in part to alterations in cholesterol metabolism leading to an impairment in the supply of cholesterol for steroidogenesis as well as reduction in 3βHSD activity.

1941 CHOLESTEROL CONCENTRATION AND SIDE-CHAIN CLEAVAGE ACTIVITY IN MITOCHONDRIA ISOLATED FROM THE OUTER AND INNER ZONES OF THE GUINEA PIG ADRENAL CORTEX.

T. Obara* and C. A. Strott, NIH, Bethesda, MD 20205, U.S.A.

The physiological role of the zona reticularis of the adrenal cortex is not well understood. We have used the guinea pig as an animal model: the adrenal cortex is composed of a brown inner zone (reticularis) and a yellow outer zone (fasciculata/glomerulosa). We have previously reported that, in contrast to cells isolated from the outer zone, cells isolated from the reticularis have a low basal production of steroids (cortisol, progesterone, etc.) and that there is little or no steroid response to either ACTH or cAMP. In order to investigate this finding in more detail, mitochondria were isolated from the two zones and examined for cholesterol content and side-chain cleavage (SCC) activity. SCC activity using endogenous substrate was approximately 3 times higher in mitochondria isolated from the outer zone. The concentration of total and free cholesterol was markedly reduced ($p<.001$) in the inner zone. When cholesterol was added to mitochondrial incubations, there was no essential change in SCC activity for either zone. When 25-OH cholesterol was added, there was an increase in SCC activity at late time points for both zones, but the essential difference in activity between the two zones remained the same. Ether-induced stress increased SCC activity ($p<.005$) in the outer zone but not the inner zone. Acute dexamethasone suppression had no effect. In summary, the concentration of cholesterol is markedly reduced in the zona reticularis as is cholesterol SCC activity. This results in little or no steroid production both basally and in response to ACTH. The exact basis for the low cholesterol content is the subject of ongoing studies.

1942 **ADRENAL GLOMERULOSA AND FASCICULATA RESPONSE TO LOW DOSE GRADED ACTH IN DSH**

S.E. Oberfield,* L.S. Levine, E. Stoner, S. Pang, M.I. New, The New York Hospital-Cornell Medical Center, New York 10021, USA.

The regulation of aldosterone (aldo) secretion in dexamethasone suppressible hyperaldosteronism (DSH) is not clearly understood. We previously demonstrated that the aldo response in these patients to a 6-hour ACTH infusion (cortrosyn, $ACTH^{1-24}$, 0.4 mg) is increased. We have proposed that aldo may be a product of the adrenal fasciculata, as ACTH or another pituitary peptide appears to be the predominant stimulus for aldo release. To further evaluate the sensitivity of adrenal steroids to low dose ACTH in DSH, cortrosyn was infused in 9 patients with DSH on a regular Na diet at increasing rates of 1.6-400 mIU/30 min in the supine position. For comparison, 3 normotensive (NT) and 3 hypertensive (HT) patients were also studied. 3 of the 9 DSH patients were receiving glucocorticoid therapy at the time of the infusion. The data for aldo ($\bar{X}$ ± SD) are presented below.

ACTH dose (mIU/30 min)	DSH (no Rx)	DSH (Rx)	HT	NT
0	15.6±17.0	15.0±19.2	6.0±3.6	8.8±9.4
50	68.5±38.7	65.4±19.0	7.8±6.6	13.1±5.8
100	82.8±38.4	82.7±23.3	12.4±10.9	16.4±5.6
200	96.0±35.8	91.2±32.1	34.6±35.2	15.0±8.3
400	102.4±35.5	81.6±38.1	14.5±5.2	18.1±7.5

No difference was demonstrated in the threshold of adrenal steroid responses between any groups (not shown). However, the response of aldo to ACTH in DSH patients was markedly increased and statistically significantly different by the 50 mIU/30 min dose. The responses of DOC, B, and F (not tabulated) did not differ. The aldo/F ratio was greater in the DSH patients. In DSH, the increased sensitivity of aldo to ACTH even at very low doses may explain the biochemical response to treatment with physiologic doses of glucocorticoids.

1943 EFFECTS OF O,P´-DDD, TRILOSTANE, METYRAPONE, CYANOKETONE AND SOLDACTONE ON ADRENAL STEROID SYNTHESIS. M. Ojima*, M. Saito and S. Fukuchi, The Third Department of Internal Medicine, Fukushima Medical College, Fukushima, Japan.

Effects of o,p´-DDD, trilostane, metyrapone, cyanoketone and soldactone on adrenal 11ß-hydroxylase(OHlase), 18-OHlase and 3ß-hydroxysteroid dehydrogenase(HSD) were examined in vitro using mitochondrial and microsomal fractions prepared by standard centrifugation procedures from the homogenate of bovine adrenal corteces. All these 5 drugs inhibited 3ß-HSD, 11ß-OHlase and 18-OHlase activity in vitro. Concentrations of the drugs inhibiting enzymes are shown in a Table.

Enzymes	Concentrations of drugs (M)				
	o,p´-DDD	Trilostane	Cyanoketone	Metyrapone	Soldactone
3ß-HSD	$3x10^{-3}$	10^{-7}	10^{-5}	10^{-2}	10^{-5}
11ß-OHlase	10^{-6}	10^{-5}	$3x10^{-3}$	10^{-5}	10^{-4}
18-OHlase	10^{-4}	$3x10^{-5}$	10^{-4}	10^{-7}	10^{-3}

The inhibition of o,p´-DDD, trilostane, cyanoketone and metyrapone were diminished by an addition of 0.25 - 1.0 mM of cofactor (NADPH or NAD). The results indicate that these 4 drugs may reduce NADPH or NAD utilization, resulting in the inhibition of steroidogenesis. However, the inhibitory effects of soldactone were not improved by cofactor, which suggest the difference of mechanism between this drug and above 4 inhibitors.

1944 HIGH PERFORMANCE LIQUID CHROMATOGRAPHY (HPLC) AND RADIOIMMUNOASSAY (RIA) FOR SIMULTANEOUS MEASUREMENT OF DEOXYCORTICOSTERONE (DOC), 18-OH-DOC, CORTICOSTERONE (B) AND 18-OH-B. G.Opocher, N.Sonino*, G.Carpenè, F.Pedini and F.Mantero, Institute of Semeiotica Medica, University of Padova, Italy.

The measurement of DOC,18-OH-DOC,B,18-OH-B allows a better evaluation of the separate function of adrenal zona glomerulosa and fasciculata, enzyme deficiency,adrenal tumors and some forms of hypertension. However the assays of these steroids are available only in a few laboratories because of the complex pre-RIA separation required. Aim of the study has been to set up an HPLC-RIA system for simultaneous measurement of plasma DOC,18-OH-DOC,B,18--OH-B. Method: 2-4 ml of plasma extracted by dichloromethane were processed by reverse phase HPLC: on the elution fraction of DOC,18-OH-DOC,B,18-OH-B RIA were performed by antisera of good specificity. Results: by a 46 min acetonitrile/water gradient program a mixture of 18-OH-B,aldo,F,18-OH-DOC,B S,DOC,testosterone,17-OH-progesterone was separated. The between peak interval was at least 1 min; retention times showed mean V.C. of 1.9%. The recovery was 70-80% and blancks undetectable. Results from normal subjects were in agreement with the literature. The automatic processing allowed the separation of 7 samples every 10 h. Conclusion: a combined HPLC-RIA method with high specificity for the simultaneous measurement of DOC,18-OH-DOC,B, 18-OH-B has been set up. By quick performance and automation it shows advantages compared to the methods so far employed.

1945 ADRENAL ANDROGEN 19-DESMOLASE AND 19-HYDROXYLASE. Y. Osawa* and C. Yarborough, Endo. Biochem. Dept., Medical Fndn. of Buffalo, NY 14203 USA

We recently discovered a non-aromatizing androgen 19-desmolase to produce 19-norandrogen and the involvement of 19-hydroxyandrogen in the pathway (Endocrinology, 112S Abs.664, 1983). We assessed the localization of the 19-hydroxylase activity in the dog adrenal and studied the 19-aldehyde formation from [^{14}C]androstenedione(A) in a microsomal incubation with NADPH. Standard [^{3}H]-19-hydroxy-A(19-OHA) or [^{3}H]-3,17-dioxo-4-androstene-19-al(19-OXOA) was added at the end of [^{14}C]A incubation and the product was purified to a constant $^{3}H/^{14}C$ ratio through TLC's, acetylation, and countercurrent distribution. Dissected zona reticularis showed a 3.5-fold higher specific activity of 19-OHA formation (9.0pmol/min/mg protein) than zona fasciculata plus glomerulosa and it was also 1.3 times higher than that of the total slice of the adrenal cortex. On sedimentation of the tissue homogenate the majority of 19-hydroxylase activity (78%) was found to belong to the 12,000xg supernatant fraction with minor activity in the 1,200xg pellet (7%) and the mitochondria (15%) fractions. Due to its instability the aldehyde was reduced with $NaBH_4$ immediately after its separation from [^{14}C]-19-OHA by TLC. The aldehyde was thus converted to 19-OHA in a high yield and rigorously purified. Specific activity of the microsomal 19-OXOA formation was 0.5pmol/min/mg. The results indicate that androgen 19-hydroxylase predominately resides in zona reticularis and belongs to the 12,000xg non-sedimental fraction. The 19-aldehyde formation suggests that the first two steps of the 19-desmolation may be identical with those of estrogen biosynthesis and the difference may reside in the third step. Supported by DHHS HD18492 and RR05716.

1946 EVIDENCE OF PANADRENOCORTICAL ADAPTATION TO SEVERE ILLNESS.
Lawrence N. Parker*, Ellis R. Levin, Eric T. Lifrak, U. of California, Irvine - VA Medical Center, Long Beach, California, USA.

During serious illness, there are characteristic increases in serum cortisol concentrations and urinary cortisol excretion. In the present studies we investigated these changes in glucocorticoid metabolism in relation to adrenal androgen metabolism as measured by RIA of cortisol, dehydroepiandrosterone (DHA) and DHA sulfate (DHAS). A group of seriously ill (SI) men were compared with an age-matched control group and the following changes were noted in the SI group: (1) basal serum cortisol concentrations were elevated, (2) basal serum DHA and DHAS concentrations tended to be lower, (3) basal serum DHA/cortisol and DHAS/cortisol ratios were markedly decreased, (4) ACTH-stimulated serum cortisol concentrations increased by the same absolute amount in both groups, whereas the increase in stimulated DHA concentration was 57.2% less in the SI group, and (5) basal urinary unconjugated DHA/cortisol ratios were 63.6% lower reflecting a combination of decreased excretion of DHA and increased excretion of cortisol.

Recently, Zipser et al (JCEM 53:867, 1981) described the entity of Hyperreninemic Hypoaldosteronism in the SI, which is a syndrome with normal cortisol dynamics. Their findings combined with our own indicate a relative shift in the metabolism of adrenal pregnenolone in the SI towards glucocorticoids and away from mineralocorticoids and adrenal androgens. The etiology of this dissociation is unknown. We speculate that this shift of relative biochemical pathway predominance may be a factor necessary for survival of chronic severe stress.

1947 THE EFFECTS OF EXOGENOUS CORTISONE (E) ON THE INTERCONVERSION OF CORTISOL (F) AND E IN THE BABOON. Gerald J. Pepe* and Eugene D. Albrecht. Department Physiology, Eastern Virginia Medical School, Norfolk, VA and Department OB/GYN, University of Maryland School of Medicine, Baltimore, MD USA

In the fetus, the conversion of F to E (80%) exceeds the reverse reaction (15%). Since the fetus is exposed to high quantities of E throughout most of pregnancy, we determined whether F-E interconversion is altered following acute changes in serum E. Adult female baboons (N=3) were sedated with ketamine, constantly infused for 180 min via an antecubital vein with 15 μCi[^{14}C]F and 20 μCi[^{3}H]E, and saphenous vein blood samples obtained at 70, 80 and 90 min. At 90 min, an infusion of E (166 μg/min) was initiated and blood samples obtained at 160-180 min. This protocol was repeated in the same animals treated 24 and 3 h prior to infusion with 3 mg betamethasone (Beta). Metabolic clearance (MCR), transfer constants (%) and serum levels (μg/dl) of F and E were determined. Results ($\bar{x}$±SE):

Treatment	MCR-F	MCR-E	%E to F	%F to E	F	E
None	250±16	562±29	55±7	66±5	31±4	8±1
None+E	237±7	704±56	62±5	60±6	54±7	21±2
Beta	171±15	271±61	76±5	66±9	4±2	1±0
Beta+E	199±7	369±80	70±4	45±6	41±6	34±8

E increased (P<0.05; paired "t") MCR-E and serum F and E levels in control and Beta-treated baboons. E also decreased %F to E in Beta but not control animals. These findings suggest that acute changes in serum E alter MCR-E, do not influence the conversion of E to F and may decrease the conversion of F→E. Therefore, we suggest that the high conversion of F to E in the fetus is probably not the result of the elevated E concentrations in fetal blood. Supported by NIH HD13294.

1948 IMMUNOCHEMICAL CHARACTERIZATION OF HCG-LIKE SUBSTANCE IN MENOPAUSAL WOMEN'S URINE. S.J. Silverberg*, E.G. Armstrong, J.P. Schlatterer, and R.E. Canfield, Departments of Medicine and Pathology, College of Physicians and Surgeons of Columbia University, New York, NY 10032.

An hCG-like substance has been detected in the urine of normal nonpregnant individuals utilizing highly sensitive and specific immunoradiometric assays (IRMA). The assays use solid phase coupled monoclonal antibodies to either the hCGβ or α subunit for extraction of hormone from urine, and a purified, radiolabeled antiserum to the unique COOH-terminal peptide region of the β subunit (βCTP) for quantification of the extracted hCG. The monoclonal antibody to the β subunit (B101) binds highly purified free β subunit 13% as efficiently as dimeric hCG, whereas the monoclonal antibody to hCGα (A102) exhibits negligible binding of free β subunit. While only a minority of normal male and nonpregnant females of reproductive age had detectable levels of hCG immunoreactivity, all twenty normal menopausal females studied had significantly elevated levels (mean = 0.123 ng hCG/mg creatinine). Dilution curves of a commercial preparation of postmenopausal women's urinary gonadotropins (Pergonal), and immunoaffinity purified material from a menopausal woman's urine, were parallel to the hCG standard curve in the IRMA utilizing B101. Parallel analyses of six menopausal women's urine by the IRMA's utilizing B101 and A102 indicated that a large proportion of the immunoreactive substance contained both α subunit and βCTP epitopes. In conclusion, a substance which possesses the immunodeterminants for monoclonal antibodies to the hCG α and β subunits, as well as an antiserum to βCTP has been identified in menopausal women's urine. This substance is likely to be, at least in part, dimeric hCG.

1949 SPONTANEOUS TAIL SKIN TEMPERATURE SURGES IN AGING FEMALE RATS: DEPENDENCE ON REPRODUCTIVE STATE AND AMBIENT TEMPERATURE. J.W. Simpkins*and M.J. Katovich. College of Pharmacy, University of Florida, Gainesville, FL 32610.

We have recently observed spontaneous tail skin temperature (TST) surges in old anestrous and constant estrous (CE) rats, but not in old repeatedly pseudopregnant (PP) or young normally cycling (NC) rats. In the present study, we evaluated a larger population of aging Long-Evans female rats for the incidence and characteristics of these tail skin flushes. Young (5-7 months) and old (19-29 months) rats were placed in an environmentally controlled room with ambient temperatures maintained at 24-25°C or 29-30°C and TST were monitored by means of a surface thermistor every 5 min for a 2 hour period. While in young NC and old PP rats the incidence of flushing was low at 24-25°C (8 to 17%) and at 29-30°C (28-33%), old CE rats exhibited a flushing incidence of 21% and 74% at 24-25°C and 29-30°C, respectively. The observed flushing episodes did not differ among groups with respect to their onset (16.4±1.5 min) duration (24.6±1.5 min) or amplitude (1.5 to 2.0°C). However at both low and high ambient temperatures, the frequency of flushes were significantly greater in old CE rats than in young NC or old PP animals. Collectively, these data indicate (i) that reproductive status, rather than age per se is an important determinant of the propensity for TST instability, (ii) that increasing ambient temperature increase the frequency but not other parameters of flushes and (iii) that the spontaneous TST surges in old CE rats are similar in several respects to the hot flushes observed in menopausal women. (Supported in part by NIH Grants AG02021 and HD18133).

1950 HYPOTHALAMIC NEUROTRANSMITTER CONTENT AND *IN VITRO* LHRH RELEASE IN AGING MALE F344 RATS. R.W. Steger*, L. DePaolo, A. Johns and A. Shepherd, Dept. of Obstetrics and Gynecology, Physiology, and Clinical Pharmacology, Univ. of Texas Health Science Center at San Antonio, TX 78284, USA.

In order to elucidate possible mechanisms accounting for age-related reductions of serum LH and testosterone (T) levels in male F344 rats, we measured hypothalamic norepinephrine (NE), dopamine (DA), serotonin (5-HT) and 5-hydroxy indole acetic acid (5-HIAA) content and *in vitro* median eminence LHRH release in 4-, 11-, 18- and 27-month-old rats. Serum LH, T and prolactin levels declined progressively and significantly between 11 and 27 months. During the same time period, hypothalamic NE and DA levels were significantly decreased and 5-HT and 5-HIAA levels increased significantly. However, the 5-HT/5-HIAA ratio was unchanged, suggesting that 5-HT turnover remained constant. Basal LHRH release also increased significantly with age and, although the percent increase in LHRH release after stimulation with 60 mM NE tended to decrease with age, this decrease was not significant. The *in vitro* pituitary response to LHRH (10^{-8}M) stmulation was likewise unaffected by advancing age. Thus, it appears that changes in serum LH levels in aging male F344 rats are due to changes in hypothalamic neurotransmitter metabolism rather than to the inability of LHRH neurons to respond to noradrenergic stimulation or pituitary gonadotropes to respond to LHRH stimulation.

1951 TESTOSTERONE, LH, FSH, PROLACTIN AND SPERM IN AGING HEALTHY MEN. P.D. Tsitouras* and T.C. Hagen. Dept. of Medicine, Medical College of WI and Wood VA Med. Ctr., Milwaukee, WI, Dept. of Medicine, NY Medical College, Valhalla, NY and Coler Hosp., Roosevelt Isl., NY, USA.

We have reported that PM serum testosterone (T) does not decline, but LH and FSH increase with age in healthy upper-middle class men from Baltimore (BL). AM T was reported to be diminished or unaltered with age. In a small number of healthy men AM but not PM T was reported to decline with age. To further clarify the issue we studied 63, 21-85 yr. old, lower-middle class, laborers or farmers from Wisconsin (W), screened for health as in BL. T, LH, FSH and prolactin (PRL) were determined in 4 samples drawn from 8-9 AM and 4 from 2-3 PM. Many also gave a sperm sample. Results were analyzed by linear regression and t-test (young, 21-40, n=22, vs. old, 61+, n=24). We found a significant correlation between age and AM T (r=-.68, p<.001) or PM T (r=-.61, p< .001). AM T was higher in young, 743±42 ng/dl ($\bar{x}$±SE), than old, 430±21 (p<.001), as was PM T, 595±45 vs. 354±15 (p<.001). Nonetheless, all but one old had T within the normal range. FSH increased with age, AM: r=.42, p<.001; PM: r=.33, p<.05. LH and PRL did not change with age. Sperm concentration did not change, but older men have lower ejaculate volume (p<.005), motility (p<.001) and more abnormal spermatozoa (p<.001). T in W young was 55% higher than BL young, while T in W old was 25% lower than BL old. The data from the present population indicate that both AM and PM T levels decline with age. LH and PRL do not change. The FSH increase observed is associated with an age-related spermatogenic defect. Factors other than health, i.e. socioeconomic or sampling variables (BL men were hospitalized) may also determine whether observed serum T declines with age.

1952 HORMONAL AND HEMODYNAMIC EFFECTS OF GRADED CALCITONIN INFUSIONS IN HYPERTENSIVE MAN. L.M. Resnick, F.B. Müller, J.P. Nicholson, J.H. Laragh, Cardiovascular Center, Cornell Univ. Medical Center, New York, N.Y., USA

To further investigate previous reports of deviations in serum levels of calcium regulating hormones in essential hypertension (EH) (Resnick & Laragh, 1984), we assessed hemodynamic, metabolic and hormonal responses to graded i.v. bolus infusions of salmon calcitonin (sCT, 10^{-3}-10 U.) in 15 supine, fasting EH inpatients in metabolic balance. sCT caused a dose-dependent increase in peripheral forearm blood flow (FAF) concurrently with a suppression of both plasma renin activity (PRA) and aldosterone(PA). Serum ionized calcium (Ca^{++}) fell significantly only with maximal doses. The results indicated (mean±S.E.M.):

	Ca^{++} (mEq/L)	PRA (ng/ml/h)	PA (ng%)	FAF (ml/min/100 ml)
Control	2.40	4.27	18.0	3.37
	±0.03	±1.08	± 3.8	±0.45
10^{-3} U.	2.36	3.48	12.2*	3.68*
	±0.03	±0.88	± 2.8	±0.38
10^{-1} U.	2.31*	3.22*	10.8 ***	4.92**
	±0.03	±0.85	± 2.7	±0.84

*p<0.05, **p<0.01, ***p<0.005 vs. control (Wilcoxon)

Calculated TPR fell 17% (10^{-3} U., p<0.05) and 42% (10^{-1} U., p<0.005).

We conclude: 1) calcitonin has vasoactive properties in hypertensive man, 2) calcitonin also suppresses both PRA and PA, but PA to a greater extent. These results raise the possibility that endogenous CT may modify peripheral vasoconstrictor tone as well as the activity of the renin-aldosterone system in essential hypertension.

1953 THE NATURAL HISTORY OF SALT-WASTING DISORDERS OF ADRENAL AND RENAL ORIGIN.

Ariel Rösler*, Endocrinology and Metabolism, Hebrew University-Hadassah Medical Center, Jerusalem, Israel.

21 patients with hypoaldosteronism due to type 2 corticosterone methyl-oxidase defect(HA) and 7 with pseudohypoaldosteronism(PHA), studied during extended periods of life, showed with age a spontaneous and progressive normalization of Na^+ balance. The clinical severity varied from acute salt-wasting crisis in infancy and short stature in childhood, to an asymptomatic state in adults detectable only by biochemical methods. Infants with HA had high plasma renin activity(PRA;70-650 ng-AI/ml/hr) which decreased with age, and became normal in adults. Cortisol followed a similar pattern, but marked elevations of deoxycorticosterone(DOC;28-550 ng/dl) and 18-OH-corticosterone(18-OHB;650-6500 ng/dl) relative to aldosterone(A;3-29 ng/dl) persisted throughout life in all untreated patients. The 18-OHB/A ratio, normally 6.2±3.5, ranged between 160-760. Patients with PHA had PRA(70-685 ng-AI/ml/hr); DOC(56-1201 ng/dl); 18-OHB(650-6800 ng/dl) and A (150-2000 ng/dl) which remained all very elevated, but kept a normal 18-OHB/A ratio (6.9±5.1) PRA, DOC and 18-OHB correlated significantly with each other during all variations in Na^+ balance. Na^+ repletion partially suppressed these parameters, but total normalization could only be achieved in HA, when a mineralocorticoid was added. IV angiotensin II and K^+ increased DOC and 18-OHB but dexamethasone failed to suppress them, indicating that these steroids originated from the glomerulosa zone. Normalization of Na^+ balance is not due to differences in steroid secretion with age since the basic abnormalities remain unchanged. Improvement in renal responsiveness, a major compensatory mechanism in PHA, is also operative in HA.

1954 ALTERATION OF ALDOSTERONE SECRETION IN CHRONIC RENAL FAILURE(CRF)DUE TO A DERANGED TONIC DOPAMINERGIC INHIBITION. RECOVERY AFTER RENAL TRANSPLANTATION(Tx).

L.Ruilope, R.Garcia-Robles,* J.Parada, C.Prieto, J.Nieto, J.Sancho, and J.L.Rodicio. 1º de Octubre & Ramón y Cajal Hospitals & Dept.Exptl.Endocrinol. University Complutense, Madrid. Spain.

It is well known the existence of an increased aldosterone secretion in CRF.We invesigated the role of the tonic dopaminergic inhibition of A secretion in CRF.A group of 16 normotensive patients in hemodialysis program(HP),8 Tx and 5 normotensive volunteers(NV)were studied.In a first step PRA and plasma A(PA) were measured both basal and after sodium depletion induced by isolated ultrafiltration (15 ml/kg/1h)in HP and by furosemide (80 mg.orally) in Tx and NV.In HP the basal values of PA were higher($p < 0.05$)and those of PRA lower($p<0.05$) than in Tx and NV, but both parameters were closely correlated($r=0.627$; $p<0.01$).In a second step the response of PRA, PA, plasma potassium, cortisol and prolactin(PRL) to metoclopramide (10 mg iv)administration have been measured at -15',0,10',15',20',30', and 60 min.In HP, Tx and NV no variation of PRA, potassium and cortisol was observed.Basal PRL was higher in HP($p<0.02$),but its response as well as that of PA was blunted when compared to Tx and NV($p<0.01$).The response of PA was similar in Tx and NV. In HP the tests were repeated after treatment with Lisuride(0.025 mg/8h/15d) a dopamine agonist.A decrease of PA both basal and after ultrafiltration and metoclopramide together with a diminution of basal PRL were observed($p<0.05$-0.01).We concluded that there is an alterations in the dopaminergic control of A secretion in CRF. This alteration disappears after a successful renal transplant.

1955 SALINE INFUSION IN ESSENTIAL HYPERTENSIVES - RESPONSE OF RENIN-ALDOSTERONE AXIS AND SODIUM EXCRETION BEFORE AND AFTER CONVERTING ENZYME INHIBITION.

L.L. Rydstedt*, N.K. Hollenberg and G.H. Williams, Depts. of Medicine and Radiology, Brigham and Women's Hospital, Boston, MA U.S.A.

Previous studies in hypertensive(HTN) patients have shown that during saline(Na) infusion, 60% of HTN patients have a delayed suppression of plasma renin activity(PRA) and plasma aldosterone(PA). To further elucidate this phenomenon, PAH clearance and Na excretion rates in response to a 62 mEq Na load intravenously were measured in 16 essential HTN and 9 normotensives(NT) on a 10 mEq Na/100 mEq K diet before and after receiving a converting enzyme inhibitor(CEI) for 3 days. The HTN patients could be divided into two groups when compared with the NT subjects based on their PRA-PA suppressibility with the Na load. The non-suppressors(NSup) (n=7) had a change in PRA-PA of less than 20% while the NT and suppressor hypertensive(Sup) (n=9) responses were greater. The effect of CEI on Na excretion (mEq/9 hrs) and PAH clearance (ml/min/1.73 m^2) was (mean±SEM):

	NT	Sup	NSup		NT	Sup	NSup
Na excretion				PAH clearance			
Pre-CEI	24±4	22±5	12±2	Pre-CEI	581±16	596±18	560±38
Post-CEI	--	25±4	26±7	Post-CEI	718±27	581±41	709±20

The NSup had significantly less ($p<0.02$) Na excretion prior to CEI than NT and Sup. CEI significantly ($p<0.03$) increased both Na excretion and PAH clearance in the NSup but had no effect in the Sup. Thus, NSup have a decreased ability to excrete Na and, therefore, may have Na sensitive hypertension. Furthermore, short-term CEI appears to correct this abnormal Na handling.

1956 PREOPERATIVE EVALUATION OF THE POSTOPERATIVE PROGNOSIS OF HYPERTENSION IN PRIMARY ALDOSTERONISM

T. Saruta*, I. Saito, T. Yasui, H. Suzuki, Y.Igarashi and M. Kawamura Department of Internal Medicine, Keio University School of Medicine, Tokyo, Japan.

Postoperative prognosis of hypertension was evaluated preoperatively in 39 patients with primary aldosteronism due to adenoma by examining the degree of hypertension, hypertensive disposition, the age of the patients, duration of the hypertension, hypertensive vascular changes, renal function, plasma renin activity (PRA), plasma aldosterone (PA) and effectiveness of 100 mg/day of spironolactone for 2 weeks on blood pressure (BP). Furthermore, renal biopsy was done to see vascular changes and the juxtaglomerlar apparatus at operation for adrenalectomy.

In 31 of 39 patients BP was reduced below 160/100 mmHg within a year after adrenalectomy. In the other 8 patients the BP was not reduced markedly and it remained over 160/100 mmHg. There was no significant differences in the age of the patients, hypertensive disposition, the degree of hypertension, renal function, EKG changes, PRA, and PA between these two groups. However, there was a significant difference in the effectiveness of spironolactone between these two groups. That is to say, the BP in the group in which postoperative reduction in BP was observed was reduced over 20 mmHg systolic and 10 mmHg diastolic or over 13 mmHg in mean BP by the administration of spironolactone. Hypertensive changes in optic fundi and arteriosclerosis in renal specimens were remarkable in the group in which postoperative reduction in BP was not observed. Effectiveness of spironolactone on BP was superior to the observation of vascular changes in evaluating postoperative prognosis of hypertension in primary aldosteronism.

1957 SLOW CALCIUM CHANNEL (SCC) NUMBER OF THE ADRENAL ZONA GLOMERULOSA (ZG) AND VASCULAR SMOOTH MUSCLE (VSM) ARE INFLUENCED BY DIETARY NaCl CONTENT. R. Schiebinger, Endocrinology, Hypertension and Metabolism Section, University of Oklahoma, Oklahoma City, OK, USA 73190.

During NaCl restriction, plasma angiotensin II (AII) is elevated, aldosterone secretion by the ZG is enhanced, and VSM reactivity is blunted. The opposite is true during NaCl loading. AII binding during NaCl restriction is increased in the adrenal ZG and decreased in VSM. A reciprocal response is observed during NaCl loading. Thus, the responsiveness of the two tissues to AII parallels that of AII binding. Since AII stimulation is dependent on calcium influx through the SCC, we asked the question whether membrane SCC number in the adrenal ZG and VSM are influenced by dietary NaCl content. Rats were placed on a high (+) or low (-) NaCl diet. After two weeks, the adrenal capsule containing the ZG and aorta were harvested. Membranes were prepared by differential centrifugation. SCC binding studies were performed using ^{3}H nitrendipine. Binding was examined at seven different concentrations for the adrenal and five for the aorta from 0.1-2 nM in triplicate. The results from two separate studies are presented below (mean ± SEM).

	ZG		VSM	
	+NaCl	-NaCl	+NaCl	-NaCl
K_d (nM)	.78 ± 14	.78 ± 16	.77 ± 26	.81 ± 23
B_o (fmol/mg prot)	66 ± 3	97 ± 9	68 ± 6	39 ± 9

We conclude that: 1) the NaCl content of the diet significantly influences membrane SCC number (B_o) in the adrenal ZG and VSM without changing the K_d, 2) changes in SCC number parallel that of AII binding in the adrenal ZG and VSM, 3) changes in SCC number may influence the responsiveness of these tissues to AII, and 4) the AII receptor may be linked to the SCC.

1958 19-OXO-ANDROSTENEDIONE AS A NEW HYPERTENSINOGENIC AGENT. H. Sekihara*, The Third Department of Internal Medicine, University of Tokyo Faculty of Medicine, Hongo, Tokyo 113, Japan.

In a previous paper, we demonstrate that 19-hydroxyandrostenedione is an amplifier of the action of aldosterone and a potent hypertensinogenic agent (Endocrinology 113:1141, 1983). We also reported that 19-oxo-androstenedione (19-oxo-AD) amplifies the action of aldosterone. In bioassays using adrenalectomized rats, 19-oxo-AD did not cause any significant change in urinary sodium and potassium excretion. However, urinary sodium excretion of rats pretreated with 19-oxo-AD and given aldosterone was significantly lower than that of rats given aldosterone alone. In addition, the administration of 19-oxo-AD to rats with the adrenals caused a significant decrease in urinary sodium excretion. To elucidate further the biological activities of this steroid hormone, we evaluated the hypertensinogenic effects of 19-oxo-AD in the present study. 100 µg or 1 mg of 19-oxo-AD dissolved in 1 ml of sesame oil was injected into 5 rats with both adrenals and kidneys drinking water once a week for 4 weeks and the changes in blood pressure were evaluated. For controls, 1 ml of sesame oil was injected. The administration of 100 µg of 19-oxo-AD caused no significant changes in blood pressure. However, the administration of 1 mg of 19-oxo-AD caused a significant elevation of blood pressure in the 2nd week and showed significantly higher levels thereafter. The blood pressure of controls and the 19-oxo-AD-treated rats in the 4th week was 122±4 (SE) and 137±2 mmHg, respectively. These results indicate that 19-oxo-AD works as a hypertensinogenic agent in the presence of the adrenal cortex.

1959 CHLORBUTOL, A NEW INHIBITOR OF ALDOSTERONE BIOSYNTHESIS IDENTIFIED DURING EXAMINATION OF HEPARIN EFFECT ON ALDOSTERONE. S. Sequeira* and T.J. McKenna, Dept. of Endocrinology, St. Vincent's Hosp., Dublin, Ireland.

Since routine heparin (H) therapy inhibits aldosterone production (AP) in the adrenal (J Clin Endocrinol Metab 56:108-112, 1983), we examined its mechanism of action using bovine adrenal glomerulosa cell suspensions. Pure H had no significant effect on AP whereas a commercial solution of H containing the preservative chlorbutol (CB), 2.8 X 10^{-2}M, grossly inhibited AP. CB, in a dose dependent manner, suppressed basal AP from 4300 ± 985 pM/l (mean ± SE) to 878 ± 423 pM/l, $p<0.001$, and suppressed angiotensin-II-stimulated AP from 13750 ± 2012 pM/l to 1637 ± 714 pM/l, $p<0.001$. To elucidate the inhibitory action of CB we utilized trilostane (TS) an inhibitor of pregnenolone (Δ5P) to progesterone conversion, and aminoglutethimide (AG) an inhibitor of cholesterol to Δ5P conversion. AP was completely suppressed by each inhibitor. Δ5P fell from 30.60 ± 5.25 nmol/l in TS-treated cells to 4.42 ± 0.88 nmol/l in cells incubated with both TS and CB. AP from exogenously added corticosterone (2.5 X 10^{-7}M) fell from 1985 ± 268 pM/l in AG-treated cells to 968 ± 164 pM/l in cells incubated with both AG and CB. CB, 2.8 X 10^{-3}M and AG, 7.6 X 10^{-5}M inhibited AP to the same extent. Thus CB is a potent inhibitor of AP in vitro; the early phase of the aldosterone biosynthetic pathway is inhibited almost completely, and the late phase partially. Since CB is a widely used pharmaceutical preservative and has a slow metabolic clearance, $t_{\frac{1}{2}}$ = 14 days, these findings may prove to be of major toxicological and therapeutic significance and may account for the clinical inhibition of AP previously attributed to heparin.

1960 THE EFFECT OF DDAVP ON LEARNING AND MEMORY IN AMNESIA DUE TO CLOSED HEAD INJURIES. P. Johnson*, R. Ehrlich and J. Kershner, The Hospital for Sick Children, Division of Endocrinology, Ontario Institute for Studies in Education, University of Toronto, Toronto, Ontario M5G 1X8, Canada.

A double blind crossover design study was performed on 14 subjects aged 18-25 who had suffered a severe closed head injury. Coma had lasted from 2 wks to 6 mnths. All had anterograde amnesia. All subjects had an IQ of >80, were at least 1 yr post coma, had normal drinking habits, urine concentration and on no other medication. There were 10 males and 4 females. A variety of tests measuring short term, long term and working memory as well as learning and forgetting curves were administered. The tests were given before, 2 wks after starting the DDAVP (D) or the vehicle without drug (P), and 8½ wks after stopping either D or P and following the crossover. D was self-administered intranasally, 10 μg twice a day for 7 days and then 20 μg/day for a further 7 days. P was given in the same volume and schedule as D. The first 6 subjects were studied in hospital. Since there were no adverse effects on body weight, fluid intake, urine concentration and serum electrolytes, the remainder were studied at home. The D or P administration was always supervised. Three subjects dropped out. In the first 7 to complete the study, ANOVA showed a significant effect of D on working memory. Raw scores on other memory tests indicated a D effect. Effects were evident by 2 wks but gone by 8½ wks. P had no effect. Subjects could correctly tell when on D. Ongoing testing is being carried out with the remaining 4 subjects.

Conclusion: These preliminary results suggest that DDAVP has a significant effect on memory in post head injury subjects.

1961 PSYCHOLOGICAL CHARACTERISTICS IN HIRSUTISM. A.Kocijancic[+], J.Prezelj and M.Tusak,Department of Endocrinology, University Medical Centre, Zaloška 7, 61000 Ljubljana, Yugoslavia.

It is a known fact that emotional stress may induce the devolopment of hirsutism and enhance the rate of growth of body hair. A study was made on psychological characteristics of 30 women with idiopathic hirsutism. The Freiburg personal inventory, assessment of emotional relationships within the family, the draw a tree test, self-localisation in space, Luchers's colour test and Rohrschach's test were used. The results showed a significantly increased incidence of symptoms of regression. The mother was found to be the dominant person in the primary family of the tested women. Most of the negative emotions were attached to the father. The distribution and density of body hair was found to be correlated to the degree of aggression, anxiety, emotional instability and depression. Presently it is not possible to conclude whether the described psychological characteristics represent a reaction to the disagreable body appearance or may be one of aetiological factors in primary hirsutism. A long-term prospective study has been designed to answer this question.

1962 STEROID THERAPY : EFFECTS ON CALCIUM ABSORPTION AND EXCRETION AND BONE RESORPTION. A.G. Need*, J.C. Philcox, B.E.C. Nordin. Institute of Medical and Veterinary Science and Royal Adelaide Hospital, South Australia

Glucocorticoid therapy is a well recognized cause of osteoporosis but the pathogenesis is poorly understood. We therefore studied 39 patients (22 female) treated with prednisolone (PDN)(mean 18.4 mg/d $\pm$3.5SE) for periods from 0.1 to 23 years (mean 7.2$\pm$1.2). We measured radio-calcium absorption (α), plasma calcium (Ca)mmol/ℓ, fasting urinary calcium/creatinine (Ca/Cr), tubular maximum for calcium reabsorption (TmCa)mmol/ℓGF and, as a measure of bone resorption, fasting urinary hydroxyproline/creatinine (OHPr/Cr). Spine x-rays were performed in 36 patients and used to group patients as normal (N,13), ?osteoporotic (?OP,9) or osteoporotic (OP,14). α was lower in the OP than the N group (.41$\pm$.05 vs .88$\pm$.03, $p<.001$), Ca was similar in both groups, Ca/Cr was higher in the OP than the N group (.48$\pm$.08 vs .19$\pm$.05, $p<.01$), TmCa was lower in the OP than the N group (1.85$\pm$.06 vs 2.22$\pm$.09, $p<.005$) and OHPr/Cr was high in the OP than the N group (25$\pm$12 vs 13$\pm$5, $p<.005$). The dose of PDN was not significantly different between the 2 groups (OP 15$\pm$2 and N 12$\pm$2) nor was the duration of therapy (OP 6.4$\pm$1.9, N 8.9$\pm$2.3). Results for the ?OP group lay in between the OP and N groups. In all 39 patients multiple linear regression (MLR) showed α ($p<.005$) and TmCa ($p<.01$) were negatively related to OHPr/Cr with age being non-significant (multiple R .68). Further MLR showed α to correlate negatively with dose of PDN ($p<.02$) and age ($p<.01$). TmCa correlated negatively with dose of PDN ($p<.05$) but not with age. These results indicate that bone loss during steroid therapy is caused by decreased intestinal calcium absorption and decreased tubular reabsorption of calcium and that both abnormalities are related to the dose of PDN.

1963 OPIOID INHIBITION OF SYNAPTOSOMAL VOLTAGE-DEPENDENT Ca^{++} INFLUX.

M. Murayama*, K. Kamikubo, H. Murase, K. Yasuda and K. Miura
Department of Internal Medicine (III), Gifu University School of Medicine, Gifu 500, Japan.

The present study was undertaken to investigate the mechanism underlying the opioid inhibition of Ca^{++}-dependent neurotransmitter release from presynaptic terminals. Synaptosomes prepared from male Wistar rat brains were incubated with opioid and $^{45}CaCl$ at 30°C. Opioid agonist such as morphine showed no effect on basal synaptosomal $^{45}Ca^{++}$ accumulation at 5mM KCl (0.85 ± 0.06 nmole/mg protein). High K^{+} (70mM) -induced depolarization evoked 3-fold increase in the synaptosomal $^{45}Ca^{++}$ accumulation. Opioid agonists inhibited the depolarization-dependent $^{45}Ca^{++}$ uptake in a dose-dependent manner. ED_{50} for the morphine inhibition of the depolarization-dependent $^{45}Ca^{++}$ uptake was 10-100nM. The maximum inhibition by opioid was approximately 50%. Naloxone reversed the opioid inhibition of the depolarization-dependent $^{45}Ca^{++}$ uptake. These results provide evidence that opioids inhibit the neurotransmitter release by reducing voltage-dependent Ca^{++} influx to presynaptic terminals.

1964 HUMAN LEUMORPHIN-SPECIFIC RIA AND DISTRIBUTION OF IMMUNOREACTIVE LEUMORPHIN IN HUMAN BRAIN.

K. Nakamura*[1,2], C. Yanaihara[1], J. Itoh[2], M. Irie[2], H. Imura[3] and N. Yanaihara[1], [1]Shizuoka College of Pharmacy, Shizuoka 422, [2]Toho University School of Medicine, Tokyo 143, and [3]Kyoto University School of Medicine, Kyoto 606, Japan.

Leumorphin is a putative opioid peptide which constitutes the C-terminal nonacosapeptide sequence of preproenkephalin B. Human leumorphin was synthesized by the solid-phase method and using this, a human leumorphin-specific RIA (anti-human leumorphin serum R0014) was developed. The RIA was shown to recognize the central to C-terminal portion of the peptide and have no crossreactivity with rimorphin, enkephalins and endorphins at all. Leumorphin-like immunoreactivity (IR-LM) detectable by the RIA was contained in corpus striatum, mid brain, pallidum and pons in the highest concentrations (186 - 300 pg/mg wet weight of tissue, n=4) and in medulla oblongata, hypothalamus, thalamus, pituitary, cerebellum and frontal lobe in moderate concentrations (62 - 96 pg/mg, n=4). No detectable IR-LM was found in hippocampus and amygdaloid nucleus. The IR-LM in the mid brain was found to comprise mostly a leumorphin C-terminal fragment-like peptide suggesting the existence of rimorphin in the tissue, while a part of IR-LM in the pituitary was attributable to a leumorphin-like peptide. Synthetic human leumorphin exhibited a dose-dependent opiate effect (ED_{50} 2.49 nM) on electrically stimulated contraction of the guinea pig ileum and caused significant analgesia (ED_{50} 4.47 nmol/mouse) in mice. The present results demonstrate the distribution of leumorphin-related peptides in human brain in such a way to support physiological significance of leumorphin or/and rimorphin as a new family of opioid peptide.

1965 INHIBITORY ACTION OF LEUPEPTIN ON PARATHYROID HORMONE DEGRADATION. E. Shimizu*, M. Moriyama, Y. Okamoto, K. Ota, J. Maeda and L.M. Sherwood. Division of Gerontology, Department of Medicine, Wakayama Medical College, Department of Laboratory Medicine, Wakayama Medical College, Japan and Albert Einstein College of Medicine, New York.

Parathyroid hormone (PTH) is well known to be capable of secreting with time dependency and rapidly facilitating intracellular degradative process of PTH in higher calcium medium. Our study is focussed on the action of PTH degradation at the stimulus of PTH secretogogues and the mechanism of inhibitory PTH secretion in higher calcium medium, using the well established perifusion method. When calcium concentration in perfusate was changed 1.25 mM Ca into 3.0 mM Ca, using perifusion system, PTH secretion was inhibited but however, increased in addition of leupeptin in higher calcium perfusate. Furthermore the epinephrine or dopamine induced PTH secretion was enhanced by addition of leupeptin in perfusate, mediated via PTH degradative process but not adenylate cyclase system. The results indicated that the degradative process of PTH in parathyroid glands was played important roles for regulating PTH in higher calcium condition medium and sustaining an increment of PTH at the stimulus of PTH secretogogues which was not mediated via adenylate cyclase system.

1966 PAROTID GLAND: A NEW TARGET ORGAN OF PARATHYROID HORMONE. M. SHIRAKI*, G. S. ROTH, M. GEE AND B. J. BAUM[a]. Endocrinology Section, Clinical Physiology Branch, Gerontology Research Center, NIA, NIH, Baltimore, MD, USA and a Clinical Investigations and Patient Care Branch, NIDR, NIH, Bethesda, MD, USA.

It has been reported that the parotid gland can respond to parathyroid hormone (PTH) *in vivo*. However, to date, direct demonstration of PTH actions in parotid cells has not been asccomplished. Therefore, we have studied the direct effects of PTH in rat parotid cells *in vitro*.

Enzymatically dispersed parotid cell aggregates (PCA) were obtained from male Wistar rats in a manner similar to that described by Ito et al. (JBC 257, 9532, 1982). The PCA were incubated with 0.2μCi/ml of $[^{32}P]H_3PO_4$ for 60 min. and then were incubated with vehicle, 1-34human or 1-34bovinePTH. After 15-30 min. incubation, significant ^{32}P release(150-200% of control) from PCA was observed in the hormone treated groups. This phosphate release from PCA showed dose dependency for PTH (1.3×10^{-7}-6.8×10^{-6}M) as well as for media $PO_4^{=}$concentration (0.7-7.0mM). PCA treated with PTH also showed dose dependent cyclic AMP release (control = 0.17, maximum PTH = 11.4 pmole/mg protein). The phosphate release induced by PTH significantly correlated with cyclic AMP release (r = 0.97).

These findings strongly suggest that parotid cells may be a target for PTH.

1967 INCREASED SUCCINIC DEHYDROGENASE ACTIVITY IN CELLS OF THE RAT KIDNEY IN CALCIUM DEFICIENCY S.F.Silverton*, E.V. Adlin, B.J. Channick, Dept. of Endocrinology, Temple University Hospital, Phila, Pa. 19140 USA.

Unlike steroid hydroxylation by the P-450 system in the liver, it has been suggested that hydroxylation of 25-OH D_3 in the kidney requires mitochondrial dehydrogenases. Utilizing quantitative cytochemical techniques, changes in mitochondrial dehydrogenases in the pars recta of kidney tubules as demonstrated by succinic dehydrogenase was investigated in a rat model of calcium deficiency. Generation of total reducing equivalents, as well as hydrogen passed along mitochondrial cytochromes, 'Type I hydrogen', was studied using succinate as substrate. Fresh frozen tissue sections were incubated with polyvinyl alcohol as enzyme stabilizer and neotetrazolium chloride as proton acceptor. Reaction product was measured in individual cells with a scanning integrating microdensitometer. Compared to calcium replete animals, calcium deficient animals were shown to have increased Type I hydrogen in cells of the pars recta of the kidney (48.71 ± 6.64 O.D. units x 10^2 vs 31.69 ± 4.52 O.D. units x 10^2, $p<0.01$). Total hydrogen equivalents were not significantly different (107.11 ± 5.89 vs 104.90 ± 8.40, n.s.). Increases in Type I hydrogen, which is assumed to provide hydrogen for steroid hydroxylation are consistent with increased 1-hydoxylation in calcium deficiency.

1968 ANALYSIS OF HUMAN CALCITONIN mRNA AND THE HUMAN CALCITONIN GENE.
P.H. Steenbergh*, J. Zandberg, H.S. Jansz and C.J.M. Lips, Institute of Molecular Biology, Laboratory for Physiological Chemistry and Department of Internal Medicine, State University Utrecht, Utrecht, The Netherlands.

The structure of the mRNA encoding calcitonin (CT) in man has been studied by cDNA cloning and nucleotide sequence analysis. mRNA was isolated from medullary carcinoma of the thyroid (MTC). These tumors, originally from the thyroidal C-cell, are associated with excessive CT levels. Northern blots of this mRNA show hybridization of a 1000-nucleotides-long RNA with a CT-specific probe. In addition, some longer minor species (up to 5000 nucleotides) are detected with this probe in these tumors. Nucleotide sequence analysis of cDNA clones obtained from the tumor RNA revealed the sequence of the entire precursor protein for CT containing 141 aminoacids. As in the case of rat CT, human CT is excised from this precursor leaving N- and C-terminal peptides. One cDNA clone was isolated showing the sequence of an incompletely or incorrectly processed mRNA molecule, probably originating from one of the longer RNA species seen in the Northern blots. In rats, tissue specific alternative splicing of CT gene transcripts has been described resulting in a different peptide, calcitonin gene related peptide, in neural tissues. To study the human CT gene organization cosmid clones containing this gene were isolated from a human gene library. The analysis of these clones is in progress. This investigation was supported by the foundation for Medical Research (FUNGO).

1969 COMPARISON OF THE INFLUENCE OF OVARIAN FUNCTION AND AGE ON CALCIUM METABOLISM IN WOMEN.

J.C. Stevenson*, G. Abeyasekera, C.H. Myers, G. Lane, M. Padwick, J.A. Endacott and M.I. Whitehead. Endocrine Unit, Royal Postgraduate Medical School, London U.K. and Academic Dept. of Gynaecology, King's College Hospital, London U.K.

Although osteoporosis is far more common in women than in men, the relative contributions of the menopause and the aging process are still questioned. Both processes may lead to changes in calcium regulating hormones. We have therefore measured levels of these hormones in 13 young premenopausal women (mean age 30 years, age range 16-44), 15 young women without ovarian function (mean age 27 years, age range 16-39) and 17 middle-aged postmenopausal women (mean age 50 years, age range 43-55). Calcium (Ca), phosphate (P), alkaline phosphatase (ALP), parathyroid hormone (PTH), calcitonin (CT), 1,25 dihydroxyvitamin D (1,25$(OH)_2$D) and 25 hydroxyvitamin D (25OHD) were measured in fasting venous blood samples. In addition, CT reserve was assessed by a 1 minute intravenous calcium infusion (2mg/kg body weight). Comparison of young women with and without ovarian function showed in the latter group lower basal and peak CT levels, lower 1,25$(OH)_2$D levels, higher ALP levels, slightly higher Ca and P levels, and slightly lower PTH and 25OHD levels. Comparison of young and old women without ovarian function showed in the latter group, lower basal CT levels, lower P levels, slightly lower calcium levels, and slightly higher PTH and 25OHD levels. Whilst age and ovarian function both affect calcium homoeostasis, we conclude that the latter is of more importance in determining calcium and bone metabolism in the normal postmenopausal woman.

1970 SHORT-TERM ESTROGEN TREATMENT IN POSTMENOPAUSAL WOMEN INCREASES SERUM 1,25-DIHYDROXYVITAMIN D, YET DECREASES SERUM PARATHYROID HORMONE.

J.L. Stock*, J.A. Coderre, and L.E. Mallette, Worcester Memorial Hospital and the University of Massachusetts Medical School, Worcester, MA 01605 and V.A. Medical Center, Houston, TX 77211, U.S.A.

Previous studies have suggested that months of estrogen administration lead to an increase in circulating immunoreactive parathyroid hormone (iPTH) which stimulates renal synthesis of 1,25-$(OH)_2$D. We measured iPTH in serum from 10 postmenopausal women before and after 14 days of 50ug ethinyl estradiol, using a sensitive radioimmunoassay (RIA) directed at the midregion of the PTH molecule. The assay utilizes antiserum generated in a goat against human PTH and ^{125}I-labeled tyr^{43}-hPTH-(43-68) as radioligand, and detects hormone in >99% of normal persons. Levels of iPTH were detectable and in the normal range in all women and after treatment decreased in 9 of 10 subjects from a mean of $0.53 \pm .15$ to $0.41 \pm .12$ ng/ml ($p < .001$). Fasting urinary calcium and hydroxyproline and serum calcium, phosphorus, and albumin were all significantly lower, and serum 1,25 $(OH)_2$D was higher (from 60 ± 16 to 92 ± 26 ng/ml, $p < .005$). Similar decrements in iPTH were found in the same samples utilizing a different midregion-specific RIA. When the study was repeated in 6 women, serum iPTH was significantly lower at 4 weeks but unchanged after 8 weeks of estrogen compared to pretreatment levels. This unexpected decline in serum iPTH may be related to the short course of treatment compared to previous studies or to differences in immunologic activity detected by our assays. The fall in iPTH in the face of rising 1,25 $(OH)_2$D suggests that the changes in vitamin D induced by estrogen are not simply secondary to changes in PTH.

1971 ISOLATION AND CHARACTERIZATION OF A NEW ENDOGENOUS VITAMIN D IN RAT AND HUMAN SKIN. M. St. Lezin, S.A. Holick and M.F. Holick*, Department of Nutrition and Food Science, Massachusetts Institute of Technology, Cambridge, MA and Vitamin D Laboratory, Massachusetts General Hospital, Boston, Massachusetts, U.S.A.

It is well established in mammals including man, that exposure to sunlight results in the cutaneous synthesis of vitamin D_3 (D_3) from provitamin D_3 (pro-D_3). To date, it has been assumed that D_3 is the only natural form of vitamin D that is produced in mammalian skin. We now have unequivical evidence for the existence of another naturally occurring cutaneous pro-D in rat and man that is converted to a new vitamin D after exposure to simulated sunlight. Lipid extracts from skin of 14-day old rats were chromatographed on a straight phase hplc system and the pro-D peak was collected. The pro-D was dissolved in MeOH and chromatographed on a C-18 reverse phase column. The eluant was monitored at 282 nm and a UV absorption spectrum was determined for each peak with an in-line hplc spectrophotometer. This system revealed that the apparent homogenous pro-D peak recovered from straight phase hplc contained an additional sterol that had a UV spectrum (λ_{max}295, 282 and 271 nm) which is characterisic for pro-D. Mass spectrometry, UV spectroscopy, UV sensitivity, and cochromatography analyses strongly suggest that the structure of this new pro-D is cholesta-5,7,24-triene-3β-ol. During exposure of this new cutaneous pro D to simulated sunlight, it is converted to 24-dehydropre-D_3 which, in turn, thermally isomerized to 24-dehydrovitamin D_3. An analysis of human skin also revealed the presence of the 24-dehydrovitamin D_3 precursor. Therefore, at least two vitamin Ds are made in rat and human skin.

1972 EFFECTS OF HUMAN PARATHYROID HORMONE (hPTH) ANALOGUES ON CYCLIC AMP PRODUCTION OF RAT RENAL CORTICAL CELLS IN PRIMARY CULTURE. T. Takano*, M. Yoneda, M. Tsukada, K. Takatsuki and A. Tomita, 1st Department of Medicine, Nagoya University School of Medicine, Nagoya, Japan.

The structure-function relationship of human PTH was studied using rat renal cortical cells. Monolayer cultured cells were incubated with or without hPTH 1-34 in Dulbecco's modified Eagle medium containing 2 mM 3-isobutyl-1-methyl-xanthine. To this medium, Tyr^{34}hPTH 3-34 NH_2 (3-34), Tyr^{34}hPTH 5-34 NH_2 (5-34), Tyr^{34}hPTH 7-34 NH_2 (7-34), Tyr^{34}hPTH 8-34 NH_2 (8-34) or Tyr^{34}hPTH 9-34 NH_2 (9-34) were added to examine their agonistic or antagonistic properties. After 60 min of incubation, cAMP in the medium and the cells were determined by radioimmunoassay. The stimulative effect of hPTH 1-34 (2.43×10^{-8}M) on cAMP production was almost completely inhibited in cells exposed to 3-34 (2.43×10^{-5}M), although 3-34 by itself showed a slight agonist potency at the same concentration. On the other hand, 5-34, 7-34, 8-34 and 9-34 at 2.43×10^{-5}M caused marked increase in cAMP production both in the presence (2.43×10^{-8}M) and absence of hPTH 1-34. The data demonstrate that deletion of the first two amino acid residues of hPTH 1-34 definitely reduces hormonal activity resulting in a peptide with antagonist property, but deletion of additional 2-6 residues creates peptides that behave rather as agonists. This paradoxical phenomenon might be explained by differently altered tertiary structure in the biologically active domain of the molecules.

1973 CHARACTERIZATION OF VOLTAGE SENSITIVE CALCIUM CHANNELS IN A CLONAL PITUITARY CELL LINE. Gary A. Shangold* and Richard J. Miller, Depts. of Obstetrics and Gynecology and Pharmacological and Physiological Sciences, Univ. of Chicago, Chicago, IL 60637, U.S.A.

Electrophysiological studies have demonstrated the existence of voltage sensitive calcium channels (VSCC) in anterior pituitary cells. The purpose of our investigation was to characterize the VSCC involved in the release of anterior pituitary hormones. We studied $^{45}Ca^{+2}$ fluxes in a clonal rat anterior pituitary cell line, GH_3, known to synthesize and secrete prolactin and growth hormone. When the K^+ concentration of the medium was raised to 70 mM from 5 mM, there was an immediate (< 2 min) increase in net Ca^{+2} influx. This increase was apparent over the total assay period of 15 min. Ca^{+2} uptake was stimulated approximately 10-fold over basal levels. Stimulation of Ca^{+2} influx was not blocked by tetrodotoxin (10^{-6}M) or by total substitution of choline for Na^+ in the assay medium. This indicates that Ca^{+2} influx did not occur via sodium channels or as a result of Na^+/Ca^{+2} exchange. However, Ca^{+2} uptake was inhibited by several substances that act as VSCC blockers in other tissues. The organic VSCC blockers nitrendipine, nisoldipine, D-600 and diltiazem blocked the stimulation of Ca^{+2} uptake. (-)-Nimodipine was more potent than (+)-nimodipine. The organic VSCC blocker Cd^{+2} also inhibited the stimulation of Ca^{+2} influx. The novel dihydropyridines BAY K8644 and CGP 28392 have been shown to activate rather than block VSCC in other tissues. In GH_3 cells, both of these compounds further enhanced Ca^{+2} influx stimulated by 70 mM K^+. The effects of BAY K8644 could be blocked by the antagonist nitrendipine. These results indicate that voltage dependent influx of Ca^{+2} into GH_3 cells occurs via VSCC and that these channels have high affinity for organic VSCC blocking drugs.

1974 THREE-DIMENSIONAL (3-D) CULTURE OF BONE CELLS IN COLLAGEN GELS. Deanna J. Talley*, Div. Biochem., Marquette Univ. Sch. Dentistry, Milwaukee, WI, USA.

Previous attempts at long-term culture of bone cells which maintain functional activity equal to that in corresponding cells *in vivo* have met with limited success, due in part to failure of cells in monolayer to form an architecture similar to cells *in vivo*. In the present study, 3-D cultures were employed to determine if bone cells would maintain functional activity at *in vivo* levels for 3 wks in culture. Cells were isolated from calvariae of neonatal ICR mice by trypsinization and inoculated in dishes containing 0.1% agar in culture medium. Cells also were inoculated as monolayers. After 24 h, the suspension of cell aggregates (10-15 cells) in agar dishes was removed and inoculated in a cold solution of collagen: medium and permitted to form gels. Culture medium containing 10mM β-glycerophosphate was added and changed each 2-3 days. Alkaline phosphatase activity in cell homogenates was measured by colorimetric assay of the hydrolysis of ρ-nitrophenylphosphate. Cells cultured as monolayers exhibited 90-100% attachment and at low cell density (10^5 cells ml^{-1}) doubled in cell number in 24-36 hours. Alkaline phosphatase activity per cell was less than one-fifth the *in vivo* level and declined to immeasurable levels after 5-7 days in culture. In contrast, cells cultured as aggregates in collagen gels maintained enzyme activity at the *in vivo* level for 3 weeks in culture. Removal of 10mM β-glycerophosphate from medium resulted in a 50% decline in cellular alkaline phosphatase activity. These results show that culture of bone cell aggregates in collagen gels provides a model system similar to conditions *in vivo*. This should be useful to elucidate mechanisms regulating mineralization as well as to study bone diseases.

1975 STEROID RECEPTORS IN CHEMICALLY-INDUCED COLON CARCINOGENESIS.
Emi Odagiri*, Kazuko Jibiki, Saeko Nakamura, Reiko Demura and Hiroshi Demura. Department of Radioassay, Tokyo Womens' Medical College, Tokyo, Japan

It has been reported that the incidence of dimethylhydrazine (DMH) induced colon cancer is different between male and female BD rat. We have measured steroid receptors in DMH-induced colonic neoplasm to study whether steroid hormone is involved in the growth of these tumors. Beginning at either 30 or 60 days of age, BD-IX rats received 20 mg of 1,2-DMH per kg BW, once a week for 20 weeks. Fifty-seven rats were killed at 40-45 weeks after the initial injection. For the measurment of AR,ER and PR, the cytosol was incubated with ^{3}H-R1881,^{3}H-E_2 or ^{3}H-R5020 in the presence or absence of a 100-500 fold excess of unlabeled hormones. The incidence of colonic neoplasm was 100% and 96% in male and female rats, respectively. The total number of colonic neoplasms was 263 among 57 rats. The mean number of colonic neoplasms was 5.6 in male and 3.5 in female rats, respectively. Seventy-eight colonic neoplasms were larger than 1 cm diameter, of which 58 (74%) were seen in male rats. AR was found in 50.9% of colonic neoplasms and the number of binding sites ranged from 3-62.7fm/mg protein. The incidence and the levels of AR were higher in male(60.5%,16.9$\pm$3.6 fm/mg protein) than in female rats(35.3%, 4.6$\pm$o.8 fm/mg protein). These tumors also bound ^{3}H-E_2 and ^{3}H-R 5020, but the levels were lower than that of AR. These results suggest that sex steroid involves in DMH-induced colon tumorigenesis.

1976 ENOLASE ISOZYMES (α-, β-, γ-ENOLASE) IN THE ENDOCRINE TUMORS.
S. Ohtani*, K. Iwase, K. Kato°, A. Nagasaka, K. Miura, K. Kawase, A. Nakai, T. Aono, T. Ohyama, I. Nagatsu, H. Nakagawa, K. Kataoka and H. Hasegawa, Fujita-Gakuen Univ. School of Medicine, Toyoake, Aichi 470-11 and ° Institute for Deveropmental Research, Aichi Pref, Colony, Kasugai, Aichi 480-03, Japan.

The glycolytic enzyme enolase is composed of three subunits(α, β, γ). The γ-enolase found in nerve cell bodies, axons and neuroendocrine cells is called the neuron-specific enolase(NSE). We measured the tissue and serum enolase isozymes in various endocrine tumors and immunostained the isozymes in those tissues by the unlabeled antibody peroxidase anti-peroxidase method. 21 cases of endocrine tumors(thyroid;13, parathyroid;1, adrenal;4, islet cell;2 and pituitary;1) were examined. Serum samples were obtained before and after the operation. The assay for human enolase isozymes carried out by a sandwich enzyme immunoassay system using antibody labeled with β-D-galactosidase. In all the tumors, large amounts of α-enolase were detected as in the other tissues, whereas β-enolase was scarcely detected. Thyroid medullary carcinoma, pheochromocytoma and pituitary eosinophilic adenoma (acromegaly) contained large amounts of NSE. Thyroid papillary or follicular carcinoma and adenoma and adrenocortical adenoma contained only small amounts of NSE. Serum NSE values were closely related with those of tissue NSE. The immunohistochemical study showed strongly stained NSE in medullary carcinoma, phaochromocytoma and pituitary eosinophilic adenoma. These data imply that there are large amounts of NSE in APUDomas and that serum NSE measurement is a valuable diagnostic test for routine screening and a subsequent therapeutic monitoring of tumors.

1977 EFFECT OF THYMOSIN FRACTION 5 ON T-LYMPHOCYTE ROSETTE FORMATION IN NIGERIAN PATIENTS WITH DIFFERENT TYPES OF CANCER. S. O. Olusi*, S. F. Oluwole and W. O. Odesanmi. Faculty of Health Sciences, University of Ife, Ile-Ife, Nigeria.

Since the thymus plays a dominant role in the host's immunological defensive mechanisms, the role of thymosin in the treatment of malignancies has been the subject of extensive investigations. We have studied the effects of thymosin fraction 5 in vitro on T-lymphocyte rosette formation in 14 patients with hepatocellular carcinoma, 21 with Burkitt's lymphoma, 13 with Hodgkin's disease and 15 with breast cancer. It was found that thymosin fraction 5 caused statistically significant increases in percentages of E-rosettes in 19 out of 21 patients with Burkitt's lymphoma, all of patients with Hodgkin's disease but in only 2 out of 14 patients with hepatocellular carcinoma and 2 out of 15 patients with breast cancer. Based upon this in vitro study, we propose that a clinical trial with thymosin in children with Burkitt's lymphoma is warranted.

1978 USE OF FLOW CYTOMETRY FOR THE DETERMINATION OF ESTROGEN RECEPTORS IN BREAST CANCER. M. Pagé*, A. Daver, H. Coic, A. Chassevent, G. Bertrand, F. Larra, Dép. Biochimie, Fac. Médecine, Université Laval, Qué., Canada*; Centre Paul Papin, Angers, France.

There is an increasing emphasis on early detection of primary breast cancers and methods which require only small number of cells. Biochemically determined estrogen receptors (ER) in tissue homogenates may give misleading results because of tumour heterogeneity. Many histochemical and immunohistochemical methods do not always satisfy the criteria for demonstrating high affinity cytosolic receptors due to their lack of specificity. We have developed a flow cytometric method for the measurement of ER in monodispersed cells obtained from tumour masses after surgery or from cells from breast cancers obtained by needle aspiration. High affinity specific binding of ER type I was demonstrated by incubating single cell suspensions of ER positive human mammary adenocarcinoma cells (MCF-7 and ZR-75-1) with nanomolar concentrations of fluoresceinated estrone (17 FE); ER negative cells were used as controls. Cells were also preincubated with a 100 fold excess of diethylstilbestrol to block 17 FE binding. The specificity of 17 Fe binding was demonstrated by showing fluorescence in ER positive cells only and inhibition by preincubating with a 100 fold excess of DES. Similar studies were performed in breast cancer cell suspensions obtained after surgery and from needle aspirates. We found 75% correlation between the FCM assay described and estrogen receptor binding assay used in the clinical laboratory. This FCM assay offers many advantages since it is rapid and requires less than 10^5 cells.

1979 THE EFFECT OF ANABOLIC STEROIDS (19-NORTESTOSTERONE, 19-NORANDROSTENEDIONE) ON GROWTH AND AROMATASE ACTIVITY IN CULTURED HUMAN BREAST CARCINOMA CELLS. E. Perel*, L.Kharlip, M. Blackstein, and D.W. Killinger, Department of Medicine and Institute of Medical Sciences, University of Toronto, Toronto Canada M5R 1A8.

The effects of 19-nortestosterone (nor-T) and 19-norandrostenedione (nor-A) on cell growth and aromatase activity, were studied in cultures of a human breast carcinoma cell line derived from a primary tumour (MD). Growth curves were examined in α-MEM with 15% fetal calf serum, alone, or in the presence of 10^{-6}M nor-T or nor-A. Studies on aromatase activity were carried out on cells in the late exponential growth phase, preincubated for 24 hrs with or without nor-T or nor-A at concentrations of 10^{-8}, 10^{-7} or 10^{-6}M. There was no effect of either nor-T, or nor-A on the rate of cell growth. There was however, a marked effect of both compounds on aromatase activity. The formation of E_1 was inhibited by 50% at a concentration of 10^{-8}M and 90% at a concentration of 10^{-7}M or greater. Estradiol formation was inhibited by 50 to 100% at 10^{-6}M. Under similar conditions, aminoglutethamide (10^{-6}M) inhibited estrone formation by 25 to 50%. These studies indicate that the anabolic steroids nor-T and nor-A are effective inhibitors of aromatase activity at concentrations as low as 10^{-8}M and warrant further study of their clinical value in the treatment of breast carcinoma.

1980 A RELATIONSHIP BETWEEN ESTROGEN AND DEHYDROEPIANDROSTERONE SULFURYLATION AND ESTROGEN RECEPTOR STATUS IN HUMAN MAMMARY CARCINOMA. T. Pewnim* and J.B. Adams, School of Biochemistry, The University of New South Wales, Kensington, N.S.W. 2033, Australia, and Faculty of Science, Silpakorn University, Nakornpathom 73000, Thailand.

A great many studies have now shown that the levels of estrogen receptor (ER) in human breast cancer tissue are related to response to hormone ablative, or hormone additive, treatments. One other biochemical parameter which is also related to prognosis and response to hormone ablation is the assessment of steroid sulfurylation (Dao *et al.*, Nat. Cancer Inst. Monographs, 34 : 205, 1971). We later demonstrated the existence of a relationship between estrogen sulfurylation and ER status in 62 breast tumors (Pewnim *et al.*, Steroids, 39 : 47, 1982). We now wish to report a relationship between both estrogen and dehydroepiandrosterone (DHEA) sulfurylation and ER status. Cytosol fractions of 69 mammary carcinoma specimens were assayed for [^{35}S]estradiol-3-sulfate (ES) and [^{35}S]DHEA-3-sulfate (DHEAS) formation and ER content. A positive correlation was found between ES and DHEAS formation having a correlation coefficient of 0.86 ($p<0.001$). The formation of ES and DHEAS in ER positive tumors were significantly higher than ER negative tumors [74±10 and 50±7 (mean±S.E.M.) *versus* 30±9 and 20±6 pmole per mg protein per 2 hr, respectively, $p<0.001$ in both cases]. By selecting discriminating values for ES of 40 and for DHEAS of 50 pmole per mg protein per 2 hr, then 20/22 (91%) of the ER negative tumors were below these points. In conclusion we can state that the assessment of estrogen and DHEA sulfotransferase activities may be an alternative method for the evaluation of hormone responsiveness in mammary cancer.

1981 PROLACTIN (PRL), ESTRADIOL (E) AND PROGESTERONE (Pg) RECEPTOR (R) LEVELS IN HUMAN BREAST CANCER AFTER BROMOCRIPTIN TREATMENT. JP. Peyrat, Ph. Vennin, B. Vandewalle, J. Bonneterre, J. Djiane (2), J. Lefebvre, Laboratoire d'Endocrinologie Expérimentale, Centre de Lutte Contre le Cancer de la Région Nord, BP 307, 59020 LILLE CEDEX (France), (2) Laboratoire de Physiologie de la Lactation CNRZ-INRA 78350 JOUY-EN-JOSAS

The levels of PRLR in breast cancers are low and difficult to detect. Since specimens are obtained at surgery, the raise of PRL plasma levels during general anesthesia could lead to the blocking of available receptor sites. We have previously shown that in vitro desaturation of PRLR by MgCl2 3 M induced an increase of PRLR positive tumors and of PRLR levels (Peyrat et al. 1981 Breast Cancer Res. Treat. 1:369). The current study investigates the effect of bromocriptin (CB 154, Sandoz), a prolactin lowering drug, on PRLR, ER and PgR levels in human breast cancers. Bromocriptin was given 2,5 mg per os twice daily for four days. The results obtained for the treated population (n = 30) was compared to those obtained for the untreated population (n = 120) during the same period. There was 52 % PRLR positive tumors in the treated population (PRL = 2.45 ± 0.39 (SEM) ng/ml) and 49 % in the untreated one (PRL = 79 ± 5 (SEM) ng/ml). PRLR levels, respectively 1.9 % (± 0.12 SEM) and 2.4 % (± 0.14 SEM), were not statistically different. MgCl2 treatment led in both cases to an increase in PRLR positive tumors and in PRLR levels. The number of ER positive tumors was significantly increased after treatment with bromocriptin in premenopausal women. Neither the rate of positivity nor the levels of PgR were changed by the treatment. The inefficiency of bromocriptin in unmasking prolactin receptors in breast cancers in vivo is clearly demonstrated.

1982 REPORT OF A HYDATIDIFORM MOLE CONTAINING RENIN, INACTIVE RENIN, PROGESTERONE AND HCG. A. M. Poisner*, H.C. Cheng, T. Tomita, R. Poisner and C. R. King, Depts. of Pharmacology, Toxicology & Therapeutics, Obstetrics & Gynecology and Pathology & Oncology, Univ. of Kansas Medical Center, Kansas City, KS 66103, USA.

Renin has been localized in trophoblasts in chorion laeve and has been suggested as a possible marker of trophoblastic tumors (Endocrinology 109: 1150, 1981). We report here the presence of high concentrations of renin in a hydatidiform mole, together with progesterone and HCG. The patient had a preoperative HCG level of 286,000 mIUnits/ml at 15 weeks. One week after D & C, the level was 9,000 and it subsequently fell to 10.5. There were no signs of hypertension during the clinical course. An extract of the molar tissue was assayed for renin and inactive renin, progesterone and HCG. The concentrations in the mole were (per gm tissue): active renin= 2.31 mU; inactive renin=17.35 mU; total renin=19.66 mU; HCG= 4411 Units; progesterone=3.10 ug. For comparison, the total renin content (mU/gm) in term chorion laeve was 21.0 (n=9) and in placenta was 0.02 (n=4). Immunoperoxidase study using antiserum to pure human kidney renin revealed renin in the principal tumor cells. The results support the suggestion that renin and inactive renin are markers of trophoblasts and may be useful in diagnosing and monitoring the course of trophoblastic disease. Supported by N.I.H. Grant HD 16552.

1983 NEUTRALIZATION BY AN ANTIANDROGEN OF THE STIMULATORY EFFECT OF ADRENAL STEROIDS ON THE RAT PROSTATE. P. Poyet*, J. Hamel, P. Gagnon and F. Labrie, MRC Group in Molecular Endocrinology, CHUL, Quebec G1V 4G2, Canada.

The role of adrenal androgens on the growth of human prostatic adenocarcinoma has recently been demonstrated. In order to further characterize the action of adrenal steroids on the prostate, adult castrated male rats were treated for 14 days with dehydroepiandrosterone (DHEA) or DHEA-sulfate (DHEAS). While DHEAS had no effect, DHEA increased ventral prostate weight by 2.5- and 5-fold at the twice daily doses of 0.5 and 2 mg, respectively ($p < 0.01$). Two other adrenal steroids, namely androst-5-ene-3β,17β-diol (Δ^5-diol) and androstenedione (Δ^4-dione), did also increase ventral prostate weight in a dose-dependent manner. At the highest dose studied (0.5 mg, twice daily), Δ^5-diol and Δ^4-dione increased ventral prostate weight by 5- and 6-fold, respectively ($p < 0.01$). Concomitant administration of a pure non-steroidal antiandrogen (RU 23908, 5 mg, twice daily), while having no effect by itself, completely blocked the stimulatory action of adrenal androgens on secondary sex organ weight. The effectiveness of the antiandrogen was further assessed by treating castrated males with testicular androgens. The 3- to 4-fold stimulation of ventral prostate weight induced by a low dose of dihydrotestosterone or 5α-androstane-3α,17β-diol (0.05 mg, twice daily) was completely prevented by simultaneous treatment with the antiandrogen. The present data indicate that steroids of adrenal origin can have adverse effects in cancer of the prostate and demonstrate that the use of a pure antiandrogen can efficiently prevent the action of these steroids.

1984 BOMBESIN-LIKE IMMUNOREACTIVITY IN HUMAN PLASMA. Janet Price*, G.M. Besser and Lesley H. Rees, Departments of Chemical Endocrinology and Endocrinology, St. Bartholomew's Hospital, London, EC1A 7BE, U.K.

In man bombesin-like immunoreactivity (BLI) occurs in some endocrine tumours, but it is not clear if such tumours secrete BLI in vivo. Indeed, little is known about circulating BLI. Tracer degradation and insensitive RIA have made it difficult to study. We have developed an extracted RIA which eliminated tracer damage and increased the assay sensitivity. Plasma BLI was extracted onto Vycor glass (50mg), washed sequentially with H_2O and 1M HCl and eluted with 80% aqueous methanol. The eluate was dried down under N_2 at 60°C, the residue reconstituted in a minimal volume of buffer and assayed using an antiserm directed towards the C-terminus of bombesin. The mean recovery of standard bombesin was 60% (n=10); the intra-assay C.V. was 7% (mean, 186pg/ml; n=20) and the inter-assay C.V. was 10.5% (mean, 173pg/ml; n=8). The minimum detection limit was 20pg/ml. BLI was undetectable in normal subjects (n=10), however RIA of an extract of a plasma pool (90ml) indicated a level of approx. 4pg/ml. 8/157 subjects with diverse pathologies had detectable BLI levels (25-330pg/ml) and these were associated with various malignancies (carcinoids of the thymus (n=1), lung (n=2), medullary carcinoma of the thyroid (n=1), small cell carcinoma of the lung (n=4)). 5 subjects also had ectopic ACTH secretion. Significant tumour BLI concentrations were detected in 3 subjects and in one of these a BLI level of 191pg/ml was seen in the mediastinal vein draining tumour metastases. Our results indicate that although normally undetectable, plasma BLI is elevated in some malignant conditions and may be associated with multiple hormone producing tumours.

1985 POTENT INHIBITORY EFFECT OF A PURE ANTIANDROGEN ON THE GROWTH OF THE DUNNING R3327 TUMORS IN THE RAT.

L. Proulx, F. Létourneau* and F. Labrie, MRC Group in Molecular Endocrinology, CHUL, Quebec G1V 4G2, Canada

Daily treatment of male (Copenhagen x Fisher) F_1 rats bearing the Dunning R3327 tumor with 1 μg of the LHRH agonist [D-Ser(TBU)^6, des-Gly-NH_2^{10}] LHRH ethylamide for 20 weeks decreased by 35, 52 and 30% the weights of ventral prostate, seminal vesicles and testes respectively but had no significant effect on tumor growth as evaluated by measures of tumor volumes up to 20 weeks of teatment. When the antiandrogen Anandron was administered daily at the dose of 10 mg per animal concomitantly with 1 μg of the LHRH agonist, the weights of ventral prostate, seminal vesicles and testes were decreased by 73, 59 and 66%. More importantly, a complete arrest of tumor growth was observed in the LHRH agonist + antiandrogen-treated animals, the tumor volumes at 20 weeks being 49 ± 12, 52 ± 18 and 4 ± 2 cm^3 in the control, LHRH agonist-treated and LHRH agonist + antiandrogen-treated groups. After 20 weeks of treatment, the increase in tumor volume was 17-fold in the control group, 18-fold in the LHRH agonist-treated group and 3-fold in the LHRH agonist + antiandrogen-treated group. The present data clearly show that unlike castration which has been shown to cause a transient arrest of growth of the Dunning R3327 tumor, combined treatment with an LHRH agonist and a pure antiandrogen causes a prolonged remission with no sign of relapse up to at least 20 weeks.

1986 INTERACTION OF EQUINE ESTROGENS WITH HUMAN SERUM PROTEINS.

C.C. Pan*, C.A. Woolever and B.R. Bhavnani. Dept. Obs./Gyn., McMaster University, Hamilton, Ontario. Canada.

Equilin sulfate (EqS) is one of the major components of conjugated equine estrogen preparations such as Premarin^R and we have reported that the metabolic clearance rate (MCR) of EqS was only 6-8% that of equilin (Eq),(JCEM 56: 1048, 1983). Since binding of steroids to serum proteins appears to influence their MCR, we have studied the binding of EqS, Eq, to human serum proteins and have compared this to the serum protein binding of E_1, E_1S, E_2 and DHT. Undiluted serum (0.5 ml) obtained from postmenopausal women was incubated with 5 pmoles of the above ^{3}H-steroids at 37°C for 30 min., and then subjected to gel filtration (Sephadex G-150) at 4°C. With Eq, E_1, E_2 and DHT two peaks of radioactivity were associated with proteins having mol. wts. of 130,000 (SHBG) and 67,000 (albumin) daltons, respectively. In the case of ^{3}H-EqS and ^{3}H-E_1S, binding to SHBG was not detectable, however, the major peak of radioactivity was associated with albumin. Binding to SHBG and albumin was confirmed by removing SHBG or albumin from the serum with specific affinity matrices Con-A-sepharose 4B gel or (CM Affi-Gel Blue), respectively. The relative binding affinities of the above steroids to SHBG at 37°C determined by competitive Scatchard analysis using the DEAE filter assay and ^{3}H-DHT were 1.4, 0.7, 2.0 and 46.0 ($10^8 M^{-1}$) for Eq, E_1, E_2 and DHT respectively. These results indicate that the equine estrogens bind to SHBG and albumin in a manner similar to the classical estrogens E_1 and E_2 and that the low MCR of EqS may be due to its binding with albumin.

Supported by The Medical Research Council of Canada #MT-3724.

1987 **HIRSUTISM DUE TO GONADOTROPIN-DEPENDENT ANDROGEN SECRETING LIPOID CELL OVARIAN TUMOR**

S. Pang, *R.L. Leibel, W.J. Sweeney III, M.I. New, The New York Hospital-Cornell Medical Center, New York, NY 10021 U.S.A.

We report a 39-year-old female who presented with a 22-year history of slowly progressive hirsutism and secondary amenorrhea and was found to have a non-metastatic ovarian tumor secreting gonadotropin-dependent androgens. Baseline LH levels were in the range seen in normal females during the late follicular stage of the menstrual cycle, despite markedly elevated Δ-4-androstenedione (Δ4-A) and testosterone (T). LHRH administration (100 μg IV bolus) increased LH four-fold (from 20 to 88 mIU/ml) at 45" post injection, with a two-fold increase in Δ4-A (from 1263 to 2528 ng/dl). The Δ4-A, T and 17-hydroxyprogesterone (17-OHP) secretion by the tumor were neither ACTH-stimulable nor dexamethasone-suppressible, while cortisol (F) dynamics were normal. However, markedly elevated Δ4-A and T and moderately elevated 17-OHP were markedly decreased following 3 days of Norlutin administration, and hCG administration markedly increased 17-OHP, Δ4-A and T. Tumor site ovarian vein concentrations of Δ4-A (52,490 ng/dl) and T (2,547 ng/dl) were extremely high. The contralateral ovary was normal both grossly and microscopically. Upon removal of the tumor, androgen levels fell to either low normal or below the normal range. Pathology of the tumor was consistent with a lipoid cell tumor of the ovary. The in vivo hormonal data suggest that hormonal secretion of the ovarian tumor was gonadotropin-dependent and that the slowly growing tumor was most likely the cause of the long-term, slowly progressive hirsutism in this patient.

	mIU/ml		ng/dl	μg/dl	ng/dl			
	LH	FSH	DHA	F	17-OHP	Δ4-A	T	E_2
Baseline	12-20	5	446	11	658	1345	261	4
Post ACTH (40 U IV)			761	33	526	1344	184	4
Post Dex (2 mg/d x 5d)			218	<0.1	1300	2735	337	<2
Post Dex x 12d + Norlutin (30 mg/d x 3d)	<3		65	<0.1	197	434	50	<2
Post Dex x 17d + hCG (5000 U/d IM x 3d)			193	<0.1	3800	3245	786	6
Post op (3rd day)			274			87	8	<2

1988 EVALUATION OF GONADAL FUNCTION FOLLOWING LONG-TERM TREATMENT FOR ACUTE LYMPHOBLASTIC LEUKEMIA IN GIRLS. T. Pasqualini*, M.E. Escobar, H. Domené, F. Sackmann Muriel, S. Pavlovsky and M.A. Rivarola. CEDIE and Unidad de Hematología, Hospital de Niños, Buenos Aires, Argentina.

Twenty-three girls following long-term treatment($\bar{X}$:51 months)for acute lymphoblastic leukemia were studied;13 prepubertal(5,3-8,6 years old)and 10 pubertal(9,2-13,2 years old):5 at genital stage (G)II, 1 at G III,2 at G IV and 2 at G V;the G IV and G V girls were postmenarchal. Follow up during the study ranged from 2 months-6,2 years($\bar{X}$:2 years). At the end of the study 8 patients were still prepubertal,2 patients were in G II,4 in G III,1 in G IV 8 in G V;10 were postmenarchal. Thirteen out 15 patients had sexual development at chronological ages before the normal mean and 8 out/10 reached menarche before mean normal age. In 5/19 patients bone age was significantly accelerated. Twelve of the 15 pubertal patients had received cranial cobaltotherapy.Serum gonadotrophins response to LH-Rh was normal in 12 prepubertal girls.Basal(b)LH($\bar{X}$ ± SD)13 ± 3 ng/ml LeR 907,maximal response(MR)62 ± 34; b FSH 73 ± 26,MR 304 ± 135;and in pubertal patients b LH 34 ± 20(n=15),MR 171± 90(n=14),b FSH 140 ± 92 (n=15), MR 310 ± 172 (n=14). Serum estradiol values were normal.Two of 4 patients studied had ovulatory values of serum progesterone (19 and 12 ng/ml),these were the patients with more advanced gynecology cal age.This study suggests that neither the disease nor the long-term antileukemic therapy seems to injure gonadal function in girls.Tendence to early sexual development was observed,probably related with cranial cobaltotherapy

1989 EFFECT OF BROMOCRIPTINE ON POLYCYSTIC OVARY SYNDROME

J. J. Pehrson*, C. L. Longcope, G. Orczyk and J. L. Vaitukaitis, Department of Medicine, Boston University School of Medicine, Boston, MA 02118. U.S.A.

Polycystic ovary syndrome (PCOS) is a common disorder affecting approximately 5% of women during their reproductive years. In view of evidence supporting altered dopaminergic modulation of LH and prolactin secretion among affected women, 37 women with PCOS were treated with a dopamine agonist, bromocriptine. Women with either normal or elevated prolactin levels (>26 ng/ml) received 2.5 mg twice daily for up to two years. No patients had neuroradiologic evidence of a pituitary tumor or biochemical evidence of partial enzymatic steroidogenic defects. All patients were studied during states of prolonged amenorrhea or in the early follicular phase. When compared to normal women studied in their early follicular phase, women with PCOS had significantly higher LH/FSH ratios and blood production rates of testosterone and androstenedione. Bromocriptine treatment was associated with a markedly improved menstrual pattern in 31 of the 37 women - 19 of 21 with normal basal prolactin levels prior to therapy and in 12 of 16 with abnormally high basal prolactin levels prior to therapy. Changes in androgen metabolism were less striking and remained abnormally high among several women who resumed regular menses. The reason for that disparity is not readily apparent but may reflect normalization of either an idiopathic or sex steroid induced alteration of hypothalamic function with bromocriptine. Dopamine agonists may be an effective nonhormonal form of therapy for women with polycystic ovary syndrome whether they present with normal or elevated basal prolactin levels.

1990 TREATMENT OF PRECOCIOUS PUBERTY WITH LHRH ANALOG: REVIEW OF THE NIH EXPERIENCE. O. Pescovitz*, K. Barnes, A. McNemar, K. Hench, C. Foster, D. Kenigsburg, D. L. Loriaux, G. B. Cutler, Jr., and F. Comite. DEB, NICHD, NIH, Bethesda, Md. 20205

Since 1979, 124 children have been referred to NIH for evaluation of precocious puberty and for treatment with the LHRH analog, D-Trp^{6}-Pro^{9}-NEt-LHRH (LHRH$_{a}$). The children were given the following diagnoses: idiopathic precocious puberty (IPP), hypothalamic hamartoma (HH), other CNS lesions (CNS), congenital adrenal hyperplasia and true precocious puberty (CAH/TPP), McCune-Albright Syndrome (MAS), and familial male precocious puberty (FPP). Their mean pretherapy data are shown below (BA/CA = Bone age/age):

	Male/ Female	age (y)	Tanner Stage	BA/CA	Basal LH/ FSH mIU/ml	LH/FSH p LHRH	E_2(F) ng/l	T(M) ng/dl
IPP	1/50	5.7	2.5	1.7	9.9/8.5	73/28	31	594
HH	9/14	4.1	2.9	2.3	10.7/10.5	137/31	41	438
CNS	7/15	6.3	3.0	1.5	7.7/7.2	52/24	47	422
CAH/TPP	8/1	8.3	3.3	1.6	8.3/8.5	54/19	40	165
MAS	0/8	5.4	2.6	1.6	3.5/3.5	30/9	54	---
FPP	9/0	4.9	2.7	2.0	1.8/0.9	3.5/3.6	--	325

Patients with HH were the youngest and had the most advanced bone age and highest gonadotropins of the 4 groups with TPP. The patients with IPP, CNS, HH, and CAH/TPP responded to LHRH$_{a}$ with regression of clinical signs of puberty, a decrease in basal and LHRH-stimulated gonadotropins and sex steroids, and normalization of growth rate and the rate of bone age maturation. Patients with FPP and most patients with MAS did not not respond to LHRHa therapy which suggests that gonadal function in these patients was independent of hypopothalamic-pituitary activation.

1991 PITUITARY-TESTICULAR AXIS IN DIABETIC MEN. R. Quadri*, R.Giannella, P. Carpano Maglioli, M. Manenti, G. Bellomo, M. Veglio, D. Fonzo, Patologia Medica E, Istituto di Medicina Interna, via Genova 3, 10126 Torino, Italy.

The aim of this study has been the evaluation of the pituitary-testicular axis and of the prevalence of sexual dysfunctions in twenty seven diabetic men randomly selected from an out-patient diabetic clinic. Erectile failure was the most common abnormality (40.7%) followed by loss of libido (14.9%) and premature ejaculation (11.1%). Patients have been divided in different groups according to the type of diabetes (1 or 2) and the presence or absence of sexual dysfunctions. Plasma basal testosterone, FSH, LH and prolactin have been measured. FSH, LH and prolactin concentrations in plasma have also been measured after stimulation with 100 mcg LHRH and 200 mcg TRH. Hormonal levels did not significantly differ between the different groups considered (control vs diabetes type 1 vs type 2, presence vs absence of sexual dysfunctions) both in basal conditions or after stimulation. The present study supports the view that hormonal derangements have little if any influence on the pathogenesis of impotence in diabetic patients. We suggest that sexual dysfunctions in such subjects are mainly due to neurological or vascular imbalance.

1992 **DIAGNOSTIC APPROACH IN PATIENTS WITH HYPERANDROGENISM.** T. Rabe*, L. Kiesel, K. Mössler, K. Grunwald and B. Runnebaum, Dept. OB/GYN, Division of Gynecological Endocrinology, Universitäts - Frauenklinik, Voßstr. 9, D-6900 Heidelberg, West Germany

Hirsutism, alopecia, acne and seborrhoea and virilism in the female are clinical symptoms of hyperandrogenism. Clinical signs and laboratory data (testosterone, free testosterone, dihydrotestosterone, dehydroepiandrosterone sulfate, 17a-hydroxyprogesterone, cortisol, dexamethasone, LH, FSH, prolactin and 17-ketosteroide in urine) are evaluatated to exclude an androgen producing tumor of the adrenal gland and of the ovary. In a prospective study with 50 premenopausal patients short time fluctuations of hormones in serum were determined at day 3 - 5 of the menstrual cycle (test day 1) and the cortisol day rhythm (8.00 a.m.,10.00 p.m.) was controlled. At 10 p.m. dexamethasone (DXM) (3 mg) was given orally and hormones were analysed the next morning (8.00 a.m.). ACTH stimulation was checked at day 7. From day 8 to 11 DXM (4x0.5 mg) was given and continued from day 12 to 21 to exclude a late onset of the adrenal depression. From day 22 to 25 a higher DXM dose (4x2 mg) showed result in a complete inhibition of the adrenal gland. From day 26 a continuous low dose DXM (0.5 mg at 8.00 p.m.) treatment was initiated for 12 weeks and followed by a hCG (5.000 IU im.) ovarian stimulation test. By these tests a cushing disease was found in two, a polycystic ovarian disease in four and enzyme defects or diminuished enzyme activity in the adrenal cortex was found in five patients. The interdepence of steroids and proteohormones in respective blood samples was analysed in respect to a correlation between the severity of the disease and changes in hormonal pattern. The results of the tests are interpreted and different treatment regimen are discussed. Furthermore the efficiency and side effects of a randomized treatment with cyproterone acetate versus spironolactone in hirsute patients (n=25) is analysed.

1993 Comparative evaluation of Estriol (E_3), Cystine amino peptidase (CAP), human Placental Lactogen (hPL) and Estradiol-17 beta (E_2) as predictors of fetal well being.

*Rajakumar, G., Raghavan, K.S., Sinha, M.K., Mathur, V.S. and Gupta, A.N. Departments of Pharmacology and Obstetrics & Gynecology, Post Graduate Institute of Medical Education and Research, Chandigarh-160 012 India.
*Presenting author, present address: Department of Neurosciences, 4N73, Health Sciences Centre, McMaster University, Hamilton, Ontario, Canada L8N 3Z5.

IUGR have been reported even in the absence of any maternal complications. In the present study, a battery of biochemical indices of fetal well being in a longitudinal study were evaluated. Thirty-one patients (with known LMP) during the first antenatal visit to the hospital were chosen at random and serial maternal blood samples were drawn at different weeks of gestation. Biochemical markers such as CAP (colorimetrically), hPL, E_2 and E_3 (Radio immunoassay) have been estimated in the plasma. All the 31 patients delivered live IUGR babies, without maternal complications during the antenatal period. (URGR - Intra uterine growth retardation).

While correlating the antenatal maternal values of the biochemical parameteres with the fetal outcome, it was found that the plasma estriol (a product of the fetal placental unit) was the best predictor of fetal well being/outcome rather than plasma CAP, hPL and E_2 (products of placental unit alone. According to the rank order of sensitivity, E_3 (93%) was followed by CAP (45%) hPL (29%) and E_2 (13%).

It is recommended that E_3 be included in any battery of tests for fetal well being. (This study was supported by the Indian Council of Medical Research).

1994 A RANDOMIZED DOUBLE-BLIND CONTROLLED STUDY ON THE USE OF BROMOCRIPTINE FOR THE TREATMENT OF CYCLIC MASTODYNIA, John H. Reynolds*, Maire T. Buckman, and Glenn T. Peake. Dept. of Medicine, Univ. of New Mexico and the Albuquerque VA Hospital, Albuquerque, N.M. 87131.

Fifteen normally cycling young women with normal serum prolactins consented to be enrolled. All were healthy, except for having cyclic mastodynia (premenstrual breast pain and tenderness, ameliorated at the onset of menses). Eight subjects received bromocriptine 2.5 mg bid and 7 a placebo in a randomized double-blind controlled fashion for 4 cycles. Four women who received bromocriptine experienced complete resolution of tenderness on breast exam by the last cycle, 3 had partial improvement, and 1 was unchanged. Two subjects had no side effects from the drug, and 6 reported mild side effects. The commonest complaint was nausea, most adverse reactions were significantly diminished or resolved by the end of the study, and all volunteers completed the study. In contrast, 3 members of the placebo-treated group experienced no change in their mastodynia, 2 had partial resolution, and only 1 had complete amelioration by the end of the study. The seventh member of this group was excluded because of accidental pregnancy. We conclude that bromocriptine was an effective and well-tolerated agent for the treatment of these euprolactinemic women with cyclic mastodynia. The mechanism for this effect of bromocriptine is unknown, but suppression of prolactin to low levels may play a role in resolution of the breast tenderness.

1995 TESTOSTERONE (T) CONCENTRATION IN SALIVA OF PATIENTS WITH CONGENITAL ADRENAL HYPERPLASIA (CAH). I. Rezvani*, A.M. DiGeorge, W.P. Slomiany, W.C. Rossi, T.H. Lipman, R.L. Joshlin, Dept. of Pediatrics, Temple Univ. Sch. Med., St. Christopher's Hospital for Children, Phila., PA 19133, USA

Salivary concentrations of steroid hormones are believed to reflect the free nonprotein-bound fraction of the hormone. We have measured the levels of T in 24 paired samples of sera and saliva from 20 patients (6 males, 14 females) with CAH (21-hydroxylase deficiency) ranging from 3 to 20 years of age. These results were compared with those from 20 normal adult males (24-34 years of age). Levels of T in saliva correlated well with T in serum in normal adults ($r=0.7$) and in patients with CAH ($r=0.9$). The mean level of T in saliva was significantly higher in patients with CAH than in normal adult males ($p < 0.01$) despite significantly lower mean levels of T in serum in patients with CAH ($p < 0.03$). Female patients with serum levels of T between 95 and 150 ng/dl had levels of T in saliva (17 to 35 ng/dl) equal to or greater than levels we found in normal adult males. Male patients had salivary levels of T as high as 10 times the mean level for normal males. Our data indicate that although concentration of T in saliva reflects the degree of therapeutic control of patients with CAH, salivary levels are higher than expected for the level of T in serum in patients whose disease is not under good control. The reason for this disproportionate elevation of T in saliva is unclear and is being investigated further.

1996 THE ENDOCRINE PROFILE DURING GESTRINONE TREATMENT. C. Robyn*, P. Bourdoux and G. Copinschi, Clinique d'Endocrinologie Sexuelle, Laboratoire de Médecine Expérimentale, Université Libre de Bruxelles and Laboratoire des Radioisotopes, Hôpital Saint-Pierre, 322 rue Haute, 1000-Bruxelles, Belgium.

Gestrinone (2.5 mg orally twice a week) is an anti-progesterone now used in the treatment of endometriosis. The purpose of this study was to investigate the effects of this steroid on serum levels of pituitary, ovarian, adrenal and thyroid hormones as measured by radioimmunoassays in six regularly menstruating volunteers tested daily during a control cycle, the first and third months of treatment. Mean levels of GH, DHEA-S and prolactin remained unchanged while those of total oestradiol, androstenedione, testosterone, cortisol, T3 and T4 were significantly reduced by 30-50% during Gestrinone administration. In addition, episodic increases in oestradiol took place; they were occasionally followed by very small LH peaks and by short and transient progesterone rises. Indeed LH and FSH secretions were not abolished as revealed by LH-RH tests performed at the end of the third month of treatment. Thus, Gestrinone at a dose effective in the treatment of endometriosis, reduces the serum levels of the total androgens and thyroid hormones and induces partial suppression of the ovarian activity. The effects of this steroid on the hormone binding proteins remain to be elucidated.

1997 INHIBITION OF THE KALLIKREIN-KININ SYSTEM AND VASCULAR REACTIVITY IN BARTTER'S SYNDROME. J.A.Rodríguez*, J.M.López and D.Mahana. Department of Endocrinology, School of Medicine, Catholic University of Chile. Casilla 114-D. Santiago-Chile.

To study the significance of the increased activity of the kallikrein-kinin system described in patients with Bartter's syndrome, the pressor response to infused angiotensin II (AII) was investigated in four patients with the syndrome receiving no treatment and during the administration of aprotinin and of indomethacin. All patients had increased urinary kallikrein; prostaglandin E_2 was high in all patients in whom it was measured (3/4). Aprotinin significantly ($p<0.05$) decreased the dose of AII required to induce a 20-mmHg increase in diastolic blood pressure, from 135±57 to 70±25 ng/kg/min (mean±SD), without significantly changing plasma renin activity, serum potassium, mean blood pressure or urinary prostaglandin E_2. Indomethacin normalized the pressor response to AII (pressor dose 10 ng/kg/min) in 3 patients who had been pre-treated for 4 days but not in one patient who received a single oral dose of indomethacin 5 hours before the test. Our results suggest that inhibition of the kallikrein-kinin system alone accounts for approximately a 50% decrease in vascular resistance to the pressor effect of AII in Bartter's syndrome, while additional suppression of prostaglandins entirely normalizes the vascular response to AII. These observations underscore the importance of the kallikrein-kinin system as a vasodilator in Bartter's syndrome and support the concept that this system may contribute to the regulation of blood pressure in man.
Funding: Grant 100/82 DIUC.

1998 RESULTS OF TRANSSPHENOIDAL SURGERY IN 60 ACROMEGALICS, F. Roelfsema*, M. Frölich and H. van Dulken. Dept. Endocrinology, Dept. Chemical Pathology and Dept. Neurosurgery. University Hospital, Leiden, the Netherlands.

We evaluated the results of transsphenoidal surgery in 60 acromegalics. Preoperative plasma GH levels varied from 8-600 mU/l. Postoperative levels normalized (i.e. $\leqq$ 5 mU/l = 2.5 ug/l) in 37 patients. A preoperative paradoxical increase of GH after TRH injection present in 33 patients normalized in 17 patients of whom 15 had postoperative GH levels $\leqq$ 5 mU/l. Most of the patients who had still increased GH levels or a paradoxical reaction to TRH postoperatively, received pituitary irradiation. Follow-up studies during 1-6 years (mean 3.2 years) of 16 non-irradiated patients with GH levels $\leqq$ 5 mU/l (of whom 10 had a normalized paradoxical response to TRH) showed no clinical and biochemical recurrence. In 22 postoperative irradiated patients the plasma GH level decreased during follow-up studies (duration 1-5 years, mean 2.2 years) and no recurrence occurred. However, 4 non-irradiated patients with either a plasma GH level > 5 mU/l or a paradoxical response to TRH postoperatively, showed a gradual increase of plasma GH, associated with clinical active acromegaly, during the follow-up period.

This study demonstrates that patients with postoperative plasma GH levels $\leqq$ 5 mU/l, particularly when associated with a normalized paradoxical GH response to TRH, have a favourable outcome. However, patients with postoperative GH > 5 mU/l, or with a persistent paradoxical response to TRH may show relapse during follow-up studies and in these cases additional pituitary irradiation is indicated.

1999 DIFFERENT PATTERNS OF PRL AND TSH RESPONSES AFTER DOPAMINE ANTAGONIST(DOMPERIDONE)AND TRH ADMINISTRATION IN PATIENTS AT DIFFERENT STAGES OF ANOREXIA NERVOSA.

M.Rolla*,A.Andreoni,D.Belliti,G.Andreani,S.Devescovi,M.Ceragioli, R.Paolicchi,A.Clerico,I Clinica Medica-Laboratorio Fisiologia Clinica CNR-Pisa, Italy.

PRL and TSH responses to Domperidone(DMP)(10mgr.i.v.)and to TRH(200μg i.v.) were evaluated in 15 female adolescents(age-range 14-18years)affected by anorexia nervosa(AN)and in 10 age-matched subjects as a control group. Patients(pts) were classified into 2 groups:group a)10 pts with 25-36% reduction of ideal body weight,prepubertal-like response to LHRH test, delayed TSH maximum response to TRH, serious psychological and eating behaviour disturbances;group b)5 pts in partial remission of the psychological disturbance,with normal weight and pubertal-like response to LHRH test.All pts were drug free.Group a)Mean basal PRL levels($5,6\pm1,3$ng/ml vs $12\pm6,5$ng/ml) and its increase after DMP administration($63,4\pm20,4$ng/ml vs $195\pm87,3$ng/ml)were found to be significantly($p<0,01$)lower as compared to the controls.No differences were observed in basal TSH levels;after DMP a TSH increase was observed only in subjects of the control group. Group b)The PRL and TSH responses to DMP were not different from those of the controls. No differences were observed in PRL and TSH responses to TRH between AN pts(groups A,B) and the controls. In agreement with the hypotheses of other authors our data suggest that dopamine activity in AN subjects is modified at least in the more severe stages of the disease. Further studies are necessary.

2000 REPRODUCTIVE DYSFUNCTION IN FEMALE BROOK TROUT FROM ACIDIFIED NORTHERN ONTARIO LAKES.

R.J.J. Roy*and W.H. Tam, Dept. of Zoology, University of Western Ontario, London, Ontario, N6A 5B7, Canada.

Published results from laboratory studies suggest that low pH could affect fish reproduction. This study examines the effects of low pH on reproduction of brook trout (Salvelinus fontinalis). Four neighbouring lakes in northern Ontario (approx. 83° W, 43° N) were sampled from June to November for two years. Lake size, temperature, photoperiod and food supply were similar for all lakes. The specific objective of the study is to determine if pH could influence aspects of the reproductive physiology of brook trout. The secondary growth phase of oogenesis was studied using histology, timing of ovulation and spawning determined by on-site observations, and plasma estrogens determined by RIA. Results show that rapid oogenesis began in mid-June in neutral lakes (NL), * whereas in acidic lakes (AL), it began in mid-July. Once commenced, the rate of oogenesis of fish from AL equalled or surpassed that of fish from NL, and no qualitative or quantitative differences in the ovary could be detected prior to ovulation. Ovulation and spawning in NL occurred by the first and second week of October, respectively, whereas trout from AL did not ovulate until the third week, and the majority of fish had not spawned by mid-November when all the lakes began to freeze over. Plasma estrogen levels of trout from NL and AL rose with rapid oogenesis and fell with ovulation and spawning. Thus, the acidity of lake water delayed the onset of oogenesis, ovulation and spawning of brook trout. This delay may affect the survival of trout embryos and alevins, and could alter the lake population. This study was supported by the Ontario Ministry of the Environment. *NL pH=7.2; AL pH=5.5

2001 PARTIAL PRIMARY STRUCTURE OF COHO SALMON GROWTH HORMONE (sGH).

S. Steiny*, D. King, R. Nishioka, P.W. Schilling and C. S. Nicoll, Depts. of Physiology Anatomy, Genetics, Zoology and the Cancer Research Lab., University of California, Berkeley, CA 94702 and California Biotechnology Inc., Mountain View, CA 94043, USA.

In order to obtain secreted salmon GH (sGH) for biological and chemical characterization the growth hormone cell region of pituitaries from coho salmon (Oncorhynchus kisutch) were incubated in organ culture at 14°C for five days. The sGH was purified from the culture medium using reverse phase liquid chromatography (HPLC). The GH fraction was lyophilized and tested for purity by HPLC and sodium dodecyl sulfate slab gel electrophoresis (SDSGE). The sGH was homogeneous and had a molecular weight of about 22,500 daltons by SDSGE, with a single NH_2-terminal residue. The first 41 NH_2-terminal amino acids were sequenced and were found to be NH_2-Ile-Glu-Asp-Glu-Arg-Leu-Phe-Asp-Ile-Ala-Val-Ser-Arg-Val-Glu-His-Leu-His-Leu-Leu-Ala-Glu-Try-Pro/Met*-Phe-Asn-Asp-Phe-Asp-Gly-Thr-Leu-Leu-Pro*/Met-Asp-Glu-Arg-Arg-Glu-Leu-Asn-. This sequence was compared to those of human (h) and bovine (b) GH, and with chum salmon prolactin (sPRL) (Kawauchi, Gen. Comp. Endocr. 49: 1983). The sequences were aligned to obtain maximal homology. Thus, the NH_2-terminal amino acid of sGH was aligned with the first one of sPRL, and with the fourth and fifth NH_2-terminal amino acids of hGH and bGH, respectively. In this sequence comparison 65% of the amino acids of the mammalian GH's are identical. sGH had 40% identical amino acid homology with hGH and bGH but only 28% identical homology with chum salmon PRL. Thus, in terms of structure the presumptive sGH is more closely related to mammalian GH's than it is to salmon PRL.

Supported by the California Sea Grant College Program, Project R/F-78.

2002 Plasma cortisol levels in Rusa deer (Cervus timorensis) after ACTH administration.

T.Stelmasiak*, S.van Mourik Attwood IVR Westmeadows Vic. Australia.

The activation of pituitary-adrenal system is a sensitive indicator of stress. The secretion of cortisol can be stimulated as effectively by environmental stressors as by administration of synthetic ACTH. The extent of the adrenal stimulation in response to stress or ACTH administration appears to be different in different species of animals. Rusa deer represent one of the most recently domesticated animals in Australia and many physiological parameters are unknown. We investigated the effect of different doses of ACTH on adrenal activity in Rusa deer. Mature stags (appr.BW 100 kg) were immobilized$^{\Delta}$ for a total of 2.5 hours, cannulated and blood samples were taken at 10 minute intervals. The animals were challenged with different doses of synthetic ACTH i.v.(0(n=2), 0.37(n=2), 0.75(n=3), 1.5(n=3), 3.0 (n=3), 6.0(n=3) i.u./stag). Cortisol levels were measured using a double antibody RIA. Maximum cortisol levels recorded for different ACTH doses were: 0.37:45.31±8.3;0.75:85.64±16.2;1.5:68.69±21.8;3.0:90.52±5.3;6.0;125.94±16.7 ng/ml±SD. The areas under the response curve, after substracting baseline values, for each dose were: 11.0±1.4;28.9±7.5;45.5±20.6;62.2±6.2; 85.0±11.8 respectively. The regression equation for logdose of ACTH was Y (area)=60.02* logdose+36.03 (r=0.99). In comparison with results for other species (sheep; Fulkerson and Jamieson, 1982; pigs: Moss, 1981) Rusa deer appear to be extremely sensitive to ACTH administration. Further investigations are being conducted in order to establish whether this phenomenon is characteristic to Rusa species or rather is associated with wild animals in general. Fulkerson, W.J., Jamieson P.A.(1982) Aust.J.Biol.Sci.35:215. Moss B.W. (1981) in: Current topics in Vet.Med.and Anim.Sci.Vol.11:112.
ΔRompun 50mg Bayer AG W.Germany, Fentaz 0.6ml Ethnor Pty.Ltd. Australia.

2003 MECHANISM OF EPINEPHRINE DERIVED DRUGS ON LONG LASTING PARATHYROID HORMONE (PTH). E. Shimizu, Y. Okamoto, K. Ota* and J. Maeda. Division of Gerontology, Department of Medicine, Wakayama Medical College, Department of Laboratory Medicine, Wakayama Medical College, Japan.

Since the epinephrine-induced Parathyroid Hormone (PTH) secretion is only short-lasting and immediatly followed desensitization. Attempt is made to prolong PTH release, mediated via adenylate cyclase system and the mechanism of desensitization on PTH release by the action of epinephrine. Using bovine parathyroid cell test tube incubation, the well defined bovine tissue perifusion system and the infusion study in male wistar rats, our synthesized drugs were confirmed to have long activating PTH release via high affinity of them to cells and activation of adenylate cyclase activity, as described herein. These drugs were derived from epinephrine tagged to 15 fatty acid to ethanolamine of epinephrine. The action of epinephrine was suggested to be rapidly disappeared by the conversion of epinephrine into adenochrome in cell membrane and to sustain the long lasting epinephrine like action by the stimulus of those drugs, by which was caused by the protection from binding H^+ in ethanolamine with OH^- in benzene ring attaching 15 fatty acid to epinephrine.

2004 ACTIVATION, DESENSITIZATION AND RECYCLING OF FROG ERYTHROCYTE β-ADRENERGIC RECEPTORS: DIFFERENTIAL PERTURBATION BY IN SITU TRYPSINIZATION.
B. Strulovici* and R.J. Lefkowitz, Depts. of Medicine and Biochemistry, Duke University Medical Center, Durham, North Carolina 27710 U.S.A.

We have utilized limited in situ trypsinization of the adenylate cyclase coupled β-adrenergic receptor of frog erythrocytes to probe the processes of receptor activation, desensitization and recycling. Treatment of intact erythrocytes with trypsin (1 mg/ml) for 1 hour at 20°C converts all the receptor peptides (identified by photoaffinity labeling with p-azido-^{125}I-benzylcarazolol) from a ∿ 58,000 M_r to a ∿ 40,000 M_r species. Nonetheless, the trypsinized β-adrenergic receptors bind agonists and antagonists with unaltered affinity and with no change in the number of binding sites. Moreover, the ability of the proteolyzed receptors to interact with the nucleotide regulatory protein to form a high affinity guanine nucleotide sensitive state and to activate adenylate cyclase were also unaltered. However, upon exposure of intact cells to the agonist isoproterenol, trypsinized β-adrenergic receptors were more rapidly and more completely cleared from the plasma membranes ("down-regulated") than untrypsinized receptors . Whereas down-regulated receptors from non-trypsinized cells appear to recycle to the cell surface after removal of the agonist, internalized trypsinized β-adrenergic receptors do not recycle to the plasma membrane and appear to be degraded within the cell. These data suggest that in situ proteolysis of the receptors might serve as a physiological trigger for their internalization and degradation.

2005 REGULATION OF RAT KIDNEY ADENYLATE CYCLASE BY FORSKOLIN. S. Sulimovici*, C.A. Breyer and M.S. Roginsky, Nassau County Medical Center, East Meadow, NY 11554 U.S.A.

The effect of forskolin on the activation of adenylate cyclase by guanyl nucleotides, fluoride ion and parathyroid hormone (PTH) was studied in rat renal membranes. In this system forskolin produced a 10-12 fold increase in the specific activity of renal adenylate cyclase with an apparent K_m value of 5 μM. The adenylate cyclase response to bovine PTH (1-34), GTP or its analog guanyl-5'-yl imidodiphosphate (Gpp(NH)p), sodium fluoride (NaF), as well as combined PTH and the guanyl nucleotide, was increased by the addition of diterpene. Forskolin (10 μM) with Gpp(NH)p (10 μM) and with the combination of PTH (2.5 U) and GTP (10 μM) caused a synergistic effect on adenylate cyclase activity, while similar concentrations of forskolin with GTP, NaF (5 mM) or PTH and PTH with Gpp(NH)p produced an additive effect. Extraction of the guanine nucleotide-binding regulatory component (G/F) from the kidney membranes with 1% sodium cholate did not affect the stimulation of adenylate cyclase by forskolin (28.5 ± 3.1 to 182.9 ± 10.4 pmoles/mg protein/min). Uncoupling of the G/F component, by treating membranes with 30 mM $MnCl_2$, did not affect forskolin stimulation but did abolish the effects of the guanyl nucleotides. The present data indicate that: 1) forskolin interacts with various stimulators of adenylate cyclase by potentiating activation in both synergistic and additive manners; 2) forskolin stimulates the adenylate cyclase system by acting mainly at the catalytic site of the enzyme, a mechanism which is different from that of hormones, guanyl nucleotides or NaF.

2006 THE HORMONE DISTRIBUTION PROGRAM OF NIH - NIADDK. Robert A. Tolman*, Salvatore Raiti and Albert F. Parlow. NIADDK, NIH, Bethesda, MD; National Hormone and Pituitary Program, Baltimore, MD; and Pituitary Center, Harbor - UCLA Medical Center, Torrance, CA.

In the early 1960's, the National Institute of Arthritis, Diabetes and Digestive and Kidney Diseases (NIADDK), one of the Institutes of the National Institutes of Health (NIH), established a hormone distribution program for the purpose of supplying hormones for clinical and basic research. From an initial inventory of 14 animal hormones plus human growth hormone, this program has expanded to the point where 60 or more hormone preparations and subunits are prepared and distributed. Eleven species of animals, including humans, are represented. In addition, antisera to many of these materials have been developed and are available for radioimmunoassay, immunocytochemistry and immunoprecipitation. The hormone and antiserum production portion of the program isolates highly purified pituitary and other hormones, as well as polyclonal antibodies with high afinity, specificity and sensitivity. Hormones and antisera elaborated as well as outlines of some extraction methods will be discussed.

2007 EFFECT OF CONTINUOUS GNRH AGONIST TREATMENT ON SERUM LH AND TESTOSTERONE: RESPONSE TO GNRH AND TESTICULAR HISTOLOGY IN MALE RHESUS MONKEYS. D.R. Mann*, K.G. Gould, M. Smith and D.C. Collins, Morehouse School of Medicine, Yerkes Primate Research Center, Emory University School of Medicine/VA Medical Center, Atlanta, GA 30310, USA.

Three adult male rhesus monkeys were treated continuously (osmotic minipump) for 20 wk with a GnRH agonist (Ag, Wyeth Labs; Wy-40972; 25 µg/day). Ag treatment led to a transient rise (first two days) followed by a precipitous fall in serum levels of LH and testosterone (T). Basal levels of serum LH and T fell below pretreatment values within two wk of beginning Ag treatment where they remained throughout Ag administration. Responses of serum LH and T to 50 µg GnRH were abolished by four wk of Ag treatment. Testicular volume decreased to 10% of pretreatment values over the 20 wk of Ag administration. Testicular histology (needle biopsies) at 20 wk of Ag treatment showed a complete arrest of spermatogenesis in two animals. Seminiferous tubules were atrophied. Germinal cell division and mature spermatids were absent. The third animal exhibited an incomplete block of spermatogenesis. Germinal cell division was evident in this animal, but few, if any, mature spermatids were present in the seminiferous tubules. There was no sign of a focal block of spermatogenesis or calcification of tubules in any animals. A complete restoration of testicular volume and spermatogenesis occurred by three mo posttreatment. Our data suggest that continuous Ag administration is an effective and reversible method of blocking spermatogenesis in the male rhesus monkey. Supported by Wyeth Laboratories, NIH Grants RR-08006 and RR-00165 and NSF Grant PCM-81-19793.

2008 SUPPRESSION OF PITUITARY AND TESTICULAR FUNCTIONS IN HEALTHY MEN BY CONSTANT GNRH AGONIST INFUSION. Th. Schürmeyer, U.A. Knuth, H.P. Lange, C.W. Freischem, J. Sandow (x), F.Bint Akhtar and E. Nieschlag*, Max Planck Clinical Research Unit for Reproductive Medicine, Steinfurter Straße 107, D-4400 Münster and (x) Hoechst AG, D-6000 Frankfurt, F.R. Germany.

In a trial for male fertility control the effects of constant GnRH agonist (buserelin) infusion on pituitary and testicular function were investigated. The agonist was administered subcutaneously over 12 weeks to two groups of healthy young men from osmotic minipumps worn extracorporally. Seven men received 118 $\pm$ 24 µg/day from pumps changed biweekly, four men received 230 $\pm$ 27 µg/day from pumps changed weekly. After an initial rise serum LH, FSH and testosterone decreased. The decrease occurred faster in the higher dose group in whom the LH response to acute GnRH stimulation was lost under treatment, while the response was drastically reduced in the other group. Androgen substitution with testosterone undecanoate (80-120 mg p.o.) daily was initiated when the subjects complained about decreased libido and/or potency or when serum testosterone fell below 10 nmol/l, on average in the fifth week. Sperm counts decreased significantly and below the lower normal limit of 20 mill./ml. The nadir was reached in week 12 of treatment in the higher dose group, and in week 4 post treatment in the lower dose group. Constant infusion of the GnRH agonist was very effective in terms of desensitization of the pituitary and suppression of endocrine testicular function. However, a higher dose appears to be required to achieve azoospermia.

2009 EFFECT OF BREAST VS FORMULA FEEDING ON CIRCULATING THYROXINE LEVELS IN PREMATURE INFANTS.

L.V. Oberkotter*, G. Pereira, M.H. Paul, H. Ling and M. Farber, Dept. of Gynecology and Obstetrics, Albert Einstein Med. Ctr., N.D., and The Children's Hosp. of Phila., Philadelphia, PA, U.S.A.

Circulating thyroxine levels at initial (T_4-1) and follow-up (T_4-2) screening for congenital hypothyroidism were measured in two groups of premature infants (750-2000 g) receiving either breast milk (BF,n=11) or formula feeding (FF,n=19) with varying degrees (0-60%) of caloric intake as hyperalimentation (HAL). Initial T_4 levels were equally depressed in BF (3.17 $\pm$ 0.38 μg T_4/dl;mean $\pm$ SD) and FF (3.27 $\pm$ 0.29 μg/dl) infants. At follow-up, pronounced increases in T_4 levels occurred in both groups ($p<0.001$); T_4-2 levels in the breast milk-fed group were, however, significantly higher (8.69 $\pm$ 0.60 μg/dl) than those of their formula-fed counterparts (6.76 $\pm$ 0.68 μg/dl, $p<0.03$). Further, no BF infants had T_4-2 levels <6.0, whereas 47% of T_4-2 levels in FF infants were <6.0; birth weight, gestational age, and post-partum age at the time of T_4-2 were not significantly different. The observed differences in T_4-2 levels persisted when the groups were subdivided on the basis of % calories received as HAL, and were most pronounced in the group receiving >10-60% HAL (7.40 $\pm$ 0.58 μg/dl BF vs 4.99 $\pm$ 0.71 μg/dl FF, $p<0.025$). The resulting data are in agreement with previous reports of the presence of thyroidal substances in breast milk and their influence upon thyroid economy in the full-term neonate. The data further indicate that mode of nutrition can influence thyroid hormone status in premature infants, and that T_4 levels in breast milk-fed premature neonates at 3-4 wks of life are high compared with those of their formula-fed counterparts.

2010 ONTOGENY OF MULTIPLE MOLECULAR WEIGHT FORMS OF IMMUNOREACTIVE (IR) ACTH IN THE HUMAN PITUITARY GLAND.

C.R. Parker, Jr.* and J.C. Porter, Dept. of Obstet. and Gyn., Univ. Texas Southwestern Med. School, Dallas, 75235, TX, USA.

The factor(s), other than ACTH 1-39, that regulates growth and steroidogenesis in the fetal adrenal cortex is unknown. Inasmuch as there are multiple products that are derived from the precursor of ACTH, and since such products may influence adrenal function, we investigated the ontogeny of ACTH and structurally related peptides in the human pituitary. Anterior pituitary glands were obtained at autopsy (1-20 hr postmortem) from fetuses, infants, and adults. Tissues were extracted in 5 M acetic acid according to the methods of Eipper and Mains (Endo. Rev., 1:1, 1980). Extracts were brought to 8 M urea and were chromatographed on columns of Sephadex G-75. Column fractions were evaporated, suspended in PBS, and assayed for ACTH by RIA (mid-portion antiserum). Of the 5 distinct forms of IR-ACTH detected, one had a fractional elution volume (Kd) identical to that of ACTH 1-39 (0.62); the others were apparently larger and comprized about 20% of the total IR-ACTH. Whereas the relative amounts of ACTH 1-39 were similar in each age group, those of the 3 largest IR-ACTH forms differed ($P<0.005$) among these groups. Fetuses had the most (9.0% of total IR-ACTH) of the largest IR-ACTH form (Kd=0.07) and the least amounts of IR-ACTH having Kds of 0.18 (3.9%) and 0.27 (1.2%). Values for infants were intermediate between those of fetuses and adults. We conclude that processing of the ACTH precursor is altered during development and that such changes may play a role in adrenal maturation. Supported by HD 14513.

2011 BIOLOGICAL RESPONSES OF ESTRIOL, ESTRIOL-3-SULFATE AND ESTRIOL-3-SULFATE + TAMOXIFEN IN THE FETAL AND NEWBORN UTERI OF GUINEA PIG. J.R. Pasqualini* and B.-L. Nguyen, C.N.R.S. Steroid Hormone Research Unit, Foundation for Hormone Research, 26 boulevard Brune, 75014 Paris, France.

After administration of estriol (E_3) (1 mg/Kg/day) or estriol-3-sulfate (E_3-S) (1.4 mg/Kg/day) to pregnant guinea pigs (49-60 days of gestation) for 6 consecutive days a similar uterotrophic effect is observed in the fetal uterus for both treatments ; the weight increases 1.8-2.5 times in relation to the non-treated animals. In the same fetal tissue the stimulation is very intense for the progesterone receptor : 7-12 times in relation to the control animals. In another series of experiments newborn guinea pigs (2-days-old) were treated with : E_3 (100 μg/animal), E_3-S (140 μg/animal) or E_3-S + tamoxifen (T) (140 μg + 300 μg/animal) for 2 days (Experiment A) or 12 days (Experiment B). In relation to the non-treated animals in Experiment A, the weight of the uterus increases by 65, 130, 110 % respectively, the PR increases respectively 1.3, 1 and 1.5 times per mg of DNA. In Experiment B, the weight of the uterus increases by 310, 350, 540 % respectively and the PR increases 0.7, 0.7 and 1 times respectively. Histological studies show an intense hypertrophic effect, particularly in the epithelium of the endometrium of the fetal and newborn uteri after the different treatment with E_3, E_3-S or E_3-S + T. In the newborns an intense uterotrophic effect is also observed on the uterine glands. It is concluded that : I) the uterotrophic effect of E_3 or E_3-S is very intense both before and after birth, II) the stimulatory effect on PR decreases very significantly after birth, III) E_3-S can act as a potent estrogen precursor, IV) tamoxifen does not antagonize the effects provoked by E_3-S.

2012 NATURE AND PROPERTIES OF MATERIAL BOUND TO SEX HORMONE BINDING GLOBULIN (SHBG) IN PREGNANCY SERUM. A. Philip* and B.E. Pearson Murphy, Reproductive Physiology Unit, Montreal General Hospital and Reproductive Centre, McGill University, Montreal, Canada.

The 'total androgen' levels as measured by competitive binding to SHBG in late pregnancy serum are about 15-fold higher than in non-pregnant serum, yet the levels of testosterone and other known ligands rise only slightly or not at all during pregnancy. When maternal serum extract was fractionated on a Sephadex LH-20 column, the bulk of SHBG-bindable material eluted in the region of low polarity and consisted of 3 major peaks which did not correspond to any of the known sex steroids. Peak 1 has been tentatively identified as 5α-pregnane-3,20-dione and peak 3 as 2-methoxyestrone on the basis of their elution patterns, cross-reactivity data in various assays and their known plasma levels. Peak 2 remains unidentified; its levels are variable in early gestation, continue high through late pregnancy, and fall towards term, being undetectable at the time of spontaneous labour, whether premature or term. Peak 2 appears to be of placental origin since placental levels were 5-10 fold higher than but parallel with those of serum, while they were undetectable in other fetal tissues (ovary, testis, liver and adrenal); it is strongly bound to SHBG, having an affinity close to that of testosterone under physiological conditions (37°C, undiluted serum). In summary, about half the material bound to SHBG in pregnancy consists of substances not previously recognized as SHBG ligands, viz. 5α-pregnane-3,20-dione, 2-methoxyestrone, and a still unidentified compound which appears to be placental in origin and falls in association with premature and term labour.

2013 PERSISTENCE OF MULLERIAN DUCTS IN MALE RABBITS PASSIVELY IMMUNIZED AGAINST ANTI-MULLERIAN HORMONE DURING FETAL LIFE. J.Y. Picard*, D. Tran, B. Vigier and N. Josso, Unité de Recherches de Génétique Médicale INSERM, Hôpital des Enfants Malades, 75743 Paris Cedex 15, France.

Male differentiation of the genital tract is characterized by regression of Müllerian ducts, produced by anti-Müllerian hormone (AMH), synthesized by fetal Sertoli cells, and by stabilization of Wolffian ducts and masculinization of the urogenital sinus and external genitalia, induced by testosterone or by its reduced metabolite. Dissociation between events mediated by either AMH or testosterone occurs in human patients in whom the biosynthesis or peripheral effect of one of the hormones is impaired, usually through a congenital error of metabolism. For instance, persistence of Müllerian derivatives in normally virilized males is genetically transmitted as an X-linked condition, which affects the biosynthesis of either AMH or its putative Müllerian receptor. We have obtained the same result in rabbits by blocking endogenous testicular AMH through transplacental passage of anti-AMH antibodies induced in the mother. A female rabbit was repeatedly injected with 12 µg AMH, and developed anti-AMH antibodies detectable by ELISA. She was then mated, and a booster injection of 24 µg administered at the 8th day of pregnancy, allowing peak levels of circulating antibodies to develop at 14 days, the time when the rabbit fetal testis first begins to produce AMH detectable by immunocytochemistry. Three successive litters were obtained in similar conditions, producing a total of 13 males. Only 3 had normally regressed Müllerian ducts, in all the others Müllerian ducts were present, although Wolffian and prostatic development were similar to that of normal male controls. Testicular position and structure were apparently normal. The present data confirm the dual nature of fetal testicular secretion and indicate that AMH is not required for testicular descent in fetal life.

2014 THE INFLUENCE OF LACTATIONAL HORMONES ON MAMMARY GLAND BIOLOGY IN RATS TREATED WITH 7,12-DIMETHYLBENZANTHRACENE (DMBA) DURING GESTATION. H.S. Pitkow*, M. Goldman, and W. Urbas, Penna. Col. of Podiatric Med. and Hahnemann Med. Col., Phila., PA., 19107, U.S.A.

We have reported that DMBA administered to pregnant rats caused a significant decrease in mammary gland nucleic acid contents on day 1 post-partum. No significant differences were found on days 6 and 11. The retarded litter weight on day 6 was normal by day 11. In order to determine the effects of DMBA on hormones essential for lactation, female adult virgin Long Evans rats (12 animals/group) were intraperitoneally injected daily with 1 mg DMBA in 0.2cc sesame oil on days 8 through 12 of pregnancy. On days 1, 3, and 8 postpartum prolactin or corticosterone serum levels were determined by radioimmunoassay. On day 1 of lactation we observed a significant decrease in corticosterone levels (32.8 ± 2.7 µg/100ml) in DMBA rats when compared to controls (55.9 ± 5.2 µg/100ml). No significant differences were found in corticosterone levels on day 8 nor prolactin levels on day 3. Our data suggests that DMBA in pregnancy suppresses the normal increase in corticosterone levels in early lactation thereby depressing mammary gland growth (i.e., DNA) and secretion (i.e., RNA). We believe the normalization of corticosterone levels by day 8 between control and DMBA groups account for the mammary gland rebound phenomenon.

2015 INSULIN RECEPTORS IN HUMAN BRAIN. ONTOGENIC STUDY.

N. Potau*, E. Riudor and A. Ballabriga. Ciudad Sanitaria Valle de Hebrón, Hospital Infantil, Universidad Autónoma. Barcelona, Spain.

Little information is available concerning the ontogeny of the receptor for insulin in human beings. The following study attempts to contribute with new data on insulin receptors in C.N.S. Synaptosomal membrane fraction was obtained from infants, between 12 to 24 hours post-mortem. Fraction heterogeneity was assesed by electronic microscopy and enzymatic determinations: 5'mononucleotidase and Na^+ K^+ ATPase. Specific ^{125}I-insulin binding has been detected in all regions of the C.N.S. studied wich was greater in the cerbrum, 20 %/mg than in the cerebellum and thalamus, 12.2 %/ mg and 16.3 %/mg respectively. Binding constants of insulin receptors in human brain were obtained by a computerized aproach assumming two classes of binding sites. Insulin receptors were present as early as 14 weeks of gestation with important decreases around 30th weeks of gestation and after birth. Mean value of receptor number was 6 pmol/mg before 20th weeks of gestation and 0.6, 0.3 pmol/mg after birth and in adulthood respectively. The early appearance of insulin receptors in a high concentration in human brain may be related to maturation of this tissues in coincidence with a critical point around 30th weeks of gestation.

2016 THE EFFECT OF EGF AND DEXAMETHASONE ON SOMATOMEDIN SECRETION BY FETAL HEPATOCYTES.

Robert A. Richman*, Mark R. Benedict, James R. Florini, Barbara A. Toly and Ira H. Ames. Department of Pediatrics and Anatomy, SUNY Upstate Medical Center, and Department of Biology, Syracuse University, Syracuse, NY 13210, U.S.A.

To determine which hormones might regulate fetal somatomedin (SM) secretion, we measured SM levels in conditioned medium from primary cultures of fetal rat hepatocytes. We employed a displacement assay (competition for binding of radiolabeled multiplication stimulating activity (MSA) to the SM binding protein) for total SM and the radioimmunoassay for SM-C. EGF and dexamethasone (DEX) were the most active hormones tested, as measured by the displacement assay, stimulating SM levels 2-3 times above the control. Rat growth hormone (GH) was much less stimulatory. Human placental lactogen (hPL), glucagon and insulin had little effect. Stimulation of SM secretion by both EGF and DEX was time- and dose-dependent. The maximal response occurred at 48 hours, at a concentration of about 1×10^{-7} M of either hormone. EGF also altered the surface characteristics of the fetal hepatocytes in a time- and dose-dependent manner. Using scanning electron microscopy, we found that both EGF-treated and control hepatocytes formed cellular aggregates within 6 hours. After 48 hours, the EGF-treated cells were considerably different. The cellular aggregates were thicker, the intercellular boundaries were more easily discernible, cell surfaces had ridges, numerous microvilli, and cytoplasmic excrescences or blebs suggestive of secretory activity. We conclude that EGF and DEX, but not GH or hPL, stimulated the secretion by fetal hepatocytes of a fetal SM which resembled MSA. The effects of EGF on fetal hepatocyte SM secretion and morphology may be related.

2017 DOES THE FETAL LUNG PRODUCE ACTH?

R.Riquelme,M.Serón-Ferré,A.Germain,and A.Llanos*.Dept Preclin Div.Oriente,Fac.Med,U de Chile.& Rep Endocr Ctr,UCSF,SF,CA.

Since ectopic ACTH is found in lung carcinoma and in placenta we investigated 1) the content of immunoreactive ACTH (iACTH) in human fetal lung and placenta and 2) whether fetal lung iACTH is secreted into amniotic fluid (AF). iACTH content was measured in 6 human fetal lungs and placentas (GA 15-20 wks) obtained from Path Dept,UCSF. iACTH was extracted with silicic acid and measured by RIA using a kit from Immuno Nuclear Co. iACTH content was 0.23±0.09 pg/mg wet tissue ($\bar{x}$±SE) in lung and 0.29±0.06 in placenta. 3 ewes were operated at 80% of gestation. Catheters were placed into the fetal vessels,amniotic cavity and in the fetal trachea to prevent pulmonary fluid (PF) from reaching AF. Fetal plasma, AF and PF were collected daily. Tracheal obstruction was started after 2 days of control sampling and lasted 13 days. iACTH was undetectable in PF. AF iACTH did not change during tracheal obstruction. In contrast,fetal plasma iACTH increased from 38±5 to 150±40 pg/ml ($p<0.025$). These results show that fetal lung contains iACTH,but is not secreted into the PF and AF. The increase in iACTH in fetal plasma after tracheal obstruction is unlikely to be a response to stress since blood gases were normal in the obstructed fetuses. Therefore it is possible that fetal lung ACTH is secreted into the fetal circulation.
(Supported by grant B-904-8344,DDI,U.de Chile)

2018 SPECIFIC CORTISOL BINDING IN HUMAN FETAL MEMBRANES, AMNIOTIC FLUID AND SERUM. L. Riopel*, J.C. Kossmann, J.C. Lavoie, R.J. Gauthier and W. Gibb. Research Unit on Reproductive and Developmental Biology, Centre de Recherche Pédiatrique, Hôpital Sainte-Justine and Dept. Obs/Gyn, University of Montreal, Montreal, Quebec, Canada.

A transcortin-like protein which binds cortisol and progesterone has been described in human fetal membranes and appears to be extracellular. Because of the importance of these tissues in relation to the onset of labor and the importance of cortisol and progesterone in parturition of various species, we have attempted to further characterize the properties and distribution of this protein. With fetal membranes obtained from dichorionic twin pregnancies specific binding was found in the area of the membranes not in contact with decidua, indicating that the presence of the protein in the membranes is unlikely due to serum contamination. Certain physico-chemical characteristics of the specific cortisol binding in amnion, amniotic fluid and serum were then compared. The binding protein(s) in the three tissues had the same electrophoretic properties. In both term amniotic fluid and amnion the interaction of the protein(s) with Concanavalin A was less than in pre-term amniotic fluid and plasma ($p < 0.05$), indicating that the protein in term amniotic fluid and amnion differs in its state of glycosylation from serum transcortin. This, and the presence of the protein in the area of the membranes of dichorionic twin pregnancies not in contact with decidua, are consistent with the specific cortisol binding in human fetal membranes being of amniotic fluid origin.
Supported by M.R.C. (Canada).

2019 SOMATOSTATIN DEPLETING ACTIVITY OF CYSTEAMINE-RELATED THIOLS AND AMINES IS A DETERMINANT OF THEIR DUODENAL ULCEROGENIC POTENCY. Sandor Szabo* and Seymour Reichlin. Brigham and Women's Hosp., Harvard Med. Sch. and Tufts-New Engl. Med. Center, Boston, Mass. U.S.A.

Cysteamine ($HS-CH_2-CH_2-NH_2$), a potent duodenal ulcerogen (DU) stimulates gastric acid and gastrin secretion, and depletes immunoreactive somatostatin (IRS) from the gut and hypothalamus of the rat (Endocrinology, 109, 2255, 1981). To elucidate the structural requirements for this effect we compared the DU potency of a series of cysteamine analogues with their IRS depleting activity. Adult female Sprague-Dawley rats were killed 4 hr after p.o. dose of the test chemicals given in molar equivalents to 30mg/100g of cysteamine-HCl. IRS depleting activity in gastric mucosa, expressed as % of controls is listed in descending order with Duodenal Ulcerogenic Index (DUI) (J. Pharm. Exp. Ther., 223, 68, 1982): cystamine (55%, 2.0); cysteamine (59%, 2.4); 2-dimethylaminoethanethiol (59%, 0.4); ethylamine (66%, 1.2); 1,3-propanedithiol (70%, 0.4); propylamine (75%, 0.5). The following thiols and amines had no IRS depleting effect (>80% of controls) and DUI (0-0.3): L-cysteine, ethanethiol, 1-propanethiol, penicillamine, dimercaprol, 1,4-dithiothreitol, ethanolamine. The DU potency of cysteamine-related chemicals is significantly ($p<0.01$) correlated with their IRS depleting activity ($r=-0.738$). IRS depletion is hence essential for DU activity of thiols and amines. Structural requirements are the presence of either -SH or $-NH_2$ on a 2-3 carbon alkyl molecule. Both radicals together increase potency, insertion of a carboxyl group next to amine in cysteamine (i.e., cysteine) abolishes both IRS depleting and DU potency. Thus, IRS depletion and induction of duodenal ulcer is an unique and correlated property of cysteamine and its close derivatives.

2020 GIP RESPONSE TO GLUCOSE IN STZ AND VMH RATS *IN VIVO*. J. Takemura*, Y. Seino, S. Matsukura and H. Imura, Second Division, Department of Internal Medicine and Clinical Nutrition, Kyoto University School of Medicine, Kyoto 606, Japan.

Since a close relationship between insulin (Ins) and gastric inhibitory polypeptide (GIP) has been suggested, GIP response to glucose from a rat intestinal perfusion *in vivo* was measured in both streptozotocin diabetic rats (STZ) and ventromedial hypothalamic lesioned rats (VMH). Male Wistar rats were administered iv 60mg/kg streptozotocin. Control rats were given saline alone. VMH nuclei of female Wistar rats were destroyed electrically. Rats sham-operated without current served as controls. After 4-5 weeks, the perfusion study was performed. Under anesthesia, the lumen of the small intestine was perfused with saline at a rate of 2ml/min from a point just below the pylorus to the ileal end, through which the contents were allowed to drain. 50mM glucose was introduced into the lumen over a 30min period. Blood was collected from the jugular vein each 10min over a 50min period. Plasma glucose levels were remarkably high and the Ins response to glucose was very poor in STZ. The basal plasma GIP in STZ was significantly elevated compared to controls. However, the mean peak values of GIP after glucose loading were not different from each other. The $\Sigma\Delta$GIP during a 30min period demonstrated a significantly diminished GIP response in STZ compared to normals. Plasma Ins concentrations in VMH were 4-9 fold higher than controls over the entire study period. Both basal GIP and glucose-induced GIP secretion was markedly higher in VMH than in controls. These results suggest that Ins has no suppressive effect on GIP release and that metabolic derangement affect GIP secretion.

2021 β-ENDORPHIN LIKE IMMUNOREACTIVITY IN HUMAN NORMAL AND PATHOLOGICAL GASTRO-INTESTINAL TISSUES. A. Tari*, Y. Miyachi and A. Miyoshi, Department of Internal Medicine, University of Hiroshima, Hiroshima and Shizuoka General Hospital, Shizuoka, Japan.

Effects of β-Endorphin(β-EP) on gastrointestinal functions were known, however, little information was available concerning the presence and characteristics of β-EP like immunoreactivity(β-EP-LI) in the human normal and pathological gastrointestinal tissues. Mucosal and muscle layer from gastric antrum and fundus, gastric carcinomas and intestinal tissues were extracted with boiling 1Nacetic acid, treated by Heparin-Mn^{++} in order to exclude lipoprotein and then subjected to specific β-EP radioimmunoassay and also to gelchromatography on Sephacryl G-50 superfine column(0.9x90cm). β-EP-LI in mucosal and muscle layer of gastric antrum and fundus, and in intestines were 10 -50ng/g tissue. In moderately differentiated gastric adenocarcinoma β-EP-LI is high, especially in two cases it was more than 300ng/g tissue. In contrast, β-EP-LI was low in poorly differentiated gastric adenocarcinoma. β-EP-LI in the normal gastric mucosa and muscle was eluted mainly in the position corresponding to β-Lipotropin(β-LPH), while in the gastric adenocarcinoma in the position of β-EP. The degradation of β-EP in vitro by the tissue homogenates was very rapid, less than 25% being left in 5 min incubation with both gastric mucosa and moderately differentiated adenocarcinoma. The high β-EP-LI in the moderately differentiated gastric adenocarcinoma and the low in the poorly differentiated adenocarcinoma with the characteristic elution profiles on Sephacryl G-50 suggest the different processing of β-EP synthesis in the tumor tissues and some role of β-EP in the differentiation and proliferation of carcinoma.

2022 COXSACKIE B VIRUS SPECIFIC IgM RESPONSES, COMPLEMENT-FIXING ISLET CELL ANTIBODIES, HLA DR ANTIGENS AND C-PEPTIDE SECRETION IN 94 NEWLY DIAGNOSED TYPE I DIABETICS. G.Schernthaner*, J.E.Banatvala, W.Scherbaum, W.R.Mayr, M.Borkenstein, E.Schober. Universities of Vienna and Graz, Austria, Department of Virology, St.Thomas'Hospital, London, University of Tübingen, FRG.

Genetically determined disease susceptibility, viral infections and autoimmune mechanisms are thought to be involved in the pathogenesis of type-I diabetes. However, no information exists concerning a possible interrelation among these factors. We report on a one-year prospective follow-up study of 94 newly diagnosed type-I diabetics, whereby CB-virus specific-IgM responses (CB-V-IgM-R), complement-fixing islet cell antibodies (CF-ICA) and C-peptide were studied at diagnosis and two wk thereafter. All patients (pat) were characterized by HLA DR phenotypes.

Results: 1) CB-V-IgM-R were observed in 15 of 68 (22%) pat with early onset, but in only 1 of 26 pat with late onset above 20 yrs. Interestingly, 4 of these 16 sera were only positive two wk after, but not at diagnosis. 13 out of 16 pat showing CB-V-IgM-R were DR4 positive. 2) CF-ICA (IgG-ICA)were dedected in 48%(60%) of the sera at diagnosis and were not correlated to CB-V-IgM-R. Interestingly, 3 pat showed CF-ICA two wk before CB-V-IgM-R could be dedected. 3) C-peptide at diagnosis did not correlate with CB-V-IgM-R, presence or absence of CF-ICA and HLA DR phenotypes.

The data of this study indicate that 20% of type-I diabetics (predominantely DR4 positives) with early onset show CB-V-IgM-R. The fact that CF-ICA were detectable in 3 newly diagnosed pat two wk before CB-V-IgM-R were noted, may indicate that the superimposed viral infection may have precipitated but not caused the beta-cell damage.

2023 ROLE OF FSH IN FOLLICULAR DEVELOPMENT IN THE BONNET MONKEY: STUDIES USING AN ANTISERUM TO FSH. C.S. Sheela Rani*, N. Ravindranath, and N.R. Moudgal, Dept. of Biochemistry, Indian Institute of Science, Bangalore-12, India.

The effect of injecting a highly specific and potent antiserum to FSH (a/s) produced in a donor bonnet monkey,at desired periods of the menstrual cycle on follicular maturation was studied. Upon injection of 1 ml of a/s on day 1 of cycle (=first day of menstrual bleeding), the serum showed the presence of FSH antibody (monitored by the binding of ^{125}I-labelled hFSH) for nearly 15 days,after which it became undetectable. The cycle length in these monkeys was extended to nearly 45 days. However, they exhibited increases in estradiol (E_2) and progesterone (P) levels typical of normal follicular and luteal phases, except that day 1 of cycle was postponed; the latter coincided with the time when the circulating antibody showed clearance. It thus appeared that the onset of follicular maturation occurred only when normal level of FSH was restored. The period for which FSH was neutralized could be varied by altering the volume of the a/s. Further, injecting 25 µl of a/s on day 7 of cycle (mid-follicular phase) caused atresia of the growing follicle as indicated by a sharp fall in serum E_2 level. In these monkeys, another follicle developed soon thereafter as indicated by peak E_2 values seen 9-10 days later. However, injection of a/s during the luteal phase had no effect on serum P levels as well as on the length of the cycle. It is concluded that FSH is absolutely essential for initiation and progression of follicular maturation and that it has no role in luteal function in the primate. Also in contrast to other methods used for suppression of FSH levels, use of an a/s provides a better approach to define the role of FSH in ovarian processes (supported by grants from the WHO, Geneva and ICMR, New Delhi).

2024 "IN VITRO" GLYCOSYLATION OF BIOACTIVE RAT LH: REGULATION BY LH-RH. A.R. Solano*, M.L. Sardañons and E.J. Podestá. Centro de Investigaciones Endocrinológicas. Hospital de Niños. Gallo 1330. (1425) Buenos Aires. ARGENTINA.

The regulation of rLH bioactivity (B-LH) and its correlation with molecular forms "in vitro" labelled with carbohidrates was studied in presence and absence of LH-RH. The incorporation of ^{3}H-mannose, ^{3}H-galactose and $^{35}SO_4$ to rLH, released from isolated pituitaries and stored in the gland was evaluated by immunoprecipitation and, isoelectrofocusing (IEF). LH-RH increases the release of B-LH (86 $\pm$ 6.3 vs 20.5 $\pm$ 1.7 ug) and the rLH measured by RIA (I-LH = 36 $\pm$ 2.7 vs 10.5 $\pm$ 0.9 ug). Moreover the pituitary LH content before LH-RH is lower than post LH-RH (562 vs 600 ug/gland) while I-LH is higher (394 vs 343 ug/gland). Since the I-LH is a parameter of the mass of rLH, these results suggest that LH-RH controls the pituitary conversion of a inactive LH to a B-LH, rather than "de novo" synthesis,otherwise similar changes would be observed in B-LH as well as I-LH. Incorporation of 2-^{3}H mannose to released rLH without and with LH-RH was 1281 $\pm$ 50 vs 764 $\pm$ 38 dpm/ug respectively, with a pI = 8,2 in IEF (pI of the highest B-LH). In the pituitary rLH the results were 1454 $\pm$ 61 vs 2063 $\pm$ 57 dpm/10 ug respectively, with peaks of radioactivity at pI = 8,2 and 9 - 9,5 (lowest B-LH). These results suggest that LH-RH stimulates the pituitary mannose incorporation into rLH, being part of these residues splitted before to be released. Galactose incorporation for released rLH was 2770 $\pm$ 30 increased after LH-RH to 3554 $\pm$ 56 dpm/ug while $^{35}SO_4$ was 958 $\pm$ 75 vs 1735 $\pm$ 180 dpm/ug respectively. $^{35}SO_4$ was incorporated only in rLH of pI 8,2 in both released and stored rLH, suggesting that sulfated complex oligosaccharide may be important for expression of full biological activity.

2025 CHROMATOGRAPHY OF HUMAN PITUITARY LUTEINIZING HORMONE BY FPLC.

A. Stockell Hartree*, J.B. Lester and R.C. Shownkeen, ARC Animal Research Station, Cambridge CB3 OJQ, UK.

We have studied the chromatographic behavior of a purified preparation of hLH (DEAE-I) on a column of Mono Q (1 ml total volume) in the Pharmacia FPLC system. The starting buffer employed was 0.01 M Tris at pH 7.8, and NaCl was incorporated in a linear gradient for elution of protein. Although a small amount of unadsorbed protein was eluted with starting buffer, most of the hLH was adsorbed to the column and was eluted over a broad range of ionic strength (from 0.028 M to 0.175 M NaCl). When the procedure was scaled up to repeatedly fractionate 10 mg of hLH at a time into 14 sub-fractions, there was 84.5% recovery by weight of the hormone applied to the column. Each of these sub-fractions was heterogeneous on polyacrylamide gel electrophoresis (PAGE) at pH 8.9, but the relative amounts of the more negatively charged bands increased with ionic strength of eluting buffer. Sub-fractions tested by FPLC were also heterogeneous, although each was eluted over a narrower range of ionic strength than was DEAE-I. The unadsorbed sub-fraction was recovered in a yield of 9.5% by weight of the DEAE-I starting material. It stained weakly on PAGE, was less acidic than the other sub-fractions, and by rat Leydig cell receptor assay was nearly twice as active as DEAE-I. Other hLH sub-fractions had receptor-binding potencies between 65% and 208% of DEAE-I. We conclude that FPLC provides a convenient and efficient method for separating molecular species of hLH which may differ in their biological properties.

2026 EFFECT OF NICOTINE AND CIGARETTE SMOKE INHALATION ON HORMONAL ALTERATIONS IN THE FEMALE RAT V. V. Subbarao Department of Physiology, College of Medical Sciences, Bendel State University, Ekpoma, Nigeria.

Many clinical reports have suggested that the inhalation of tobacco smoke has delterious effects on the physiology of reproduction. Studies in experimental animals have both confirmed and denied this observation. The purpose of the present investigation is to find the nicotine induced hormonal disturbances. Female albino rats were exposed to tobacco smoke inhalation and oral feeding of nicotine extract. The serum levels of follicle stimulating hormone (FSH), leutinizing hormone (LH) and estradiol were estimated by RIA methods. Both cigarette smoke inhalation and nicotine extract oral feeding resulted in the reduction of FSH and LH levels and the estradiol level is elevated. This indicates, tobacco smoke inhalation and nicotine oral feeding alters the production of gonadotrophins by exerting their influence on the hypothalamo-pituitary-gonadal axis resulting in the reproductive dysfunction.

2027 DIFFERENTIAL EFFECT OF GLUCOCORTICOIDS ON SECRETION OF FSH AND LH AND RESPONSIVENESS TO GNRH BY RAT PITUITARY CELLS IN VITRO. D. E. Suter* and N. B. Schwartz, Dept. of Neurobiology and Physiology, Northwestern University, Evanston, IL 60201.

Because high levels of glucocorticoids (G) are deleterious to reproduction, we sought to determine if this effect is exerted directly on the pituitary. Dispersed pituitary cells from adult female rats were divided into the following treatments: 1) controls (no G), 2) cells receiving 60 or 600 ng/ml corticosterone (B) or hydrocortisone (F) during a 48h pre-incubation and a 48h challenge incubation, and 3) cells receiving no G during the 1st 48h and 60 or 600 ng/ml B or F during the 2nd 48h. These levels of B represent low and high values within the physiological range. During the 2nd 48h, some cells from each group were treated with GnRH (1.7×10^{-12} - 4.6×10^{-9} M). FSH and LH in media were measured by RIA. Treatment with B for 96h increased basal secretion of FSH 2-fold ($P<.05$). Other treatments resulted in basal FSH levels that were between control and 96h of B. Maximal secretion of FSH in response to GnRH was 68% higher in cells treated for 96h with 600 ng/ml B than in controls ($P<.05$). Again, other treatments resulted in intermediate levels of FSH. In contrast, B or F decreased ($P<.05$) basal LH secretion with no effect on maximal LH secretion. There was no consistent effect of G on the slope of the GnRH dose-response curve for FSH, but 96h treatment with F increased ($P<.05$) the slope of the dose-response curve for LH. Although basal LH is suppressed, normal or enhanced response of LH to GnRH suggests that negative effects of G on reproduction are not exerted directly on LH secretion. Divergent effects of G on basal FSH and LH suggest a novel aspect of differential regulation of the gonadotropins. (Supported by NIH HD06416 and HD07504).

2028 THE INFLUENCE OF STRESS ON RELEASE OF GONADOTROPINS IN FEMALE ALBINO RATS DURING DIFFERENT PHASES OF THE OESTROUS CYCLE.

A. TAHA*, L.A. BASHA AND BADAWI, M.M.
*FACULTY OF VETERINARY MEDICINE, ZAGAZIG UNIVERSITY, ZAGAZIG, EGYPT.

The effect of ether anaesthesia on serum gonadotropins was determined throughout the oestrous cycle of female Albino rats. Animals were anaesthetised repeatedly and blood samples were taken at time intervals of 5, 10, 30, 45, 90 and 120 min. Compared to decapitation, ether anaesthesia induced a significant increase in serum gonadotropin levels throughout the period of study during the oestrous cycle. On the afternoon of proestrus, no further increase in already elevated levels of gonadotropins was observed.

It is thus concluded that ether anaesthesia as a stress factor can induce a rapid release of FSH and LH during the different stages of rat oestrous cycle except at the afternoon of proestrus.

2029 EVIDENCE FOR THE DIVERGENT EFFECTS OF ESTROGEN ON THE 1ST AND 2ND POOLS OF PITUITARY GONADOTROPIN. T. Tamada*, S. Araki, K. Chikazawa and M. Motoyama, Dept. of OB/GYN, Jichi Medical School, Tochigi, JAPAN 329-04

Functional characterization of the gonadotrophs in the presence or absence of estrogen was determined in 8 women with hypergonadotropic hypogonadism and 12 normally menstruating women. These subjects were divided into 2 groups. In one group, various amounts of LHRH (0.625-10 μg/hr) were administered at a constant rate for 66 hr. In the other group low doses of LH-RH (0.625-2.5 μg/hr) was given concomitantly with estradiol (500 μg/24 hr) which started 6 hr before the onset of LHRH infusion. Blood samples were obtained at the intervals of 3-6 hr throughout the experiments for the analysis of LH, FSH and estradiol. In hypergonadotropic subjects with lower estradiol levels, LH increased promptly in response to LHRH. However, the drastic elevation was not sustained for more than 18 hr, culminating in a narrow peak of LH. On the contrary LH responses were lower, but prolonged in the early follicular phase. An initial peak was observed at 3-6 hr followed by a broad secondary increase which sustained for around 42 hr. Although sole administration of estradiol (administered at the perovulatory secretion rate for 66 hr) failed to induce a positive feedback effect on LH release in the early follicular phase, the concomitant administration of minimal dose of LHRH brought on a remarkable increase in LH following a certain lag phase. This LH release was composed of two main peaks which occured at several hr interval. The latter peak might reflect a newly synthesized pool which could be built up by estrogen. The present data may provide a favourable explanation for the mechanism of prolonged activation of the pituitary in a preovulatory phase.

2030 EFFECT OF TESTOSTERONE (T) ON GONADOTROPIN RESPONSE TO $N^6,O^{2'}$-DIBUTYRYL ADENOSINE 3',5'-CYCLIC MONOPHOSPHATE (DBcAMP), cAMP BINDING AND cAMP PRODUCTION IN PITUITARY CULTURES. L.K. Tang*, A.C. Martellock, and F.Y. Tang. Dept. OB/GYN, U. Rochester, Rochester, New York, 14642, USA.

The role of testosterone (T) in modulation of pituitary FSH and LH responses to DBcAMP was examined in the pituitary cultures prepared from intact young female rats. Hormone contents in media and cell homogenates were determined by radioimmunoassays. Incubation with 8 mM DBcAMP for 4 h consistently induced a significant ($P<0.05$) increase in both FSH and LH release. Pretreatment with 10 nM T for 4 days augmented the DBcAMP-induced FSH release (160% of non-T-treated control), but had no effect on the DBcAMP-induced LH release. Data indicate that T treatment for 4-7 days stimulated FSH production (sum of hormone contents in medium and cells) without any effect on LH production. T pretreatment further augmented the DBcAMP stimulation of FSH production without any effect on LH production. Intracellular cAMP was significantly increased to 3- to 8-fold of control after T treatment for 3 or 6 h, respectively. Furthermore, cAMP-binding activities were significantly increased after T treatment for 1-10 days (130-174% of control). Our previous data indicate that estrogen stimulates LH production, cAMP binding, cAMP production, and LH response to DBcAMP whereas these data indicate that T exerts stimulatory effects primarily on FSH in a similar fashion. These results support the concept of a unified mechanism to regulate two gonadotropins via different gonadal steroids. (Supported by NIH grants HD-10837, CA-25455, and HD-00288).

2031 SOMATOMEDIN-C (Sm-C) IN BLOOD AND TISSUES FOLLOWING PARTIAL HEPATECTOMY IN THE RAT: PREDOMINANT ROLE OF NUTRIENT INTAKE. W.E.Russell*,L.E.Underwood& A.J.D'Ercole, Dept. of Pediatrics, Univ. of North Carolina, Chapel Hill,USA

We measured Sm-C (RIA) in blood and tissues of rats following partial hepatectomy (PH) to determine a possible regulatory role for this growth factor in liver regeneration. Male Sprague-Dawley rats (200-250gm) underwent a 68% PH. From a mean pre-PH value of 0.66 U/ml±0.19(SD), the serum Sm-C rose 1.7 fold to 1.09±0.08 one hour after PH ($p<0.001$ compared to sham hepatectomized [SH] values). Concurrently there was a 2.0 fold rise in serum Aspartate Amino Transferase (AST, SGOT), suggesting that Sm-C rose because of hepatocellular injury rather than a specific secretory event. In the subsequent 22 hr, serum Sm-C fell to 0.31±0.06 U/ml, while ad lib fed SH rats were 0.73±0.03 U/ml. During this time, liver tissue levels of Sm-C also declined to 30% of basal, but lung and kidney remained unchanged. Despite depressed Sm-C in blood and liver at 22 hr, hepatic DNA synthesis was elevated 10 fold. Since nutrition is a major determinant of Sm-C, we measured food consumption of PH rats and found it to be greatly depressed in the first 22 hr (20.8±2.6 vs 4.33±2.9 gm/d; $p<0.001$). Serum Sm-C in SH rats which were post-operatively pair fed with PH rats was indistinguishable from that of PH rats at 22 hr (0.35±0.11 vs 0.31±0.06 U/ml). We conclude that: a) the early rise in serum Sm-C following PH reflects non-specific liver damage, while the subsequent fall is due to diminished food intake and not diminished liver mass; b) nutrient deprivation lowers Sm-C in liver before other tissues in keeping with the liver's central role in the regulation of nutrient utilization and somatomedin production; and c) Sm-C is unlikely to play a major regulatory role in liver regeneration.

2032 SOMATOMEDIN LEVELS OF TALL ADOLESCENTS UNDER BROMOCRIPTINE TREATMENT AND BROMOCRIPTINE INTERFERENCE IN SOMATOMEDIN BIOASSAYS. R.M. Schimpff *, D. Evain Brion, J.C. Job. Inserm U 188, 75014 Paris - France.

Somatomedin and bromocriptine levels were measured before and after 3 months of bromocriptine (BC) treatment 5 mg/day in the sera of 16 tall adolescents with excessive adult height prediction. Somatomedin was measured both by RIA for Sm C and by 2 bioassays: sulfate uptake into chick embryocartilage (SU) and thymidine incorporation into human lectin-activated lymphocytes (TI). RIA was used for BC. Results were:

	Sm C U/ml	SU U/ml	TI U/ml	BC ng/ml
Before	1.34 ± .17	1.10 ± .11	1.45 ± .17	
After 3 ms	1.40 ± .14	1.10 ± .07	1.12 ± .19	0.61 ± .08

thus showing a significant drop of TI ($p < .002$) without decrease of Sm C and SU. In vitro, BC 0.1 to 100 nM added to the media inhibits the stimulating effect of normal serum on bioassays, by 20 to 80% for TI and 20 to 50% for SU. These in vivo and in vitro effects of BC upon growth-promoting activity of serum could contribute to explain discrepancies between clinical and hormonal effects of BC in acromegaly.

2033 GROWTH HORMONE-DEPENDENCE OF SOMATOMEDIN-C (SM-C) PRODUCTION BY ADULT RAT HEPATOCYTES. Carolyn D. Scott* and Robert C. Baxter. Dept. of Medicine, University of Sydney and Dept. of Endocrinology, Royal Prince Alfred Hospital, Sydney, Australia.

To quantitate the contribution of the liver to circulating SM-C levels we have measured immunoreactive rat SM-C in extracted medium conditioned by primary monolayer cultures of adult rat hepatocytes. Since neither acid-ethanol extraction nor SP-Sephadex anion exchange quantitatively removed SM binding protein, samples were separated by high pressure gel chromatography (Waters I-125) in 0.2M acetic acid, 0.1M trimethylamine, pH 2.7. SM-C (retention volume 10.5ml) was measured in neutralised fractions using specific antiserum Tr4. Recovery of SM-C was independent of the amount of binding protein in the original sample. Normal adult rat hepatocytes ($2x10^6$ cells in 2.5ml serum-free modified Waymouth medium) released SM-C (pI 8.75) at a linear rate equivalent to 1.4±0.3ng human SM-C/mg cell protein/h from 24h in culture to at least 96h. Bovine GH (200ng/ml), increased this rate by 58±26% (n=6, $p<0.001$), cycloheximide (15μg/ml) reduced synthesis by 90% ($p<0.001$) and actinomycin D (0.1μg/ml) caused a 50% decrease (p=0.01) SM-C production was undetectable in hepatocytes isolated from hypophysectomised rats and was restored by pretreatment in vivo for 6 days with bovine GH (150μg/day). Assuming a half-life of 3h for serum SM-C the measured production rate by hepatocytes is sufficient to account for circulating rat SM-C levels (700-800ng/ml). Since SM-C production shows GH dependence in vivo and in vitro we conclude that the liver is the major source of circulating SM-C. Supported by the NH&MRC.

2034 PROFILE OF SERUM IMMUNOREACTIVE BASIC SOMATOMEDIN (IRSM) DURING GESTATION. M.S. Sheppard*, B. Bhaumick and R.M. Bala. Dept. of Medicine, Univiversity of Saskatchewan, Saskatoon, Saskatchewan, S7N OXO, Canada.

As basic somatomedin, one of the Type I or basic group of somatomedins may have a role in pregnancy, we measured serum levels of IRSM during gestation in two strains of Wistar rats. In inbred Wistar rats a complex gestational profile of IRSM was found (acidifed sera, N = 5 or 6). Values at day 1 were not different than controls (1 U/ml). IRSM values rose and peaked at day 9 (1.6 ± 0.11, Mean ± SEM, U/ml) then fell to 0.72 ± 0.10 at day 15, 0.47 ± 0.06 at day 20 and 0.20 ± 0.07 at day 21 and returned to control levels post partum. The same values were found when measured by radioreceptor assay. Acid-ethanol extraction prior to assay yielded a similar profile - IRSM was elevated at day 9 and decreased to very low levels at day 22. In studies with Wistar rats (purchased from Canadian Breeding Farms and Laboratories, Montreal) IRSM levels were similar to those found previously although the decrease at day 21 was not as marked (0.57 ± 0.08, N = 11). The differences found in the two strains may be due to slight differences in the length of gestation as IRSM changes rapidly from day 19-22 in the inbred strain or may be real differences in serum IRSM levels. In serum samples taken from pregnant women during the last trimester of pregnancy IRSM levels were slightly elevated compared to controls. These studies emphasize the levels of IRSM in Wistar rats change during gestation and that serum IRSM responds differently to gestation in the rat compared to the human. Supported by the M.R.C. M.S. Sheppard is a Scholar of the Canadian Liver Foundation.

2035 MEASUREMENT OF INSULIN-LIKE GROWTH FACTOR II IN HUMAN SERUM BY AN HOMOLOGOUS RADIORECEPTOR ASSAY. G.L. Spadoni*, M. Tally, G. Enberg and K. Hall, Instituto di Clinica Pediatrica, Viale Regina Elena 324, 00161 Roma, Italy. Department of Endocrinology, Karolinska Institutet, Stockholm, Sweden.

A homologous radioreceptor assay for IGF II utilizing the human erytroleukemia cell line K562 was developed. These cells have binding sites for insulin and IGF II but not for IGF I (Tang 1983, in press, Tally in prep). In competing with labelled IGF II on its receptor IGF I was shown to be 10 times less potent than IGF II while insulin does not compete at all. This new RRA was applied to serum from normal adults, hypopituitary, acromegalic and nephropatic patients. All serum specimens were prepared by gel filtration (on a Sephadex G50 medium column) at acidic pH in order to dissociate and separate IGF II from its carrier protein.

The K562 cells provide a useful RRA system for IGF II. In 3 normal adults we found IGF II levels ranging from 979 to 1076 ng/ml with a mean value (+SE) of 1024+28 ng/ml. In 4 sera from hypopituitary patients we found significantly lower levels with a mean value of 278+33 ng/ml. Three patients with acromegaly were found to have normal levels of IGF II with a mean value of 1021+185 ng/ml. In 3 patients with nephropatic uremia we did not find elevated levels of IGF II (mean value 720+42) in contrast to what others have found with a different RRA (Goldberg 1982, JCEM 55, 1040). No elevation was found in a patient with tumour-induced hypoglycemia.

2036 ISOLATION OF THE HUMAN PLASMA CARRIER PROTEIN FOR SOMATOMEDIN. E. Martin Spencer* and W.-C. Tseng, Children's Hospital, San Francisco, CA 94118.

The somatomedins (SMs) are the only polypeptide hormones transported in plasma bound to a carrier protein(s). The carrier protein (CP) serves to prolong the half-life of the SMs and maintains them in an inactive state, but could also have other important physiologic properties. An acid stable subunit was isolated from Cohn fraction IV by a sequential scheme involving two different fractional precipitation steps, ion exchange chromatographies on CM-cellulose and SP-Sephadex, Sephadex G-100 gel filtration, affinity chromatography, and Sepahdex G-100 gel filtration. The molecular weight of the starting CP was primarily 150,000 daltons with a small amount of 50,000. After SP-Sephadex chromatography at an acidic pH, the molecular weight fell to 50,000. The final product gave a single band of binding activity in two different analytical systems, SDS-PAGE and isoelectric focusing, and had a molecular weight of approximately 50,000 daltons. SDS-PAGE of the purified acid stable subunit under reducing conditions resulted in the loss of the 50,000 band and the appearance of prominent bands of about 18,000 and 25,000 with a minor band at 30,000 daltons. The amino acid, phosphate, and sugar compositions of the 50,000 dalton carrier protein and its reduced chains will be determined. This infomation suggests that the 50,000 dalton acid-stable CP subunit is composed of 2 or more chains which could come from different CPs or result from the proteolytic activity found in association with the CP. Their relationship to the intact subunit will be assessed by N-terminal microsequence analysis. Supported by HD 14506.

2037 DEMONSTRATION OF SOMATOMEDIN C/INSULIN-LIKE-GROWTH FACTOR I (SM-C/IGF I) IN FETAL RAT BONE IN ORGAN CULTURE.

H. Stracke[+], S. Rossol, A. Bungartz and H. Schatz, Center of Internal Medicine, University of Giessen, D-63oo Giessen, F.R.G.

The influence of growth hormone (GH) and thyroid hormones on bone growth is thought to be an indirect one. Tibiae of 16-18 day old rat embryos were incubated (according to RAISZ) for 5 days in a specific culture medium with the addition of either 4 U or 8 U of GH per 1oo ml medium, or 1oo ug T3 or 5oo ug T4 per 1oo ml medium. Measurement of the alcaline phosphatase (AP) in the culture medium served as functional parameter of bone formation. SM-C/IGF I was measured radioimmunologically in culture medium. After the first 6 days of culture AP was elevated to 53 % over the initial value. Stimulation of the osteoblasts by addition of GH and T3 to the culture medium showed an increase of AP dependent on concentration and bone-age, while this increase was not seen after addition of T4. Four days after the addition of GH SM-C/IGF I was increased within the medium for about 16o percent compared to the control cultures without GH. SM-C/IGF I was also measurable in fetal bone extracts. Conclusion: The increase of SM-C/IGF I in the culture medium of rat bone after addition of GH supports the hypothesis that the influence of GH on bone formation is mediated by growth factors, however such growth factors appear to be synthesised also locally within the bone.

2038 THE ORGANIZATION OF THE GENE ENCODING HUMAN INSULIN-LIKE GROWTH FACTOR I.

J.S. Sussenbach[1]*, P. de Pagter-Holthuizen[1], J.W.M. Höppener[2], C.J. Lips[2], F.M.A. van Schaik[1], M. Jansen[3] and J.L. Van den Brande[3]. [1]Laboratory for Physiological Chemistry, [2]Department of Internal Medicine and [3]Department of Pediatrics, State University of Utrecht, Utrecht, The Netherlands.

Recently, we have reported the isolation of cloned cDNA encoding insulin-like growth factor I (IGF-I) from a human liver cDNA library (M. Jansen et al., Nature 306 (1983) 609). Nucleotide sequence analysis of this cDNA (777 nucleotides) indicated that IGF-I (70 amino acids long) is synthesized as a precursor molecule consisting of the IGF-I sequences flanked by an N-terminal peptide of at least 25 and a C-terminal peptide of 35 amino acid residues.

The cDNA clone encoding IGF-I precursor was used to study the location and the organization of the IGF-I gene in detail. Restriction enzyme analysis of DNA from human/chinese hamster somatic cell hybrids showed that the human IGF-I gene is located on chromosome 12. From a cosmid library of human DNA a number of clones were isolated, which cross-hybridized with the IGF-I cDNA clone. Further characterization of the cosmid clones indicated that they probably do not represent the IGF-I gene itself, but closely related sequences. Their precise nature is under investigation. Using total human DNA digested with various restriction endonucleases and characterized by Southern blotting and hybridization with IGF-I cDNA under stringent conditions it could be shown that the IGF-I gene extends over a region of about 20 kd. This suggests that multiple IGF-I genes exist or that the IGF-I gene contains introns.

2039 LOCAL INJECTION OR INFUSION OF HUMAN GROWTH HORMONE STIMULATES UNILATERAL EPIPHYSEAL GROWTH IN HYPOPHYSECTOMIZED RATS.

S.M. Russell*, N.L. Schlechter, E.M. Spencer and C.S. Nicoll, Dept. of Physiology-Anatomy and Cancer Research Lab., University of California, Berkeley, CA 94720 and Children's Hospital, San Francisco, CA 94119, USA.

Evidence for mediation of the growth-promoting activity of GH by somatomedin(s) (SM) was provided by Schoenle et al. (Nature 296:252, 1982), who showed that infusion of SM-C caused growth in hypophysectomized (HX) rats. However, Isaksson et al. (Science 216: 1237, 1982) demonstrated accelerated unilateral bone growth in HX rats given local injections of human GH (hGH). We have confirmed the results of Isaksson et al. using two different methods. Four daily injections of 0.6 or 6.0 μg hGH in a volume of 10 μl were given directly into the right proximal tibial epiphyseal growth plate of ether-anesthetized rats that had been HX 14 days previously. Saline was similarly injected into the left tibial plate. The saline-injected left epiphyseal plates had a width of 143 ± 5 μm, and the low and high doses of GH increased the widths to 172 ± 12 and 168 ± 7 μm, respectively. These increases were significant ($p < 0.05$ and 0.001, respectively), but no dose-response effect was seen. Neither saline nor 6.0 μg hPRL/day into the right tibial growth plate stimulated epiphyseal growth compared to the saline-injected left side. In preliminary studies, infusion of 2.0 μg hGH/day into the right femoral artery of HX rats caused striking unilateral right tibial growth. We are currently testing the effects of local injections and infusion of purified SM-C, alone and in combination with GH. These studies should help clarify the roles of GH and SM in promoting growth. Supported by NSF grant 8203583 and NIH grant HD 14506.

2040 RAPID RIA OF PLASMA GH AND ITS APPLICATION TO BETTER TREATMENT OF ACROMEGALY.

S. Sato*, K. Hanew, A. Sasaki, Y. Shimizu, H. Ikeda, R. Katakura, H. Niizuma and K. Yoshinaga, II nd Department of Medicine and Neurosurgery, Tohoku University School of Medicine, Sendai 980, Japan

To improve the surgical results in patients with acromegaly, rapid RIA of plasma GH was developed. At first, the best reaction temperature was studied. Among 20, 30, 40, and 50°C, 40°C gave the best data. Secondly, the shortest incubation time was studied, and rapid RIA was performed within 16 min. Namely, standard GH (100 μl) and Ist antibody (AB)(200 μl) were incubated for 4 min, then ^{125}I-HGH (200 μl) was added and incubated for 8 min, and finally II nd AB with polyethylene glycol (600 μl) was added and incubated for 4 min. The Bo/T was 21.4% and B/T was 6% at the concentration of 80 ng/ml. The GH values obtained by this method and the usual method correlated well ($r=0.9$, $P <0.001$). Using the rapid RIA it became possible within 35 min after the hypophysectomy to report the data to the neurosurgeon. This RIA method was applied to 8 patients with acromegaly. In two cases plasma GH decreased markedly (62 - 71% from preoperative values) at the termination of the hypophysectomy, and later fell to normal ranges. The remaining 6 cases showed only slight decreases (8 - 34%), and were judged as unsuccessfully operated. In three of these further removal of residual tumors led to steep declines in plasma GH. In the other 3 cases no further surgery was performed because the surgeon believed that the pituitary adenoma was removed completely (two cases) or further removal was made impossible by marked tumor invasion (one case). Therefore, adequate GH decreases were not obtained in these cases. In conclusion, plasma GH is rapidly measurable within 16 min and this rapid RIA method has practical value improving the surgical results in acromegalic patients.

2041 THE EFFECTS OF LONG TERM hpGRF (I-40) TREATMENT ON GH SYNTHESIS AND SECRETION IN VITRO. M.F.Scanlon*, C.Dieguez, S.M.Foord, J.R.Peters and R.Hall. Department of Medicine, Welsh National School of Medicine, Heath Park, Cardiff CF4 4XN, Wales, United Kingdom.

Potent GH releasing peptides isolated and characterised from human pancreatic tumours (hpGRFs) may be substantially the same as GH releasing hormone of hypothalamic origin. We have investigated the effects of hpGRF (I-40) on the synthesis and secretion of GH by 3 day primary cultures of male rat anterior pituitary (AP) cells over a period of 30hrs. Dispersed AP cells were prepared by conventional enzymic methods and plated at a density of IO^5/ml/well. Culture medium was semi-synthetic as described by Brazeau et al. I982. 24hr hpGRF treatment increased total GH (cell content + secretion) 2-fold (ED_{50} 0.02nM) and GH release 3-fold (ED_{50} 0.008nM). Responses were maximal at IO^{-9}M. Pretreated cells were then subject to further stimulation with either hpGRF or the Ca^{2+} channel ionophore A23I87 (IO^{-6}M). The amount of GH released by either compound fell according to the previous dose of hpGRF (eg I.9±0.Iug after saline, I.2±0.07ug after IO^{-II}M hpGRF, 0.69±0.05ug after IO^{-9}M hpGRF and 0.47±0.03ug after IO^{-7}M hpGRF in the case of IO^{-9}M hpGRF). However in proportion to the amount of GH available for release (cell GH content) hpGRF dose response curves had the same B_{max} and ED_{50}. If the dose response curves were corrected accordi- to the amount of GH released by A23I87 rather than cell GH content hpGRF appeared to enhance subsequent hpGRF responsiveness. Similar data were obtained when pretreatment was for 3 or I2hrs. Under similar conditions and using the same protocol LH responses to LHRH were markedly desensitized. The data suggest that hpGRF does not desensitize in vitro.

2042 GROWTH HORMONE GENES IN THE SYNDROME OF BIOINACTIVE GROWTH HORMONE. L. Sexton, V. Vigil and J. Parks*. Department of Pediatrics, Emory University School of Medicine, Atlanta, Georgia, USA.

The syndrome of bioinactive growth hormone (BGH), as described by Kowarski, suggests a primary abnormality of GH structure. Low circulating levels of GH preclude amino acid sequencing as a direct test of the model. We have examined restriction patterns of the GH family of genes to identify potentially abnormal GH genes for cloning and sequencing. Our sample consists of Kowarski's original patient, 9 BGH patients studied at Emory University, their parents and siblings. DNA specimens were digested with the enzymes Bgl II, Bgl II + Bam HI, Hinc II and Msp I which characterize 5 polymorphic sites within the 55 kb GH gene cluster. The combination of site presence or absence within a single cluster defines a GH restriction haplotype. The 10 patients showed no abnormalities of GH restriction fragment size. Distribution of the 3 most common haplotypes among the patients did not differ from the distribution in a reference sample of persons of normal stature. There were no families in which a sibling of normal height and a patient had definitely inherited the same pair of GH genes from their parents. Thus, we could not exclude autosomal recessive inheritance of abnormal GH genes in any of the pedigrees. Kowarski's patient was homozygous for a rare haplotype which was present only in his family and in one of the reference sample of 30 chromosomes. If other patients with the syndrome of BGH are also found to be homozygous for the rare haplotype, then this may serve as a marker for a particular mutation responsible for BGH.

2043 *RECEPTOR BINDING AND DOWNREGULATORY PROPERTIES OF HUMAN GROWTH HORMONE 22K AND ITS NATURAL 20K VARIANT ON IM-9 HUMAN LYMPHOCYTES.* *J. Smal*, J. Closset, G. Hennen and P. De Meyts. Endocrinologie, Univ. de Liège, C.H.U. B23, B-4000 Liège and HORM UNIT, U.C.L. 7529, Av. Hippocrate 75, B-1200 Bruxelles BELGIQUE.*

Our earlier binding studies of the 22K and 20K variants of hGH to pregnant rabbit liver and mammary receptors (Biochem. J., 1983, 214, 885-892) suggest that the 20K variant was a low affinity analogue of the 22K. Since the receptor population in these tissues is not fully characterized, we have now investigated their binding to the well characteried and highly specific hGH receptor of the human lymphocyte IM-9 cell-line. The maximum bindability of radioiodinated 22K and 20K to IM-9 cells was 60% and 45% respectively. Both hormone variants have essentially the same binding characteristics : slow association (equilibrium reached in 8-10 hrs at 30°C), poor reversibility ("tight binding"), linear Scatchard plot, same specificity as shown by lack of competition by bGH, pGH, eGH or fragments 32-46 (missing in the 20K variant) 1-134, and 140-191. Both unlabeled hormones inhibit binding of both tracers completely, with the 20K variant being only half as potent as the 22K. The affinity is 2.8 X $10^9 M^{-1}$ for 22K and 1.6 X $10^9 M^{-1}$ for 20K. This decreased affinity of the 20K appears to be due to a lower association rate constant. Concentrations (5 ng/ml) of the two variants that occupy about 15% of the total sites induce a marked downregulation of the receptors after 18 hrs incubation but the 20K variant (50% decrease) has a smaller effect than the 22K (75% decrease). Thus the only consequence of the 32-46 deletion in 20K is a lower association rate and affinity for the IM-9 lymphocyte hGH receptor, possibly due to a conformational change. However, it is well documented that the major biological difference between 22K and 20K forms of hGH is the absence of the early insulin-like activity of the 20K variant. The close binding characteristics reported here for the two forms suggest that differences in the insulin-like effects of both variants could probably not be explained by differences in the nature of their interaction with the hGH receptor.

2044 DOES GROWTH HORMONE SECRETION INCREASE DURING PUBERTAL DEVELOPMENT? B.E. Spiliotis*, A.W. Root and B.B. Bercu, Pregnancy Research Branch, NICHD, NIH, Bethesda, MD, U.S.A. 20205 and All Children's Hospital, University of South Florida, St. Petersburg, Florida, U.S.A. 33701.

Whether growth hormone (GH) secretion increases during pubertal development in humans remains controversial. To further assess this issue we used a nonhuman primate model. Thirty-two male macaques (rhesus and cynomologous) from prepubertal through adult life were studied. Both intact and castrate monkeys were evaluated. Twenty-four hour (or longer) sampling was done in unesthesized animals which were in a mobile vest and tether assembly. Blood was removed either at 15 minute intervals for 24 hours or at 25 or 30 minute intervals for up to 54 hours through a femoral venous catheter. Pubertal development was assessed on the basis of gonadotropin and testosterone secretion, testicular volume, hCG challenge tests and skeletal age. The results of the intact monkeys are summarized below:

Developmental age group	n	Mean 24h GH conc. (ng/ml)	$\bar{X}$ peak GH conc. (ng/ml)	# GH pulses ≥ 5ng/ml
prepubertal	4	9.8 ± 2.5*	20.3 ± 3.1	13 ± 1
pubertal	6	8.0 ± 1.7	16.3 ± 2.3	12 ± 2
adult	8	7.8 ± 0.9	15.7 ± 2.2	11 ± 1

*mean ($\bar{X}$ ± SE) for all data.

There were no statistical differences between the above groups. These data agree with our observations in humans that 24 hour GH output does not increase during pubertal development.

2045 DIFFERENTIAL STIMULATION OF STORED AND NEWLY SYNTHESIZED GROWTH HORMONE RELEASE BY GROWTH HORMONE RELEASING HORMONE (GHRH, 1-44) IN VITRO.

M.E. Stachura*, J.M. Tyler, P.K. Farmer, P.G. Kent, and Y.H. Lee, Department of Medicine, Medical College of Georgia and VA Medical Center, Augusta, Georgia 30910, U.S.A.

Using rat pituitary fragments in static incubation and in perifusion, the effects of synthetic GHRH (1-44) were examined using a double-label, specific immunoprecipitation protocol which permitted simultaneous study of growth hormone (GH) synthesis, as well as release of both stored and newly synthesized hormone. Activity of the GHRH was first checked by confirming other reports: (1) dose responsivity in perifusion (0.1-10 nM; maximum, 647% of basal GH release); (2) in vivo effectiveness (specific stimulation to 1650% of base); and (3) lack of response by GH_3 tumor cells. Using the double-isotope protocol in the experiments reported here, we observed: (a) GHRH (0.3-3 nM) stimulates stored GH release (139-240% of control); (b) simultaneous stimulation of newly synthesized GH release was significantly greater (176-610% of control); and (c) these effects occurred without altering the rate of GH synthesis (92-102% of control). In parallel, 1 mM $(Bu)_2$cAMP stimulated release of new (770%) in preference to stored GH (273%) without altering synthesis (111% of control). Unexpectedly, GHRH was observed to stimulate stored prolactin (PRL) release slightly (but significantly) without altering either release of new PRL or PRL synthesis. Conclusions: GHRH differentially stimulates GH release from separate intracellular compartments by modifying intracellular movement of newly synthesized GH and exhibits cross-over stimulation of PRL release.

2046 THE MOLECULAR NATURE OF CIRCULATING HUMAN GROWTH HORMONE: A COMPARISON OF SECRETORY STIMULI.

M. Stolar and G. Baumann,* Center for Endocrinology, Metabolism and Nutrition, Northwestern University Medical School, Chicago, Illinois, USA.

Plasma growth hormone (hGH) in man consists of several monomeric molecular forms, namely the 22,000 dalton form (22K), the 20,000 dalton variant (20K) and one or more acidic forms (acetylated, deamidated or cleaved hGH). It is not known whether the release of the various hGH forms from the pituitary gland varies with the type of secretory stimulus. We therefore compared the plasma hGH patterns after several pharmacological stimuli, under conditions of physiological release in normal man and during pathological secretion in acromegaly (N=20). Pharmacological stimuli examined included L-DOPA, propranolol, estrogen and TRH. Physiological stimuli included sleep, exercise and spontaneous secretory spikes occurring at random times. hGH was extracted from plasma by immunoaffinity chromatography and analyzed by polyacrylamide gel electrophoresis and isoelectric focusing. In all cases, the 22K form was the predominant circulating species (∿85%), with 20K as the next most prevalent form (∿10%), and acidic forms present in small amounts (<5%). Patterns of plasma hGH were similar after all stimuli. The distribution of hGH forms in plasma largely reflected that seen in pituitary extracts.

Conclusions: 1) hGH secreted in response to exogenous and endogenous stimuli consists of the same molecular species in similar proportions. 2) Secretory stimuli appear non-selective with respect to individual hGH forms. 3) It seems likely that, in response to any stimulus, the contents of the pituitary secretory granule are released in a non-specific manner.

2047 ANTIESTROGEN ACTION ON HYPOTHALAMIC NERVE CELLS. R.L. Moss* and C.A. Dudley. Department of Physiology, UTHSCD, Dallas, Texas 75235.

In order to study the possibility that recognition of estradiol may occur at the surface membrane level of hypothalamic nerve cells, the action of antiestrogen on membrane excitability was examined. Twenty-four hours after subcutaneous administration of saline, estradiol benzoate (EB), CI-628 (a steroidal antiestrogen) or EB in combination with CI-628, extracellular action potentials were recorded and 17-β-estradiol hemisuccinate ($17\beta E_2S$) was iontophoresed via micropipettes, placed in the medial-preoptic-septal (MPO-S) area of urethane-anesthetized, ovariectomized female rats. Two parameters, namely, the spontaneous firing rate (FR) and membrane responsiveness to $17\beta E_2S$ were compared over the various pretreatments. To date, the electrical activity of 271 MPO-S neurons has been recorded and 34% of these neurons have been found to be responsive to $17\beta E_2S$. Higher mean (M) FRs were observed in animals pretreated with EB (MFR=4.16 spikes/sec; n=125), CI-628 (MFR=4.89 spikes/sec; n=42), and EB in combination with CI-628 (MFR=6.12 spikes/sec; n=28) than with saline (MFR=3.91 spikes/sec; n=76) suggesting that the antiestrogen, CI-628, is capable of exerting an agonistic action on spontaneous activity. The number of MPO-S neurons found to be sensitive to the direct application of $17\beta E_2S$ was decreased by approximately 50% in animals pretreated with EB plus CI-628 (27% of the neurons were estrogen-sensitive) as compared to animals pretreated with either saline, EB or CI-628 (on the average 43% of these neurons were estrogen-sensitive). The present findings suggest 1) that alterations in the genome can result in surface membrane changes and/or 2) the existence of specific estrogen-sensitive postsynaptic sites. NIH #NS10434.

2048 DIFFERENTIATED EFFECTS OF MET- AND LEU-ENKEPHALIN ON LH-SECRETION. N. Parvizi* and F. Ellendorff, Institute for Animal Science and Animal Behaviour (FAL), Mariensee, 3057 Neustadt 1, F.R.G.

Seventeen adult castrated male Göttingen miniature pigs were bilaterally provided with guide 22 G stainless steel tubings bearing a 28 G inner tubing in the amygdala (AMY) and mediobasal hypothalamus (MBH). A silastic catheter was inserted into the jugular vein 5 days prior to the onset of the experiment. On different experimental days 30 ng of Met-enkephalin (Met), 30 ng Leu-enkephalin (Leu) or 1 µl saline (0.7%) were bilaterally microinjected into the AMY, MBH or AMY and MBH. Blood samples were taken from 90 min before to 180 min after the microinjection in 10 min intervals. The microinjection of Met had no significant effects on plasma LH-levels, however, it resulted in a dramatic change in the pattern of LH-secretion, when it was microinjected into the MBH. In contrast, microinjection of Leu into the MBH decreased ($P < 0.01$) plasma LH-levels without having any effect on the pattern of secretion. Microinjections into the AMY had no effects. In conclusion, the results indicate that the enkephalins play a differentiated role in the regulation of rate and mode of the LH-secretion.

2049 THE STIMULATION OF PHAGOCYTIC ACTIVITY OF THE RETICULO-ENDOTHELIAL SYSTEM BY SYNTHETIC AND NATURAL METHYL-ESTROGENS.

N. Mendoza-Patiño*, J.J. Mandoki, C. Rubio-Póo, C. Lemini, E. Zavala, and G. Silva. Departamento de Farmacología, Facultad de Medicina, and Escuela Nacional de Estudios Profesionales Zaragoza, Universidad Nacional Autónoma de México, 04510 México D.F., México.

The purpose of the study was to assess the influence on the phagocytosis-stimulating-action of estrogens with methyl groups replacing hydrogen atoms at various positions of the molecule. The following estrogens were studied: 1-methyl-estradiol-17β, 2-methyl-estradiol-17β, estradiol-17β-3-methyl ether, 7α-methyl-estrone, 8β-methyl-estradiol-17β-3-methyl ether, meprane dipropionate, benzestrol, and mirestrol. Phagocytic activity was estimated by the rate of intravascular clearance of colloidal carbon, according to the method of Biozzi et al. (1954), modified by us. CD1 male mice received intravenously a colloidal carbon suspension (30 mg of carbon per 100 g of body weight). Three minutes after the injection, a sample of blood was obtained and the carbon concentration of the hemolyzed blood was estimated spectrophotometrically. The methyl group at the 8β position decreased the phagocytosis-stimulating-action in a marked manner. A methyl group attached to the carbon atom 2, decreased the response moderately. Methyl groups at positions 1, 11α, and 11β did not affect the response significantly.

2050 IDENTIFICATION OF THE HUMAN RENIN GENE AND STUDIES OF RENIN GENE EXPRESSION

B.J. Morris*, D.F. Catanzaro, J. Hardman, N. Mesterovic, J. Tellam, Y. Hort and J. Shine, Molecular Biology & Hypertension Laboratory, The University of Sydney, Sydney, N.S.W., 2006 and Centre for Recombinant DNA Research, The Australian National University, Canberra, A.C.T., 2601, Australia.

The complete sequence of the gene coding for human renin was obtained from positive colonies identified in the human genomic DNA library of Maniatis, using mouse renin cDNA as a hybridization probe. The coding regions were found on 9 exons which were interrupted by 8 introns occupying the bulk of DNA in the gene. Overall homology of exons with mouse cDNA was 75%. The sizes of the exons and positions of the introns were similar to those in the human pepsin gene described recently. Homology with human pepsin, which belongs to the same (aspartyl protease) family as renin, was 33%. Human renin, like mouse renin, had pre and pro regions and other features associated with its highly specialized hydrolysis of angiotensinogen in the bloodstream. Residues involved in recognition and binding to substrate deviated subtly in human renin to accommodate the unique Val^{11} residue at S_1' of human substrate. Hybridization histochemistry localized renin mRNA in the juxtaglomerular cells of the kidney and granular duct cells of the mouse submandibular gland (SMG). A hybri-dot assay was developed to measure renin mRNA. In studies of gene expression concommitant increases in renin mRNA and renin were seen in SMG during the onset of sexual maturity in male mice, reaching values 40x pre-pubertal. The amounts in females were initially lower, increased to a smaller extent during development, and could be stimulated by testosterone. Castration of males reduced renin mRNA in SMG and sodium depletion increased renin mRNA in kidney.

2051 GROWTH HORMONE RESPONSE TO hpGRF IN CHILDREN WITH GROWTH DISORDERS

Pintor C.*, Loche S., Puggioni R., °Locatelli V., °Cella S.G., °Müller E.E.
Dept. of Pediatrics,University of Cagliari and ° Dept of Pharmacology,University of Milano,Italy

We present data on the clinical use of GRF (hpGRF1-40,Bachem Bubendorf Switzerland;1 ug/Kg i.v.) in normal children(N),constitutional short stature(CSS),idiopathic GH deficiency(IGHD),subjects operated for chraniopharyngioma(CP)and affected by thalassemia major.CSS showed a reduced and delayed response,IGHD showed a slight but significant response,T subjects showed different responses while CP did not respond.Our data confirm the suitability and specificity of hpGRF.They also suggest that IGHD is due to a hypothalamic disorder and that a central disorder is present in T and CSS.From these data it appears that hpGRF might be a valid diagnostic tool and a possible therapeutical agent for growth disorders. (hGH by RIA, ng./ml.)

Time(min)	0	15	30	45	60	90	120
N(n=7) $\bar{M}$	2.1	36.8	34.8	27.0	20.5	7.5	5.2
± SD	1.1	12.8	13.9	16.3	13.6	4.5	4.5
CSS	0.2	4.1	4.3	3.3	1.9	0.9	13.4
CSS	0.4	3.8	6.9	20.4	13.6	3.4	1.1
CSS	0.9	4.4	1.8	2.0	9.7	10.0	2.2
CSS	1.1	5.0	4.3	1.8	3.6	13.7	4.4
CSS	1.8	3.6	1.7	13.2	7.7	4.4	1.0
CSS	0.9	4.8	5.2	1.2	0.8	8.1	7.8
T	0.9	8.8	5.8	4.5	4.2	2.8	1.6
T	1.4	19.6	46.7	12.7	7.8	4.9	3.2
T	0.6	7.4	4.1	2.9	1.2	0.5	0.6
T	2.3	2.0	1.1	0.7	0.7	0.6	2.5
T	2.9	21.9	11.5	5.2	2.7	1.1	0.6
CP	0.4	5.1	4.3	2.7	2.4	1.7	0.8
CP	0.4	0.9	0.7	0.9	0.5	0.4	0.4
IGHD $\bar{M}$	0.7	9.7	4.7	2.8	2.4	2.0	1.4
±SD(n=7)	0.3	3.9	5.0	3.5	2.9	1.6	1.4

2052 CORTICOTROPIN-RELEASING FACTOR (CRF) INHIBITS SECRETION OF ARGININE VASOPRESSIN (AVP) AND OXYTOCIN (OT) INTO RAT HYPOPHYSIAL PORTAL PLASMA.

P.M. Plotsky*, T.O. Bruhn and S. Otto. Peptide Biology Laboratory, The Salk Institute, La Jolla, CA.

We have recently been investigating central interactions among putative adrenocorticotropin (ACTH)-releasing agents and have previously reported that central administration of AVP inhibits secretion of immunoreactive CRF (irCRF) into rat hypophysial portal plasma in a dose-dependent manner. Male Sprague-Dawley rats (350-450g) were prepared for portal blood collection under urethane anesthesia (1.1g/kgBW,ip). We now report that third-ventricular injection (1.0 μL) of 100 pmoles synthetic ovine CRF significantly inhibits ($p < 0.001$) secretion into the portal circulation of both irAVP by 83.5 ± 3.5% (n=6) and irOT by 70.1 ± 10.7% (n=6). Preinjection concentrations of irAVP and irOT were 527.3 ± 89.7 and 1814 ± 508.1 pg ml^{-1}, respectively. Short-term exposure (< 60 min) to central ovine CRF, which exhibits no cross-reactivity in our homologous rat CRF assay using antiserum rc 68, was without effect on portal plasma irCRF concentrations (623.5 ± 145 pg ml^{-1}, n=6). Vehicle injection did not alter portal levels of irCRF, irAVP, or irOT. We conclude that central CRF may modulate hypothalamic secretion of both AVP and OT, a hormone of stress, into the portal system. Furthermore, central AVP and CRF appear to have reciprocal effects on secretion of one another into the portal system. Finally, hypophysial portal and neurohypophysial secretion of AVP and OT may be differentially regulated, as suggested by the observations of Bruhn et al. that central CRF elevates systemic OT levels.

2053 REGULATION OF THE PITUITARY-GONADAL AXIS FUNCTION BY AN GnRH ANTAGONIST IN MALE RATS. M. Puente*and K.J. Catt. ERRB, NICHD, NIH, MD. 20205, U.S.A.

The effects of a potent GnRH antagonist (GnRHa) on the inhibition of the pituitary-gonadal function were investigated in normal and castrate male rats. For this purpose, 40-46 day old rats were injected with increasing doses of the (Ac-D-pClPhe^{1,2},D-Trp^{3},D-Arg^{6},D-Ala^{10})GnRH analog and killed 12, 24 or 48 hours later. In each animal, pituitary GnRH receptors and gonadal receptors for LH, FSH and PRL were measured and compared with changes in plasma gonadotropins, PRL and testosterone (T). Treatment of the intact rats with the lower doses of GnRHa (1, 5 or 10 µg) reduced the GnRH receptor concentration to 30, 15 and 9% of the control values respectively, without affecting the serum gonadotropin, PRL or T levels. Such effects have been consistently found at 12, 24 and 48 hours after GnRHa injection. After treatment with higher doses of GnRHa (100 and 500 µg), there were more marked decreases in GnRH binding, to 8% and 4% of the control values, accompanied by a dose-related decrease of serum LH and T with complete suppression by 500 µg of GnRHa. Of the testicular receptors assayed, those for PRL were reduced by about 60% in the 500 µg treated animals. In contrast, in castrate rats the LH values are reduced to hypophysectomized levels with a decrease of only 70% in the pituitary GnRH receptor level, an effect which is obtained with 100 µg of GnRHa. These data suggest that extensive or complete occupancy of the pituitary GnRH receptor population is necessary to reduce plasma LH and T values in intact rats, in which compensatory changes in endogenous GnRH secretion are presumably rapidly induced by decreased testicular steroid secretion, whereas in castrated animals partial occupancy of the available receptor sites is able to inhibit the elevated rate of gonadotropin secretion.

2054 MODE OF FOLLICULAR FLUID ADMINISTRATION RESULTS IN DIFFERENTIAL EFFECTS ON HYPOTHALAMIC LHRH CONTENT. V. Rettori*, R. Reynoso, A. Seilicovich, E. Quaglia and R. Steger, Centro de Investigaciones en Reproducción, Facultad de Medicina, U.B.A. and Dept. of Ob/Gyn, Univ. of Texas Health Sci. Center, San Antonio, TX 78284, USA.

Porcine follicular fluid (PFF) from which the steroids have been removed by charcoal extraction has been documented to selectively lower serum FSH levels by a direct action on the pituitary gland. However, it may also be possible that PFF lowers FSH levels by disrupting the normal release of hypothalamic LHRH. In the present study, PFF was shown to selectively reduce serum FSH levels without affecting LH levels in immature and/or mature rats, whether given acutely (200 µl/100 g s.c.), chronically (200 µl/rat, twice-daily for 5 days), or by infusion (200 µl/rat/2 h). The acute s.c. injection of PFF resulted in a four-fold increase in hypothalamic LHRH levels as measured by RIA. The 2 h infusion of PFF likewise resulted in doubling of hypothalamic LHRH levels. In contrast, chronic PFF treatment resulted in a significant decline in LHRH levels as compared to the saline-treated controls. Although the amount of LHRH released by the hypothalamus cannot be ascertained by simply measuring LHRH content, the present data suggest that PFF may have both pituitary and hypothalamic sites of action.

2055 TREATMENT OF PROSTATIC TUMORS BY THE LH-RH AGONIST D-Trp6-LH-RH : EFFICIENCY OF A LONG-ACTING FORM UPON TESTOSTERONE, LH AND D-TRP6-LH-RH PLASMA LEVELS. M. Roger*, J. Duchier, N. Lahlou, R.Y. Mauvernay, A.V. Schally, Fondation de Recherche en Hormonologie, BP 110, 94268 Fresnes, France.

The levels of LH, Testosterone (T) and D-Trp6-LH-RH (Trp6) were compared in two groups of men with prostatic tumors, aged 65 to 75, submitted to different regimens of Trp6 administration. Trp6 was measured by RIA after ethanol extraction. The detection limit was 150 pg/ml. 4 patients were given 500 µg subcutaneously (SC) daily for 7 days (d). Plasma T (ng/ml)and LH (ng LER 907/ml) levels rose respectively from 1.6-9.3 and 25-290 at d0 to 2.9-12 and 310-690 at d2, fell to 0.5-2.1 and 48-70 at d14, then rose gradually to 3.1-12 and 90-500 at d25-28. Plasma Trp6 levels (pg/ml) peaked at d2 (2700-4800), were still detectable at d12 (150-300) but became undetectable after that. Five patients were given the same SC regimen, then received at d8 and d28 3 mg intramuscularly (IM) of a long acting preparation designed for releasing 100 µg Trp6 per 24 h. The same pattern as in the 1st group was seen in all 5 subjects until d13. In 3 of them T and LH levels decreased further on until d28 (respectively 0.10-0.15 and 33-46 ng /ml). The 2nd IM injection at d28 did not induce any new stimulatory response. Detectable Trp6 levels (0.4-3.2 ng/ml) were found not only during SC treatment, but also after IM administration. In the other 2 subjects, both T and LH levels increased from d13 to d28 and the 2nd IM injection induced a transient response of LH and T in both. In these 2 subjects Trp6 levels were below the detection limit at d13 and d21 in one, from d13 to d28 in the other one. This study demonstrates the ability of IM long acting D-Trp6-LH-RH to sustain pituitary and/or testicular desensitization.

2056 STUDIES WITH HUMAN PANCREATIC TUMOR GROWTH HORMONE RELEASING FACTOR (hpGRF-40) IN FOUR FAMILIES WITH GENETIC HYPOPITUITARISM. A. Rogol*, T. Foley, R. Furlanetto, M. Thorner, and R. Blizzard, Univ of VA School of Medicine, Charlottesville, VA, Univ of Pittsburgh School of Medicine, Pittsburgh, PA and Children's Hospital of Philadelphia, PA.

There are at least 6 single gene disorders which are associated with diminished or absent growth hormone (GH). Four (Types IA, IB, II and III) are characterized by isolated GH deficiency (IGHD) and two are characterized by panhypopituitarism (Types I and II, PD). We have studied the GH release to hpGRF and other tests in 4 families encompassing 3 of the types to better understand, if possible, the site of the defect and the variability of responses that might occur with hpGRF.

Family	Genetic type	Generations Tested	Persons Tested	Max GH response to hpGRF (ng/ml)	Other
#1	II IGHD-AD	4	4	3.5	3.0
#2	IB IGHD-AR	1	2	11	4.1
#3	I PD-AR	1	2	6.8	3.7
#4	I PD-AR	1	3	>10	1.3

Two of the individuals in family #1 were given hpGRF (0.33 ug/kg) q 3 h IV 32 times. Somatomedin-C determinations did not increase as is characteristic with this stimulus in most patients with IGHD. This priming also did not increase the GH release to a large challenge of hpGRF (10 ug/kg). These results indicate that patients with Type II IGHD probably have a pituitary defect accounting for their GH deficiency, while patients with Type IB IGHD or Type I PD probably have a suprapituitary defect accounting for their GH deficiency. hpGRF conceivably could serve as a therapeutic agent in these latter 2 types.

2057 RADIOIMMUNOASSAY (RIA) OF HUMAN PANCREATIC GROWTH HORMONE RELEASING FACTOR (hpGRF)-44. A. Root*, M. Sweetland, G. Duckett, M. Root, University of South Florida College of Medicine, Department of Pediatrics, Tampa, and All Children's Hospital, St.Petersburg, FL, USA.

In order to measure hpGRF-44 an RIA was established. HpGRF (Bachem) was labeled with ^{125}I by the chloramine-T method and purified on a 0.9x50 cm column of Sephadex G50-fine, equilibrated and eluted with 0.1 M HAc, 0.1% HSA. Three radioactive peaks were eluted. The mid-peak was ^{125}I-hpGRF-44 which was 95% precipitable by 10% trichloracetic acid, 90% bound by talc and 80-90% precipitable by excess anti-hpGRF-44 serum. Radiolabeled ^{125}I-hpGRF-44 was stable in buffer at room temperature for 120 hours. Four rabbits were immunized with hpGRF-44, conjugated to BSA by carbodiimide, in complete Freund's adjuvant, injected intradermally at multiple sites. Three months after the second injection two satisfactory antisera were obtained. Neither antiserum recognizes SRIF, TRH, CRF, GnRH, hGH, rGH or a number of other peptides. Anti hpGRF-44 serum R3 (final concentration 1/140,000, B_0-30%) is highly specific for the 44 amino acid peptide (B_{50}:hpGRF-44:0.62 ng/tube; hpGRF-40:16.9; hpGRF-37:75.7) and binds $<$6% radiolabeled hpGRF-40 or hpGRF-37. Anti-hpGRF-44 serum R2 (final dilution 1/70,000, B_0 30%) recognizes all three species of hpGRF (B_{50}:hpGRF-44:0.32 ng/tube; hpGRF-40:0.06; hpGRF-37:0.02) and binds 20% of radiolabeled hpGRF-40 or hpGRF-37. At room temperature human serum and EDTA plasma slowly degrade ^{125}I-hpGRF-44 (40-50% in 6 hours). Rat serum rapidly degrades ^{125}I-hpGRF-44 (40-50% in 30 minutes). HpGRF was not detectable in methanol extracts of rat hypothalamus in this RIA employing anti hpGRF-44 serum R3.

2058 NEURONAL RESPONSIVENESS TO GONADOTROPIN-RELEASING HORMONE (GnRH) AND ITS CORRELATION WITH SEXUAL RECEPTIVITY IN THE RAT. J.M. Rothfeld* and D.S. Gross*, Departments of Physiology and Human Anatomy, University of California School of Medicine, Davis California 95616.

Infusion of GnRH within preoptic-septal regions (POA/S) facilitates mating behavior in the female rat. Moreover, iontophoretic application of GnRH exerts both excitatory and inhibitory effects on the spontaneous discharge rates of individual neurons in the POA/S. In the present study, an attempt was made to correlate the responsiveness of individual POA/S units to iontophoretically applied GnRH with the onset of sexual receptivity. In both behavioral and electrophysiological studies, ovariectomized, estrogen-primed rats were used. In behaviorally tested rats, lordosis quotients (LQ) were determined at varying times following progesterone (P) injection. For electrophysiological studies, P was given 1 hr after the start of recording. GnRH was iontophoretically applied for 30 sec at 16 nA on spontaneously discharging cells. A unit was deemed excited (↑) or inhibited (↓) if a repeatable 30% change in discharge rate was observed. From 0-3 hr, as receptivity increased rapidly (from an LQ of 0 to 68) excitatory responses predominated, with 13% of total units tested (n=49) ↑ and 5.3% ↓ by GnRH. From 4-6 hr, as receptivity increased only slightly (from an LQ of 71 to 88) inhibitory responses predominated, with 11.3% of units tested (n=38) ↑ and 23.3% ↓ by GnRH. From 7-9 hr, as receptivity reached a plateau (LQ from 90 to 92) excitatory responses predominated, with 26% of units tested (n=26) ↑ and 4.2% ↓. These findings confirm the E/P biasing effect on POA/S unit responses to GnRH. Moreover, they suggest that a dynamic relationship exists between GnRH responses at the cellular level and sexual behavior throughout the course of steroid-induced receptivity.

2059 INTRANASAL TRH: AN EFFECTIVE STIMULATION OF PITUITARY AND THYROID RESERVE.
A. Ryff-de Lèche*, J.J. Staub, S. Paul, J. Girard, B. Polc, B. van der Owe, Div. of Endocrinology, Dept. Medicine, University Hospital, CH-4031 Basle.

Polypeptide hormones (LHRH, DDAVP, GHRF) are effective after intranasal administration and have proven to be diagnostically and therapeutically efficacious. Recently TRH has been developed for nasal application. We studied the TSH, free T4-(fT4) and T3-response after nasal TRH (TRH Hoechst) and compared the results to iv and oral TRH. 18 healthy euthyroid subjects (23-26 years) received 40mg TRH orally and 2mg TRH intranasally. 13 subjects also received 200μg TRH iv.-TSH, fT4 and T3 serum levels were determined by RIA at 0, 20, 30, 60, 120 and 180 min. Results and conclusions: The mean TSH peak after nasal TRH (14.7 ± 1.6 mU/l) is significantly higher than for iv. TRH (8.4 ± 1.4 mU/l, $p<0.005$) and lower than for oral TRH (23.1 ± 4.4 mU/l, $p<0.005$). Time response analysis shows a similar prompt stimulation in nasal and iv TRH (peak at 20' and 30' respc.) contrary to oral TRH (peak at 180'), but the duration of the stimulatory effect is prolonged compared to iv. administration. T3 increment at 180' was 45.3%, which is somewhat lower than in oral TRH (52.9%, $p<0.005$), and equivalent to iv. TRH (43%, p = ns). Stimulation of fT4 at 180' is identical for nasal and iv. TRH (28.2% and 29.2% respc.). Due to the delayed TSH increase after oral TRH, the fT4 response is not yet fully stimulated at 180' (18.9%). Nasal mucous membrane tolerance is excelent and systemic side effects are comparable to iv. TRH. The present data demonstrate that intranasal TRH, by way of direct resorption into the venous circulation, stimulates TSH and thyroid hormone secretion effectively.

2060 DECREASE IN CORTICOTROPIN-RELEASING FACTOR (CRF)-LIKE IMMUNOREACTIVITY IN RAT INTERMEDIATE AND POSTERIOR PITUITARY LOBES AFTER STALK SECTION.
J.M. Saavedra,* C.Rougeot, J. Culman, A. Israel, M. Niwa, M.C. Tonon, F. Dray and H. Vaudry, Section on Clinical Psychopharmacology,Laboratory of Clinical Science, NIMH, Bethesda, Md. 20205,USA.

Corticotropin Releasing Factor (CRF) stimulates α-MSH secretion from rat intermediate pituitary lobe (Proulx-Ferland et al, 1982). CRF fibers are present in the neurohypophysis (Burlet et al, 1983). We determined CRF-like immunoreactivity by RIA in intermediate and posterior pituitary lobes of stalk sectioned rats and sham operated controls. The antigenic determinant read by the CRF antibody used (231-0607, from H. Vaudry) was contained within the Gln^{26}- Leu^{37} region of the molecule. Both the intermediate and posterior lobes of control rats contained similar amounts of CRF (591 ± 78 and 487 ± 34 pg/mg protein, respectively).Transection of the pituitary stalk produced a marked decrease in CRF-like immunoreactivity in both structures. The CRF content of the intermediate lobe after stalk section was 62 ± 17 pg/mg protein, a decrease of 90%, and that of the posterior lobe was 90 ± 13 pg/mg protein,an 83% decrease. Our results suggest that most of the CRF-like immunoreactivity in the rat intermediate and posterior pituitary lobes is contained in nerve fibers of brain origin and support the hypothesis of a role of CRF in the release of intermediate and posterior lobe peptides.

2061 EVIDENCE FOR EXISTENCE OF SOMATOSTATIN-LIKE IMMUNOREACTIVITY IN CATECHOLAMINE STORAGE GRANULES OF BOVINE ADRENAL MEDULLA. H. Saito*, S. Saito, T. Ohuchi and M. Oka, Departments of Laboratory Medicine, Internal Medicine and Pharmacology, University of Tokushima, Tokushima 770, Japan.

We have previously reported somatostatin(SRIF)-producing adrenal pheochromocytoma and pointed out a possibility that SRIF and catecholamine(CA) are located in the same tumor cells. In the present study, we investigated the relationship between SRIF and CA release from normal bovine adrenal medulla, and subcellular storage site and mode of existence of SRIF. A fresh bovine adrenal gland was perfused in a retrograde manner with 100 % O_2-saturated 20 mM Tris-HCl buffer(pH 7.4) at 37°C, at a rate of 4 ml/min. After 60 min-preperfusion, 1 ml of 10 mM acetylcholine(ACh) was infused and the perfusate was collected at intervals of one min. On the other hand, a soluble lysate of chromaffin granules was prepared by sucrose density gradient and the molecular heterogeneity of immunoreactive somatostatin(IR-SRIF) in the extract of it was analysed by gel-filtration chromatography. Although the concentration of IR-SRIF in samples during the period of preperfusion was below 5 pg/ml, an excessive release(35.5 pg/ml) was observed between 1-2 min after the stimulation with ACh, and thereafter, release of IR-SRIF continued over 6 min. A similar result was obtained in the series of CA determination. Chromatographic study on the extract of chromaffin granule lysate revealed three IR-SRIF components corresponding to prepro-SRIF(76.8 %), SRIF-28(14.1 %) and SRIF-14(9.1 %). These findings suggest that SRIF with molecular heterogeneity is stored in the adrenal chromaffin granules and released into the circulation with CA by exocytotic secretion.

2062 PROLACTIN (PRL) INHIBITS LUTEINIZING HORMONE RELEASING HORMONE (LHRH) SECRETION INTO PITUITARY STALK BLOOD: A POSSIBLE ROLE FOR β-ENDORPHIN AS A MEDIATOR. Dipak K. Sarkar*, S.S.C. Yen, Dept. of Reproductive Med., Univ. of California, San Diego, La Jolla, CA 92093 USA.

Hyperprolactinemia can reduce gonadotropin secretion in rats, but the mechanism of this effect of PRL is not clear. We have investigated 1) the action of PRL on LHRH secretion and 2) the interaction between PRL, opiates and LHRH. The effect of PRL on LHRH secretion was studied after transplanting 4 anterior pituitaries to the kidney capsule of ovariectomized female rats for 2-3 weeks. The level of PRL in rats with pituitary transplants (PT) was approximately 5-fold higher than in control rats. Pituitary stalk plasma LHRH in rats with PT was approximately 4 times lower than in rats without PT. Since opiates inhibit the secretion of LHRH, we have tested whether the reduced secretion of LHRH in rats with PT is associated with an increase in the opiate activity. This was studied by measuring 1) the concentration of plasma β-endorphin and 2) the response of LHRH to opiate antagonist naloxone. β-endorphin level in pituitary stalk plasma was approximately 4-fold higher in rats with PT than in rats without PT. Peripheral plasma β-endorphin levels were similar in both groups but were significantly smaller (20- to 80-fold) than those in pituitary stalk plasma. Naloxone (10 mg/kg, s.c.) increased pituitary stalk plasma LHRH in both groups, but the % change of LHRH was higher in rats with PT. The present results demonstrate that hyperprolactinemia can reduce LHRH release. The negative correlation between hypothalamic LHRH and β-endorphin secretion in hyperprolactinemic rats suggests a possible involvement of β-endorphin in PRL action on LHRH.

2063 CORTICOTROPIN-RELEASING FACTOR(CRF)-LIKE MATERIAL IS PRESENT IN HUMAN(h) PLACENTA AND THIRD TRIMESTER PREGNANCY PLASMA. A. Sasaki*, A.S. Liotta, M. Luckey, and D.T. Krieger, Div. of Endocrinology, Mt. Sinai Medical School, New York, NY 10029

The presence and nature of CRF-like material in human placenta and plasma was investigated. Two radioimmunoassays were employed using rat(r)CRF as std and tracer(cDNA sequencing predicts hCRF is identical to rCRF). Dispersed rat anterior pituitary cells were used to assess bioactivity(BIO), and gel filtration and reverse phase HPLC were used for physicochemical characterization. Three immunoreactive(IR) size classes were detected in term placental extracts:I,MW>10000;II,>5000;III,rCRF(1-41)-sized. Peak II was a minor component, while peak I(putative precursor) was c. 60% as abundant as peak III. Peak III was indistinguishable from rCRF in its IR-to-BIO potency estimates, and eluted with the same retention times as rCRF in two different HPLC systems that display differing selectivities for ovine and rCRF. The apparent concentration of IR placental CRF was greater in trophoblastic-enriched tissue(c. 9 pmol/g) than in total placenta(c. 5 pmol/g). BIO and IR CRF was detected in third trimester plasma(c. 15 fmol/ml), but not in first or second trimester or nonpregnant female plasma(<1.2 fmol/ml), or in patients with Nelson's or Cushing's disease, or with pheochromocytomas(< 2.5 fmol/ml). In addition IR CRF was not detectable in basal or stressed rat plasma(< 5 fmol/ml). These data suggest that human placenta synthesizes CRF(probably in trophoblasts from a larger precursor); such material may have a role in the regulation of the placental pro-opiomelanocortin-like system as well as being secreted into the maternal circulation.

2064 DIURNAL ADMINISTRATION OF SOMATOCRININ (hp GRF 1-44 NH_2 or GRF) DOES NOT MODIFY THE SLEEP-RELATED GROWTH HORMONE SECRETION. G. Sassolas*, B.ROUSSEL, P. GARRY, J.P. BOISSEL, R. COHEN, S. BIOT-LAPORTE, A. ELM CHARFI and M. JOUVET, Centre de Médecine Nucléaire, B.P. Lyon Montchat, 69394 LYON Cedex 3, France.

Exogenous growth hormone (GH) administration to normal subjects induces a decrease in the nocturnal GH secretion related to sleep. In order to determine whether the GH rise induced by GRF would exert such an effect, we studied GH secretion during the nights preceding and following GRF administration.

Six normal young men (22-26 Y.O.) were given 50 µg GRF one day at 08.00 h and another day separated by one week at 20.00 h each. Blood samples were drawn for GH determinations every twenty minutes all over the nights and at usual times after iv GRF. The sleep-waking cycle was classicaly recorded by EEG and EOG electrodes chronically attached.

Our results show :

1) the chronology of the sleep-related GH peaks is not modified by GRF, intravenously administered in the morning or in the evening before the sleep onset.
2) the magnitude of the sleep-related GH peaks is not modified by GRF even when administered in the early evening.
3) the magnitude of the spontaneous nocturnal GH peaks is related to the magnitude of the GRF induced GH peaks.

2065 EFFECTS OF ADRENERGIC AGENTS ON RAT GROWTH HORMONE (rGH) RESPONSES TO HUMAN PANCREATIC GH RELEASING FACTOR(hpGRF-44). S. Sawano*, T. Kobayashi, Y. Fukushima, S. Ozaki, M. Mori, T. Takaoka and S. Ohashi, Dept. Endocrinol., Toranomon Hosp.; Okinaka Memorial Inst. for Med. Res.; Asahi Life Inst. for Adult Diseases; Res. Center of Tissue Culture, Dokkyo Univ. Sch. Med.; and Res. Inst. for Polymers and Textiles., Tokyo 105, Japan.

In vivo and *in vitro* effects of adrenergic agents on rGH responses to GRF were investigated. Under nembutal anesthesia, isoproterenol(IS, 3μg), propranolol(PR, 750 μg), IS+PR, norepinephrine(NE, 30μg), phentolamine(PH, 750μg) or NE+PH was dissolved in 3 ml saline and infused for 45 min. A single iv injection of GRF(200ng) was performed 15 min after initiation of the infusion of these agents, and blood was drawn immediately before and 3, 6, 12 and 24 min after GRF. During infusion of saline, GRF promptly stimulated serum rGH release from the base line level of 190 ± 22 (mean ± S.E.) ng/ml to the peak value of 1,601 ± 153 ng/ml at 3 min, which was inhibited by IS infusion (626 ± 93 ng/ml, $p<0.01$). This inhibitory effect of IS was completely canceled when IS was infused together with PR (1,408 ± 296 ng/ml). On the other hand, neither NE nor PH affected rGH response to GRF, but a concomitant infusion of NE and PH resulted in a decrease in rGH level to 1,078 ± 91 ng/ml ($p<0.01$). In monolayer cell cultures of rat pituitaries, IS, PR, NE or PH did not affect either the basal or GRF-stimulated rGH secretion. These results clearly show that the β-adrenergic agonism inhibits GRF-induced serum rGH rise. Considering together with *in vitro* results, it is suggested that the inhibitory effect of IS is not caused by changing the responsiveness of the pituitary to GRF, but presumably by mediating the increased secretion of somatostatin.

2066 EFFECT OF MULTIPLE PULSES OF GRF-44 ON GH RELEASE IN GH DEFICIENT PATIENTS. E.A. Schriock*, J.A. Hulse, D.A. Harris, S.L. Kaplan, M.M. Grumbach, Department of Pediatrics, University of California San Francisco, CA, USA

The GH response to a single IV pulse of synthetic, amidated GRF-44 may be blunted or absent in patients with GH deficiency (GHD) (Schriock, Lustig, Kaplan, Grumbach, unpublished data). To determine if multiple pulses of GRF-44 enhance the GH response to GRF, 10 GHD patients (4 idiopathic, 4 organic, 2 familial) were given GRF-44 IV every 2 hours for a total of 4 to 12 pulses (first and last, 5 μg/kg; others, 1 μg/kg). Studies were begun at 0800-0900h in 8 patients and 1900-2000h in 2 patients. Seven of the 10 patients responded to the initial GRF pulse with an increase in plasma GH concentration (mean peak GH ± SE; 9.0 ± 2.2). Two of the 3 nonresponders had familial GHD and did not respond to any of four doses administered. The third patient began to respond with the fourth pulse and achieved a maximum GH concentration of 7.8 ng/ml after the seventh pulse. Six patients had an increase in plasma GH after each pulse of GRF. Eight patients had their highest response (22.3 ± 7.2 ng/ml) after 4 to 12 pulses of GRF; these occurred between 1800 and 0300h and were unrelated to sleep in 5 of the patients. In the 8 patients the integrated GH response area between 2000 and 0800h (2651.8 ± 785.19 ng·min/ml) was greater than that between 0800 and 2000h (1467.4 ± 521.7 ng·min/ml; $p<0.01$) regardless of when the individual's study began. CONCLUSIONS: Multiple IV pulses of GRF-44 can induce GH secretion in GHD patients unresponsive to a single GRF pulse and increase the responses of other GHD patients; this suggests a priming effect of GRF-44 on the somatotrope and the presence of hypothalamic GRF deficiency. Responsiveness to GRF-44 appears to be greater at night and not consistently related to sleep.

2067 HUMAN CORTICOTROPIN RELEASING FACTOR (hCRF) IS METABOLIZED MORE RAPIDLY THAN OVINE CORTICOTROPIN RELEASING FACTOR (oCRF) IN MAN. T.H. Schuermeyer, T.P. Tomai, P.W. Gold, P.C. Avgerinos, H.M. Schulte, G.B. Cutler Jr., D. L. Loriaux and G.P. Chrousos*, NICHD and NIMH, NIH, Bethesda, Md, 20205, U.S.A.

The recently sequenced human corticotropin releasing factor (hCRF) is a 41 amino acid peptide which differs from ovine corticotropin releasing factor (oCRF) by 7 amino acids. When hCRF is given as an i.v. bolus to normal men it causes briefer plasma ACTH and cortisol elevations than those elicited by ovine corticotropin releasing factor (oCRF), which acts as a long-acting CRF analog in man. The prolonged effectiveness of oCRF can be explained by its long half-life and low metabolic clearance rate (MCR), which is only about 2 ml/kg/min in man. To investigate whether hCRH is metabolized more rapidly than oCRF, we measured plasma IR-hCRF levels after an i.v. bolus injection of 1 and 5 ug/kg of synthetic hCRF in 18 healthy volunteers using a specific radioimmunoassay (antibodies raised in rabbits against a hCRF-BSA conjugate). Plasma IR-hCRF concentrations decayed much faster than those of IR-oCRF. After injection of 1 and 5 ug/kg of hCRF, plasma concentrations of IR-hCRF were undetectable (<80 pg/ml) after 90 and 120-150 min, respectively. The calculated MCR (mean ± SD) was 15.1 ± 5.9 ml/kg/min after the higher dose (n=8) and 24.1 ± 9.1 ml/kg/min after the lower dose (n=10). Thus, the calculated MCR of hCRF is about 10 times greater than that of oCRF and in the range of other releasing factors and peptide hormones. We conclude : The different MCRs of hCRF and oCRF in man may explain their different duration of effect.

2068 HUMAN CORTICOTROPIN RELEASING FACTOR (hCRF): DOSE-RESPONSE AND TIME-COURSE OF ACTH AND CORTISOL SECRETION IN MAN. T.H. Schuermeyer*, P.C. Avgerinos, P.W. Gold, T.P. Tomai, W.T. Gallucci, G.B. Cutler Jr., D.L. Loriaux and G.P. Chrousos, NICHD and NIMH, NIH, Bethesda, Maryland, 20205, U.S.A.

Human corticotropin releasing factor is a recently sequenced 41 amino acid peptide, 17 % different from ovine CRF (oCRF) (EMBO Journal 2: 775, 1983). We investigated the response of plasma ACTH and cortisol concentrations to graded doses of hCRF given as an i.v. bolus to normal volunteers at 2000. Dose-dependent elevations of plasma ACTH and cortisol were observed (mean±SE). The time-course patterns of these responses were monophasic and significantly shorter than those after oCRF.

Dose	n	plasma ACTH (pg/ml)			plasma cortisol (ug/dl)		
ug/kg		0 min.	30 min.	180 min.	0 min.	30 min.	180 min.
0.01	3	6.6 ± 1.7	4.8 ± 0.9	4.4 ± 0.9	5.2 ± 2.6	4.1 ± 1.7	4.1 ± 1.3
0.05	3	7.1 ± 1.8	6.0 ± 0.3	3.8 ± 0.1	6.6 ± 3.5	6.4 ± 2.5	2.2 ± 0.6
0.1	6	7.7 ± 1.0	7.9 ± 0.9	6.8 ± 1.3	5.8 ± 1.3	6.4 ± 1.1	3.7 ± 1.3
0.5	9	9.2 ± 1.3	15.7 ± 2.1	6.3 ± 0.5	6.4 ± 0.8	10.2 ± 1.6	3.0 ± 1.1
1	15	7.4 ± 0.5	16.1 ± 1.6	5.9 ± 0.7	5.2 ± 0.5	13.1 ± 0.9	5.0 ± 1.0
5	5	8.0 ± 1.9	37.3 ±13.2	15.9 ± 3.1	6.2 ± 2.1	13.5 ± 1.7	11.3 ± 1.7

Heart rates increased slightly (+ 26%) at the highest dose without any significant changes in blood pressure. A facial flush was experienced by all subjects receiving this dose and by 5 subjects, who received 1 ug/kg. We conclude: (1) Synthetic hCRF caused brief ACTH and cortisol increases, more similar to those occurring spontaneously or under stress than those observed after oCRF. Thus, oCRF acts as a long-acting CRF analog in man. (2) No serious side-effects were observed up to a dose of 5 ug/kg.

2069 A STUDY IN THE RAT OF THE CONTRIBUTION MADE BY ITS COMPONENTS TO THE CIRCADIAN RHYTHM OF THE HYPOTHALAMO-PITUITARY-ADRENOCORTICAL AXIS.

S. A. Nicholson*, J-H Lin, S. N. Mahmoud, E. A. Campbell, B. Gillham and M. T. Jones, Departments of Gynaecology and Biochemistry, St. Thomas's Hospital, London SE1 7EH, U.K.

Female rats were maintained for several weeks on a fixed lighting schedule (lights on 0600 to 1800h). Groups were decapitated at various times of the day and tissues of the HPA axis removed and incubated *in vitro*. Basal secretion of corticotrophin-releasing factor (CRF) from the isolated hypothalamus *in vitro* was slightly but significantly elevated from tissues removed in the evening (1700h) compared to that from those removed in the morning (0800h). There was no significant change with time of day in the CRF response *in vitro* to excitatory neurotransmitters (acetylcholine and serotonin). CRF content was significantly higher in the evening, as measured by bioassay (BA) and radioimmunoassay (RIA). In contrast, pituitary responsiveness to ovine CRF (by RIA) and hypothalamic extract (HE, by BA) *in vitro*, and to injection of the HE *in vivo* (by BA) was considerably greater in the evening. Adrenal responsiveness to ACTH, given *in vivo* or *in vitro*, was also enhanced in the evening. Placement of electrolytic lesions in the mediobasal hypothalamus markedly reduced the diurnal variation in pituitary responsiveness, but completely reversed the normal variation in adrenal responsiveness (that is, the response to ACTH was lower in the evening than in the morning). It is concluded that the frequency of the circadian rhythm is determined by the hypothalamus (or higher centres), and the amplitude by changes in the responsiveness of the pituitary and adrenal glands.

2070 EFFECTS OF NEONATAL MSG TREATMENT AND ANTERIOR HYPOTHALAMIC DEAFFERENTATION ON LH SECRETION IN THE OVARIECTOMIZED RAT.

P. A. Rose and R. F. Weick*, Department of Physiology, University of Western Ontario, London, Canada.

Previous research showed that electrolytic lesions of the arcuate nuclei and anterior hypothalamic deafferentiation (AHD) blocked pulsatile LH release in the ovariectomized rat, but that neither lesion was sufficient by itself. This led to the hypothesis that two separate neural pathways are capable of effecting pulsatile LH release, which we tested in a different way. Newborn rats were treated with monosodium glutamate (MSG), which damages the arcuate nuclei, or NaCl of the same osmolarity as a control. As adults, the rats were gonadectomized, and 2 weeks later AHD or sham AHD was performed. One week after that, the rats were catheterized, and small blood samples were taken every 5 min for 3 h and the plasma assayed for LH. Neither MSG alone, AHD alone, nor the combination affected the numbers of animals with pulsatile LH patterns, mean LH levels, or LH pulse amplitude or frequency. Group sizes ranged from 8 to 13 rats. We interpret these results to mean that MSG spares those elements of the arcuate nuclei which are important for LH secretion, that electrolytic lesions of the arcuate destroy the fibers of passage which are important for LH secretion, or that functional reorganization of the systems controlling LH secretion occurs following neonatal MSG treatment.

Supported by MRC of Canada.

2071 MEDIAL BASAL HYPOTHALAMUS LESIONS (MBHL) AND PITUITARY STALK SECTIONS (SS) BLOCK THE PROGESTERONE-INDUCED LH SURGE IN OVARIECTOMIZED RHESUS MONKEYS.

R.R. Yeoman*, R.L. Norman†, E. Terasawa. Wis. Reg. Primate Res. Ctr., Univ. WI 53715, †Dept. Anat. Texas Tech U. Sch. of Med., Lubbock, TX 79430.

In rhesus monkeys progesterone (P) administration after a small dose of estradiol benzoate (EB) induces an LH surge with short latency (∿7 hr) and short duration (∿18 hr). In the present experiment the sites of positive feedback action of P were investigated using two methods, MBHL and SS, which are known to eliminate endogenous LHRH reaching the pituitary. Five ovariectomized animals received radiofrequency lesions in the arcuate nucleus and median eminence. The other 5 received SS with insertion of a teflon barrier. P effects after surgery were tested under LHRH pulsatile infusion (1μg/min for 6 min/h). The basic protocol for P (2.5mg) administration following EB (30μg) was described elsewhere. In 3 of 5 MBHL animals the P-induced LH surge was entirely abolished. In the remaining 2 MBHL animals a markedly attenuated LH surge (1/10 amplitude of the prelesioned control) was observed but in histological examination after sacrifice it was found that substantial tissue of the MBH remained in these 2 animals. In 4 of 5 SS animals the P-induced LH surge was completely eliminated, while in 1 of 5 SS animals an attenuated LH surge was observed. Although no histological examination has been performed yet, in the last animal we observed a pituitary tumor extending above the roof of the sella turcica during SS surgery. Therefore, an intact MBH with connection to the pituitary is essential for the P-induced LH surge. This indicates that P with a small priming dose of EB stimulates the release of LHRH from the brain. (Supported by grants RR00167, HD11355, and HD15433.)

2072 CYTOPLASMIC TRANSLATION OF CYTOCHROME OXIDASE UNITS IN THE MOUSE BLASTOCYST IS AN EARLY EVENT IN ACTIVATION FROM DELAYED IMPLANTATION.

C. Magnusson*, B. Einarsson & B.O. Nilsson,
Dept. of Physiology, Göteborg and Dept. of Human Anatomy, Uppsala, Sweden.

Blastocysts from mice, ovariectomized three days after mating and substituted with progesterone, attain a state of low metabolic activity, "delayed implantation". When activated by an estrogen injection the blastocyst rapidly doubles its O_2 consumption and the cytochrome oxidase enzyme is activated (Nilsson et al 1982, J Embryol exp Morph 71:75). In a culture system known to permit trophoblast outgrowth, a process regarded analogous to implantation, O_2 consumption also increased. To see whether activation of cytochrome oxidase needs synthesis of new protein or just activation of enzyme precursors, inhibitors of transcription (cytosine arabinoside and α-amanitin) and RNA translation in the cytoplasm (cycloheximide) and mitochondria (chloramphenicol) were added to blastocysts cultured for 4-6 h in Brinster medium. O_2 consumption was measured spectrophotometrically using hemoglobin as O_2 tension indicator (Hultborn 1974, Acta Physiol Scand Suppl 404).

After 6 h culture blastocyst O_2 consumption had increased by 50%. Cycloheximide (1 μg/ml) inhibited this increase while the other inhibitors all were without effect. This suggests that cytochrome oxidase activation involves translation of preformed RNA templates in the cytoplasm, while the part of the enzyme that is synthesized in the mitochondria is already present. Thus, we believe that the trophoblast control of oxidative phosphorylation lies post-transcriptionally.

2073 HUMAN CHORIONIC GONADOTROPIN (hCG) DETECTION BY RADIOIMMUNOASSAY, ENZYME-LINKED IMMUNOSORBENT ASSAY (ELISA) AND BY HEMAGGLUTINATION INHIBITION (HAI) DURING EARLY, MIDDLE AND LATE PREGNANCY. W.E. Nixon*, O. Pescovitz, R. Reid, J. Lunney, R. Leslie, B. Nisula, D.L. Loriaux. Developmental Endocrinology Branch, NICHD, NIH, Bethesda, Maryland.

The enzyme-linked immunosorbent assay (ELISA) offers a rapid, inexpensive and less hazardous methodology for determination of hormones. We present preliminary experiments in the development of an hCG ELISA and comparisons with results in an established RIA (SB_6) and an hemagglutination inhibition assay (β-Neocept). Plasma inhibited binding of antisera to hCG-coated microtiter plates nonspecifically; however, Cancanavalin A extraction eliminated that inhibition. Subsequently, pre-incubation of hCG-coated microtiter plates with ovalbumin (1%) was used to eliminate this nonspecific plasma interference and LH and FSH crossreactivity. ELISA characteristics include: 1) range of detection, 50-0.78 ng (CR 121); sensitivity, 0.8-1.0 ng; 3) crossreactivity with LH and FSH, not detected (<1.0%); 4) intra-and interassay coefficient of variation, 9.4% and 10.6%, respectively. HCG standard curves and doubling dilutions of urine and serum from each trimester of pregnancy exhibited regions with parallel slopes; these regions were used for potency determinations. During peak hCG excretion (days 50-80), RIA values in urine (20 μg/ml) were greater than ELISA values (10 μg/ml). Prior to day 50 and following day 80, RIA and ELISA values were comparable. In serum, RIA values tended not to exceed ELISA values; however, at the day 50 peak (11.5 μg/ml), values in RIA and ELISA were indistinguishable. We conclude that with the use of ovalbumin to eliminate nonspecific interference this ELISA for hCG yields results similar to an established RIA.

2074 LHRH TREATMENT OF MALE HYPOGONADOTROPIC HYPOGONADISM. S. J. Nillius*, G. Skarin and L. Wide, Departments of Obstetrics and Gynecology and Clinical Chemistry, University Hospital, Uppsala, Sweden.

Chronic pulsatile subcutaneous LHRH therapy was given to four males, aged 18-29 years, with hypogonadotropic hypogonadism. They had very low pretreatment levels of gonadotropins and testosterone in serum. The LHRH therapy was given by means of a small automatically-timed infusion pump (Zyklomat, Ferring). The pump infused 1, 5 or 20 μg LHRH subcutaneously once every 90 min through a chronic indwelling catheter in the lower abdominal wall or the ventral part of the upper thigh. The long-term (90-328 days), out-patient treatment was safe and very well accepted by the patients.

Puberty was induced in an 18-year-old boy who had developed panhypopituitarism after surgery of a craniopharyngeoma. The pulsatile LHRH therapy induced normal gonadotropin and testosterone secretion within one month. Rapid growth of penis and pubic hair to adult size and type occurred during the 328-day-long therapy. The testis volume increased from 2 to 12 ml. Nocturnal emissions occurred after 38 weeks of pulsatile LHRH treatment and sperms were found in the ejaculate after 43 weeks.

Potency and spermatogenesis were induced in the three infertile hypogonadotropic men with hypothalamic dysfunction. Normal gonadotropin and testosterone serum concentrations were restored within 10 days of therapy. Libido and potency returned. The first ejaculates contained no sperms. Spermatogenesis was induced and normalized with continued treatment. The wifes of two men conceived after 6 and 7 months of LHRH therapy, respectively. Two healthy girls have been born and paternity tests were positive. The third man has only been treated for 3 months at present.

2075 EFFECT OF DANAZOL ON SERUM FSH, LH, PROLACTIN AND CORTISOL LEVELS IN POSTMENOPAUSAL AND OOPHORECTOMIZED WOMEN. T.Okamura*, T.Takeuchi, T.Yaginuma and T.Kobayashi, Dept of Obstet and Gynecol, Faculty of Med, Univ of Tokyo at Mejirodai, Tokyo, Japan

The present study was performed by serial blood samplings through an indwelling catheter into the cubital vein every 20 min for 2 hours for hormone assay before and after the administration of Danazol(D) at a daily dose of 400mg in 4 women and 600mg in 5 women. The time-course of FSH, LH and prolactin levels was shown not to correlate with that and each value of cortisol levels in individuals before D, expressing stress if caused by blood sampling. In comparison between mean hormone levels of 7 serum samples before and after D, (1) FSH levels lowered in all women after D of 400mg and 600mg ($P<0.01$ and $P<0.005$, respectively), (2) LH levels lowered in only one woman after D of 400mg ($P<0.01$) and in 4 women in a dose of 600mg ($P<0.01$), (3) prolactin levels lowered in 2 women of D of 400mg ($P<0.001$) and in one woman of D of 600mg, but increased in one woman of D of 600mg ($P<0.001$), (4) cortisol levels lowered in only one woman after D of 400mg ($P<0.01$) and in 4 women after D of 600mg ($P<0.01$). These results suggest that blood samplings, which might cause stress, do not influence blood FSH, LH and prolactin levels and indicate that D suppresses FSH and LH release and cortisol secretion in the comparably larger dose, but does not constantly prolactin release.

2076 COMBINED ENDOCRINE AND ULTRASOUND ASSESSMENT OF OVULATION: IDENTIFICATION OF A GROUP OF INFERTILE WOMEN WITH PERSISTENT HIGH LH, AND LUTEINIZATION WITHOUT OVULATION. P. Petsos, C. Chandler, M. Oak, W. Ratcliffe, R. Wood & D.C. Anderson*. Departments of Medicine, Obstetrics and Gynaecology, Chemical Pathology and Radiology, Hope Hospital, Eccles Old Road, Salford UK

We have examined the possibility that in a significant number of couples with unexplained infertility the woman may have a subtle endocrine defect leading to anovulation, despite regular menstrual cycles with luteinization. Detailed serial profiles of serum LH, FSH, progesterone and oestradiol, were combined with ultrasound, during 43 cycles in 33 women. Two were normal volunteers, one other was studied during a conception cycle, 7 had a probable non-hormonal cause of infertility, and 23 had long-standing infertility that had remained unexplained after extensive previous investigation. Of 37 cycles suitable for analysis, 22 showed undoubted ovulation by all criteria, including development and collapse at mid-cycle of a single follicle. Of the remainder, 6 cycles from 4 women showed a pattern of persistent high LH throughout, and luteinization of a cyst or cysts without ovulation. A similar endocrine profile was seen in 3 other infertile women, in whom ultrasound was not performed. Preliminary studies indicate that whereas in women with classical polycystic ovarian syndrome (PCOS) the high LH levels suppress with the progestogen medroxyprogesterone acetate (10mg/day for 14 days), they do not do so in the syndrome of infertility, high LH and pseudo-ovulation. We postulate that the underlying defect may be an inability of the gonadotrophe to switch from an LH to an FSH-secreting mode in response to the normal cyclical changes in GnRH pulse frequency and circulating steroid concentrations.

2077 STUDIES ON THE PARACRINE ACTIONS OF INSULIN ON SOMATOSTATIN RELEASE AND ON INTRAINSULAR TRH. G. Schäfer*, A. Heyer, A.Ferdussian, S.Ahuja and H. Schatz, Center of Internal Medicine, University of Giessen,F.R.G.

The influence of insulin on somatostatin release is still an unsettled question as well as the role of intrainsular TRH. Collagenase-isolated rat pancreatic islets were studied under static conditions and also during perifusion, both freshly after isolation and after culture. A significant inhibition of somatostatin release by exogenous insulin was observed only in precultivated and not in freshly isolated islets. Unexpectedly, perifusion with anti-insulin serum resulted in a significant inhibition of somatostatin release. Islets of newborn rats contained much more TRH compared to adult islets (14.5 ± 6.4 and 0.44 ± o.88 pg TRH/islet, respectively, $\bar{x}$ ± SEM). Augmentation of insulin release by TRH and its decrease by anti-TRH-serum were only borderline significant. A significant inhibition of glucagon release was observed, however, by anti-TRH antiserum. Conclusion: Restitution during culture of altered insulin receptors of the D cells may explain the inhibitory action of insulin on somatostatin release after precultivation. The inhibitory action of antiinsulin serum might be due to an insulin-like action of immunoglobulins or of anti-idiotypic insulin antibodies.
A paracrine role of intrainsular TRH (present in high amounts in the perinatal period) has to be discussed.

2078 STUDIES ON PERIPHERAL T LYMPHOCYTE SUBSETS IN THE DIABETICS. M. Shimizu*, K. Okano, Y. Nozawa, S. Kou, T. Kato, K. Hoshi, T. Sano and K. Someya, Third Department of Internal Medicine, St. Marianna University School of Medicine, Kawasaki, Japan.

In order to elucidate immunological abnormalities in the diabetics, peripheral T lymphocyte subsets of 10 patients with insulin-dependent diabetes mellitus (IDDM), 12 with noninsulin-dependent diabetes mellitus (NIDDM) and 16 normal subjects, were analyzed by Cell Sorter (JASCO, FCS-1) using Ortho-mune OK series monoclonal antibodies: OKT3 (pan T cell), OKT4 (helper-inducer T cell), OKT8 (suppressor-cytotoxic T cell), OKIa1 (B cell, activated T cell). There was a significant positive regression between age and $OKT4^{+}T$ cell/$OKT8^{+}T$ cell ratio only in the normal subjects (Y=0.161 + 0.034X, r=0.70, $p<0.01$). $OKT3^{+}T$ cell was significantly increased in IDDM group (71.2 ± 7.7 %) compared to its age-matched normal group (59.9 ± 11.6 %) ($p<0.05$). $OKT4^{+}T$ cell in the IDDM group (41.6 ± 13.0 %) also showed a significant increase compared to its age-matched normal group (26.9 ± 8.7 %) ($p<0.05$). $OKT8^{+}T$ cell, however, showed no significant differences among the IDDM group, NIDDM group and their age-matched normal groups. $OKT4^{+}T$ cell/$OKT8^{+}T$ cell ratio in the IDDM group (1.71 ± 0.95) significantly increased compared to its age-matched normal group (0.94 ± 0.35) ($p<0.05$). $OKIa1^{+}$ cell showed no significant differences among these groups. These lymphocyte subsets or their ratio showed no significant correlations with diabetic duration, HbA_1, plasma glucose or HDL-cholesterol in the IDDM group and NIDDM group. These data suggest that there exist alterations in immuno-regulatory mechanism in IDDM.

2079 NALOXONE EFFECT ON INSULIN SECRETION IN OBESITY

N. Sicolo°, E. De Palo, C. De Palo, C. Martini, R. Gatti, R. Vettor
Istituto di Semeiotica Medica, Cattedra di Patologia Medica III^; Università di Padova, Italy

Obese patients show a hyperinsulinism which may play an important role in the developement and/or maintenance of obesity itself. Data obteined in genetically obese rats showed an increase in endorphyn brain concentration; moreover Naloxone administration is able to correct feeding behaviour in 2-Deoxy-glucose treated rats. Since opioid peptides seem to stimulate insulin secretion both in vivo and in vitro, we carried out an investigation to verify whether the obese patient's hyperinsulinism may be modified by opioid receptor antagonist administration.

Blood glucose and plasma insulin responses to OGTT and Arginine infusion were measured before and during Naloxone administration in two groups of obese and control subjects. Naloxone alone did not modify basal blood glucose and insulin levels both in obese and in control subjects. Glucose-induced insulin response was significantly reduced by Naloxone administration in obese subjects (80 ± 10 vs 48 ± 4 μU/ml at 30'; 84 ± 7 vs 71 ± 4 at 60'; 81 ± 13 vs 70 ± 7 at 90'; 89 ± 8 vs 61 ± 9 at 120'; $p < 0.001$)but not in controls without changes in glycaemic pattern. Opioid antagonist administration did not modify insulin response to arginine in obese and control group.

Our results support the hypothesis that opioid-like peptides may play a role in the beta-cell hyperresponsiveness to glucose in obesity.

2080 PROISLET ISOTRANSPLANTATION - FUNCTIONAL STUDIES.

Charmaine J. Simeonovic, K.J. Lafferty, S.P. Haynes and J.D. Wilson* Transplantation Biology Unit, John Curtin School of Medical Research, Australian National University and Department of Endocrinology, Woden Valley Hospital, Canberra, Australia.

Proislets consist of undifferentiated tissue elements which have the capacity to develop into fully differentiated islets following transplantation.[1] They are prepared by collagenase digestion of foetal pancreas followed by culture of the digested tissue in 10% CO_2 95% air for 4 days. In this study CBA mice, rendered diabetic by intravenous injection of 250 mg/kg streptozotocin, were transplanted with proislets derived from foetal pancreases removed from CBA foetuses at 17 days gestation. Four groups of mice received proislets derived from 8, 6, 4 and one foetus respectively. Normoglycaemia (blood sugar < 11 mmol/l) was restored 25-230 days after transplantation. All mice reverted to the diabetic state after removal of the grafts. Oral glucose tolerance tests (50 mg) were performed on all mice after restoration of normoglycaemia and the glucose and insulin responses compared to those in 4 age and sex matched normal CBA mice. The glucose response (increase in area under glucose curve) was not significantly different in any of the groups of transplanted mice compared to the normal mice. The insulin response in all transplanted mice was significantly diminished suggesting an increased sensitivity to insulin in these animals. Proislets are much less immunogenic than cultured foetal pancreas and therefore may offer possibilities for clinical pancreatic islet transplantation. This work was supported in part by P.H.S. Grant AM28126.

[1]Simeonovic C.J. and Lafferty K.J. Aust. J. Exp. Biol. Med. Sci., 60, 383, 1982.

2081 INSULIN AS A SIGNAL TO THE BRAIN. G.A. Smythe*, J.E. Bradshaw, H.S. Grunstein and L.H. Storlien. Garvan Institute of Medical Research, St. Vincent's Hospital, Sydney, 2010, Australia.

The questions whether insulin has a role in signalling the brain or in mediating brain glucose uptake are controversial. In view of the proposal that the brain glucose control system is mediated via central noradrenergic neuronal activity (NNA), we investigated the effects of insulin administration on medial basal hypothalamic (mbh) NNA in fasted and fed rats. Computerized GC/MS was used to assess NNA from the ratio of the mbh concentration of 3,4-dihydroxyphenylethyleneglycol to that of norepinephrine. Following insulin administration (2U/kg; blood glucose -44% at 10min) NNA was suppressed ($p < 0.005$) by 10min and remained down for a further 10min. However 30min after insulin NNA exhibited the expected stress response to hypoglycemia and rose again to be significantly higher ($p < 0.05$) than in saline controls and at 45min was highly significantly elevated. While serum ACTH and corticosterone levels after insulin were positively and highly significantly correlated with NNA at all times, plasma glucagon remained unaltered initially but increased >2-fold by 45min, raising the possibility that glucagon release may be neurally stimulated by NNA. The NNA responses after insulin were unaffected by feeding or fasting; this result and further data indicating brain glucose utilisation was reduced ($p < 0.01$) 5-10min after insulin suggest that insulin exerts rapid effects on mbh NNA as a signal to the brain - perhaps via cellular potassium shifts - rather than by increasing brain glucose uptake. This study was supported by the NH&MRC of Australia.

2082 THE RELATIONSHIP OF THYROID FUNCTION TESTS (TFT) AND METABOLIC PARAMETERS IN PATIENTS WITH DIABETIC KETOACIDOSIS (DKA). J. Spencer*, A. E. Kitabchi, M. B. Murphy, M. Mojallali, J. Karas and R. Matteri, Dept. of Med. and Clin. Res. Cntr., Univ. of TN Cntr. for Health Sci., Memphis, Tennessee, U.S.A.

It has been suggested that alteration of CHO metabolism affects TFT in man. We have studied TFT (T_3, FT_4, TSH) in 32 consecutive cases of DKA and correlated their values at 0, 12, 24 and 48 hrs after insulin therapy with the following parameters: temperature, glucose, HgA_1, HCO_3, pH, ketone bodies and cortisol. Whereas T_3 values were significantly below normal at the time of admission (66.3 ± 4.6 ng/dl) with values of 46, 58 and 83 ng/dl at 12, 24 and 48 hrs respectively, TSH and T_4 values were within normal limits at admission and after therapy. No significant correlation was noted between initial levels of T_3, FT_4 (1.18 ± 0.05) and TSH (2.8 ± 0.36) with cortisol (64.8 ± 8.89), glucose (494.4 ± 36.2), ketone bodies (12.12 ± 0.86), pH (7.09 ± 0.02), HCO_3 (5.67 ± 0.43) or temperature (97.9 ± 0.29). A significant negative correlation ($r=-0.40$, $P<.03$) between initial T_3 (but not FT_4 or TSH) and HgA_1 ($13.25 \pm 0.4\%$) was observed. T_3 correlated negatively with body temperature at 48 hrs of therapy ($r=-0.48$, $P<.02$). We conclude that in DKA the most significant correlate of thyroid function is the relationship of T_3 and chronic glycemic control as assessed by HgA_1 and that body temperature is negatively correlated with the level of T_3 during the recovery phase.

2083 EFFECTS OF EXPERIMENTAL DIABETES ON HYPOTHALAMIC CATECHOLAMINES.
Jennifer Stewart*, Donald Workman and John Althaus, Virginia Commonwealth University, Richmond, VA. and University of Virginia, Charlottesville, VA., U.S.A.

We have studied the effects of short-term streptozotocin diabetes (4 days duration) on the steady state concentrations and the rate of turnover of catecholamines in the hypothalamus of rats. Catecholamine concentrations were measured with high pressure liquid chromatography and electrochemical detection. We calculated rate constants of amine loss, catecholamine turnover time, and turnover rates from the decline of amine levels induced for 4 hrs by treatment with alpha-methyltyrosine (mpt). Five control and 5 or 6 diabetic animals were evaluated after saline and at each time point after the initial injection of mpt. Mean basal concentrations of epinephrine were lower ($p<0.01$) in the hypothalamus of diabetic animals (31.6 ± 2.6 ng/g) than in that of non-diabetics (44.7 ± 2.8 ng/g). Whereas steady state concentrations of dopamine and norepinephrine did not differ significantly in diabetics and non-diabetics, a reduction ($p<0.05$) in the mpt-induced depletion of these amines was associated with diabetes. Also, the rate of restoration of dopamine concentrations, measured 6 hrs after mpt treatment, was lower in diabetic than non-diabetic rats ($p<0.02$). The turnover rate of epinephrine in the hypothalamus of control animals was approximately 5 ng/g/hr, but the rate was too slow in diabetic animals for a meaningful estimation. These findings provide evidence that the early onset of diabetes may alter the availability of catecholamines in the hypothalamus.

2084 POTENCY OF SOMATOSTATIN-28 (SS-28) IN THE DOG AND ITS PHYSIOLOGIC ROLE IN THE RELEASE OF INSULIN.
G.J. Taborsky, Jr.*, and T.L. Paquette, VA Med Cntr, U. Wash., Seattle, WA, and Salk Inst., La Jolla, CA, U.S.A.

SS-28 has been found to be 10 times more potent than SS-14 on rat insulin (I) release. This, coupled with the discovery of SS-28 circulating in arterial blood, suggested that SS-28 may hormonally modulate I secretion. To test this hypothesis, we infused SS-28 IV into anesthetized dogs, measured SS-like-immunoreactivity (SSLI) in arterial plasma and its effect on basal I and glucagon (GG) output from the in situ pancreas. SS-28 infused IV at 0.51 nanomoles (nm)/min raised arterial SSLI by $1{,}122 \pm 143$ femtomoles (fm)/ml and produced a moderate inhibition of I output ($\Delta = -39 \pm 6\%$ of basal; $p < 0.0005$, n=7) with no change of GG output ($\Delta = +13 \pm 20\%$). Surprisingly, a dose of SS-14 (0.102 nm/min), which caused a 10-fold smaller rise of arterial SSLI ($\Delta = +108 \pm 16$ fm/ml), produced comparable inhibition of I output ($\Delta = -45 \pm 8\%$ of basal; $p < 0.0005$; n=9) and slight inhibition of GG output ($\Delta = -18 \pm 8\%$ of basal; $p < 0.05$; n=9). Thus, circulating SS-28 appears 10-fold less potent than SS-14. Furthermore, increments of endogenous, arterial SSLI ($\Delta = +32 \pm 5$ fm/ml; n=6 or $\Delta = +34 \pm 7$ fm/ml; n=8) achieved during strong stimulation of SS secretion by either IV isoproterenol or CCK-8 were 10-fold lower than those ($\Delta = +355 \pm 33$ fm/ml) achieved by the minimally effective dose (0.17 nm/min) of SS-28 (ΔI output = $-13 \pm 8\%$ of basal; $0.05 < p < 0.1$; ΔGG output = $+22 \pm 14\%$ of basal, n=7). Thus, endogenous levels of SS-28 in arterial plasma are incapable of inhibiting insulin release. **Summary:** 1) circulating SS-28 is 10-fold less potent than SS-14 on canine insulin release; 2) stimulated levels of endogenous, arterial SSLI are 10-fold lower than those of SS-28 that barely inhibit I release. **Conclusion:** SS-28 is not a hormonal modulator of I release in the dog. (in coll. w. J. Rivier)

2085 NATURAL COURSE AND EFFECT OF SEX HORMONE ON ISLET CELL SURFACE ANTIBODIES (ICSA) IN NOD MICE. I. Takei*, T. Maruyama, K. Kataoka and S. Matsuki, Department of Internal Medicine, School of Medicine, Keio Univ., Tokyo, Japan.

The NOD mouse is an animal model of insulin-dependent diabetes mellitus (IDDM), and the incidence of onset of diabetes shows a remarkable predominance of females. As ICSA are closely related to the pathogenesis of IDDM, we examined ICSA of male and female NOD mice from afterbirth, and the effect of sex hormones on ICSA.
The female NOD mice were classified into 3 groups; (1) non-treatment (2) testosterone administrated and (3) castrated groups, while the male NOD mice were classified into (1) non-treatment, (2) progesterone + estrogen administrated and (3) castrated groups. Blood was taken from the orbital vein of each mouse every 4 weeks from 3 weeks to 19 weeks old of age. Each sex hormone was administrated subcutaneously once a week. ICSA were determined using pancreatic beta cells of CD-1 mouse as the antigen and were measured by ^{125}I-Protein A radioligand assay.
In the case of female NOD mice, the non-treatment group showed a gradual increase of ICSA until the peak at the 11th week, then a further gradual increase. However, the values of the testosterone group were suppressed. Males in the non-treatment group showed the peak at the 7th week and there were lowes leves of ICSA in males than in females at the 19th week in the non-treatment group. The progesterone + estrogen group showed no peak at the 7th week.

2086 BENEFICIAL EFFECT OF PHYSICAL TRAINING ON EXPERIMENTAL DIABETES MELLITUS: A TIME-COURSE STUDY. G. Tancrède*, A. Nadeau, S. Rousseau-Migneron, C. Jobidon and D. Trudel. Laboratoires de Recherche en Endocrinologie et Métabolisme, CHUL, Québec, G1V 4G2, Canada.

We have previously reported that a ten-week program of physical training can improve experimental diabetes in the rat (Diabetes 31:406, 1982). To better characterize this model, a time-course study was performed by measuring overnight glucosuria (16h - 8h) once a week. Diabetes was induced in male Wistar rats (±200g) by the I.V. injection of streptozotocin (45 mg/kg). Seven days later, blood glucose was determined after a four-hour fast; rats with values between 250 and 400 mg/dl were either trained (n = 57) or kept sedentary (n = 60). Training was done progressively on a treadmill, twice daily, five days per week, according to the following program: 10 min at 22m/min for 3 weeks, 40 min at 28m/min for 3 weeks and 60 min at 31m/min for 3 weeks. In sedentary rats, glucosuria increased progressively during the experimental period while it tended to plateau in the trained group. After 3, 6 and 9 weeks, glucosuria had disappeared respectively in 9, 14 and 15 trained rats, and only in 1, 2 and 2 sedentary rats; differences between groups were significant at $p < 0.01$ by X^2. These data suggest that the beneficial effect of physical training in this model is obtained progressively and mostly during the first 6 weeks of the conditioning program. These results shall permit to shorten the training program in studies directed at elucidating the mechanism by which physical training improves diabetes mellitus.
Supported by MRC and CDA.

2087 IMPROVEMENT IN DIABETIC NEPHROPATHY : RELATION TO METABOLIC CONTROL.
A.C. Thai*, P.P.B. Yeo, K.W. Wang, L. Chan, K.F. Lui, J.S. Cheah and B.Y. Tan, Department of Medicine, National University of Singapore, Singapore General Hospital, Outram Road, Singapore.

The important relation between glycaemic control and chronic complications of diabetes remains unresolved. We conducted a prospective one-year study on 78 diabetic patients who are participants of a home-blood glucose monitoring programme to study the effect of glycaemic control upon nerve, eye and renal complications. Retinopathy was assessed by florescein angiography, neuropathy by nerve conduction, and nephropathy by urine Albustix and serum β2 microglobulin measurements. Patient performed 6 point glucose profile one day of the week and HbA_1 concentration was determined at 3-monthly interval. The frequency of complications at onset of study was 17% (nerve), 24% (eye) and 44% (renal). Interim data at 6 month showed a significant fall in HbA_1 at 3 month ($p < 0.02$) but not at 6 month. There was no significant change in eye and nerve complications. An interesting finding was observed for renal function. 34 patients had proteinuria and/or raised β2 microglobulin at onset. Of these, 22 (65%) became Albustix negative with a concommittant fall in β2 microglobulin level ($p < 0.01$) at 6 month. The remaining 12 (35%) patients showed persistent proteinuria during the study with no change in β2 microglobulin. HbA_1 concentration at 6 month was significantly lower for the group with improved renal function compared to the group which did not improve ($p < 0.01$). Our study suggests that good long term metabolic control may reverse diabetic nephropathy.

2088 ANTERIOR PITUITARY HORMONE BINDING PROTEINS IN SERA FROM SPONTANEOUSLY DIABETIC BB RATS.
T. Togane* S. Yagihashi[1], A.A.F. Sima[1] and H.G. Friesen, Depts. of Physiology and Pathology[1], University of Manitoba, Winnipeg, Manitoba, Canada R3E 0W3.

Autoantibodies to anterior pituitary cells have been identified in sera from Type I diabetic patients. In the present study we have looked for autoantibodies to pituitary hormones in spontaneously diabetic BB rats. Sera from prediabetic BB rats (PD), acute diabetic BB rats (AD) and age-matched non-diabetic Wistar rats (controls) were examined for binding to rat prolactin (rPRL) and/or rat growth hormone (rGH). Under the assay conditions used, the percentage binding of ^{125}I-rPRL was 18.3 ± 2.0 (mean ± SD) (n = 15) in controls; 18.9 ± 3.5 in PD; and 25.1 ± 6.6 (n = 12) in AD rats ($P < 0.002$ vs control and PD). Similarly the percentage ^{125}I-rGH bound was 13.6 ± 1.3 (n = 13) in controls; 15.5 ± 1.5 (n = 13) in PD rats; and 21.7 ± 11.5 (n = 10) in AD rats ($P < 0.02$ vs control). In AD rats 5 of 12 sera bound ^{125}I-rPRL more than 2 S.D. above the mean of controls, and 4 of 10 sera bound ^{125}I-rGH more than 2 S.D. above the mean of controls. Not all rat sera which bound ^{125}I-rPRL bound ^{125}I-rGH. After gel filtration of rat serum, hormone binding activity eluted in fractions containing macroglobulins (i.e. IgM). In conclusion, the presence of serum binding proteins for rPRL and rGH was demonstrated in diabetic BB rats providing further evidence of an immunologic disorder in these animals.

2089 EFFECTS OF β-RECEPTOR STIMULATION AND BLOCKADE ON THERMOGENESIS. K. Scheidegger*, R. Woo and E. Danforth Jr., Metabolic Unit, Dept. of Medicine, University of Vermont, Burlington VT 05405, USA

β-adrenoceptor agonists stimulate metabolic rates (MR) and are therefore of potential value in the treatment of obesity. We have studied the thermogenic effect of terbutaline sulfate (TS) after acute (5mg) and prolonged (5mg tid for 2 weeks) oral administration in 7 healthy, normal weight males aged 27±2 years. Basal MR increased after prolonged treatment with TS from 5.42 ± 0.17 to 5.66 ± 0.22 kJ/min ($p<0.05$). However, the acute thermogenic response to the drug was markedly blunted after 2 weeks with the $\Delta\dot{V}O2$ (area under the curve for 4hrs) being 35 ± 4 before and 9 ± 3 ml/min after treatment ($p<0.001$). Acute beta-blockade with propranolol (3mg bolus and 0.08mg/min inf) decreased basal MR initially by 0.14 ± 0.04 kJ/min ($p<0.02$ vs. basal) and after chronic β-receptor stimulation by 0.18 ± 0.04 kJ/min ($p<0.01$ vs. basal). Thus, the effect of beta-blockade on MR was not different before and after chronic TS. Conclusion: The acute thermogenic effect of a single dose of TS is decreased during prolonged administration of the drug, although basal MR are increased, indicating development of tolerance. We previously have reported changes in the serum concentrations of triiodothyronine and thyroxine after chronic administration of TS and suggested a role for the thyroid hormones in the observed changes in basal MR. This study confirms that other mechanisms than β-stimulation are involved in the chronic thermogenic effect of TS, since the increase in MR after chronic β-receptor stimulation could not be entirely blocked by propranolol.

2090 CONTROL OF SUPERFUSED ADRENAL CELLS BY ACTH AND cAMP PULSES: EVIDENCE FOR POST-RECEPTOR DESENSITIZATION. D.Schulster*, R.Clarke, B.Rafferty and B.Williams~, NIBS&C Holly Hill, London NW3 6RB and ~Dept.Med., Western Gen. Hosp., Edinburgh EH4 2XU.

In vitro superfusion allows study of dynamic responses of cells under conditions that approach physiological. Corticosterone(B) and cAMP outputs from rat adrenal fasciculata cells were determined in a Teflon column superfusion system, following pulsed treatment with ACTH agonists. Repeated small identical 80sec. pulses of (1-39)ACTH or (5-24)ACTH initially sensitized, but then desensitized the cells. Repeated injections of 0.4 pmoles (1-39)ACTH generated maximal outputs of 361, 444, 387, 337, 317, 241, 178 ngB/min. A final dose of 8 pmoles ACTH restored maximal responsiveness; cell loss or death could thus not account for the desensitization effect. Furthermore only sensitization of the cells was observed following repeated 60sec pulses of 5 µmoles cAMP with responses of 22, 45, 60, 68, 102, 115 ngB/min. It was concluded that the desensitization lesion occurred prior to cAMP production. Binding studies with isolated cells using I-125 labelled ACTH suggest a post-receptor event and that this 'lesion' probably lies between hormone receptor and adenylate cyclase. Dissimilarities were revealed when the ratios of the steroid and cAMP outputs elicited by (1-39)ACTH and (5-24)ACTH were examined. Peak ratios for B were >1 (ie 1.2, 1.1 and 1.3) whereas the peak ratios for cAMP were considerably < 1 (ie .55, .39 and .78). These differences emphasize the lack of correlation between steroidogenesis and cAMP output. We conclude that i) nucleotide-regulatory protein is implicated in the desensitization and ii) more than one receptor mechanism for ACTH-induced steroidogenesis operates.

2091 EFFECT OF THYROID HORMONE ON TISSUE CALMODULIN CONCENTRATION IN THE RAT.
J. Segal*, A. Coppens and S.H. Ingbar, Beth Israel Hospital, Boston, MA

Calmodulin influences the activity of numerous metabolic systems, some of which are also influenced by thyroid hormones. Therefore, we have performed studies to determine whether thyroid hormones, unlike the many other classes of hormone which have been shown to have no effect, would influence tissue calmodulin content. Total calmodulin concentrations in the thymocytes, liver, heart, brain, and skeletal muscle of female rats 35 days of age were measured by RIA in the following treatment groups: control (intact or sham-operated); hypothyroid (thyroidectomy at 21 days or 2% $KClO_4$ in water at 28 days); thyrotoxic (2 ug T_3/100 g s.c. daily, or either 3 ug T_3 or 3 ug T_3 + 4 ug T_4/100 g s.c. twice daily, starting at age 28 days). Compared with control values (100%), calmodulin content in animals given T_3, with or without T_4, was increased significantly ($p<0.02$) in thymocytes (147-154%), liver (160-203%), heart (140-150%), and brain (140-161%), but not in skeletal muscle. Calmodulin concentrations of tissues in both hypothyroid groups did not differ from those in their respective controls. Conclusions: These findings are apparently the first demonstration of a hormonal effect on tissue calmodulin concentrations, and they support the possibility that certain of the metabolic effects of thyroid hormones are calmodulin-mediated.

2092 ADENOSINE POTENTIATES THE EFFECTS OF LH AND ISOPROTERENOL ON ISOLATED LUTEAL CELLS BUT NOT ON WHOLE CORPORA LUTEA. Monica Sender-Baum* and Kurt Ahrén, Department of Physiology, University of Göteborg, Sweden

It is known that adenosine (Ads) potentiates the effect of LH on cyclic AMP (cAMP) and progesterone production in isolated cells from heavily luteinized rat ovaries (Behrman et al, J Steroid Biochem 19,789,1983). We have now studied whether Ads potentiates the effects of LH and isoproterenol (Iso) on whole rat corpora lutea (CL) and on isolated cells from individual CL.

Immature rats were injected with 8 IU PMSG on day 26 leading to ovulation 3 days later with subsequent formation of a normal number of CL functioning for 10-12 days (Herlitz et al, Europ J Obstet Gynec Reprod Biol 6/4,175, 1976). Individual CL were extirpated 5 days after ovulation (10-12 from each rat). Whole CL (2 in each flask) were incubated for 30 min with LH (1 ug/ml; NIH-S24), 1 uM Iso, LH + 50 uM Ads and Iso + 50 uM Ads. Both LH and Iso stimulated cAMP production markedly. Ads did not potentiate these effects. Luteal cells were enzymatically dispersed from the same typ of CL (appr. 100 CL for each isolation) as described by Behrman et al (Endocrinology 107, 656, 1980). The cells were incubated for 60 min with LH, Iso and Ads as described above. Both LH and Iso stimulated cAMP production. Ads potentiated markedly the effects of both LH and Iso.

It is possible that the isolation procedure depletes the luteal cells of factors (e g Ads) necessary for optimal cAMP production. In the rapidly excised intact CL this depletion might not be as pronounced. Another possibility, less likely, is that Ads does not penetrate freely into the intact corpus luteum.

2093 STIMULATION OF POLY(ADP-RIBOSE) SYNTHESIS BY ESTROGEN IN RAT ANTERIOR PITUITARY. H. Seo*, N. Suganuma, K. Sueda and N. Matsui, The Research Institute of Environmental Medicine, Nagoya University, Nagoya, Japan.

It is well known that estrogen (E) stimulates cellular proliferation and PRL synthesis in rat anterior pituitary. Because cellular functions such as DNA synthesis, transcription and differentiation is altered by poly ADP ribosylation of chromatin proteins, we investigated whether the effect of E on the pituitary could involve an alteration of poly(ADP-ribose) synthesis from NAD.

Anterior pituitaries from male Wistar rats were obtained at 12, 24, 48 and 72 hours after single injection of 500 ug estradiol dipropionate. Poly(ADP-ribose) synthesis was assessed by incubation of purified nuclei with ^{14}C-NAD and subsequent TCA precipitation. The product could be digested with phosphodiesterase I from snake venom but not with DNase nor with RNase, demonstrating the authenticity of poly(ADP-ribose) synthesis. E stimulated the rate of poly(ADP-ribose) synthesis twice the control level after 12 hours and gradually increased up to three times at 72 hours. This increase was demonstrated in the presence of inhibitors of poly(ADP-ribose) degrading enzymes, namely NaF and NAD, suggesting that E increased the amount or the activity of poly(ADP-ribose) synthetase. The increase of DNA synthesis and PRL mRNA activity followed that of poly(ADP-ribose) synthesis. Thus, it was suggested that enhanced poly(ADP-ribose) synthesis may mediate some effect of E on the anterior pituitary. Supported in part by Grant-in-Aid for Cancer Research from the Ministry of Education, Japan (No. 57010034).

2094 EFFECT OF GLUCOCORTICOID ON CORTICOTROPIN-RELEASING FACTOR (CRF) INDUCED cAMP PRODUCTION IN RAT ANTERIOR PITUITARY CELLS IN VITRO. N. Shimizu*, S. Miyabe, K. Tanaka, T. Watabe, T. Horiuchi and M. Hasegawa, First Department of Medicine, Teikyo University School of Medicine, Tokyo 173, Japan.

Although the suppressive effect of glucocorticoid on ACTH release is well established, the exact mechanism of this inhibitory effect is not fully understood. The present experiment was undertaken to evaluate the effect of glucocorticoid on cAMP production stimulated by CRF. Cultured rat anterior pituitary cells were preincubated with 100 nM dexamethasone (Dex) for 18 hrs with or without cycloheximide (CX, 10 μg/ml) or actinomycin D (AD, 2 μg/ml) at 37°C under 95 % air-5 % CO_2. Cells were then incubated with synthetic ovine CRF (10 nM). ACTH in the medium and intracellular cAMP were determined by RIA immediately before, 30 and 240 min after the addition of CRF. CRF caused a significant increase in both cAMP production (mean ± SE, 0.67 ± 0.06 and 4.97 ± 0.21 pMol/ml before and at 30 min after CRF, respectively) and ACTH release (mean ± SE, 3.7 ± 0.9 and 37.8 ± 1.5 ng/ml, before and 240 min after CRF, respectively). Pretreatment of the cells with Dex suppressed CRF-induced ACTH release and cAMP production to 50.7 ± 3.1 and 71.2 ± 2.3 % of the control levels, respectively. However, cAMP production was not suppressed when the cells were preincubated with both Dex and CX or AD. These results suggest that the inhibitory effect of glucocorticoid on ACTH release is mediated at least in part by suppression of cAMP production, which results from the new protein synthesis induced by glucocorticoid in rat anterior pituitary cells.

2095 PHOSPHORYLATION OF RAT LIVER GLUCOCORTICOID RECEPTOR. V. Singh, T. Eessalu, S. Ghag and V. Moudgil*, Biological Sciences, Oakland University, Rochester, Michigan 48063 USA.

Phosphorylation of rat liver glucocorticoid receptor was performed by incubating a liver mince with [^{32}P]-orthophosphate. The tissue mince was then homogenized and centrifuged at 150,000xg for 60 min. The "cytosol" was fractionated with 40 % $(NH_4)_2SO_4$ and incubated with 40 nM [^{3}H]-dexamethasone mesylate for 3 h at 0°C. In parallel experiments, the tissue mince was incubated with unlabeled orthophosphate and [^{3}H]-dexamethasone mesylate, or with [^{32}P]-orthophosphate and unlabeled dexamethasone mesylate. The glucocorticoid-receptor complex was purified about 2,000-fold by $(NH_4)_2SO_4$ fractionation, phosphocellulose and DNA-cellulose chromatography. SDS polyacrylamide gel electrophoresis of the purified glucocorticoid receptor revealed the presence of two ^{32}P-containing bands with apparent molecular weights of 90,000 and 50,000 daltons. Some preparations yielded only the 90,000 dalton protein suggesting that the 50,000 dalton molecule may be a proteolytic fragment of 90,000 dalton species. Samples labeled with [^{3}H]-dexamethasone mesylate and purified as above co-migrated with ^{32}P-containing bands. Both the 90,000 and 50,000 dalton bands appeared to possess the steroid binding, DNA binding and phosphorylation site(s). The purified phosphorylated receptor sedimented as 3.8S in sucrose gradients. We also observed that rat liver glucocorticoid receptor phosphorylation is divalent cation (Mg^{++}) dependent . Our results suggest that rat liver glucocorticoid receptor is a phosphoprotein.

These studies were supported by NIH grant AM 20893·

2096 CHARACTERIZATION OF THE NUCLEAR ACCEPTOR SITES FOR THE AVIAN OVIDUCT PROGESTERONE RECEPTOR. Spelsberg, T., Gosse, B., Rasmussen, K., Toyoda, H., Seelke, R. and Littlefield, B.* Dept. Cell Biology, Mayo Foundation, Rochester, Minnesota 55905.

Evidence has previously been reported that the nuclear acceptor sites for the avian oviduct progesterone (PR) and estrogen (ER) receptors are composed of specific fraction of chromosomal protein(s) tightly bound to the DNA. Many of these sites appear to be "masked" by other proteins in intact chromatin. Conditions and methods have been developed to reconstitute native-like acceptor sites using the isolated "acceptor proteins" (AP) and hen DNA. The reconstituted acceptor sites display the same receptor dependency, saturation, and patterns of binding as demonstrated in vivo and in vitro for the native undissociated acceptor sites. In contrast, pure DNA does not display saturable binding or the in vivo-like patterns of binding. The acceptor activity when dissociated from DNA appears to be a protein, displaying a density of 1.24 g/cc and a lability susceptibility to proteases but not nucleases. This activity in the AP have molecular sizes in the range of 14,000 to 20,000, isoelectric points of pH 5.3 and pH 6.4 and are very hydrophobic. The activity has been purified ∿100,000-fold from whole tissue. Interestingly, a limited number of acceptor sites can be generated on the hen DNA even when excess AP is used in the reconstitution process. The DNA from other animals (e.g., human, dog, cow) including frogs also can generate similar acceptor sites using hen oviduct AP and PR. However, the DNA from other organisms, e.g., insects, plants, certain fish and prokaryotes, cannot generate the acceptor sites. A correlation exists between the presence of these sequences in an organism's genome and the presence of a functional PR in that organism.

2097 LACK OF A DIRECT EFFECT OF EXOGENOUS INSULIN ON THE B-CELL. J. Stagner, E. Samols[A] and K. Polonsky, VA Medical Center and Univ. of Louisville, Louisville, KY and Univ. of Chicago, Chicago, IL, USA.

It has been established that exogenous insulin may inhibit endogenous insulin, but whether this is a direct or indirect effect upon the islet is not certain. We therefore examined the effect of exogenous insulin on insulin release from the isolated dorsal lobe of the canine pancreas *in vitro* (N=6). Endogenous insulin (I) was measured frequently both directly by RIA and indirectly as the increment of change of total insulin from its respective baseline during an insulin infusion of 1.2 or 12 mU/ml/min as was canine C-peptide (C-pep). An arginine 10mM stimulation was used to define the increment (ASΔI) of insulin release above each respective baseline. During basal perfusions (88mg/dl glucose) there was excellent correlation between C-pep and I (R=.94, N=90, $p<0.0005$, mean basal C-pep 0.72±.14 pM/ml, I 405±79 uU/ml) as well as the increase during arginine stimulation (R=.93, $p<0.0125$, increment I 593±136 uU/ml, C-pep 3.79±1.26 pM/ml). During the infusion of insulin 1.2 mU/ml/min, there was correlation between the mean ASΔI of 564±53 uU/ml and the ASΔC-pep of 3.87±1.02 pM/ml (R=.59, $p<0.0005$). Infusion of 12 mU/ml/min I produced an ASΔI of 566±387 uU/ml and an ASΔC-pep of 3.75±1.89 pM/ml. During the infusions of 1.2 and 12 mU/ml/min I, C-pep did not suppress from basal levels, but appeared to increase (1.43±.33 and 1.33±53 pM/ml, respectively). During arginine infusions following exogenous insulin, 1.2 and 12 mU/ml/min there was no significant suppression of ASΔI 564±53 and 566±368 uU/ml nor the ASΔC-pep of 3.87±1.02 and 3.75±1.89 pM/ml ($p<0.45$) from basal levels. These observations strongly suggest that exogenous insulin does not directly suppress the B-cell; the suppression of endogenous insulin *in vivo* is presumably an indirect effect.

2098 LOCALIZATION OF INSULINOMA BY PERCUTANEOUS TRANSHEPATIC SAMPLING OF BLOOD IN THE PORTAL VENOUS SYSTEM (TPVS) DURING GLUCAGON INFUSION (GI)
J.L. Richard, D. Mirouze, J. Bringer, M. Rodier, J. Marchal, A. Orsetti, J. Mirouze. Endocrinology, Saint Eloi Hospital, F-34059 MONTPELLIER.

TPVS is a reliable mean to localize small insulinomas but may be inefficient when insulin (I) gradients are missing. To optimize this procedure, TPVS was repeated during an IV GI in 2 men suspected of insulinoma but with negative abdominal scan and pancreatic arteriography. Serial blood samples were withdrawn from splenic, portal, and superior mesenteric veins during TPVS. The first sampling was obtained in basal state and the second one 20 min. after the begining of GI in an antebrachial vein at a constant rate (22 µg/min.). No gradient of basal I was found in the 2 patients. During GI both patients showed a dramatic increase of I in the mid-splenic vein. In patient A insulinoma was found in the pancreatic body according to the gradient. In patient B tumor was intragastric ; this apparent discrepancy was due to the drainage of the tumor in the mid-splenic vein through the gastro-epiploic vein.

	Site of the tumor		Mean of I levels at the sites of TPVS (µU/ml)				
			Splenic vein			Portal	Sup.Mesenteric
			Distal	Mid	Proximal	vein	vein.
Case A	Body of	Basal	19.7	52.0	57.0	35.3	13.5
(50 yrs)	Pancreas	GI	44.0	256.3	106.0	104.3	42.5
Case B	Intra-	Basal	19.0	29.3	22.5	29.0	14.0
(73 yrs)	Gastric	GI	27.0	196.0	85.5	114.0	52.0

When TPVS is negative or doubtful GI might be performed to improve the accuracy of this localization procedure.

2099 IN VIVO AND IN VITRO ANTIKETOGENIC EFFECT OF GLUCOSE PER SE. J.P. Riou*, M. Beylot, G. Sautot, M. Delinger and R. Mornex, INSERM U.197, Faculté de Médecine A.Carrel and Hôpital de l'Antiquaille, 69 Lyon, France.

The in vivo effect of glucose per se on blood ketone body and NEFA has been studied in 4 normal men starved for 60 h (250 kcal/kg/day) receiving a somatostatin (SRIF) infusion (500 μg/h). When glycemia was raised by exogenous IV glucose infusion, 90 min after starting SRIF, from 3.3±0.2 to 12± 1 mMol/l for 180 min neither insulin nor c peptide increase. NEFA dropped acutely in 30 min from 1.7±0.2 mM to 1±0.15 mM ($p < 0.01$) and remained stable. Ketone body decreases thereafter in a time-related manner from 2.2±0.4 to 1.2±0.4 mMol/l ($p < 0.01$).

In order to ascertain whether glucose has been acting only on lipolysis or also on the liver ketogenic capacity, its effect was studied in vitro on isolated liver cells from 24 h starved rats incubated with various amounts of Na-palmitate. Glucose (30 mM) did not affect the maximal ketogenic capacity (80 μMol/g (w/w)/hour) measured with 1.6 mM Na-palmitate but decreases the apparent Na-palmitate K 0.5 for ketogenesis from 0.18 to 0.35 mM. At physiological free fatty acids concentration (0.22 mM) glucose decrease ketogenesis by 90 %. The effect was time-dependent, maximum after 30 min of incubation. Half maximum inhibition by glucose was obtained at 6 mM, a concentration at which lactate production was unaffected.

These results show that glucose per se inhibits ketogenesis in vivo by acting probably both on lipolysis and on liver ketogenic capacity.

2100 PAIRED STUDY OF INSULIN-INDUCED HYPOGLYCEMIA DURING CONTINUOUS SUBCUTANEOUS INSULIN INFUSION OR CONVENTIONAL INSULIN THERAPY.
N. W. Rodger*, J. Dupre, University of Western Ontario, London, Canada.

Although techniques of insulin administration maintaining near-normoglycemia are attended by increased risk of hypoglycemia, enhanced efficiency of the glucoregulatory response might offset this hazard. During a crossover trial of continuous subcutaneous (SC) insulin infusion (CSII) or conventional insulin therapy (CIT), we investigated the immunoreactive glucagon (IRG, antibody 30 K) response to hypoglycemia induced by an SC insulin bolus (0.1 U/kg) in the abdomen from the infuser during CSII, or by injection during CIT. Eight normal-weight volunteer subjects were studied. Five had basal C-peptide (Cp) <0.01 pmol/ml (Cp negative): all had evidence of abnormal autonomic function (heart rate response to standing and/or deep breathing). Symptoms of hypoglycemia were noted in all subjects. Responses were compared using paired t or paired difference tests. Decrease in glycemia (decrement as % of baseline, 0-180 min, mean ±SE) was 65±3 (CSII) vs 60±3 (CIT) ($p<0.05$). Free immunoreactive insulin (FIRI)(μU/ml, polyethylene glycol extraction) at 30 min was 19±4 (CSII) vs 9±4 (CIT)($p<0.05$) and from 0-60 min as % of 0-180 min increment under the curve was 39±7 (CSII) vs 20±3 (CIT)($p<0.05$). IRG increment 60-180 min did not differ between CSII and CIT. Enhanced hypoglycemia during CSII relative to CIT can be attributed to more rapid absorption of insulin bolus during CSII. IRG response, which did not increase during CSII even with a greater hypoglycemic stimulus, may be limited by autonomic neuropathy, insensitivity to the measured differences in glycemia during CIT or CSII, or be inhibited by characteristics of insulinemia during CSII.

2101 IDENTIFICATION OF DIFFERENT GONADOTROPHS IN THE HUMAN PITUITARY USING SPECIFIC MONOCLONAL ANTIBODIES TO GONADOTROPHINS.

A.N.THAKUR*, R.MIRAKIAN¶, A.O'SHEA, C.A.RICHARDSON¶, A.SESAY and R.P.EKINS. Department of Molecular Endocrinology and ¶Department of Immunology, The Middlesex Hospital Medical School, Mortimer Street, London W1, U.K.

Considerable controversy exists regarding whether both LH and FSH are secreted by the same gonadotrophic cell type. We have attempted to resolve this question by the use of highly specific monoclonal antibodies (McAbs) to glycoprotein hormones. Hybridoma secreting McAbs to hLH, hFSH and hTSH were raised by fusing mouse myeloma cell line JK-Ag,8 with spleen cells from BALB/c mice immunised with the appropriate hormone. McAbs derived were screened for specificity and binding affinity for the antigen. Immunologically specific antibodies were further screened for their ability to neutralise the biological activity of the corresponding hormone. In the present study these immuno- and biologically specific McAbs have been used. Frozen sections of normal human pituitary were studied by indirect immunofluorescence (IF), using an Avidin-Biotin system. With 3 anti-gonadotrophic McAbs and one anti-TSH McAb positive isolated granular cells were detected. Preliminary results obtained by double IF technique revealed heterogeneity of gonadotrophs: the majority of positive cells reacted with both anti-LH and FSH McAbs although selected cells stained specifically either with anti-LH or anti-FSH antibodies. Specific anti-TSH McAb did not stain FSH positive cells in double IF staining. Thus, this study demonstrates the presence in the human pituitary of three subsets of gonadotrophic cells secreting/storing only FSH or LH and both FSH and LH.

2102 HIGHLY SPECIFIC AND SENSITIVE HYBRIDOMA ANTIBODIES FOR THE FREE α-SUBUNIT OF HUMAN GLYCOPROTEIN HORMONES.

N.R. THOTAKURA AND O.P. BAHL*, Department of Biological Sciences, SUNY at Buffalo, Amherst, NY 14260, USA.

The free α-subunit of human chorionic gonadotropin (hCG-α) has been detected in various physiological and pathological conditions. Besides being produced during pregnancy, it is secreted by gonadal and gastrointestinal tumors, in breast carcinoma, choriocarcinoma and bladder cancer. In order to facilitate the detection of these tumors, we have by hybridoma technology developed very sensitive and highly specific antibodies to hCG-α (A2-58, monoclonal and A2D4, polyclonal). Their specificity is further shown by their failure to inhibit labelled hCG binding to ovarian hCG/hLH receptor. Interestingly, A2D4 antibody was found to be 100-200 times more sensitive in detecting deglycosylated hCG-α than native hCG-α. Employing these antibodies assays were developed to detect the free α subunit at concentrations as low as 40pg. These assays have insignificant cross reactivity with intact hCG, hLH and other glycoprotein hormones (A2-58 has 0.86% and A2D4, 0.17% cross reactivity) and can be used for the assay of hCG-α in the presence of intact hCG. Thus, they have potential in the clinical diagnosis of α-subunit producing tumors. These hCG-α antibodies are prepared in homogenous form by a combination of DEAE-affigel blue chromatography, gel filtration and affinity chromatography. For further characterization, their Fab fragment have been prepared. Both these antibodies have been found to belong to IgG1 subclass.

Supported by USPHS grant #HD 08766.

2103 Effects of β-casomorphin on thyrotropin secretion in rats.
T. Mitsuma*, M. Chaya, T. Mogimori and K. Sahashi, 4th Dept. of Internal Medicine, Aichi Medical University, Nagakute, Aichi 480-11, Japan.

Effects of β-casomorphin on thyrotropin (TSH) secretion in rats were studied. β-casomorphin (300 μg/kg) was injected iv, and the rats were serially decapitated. Thyrotropin-releasing hormone (TRH), TSH and thyroid hormone were measured by radioimmunoassay. The hypothalamic immunoreactive TRH (ir-TRH) contents increased significantly after β-casomorphin injection, whereas its plasma concentrations tended to decrease. The plasma TSH levels decreased significantly in a dose-related manner with a nadir at 40 min after the injection. The plasma thyroid hormone levels showed no change. The plasma ir-TRH and TSH responses to cold were inhibited by β-casomorphin, but the plasma TSH response to TRH was not. Naloxone partially blocked the inhibitory effect of β-casomorphin on TSH levels. In the haloperidol-pretreated group, the inhibitory effect of β-casomorphin on TSH levels was prevented, but not in the L-DOPA-, para-chlorophenylalanine- or 5-hydroxytryptophan-pretreated group. These drugs alone did not affect plasma TSH levels in terms of the dose used. The findings suggest that β-casomorphin acts at the hypothalamus to inhibit TRH release, and its effects are modified by a dopaminergic system and opioid receptor.

2104 **IDENTIFICATION OF ENZYMATIC ACTIVITY PRODUCING α-AMIDATED PEPTIDES IN RAT TISSUES.**
A. Myers, R. Mains, B. Eipper*, Neuroscience Dept., The Johns Hopkins University School of Medicine, Baltimore, MD 21205, U.S.A.

Precursors to α-amidated peptides contain a glycyl residue to the carboxyl terminal side of the residue to be α-amidated. Secretory granules from pituitary and hypothalamus contain an enzymatic activity capable of converting the model substrate ^{125}I-D-Tyr-Val-Gly into ^{125}I-D-Tyr-Val-NH_2; the activity is dependent on copper, ascorbate and molecular oxygen. The specificity of the enzyme is broad and a similar enzyme could be involved in synthesis of many bioactive α-amidated peptides. A similar copper and ascorbate stimulatable enzymatic activity was detected in extracts of several tissues with levels (pmol/mg protein/h) varying in the order: anterior pituitary $\geq$ neurointermediate pituitary > hypothalamus > submaxillary gland > thyroid $\simeq$ rest of brain. No detectable activity (<3 pmol/mg protein/h) was found in extracts of cerebellum, adrenal, pancreas, testes, duodenum, antrum, spleen, liver, lung, skeletal muscle, or kidney. Rat serum contained a similar enzymatic activity (87 ± 20 [SD] pmol/ml/h at 0.5 μM peptide substrate; n=17). Addition of 25 μM $CuSO_4$ stimulated activity 18-fold. Addition of 2.5 mM ascorbate stimulated activity 10-fold. Activity in serum was linear in time for 3h and in amount of serum to 6 μl serum/40 μl assay; the pH optimum was 7-8. The source of α-amidation activity in rat serum was investigated by examining α-amidation activity in serum from hypophysectomized, adrenalectomized, castrated, ovariectomized, thyroidectomized, sialectomized, and thymectomized rats. Supported by AM-32949, DA-00266, and McKnight Fdn.

2105 ENDOCRINE ASPECTS OF ELECTROCONVULSIVE TREATMENT IN MENTAL ILLNESS.

D.Nerozzi*, S.Graziosi, A.Magnani, S.Murgiano, M.Amalfitano, G.Cozza and G.Frajese, Neurophysiopathology Chair and 5th Medical Clinic, University of Rome, 00100 Rome, Italy.

Electroconvulsive treatment (ECT), an effective therapy for severe depression, can be considered a model of acute stress. After TRH injection (200 mcg i.v.), PRL and TSH patterns were evaluated in basal conditions, after the first ECT and then again at the end of a therapeutic course of 8 ECT's in 8 severely Depressed patients and in 8 Schizophrenics as controls. Results obtained after the first ECT evidentiated a rise in PRL and a decrease in TSH values in both Depressed and non-Depressed patients suggesting an aspecific stress response. At the end of the therapeutic course TSH values increased significantly ($p < 0.02$) in Depressed patients, while they returned to basal values in the other group. PRL levels presented a moderate rise both in Depressed and non-Depressed patients (the peak shifted from 15' to 30' in Control patients). The different response of the Control group in comparison to that of the Depressed patients suggest that the action mechanism of ECT becomes more specific when it is repeated and differs according to the organic substrate underlying different affective disorders. The data obtained also suggest the existence of a direct action of the Noradrenergic System on the pituitary thyrotrophs under stress condition.

2106 THE EFFECT OF Δ^1TETRAHYDROCANNABINOL (THC) ON LUTEINIZING HORMONE (LH) RELEASE IN CASTRATED AND HYPOTHALAMIC DEAFFERENTED (CHD) MALE RATS.

I. Nir* and M. Puder, Hebrew University Schools of Medicine and Pharmacy, Jerusalem, Israel.

THC acutely suppresses tonic serum LH and prolactin levels in adult male rats. The exact site of its suppressive action has not been identified. We have performed a complete hypothalamic deafferentation which disrupts the medial basal hypothalamus (MBH) from the rest of the CNS, and did not abolish the ability of THC to suppress hypothalamic-pituitary response in gonadectomized male rats. This was evidenced by the equally reduced plasma levels of LH and prolactin before and after CHD. Previous results obtained by us eliminate the pituitary as a reasonable site for THC action in suppressing LH and prolactin secretion. Present results indicate THC is able to act inside the MBH and that the MBH-pituitary axis remains responsive to its inhibitory effect despite interruption of neural connection between the MBH and extrahypothalamic areas. However, the CRF neurons in the MBH appear functionally impaired through the transection and become unresponsive to the THC stimulation normally produced. Different patterns of action seem to rule the various hypophyseal hormones controlled by the hypothalamus, suggesting a possibility that a continuous release of LH-RH and PIF is maintained by the activity of noradrenergic and dopaminergic neurons surviving inside the island.

2107 EFFECT OF SOME PUTATIVE NEUROTRANSMITTERS ON EXCITABILITY OF IDENTIFIED TUBEROINFUNDIBULAR NEURONS IN RAT HYPOTHALAMIC SLICES. M. Nishihara*, T. Matsukawa and F. Kimura, Department of Physiology, Yokohama City University School of Medicine, Yokohama 232, Japan.

It is suggested that some monoamines and amino acids are involved in the control of anterior pituitary hormone secretion as neurotransmitters in the hypothalamus. We examined the effect of γ-aminobutyric acid (GABA), glycine, serotonin (5-HT), dopamine (DA) and norepinephrine (NE) on excitability of tuberoinfundibular (TI) neurons in hypothalamic slices of ovariectomized rats. By electrical stimulation of the median eminence, 138 antidromically activated TI neurons were recorded in the arcuate and its adjacent area. GABA and glycine (0.1-1.5 mM) inhibited the antidromic propagation into the soma and dendrites, but not the initial segments, in 31 of the 83 and 10 of the 32 cells tested, respectively, suggesting that these amino acids hyperpolarized the membrane of soma and dendrites. On the other hand, 5-HT, DA and NE (10-100 μM) inhibited the somatodendritic spike in less than 5% of cells tested. Spontaneous discharge was observed in about 40% of antidromically identified TI neurons. The effect of drugs on spontaneous unit activity is summarized in Table 1. The present data demonstrate that GABA and glycine have an inhibitory effect and 5-HT has a facilitatory effect on excitability of TI neurons in the arcuate.

Table 1.

	Total	Facilitation	Inhibition	No effect
GABA	34	0 (0.0%)	31 (91.2%)	3 (8.8%)
Glycine	23	0 (0.0%)	17 (73.9%)	6 (26.1%)
5-HT	29	16 (55.2%)	5 (17.2%)	8 (27.6%)
DA	20	6 (30.0%)	8 (40.0%)	6 (30.0%)
NE	21	6 (28.6%)	7 (33.3%)	8 (38.1%)

2108 MODIFICATION BY ALFA-METHYL-P-TYROSINE OF CIRCULATING THYROID HORMONE AND TSH AS WELL AS CATECHOLAMINES IN THE CNS OF RATS. T. Ohtsuka, N. Koibuchi and M. Suzuki*, Dept. of Physiology, Inst. of Endocrinology, Gunma University, Maebashi, 371, Japan.

Although there is ample evidence on a stimulating effect of norephinephrine centrally given on TSH release in rats, administration of alfa-methyl-p-tyrosine (α-MT), an inhibitor to catecholamine biosynthesis produces many contradictory findings. Thus the aim of this study is to find α-MT effect on plasma hormones. Male Wistar rats weighing about 350g were ip given α-MT (250 mg/kg) and blood samples were collected from indwelling jugular cannulae of conscious unrestraint rats. Plasma TSH decreased rapidly to 62 % by 3 hr after α-MT injection and then slowly recovered. Whereas plasma T4 and T3 levels were reduced rapidly and contineously to 17 and 36 % by 12 hr respectively. Hypothalamic catecholamine contents decreased clearly and continuously to 68 % (NE) and 32 % (DA) by 3 hr and to 21 and 17 % by 12 hr respectively. Simultaneously T3-binding capacity index of sera from α-MT injected rats was also decreased by 12hr, indicating a displacement by the drug of plasma T4 and T3 from their binding sites of plasma protein. Then we measured metabolic clearance rate (MRC) of 125-I-T4. Alfa-MT administration stimulated from 8.12 ml/hr (125-I-T4) to 13.95 (125-I-T4) and 14.36 (127-I-T4) respectively, and reduced t1/2 (half life time) from 11.56 hr (125-I-T4) to 6.56 (125-I-T4) and 6.40 (127-I-T4). These results indicate that α-MT affected not only hypothalamic catecholamine contents but also MCR of T4 and T3, probably displacing them from plasma protein, and further inhibited completely thyroid hormone release.

2109 DIFFERENTIAL EFFECTS OF ETHANOL UPON STIMULATION OF ADENYLYL CYCLASE IN HUMAN CORPUS LUTEUM MEMBRANES. F.J. Rojas* and R.H. Asch, Dept. Ob-Gyn, The University of Texas Health Science Center at San Antonio, Texas, 78284, U.S.A.

Ethanol has been shown to affect hCG and LH stimulation of Adenylyl cyclase (AC) in homogenates from rat and rabbit corpora lutea (CL). The mechanism by which ethanol exerts this action, however, remain unresolved. Since we have previously characterized AC activities present in membranes fractions from human CL from midluteal phase it was of interest to investigate the effects of ethanol in this enzyme system. Ethanol up to a concentration of 5% (v/v) was without effect on basal luteal AC but markedly potentiated NaF and hCG + GMP-P(NH)P stimulation in a dose-dependent manner. In contrast, ethanol progressively inhibited forskolin stimulation at the same range of ethanol concentrations. Maximal NaF or hCG + GMP-P(NH)P stimulation of AC activity were observed at 5% ethanol and reached values $\sim$ 100% higher than controls without ethanol. However, at the same ethanol concentration, forskolin-stimulated AC activity was reduced by 40% relative to controls. Equilibrium binding studies involving $[^{125}I]$ hCG interaction with the luteal membranes in the presence of 5% ethanol showed an increase of 10% ($P<0.01$) in specific hCG binding without appreciable effect on the affinity for hormone. Thus, although ethanol significantly increased gonadotropin binding sites on membranes, this increase was not proportional with the extent at which ethanol potentiated the gonadotropin-stimulated AC. The present data indicate that the acute effects of ethanol cause specific and well differentiated changes on the human luteal AC and that the synergistic interaction of ethanol and gonadotropin stimulation of AC is at least in part due to an increase in the coupling process by which the AC components affect enzyme activation. (Supported by UTHSCSA Grant SO7-RR05654).

2110 DISSOCIATION BETWEEN LUTEINIZING HORMONE (LH) ACTION AND INTERNALIZATION. E.A. Rorke*, G. Faircloth, and J.L. Vaitukaitis, Departments of Medicine and Physiology, Boston University School of Medicine, Boston, MA 02118, U.S.A.

LH not only accumulates more rapidly within pseudopregnant rat ovarian cells but also is metabolized more rapidly than human chorionic gonadotropin (hCG) in those cells. Since it was unclear whether the different rates of internalization and intracellular metabolism affected biological activities, studies were undertaken to determine if the metabolism of LH and its biologic effects could be dissociated under conditions in which high intracellular levels of LH were maintained. Pseudopregnant rats received two 1.0 μg (11IU) injections of LH, separated by one hour. Cytosolic LH was characterized by radioimmunoassay and bioassay. In addition, ovarian responsiveness was ascertained by measuring cAMP dependent protein kinase (CDPK) activity and cAMP concentrations after LH stimulation. Cytosolic LH levels increased rapidly following the first injection, peaked at one hour and declined thereafter. After the second LH injection, a 35% increase in peak cytosolic LH concentrations resulted. Following the second injection, LH biologic potency was higher than that present in ovarian cytosol after the first LH injection. Ovarian responsiveness was blunted following initial LH stimulation since no significant increase in cAMP levels was observed and the LH-induced CDPK activity was only a small fraction of that present after the first LH injection. In contrast, significant LH internalization occurred after the second LH injection. The foregoing observations suggest independent subcellular mechanisms for inducing LH biologic effects and internalization.

2111 IDENTIFICATION OF β-ENDORPHIN IN OVARIAN INTERSTITIAL CELLS: ITS STIMULATION BY LH. M. Rothrock, D. Sarkar and G.F. Erickson,* Dept. Reproductive Med., Univ. of California, San Diego, La Jolla, CA 92093 U.S.A.

There is now substantial evidence that many regulatory peptides are present in both central and peripheral tissues. Recently, the pituitary/neuropeptide, β-endorphin, has been found to occur throughout the male reproductive tract, including the cytoplasm of testicular Leydig cells. We have now investigated here the possible presence of β-endorphin in the ovarian interstitial cells. The antisera to β-endorphin was kindly provided by Professor S.S.C. Yen. Immunocytochemical analysis of ovarian sections of immature hypox. rats (employing the peroxidase-antiperoxidase technique) revealed intense β-endorphin-like immunoreactivity in the cytoplasm of the secondary interstitial cells. β-endorphin-like material was also distributed throughout the germinal epithelium of the ovary, but no immunostaining of β-endorphin was seen in the ova, granulosa or thecal cells. Interestingly, pre-treatment for 2 days with hCG (10 μg injections twice daily) *in vivo* caused dramatic increases in the amount of β-endorphin-like material distributed in the IC. Radioimmunoassay of pooled extracts of ovaries of hypox. rats revealed the presence of significant amounts of β-endorphin-like material. In agreement with our immunocytochemical studies, the amount of radioimmunoassayable β-endorphin was markedly increased in hCG-treated ovaries. Similar increases in β-endorphin-like material was obtained when dispersed IC were treated with LH in serum-free cell culture. These results suggest that ovarian androgen producing cells contain β-endorphin and that its production is stimulated by LH. The existence of β-endorphin-like material in ovarian IC has new implications for female reproductive regulation.

2112 AN ENZYMATIC METHOD FOR DISSOCIATING PRIMARY TO ANTRAL FOLLICLES FROM THE HAMSTER OVARY. S.K. Roy* and G.S. Greenwald. Dept. of Physiology, Univ. of KS Medical Ctr., Kansas City, KS 66103.

Ovaries from 6 hamsters on each day of the cycle (Day 1=ovulation; Day 4=proestrus) were collected, C.L. and large antral follicles (Stage 10) dissected and the ovaries then incubated with collagenase, DNAase and pronase to disperse intact follicles. Histological studies with 2462 isolated follicles showed that 14% of the follicles were atretic with 50% of the total having 1-3 layers of granulosa cells (Stages 1-3) and a second peak of 18% in antral follicles (Stages 8-10). Thecal cells did not appear until the follicles had 7-8 layers of granulosa cells (Stage 6) and this presumably accounts for reduced atresia in this class and beyond. Ultrastructurally, Stage 3 follicles showed normal morphology which was not disrupted by exposure to enzymes; moreover there were prominent signs of potential steroidogenesis. The number of Stage 1-10 follicles was constant throughout the estrous cycle; e.g. on Day 1 there were 444±31 follicles per animal and on Day 4: 463±30. Follicle distribution in different stages showed rhythmic fluctuations throughout the cycle. Stage 1-5 follicles showed the most dramatic changes in numbers between 0900 and 1500h and this was especially clear cut for the Stage 1 follicles. This method is applicable to problems involving small follicles. For example, follicle kinetics: removal of one ovary at 0900h on Day 3, results 6h later in conversion of Stage 4 follicles (quadrilaminar granulosa cells) into Stage 5 follicles; hormone binding: Stages 1-10 follicles bind FSH and PRL but hCG binding is first noted in Stage 5 & 6 follicles; DNA activity: ^{3}H thymidine incorporation into all stages of follicles is maximal on Day 1, 1500h in response to the 2nd FSH surge.

2113 HCG INCREASES 3β-HSD ACTIVITY IN THE INCUBATIONS OF DISPERSED RAT OVARIAN CELLS. Y.Sano*,A.Kambegawa,S.Okinaga and K.Arai, Department of Obstetrics and Gynecology,Teikyo University Scool of Medicine, Kaga 2-11-1, Itabashiku Tokyo 173 Japan.

Progesterone(P_4) production in ovary increases at preovulatory phase and this is considered to be due to the LH effect to stimulate ovarian cholesterol side chain cleavage enzyme (CSCC) activity. Δ^5-3β-Hydroxysteroid dehydrogenase (3β-HSD) seems also to be enhanced by the gonadotropin. In this experiment, the regulation of 3β-HSD by hCG wasstudied in the incubations of dispersed rat ovarian cells. Ovaries were obtained from immature female rats injected with 10IU PMSG 2 days before the experimentand dispersed with collagenase and DNase. The dispersed ovarian cells were suspended in Ham F12 medium containing 10mM HEPES, and then incubated with or without hCG (100IU/ml) or dibutyryl cAMP(0.5mM) at 37C in 5% CO_2in air. After each incubation period, the medium was changed for a new one containing 10nmol of ^{14}C-pregnenolone(P_5) and then incubated for 1hr. The metabolites of ^{14}C-P_5 were extracted,separated andidentified. 3β-HSD activity was expressed as the sum of the amounts of P_4 and 20α-dihydroprogesterone formed from ^{14}C-P_5. P_4concentration in the changed medium was measured by RIA. Addition of hCG or dibutyryl-cAMP to the medium increased the P_4concentration approximately 6-fold after 5 hr of incubation. 3β-HSD activity was also increased after an addition of hCG or dibutyryl-cAMP.After 5 hr of incubation, 3β-HSD activity in hCG treated cells was 1.3-fold higher than controls and 1.7-fold at 7 hr of incubation. Dibutyryl-cAMP caused a 1.7-fold stimulation of 3β-HSD at 5 hr of incubation. The present data demonstrate that hCG increases not only CSCC but also 3β-HSD in preovulatory rat ovarian cells and suggest that the effect is mediated by cAMP.

2114 POSTPARTUM HYSTERECTOMY IN CATTLE AND RESULTING HYPOPHYSEAL, OVARIAN AND UTERINE HORMONE SECRETION. E. Schallenberger*, H.H.D. Meyer, D. Schams, H.-J. Breitinger, S.J. Oschmann, G. Enzenhöfer and D.L. Walters, Institut für Physiologie, TU München, 8050 Freising-Weihenstephan, FRG.

Six heifers received immediately after parturition catheters in the aorta and the vena cava caud. to get access to the ovarian and uterine blood supply and drainage. Three animals were hysterectomized thereafter. Luteal function started between days 11-15 pp. Series of frequent samplings were performed every other day. Results are as follows: 1) Frequency and amplitude of LH but not of FSH release from the pituitary increase after hysterectomy. 2) There is no negative feedback of progesterone on LH during the first 2 weeks of the luteal phase in hysterectomized heifers. Progesterone increases in the hysterectomized animals after this period when luteolysis occurs in the controls. 3) Estradiol-17ß concentrations including the preovulatory ones are low during the first 3-4 weeks pp. 4) Ovarian oxytocin vanishes after about 2 weeks of luteal function independently of the presence of the uterus. 5) Prostaglandin $F_{2\alpha}$ and its 13,14-dihydro-15-keto--metabolite are secreted in high concentrations (15 or 50 pmol/ml, respectively) immediately after parturition from the uterus into the vena cava and decrease after hysterectomy to about 1/10th within 30 min and to 1/40th within 12 h. These low levels are reached about 14 days later in the intact controls. PgFM as well as $PGF_{2\alpha}$ are lower in the aorta than in the vena cava. We conclude that an intact ovarian-uterine unit is able to inhibit pituitary function in the dairy cow for about 2 weeks pp. Prostaglandin F may be involved but its specific role remains to be defined. Supported by the DFG. D.L.Walters was an A.-v.-Humboldt fellow.

2115 FOLLICLE STIMULATING HORMONE (FSH) STIMULATES APOLIPOPROTEIN E (APO E) PRODUCTION BY CULTURED RAT OVARY GRANULOSA CELLS (GC). J. Schreiber* , D. Driscoll , and G. Getz , University of Chicago, Chicago, Il. 60637 USA

We report the first demonstration of apo E synthesis and gonadotropic stimulation of its production by ovarian steroidogenic cells. Apo E is a surface constituent of several classes of plasma lipoproteins (LP) and plays a critical role in the recognition and uptake of LP by cells. In an examination of the control of apo E synthesis by extrahepatic steroidogenic tissue, we cultured ovary GC from DES-stimulated hypophysectomized immature rats for 30 hrs in serum-free McCoy's medium (with & without added FSH &/or androgen). After incubating the GC an additional 18 hrs with ^{35}S-methionine, apo E in the medium was immunoprecipitated by a monospecific goat-anti rat apo E antibody, isolated by binding to Protein A sepharose, and electrophoresed on SDS/5-22% polyacrylamide gel. ^{35}S-proteins were located by fluorography and bands quantified by scanning densitometer. GC produced a protein band (0.1 % of total secreted protein) which was identified as apo E by electrophoretic mobility, immunoprecipitation by monospecific antibody, and limited proteolysis mapping by S. aureus V8 protease. Addition of 50 ng/ml oFSH to the culture medium stimulated a 3-fold increase in apo E secretion. Apo E synthesis is not tightly coupled to steroidogenesis because the addition of 10^{-7} M androgen plus FSH stimulated a marked increase in progestin synthesis over FSH alone, but added androgen had little effect on apo E secretion. The physiologic role of GC apo E is unknown, but could be important in cholesterol transport, cellular LP uptake, and/or cellular phospholipid synthesis and metabolism. Supported by grants HL 15062, GM 07197, and HD 17753.

2116 NON-AROMATIZABLE ANDROGENS STIMULATE ESTRADIOL-17β (E_2) PRODUCTION BY PORCINE OVARIAN GRANULOSA CELLS. M. Schweitzer and C. St.G. Hall*, Lady Davis Institute for Medical Research, Sir Mortimer B. Davis - Jewish General Hospital and the Department of Medicine, McGill University, Montreal, Quebec, Canada H3T 1E2.

We have studied the effect of non-aromatizable androgens on estradiol-17β (E_2) production by porcine granulosa cells obtained from small, medium and large ovarian follicles. Granulosa cells were incubated in air at 37°C for 16 hrs. 10^{-3} M dihydrotestosterone (DHT) and methyltrieneolone (R-1881) a potent non-aromatizable synthetic androgen increased E_2 production 10-20 fold over control values. There was no difference in maximum E_2 production in cells obtained from small, medium or large follicles though basal E_2 production of cells obtained from large follicles was twice that of cells from small follicles. Addition of 10^{-6} M testosterone to either 10^{-3} M DHT or 10^{-3} M R-1881 did not further increase E_2 production. The addition of 10^{-3} M flutamide, an anti-androgen, to the incubation media resulted in a 40-50% decrease in E_2 production. When 10^{-4} M testolactone, an aromatase inhibitor was added, a 30-50% decrease in E_2 production occurred. Inhibitors of protein synthesis, cycloheximide 4 mg/ml, puromycin 10 μg/ml and actinomycin D 0.2 μg/ml did not significantly affect DHT stimulated E_2 production, although progesterone production stimulated by follicle stimulating hormone (FSH) 100 ng/ml and lutenizing hormone (LH) 100 ng/ml was inhibited by 65-90%. The present data demonstrate that high concentrations of non-aromatizable androgens will stimulate E_2 production by porcine granulosa cells throughout follicular development and suggest that this effect is not mediated through new protein synthesis.

2117 INAPPROPRIATE HIGH SECRETION OF VASOPRESSIN IN HEART FAILURE INFLUENCES ON PERIPHERAL VASCULAR RESISTANCE AND FORMATION OF EDEMA. A.J.G. Riegger*, E. Bauer and G. Liebau, Medizinische Universitätsklinik, D 8700 Würzburg, F.R.G.

Beside its water retaining properties vasopressin (AVP)has powerful vasoconstrictor effects and may contribute to the increase of peripheral vascular resistance (PVR) in heart failure. We studied AVP in an animal model of high output heart failure (60 days) in rats with an aorto-caval fistula (n=28). 18 sham operated rats served as controls. Cardiac output was measured by thermodilution, BP in the aorta and plasma AVP by RIA.The vasoconstrictor effect of AVP was tested by using a specific AVP-inhibitor. The controls showed the exspected positive correlation between plasmaosmolality (Posm)and AVP(12.8±5.1 pg/ml)(r= 0.65; $p<0.01$)(Posm 291±10). The rats with heart failure had elevated AVP-levels (33.5± 24.1 pg/ml) and lower Posm (286±11 mosmol/kgH_2O)and a negative correlation between Posm and AVP (r= -0.70; $p<0.001$), 7 animals had severe edema. The bolus injection of AVP-inhibitor resulted in no effect on BP and PVR in both groups, including animals with AVP-levels up to 86 pg/ml. In conclusion AVP did not contribute to an increase of PVR in heart failure or its effect was counterbalanced by central regulating systems. It seems that the inappropriate high secretion of AVP plays an important role in the formation of edema and of the "dilutional hypoosmolality" by enhanced water reabsorption.

2118 A SIMPLE AND HIGHLY SENSITIVE RADIOIMMUNOASSAY FOR 8-ARGININE VASOPRESSIN IN HUMAN PLASMA USING AN ODS-SILICA MICROCOLUMN TECHNIQUE. H. Sakurai*§, F. Kurimoto§, A. Kanai§§, H. Ohno§§, K. Nomura§§§, H. Demura§§§, K. Shizume §§§, § Mitsubishiyuka Lab. of Medical Science, §§ Mitsubishi Petrochemical Co., §§§ Tokyo Women's Medical College, Itabashi-ku, Tokyo, 175, JAPAN.

A highly sensitive and simple radioimmunoassay for the measurement of 8-Arginine vasopressin (AVP) in human plasma has been developed. Dose response curve ranges from 0.025 to 8 pg/tube. This simple extraction technique employing an ODS-silica microcolumn recovered 83.7 ± 10.4 (SD) % of AVP in the range of 1 - 20 pg/ml added to 0.5 ml plasma. Determination of AVP in each fraction of plasma which was gel-filtrated through Sephadex G25 (1 x 80 cm) found that the fraction of plasma AVP was superimposed on that of authentic AVP and interference of non-specific substances was completely eliminated by ODS-silica microcolumn. Using the assay, 13 of 16 patients with DI showed plasma AVP concentrations ranging from 0.03 to 0.21 pg/ml and the other 3 patients had less than 0.03 pg/ml. The AVP concentrations of DI were clearly discriminated from those obtained in normal subjects (0.30 - 4.20 pg/ml, n=65). The within and between assay variability was about 10 % each. Plasma AVP concentrations of normal subjects (n=6) standing, sitting and supine after 8 hr. of fluid deprivation were 2.41 ± 1.15 (SD), 1.95 ± 0.85 and 0.97 ± 0.48 pg/ml (30 min after) respectively. Plasma AVP concentrations of normal subjects (n=6) after water loaded (20 ml/Kg wt) were clearly reduced from 1.89 ± 1.00 (before) to 0.42 ± 0.21 (stnding for 60 min)and also from 0.89 ± 0.41 to 0.40 ± 0.22 pg/ml (supine for 60 min).

2119 OXYTOCIN INHIBITS RECOVERY OF OVARIAN ACTIVITY IN SOWS AFTER WEANING. W. Schaekel*, F. Ellendorff, Institute of Animal Science and Animal Behaviour (FAL), Mariensee, 3057 Neustadt 1, F.R.G.

Ovarian oxytocin secretion has revived interest in a possible role of oxytocin in the regualtion of ovarian function. Our experiment studied the effects of oxytocin on the induction of ovarian activity subsequent to lactational anestrus in sows. Pulsatile oxytocin [Oxy (25 mU/ml)] or sham injections [solvent or NaCl] were given via indwelling catheters into the external jugular vein every 45 min (3 ml each) for 3 weeks to mimick suckling-induced oxytocin release. Every second day plasma progesterone (P_4) was analyzed for 1) untreated control sows (C, n = 7 sows), 2) shams (S, n = 12 sows), 3) oxytocin (Oxy, n = 17 sows). All oxy sows remained below 1 ng/P_4/ml plasma throughout the experiment, whereas in both, C and S sows P_4 was significantly elevated from day 5 after weaning (i.e. day 5 after the start of the experiment). C and S had mean peak levels of P_4 of 24 ng P_4/ml in plasma on day 17. The data suggest, that oxytocin is responsible for the absence of ovarian activity during lactation.

2120 OCCURRENCE OF OXYTOCIN, VASOPRESSIN AND NEUROPHYSINS IN PERIPHERAL NERVES. R.P. Sequeira* and I.M. Chaiken, Laboratory of chemical Biology, NIADDK, National Institutes of Health, Bethesda, MD 20205 USA.

Axons containing hypothalamo-neurohypophyseal peptides have been found in various extrahypothalamic sites within the central nervous system. Given current interest in the occurrence of bioactive peptides in peripheral autonomic fibers, we have analyzed both cervical vagus and sciatic nerves for the presence of oxytocin, arginine vasopressin (AVP), and their respective common biosynthetic precursor protein components, neurophysin-I (NP-I) and neurophysin-II(NP-II). Cat vagal extracts were fractionated by reverse phase high performance liquid chromatography(RP-HPLC), with molecular species quantitated by radioimmunoassay(RIA). Roughly equal amounts of the two hormones were detected. This also was observed for the NP's, although molar amounts of the latter were larger compared to those of hormones. Analysis of rabbit vagal NP's was performed by affinity chromatography of tissue extracts on lysine vasopressin(LVP)-Sepharose and RP-HPLC of LVP-binding proteins. UV-Detectable peaks observed at positions corresponding to those of authentic bovine pituitary NP's indicated the presence of approximately equal amounts of oxytocin- and AVP-associated NP's. Affinity chromatography/RP-HPLC analysis also allowed detection of approximately equal amounts of the two major NP's in rabbit sciatic nerve. And, both hormones were detected in sciatic nerve by RIA. The biosynthetic origin, cellular localization and physiological functions of neurohypophyseal peptides in peripheral nerves are yet to be defined, as is the relationship of peripheral neuronal pathways to the occurrence of hormones and NP's in other peripheral sites, such as the ovary.

2121 ARGININE VASOPRESSIN AND ACTH RELEASE: CORRELATION BETWEEN BINDING CHARACTERISTICS AND BIOACTIVITY IN ANTERIOR PITUITARY DISPERSED CELLS.

E. Spinedi and A. Negro-Vilar*, Reprod. Neuroendoc. Sect., Lab. Reprod. Devel. Tox., NIEHS, NIH, Research Triangle Park, NC 27709 USA.

The binding characteristics of arginine vasopressin (AVP) were evaluated and correlated with its biological activity using rat anterior pituitary dispersed cells. AVP released ACTH in a concentration-dependent fashion, with a minimal effective dose of 10^{-10} M. ^{3}H-AVP, used as ligand for binding studies, showed full biological activity at different concentrations. Saturable and high affinity binding sites for ^{3}H-AVP have been obtained using intact cells. Specific binding reached equilibrium by 180 min at 22 C and rapid and complete dissociation was obtained with an excess of AVP. Scatchard analysis showed a single class of binding sites, with an apparent K_D of 1.63 nM and a binding capacity (B_{MAX}) of 10.7 fmol/10^6 cells, at 37 C. At 22 C, K_D and B_{MAX} values were within the same order of magnitude. AVP displaced ^{3}H-AVP binding with an IC50 of 1.5 x 10^{-7} M, while oxytocin showed a somewhat higher IC50 (0.9 x 10^{-6} M) and did not achieve complete inhibition of binding. An AVP analog with a ring substitution (Asu^{1,6}-AVP) showed decreased displacement capacity. Both oxytocin and the AVP analog showed weak ACTH-releasing activity, indicating that changes in the tail and/or ring portion of the AVP molecule reduce both the binding affinity and the ACTH-releasing activity of these peptides. Rat corticotropin-releasing factor and angiotensin II had no affinity for AVP binding sites. The results indicate that specific AVP binding sites in anterior pituitary cells are closely correlated with the intrinsic ability of the peptide to elicit ACTH release.

2122 CIRCADIAN MODULATION BY MELATONIN OF MURINE ACTH SECRETION & CORTICOSTERONE PRODUCTION IN VITRO.

S. Sanchez de la Pena*, F. Halberg, E. Haus, D. Lakatua, E. Halberg and F. Ungar, Univ. of Minnesota, Mpls, MN, USA

Pineal homogenate modulates in a rhythmic sequence (feed-sideward), i.e., attenuates, leaves unaffected & amplifies the effect of ACTH 1-17 on corticosterone production in vitro (Brain Res. Bull. 11:117, 1983). Melatonin may contribute to this modulation & also acts without ACTH addition, as demonstrated herein. 72 female CD2F$_1$ mice, 8 wks old, 2/cage, were standardized for >1 week in L06^{00}18^{00}D18^{00}-06^{00}. 12 mice were decapitated every 4 h during 24 h. At each of 6 circadian stages, adrenals were cleaned, bisected and transferred into plastic wells containing 0.5 ml Krebs-Ringer buffer (pH 7.35) with 0.01 M glucose and albumin (1%) added (KRB) in 95% O_2 and 5% CO_2 at 37±1°C. 4 adrenal halves were incubated in each well for 30 min & the fluid discarded. During the ensuing 3 h, plates were incubated with or without melatonin (10^{-7} M). Corticosterone was determined fluorometrically: the differences in mean values from incubations in KRB with & without melatonin & ± ACTH were analyzed by the single cosinor method by which the "no-rhythm" assumption was rejected (P<.001). The acrophase (ϕ), indicating the time of amplification of corticosterone production by melatonin was at -204° (360°≡24h; 0°=light onset). Melatonin action by itself (in the abrence of exogenous ACTH) may contribute to a direct pineal effect exerted upon adrenocortical function by action upon (its own or) ACTH receptors or some other internal mechanism. Parallel studies in vitro also indicate a direct melatonin effect upon pituitary ACTH secretion in the absence of the hypothalamus. Such time-dependent neuroendocrine mechanisms may underlie differences between enhancement or inhibition of malignancy by the same total dose of melatonin. SUPPORT: USPHS (GM-13981); NCI (CA-14445).

2123 PINEAL GLAND AND HYPOTHALAMUS-PITUITARY-GONADAL SYSTEM OF MALE GOLDEN HAMSTERS DURING AN ARTIFICIAL WINTER SEASON IN A CLIMATIC CHAMBER. Y. Shiotani*, H.J. Cho, S. Shiosaka, K. Tasaka#, A. Miyake# and T. Aono#. Dept. of Neuroanat., Inst. of Higher Nervous Activity, and Dept. of Obstet. and Gynecol.(#), Osaka Univ. Med. School, 4-3-57, Nakanoshima, Kitaku, Osaka, Japan.

Male golden hamsters were exposed gradually to low temperature and short photo-period in a climatic chamber, and kept finally in 5°c: 3 hr light / 21 hr darkness for more than 5 weeks. After the experiment, 1) most of the pinealocytes showed the signs of enhanced cellular activity, such as well-developed sER or Golgi apparatus. 2) LH-RH neuron system in the septal or preoptic area was immunostained more abundantly than the control group, coincident with RIA of hypothalamic LH-RH. 3) Pituitary gonadotrophs contained accumulated granules, lysosomes and ill-developed cell organelles, indicating suppressed cellular function, whereas mammotrophs showed the signs of stimulated function. 4) Testes and accessory sex organs involuted strikingly, weighing 13% and 39% of those of the controls respectively. Seminiferous tubules atrophied and no sperm was observed. Leydig cells were shrunken and cell organelles other than mitochondria were rarely seen. It would be suggested that increased pineal hormones during the experiment suppressed discharge of the hypothalamic LH-RH, resulting in hypofunction of pituitary gonadotrophs and subsequent gonadal atrophy.

2124 THE EFFECTS OF PROLACTIN (PRL) ON RAT TESTICULAR STEROIDOGENIC ENZYME ACTIVITIES. A.K. Munabi*, V. Mericq, M.C. Gelato, S. Malozowski, R. D'Agata, M.M. Koppelman, B.D. Albertson, F. Cassorla, and D. Lynn Loriaux DEB, NICHD, NIH, Bethesda, MD 20205

We examined the effects of PRL on testicular microsomal 3β-hydroxysteroid dehydrogenase (3β-HSD) 17-hydroxylase (17-OH), 17,20-desmolase (17,20-D), 17-ketosteroid reductase (17-KSR) and aromatase activities in hyperprolactinemic rats and controls. Adult hypophysectomized, gonadotropin replaced Fisher rats were rendered hyperprolactinemic by isografting pituitaries under the kidney capsule. The controls received skeletal muscle. All rats were sacrificed 7 days later and serum PRL was measured in each. The testes were resected, pooled according to PRL levels, and microsomes were prepared from each pool. The activities of the 3βHSD, 17-OH, 17,20-D, 17-KSR and aromatase were measured using as substrates ^{14}C dehydroepiandrosterone, progesterone, 17-hydroxyprogesterone, androstenedione, and testosterone respectively. Results are shown below.

	Control	Hyperprolactinemic	
Serum PRL (ng/ml)	4.3 ± .6*	198 ± 14	
3β-HSD †	217 ± 20*	124 ± 11	† = pmol/mg protein/min
17-OH †	358 ± 30*	86 ± 9	
17,20-D †	147 ± 13*	87 ± 7	* = p<0.01
17-KSR †	107 ± 3*	69 ± 7	
Aromatase †	76 ± 16*	16 ± 5	n = 14

We conclude that hyperprolactinemia is associated with decreased activities of 5 key testicular steroidogenic enzymes. This is consistent with decreased testicular steroid secretion, and may explain some of the abnormalities found in patients with hyperprolactinemia.

2125 STIMULATION OF rGH RELEASE BY 12-O-TETRADECANOYLPHORBOL-13-ACETATE (TPA) IN PRIMARY PITUITARY CELL CULTURE - INTERACTION BETWEEN TPA AND SOMATOSTATIN OR hpGRF(1-44). E. Ohmura* and H.G. Friesen, Dept. of Physiology, University of Manitoba, Winnipeg, Manitoba, Canada R3E OW3.

Specific binding sites for phorbol esters have been reported in a pituitary cell line (GH_4C_1 cell). In the present study, we examined the effect of TPA on rGH release in rat primary pituitary cell cultures. TPA stimulated rGH release in a dose dependent manner. (ED50 = 1.1 x 10^{-9}M). Maximum stimulation (3.2 - 4.5 fold above control) was achieved at a dose of TPA, 8.1 x 10^{-9}M. On the other hand, rPRL release did not change significantly, but there was a small increase in rTSH release by TPA (0.8 fold above control). Somatostatin-14 (10^{-9}M) suppressed rGH release induced by various doses of TPA. The different Km values (in Lineweaver-Burk plot) between TPA alone (Km = 0.42 x 10^{-9}M) and TPA + somatostatin (Km = 1.6 x 10^{-9}M), suggest that the two agents act competitively on the cells. When various doses of TPA and hpGRF-44 (0.1, 1 ng/ml) were added simultaneously, there were clear additive effects on rGH release at all doses of TPA including maximally stimulatory doses of TPA. These results suggest that the two substances act on rGH release through different pathways. However, when both agents were added Km values decreased compared to that using TPA alone, suggesting that the two factors, at least in part, act competitively on the somatotrophs. In conclusion, the data are consistent with the hypothesis that TPA competes with GRF and somatostatin on the somatotroph perhaps through a common mediator protein kinase C.

2126 PREOPERATIVE LATERALIZATION OF ACTH-SECRETING PITUITARY MICROADENOMAS BY BILATERAL AND SIMULTANEOUS INFERIOR PETROSAL VENOUS SINUS SAMPLING. E. Oldfield*, G. Chrousos, H. Schulte, M. Schaaf, P. McKeever, A. Krudy, G. Cutler, Jr., D. Loriaux, and J. Doppman, SNB, NINCDS*, DEB, NICHD and Diagnostic Radiology Dept., NIH, Bethesda, MD 20205

Surgical treatment of Cushing's disease may fail because of the surgeon's inability to find and excise pituitary microadenomas 5 mm or less in diameter. Preoperative determination of the side of the pituitary gland in which a microadenoma resides may improve the results of surgery by permitting the surgeon to find smaller tumors or, if a tumor is not found, to excise the half of the pituitary gland thought to harbor the microadenoma. We performed simultaneous bilateral inferior petrosal sinus (IPS) and peripheral vein sampling in 7 patients with Cushing's disease for determination of plasma ACTH concentrations in an attempt to localize the source of ACTH secretion. In the patients with normal computed tomographic studies and pituitary microadenomas, IPS ACTH levels were higher on the side where a microadenoma was later found and removed during transsphenoidal surgery. Two of these patients, in whom no adenoma was found at surgery, experienced clinical and hormonal cure after removal of half of the gland ipsilateral to the IPS with the greatest ACTH gradient. In 3 patients ACTH levels in the IPS contralateral to the adenoma were similar to peripheral levels, and if sampled alone, would have suggested a peripheral source of ACTH. The 7th patient, who had corticotroph cell hyperplasia, had symmetrical IPS ACTH gradients. Thus, bilateral simultaneous IPS and peripheral vein sampling for determination of plasma ACTH concentrations predicted the position of an ACTH-secreting microadenoma in the pituitary gland.

2127 β_2-ADRENERGIC CONTROL OF GROWTH HORMONE (GH) SECRETION BY RAT ANTERIOR PITUITARY CELLS (AP). S.N. Perkins*, W.S. Evans, M.O. Thorner and M.J. Cronin. University of Virginia School of Medicine, Charlottesville, VA., U.S.A.

We recently demonstrated that β-adrenergic (β) agonists can stimulate GH release by a direct action on rat AP (NEUROENDOCRINOLOGY 37:473, 1983). We confirmed and extended this observation by monitoring dynamic hormone secretion by perifused dispersed AP, by measuring β receptors directly in crude AP membranes with [^{125}I]-iodocyanopindolol (ICYP) and by assessing cellular cAMP accumulation in AP monolayers. Perifused AP were exposed to 5 min pulses of at least 4 concentrations of adrenergic agonists in randomized order. The half-maximal agonist concentrations for stimulation of GH release were characteristic of a β_2 receptor (EC_{50}'s, mean $\pm$ SEM, n=4): l-isoproterenol (ISO, 14 $\pm$ 2 nM), l-epinephrine (EPI, 160 $\pm$ 30 nM) and l- norepinephrine (NE, >1 µM). β agonists had no apparent effect on the release of prolactin or luteinizing hormone. Subtype-selective β drugs inhibited ICYP binding to AP membranes with potencies also consistent with a β_2 receptor (inhibition constants at [ICYP] = 20-30 pM, mean $\pm$ SEM, n=3): IPS-339# (4.3 $\pm$ 1.6 nM), zinterol (120 $\pm$ 20 nM), metoprolol (6.2 $\pm$ 0.5 µM), and practolol (230 $\pm$ 20 µM). cAMP accumulation by AP incubated for 5 min with 1 µM ISO was 2-4 fold greater than control ($P < 0.001$, n=3). The stimulation of cAMP levels by ISO was rapidly down-regulated and completely abolished after 30 min of incubation. These data suggest that the rat AP contains β_2 receptors and that their activation can amplify the rate of GH release. If this is the case, then EPI must be denoted as a GH releasing factor and hypothesized to have physiological significance in the rat. #IPS 339 (t-butyl-amino-3-ol-2-propyl)oxmino-9-fluorene HCl. (NSF Fellowship, CI A HD00439, HD13197 AM32632, RCDA 1K04NS500601, HD18409, AM22125)

2128 ASPECTS OF THE CHOLINERGIC CONTROL OF GH AND ADRENOCORTICAL HORMONE SECRETION IN MAN. L.Portmann *, Ioana Lancranjan,E.Maeder and J.P.Felber,Division of Endocrinology,CHUV,Lausanne,Switzerland.

Evidence has accumulated that the cholinergic stimulation increases the secretion of GH,ACTH and corticosteroid hormones in animals.Cholinergic agonists administered intraventricularly stimulate corticoid secretion in the rat,whereas atropine implanted in the hypothalamus blocks it,as well as the stress-stimulated corticosterone secretion(Kaplariski and Smelik,1973).In cats the diurnal rise in cortisol is specifically and completely suppressed by small doses of atropine(Krieger and Krieger,1967). In vitro acetylcholine stimulates the synthesis and release of CRF,effect which is blocked by nicotinic and muscarinic receptor antagonists(Buckingam and Hodges,1979).In the rat,atropine suppresses also GH secretion(Bruni and Meites,1978).We investigated in man the role of the cholinergic control of GH,ACTH and cortisol secretion by testing the effect on resting,circadian pattern and insulin stimulated plasma levels of these hormones by a new compound,106-689,which is a potent central anticholinergic(inhibitory effect on EEG arousal reaction caused by arecoline and on H-QNB binding on calf cortex).Cortisol resting plasma levels decreased significantly after the administration of 106-689,with nadir levels of 9.4$\pm$1.3;4.4$\pm$ 0.9 and 2.7$\pm$0.3 µg/dl($p<0.001$) after respectively placebo,106-689 10 and 25 mg dose.The 7 days' treatment with 10 mg daily 106-689 was followed by a decrease in morning cortisol levels(16.0$\pm$0.9 vs 14.4$\pm$1.9 µg/dl,n.s.).No impairment in ACTH and cortisol resposes to hypoglycemic stress(ΔACTH:102.5$\pm$18.7 pg/ml and Δcortisol 24.1$\pm$ 1.2 vs 23.1$\pm$1.4 µg/dl respectively after placebo and 106-689 treatment)and circadian rhythm(diurnal peak of cortisol:17.5$\pm$1.5 vs 18.7$\pm$3.2,n.s.)was found after 7 days' treatment with 106-689.Conversely,GH resting plasma levels were not influenced by 106-689,whereas GH secretion stimulated by insulin induced hypoglycemia-stress(ΔGH 34.9$\pm$4.2 vs 25.0$\pm$3.4,*p<0.01)and sleep induced GH peak(15.9 vs 11.4,*p<0.05)were significantly decreased by 106-689 administration.These data suggest that in normal man the cholinergic system has a tonic stimulatory effect on basal ACTH-cortisol secretion but it is not involved in the control of stress-induced and morning rise of these hormones,whereas it controls both stress and sleep-induced GH release.

*ng/ml

2129 IMMUNOCYTOCHEMICAL STUDY OF THE HUMAN PHARYNGEAL HYPOPHYSIS. L.A.Puy*, A.O.Stati and D.R.Ciocca, Laboratorio de Reproducción y Lactancia (LARLAC), Casilla de Correo 855, Mendoza 5500, Argentina.

The human pharyngeal hypophysis is a constant formation found in the periostium situated at the conjunction of the sphenoid and the vomer bones. Identification of the cell types present in this gland and morphologic response of these cells to endocrine disorders have not been adequately documented. Ten autopsy pharyngeal hypophyses were studied by immunocytochemistry at light microscopic level. Seven of the pharyngeal hypophyses were obtained from patients without endocrine abnormalities and the other three from patients with disturbed endocrine function. In the seven normal glands tested, ACTH, β-LPH, β-FSH, β-LH, β-TSH,PRL and GH cells were identified. No predominance of a particular cell type was observed, most of them were present in moderate number or as occasional cells. On the other hand, the pharyngeal hypophysis of a patient treated with metoclopramide, a dopamine-receptor-blocking drug, showed PRL cell hyperplasia; while the pharyngeal hypophysis of a patient with chronic hepatic cirrhosis showed numerous PRL and GH cells. The pharyngeal hypophysis of a patient with hypothyroidism appeared hypertrophied, with TSH cell hyperplasia. These data show the capacity of the pharyngeal hypophysis to produce hormones and to respond with hypertrophy and/or hyperplasia of definite cell types to endocrine disorders.
This study was supported by the CONICET.

2130 EFFECTS OF FORSKOLIN ON PROLACTIN AND GROWTH HORMONE SECRETION FROM OVINE PITUITARY CELLS. K.P. Ray*, J.J. Gomm and M. Wallis, Biochemistry Laboratory, University of Sussex, Falmer, Brighton BN1 9QG, U.K.

Previous studies of prolactin and growth hormone (GH) secretion suggest that cyclic AMP may be involved as a second messenger in the actions of some releasing factors such as vasoactive intestinal polypeptide and GH releasing hormone. In this study we used forskolin, a non-selective activator of adenylate cyclase, to investigate the effects of raising pituitary cell cyclic AMP concentrations on prolactin and GH secretion from ovine pituitary cell cultures. Inhibitory effects of dopamine on forskolin-induced secretion and cyclic AMP accumulation were also studied. Incubation of pituitary cells with forskolin (0.1-10μM; 30 min) produced a modest dose-related rise in prolactin release (to 180% of basal) but a greater stimulation of GH secretion (to 400% of basal). Cellular cyclic AMP concentrations were also increased up to 15-fold under these conditions. Dopamine (0.1μM) in the presence of forskolin inhibited prolactin secretion to below the basal level and considerably attenuated the stimulation of GH release. There was a small but significant inhibition ($p<0.02$; Students t test) by dopamine of cyclic AMP levels measured in the presence of 10μM forskolin. Forskolin (10μM) stimulated secretion of prolactin (to 160% control) and GH (to 490% control) by 15 minutes and this stimulation was maintained for at least 1 hour. These results indicate that raising cellular cyclic AMP concentrations stimulates the secretion of both prolactin and GH. The relatively large stimulatory effects of forskolin on GH secretion compared with those on prolactin release suggest that modulation of cyclic AMP may be more important in the acute regulation of somatotrophs.

2131 A MODEL FOR STUDYING NEGATIVE FEEDBACK OF THE PITUITARY-ADRENOCORTICAL AXIS IN MAN - A PRELIMINARY REPORT. P.M.Rosman*, C. Goldstein, and J. Habas, Endocrine Section, V.A. Medical Center, and Division of Endocrinology/Diabetes, S.U.N.Y., Downstate Medical Center, Brooklyn, New York 11209 and 11203.

We developed a model to study level-sensitive negative feedback (NF) of the pituitary-adrenocortical axis in man when plasma (P) cortisol (F) levels are in the physiologic range. We collected blood samples every 20 minutes between midnight and 10 AM in a sleep entrained subject during 7 studies done 1 to 2 weeks apart. The subject underwent one night of sleep deprivation before each study. Lights off was at midnight, subjective sleep latency was 5 minutes, and arousal was at 7:20 AM. Plasma F levels were measured by RIA. The timing and basal values of F secretion were reproducible for five consecutive secretory episodes in two studies done 1 week apart. To study the effect of level-sensitive NF on arousal-associated F secretion, hydrocortisone (HC) was infused intravenously during a 4 hour period before awakening. During dexamethasone suppression, endogenous hormone secretion was mimicked using a HC dose calculated from the F metabolic clearance rate obtained in this subject. In subsequent studies, 4 hour infusions of HC were performed at a rate of 2 mg/hr without dexamethasone suppression and P total F levels were measured every 3 minutes during the hour before and after awakening. P free F and ACTH were measured by equilibrium dialysis and by RIA, respectively, during the same time period. When HC was begun either 4 or 5 hours before arousal, the P total and free F levels increased after awakening as they did during baseline studies where no infusions were done. However, after the infusions P ACTH levels were decreased by over 50% compared with baseline studies during the post-arousal period. In conclusion, reproducibility of the timing and basal state of F secretion can be elicited in a sleeping, entrained, human subject. In preliminary studies, arousal-associated ACTH secretion appeared to respond to level-sensitive NF when F levels were in the physiologic range.

2132 PRESENCE OF PROLACTIN RECEPTORS AND COUPLING TO ORNITHINE DECARBOXYLASE ACTIVITY IN HUMAN PERIHERAL BLOOD LYMPHOCYTES. D.H. Russell*, R. Kibler, D.F. Larson, B. Poulos and B.E. Magun, Univ. of Arizona, Tucson, AZ 85724.

We have demonstrated prolactin receptors on human peripheral blood lymphocytes and these receptors are coupled to the induction of ornithine decarboxylase, a key growth regulatory enzyme. The dissociation constant was K_D app = 1.66 x 10^{-9} M and the receptor number was 600 receptors/cell. The receptor was specific for prolactin in the presence of a large excess of growth hormone, insulin, or epidermal growth factor. Studies in rats as well as in mixed populations of lymphocytes demonstrated that binding of [^{125}I]prolactin to the receptor was blocked by the presence of cyclosporine (10^{-6} M, Sandimmune®, i.v. solution). In rats, the rapid induction of ornithine decarboxylase (4-6 h) in response to prolactin was blocked by 10^{-6} M cyclosporine. Cyclosporine did not affect the binding of [^{3}H]dihydroalprenolol, a β-adrenoceptor antagonist, to lymphocytes, suggestive again of the specificity of the drug for prolactin receptors. Preliminary studies on purified populations of T-cells, B-cells and monocytes indicate that both T-cells and B-cells contain prolactin receptors. Monocytes did not exhibit any specific binding of [^{125}I]prolactin. T-cells demonstrated enhanced binding of [^{125}I]prolactin at 10^{-9} and 10^{-8} M cyclosporine, partial inhibition at 10^{-7} M and complete inhibition of binding at 10^{-6} M cyclosporine. Specific binding of [^{125}I]prolactin to B-cells was only partially blocked by 10^{-6} M cyclosporine, in contrast to the complete inhibition of binding to T-cells. Prolactin receptors may be important in the regulation of certain lymphocyte immune functions, and cyclosporine may exert its immunosuppressive action via these receptors.
(Supported by USPHS Research Grant CA-14783 from the NCI)

2133 THE HYPOPROLACTINEMIC RAT (IPL) : PITUITARY AND SEX STEROIDS HORMONES DURING THE ESTROUS CYCLE AND GESTATION. I.Sabbagh+, P. Guillaumot, J. Bertrand and H. Cohen. Institut Pasteur, 77 rue Pasteur, 69007 Lyon, France. INSERM-U.34, Hôpital Debrousse, Lyon, France.

IPL nude rats are characterized by a delayed puberty and absence of lactation. In these rats, serum prolactin (PRL) is low (RIA and BioA) while pituitary content is normal. In adult IPL males serum LH and FSH are in addition somewhat reduced and serum testosterone (T) is half normal. In this study, we have measured serum levels of estradiol (E_2), progesterone (P), LH, FSH and PRL in IPL and normal female rats, during estrous cycle and pregnancy. On diestrus (DE) and estrus (E) days, decapitation was done at noon. On the day of proestrus (PE) rats were sacrificed at 10.00, 12.00, 16.00 and 19.00. Serum PRL was significantly lower in the groups of IPL than in normals rats, except on PE at 16.00. However, E_2 and P were similar in the 2 groups of rats. Surprisingly, in IPL rats serum LH was significantly higher than normal at DE. Pregnant rats were studied either longitudinally (individual blood obtained by cardiac puncture in the same rat throughout gestation) or in groups of 6-8 rats sacrificed at different days of gestation, the day of sperm being assigned as day 0. Serum PRL levels were significantly lower in IPL than in normal throughout gestation, those of FSH and E_2 were lower only at days 21 and 22. No difference was found in P levels. It is concluded: 1) that hypoprolactinemia does not appear to affect adrenal and ovarian steroidogenesis in the female IPL rat, in contrast to what observed in the male (decreased T). 2) The abnormal rise in E_2 at the end of gestation together with hypoprolactinemia may be responsible for the absence of lactation observed in the IPL rats.

2134 ANTITUMOR EFFECT OF BROMOCRIPTINE ON PROLACTINOMAS. Y. Saitoh*, H. Mori, S. Mori, K. Matsumoto and T. Uozumi#, Department of Neurosurgery and Pathology, Osaka University Medical School, 1-1-50 Fukushima, Fukushima, Osaka, Japan, # Department of Neurosurgery, Hiroshima University

To clarify the mechanism of antitumor action of bromocriptine(CB) on prolactinomas(PRLomas). PRLomas treated with CB were studied by light microscopic morphometry and electron microscopy. CB was administered to 11 patients 10 mg/day for 2 weeks, preoperatively. PRLomas from 6 patients were removed immediately after the treatment with CB (Group 1), whereas those from 5 patients were removed 1 week after treatment (Group 2). All CB-treated patients demonstrated a decrease in serum PRL levels, and 2 patients demonstrated reduction in tumor size on CT scan. In Group 1, in addition to decrease in size of individual tumor cell (905 μm^3 on average, as compared with 1,500 μm^3 of untreated tumors), degeneration and necrosis of the tumor cells were observed. Membranous structures of degenerated tumor cells accumulated in the stromal tissue, which increased to be 23% of the whole tumor volume, as compared with 10% of the untreated tumors. The tumors from Group 2 consisted of fibrotic and regrowing parts. In the fibrotic part, necrosis of tumor cells were more prominent with an increase in stromal volume up to 43% of the whole tumor volume. The regrowing part showed a histology resembling to untreated PRLomas. It is suggested that the size reduction of PRLomas treated with CB results from the reduction in size as well as necrosis of individual tumor cell. PRLomas seem to consist of two populations. One is sensitive to cytocidal action of CB, and the other is resistant. Cessation of CB treatment seems to allow the resistant population to proliferate.

2135 INDIRECT EVIDENCE OF THE DOPAMINE (DA) INFLUENCE ON GNRH NEURONS IN CHRONIC ANOVULATION SYNDROMES. C.Salazar*,H.Porias,A. Hernández Bueno,(Spon:V.Cortés Gallegos).Reproductive Endocrinology. Hospital General de México, SSA, Mexico City (Durango 290-607, México 06700, DF).

High DA concentration in the tuberoinfundibular system has an inhibitory influence on the GnRH neurons, e.g.Prolactinoma.By using metoclopramide(MCP)in an attempt to evaluate indirectly its influence in other conditions, we selected four groups of patients with chronic anovulation.I:Polycystic ovary(n=7);II: Hyperprolactinemia without evidence of tumor(n=5);III Polycystic ovary with hyperprolactinemia(n=5);and IV:Prolactinoma(n=4 After three basal samples MCP(10mg as a single bolus)was administered and peripherial blood samples were taken every 15 minutes, during one hour.Basal LH(mIU/ml)of 61 ± 54($\bar{x}\pm$SD)(I)and 33 ± 7(III)was different(p 0.001)from those found in II and IV, whose highest level was 15.9mIU/ml.Basal prolactin(PRL)levels (ng/ml)were:I:11.4 ± 4;II:51.3 ± 27; III:37.3 ± 9 and IV:130 ± 114. After MCP the maximal response for LH and PRL(expressed asΔ%) was respectively I: 12and2962;II: 43and800;III:79and189;IV:120 and5. These data indicate that DA exerts an inhibitory effect on GnRH secretion,which depends on its concentration in the hypothalamus and it seems to be influenced by the estrogen concentration in the same site.The PRL behaviour may depend on the availability of DA at the lactotroph and the response to MCP could also be mediated by the estrogen environment.

2136 PROSTAGLANDIN SYNTHESIS INHIBITION PREVENTS PRL-INDUCED STRUCTURAL LUTEOLYSIS IN THE RAT. J.E. Sanchez-Criado *, K. Ochiai, and I. Rothchild. Department of Reproductive Biology, Case Western Reserve University, Cleveland, Ohio 44106, USA.

Preliminary experiments showed that the PRL secreted between days 15 and 22 by the autotransplanted pituitary of cyclic rats hypophysectomized on day 2 (metestrus), after the temporary depression of PRL secretion by sc treatment on days 12 to 14 with CB-154 (0.4 mg/rat/day), reduced mean corpus luteum (CL) weight on day 22 to 0.98 ± 0.07 mg (N=17) from the control weight of 1.47 ± 0.08 mg (N=15) in rats in which PRL secretion was continually depressed by treatment with CB-154 from days 12 to 22. The CB-154 treatment reduced the serum progesterone level from >110 ng/ml before treatment to < 10 ng/ml by day 15, and the PRL level from >35 ng/ml to $<$ 10 ng/ml by day 13. To see whether the luteolytic action of PRL was associated with prostaglandin (PG) production, indomethacin (IM)-containing silastic capsules, or blank capsules, were inserted on day 12 into the ovarian bursae of pituitary autotransplanted rats. The rats were then treated either with CB-154 on days 12 to 14 and with the vehicle from days 15 to 22, or with CB-154 from days 12 to 22. In the presence of IM and the short treatment with CB-154, mean CL weight on day 22 was 1.35 ± 0.09 mg (N=12); it was 0.90 ± 0.10 (N=13) in those bearing blank capsules. IM had no effect in the rats treated with CB-154 from days 12 to 22. We interpret these results to mean that the PRL-induced structural luteolysis is itself induced by, or requires the action of, PGs produced within the CL. (Supported in part by Ford Foundation TG 670-0135C and by NIH RG 07640).

2137 NO EVIDENCE FOR DISULFIDE-LINKED OLIGOMERS OF PROLACTIN IN THE RAT PITUITARY GLAND. Jonathan G. Scammell* and Priscilla S. Dannies, Department of Pharmacology, Yale University School of Medicine, New Haven CT 06510.

Poorly immunoreactive, disulfide-linked oligomeric forms of prolactin (PRL) exist in secretory granules isolated from bovine pituitary gland (Endocrinology 112, 1880). Hence, PRL detectability by RIA is greatly enhanced by thiols and inhibited by divalent cations and cysteamine. We have examined PRL detectability in the rat pituitary using: 1) Primary cultures of either normal male rat pituitary cells or E_2-induced pituitary tumors from female Fischer 344 rats; 2) Secretory granules isolated from Fischer pituitary tumors. Sonication and incubation of cells with either 1 mM $ZnCl_2$ or EDTA or 5 mM glutathione (GSH), β-mercaptoethanol (MCE) or dithiothreitol (DTT) did not alter PRL detectability by RIA, while the loss of PRL immunoreactivity in CSH-treated cells was completely reversed by DTT (0.5-5 mM) under the same conditions. Sonication and incubation of secretory granules, isolated by isotonic Percoll density gradient centrifugation, with 1 mM $ZnCl_2$ or EDTA did not alter PRL detectability, while GSH (0.5 to 5 mM) or MCE (0.1 to 3 mM) slightly inhibited PRL detectability. No treatment interfered with the PRL RIA. In addition, we labelled cultures of Fischer tumor cells with [^{3}H]leucine for 8 hr and measured [^{3}H]PRL in solubilized cells by SDS-PAGE under both reducing and non-reducing conditions. There was no difference between cpm in the [^{3}H]PRL peaks under the two conditions. We have found no evidence for disulfide-linked oligomeric forms of prolactin in the rat pituitary gland.

2138 THE GENE FOR PLACENTAL LACTOGEN IN THE COW APPEARS TO HAVE EVOLVED FROM PROLACTIN RATHER THAN GROWTH HORMONE. L.A. Schuler*, W.L. Hurley, and Jack Gorski. Depts. of Structural and Functional Sciences and Biochemistry, Univ. of Wisc., Madison, WI 53706 and Dept. of Dairy Science, Univ. of Ill., Urbana, IL USA

Placental lactogen, or chorionic somatotropin, is a member of the growth hormone gene family. The protein products of these genes are similar in size and amino acid composition in all species, but in the bovine, the placental lactogen protein is about 50% larger. We have prepared a cDNA from messenger RNA (mRNA) isolated from bovine cotyledonary tissue which is homologous to, yet distinct from bovine prolactin, and much less like bovine growth hormone. This contrasts sharply with human chorionic somatotropin, which is very closely related to growth hormone. While expressed by the placenta, the placental lactogen gene is not transcribed by the pituitary or liver of the bovine. The mature mRNA is about 1100 nucleotides in length, larger than the mRNAs of the other members of this gene family, which is consistent with the reported size of the protein. Sequence analysis of the 3' portion of the cDNA indicates about 75% homology to prolactin at the level of nucleotide sequence, and 39% at the level of amino acid sequence. We conclude that a new member of the growth hormone gene family, bovine placental lactogen, appears to be evolutionarily derived from prolactin rather than growth hormone as is the case in man. This study was supported by NIH grants CA-18110 and HD-07118-04.

2139 ESTROGEN STIMULATES PROLACTIN GENE TRANSCRIPTION IN PRIMARY PITUITARY CELL CULTURES. J. D. Shull*, J. H. Walent, M. L. Lieberman and J. Gorski, Departments of Biochemistry, Animal Sciences and Human Oncology, University of Wisconsin, Madison, Wisconsin, U.S.A.

It has previously been shown that a single injection of 17ß-estradiol (E_2) rapidly stimulates (within 30 min) the transcription of the rat prolactin (Prl) gene, and that this stimulation can be observed under conditions of inhibited pituitary protein synthesis. To study further the mechanisms by which E_2 regulates Prl gene expression, we are now examining the effects of this steroid hormone on Prl transcription in nuclei isolated from cultured pituitary cells. In cells prepared from male rats, a 24 hr exposure to E_2 (10^{-9} M) results in a 5 to 8-fold increase in Prl transcription. Significant increases in Prl transcription have been observed after as little as 6 hr of E_2 treatment. In contrast, the transcription of the closely related growth hormone gene was not effected by E_2. In one preliminary experiment, E_2 induced Prl transcription in cultures in which cycloheximide treatment had inhibited protein synthesis by more than 95%. In cells derived from female pituitaries, E_2 (24 hr exposure) stimulated Prl transcription by approximately 10-fold. These results indicate that E_2 is a direct regulator of Prl gene expression acting at the level of transcription. Supported by NIH grants HD-08192, CA-18110 (J.G.); 5 T32 HD07007-05 (J.D.S.); AM-25694 (M.E.L.).

2140 REGULATION OF PROLACTIN GENE TRANSCRIPTION IN VIVO: ROLES OF ESTROGEN AND DOPAMINE. J. D. Shull, S. R. Mellon and J. Gorski*, Departments of Biochemistry and Animal Sciences, University of Wisconsin, Madison, Wisconsin, U.S.A.

The short-acting estrogen 16α-estradiol stimulates prolactin (Prl) transcription in the pituitary of the male rat in a biphasic manner. The first phase is observed within 30 min of treatment and persists through 2 hr while the second phase is observed by 6 hr and continues through 24 hr. To test the hypothesis that this second phase is mediated through either an alteration in dopamine release from the hypothalamus or an alteration in the responsiveness of the pituitary to dopamine, we are examining the effects of various dopamine agonists and antagonists, alone and in combination with estrogen, on Prl transcription. Pimozide (0.63 mg/kg) stimulates Prl transcription approximately 2-fold within 1 hr of treatment, and this stimulation persists for at least 24 hr. Pimozide does not effect the transcription of the closely related growth hormone gene. In a preliminary experiment, haloperidol (0.63 mg/kg) also stimulated Prl transcription approximately 2-fold. In contrast, the dopamine agonist α-ergocryptine (0.8 to 4.0 mg/kg) inhibits Prl transcription by approximately 50% within 1 hr and through at least 8 hr following treatment. Experiments are presently in progress to determine: 1) the effectiveness of these compounds in occupying the dopamine receptor and 2) the effects of estrogen on Prl transcription when the pituitary dopamine receptors are blocked by these compounds. Supported by NIH grants HD-08192, CA-18110 (J.G.) and S T32 HD07007-05 (J.D.S.).

2141 Catecholestrogen Regulation of Prolactin Synthesis in Pituitary Cell Culture. M.A. Shupnik*, A. Klibanski, C. Longcope and E.C. Ridgway, Thyroid Unit, Massachusetts General Hospital, Boston, MA 02114, U.S.A.

The 2-hydroxycatecholestrogens (CEs), 2-hydroxyestrone (2-OHE_1) and 2-hydroxyestradiol (2-OHE_2) were tested for their ability to directly alter prolactin (PRL) production and PRL mRNA levels in rat pituitary cell culture. When cells were treated with either 10^{-8}M 2-OHE_1 or 2-OHE_2, increases in secreted PRL were noted at 4 h and 24 h (20% and 110% over control, respectively) but not at 30 min. In parallel cultures, metabolism of radioactive CEs showed that the major metabolite at all times for both CEs was the 2-CH_3 derivative. Even at 24 h nearly 50% of each compound was the original CE, and at no time was there any detectable conversion to parent steroid. Treatment of cells for 48 h with increasing concentrations either CE resulted in a biphasic dose response. Between 10^{-10} and 10^{-8}M, PRL production was increased 7-fold for 2-OHE_1 and 3-fold for 2-OHE_2 with ED_{50}s of 8X10^{-9}M. Above 5X10^{-8}M however, both compounds decreased PRL levels until at 10^{-6}M PRL production was 60% of control. Changes in PRL mRNA levels paralleled those of production. Treatment with 10^{-8}M of either 17-β estradiol (E_2), 2-OHE_1, or 2-OHE_2 resulted in 2 to 5-fold increases in translatable and hybridizable PRL mRNA. At 10^{-6}M 2-OHE_1 or 2-OHE_2 there was a decrease of 35-80% in PRL mRNA. This concentration of 2-OHE_1 also inhibited the action of 10^{-8}M E_2 on PRL mRNA. However, 10^{-6}M 2-OHE_2 + 10^{-8}M E_2 together increased PRL mRNA levels as much as with E_2 alone. Thus CEs at low concentrations act on the pituitary as E_2 agonists to increase PRL synthesis, but at high concentrations act as inhibitors of PRL production.

2142 ROLE OF PROSTAGLANDINS IN FROG ADRENAL STEROIDOGENESIS. I. Perroteau*, P. Netchitailo, F. Homo-Delarche§, C. Delarue and H. Vaudry. ERA CNRS 891, Fac. Sci. Rouen, 76130 Mt-St-Aignan, France, § INSERM-U7, Physiol. Pharmacol. Vasc. Ren., Hôp. Necker, 161 rue de Sèvres, 75015 Paris, France.

The role of prostaglandins (PGs) in the regulation of corticosteroid production by the frog interrenal gland has been investigated in vitro using perifusion technique. Steroids and PGs were measured by radioimmunoassays. Administration of graded doses of PGs (8.8nM to 2.8μM) led to a dose related increase in corticosteroid output in the following order of potency: PGE1 PGI2 PGE2 PGB2 PGB1 PGF2α PGF1α. PGE1 (8.8nM) increased corticosterone and aldosterone productions by 200 and 250%, respectively. Four pulses of PGE1 within the same experiment led to similar secretory responses and a prolonged administration (6Hrs) gave rise to a stable stimulation of corticosteroid secretion. The requirement of endogenous PGs in the spontaneous corticosteroid biosynthesis was demonstrated by the inhibition of corticosterone and aldosterone production induced by indomethacin (IDM, 5μM, 4Hrs) or meclofenamic acid (10μM, 4Hrs), two inhibitors of PG biosynthesis. ACTH increase corticosteroid release without affecting PG biosynthesis and IDM or meclofenamic acid did not impair the response of adrenal glands to ACTH or dbc AMP. In contrast, angiotensinII (AII) stimulated PGE2 and PGI2 productions prior to the increase of corticosteroid productions. In addition, PG synthetase inhibitors were responsible for a clear inhibition of AII induced corticosteroid biosynthesis. These results provide evidence that corticosteroidogenic actions of ACTH and AII are mediated by different mechanisms. They indicate that, in amphibians, PGs contribue to spontaneous corticosteroid biosynthesis and act as mediators for AII action.

2143 PROSTAGLANDIN FORMATION IN HUMAN MYOMETRIAL CELLS IN CULTURE: EFFECT OF GLUCOCORTICOSTEROIDS AND ARACHIDONIC ACID.
Marilyn Richardson*, Murray D. Mitchell, Paul C. MacDonald, and M. Linette Casey, Cecil H. and Ida Green Ctr. for Reprod. Biol. Sci., Univ. of Texas Southwestern Medical School, Dallas, TX 75235 U.S.A.

With respect to prostaglandin (PG) formation and the secretion of cortisol in women during labor, there appears to be a physiologic paradox. The dramatic increase in cortisol in women in labor could be expected to act to decrease PG formation in amnion and decidua, tissues that are believed to be sites of origin of PGs during labor. We found, however, that amnion and decidua are immune to this action of cortisol. In myometrium, PGI_2 and PGE_2 are produced, and PGI_2 is believed to cause uterine quiescence. We found that treatment of human myometrial cells in culture with dexamethasone (DEX, 10^{-8} M) caused an 80% reduction in PG formation. Cortisol (10^{-8} - 10^{-6} M) also acted to inhibit PG formation, and cortisol mesylate (10^{-6} M) attenuated the inhibition of DEX. When arachidonic acid (AA, 10^{-8} M) was added to these cells there was a 3-fold increase in the production of PGI_2 and PGE_2. In the presence of DEX (10^{-8}) and AA (10^{-8}), there was no increase in PG formation over that produced by cells treated with DEX alone. Thus, we conclude that the "flight or fight" phenomenon that is associated with fear and pain of labor and that causes increased cortisol secretion by the adrenal may act to perpetuate labor since amnion and decidua are immune to suppression of PG formation by cortisol but myometrial PGI_2 production is suppressed by cortisol. Moreover, it appears that the action of glucocorticosteroids in myometrium is not by way of inhibition of AA release but rather by way of inhibition of cyclooxygenase activity.

2144 FURTHER STUDY ON THE CAUSAL RELATIONSHIP BETWEEN DEVELOPMENTAL CHANGES IN LH RELEASE AND THE ONSET OF PUBERTY IN FEMALE RHESUS MONKEYS: EFFECTS OF POSTERIOR HYPOTHALAMIC LESIONS.
N.J. Schultz* and E. Terasawa, Wis. Reg. Primate Research Ctr., Univ. of Wis., Madison, WI 53706, U.S.A.

Previously, we have hypothesized that alteration of the LHRH release pattern, but not resetting of the gonadostat, is the key factor controlling the onset of puberty. This is based on our results in female monkeys demonstrating that 1) alteration of the LH secretory pattern occurs in association with puberty, 2) this LH alteration also occurs in neonatally ovariectomized subjects with the same time course, and 3) lesions of the posterior hypothalamus (PH) advance the ages of menarche and first ovulation. In order to test this hypothesis we made radiofrequency lesions in the PH of ovariectomized monkeys at age 17 months (mo) and observed LH changes between ages 12 and 40 mo. 1) In animals with PH lesions basal LH had already increased by 1 mo postoperatively, and reached a maximum at age 25 mo, while in control animals it remained low until age 25 mo after which it started to increase, reaching a plateau at age 30 mo. 2) In lesioned animals diurnal LH fluctuations with nocturnal increases began to appear by 1 mo postoperatively, while in controls they were not demonstrable until age 26 mo. 3) At age 21 mo a much higher amplitude of pulsatile LH in lesioned animals was observed when compared to that in controls. Thus, lesions of the PH resulted in an earlier occurrence of the pubertal changes of LH release. These results, together with our previous observations in intact animals, suggest that precocious puberty induced by PH lesions is due to the advancement of LH release during development. The evidence supports the hypothesis that facilitation of LHRH release with maturation of the hypothalamus is crucial for the onset of puberty. (Supported by Grants RR00167, HD11355 and HD15433.)

2145 NALTREXONE DELAYS THE ONSET OF PUBERTY IN RATS: IS A SENSITIZATION MECHANISM INVOLVED? G.E. Simpson*, J.R. Murphy, M.S. Blank. Yerkes Regional Primate Research Ctr. of Emory University, Atlanta, Georgia, 30322, U.S.A.

Although opiate antagonists regulate LH secretion acutely in a variety of species and physiological circumstances, including sexual maturation of the female rat, the effect of their chronic administration has not been studied. Naltrexone base (30 mg) (N) or placebo (P) pellets were implanted (sc) in 21-day-old female rats. Once regular estrous cyclicity was attained, the ovaries were removed at metestrus and fresh pellets implanted. Although there was no significant difference in weight gain between the two groups before puberty, naltrexone delayed the appearance of vaginal opening by three days (P=34±.5, N=37±1 days). After puberty, naltrexone augmented the serum LH (ng RP-1/ml) response to ovariectomy, as shown below:

PELLET GROUP	N	WEEKS AFTER OVARIECTOMY 1	2	3	6
NALTREXONE	7	2105±125(SE)*	3193±589*	3026±452	4940±596*
PLACEBO	8	1114±234	1451±180	3533±365	2638±401

Morphine (10 mg/kg) administered on the seventh week after ovariectomy produced a 35±14% decrease in LH levels in the P group, but a 71±5% decrement in the N group. Thus, chronic treatment with the opiate antagonist naltrexone delays the onset of puberty. Since rats treated chronically with naltrexone are supersensitive to the LH-lowering effects of morphine, sensitization of endogenous receptors might also mediate the delay in sexual maturation. Supported by NIH HD15073 and RR00165.

2146 A CLINICAL TEST USING PULSATILE GnRH FOR THE DIFFERENTIATION OF MALE HYPOTHALAMIC HYPOGONADISM (HH) FROM CONSTITUTIONAL DELAY OF PUBERTY (CD). W.G. Sippell*, C.J. Partsch, M. Hermanussen and F. Lorenzen, Pediatric Endocrinology Unit, Univ. Dept. of Pediatrics, D-2300 Kiel, W-Germany.

To date, it is not possible to differentiate reliably between HH and severe CD on the basis of a standard GnRH bolus test (GBT) or other known endocrine or clinical parameters. We studied, therefore, 17 hypogonadal males, 9 with a presumptive diagnosis of HH (age 14.5 - 41, bone age 12.5 - 19 yrs, testes 1 - 5 ml) including 4 with Kallmann syndrome, and 8 with suspected CD (age 14.5 - 18.3, BA 11.5 - 15 yrs, testes 1.5 - 11 ml). Basal and peak LH and FSH levels after GBT were greatly overlapping between the two groups. In each patient, a spontaneous nocturnal plasma profile of LH and FSH, sampled every 20 min, was followed by a pulsatile GnRH stimulation (5 µg iv every 90') via a portable minipump (Zyklomat®, Ferring, Kiel) for 36 hrs. Before and after this pumping, a GBT (100 µg iv) was performed and plasma testosterone (T), androstenedione (Δ^4) and DHAS were measured. Pulse analysis revealed 0 - 6 (25 in total) spont. noct. LH peaks in the CD but none in any of the HH pts. GBT after pumping showed signif. higher (P<0.001) LH increments in CD than in HH pts with almost no overlap (range 4.1 - 13.6 vs 0.8 - 4.2 mU/ml). Similarly, T rose signif. during pumping from 114 ± 43 to 285 ± 92 ng/dl in the CD boys, but did not change signif. in the HH group (29 ± 10 vs 41 ± 11 ng/dl). Δ^4 and DHAS did not change signif. in either group. Conclusion: The sequence of noct. LH profile, 36 hrs of pulsatile GnRH, and GBT differentiates CD and HH far more exact than previously possible: males with permanent HH (in contrast to those with CD) are characterized by (1) absence of signif. noct. LH pulses, (2) signif. higher pituitary LH depletion and (3) no rise of T after short term priming of the pituitary by pulsatile GnRH.

2147 MOLECULAR PROPERTIES OF THE UTERINE CYTOSOLIC ESTROGEN RECEPTOR (ER) OF THE VERVET MONKEY (CERCOPITHECUS AETHIOPS PYGERETHRUS). HC Potgieter, T Klein, JH Spies, M Thierry, *C van Aswegen & JJ van der Watt, Nucor Inst. of Life Sciences & *Dept. of Biochem., Fac. of Med., Univ. of Pretoria, 0002, RSA.
The uterine cytosolic ER from the Vervet monkey has been partially characterized by means of competitive protein binding studies, sucrose density gradients, gel permeation chromatography (Ultrogel AcA-22 and Waters I-250 HPLC column), electrophoresis and iso-electric focussing. Mean concentration of ER (Bmax) for a batch of 21 uteri was found to be 327±165 femtomoles per mg protein while a dissociation constant (K_d) of $3.15\pm1.4\times10^{-10}$M could be illustrated for the same batch of uteri. The mean sedimentation coefficient (Beckman VTi-80 rotor) in low ionic strength media in the absence or presence of 10mM sodium molybdate was 8.4±0.4 S. A marked protective effect by sodium molybdate on the ∿8S component could be illustrated. Exposure of the charged cytosolic ER complexes to 0.4M KCl rendered a time dependent loss of the ∿8S moiety with a resultant formation of more than one entity in the 3-5S range. Chromatography on Ultrogel AcA-22 columns yielded large components in low ionic strength buffers: 4.68×10^5 daltons with a Stokes radius of 63.2A in the absence of sodium molybdate and 3.87×10^5 dalt. with a Stokes radius of 60.0A in the presence of sodium molybdate. On the same column but in higher ionic strength buffers a much smaller component was observed: 8.61×10^4 daltons with a Stokes radius of 41.8A in 0.154M KCl and 9.22×10^4 dalt. with a Stokes radius of 42.3A in buffers containing 0.4M KCl. HPLC on a Waters I-250 gel column rendered high molecular mass entities (4.85×10^5 and 2.01×10^5 dalt.) in low ionic strength buffers not containing sodium molybdate, while only the 2.01×10^5 dalt. appeared in buffers containing 10mM sodium molybdate. Upon chromatography in Tris buffer containing 100 mM KCl only one macromolecular component (2.11×10^5 dalt.) appeared to be present. High ionic strength conditions (0.4M KCl) rendered high molecular mass aggregates (7.2×10^5 dalt.) in the absence of sodium molybdate and only one macromolecular entity of 1.52×10^5 dalt. in the presence of sodium molybdate. Disc gel electrophoresis on polyacrylamide gels yielded only one symmetrical peak displacable with 100 times excess levels of diethylstilbestrol. Upon iso-electric focussing on Agarose gels two peaks were obtained: a major peak with a pI of 6.6±0.2 and a minor peak at pI= 5.5±0.3.

2148 PEPTIDE MAPPING ANALYSIS OF AVIAN PROGESTERONE RECEPTOR. R. K. Puri and D. O. Toft*, Department of Cell Biology, Mayo Clinic/Foundation, Rochester, Minnesota 55905.

Two 8S forms (I and II) of progesterone receptor from the chicken oviduct were isolated to near homogeneity. SDS-gel electrophoresis showed that receptor form I contains a peptide of Mr = 75,000 and form II contains a peptide of Mr = 110,000. These are believed to be the A and B receptor subunits that were described previously. In addition, both receptor forms contain a peptide with Mr = 90,000 that does not bind steroid. To investigate the possibility that these subunits are structurally related, they were isolated by preparative SDS-gel electrophoresis and subjected to peptide mapping analsysis. The proteolytic enzymes, V8 protease, pappain and α-chymotrypsin, were used to cleave the receptor subunits to generate their fragmentation patterns. Receptor subunits from tissue labeled with [^{32}P]orthophosphate were also subjected to peptide mapping analysis where the ^{32}P-labeled peptides were identified by autoradiography.

The electrophoretic patterns of peptide fragments (phosphorylated and nonphosphorylated) of the 90,000 dalton protein from receptor forms I and II were identical but were clearly different from the peptide patterns from A and B subunits. The enzymatic digestion of subunits A and B generated similar peptide patterns. Some minor differences were observed which could result either from a different genetic origin of these peptides or from post-translational modification. However, in comparing the phosphopeptide patterns from subunits A and B, more differences were observed than existed in their patterns of total peptides. This suggests that the two peptides are not phosphorylated in identical fashion.

2149 DIETHYLSTILBESTROL IS AN INTERNALLY MOBILE MOLECULE: ^{13}C-N.M.R. EVIDENCE.
J.I. Quivy, J. Poupaert+, P. Dumont+ and G.G. Rousseau*, Departments of Medicinal Chemistry+ and of Biochemistry and Cell Biology, Louvain University Medical School, B-1200 Brussels, Belgium.

Examination of the conformation of diethylstilbestrol (DES) has so far been restricted to theoretical calculations and X-ray diffraction studies. To investigate the conformational behavior of DES in solution, we have undertaken a ^{13}C-N.M.R. study in three solvent systems ($CDCl_3$ + CD_3COCD_3, CH_3OD, and CD_3SOCD_3, at 38° C). The chemical shifts were assigned to the different carbons by the OFF-RESONANCE and J-modulated SPIN-ECHO techniques. Spin-lattice relaxation times (T_1) and nuclear Overhauser enhancement (NOE) factors were determined by the inversion-recovery and inverse-gated decoupling techniques, respectively. The high values of NOE factors indicated a fully dipolar relaxation mechanism. The T_1 values of the meta and ortho carbons were identical and much shorter than the ipso and para carbons, indicating that the system has a rotational symmetry along the ipso-para axis. Moreover, the methylene carbon of the ethyl moiety had a T_1 value significantly shorter than the methyl group, suggesting that extra relaxation is offered by concerted rotation of the methylene group and of the phenol moiety. This is consistent with the existence of different minimum energy conformations. In conclusion, DES appears in solution as an internally mobile molecule which can, therefore, accomodate easily the geometry requirements of the estrogen receptor binding site. This model is compatible with the hypothesis (Hospital et al., J. Steroid Biochem. 6: 221-225, 1975) that the receptor-binding conformation of DES is 'asymmetrical with crossed cycles'. Study supported by the Ford, Mellon, and Rockefeller Foundations.

2150 DOES THE sRNA PLAY A ROLE IN THE REGULATION OF ESTROGEN TRANSPORT INTO THE NUCLEUS? B. Ramanath Rao*, L229 Meander, AZVU, De boelelaan 1117, 1007 MB Amsterdam,The Netherlands.

Rabbit uterine cytosol incubated with ribonuclease (RNase) reduced ^{3}H-estradiol-17B ($^3H-E_2$) binding to estrogen receptors (ER). Reduction in $^3H-E_2$ binding varied in different uterine cytosol preparations (0-29%). Rabbit uterine soluble ribonucleic acid (sRNA) prepared by phenol extraction method had no detectable $^3H-E_2$binding activity. Additionally, there was no increase in $^3H-E_2$ binding to uterine cytosol ER when sRNA from the uterus or the commercially obtained yeast RNA was added to the incubation mixture. Sedimentation values of $^3H-E_2$-ER complex was reduced in the RNase treated compared to untreated or sRNA added samples from 4S to slightly lower than 4S. Incubation at 30°C of nuclei (prepared without surfactant agents) in the presence of $^3H-E_2$ with a) uterine cytosol, b) ER enriched uterine cytosol using 30% $(NH_4)_2SO_4$, c) uterine cytosol plus RNase,d) uterine cytosol plus uterine sRNA added, showed that the highest nuclear $^3H-E_2$ uptake was observed in samples incubated with uterine cytosol and RNase compared to others. No qualitative change in the sedimentation values was observed between the nuclear ER isolated from these samples.

Conclusion: sRNA may regulate $^3H-E_2$-ER translocation process from the cytoplasm into the nucleus.

2151 CONTROLLED REVERSIBILITY OF THE PREFERENTIAL CONVERSION OF TYPE Y ESTROGEN RECEPTOR BETWEEN THE STEROID BINDING AND NON-STEROID BINDING FORMS.
William J. Raymoure*, Reid W. McNaught and Roy G. Smith, Baylor College of Medicine, Dept. of Urology, Houston, TX 77030 USA.

Two high affinity estrogen receptors (X, Kd 0.1 nM; Y, Kd 1 nM) have previously been identified in the chick oviduct. We have now demonstrated that in oviduct cytosol from chicks stimulated 14d with DES and then withdrawn 4d, Y but not X exists in a non-steroid binding form (Ynb). Ynb can be converted to Y during assay under exchange conditions (30°C, 3h) in the presence of 5 mM ATP, ADP, and to a lesser extent, GTP. Scatchard analysis demonstrated a specific increase of 3-7 fold in receptor Y, which was confirmed by steroid binding specificity assays. Conversion was dependent upon Mg^{2+}, with an optimal concentration of 3-5 mM, but not Ca^{2+} or Mn^{2+}. Neither cAMP nor cGMP in the presence of isobutymethylxanthine converted Ynb to Y, nor did they alter the ATP effect. Incubation with blocked ATP and ADP derivatives AMP-PCP, AMP-CPP, and AMP-CP did not increase [Y]. The nucleotide mediated increase in Y was not a protective effect against loss due to elevated temperature since after Y was destroyed in cytosol under controlled conditions (37°C, 15 min) 50-65% of the Y could be recovered by subsequent treatment with ATP. This is the first report of the controlled preferential interconversion of a single estrogen receptor type between a steroid binding and a non binding form (Y↔Ynb) in a tissue which contains two estrogen receptors. This interconversion does not appear to be mediated by cyclic nucleotides.

Supported by NIH Grant #HD17727 and Robert A. Welch Foundation Grant AU844.

2152 STRUCTURE OF THE "NON-TRANSFORMED" "8S" PROGESTERONE RECEPTOR OF THE CHICK OVIDUCT.
J.M. Renoir, J. Mester*, T. Buchou, C. Radanyi and E.E. Baulieu, INSERM U 33, Lab. Hormones, 94270 Bicêtre, France.

Highly purified forms I and II of non-transformed, molybdate-stabilized, 8S progesterone receptor (PR), were resolved by DEAE-sephacel chromatography. SDS-PAGE revealed by silver staining indicated the presence of subunit A (79kDa) and 90K protein in I, and of subunit B (110kDa) and also 90K protein in II. Scanning of the gels indicated that 90K is $\sim$ 2 times more abundant than either A or B in each form. Immunoblotting and density gradient studies with anti-8S-PR and anti-B polyclonal antibodies, and with an anti-90K monoclonal antibody confirmed these results. Anti-B antibodies reacted with A, but no immunological cross-reactivity was found between A or B and the 90K protein. Affinity labeling of purified 8S-PR and of isolated subunits with ^{3}H-R 5020 confirmed that A and B are hormone binding proteins, contrary to the 90K protein. After cross-linking of I and II 8S-PR forms with 0.4 % glutaraldehyde, $s_{20,w}$ was found $\sim$ 8S, Rs was $\sim$ 7 nm, and after silver staining of SDS-PAGE, Mr was found $\sim$ 260kDa. From these results and specific activity of the purified 8S-PR, we concluded that I and II forms include 1 molecule of hormone binding subunit (A or B) and 2 molecules of the non-hormone binding 90K protein.

2153 CYTOPLASMIC ANDROGEN RECEPTOR CONTENT IN CANCER OF THE LARYNX.

Ž.Reiner,* V. Petric, D. Cvrtila, Departments of medicine, ORL and nuclear medicine Dr. M. Stojanović University Hospital, 41000 Zagreb, Yugoslavia

There are many data which suggest that the larynx is a target organ for androgens. Since carcinoma of the larynx occures much more often in males, androgens could be growth-stimulating factor for this tumor. Therefore tumor tissues of 27 patients (25 males and 2 females) obtained by total laryngectomy were tested for the presence of androgen (AR) and estrogen (ER) receptors. In 8 cases progestin (PgR) receptor levels were quantitated too. We used chromatofocusing of the receptor proteins and dextran-coated charcoal technique. ^{3}H-DHT and R1881 were used as ligands for the measurement of AR, ^{3}H-estradiol and R2858 for ER and R5020 for PgR. Our results showed that all tumors contained AR discriminating the patients into two groups: one (13 males and 1 female) having lower AR levels (23,1-150 fmoles/mg protein) and the other (12 males and 1 female) with higher AR levels (more than 250 fmoles/mg protein - the highest value was 859). Almost all of the patients from this second group had an infiltrative growth and large volume of tumor and 8 of them had a recidive. On the other hand, all the patients from the group with lower AR values had smaller localized tumors and only 3 of them had a recidive. All of the analyzed tumors lacked PgR, and we could demonstrate the presence of ER just in 3 male patients but the ER values were so low (6-7,4 fmoles/mg protein) that their importance should be questioned. The results presented suggest that at least some of the carcinoma of the larynx might be hormone dependent so that the patients might be managed by endocrine therapy and that AR analysis could be of prognostic value.

2154 TRANSFORMATION PROPERTIES OF ANDROGEN RECEPTOR FROM DUNNING PROSTATIC TUMOR.

D.R.Rowley*, R.T. Premont, C.H. Chang, and D.J. Tindall, Dept. Cell Biology, Baylor College of Medicine, Houston, TX 77030, U.S.A.

The mechanism of androgen receptor transformation to a DNA binding state has not been fully determined. To better understand this process we have defined several properties and molecular forms relative to transformation. Cytosol was prepared from rat Dunning prostatic tumor either with or without 10 mM Na_2MoO_4 (transformation inhibitor) and was labeled with [^{3}H]-dihydrotestosterone. Transformation was determined by DNA-cellulose column chromatography. Cytosol was incubated with varying concentrations of KCl (transformation inducer) for various periods of time. Maximal transformation (>80% specific activity bound to DNA-cellulose) was achieved by 30 min in the absence of Na_2MoO_4 and required 200 mM KCl. In cytosol containing Na_2MoO_4 maximal transformation was possible but required 18 h of incubation with 500 mM KCl. Sucrose density gradient analysis indicated that an aggregated 9 S form (non DNA binder), disaggregated to a 4.4 S form when incubated with KCl. The 4.4 S form subsequently reaggregated to a 7-8 S form (DNA binder) when KCl was removed. The 4.4 S form was retained under low salt conditions if it were first chromatographed on phosphocellulose. The 4.4 S form also bound to DNA-cellulose. These data suggest that salt-induced transformation is accompanied by a disaggregation, reaggregation phenomenon. The reaggregated 7-8 S form as well as the partially purified, disaggregated 4.4 S form will both bind to DNA. In addition, the Na_2MoO_4 stabilized receptor required greater energy to induce disaggregation, and the molecular forms are identical to that in the absence of Na_2MoO_4.

2155 EVIDENCE FOR AN ANDROGEN RECEPTOR IN HUMAN PLACENTAL CYTOSOL FROM VARIOUS PERIODS OF GESTATION. N.Saito*, S.Kanasugi, S.Kawagoe, and M.Hiroi, Department of Obstetrics and Gynecology, Yamagata University, School of Medicine, Yamagata city, Japan.

It is said that human placenta is a target organ for androgen action,and androgen receptor is present in it. But, the characterization of the androgen receptor in human placenta is poorly understood. Androgen receptor binds dihydrotestosterone(DHT) and methyltrienolone(R1881). In first trimester of gestation,Scatchard analysis of hormone-stripped human placental cytosol contains high affinity binding population with dissociation constants(Kd) of 3.3×10^{-9} M for DHT and Kd's 2.7×10^{-9} M for R1881. concentration of binding sites was 86 to 134 fmoles/mg protein for R1881. While, in third trimester, placental cytosol has two DHT binding compornents with Kd's of 1.5×10^{-10} M and 3.7×10^{-9} M, and single R1881 binding compornents with Kd's of 1.9×10^{-9} M. Concentration of binding sites was 210 to 390 fmoles/mg protein for R1881. DHT and R1881 binding in human placental cytosol are demonstrated by isoelectric focusing(IEF) technique. Placental cytosol preincubated with $20nM\ ^3H$-DHT on IEF reveals specific binding peaks at elution pH's(EpH) of 4.0 and 5.2 in first trimester, and EpH of 4.6, 5.3 and 6.0 in third trimester. While, preincubated with $50nM\ ^3H$-R1881 reveals peaks at EpH of 4.2 in first trimester, and EpH of 4.4 and 5.2 in third trimester. DHT binding at EpH's 5.3 contains a heat stable population. These studies demonstrates that androgen receptor changes biochemical characterization in various periods of gestation. R1881 and DHT binding sites increase with the progress of gestational periods.

2156 IDENTIFICATION AND CHARACTERIZATION OF A HUMAN CORTICOSTEROID BINDING GLOBULIN VARIANT. P. A. Robinson and G. L. Hammond*, Hope Hospital, Salford, 6, U.K.

A corticosteroid binding globulin variant (CBG_v) has been identified in a serum sample taken from an apparently healthy woman during late pregnancy. Identification was based on the observation that the CBG_v exhibited approximately half of the cortisol binding capacity expected when compared to its concentration measured by radioimmunoassay (RIA). Affinity purification of CBG_v excluded the possibility that this anomaly was caused by assay interference and demonstrated that immuno-reactive CBG_v was capable of binding cortisol. The CBG_v has a molecular weight (63,800 daltons) similar to normal CBG, and no evidence of molecular aggregation was found by gel filtration. Although the electrophoretic mobility, isoelectric profile and immunochemical identity of CBG_v appear to be similar to normal CBG, it focussed as two distinct bands (pI 5.48 and pI 5.53) after desialylation with neuraminidase, unlike normal CBG which focusses only at pI 5.48. Investigation of the steroid binding characteristics of CBG_v revealed a reduced association-rate constant ($K_a = 1.05 \times 10^9$ L/mol) and half-time of dissociation ($t_{\frac{1}{2}} = 12.5$ min) when compared with normal CBG ($K_a = 1.39 \times 10^9$ L/mol and $t_{\frac{1}{2}} = 25$ min) at 0° C, but an apparently normal steroid-binding specificity. No other CBG variants were identified among other normal controls (n= 66) or 9 patients with Cushing's syndrome. It is suggested that binding capacity and RIA measurements of CBG will reveal other variants of CBG, and lead to a greater understanding of their physiological significance. This study was supported by the MRC (U.K.).

2157 A NEW APPROACH FOR STUDYING STEROID RECEPTORS: COMBINATION OF IN VITRO BINDING WITH AUTORADIOGRAPHIC LOCALIZATION OF ^{3}H-CORTICOSTERONE IN RAT BRAIN SECTIONS.
W.H. Rostène*, A. Sarrieau, D. Philibert, M. Moguilewsky and M. Vial, INSERM U.55, Hôpital Saint-Antoine, 75012 Paris and Roussel-Uclaf, 93230 Romainville, France.

The aim of the present study is to describe a new methodology which allows us to study the specific binding of ^{3}H-corticosterone (^{3}H-CS) on frozen unfixed brain sections of adrenalectomized (ADX) rats without using conventional cytosolic and/or nuclear preparations. Sections at the level of the hippocampus were incubated at room temperature with 5 mM ^{3}H-CS (total binding) + 50 μM CS (non specific binding). The *in vitro* specific binding of ^{3}H-CS represented 70% of the initial binding and reached equilibrium after 15 min. Scatchard analysis showed that ^{3}H-CS bound to a single class of receptors with a dissociation constant (Kd) of 10^{-8} M and a number of binding sites (B_M) of 100 fmoles/mg protein. Various steroids were able to compete with ^{3}H-CS binding: CS>progesterone>dexamethasone,RU 26988 (glucocorticoid agonist),RU 38486 (antagonist), aldosterone>estradiol and testosterone. The binding of ^{3}H-CS increased after ADX, whereas Kd's did not change, and reached a maximum after 14 days. On the contrary, CS replacement after ADX induced a decrease in ^{3}H-CS binding. Some sections were incubated under similar conditions and apposed to a ^{3}H-Ultrofilm, LKB. Autoradiograms obtained after 6 months exposure showed that the highest concentrations of ^{3}H-CS binding sites were found in the hippocampus in agreement with previous *in vivo* autoradiographic studies. This rapid and reliable technique gives promise of facilitating new developments in the study of steroid action. This work was supported by INSERM (PRC 133044).

2158 BINDING OF [^{3}H]TRIAMCINOLONE ACETONIDE-RECEPTOR COMPLEXES TO CHROMATIN FROM THE B-CELL LEUKEMIA LINE, BCL_1.
Mary F. Ruh*, Raj K. Singh, C.J. Bellone, T.S. Ruh. Departments of Physiology & Microbiology, St. Louis University School of Medicine, St. Louis, MO 63104 U.S.A.

The binding characteristics of partially purified glucocorticoid receptor complexes from hormone sensitive, non-differentiating BCL_1 cells to sequentially deproteinized BCL_1 chromatin-cellulose were investigated. [^{3}H]Triamcinolone acetonide (TA)-receptor complexes were purified (approximately 30-fold) from DEAE-cellulose columns by salt elution which allowed receptor activation only in the absence of molybdate. Addition of 10 mM molybdate to receptor preparations completely blocked salt activation by 0.3 M KCl. The binding pattern of the activated [^{3}H]TA-receptor complexes to chromatin-cellulose extracted with 0-8M GuHCl revealed three regions of increased binding activity (acceptor sites) at 2, 5 and 7M GuHCl. These acceptor sites were made available by unmasking of non-histone proteins which could be removed by higher concentrations of GuHCl, i.e., 3,6 and 8M. Non-activated receptor complexes demonstrated very low binding to deproteinized chromatin. It was also shown that chromatin binding required intact glucocorticoid receptors. Scatchard analysis demonstrated that BCL_1 chromatin possesses multiple, high-affinity binding sites which differ in their affinity for the glucocorticoid receptor (Kd=0.38 nM for 5M GuHCl- and 0.70 nM for 2M or 7M GuHCl-extracted chromatin). However, the number of binding sites per cell was the same (i.e., 15,000). This study provides a baseline for future studies comparing changes in sensitivity to glucocorticoids to acceptor site activity in mitogen-stimulated BCl_1 cells at various stages of differentiation. Supported by the McBride-Love Foundation.

2159 INSULIN RECEPTOR AFFINITY REGULATION IN A MINIMAL DEVIATION HEPATOMA CELL LINE. R. Lotan*and M. Lender, (SPON: B. Draznin). Departments of Surgery and Medicine, Loyola University, Maywood, Illinois, 60153, USA.

Scatchard analysis of binding data indicated that wheat germ agglutinin (WGA) mediated increase in insulin binding to hepatoma cells (4-II-E-C3) was due to a 10 fold increase in the receptor affinity, (Hofmann, C. et al. Clin. Res. 30: 742A, 1982). The purpose of the present studies was to investigate various conditions modulating the affinity of the insulin receptor, using these cells. Trypsin treatment of H4 monolayer cell cultures prior to measuring binding of ^{125}I-insulin in the presence of increasing concentrations of native insulin resulted in a leftward shift of the competition curve, thus indicating an increased affinity of the receptor to insulin. Immunological detection of plasma membrane insulin receptors in intact cells was accomplished by incubation of monolayer cultures with rabbit serum containing antibodies to purified insulin receptors. Cell-bound antibodies were detected by a secondary incubation with ^{125}I-labeled protein A. Treating H4 cells with WGA did not change cell associated radioactivity, thus immunologically confirming the lack of WGA effect on the presence of insulin receptor in H4 cells. Treatment with trypsin (5 μg/ml) increased ^{125}I-insulin binding by 50% above control level, further exposure to WGA (5 μg/ml) did not result in increase in affinity. Since the effects of WGA and trypsin on the receptor affinity were not additive, both were probably acting by a similar mechanism. These results suggest that WGA or trypsin may decrease the interaction between insulin binding and receptor affinity regulating component, increasing the affinity of the plasma membrane insulin receptors for insulin.

2160 PROCESSING OF THE INSULIN RECEPTOR IN CHINESE HAMSTER OVARY (CHO) CELL GLYCOSYLATION MUTANTS. A. McElduff*, J.M. Podskalny, R.W. Rees-Jones, M. Quarum, A. Robbins, J. Roth, and P. Gorden. Diabetes Branch, NIADDK, National Institutes of Health, Bethesda, Maryland 20205.

To determine the role of receptor glycosylation in post-translational processing of the insulin receptor, we have studied two mutant CHO cell lines with specific defects in protein glycosylation. B421 cells are unable to synthesize mannosylphosphoryldolichol resulting in the transfer of an incomplete high mannose carbohydrate during core glycosylation. Lec 1.3c cells lack N-acetylglucosamine transferase I activity and as a result cannot synthesize complex type glycoproteins. Surface iodination of the cells demonstrates the α and β subunits of the insulin receptor. In the Lec 1.3c cell line, both subunits migrate with lower apparent molecular weights in SDS gels than either wild type or B421 cells. Affinity cross-linking with ^{125}I-insulin labeled the α subunit in both mutants; insulin stimulated the incorporation of ^{32}P from γ^{32}P-ATP into the β subunit in both mutants. Biosynthetic labeling with mannose identified the 190K precursor in both wild type and mutant cells. All cell lines appeared to process the high molecular weight precursor normally.

We conclude that, despite marked disturbances in protein glycosylation, complete, but possibly qualitatively abnormal processing, of the 190K precursor of the insulin receptor to the mature α and β subunits can occur. These mature subunits retain the properties of insulin binding albeit with altered affinity (Podskalny, et al., abstract).

2161 INSULIN RECEPTOR AND ITS PROGNOSTIC FACTOR AMONG OBESE CHILDREN.
H. Nemoto*, Y. Yamazaki, M. Murata, Dep. Pediatrics, Tokyo Women's Medical College Second Hospital, Arakawa, Tokyo, Japan.

We measured *I-insulin binding to erythrocytes in fasting states and oral glucose torelance tests from 7 obese children(male 6, female 1,9-14 years old) with type 1 D.M. and hyperlipidemia(group 1),20 obese children (male 16, female 4,9-15 years old) with hyperlipidemia(group 2) and 22 obese children(male 19,female 3,8-15 years old) without these abnormalities (group 3). In the group 3, *I-insulin binding to erythrocytes and obese index($Y=7.427-0.025X, R=-0.721, P<0.01$), *I-insulin binding and IRI($Y=8.043-0.070X, R=-0.776, P<0.01$), *I-insulin binding and ΣIRI, IRI and ΣIRI were all correlated even in severe cases. But in the group 2, the disparity of obese index, *I-insulin binding, IRI and ΣIRI were often found even in mild obese cases. In the group 1, we found no correlation between *I-insulin binding, IRI, ΣIRI, and obese index. In the oral glucose torelance tests of 4 cases of group 1, *I-insulin binding were depressed markedly within 30 min($P<0.01$). This phenomenon was not observed in the other groups. The depressed *I-insulin bining of the other groups was observed later than two hours even in severe hyperinsulinemia cases. After reduced their weight, group 1 and 2 patient's binding, IRI and ΣIRI has improved and moved to group 3's correlation lines. No immediate depressed *I-insulin binding were observed in them.

We recommend to check not only the weight but also IRI and insulin binding level. We hypothesed insulin down regulation doesn't work well in group 1 and 2. They may involve postreceptor defect.

2162 PHOTOAFFINITY LABELING OF GONADOTROPIN-RELEASING HORMONE (GnRH) RECEPTORS
K. Nikolics* and J. Ramachandran, Hormone Research Laboratory, University of California, San Francisco, CA 94143 and Institute of Biochemistry*, Semmelweis University Medical School, Budapest, Hungary

Photoreactive derivaties of GnRH have been prepared and characterized. These were tested in rat pituitary monolayer cell cultures for their effectiveness in terms of LH release in the dark and after exposure to long-wave ultraviolet light. The photoreactive 2-nitro-4(5)-azidophenylsulfenyl group [2,4(5)NAPS] was incorporated into different positions of the decapeptide. Introduction of the 2,4-NAPS group in the side chain of Trp^3 caused complete loss of LH releasing activity in vitro and the peptide did not act as an inhibitor either. After photolysis, the analog remained inactive and did not inhibit the action of GnRH. $[D\text{-Lys}(2,4\text{-NAPS})]^6$-GnRH-(1-9)-NHEt was found to be a very potent agonist of the releasing hormone and after photolysis, caused nearly maximal release of LH in vitro. $[Orn(2,4\text{-NAPS})]^8$-GnRH and $[Orn(2,5\text{-NAPS})]^8$-GnRH were full agonists with a lower ED_{50} value than that of GnRH. However, after photolysis, the 2,4-NAPS analog released maximal levels of LH and FSH, whereas the 2,5-NAPS analog was inactive. Prolonged activation of LH release induced by the $[Orn(2,4\text{-NAPS})]^8$-analog and the [D-Lys(2,4-NAPS)]-analog after photoaffinity labeling caused desensitization of pituitary gonadotrophs; the former at a more rapid rate than the latter. These results suggest that $[Orn(2,4\text{-NAPS})]^8$-GnRH is a very effective probe for the direct labeling of GnRH receptors. Supported by a grant from the National Science Foundation (INT-8217048).

2163 INSULIN ACTIVATES THE APPEARANCE OF IGF-II RECEPTORS ON THE ADIPOCYTE CELL SURFACE. Y. Oka* and M. P. Czech, Department of Biochemistry, University of Massachusetts Medical School, Worcester, MA 01605.

In order to evaluate the mechanism of insulin action to increase rat ^{125}I-insulin-like growth factor II (IGF-II) binding to rat adipocytes, a potent rabbit antiserum was raised using purified IGF-II receptors from rat placental membranes. The antiserum elicited a positive ELISA reaction against purified IGF-II receptor at 5,000 fold dilution, and markedly inhibited ^{125}I-IGF-II binding to adipocyte plasma membranes when added prior to the growth factor. Similar precipitation lines formed between agar wells containing antiserum versus IGF-II receptor in the presence or absence of 1μM IGF-II, indicating that binding of anti-receptor immunoglobulin (Ig) to the IGF-II receptor is not affected by occupancy of the IGF-II binding site. Intact adipocytes treated with or without insulin were incubated with anti-IGF-II receptor Ig, washed and further incubated with ^{125}I-goat anti-rabbit IgG to monitor the amount of anti-receptor Ig bound. Insulin induced parallel increases in anti-IGF-II receptor Ig binding (2.4 fold) and ^{125}-IGF-II binding (3 fold) to the adipocytes, indicating the exposure of new receptors on the cell surface in response to hormone. When adipocytes were incubated with ^{125}I-IGF-II for 5 min at 10°C, washed, and homogenized before or after further incubation at 37°C, the amount of ^{125}I-IGF-II associated with low density microsomes increased with time at 37°C, while that with plasma membranes decreased. Insulin did not affect on this endocytotic process. These data demonstrate that insulin increases the number of IGF-II receptors in an exposed position on the adipocyte cell surface. The data suggest that the site of insulin action is the rate of exocytosis of IGF-II receptors.

2164 DIFFERENTIATION OF AGONIST AND ANTAGONIST SPECIFIC FORMS OF SOLUBILIZED ANGIOTENSIN II RECEPTORS BY HPLC. H. Ong*, J. Gutkowska, P.W. Schiller, N. McNicoll and A. De Léan. Faculté de Pharmacie, Université de Montréal and Institut de Recherches Cliniques de Montréal, Montréal, Québec, H2W 1R7, Canada.

Previous competitive binding studies of bovine adrenal glomerulosa membrane receptor revealed that agonists discriminate two interconvertible forms of angiotensin II receptor. This receptor was reversibly labelled with the agonist [^{131}](Sar^{1})angiotensin II ([^{131}]SARANG) or with the antagonist [I^{125}](Sar^{1}Ile^{8})angiotensin II ([I^{125}]SARILE) under various conditions: with guanosine-5'-γthio-triphosphate (GTPγS), or with bile salt (cholate), or with different concentrations of angiotensin II (10^{-5}-10^{-8}M), and then solubilized with the non ionic detergent octylglucoside. The solubilized receptor was then processed through a purification step on DEAE ion exchange followed by an HPLC steric exclusion chromatography. GTPγS enhanced the dissociation of [I^{131}]SARANG from solubilized receptor while it did not affect [I^{125}]SARILE binding to the receptors. Cholate destabilized [I^{131}]SARANG binding presumably by disrupting protein-protein interactions. Estimation of the apparent molecular size of agonist- and antagonist-occupied receptor reveals that the agonist-occupied receptor behaves as a protein 45,000 daltons larger than the antagonist-occupied receptor. This suggests that the agonist-occupied angiotensin II receptor is associated with a guanine nucleotide binding protein regulating its affinity for the hormone.
(Supported by grant from Medical Research Council of Canada).

2165 RAT PITUITARY LHRH-RECEPTORS AFTER ACUTE AND CHRONIC TREATMENT WITH A LHRH AGONIST OR ANTAGONIST. S. Pavlou*, R. Thau, and K. Sundaram, The Population Council, New York, N.Y. 10021

Pituitary LHRH-receptors have been shown to increase after intermittent treatment with LHRH agonists and decrease after LHRH antagonists. In order to better understand these changes we investigated changes in LHRH-receptor concentration using ^{125}I-labelled agonists and antagonist. The agonist [(imBzl)-D-His^6,Pro^9-NEt]LHRH (AgI) or [D-Ser(TBU)^6,Pro^9-NEt]LHRH (AgII) and the antagonist [Ac-DNAL(2)^1,4FDPhe^2,DTrp^3,DArg^6]LHRH (Ant) were iodinated by the chloramine T method, purified on HPLC and the mono-iodinated fraction collected. When tested with rat pituitary membranes these preparations were found to have high specific activities (1200-1500 Ci/g), high affinities (4.9$\pm$.8, 2.1$\pm$.4, and 0.8$\pm$.1 nM^{-1} for AgI, AgII, and Ant, respectively), and 50-60% binding in the presence of excess receptors. At 2, 4, and 24 hrs after a single dose of Ant (350ug/kg), the Ag binding was 20, 18, and 44% of control while that of the Ant was 67, 62, and 51% of control, respectively. 24 hrs following 8 days treatment with Ant (625ug/kg), Ag binding was 8.4% and Ant binding was 43.7% of control. At 2, 4, 6, 24, and 48 hrs after a single dose of Ant-I (40ug/kg), the Ag binding was 83, 30, 29, 183, and 128% of control, respectively, while that of the Ant remained unchanged (97, 95, 80, 106, and 97% of control) for the same time period. 24 hrs following 7 days treatment with AgI (40ug/kg), Ag binding increased to 140% of control but there was no change of Ant binding (99% of control). These observations suggest that following treatment of rats with LHRH analogs there may be quantitative as well as qualitative changes in pituitary LHRH receptors.

2166 Purification and Characterization of the porcine ovarian LH/hCG receptor. J. Wimalasena*, J.P. Wiebe and J.H. Abel,Jr. Hormonal Regulatory Mechanisms Laboratory, Department of Zoology, University of Western Ontario, London, Ont. Department of Zoology, University of Tennessee, Knoxville, TN

The major part of porcine corpus luteum (CL) LH/hCG receptor (LH/hCGR) activity was localized in the crude plasma membrane (PM) fraction. Detergent soluble LH/hCGR (DSR) with an 80% yield was extracted from PM by Triton X100 in the presence of 25% glycerol and protease inhibitors. DSR was stable at -60° for 60d. The equilibrium association constant (K_A) for homogenate, PM, DSR, were $2.0x10^{10}M^{-1}$ and the specific binding capacity (SBC) were 50-70 fmoles/mg. Glycerol increased K_A and SBC of DSR. DSR is glycoprotein in nature and could be resolved to complexes M_r 2.7,5.4x10^5. Purification of DSR by two cycles of hCG-sepharose affinity chromatography gave a yield of 30%, K_A=2.8x$10^{10}M^{-1}$, SBC-1400 pmoles/mg, a purification of 20,000 fold. Pure LH/hCGR when analysed on sodium dodecyl sulfate polyacrylamide gel electrophoresis (SDS/PAGE) and silver staining demonstrated a predominant band at M_r 68K and a faint band M_r 45K. Autoradiography of ^{125}I LH/hCGR showed one band at M_r 68K. Incubates of ^{125}I LH/hCGR and highly purified hCG or hFSH, 2.5μg/ml or BSA 5μg/ml, were analysed on disc gels. While addition of hCG lead to appearance of M_r 120K peak and a reduction in the M_r 64K peak, only the M_r 64K peak was apparent with hFSH and BSA. These results suggest that highly purified LH/hCGR has a M_r 68K subunit which can specifically interact with hCG.

Supported by N.I.C.H.D.(USA) and NSERC (Canada).

2167 PROTEIN A AS A MODEL TO STUDY COOPERATIVE SITE TO SITE INTERACTION AMONG HORMONE RECEPTORS.

GJM Tevaarwerk* and WF Clark, University of Western Ontario, London, N6A 5B8, Canada.

Site to site interaction (cooperativity) among neighbouring receptors has been postulated for several hormones. We have attempted to develop a simple model to study the mechanism of cooperativity. Protein A, found on the surface of Staphylococcus aureus (Cowan 1 strain) bacteria, was used as a source of oligomeric Fc receptors and human IgG as the ligand. An aliquot of IgG was labelled with ^{125}Iodine and used as a tracer. Dose response curves were determined and revealed concave curvilinear graphs on Scatchard analysis, indicating either receptor heterogeneity or negative cooperativity. Labelled IgG, previously allowed to bind to protein A, was incubated in excess buffer and the rate of dissociation of ^{125}I-IgG from protein A determined. It was found that if unlabelled IgG was added to the buffer dissociation of ^{125}I-IgG was markedly accelerated. The rate of dissociation was significantly greater at high receptor occupancy. The phenomenon could not be shown to be due to competition between labelled and unlabelled ligand for receptor sites during re-association. We conclude that the Fc receptors of protein A exhibit negatively cooperative site to site interaction. As such it may prove to be a useful tool in attempts to elucidate the mechanism of cooperativity among hormone receptors.

2168 A HIGH AFFINITY THYROID HORMONE BINDING SITE ON RAT LIVER NUCLEAR ENVELOPES.

J.T. Venkatraman* and Y.A. Lefebvre, Department of Medical Biochemistry, Faculty of Medicine, The University of Calgary, Calgary, Alberta, T2N 4N1, Canada.

Much evidence suggests that thyroid hormone action is initiated by the binding of L-triiodothyronine (L-T_3) to non-histone receptors within the nucleus. We wish to elucidate the mechanism by which L-T_3 traverses the nuclear envelope during its translocation from the cytoplasm to the nucleus. We have reported the characteristics of a class of T_3 binding sites on the nuclear envelope having a K_D of 86nM. We now report the properties of a class of higher affinity binding sites. Nuclear envelopes were prepared from male rat liver after treatment of purified nuclei with DNAse at pH 8.5. Phase contrast examination of the membrane material revealed the presence of intact nuclear ghosts and sheets of torn envelope. Maximum specific binding of L-T_3 to nuclear envelopes occurred after incubation of ^{125}I-T_3 with 10-20 μg nuclear envelope protein at 20°C for 3h. Scatchard analysis revealed a class of binding sites with a K_D of 5nM and a maximum binding capacity of 37 pmol/mg nuclear envelope protein. Tri-iodothyroacetic acid and reverse-T_3 competed as effectively for binding of ^{125}I-T_3 as L-T_3, indicating that this site differs from described cytosolic and nuclear receptors. $MgCl_2$ and $CaCl_2$ at concentrations of 1 and 2 mM enhanced the binding of L-T_3 to nuclear envelope preparations, while 2 mM EDTA inhibited the binding. Dithiothreitol from 0.1 mM inhibited the binding. We now wish to determine whether this nuclear envelope binding site plays a role in regulating the concentration of T_3 within the nucleus.
This study was supported by the MRC and AHFMR.

2169 A COMPARISON OF AROMATASE ACTIVITY FOR C-19 STEROIDS IN FETAL LIVER, ADULT LIVER AND HEPATOMA TISSUES OF HUMAN SUBJECTS.

C. Sakai*[1], T. Yamamoto[1], H. Okada[1] and Y. Osawa[2], [1] Dept. of OB/GYN, Kyoto Pref. Univ. Med., Kyoto 602, Japan and [2] Medical Foundation of Buffalo, Inc., Buffalo, U.S.A.

Although the in vitro study has shown that human fetal liver contributes significantly to the aromatization of androgen, it has thought that liver in adult has none or low level of aromatase activity. We have investigated whether or not human adult liver, hepatoma and hepatic hemangioma are able to aromatize various C-19 steroids (A,T,DHEA,DHEAS) and have examined the stereospecific disposition of 1β-H and 2β-H of A-ring during the process of aromatization. After incubation of the tritiated C-19 steroids (10 μCi) with human liver homogenates (1 g w.w in 10 ml of 0.1M-PBS, pH7.4) and NADPH (5mg) at 37°C for 2h in air, E_1, E_2 and E_3 were isolated and identified after a series of purification steps involving Bio-Rad AG1-X2 column chromatography, T.L.C. and co-crystallization. The findings indicated that the human fetal liver extensively aromatized various C-19 steroids to estrogens (E_1, E_2, E_3), whereas human adult liver and hepatoma tissues exhibited very low to almost no aromatization. Hepatoma tissues biosynthesized E_1 (~0.08 pmol/h/g) at a slightly higher rate than normal liver tissues (~0.04 pmol/h/g). No estrogen, however, was transformed from A by the hemangioma tissue. Therefore, it apears likely that in the fetus, mainly liver contributes to estrogen biosynthesis but in the adult, extrahepatic tissues are responsible for aromatization. Furthermore, the aromatization by fetal liver involves the removal of cis C-1β and -2β hydrogens of A.

2170 3α ANDROSTANEDIOL (3αAd) CONCENTRATIONS IN OVARIAN AND ADRENAL BLOOD EFFLUENTS IN NORMAL AND HIRSUTE WOMEN.

F. Sciarra*, V. Toscano, D. Casilli, M.V. Adamo, M. Maroder and C. Conti, Istituto di V Clinica Medica Generale, Università di Roma 00100 Rome Italy

3αAd derives almost exclusively from the peripheral extrahepatic metabolism: a possible glandular secretion must be excluded.3 normal menstruating women, 2 with PCO syndrome and 2 with hirsutism,normal menses and an isolated increase in plasma 3αAd were studied.Testosterone(T),Androstenedione (A),Dihydrotestosterone (DHT),3αAd and 3βAd were evaluated in peripheral,ovarian and adrenal vein blood,collected with simultaneous selective catheterization. RIA was used after celite chromatography.A significant increase in plasma 3αAd (17-19 ng/dl) was found in all cases of hirsutism,but no ovarian or adrenal gradient was observed for this compound.A gradient for A and/or T was found in all subjects,particularly in those with PCO syndrome.These results exclude an ovarian,adrenal Androstanediols secretion both in normal and in hirsute women. The isolated increase in plasma 3αAd found in some hirsute females accounts for an active extraglandular formation of this metabolite.A form of peripheral hirsutism may be advanced in these cases

2171 INTERACTION OF NITROXIDE SPIN-LABELED SUBSTRATES AND INHIBITORS WITH CYTOCHROME P-450$_{scc}$.

D. Seeley, H. Schleyer, D. Seitz, D. Cooper, K. Kashiwagi and H. Salhanick*. Dept. Pop. Sci., Harvard Univ., Boston, MA 02115. USA, Dept. Surg. Res., Univ. of Pennsylvania, PA 19104, USA and Dept. Chemistry, Northeastern University, Boston, MA 02115. USA.

Substrate analogs and inhibitors which bind to cytochrome P-450$_{scc}$ yield either Type I, Type II or Reverse Type I spectral changes in the Soret region. Substances containing nitroxide spin-labels demonstrate a broadening of the nitroxide triplet when immobilized on a protein. Nitroxide spin-labeled analogs of cholesterol and aminoglutethimide were studied by optical and EPR spectroscopy for affinity to the cytochrome P-450 associated with cholesterol side-chain cleavage. A nitroxide spin-labeled analog of 11-deoxycortisol was identified which formed a Reverse Type I complex with purified cytochrome P-450$_{scc}$ and had a dissociation constant of about 1 µM by both optical and EPR spectroscopy. A spin-labeled analog of aminoglutethimide elicited a Reverse Type I spectrum (aminoglutethimide causes Type II spectra) and had a dissociation constant of about 10 µM as determined by optical and EPR spectra. Purified cytochrome P-450$_{scc}$ stripped of the heme prosthetic group bound both the cholesterol analog and the aminoglutethimide analog as well as did intact cytochrome P-450. This demonstrates that the heme is not a required component of the substrate binding site and implies that enzymatic inhibition by aminoglutethimide may not result from interaction with the heme. The best estimate of the number of binding sites of the substrate and inhibitor analogs is one binding site per molecule cytochrome P-450.

2172 INHIBITION OF THE CYTOCHROME P-450$_{scc}$ SYSTEM ELECTRON TRANSPORT BY A SITE SPECIFIC ANTIBODY.

D. Seeley*, A. Wolfson, J. Hourihan, H. Schleyer, K. Kashiwagi and H. Salhanick. Dept. Pop. Scis., Harvard University, Boston, MA 02115, USA and Dept. Surg. Res., University of Pennsylvania, Philadelphia, PA 19104, USA.

The mechanism of inhibition of cholesterol side-chain cleavage by a specific active site-directed antibody to cytochrome P-450$_{scc}$ has been elucidated. The antibody had no effect on the substrate binding site as determined spectrally. It did not modify the heme environment insofar as can be detected by EPR. It did not bind to or affect the function of either the iron-sulfur protein or its reductase. Although the antibody had no effect on chemical reduction of the P-450 or on P-450-CO complex formation, it did inhibit the NADPH-dependent reduction of P-450 and the subsequent formation of the P-450-CO complex. This inhibitory effect is concentration-dependent, and is correlated with the inhibitory effect of the antibody on enzymatic cholesterol side-chain cleavage. Similar results were obtained using the F_{ab} fragments. These results indicate that the antibody most probably inhibits side-chain cleavage by binding to a region close to the iron-sulfur protein binding site, thereby either preventing transfer of reducing electrons to the cytochrome P-450 or preventing a conformational change necessary for reduction.

2173 RESPONSIVENESS OF MOUSE MAMMARY ADIPOSE TISSUE TO ESTRADIOL

G. Shyamala* and A. Ferenczy. Lady Davis Institute for Medical Research and Department of Pathology, Sir Mortimer B. Davis - Jewish General Hospital and McGill University, 3755 Cote Saint-Catherine Road, Montreal, Quebec, Canada H3T 1E2.

In the female mouse, the mammary epithelium is embedded in a pad of adipose and connective tissue commonly known as the mammary fat pad. Previously we have shown that the mammary glands of castrated virgin mice respond to estradiol (E_2) in vivo by several metabolic criteria including a marked increase in the rate of DNA synthesis (Endocrinology 110:1249, 1982). We have now examined the effect of E_2 on the rate of DNA synthesis among the various cell types in the mammary glands of castrated virgin mice using the technique of histoautoradiography. Our studies show that in addition to the epithelium, the adipose tissue is also responsive to E_2. In fact an analysis of the temporal relationship between E_2 treatment and E_2 mediated increase in DNA synthesis reveal that the responsiveness to E_2 may occur in the adipose tissue earlier than in the epithelium. These present observations taken together with our previous observations that the de-epithelialized mammary fat pad contain estrogen receptors (Endocrinology 108:825, 1981) lead us to conclude that mammary adipose tissue is a target site for estrogen action. (Supported by a grant from the National Cancer Institute of Canada.)

2174 ETHANOL DIRECTLY STIMULATES DIHYDROTESTOSTERONE (DHT) CONVERSION TO 5α-ANDROSTAN-3α,17β-DIOL (3α-DIOL) AND 5α-ANDROSTAN-3α,17β-DIOL (3β-DIOL) IN RAT LEYDIG CELLS (LC).

E. P. Murono* and V. Fisher-Simpson, Research Service, WJBD Veterans Hospital and Departments of Medicine and Physiology, Univ. South Carolina Sch. Medicine, Columbia, SC 29201, USA

The direct effect of ethanol on [^{3}H]-DHT (10 μM) conversion to 3α-diol and 3β-diol ((3α+3β)-diol) in rat Leydig cells purified by metrizamide density gradients was examined. When intact LC were incubated in the presence of varying amounts of ethanol (2.2-652 mM), the lower ethanol concentrations which would be expected in the circulation of alcoholic males (2.2-65 mM) increased [^{3}H]-DHT conversion to (3α+3β)-diol, in direct relation to the dose of ethanol added. The stimulation at 65 mM ethanol was 2-fold over control. Higher ethanol concentrations also increased [^{3}H]-DHT conversion to (3α+3β)-diol, but this was lower than the peak stimulation observed at 65 mM ethanol. The addition of 4-methylpyrazole (1 mM), an alcohol dehydrogenase inhibitor, blocked the stimulatory effect of ethanol. Furthermore, when 10,000xg supernatants of LC were incubated with limiting NADH (0.0005 mM) and NAD^+ (0.001 mM) concentrations, ethanol (2.2-65 mM) increased [^{3}H]-DHT conversion to (3α+3β)-diol; however, with a saturating level of NADH (0.2 mM) and 0.001 mM NAD^+, ethanol had no effect. These studies demonstrate for the first time that concentrations of ethanol present in the circulation of alcoholic males, increase DHT conversion to (3α+3β)-diol, and that this effect is probably mediated by LC alcohol dehydrogenase activity which increases the level of NADH. These results may have significant impact in DHT sensitive tissues since ethanol may decrease DHT availability.

2175 DOMINANT INFLUENCE OF ANDROGEN IN THE MULTIHORMONAL INDUCTION OF α_{2u} GLOBULIN mRNA IN RAT LIVER. C.V.R. Murty*, B. Chatterjee and A.K. Roy, Oakland University, Rochester, MI 48063, U.S.A.

Multihormonally regulated synthesis of α_{2u} globulin begins only after puberty in the male rat and in the mature male its hepatic synthesis is drastically reduced after castration. However, based on the results of gene transfection and other studies it has recently been suggested that either glucocorticoid alone or pulsatile growth hormone secretion mediated by the androgen can induce secretion of α_{2u} globulin. We therefore, have examined the effect of various hormone combinations on the hepatic levels of α_{2u} globulin mRNA in hypophysectomized male rats and in female rats after ablations of adrenals and ovaries. Hepatic concentration of α_{2u} globulin was assayed by RIA and the hepatic level of α_{2u} globulin mRNA was determined by hybridization with a cloned cDNA probe. Treatment of female rats, that lacked both ovaries and adrenals, with glucocorticoid alone did not induce α_{2u} mRNA. Whereas, treatment of these animals with both glucocorticoid and androgen resulted in the induction of α_{2u} globulin and its mRNA to about 50% of the normal male. Treatment of hypophysectomized male rats with a combination of glucocorticoids, growth hormone and DHT resulted in the induction of α_{2u} mRNA to about 80% of the normal male. However, inclusion of estradiol-17β to this combination almost completely blocked the inductive effect. Furthermore, reversal of the episodic to pulsatile pattern of growth hormone secretion in the old male rat with L-dopa failed to induce α_{2u} mRNA. We conclude that androgen is the dominant hormone and neither glucocorticoid nor the pulsatile pattern of growth hormone secretion alone can turn on the gene for α2u globulin. Supported by the NIH.

2176 METABOLISM OF DHT TO ANDROSTANEDIOLS BY SHEEP ERYTHROCYTES. C.D. Nancarrow* and P.J. Connell, CSIRO, Division of Animal Production, P.O. Box 239, Blacktown, 2148, Australia.

Erythrocytes of fetal and adult sheep rapidly metabolise DHT to both 5α-dihydroandrostane-3α,17β-diol (3α-AD) and its 3β-isomer (3β-AD). Some parameters of these activities were estimated on blood obtained from 3 groups of fetal sheep and 2 groups of lambs representing 5 ages (Table 1). The equilibrium position of the reaction(s), the proportion of 3α-AD in the reduction products and the rate of DHT reduction (3α-AD + 3β-AD) were estimated by incubating 0.02-1.0 ml whole blood with labelled DHT for 5-60 min. The steroids were separated by thin layer and paper partition chromatography. The results in Table 1 show that DHT is almost quantitatively reduced by erythrocytes with 3β-AD the major fetal product and 3α-AD the major adult product. The rate of DHT reduction was slower in lamb than fetal blood. The evidence suggests that erythrocytes of sheep act as a secondary endocrine organ by modifying the circulating levels of androgens.

Table 1. DHT metabolism by sheep erythrocytes (mean ± S.D.; n).

Age (days)	Equilibrium (%)	3α-AD (%)	Rate DHT reduction µmol/ml erythrocytes/h
* 51--54	96.8 ± 1.0 (8)	9.9 ± 3.8 (8)	7.57 ± 2.76 (7)
98-119	96.1 ± 3.6 (17)	10.3 ± 6.2 (17)	5.09 ± 2.10 (17)
141-145	96.4 ± 1.1 (11)	12.3 ± 9.4 (11)	3.75 ± 2.12 (10)
** 0---3	96.0 ± 1.7 (38)	33.6 ± 20.8 (34)	1.89 ± 1.03 (37)
50--60	93.8 ± 4.0 (18)	94.3 ± 5.0 (19)	0.98 ± 0.46 (18)

*Fetal age. **lamb age.

2177 AN ANIMAL MODEL FOR THE STUDY OF LEAD TOXICITY ON THE HYPOTHALAMIC-PITUITARY-TESTICULAR AXIS. RZ Sokol,* C. Madding, and R.S. Swerdloff, Department of Medicine, Harbor-UCLA Medical Center, Torrance, CA.

Environmental exposure to toxic levels of lead (Pb) occurs in a number of industries with potential adverse effects on the reproductive capacity of exposed men. In order to ascertain if reproductive abnormalities occur in experimental animals when exposed to low levels of Pb, 52 d old animals were treated with water containing a) 0% Pb acetate (PbA) b) 0.1% PbA, c) 0.3% PbA for 30 d. Serum Pb, FSH, LH, testosterone (T), intratesticular T, and sperm counts were measured.

Group	Control	0.1%	0.3%
Lead levels (μg/dl)	<6.0	34.3±2.5[d]	59.5±4.0[d]
Sperm Counts (10^6/testis)	102.5±7.9	69.8±2.1[a]	48.3±1.6[d]
LH (ng/ml)	53.5±11.5	42.9±8.6	39.4±8.3
FSH (ng/ml)	348±24.2	271±21.1	264±23.4
Serum T (ng/dl)	607.1±108.8	311.3±52.1[a]	168.3±24.4[c]
Intratest. T (ng/gm)	920.6±138.5	817.9±36.0[b]	679.8±70.3[d]

[a] $p<.05$, [b] $p<.02$, [c] $p<.01$, [d] $p<.001$

Increased serum lead concentration was negatively correlated with sperm counts (r=-0.8000; p<.001) and intratesticular T levels (r=-0.6114, p<.001).

Similar results were obtained in 70 d old rats. Conclusions: 1) Dietary exposure to Pb results in inhibition of testicular function as manifested by suppressed spermatogenesis and decreased serum and intratesticular T levels. 2) The predominant mechanism of action appears to be suppression of the hypothalamic-pituitary axis, although direct testicular toxicity may also occur. 3) Alterations in the hypothalamic-pituitary-testicular axis occur in a dose/response fashion. 4) Our experimental design can serve as an animal model for the study of environmental exposure to lead.

2178 THE EFFECT OF THE INDAZOLE CARBOXYLIC ACID DERIVATIVE, TOLNIDAMINE, ON TESTICULAR FUNCTION IN THE RAT. I.M. Spitz*, G.L. Gunsalus, J.P. Mather, R. Thau, and C.W. Bardin, The Population Council, New York, N.Y.

Tolnidamine (TOL) inhibits spermatogenesis in rats, rabbits and monkeys. Previous studies have described its effects on germ cell morphology and Leydig cells but there are no reports on Sertoli cells. In this study we used androgen binding protein (ABP) secretion as an index of Sertoli cell function. We first determined the effect of increasing concentrations (25 ng-2.5 ug) of TOL on ABP secretion from isolated Sertoli cell cultures from 20 day old rats. In these experiments TOL produced no apparent change in ABP secretion. Oral administration of TOL (250 mg/kg) in a single dose to mature male rats produced a significant decrease in testicular and epididymal weights by 5 days. There were no changes in plasma testosterone. Serum ABP levels were significantly increased by 16 hrs and maximum levels were observed after 32 hrs. Serum ABP levels were persistently elevated during 12 days of observation. Epididymal ABP content showed a steady decrease which was already evident by 7 hrs and lowest values occurred at 12 days. Testicular ABP content increased by 160% at 16 hrs and remained persistently higher than control values for the full 12 days. The decline of epididymal ABP content without an increase in testicular weight suggests that TOL inhibits ABP transport to the epididymis. This results in accumulation of testicular ABP with a rise of this protein in blood and implies that TOL does not inhibit the release of ABP from the base of the Sertoli cell into the blood. In contrast to the effect of TOL on Sertoli cells, Leydig cells do not appear to be compromised.

2179 TEMPERATURE SENSITIVITY OF PROGESTERONE-BINDING CYTOCHROME P450 FROM RAT TESTIS MICROSOMES. W.Staib[+], J.Rediger and N.Kühn-Velten, Institut f. Physiologische Chemie II, Univ., Moorenstr.5, D-4000 Düsseldorf, Germany.

Surgically induced cryptorchidism results in an inhibition of testicular C-17,20-lyase activity within seven days (Acta endocrinol.101 (1982), 301-306). In accordance with this observation, a reduced testosterone response on LH stimulation in vivo occurs after heating of testes (Andrologia 12 (1980), 12-19). The present study was undertaken to elucidate temperature sensitivity of microsomal progesterone-binding cytochrome P450 which is an essential component of the 17a-hydroxylase/C-17,20-lyase complex in rat testis. Either whole testes or testis microsomes were incubated at various temperatures and progesterone-induced spectral changes of microsomal cytochrome P450 were measured (FEBS Lett.54 (1983),70-74). An 18.5% loss of apparent progesterone binding sites can be observed after 3 hours of incubation at 32°C (the normal scrotal temperature of the rat) whereas a 33.8% loss is observed after incubation at 36°C. If isolated microsomes from rat testis are incubated, a diminution by 12.5% occurs within 3 hours at 32°C whereas a loss by 18.9% results after 3 hours at 36°C. A linear dependence of diminution of cytochrome P450 with time is obvious both at 32°C and 36°C and the regression coefficients (slopes) are different with $p < 0.005$. If testis microsomes are washed three times and then incubated at 36°C for 3 hours, the apparent loss of cytochrome P450 amounts only to 10.8%. This difference can be attributed to the effect of contaminating cytosol components (proteases?). In conclusion, the short-termed decrease of testosterone formation by heat-treated testes may at least partly be due to temperature effects on microsomal cytochrome P450.

2180 BINDING OF SERTOLI CELL SECRETORY PROTEINS BY TESTICULAR GERM CELLS. Anna Steinberger*, Rajan Dighe and Julio Diaz, Department of Obstetrics, Gynecology and Reproductive Sciences, University of Texas Medical School, Houston, Texas 77030.

Differentiation of germ cells during spermatogenesis may require specific products secreted by the Sertoli cells. Since the Sertoli cells secrete a large number of proteins, we investigated whether some of these proteins are specifically bound by the germ cells at certain stages of differentiation. Incubation of isolated rat germ cells for 1h at 34C with ^{125}I-rat transferrin showed binding of radioactivity which was saturable and could be displaced to a large extent by an excess of unlabeled transferrin. Autoradiography of the germ cells following the incubation revealed most intense labeling of the spermatocytes with some label being associated with the round spermatids. A similar binding pattern was observed when the germ cells were incubated with dialyzed media from Sertoli cell cultures which were prelabeled with ^{3}H-leucine. The nature of the bound radioactivity is under investigation. These results suggest that germ cells, particularly the spermatocytes, bind and may utilize certain Sertoli cell secretory proteins which may be required for the meiotic division.

This study was supported by NIH grant HD-17802.

2181 INFLUENCE OF PROLACTIN AND BROMOCRIPTINE ON MALE GONADAL FUNCTION DURING SEXUAL MATURATION. M.Suescun, S.Gonzalez, M.de las Heras, V.Chiauzzi and R. Calandra*. Instituto de Biología y Medicina Experimental, Obligado 2490, 1428 Buenos Aires, Argentina.

Prolactin (PRL) acts on testis by increasing the number of LH receptors and its sensitivity to LH. A controversial information exists concerning to PRL and Bromocriptine (Br) on remainder aspects of testicular function. In the present study we evaluated the effects of PRL and Br during gonadal maturation. Mild hyperprolactinemia (85 ± 32 vs 25 ± 8 ng/ml) induced by pituitary homografts during 40 days, results in a pronounced enhancement (98%) in the testicular 5α-reductase activity ($p<0,05$) in homogenate and microsomes.When PRL ($5x10^{-8}$M) was incubated with decapsulated testes, a significant stimulation of this activity was observed in isolated seminiferous tubules (ST). Previously, we have shown that Br reduced the 5α-reductase in ST (Endocrinology 109;2188,1981). Daily administration of Br (0,75; 1; 3 mg/kgBW) for 10 days, starting at 30 days of age, suppressed PRL without changing LH levels. Br at all doses tested, markedly depressed sera testosterone (T) and 5α-androstanediol(A-diol). Intratesticular T and A-diol levels were diminished (25 and 35%) during hypoprolactinemia ($p<0,05$). Basal and sub-maximal hCG-stimulation of androgen production (AP) by decapsulated testes and dispersed Leydig cells, showed a significant diminution in Br groups in comparison to the controls. Maximal testicular response was not altered. In contrast,Br (10^{-5}-10^{-7}M)incubated with decapsulated testes, raised basal and sub-maximal hCG-stimulated AP ($p<0,05$). Thus, during puberty PRL influence testicular steroidogenesis in rat testis. Some evidence of a direct effect of PRL and Br are presented. (Sup.CONICET-Fund.Roemmers).

2182 LOCALIZATION OF A HAMSTER SPERM MEMBRANE PROTEIN WITH AN AFFINITY FOR THE ZONA PELLUCIDA. R. Sullivan*, K.D. Roberts, A. Chapdelaine, S. Chevalier and G. Bleau. Maisonneuve-Rosemont Research Center, Montreal, Canada.

Species specificity of fertilization is ensured at the level of sperm-egg interaction (the zona pellucida (z.p.) is in part responsible for this specificity). Using hamster gametes, we have developed a system in which electrophoretic patterns of sperm membrane proteins are electrophoretically transfered to a nitrocellulose membrane ("western blot"). An autoradiogram of this nitrocellulose membrane, preincubated with solubilized-radiolabelled z.p., revealed a 26.4 Kd sperm protein which binds z.p. proteins in a species specific manner. In order to further characterize this sperm protein we have submitted epididymal spermatozoa to detergent treatment. Electrophoretic patterns of sperm proteins extracted with 3% Triton X-100 or 0.5% Nonidet p-40 revealed essentially the same bands including that corresponding to the protein with an affinity for the z.p. proteins. At the electron microscopic level, these treated spermatozoa exhibited a loss of the plasma membrane and acrosome. When spermatozoa were exposed to Triton X-100 at a concentration of 0.04%, the 26.4 Kd protein was not extracted. Electron micrographs of these spermatozoa revealed that only the plasma membrane of the post-acrosomal region resisted this treatment. During the process of fertilization, it is precisely this region which is involved in the contact with the z.p. It is proposed that the 26.4 Kd sperm membrane protein of the post-acrosomal region be considered as a z.p. receptor implicated in sperm-egg recognition. Supported by MRC and FCAC

2183 **THE ACUTE EFFECT OF THYROID STIMULATING HORMONE (TSH) ON GUINEA-PIG THYROID METABOLISM.** H. Perrild *[1], N. Loveridge[2], S.Reader [3] and W. Robertson [3]. Dept. Int. Med. Herlev Hosp. 2730 Herlev, Denmark. [1] Kennedy Inst. of Rheumatology, London W6.[2] Univ. Manchester, Dept. Chem. Path., Hope Hospital, Salford M6 8HD, U.K.[3].

Quantitative cytochemistry has been used to study acute effects of TSH(1mU/L) on thyroid metabolism using thyroid segments in organ culture. We examined the enzymes involved in NADPH production [NAD^+ kinase (NKase), glucose-6-phosphate dehydrogenase (G-6-PDH)] and reoxidation (microsomal respiratory pathway), and iodine organification (peroxidase). Lysosomal function was studied using leucyl-napthylamidase (LNAase) as a marker of membrane permeability and N-acetyl-β-glucosaminidase (NAG) as an indicator of thyroglobulin processing. After TSH stimulation there was a 60% increase in NKase activity which peaked at 10 min and preceded changes in the reoxidation of NADPH (up 35% by 30 min). G-6-PDH activity was unaffected. Peroxidase activity rose by 120% after 30 min. TSH induced changes in LNAase activity were biphasic peaking at 6 and 25 min (42 and 58% increases) respectively. NAG activity increased by 40% after 30 min. In conclusion, quantitative cytochemistry offers new insights into the mechanism of TSH action, with direct effects on NKase peroxidase and NAG activities being shown for the first time. The timing and magnitude of the changes in NKase activity (itself inhibited by NADPH) may indicate a regulatory role for this enzyme. Finally, the lysosomal effects are consistent with an early fusion of endocytotic vesicles and a later proteolytic breakdown of thyroglobulin.

2184 HIGH DOSE CARBIMAZOLE(CBZ)THERAPY IN GRAVES' DISEASE:IN VIVO AND IN VITRO STUDIES. P.Pozzilli*,R.Kennedy,U Di Mario,M.Sensi,A.Signore,K.Guy, D.Andreani, Cattedra di Endocrinologia(I), university of Rome, Italy.

It is now recognised that CBZ,in addition to its known antithyroid effect has immunosuppressive properties. We have phenotyped activated T cells with monoclonal antibodies(4F2,TAC,anti-DR panel)in 18 patients with Graves' disease at diagnosis and during 12 months therapy with initially 60mg CBZ followed by 20mg maintenance dose + thyroxine. 10 patients received standard CBZ doses. The in vitro effect of 30,60,120 and 250µmol/l CBZ on activated T cells(mitogen or spontaneous)was studied in patients and normal controls. Patients treated with high doses did not show any side effect. Preliminary results indicate that clinical remission times were comparable in both groups of patients. T cells showing one or more activation antigens were found in nearly all patients at diagnosis,but they disappeared more rapidly in patients treated with high CBZ doses. In vitro studies showed that activated TAC^+ (anti-T cell growth factor receptor) T cell number could be reduced earlier by 30µmol/l CBZ; with higher doses T cell activation was inhibited. This study indicates:a) activated T cells are a common feature in patients with Graves' disease at diagnosis;b) they tend to disappear more rapidly from circulation following CBZ therapy;c) CBZ is capable of impairing the expression of lymphocyte differentiation antigens in vitro;d) this property of CBZ should be considered for the treatment of other autoimmune endocrinopathies characterised by increased levels of activated T cells.

2185 SERUM PROTEIN BINDING OF THYROXINE (T_4) DURING T_4 TREATMENT IN A PATIENT WITH FAMILIAL DYSALBUMINEMIC HYPERTHYROXINEMIA (FDH).

B. N. Premachandra*, J. Wortsman and K. Williams, VA Medical Ctr., Jefferson Barracks, St. Louis, Missouri and SIU School of Medicine, Springfield, Illinois

Graded levels of T_4 (0.2, 0.4 and 0.6 mg/day) were administered each for 2 weeks to a subject having familial dysalbuminemic hyperthyroxinemia (FDH). Following the initial 2 weeks of treatment (0.2 mg/day), ^{125}I-T_4 tracer binding by TBG was reduced from 42.8% to 30.1% (paper electrophoresis). TBG-RIA showed an 8% decrease from the pre-treatment value of 3.7 mg/dl. T_4 tracer transport in the albumin region increased from 24.2 to 37.9%. Carriage by pre-albumin was unchanged (33% vs. 31.9%). From the beginning of 0.4 mg to 0.6 mg T_4/day termination, % tracer T_4 binding remained constant at all three T_4 protein binding regions (albumin = 41.8%, pre-albumin = 38.5%, TBG = 19.9%). Relative to initial values % T_4 carriage showed albumin = 72.7% increase; pre-albumin = 16.7% increase; TBG = 53.5% decrease. TBG concentration as determined by RIA showed a decrease of 16.2% at the end of T_4 treatment relative to pre-treatment values. These data indicate that alterations in T_4 binding protein in the FDH proband during exogenous T_4 treatment were mediated principally by TBG and the abnormal albumin fraction. The lesser rate of T_4-pre-albumin binding increase might have been due to the reported negative cooperativity of the 2 molecular binding sites of TBPA.

2186 PRIMARY HYPERPARATHYROIDISM IN PREGNANCY.

R. Rajabian*, M.A. Taghinia, A. Farzad, A.H. Tavakolizadeh and F. Sharifian, Ghaem Medical Center, University of Mashhad, Iran.

Hyperparathyroidism or Von Recklinghousen's disease is seldom observed in association with pregnancy. We are presenting and discussing 2 cases of primary hyperparathyroidism in pregnancy. These patients presented with bone pain, osteitis-fibrosa cystica and pathologic fractures. Both patients had parathyroid adenoma removed successfully during pregnancy and gave birth to a normal baby by cessarean section.

2187 STUDY OF CARBOHYDRATE AND LIPID METABOLISM IN GRAVE'S DISEASE. JP. Randin*, B. Scazziga, E. Jéquier, JP. Felber. Division d'Endocrinologie et Biochimie Clinique, CHUV ; Institut de Physiologie, 1011 Lausanne, Switzerland.

In an attempt to clarify some conflicting data on carbohydrate and lipid metabolism in hyperthyroidism, 12 patients (5 men, 7 women) with Grave's disease have been studied for 3 h during an OGTT (100 g) by using continuous indirect calorimetry. Impaired glucose tolerance was observed with significantly increased fasting plasma glucose (5.3 ± 0.1 vs 4.7 ± 0.1 mmol/l $p<0.001$). The insulin plasma concentrations were significantly elevated only at 30 min after the oral glucose load (127 ± 26 vs control 77 ± 7 µU/ml, $p<0.02$). In the fasting state, the free fatty acid concentrations were significantly higher (828 ± 70 vs 581 ± 47 µmol/l, $p<0.01$), decreasing to control values after 30 min. Glucose oxidation was not different in the fasting state (14 ± 3 vs 16 ± 0.9 g/3 h). On the contrary, lipid oxidation was significantly elevated (20.6 ± 1.3 vs 9.0 ± 0.5 g/3 h, $p<0.001$). After the glucose load, total glucose oxidation increased to 47.1 ± 2.0 vs 33.4 ± 1.4 g/3 h, $p<0.001$) while lipid oxidation fell to normal values after 60 min. Glucose storage was clearly lower (49.2 ± 3 vs 67.0 ± 1.2 g/3 h, $p<0.001$). The present study demonstrates that the well-known increase of the energy expenditure in Grave's disease results in an important increase of lipid oxidation in the fasting state, and in an increase of glucose oxidation after an oral glucose load. If one considers glucose oxidation, insulin resistance cannot therefore be evoked as a cause of the impaired glucose tolerance in hyperthyroidism.

2188 SPECIFIC IMMUNOPRECIPITATION BY THYROID STIMULATING IMMUNOGLOBULIN-CONTAINING SERUM OF A THYROID MEMBRANE SURFACE PROTEIN WITH CHARACTERISTICS OF THYROGLOBULIN. B. Rapoport*, P. Seto and R. Magnusson, Dept. of Medicine V.A. Hospital and U.C.S.F., San Francisco, CA. 94121 U.S.A.

Characterization of the antigen (Ag) to thyroid stimulating immunoglobulin (TSI), presumably the TSH receptor, remains elusive. We therefore attempted immunoprecipitation of the TSI Ag using cultured human thyroid cells radiolabeled to high specific activity by 35S-methionine (all proteins labeled) or by 125I + lactoperoxidase (only cell surface proteins labeled). Both techniques produced similar results. Crude membrane preparations from the labeled cells were solubilized in buffer containing 1% Triton, and were then incubated with TSI-containing or control serum. IgG was precipitated with goat anti-human IgG, and was subjected to SDS-polyacylamide gel electrophoresis and autoradiography. About 30 proteins were immunoprecipitated by both normal and control serum. However only one protein (~320,000 Mr) was preferentially selected by TSI containing serum (6/6 tested). This protein constituted only a minute amount of membrane protein because it was not apparent on electrophoresis of the membrane extract prior to immunoprecipitation. It corresponded (in migration) to a human thyroglobulin (Tg) standard. Tg also inhibited immunoprecipitation of the 320 K Mr band. Anti-Tg antibodies were detected in some, but not all, TSI-active sera that immunoprecipitated the 320,000 Mr band.

These data indicate that: 1) TSI-containing serum interacts specifically with a single protein component, either embedded in or adsorbed to the outer surface of the thyroid plasma membrane. 2) This protein is, or is related to, Tg. 3) Surprisingly, TSI did not immunoprecipitate any protein consistent with the variously reported sizes of the TSH receptor.

2189 RADIOIMMUNOASSAYS SPECIFIC FOR THE TERTIARY AND FOR THE PRIMARY STRUCTURE OF THYROXINE-BINDING GLOBULIN (TBG): MEASUREMENT OF DENATURED TBG IN SERUM. S. Refetoff*, Y. Murata, G. Vassart, V. Chandramouli and J.S. Marshall, Dept. of Medicine, Univ. of Chicago, IL USA; IRIBHN, Free Univ. of Brussels, Belgium; and Case Western Reserve Univ., Cleveland, OH USA.

Current methods for measurement of TBG in serum are based on either its immunoreactivity or bioactivity (T4-binding). Using two subpopulations of antibodies, we were able to develop radioimmunoassays (RIA) specific for native TBG and denatured TBG (DN-TBG). The TBG RIA, using ^{125}I-TBG as tracer, measured equivalent amounts of TBG, desialylated TBG (STBG) and deglycosylated TBG (dg TBG), but did not cross react with DN-TBGs. The DN-TBG RIA using ^{125}I-reduced pyridylethylated-TBG (RP-TBG), measured equivalent amount of RP-TBG, heat denatured TBG (ΔH-TBG) and acid denatured TBG (AC-TBG) but did not cross react with TBG, STBG or dg TBG. Heat and acid treatments of serum TBG produced a progressive loss in TBG measured by RIA and T4-binding capacity with a reciprocal and quantitative increase in DN-TBG, devoid of T4-binding activity. DN-TBG was detected in all normal sera (mean $\pm$ SD: 6.05 $\pm$ 2.25 µg/dl). Mean concentrations were not different in 8 pregnant women, 5 subjects with familial low TBG, 15 hypothyroid, 15 hyperthyroid, 7 hepatic failure and 8 renal failure patients. Mean values, 2.43 $\pm$ 0.88 and 2.89 $\pm$ 1.54 µg/dl, were lower ($p<0.01$) in 12 cord sera and in 7 neonates, respectively. No DN-TBG was present in serum of subjects with inherited TBG absence. In conclusion, TBG and DN-TBG can be measured specifically in samples containing both forms. DN-TBG is a normal constituent of serum, the concentrations of which do not correlate with those of TBG. Supported by USPHS Grant AM-15070.

2190 REGULATION OF TSH SECRETION IN THE TRAINED CONSCIOUS DOG. G. E. Richards* and T. S. Farris, Department of Pediatrics, University of Texas Medical Branch, Galveston, Texas, USA.

Experiments in humans and rats have suggested that dopaminergic, serotoninergic and α1 adrenergic neurotransmitter systems may play a role in regulation of TSH secretion. To determine whether TSH secretion in dogs is mediated by CNS neurotransmitters, we measured cTSH after administration of clonidine, 5-hydroxytryptophan, haloperidol and morphine. Five male mongrel dogs were trained to stand in a sling for repeated blood sampling through an indwelling venous catheter. Blood was drawn at frequent intervals during a 1½ hour control period and 2 hours after administration of the pharmacologic stimuli. Plasma TSH was measured using a cTSH kit prepared by CANAM Diagnostics, based on the method of Quinlan (Endocr. 108:937, 1981). Assay sensitivity was 0.5 ng/tube interassay variation 11% and intraassay variation 9.3% at approximately 50% displacement. There was approximately 1% cross reactivity with cPRL and 2% with cGH (kindly provided by Dr. A. F. Parlow through the National Hormone and Pituitary Program). Mean basal TSH was 5-10 ng/ml in the group of 5 dogs in 4 different experiments. Intravenous administration of clonidine 2.5 µg/kg as a bolus, 5-hydroxytryptophan 10 mg/kg given over 15 minutes, haloperidol 2 mg as a bolus and morphine 0.5 mg/kg as a bolus did not significantly change plasma cTSH concentration. We conclude that α2 adrenergic, serotoninergic and dopaminergic systems do not play a dominant role in TSH regulation in the dog. To completely exclude the role of opiates, other analogs with differing receptor specificities must be tested.

2191 EVALUATION OF MUSCULAR CATABOLISM IN HYPOTHYROIDISM BY 3-METHYLHISTIDINE EXCRETION (3MH). M. RODIER*, J.L. RICHARD, L. BALDET, C. JAFFIOL, J. MIROUZE
Endocrinology, Saint Eloi Hospital, F-34059 MONTPELLIER.

Myofibrillar catabolism is controlled by nutritional and hormonal status. In an attempt to evaluate the role of thyroid hormones, we study the protein breakdown in hypothyroidism, using urinary 3MH, 3MH/body weight (3MH/BW), and 3MH/urinary creatinine (3MH/Cr) ratios. 21 hypothyroid patients (18 women, 3 men ; 20-79 yrs) are investigated at diagnosis ; 4 are restudied after 3-6 months of substitutive therapy. 21 healthy volunteers (10 women, 11 men ; 24-60 yrs) serve as controls. 24-hr urine is collected during the last 3 days of a 6-day meat-free diet ; 3MH is measured according to Spackman and Cr to Jaffé ; FT_4I, T_4 and T_3 are determined by RIA. The Student's t test and the least squares method are used for the statistical analysis. 3MH and Cr, 3MH/BW and 3MH/Cr are significantly lower in hypothyroid patients (table ; mean ± SEM). There is no correlation between 3MH, 3MH/BW, 3MH/Cr and hormonal parameters. There is no significant increase of 3MH, Cr, 3MH/BW and 3MH/Cr after treatment, however only 4 patients are restudied.

	3MH(μmol/d)	Cr(mmol/d)	3MH/BW(μmol/kg/d)	3MH/Cr(molar)
Patients	86.1 ± 8.7	8.58 ± 0.72	1.31 ± 0.13	9.79 ± 0.85
Controls	193.3 ± 13.9	13.11 ± 0.89	3.16 ± 0.19	14.99 ± 0.88

3MH is claimed to be a valuable index of myofibrillar breakdown ; in our patients, the reduced 3MH excretion may be explained by the catabolic effect of thyroid hormones. Since there is no correlation between 3MH, 3MH/Cr and thyroid parameters, others factors are suspected : the renal function may be implicated since Cr which is initially reduced increases along with the 3MH excretion during treatment.

2192 THYROID AUTOANTIBODIES IN 71 FAMILIES WITH 194 HLA CHARACTERIZED CHILDREN. S.H. Roman*, M.E. Witt, P. Rubinstein, F. Ginsberg-Fellner and T.F. Davies, Departments of Medicine and Pediatrics, Mount Sinai School of Medicine and New York Blood Center, New York, N.Y., USA.

Autoimmune thyroid disease has been HLA associated yet the relationship of HLA antigen expression to thyroid autoantibody (TA) production is uncertain. We have screened the children (age 2-23 yrs) from 71 families at risk for autoimmune endocrine disease because of a Type 1 diabetic child proband for thyroid autoantibodies (Ab) to thyroglobulin (Tg) and microsomal antigen (M) using highly sensitive ELISAs. 42.3% of this population possessed Tg-Ab and/or M-Ab ($r=0.68, p<0.001$ between Abs). 23.2% of children positive for TA expressed DR5 in contrast to 10.7% in the group negative for TA ($p<0.03$). The frequency of DR5 in those subjects possessing high TA levels (ELISA Index>1.0) was 28.3%. Within family analysis of HLA identical siblings (n=40 pairs) indicated 42.5% discordance between members of sib pairs for TA. Examination of HLA non-identical sibs (n=18 pairs) demonstrated one sib pair with concordance for TA positivity. In conclusion: (1) The prevalence of TA in this selected population is unusually high; (2) DR5 is one significant risk factor for development of TA; and (3) The high discordance in HLA identical sibs for TA provides strong evidence for additional non-HLA factors in the expression of TA secretory potential.

2193 REGULATION OF THYROGLOBULIN (Tg) GLYCOSYLATION. C. Ronin*, E. Fenouillet, S. Hovsepian+ and G.Fayet+, U 172 INSERM, Bd. P. Dramard, 13326 Marseille and +U 38 INSERM, Bd. J. Moulin, 13385 Marseille, France.

Since glycosylation could play a role in Tg secretion, we have examined Tg glycosylation in follicular-associated thyroid cells under basal and thyrotropin (TSH)-stimulatory conditions. Porcine thyroid follicles in serum-free, iodine-free medium (J. Cell. Biol. 1982, 93, 479-488) were stimulated or not by TSH (200 U/ml) on day 4 and incubated with ^{3}H-glucosamine (1mCi) for 24hrs on day 6. Extrafollicular Tg was purified, digested with pronase and the labeled glycopeptides analyzed by sequential affinity chromatography on immobilized lectins. 91% of the glycopeptides from TSH-stimulated cells were unretained on Concavalin A-Sepharose(ConA-Seph), 8% and 1% eluted at low and high concentration of sugar respectively. This is at variance with chemically labeled oligosaccharides from iodinated colloidal Tg for which 49% were unbound, 41% and 10% bound to ConA-Seph respectively. ConA-retained glycopeptides from stimulated cells were also largely retained on lentil-Sepharose, indicating a typical fucosylated biantennary carbohydrate (CHO) structure. The ConA-unretained glycopeptides were not retained on lentil-Sepharose, 42% of them being retarded on E-phytohemagglutinin(PHA)-Agarose and 35% on L-PHA-Agarose, suggesting heterogeneous triantennary CHO structures. Similar results were obtained for glycopeptides from non-stimulated cells. Thus, glycosylation of extrafollicular Tg is not modified by TSH in serum-free, iodine-free cell culture but the resulting CHO chains are of more complex structure than those of iodinated colloidal Tg.

2194 PURE α-SUBUNIT-PRODUCING TUMOR DERIVED FROM A THYROTROPIC TUMOR: ABNORMAL REGULATION OF α-SUBUNIT AND ITS mRNA BY T4. D.S. Ross*, J.D. Kieffer, M.A. Shupnik, W.W.Chin, and E.C. Ridgway, Thyroid Unit, Massachusetts General Hospital, Boston, Massachusetts 02114.

Mouse thyrotropic tumors are a useful model for studying TSH and subunit biosynthesis. We have recently documented the spontaneous conversion of a mouse thyrotropic tumor to a pure α subunit-producing tumor in which both free TSH-β subunit and intact TSH are absent (Endocrinol. 1983; 113:1587). Our current studies compare the regulation of α-subunit biosynthesis by thyroid hormones in thyrotropic tumors (TtT-97) and the pure α-subunit-producing tumors (MGH 101A). The α-subunit secretion from MGH 101A and TtT-97 tumors have shown clear differences in responsiveness *in vivo* to T4 (10 μg/100 g/day, ip, for 12 days). Plasma α-subunit concentrations in mice bearing MGH 101A were not decreased by T4 treatment, while the plasma α-subunit levels in mice bearing TtT-97 were reduced to less than 10% of control. Steady-state levels of mRNA encoding for pre-α-subunits in MGH 101A and TtT-97 were measured by hybridization with a specific cDNA probe. T4 treatment did not change the α-subunit mRNA levels in MGH 101A, while those in TtT-97 were reduced to 15% of control. Other studies using a cDNA specific for TSH-β mRNA revealed that MGH 101A tumors did not produce detectable TSH-β mRNA. In TtT-97 tumors TSH-β mRNA was easily detected and fell to undetectable levels after 12 days of T4. We conclude that the pure α-subunit-producing tumor MGH 101A (1) displays abnormal α-subunit responses to T4 regulation *in vivo* at both transcriptional and secretory levels, and (2) it is characterized by an absence of both the apoprotein and mRNA encoding the TSH-β subunit.

2195 HYPOTHALAMO-PITUITARY-THYROID AXIS IN INFANTS* AND CHILDREN DURING HYPOTHERMIC CARDIOVASCULAR SURGERY.

I. Rozenberg.:, Ph. Manchon..., C. Oliver., J. Aubert., J.P. Couvely., M. Carcassonne., J. Vague., . Fac. Med. Marseille, .. Fac. Med. Créteil, ... CNAM-Paris, France.

In man, thyroid response to chronic cold exposure is demonstrated but little is known about involvement of thyroid function during acute cold exposure. Hypothalamo-pituitary-thyroid axis (TRH, TSH, T4, T3) was studied in infants and children undergoing hypothermic cardiovascular surgery. Patients were dividen in 2 groups : group 1 deep hypothermia -rectal temperature range 18°5-25° - n = 4 - age range 4-18 months ; group 2 mild hypothermia-rectal temperature 28°-34°-n=5-age 14 months-12 years. Plasma samples were collected during the course of surgery. Hormone levels were assessed by RIA and values were corrected according to body surface. Data were analyzed using analysis of covariance. Group 1 was characterized by initially high TSH and low T4, T3 levels which significantly increased during the course of surgery. TRH values were not modified except for the youngest infant which exhibited concomitantly striking rise of TRH levels and indetectable plasma ACTH values. Plasma ACTH was increased in 1 child. Group 2 was characterized initially low T4,T3 levels which significantly increased during the course of surgery. TSH and TRH values were not significantly modified. Plasma ACTH levels rose in 3 children. In conclusion, acute cold exposure in infants and children undergoing hypothermic cardiovascular surgery provoked an initial fall of T4 and T3 levels, followed by a significant increase during the course of surgery. Deep hypothermia, a procedure for the youngest patients, did not modify TRH values except for the youngest infant but induced an elevation of TSH levels.

2196 Auto-and heteroantibodies against human thyroglobulin present the same heterogeneity and fine specificities.

J. Ruf, P. Carayon* and S. Lissitzky
Biochimie Médicale- U 38 INSERM Faculté de Médecine, F 13385 Marseille Cédex 5 France.

Circulating antibodies reflect, at least in part, the regulatory activities of the immune system. Hence, the study of the repertoire of autoantibodies present in various situations may distinguish the several mechanisms of maintenance and loss of tolerance. By using well characterized monoclonal antibodies directed against human thyroglobulin*, the fine specificity of anti-thyroglobulin autoantibodies from normal subjects, Graves'patients and patients with thyroid carcinoma was studied and compared to that of antibodies from rabbits immunized with thyroglobulin prepared from different species. While the fine specificities of anti-human thyrogloublin antibodies were found identical in the three groups of human subjects and in rabbits immunized with human thyroglobulin, autoantibodies in Graves'patients consistently showed a predominant interaction with one of the antigenic determinants of human thyroglobulin. By contrast, autoantibodies in patients with thyroid carcinoma only differed from those in normal subjects by an increase in serum concentrations. Our data suggest that the repertoire of anti-human thyroglobulin autoantibodies is similar in various species and in normal and pathological conditions and that loss of tolerance results in specific increase of autoantibody concentration.

*EMBO J. 1983, 2, 1821

2197 LYMPHOCYTOTOXIC ANTIBODIES IN AUTOIMMUNE THYROID DISEASE. M. Ryan*, V.Sridama, and L.J. DeGroot. Thyroid Study Unit, Department of Medicine, The University of Chicago, Chicago, IL. U.S.A.

An increased incidence of cold-reactive lymphocytotoxic antibodies (LCTA) has been demonstrated in sera of patients with Graves' disease and Hashimoto's thyroiditis. The cell targets and functional significance of these LCTA have been in dispute. We detected cold-reactive LCTA activity by microcytotoxicity assay in sera from 18 of 79 (24%) Graves' patients, 6 of 21 (29%) Hashimoto's patients, and 5 of 42 (12%) normal controls. LCTA activity was the same in euthyroid treated (23%) and toxic untreated (29%) sera, and among patients treated with surgery, RAI, or antithyroid drugs. There was no correlation between the presence of LCTA activity and age, sex, MCHA titer, TGHA titer, or FTI. Of 19 LCTA positive Graves' sera, 13 (69%) were reactive with B cells alone, 5 were reactive with both B and T cells (26%), and 1 was reactive with T cells alone. In the 6 LCTA positive Hashimoto's sera, 3 were reactive with B cells, and 3 were reactive with both B and T cells, and none with T cells alone. Both suppressor-cytotoxic (OKT8) and helper (OKT4) T-cell subsets were targets of LCTA activity in sera with T-directed lymphocytotoxicity. The OKT4:OKT8 ratio in blood in patients with LCTA was the same as in patients without LCTA. Binding of antilymphocyte IgG, detected by ^{125}I-labeled protein A, did not correlate with LCTA. Lymphocytes from patients with toxic Graves' disease were as susceptible to lysis by lymphocytotoxins as normal lymphocytes. We conclude that antilymphocyte antibodies are: 1) increased in patients with autoimmune thyroid disease, 2) not correlated with age, sex, clinical parameters, or type of treatment, 3) directed primarily against B lymphocytes, 4) presumably IgM antibodies, and 5) equally reactive with normal lymphocytes and toxic Graves' lymphocytes.

2198 HYPERTHYROIDISM INDUCED IN RATS BY LONG-TERM INFUSION OF THYROTROPIN RELEASING HORMONE (TRH). J. Sandow*, W. von Rechenberg, G. Jerabek-Sandow and S. Kille. Hoechst AG, Pharmacology H 821, D-623 Frankfurt/Main 80, Germany, F.R.

The secretion of TSH is activated by hypothalamic TRH, and controlled by long-feedback via thyroid hormone secretion. In adult male rats, the effect of continuous exposure to long-term TRH stimulation was investigated by implanting osmotic minipumps s.c., delivering a daily dose of 0.1-1.0 mg/rat for one or two weeks. Blood samples for hormone determinations (TSH, T3, T4, GH) were taken from jugular catheters, and the tissue content of TRH, TSH, prolactin, GH, ACTH and corticosterone was determined. Biological integrity of TRH in the minipumps was ascertained by the TSH response in recipient rats, at the end of infusion period. Results: Continuous exposure to TRH for one or two weeks caused a significant dose-dependent increase in thyroid weight, serum TSH, T3 and T4. Serum GH was markedly stimulated during the first weeks of infusion. Pituitary content of TSH was dose-dependently depleted, GH content was slightly increased, and prolactin content was unchanged. Pituitary ACTH and adrenal corticosterone content were dose-dependently suppressed. This finding is at variance with the stimulatory effect of TRH on pituitary ACTH content in thyroidectomized male rats. Hypothalamic TRH content did not change with treatment. Conclusions: TRH stimulation by long-term infusion in intact rats enhances TSH secretion, partly depletes pituitary TSH content, and induces hyperthyroidism and goitre formation. Long-term TRH infusion overrules target organ feedback by thyroid hormones, and consistently activates pituitary TSH secretion for 14 days.

2199 THYROXINE UPTAKE BY CULTURED HEPATOCYTES: A MODEL OF BIOAVAILABLE THYROID HORMONE. D. Sarne*, S. Refetoff, A. Horwitz and N.H. Scherberg, Depts. of Medicine and Pediatrics, Univ. of Chicago, Chicago, Illinois USA 60637.

Serum thyroxine (T4) is highly bound to thyroxine-binding globulin (TBG), but only the unbound hormone is thought to be available for cellular uptake. Several laboratory methods have been used to estimate this free T4 fraction. We have examined T4 uptake in cultured hepatocytes and report our findings in this model of bioavailable thyroid hormone. Confluent Hep G2 cells (a human hepatocellular carcinoma cell line) were incubated with medium containing human serum samples and tracer [^{125}I]-T4. Following removal of the medium, the cells were washed and harvested, and the [^{125}I]-T4 taken up by the cells was measured. Cellular uptake of T4 (CT4) was calculated as the product of the fractional uptake of [^{125}I]-T4 by the cells and the total T4 in the medium. Decreasing the amount of TBG or heat inactivation of serum TBG resulted in an increase of CT4. Addition of exogenous T4 also increased CT4. Serum from normal volunteers and patients with hypothyroidism and hyperthyroidism were evaluated in the culture system. Free T4 by equilibrium dialysis (FT4) and a free thyroxine index (FTI) calculated as the product of total T4 and a normalized resin T4 uptake were also determined for the same samples. CT4 correlated with both the FT4 ($r = 0.90$) and the FTI ($r = 0.87$). We conclude that thyroxine uptake in this model 1) reflects the amount of thyroxine available to cells and 2) offers the potential for evaluating factors which may modify the availablility of serum thyroid hormones to tissues. Supported by USPHS Grant AM 06169.

2200 Induction of iodothyronine-5'-deiodinating activity by thyroid hormone, hydrocortisone, and insulin in cultured fetal liver of mouse. K.Sato H.Mimura,* H.D.Chol, T.Tsushima, & K.Shizume. The Second Dep of Int Medicine, Tokyo Women's Medical College, Ichigaya-Kawadacho, Shinjukuku, Tokyo, Japan.

To elucidate the regulatory mechanism of ontogenetic development of iodothyronine-5'-deiodinating activity(IT-5'-DA) in the perinatal period, fetal liver of mice on the 19th day of gestation, in which no IT-5'-DA was detected, was cultured in Dulbecco-Vogt medium supplemented with 10 % fetal calf serum which had been depleted of thyroid hormones by treatment with AG-1X-10 resin. Without addition of hormones, no enzyme activity was detected even though liver cells were cultured for 1 month. Insulin(I) T4, hydrocortisone(HC) alone could not induce the enzyme activity. However, when T_4(10^{-7}M) together with HC(0.1 - 1.0 μg/ml) was supplemented, the enzyme activity was detected. I(1 μg/ml) further enhanced the enzyme activity induced by T_4 and HC. IT-5'-DA was detectable after 3 day culture, peaked at 2 - 3 weeks, and then gradually decreased. The increase in the enzyme activity was due to an increase in Vmax, whereas Km value was not altered. T_3 was more efficacious in inducing the enzyme activity than T_4, whereas rT_3 elicited no biological activity. Half maximal concentrations of T_3 and T_4 in inducing IT-5'-DA were 2×10^{-9} and 7×10^{-8} M, respectively. Free T_3 and T_4 were on the order of 10^{-11} and 10^{-10} M, respectively. The optimum HC concentration for inducing the enzyme activity was 0.4 μg/ml.

These findings suggest that ontogenetic development of iodothyronine-5'-deiodinase in fetal mouse liver is induced by physiological concentrations of thyroid and glucocorticoid hormones and that insulin plays a permissive role in inducing the enzyme activity.

2201 THYROID GROWTH STIMULATING IMMUNOGLOBULINS ESTIMATED BY ^{3}H-THYMIDINE INCORPORATION INTO ISOLATED PORCINE THYROID FOLLICLES IN PATIENTS OF AN IODINE-DEFICIENT GOITER REGION.

H.Schatz*, F.H.Beckmann and M. Floren, Center of Internal Medicine, University of Giessen, F.R.G.

Thyroid growth stimulating immunoglobulins (TGI) appear to act a part in pathogenesis of some forms of goiter. We tried to set up a simple, radiometric TGI assay using ^{3}H-thymidine incorporation into isolated porcine thyroid follicles which are easy to isolate in large amounts from porcine thyroid glands obtained from the slaughter house. After a 24h-culture period for reaggregation, TSH in standard concentrations or patient's immunoglobulins were added for another 24 hrs, together with ^{3}H-thymidine. The normal range for thymidine incorporation (mean $\pm$ 2 standard deviations) was derived from healthy controls. Among 15 patients with the diagnosis " simple (recurrent) goiter", 3 exhibited TGI activity, the highest value for thymidine incorporation was found in a patient who developped a large goiter in spite of a therapy with 15o ug T4. TGI was also detected among goitrous patients with Graves' disease. Conclusions: Porcine thyroid follicles can be used for a simple radiometric TGI-assay. Although Giessen is situated in a region with iodine deficiency, TGI should be considered as a possible cause of " simple (recurrent) goiter" also in this endemic goiter area. For evaluating the clinical significance of TGI, however, larger series of patients have to be studied also longitutionally in our district.

2202 ULTRASONOGRAPHY OF THE ORBIT IN GRAVES' DISEASE.

E.Schifferdecker*, P.M. Schumm, F. Schulz, K. Schöffling. Center of Internal Medicine, Dept. of Endocrinology, University of 6000 Frankfurt a.M., Theodor-Stern-Kai 7, FRG.

Today, computed tomography is the method of choice to examine the retroorbital space for signs of endocrine ophthalmopathy (e.o.) in patients with Graves' disease, but orbital sonography, though less accurate, has some advantages (less expensive, no radiation, easily available) and is therefore suitable as a routine screening method for early e.o. in patients with diffuse hyperthyroidism. Orbital sonogramms were performed in 41 individuals, 15 with apparent e.o., six with diffuse thyrotoxicosis without clinical eye signs, and 20 controls. The Toshiba Ultrasonoskop SAL 20A for B-scans with the PL 50B 5 MHz transducer normally employed for thyroid scans was used; because of its size of 70x22 mm allowing only horizontal scans when placed on the bulbus. In the controls, diameters of medial rectus muscles ranged from 3-6 mm (median 4 mm), diameters of lateral rectus muscles from 2-6 mm (median 3 mm). In the e.o. group, corresponding values were 4-9 mm (median 6 mm) and 3-8 mm (median 6 mm). In nearly all patients with e.o. at least one muscle was 6 mm in diameter; in only two controls one out of the four muscles was 6 mm. The results in hyperthyroid patients without eye signs were heterogenous. Our findings show that with the employed method eye muscle diameters exhibit different distributions in normals and patients with clinically apparent e.o., so a clear distinction between "normal" and "pathological" seems possible, if all muscles would be included in the analysis. However, an improved technique, especially a smaller, better placeable transducer allowing examination of all outer eye muscles is necessary to reach this aim.

2203 EFFECT OF THYROXINE (T4) AND/OR TESTOSTERONE (T) ON EPIDERMAL GROWTH FACTOR (EGF) CONCENTRATIONS IN A CONGENITALLY HYPOTHYROID MOUSE MODEL. S.M. Scott*, J. Lakshmanan, G.G. Buenaflor, and D.A. Fisher. Harbor-UCLA Medical Center UCLA School of Medicine, Torrance, CA 90509

Using a congenitally hypothyroid mouse model (hyt/hyt), we studied the effects of T4 and/or T on submandibular gland (SMG) EGF levels at 20 and 30 days. Male pups were placed into one of 4 groups: A=untreated; B=T treatment (0.5 mg at 7 and 14 days); C=T4 treatment started at birth (0.05 µg/d x 3d, 0.10 µg/d x 3d, 0.25 µg/d x 3d, 0.5 µg/d x 3d, 1.0 µg/d); D=T + T4; Group E was composed of pups from euthyroid control animals. Tissues were homogenized in PBS, 4°C and the 25,000g supernatant was used in a mouse EGF RIA. T4 values are expressed as µg/dl, SMG wt as gm/100 gm BW, and EGF values as ng/mg protein. Results are expressed as Means ± SEM:

	20 days			30 days		
Group	T4	SMG wt	EGF	T4	SMG wt	EGF
A	<0.5	0.70±.03	$0.1\pm.07^{0}$	<0.5	0.76±0.04	26±20*
B	<0.5	0.79±.04	15.1±9	<0.5	0.86±0.09	206±70
C	6.2±.5	$0.99\pm.09^{a}$	6.1±9	5.5±.6	1.05 ± 0.01^{b}	108±50
D	5.8±.8	$1.02\pm.09^{a}$	$32.8\pm10^{\delta}$	6.0±.7	1.10 ± 0.03^{b}	250±100
E	5.7±.8	0.81±.06	1.6±5	4.2±.8	0.79±.04	260±120

By ANOVA: ^{0}*(B-E) > A, δ(D > B, C, E); ^{a,b}(C, D) > (A, B, E); $p<0.05$
In summary: 1) SMG-EGF is markedly reduced in hyt/hyt mice; 2) T4 or T increases SMG-EGF in hyt/hyt mice at 20 and 30 days; 3) At 20 days, T significantly stimulates SMG-EGF without prior exposure to T4 although (T + T4) > T or T4; 4) T4 and T + T4 increases SMG/BW > T.

2204 THE MEASUREMENT OF THYROIDAL IODINE CONCENTRATION BY IN VIVO X-RAY FLUORESCENT ANALYSIS AND ITS CLINICAL IMPLICATION. N. Sekita*, K. Okano, K. Someya, K. Imamura, M. Fujii and Y. Sasaki, Third Dept. of Internal Medicine and Dept. of Radiology, St. Marianna University School of Medicine, Kawasaki, Japan, Dept. of Radiology, Toho University School of Medicine, Tokyo, Japan

With the purpose of evaluating the clinical usefullness of measuring thyroidal iodine concentrations, a simple apparatus was designed and constructed for in vivo x-ray fluorescent analysis. The apparatus consists of an Am-241 exciting source and pure Ge detector($50mm^2$x5mm) for measuring $K\alpha$ fluorescent x-rays emitted from exited iodine. A diversing collimator was so designed that most of one lobe of the thyroid is within the field of view. Iodine concentrations measured in 34 normal thyroids resected at autopsy were 0.53 ± 0.25 mg/g. Iodine concentrations measured on each lobe of the thyroid from 30 healthy volunteers revealed 0.53 ± 0.29mg/g. Iodine concentrations were low in 7 chronic thyroiditis and 7 subacute thyroiditis. Most of 33 patients with Graves' disease showed normal or low iodine concentrations regardless of status of treatment or thyroidal function. Nodule/Gland ratio of I-127 concentration was 0.77 ± 0.46 in 27 patients with cold nodule and 1.56 ± 0.25 in 5 with hot nodule. When thyroidal iodine concentrations were compared with CT units (Hounsfield unit) of the thyroid glands in computed tomography, there was significant positive correlations both in normals and the patients with thyroid diseases. This method for the measurement of thyroidal iodine concentration is much lower than that of computed tomography in exposure dose and seems to be useful especially for the diagnosis of thyroid carcinoma.

2205 PLASMA β-ENDORPHIN, DEXAMETHASONE NON-SUPPRESSIBILITY AND MOOD CHANGES IN THE PUERPERIUM.

R. Smith*, M. Brinsmead, B. Singh, P. Owens, T. Lewin and C. Hall. Faculty of Medicine, University of Newcastle, Newcastle, N.S.W. Australia.

This study was performed to determine the relationship between the hypothalamic-pituitary-adrenal axis and the mood disturbances of the puerperium. In 13 pregnant women plasma β-endorphin, cortisol and mood status was assessed before, during and after labour. Overnight Dexamethasone Suppression Tests (DST) were performed at 4 days post partum and from 1 to 5 months later. The DST was also performed in 11 patients presenting with post partum psychiatric states. Results of the DST in these two groups were compared with control subjects (depression, psychosis, normal women, women on oestrogens and men). Plasma β-endorphin and cortisol rose dramatically at the time of labour and was related to the type of obstetric analgesia. Plasma β-endorphin and cortisol returned to normal by 4 days post partum. Post-partum women showed a brief period of elevated mood up to the 3rd day followed by a depression of mood. On the 5th day post partum plasma cortisol (at 4 pm) after dexamethasone was dramatically elevated compared to the control groups but had returned to normal in the majority of patients when repeated at 1 to 5 months. In the 11 patients with post partum psychiatric states the plasma cortisol failed to suppress normally in 7. The previously unreported abnormalities of the post partum DST may be related to limbic-hypothalamic system dysfunction, to disturbances of cortisol binding or to altered dexamethasone metabolism. The peri-partum changes in β-endorphin may help to explain the phenomenon of the 'post-partum blues".

2206 MAJOR AFFECTIVE DISORDERS:FURTHER EVIDENCE FOR DYSFUNCION OF THE HYPOTHALAMIC PITUITARY ADRENAL AXIS.

C.Stefanis[1], J.Chan[2], N.Seidah[2], M.Chrétien[2] and G.Tolis*[3,4], Eginition[1] and Hippokrateion[3] Hospitals,Athens,Greece, Clinical Research Institute[2] and McGill University[4],Montreal,Quebec,Canada.

Radioimmunoassayable cortisol and N-POMC were measured in serum samples obtained from 27 patients with major affective disorders (unipolar n:19,bipolar n:8,DSM-III class.).Blood was drawn at 0800 and 2300 h prior to and at 0800,1600 and 2300 h after the administration of 1 mg dexamethasone.

Patients with values of N-POMC >100pg/ml or cortisol > 5 ug/dl were considered as non-suppressors.

Absence of circadian periodicity and suppressibility of plasma cortisol was found in 46% and 32% of patients respectively. N-POMC values were elevated at 2300 h prior to Dex in 77% of patients (mean 235.3,range 117-326 pg/ml. Following the administration of Dexamethasone plasma N-POMC values suppressed in 40% of patients at 0800 h but only in 24% at 1600 h and in 21% at 2300 h indicative of an escape phenomenon. In 62% of cortisol suppressors N-POMC values were in excess of 150 pg/ml.

No correlation was found between basal cortisol or N-POMC values and rating of the depressive symptoms with Hamilton scale.

The above data suggest that in major affective disorders there is a considerable dysfunction of the hypothalamic pituitary adrenal axis as far as the circadian periodicity and suppressibility to Dexamethasone. The dissociation between cortisol and N-POMC dynamics in depressive disorders deserves further investigation.

2207 LEUMORPHIN IS A NOVEL ENDOGENOUS OPIOID PEPTIDE IN MAN. M. Suda*, K. Nakao, M. Sakamoto, T. Yoshimasa, N. Morii, Y. Ikeda, S. Oki, I. Tanaka, C. Yanaihara, N. Yanaihara, S. Numa, and H. Imura, 2nd Division, Department of Medicine and Department of Medical Chemistry (S.N.), Kyoto University Faculty of Medicine, Kyoto 606, Shizuoka College of Pharmacy, Shizuoka (C.Y.) and National Institute for Physiological Sciences, Okazaki (N.Y.), Japan.

Leumorphin corresponds to amino acid residues 228-256 of preproenkephalin B, a common precursor of neo-endorphin and dynorphin. Leumorphin is a potent κ opioid receptor agonist (Suda et al. Life Sci. 32, 2769, 1983) and exists in porcine pituitaries (Nakao et al. BBRC in press). Currently, the gene sequence analysis of human proenkephalin B shows that human leumorphin differs in 3 amino acid compositions from porcine leumorphin (Horikawa et al. Nature in press). We now report the opioid activity and the endogenous existence of human leumorphin. In the guinea pig ileum assay, synthetic human leumorphin was 150 times more potent than Leu-enkephalin. This peptide inhibited the contraction of the rabbit vas deferens known to have only the κ opioid receptor. Reverse phase HPLC and gel permeation chromatography coupled with a RIA for leumorphin and rimorphin revealed that leumorphin-like immunoreactivities (LM-LI) in extracts from human striatum emerged at the same elution positions as those of synthetic leumorphin and rimorphin. LM-LI and dynorphin-LI distributed in parallel throughout the brain. These observations along with the recent evidence of the predominance of κ opioid binding sites in the human brain suggest that human leumorphin plays an important physiological role in the human central nervous system.

2208 EFFECTS OF EXOGENOUS BETA-ENDORPHIN ON THE PITUITARY AND ADRENAL GLANDS. S. Tan*, Loma Linda University, Loma Linda, California 92350, U.S.A.

Since the discovery of opiate receptors in the brain, pituitary and adrenal glands, the role of opioids as neurotransmitter and hormone modulator has been postulated. This study investigates the effect of beta-endorphin (β-EP) on the pituitary and adrenal hormones. Intravenous administration of β-EP (25 μg/kg) to normal men causes an increase in prolactin (peak Δ of 16±4.2 ng/ml over basal levels, $p<0.001$), plasma renin activity (PRA, Δ 4.3±1.2 ng/ml/h, $p<0.02$) and plasma aldosterone (Δ 4.5±2.6 ng/dl, $p<0.05$), but decreases LH (nadir ∇ -4.4±0.5 mIU/ml below basal levels, $p<0.02$) and cortisol (∇ -9.7±1.0 μg/dl, $p<0.001$) levels. There are no significant change in ACTH, FSH, growth hormone and TSH levels. Intravenous administration of 2 mg naloxone 15 min prior to β-EP injection followed by naloxone infusion (1 μg/kg/min for 120 min) abolish the prolactin rise, blunt the PRA and aldosterone increase, produce a paradoxical rise in ACTH (Δ 12±3.7 pg/ml, $p<0.01$), and increase LH (Δ 8.4±2.0 mIU/ml, $p<0.01$) and cortisol (Δ 6.5±3.5 μg/dl, $p<0.05$) levels. Administration of naloxone injection and infusion without β-EP produces similar rise of LH and cortisol, but stimulates greater ACTH rise (Δ 35±7.4 pg/ml, $p<0.001$). Oral ingestion of 0.3 mg clonidine 1 h prior to β-EP injection enhances the PRA rise (Δ 9.8±2.1 ng/ml/h, $p<0.005$) and naloxone fails to blunt this rise. These data suggest that the actions of β-EP on the pituitary and adrenals are mediated through opioid receptors, and the action on renin secretion is modulated by the sympathetic nervous system.

2209 ENKEPHALIN-CONTAINING PEPTIDES OF PHEOCHROMOCYTOMA. Glen R. Van Loon* and Shaker Mousa, Veterans Administration Medical Center and Department of Medicine, University of Kentucky, Lexington, Kentucky 40511.

Enkephalin-containing peptides have been localized in chromaffin cells of the adrenal medulla and in pheochromocytoma. It remains unclear to what extent processing of the precursor molecule, proenkephalin A, occurs in pheochromocytoma. In this study, we have used high pressure liquid chromatography with electrochemical detection to specifically quantitate the enkephalin-containing peptides in adrenal pheochromocytomas from two patients. We quantitated not only free [Met] and [Leu]enkephalin, but also [Met]enkephalin sulfoxide and a number of extended enkephalin peptides. These included [Met]enkephalin-Arg^{6}-Phe^{7} which represents the carboxy terminus of proenkephalin A, [Met]enkephalin-Arg^{6}-Gly^{7}-Leu^{8}, an internal sequence, and peptide E, a pentacosapeptide sequence containing both a [Met]enkephalin and a [Leu]enkephalin residue. However, the concentrations and molar ratios of these peptides in the two tumors differed. Although the [Met]enkephalin residues of proenkephalin A are flanked by paired basic amino acid residues, incubation of tumor tissue with trypsin did not increase the concentration of free [Met]enkephalin. Thus, processing of proenkephalin A in pheochromocytoma yields a number of enkephalin-containing peptides similar to those identified in bovine adrenal medulla, but processing may differ considerably in these tissues.

2210 CONTROL OF α-MSH RELEASE FROM THE PARS INTERMEDIA OF THE AMPHIBIAN XENOPUS LAEVIS; A MICROSUPERFUSION STUDY. B.M.L. Verburg-Van Kemenade*, B.G. Jenks, M.C. Tonon, H. Vaudry and A.P. van Overbeeke, Dept. Zoology, Cath. Univ., Nijmegen, The Netherlands and Groupe Recherche Endocrinol. Moléc., Univ. Rouen, Mt-St-Aignan, France.

In amphibians the pars intermedia plays an important role in color adaptation of the skin. In black background adapted clawed toads, Xenopus laevis, this gland exhibits high rates of biosynthesis of pro-opiomelanocortin (POMC), processing of POMC to a number of peptides, including α-melanocyte stimulating hormone (α-MSH), and release of these peptides. In white-adapted animals biosynthetic activity and hormone release are very low. The purpose of the present study was to analyse the role of a number of potential secretagogues on the release of α-MSH. Individual neurointermediate lobes of Xenopus were superfused in a microsuperfusion system up to 6 hours, during which period pulses of secretagogues were administered. Fractions of the superfusate were collected and their α-MSH content measured by radioimmunoassay. In lobes of black-adapted animals, dopamine (conc. ranging from 10^{-8} to 10^{-6} M) caused a dose-dependent, reversible inhibition of α-MSH release. There was no desensitization of the tissue to dopamine. Gamma-aminobutyric acid (GABA) (conc. ranging from 10^{-5} to 10^{-4} M) also inhibited α-MSH release in a dose-dependent manner. No effects were obtained with phenylephrine and isoproterenol (an α- and a β-adrenergic receptor agonist, resp.), with corticotropin releasing factor (CRF), with serotonin or with melatonin. Thyrotropin releasing hormone (TRH) did not affect α-MSH release from lobes of black-adapted animals, but stimulated α-MSH release from lobes of white-adapted toads.

2211 THE ROLE OF CYCLIC AMP (CAMP) ON CORTICOTROPIN RELEASING FACTOR (CRF) MEDIATED ACTH SECRETION. S. Vernigor* and D. Sobel, Naval Hospital Bethesda & USUHS, Departments of Medicine & Pediatrics, Bethesda, MD 20814, USA.

CAMP many be an important mediator of ACTH secretion by the observation that CRF stimulates pituitary intracellular CAMP(Labrie 1982). To further investigate the role of CAMP as a mediator of CRF stimulated ACTH release, we studied 1)the action of 3 phosphodiesterase inhibitors, caffeine, theophyllin and isobutylmethylxanthine (IBMX),stimulators of intracellular CAMP, on CRF mediated ACTH release 2)the effect of ^{8}Br-CAMP on CRF mediated ACTH release 3)the generation of intracellular CAMP induced by CRF. Anterior pituitaries were dispersed to single cells in trypsin. Culture dishes with $3.5x10^{5}$cells were incubated 3 days, washed, and replaced with test media for 3.5 hrs. Intracellular CAMP and culture media ACTH were determined by RIA. A nonstimulatory dose of caffeine(0.5mM) increased CRF(10nM) induced ACTH release from 3.83±0.20 (no caffeine) to 4.73±0.21ng/dish($p<0.05$). CRF mediated ACTH release of 3.17±0.08ng/dish was augmented to 4.98±0.34ng/dish with the addition of a nonstimulatory dose of theophyllin(50μM)$p<0.01$. A nonstimulatory dose of IBMX increased CRF (10nM) mediated ACTH release from 3.51±0.18ng/dish to 4.63±0.15($p<0.05$). ACTH release induced by a maximal stimulatory dose of CRF(100nM)(20.86±0.70ng/dish) was not altered with the addition of a maximal stimulatory dose of ^{8}Br-CAMP(7mM) (21.25±0.20ng/dish). CRF(10nM) induced a 150% increment of intracellular CAMP over control cells. Summary: 1) caffeine, theophyllin and IBMX potentiate CRF mediated ACTH release in primary rat pituitary cell culture 2) ACTH release induced by a maximal stimulatory dose of CRF is not increased by CAMP 3) CRF (10nM) stimulated intracellular CAMP is confirmed. This data provides further evidence that CRF stimulated ACTH release is mediated by CAMP.

2212 REGULATION OF BRAIN β-ENDORPHIN BY SEX STEROIDS: DIFFERENCES BETWEEN MALES AND FEMALES. Sharon L. Wardlaw* and Andrew G. Frantz, Dept. of Medicine, Columbia University College of Physicians and Surgeons, New York, N.Y.

We have previously reported that the concentration of hypothalamic β-endorphin (β-EP) in cycling female rats is unchanged by ovariectomy. However, chronic treatment of ovariectomized rats with physiological levels of estradiol lowers hypothalamic β-EP, possibly by increasing β-EP release in the presence of constant rather than fluctuating levels of estradiol. The present study was designed to compare brain β-EP in males and cycling females and to examine the effect of orchiectomy and testosterone replacement on brain β-EP. Hypothalamic β-EP was measured in 3 groups of 16 rats each: 1) male compared to female rats of the same weight; 2) intact vs. castrated males (4 weeks); 3) castrated males treated for 4 weeks with either testosterone or sham silastic capsules. The medial basal hypothalamus (MBH), median eminence (ME), and anterior hypothalamus (AH) were homogenized in 0.2N HCl and assayed for β-EP by RIA. In the MBH the β-EP content in males was 6.97 ± .70 (SEM) ng compared to 9.17 ± .54 ng in females ($p<.025$). After orchiectomy, the β-EP content of the MBH rose from 7.15 ± .35 ng in the intact males to 9.08 ± .43 ($p<.005$). In another group of orchiectomized rats, the β-EP content fell to 6.91 ± .18 ng with testosterone compared to 10.8 ± .39 ng without testosterone replacement ($p<.001$). Increases were also seen in the ME and AH after orchiectomy which were reversed by treatment with testosterone. We conclude that testosterone as well as estradiol affects brain β-EP. In addition, the effect on brain β-EP depends on whether the steroids are secreted constantly as in the male or fluctuate as in the cycling female.

2213 MALE PSEUDOHERMAPHRODITISM AND ADRENOCORTICAL HYPERPLASIA DUE TO COMBINED 17,20 DESMOLASE, 21 HYDROXLYASE DEFICIENCY. R. Peterson*, J. Imperato-McGinley, T. Gautier, C. Shackleton, Cornell University Medical College, NY, University Pedro Henriquez Urena, Dominican Republic, and University Calif., Berkeley.

A 4.5 y 46XY child with pseudovaginal perinealscrotal hypospadias and cryptorchidism was evaluated at 7 and 16 mos. Basal plasma concentrations (specific RIA's) of androstenedione, testosterone (T) dehydroepiandrosterone and its sulfate were low-normal before and after ACTH stimulation (6 hr iv). Basal plasma levels of progesterone (P 0.5-2.0 ug%), 17αhydroxyprogesterone (17P 0.19 ug%), corticosterone (B 2.4-4.0 ug%) and (desoxycorticosterone (DOC 0.026-0.04 ug%) were elevated. Plasma cortisol was (F 8-13 ug%). hCG stimulated plasma testosterone (T) was only 32 ng%. ACTH (6 hr iv) stimulated plasma B (10 ug%) and 17P (2.26 ug%) were abnormally increased. Gas liquid chromatography of basal and ACTH urines demonstrated elevated B metabolites but no 11-oxo or 11-deoxo C19 steroids. At 3.7 y plasma levels of P (2.0 ug%), B (4.8 ug%), DOC (0.06 ug%), 17P (0.86 ug%), pregnenolone (0.29 ug%), 17α hydroxypregnenolone (0.11 ug%) were elevated. hCG (12 days) modestly increased these steroids, but plasma T rose only to 64 ng%. ACTH (14 hr iv) increased levels of all C21 steroids but not C19 steroids. At 4.5 y plasma P was 6.0 ug%, F and B 6.0-9.6 ug% and 17P 1.5 ug%. Plasma levels of ACTH (pm x5) were high at 475-850 pg/ml. All plasma steroid levels were suppressed below normal by dexamethasone. This is first report of male pseudohermaphoroditism due to 17, 20 adrenal and gonadal desmolase deficiency, combined with partial adrenal 21-hydroxylase deficiency and adrenocortical hyperplasia secondary to deficient cortisol secretion.

2214 POTASSIUM MODULATION OF CORTISOL SECRETION FROM PERIFUSED NORMAL AND HYPERFUNCTIONING HUMAN ADRENAL CELLS. L. M. Robertson,* D. Cook, L. D. Keith, and J. W. Kendall, Research Service, VA Medical Center and Dept. of Medicine, Oregon Health Sciences University, Portland, OR 97201, U.S.A.

Recently we demonstrated that extracellular potassium (K^+) concentrations modulate secretion of corticosterone (B) from perifused mouse adrenal cells. In the present study, we examined the effect of variations in K^+ concentration on secretion of cortisol (F) from normal and hyperfunctioning (hyperplastic, adenomatous) human adrenal tissues. Each tissue was dispersed with collagenase and perifused (1 ml/min) with Dulbecco's Modified Eagle Medium supplemented with 0.1 % BSA (DMEM). F concentration in two-min fractions was determined by radioimmunoassay. The antiserum has less than 1 % crossreactivity with B and aldosterone. In normal cells, a 10-min exposure to 54 mM K^+ DMEM elicited a significant increase in F secretion ($p<0.01$). The response was equal to that obtained with a two-min exposure to 20 pg/ml ACTH and comparable to that found with normal mouse adrenal cells. Variations in K^+ concentration did not modulate basal secretion in the adenomatous cells. In hyperplastic cells, the response to 10 min of 54 mM K^+ DMEM was significantly smaller than that obtained with two min of 20 pg/ml ACTH ($p<0.01$). In all hyperfunctioning cells the response to 20 pg/ml ACTH was diminished in the presence of K^+-free DMEM. CONCLUSIONS: 1) variations in K^+ concentration modulate basal F secretion from normal human adrenal cells; 2) there are qualitative differences between normal and hyperfunctioning human adrenal cells in response to variations in K^+ concentration. These results are consistant with the hypothesis that ions are involved in the etiology of human adrenocortical hyperfunction.

2215 USEFULNESS OF URINARY 6β-HYDROXYCORTISOL (6βOHF) EXCRETION IN THE DIAGNOSIS OF CUSHING'S SYNDROME. P. Saenger*, R.E. Peterson, Dept. Peds., Montefiore Med. Ctr., Dept. Med., Cornell Univ. Med., New York.

Rapid and simple laboratory diagnosis of cortisol excess due to Cushing's syndrome is highly desirable. To date chronic overproduction of cortisol and loss of diurnal cortisol variation are considered to be the most consistent metabolic abnormalities in Cushing's syndrome. Nonetheless free urinary cortisol (F) and plasma cortisol levels may yield false negative results. We therefore applied a recently developed RIA for 6βOHF. 6βOHF is the major unconjugated urinary metabolite of cortisol. In the evaluation of 33 adolescents and young adults for Cushing's syndrome near normal 17OH corticosteroids (<14mg/24h and/or F (<120μg/24h) were found in 6 patients. 6βOHF was at least 10 times above nl in all 33 patients (mean: 8.11mg/24± 2.01(SE)mg/24h vs nl 0.4±0.1mg/24h). The ratio of 6βOHF/F was also markedly elevated (mean 14.8±3.3; vs nl 6.7±1). The highest 6βOHF excretion was seen in patients with ectopic ACTH production and adrenal cancer (35 and 75mg/24h respectively). The data show that 6βOHF is a rapid and reliable test for hypercortisolemia due to Cushing's syndrome. 6βOHF proved to discriminate better than either 17OH corticosteroids or F; no false negative or positive cases were seen in the present series. Our data suggest further that excess ACTH indirectly and cortisol directly induce 6β-hydroxylase activity causing highly diagnostic increases in 6βOHF excretion. Measurement of urinary 6βOHF is therefore suggested as a new, clinically useful test in the evaluation of hypercortisolemic states in adolescence.

2216 THE EFFICACY OF 131-I-METAIODOBENZYLGUANIDINE (MIBG) SCINTIGRAPHY FOR LOCATION OF PHEOCHROMOCYTOMAS; EXPERIENCE IN 400 CASES. B. Shapiro*, J. Copp, J. Sisson, P. Eyre and W. Beierwaltes. University of Michigan, Ann Arbor, Michigan, 48109, USA.

The radiopharmaceutical 131-I-MIBG follows the pathway of norepinephrine into adrenergic tissues and thus permits the location of pheochromocytomas varying widely in type and site. This is noninvasive and allows the entire body to be screened in a single procedure. The results in 400 cases referred for suspected pheochromocytomas were reviewed and the scan results classified as true positive, true negative, false positive, false negative, equivocal positive and equivocal negative on the basis of plasma and urine catecholamines; CT scan, angiography and other radiological procedures; surgical exploration and histology; and follow up. There were 30 sporadic adrenal, 17 sporadic extra-adrenal (9 intrathoracic and 9 intrabdominal), 47 malignant metastatic and 12 familial adrenal case. In 207 cases pheochromocytoma was definitely ruled out and in 80 cases probably ruled out.

Group	Sensitivity %	Specificity %
Sporadic Benign	81.1	98.9
Malignant	93.3	NA
Familial	80.0	100

Thus where available 131-I-MIBG scintigraphy is the technique of choice for initial location of pheochromocytomas.

2217 ETOMIDATE ANESTHESIA INHIBITS THE CORTISOL RESPONSE TO SURGICAL STRESS

B. Sherman*, M. Mehta and M. Ghoneim, Departments of Internal Medicine and Anesthesiology, University of Iowa, Iowa City, IA, USA 52242

Etomidate, R-(+) ethyl-1(Phenylethyl)-IH-imidazole-5 caroxylate is a potent, short-acting hypnotic used for total intravenous anesthesia. Increased mortality associated with surprisingly low plasma cortisol levels was reported in critically ill patients who received etomidate for sedation in an intensive care setting. We measured plasma cortisol and ACTH during and following surgery in 18 patients undergoing routine gynecologic procedures, 9 of whom received etomidate and 9 methohexital, a rapidly-acting barbiturate. The mean plasma cortisol and ACTH concentrations before anesthesia were not different in the two groups, 11.1±1.5 vs 12.1±1.6 μg/dl and 26.2±5.6 vs 25.4±5.8 pg/ml respectively. After the start of surgery, the mean plasma cortisol concentration increased to 25-30 μg/dl in the methohexital group. Cortisol levels did not increase in any patient in the etomidate group, remaining between 6-8 μg/dl. Plasma ACTH rose in both groups, reaching 404±115.6 pg/ml in the etomidate group and 572.3±189.4 pg/ml in the methohexital group. The rise in plasma prolactin and growth hormone was equivalent in the two groups. Etomidate appears to be a rapidly-acting, previously unrecognized inhibitor of adrenal steroidogenesis. The absence of clinical consequences associated with the blunted adrenal response suggests that a major increase in adrenal hormone production may not be necessary to cope satisfactorily with the stress of surgery. However, prolonged use for the purposes of sedation could result in complete inhibition of adrenal function and the consequences of adrenal insufficiency.

2218 A NEONATAL MASS-SCREENING FOR CONGENITAL ADRENAL HYPERPLASIA(CAH) DUE TO 21-HYDROXYLASE DEFICIENCY IN JAPAN.

K.Shimozawa*, S.Saisho, N.Saito, N.Sakurada, J.Yata, Y.Hikita, K.Kawanami, A.Takehiro, Y.Igarashi, K.Okada, Y.Harada, Y.Hyodo and M.Irie. Dept. of Pediatr., Sch. of Med., Tokyo Med. & Dent. Univ. ; Dept. of Pediatr., Sch. of Med., Hamamatsu Univ.; Obstetricians' Associ. in the West of Shizuoka Prefecture; The 1st Dept. of Intern. Med., Sch. of Med., Toho Univ., Tokyo, Japan.

We devised a simplified radioimmunoassay method for 17-OH-progesterone (17-OHP) using a 3 mm disc of dried blood on filter paper. Using this method, a pilot neonatal mass-screening study for CAH had been carried out for a period of 30 months in Shizuoka Prefecture, Japan. During this period 34,314 neonates were screened, and the mean "Disc-17-OHP" value and S.D. were 19.8 and 9.54 pg/disc, respectively. We tentatively decided the 99th-percentile value as a recalling point, resulting 335 neonates(0.98%) were candidates for recall. Out of them, 208 infants who responded to recall were evaluated by physical examinations, plasma electrolytes, plasma 17-OHP and 21-deoxycortisol concentrations as well as pregnanetriol and pregnanetriolone values in spot urine specimen and in a part of responders plasma 17-OH-pregnenolone and its sulfate were also examined. As a result, 3 infants(2 salt-losers and 1 simple-virilizer) were proved to have CAH and incidence of CAH and its heterozygous carrier were calculated to be 1/11,438 and 1/54, respectively, in Japan.

Althouth there are yet several problems to be solved, the present study demonstrates the good feasibility of neonatal mass-screening program for CAH and indicates that the incidence of CAH is probably much greater than that previously reported by case-assessment in Japan(1/43,764).

2219 The In Vivo Effect of Ovine Prolactin (oPRL) on Adrenal Steroidogenic Enzyme Activities in the Female Rat. M.L. Sienkiewicz*, J. Karanian, S. Liu, D. Bolt+, R. Knazek, D.L. Loriaux and B.D. Albertson. +USDA Research Center, Beltsville, Md., and DEB, NICHD, NIH, Bethesda, Md.

To explore the effect of prolactin on adrenal cortical function, graded doses of purified oPRL (0, 1.0, 10.0 & 100.0 ug) were injected subcutaneously into hypophysectomized, PMSG and HCG treated rats every 4 hours for 4 days. The animals were decapitated, adrenal glands weighed and mitochondria and microsomes purified by previously described techniques (JCI 67: 1177, 1981). Adrenal 3β-hydroxysteroid dehydrogenase/isomerase (3β-HSD), 17-hydroxylase (17-OHase), 21-hydroxylase (21-OHase) and 11-hydroxylase (11-OHase) were measured using 14C-labelled DHA, Progesterone and DOC, respectively, as substrates. Steroid products were verified by derivative formation. Adrenal weight and histology in the oPRL treated animals did not differ from vehicle treated animals. Adrenal enzyme activities are given as nM or pM product formed/min/mg protein.

Dose oPRL ug	Plasma oPRL ng/ml	3β-HSD nM/min/mg P	17-OHase pM/min/mg P	21-OHase nM/min/mg P	11-OHase pM/min/mg P
0	4.5± 0.5	9.4±0.5	1397.4±116.1	11.3±0.7	259.0±24.1
1.0	3.7± 0.6	4.0±0.2§	381.3± 40.1§	5.2±0.5§	63.1± 4.1*
10.0	23.1± 6.8*	3.9±0.1	270.0± 20.5*	4.7±0.3	166.2± 9.5†
100.0	134.4±30.3†	2.0±0.1	274.3± 16.6	2.9±0.2§	20.1± 4.4§

* p<.05 † p<.01 § p<.001 vs previous dose

We conclude that oPRL administered to hypoxed, gonadotropin replaced female rats produces a decrease in adrenal 3β-HSD, 17-OHase, 21-OHase and 11-OHase in a dose dependent manner.

2220 EFFECTS OF HEMODIALYSIS (HD) ON CIRCULATING LEVELS OF ADRENAL ZONA GLOMERULOSA (ZG) AND FASCICULATA (ZF) STEROIDS. C.T. Spalding,* P.G. Zager, H.J. Frey and M. Brittenham, Univ. of New Mexico, Albuquerque, New Mexico, USA.

We compared the responses of circulating levels of ZG and ZF steroids to HD (n=8). Plasma levels of ZG steroids, e.g., 18-hydroxycorticosterone (18-OH-B) and aldosterone (Aldo) and ZF steroids, e.g., corticosterone (B), cortisol (F), 11 deoxycorticosterone (DOC) and 18-hydroxy-11-deoxycorticosterone (18-OH-DOC) were measured immediately before and after a 4h HD.

	18-OH-B ng/dl	Aldo ng/dl	B ng/dl	F µg/dl	DOC ng/dl	18-OH-DOC ng/dl
Pre	88 ± 41	34 ± 15	304 ± 89	16 ± 2	4.8 ± 0.9	8.2 ± 2.2
Post	35* ± 19	13** ± 7	276 ± 104	13 ± 2	3.5 ± 0.9	5.9 ± 1.2

*p = .05 post vs. pre
**p < .05

HD decreased plasma levels of ZG but not ZF steroids. Measurements of Aldo and 18-OH-B in blood and dialysate sampled before and after passage through the artificial kidney revealed no significant dialysance of either steroid. HD removed 1.1 ± 2.4 L of extracellular fluid and decreased plasma potassium from 5.1 ± 0.3 to 3.7 ± 0.3 mEq/L (p < .001). Conclusions: Circulating levels of ZG steroids decreased during HD despite significant ultrafiltration and no changes in plasma levels of ZF steroids and presumably ACTH. Plasma potassium is a major factor in the regulation of plasma 18-OH-B and Aldo during HD.

2221 THE MAINTENANCE OF STRUCTURE AND FUNCTION OF ADRENAL ZONA GLOMERULOSA CELLS IN LIPOPROTEIN-DEFICIENT RATS. D.Szabó,[x] K.Sz. Szalay and I.E. Tóth, Institute of Experimental Medicine Hungarian Academy of Sciences 1450 Budapest, P.O.B. 67., Hungary.

Lipoprotein deficiency was maintained for 48 hours by applying 4-aminopyrazolo-(3,4-d)-pyrimidine in male albino rats and the effect on the structure and function of isolated adrenocortical cells was investigated. Neither the morphology nor the steroidogenic response of zona glomerulosa cells changed; however, in the zona fasciculata cells a marked reduction in the quantity of lipid droplets was associated with a decreased steroidogenic response to ACTH. The results indicate that despite of lipoprotein deficiency, zona glomerulosa cells contain a reserve of intracellular cholesterol, thus retaining their responsiveness to stimulation. The fact that the lipoprotein deficiency does not affect lipid droplets located in the glomerulosa cells and in the fasciculata cells in a similar manner, is probably due to the differences in their physical state and chemical composition.

2222 DELAYED AGING OF PITUITARY-THYROID FUNCTION IN TRYPTOPHAN-DEFICIENT AND FOOD RESTRICTED FEMALE LONG EVANS RATS. A. Vallerga* and P.S. Timiras. Dept. of Physiology/Anatomy, Univ. of Calif., Berkeley, CA, 94720, U.S.A.

Juvenile rats fed diets restricted in the essential amino acid tryptophan experience a delay in growth and maturation similar to rats on a food restricted regimen. At late ages, when the tryptophan-deficient rats are provided a normal diet, they show a delay in age-related impairment of homeostatic response to cold, reproductive competence and coat quality and postponed onset of tumoregenesis and mortality. In view of the importance of thyroid hormones as putative modulators or pacemakers for growth, development and aging, we have measured serum and pituitary TSH, total serum T4 and T3 levels throughout the lifespan in control, tryptophan-deficient and food restricted female Long-Evans rats. In controls, total T4 and TSH first decreased by 12 months; at 24 mos.T4 remained low while serum TSH markedly increased as compared to 4 month levels; total T3 was unchanged. In tryptophan-deficient rats, T4 only slightly decreased at 24 mos.; TSH increased early and remained high; T3 was low at 2 and 4 mos. but increased thereafter. In food restricted rats, total T4 also remained essentially unchanged with age as compared to 4 mos. controls; TSH levels were similar to the tryptophan-deficient rats; total T3 was high between 2 and 4 mos. but declined to low levels by 12 mos. and remained unchanged at 24 mos. These data show that T4 levels do not undergo the changes induced by age as in control rats when the animals are maintained from weaning on restricted diets; it is speculated that persistence in normal thyroid function in these restricted animals may explain the delay in aging reported after tryptophan and food restriction. Aided by NIH Grant AG-00043.

2223 AGE-RELATED CHANGES IN THE DISTRIBUTION OF FORMS OF β- AND γ-ENDORPHINS IN THE BRAINS OF RATS. Charles W. Wilkinson* and Daniel M. Dorsa, GRECC, VA Medical Center, and Univ. of Washington, Seattle, WA, USA.

We investigated age-associated changes in regional concentrations and structural forms of β-endorphins (βE) and γ-endorphins (γE) in the brains and pituitaries of rats using a combination of reverse phase high performance liquid chromatography (HPLC) and radioimmunoassay. Ten 8-month old and ten 24-month old male Fischer 344 rats were decapitated. Brains and pituitaries were quickly removed, dissected into 12 areas, and frozen on dry ice. Tissues were boiled in 1 M acetic acid, sonicated, and the peptides were eluted from ODS-silica cartridges using 80% acetonitrile (ACN) containing 0.1% trifluoroacetic acid (TFA). The peptides were separated on a 5 μ, 330 Å pore, C_{18} reverse phase column using a gradient of 80% ACN containing 0.1% TFA against 0.11% TFA in water with detection at 210 nm. Fractions were collected and assayed for γE-like immunoreactivity (γE-LI) and βE-LI. The predominant form of βE-LI in the hypothalami of young rats co-eluted with βE 1-31 standards. Less than 2% of the total βE-LI was present in fractions co-eluting with α-N-acetylated forms. Total βE-LI and βE 1-31 concentrations were lower in hypothalami of old rats than in young rats. Although distribution of forms was highly variable in the old rats, as much as 10 times the amount of acetylated forms of βE 1-31, 1-27, and 1-26 was found in the hypothalami of old rats relative to that in young rats. Similar age-associated differences were found in the distribution of γE-LI. As much as 40% of γE-LI in old rat hypothalami was found in fractions co-eluting with α-N-acetylated γE. Only trace amounts of γE-LI co-eluting with acetylated γE could be found in young rat hypothalami. Distribution of γE- and βE-related peptides in rat hypothalamus changes with age with a tendency toward a relative increase in acetylated forms.

2224 CYCLIC NUCLEOTIDE REGULATION OF GnRH RECEPTORS IN VITRO: DEPENDENCE ON CALCIUM AND MICROTUBULE FUNCTION. L. S. Young*, S. I. Naik and R. N. Clayton, Department of Medicine, University of Birmingham, B15 2TH, England

Exogenous cyclic adenosine nucleotides increase GnRH receptors (GnRH-R) in intact cultured rat pituitary cells in a similar manner to that observed with GnRH itself. Pituitary cells were cultured in Ca^{2+} and serum-containing medium for 60 hr prior to treatment with dibutyryl cAMP (dbcAMP, 1 mM), GnRH (1 nM), or KCl (58 mM) for 10 hr. Cells were harvested, washed x 3, and incubated with ^{125}I-GnRH-agonist (GnRH-A) to determine receptor content. Under these conditions all three agents increased GnRH-R by 50-100%. Incubation of pituitary cells with 3 mM EGTA for 10 hr reduced unstimulated receptor levels by 20% and completely prevented the stimulation of GnRH-R by either dbcAMP, GnRH or KCl (control = 5.6 ± 0.4, EGTA = 4.6 ± 0.5, dbcAMP = 14.7 ± 0.7, dbcAMP + EGTA = 3.25 ± 0.1 fmol/10^6 cells). Similarly, Co-incubation of pituitary cells with these stimulators and verapamil (100 μM) prevented GnRH-R increases. Calcium ionophore (A23187) increased GnRH-R at low concentrations (control = 8.3 ± 0.4, 10 nM A23187 = 11.8 ± 1.2, 100 nM A23187 = 13.3 ± 0.2 fmol/10^6 cells). Treatment with vinblastine for 10 hr (VIN, 100 μM) reduced basal GnRH-R by 60%. However, 1 μM VIN did not affect basal receptor levels but markedly reduced the increase in GnRH-R stimulated by all three agents (control = 6.7 ± 0.1, VIN = 6.9 ± 0.7, dbcAMP = 13.0 ± 1.5, dbcAMP + VIN = 7.2 ± 0.9 fmol/10^6 cells). These results indicate that receptor stimulation by dbcAMP, GnRH and KCl is a calcium dependent process requiring the integrity of the microtubule system and further suggest that endogenous cAMP may be involved in GnRH action.

2225 AGING DOES NOT AFFECT STIMULATION EVOKED FATIGUE OF VASOPRESSIN RELEASE FROM THE NEUROHYPOPHYSIS. V.K.Zbuzek*, V.Zbuzek and W.Wu. Dept. Anesthesiology, UMDNJ, New Jersey Medical School, Newark, NJ 07103, USA

Recent studies have suggested that vasopressin (VP) release as a response to a repeated electrical and/or chemical stimulation declines as the gland becomes fatigued. Our previous study demonstrated that VP release decreases during the aging process, therefore we asked the question: Is fatigue of VP release more severe in the old rats? Forty eight neurohypophyses (NH) without pars intermedia of Fisher 344 male rats differing in age (2, 12 and 30 months) were individually superfused with Medium TC 199 for 3½ hrs. Following the initial traumatic release, the glands were stimulated three times for 10 min with 56 mM K^+ Locke's solution with a resting periods of 35 min between stimulations. Fractions were collected in 5 min intervals and VP was measured by RIA. Old glands secreted about one half of VP (expressed per mg NH) than the young ones, during traumatic and basal release as well as following chemical stimulations. Adult glands released similar amount of VP as the young glands during the traumatic and basal release, but their responses to the chemical stimuli were as low as those of the old glands. The responses to the chemical stimuli expressed as % change related to the first response were identical in all three ages. These data indicate that during the aging process: 1) basal and stimulated VP release is impaired, 2) a fatigue of VP release, evoked by repeated chemical stimulation of NH, is not more severe in aged rats as compared to younger rats. Supported by NIA grant R01 AG02778.

2226 REGULATION OF LIVER ANGIOTENSIN II (AII) RECEPTORS BY INTRAVENOUS AII AND Na^+ RESTRICTION. C. Sernia*, L.B. Sinton and W.G. Thomas, Department of Physiology & Pharmacology, Uni. of Queensland, St. Luica 4067, Australia.

AII receptors are present in the rat liver [Campanile *et al.* (1982) *J. Biol.Chem.*, 257, 4951]. We have examined the regulation of these receptors by (a) intravenous Ile^5-AII infusion (Alzet minipumps; 25 ng/kg/min, 4-7 days) and (b) low dietary Na^+ (< 8 mmol/100g, 3-4 weeks). Liver membranes from control male Wistar rats bound AII with an affinity (K_a, 20°C) of 4.00±0.24 nM^{-1} (mean±s.e.m., n=21) and a receptor concentration (R_o) of 35.8±2.5 pmol/g tissue. Specific binding was enhanced by Mg^{2+} (50 mM^{-1}) and Na^+ (150 mM^{-1}) but was inhibited by EDTA (5 mM^{-1}) and DTT (5 mM^{-1}). Peptides were bound in decreasing order of affinity: Val^5-AII > Ile^5-AII > des-Asp-Ile^5-AII > Sar^1-Ala^8-AII > Ile^5-AI > des-Asp-Ile^5-AI >> neurotensin = LHRH ≅ 0. AII infusion increased the R_o by 25% compared to paired control values of 31.0±3.7 (n=8) pmol/g tissue ($p<0.05$, paired *t*-test), while the K_a did not change significantly from control (4.15±0.34 nM^{-1}). In contrast Na^+ restriction decreased the K_a from a control value of 3.85±0.26 nM^{-1} to 3.31±0.15 nM^{-1} (n=11) ($p<0.05$) without changing the R_o. Water intake (26.6±1.1 ml/rat/day) was not altered by AII infusion but sodium restriction decreased it to 21.7±1.2 ml/rat/day ($p<0.01$). Plasma renin activity (ng AI/ml/h) was also measured (control: 13.6±1.8; AII infusion: 9.0±1.2; and Na^+ restriction: 47.2±5.9). It was concluded that the liver contains a high concentration of specific AII receptors which are affected by changes in AII levels and Na^+ restriction. The difference in response to these two factors appears to support the view that changes induced by low Na^+ are not simply due to increases in AII concentrations.

2227 JUVENILE HYPERTENSION WITH ABNORMAL STEROID CATABOLISM: FAMILY STUDIES OF FOUR PATIENTS. C.H.L. Shackleton[1*], E. Arteaga[2,3], J. Rodriguez[2], and J.S.D. Winter[4]. [1]Children's Hospital Medical Center of Northern California, Oakland, CA 94609, [2]Medical Service, San Francisco General Hospital, San Francisco CA 94110, [3]Universidad Catolica de Chile, Santiago, Chile and [4]Children's Hospital, Winnipeg, Manitoba, Canada R3E OW1.

A rare form of low-renin hypertension in children is associated with abnormal terminal metabolism of steroids. This is most apparent in the incomplete metabolism of cortisol where little conversion to urinary tetrahydrocortisone (THE) takes place. Thus, it is possible that the primary defect is a deficiency of 11β-hydroxysteroid oxido-reductase. The connection between the steroid catabolic disorder and the hypertension has yet to be explained. We report here details of the plasma and urine steroid profiles of four new patients (aged 1.5-14 yrs) with the disorder. At the time of initial investigation the patients had normal plasma values of corticosterone, cortisol, deoxycorticosterone, and 18-hydroxydeoxycorticosterone but subnormal 18-hydroxycorticosterone and aldosterone concentrations. In these patients the excretion of THE was only 3-5% of the combined excretion of tetrahydrocortisol + allotetrahydrocortisol (normal 70%).

Studies are being carried out on two of the families. In one case neither two normotensive siblings nor the parents had abnormal urinary steroid profiles. In another family, one child died (aged 6 years) from a stroke and both living children are affected. The parents are normotensive and analysis of their urinary steroids (baseline and during ACTH administration) has yet to be completed.

2228 EVIDENCE THAT 5-HYDROXYTRYPTOPHAN-INDUCED STIMULATION OF ALDOSTERONE IS MEDIATED THROUGH THE CNS. Y. Shenker*, M. D. Gross, R. J. Grekin, Divisions of Endocrinology and Metabolism and Nuclear Medicine, VA Medical Center and the University of Michigan, Ann Arbor, MI 48109 U.S.A.

5-hydroxytryptophan (5HTP) and serotonin both stimulate aldosterone (aldo) secretion in man. To determine if this stimulation is mediated through the CNS, we administered 200 mg 5HTP orally to six healthy volunteers on two occasions. Subjects were pretreated with dexamethasone, 2 mg daily for three days. During stage B, they were also pretreated with carboxydopa, a peripheral decarboxylase inhibitor, 25 mg tid for three days. Carboxydopa blocks peripheral conversion of 5HTP to serotonin, and should increase levels of 5HTP and serotonin in the CNS. No changes were observed in blood pressure, pulse, or plasma levels of sodium, potassium, renin, ACTH, cortisol or serotonin. Plasma 5HTP increased from 7.1±3.2 to 170.4±96.7 ng/ml at 180 min and from 41.3±24.5 to 811.9±340.6 ng/ml during stage A and B respectively ($p < 0.05$ basal vs 180 min for both stages and stage A vs stage B at 180 min). Aldo levels are shown in ng/dl:

	Basal	120	180	240	360
Stage A	4.2±0.9	13.4±3.3*	9.0±2.1	7.0±1.4	4.9±0.9
Stage B	4.7±0.7	15.4±1.7*	19.4±1.8*α	15.6±1.0*α	10.1±1.2*α

* $p < 0.01$ compared to basal   α $p < 0.0025$ compared to stage A

In summary 1) Carboxydopa increases plasma levels of 5HTP without affecting plasma serotonin. 2) Carboxydopa enhances the aldosterone stimulating effect of 5HTP. These results suggest that the effect of 5HTP upon aldosterone is mediated through the central nervous system. A direct adrenal effect of 5HTP cannot be excluded.

2229 A MODEL FOR RENIN PRECURSOR PROCESSING. F.Soubrier*, MT. Corvol, F.X.Galen, C.Devaux, J.Menard and P.Corvol. INSERM U36,17 rue du Fer a Moulin,75005 Paris, France.

A single human renin gene codes for renal and extra-renal renins. cDNA cloning has shown that human renal renin precursor is translated from a unique mRNA into a preprorenin of 45KD with 2 N-glycosylation consensus sequences. By structure analogy with processing of mouse Submaxillary gland preprorenin into active renin,human preprorenin likely follows several processing events:1)Removal of a presegment 2)Activation of renin by cleavage of the prosegment after paired basic residues and 3)Glycosylation.The biosynthesis of human renin has been studied in chorionic cells and juxta-glomerular(JG) tumoral cells.1)In chorion, incorporation of ^{35}S-methionine into immunoprecipitable renin showed that renin was biosynthetized as an inactive enzyme.2)In the JG tumoral tissue, pulse-chase experiments showed that renin was processed from an inactive 55KD precursor into an active 44KD protein.In cultured tumoral cells,renin was present as an inactive 55KD form and no processing into an active form could be shown. In the tumoral tissue,endocrine secretory renin granules were observed as in the normal kidney,however in the chorionic cells and in the cultured tumoral cells,no renin granules could be detected.Therefore the absence of granules was associated with the loss of capacity of packaging and processing 55KD renin into the active 44KD form. After removal of the signal peptide, prorenin could follow 2 pathways:1)Complete intracellular processing associated with packaging within the secretory granules.2)No further processing of the inactive proform due to the absence of renin granules.

2230 EVIDENCE FOR A D_2 DOPAMINERGIC RECEPTOR IN THE ADRENAL ZONA GLOMERULOSA. N. Stern*, C. Wiedeman, F. Krall and M. Tuck, UCLA School of Medicine, VAMC, Sepulveda, California, U.S.A.

Whereas the mechanisms by which dopamine affects the secretion of aldosterone remain unknown, its effects on a number of other endocrine functions are mediated by specific membrane bound receptors. We now report the identification of D2 dopaminergic receptor in the adrenal zona glomerulosa (AZG) using [^{3}H] spiperone (*S), a radioligand with high affinity for dopaminergic receptors. *S binding was specific (defined as binding displacable by (+)d-butaclamol, 5 μM), saturable and of high affinity in the capsular portion of the rat adrenal (Kd 1.5±0.5 nM) and in partially purified 45000 g membrane preparations derived from bovine (Kd 1.1-3.0 nM) and human (Kd 3.7 nM) AZG. Affinity and receptor concentration (Bmax= 38±8 fm/mg protein) were not affected by coincubation with angiotensin II (2.4x10^{-8}M) or K+ (8mM)(bovine preparation). Evidence suggesting the classification of this receptor as D_2 includes: a) higher affinity of the specific D_2 agonist LY 171555(IC_{50}=18±3 nM) compared to the specific D_1 agonist SKF 38393 (IC_{50} 251±50 nM); b) high affinity of the specific D_2 antagonist domperidone (IC_{50_1}=1.9 nM, IC_{50_2}=900 nM; a biphasic competition curve); c) inability of dopamine, 10^{-4} M, to stimulate cyclic AMP generation in bovine and human AZG membrane preparations. Identification of a specific dopaminergic receptor in AZG supports a direct effect of dopaminergic agonists and antagonists on aldosterone production in the adrenal.

2231 PRIMARY ALDOSTERONISM CAUSED BY ALDOSTERONE-PRODUCING ADENOMA IN 18 CONSECUTIVE CASES SELECTED FOR OPERATION. G.S. Stokes*, and R. Campbell, Sydney Hospital, Sydney and Royal North Shore Hospital, St. Leonards, N.S.W. 2065, Australia.

Pre-operative findings were reviewed in a consecutive series of 18 patients (5 male, 13 female; age range 26-57 yr.) who were submitted to bilateral adrenal exploration after investigation for hypertension and hypokalemia. Although radiographic or other evidence of a discrete adrenal tumor site could be elicited pre-operatively in only 8 of these cases, all proved to have an aldosterone producing adenoma (APA) and not adrenal hyperplasia. Homeostasis of aldosterone secretion had been tested in 11 cases by sodium depletion followed by a 4-hour intravenous infusion of 2 litres 0.9% saline on each of 2 successive days. In contrast to a control series of 10 patients with essential hypertension, in whom urinary aldosterone excretion was suppressed to normal by the sodium load, there was a failure of suppression in these 11 cases. A marked fall in serum K concentration after the first saline infusion, precluding the completion of the full test, was correctly predictive of APA in another 5 cases. Conversely, each of the following criteria was found to have produced some false-negative predictions:- suppression of aldosterone excretion by DOCA administration (17% false), stimulation of plasma renin activity with low-sodium diet (18%), adrenal scintiscans (50%), adrenal phlebograms (55%), and lack of blood pressure control with spironolactone (60%). Of the various diagnostic approaches used, the criterion of lack of aldosterone suppression with intravenous sodium loading proved the most reliable in positively indicating a diagnosis of APA.

2232 MECHANISMS IN GLUCOCORTICOID-REMEDIABLE ALDOSTERONISM. Stanley Ulick*, Michael D. Chu and Marianne Land. V.A. Hospital, Bronx, NY 10468 U.S.A.

The biochemical mechanism operating in a form of mineralocorticoid hypertension known as glucocorticoid-remediable aldosteronism, first described by Sutherland, Ruse and Laidlaw in 1966, has not been elucidated. The diagnosis has generally been established by the autosomal-dominant mode of transmission and the marked sensitivity of aldosterone secretion in the disorder to ACTH. In the course of a study of the urinary steroid pattern by gas chromatography/mass spectrometry in two brothers with this disorder, we noted the abundant presence of two new steroids, unconjugated 18-hydroxycortisol, and a tetrahydro metabolite of 18-oxocortisol. This pattern of overproduction of the two C-18-oxygenated cortisols was otherwise observed only in the aldosteronoma of Conn's Syndrome. The formation of these C-18-oxygenated cortisols serves as a biochemical marker for the disorder and provides insight into the mechanism. A study of their biogenesis revealed that cortisol was the precursor and that the enzymatic locus of formation was corticosterone methyloxidase. The C-18-oxygenated cortisols, however, are not normal secretory products *in vivo*. The two major manifestations of the disorder are explained by a derangement in adrenocortical zonal separation such that fasciculata zone products become available in high local concentration at sites of aldosterone biosynthesis. The utilization of cortisol by corticosterone methyloxidase leads to the overproduction of C-18-oxygenated cortisols of which the 18-oxo derivative, a mineralocorticoid agonist, very likely contributes to the clinical manifestations of the disorder. The utilization of the fasciculata zone ACTH-dependent corticosterone pool by the same methyloxidase leads to ACTH-dependent hypersecretion of aldosterone.

2233 FUROSEMIDE-INDUCED ALTERATIONS IN THE ACTIVATION OF THE PRORENIN-RENIN SYSTEM IN DOG PLASMA. E.A. Wilczynski* and D.H. Osmond, Dept. of Physiology, Univ. of Toronto, Toronto, Canada.

Plasma renin activity (PRA) is raised by furosemide (F) administration, but the effects on prorenin and its 'convertase' are less clear. Dogs were treated either with F, 15 mg/day, or placebo for 7 days. PRA and prorenin (activated with 2-5 mg trypsin/ml plasma) were measured in terms of angiotensin I generation. PRA rose significantly by 130% of normal on days 1-4 of F treatment, and had returned to control levels by day 7. 'Total' prorenin fell after F to 52-74% of normal, where 100% is the maximal derived amount in the placebo group using 5 mg/ml trypsin. The data represent % of this maximum.

	Day 1			Day 4			Day 7		
Trypsin (mg/ml)	2	3	5	2	3	5	2	3	5
Placebo	17	67	100	21	66	100	22	63	100
Furosemide	29*	45*	67*	27*	49*	52*	33*	63	74

The data suggest that while total plasma prorenin appears to be suppressed by F, prorenin 'convertase' is enhanced, since (a) the lower prorenin is accompanied by higher circulating renin, (b) low trypsin, aided by this extra convertase developed after F, activates prorenin more effectively, and (c) 3 mg trypsin/ml plasma becomes as effective as 5 mg/ml after F. Thus, the increased PRA due to F is apparently associated with increased 'convertase' and may be partly due to systemic conversion of prorenin.

Supported by the Ontario Heart Foundation.

2234 BEHAVIOUR PROBLEMS AND PSYCHOLOGICAL DISTURBANCES IN SCHOOL CHILDREN SUFFERING FROM HYPOTHYROIDISM. Rita Landau* and Baruch Landau, Mental Health Clinic, Natanya, and Dept. of Endocrinology, Beilinson Medical Center, Petah Tikva, and Tel Aviv University Medical School, Israel

Six children were referred to the Mental Health Clinic because of behaviour disorders characterized by sluggishness, diminished activity, irascibility, a very short attention span, failure in scholastic achievement and aggressiveness against peers in school. Hypothyroidism was diagnosed. Two had a sublingual thyroid, one Hashimoto's disease and three primary idiopathic hypothyroidism. Following institution of thyroid therapy there was a definite clinical and scholastic improvement. The psychopathology and severe behaviour disorders accompanying marked hypothyroidism will be discussed.

2235 THE 24-H PROFILE OF ACTH AND CORTISOL IN UNIPOLAR AND BIPOLAR DEPRESSION.
P. Linkowski*, E. Van Cauter, M. Brasseur, R. Leclercq, J. Golstein, G. Copinschi and J. Mendlewicz, Free University of Brussels, Belgium.

Plasma ACTH and cortisol (F) were measured every 15-min for 24 hrs in 19 untreated depressed patients [20 unipolars (UP), 9 bipolars (BP), ages 31-61] and in 9 age-matched controls (C). All were males without any physical disorder or clinical evidence of Cushing's. For each profile, the circadian variation was quantified by a best-fit curve and the overall pulsatile activity was estimated by summing up the increments of all significant spikes. The quiescent period (QP) of ACTH-F secretion was defined as the time intervals with concentrations lower than 50% of the 24-h mean. In depressed patients, the 24-h mean ACTH levels were within the normal range while the mean F levels were significantly elevated (UP: 14.7 $\pm$ 3.7 μg/dl; BP: 15.3 $\pm$ 4.8 μg/dl; C: 9.3 $\pm$ 1.5 μg/dl; $p<.001$), due to enhanced overall pulsatile activity ($p<.05$). The circadian rhythm of F persisted in all patients but was set at a higher level with an elevated morning acrophase (UP: 21.4 $\pm$ 4.1 μg/dl; BP: 22.7 $\pm$ 5.1 μg/dl; C: 16.0 $\pm$ 2.1 μg/dl; $p<.001$) and a shorter evening QP (UP: 141 $\pm$ 134 min; BP: 158 $\pm$ 119 min; C: 283 $\pm$ 96 min; $p<.05$). Moreover, the QP ended, on the average, 2 hrs earlier in depressed patients ($p<.02$) with no change in timing of the morning maximum. F changes paralleled ACTH changes. No UP-BP differences could be demonstrated. These results show 1) that clinical signs of Cushing's do not develop with F levels increased by up to 100% when pulsatile secretion is enhanced rather than blunted 2) that depression is associated with desynchronization of the mechanisms controlling the morning maximum and the QP of the adrenocorticotropic rhythmicity.

2236 Production of bone resorbing factor by a colony-stimulating factor(CSF)-producing cell line(T3M-1) derived from a patient with granulocytosis and hypercalcemia. K.Sato*, H.Mimura, T.Okabe#, and K.Shizume. The Sec Dep of Int Med, Tokyo Women's Medical College, Ichigaya-Kawada-cho 10, Shinjukuku, Tokyo, and #the Third Dep of Int Med, University of Tokyo, Tokyo, Japan.

A squamous cell carcinoma from a patient who developed marked leukocytosis and hypercalcemia was transplanted into nude mice in which severe hypercalcemia and leukocytosis also developed. This tumor(LJC-1-JCK) made a cyst in the tumor, in which colony-stimulating activity(MW: ~30,000) as well as bone resorbing activity(MW:10,000 - 20,000) was demonstrated. Recently a cell line producing colony-stimulating factor(CSF) was established from this tumor.

To elucidate whether this cell line(T3M-1) produces bone-resorbing activity, conditioned medium of the cell culture was concentrated by PM-10 ultrafiltration, and applied to Sephadex G-100 column chromatography. Each eluate was dialysed against BGJ medium and colony-stimulating activity and bone resorbing activity were assessed simultaneously.

Powerful bone resorbing activity was eluted at the molecular weight of 10,000 - 20,000, whereas colony-stimulating activity was eluted at the M.W. of ~30,000, suggesting that both activities are due to different macromolecular factors. The bone resorbing activity could not be accounted for by EGF, osteoclast activating factor, prostaglandins, or vitamin D metabolites. Furthermore, when the cells were transplanted into nude mice, marked hypercalcemia and leukocytosis developed. Since there are several similar case reports in Japan, we presume that hypercalcemia associated with CSF-producing tumors is a new type of humoral hypercalcemia of malignancy.

2237 CARDIOVASCULAR ACTIONS OF CENTRALLY APPLIED NEUROHYPOPHYSIAL PEPTIDE ANALOGS. Q.J. Pittman* and L. Wahler, Dept. of Pharmacology and Therapeutics, Faculty of Medicine, University of Calgary, Calgary, Canada.

The presence of nerve fibres immunoreactive for arginine vasopressin (AVP) or oxytocin in areas of the brain known to be involved in cardiovascular control suggests a potential role for these peptides in the central control of blood pressure. We have reported that intracerebroventricular (icv) injections of picomole quantities of AVP caused short-latency, dose-related pressor responses in anesthetized rats. The present series of experiments examines the pressor effects of analogs of AVP applied icv. Male Sprague-Dawley rats anesthetized with urethane were prepared with carotid or femoral catheters for blood pressure measurements. Peptides were stereotaxically injected into a lateral cerebral ventricle in a volume of 5 μl of sterile artificial cerebrospinal fluid. Each rat received one injection and each dose of peptide was tested in 5 rats. AVP (0.05-0.5 pmoles) was without effect on blood pressure whereas 5-500 pmoles AVP caused dose-dependent, short-latency pressor responses. Injections of arginine vasotocin (0.05-500 pmoles) were equipotent to AVP whereas oxytocin was approximately 100 x less potent. MSH-release-inhibitory factor (the tail of the oxytocin molecule) and 1-desamino-8-D-arginine vasopressin (ddAVP) were ineffective at a dose of 500 pmoles following central injection. These studies support the idea that the central receptor for the pressor action of AVP resembles the peripheral vasoconstrictor receptor.

Supported by MRC and CHF.

2238 DIFFERENT EFFECTS OF INTRACEREBROVENTRICULAR ADMINISTRATION OF MORPHINE ON PROLACTIN RELEASE IN NORMAL AND CASTRATED MALE RATS. F. Piva*, R. Maggi, P. Limonta and M. Motta, Department of Endocrinology, Via A. del Sarto, 21, 20129 Milano, Italy.

It has been recently shown in this laboratory that morphine injected intraventricularly (i.v.t.) inhibits LH secretion in long-term castrated males, but stimulates LH release in normal male rats (Limonta, Giudici, Piva, Martini, Program 64 Meet. Endocrine Soc., 1982, p. 389). We have now analyzed whether the presence or absence of endogenous androgens might also modify the effects exerted by morphine on prolactin release. Normal and long-term (3 weeks) castrated adult male rats were injected i.v.t. with 200 ug/rat of morphine. The animals were killed at different time intervals after treatment (from 5 min. up to 3 hours) by decapitation; blood was collected and serum levels of prolactin were measured by RIA. Animals i.v.t. injected with saline and killed at the same time intervals served as controls. The results show that morphine induces a significant enhancement of serum levels of prolactin in normal rats 10, 20, 40 and 60 min. after i.v.t. injection. In castrated animals the administration of morphine did not induce any significant alteration of serum prolactin levels, except for a small enhancement of prolactin observed at 90 min. These results suggest that the presence of endogenous androgens is essential to permit to intracerebrally administered morphine to develop its effects on prolactin release in adult male rats. (Supported by CNR through the Project "Preventive and Rehabilitative Medicine").

2239 Effect of $1,25(OH)_2D_3$ on insulin secretion, direct or mediate. Y. Tanaka*, Yo. Seino, M. Ishida, K. Yamaoka, K. Satomura, H. Yabuuchi, H. Ishida[1)], Yu. Seino[1)] and H. Imura[1)], Department of Pediatrics, Osaka University School of Medicine, Osaka 553, Japan, [1)] Department of Internal Medicine, Kyoto University School of Medicine, Kyoto 606, Japan.

To ascertain whether vitamin D (D) directly acts on insulin release or mediately through plasma calcium (Ca), we designed two experiments. In Experiment I, we studied glucose-induced insulin secretion in D-deficient rats (reared on a D and Ca deficient diet), D-replete rats (reared on the same diet and given 250 ng of $1,25(OH)_2D_3$ i.p. for 3 days) and Ca-replete rats (reared on the same diet and given 72 mg of Ca i.p. for 3 days), using the isolated perfused rat pancreas.
In Experiment II, the isolated D-deficient rat pancreas was perfused with and without $1,25(OH)_2D_3$ for 90 minutes to study the direct effect of $1,25(OH)_2D_3$ on insulin release. We found in Experiment I that glucose-induced insulin release from D-replete and Ca-replete rat pancreas was increased compared to that from D-deficient rats but there is no significant difference between the D-replete and the Ca-replete rats. In Experiment II, glucose-induced insulin release from the D-deficient pancreas perfused with $1,25(OH)_2D_3$ was not increased compared to that from the pancreas perfused without $1,25(OH)_2D_3$. These results indicate that D acts mediately on insulin secretion through plasma Ca, at least in part, and has no acute, direct effect on insulin release.

2240 HUMAN CALCITONIN SECRETION RATE HAS BEEN SERIOUSLY OVERESTIMATED. R. Tiegs*, H. Heath III, Division of Endocrinology and Metabolism, Mayo Clinic and Mayo Medical School, Rochester, Minnesota, 55905, USA.

Heterogeneity of circulating calcitonin (CT) has confounded prior attempts to define the physiology of CT and may have led to serious overestimates of CT secretion rates (SR). Therefore, we have applied a new silica extraction method (JCEM 57:5, 1983), with markedly improved specificity for biologically active monomeric CT (hCT-M), to study metabolic clearance rates (MCR) and SR for hCT-M in 5 male and 5 female normal volunteers aged 20-29. MCR was determined by infusion of Ciba hCT-M to constant plasma concentration. SR of hCT-M was calculated from basal extractable iCT and MCR values.

	Plasma extractable iCT, pg/ml		MCR	SR
Subjects	Basal	Infusion	ml/min·kg	ng/d·kg
Male (n=5)	3.6 ± 0.8	178 ± 14.9	8.4 ± 1.1	40.5 ± 7.6
Female (n=5)	2.4 ± 0.2	197 ± 18.2	7.9 ± 0.4	27.1 ± 1.4

In these small groups, the MCR does not appear to differ between the sexes. These preliminary data suggest that higher plasma iCT concentrations in men result from increased secretion. CONCLUSIONS: 1) Basal SR for hCT-M are remarkably low (<1 MRC-B Unit/d), 1/40th-1/100th of prior estimates; and 2) CT doses used in experimental treatment of osteoporosis (up to 100 U/d) have been vastly in excess of basal SR.

2241 EFFECTS OF VITAMIN D DEFICIENCY ON ESTRADIOL-17β METABOLISM IN THE LAYING HEN.
C.P.W. Tsang* and A.A. Grunder, Animal Research Centre, Agriculture Canada, Ottawa, Ontario, K1A 0C6, Canada

Evidence is presented that there are aberrations of estrogen metabolism in vitamin D-deficient laying hens. Five White Leghorn hens, 35 weeks of age, all laying soft-shelled eggs as a result of complete withdrawal of supplemental dietary vitamin D_3, were found to have a 3-fold higher molar ratio of plasma estradiol-17β-3-sulfate ($E_2β$-3S) to estradiol-17β ($E_2β$) compared to 5 control laying hens fed a vitamin D_3-supplemented diet. A study of the disappearance of [^{3}H]$E_2β$ administered iv revealed abnormally high accumulation of [^{3}H]$E_2β$-3S in plasma and concomitantly, markedly reduced formation of [^{3}H] estradiol-17α-3-sulfate ([^{3}H]$E_2α$-3S) compared with the control hens. This suggests a block in the conversion of [^{3}H]$E_2β$-3S to [^{3}H]$E_2α$-3S via [^{3}H] estrone sulfate ([^{3}H]E_1S), previously shown to be a major pathway for $E_2β$ metabolism ($E_2β \rightleftharpoons E_2β$-3S $\rightleftharpoons E_1S \rightleftharpoons E_2α$-3S). As a result, the metabolic clearance rate of [^{3}H]$E_2β$ from the plasma of the vitamin D_3-deficient hens was 15% below normal. The estimated $E_2β$ production rate was reduced by 60%. However, the reduced production rate of $E_2β$ may have been related to the lenghtening of the ovulatory cycle during vitamin D deficiency. We conclude that vitamin D deficiency affects the biosynthesis and catabolism of $E_2β$ in the laying hen.

2242 THE INTERACTION BETWEEN 25-HYDROXYCHOLECALCIFEROL AND CALMODULIN.
H. Van Baelen*, H. Van Belle, F. Wuytack and R. Bouillon, Laboratorium voor Experimentele Geneeskunde, Rega Instituut, 3000 Leuven and Laboratory of Biochemistry, Janssen Pharmaceutica, 2340 Beerse, Belgium.

As recently shown by Reddy and Johnson (1) dansylchloride labeled calmodulin (CDR) strongly binds 25-hydroxycholecalciferol (25-OH-D_3). Using the CDR-dependent phosphodiesterase (PDE) assay this interaction could be confirmed. The I_{50}-value, which is the concentration for 50% inhibition, was 4×10^{-7} M at 6 nM CDR. Under the same experimental conditions the I_{50}-values for R 24571 - the most potent inhibitor known up till now - and for trifluoperazine - the CDR antagonist of preference - were 10^{-8} M and 2×10^{-6} M, respectively. The presence of 8×10^{-7} M pure human vitamin D-binding protein (DBP) in the PDE assay completely abolished the inhibitory effect of 25-OH-D_3 at concentrations not exceeding the DBP concentration. The I_{50}-value was 1 μM. Further evidence for an interaction between CDR and 25-OH-D_3 was obtained using CDR linked to Sepharose 4B. Radioactive 25-OH-D_3 was retained by the matrix but could easily be eluted by solutions containing DBP. Using sucrose gradient ultracentrifugation of pure CDR and of a mixture of CDR and DBP (molar ratio 100:1), previously incubated with radioactive 25-OH-D_3, binding to CDR could be demonstrated only in the absence of DBP. It is concluded that 25-OH-D_3 is one of the better inhibitors of CDR-dependent PDE by binding to CDR but that the affinity is low compared to DBP.
(1) Reddy, G.S. and Johnson, J.D., VIII Int. Conf. on Calcium Regulating Hormones, Abstract P-4, Workshop Tokyo, Japan, Oct. 1983.

2243 CHANGES OF PLASMA CONCENTRATIONS OF VITAMIN D METABOLITES DURING GLUCOCORTICOID(GC) ADMINISTRATION. H.Yamada*, Y.Suzuki, Y.Ichikawa, K.Arikawa, S.Kawai, H.Oshima, T.Shinozawa, T.Yoshida, H.Tanaka, and M.Homma, School of Medicine, Keio University, Tokyo 160, Japan.

Since there have been contradicting reports about vitamin D metablism in patients under GC therapy, we have studied the plasma concentrations of 25-hydroxy-vitamin D(25OHD) and 1α,25-dihydroxy-vitamin D(1,25(OH)$_2$D) in 22 patients with systemic lupus erythematosus(SLE) under GC therapy(GC group), in 8 patients with SLE not under GC therapy(non-GC group), and in 14 normal subjects. Means of plasma 25OHD in both GC group(9.2±3.2(mean±SD)ng/ml) and non-GC group(11.6±4.1) were significantly lower than that in normal subjects(18.5±4.4)($p<0.001$, $p<0.01$, respectively), probably because of insufficient exposure to the sunlight or poor nutrition in these patients. The mean of plasma 1,25(OH)$_2$D in GC group(mean prednisolone dosage 30 mg/day, mean administration period 1 year)(27.3±7.9 pg/ml) was significantly lower than those in normal subjects(41.2±5.0) and in non-GC group(35.6±9.2)($p<0.001$, $p<0.02$). Plasma 1,25(OH)$_2$D correlated inversely with total prednisolone dosage for the preceding three months($r=-0.546$, $p<0.05$). 9 patients studied before and every week after the start of GC administration showed a significant increase after one week and the subsequent decrease in the plasma 1,25(OH)$_2$D. 8 patients studied before and after two months of GC therapy showed a significant decrease in the plasma 1,25(OH)$_2$D, whereas the mean of plasma 25OHD did not change from the initial value. The present study suggests that the plasma 1,25(OH)$_2$D transiently increases one week after the start of GC administration, but it decreases after the long-term GC therapy.

2244 CALCIUM METABOLISM IN THYROID DISEASES--LOW SERUM VALUE FOR 1,25-DIHYDROXYVITAMIN D IN HYPERTHYROIDISM-- K.Yamada*, Y.Iida, S.Yamamura, J.Aoki, M.Hino, C.Shigeno, I.Yamamoto, J.Konishi, and K.Torizuka, Kyoto University, Kyoto, Japan.

Abnormal thyroid functions are often accompanied with abnormal calcium metabolism. To investigate calcium metabolism in abnormal thyroid functions, we measured various calcium regulating hormones in 60 patients of abnormal thyroid function. Values for serum calcitonin, phosphorus, and 25-dihydroxyvitamin D were not different between in patients with hyperthyroidism and in those with hypothyroidism. However, values for serum calcium and parathyroid hormone (PTH) are slightly lower in patients with hyperthyroidism than in those with hypothyroidism, although all values remain within normal ranges. Furthermore, values for 1,25-dihydroxyvitamin D are significantly low (20±14 pg/ml, mean±s.d) in patients with hyperthyroidism, while those in hypothyroid patients ranged within normal (40±19 pg/ml). Low values for 1,25-dihydroxyvitamin D in hyperthyroidism explain the significantly low calcium absorption from the intestine, estimated by ^{47}Ca measurement with a whole body counter, which is performed in several patients with hyperthyroid function. The reason why serum values for 1,25-dihydroxyvitamin D are low in hyperthyroidism remains unclear, but it may be attributable to decreased activity of 1 -hydroxylase in the kidney due to slight hypoparathyroidism.

2245 CIRCADIAN RHYTHM IN CALCIUM REGULATING HORMONES.
K. Yamada*, S. Yamamura, J. Aoki, M. Hino, C. Shigeno, I. Yamamoto and K. Torizuka, Kyoto University, Kyoto, Japan.

To clarify diurnal variations in calcium regulating hormones, we examined in four healthy men with each hour bleeding, and measured serum parathyroid hormone (PTH), calcitonin and vitamin D metabolites in addition to determination of serum calcium, phosphorus and ionized calcium. PTH was determined by two different methods; one is by C-terminal assay and the other is by a method which estimates intact PTH in the plasma. Ionized calcium showed clear diurnal rhythm having its nadir in the midnight and its zenith in the afternoon. Serum phosphorus also showed diurnal rhythm, possessing two peaks in a day; one is around noon and the other is in the midnight. Calcitonin and 25-hydroxyvitamin D showed no diurnal variations. PTH showed no diurnal rhythm when it was determined by C-terminal assay, but the assay for intact PTH revealed significant increases in PTH secretion at mid-night, having a good contrast to ionized calcium. 1,25-dihydroxyvitamin D showed no diurnal variation and, furthermore, no pulsatile variation was found by measurement of samples taken every three minutes for one hour. Thus, our results confirm increases of secretion of PTH in mid-night and deny diurnal variation of 1,25-dihydroxyvitamin D.

2246 INHIBITORY INFLUENCE OF PROSTAGLANDIN E_2 ON THE RENAL EFFECTS OF CALCITONIN IN RATS.
M. Yamada, T. Matsumoto*, N. Takahashi, T. Suda and E. Ogata, Fourth Department of Internal Medicine, University of Tokyo School of Medicine, and Department of Biochemistry, Showa University School of Dentistry, Tokyo, Japan.

The influence of prostaglandin E_2 (PGE_2) on the effects of PTH and calcitonin (CT) was examined in order to investigate the possible role of PGE_2 in modulating the renal effects of these hormones. As reported previously (Biochem. J. 216:237, 1983), intraarterial infusion of 20μg/h PGE_2 alone into vitamin D-deficient thyroparathyroidectomized (TPTX) rats caused a stimulation of *in vivo* conversion of $[^3H]25(OH)D_3$ into $[^3H]1,25\text{-}(OH)_2D_3$ from 12.2 ± 0.6 pmol/100ml to 19.5 ± 1.1 pmol/100ml ($p<0.01$). When 20μg/h PGE_2 was infused along with 500mU/h CT, the stimulatory effect of CT on plasma accumulation of $[^3H]1,25(OH)_2D_3$ was significantly inhibited to a level similar to that with PGE_2 alone. Furthermore, when PGE_2 was administered along with CT to vitamin D-replete TPTX rats, the marked stimulatory effect of CT on renal Pi excretion was significantly inhibited. The same amount of PGE_2 caused no significant changes in PTH-induced stimulation of plasma $[^3H]1,25(OH)_2D_3$ accumulation or renal Pi excretion. These data demonstrate that PGE_2 has a specific inhibitory influence on the effects of CT on $25(OH)D_3$ metabolism and Pi excretion in rats. The present results are consistent with the notion that PTH and CT cause the stimulation of 1α-hydroxylase and phosphaturia by acting at different renal tubular segments through different mechanisms.

2247 MARKED INHIBITION OF THE GROWTH OF SC115 TUMOR CELLS BY A PURE ANTIANDROGEN.
L. Proulx*, G. Leblanc, F. Létourneau and F. Labrie, MRC Group in Molecular Endocrinology, CHUL, Quebec G1V 4G2, Canada

The growth of the SC115 mammary carcinoma in mice is androgen dependent. When castration was performed three days before the inoculation of tumor cells (SC115), the appearance of tumors wad delayed by 15 days (as compared to intact animals). In an intact group, the incidence of animals bearing tumors reached 100% between 10 and 14 days following inoculation while, in the castrated group, a 30% incidence was observed after 25 days and 100% of the animals had tumors at 66 days. Daily treatment with 0.5 mg of the pure antiandrogen Anandron had no effect when administered in intact animals. However, daily treatment with 0.2 mg of the antiandrogen started the day of castration led to an incidence of 11% of animals having tumors at day 42 with a maximum of 44% at day 120. Measurements of cytosolic androgen receptor levels with [^{3}H]R1881 show values of 30 ± 10 and 70 ± 15 fmoles/mg protein in the tumors of castrated and intact animals, respectively. The present data show that castation of male mice does not prevent but only delays the appearance of mammary tumors while addition of the antiandrogen in castrated animals not only delays but also decreases the incidence of the tumors by 56% at 120 days. Since mouse adrenal glands secrete low amounts of adrenal androgens, such data suggest that androgen receptors free of ligand are biologically active, and can be, at least partly, blocked by a pure antiandrogen.

2248 FORMATION OF CATECHOL ESTROGENS BY HUMAN BREAST CANCERS AND THEIR BINDING TO ESTROGEN RECEPTOR (ER).
R. H. Purdy*, C. van Aswegen and J. L. Wittliff, Southwest Foundation for Biomedical Research, San Antonio, TX 78284, and the James Graham Brown Cancer Center, School of Medicine, University of Louisville, Louisville, KY 40292, USA.

Estradiol is metabolically activated by microsomes from human breast cancers to the catechol estrogens, 2-hydroxyestradiol (2-OHE$_2$) and 4-hydroxyestradiol (4-OHE$_2$). The rates of formation of these catechol estrogens by microsomes from 16 ER+ malignant breast tumors has been measured using a radioenzymatic assay with product identification by HPLC. The ratio of the rates of formation of 2-OHE$_2$/4-OHE$_2$ ranged from 4 to 67 with a mean of 20. Thus, *in vitro*, estradiol is principally converted to 2-OHE$_2$. The physiological significance of the formation of these catechols by breast cancers has been explored by measuring their interactions with ER isolated from a pool of ER+ tumors. The displacement of [^{3}H]-estradiol from ER by the catechols was assayed using 0.33 mM ascorbic acid to prevent oxidation of the catechols. The relative affinities compared to estradiol (100) were 89 for 2-OHE$_2$ and 154 for 4-OHE$_2$. The relative affinities of two epoxyenones, which are possible intermediates in the formation of 4-OHE$_2$, was 2.7 for 4α,5α-epoxy-17β-hydroxyestra-1-en-3-one and 0.01 for 4β,5β-epoxy-17β-hydroxyestra-1-en-3-one. These results suggest that metabolic activation of estradiol to catechol estrogens within ER+ breast cancers may serve to further stimulate their growth. This study was supported by Grants CA-24629 and CA-19657 from the National Cancer Institute, DHHS, and the Southwest Foundation Forum.

2249 DEMONSTRATION BY MASS SPECTROMETRY OF LONG CHAIN FATTY ESTERS OF ANDROSTERONE IN HUMAN BREAST CYST FLUID. U. Raju, M. Levitz*, S. Banerjee, A. Bencsath and F.H. Field, N.Y.U. Medical Center, New York, N.Y. 10016, and The Rockefeller University, New York, N.Y. 10021, U.S.A.

Incubation of ^{3}H-androsterone (A) in homogenates of human breast tumors results in long chain fatty esters of A(3-48%). Breast tumor tissue homogenates were incubated with androsterone; then submitted to solvent extraction, Celite chromatography, high performance liquid chromotography (HPLC) and OH^- negative chemical ionization mass spectrometry (MS). The $(M-1)^-$ ions of the stearate, oleate, palmitate, palmitoleate and linoleate esters of A in decreasing order of predominance were produced. Appropriate blanks were negative. Since patients with fibrocystic disease are at risk for developing breast cancer, we analyzed human breast cyst fluids for the presence of fatty esters of A. The fluids were extracted with chloroform-methanol, and from the organic phase A-esters were separated from A by Celite chromatography and hydrolyzed with methanolic KOH. The liberated A was purified on Celite and estimated by radioimmunoassay. The eight cyst fluids analyzed had 0.5 - 3.0 ng/ml of fatty esters measured as A. One specimen after initial purification was purified further by reverse phase Celite chromatography and HPLC. Individual fractions from the latter were analyzed by MS. The palmitoleate of A was the predominant ester. However, the possibility that dehydroisoandrosterone palmitate, an ester with the same mass ion is also present is being investigated. The methodology permits correlations to be made between the ester profile and the course of fibrocystic disease and with a variety of characteristics of breast tumors.

2250 REGRESSION OF LUNG METASTASES IN A PATIENT WITH PROSTATIC CARCINOMA DURING THERAPY WITH D-TRP-6-LHRH. A. Ramalho, A.M. Comaru-Schally*, P.R. Leitao and A.V. Schally. Urology Clinic, General Hospital - INAMPS Fortaleza-CE, Brazil and V.A. Med. Center and Tulane Univ. Sch. Med., New Orleans, LA 70146, USA.

Six patients with biopsy-proven prostatic carcinoma, 3 with stage C and 3 stage D disease were treated with LHRH Agonist, D-Trp-6-LHRH. One patient with stage D-2 had widespread lung metastases. Two patients presented with signs of prostatism. The analog was given s.c. once daily at a dose of 500µg for the first 7 days. Subsequently the dose was reduced to 100µg/day during the following 6 to 9 months. In all patients plasma testosterone concentrations decreased after the first month and remained at castration levels. A tendency for the normalization of plasma acid phosphatase levels was observed in all patients, and the same was true for the plasma prostatic phosphatase concentrations. Objective and subjective signs of regression of disease were seen in all patients. In a patient who had an indwelling catheter for relief of urinary outflow obstruction, the catheter was removed after the third week of therapy. One patient with stage D-2, who was bedridden due to severe bone pain and dyspnea caused by widespread metastatic lung disease, showed dramatic clinical response and a complete remission of the lung metastases on X ray after 4 months of therapy with LHRH Analog. This patient has resumed all his activities. Our findings extend previous reports on successful treatment of patients with P.C. with Analogs of LHRH. Moreover, these may be the first observations of a complete regression of lung metastases in a patient with P.C. during therapy with D-Trp-6-LHRH.

2251 TAMOXIFEN RESISTANCE AND PLOIDY OF ESTROGEN RECEPTOR(ER)-POSITIVE SUBLINES OF T-47D HUMAN BREAST CANCER CELLS. R. Reddel*, L. Murphy and R. Sutherland. Ludwig Institute for Cancer Research (Sydney Branch), University of Sydney, N.S.W., 2006, Australia.

A considerable proportion of ER-positive breast tumors are resistant to tamoxifen and many which are initially sensitive become resistant during treatment. In order to find suitable models of ER-positive, tamoxifen-resistant breast cancer we have studied several spontaneously arising sub-lines of T-47D breast cancer cells in vitro. Cells were grown in RPMI 1640 medium supplemented with 10% fetal calf serum and passaged weekly by tryp-sinization, with inoculation densities being adjusted to maintain contin-uously exponential growth; no other selection pressures were used. Four successive cultures derived from 4 vials of the same batch of cryopreserved cells underwent distinct morphologic changes and decreases in population doubling times. Ploidy was monitored by DNA flow cytometry and karyotype analysis. If wild type T-47D cells are arbitrarily designated as diploid, then the sublines are diploid (T-47D-4), hypertetraploid (T-47D-5), a mixture of diploid and tetraploid (T-47D-6), and tetraploid (T-47D-8). Each of these sublines had ER and antiestrogen binding site contents similar to those of the wild type. The sensitivity of T-47D-4 to tamoxifen was similar to that of the wild type, but T-47D-5 had a >25-fold resistance, being indistinguishable from ER-negative breast lines in this regard. T-47D-8 and a cloned tetraploid subline of T-47D-6 had intermediate sensitivities. There thus appears to be some correlation in this system between ploidy and tamoxifen resistance. The relevance of this to tamoxifen resistance in vivo remains to be determined.

2252 THE EFFECT OF LIPIDS ON PLASMA FREE OESTRADIOL IN VITRO AND IN VIVO. M.J. Reed, R.W. Cheng, P.A. Beranek and V.H.T. James. Department of Chemical Pathology, St. Mary's Hospital Medical School, London W2 1PG, UK.

The biologically free oestradiol (E2) fraction in plasma is elevated in postmenopausal women with breast cancer (Moore et al., 1983; Reed et al., 1983) although the reason for this increase is not known. As it has been suggested that lipids may be able to alter the binding of E2 to plasma proteins, we have studied the effect of the addition of free fatty acids on the binding of E2 to plasma proteins in vitro and the effect of eating a high fat content meal on the free E2 fraction in plasma. We have also examined the relationship between the free E2 fraction and plasma levels of triglycerides in postmenopausal women with breast cancer. Addition of 2 mmol/l oleic acid, but not linoleic acid, produced a significant increase (48%) in the free E2 fraction. At higher concentrations of both oleic and linoleic acid (5 mmol/l) the free E2 fraction increased by 87% and 72% respectively. After eating a high fat content meal, although triglyceride levels increased significantly, no increase in the free E2 fraction was detected. So far no significant correlation has been found between the free E2 fraction and plasma levels of triglycerides in postmenopausal women with breast cancer. From these studies it is concluded that although free fatty acids can alter the binding of E2 to plasma proteins, any such role that free fatty acids or triglycerides may have in vivo remains to be established. This work was supported by a grant from the Cancer Research Campaign.

Moore et al., (1983), Int. J. Cancer, 29: 17.
Reed et al., (1983), Cancer Res., 43: 3940.

2253 STEROID HORMONE PROFILES IN MEN TREATED WITH MEDICAL ADRENALECTOMY FOR ADVANCED PROSTATE CANCER. E. Samojlik*, M. Kirschner, N. Ertel, A. Lippman and Y. Park, Newark Beth Israel Medical Center, Newark, N.J. and V.A. Medical Center, East Orange, N.J., U.S.A.

Fifteen orchiectomized men with advanced prostate cancer (Stage D) were treated with 1,000 mg/day Cytadren (AG) along with 40 mg. cortisol (HC). Hormonal profiles were obtained in urine and blood prior to therapy and then monthly thereafter. The following were observed:

URINARY METABOLITES	Before	During	P Values
Estrone (μg/day)	2.24 $\pm$ 0.34	0.13 $\pm$ 0.03	<0.01
Estradiol (μg/day)	0.39 $\pm$ 0.06	0.05 $\pm$ 0.006	<0.01
Testosterone-G (μg/day)	6.71 $\pm$ 0.98	3.31 $\pm$ 0.35	<0.01
6_{β}-OHF (μg/day)	338.7 $\pm$ 70.2	2673 $\pm$ 364	<0.001
17-OHCS (mg/day)	4.06 $\pm$ 0.39	12.3 $\pm$ 0.61	<0.01
17-KS (mg/day)	3.74 $\pm$ 0.32	4.30 $\pm$ 0.37	N.S.

Plasma levels of E_1, E_2, DHT, T decreased to approximately 1/2 basal levels, except DHEAS which fell from 452 $\pm$ 72 to 80 $\pm$ 8.2 ng/ml. Plasma 6_{β}-OHF rose 2-fold over basal levels, compared to the 8-fold increase in urine.

Our data demonstrate that AG + HC therapy for prostate cancer (Stage D) results in significant decreases in both plasma and urinary androgens and estrogens. In contrast, the ratio of 6_{β}-hydroxy to other metabolites of cortisol are increased by this therapy, reflecting the action of AG on liver microsomal enzymes.

Analysis of these data suggests no differences in response of plasma or urinary androgens and estrogens in men who responded vs. non-responders.

Quebec, Canada G1V 4G2

2254 DECREASED LH BIO/IMMUNO RATIO DURING TREATMENT WITH THE SUPERAGONIST ANALOG OF GnRH, LEUPROLIDE, FOR PROSTATE CARCINOMA. R. Santen,* B. Warner, and M. Dufau, Division of Endocrinology, The M.S. Hershey Medical Center, The Pennsylvania State University, Hershey, PA 17033, and NICHD, National Institutes of Health, Bethesda, MD. 20214.

The medical equivalent of surgical castration can be induced by administration of a potent agonist analog of gonadotropin releasing hormone, Leuprolide (D-Leu^6-GnRH-proethylamide), 1-10 mg daily in men with prostate cancer. Plasma testosterone (T) after one year of treatment with Leuprolide was 16±2.1 ng % (mean±SEM, n=21) compared to 11±0.9 ng % in response to castration (n=25). This 95% decline in T (i.e., 320 to 16 ng %) paralleled a 98% decrease in LH measured by bioassay (61 mIU/ml to 1.7 mIU/ml) but exceeded the 76% decrease in LH by RIA (26 mIU/ml to 6.2 mIU/ml). This greater fall in biologically active LH suggested that Leuprolide might qualitatively alter the nature of the LH molecule secreted. We addressed this question by using the bio/immuno (B/I) ratio as an indirect marker for qualitative changes in circulating LH as in previous studies from our laboratory. In 18 intact men with prostate cancer, the basal B/I ratio was 2.63±0.28 and fell dramatically during treatment to 0.16±.09 ($p<.01$). This change could have resulted from a decline in T or a direct pituitary action of Leuprolide. To distinguish between these possibilities, we also studied 8 castrate men. Their B/I ratio also decreased from a basal value of 1.54±.19 to 0.63±.25 ($p<.05$), suggesting a direct pituitary effect of Leuprolide. These results suggest that Leuprolide, through a direct pituitary action, may alter the qualitative nature of the LH molecule secreted.

2255 INCREASED EFFICACY OF D-TRP^6-LH-RH MICROCAPSULES COMBINED WITH CYCLOPHOSPHAMIDE IN THE TREATMENT OF PROSTATE TUMORS IN RATS. A.V. Schally and T.W. Redding*, VA Med Center and Tulane Med Sch, New Orleans,LA 70146 USA.

The demonstration of inhibition of prostate tumor growth in rats by D-Trp^6-LH-RH and a significant clinical improvement seen in prostate cancer patients treated daily with this and other superagonists of LH-RH, prompted us to develop more convenient methods of therapy as well as investigate the combination with cyclophosphamide (Cytoxan) in order to enhance therapeutic response. Microcapsules of D-Trp^6-LH-RH,formulated from poly(d,l,-lactide-co-glycolide) for controlled release, were provided by Dr. T.Tice, Southern Research Inst.,AL. Treatment was started 60 days after the transplantation of the Dunning R3327H prostate tumor. D-Trp^6-LH-RH microcapsules, equivalent to a dose of 25 μg/day, were injected i.m. once a month for 3 months. Cytoxan (5 mg/kg) was injected i.p. twice a week. After 90 days rats were sacrificed, tumors and organs removed, and weights recorded.

The table below summarizes our results: Mean ± S.E., * p=<.01

	Tumor Wt. gm	Tumor Vol. mm^3	Testes Wt. gm	V. Prostate Wt. mg
Control	14.89 ± 2	17543±2996	3.18±.08	467±12
D-Trp^6-LH-RH	0.17 ± .06*	883±406*	0.41±.01*	25±.9*
Cytoxan	2.26 ± .74*	3016±787*	3.10±.05	407±37
D-Trp^6-LH-RH + Cytoxan	0.019± .008*	31±10*	0.44±.007*	33±4*

These preliminary results in rats strongly suggest that combination of once a month controlled delivery system of D-Trp^6-LH-RH with Cytoxan could further improve therapeutic response obtained with this agonist of LH-RH in men with prostatic cancer. This study was supported by VA and NIH.

2256 ETIDRONATE FOR THE RELIEF OF METASTATIC BONE PAIN. Walter Schnur*, Greenhills, Ohio, U.S.A.

This report describes unexpectedly gratifying results in the treatment of bone pain from osseous metastases arising from primary prostate (two patients), lung (one patient) and breast (three patients) cancer. All patients had previously received appropriate treatment, that is surgery, radiotherapy and/or chemotherapy. When treatment with etidronate was started, all patients were receiving varying doses of analgesics, including codeine, meperidine, morphine, and hydromorphone. Treatment consisted of a single daily dose of etidronate disodium (Didronel), 5mg/kg to 7mg/kg. The condition of all patients improved within three weeks. This improvement was demonstrated by a decreased number of requests for analgesics. Three patients have since died, the first two with breast carcinoma but without bone pain. The third who had lung cancer, developed pain from nervous system involvement, but his osteolytic lesions remained pain-free. The condition of the patients with prostatic cancer had worsened on hormonal therapy. After treatment with etidronate, the condition of both patients improved to the extent that all analgesia was discontinued except for an occasional acetaminophen tablet at bedtime. One patient after six years of slowly progressive disease has returned to managing his business affairs. X-ray films of his widespread extensive spinal metastases have shown no extension in more than two years, and his acid phosphatase level has returned to normal. The second patient, who had been chair-bound, was able to place Christmas decorations on his housetop and is pain-free.

2257 LONG-TERM SUPPRESSION OF GONADOTROPHIN SECRETION WITH LHRH-ANALOGUE ICI 118630. Shalet, S.M.* Ahmed, S.R., Brooman P.J.C., Howell, A. and Blacklock, N. J. Departments of Endocrinology, Urology & Oncology, Christie & Withington Hospitals, Manchester.

In man LHRH-analogue ICI 118630 (D-Ser $(Bu^{t})^{6}$ $Azgly^{10}$) will reduce testosterone concentrations into the castrate range within 4 weeks of treatment[1], however the long-term hormonal effects of such treatment are unknown. We have now treated 18 patients with advanced prostatic cancer with ICI 118630. Ten patients, aged 58-84 years, have received a once daily subcutaneous injection of 250 μg. (maintenance dose) of ICI 118630 for between 6-18 (median 12) months. The testosterone level was between 10.3 - 24 nmol/l (mean 15.4 nmol/l) before treatment, < 2 -3.6 nmol/l after 4 weeks and was undetectable (< 2 nmol/l) in all patients after 1 year of treatment. The mean basal FSH and LH concentrations were 7 mU/ml and 11.8 mU/ml before treatment, 3.3 mU/ml and 2.4 mU/ml after 4 weeks and 2.9 and 2.8 mU/ml after treatment for 6 months. However, in 3 patients, FSH but not LH levels were only partially suppressed after 9 months' treatment with ICI 118630. Conclusions: LHRH-analogue ICI 118630 will maintain the testosterone level in the castrate range after 1 year of continuous therapy. The major effect of ICI 118630 is at the level of the pituitary[1] and there appears to be a different threshold for suppression of FSH and LH.

1. Ahmed, S,R., Brooman, P.J.C, Shalet, S.M., Howell, A., Blacklock N.J. and Rickards, D. (1983) Lancet: ii, 415.

2258 GYNECOMASTIA IN LEPROMATOUS LEPROSY IS ASSOCIATED WITH PRIMARY TESTICULAR FAILURE BUT NOT WITH ELEVATED SERUM ESTRADIOL. R. Rolston*, M.R. Hopton† and P.M. Taylor, SLRT Center, KARIGIRI, India 632106 and †Department of Biochemistry, City Hospital, DERBY, DE3 3NE, U.K.

Gynecomastia in lepromatous leprosy is well recognized, but its endocrine basis has been insufficiently investigated. We have studied age matched groups of 10 patients with lepromatous leprosy and gynecomastia (LL + G), 10 with lepromatous leprosy but no gynecomastia (LL), 10 with tuberculoid leprosy (TT) and 10 healthy male volunteers (HV). No subject showed clinical or biochemical signs of liver disease. Mean basal serum hormone concentrations (± SEM) were as follows:-

	LH (U/l)	FSH (U/l)	Testosterone (nmol/l)	Estradiol (pmol/l)	Prolactin (mU/l)
LL + G	30 ± 5 a) d)	19 ± 1 b) e)	14 ± 2 c)	221 ± 17	163 ± 48
LL	18 ± 6	11 ± 2	22 ± 2	207 ± 16	114 ± 21
TT	9 ± 2	4 ± 1	27 ± 1	215 ± 27	106 ± 12
HV	5 ± 1	3 ± 1	25 ± 1	193 ± 20	68 ± 8

a) $p < 0.05$ v LL; $p < 0.001$ v HV; b) $p < 0.001$ v LL and HV; c) $p < 0.01$ v LL; $p < 0.001$ v HV; d) $p < 0.05$ v HV; e) $p < 0.01$ v HV.

LH and FSH responses to GnRH were greater in LL + G and LL than in HV. These results suggest that gynecomastia in lepromatous leprosy is not, as hitherto supposed, caused by a rise in serum estrogens consequent to an impairment of liver metabolism, but is directly related to failure of the infiltrated testes to secrete testosterone in the presence of a normal pituitary feedback control mechanism.

2259 THE ROLE OF PITUITARY GONADOTROPINS IN FOLLICULAR STIMULATION AND OOCYTE MATURATION IN THE HUMAN. Z. Rosenwaks*, J.E. Garcia, S. Muasher, and G.S. Jones, Howard and Georgeanna Jones Institute Of Reproductive Medicine, Department of Obstetrics and Gynecology, Eastern Virginia Medical School, Norfolk, Virginia 23507

The role of gonadotropins follicle stimulating hormone (FSH) and luteinizing hormone (LH) in follicular development and oocyte maturation was investigated in 12 normally ovulating patients during in vitro fertilization. Response to menopausal gonadotropin (HMG)+ stimulation was compared to response with FSH° in each patient. Follicular development was assessed by daily estradiol (E_2) assays and number of follicles developed; oocytes were assessed by morphology. Follicular E_2 values were similar for each patient after either FSH or HMG. Endogenous LH levels appeared to be suppressed 16 hours after I.M. administration for both preparations. Oocyte status after aspiration and pregnancy rate are compared in the following table: data presented as mean ± S.E. for 12 patients

	Follicles	# Oocytes	Preovulatory Oocytes	Immature Oocytes	# Embryos Transferred/ Cycle	Pregnancies/ Transferred Cycle
HMG	5.6±0.67	4.7±0.51	1.75±0.51	1.83±0.50	2.3±0.35	0
pure FSH	9.1±1.18*	8.0±1.12*	2.9±0.62	4.3±1.26	3.4±0.56	6

The data suggest that exogenous LH is not required for follicular E_2 synthesis or maturation of the oocyte. The excellent hormonal E_2 response and the high pregnancy rate with pure FSH suggests that FSH and not LH may be the critical gonadotropin which insures follicular development and oocyte viability.

*- $p < 0.05$ paired student test
\+ - HMG-Pergonal, 75 IU FSH & LH ° - Metrodin, Serono 75 IU FSH

2260 PROSPECTIVE CLINICAL AND BIOCHEMICAL STUDY OF HIRSUTISM, USING TWO TREATMENTS AND INVOLVING 60 PATIENTS DURING TWELVE MONTHS.
R.Rubens*, A. Vermeulen; Dept. Endocrinology, R.U.G., Ghent, Belgium.

Data concerning clinical and biochemical evolution of hirsutism being scarce, we performed a study on 60 hirsute women during twelve months. Selection of treatment was based on two androgen profiles (Testosterone (T), free testosterone (FT), androstenedione, dihydrotestosterone, 5α-androstane 3α,17β-diol, dehydroepiandrosterone, 5-androstene-3β,17β-diol, dehydroepiandrosterone sulphate) under basal conditions and after five days (3 x 1 mg) dexamethasone (DXM) respectively. Severity of hirsutism was graded according to Ferriman & Gallway (H.G. = score). Patients were treated by : 1) DXM (0.5 mg at 11 p.m.) when the DXM test revealed exclusive adrenal androgen hypersecretion (n=25). 2) Cyproterone acetate 50 mg a day (5th to 16th day of cycle) combined with ethinyl-oestradiol 50 ug a day (5th to 26th day) (CA & EE2) when a non DXM suppressible hyperandrogenism was present (n=35). Both groups were comparable as well clinically (H.G. DXM 12.88 ± 4.50 and H.G. CA & EE2 12.34 ± 5.47 respectively) as biochemically except for T and FT levels which were significantly higher in the CA & EE2 group.
After twelve months of treatment H.G. decreased significantly in both groups, but mean score (6.39 ± 5.74) in the CA & EE2 group was significantly lower than in the DXM group (9.45 ± 5.16). Nevertheless androgen levels including FT were lower in the DXM group than in the CA & EE2 group. These data indicate CA & EE2 to be the more active treatment, acting in distinction with DXM both at the pituitary and the target level.

2261 MAGNESIUM DEFICIENCY IN A MEDICAL INTENSIVE CARE UNIT POPULATION. E. Ryzen*, P.W. Wagers, F.R. Singer, and R.K. Rude, Department of Medicine, University of Southern California School of Medicine, Los Angeles, CA. USA

Magnesium (Mg) deficiency may develop in a variety of clinical conditions, including diarrhea, alcoholism, hypercalcemia,and hypophosphatemia, as well as with parenteral fluid, aminoglycoside, and diuretic therapy. Mg depletion can cause weakness, seizures, cardiac arrhythmias, mental status changes, hypocalcemia, and hypokalemia. We have previously reported that approximately 10% of patients (pts.) admitted to an acute care hospital have frankly low serum Mg (sMg) concentrations (REF: Am. J. Clin. Pathol. 1983, 79:348). In this study we monitored daily sMg in all pts. with serum creatinine of 1.1mg/dl or less who were admitted to the Los Angeles County medical intensive care unit (ICU) over a 36-day period. 33 pts. were studied. Of these, 22 (67%) had hypomagnesemia either on admission to the ICU or during their stay in the ICU. The sMg in the hypomagnesemic population was 1.1 meq/l ± .02 (mean±SEM) with a range of 0.4-1.4meq/l. 5 pts. had hypocalcemia which resolved with Mg therapy. 9 other pts. had conditions that may have been aggravated by Mg deficiency but could not be attributed to Mg depletion alone (5 pts. had arrhythmias, 4 seizures). We conclude that ICU pts. have a very high incidence of hypomagnesemia and suggest that the sMg be monitored on a regular basis in such pts.

2262 THE RESPONSE OF PAINFUL BENIGN BREAST DISEASE TO TRI-IODOTHYRONINE. M. Saikia and Ivor H. Mills*, Department of Medicine, University of Cambridge, Cambridge CB2 2QQ, England.

The effect of tri-iodothyronine 20 micrograms twice daily for 12 months was assessed in 42 menstruating women who complained of breast pain associated with fibro-cystic disease of the breasts. Their ages ranged between 22 and 45 years and none was on any hormonal treatment: previously they had had a variety of unsuccessful treatments. The scoring and the results are shown in the Table.

Mean symptom score at 3, 6, 9 and 12 months of treatment

	Score	3 months	6 months	9 months	12 months
Worse	-1	5	5	4	3
No change	0	17	11	7	7
Improved	1	12	14	8	5
Much improved	2	7	11	14	12
Excellent	3	1	1	9	15
Mean score		0.57	0.81	1.41	1.69

By the end of one year of treatment 76% had had improvement in their breast pain. The mean initial serum prolactin was 294±32 mU/l. On treatment 28 women had a mean prolactin of 247±25 mU/l which was a mean fall of 140±42 from their control values. Serum thyroxine fell from 102±3.0 to 36±3.9 nmol/l (P<0.001) and the tri-iodothyronine rose from 1.9±0.1 to 4.1±0.2 nmol/l (P<0.001). Tri-iodothyronine is effective treatment for 76% of the women with painful breast disease.

2263 PREDICTIVE VALUE OF TSH RECEPTOR ANTIBODY (TRAb) FOR NEONATAL HYPOTHYROIDISM IN PATIENTS WITH HYPOTHYROID AUTOIMMUNE THYROIDITIS (HAT).
H. Saito*, N. Momotani, K. Arikawa, and K. Ito, Ito Hospital, and Department of Internal Medicine, School of Medicine, Keio University, Tokyo, Japan.

Recently, the transplacental passage of TRAb which inhibits the stimulating activity of TSH has been assumed to play a role in transient neonatal hypothyroidism in the infants from mothers with HAT. However, neonates from TRAb positive mothers with HAT are not always suffering from hypothyroidism. In the present study we measured TRAb in 10 immunoglobulin Gs (IgGs) from 8 patients with HAT in the 10 pregnancies and thyroid status of each neonate. All the patients had antimicrosomal antibodies. TRAb was measured with 1 mg IgG (Smith's kit). TRAb was detected in 6 of 10 IgGs. Of these 6, 5 had strongly positive TRAb (range: 71-97%). TRAb in IgGs from cord sera was almost identical with that of each patient. 8 of the 10 neonates were euthyroid biochemically as well as clinically. Two instances of transient neonatal hypothyroidism occurred to a mother whose TRAb in both pregnancies was the most positive of all. Even with 10 μg IgG, her TRAb was strongly positive. Moreover, her IgGs definitely inhibited adenylate cyclase (AC) stimulation induced by TSH. As for the other patients with strongly positive TRAb, the IgG only moderately inhibited AC stimulation by TSH, and the TRAb was only slightly positive when measured with 10 μg IgG.
Conclusions: 1) Strongly positive TRAb with 1 mg IgG in maternal sera is not always a marker of neonatal hypothyroidism. 2) The TRAb, if strongly positive even with 10 μg IgG may increase suspicion of neonatal hypothyroidism.

2264 SCREENING PROGRAM FOR CONGENITAL HYPOTHYROIDISM (CH) IN NOVA SCOTIA.
S. Salisbury*, M. Givner, C. Smith, S. Lovitt, A.C. Allen, J.T.R. Clarke and M. Spence, I.W.K. Hospital for Children and Victoria General Hospital, Departments of Pediatrics and Pathology, Dalhousie University, Atlantic Research Centre for Mental Retardation, Halifax, Nova Scotia, B3J 3G9, Canada.

In 1979 a province-wide neonatal screening program, reaching 99.8% of this population, was initiated to determine the incidence and effectiveness of early recognition and treatment of CH. Heel prick filter paper dot thyroxine (T4) was measured by radioimmunoassay on samples obtained between day 3 and 5. If the T4 value fell within the lowest 10% of the assay, the T4 dot was repeated and thyrotropin (TSH) measured. Dot recalls (rate=0.6%) were requested if paper was undersaturated. If the dot TSH was borderline or elevated a serum recall (0.2%) was initiated. Where the dot TSH was definitely elevated the infant was examined, T4 and TSH assayed and treatment started with 25 ug T4 while waiting for confirmation. Over a 53 month period, 53,529 infants were screened: 16 cases of CH were detected (incidence 1:3,346), including 3 goitres, 5 ectopic thyroids, 6 thyroid agenesis and 1 Down syndrome. Since 1980 the average age at onset of treatment has been 16 days with the exception of the patient with Down syndrome and a child who had diabetic embryopathy with ectopic thyroid, both of whom had borderline TSH results. Prior to the screening program only 4/24 infants referred to our centre were diagnosed and treated under age 1 month. The program has been successful in providing complete screening of our Maritime population. No child with CH due to ectopic thyroid, goitre, or agenesis has been missed using a primary T4 screen backed up by TSH. Supported by the Nova Scotia Department of Health

2265 COMPARISON OF AEROSOLIZED INSULIN IN TYPE I AND TYPE II DIABETICS: EFFECTS ON ON PREVENTING POSTPRANDIAL HYPERGLYCEMIA.

R. Salzman*, G. Griffing, J. Manson E. Stoltz, J. Armstrong, A. McCall, N. Ruderman, and J.C. Melby, Evans Memorial Department of Clinical Research and the Department of Medicine, University Hospital and Boston University School of Medicine, Boston, Massachusetts 02118

Prior studies have shown that insulin administered intranasally (INI) closely mimics the physiologic pattern of insulin secretion following a meal. To determine whether INI can control postprandial hyperglycemia, it was administered to type I and II diabetics just prior to ingestion of a mixed meal (10 cal/kg, 50% CH_2O, 20% protein, 30% fat) eaten at 0800 h following an overnight fast and discontinuation of insulin for 24 hours. The same meal was eaten after an intranasal placebo on another day. As shown below, INI (1.0-1.5 U/kg) diminished postprandial hyperglycemia in both groups. The effect was evident within one hour and persisted throughout the four hours of the study. On a per-weight basis, INI was slightly more effective in type I patients. These studies suggest that INI can normalize postprandial glucose increments in patients with both types I and II diabetes.

Subjects		Type I			Type II		
Treatment	Placebo	Placebo	1 U/kg	1.5 U/kg	Placebo	1 U/kg	1.5 U/kg
(time-hr)	n=6	n=17	n=16	n=10	n=8	n=8	n=7
0	95 ± 8	213 ± 22	230 ± 25	191 ± 20	140 ± 13	158 ± 21	151 ± 28
1	102 ± 11	364 ± 28	250 ± 29	129 ± 20	229 ± 21	215 ± 34	148 ± 34
2	86 ± 9	404 ± 18	285 ± 28	146 ± 27	252 ± 26	236 ± 33	171 ± 37
3	95 ± 4	391 ± 19	295 ± 25	150 ± 30	228 ± 24	226 ± 33	178 ± 36
4	99 ± 7	367 ± 20	283 ± 25	167 ± 28	193 ± 28	200 ± 34	170 ± 34

2266 VISUALIZATION OF FUNCTIONNING LUNG METASTASES OF DIFFERENTIATED THYROID CARCINOMA BY CHEST COMPUTED TOMOGRAPHY (CT).

M. Schlumberger*, P. Fragu, J.D. Piekarski, C. Parmentier Institut Gustave-Roussy - 94805 Villejuif Cedex France.

25 studies were carried out in patients with differentiated thyroid carcinoma, having lung metastases proven by a recent radioiodine test. They were explored by a chest radiograph and a CT scan. In 6 of these patients CT scans were repeated after treatments with ^{131}I. All the radiologic examinations have been bindly reviewed by 3 independant observers. In 6 patients, the chest radiograph showed metastatic micronodules which were confirmed by CT. In 19 cases chest radiograph was normal or questionable : in 14 of them, CT clearly detected micronodules, and no discrepancy existed between the 3 observers. After radioiodine treatments, CT showed a decrease in the number of the chest nodules. A close relationship has been found between the number of the chest nodules and Tg levels in the serum but no such relationship existed with ^{131}I uptake in the lungs. It must be stressed that CT exclusively visualized peripheral nodules, but was unable to distinguish central nodules from vascular normal structures. The characterization of the pulmonary intersititium by density measurements on the CT scans was unsuccessful. This work points out the improvement brought by the use of CT in the difficult diagnosis and follow up of micronodular lung metastases of differentiated thyroid carcinoma.

2267 DELAYED RESPONSE IN OVULATION INDUCTION WITH PULSATILE LRH - TREATMENT

J. Schoemaker*, H. v. Kessel and T. Korsen, Division of Reproductive Endocrinology and Fertility, Department of Obstetrics and Gynecology, Academic Hospital of the Vrije Universiteit, Amsterdam, The Netherlands.

Induction of ovulation with pulsatile administration of LRH in hypogonadotropic patients has been shown to be highly effective. However, some patients show a definitely delayed response. We studied the endocrinology of 7 such patients (2 olfacto-genital syndrome, 2 idiopathic hypogonadotropic hypogonadism, 1 delayed puberty, 1 hypothalamic multiple sclerosis and 1 secondary amenorrhea of unknown origin) during induction of ovulation with LRH.

In 2 cycles in 2 patients no increase in estrogen excretion was observed. In 1 of these patients follicular growth, followed by ovulation could be induced with a different treatment schedule. In 2 cycles in 2 patients a gradually increasing estrogen excretion was observed without a clear estrogen surge. In 1 of these cycles 2 minor LH peaks were observed. In 1 patient ovulation could be induced with a different treatment schedule without further delay; in the other by treatment for 51 consecutive days in which the ovulatory cycle was preceded by an anovulatory one. In 4 more cycles in 3 patients a clear estrogen surge was obtained without subsequent ovulation. One of these patients ovulated after a different dose schedule and 1 after the addition of hCG.

It is concluded that under prolonged pulsatile LRH treatment, as is the case in normal pubertal development, the institution of ovulatory cycles may be preceded by the occurrence of all types of anovulatory ones.

2268 SHORT- AND LONG-TERM CONTINUOUS INFUSIONS OF CORTICOTROPIN RELEASING FACTOR (CRF) IN MEN AND NONHUMAN PRIMATES : PHYSIOLOGIC AND CLINICAL IMPLICATIONS

H.M. Schulte*, G.P. Chrousos, D.L. Healy, P.W. Gold, E.H. Oldfield, J.D. Booth, G.B. Cutler Jr., and D.L Loriaux. Dept. of Medicine, Univ. Essen, FRG and DEB, NICHD, National Institutes of Health, Bethesda, Md. 20205, USA

To evaluate the response of the hypothalamic-pituitary-adrenal(HPA) axis to continuous stimulation of the corticotroph cell, we infused ovine CRF iv over 8 and 24h in normal volunteers and over 2 weeks in rhesus monkeys. For comparison, ACTH (0.5 μg/kg/h) and normal saline (NS) infusions were given. Plasma IR-ACTH during continuous 8 h CRF infusions to men, at 3 different doses(0.5, 1, 3 μg/kg/h), reached plateau levels of 15-20 pg/ml by 3h. Plasma cortisol levels were higher (14-23 μg/dl) than those during NS infusion but did not reach the levels observed during continuous ACTH infusion. 24-Hour infusion of CRF (1 μg/kg/h) also caused only mild elevations of plasma and urinary free cortisol, which were much lower than those observed with continuous ACTH infusion. The circadian rhythms of plasma ACTH and cortisol persisted during CRF. Urinary free cortisol values(173 ± 43 μg/d) were comparable to those seen in depression but never reached levels seen in Cushing's disease. Continuous infusion of CRF in nonhuman primates over 2 weeks resulted in mild elevations of plasma IR- ACTH, cortisol, and urinary free cortisol (compared to NS infusion) that were much less than those obtained during ACTH infusion. These data suggest that continuous stimulation with CRF *in vivo* does not desensitize or hypersensitize the corticotroph. The stimulatory activity of CRF is apparently harnessed by the negative feedback exerted by the elevated circulating cortisol upon the corticotroph. The circadian periodicity of the HPA axis during CRF infusion suggests that factors other than CRF contribute to the adrenal circadian rhythm.

2269 HYPERPROLACTINEMIA ASSOCIATED WITH ACANTHOSIS NIGRICANS AND FAMILIAL INSULIN RESISTANCE. F. Schwenk*, A. Hayles, and M. Haymond, Mayo Clinic and Foundation, Rochester, Minnesota, 55905, USA.

Acanthosis nigricans, acral hypertrophy, and insulin resistance were observed in a mother and 3 daughters. Oral glucose tolerance was normal, but peak post-glucose plasma insulin (IRI) concentrations were elevated (244 to 1010 uU/ml; normal 90±12 uU/ml). Two monozygotic twin daughters had hyperprolactinemia (HP)(31-71 ng/ml; normal < 23 ng/ml) and elevated urinary ketogenic steroids but not the mother or the other sibling. To determine if the increased ketogenic steroids were the result of HP alone or endogenous ACTH, both twins underwent IV ACTH stimulation, and then one twin received dexamethasone (Dex) (0.75 mg daily X 3 weeks) and the other bromocriptine (Brc)(increasing dose up to 2.5 mg TID by week 3). ACTH increased plasma steroids similar to normals in both. Baseline urinary androsterone (Andr) (6.9 and 5.8 mg/24 hrs) and etiocholanolone (Etio) (3.2 and 5.2 mg/24 hs) were elevated (normals 0.5 to 2.4 and 1.1 to 3.0 mg/24 hrs, respectively). Dex decreased both Andr and Etio to 1.1 mg/24 hrs but HP persisted and insulin resistance was unchanged. Brc normalized plasma prolactin (6 ng/ml) as well as Andr and Etio (1.2 and 1.1 mg/24 hrs, respectively), whereas peak IRI following oral glucose increased (244 to 453 uU/ml). Both girls were then treated with Brc 2.5 mg TID but after 3 months again had HP, with even higher peak post-glucose IRIs (244 to 620 uU/ml and 655 to 6100 uU/ml). SUMMARY AND CONCLUSION: 1) A familial incidence and HP should be sought in the clinical setting of acanthosis nigricans and insulin resistance; 2) the abnormal adrenal androgen production observed in this syndrome may be, in part, the result of hyperprolactinemia; 3) the relationship between Brc and observed increased post-glucose IRI remains to be determined.

2270 INTERMITTENT ECTOPIC CUSHING'S SYNDROME: LOCALIZATION OF AN OCCULT ACTH SOURCE BY SELECTIVE BRONCHIAL LAVAGE FOR ACTH. T.P.Segerson*, H.Raff, M.N.Katzoff, S.A.Levy, and J.W.Findling. Dept. of Medicine, Medical College of Wisconsin-St. Luke's Hospital, Milwaukee, WI 53215

Intermittent ectopic Cushing's Syndrome (CS) is not well recognized. The absence of a discernible ectopic source of ACTH may lead to an incorrect diagnosis of pituitary Cushing's Disease. We describe a patient with intermittent cortisol excess and features of ectopic CS. We propose possible localization of the ectopic source of ACTH by selective bronchial lavage. A 71 yr old woman presented with weakness, confusion, edema, hypertension, and hypokalemia. Evaluation showed dexamethasone nonsuppressible hypercortisolism, elevated ACTH, and metyrapone unresponsiveness. Reevaluation 3 months later showed a remission. Patient was well without therapy until 21 months later when she again presented with CS. CT scans showed a normal pituitary and bilateral adrenal enlargement. Selective venous sampling showed a petrosal sinus to peripheral ACTH ratio of <2.0. Chest radiographs to date have not identified a lesion. Selective bronchoscopic lavage for ACTH gave the following:

Bronchus	ACTH (pg/ml of lavage fluid)
LLL Superior	1000
LLL Basilar	48
Lingula and RUL	86-93
RML & RRL	<50

Eucortisolemia has been maintained for 15 months with aminoglutethimide and metyrapone. Conclusions: Intermittent hypercortisolism may be a feature of ectopic CS. In the absence of a radiographic lesion, selective lobar bronchial washings may localize an occult ACTH-secreting pulmonary neoplasm.

2271 HORMONAL RESPONSES TO EXTREME EXERCISE. C G Semple*, J A Thomson, and G H Beastall. Departments of Medicine, Victoria Infirmary and Royal Infirmary, and The Department of Pathological Biochemistry, Royal Infirmary Glasgow, Scotland.

Endocrine responses to extreme effort were investigated in ten healthy adult males (age range 23-49 years) who successfully completed the Glasgow marathon. Blood was withdrawn during the week prior to the marathon at the estimated time of completing the race and as soon as possible after the end of the race. Fluids were freely available during the race. The microhaematocrit of the runners did not change after the marathon making it unlikely that haemoconcentration would have any significant effect on results. Serum was stored at $-20^{\circ}C$ until assay and to avoid interassay variation each pair of samples was measured in the same assay system. T4, T3, TSH and FT4 showed no significant change. Serum cortisol rose from 338 ± 147 (mean $\pm$ SD) to 1640 ± 884 nmol/l ($p < 0.01$). Androstenedione, DHAS, and oestradiol levels also increased ($p < 0.01$) but serum testosterone fell from 18.9 ± 5.0 to 14.9 ± 3.6 nmol/l ($p < 0.01$). SHBG levels did not change. The fall in testosterone levels was accompanied by a decrease in LH from 4.1 ± 1.9 to 2.5 ± 1.2 U/l ($p < 0.05$). FSH levels were unchanged but serum prolactin rose from 139.8 ± 100.8 to 333.5 ± 283.6 mU/l ($p < 0.01$). It is proposed that the fall in LH and consequently testosterone is due to suppression by increased levels of either cortisol or endogenous opioid peptides both of which increase with physical exertion.

2272 LUTEINIZING HORMONE-RELEASING HORMONE (LHRH)-LIKE AND THYROTROPIN-RELEASING HORMONE (TRH)-LIKE SUBSTANCE(S) FOUND IN THE HEPATOPANCREAS OF GRASS SHRIMP (*Penaeus monodon*). W. C. M. Wan*, M. C. Fann, and P. S. Wang, Institute of Zoology, Academia Sinica and Department of Physiology, National Yang-Ming Medical College, Taipei, Taiwan, (115), Republic of China

The acid extract of the hepatopancreas of grass shrimps (SHE) subjected for a double radioimmunoassay (RIA) of LHRH and TRH. In these RIA systems, the synthetic LHRH and TRH were utilized as standards and for radioiodination, and the antisera for LHRH and TRH were obtained from rabbits immunized by hormone-bovine serum albumin conjugates. Increasing of the SHE in both of RIA systems demonstrated that the dose response curves are paralleled with the standard curves respectively. Both radioimmunoassayable TSH and LH can be induced by SHE in perifusion and static incubation systems with rats pituitaries as target tissues. Immunoprecipitation of SHE with individual antiserum or both , significantly decreased the hormones in the supernatants as measured by RIA, and its inducing of LH and TSH release in incubation systems also significantly decreased. Hypothalamic hormone-like substances were undetectable in tissues such as the muscle of the body, heart, nerve trunks, eye and eye stalk.The present data indicated that there are substances in the shrimp with an immunoreactivity of TRH and LHRH.

2273 CATECHOLAMINE-MEDIATED PRESSOR RESPONSES TO GONADOTROPIN-RELEASING HORMONE IN TOADS. J.X. Wilson*, B.N. Van Vliet and N.H. West, Department of Physiology, College of Medicine, University of Saskatchewan, Saskatoon, Sask. S7N OWO Canada.

Gonadotropin-releasing hormone (GnRH) is thought to regulate reproductive function in amphibians because the administration of synthetic GnRH increases circulating levels of luteinizing hormone and androgens. However, immunoreactive GnRH or GnRH-like peptides also are putative transmitters in amphibian brain, sympathetic ganglia and adrenal glands. We injected synthetic GnRH intravenously into conscious, adult toads (Bufo marinus) to elucidate the nervous and cardiovascular actions of the hormone. GnRH (0.001 - 1.0 nmol/kg) produced dose-dependent increases in mean arterial blood pressure and pulse pressure within 3 min post-injection. These pressor responses to GnRH were specific to the hormone since they could be inhibited reversibly by [D-pGlu^{1} D-Phe^{2}, D-Trp^{3,6}]-GnRH. Arterial plasma concentrations of unconjugated catecholamines increased simultaneously with the rise in blood pressure following GnRH injection: the half-maximal pressor dose of GnRH (0.1 nmol/kg) caused a 3-fold increase in plasma epinephrine and a 20-fold increase in plasma norepinephrine concentrations. Pretreatment of toads with an alpha-adrenergic antagonist, prazosin, and a beta-adrenergic antagonist, propranolol, abolished the pressor responses to GnRH. We conclude that GnRH mobilizes catecholamines, which act through alpha- and beta-adrenergic mechanisms to raise blood pressure. Thus, endogenous GnRH or GnRH-like peptides may coordinate the pituitary, nervous and cardiovascular mechanisms which prepare toads for seasonal reproductive activity. This study was supported by NSERC, Saskatchewan Health Research Board and MRC.

2274 EFFECTS OF A PHASE-ADVANCE OF DARKNESS ON THE OVULATORY CYCLE OF THE HEN. S.C. Wilson, Department of Physiology & Biochemistry, University of Reading, Whiteknights, Reading RG6 2AJ, England.

Hens maintained under continuous light can ovulate at times throughout the 24 h day. In contrast, under standard conditions of light and darkness the occurrence of ovulation is restricted to an 8-10 h period of the day. It is therefore possible that hormonal changes associated with darkness are important in determining the temporal distribution of ovulations. To investigate this possibility hens maintained on 16 h light:8 h darkness were subjected to an abrupt advancement of darkness. When advanced darkness occurred at less than 6-8 h after a mid-sequence ovulation the next expected preovulatory release of LH and ovulation was usually delayed or blocked in association with a reduction in effectiveness of injected ovine LH to stimulate the secretion of progesterone. When advanced darkness occurred at greater than 6-8 h after a mid-sequence ovulation the next expected preovulatory release of LH and ovulation was generally advanced in association with an increased LH response to injected progesterone. Advancement of darkness by 4-7 h brought about changes in the tonic secretion of LH and an advancement of the circadian increase in secretion of corticosterone regardless of whether ovulation was advanced or delayed. These results suggest that events associated with darkness may normally advance or delay follicular maturation depending on the state of development of that follicle at the onset of darkness. This study was supported by the Agricultural Research Council.

2275 CHANGES IN cAMP LEVELS DURING IN VITRO CAPACITATION OF HAMSTER SPERMATOZOA.
J.G. Tezon* and C.W. Bardin, The Population Council, New York, N.Y. 10021.

The adenylate cyclase system in spermatozoa is believed to be refractory to hormones. As a consequence alternative mechanisms were sought for the modulation of cAMP levels in these cells. In this study we have investigated how the factors required for in vitro capacitation of hamster spermatozoa influenced the content of cAMP. Washed epididymal sperm were incubated in Tyrode's modified medium (TALP, 0.3% BSA, 0.1% PVA, 10 μM Hypotaurine) under oil. Immunoassayable cAMP declined (85%) within the first 10 min of incubation and 0.1 mM MIX in the medium allowed recovery of cAMP to control levels after 1 hr. The effects on cAMP levels of epinephrine and isoproterenol, known to facilitate capacitation in vitro, were studied after 1 hr incubation in the presence of MIX. Both compounds showed a dose response effect with maximal (2 fold) stimulation at 10 μM concentration. Other components necessary for in vitro capacitation such as the chelators, penicillamine or 4,5 dihydronaphthalene 2,7-disulfonic acid, increased cAMP by 8 fold. Since protein carboxyl methylation (PCM) is linked to the acquistion of activated motility, the effects of the inhibitor homocysteine (0.1 mM) was next investigated. Low PCM activity was associated with increases in both basal and catecholamine induced cAMP. Finally Ca++ is required for the acrosomal reaction, another component of capacitation. This ion at a concentration of 2 mM increased the cAMP response to both catecholamines and chelators. Conclusion: Cyclic AMP accumulation in spermatozoa is regulated by hormones and other factors that are required for in vitro capacitation.

2276 ACTIVATION OF THE RAT PLATELET cGMP-BINDING PHOSPHODIESTERASE BY cAMP-DEPENDENT PROTEIN PHOSPHORYLATION. Johanne Tremblay* and Pavel Hamet. Clinical Research Institute Montreal, Quebec H2W 1R7, Canada.

Platelets contain a cGMP phosphodiesterase which binds cGMP with high affinity at a site that seems different from the catalytic site. An allosteric interaction occurs between the catalytic and the binding sites: Several competitive inhibitors of PDE appear to increase the apparent affinity of cGMP binding. We have previously reported that PDE activity and binding of cGMP are increased by exposure of washed platelets to agents that increase cAMP levels (forskolin, PGE_1, PGI_2) and by phosphodiesterase inhibitors (MIX, indomethacin, dipyridamol). We present here evidence that cAMP-dependent phosphorylation is involved in this process. When supernatant of washed platelets was preincubated with agents promoting phosphorylation (ATP, $MgCl_2$, cAMP) followed by appropriate dilution for the measurement of PDE activity no effect was observed. However when MIX was added to the incubation mixture a significant increase of cGMP-PDE activity was obtained. The PDE activation was inhibited by a non-hydrolysable analog of ATP, AMP (PNP). The maximal stimulation was reached after 5 min of incubation and was observed only in presence of MIX. The effect of MIX is not due to preservation of cAMP from hydrolysis but increases the susceptibility of the cGMP-binding PDE to phosphorylation. Finally, prior exposure of intact platelets to forskolin and MIX prevented further activation by in vitro phosphorylation. The results suggest that the hydrolysis and binding of cGMP by the cGMP-binding phosphodiesterase can be increased in intact platelets by phosphorylation. Supported by MRC,NIH AM 2199,CHF.

2277 **A NEW VARIANT OF ACANTHOSIS NIGRICANS, VIRILISM WITH HYPERINSULINEMIC GLUCOSE INTOLERANCE ASSOCIATED WITH NORMAL RBC INSULIN RECEPTORS AND EXOGENOUS INSULIN RESPONSIVENESS.** **B.L.Wajchenberg+, A.C.Lerário, B.B.Mendonça, W.Bloise, J.A.M.Marcondes, R.DiDio, H.Tager and L.G.Heding, Diabetes and Adrenal Unit, Hospital das Clinicas and CRIESP, S.Paulo, Brazil; Dep. Biochemistry, Univ. Chicago and Novo Research Institute, Bagsvaerd, Denmark.**

Two negro females(nº1:20 yr and nº2:15 yr)with Acanthosis nigricans, virilism, polycistic ovaries and secondary amenorrhea with the absence of antibodies to insulin receptor are presented. Excess testosterone and androstenedione production was secondary to ovarian hypersecretion as suggested by prolonged dexamethasone supp. test(nº1) and also by simultaneous ovarian and adrenal vein catheterization(nº2). Greatly elevated basal and stimulated insulin levels were associated with severe(nº1) and mild glucose intolerance(nº2). No elevations of known circulating insulin antagonists were detected including GH, F, glucagon or insulin antibodies. No structurally abnormal insulin was detected in plasma of both patients by reverse-phase HPLC. High basal proinsulin levels corresponded to the increased insulin values.

Significant receptor and postreceptor defects were excluded by normal interaction of insulin to its RBC receptors and normal responses to porcine I.V. insulin.

These findings were consistent with a defect in circulating insulin action.

2278 INHIBITORY EFFECTS OF THE ANTIPROGESTERONE STEROID RU 486 ON GONADOTROPIN SECRETION IN WOMEN. G. Schaison*, M. George, N. Lestrat, M. Lagoguey and E.E. Baulieu. Service d'Endocrinologie et des Maladies de la Reproduction and INSERM U33 Hôpital de Bicêtre, 94270 Bicêtre, France.

In women, the antiprogesterone steroid RU 486 administered in the luteal phase of the cycle induces uterine bleeding and is promising as a new agent for fertility control. In order to study its mechanism of action, the drug was administered orally to 18 normally cycling and 6 postmenopausal women. In cycling women, 25, 50 or 100 mg daily were given for 4 days starting on the 4th day after basal body temperature shift. Uterine bleeding occurred in all cases on the 3rd day of RU 486 administration. Plasma LH levels were measured daily at 15 min intervals for 4 hrs. In the 10 women treated either with 25 or 50 mg/d, no significant change of LH was observed. In the 8 subjects receiving 100 mg/d, mean ($\pm$ SE) levels decreased significantly ($p < 0.01$) from 3.2 ± 0.6 to 1.1 ± 0.2 mIU/ml. Computerized LH pulsatility disappeared during treatment. In post menopausal women, RU 486 (200 mg daily) was given during the last 6 days of a 15 day treatment with estradiol benzoate (EB) 625 µg/d, while 6 other postmenopausal women received EB alone. LH and FSH levels were found to be 2.6 ± 0.8 and 6.5 ± 1.9 mIU/ml after the combined treatment and 14.1 ± 1.0 and 17.3 ± 2.2 mIU/ml after EB alone. The difference was significant for both hormones ($p < 0.001$). Conclusions : 1) 25 mg and 50 mg/d of RU 486 given in the luteal phase, constantly induce uterine bleeding and do not alter gonadotropin secretion in cycling women, confirming its direct effect upon endometrium. 2) 100 and 200 mg/d of the drug impair gonadotropin secretion in both normally cycling and postmenopausal women.

2279 EFFICACY OF SUBCUTANEOUS IMPLANTS OF NORETHINDRONE (NET) PELLETS AS A LONG ACTING CONTRACEPTIVE.

M. Singh,* B.B. Saxena, G.N. Gupta, R. Landesman, and W.J. Ledger, Division of Reproductive Endocrinology, Department of Obstetrics & Gynecology, Cornell University Medical College-The New York Hospital, New York, New York 10021

Forty-two fertile, sexually active women of 20-35 years were enrolled in the study. On the 5th day of the menstrual cycle, three or four 5x3x2.6 mm pellets of 35 mg NET each were implanted by a trocar through a 3 mm incision on the ventral surface of the forearm under local anesthesia as an out-patient procedure. Blood samples were collected at mid-cycle and luteal phase during the control cycle and once a month during the post-implant period for E_2, P, and NET determinations. During the control and every 3rd menstrual cycle, serum LDL-HDL ratio and SMAC's were determined; PAP smear and complete physical and pelvic examinations were also performed. No pregnancy occurred in 15 women with four pellets up to a period of 11 months. In 27 women with three pellets, one pregnancy occurred at the 6th month. Intermenstrual bleeding occurred in 28% of the women during initial cycles which subsequently normalized. Only 14% of the cycles were ovulatory with three pellets (serum NET levels 0.4-0.5 ng/ml) and 11% with four pellets (serum NET levels 0.6-0.7 ng/ml). There were no significant changes in the serum LDL-HDL ratio and SMAC's during the post-implant period. There was an ameliorating effect on dysmenorrhea and pre-menstrual syndrome. These observations indicate that NET pellets are safe, low-dose, convenient, inexpensive, and a reversible form of long acting contraception with a high degree of acceptability as the first choice of contraception by the volunteers. (Support - PARFR, Endocon, Inc., The Rockefeller Foundation)

2280 SOMATOMEDIN AND NONSUPPRESSIBLE INSULIN-LIKE ACTIVITY (NSILA) IN PREGNANT MOTHERS AND THE UMBILICAL CORD BLOOD OF MATURE AND PREMATURE INFANTS.

N.A. Samaan*, R.V. Sellin, P.N. Schultz, M.E. Rivera, and B. Held. Endocrinology, Univ. of Texas M.D. Anderson Hosp. and OB-GYN, Univ. of Texas Med. School at Houston, Houston, Texas 77030.

This study was undertaken to determine the possible significance of the changes in the immunoreactive growth hormone (hGH), human chorionic somatomammotropin (HCS), somatomedin-C (SM-C,RIA), somatomedin activity (SMA) by the rat costal cartilage, and NSILA measured by fat pad bioassay in pregnancy and neonates. Sera from 15 normal women at term (Group A) and 15 normal women who delivered prematurely (Group B) were compared with 10 normal nonpregnant women matched for age (Group C). Umbilical cord blood was obtained from Groups A & B at delivery. Basal hGH levels were not elevated in Groups A or B mothers. The HCS levels in Groups A & B mothers were high but unmeasurable in the infants or in Group C. The SM-C,RIA in Groups A & B mothers was higher than in Group C ($p < 0.001$). The SMA in Groups A & B mothers was higher than in Groups A & B infants and Group C. The NSILA in Groups A & B mothers was higher than Group C ($p < 0.001$). The hGH level in Group B infants was higher than Group A infants ($p < 0.001$) and both were higher than Group C ($p < 0.01$). In contrast SMA,RIA in Groups A & B infants were less than Group C ($p < 0.001$). NSILA in Group B infants was less than Group A ($p < 0.01$). We conclude that 1) There is correlation between somatomedin, NSILA and HCS but not with hGH in pregnant mothers. 2) There was correlation between NSILA, somatomedin and the fetal age. 3) There was marked discordance between hGH and somatomedin in premature and mature neonates.

2281 DIFFERENTIATION OF EMBRYONIC NEUROBLAST CELLS INTO NEURONS IN VITRO. M. Sanyal,* C. Leranth, W. Biggers and F. Naftolin. Dept. of Ob/Gyn, Yale University School of Medicine, New Haven, CT 06510

A system of neural tissue culture utilizing neural tube fragments of rat embryos of pregnancy day 12 (Witschi stage 17/18) has been developed. In this system neural tube tissues were dissected, dispersed into fragments and cultured over a Vitrogen (collagen) surface with MEM culture medium containing 10% horse and 10% calf sera in 10% CO2 and air at 37°C. Within 3 days of culture neuroblast cells differentiate, with branching processes emerging from neural tube fragments, with number and length proportional to fragment size and duration of culture, respectively. Two differentiated neuronal cell types with neurite outgrowths were distinguished: (I) neuroblast cells extending long, thin branching processes and remaining within neural tube tissue mass, and (II) neuroblast cells migrating out of the neural tube tissue mass and developing unipolar or multipolar thick processes. With immunoperoxidase histochemical methods they could be further characterized: type I neuroblast cells within the tissue mass and their neurites stained intensely for glutamic acid decarboxylase (GAD), and type II migrating neuroblasts with noradrenalin antibodies. At the initiation of culture, neuroblast cells were undifferentiated, and culture conditions permitted progressive differentiation into neurons. Since catecholamine positive cells will presumably develop into ganglion or medullary neurons, and GAD containing cells into inhibitory interneurons, it is likely that these cell types represent the initial differentiation stages of neuroblast cells produced under the culture conditions utilized. (Supported by NIH HD14587 and Mellon fellowship grants)

2282 EARLY HORMONAL POTENTIALITIES AND INITIAL SEX DIFFERENTIATION IN QUAIL GONADS. D.Scheib*, M.Reyss-Brion, Th.M.Mignot and A.Guichard. Institut Embryologie CNRS et Collège de France(Nogent sur Marne) and Laboratoire de Chimie Hormonale Port-Royal (Paris),France.

The present investigation was performed on sex-linked quail embryos. The early hormonal potentialities of their gonads were controlled in vitro by RIA, at 51/2-61/2 days,in absence and in presence of steroid precursors. Undifferentiated male and female gonads displayed at 51/2 days divergent steroidogenic potentialities before any apparent sexual feature. At both ages,female gonads were more active than male gonads and produced estradiol; male gonads had only a weak aromatizing capacity and produced mainly testosterone. The in vitro hormonal biosynthesis was greatly enhanced in presence of steroid precursors. In female gonads,left-right differences in steroid levels were already obvious by 51/2 days, concomittant with an asymmetry in their protein levels; such a divergence was not evident for male gonads.These results show that a molecular difference(specific enzymes) precedes cellular organization as previously suggested by histoenzymological observations.Moreover they emphasize the feminizing role of estrogens and corroborate the hormonal patterns found for differentiated quail gonads.

2283 STUDIES ON THE ROLES OF MILK PRL AND INSULIN (I) IN THE SUCKLING RAT.
N.L. Schlechter*, S.M. Russell, A. Lim and C.S. Nicoll, Dept. of Physiology-Anatomy and Cancer Research Lab, Univ. of California, Berkeley, Ca. 94720

Hypophysectomized (HX) rat pups continue to grow at 50% of normal. Thus, we studied whether growth-promoting hormones are transferred from mother to pup via milk. PRL is present in high concentration in milk, and it is taken up across the infant gut into serum. However, HX pups given high doses of PRL either by SC injection or intragastrically showed no increase in growth rate. The possibility that I in milk may function as a growth factor for pups was also studied because we found that rat milk contains high concentrations of I (11-25ng/ml). We also found that IV injection of 1U of porcine I (pI) into lactating females resulted in a 21-fold increase in milk I within 15 min and a 36-fold increase after 1 hr. Also, streptozotocin (STZ)-injected infants show variable patterns of glycosuria (GU). Of 31 pups given STZ, 19% showed no GU and only 6.5% showed persistent GU; 35.5% had GU for only 1 to 2 days after injection with a resumption of GU within 2 days after weaning, and 39% of the pups displayed only the post-weaning GU. These results suggest a milk factor is responsible for the pups' resistance to GU. Sera from pups suckling on mothers which were injected with 1U pI showed no difference in I concentration from sera of pups suckling on saline-injected mothers. Similarly, pups intubated with cow milk containing up to 30 mU of pI/ml showed no difference in serum I concentration from pups fed untreated cow milk. Since I does not appear to be absorbed across the infant gut, milk I cannot account for continued growth of HX pups or the apparent resistance of some pups to STZ-induced GU.

2284 SYNTHESIS OF ADRENOCORTICAL STEROIDS BY HUMAN PLACENTA. M.J. Schofield*, and F.J. Auletta, University of Vermont College of Medicine, Depts. of Ob/Gyn and Biochemistry, Burlington, Vermont 05405, U.S.A.

Following initial studies by this laboratory indicating the ability of ovine placenta to synthetize cortisol (F) from 11-deoxycortisol (S) and 17^{α}OH-progesterone (17OH-P), similar studies were conducted examining human term placental tissue. Intact placentas were obtained from both normal and caesarean deliveries, and maintained at 4°C throughout the preparation procedures. Subcellular fractions were prepared by centrifugation of tissue homogenates in 0.25 M sucrose and the corresponding mitochondrial (800-15,000 x g) and microsomal (15,000-105,000 x g) fractions isolated and incubated in a Krebs-Ringer bicarbonate buffer containing 2 mg/ml glucose and a NADPH generator system, at 37°C in a Dubnoff-type shaking bath for 1 hour. Synthesis from added precursors was determined using tritiated tracers following ethyl acetate (EtAc) and methylene chloride (MeCl) extraction and 3-one dimensional TLC in the solvent systems: 7:3 EtAc/ isooctane, 4:1 MeCl/diethyl ether, and 9:9:2 EtAc/isooctane/aceticacid. Conversions from progesterone to 17OH-P and S, and 17OH-P to S were observed in the microsomal preparations. To a lesser extent, conversion of S to a compound which migrated on TLC with F/cortisone was seen in the mitochondrial fraction. The former finding is consistent with the reports of placental 17OH-P production at term. The additional 11^{β}-hydroxylase activity may serve to explain the origin of increasing S secretion from the feto-placental unit approaching labor. These findings strongly suggest that the human placenta at term has the capability of synthesizing glucocorticoids.

2285 CIRCADIAN VARIATION OF PLASMA OXYTOCIN IN THE LATE GESTATION RHESUS MONKEY.

M. Serón-Ferré*, N.F. Taylor, M.C.Martin, R.D. Leake and D.B.Fisher. Rep. Endo.Ctr.,Dept.Ob.Gyn.& Rep.Sci.UCSF, SF, CA, and Dept.Ped.UCLA, Sch.Med., Harbor/UCLA Med.Ctr. Torrance, CA.

The rhesus monkey shows a marked circadian variation of uterine electromyographic activity (EMG) the last 10 days of gestation. We decided to investigate whether there is a concomitant circadian variation of oxytocin at this time. To that effect we inserted femoral catheters in 4 pregnant rhesus monkeys (110 d GA) acclimated to restraint chairs. EMG was monitored continuously until delivery. Animals were kept with lights on from 0600 to 1800 h. Weekly maternal samples were collected every 2 hours for 26 h in 2 animals during the 6 wks prior to delivery. The other 2 animals were sampled 1 and 3 wks before delivery. All animals delivered at term (168+7 d). Blood was centrifuged immediately, plasma was removed, snap frozen and kept at -20°C until analysis. Oxytocin was measured by RIA after acetone extraction. Daily mean plasma oxytocin concentrations were similar in all animals. Samples taken 7 days prior delivery showed a marked circadian variation (peak 2,5 times mean) in all animals. The increase starts at 1800, peaks at 2000 and wanes by 0200. This peak in plasma oxytocin concides with the circadian peak of EMG found during the last 10 days of gestation. This data suggests that circadian surges of oxytocin may contribute to regulate uterine contractions.

Supported by NIH HD-08478.

2286 EFFECTS OF MATERNAL CIRCADIAN RHYTHMS ON FETAL OSCILLATION UNDERLYING THE CIRCADIAN RHYTHM OF PLASMA CORTICOSTERONE IN RATS.

T. Shirakawa*, S. Honma, K. Honma, and T. Hiroshige, *Department of Pedodontics, School of Dentistry, and Department of Physiology, School of Medicine, Hokkaido University, Sapporo Japan.

Our previous experiments (J.Physiol. 325,521,1982) suggested that the circadian oscillation underlying the corticosterone rhythm was initiated prenatally and the phase of oscillation was determined by mother circadian system before birth. However, the onset time of entrainment during gestation remains unknown. In this study, circadian rhythms of locomotor activity and corticosterone level in pregnant rats were eliminated by bilateral lesions of suprachiasmatic nuclei(SCN) at day 3 or 10 of gestation and the postnatal manifestation of corticosterone rhythm was examined in individual pups. Effective lesion of SCN at day 3 of gestation resulted in an abortion. But rats whose SCN were lesioned at day 10 of gestation maintained pregnancy, and the pups born to and nursed by their original mother were optically enucleated immediately. At the 4th, 5th and 6th postnatal weeks all pups showed circadian free-running rhythms of plasma corticosterone level with similar phase angles. However, the circadian rhythm of the pups born to operated mothers was phase delayed by about 4 hours to that of blind control pups born to unoperated mothers. It is concluded that the circadian oscillation underlying corticosterone rhythm of rats has entrained to the maternal circadian system during fetal life. Furthermore, it is suggested that the entrainment occurs before day 10 of gestation.

2287 TRANSPORT OF STEROIDS FROM FETAL MONKEY PLASMA INTO THE RAT BRAIN. S. Sholl*, Wisconsin Regional Primate Research Center, University of Wisconsin, Madison, Wisconsin 53715-1299 U.S.A.

In the fetal primate, sex steroids which have been found in the circulation may influence the development of the brain. The extent to which these hormones are accessible to neuronal cells may be influenced by binding proteins in fetal blood. The effect of these plasma components on the accessibility of testosterone (T), dihydrotestosterone, estradiol and estrone was evaluated in fetal monkeys (Macaca mulatta) on Days 135-162 of gestation using the technique of Oldendorf (Brain Res. 24:372, 1970). The rat was used as the test-subject. Monkey fetal plasma (200 µl), equilibrated with [^{3}H]-labeled steroids and ^3H_2O (as a readily diffusible reference), was rapidly injected into the rat carotid artery. The brain was removed within 15 s of injection and the BUI estimated. (BUI = [^{3}H]steroid/^3H_2O ratio in brain/ratio in test-sample x 100.) BUI was greatest for T-male, female plasma (102%, 81%, respectively), while uptake for the other steroids examined was approximately 55-60%. Sex differences in BUI were not evident. These data indicate that blood-brain transport of T is not reduced by protein in monkey fetal plasma, while the transport of estrogens is retarded. The retardation in estrogen transport may help to protect the fetal female brain from potential masculinization.

2288 REGULATION OF 3β-HYDROXYSTEROID DEHYDROGENASE ACTIVITY IN HUMAN FETAL ADRENOCORTICAL CELLS BY ACTH AND TRIIODOTHYRONINE (T3). M.H. Simonian*, Dept. Physiology and Biophysics, The University of Iowa, Iowa City, IA 52242, U.S.A.

The functional zonation of the human fetal adrenal cortex is characterized by a lower 3β-hydroxysteroid dehydrogenase, $\Delta^{4,5}$-isomerase (HSD) activity in fetal zone (FZ) cells relative to that in definitive zone (DZ) cells. Chronic treatment of FZ cell cultures with ACTH in serum-supplemented medium induces the HSD activity to the same level as in DZ cells. Using serum-free conditions, cell cultures from DZ and FZ were treated without and with ACTH for 48h and the HSD activity assayed in whole cells by the conversion of [^{3}H]dehydroepiandrosterone to androstenedione. The basal activity of HSD was 3-to-5 fold higher in DZ cells than the homologous FZ cells (P<.001) from two midgestation fetuses. Treatment of FZ cells with 10nM ACTH and assayed in the absence of ACTH, increased the HSD activity 5-fold. This maximal stimulatory effect of ACTH on the HSD activity required the presence of 1nM T3 (ED_{50}=31pM). In the absence of T3, the effect of ACTH was only one-half of that observed in the presence of T3. T3 had no effect on the ED_{50} of ACTH (0.3nM) for the induction of the HSD activity and T3 alone had a minimal stimulatory effect of 30-50% (P<.01). T3 had the same synergistic effect on ACTH-induction of HSD activity in DZ cells maintained in culture for two weeks in serum to allow the basal HSD activity to decrease prior to the serum-free treatment and assay. Thus, the maximal trophic effect of ACTH on HSD activity and the induction of this activity in FZ cells to the basal level observed in DZ cells requires the presence of T3.

2289 THE RELATIONSHIP BETWEEN SERUM TRIIODOTHYRONINES LEVELS AND THE EXTRATHYROIDAL THYROXINE MONODEIODINATION DURING THE NEONATAL PERIOD IN THE PIG. A.B. Ślebodziński, E. Brzezińska-Ślebodzińska and R. Drews*, Department of Experimental Pathology of Animals, PAN, ul. Grunwaldzka 250, Poznań, Poland.

Paralleled studies on profiles of serum T_4, T_3 and rT_3, and on the T_4 5′- and 5- monodeiodination in the extrathyroidal tissues (liver, kidney, muscles, brain) in newborn pigs have been performed. It has been found that an individual hormone profile is biphasic i.e. displays a peaks within the first 6-12 h postnatally, a nadir at about day 3-5 and a rise during the 2nd week of life, particularly in rT_3 concentration. This profile is somewhat different from that found in newborn infants of corresponding age in which a gradual rise in T_3 and a fall in rT_3 are generally observed. The amount of T_3 and rT_3 generated from exogenous T_4 per mg of tissue protein were the lowest during the most marked iodothyroninemia on the 1st postnatal day. $T_4 \rightarrow T_3$ and $T_4 \rightarrow rT_3$ conversions in the liver increased to peak levels on the day 3, then gradually decreased to a low 1st day level. Concomitant, biphasic rise in the kidney 5- and 5′- monodeiodinase activity (at about day 3 and 14) was observed. It is concluded that the immediate postnatal iodothyroninemia is due to a rapid hormone discharge from thyroid gland, whereas the 2nd serum hormone rise may reflect the intensity of the peripheral T_4 monodeiodination.

2290 PHYSALAEMIN-LIKE IMMUNOREACTIVE MATERIAL (PLIM) FROM RABBIT STOMACH: PARTIAL PURIFICATION AND CHARACTERIZATION. W. E. Wilson*, B. J. Irons, D. L. Carlton, L. H. Lazarus, and V. Erspamer (Rome, Italy), LBNT, NIEHS, NIH, P.O. Box 12233, Research Triangle Park, NC 27709.

PLIM has been extensively purified from rabbit stomach. The purification of an ethanol-formic acid extract included (a) removal of ethanol and concentration, (b) passage through strong anion and cation exchange resins (most of the PLIM did not adsorb to either resin), (c) C-8 reverse phase LC using stepwise elution with ethanol, (d) HPLC on silica gel, and (e) HPLC on ODS and diphenyl reverse phase columns. PLIM in rabbit stomach contains several components; the most prominent, PLIM-A, has been purified to apparent homogeniety by HPLC on ODS and diphenyl reverse phase columns by using a propanol-water-sodium sulfate mobile phase. PLIM-A possesses no ionizable functional groups. The affinity of PLIM-A for the hydrophobic surface of the various reverse phase column packings is markedly influenced by the ionic strength of the HPLC mobile phase. Immunoreactivity of PLIM-A is destroyed by thermolysin. Gel filtration indicates that the Mr of PLIM-A is 1200-2000. A partially purified preparation of PLIM-A exhibited tachykinin bioactivity characterized by an increase in tonus and phasic motility of guinea pig illial smooth muscle, with slower onset and relaxation than amphibian physalaemin. In rabbit large intestine, PLIM-A inhibited tone and motility; this inhibition was reversed by amphibian physalaemin.

2291 RAT GROWTH HORMONE (GH) GENE EXPRESSION IS CORRELATED WITH A SPECIFIC HYPO-METHYLATED SITE. J. Strobl*[1], P.Dannies[2], and E.B. Thompson[3], Pharmacology and Toxicology[1], West Virginia University, Morgantown, WV, Pharmacology[2], Yale University, New Haven, CT, and Laboratory of Biochemistry[3], NCI, NIH, Bethesda, MD, U.S.A.

Tissue-specific expression of some genes is correlated with the absence of 5-methylcytosine (5meC) at specific sites in these genes. We compared the distribution of 5meC in rat GH genes in DNA isolated from 7 clones of GH-producing rat pituitary adenoma tissue culture cells (GH_3), GH-non-producing GH_3 X mouse fibroblast hybrid cells, rat liver, spleen and brain to determine if this is also true of the rat GH gene. DNA was purified, digested with restriction enzymes (r.e.), electrophoresed in agarose gels, and transferred to nitrocellulose paper; GH DNA fragments were detected by autoradiography after hybridization with GH cDNA labeled with ^{32}P by nick-translation. DNAs were digested with HindIII or EcoRI to yield respectively, 5.6 or 9kbp DNA fragments containing the rat GH gene. Digestion with a second r.e., HpaII, AvaI, or ThaI was dependent upon the DNA methylation state: sequences within the coding+3'flanking DNA (HpaII) or 5'flanking DNA (AvaI or ThaI) were cleaved when cytosine but not 5meC was present in the r.e. recognition sequence. The presence of 5meC within these sequences was evident by the size of the GH DNA fragments. 5meC was randomly distributed among HpaII and AvaI r.e. sites in the rat GH genes in GH_3 and hybrid cells. In contrast, the DNA of all GH_3 clones and rat brain was unmethylated at a ThaI site in the 5'flanking DNA which contained 5meC in the hybrid cell, rat liver and spleen DNA. We conclude that hypomethylation of this site is correlated with rat GH gene expression.

2292 ONLY ONE GENE ENCODES THE BETA SUBUNIT OF A LH/CG-LIKE GONADOTROPIN IN THE RAT. M.A.Tepper* and J.L.Roberts, Department of Biochemistry and Center for Reproductive Sciences, Columbia College of Physicians and Surgeons, New York, New York, USA 10032

The presence of a chorionic gonadotropin(CG) in the placenta has been well documented in only a few mammals, namely human, baboon and horse. In the rat, the presence of a placental LH/CG-like molecule remains controversial. Several investigators have reported the presence of a LH/CG-like molecule, as well as its subunits, in the rat placenta at various gestational ages. However, this molecule has not been isolated or characterized. Thus, to more directly address the question of a rat chorionic gonadotropin, we investigated the presence of any potential gene or mRNA which could encode the beta subunit of a LH/CG-like molecule in the rat genome and placenta, respectively. Southern blot analysis of rat genomic DNA, using multiple restriction enzyme digests, revealed only one fragment per digest which hybridized to a rat LH beta cDNA probe. Thus, our data suggest that the rat haploid genome contains only one gene which encodes for the beta subunit of LH and no genes which encode for a LH/CG-like beta subunit. These data further suggest that the rat placenta does not have a mRNA that can encode for the beta subunit of either LH or a CG-like molecule.

2293 REGULATION OF BETA LH GENE EXPRESSION DURING THE ESTRUS CYCLE AND CASTRATION IN THE RAT.

M.A. Tepper, F.T. Dionne*, J.H. Eberwine, J.N. Wilcox, and J.L. Roberts, Dept. of Biochemistry and Center for Reproductive Sciences, Columbia College of Physicians and Surgeons, New York, New York, USA 10032.

In order to better understand the molecular mechanisms involved in the regulation of beta LH gene expression, we have used a cloned beta LH cDNA to analyze steady state beta LH mRNA levels, as well as transcription rates of the beta LH gene. Rats were sacrificed at different stages of the estrus cycle and the anterior pituitary was removed for either cytoplasmic RNA quantitation or nuclear transcription assays. RNA dot blots of cytoplasmic RNA isolated from rats at different stages of the estrus cycle, revealed that steady state beta LH mRNA levels do not change significantly during the 4 day cycle. Nuclear transcription assays, however, showed a change in the transcription level of the beta LH gene from a maximum of 50ppm during metestrus to a minimum of 12ppm during proestrus. In similar experiments using ovariectomized rats, a 4 fold increase in beta LH mRNA was seen after 4 weeks of ovariectomy. Three days of estradiol treatment of 3 week ovariectomized rats, resulted in a decrease in the beta LH mRNA levels back to control levels. We are presently performing the nuclear transcription experiments on ovariectomized and steroid replaced rats. These studies, taken together, suggest that estradiol decreases beta LH mRNA levels through an effect on beta LH gene expression.

2294 EFFECTS OF 17β-ESTRADIOL (E_2) AND LRH UPON THE RAT ANTERIOR PITUITARY (AP) FSH ISOHORMONES AS DISCLOSED BY CONCANAVALIN A (Con A).

A. Ulloa-Aguirre*, E. Torra, R. Scherpbier and R. Domínguez. Dept. Reprod. Biol., Instituto Nacional de la Nutrición, & U.N.A.M., Mexico 14000, D. F.

AP glands were removed from adult intact (diestrus day 2; D2) and long-term ovariectomized (Ovx) rats after specific endocrine treatments. The presence, relative ratios and biological activity (BA) of each Con A-separable AP FSH species were assessed by a specific radioimmunoassay and by an *in vitro* bioassay (aromatization by granulosa cells in culture). AP extracts from all animals exhibited 2 distinct forms of immunoactive FSH after their separation by Con A chromatography. However, the relative ratio of Con A-unbound to Con A-bound FSH species (U:B ratio) differed depending on the endocrine condition of the animal. Ovariectomy caused a dramatic decrease in the U:B ratio (D2=0.63, Ovx=0.14); AP extracts from Ovx rats under short-term (20 h) E_2 exposure (condition which decreased LRH release) exhibited the lowest ratio (0.09), while those AP glands from Ovx animals exposed to conditions which caused increased pituitary LRH exposure (immediately before the E_2-induced FSH surge at 30-34hrs, or after injection of LRH) showed an increase in their U:B ratio as compared with Ovx and Ovx + E_2-20h rats (E_2-30 h=0.14; E_2-34 h=0.21; E_2-30 h+LRH=0.25). When the *in vitro* BA of both FSH species was tested, a similar potency was found, thus suggesting that neither form of AP FSH is a subunit. These studies suggest that the existing endocrine milieu regulates the carbohydrate content and/or arrangement of the FSH molecule, and therefore, the type of FSH produced by the AP gland. (Supported by a Rockefeller Foundation Grant).

2295 GNRH AND ORCHIECTOMY DIFFERENTIALLY REGULATE LH SUBUNIT APOPROTEIN AND CARBOHYDRATE BIOSYNTHESIS. D.L. Vogel*, R.J. Sherins and B.D. Weintraub, NICHD and NIADDK, NIH, Bethesda, MD 20205, USA

We have previously shown increased synthesis of LH subunits in rat pituitaries following orchiectomy(Cx). To study regulation of specific glycosylation, we labeled pituitary quarters from adult rats 2 wk post-Cx or sham surgery(Sh) for 4 hr with ^{3}H-Glucosamine(Gln) or ^{35}S-Cystine(Cys). Incubations were done +/- 10^{-8}M GnRH. Tissue lysates(pit) and media were analyzed by SDS-PAGE for total protein (TP) and LH (material immunoprecipitated by anti-LHβ). In pit, Cx increased Cys-TP at 18K (47.8±2.7 vs 25.5±2.6*), but neither 22K nor TCA-precipitated Cys; Gln-TP did not change. In media, Cx had no effect on Cys-TP or Gln-TP. GnRH did not increase Cys-TP or Gln-TP in pit, nor did it affect Gln/Cys ratio. However, Cx increased both 22K and 18K subunits of Cys-LH in pit, but had no effect on Gln/Cys. By contrast, GnRH markedly increased Gln/Cys for 22K- and 18K-LH in Cx. In media, both Cx and GnRH increased 22K and 18K Cys-LH, but neither changed Gln/Cys.

	PIT Cys-LH* 22K	PIT Cys-LH* 18K	Gln/Cys 22K	Gln/Cys 18K	MEDIA Cys-LH* 22K	MEDIA Cys-LH* 18K
Cx+GnRH	9.9±1.2	7.3±1.5	.29±.08	.28±.14	2.9±.1	.52±.02
Cx-	12.8 .9	7.7 .6	.09 .03	.06 .02	1.3 .1	.25 .04
Sh+GnRH	3.4 .3	1.4 .4	.18 .01	.23 .05	1.3 .1	.22 .01
Sh-	4.8 .8	2.1 .7	.12 .03	.12 .05	0.8 .02	.12 .01

We conclude: 1)Relative to TP, LH incorporation of Cys and Gln is specifically stimulated by Cx, but GnRH stimulates glycosylation only; 2)Both Cx and GnRH effects are greater for the 18K(β)subunit; 3)Both Cx and GnRH stimulate release without selectively increasing glycosylation of the secreted hormone.

*dpm x 10^4 per mg protein, mean±SEM

2296 EFFECTS OF ACTH AND CORTICOSTERONE ON THE NEGATIVE FEEDBACK ACTION OF TESTOSTERONE IN THE ADULT MALE RAT. J.T.M. Vreeburg* and R.F.A. Weber. Dept. of Endocrinology, Growth and Reproduction, and Dept. of Internal Medicine III and Clinical Endocrinology, Faculty of Medicine, Erasmus University, P.O. Box 1738, 3000 DR Rotterdam, The Netherlands.

Injections of ACTH to gonadectomized male rats result in high serum levels of corticosterone and decreased levels of LH and FSH. Since administration of high doses of corticosterone to gonadectomized male rats does not inhibit the postcastration rise in LH and FSH, it has been doubted whether this steroid itself is involved in the ACTH-induced inhibition of gonadotropins, and it has been suggested that adrenal androgens might cause the reduction in serum gonadotropins. However, injections of ACTH to gonadectomized male rats did only result in a moderate increase in prostate weight, suggesting a low serum level of androgens insufficient to inhibit gonadotropin secretion. Therefore, we wondered whether high levels of corticosterone might increase the sensitivity to the negative feedback action of androgens. To study this question, adrenalectomized and gonadectomized rats received small testosterone filled capsules. Testosterone levels were too low to inhibit the postcastration rise in LH and FSH. In addition to this treatment half of the animals were injected with corticosterone acetate. The combined administration of corticosterone acetate and testosterone in doses which given separately do not affect gonadotropin levels were able to reduce both LH and FSH below the levels found normally in untreated intact male rats.

It is concluded that a high serum level of corticosterone increases the sensitivity to the negative feedback action of testosterone.

2297 CHARGE AND MCR OF HUMAN FSH IN RELATION TO SEX AND AGE. L. Wide, Department of Clinical Chemistry, University Hospital, S-751 85 Uppsala, Sweden.

The charge of FSH in extracts of individual pituitaries from 63 men and women, aged 16 to 91 years, was determined by zone-electrophoresis in agarose suspension. In each pituitary there was a spectrum of forms of FSH with different charges in a distribution close to normal. The average charge of the forms was significantly less acidic in younger women and more acidic in elderly women than in men of corresponding ages. In both men and women there was a gradual change of charge with age to more acidic forms at higher age. The average charge of the forms of FSH in serum was more acidic than that in pituitary extracts from individuals of corresponding age and sex. Half-life in plasma and metabolic clearance rate (MCR) of the different forms of human pituitary FSH were estimated by injecting whole extracts and fractions of extracts into mice. FSH of young women had significantly higher MCR than that of men and elderly women. There was a relationship between charge and MCR. FSH in pituitary extracts with less negatively charged forms of the hormone had higher MCR values. Furthermore, the more basic forms of an individual pituitary disappeared faster from the circulation than the more acidic forms. This is a likely explanation to the difference between charge of FSH in pituitary and in serum. The secretion of a spectrum of forms of FSH with different disappearance rates from the circulation may be of importance for the pulsatile stimulation of the gonads. A consequence will be a higher amplitude of short duration in combination with a prolonged stimulation at a low level. A shorter half-life of FSH of young women compared to that of men and elderly women may be important to the facilitation of the feedback control of the ovarian function.

2298 SECRETION OF A PLEIOMORPHIC FORM OF LH WITH ABNORMAL BIOLOGICAL ACTIVITY IN THE PERIPUBERTAL RAT
C.A. Wilson* and J.C. Buckingham. Dept. Obstetrics & Gynaecology, St. George's Hospital, Dept. Pharmacology, Royal Free Hospital, London, U.K.
Immature rats can be induced to ovulate by pregnant mare serum (PMS) as long as they weigh over 60g (>60g)[1] Those weighing less than 60g (<60g) do not ovulate in spite of secreting a preovulatory LH surge as measured by heterologous radioimmunoassay (RIA), and mouse Leydig cell bioassay. The latter result indicates that the LH has normal steroidogenic activity as this assay is based on the ability of LH to stimulate testosterone production. The surge cannot be measured by homologous RIA[2] or by cytochemical bioassay which is based on the ability of LH to deplete ovarian ascorbic acid; this may correlate with the fact that this LH does not induce ovulation.

In vitro studies have produced similar results in that GnRH (10ng/ml) stimulates LH secretion from pituitaries of both <60g and >60g rats as measured by heterologous RIA, but no significant release occurs from the <60g rat pituitaries according to the cytochemical assay.

Injections of either GH (20μg i/v), corticosterone (0.5 mg s/c) or triiodothyroxine (20μg i/v), before the expected LH surge induces ovulation in the <60g PMS-treated rats and converts the pleiomorphic LH to the "active" form that can be measured by cytochemical bioassay.

1. Wilson, C.A. & Endersby, C.A. Neuroendocrinology (1979).
2. ter Haar, M.B. & Wilson, C.A. J. Endocr. (1978).

2299 LH PULSE AND ESTROGEN POSITIVE FEEDBACK IN WOMEN. T.Yaginuma*, T. Takeuchi, T. Okamura and T. Kobayashi, Dept of Obstet and Gynecol, Faculty of Med, Univ of Tokyo at Mejirodai, Tokyo, Japan.

Pulsatile release of LH has been shown to be essential for estrogen positive feedback (Epf) in monkey, but not in human. Thus, we have investigated it in 25 amenorrheic women. Blood samples were obtained 7 times every 20 min for determining LH pulse through an indwelling catheter iserted into the cubital vein and at 30 min following the intravenous injection of 100 ug of LHRH and then 5mg of estradiol propionate was given intramuscularly. Blood samples were obtained to detect Epf every day for next 5 days. The mean and coefficient of variation (CV) of LH levels of 7 samples were calculated in individuals. All women responded to LHRH. Sixteen women had LH pulse as determined by the inspection of the graph of the time -course of serum LH levels and the CV above 9 %. Epf was demonstrated in all of them and the mean to be above 12 mIU/ml in 14 women. Nine women were shown to have no LH pulse by the inspection and the CV of 9 % and less. Four of them had no Epf and the mean of LH levels less than 10 mIU/ml, while the remaining 5 women showed Epf and 4 of them the mean above 12 mIU/ml. These results indicate that Epf can function without LH pulse in women particularly when mean LH levels were shown to be above 12 mIU/ml in 7 blood samples in 20 min-interval.

2300 THE BINDING OF INSULIN AND INSULINLIKE GROWTH FACTOR II TO THE ERYTROLEUKEMIA CELLINE K562. M. Tally*, Tang X.-Z., G. Enberg and K. Hall, Department of Endocrinology, Karolinska Institutet, Stockholm, Sweden.

The erytroleukemia celline K562, isolated from a patient, has specific receptors for insulin and Insulinlike Growth Factor II (IGF II) but not for Insulinlike Growth Factor I (IGF I), an advantage when studying separate binding and effect of these hormones to their insulin-and type 2 receptors. The binding kinetic differs for the two hormones. Both show a steady state at 15 min at 37°C. The insulin binding show a more sensitive displacement curve in Hepes and Tris containing buffers giving curvelinear Scatchard plots, but insensitive displacement curves in Krebs Ringer buffers giving straight Scatchard plots. The IGF II binding shows no sensitivity to the buffer composition, and has displacement curves giving straight Scatchard plots. In 10mM Hepes buffer the Ke affinity for insulin was $2.3x10^{8}M^{-1}$ and a receptor concentration of $5.3x10^{4}$ sites/cell. The affinity for IGF II, in the same buffer, was $2.4x10^{8}M^{-1}$ with a receptor concentration of $4.8x10^{4}$ sites/cell. The cross-reactivity of IGF I on the receptors was for the insulin receptor 10-50 times lower than for insulin, and on the IGF II receptor 10 times lower than IGF II. Insulin does not cross-react at all with the IGF II receptor. IGF II, however, has 12 times lower potency than insulin on the insulin receptor. Instead insulin enhance the binding of IGF II to its receptor, similarly to previous finding in rat adipocytes. The specificity of the K562 celline for IGF II makes them suitable for a specific radioreceptor assay for IGF II in human plasma.

2301 IDENTIFICATION AND CHARACTERIZATION OF TRANSFORMING GROWTH FACTORS (TGFs) IN HUMAN ANTERIOR PITUITARY GLAND. T.Tsushima,* Y.Ohba, Y.Sato, E.Obuchi, K.Sato and K.Shizume. Department of Internal Medicine, Tokyo Women's Medical College and the Institute for Growth Science, Tokyo 162, Japan

TGFs are biologically active peptides with Mr 6000-30000 which induce non-neoplastic cells to undergo anchorage-independent growth. Human pituitary glands obtained at autopsy were extracted by acid/ethanol for 18 h at 4°C, and the extract was assayed for TGF activity. Normal rat kidney(NRK, clone 48F) were seeded in 0.3 % soft agar containing test materials at a density of 10^4 cells/ml and plated in multi-well plates. Plates were incubated in a CO_2 incubator for 7 days and the number of colonies was scored under microscope. Crude pituitary extract stimulated colony formation of NRK cells dose-dependently at the concentrations of 10-400 μg protein/ml. Pituitary hormones (hGH, PRL, ACTH, LH, FSH, TSH) showed no activity at 1 μg/ml. When pituitary extract was gel-filtered on a column of Bio-Gel P-60 equilibrated with 1 M acetic acid, 90 % of TGF activity eluted as a molecule of apparent Mr 15000. Minor activities were were detected in the void volume fraction and in the position corresponding to Mr 7000. Mr 15000 species had a pI of 7.2. The TGF activity was sensitive to trypsin, heating and dithiothreitol, but not affected by DNase or RNase treatment. Partially purified TGF showed a significant activity at 1 μg/ml. TGF (Mr 15000) did not compete with ^{125}I-EGF for EGF receptors, and EGF (2 ng/ml) enhanced TGF activity only slightly. Pituitary TGF also stimulated DNA synhtesis of cultured human skin fibroblasts in a dose-related manner. In conclusion, we identified potent TGFs in human pituitary gland. The physiological significance of pituitary TGFs is not clear at present.

2302 SOMATOMEDINS (SM) AND SOMATOMEDIN INHIBITORS (SMI): COMPARISON OF BIOASSAY VS RADIOIMMUNOASSAY MEASUREMENTS. R. Vassilopoulou-Sellin* and N.A. Samaan The University of Texas M. D. Anderson Hospital, Houston, TX 77030, U.S.A.

Somatomedin (SM) levels were measured by cartilage sulfation bioassay and somatomedin-C radioimmunoassay (SM-C RIA). In normal rat serum high bioactivity coincided with high SM-C RIA potency (> 4.0 U/ml); in diabetic serum SM-C RIA revealed low but significant SM levels (1.9 ± 0.6 U/ml) despite potent cartilage sulfation inhibition. After gel-filtration, Sephadex G-75, pH 2.4 biologically equipotent SM fractions were examined. While low-mol. wt. SM in normal rat serum were very active in the SM-C RIA (> 4.0 U/ml), high-mol. wt. SM from rat liver extract had very low potency (0.03 ± 0.01 U/ml and 0.16 ± 0.06 U/ml). After gel-filtration, Sephadex G-100, pH 7.4, fractions equipotent for somatomedin inhibitor (SMI) content were also studied; while for SMI from rat liver extracts, SM-C RIA potency was extremely low (0.03 ± 0.005 U/ml), in fractions from diabetic rat serum small quantities of coexisting SM were detected(0.13 ± 0.04 U/ml and 0.15 ± 0.01 U/ml). In combination studies, addition of SMI to normal rat serum produced only a very mild reduction in expected SM-C RIA potency (85 ± 4% observed vs expected) unlike the profound inhibition previously documented in bioassays. We conclude that (1) hepatic SM, easily measured by bioassay are greatly underestimated by SM-C RIA, (2) the combination of bioassay with SM-C RIA can be used to measure coexisting SM and SMI, and (3) the disparity between bioassay and SM-C RIA measurements for liver extract SM suggests important molecular differences between hepatic and serum SM.

2303 ALTERATIONS OF TYROSINE KINASE ACTIVITY DURING RAT LIVER REGENERATION.

Kirk Ways* and H. Shelton Earp, Cancer Research Center and Dept. of Med., Univ. of North Carolina School of Medicine, Chapel Hill, NC 27514. USA

Viral transforming gene products and growth factor receptors exhibit tyrosine-specific protein kinase activity (Tyr PK). A role for this activity in regulating cellular growth has been proposed. We have examined Tyr PK using an artificial substrate, angiotensin II, as an exogenous tyrosine phosphate acceptor to determine whether its activity is elevated during regulated, *in vivo* growth as seen with rat liver regeneration after partial hepatectomy. The tissue preparation was incubated with Pipes (50mM) $MgCl_2$ (75mM), angiotensin II (25ug), and ^{32}P-ATP (3uCi, 40um) for 10 min at 30°. After termination of the reaction angiotensin II was isolated and identified using ascending thin layer chromatography and ninhydrin staining with autoradiography. Phosphate incorporation into angiotensin II was quantified by liquid scintillation counting. Tyr PK was demonstrable in normal rat liver. Its activity was augmented in the presence of increasing Mg^{++} concentrations. The majority of the activity was contained in the 100,000 x G pellet. 24 hours after partial hepatectomy (n=5) Tyr PK was elevated in the 100,000 x G pellet when compared to sham operated rats (n=5) (4.15 ± 0.5 ($\bar{x}$ ± SEM) vs. 2.68 ± 0.3 pmoles of phosphate incorporated/mg of tissue/10 min, $P < 0.01$). After partial hepatectomy Tyr PK, measured as pmoles of phosphate incorporated/mg of tissue/10 min, rose in a time dependent manner (1.62 ± 0.12 ($\bar{x}$ ± SEM) at 2 hrs, 2.34 ± 0.156 at 11 hrs, 2.93 ± 0.156 at 22 hrs, 4.55 ± 0.81 at 44 hrs, 4.15 ± 1.63 at 60 hrs). Thus, Tyr PK is elevated during controlled cellular proliferation seen with liver regeneration. The mechanisms for this elevation are unknown.

2304 LOCATION OF THE EGF RECEPTOR ON PORCINE THYROID FOLLICLE CELLS IN VITRO.

K. Westermark*, B. Westermark and L.E. Ericson, Depts of Internal Medicine and Pathology, Univ. of Uppsala, Univ. Hosp., Uppsala and Inst. of Anatomy, Univ. of Göteborg, Göteborg, Sweden.

EGF (epidermal growth factor) is a potent mitogen for porcine thyroid follicle cells in culture (Endocrinology, 1983). $|^{125}I|$ EGF binds to a high affinity receptor, (K_d 2-4x10^{-10} M); the number of receptors has been determined to 20000-25000/cell (Ann d'Endocrinologie, 1983, 44:68A). As yet, nothing has been reported on the subcellular location of the EGF receptor. Porcine thyroid follicle cells, cultured on collagen gels form an epithelial layer of polarized cells connected with tight junctions. Their basal pole faces the collagen gel and the apical pole the culture medium. Using such a culture system, Chambard et al recently found that the TSH receptor is located at the basolateral part of porcine thyroid follicle cells (J Cell Biol, 1983). In the present studies, EM autoradiographical analysis of the distribution of $|^{125}I|$ EGF bound to porcine thyroid follicle cells on floating collagen gels demonstrated that 82.5±2.5 % of the tracer was related to the basolateral and only 2.4±1.7% to the apical cell surface. The remaining radioactivity was evenly distributed over the cell. Furthermore, using the same culture system, we could demonstrate that EGF (10 ng ml^{-1}) stimulated the incorporation of $|^{3}H|$ thymidine about 5 times over the control only when gels were floating, i.e. the effect of EGF required access to the basolateral cell surface. The present data thus provide direct evidence for the asymmetrical location of functional EGF receptors on porcine thyroid follicle cells in culture to the basolateral cell surface, i.e. the surface facing the cir-

2305 INSULIN-LIKE GROWTH FACTORS AND THEIR CARRIER PROTEIN IN CEREBROSPINAL FLUID OF NORMALS AND ACROMEGALICS. U. Widmer*, J. Zapf and E.R. Froesch, Metabolic Unit, University Hospital, CH-8091 Zurich, Switzerland.

Do IGF content and IGF binding pattern in cerebrospinal fluid (CSF) of acromegalics correspond to the elevated IGF I and the increased large mol.wt. (150-200 K) IGF carrier protein in serum? Ir-IGF I and II and IGF binding patterns in CSF of 5 acromegalics were compared with those of 5 patients with intervertebral disc disease (controls): 1) Mean CSF IGF II in the acromegalics (13.6 $\pm$ 3.8 ng/ml ($\pm$ SD)) was not different from that of the controls (12.4 $\pm$ 3.2 ng/ml). 2) IGF I was not measurable in CSF of the controls; it was detectable (2.4 and 1.5 ng/ml CSF) only in the two acromegalics with the highest serum IGF I (1027 and 937 ng/ml). 3) CSF binding patterns of acromegalics and controls were identical: In contrast to serum, only one specific IGF binding peak (40-50 K) is present in CSF. It binds predominantly 125-I-IGF II, whereas binding of 125-I-IGF I is poor (ratio 10/1). Unlabeled IGF II is a more potent competitor for binding of both IGF tracers than unlabeled IGF I. The apparent capacity of the 40-50 K peak in CSF to bind 125-I-IGF II is more than 100x greater than that of the corresponding serum peak, if expressed per mg protein. Correspondingly, CSF contains 6x more IGF II/mg protein than serum. This relatively high IGF II content, the lack of IGF I in normal CSF and the fact that IGF I appears in CSF only if serum IGF I is around 1000 ng/ml may point to a specific role of IGF II and its carrier in the CNS. The absence of the 150-200 K IGF carrier complex in CSF indicates that it does not readily cross the barrier between blood and CSF.

2306 AFFINITY LABELING OF HUMAN PLASMA SOMATOMEDIN-C BINDING PROTEINS: EVIDENCE OF GROWTH HORMONE DEPENDENCE AND SUBUNIT STRUCTURE. J.R. Wilkins* and A.J. D'Ercole, Department of Pediatrics, University of North Carolina School of Medicine, Chapel Hill, NC 27514 USA.

Using disuccinimidyl suberate (DSS) we have developed a technique to covalently crosslink 125-I-labeled somatomedin-C (Sm-C) to specific binding proteins (BP's) in human plasma. 125-I-Sm-C-BP complexes with relative molecular weights (Mr's) of 24-28K and $\geq$ 90K (i.e. 90K, 110K, 135K and 160K) were most intensely labeled in acromegalic plasma and absent or nearly so in hypopituitary plasma. A 35-43K 125-I-Sm-C-BP complex was most intensely labeled in hypopituitary plasma and least so in acromegalic plasma. Reduction of samples with β-mercaptoethanol did not change the electrophoretic pattern of these 125-I-Sm-C-BP complexes. BP complexes with Mr's of 24-28K, 50K, and $\geq$ 90K were adsorbed by Concanavalin-A (Con-A). When acromegalic or normal plasma was fractionated on a Sephadex G-200 superfine column and affinity labeled, these same complexes were found in fractions which eluted near the gamma-globulin peak. On the other hand, the 35-43K complex consistently eluted after the albumin peak and exhibited no affinity for Con-A. These data indicate that the growth hormone (GH) dependent Sm-C BP's with apparent Mr's of 24-28K, 50K, 90K, 110K, and 135K may comprise the 160K gamma-globulin sized Sm-C BP. We speculate that the 24-28K complex represents the protomer which makes up each of the GH dependent Sm-C BP's while the 35-43K complex represents a different type of Sm-C BP which may serve in an auxiliary capacity.

2307 INSULIN-LIKE GROWTH FACTOR II (IGF-II) BIOSYNTHESIS IN SHORT-TERM RAT EMBRYO FIBROBLASTS: DEMONSTRATION OF Mr ~22K (PRE-PRO-) and Mr ~20K (PRO-) PRECURSORS. Y. W.-H. Yang*, J. E. Terrell, S. P. Nissley and M. M. Rechler. NIADDK and NCI, National Institutes of Health, Bethesda, MD,USA.

Recent evidence from our laboratory suggests that BRL 3A cells, a continuous cell line derived from rat liver, synthesize Mr ~22K pre-pro-IGF-II and Mr ~20K pro-IGF-II, and convert them to Mr 8.7K and 7.1K IGF-II species. The present study asks whether the same biosynthetic precursors occur in cells that have not been adapted to continuous culture. Third passage rat embryo fibroblasts (REFs), known to synthesize and secrete Mr 8.7K and Mr 7.1K IGF-II, were metabolically labeled with $[^{35}S]$cysteine in serum-free media. After 2 hours of labeling, Mr ~20K pro-IGF-II could be specifically immunoprecipitated from REF lysates. The Mr ~20K protein was precipitated by 4 antisera raised in rabbits to Mr 8.7K BRL-IGF-II, but not by non-immune serum. Immunoprecipitation of this protein was inhibited by incubation with excess unlabeled Mr 8.7K BRL-IGF-II, but not by rat insulin. The Mr ~20K protein was labeled within 10 min, but was not detected in the medium at any time (10 min-24 h). Mr 8.7K and Mr 7.1K IGF-II were present in lysates after 20 and 60 min of labeling, respectively, and in media after 3 hours. Poly A-RNA was prepared from REFs and translated in a reticulocyte lysate system with $[^{35}S]$cysteine and methionine. Mr ~22K pre-pro-IGF-II was detected in immunoprecipitates of the translated $[^{35}S]$-proteins. The Mr ~22K protein was converted to a Mr ~20K form by incubation with microsomal membranes containing signal peptidase. CONCLUSION: In REFs, as in BRL 3A cells, IGF-II is synthesized as Mr ~22K pre-pro-IGF-II and rapidly converted to Mr ~20K pro-IGF-II.

2308 PLASMA GH RESPONSES TO REPETITIVE ADMINISTRATION OF hpGRF-44 IN PATIENTS WITH IDIOPATHIC GH DEFICIENCY. K. Takano*, N. Hizuka, K. Shizume, N. Honda, M. Miyakawa, K. Asakawa and N. C. Ling. Department of Medicine, Tokyo Women's Medical College, Tokyo 162, Japan

The effect of synthetic human pancreatic growth-hormone-releasing factor (hpGRF-44) was evaluated on the GH secretion in patients with idiopathic GH deficiency (IGD). Blood samples were drawn at 5 to 15 min intervals for 2 hrs after hpGRF-44 administration. Fifty patients with IGD were administered 2 µg hpGRF-44/kg BW by single iv bolus injection. Twenty-seven patients did not respond, i.e. their plasma GH levels did not rise above 5 ng/ml; we designated these patients nonresponders (NRs). However, 23 patients responded; we designated these patients responders (Rs). Their mean GH level reached peak at 90 min with the value of 8.8 ± 0.8 (±SE) ng/ml. Their peak values ranging between 5.1 and 17.8 ng/ml.

An iv bolus injection of 100 ug hpGRF-44 was given to two NRs for four and five consecutive days and slight GH increases were observed. A hundred µg hpGRF-44 was injected im twice a day for five consecutive days to two NRs. These two patients showed plasma GH increases to iv bolus injection of 2 µg hpGRF-44/kg performed on the 6th experimental day. hpGRF-44 was infused at a dosage of 2.5 µg/min for 90 min for three to six consecutive days to 7 NRs. Four of them responded to daily GRF infusion. Further stimulated GH responses were obtained in all four Rs to repetitive administration of hpGRF-44.

These results support the concept that a majority of patients with IGD have defect in hypothalamus, and suggest that GRF administration will be useful for treatment of GH deficient children.

2309 ACTIONS OF ENDOGENOUS GROWTH HORMONE IN STREPTOZOTOCIN-DIABETIC RATS.
Jeffrey B. Tatro* and Jessica Schwartz, The University of Michigan, Ann Arbor, Michigan, USA 48109

In diabetic rats, administration of exogenous growth hormone (GH) exacerbates hyperglycemia. Hypophysectomy, on the other hand, reduces blood glucose. In normal rats, acute deficiency of endogenous GH, induced by treatment with anti-rat GH serum (ArGH), led to increased insulin-stimulated glucose oxidation (GOX) in adipose tissue in vitro. We hypothesized that in diabetic rats, endogenous GH might play an important role in glucose homeostasis by suppressing basal glucose utilization or insulin action. Thus, we examined the effects of acute GH deficiency in streptozotocin-diabetic (SZ) rats (65 mg/kg, ip, 10 days). Six hr and 3 hr prior to killing, rats received 0.5 ml ArGH or control serum, ip. ArGH-treated rats showed a small (10%; $P<.03$) but significant reduction in serum glucose, relative to that of control rats. To test whether this reflected increased glucose utilization, we measured GOX. In ArGH-treated SZ rats, basal and insulin-stimulated GOX were comparable to those of controls. Enhanced insulin-like activity of exogenous GH in vitro verified the deficiency of endogenous GH in ArGH-treated rats. We conclude that, in SZ rats: a) acute specific GH deficiency leads to a decrease in serum glucose, which suggests that endogenous GH may contribute to hyperglycemia; and b) acute GH deficiency does not affect basal or insulin-stimulated GOX in adipose tissue, whereas comparable treatment in normal rats led to increased insulin responses. Increased glucose uptake in other tissues or decreased glycogenolysis could account for the effect of ArGH on serum glucose. (Supported by NIH AM-26898 and a predoctoral fellowship from the American Diabetes Association-Michigan.)

2310 INTRAVENOUS, SUBCUTANEOUS, AND INTRANASAL ADMINISTRATION OF hpGRF-40 IN NORMAL MEN.
M.O. Thorner*, M.L. Vance, D.L. Kaiser, J. Chitwood, and W.S. Evans, University of Virginia Medical Center, Charlottesville, VA, USA.

To compare the effects of human pancreatic growth hormone (GH) releasing factor (hpGRF)-40 on GH release (ng/ml/h) above baseline when given by different routes, we determined dose-response relationships after intravenous (IV; n=7), subcutaneous (SC; n=4), and intranasal (NASAL; n=4) administration of the peptide. Dose response curves were generated following administration of IV (.003, .01, .03 and .1 ug/kg), SC (1, 3.3, and 10 ug/kg) and NASAL (3, 10, 30 and 100 ug/kg) hpGRF-40 with r^2 values of 0.36, 0.65 and 0.74, respectively. During the initial hour after IV hpGRF-40 administration both the .03 and .1 ug/kg doses elicited significant increases in GH release (3.29 ± 1.33, p=0.048 and 10.3 ± 2.98, p=0.0136, respectively; mean ± SEM) when compared to after vehicle (0.59 ± 0.32). When administered SC significant increases in GH secretion were documented after the 3.3 ug/kg (4.68 ± 0.54; p=0.0033) and 10 ug/kg (13.6 ± 2.6; p=0.014) doses when compared to vehicle (6.66 ± 2.9). When administered by the NASAL route a significant increase in GH secretion was documented with the 100 ug/kg dose (17.6 ± 1.5) when compared to vehicle (-0.38 ± 1.0) (p=0.0013). In summary, minimal doses required to stimulate GH using this paradigm in normal young men were .03, 3.3 and 100 ug/kg for the IV, SC, and NASAL routes, respectively. These results have implications in the design of therapy with hpGRF-40. Supported by AM 23632, HD 00439, HD 13197 and RR-847.

2311 DOES OPIOID PEPTIDE STIMULATE GROWTH HORMONE (GH) SECRETION VIA GH-RELEASING FACTOR (GRF)?

Y. Tonegawa*, I. Wakabayashi, T. Ihara, M. Hattori, T. Shibasaki[1] and N. Ling[2], Dept. of Med. Nippon Med. Sch. Tokyo, 113, [1]Dept. of Med. Tokyo Women's Med. Coll. Tokyo, 162 Japan and [2]Salk Institute, La Jolla, CA. 92037 U.S.A.

To examine whether opioid peptide stimulates GH secretion via GRF, we made following observations in urethane anesthetized rats. Iv injection of an analog of Met Enkephalin (Sandoz FK33-824 100ug/kg) increased plasma GH levels (ng/ml) from 11±1 to 30±7 (n=12,p<0.05) and plasma GH response to 10ug GRF (human) exceeded 2,000ng (n=5). Plasma GH response to FK33-824 was completely prevented by the prior administration of naloxone. Plasma GH response to 10ug GRF was obscured when it was given after rats had received 1ug GRF every 3min in total of 15ug (262±61 vs 285±63 n=5 NS). Under the same condition, the injection of FK33-824 increased plasma GH levels from 204±27 to 657±142 (n=10,p<0.05). In another study, either 0.6 ug GRF or saline was injected iv every 3min to rats that had received antiserum to somatostatin (ASS). Iv injection of FK33-824 immediately after rats had received the 15th GRF did not increase plasma GH levels, though plasma GH response to FK33-824 was observed in rats received saline. Pituitary GH content in GRF administered rats was reduced significantly to 70% of controls. In rats pretreated with ASS, plasma GH response to GRF but not to FK33-824 was augumented significantly as compared to previous studies.

Results show that the stimulatory effect of opioid peptide on GH secretion appears to be complex and needs further studies.

2312 A FINITE RELEASABLE GH POOL MEASURED IN MAN AFTER HUMAN PANCREATIC TUMOR GH-RELEASING FACTOR (hpGRF-40).

M.L. Vance*, M.O. Thorner, D.L. Kaiser, W.S. Evans, G. Perisutti, and L.A. Frohman, (SPON: J. T. Dunn), Univ. of Va. Medical Center, Charlottesville, VA, and Univ. of Cincinnati Medical Center, Cincinnati, OH, USA.

Previously we have shown that incremental 90 min infusions of 1, 3.3, 10, and 33 ng/kg/min of hpGRF-40 caused dose-dependent GH secretion for the 3 lowest doses. However, the stimulation of GH secretion decreased during infusion of the highest dose. To examine whether this decline was a result of a reduction in the responsiveness or of depletion of GH, we administered 6 hr infusions of vehicle or 1, 3.3, or 10 ng/kg/min hpGRF-40 on 4 occasions to 6 normal young men. At 5.5 hr each subject received hpGRF-40 3.3 ug/kg iv bolus and GH secretion was monitored for a further 2 hr. The results, as total GH released, ng/ml/hr x interval (h), are:

Dose	0 - 5.5 hr	5.5 - 7.5 hr	0 - 7.5 hr
Vehicle	10.73 ± 8.8	66.60 ± 17.4*	77.33 ± 10.5⁺
1 ng/kg/min	25.19 ± 8.3*	44.80 ± 7.6*	69.99 ± 12.0⁺
3.3 ng/kg/min	69.74 ± 30.3	28.00 ± 7.2*	97.74 ± 34.5⁺
10 ng/kg/min	45.16 ± 9.9*	21.00 ± 4.0*	66.16 ± 10.5⁺

*p < 0.02 vs baseline on same day; + p = 0.659 vs one another.

hpGRF infusions (1-10 ng/kg/min) stimulated GH secretion. The response to the 3.3 ug/kg bolus was inversely related to the previous infusion dose (p < 0.03). Total GH secreted during the infusion and bolus periods (0-7.5 hr) were indistinguishable. These results were confirmed by 24 hr infusions of vehicle or 2 ng/kg/min plus 3.3 ug/kg iv bolus of hpGRF-40 at 23.5 hr. There appears to be a finite hpGRF-40 releasable GH pool in man.

2313 SHORT AND LONG TERM STUDIES OF EFFECTS OF BIOSYNTHETIC GROWTH HORMONE IN HYPOPITUITARY PATIENTS. E. Vicens-Calvet*, N. Potau, A. Carrascosa, M. Albisu, M. Gusiñé, A. Ruibal, L. Audi, B. Strindberg and J.M. Cuatrecasas. Children's Hospital. Barcelona,Spain. KabiVitrum. Med. Department. Stockholm. Sweden.

Short term studies. Eight adolescents with growth hormone deficiency (GHD) and little possibility of further growth were studied twice: 1) When treated with human growth hormone (hGh), and 2) One month after being switched to the same dosage of biosynthetic growth hormone (BGH). Comparative data showed: a) a similar pattern in the oral glucose tolerance test with a certain degree of glucose intolerance and hypoinsulinemia, b) normal number and affinity of insulin receptors in erythrocytes and c) normal values of bioassayable somatomedin (SM). Long term studies. Four prepubertal patients with GHD, mean chronological age 9.6±3.2 yr., mean bone age 6.9±3.3 yr., were treated for six months with BGH. Results showed: a) SM increased from 0.2±0.1 u/ml to 0.9±0.2 u/ml after the first seven days and maintained similar levels throughout treatment b) mean growth velocity changed from 3.5±0.3 cm/yr., in the preceding year, to 8.5±1.2 cm/yr., during treatment, c) very little change in bone age. Throughout both studies glucose, haemoglobin $A_{1}c$, cholesterol, tryglycerides, creatinin and β_2 microglobulin remained unchanged. Growth hormone antibody titres (GHA) were absent at the beginning of studies and increased moderately after three and six months of treatment in some cases. In conclusion, BGH induces generation of SM and promotes growth in hypopituitary patients. Further study of the evolution of GHA is required.

2314 DIURNAL VARIATIONS IN PLASMA GROWTH HORMONE AND BLOOD GLUCOSE LEVELS AND THEIR RESPONSE TO EXERCISE IN INSULIN-DEPENDENT DIABETES MELLITUS (COMPARATION OF THE RESULTS OBTAINED DURING POOR METABOLIC CONTROL AND AFTER SHORT-TERM METABOLIC IMPROVEMENT)
M.Vircburger*, G.Prelević, D.Mijalković, Lj.Perić, City Clinic Hospital, Belgrade, Yugoslavia
The data about the relation between existing metabolic abnormalities in diabetes melitus and growth hormone levels are controversial. Diurnal variations in plasma GH and blood glucose levels and their response to exercise were determined before and after 2 week period of improved metabolic control on the conventional insulin therapy in 6 adult insulin-dependent diabetics. Blood samples were taken every hour during the 24 hours period starting immediately after adequate exercise overload. The results obtained enable us to differentiate two groups of patients: "responders" and "non-responders". The "responders" showed: a)GH peak during the first hours of the sleep, b)GH surge corresponded to the fall in blood glucose level even within normoglycemic range, c)significantly high GH surge was noticed when blood glucose level reached 3,5 mmol/l. The "non-responders" showed: a)normal GH peak during the first hours of the sleep, b)the absence of the GH surge after exercise overload, c)the absence of GH response to accidental hypoglycemic threshold (glucose level of 2,2 mmol/l), d)only mild GH response was observed when blood glucose level fall to the range of 1,5 mmol/l. No benefitial effect of short-term metabolic improvement on the pattern of GH secretion was observed.

2315 PLASMA GROWTH HORMONE (GH) RESPONSE TO HUMAN GROWTH HORMONE RELEASING FACTOR (GRF) IN RATS RECEIVED VARIOUS ENDOCRINE TREATMENTS. I. Wakabayashi*, Y. Tonegawa, T. Ihara, M. Hattori, T. Shibasaki[1], S. Inoue[2] and N. Ling[3], Dept. of Med. Nippon Med. Sch. Tokyo, 113, [1]Dept. of Med. Tokyo Women's Med. Coll. Tokyo, 162, [2]Dept. of Med. Yokohama City Univ. Yokohama, 232 Japan and [3]Salk Institute, La Jolla, CA. 92037 U.S.A.

Episodic GH secretion in rats poses difficult problems when the effect of GRF on plasma GH levels is assessed. We previously reported that chlorpromazine(CPZ)inhibited episodic GH secretion via factors other than somatostatin(SS)(Neuroendocrinol 30:257,1980). To examine whether GH response to GRF is modulated after hypothalamic ventromedial lesion(VMH 4wk), thyroidectomy(3wk)or T_4injection(200ug/rat,14D), rats were pretreated with CPZ(3mg/kg iv 80,20min)and antiserum to SS(ASS 1ml iv 100 min). Results:

Treatments	Basal	Peak Response (ng/ml) GRF 0.25ug/kg	1.0ug/kg	Pit.GH ug/mg protein
Control(6)	35±3]*		1351±240]*	617±41]NS
VMH(5)	24±1		589± 81	546±26
Control(8)	41±4]*	238± 25]**	3835±206]*	806±80]NS
T_4-injection(8)	23±1	95± 16	2665±381	657±44
Control(7)	25±2]*	552±102]**	1933±288]**	769±33]**
Thyroidectomy(7)	17±2	33± 2	62± 4	15± 9

*$p<0.05$,**$p<0.01$. It was ascertained that CPZ did not alter basal or GRF-stimulated GH secretion from monolayer culture of rat anterior pit. cells.

Results demonstrate that CPZ-ASS pretreatment is useful to obtain informations as to the pituitary responsiveness to GRF in vivo.

2316 ALTHESIN INTERACTION WITH PLASMA STEROID BINDING GLOBULINS. M. Pugeat+, D.Perrot, A.Mounier-Kuhn, M.J.Asensio and M.G.Forest. INSERM-U.34. Hôpital Debrousse. 69322 Lyon Cedex 05. France.

Althesin, a mixture of pregnandione derivatives, alphaxalone (AX) and alphadolone acetate (ADA), is widely used for outpatient anesthesia. Using a solid phase method (Pugeat, JCEM 53: 69,1981) we have found that AX and ADA bind with high affinity testosterone-binding globulin (TeBG)(2.8 and 2.1 x 10^9 M^{-1} respectively) and corticosteroid-binding globulin (CBG)(8.1x 10^6 M^{-1} for both). In the aim to investigate the physiological significance of these interactions, plasma TeBG and CBG binding parameters, total testosterone (T) and cortisol (F) concentrations and the percents dialysable of T and F were measured in 5 adults men during a 10' iv infusion of althesin (2-3 ml containing 9 mg/ml of AX and 3 mg/ml of ADA). Blood samples were then taken, thrice hourly before, every 10' for 1 h, and 2 h after starting the infusion. TeBG and CBG binding capacities and affinities, T levels (mean±SD)(767±415 vs 732±313 ng/dl) were unchanged, but F levels increased significantly ($p < 0.05$)(15.2±3.1 vs 19.9±2.6 µg/dl) during the 40' following althesin infusion. At the same times, the slight increase in % unbound T (from 1.90±0.32 to 2.09±0.47) and in % unbound F (from 5.40±0.52 to 5.44±0.57) were not significant. IN CONCLUSION, despite a high affinity for both TeBG and CBG, althesin does not alter the plasma distribution of T and F at the doses routinely used for short anesthesia.

2317 EFFECTS OF TRIIODOTHYRONINE ON DEVELOPMENT IN VITRO OF DOPAMINERGIC AND THYROLIBERIN HYPOTHALAMIC NEURONS. [1] J. Puymirat, [1] C. Loudes, [1] A. Faivre-Bauman, [2] C. Lassare, [2] M. Binoux and [1] A. Tixier-Vidal* , [1] Groupe de Neuroendocrinologie Cellulaire, Collège de France, 75231 PARIS Cedex 05, [2] INSERM, U. 142, Hôpital Trousseau, 75012 Paris, France.

The conditions to culture dissociated fetal mouse hypothalamic cells (16 d. fetuses) in absence of serum have been previously established (ratio neurons/glias : 5-6) (see rev. Faivre-Bauman et al, in Methods in Molecular and Cell Biology, D. Barnes et al, eds, Alan R. Liss, 1983). This permitted to study the effects of triiodothyronine (T3) (10^{-13} - 10^{-8}M) on neuron development up to 12 days in culture. Specific T3 nuclear binding sites have been detected in culture (Km : 1-10^{-11}M). T3 exerts overall effects : it increases neurite elongation and enhances in a dose dependent manner the production into the medium of IGF_s, but not of their binding proteins. T3 also exerts specific effects on dopaminergic neurons (Da n.) : it increases perikarya size, neurite branching, neurite length, DA synthesis and ^{3}H-DA uptake. In contrast it does not alter the K^+ evoked release of ^{3}H-DA (20% of content) or of TRH (4% of content). Moreover T3 acts synergistically with corticosterone (Cs) on both DA n. and TRH n., although in a different manner. On the one hand, it increases ^{3}H-DA uptake but not the % ^{3}H-DA release in response to K^+ depolarisation, and, on the other hand, it increases the K^+ evoked release of TRH (from 4 to 20%) without altering the neuron TRH content. These findings lead to the conclusion that T3 acts differentially, either alone or in synergy with Cs, at various steps of neuron development depending on the neuron specific function (supported by CNRS, MIR and INSERM grants).

2318 CARBAMYLATION OF HORMONES IN RENAL FAILURE AND THEIR BIOLOGICAL ACTIVITIES. M. OIMOMI*, S. KUBOTA, H. HATANAKA, K. ISHIKAWA, Y. YOSHIMURA, and S. BABA, The Second Department of Internal Medicine, Kobe University School of Medicine, Chuo-ku, Kobe, Hyogo, 650 Japan.

Hemoglobin A_1 (HbA_1), which is increased in patients with renal failure, is formed by carbamylation of Hb by cyanic acid derived from urea. Carbamylation is a non-enzymatic and non-specific reaction and may occur at some amino groups of proteins, other than Hb, and peptides. We previously reported that in patients with renal failure, the level of carbamylated plasma protein is elevated. In the present study, we investigated the effects of carbamylation of the biological activity of hormones in patients with renal failure. L-triiodothyronine (T_3) and neutral purified porcine insulin were incubated with varying concentrations of cyanic acid at 37°C for 48 hours to prepare carbamylated T_3 and carbamylated insulin, respectively. The resultant carbamylated T_3 and carbamylated insulin were isolated by highperformance liquid chromatography (HPLC). The biological activity of carbamylated T_3 was determined utilizing the metamorphosis of tadpoles. At a concentration of 10^{-6}mM, the biological activity of carbamylated T_3 was less than 1/10 that of T_3. Carbamylated insulin was intravenously administered in various doses to the rabbits. The percentage decrease of blood glucose increased with increased dose of carbamylated insulin. However, the percentage decrease was less than 1/10 that found with insulin. We suppose that in patients with renal failure, some hormones in the blood undergo carbamylation with resultant decreased biological activities. This is important in considering the endocrine function in patients with renal failure.

2319 IN VITRO EFFECT OF ESTROGENS ON THE PEROXIDASE ACTIVITY OF HUMAN ENDOMETRIUM.

H. Okada*, M. Nawa and J. Kimura, Dept. of OB/GYN, Kyoto Pref. Univ. Med., Kyoto 602, Japan.

It has been demonstrated that uterine peroxidase (E.C. 1,11,1.7) activity was dramatically increased by the administration of estradiol in rat. The increase of the activity was shown to be dose dependent and estrogen specific. However, the induction of uterine peroxidase in vitro has not yet been reported. In the present study, human endometrial tissue was incubated in vitro and a marked increase of peroxidase activity was demonstrated by the addition of estrogens in the incubation medium with a good dose-response relationship over a range of 1.47×10^{-8}M to 1.10×10^{-5}M. In the next experiment, estradiol and related compounds were compared in their abilities to induce peroxidase at a concentration of 10^{-7}M. From the experimental results, the ability of estrogen to induce peroxidase was 17β-estradiol > estrone > 17α-ethynylestradiol > diethylstilbestrol ≑ estriol. Progesterone, testosterone and cortisol have almost no activity. Tamoxyfen and clomiphen showed no remarkable induction of peroxidase in the experimental condition. The effect of estrogen was almost completely supressed by the addition of cycloheximide or actinomycin D in the incubation medium. The inactivity of mestranol in this system clearly indicated that the conversion of this compound to ethynylestradiol is necessary before it works in vivo.

2320 GRF: SPECIFIC HIGH AFFINITY BINDING SITES IN RAT ANTERIOR PITUITARY ARE MODULATED BY DEXAMETHASONE.

H. Seifert*, L. Bilezikjian, J. Rivier, M. Perrin and W.Vale. Peptide Biology Laboratory, The Salk Institute, La Jolla, CA 92138.

Growth hormone releasing factors from human pancreatic tumors (hpGRFs) and from rat hypothalamus (rhGRF) have been isolated previously. We describe here specific high affinity binding sites for GRFs in rat anterior pituitary homogenate and in primary cultures of rat anterior pituitary cells. An analog of hpGRF was used as radioligand: ^{125}I-[His1,Nle^{27}]-hpGRF(1-32)NH_2. Binding studies were performed in 50mM cl, pH 7-4, EoTH 2mM, $LyCl_2$ 5mM, 0.1% BSA. Binding of GRF was rapid and temperature dependent. At 37°C, maximal specific binding occurred within 10 min followed by rapid decline, whereas at 25°C, it reached a plateau after 30 min; at 4°C no measurable specific binding was obtained even after 2 hrs of incubation. Increasing the tissue concentration resulted in a corresponding linear increase of specific binding. A K_d of 0.7 ± 0.1nM and an estimated receptor density of 80 fmole/pituitary were derived from the Scatchard analysis of competition studies. The linear Scatchard curve, as well as a Hill coefficient of 1.1, are indicative of one class of high affinity binding sites. Binding affinities of GRF analogs correlate with their in vitro potencies. GRF also bound to rat anterior pituitary cells cultured in the presence of dexamethasone (5 nM), whereas there was no measureable specific GRF binding to cells cultured in glucocorticoid-free medium. Being saturable and exhibiting pharmacological specificty and high affinity for GRF peptides, the described binding site fulfills criteria of a physiological peptide receptor. Glucocorticoids may play a physiological role in regulating the sensitivity to GRF of the somatotroph.

2321 MECHANISM OF ACTION OF GROWTH HORMONE-RELEASING FACTOR AND SOMATOSTATIN: ROLE OF CYCLIC AMP. M.S. Sheppard, B.C. Moor, and J. Kraicer*, Dept. Physiology, Queen's Univ., Kingston, Ont., K7L 3N6, Canada and Dept. Medicine, Univ. of Saskatchewan, Saskatoon, Sask., S7N OXO, Canada.

The release of growth hormone (GH) from the pars distalis of the adenohypophysis is stimulated by a hypothalamic growth hormone-releasing factor (GRF) and inhibited by somatostatin (SRIF). The recent availability of synthetic GRF (human pancreatic GRF) now allows us to study the mechanisms by which the two peptides alter GH release. We use an acutely dispersed, purified (> 95%) preparation of somatotrophs obtained from rat adenohypophyses. Synthetic hpGRF-(1-40)-OH elicits a dose-related, immediate (within 2 min), reversible and repeatable increase in GH release with a concurrent or preceding increase in cyclic AMP accumulation in the somatotrophs. Cyclic GMP was not measurable (< 0.02 fmol/1000 cells) in any of our studies. SRIF (1.0 ng/ml) completely and instantly blocks the augmented release of GH induced by GRF (2.0 ng/ml) with only a small reduction in the GRF-induced increase in cyclic AMP accumulation. Low concentrations of GRF (0.1 ng/ml) and IBMX (0.02 mM, a phosphodiesterase inhibitor), which in themselves do not alter GH release, when combined, induce a significant increase in GH release. These data support the model that a) cyclic AMP is an intracellular mediator in the action of GRF and b) SRIF acts primarily at a site beyond cyclic AMP accumulation, but with a secondary action on cyclic AMP synthesis and/or breakdown. (Supported by MRC)

2322 EFFECT OF ANTI-TRH SERUM ON THE RELEASE OF PROLACTIN AND THYROTROPIN INDUCED BY SUCKLING OR ELECTRICAL STIMULATION OF THE PARAVENTRICULAR NUCLEI OR MEDIAN EMINENCE. W.J. Sheward*, H.M. Fraser† and G. Fink, MRC Brain Metabolism Unit, Edinburgh EH8 9JZ; †MRC Reproductive Biology Unit, Edinburgh EH3 9EW, U.K.

Thyrotropin releasing hormone (TRH) releases thyrotropin (TSH) and prolactin (PRL), but whether TRH is the physiological PRL releasing factor has not been established. This has been investigated here by determining the effect of injecting anti-TRH serum on the release of PRL and TSH induced by either electrical stimulation of the median eminence (ME) or paraventricular nuclei (PVN) in male rats or by suckling in lactating female rats. The animals were anesthetized with urethane for 3-4 h before application of either the electrical or the suckling stimulus. Electrical stimulation of either the ME or the PVN produced significant increases in the plasma concentration of both PRL and TSH; injection (i.v.) of anti-TRH serum, but not non-immune serum, blocked the increase in TSH but not PRL. Suckling by a minimum of 7 pups applied to the teats of mothers separated from all but one of their young overnight produced a significant increase in plasma PRL but not TSH concentration. Injection of the anti-TRH serum but not the non-immune serum significantly decreased the 'basal' concentration of TSH but did not block the increase in PRL induced by suckling. These results show that TRH does not appear to be involved in the release of PRL induced by either stimulation of the hypothalamus or suckling in the rat.

2323 GROWTH HORMONE-RELEASING FACTOR-LIKE IMMUNOREACTIVITY IN THE EXTRACTS OF NORMAL HUMAN TISSUES AND TUMORS. T. Shibasaki*, M. Nakahara, A. Masuda, T. Imaki, I. Wakabayashi[1], H. Demura, K. Shizume and N. Ling[2], Department of Medicine, Tokyo Women's Medical College, Tokyo, 162, Japan, [1]Department of Medicine, Nippon Medical College, Tokyo, [2]Laboratories for Neuroendocrinology, The Salk Institute, La Jolla, California 92037, U.S.A.

We measured growth hormone-releasing factor-like immunoreactivity (GRF-LI) in various human tissue and tumor extracts by a specific radioimmunoassay for hpGRF(1-44)NH_2 using an antiserum which recognizes the region (Met^{27}-Leu^{44})NH_2 of hpGRF(1-44)NH_2. The highest concentration of GRF-LI was detected in the extract of pituitary stalk with moderate amounts found in hypothalamus, optic chiasm and pancreas. Gel permeation chromatographic analysis of the tissue extract from hypothalamus revealed only one peak which eluted at the same position as that of hpGRF(1-44)NH_2. The extract from optic chiasm showed one peak at the same position as that of the hpGRF(1-44)NH_2 and another peak which eluted after hpGRF(1-44) NH_2. In contrast, the extract from the pancreas contained only one peak which eluted before hpGRF(1-44)NH_2. The results suggest that pro-GRF may be processed differently in different tissues. GRF-LI was detected in the extracts of two medullary thyroid carcinoma and one lung small cell carcinoma. Since these tumor extracts also contained corticotropin-releasing factor-LI and the concentrations of these peptides were significantly higher than those in normal tissues, the two hypothalamic releasing factors might be biosynthesized in the tumor cells.

2324 DESENSITIZATION OF THE RESPONSE TO GROWTH HORMONE-RELEASING FACTOR IN RAT ADENOHYPOPHYSIAL CELLS IN CULTURE. J. Simard, G. Lefèvre*, and F. Labrie, MRC Group in Molecular Endocrinology, CHUL, Québec, G1V 4G2, Canada.

During acute exposure, growth hormone-releasing factor (hpGRF-1-40-(NH_2)) induces a parallel stimulatory effect on growth hormone (GH) release and cyclic AMP (cAMP) accumulation in rat adenohypophysial cells in culture. The present study describes the detailed interaction between GRF, somatostatin (GIF) and prostaglandin E_2 (PGE_2) on GH release and cAMP accumulation in rat anterior pituitary cells in vitro. A 50% decrease in cAMP and GH responsiveness to 30 nM GRF is observed after 100 and 150 min of preincubation with 300 nM GRF, respectively. After 4h of preincubation with the neuropeptide, a 90% inhibition of both responses to GRF (1 to 7 nM) is observed. The ED_{50} value of GRF action for desensitization is similar on both GH release and cAMP accumulation. Preincubation with 300 nM GRF for 4h does not affect the ability of forskolin, cholera toxin, 8-Br-cAMP or isobutylmethylxanthine to stimulate GH release. However, a 30-40% decrease in PGE_2-induced GH release and cAMP accumulation is observed after preincubation with GRF. On the other hand, preincubation with 300 nM PGE_2 inhibits the maximal response of GH release and cAMP accumulation induced by GRF by 35 and 50%, respectively. Simultaneous preincubation with 300 nM GRF and 5 nM GIF increases by 2-fold basal GH release and blocks the decrease of GH release secondary to desensitization by GRF. The present data indicate that GRF induces a homologous desensitization of GRF action at a step preceding adenylate cyclase which is at least partly common to the site(s) of action of PGE2. In addition, GIF can at least partly protect the GRF receptor against desensitization.

2325 GLUCOCORTICOIDS AND TRIIODOTHYRONINE ARE POTENT STIMULATORS OF GROWTH HORMONE RELEASING FACTOR-INDUCED CYCLIC AMP ACCUMULATION AND GROWTH HORMONE SYNTHESIS IN ADENOHYPOPHYSIAL CELLS IN CULTURE. J. Simard, D. Michel*, C. Kreis, and F. Labrie, MRC Group in Molecular Endocrinology, CHUL, Québec, G1V 4G2, Canada.

Much experimental evidence suggests that cyclic AMP plays a major role in the control of growth hormone secretion, especially following stimulation by growth hormone-releasing factor (GRF). We have thus investigated the possible involvement of the cyclic AMP system in the stimulatory action of glucocorticoids and triiodothyronine (T_3) on GH secretion. Following preincubation of rat anterior pituitary cells with 300 nM T_3, dexamethasone, cortisol or corticosterone in an steroid- and T_3-free medium for 48 h, a subsequent incubation with a maximal concentration of hpGRF-1-40-NH_2 for 3 h increased cyclic AMP accumulation approximately 4-fold and stimulated GH release by 2-fold. On the other hand, pretreatment with T3 or glucocorticoids had no effect on basal cyclic AMP levels. In addition, preincubation with the glucocorticoids increased by 2-fold spontaneous GH release and GH cell content. GH synthesis as measured by 2-D polyacrylamide gel electrophoresis was similarly increased. The present data indicate that glucocorticoids and T_3 facilitate GH secretion by enhancing both the sensitivity of the response of the cyclic AMP system at a step preceeding cyclic AMP formation and by increasing GH cell content and synthesis.

2326 THE MECHANISM OF CALCIUM ACTION ON CORTICOTROPIN RELEASING FACTOR (CRF) STIMULATED ACTH RELEASE IN NORMAL RAT PITUICITES. D. Sobel* & H. Tao, Naval Hospital Bethesda & USUHS, Depts of Medicine & Pediatrics, Bethesda, MD,USA

The secretion of ACTH is in part controlled by a calcium dependent process. However, the site of calcium (Ca) action on normal pituicites is unknown. We studied the mechanism of Ca action upon CRF stimulated ACTH by evaluating the effects on CRF mediated ACTH secretion of 1) low Ca media 2) EGTA, a Ca chelator 3) Lanthanum, a blocker of Ca cell influx 4)Nifedipine, a blocker of slow Ca channel and 5) penfluridol, an inhibitor of calmodulin activity. Rat anterior pituitaries were dispersed in tryspin and placed in monolayer culture with $4x10^5$ cells/dish. After 3 days, the cells were washed and incubated in test media for 3.5 hrs. Media was then frozen for ACTH determination by RIA. Increasing concentrations of Ca in test media (0,1, 6mM) led to successively greater amounts of CRF (10mM) mediated ACTH release (10.63±0.55, 13.63±0.95, 16.68±0.62ng/dish respectively) EGTA (3mM) added to CRF (10nM) stimulated cells decreased the ACTH release from 16.57±1.2ng/dish to 5.28±0.4ng/dish ($p<0.01$). Lanthanum (0.5mM) inhibited CRF (10nM) induced ACTH release from 12.13±0.25 to 10.34±0.65ng/dish ($p<0.01$). This inhibition was blocked with 3mM $CaCl_2$. CRF(1nM) mediated ACTH release was reduced with the addition of nifedipine (1μM) from 6.22±0.65 to 4.59±0.09ng/dish ($p<0.01$). Penfluridol decreased CRF (10nM) induced ACTH from 10.53±0.84 to 5.92±0.12ng/dish ($p<0.01$). Summary: increasing Ca concentrations in test medium successively increases in CRF mediated ACTH release. The addition of EGTA (3mM), lanthanum (0.5mM), nifedipine (1μM), and penfluridol (1μM) inhibit CRF induced ACTH release. This data suggests that extracellular calcium, cell membrane calcium channels and calmodulin activation are involved in the mechanism of CRF mediated ACTH release.

2327 EFFECTS OF PIMOZIDE AND DES-GLY[10] [D-ALA[6]] LH-RH ETHYLAMIDE (LRH-A) ON GONADOTROPIN (GtH) RELEASE IN GOLDFISH THROUGHOUT THE REPRODUCTIVE CYCLE.
M. Sokolowska*, R.E. Peter, C.S. Nahorniak and J.P. Chang, Department of Zoology, University of Alberta, Edmonton T6G 2E9, Canada.

Previously dopamine was found to have potent GtH release-inhibitory activity in goldfish to modulate spontaneous release of GtH and to directly block the action of GtH-releasing hormone (GnRH). Pimozide (Pim), a dopamine antagonist, greatly potentiates the GtH releasing activity of LRH-A and other GnRHs in goldfish that have gonads in a prespawning condition; injection of Pim and LRH-A is highly effective at inducing ovulation, whereas injection of LRH-A alone is relatively ineffective. In the present study we investigated the variation in responsiveness of goldfish to Pim and LRH-A throughout a reproductive cycle. Injection of LRH-A alone caused no response in sexually regressed fish; fish with ovaries in late recrudescing condition had a greater response than early recrudescing, or prespawning fish. Pim potentiated the GtH release-response to LRH-A at all stages of the reproductive cycle; the greatest potentiation, in terms of levels of serum GtH produced, was in fish in late stages of ovarian recrudescence. In terms of the percentage difference between the serum GtH levels in the LRH-A vs. LRH-A plus Pim groups, the greatest potentiation was found in fish in mid-ovarian recrudescence when the acclimation temperature was 12°C, and in fish in early recrudescence at 20°C. The results indicate that dopamine inhibition on GtH release is present throughout the reproductive cycle in goldfish. The relative importance of this inhibition is influenced by stage of ovarian development and acclimation temperature. Supported by NSERC and AHFMR.

2328 CHARACTERIZATION OF RAT ADRENOCORTICAL SOMATOSTATIN RECEPTORS. C.B.Srikant* D. Lowden and Y.C. Patel, Fraser Labs, McGill University, Royal Victoria Hospital, Montreal, Quebec H3A 1A1.

We have previously shown that somatostatin (S-14) receptors in rat brain and pituitary exhibit selective ligand specificities for structural analogs of S-14 and for somatostatin-28 (S-28). In the present study we investigated the interactions of these peptides with adrenocortical S-14 receptors in order to determine whether these also exhibit distinct ligand specificities. Equilibrium binding studies using (^{125}I-Tyr^{11}) S-14 as radioligand revealed high affinity binding sites (K_d=1.1 nM and B_{max}=0.35 pmol/mg. Structural analogs of S-14 with halogenated Trp^8 moiety exhibited 4-46 fold greater binding affinity than S-14. S-28 and S-14 were equipotent (IC_{50}=0.6 and 0.75 nM) while the N-terminal fragments of S-28 were inactive. High affinity binding sites (K_d=1.2 nM;B_{max}=0.21 pmol/mg were also quantitated using (Leu^8, D-Trp^{22}, Tyr^{25}) S-28 as radioligand. The binding affinities of S-14 and S-28 determined using this radioligand were comparable (IC_{50}=1 and 1.2 nM). Extracts of adrenal cortex contained undetectable levels of S-14 like immunoreactivity. These studies confirm the presence of specific receptors for S-14 in the adrenal cortex and suggest that (1) with respect to S-14 biological activity, Trp^8 modified S-14 analogs should be more potent than S-14, S-28 equipotent with S-14, and N-terminal fragments of S-28 inactive. (2) Direct binding studies using radioiodinated (Tyr^{11}) S-14 and (Leu^8, D-Trp^{22}, Tyr^{25}) S-28 do not permit a distinction between possible separate populations of S-14 and S-28 receptors in thiss tissue. (3) In view of the absence of endogenous S-14 LI the adrenal actions of S-14 and S-28 in vivo are probably mediated through an endocrine mechanism.

2329 OVINE (o) AND HUMAN (h) CORTICOTROPIN RELEASING FACTOR (CRF) IN MAN: CRF-STIMULATION AND CRF-IMMUNOREACTIVITY. G.K. Stalla, Johanna Hartwimmer, K. von Werder, O.A. Müller. Medizinische Klinik Innenstadt, University of Munich, 8000 München 2, FRG

Nine normal volunteers received an intravenous bolus injection of 50, 100, and 200 µg oCRF. There was no dose response relationship between oCRF in this dose range and stimulated ACTH, ß-endorphin, and cortisol secretion. In addition no significant difference was observed between oCRF and oCRF together with glycine added as a stabilizer concerning ACTH and cortisol response in the 50 and 100 µg dosage. When synthetic hCRF was injected (50 and 100 µg i.v.) also no significant difference compared to the oCRF induced ACTH stimulation was observed.
In contrast to the lacking relationship between the CRF dosage and the biological response there was a clearcut dose response relationship between the amount of oCRF injected and the CRF immunoreactivity measured 15 min after injection with a specific oCRF radioimmunoassay. Though there was only 10 % cross reactivity with hCRF, CRF immunoreactivity could be detected in 53 out of 55 pregnant females and in placental extracts. Endogenous CRF immunoreactivity in humans had an identical elution profile from the Sephadex column as synthetic supporting that we are dealing with the true CRF-molecule.
Conclusion: CRF stimulation test can be performed with hCRF in the future and determination of endogenous CRF is feasible and may be of use in evaluating pituitary-adrenal diseases.

Supported by the DFG (Mu 585/2-1)

2330 **IN VIVO STUDIES ON THE EXTRACTION OF LH-RH BY HEPATIC, RENAL, AND MUSCLE TISSUE IN NORMAL SUBJECTS AND PATIENTS WITH CHRONIC LIVER DISEASE.**

M. Strohm*, H. Wernze, W. Tittor, Department of Internal Medicine, University of Würzburg and Stoffwechselklinik LVA Württemberg, Bad Mergentheim, West Germany.

Homogenates and tissue slices of liver, kidney and ovary or testis inactivate LH-RH very rapidly while other tissues e.g. muscle or lung have no effect. We measured the concentration of LH-RH by RIA in different vascular beds between 40 and 50 minutes after starting an infusion of synthetic LH-RH (Hoechst, 1,5 ug/min). Two groups of subjects were studied: gr. I six healthy persons, gr. II ten patients with hepatic cirrhosis (Ci), proven histologically. Blood samples from the femoral artery, hepatic vein, right renal and iliac vein were drawn simultaneously during diagnostic catheterization. The metabolic clearance rate was unchanged in patients with established cirrhosis (1441 ± 168 (SD) vs 1547 ± 651 ml/min) confirming previous results on patients with moderate liver dysfunction (Pimstone et al. 1977). Both groups exhibited marked extraction rates of LH-RH by leg muscles (Ci 37,2 ± 8,7 vs 46 ± 18 %, n.s.) whereas renal elimination was lower (Ci 24,7 ± 6 vs 31 ± 7,9 % n.s.) Hepatic extraction of LH-RH was rather small in both groups (Ci 12,7 ± 8,2 vs 10,8 ± 8,4 %) demonstrating that liver tissue does not play a major role in the removal of the decapeptide as suggested from in vitro studies or when organ distribution of radiolabelled LH-RH was followed after intravenous injection. Thus, our studies indicate that the skeletal muscle is an important site of inactivating LH-RH when the peptide reaches supraphysiological concentrations measurable by RIA.

2331 SOMATOSTATIN SUPPRESSION AS POSSIBLE CAUSE OF GH AND TSH SECRETORY RESPONSE TO BENZODIAZEPINES. T. Stryker,* D. Greenblatt and S. Reichlin. Department Endocrinology and Pharmacology, Tufts New England Medical Center, Boston MA

To test the hypothesis that benzodiazepines (BDZ) induce GH release by suppressing hypothalamic somatostatin (SRIF) secretion, we studied the effects of BDZ's on serum GH and TSH in man (TSH, like GH, is thought to be tonically suppressed by SRIF) and on the release of immunoreactive SRIF from fetal rat diencephalon in dispersed cell culture. 42 adult volunteers in 50 trials were given either an IV injection of 10 mg diazepam or an oral dose of 10 mg midazolam, 30 mg flurazepam or 10 mg nitrazepam. In 28% of trials plasma GH rose by 5 ng/ml or more within 90 minutes after drug administration. Males responded significantly more frequently than females (12 of 28 trials in males, 2 of 22 trials in females, $p<0.05$ by chi square test.) TSH, measured in 12 of 14 GH responders, did not significantly rise in any individual and the mean for the group showed a slight decrease when GH was at its peak (2.4 baseline vs 2.2 uU/ml at 60 minutes, $p<0.05$ by t test.) SRIF secretion by diencephalon cells in vitro was significantly suppressed by 10^{-5}M midazolam (46% decrease during 30 minute incubations, $p<0.0001$ by t test.) Secretion by cerebral cortical cells was not significantly suppressed (17% decrease, $p<0.3$ by t test) possibly reflecting regional differences in the brain for neurotransmitter control of peptide secretion. The in vitro data shows that BDZ could induce GH release by suppression of SRIF secretion but the lack of a TSH rise simultaneously with GH in vivo suggests that: 1) SRIF does not exert a tonic inhibitory effect on TSH secretion, or 2) BDZ suppresses SRIF but suppresses TSH through alternative mechanisms, or 3) BDZ releases GH through alternative mechanisms.

2332 DISTRIBUTION OF CORTICOTROPIN-RELEASING FACTOR IN HUMAN TISSUES AND ADRENAL TUMORS. T. Suda*, N. Tomori, F. Tozawa, H. Demura and K. Shizume, Department of Medicine, Tokyo Women's Medical College, Tokyo, Japan.

Distribution and characterization of immunoreactive corticotropin-releasing factor (CRF) in human tissues and adrenal tumors were examined utilizing rat CRF RIA, immunoaffinity chromatography, gel filtration chromatography and high performance liquid chromatography (HPLC). Human tissues were obtained at autopsy 3-6 h post mortem. Adrenal tumors were obtained at surgery from patients with Cushing's syndrome (n=7), primary aldosteronism (n=5) and pheochromocytomas (n=8). High concentrations of CRF were found in the hypothalamus and pituitary stalk, moderate concentrations of CRF were observed in other brain tissues, posterior pituitary and adrenal, and low concentrations of CRF were also found in other tissues outside the brain (lung, liver, stomach, duodenum, pancreas). In the adrenal, CRF was mainly localized in the medulla. CRF was also present in the adrenal tumors (pheochromocytoma > primary aldosteronism > Cushing's syndrome). Gel filtration chromatography of CRF in these tissues showed the main peak eluted at the position of synthetic rat CRF. HPLC of this main peak showed two components which eluted in the positions of synthetic rat CRF and oxidized CRF. These elution positions were the same in all tissues and identical with those in the hypothalamus. In conclusion, CRF was found in human brain, outside the brain tissues and adrenal tumors. Gel filtration and HPLC studies indicated that substantial fractions of these activities has physicochemical characteristics of authentic CRF.

2333 OVULATION INHIBITION IN THE IMMATURE RAT: BIOASSAY FOR LHRH ANTAGONISTS

K. Sundaram, F. Schmidt* and R.B. Thau, The Population Council, 1230 York Avenue, New York, N.Y. 10021

As the search for more potent LHRH antagonists continues and new antagonists are synthesized, convenient and economical methods for the evaluation of their in vivo biological potency become important. We compared the biological activity of [Ac-D-NAL(2)^1, 4FD-Phe^2, D-Trp^3, D-Arg^6]-LHRH (LHRH-A), [AcΔ^{3}Pro^1, 4FD-Phe^2, D-NAL(2)^{3,6} -LHRH (LHRH-B), and [AcΔ^{3}Pro^1, 4FD-Phe^2, D-Trp^{3,6}]-LHRH (LHRH-C) in immature female Sprague-Dawley rats maintained under a light period of 12h/day (lights on, 0630 h). All rats were given 10 IU of pregnant mare serum gonadotropin (PMSG) sc at 0930-1000 h on day 28 of age, and on day 30 an antagonist or vehicle (0.4 ml sterile water) sc at 1430-1500 h. The rats were killed on the following morning and the oviducts examined microscopically for the presence of ova. In the PMSG treated control rats the no. ovulating/no. treated (O/T) was 26/28. The antiovulatory potency of the antagonists is shown below. Doses are in μg/rat.

LHRH-A		LHRH-B		LHRH-C	
Dose	O/T	Dose	O/T	Dose	O/T
1.0	1/15	4.0	0/17	20	1/10
0.5	9/10	2.0	5/8	10	6/17
0.2	9/9	1.0	5/8	5	4/14

The order of potency, LHRH-A > LHRH-B > LHRH-C was confirmed by decreases in prostate weights and serum testosterone levels in adult male rats. It is concluded that PMSG treated immature rats provide a convenient model for rapid bioassay of LHRH antagonists.

2334 EFFECTS OF AGE ON GH RESPONSES TO HUMAN PANCREATIC GH-RF IN RATS.

J. Takahara,[1)] M. Niimi[2)], K. Kawanishi[2)] and S. Irino[1)], 1st. Department of Medicine[1)] and Central Laboratories[2)], Kagawa Medical School, Kagawa, Japan.

Response in serum GH level to human pancreatic GH-RF(hpGH-RF) in old human subjects is known to be significantly less than that in young subjects, especially children. In this study, we investigated GH responses to hpGH-RF in young and aged rats in in vitro and in vivo. Three groups rats, young rats(mean body weight:80g), middle aged rats(350g) and aged rats(600g), were used. In pentobarbital anesthetized young rats, an intravenous administration of hpGH-RF at dose of 25 ng/100g b.w. resulted in a 11.4 fold increase in serum GH level at 5 min after hpGH-RF injection. On the contrary, in aged rats the hpGH-RF at the same dose did not elicit to increase serum GH levels significantly. Isolated rat pituitary cells obtained from three groups were incubated for 3 days and an addition of hpGH-RF at dose of 5 ng/ml to cultured young rat pituitary cells caused about 11 fold increase in GH content in medium. On the other hand, the GH-RF to aged rat pituitary cells resulted in only a 5 fold increase of GH content. These results indicate that the sensitivity of sommatotrophs to hpGH-RF may be diminished with getting age.

2335 STUDY ON HUMAN PANCREATIC GROWTH HORMONE RELEASING FACTOR(hpGRF)-LIKE SUBSTANCE IN HUMAN PLACENTA. Y. Tanaka [1]*, S. Saito [2], O. Namba [1], S. Ohashi [3], S. Sawano [4] and M. Irie [1], 1) First Dept. of Med. and 2)Dept. of OB & GYN, Toho Univ. Sch. Med. Tokyo 143, Japan. 3) Res. Inst. for Polymers & Textiles, 4) Dept. Endocrinol. Toranomon Hosp., Okinaka Memorial Inst. for Med. Res., and Asahi Life Inst. for Adult Diseases.

The presence of hpGRF-like substance was examined in human placental extracts. Seven human placentas freshly obtained at the 7 to 10th week of gestation by D&C were minced and washed with saline, homogenized in 10 volumes of 2M acetic acid containing other chemicals, and centrifuged at 4,000g for 15 min at 4 C. The supernatant was filtered and lyophilized. The contents of hpGRF-like substance in the placental extracts were measured by RIA for hpGRF using an antiserum generated by sensitizing a rabbit with BSA-hpGRF-44 conjugate. In six out of seven placental extracts, hpGRF-like substance was present. These values were ranged 0.23 to 0.51 ng/mg protein. Serial dilutions of placental extracts generated competitive binding curves paralleled with that of synthetic hpGRF-44. Gel chromatography of the extracts on Sephadex G-50 column(1.6x60 cm, superfine)revealed two peaks having hpGRF-like activity. A high molecular component(s) eluted as a broad peak in and after the column void volume. A small peak of immunoreactive hpGRF-44 coeluted with synthetic hpGRF-44. The results of the present study suggest that hpGRF-like substance(s) are synthesized in the early gestational placenta.

2336 HUMAN PANCREAS GROWTH HORMONE RELEASING FACTOR (hpGRF): DIRECT CNS EFFECTS ON GROWTH HORMONE, GLUCOSE AND BEHAVIORAL REGULATION. G.S. Tannenbaum*, McGill University, Montreal, Quebec, H3H 1P3, Canada.

The hpGRF peptides have been shown to be potent and specific stimuli for the release of growth hormone (GH) when administered systemically. To determine whether hpGRF exerts any biological actions within the CNS we examined the effects of intracerebroventricular (icv) administration of hpGRF-44 (kindly provided by Dr. N. Ling) in freely-moving chronically cannulated rats. Various doses of hpGRF-44 (ranging from 0.5-10.0 µg/10 µl), or normal saline (NS), were icv injected and plasma GH, glucose and behavioral profiles were obtained over a 6-h period. Central administration of 10 µg hpGRF caused a dramatic and rapid suppression in amplitude of GH pulses (mean 6-h plasma GH level: 23.8 ± 3.2 vs 141.1 ± 21.2 ng/ml in NS controls; $P < 0.001$). The suppressive effect was dose-responsive with recovery to normal levels occurring at a dose of 1.25 µg. Administration of a specific somatostatin antiserum did not alter the depressed plasma GH profile indicating that this effect is not mediated via circulating somatostatin. A significant elevation of plasma glucose was noted 30 min post injection of 10 µg hpGRF and hyperglycemia persisted throughout the 6-h period (170 ± 9.6 vs 147 ± 1.8 mg/dl in NS controls; $P < 0.01$). Marked behavioral and motor effects characteristic of a fear response were observed following icv administration of the higher hpGRF doses. Conclusions: 1) Hypothalamic GRF, at high doses, may inhibit its own neurosecretion, and consequently that of GH, via an ultra short-loop negative feedback mechanism. 2) GRF within the CNS may play a role in glucoregulation. 3) In addition to its endocrine role as a hypophysiotrophic hormone, GRF may act as a neuromodulator affecting behavior by direct action on brain.

2337 IN VIVO ADMINISTRATION OF RAT GROWTH HORMONE-RELEASING HORMONE ANTISERUM SUPPRESSES GROWTH HORMONE RELEASE INDUCED BY ANTI-SOMATOSTATIN SERUM IN THE RAT. C.R.Thomas*, A.Arimura and P.J. Calecas, Laboratories for Molecular Neuroendocrinology and Diabetes, Department of Medicine and Anatomy, Tulane University, New Orleans, LA., U.S.A.

Previously we demonstrated the involvement of TRH in TSH release using anti-TRH serum to completely block TSH release induced by ovine anti-somatostatin serum (oA-SS). A similar experiment was conducted to examine the physiological role of rat GH releasing hormone (rGHRH) using ovine anti GHRH serum (oA-rGHRH). Urethane anesthetized rats were given intravenous injections of 1.0ml normal sheep serum (NSS) or oA-rGHRH 15min prior to a second injection of 0.5ml of NSS or oA-SS. After the second injection, jugular blood samples were taken at 10min, 20min and then every 20min for two hours and assayed for GH by RIA. Pretreatment with NSS followed by oA-SS resulted in serum GH levels of 858.1$\pm$ 127.78ng/ml at 20min which was significantly greater ($P < .01$) then controls receiving NSS only (44.3$\pm$8.66 ng/ml). Pretreatment with oA-rGHRH followed by oA-SS resulted in a significant suppression ($P < .01$) of the oA-SS induced GH release at 20min to 348.7$\pm$ 65.56ng/ml, however, serum GH levels remained significantly higher than NSS controls ($P < .01$). Additionally, oA-GHRH treatment followed by NSS decreased serum GH levels when compared to NSS controls indicating a possible role for rGHRH in basal GH release. These data support the recently isolated rGHRH as a physiological stimulator of GH release in vivo in the rat. Failure of oA-rGHRH to abolish oA-SS induced release of GH suggests either that the oA-GHRH was of insufficient amount to neutralize endogenous GHRH or that the rat may posess more than one physiologic stimulator of GH release. Supported by NIH grant AM09094.

2338 EFFECTS OF NEURAL STIMULI ON THE ACTIVITY OF IDENTIFIED NEURONES IN THE PARAVENTRICULAR NUCLEUS. D.J.Saphier and S.Feldman, Department of Neurology, Hadassah University Hospital, Jerusalem, Israel.

Recent evidence for the presence of an active corticotropin-releasing factor (CRF) within the mediodorsal parvocellular region of the paraventricular nucleus of the rat led us to examine the electrical activity of neurones in this region in response to stimulation of brain structures and sensory afferent projections known to affect adrenocortical secretion. About 15% of neurones were identified as projecting to the median eminence and the majority of these neurones were excited by stimulation of the preoptic area and the subicular cortex. Such neurones also showed an activation following photic and sciatic nerve stimulation. A high degree of convergence of responses was recorded from the population when these two peripheral neural stimuli were considered. Stimulation of the nucleus accumbens evoked inhibitory responses from 50% of the whole population and from more than 80% of those neurones excited by the other modalities. As high frequency stimulation of all these sites, except nucleus accumbens causes release of corticosterone, we conclude that these neurones found to project to the median eminence and activated by these stimuli, except for nucleus accumbens, may be candidates for the CRF-containing neurones.

2339 HYPOTHALAMO-PITUITARY (HT.P) REGULATION OF THYROID FUNCTION IN BRATTLEBORO RATS. B. Wolf*, S. Aratan-Spire, P. Czernichow, M.J. Voirol, J.N. Hugues. INSERM U 30, Hôpital Enfants-Malades Paris France ; Department of Endocrinology Hopital Avicenne Bobigny France.

Brattleboro rats with Diabetes Insipidus (DI) have altered thyroid function with elevated basal and TRH-stimulated serum TSH and decreased serum T4 as compared to normal Long Evans (LE) strain. This work was undertaken to study the HT.P regulation of thyroid function of DI compared to LE rats by measuring 1) TRH concentrations and TRH degrading activity (TRH-DA) in hypothalamus 2) Pituitary TSH content 3) 24-hour plasma TSH variations by hourly plasma sampling in chronically cannulated rats and TRH (500 ng/100 g B.W.) stimulated TSH values. TRH and TSH were determined by RIA and TRH-DA by measuring the percentage of intact TRH remaining after one hour incubation of 1 μg TRH with hypothalamic homogenats.

	TRH (pg/mg W.T)	TRH-DA (%)	PITUITARY-TSH (μg/mg W.T)	TSH (ng/ml) basal	TSH (ng/ml) post-TRH peak
DI	152,8 ± 10,4	64,3 ± 8	0,93 ± 0,1*	3,2 ± 0,7	21,9 ± 1,8*
LE	137,4 ± 11,1	66 ± 3,8	0,39 ± 0,03	2,2 ± 0,3	15,9 ± 1,1

TRH concentrations and TRH-DA were not different in both groups. Pituitary TSH and TRH-stimulated serum TSH values were significantly elevated in DI rats (respectively $p < 0{,}001$ and $p < 0{,}01$). The pattern of 24-hour of variations of serum TSH was identical in DI and LE rats. Our results are in favour of an intact HT.P regulation of thyroid function in DI rats. They are in agreement with previous studies showing primary thyroid failure in this strain of rats.

2340 STUDY ON THE EVOLUTION OF STEROIDOGENIC ENZYME AS AN INDEX OF THE PLACENTAL MATURATION. M.Ogino* and T. Jimbo, Department of Perinato-Gynecology, Kagawa Medical School, Kagawa Prefecture, Japan

The placenta produces a large amount of progesterone and estrogens and secretes them both into maternal and fetal circulations. In the present study, we have assessed the critical period by which the placenta gains the capacity to generate a significant amount of progesterone and estrogens in organ culture in vitro. For the investigation of the formation of each steroid, 14C-pregnenolone and 14C-androstenedione were used as the substrates respectively. The placenta generated a significant amount of progesterone at 6 weeks of gestation, although the placenta obtained at the same age could hardly produce a significant amount of estrone and estradiol-17β with unknown compounds formed. It was not until 7 and 8 weeks of gestation that the placenta could produce a significant amount of estrogens. The production rate of progesterone increased linearly and significantly as gestation advanced. The amount of progesterone formed in the 3rd trimester was 137.5% of that in the 1st trimester. In contrast to this, the sum of estrone and etradiol-17β produced by the placenta from 10 weeks to term was approximately 2/3 of that formed by the placenta at 7 and 8 weeks of pregnancy. Thus, it is very likely that the evolution of aromatizing enzyme system would take a different manner from that of 3β-hydroxysteroid dehydrogenase coupled with $\Delta^{5,4}$-isomerase catalyzing the formation of progesterone from pregnenolone in the course of the placental maturation.

2341 HISTOPATHOLOGIC CHANGES OF UTERUS IN GOSSYPOL-TREATED EARLY-PREGNANT RAT.
Y. Rikihisa*, Y. C. Lin and A. Walton, VA-MD Regional College of Veterinary Medicine, VPI&SU, Blacksburg, VA 24061, USA.

At laparotomy, no implantation sites were found on day-8 of pregnancy (day of sperm positive vaginal smear = day-0) in rats which had been treated with daily i.m. injections of gossypol acetic acid (GP) in 10% EtOH at 25 mg/kg starting on day-2 of diestrus and mated on day of proestrus. These studies were made to determine if implantation was inhibited or implanted conceptuses were aborted. In day-3 pregnant controls, increased glandular secretion and stromal hyperemia had become evident. At day-4, the lumen had become highly corrugated and focal closures had occurred. At day-5 closure of the lumen had occurred in all parts, and the stroma was extremely edematous and hyperemic. Small foci of decidual tissue containing many mitotic figures were present. At day-6, the decidual mass had become larger with increased mitotic figures. In treated rats, similar changes of the wall were noted at days-3 to 5; however, in the stroma just beneath the epithelium, cells were closely packed and appeared darker. On day-6, extreme hyperemia and stromal hemorrhage had occurred around well-developed decidual tissue with foci of denuded mucosal surface, and extravasation of blood into the lumen. No inflammatory reaction was noted. These results imply that GP treatment did not completely inhibit formation of decidual tissue. Absence of implantation sites noted surgically on day-8 of pregnancy might have resulted from an adverse uterine environment which would not permit survival of viable conceptuses. An early abortion process may also have been involved. Supported by NIH Grants HD 17627 and HD 16883.

2342 EVALUATION OF NORMAL CORPUS LUTEUM FUNCTION BY SERUM PROGESTERONE, ESTRADIOL AND THE PULSATILE PATTERN OF LH AND FSH.
T. Rabe*, L. Kiesel, K.-H. Jünemann, G. Rost and B. Runnebaum, Department of OB/GYN, Division of Gynecological Endocrinology, Universitäts-Frauenklinik, Voßstr.9, 6900 Heidelberg, West Germany

The luteal function was evaluated in healthy female volunteers (age 18 - 30 years) with regular menstrual cycles, normal prolactin (below 20 ng/ml) and progesterone levels (above 10 ng/ml) during luteal phase of a previous cycle. After immunological determination of urine LH surge patients (n=30) were divided into 3 groups (n=10) according to the time interval after LH surge: 4, 8 and 12 days. Serial venous blood samples were taken every 10 minutes over a period of 24 hours. Hormones were determined by means of specific radioimmunoassays. Serum progesterone and estradiol were measured every hour whereas LH and FSH pulses were analysed in blood samples withdrawn every 10 minutes. Preliminary results (n=8) indicate a day to night fluctuation of progesterone and estradiol which is evident in the middle and late luteal phase; steroid levels decreased nocturnally up to 50 % of mean daytime values. A pulsatile pattern of serum LH was observed in all volunteers. During 24 hours the frequency of LH pulses ranged from 3 to 9 pulses occuring with time intervals of 1 to 6 hours (mean: 3 h). A pulse was characterised by a two- to three-fold increase over basal LH levels in 20 minutes. Peak LH values declined towards baseline within 1.5 to 3 hours. Serum FSH showed only slight variations. Our preliminary clinical study indicates a correlation between the pattern of LH pulses and steroid secretion (estradiol and progesterone) of the corpus luteum that has been proposed for the bovine luteal phase.

2343 MENSTRUAL DYSFUNCTION AS A MANIFESTATION OF HYDROCEPHALUS. G. Redmond*, G. Gidwani, J. Bay, J. Hahn, D. Rothner, Departments of Endocrinology, Gynecology, Neurological Surgery and Neurology and the Center for Children and Youth, The Cleveland Clinic Foundation, Cleveland, Ohio

Menstrual cyclicity reflects normal functioning of a complex sequence of hypothalamic, pituitary and ovarian mechanisms. Although oligomenorrhea is a common complaint and is often due to benign conditions it may reflect serious disease of the central nervous system. We have observed two cases in which severe obstructive hydrocephalus manifested itself by menstrual dysfunction before other signs were manifest. Patient 1 presented at 20 years of age with hirsutism and amenorrhea. Initial prolactin determination was 42. Sector CT scan showed hypothalamic compression due to obstructive hydrocephalus caused by a 3rd ventricle cyst. Patient 2 presented at 17 years of age. Severe headaches had been present for several years. Prolactin level was 29.5 but hGH and cortisol were normal. Thelarche had begun at 9 years of age but menarche was delayed until 14½ and there had only been a few episodes of menstruation in the following two years. Obstructive hydrocephalus due to a 4th ventricle ependymoma was found on CT scanning. Prolactin level was unchanged postoperatively. Both patients had had withdrawal bleeding after medroxyprogesterone acetate on prior occasions.

Hypothalamic compression due to hydrocephalus can be associated with menstrual dysfunction. Hyperprolactinemia may be present but suppression of gonadotrophin release by the increased pressure may also be a factor in the pathogenesis of this condition.

2344 EARLY *IN VITRO* EMBRYONIC DEVELOPMENT FOLLOWING *IN VITRO* FERTILIZATION IN THE BOVINE. M.A.SIRARD*, R.D. LAMBERT; Laboratoire de génétique moléculaire et humaine section reproduction, CHUL, Québec, G1V 4G2, Canada.

In vitro gamete interaction has been extensively studied in numerous species but because of the very few successes in the bovine our objective was to study conditions and factors wich could improve the *in vitro* fertilization (IVF) assay. We used fertile bulls (5) and heifers treated with FSH or PMSG followed by PGF2 (and if no estrus was detected 44 hours after PGF2 , HCG was injected). Laparascopic surgery was performed 20 to 24 hours after the estimated estrus or HCG injection to obtain follicular oocytes (n=621) just prior to ovulation. After follicle aspiration, oocytes were transferred in maturation medium for 4 to 6 hours. Fresh bovine semen was treated with high ionic strength medium (380-400 MOSM/Kg) for 5 minutes and then washed and incubated for 3 to 18 hours in defined medium (DM) (Brackett, B.G. Biol. Repro. 27: 147-158. 1982). Capacitation following this treatment greatly varied from individual to another. Therefore fertilization and cleavage rates ranged from 14 to 46% and 0 to 40% respectively. Then we compared Ham-F-10 to DM for maturation, fertilization and development purposes. We obtained cleavage rates of 30% (n=38) with Ham-F-10 and 57% (n=35) with DM. *In vitro* fertilized bovine follicular oocytes reached the 2 polar body (n=39), 2-cell (n=71), 4-cell (n=40), 8-cell (n=17), 16-cell (n=2) stage after respectively 25±3, 46±3, 57±3, 74±4 and 99 hours. Those results are compatible with *in vivo* studies. This methodology could allow reproduction in numerous cows with tubal or uterine pathology once *in vivo* transfer (after IVF) is found to be successfull.

2345 PASSIVE TRANSFER OF INSULITIS TO NUDE MICE USING SPLEEN LYMPHOCYTES OF MICE TREATED WITH MULTIPLE LOW DOSES OF STREPTOZOTOCIN K. Toyama*, S. Miyake, Y. Yamaguchi, A. Takahashi, Y. Ueda, N. Kuriya, Y. Ikeda and S. Nagataki The First Department of Internal Medicine, Nagasaki University, Nagasaki 852, Japan

Low-dose streptozotocin(SZ)-induced diabetes in mice serves as a model for autoimmune insulin dependent diabetes. To elucidate the role of cell-mediated immunity, spleen lymphocytes of mice(male CD-1) given multiple low doses of SZ were injected to nude mice(male CD-1 nu/nu) and intraperitoneal glucose tolerance tests and histological examination of the islets including the examination of the islet infiltrates were performed 3 weeks after injection of spleen lymphocytes. Male CD-1 mice were given 4 successive daily doses of SZ 40mg/kg and additionally, a dose of 40mg/kg one week later. Three weeks after the first SZ injection, blood glucose levels of CD-1 mice increased significantly with histological evidence of insulitis. Similar treatment with SZ did not produce insulitis in CD-1 nu/nu mice. However the injection of spleen lymphocytes of SZ treated CD-1 mice to nude mice resulted in induction of glucose intolerance accompanied by infiltration of mononuclear cells into the islets, while thyroids and adrenals of recipient mice showed no inflammatory lesions. Histological examination of mononuclear cells in the islets revealed that Lyt-2 as well as Lyt-1 possitive cells existed in the islets which had not existed in nude mice before injection of spleen lymphocytes. However, cells stained by anti-mouse immunoglobulins antibody were rare in the islets. These results suggest that low-dose SZ-induced diabetes can be transferred passively from CD-1 to CD-1 nu/nu and major islet infiltrates are T cells.

2346 IMPROVEMENT IN INSULIN SECRETORY CAPACITY IN TRAINED DIABETIC RATS. D. Trudel*, A. Nadeau, G. Tancrède, C. Jobidon and S. Rousseau-Migneron. Laboratoires de Recherche en Endocrinologie et Métabolisme, CHUL, Québec, G1V 4G2, Canada.

A ten-week program of treadmill running improves mild diabetes mellitus induced by streptozotocin (45 mg/kg) in the rat. Although an enhanced insulin sensitivity is postulated, the exact mechanism remains to be elucidated. To assess the possibility that changes in insulin secretory capacity might be involved, plasma glucose (G) and insulin (IRI) levels were measured before, during and after a 30-min arginine infusion (50 mg/kg/min) in sedentary (SD) and trained (TD) diabetic rats and compared with sedentary controls (SC). The IRI response to arginine was estimated by planimetry. The pancreatic IRI content was also measured. TD were further divided into groups with normal (TD_1) or elevated basal G (TD_2).

	SC (n = 18)	SD (n = 15)	TD_1 (n = 8)	TD_2 (n = 8)
Basal G (mg/dl)	137 ± 3	379 ± 26	138 ± 6	351 ± 39
Basal IRI (μU/ml)	45 ± 3	24 ± 2	24 ± 3	22 ± 3
IRI area (ng/ml/min)	364 ± 52	55 ± 12	234 ± 75	58 ± 15
Pancreatic IRI (ng)	115 ± 5	8 ± 1	35 ± 7	10 ± 3

TD_1 had basal IRI levels similar to TD_2 and SD, thus suggesting an enhanced insulin sensitivity. However their pancreatic IRI content was also highly improved ($p < 0.01$), with an IRI response to arginine not different from SC ($p > 0.1$). These data suggest that partial recovery in insulin secretory capacity participates in the beneficial effect of physical training in this experimental model. Supported by MRC and CDA.

2347 ESTRIOL (E_3) INHIBITS THE DEGRADATION OF ^{125}I-INSULIN BY HUMAN PLACENTAL ENZYMES. J.C.M. Tsibris*, G. Ballejo, G. Banuelos, N.I. Cook and W.N. Spellacy. Dept. of Obstet. and Gynecol., University of Illinois at Chicago, Illinois 60612, USA.

70 μM E_3 increased by 20% the binding of ^{125}I-insulin (I) to placental plasma membranes (PPM) and decreased by 15% I degradation, assayed by acid precipitation of intact I; 0.5 mM bacitracin or 60 μM chloroquine inhibited I degradation by 30-50% but had little effect on I binding. The E_3 effect, also observed with estrone but not tamoxifen, progesterone or testosterone, was saturable and did not involve a thyroxine-like deiodination of I. The E_3 effect on I binding/degradation was more labile than the binding of I to PPM. I, made by the Bolton-Hunter method, bound to PPM only 5-10% compared to I made by the chloramine T method, but in the former the E_3-increase of I binding was greatly enhanced relative to the latter. Degradation of the two I ($\pm E_3$) did not differ greatly. The initial cleavage of I is probably done by an endopeptidase. E_3 also inhibited I degradation by placental cytosol. When the cytosol was applied on DEAE-Toyopearl 650S and eluted with a linear 0-0.4 M KCl gradient, three peaks of insulinase activity were isolated. Only the last peak (III, at 0.2 M KCl) was inhibited (50-80%) by 70 μM E_3; III was also inhibited 80% with 80 μM R24571, a very hydrophobic calmodulin (CaM) antagonist. Antibodies to CaM inhibited only III by 30%. E_3 inhibited also the degradation of ^{125}I-glucagon but not that of ^{125}I-labelled-α-casein, -human prolactin or-epidermal growth factor. After application of III on Chelating Sepharose, to remove bound Ca^{++}, 85% of the activity was recovered; addition of 70 μM E_3 ($\pm$ 1 mM Ca^{++}) to the eluates suggested that the E_3 effect on I degradation was not likely to be mediated by a Ca^{++}-dependent protease. III was not retained on Affi-Gel-CaM but in the eluates the E_3 effect was nearly doubled.

2348 Studies in Isolated Rat Islets With Linogliride Fumarate (LIN), a New Orally Effective Hypoglycemic Agent. G.F.Tutwiler,*R.W.Tuman, N.H.Wallace and W.Zawalich, McNeil Pharmaceutical, Spring House, PA. and Yale University School of Medicine, New Haven, CT

LIN [N-(1-methyl-2-pyrrolidinylidene)-N'-phenyl-4-morpholinecarboximidamide], a new orally effective hypoglycemic agent structurally unrelated to the sulfonylureas and biguanides, stimulates insulin secretion (IS) in animals and man. To evaluate its mechanism, in vitro studies were performed (perifusion or static incubation) using collagenase-isolated rat islets. LIN (0.1mM) potentiated IS in the presence of the nutrient secretagogues glucose (G,5.5mM), leucine (10mM), glyceraldehyde (2.5mM), or N-acetylglucosamine (15mM), but unlike tolbutamide, was ineffective in the absence of a nutrient or in the presence of nonstimulatory nutrients (oleic, arachidonic or pyruvic acids). Potentiation of G-induced IS was accompanied by a small increase in G-metabolism (5-^{3}H-Glucose→^{3}HOH), however blocking this increase with 2-deoxyglucose (10mM) did not alter IS. Mannoheptulose (10mM) inhibition of G-induced IS was partially prevented by LIN. Whereas verapamil (0.1mM) totally blocked G-stimulated IS, it inhibited LIN-enhanced release by only 44%. LIN did not potentiate TPA (phorbol ester) or A23187-stimulated IS. Also, trifluoperazine (10μM) inhibited (20-30%) G-stimulated IS similarly in the presence or absence of LIN. Finally, LIN did not affect G phosphorylation activity (hexokinase or glucokinase) in liver homogenates (2-^{3}H-G→^{3}HOH). In summary, linogliride stimulates insulin secretion in vitro by a nutrient-dependent process with properties suggesting a mechanism different from that of the sulfonylureas.

2349 STIMULATION BY FORSKOLIN OF ADENYLATE CYCLASE AND INSULIN RELEASE IN CALCIUM-DEPRIVED PANCREATIC ISLETS. I. Valverde*, P. García-Morales, S.P. Dufrane, A. Sener and W.J. Malaisse. Fundación Jiménez Díaz, Madrid, Spain and Lab. Experimental Medicine, Brussels Free University, Brussels, Belgium.

Forskolin (F, 0.3-30.0 μM) caused a dose-related activation of adenylate cyclase in a particulate subcellular fraction derived from rat pancreatic islets. F (5.0 μM) increased 6-fold the cyclic AMP content of intact islets, whether in the absence or presence of D-glucose (2.8 to 16.7 mM). F (5.0 μM) failed to affect significantly the oxidation of D-(U-^{14}C) glucose (11.1 mM). F (5.0 μM) also failed to affect ^{45}Ca net uptake by islets incubated in the presence of D-glucose (5.6, 8.3, 11.1 or 16.7 mM). F failed to affect insulin release at a low glucose concentration (2.8 mM), but markedly enhanced insulin output at higher glucose concentrations (5.6 to 27.8 mM). As little as 0.15 μM F was sufficient to cause a significant increment in insulin output, the maximal response being recorded at concentrations of F in the 1.5 to 15 μM range. F also augmented insulin release evoked by 2-ketoisocaproate, L-leucine, a tumor promoting phorbol ester, or Ba^{2+} (used alone or in combination with theophylline in the absence of Ca^{2+}). Whereas glucose-induced insulin release was abolished in the absence of Ca^{2+}, F enhanced insulin output from the Ca^{2+}-deprived but glucose-stimulated islets. Such an enhancing action was quite marked in media deprived of $CaCl_2$, and less pronounced but still present in media enriched with EGTA (0.5 mM). These data indicate that (i) an increase in the cyclic AMP content of the islets is unable per se to cause insulin release, (ii) the enhancing action of endogenous cyclic AMP upon insulin release evoked by either nutrient or non-nutrient secretagogues does not result from an increased net uptake of calcium, and (iii) such an enhancing action persists in the absence of extracellular Ca^{2+}.

2350 CONTINUOUS SUBCUTANEOUS GLUCAGON INFUSION (CSGI) FOR TREATMENT OF PANCREATIC α-CELL DEFICIENCY. L. Van Gaal*, R. Abs, I. De Leeuw, J. Bekaert. Dept. Endocrinology & Metabolism, University of Antwerp, Antwerp Belgium.

α-cell deficiency is a rare cause of spontaneous hypoglycemia. The diagnosis of pancreatic α-cell deficiency in a 40 years old woman with severe hypoglycemic attacks (Acta Endocrinologica, 1979, 11, 363) was established by RIA measurements of plasma glucagon levels after arginine and insulin induced hypoglycemia. Basal glucagon levels were lower than 14 pg/ml (Nl: 25-175 pg/ml). From 1976 to 1978 the situation worsened with epileptic episodes due to severe hypoglycemia with coma. Initially she was succesfully treated with Protamine Zinc-Glucagon (NOVO), 2 mg IM twice a day. After a few months she suffered from an increasing number of hypoglycemic attacks, which prompted us to augment the glucagon dose (> 15 mg daily). Variable serum glucagon levels were partially caused by local resorption problems. Due to these difficulties with several hypoglycemic attacks, a CSGI was started: the portable insulin infusion device type Microjet MC 20 (Ames) was used, because of its simplicity and the possibility to administer glucagon bolusses in square waves over an extended period of time. A mixture of 5 mg short acting glucagon initially was infused by day, 10 mg by night. With a daily meal-adapted schedule, together with 5 bolusses a day (bolus rate 0.52 cc/hr, duration 60 min.) acceptable blood glucose levels could be achieved. Gradually the concentration could be reduced; using the specific glucagon-solvens mixture, 5.077 mg glucagon was administered over a 24 hr period. HbA_1 rose from 3.1 % to 5.5. % after two months of treatment. Since 3 months no serious hypoglycemic attacks were reported in such a way that this unique way of treatment enabled her to lead a nearly normal life.

2351 SIMILAR METABOLIC EFFECTS OF PULSATILE *VERSUS* CONTINUOUS INTRAVENOUS INSULIN DELIVERY DURING EUGLYCEMIC HYPERINSULINEMIC GLUCOSE CLAMP IN NORMAL MAN. E. Verdin*, M. Castillo, A. Luyckx and P. Lefèbvre, Institute of Medicine, Univ. Liège, B-4020 Liège, Belgium.

Seven normal volunteers were studied on two different occasions where four hour pulsatile (PULS : 0.8 $mU.kg^{-1}.min^{-1}$, 7.5 min out of 15) and continuous (CONT : 0.4 $mU.kg^{-1}.min^{-1}$) I.V. infusions of human insulin (Actrapid HM, Novo) were randomly compared. A euglycemic glucose clamp was performed and a 3-^{3}H-glucose infusion was used for determination of endogenous glucose production (EGP) and metabolic clearance rate (MCR) of glucose. Plasma glucose was similar in both conditions ; plasma insulin was stable at about 28 mU/l (CONT) and fluctuated between 10 and 45 mU/l (mean: 29 ; PULS). Exogenous glucose infused was 1.137 $\pm$ 0.058 and 1.088 $\pm$ 0.099 $g.kg^{-1}.4hr^{-1}$ in CONT and PULS respectively (N.S.). EGP was totally suppressed in both conditions. Glucose MCR increased similarly to a maximum of 6.71 $\pm$ 0.19 (CONT) and 6.79 $\pm$ 0.59 (PULS) $ml.kg^{-1}.min^{-1}$ during the fourth hour. C-peptide plasma levels remained stable whereas plasma glucagon, free fatty acids and β-hydroxybutyrate were similarly suppressed in both tests. Thus, in these conditions, pulsatile and continuous insulin infusions have similar metabolic effects. These data contrast with those of MATTHEWS *et al.* (1983) who reported that, at lower plasma concentrations (5 - 19 mU/l) pulsatile insulin had greater hypoglycemic effect that continuous delivery.

2352 THE USE OF FENFLURAMINE IN INSULIN-TREATED DIABETICS: LONG TERM EXPERIENCE IN AN OUT-PATIENT CLINIC. M. Verdy*, P. Hamet and J.L. Chiasson, Division of Endocrinology, Hotel-Dieu de Montreal, Montreal, H2N 1T8, Canada.

We have already shown that acute treatment with fenfluramine in obese insulin-treated diabetics was associated with a significant decrease in blood sugar without any change in body weight. We report here our long term clinical experience with the use of fenfluramine in diabetics. Twenty one (21) obese non-insulin dependent diabetics on insulin therapy were started on fenfluramine. The medication was discontinued in 6 patients: in 2 for hypoglycemia, 2 for side effects and 2 for unrelated reasons. The 15 remaining poorly controlled patients had a mean fasting blood sugar at the last 2 clinic visits before fenfluramine of 217 ± 16 mg/dl and 231 ± 16 mg/dl respectively. They were then put on fenfluramine 60 mg HS (long acting) for a period of 1 to 22 months (mean = 7 mo.). At their first visit after the start of fenfluramine (1 wk to 2 mo), blood sugar was already down to 190 ± 16 mg/dl ($p < 0.05$) and remained decreased at 183 ± 17 mg/dl ($p < 0.01$) at their last clinic visit (1 mo to 22 mo). Insulin had to be decreased by 50% in 2 of the patients because of hypoglycemia. Mean body weight decreased slightly from 83 ± 4 kg to 81 ± 4 kg ($p < 0.05$) during the treatment period. Mean blood pressure was also lower after fenfluramine but only at the first visit: 141 ± 5/85 ± 2 to 129 ± 3/79 ± 2 mm Hg ($p < 0.02/p < 0.05$). From this experience we believe that fenfluramine can be a helpful drug in the treatment of obese non-insulin dependent diabetics who have to be put on insulin because of symptomatic hyperglycemia.

2353 INSULIN SECRETION IN MEDULLARY THYROID CARCINOMA (MTC).

R. Vettor, C. Martini, M. Manno, N. Simioni, B. Busnardo, N. Sicolo°.
Istituto di Semeiotica Medica, Cattedra di Patologia Medica III^, Università di Padova, Italy.

It is known that Ca^{++} ion plays an important role in insulin secretion and that acute administration of Calcitonin (CT) induces a blunted beta-cell response to various stimuli. To verify the effect of the constant and chronic elevation CT plasma levels, as observed in pathological conditions, in insulin secretion, we studied seven patients (F 4, M 3) with MTC, treated with different therapy (thyroidectomy 6; chemiotherapy 1) and then treated with substitutive therapy (T-3 or T-4). All patients were in satisfactory general conditions; one patient presented obesity while three patients had methastases of the liver. In MTC patients the calcium plasma level was not statistically different from controls, while CT plasma level resulted considerably higher than controls (32.3 $\pm$ 23.9 vs 0.08 $\pm$ 0.02 ng/ml). In overnight fasting MTC patients and control subjects blood glucose (BG) and plasma insulin (IRI) were assayed after oral glucose load and Arginine infusion. Our results showed a slightly, but not significantly, higher glycaemic response to OGTT in MTC patients; moreover insulin plasma levels were significantly higher ($p < 0.05$) at 30, 60 and 90 min in MTC. The insulin response to Arginine infusion was also significantly elevated.

Even though obtained under conditions of pathological and chronic elevation of CT plasma level, as observed in patients with MTC, our results show a lack of insulin inhibiting action of CT, which is evident after its acute administration. Instead they showed an enhanced insulin response to stimuli without changes in carbohydrate tolerance.

2354 FASTING TEST DURING SLEEPING PERIODS. INTEREST OF NIGHTLY AMENDED IRI/BG RATIO FOR INSULINOMA DETECTION.

C. Villaume*, B. Beck, J.M. Dollet, J.P. Pointel, P. Drouin, G. Debry. INSERM U59 - 38 rue Lionnois F-54000 Nancy

In order to get a dynamic picture of the way insulinemia abnormality as a function of blood glucose occurs in the morning in subjects with insulinoma, we measured the plasma insulin (IRI)/blood glucose (BG) amended ratio (100 IRI (µU/ml)/BG (mg/dl) - 30) during the fasting period of four sleeping subjects with insulinoma. Seven healthy subjects, two obeses, two maturity onset diabetics, two subjects with insulinoma after surgery and one with pancreatitis have been used as reference in order to determine variations during the night and to estimate the diagnostic efficiency of this ratio. Blood samples were drawn continuously in 15 or 30 minutes pools during the sleep of the subjects and BG and IRI were assayed. The mean of amended IRI/BG ratio is presented in table. Subjects with insulinoma are marked off from the other subjects by a very elevated ratio dispersion around the mean value with highly significant peaks. Mean value always remains outside of the range (7-82) which covers the totality of measured values in healthy and pathological subjects. Fasting test during the night on sleeping subjects with insulinoma makes it possible to establish in an unquestionable manner the diagnosis of insulinoma.

	NORMAL							OBESE		PANCRE-ATITIS	DIABETES		INSULINOMA				AFTER SURGERY	
Mean	39.7	59.8	11.5	22.4	17.5	27.8	23.6	28.0	35.2	15.6	16.5	18.4	181	144	88	124	28.5	33.6
SD	11.4	4.8	3.5	2.8	4.2	3.2	5.0	5.2	6.0	5.2	4.2	5.8	101	220	32	265	9.1	10.2

2355 RELIABLE LABORATORY ANALYSIS OF BLOOD GLUCOSE SAMPLED BY THE PATIENT ON FILTER PAPER. Henning von Schenck* and Staffan Wettre, Depts of Clinical Chemistry and Internal Medicine, Regional Hospital, S-581 85 Linköping, Sweden.

Reliability of blood glucose analyzed by patients at home depends on accurate handling and quality of test strips and reflectometer. Blood sampling on filter paper mailed to the laboratory for wetchemical analysis would avoid analytical uncertainty. This study reports the various analytical qualities of the paper sampling method, including effect of hematocrit and storage stability. The patient applies about 50 µl capillary blood on filter paper (Whatman 31 ET Chroma, rinsed in boric acid 0.8 mol/l). At the laboratory two more spots of EDTA blood with known glucose concentrations are applied as standards. The spot centers (6 mm ø) are punched out and eluted with continuous agitating (1 h) in 200 µl sulfosalicylic acid, 0.1 mol/l. 100 µl eluate is assayed with the routine glucose-hexokinase method (Glucostrate Improved, General Diagnostics). Intra-assay coefficient of variation, C.V., (tripl.) was between 1.2 and 5.2% and inter-assay C.V. between 4.0 and 8.2% at various levels. Accuracy (n=68) was $y = 0.96x + 0.4$ ($r=0.98$). Analytical recovery was 99 ± 4.5% (SD). Hematocrit beyond 32-49% influenced recovery. Simultaneously applied samples demonstrated good stability during 3 weeks when stored at the laboratory or mailed within town. Hence, accurate, precise and stable results were obtained with good recovery at normal hematocrit. Filter paper sampling renders thus a suitable alternative for reliable blood glucose determination in patients during every-day conditions.

2356 AUTOANTIBODIES TO HUMAN INSULIN. Terence Wilkin*, S. Nicholson and C. R. Casey, Dept. Medicine II, University of Southampton, U.K.

Antibodies to commercially prepared insulins have been recognised for many years, but autoantibodies to insulin have never gained wide acceptance. This is largely because of doubts over the specificity of the assay, exact nature of the binding factor and insulin-naivity of the subjects. We employed an immuno-specific microELISA using an anti-human IgG horseradish peroxidase conjugate to screen sera from insulin-naive non-diabetic patients with various auto-immune diseases and identified nine (three from males and six from females, ages 21 - 74) which bound insulin. Specificity was demonstrated by substituting glucagon for insulin and human gamma-globulin for test serum. Four of the sera bound human (H), porcine (P) and bovine (B) insulin, to degrees equivalent to 'moderate binding in diabetic sera, but 5 bound exclusively H insulin. 'Cold' H, P and B totally displaced, in a dose-dependent manner, the 4 sera which bound all three insulins, but only H insulin displaced the remaining 5, P and B insulins having no effect in concentrations up to 1000 mU/ml. H differs from P insulin by a single amino acid substitution. The ability of 5 out of the 9 sera to distinguish H from P suggests very limited clonality. Autoantibodies are distinct from induced antibodies, but whether they should be looked upon as natural antibodies, markers of islet-cell immunity or part expression of a polyendocrine response to viral infection is unclear.

2357 IN VIVO EFFECT OF ANDROGEN ON THE PHOSPHORYLATION OF NUCLEOLAR PROTEINS OF RAT VENTRAL PROSTATES. N.Suzuki and T.Hosoya,* Faculty of Pharmaceutical Sciences, Chiba University, Chiba 260 Japan.

Since androgen stimulates greatly the synthesis of rRNA in nucleoli of prostates and the phosphorylation of chromatin is generally considered to modify the gene expression, in vivo effect of androgen on the phosphorylation of nucelolar proteins by endogenous protein kinase was studied. Nucleoli isolated from rat ventral prostates were incubated for 10 min at 37°C with γ-[^{32}P]ATP in the presence of 100mM NaCl, 5mM $MgCl_2$ and 1mM PMSF, and proteins solublized from the nuceloli were subjected to SDS-polyacrylamide slab gel electrophoresis followed by autoradiography. Testosterone injected to 48-hr castrated rats stimulated the phosphorylation of Mr 100K protein, and to a lesser degree, Mr 160K, 77K and 36K proteins. The 100K protein resembled, in many aspects, to C23 protein of rat hepatoma nuceloli and the stimulation of phosphorylation by androgen almost leveled off at 4 hr after the testosterone administration. The phosphorylation of 100 K protein was inhibited by polyamines, especially by spermine, when the protease inhibitor (PMSF) was omitted. Although phosphorylation of several proteins other than 100K protein was somewhat enhanced by androgen, these proteins as well as the 100K protein were distinctly different from phosphoproteins contained in the preparation of partially purified RNA polymerase I. cAMP, cGMP, and Ca^{2+}-calmodulin did not affect the phosphorylation of nucleolar proteins. The present data raise the possibility that androgen may regulate rRNA gene transcription through the mediation of phosphorylation of the 100K protein, not of the subunits of RNA polymerase I.

2358 INSULIN BIOEFFECTS IN CULTURED HUMAN HEPATOMA CELLS. S. Takeda*, J.M. Podskalny, R.E. Silverman, P. Gorden. Diabetes Branch, NIADDK, National Institutes of Health, Bethesda, MD 20205.

Hep G2 cells, isolated from a human hepatocellular carcinoma, have been shown to express large numbers of insulin receptors. We now demonstrate that these cells, which maintain several normal liver functions, respond to insulin in a variety of bioassays. Glucose uptake can be increased by insulin 20-30% over basal levels with an ED_{50} of 5 ng/ml and a maximal stimulatory effect at 50 ng/ml. Likewise, the incorporation of ^{14}C-acetate into lipid is enhanced 40% by 100 ng/ml insulin and half-maximally stimulated by 3 ng/ml. The conversion of the glucose-6-phosphate dependent to the G-6-P independent form of glycogen synthase is stimulated 2-3 fold by 100 ng/ml insulin and has an ED_{50} of 10 ng/ml. When ^{3}H-uridine incorporation into acid precipitable material is measured, a two-fold increase over basal can be seen with 0.1-1 μg/ml insulin. Concentrations as low as 5 ng/ml are consistently effective in stimulating uridine incorporation. By contrast to insulin's stimulatory effects on glucose uptake, lipogenesis, glycogen synthase, and RNA synthesis, no effect of insulin on thymidine incorportation into DNA could be demonstrated. This bioeffect of insulin is thought to be mediated via growth factor, not insulin, receptors. Two such growth factors, IGF-I and MSA/IGF-II, bound poorly to Hep G2 cells. We conclude that human hepatoma cells are sensitive to low concentrations of insulin in four bioassays that measure metabolic effects of the hormone presumed to be mediated via the insulin receptor, but do not respond in an assay that measures the growth effects of insulin acting via a growth factor receptor.

2359 DUAL MECHANISM OF ACTIONS OF CORTISOL (F) ON THE SYNTHESIS OF CASEIN IN MAMMARY EPITHELIAL CELLS IN CULTURE.

Y. Taketani, M. Mizuno, S. Sakamoto and T. Oka, Dept. of OB/GY, Univ. of Tokyo, 7-3-1 Hongo, Bunkyo-ku, Tokyo, Japan and LBM, NIADDK, NIH, Bethesda, Md, 20205, U.S.A.

We have employed a primary mammary cell culture system to investigate the molecular mechanism of F involved in hormonal induction of milk protein. Mammary epithelia from lactating mice cultured on collagen gels proliferated and synthesized casein. Cell culture was carried out for 5 days with a daily change of culture medium. The amount of casein synthesized was determined by immunoprecipitation method using specific antibody against casein. The synthesis of casein was very low in culture with insulin (I) and prolactin (PRL), but increased by the further addition of F in increasing concentrations up to 3 μM. The optimal casein synthesis required the presence of 3 μM F and 5 μg/ml of I and PRL. F at a concentration of 0.03 μM caused 53% and 75% reduction in the amount of casein synthesis and translatable casein mRNA, respectively. The addition of F at both 3 μM and 0.03 μM equally increased the amount of ^{125}I-PRL binding to cells cultured with I alone, whereas the absence of F resulted in marked reduction in PRL binding. We further examined the effect of F at the level of transcription of casein mRNA using its cDNA probe. With use of the technique of RNA hybridization after pulse-labeling cells with ^{3}H-uridine, a much higher rate of casein mRNA synthesis was observed at a higher concentration of F (3 μM) compared to that at a lower concentration of F. These results indicate that F exerts its lactogenic actions by not only increasing the capacity of PRL binding to mammary epithelial cells, but also enhancing the transcriptional rate of mRNA for major milk protein, such as casein.

2360 ADMINISTRATION OF ANTI-ANDROGENS DOES NOT AFFECT PROSTATIC ACID PHOSPHATASE (PAP) ACTIVITY IN THE RAT.

M. Tenniswood,* P. Abrahams, C. Bird and A. Clark. Dept. of Biochemistry, University of Ottawa, Ottawa and Depts. of Biochemistry and Medicine, Queen's University, Kingston, Ontario, Canada.

In an attempt to develop an alternative to castration and estrogen therapy for the treatment of prostatic cancer a number of "anti-androgens" have been developed including cyproterone acetate (CA), flutamide (Flu) and Compound I (CI). However, the experimental and clinical use of these drugs has met with mixed success. To investigate the reasons for the variable results we studied the effects of these drugs on secretory acid phosphatase (SAP) activity, a sensitive marker enzyme which requires very low doses of androgen to remain active. When administered to intact adult male rats CA (10 mg/day), Flu (15mg/day), or CI (1 mg/day), cause a significant decrease in the organ weight to body weight ratios, with a concomitant rise in the specific activity of PAP. However these compounds affect neither the % inhibition of PAP by tartrate, nor the appearance of SAP on polyacrylamide gels. When administered to castrated rats given doses of 5α-dihydrotestosterone (5α-DHT) (250-750 μg/day), Flu (15mg/day) altered neither the % inhibition of PAP by tartrate, nor the pattern of activity on polyacrylamide gels, even at the lowest dose of 5x-DHT. These results suggest that these anti-androgens effect some of the androgen dependent functions of the prostate, but do not reduce the level of androgens sufficiently to curtail all of their actions. This may offer a partial explanation for the equivocal clinical results obtained with these compounds.

(Supported by the Medical Research Council of Canada)

2361 COMPARISON OF LH AND LHRH-AGONIST ACTION ON RAT LEYDIG CELL STEROIDOGENESIS.

Axel P.N. Themmen*, Jos W. Hoogerbrugge, Focko F.G. Rommerts and Henk J. van der Molen, Dept. of Biochemistry (Div. of Chemical Endocrinology, Erasmus University, P.O. Box 1738, 3000 DR Rotterdam, The Netherlands.

Stimulation of mitochondrial cholesterol side-chain cleavage in isolated Leydig cells by LH is accompanied by increased levels of cAMP, PK activation, stimulated phosphorylation of at least 6 phosphoproteins, and requires continuous protein synthesis. LHRH and LHRHa can also stimulate steroidogenesis, but the mechanism of action is unknown. A comparison of the effects of LH and LHRHa on Leydig cells showed that steroid production can be stimulated 37-fold by 100 ng/ml LH (100LH) and only 9-fold by 50 ng/ml LHRHa. Maximal stimulation of steroid production by 100LH was reached within 15 min, whereas the response to LHRHa and 0.2LH reached its maximum only after 3 hrs. The LHRH antagonist ORG30093D specifically abolished all LHRHa effects. LH stimulated cAMP production and protein phosphorylation; this could not be demonstrated with LHRHa. Both LH- and LHRHa-stimulated steroid production required extracellular calcium. The calmodulin inhibitor trifluoperazine specifically inhibited LH action, but not LHRHa stimulation of steroidogenesis. Calcium ionophore A23187 (1 μM) stimulated basal steroid production 2-fold, inhibited 100 LH action, but had no effect on 0.2LH- and LHRHa-stimulated steroidogenesis. Inhibition of 25-OH-cholesterol-dependent steroid production indicates aspecific effects of the ionophore at 10 μM. These results indicate that LHRH action on rat Leydig cell steroidogenesis is not mediated by cAMP, in contrast to LH action, while calcium appears to be important in stimulation of both hormones.

2362 STUDIES OF T_3 ACTION ON β-ADRENERGIC RECEPTOR cAMP SYSTEM IN RAT HEART MUSCLE: T_3 BINDING BY SOLUBILIZED β-RECEPTORS FROM PLASMA MEMBRANES.

H. Uchimura*, T. Mitsuhashi, K. Kubota, N. Kuzuya, and H. Ikeda. The Third Department of Internal Medicine, University of Tokyo, Hongo, Tokyo, Japan.

Adenylate cyclase(AC) responses to β-adrenergic agonists in heart plasma membranes which have been reported are presumed to be enhanced by thyroid hormones. Our study investigated T_3 effects in vitro on catecholamine-sensitive AC-cAMP in plasma membranes of rat heart muscle and T_3 binding sites of β-adrenergic receptor AC-cAMP. Heart muscle of thyroidex rats was homogenized in 0.025M Tris 0.25M sucrose buffer, pH7.6, and centrifuged at 10,000g for 15 min at 4C. Pellets were suspended with Tris buffer, pH7.6 and used as crude membranes. AC was measured by Steiner's method; cAMP was assayed by specific RIA. β-adrenergic receptor was solubilized with 0.2% Lubrol PX and purified by Ultrogel AcA34 gelfiltration. Isoproterenol(Ip) receptors were identified by binding of $[^3H]$dihydroalprenolol. Ip-stimulated AC activity was enhanced by $T_3(10^{-9}-10^{-6}M)$ dose-dependently. T_3 effects were observed within 10 min after adding T_3. AC induced by GppNHp, analogue of GTP, was also increased by T_3, but T_3 showed no effect on NaF-stimulated AC activity. T_3 effects on AC activity were also seen by using solubilized, purified receptor protein. When solubilized β-receptors were pretreated with $^{125}I-T_3$ and eluted on Ultrogel AcA34, a peak of $^{125}I-T_3$ was observed in the same position as purified β-adrenergic receptor. Purified receptors on SDS-PAGE showed several protein bands in the 40 to 60K region. These data suggest that T_3 may bind to a component of β-adrenergic receptor AC-cAMP system, affect guanine nucleotide regulatory units, and exert its effects on Ip-stimulated AC activity very quickly.

2363 REGULATION OF VITELLOGENIN GENE EXPRESSION IN MALE HEPATOCYTE PRIMARY CELL CULTURES: An Excellent Model for the Study of Steroid Hormone Action. Y. Valotaire*, C. Le Guellec, J.L. Maitre, L. Mercier and L. Dolo, Laboratoire de Biologie Moleculaire, Campus de Beaulieu, L'Université de Rennes, Rennes, France.

In most egg laying vertebrates the egg yolk proteins are synthesised in the liver as a large precursor termed vitellogenin (Vg). The regulation of Vg by estradiol (E2) has been extensively studied in Xenopus and chicken, two species which have non-seasonal reproductive cycles. Rainbow trout (Salmo gairdneri) are of particular interest since they have a seasonal reproductive cycle, a feature they have in common with most other fishes. In order to study the hormonal regulation, and other factors, which control the seasonal regulation of vitellogenesis we developed a primary cell culture system from rainbow trout liver, which offers an ideal experimental control with zero background, and a high yield of viable hepatocytes.. These hepatocytes are sensitive to estradiol and synthesise Vg (measured by an original radioimmunoassay) after induction with E2. As in other steroid target cells E2 acts via a common molecular mechanism, the binding of the hormone with high affinity to specific soluble receptor proteins (Kd 1.5×10^{-9} M). The subsequent induction of Vg gene transcription has been demonstrated using cDNA probes for Vg, albumin and globin genes, isolated from a cDNA clone library of expressed sequences from the female trout liver. That Vg genes were selectively activated by E2 was shown by hybridisation of isolated mRNA to the cloned Vg probe and compared to the induction of albumin and globin mRNA. These results show that male trout hepatocyte system offers a versatile model to study the steroid hormone action and other factors implicated in the regulation of vitellogenin gene expression.

2364 STRUCTURE AND ANDROGENIC REGULATION OF THE MOUSE RENAL β-GLUCURONIDASE GENE C.S. Watson*, B. Funkenstein, S.L. Leary, and J.F. Catterall, The Population Council and The Rockefeller University, New York, N.Y. 10021 USA

Mouse kidney β-glucuronidase is induced by androgens in a classical receptor dependent fashion and genetic regulatory mutations have been described which govern this response. In the A/J strain (Gus-r^a) the induction of enzyme activity is 3-5 times higher than in C57 black/6J animals (Gus-r^b). To study this hormonal and genetic control at the molecular level we hybridized mRNA from these two mouse strains to cloned cDNAs from the mRNAs for β-glucuronidase and the 20,000 dalton kidney androgen regulated protein (designated KAP). Female mice were treated with silastic implants which release 120 μg of testosterone/day over a 20 day time course. Induction of specific mRNA was analyzed by Northern blot hybridization of kidney poly(A) RNA. The induction of β-glucuronidase mRNA was several fold higher in the strain carrying the "a" regulatory allele while KAP mRNA induction did not differ between strains. We also demonstrated this by a more quantitative assay in which poly(A) kidney RNA was covalently bound to aminophenylthioether paper discs and hybridized to ^{32}P-nick translated cloned cDNA followed by liquid scintillation counting. The chromosomal β-glucuronidase gene was isolated from a genomic recombinant DNA library derived from the Balb/c strain which carries the "a" haplotype of the [GUS] genetic complex. We have determined the β-glucuronidase cDNA sequence which will be used to identify the 5' terminus of the structural gene. Comparison of 5'-flanking sequences of this gene with those of the "b" haplotype may lead to the identification of the cis-acting Gus-r regulatory site.

2365 ESTRADIOL STIMULATES THE SYNTHESIS OF SOLUBLE AND INTERMEDIATE FILAMENT PROTEINS (IFP) BY THE GUINEA PIG SEMINAL VESICLE STROMA. Mitchell J. Weinberger*, Elliot V. Hersh and Irene C. Sandborg, Dept. of Pharmacology, UMDNJ-New Jersey Medical School, Newark, NJ 07103 USA

The fibromuscular stroma (FMS) of the guinea pig seminal vesicle contains Type I and II estrogen binding proteins and following estrogen treatment *in vivo* the FMS exhibits increases in collagen content, wet weight and several other growth-related parameters. In order to identify specific markers of estrogen action we used SDS-PAGE and fluorography to analyze the soluble proteins synthesized by FMS *in vitro*. In previous studies we had observed that the synthesis of a 58,000 dalton (58K) peptide was unchanged following castration. In the present studies, estradiol treatment of intact animals produced a significant increase in the synthesis of the 58K peptide(7100 vs. 18500 cpm/mg protein, $p < .05$). Total incorporation was unchanged (98700 vs. 99200 cpm/mg protein). Estrogen treatment of castrate animals also increased the synthesis of the 58K peptide. This was inhibited by concomitant tamoxifen treatment. A 58K peptide was also observed in an IFP-enriched fraction prepared from the FMS. A peptide map of this band was similar to that observed by others for vimentin, a major IFP component. The time-course of appearance of the 58K peptide into the soluble and IFP-enriched fractions suggested that they might share a precursor-product relationship. Our studies suggest that estrogen produces a selective effect on FMS protein synthesis which appears to be receptor mediated. One of the proteins regulated by estrogen may be vimentin. Since the function of vimentin is presently unknown, the significance of our findings remains to be established. Supported by NIH grant HD 15681

2366 HUMAN LEUKOCYTE HMG CoA REDUCTASE ACTIVITY AS AN INDEX OF CHOLESTEROLGENESIS IN MAN. P.W. Stacpoole*, H.J. Harwood, Jr. and M. Keramidas, University of Florida, College of Medicine, Gainesville, Florida 32610.

The activity of HMG CoA reductase is rate-limiting for cholesterol synthesis (CS) in animal cells. Accurate measurement of human leukocyte (HL) reductase activity (RA) as a reflection of endogenous CS has potential advantages over classical, but laborious, methods of fecal sterol balance and radioactive tracer analysis. Using freshly isolated peripheral blood HL and cultured IM-9 human lymphoid cells, we isolated microsomal R and studied its in vitro and in vivo regulation. HL RA and IM-9 RA averaged 12.0±0.63 (SE) and 131±13 pmol mevalonate formed/min/mg microsomal protein, respectively. Insulin (10^{-8}-10^{-10} M), which stimulates rat liver RA and CS, increased IM-9 RA 2-fold following a 90 min incubation at 37°C. Dichloroacetate (DCA), which inhibits rat liver RA and CS and lowers cholesterol levels in man, inhibited IM-9 RA in a dose-dependent manner and decreased HL RA 54% following oral administration (50 mg/kg) to a normal subject. Unlike rat liver, HL RA showed no diurnal variation. Like rat liver, however, HL RA decreased with fasting and cholesterol feeding. In a normal, fed, subject HL RA averaged 10.9±1.0 pmol/min/mg and fell progressively after fasting 12h (8.1±0.7), 24h (6.3±0.2) and 36h (4.7±0.2). HL RA also decreased 56% in 2 subjects after increasing dietary cholesterol from 150 mg to 1 g/d. Conclusions: 1) microsomal HL and IM-9 RA can be accurately measured in vivo and in vitro, 2) physiologic and pharmacologic regulation of R from human white cells is similar to that found in rat liver, 3) HL RA may prove useful as an index of changes in CS in man.

2367 ABNORMAL HDL- AND LDL LIPOPROTEIN LEVELS IN PRECLINICAL HYPOTHYROIDISM: A possible coronary risk factor?

J.J. Staub*, B. Althaus, A. Ryff, A. Oberhänsli, H.B. Stähelin. Div. of Endocrinology, Dept. of Medicine, Univ. of CH - 4031 Basle

Preclinical hypothyroidism (pc hypo) (increased TSH response to TRH and normal or elevated basal TSH in the presence of normal T4 and T3 serum levels) is presently considered a risk factor for coronary heart disease (CHD). The aim of our study was to analyse the lipid profiles in this syndrome as a possible pathogenetic factor for coronary atherosclerosis. 52 women with pc hypo, 18 women with overt hypothyroidism (ov hypo) and 28 age-matched euthyroid controls were investigated. Oral TRH-tests were performed and T4, free T4, FT4I, T3 and TSH were measured by RIA as previously described (JCEM 46:26,1978). Total cholesterol (TC) and triglycerides (TG) were determinded. LDL-cholesterol (LDL-C) and HDL-C were analysed enzymatically after ultracentrifugation with precipitation, the lipoprotein (Lp) pattern by electrophoresis on agarose and densitometric analysis.

Results: ($\bar{x} \pm$ SEM) * $p<0.05$ ** $p<0.01$ *** $p<0.001$

	pc hypo (N=52)	controls (N=28)	ov hypo (N=18)	controls (N=18)
LDL (%)	52.0 ±1.0**	47.3 ± 1.2	60.4 ±3.4**	49.6 ±1.6
LDL-C (mmol/l)	4.27±0.18	3.72± 0.25	6.14±0.4**	4.3 ±0.23
HDL (%)	34.7 ±1.0*	38.4 ± 1.45	26.9 ±2.5**	35.5 ±1.71
HDL-C (mmol/l)	1.58±0.05	1.53± 0.06	1.47±0.09	1.47±0.07

A significant elevation of the LDL-Lp and a decrease of the HDL-Lp could be observed in pc hypo, thus probably representing a pathogenetic cofactor in the development of CHD.

2368 RED CELL Na,K,ATPase ACTIVITY IN OBESITY AND HYPERTHYROIDISM.

K. Suzuki*[1], T. Kadowaki [1], and R. Fujino [2], Division of Endocrinology and Metabolism, The Institute for Adult Diseases, Asahi Life Foundation [1], and Kanaji Hospital [2], Tokyo, Japan.

Although obesity (ob) and hyperthyroidism (hy) are in quite distinct metabolic status from an aspect of energy expenditure, the activity of Na, K,ATPase, which is thought to be a major determinant of cellular energy consumption, is reported to be reduced in red cells from both ob and hy. To investigate the specificity of the reduction of this membrane-bound enzyme activity, we have assessed the cytochalasin B-sensitive 14C-galactose (gal) transport activity as well as ouabain-sensitive 86Rb transport as a direct measurement of Na,K,ATPase activity. The mean values of the Vmax and Km for Rb uptake in normals were 2.0± 0.12 nmol/10^9RBC/min (SEM, n=10) and 2.0 ± 0.2 mM, respectively. The Vmax was reduced by 20% in ob (n=10) and 23% in hy (n=14). The Vmax and Km for gal uptake in normals were 86.3 ± 5.6 nmol/10^9RBC/sec and 17.4 ± 0.8 mM, respectively. These values were increased by 49% and 30% respectively in hy, whereas no change was observed in ob. Furthermore, a significant correlation (r=0.877) was found between the Vmax for Rb and gal uptake in normals, but no correlation was observed in ob and hy. The Vmax for Rb, however, correlated inversely (r= -0.732) with BMI in ob and with serum T3 (r=-0.697) in hy. The Vmax for gal uptake correlated with serum T4 (r=0.661) in hy.

These results suggest that the reduction in red cell Na,K,ATPase activity in ob is likely to be more specific than in hy, and in the latter the reduction might be a reflection of some alteration of red cell membrane.

2369 MONOCLONAL ANTIBODIES TO TSH RECEPTOR:STIMULATING AND BLOCKING ANTIBODIES

T. Yoshida*, Y. Ichikawa, K. Arikawa, T. Shinozawa, S. Kawai, H. Oshima, H. Yamada, H. Tanaka, M. Homma and K. Itoh,
School of Medicine, Keio University and Itoh Hospital, Tokyo, Japan.

It has been almost established that anti-TSH receptor autoantibodies cause hyperthyroidism and a part of hypothyroidism. In order to delineate the heterogeneity of these antibodies and their pathophysiological significance, we produced monoclonal antibodies to TSH receptor and studied their characteristics.

Four-week-old Balb/c mice were immunized with human thyroid membrane preparation, which was solubilized in Triton X-100 and purified with TSH-coupled affinity chromatography. Ten days after 4th immunization, spleens were removed and hybridoma cells were obtained by fusing spleen cells ($1x10^7$) and P3-U1 mouse myeloma cells ($1x10^6$) in the presence of polyethylene glycol according to Kohler and Milstein. Of 5400 wells seeded from 6 separate fusions, 18 antibody-producing hybridoma colonies were noted. By cloning with limiting dilution method, we constructed 5 different cell lines according to their anti-TSH receptor antibody activities. Of 4 antibodies which inhibited TSH binding to human thyroid membrane, 2 inhibited TSH (10mU/ml) stimulating thyroid adenylate cyclase (AC) and 1 stimulated AC but 1 showed no bioactivity. Another one, which did not inhibit TSH binding, stimulated AC. All of these antibodies were dependent on IgG concentration and diminished by anti-IgG antibody.

These data indicate that anti-TSH receptor antibodies are heterogeneous and may be involved in the pathogenesis of different kinds of autoimmune thyroid diseases.

2370 DOPAMINE (DA) STIMULATES RELEASE OF β- ENDORPHIN IMMUNOREACTIVITY (β-EP) FROM THE HUMAN MEDIOBASAL HYPOTHALAMUS (MBH) IN VITRO.

D.D. Rasmussen*, J.H. Liu, P.L. Wolf, and S.S.C. Yen, Depts. Reproductive Medicine and Pathology, UCSD, La Jolla, CA. 92093, USA.

Hypothalamic β-EP containing neurons have been suggested to play a role in the regulation of several hypothalamic functions, such as the release of GnRH. However, the regulatory factors which modulate hypothalamic neurosecretion of β-EP are unknown. Accordingly, a previously characterized *in vitro* perifusion system was used to investigate β-EP release from adult human hypothalami (obtained at autopsy within 12h of death) in response to DA and the DA antagonist haloperidol (HAL). β-EP concentrations (RIA) in the MBH perifusate declined during the first 2h and then stablized to a mean (± SE) basal level of 24 ± 4 pg/15 min for each 1/2 MBH (n=10). During each perifusion β-EP release increased 193 ± 94% in response to a bolus of 60 mM KCl (but not 60 mM NaCl or medium), indicating viability of the tissue. When the MBH was perifused with calcium-free medium the basal release of β-EP was suppressed and the response to 60 mM KCl was inconsistent and attenuated. Tissue viability was further confirmed by an acute increase in β-EP release (139 ± 31%, n=6) in response to a 50 mM pulse of the membrane sodium channel activator veratradine. Administration of a 10 μM pulse (15 min.) of DA consistently elicited an increase in β-EP release (85 ±5%, n=3), whereas 10 μM HAL had no effect. These studies demonstrate that DA stimulates β-EP release from the adult human hypothalamus *in vitro*.

2371 THE ATTAINMENT OF ADEQUATE DOPAMINERGIC BLOCKADE IN THYROTOXICOSIS.

F D Rosenthal*, J Vora and B P O'Malley. The Leicester Royal Infirmary, UK

The long acting dopamine antagonist metoclopramide has become well established as a pharmacological tool for investigating tuberoinfundibular dopaminergic tone in vivo and it has been generally assumed that, as a 10mgs intravenous or oral challenge, it affords complete dopamine receptor blockade, even in the hypermetabolic state of thyrotoxicosis (Sawers et al, 1982, J Clin End and Metab, 55, 175). We have considered that protracted oral loading with metoclopramide may produce more adequate dopaminergic blockade than a single oral dose in thyrotoxicosis. Seven untreated thyrotoxic patients were studied. A 13 hour serum prolactin profile was determined on a control day (day 1), after 10mgs metoclopramide orally (day 2) and after 10mgs metoclopramide orally, immediately subsequent to a 7 day regime of metoclopramide 10mgs orally 8 hourly (day 10). The mean prolactin levels of the subjects on day 2 and 10 respectively were significantly elevated as compared with mean day 1 values ($P < 0.05$; $P < 0.001$). More importantly, however, the mean prolactin levels on day 10 were significantly elevated as compared with the day 2 profiles ($P < 0.005$). In addition, the 'plateau' of peak prolactin levels over a 2 hour period, within an hour of the last dose of metoclopramide on day 10, contrasted with the shortlived rise on day 2. Thus in thyrotoxicosis a 7 day regime of metoclopramide 10mgs orally 8 hourly effects more adequate dopaminergic blockade, as assessed by serum prolactin elevations, than a single oral 10mgs dose. Our observations point to the inadvisability of assuming that a fixed dose of metoclopramide produces complete dopaminergic blockade in any metabolic context.

2372 METABOLISM OF SOMATOSTATIN-14 (S-14) BY ISOLATED PERFUSED RAT LUNGS.

Mary Doris Ruggere* and Yogesh C. Patel, McGill University, Montreal, Quebec H3A 1A1, Canada.

We have previously reported rapid *in vivo* disappearance of S-14 in rat plasma, and have shown that tissue degradation is principally responsible for this phenomenon. We have also demonstrated that S-14 is rapidly degraded in the liver by surface peptidases. Since the lung is also rich in surface-bound peptidases important in the degradation of other peptide hormones, we have investigated here S-14 degradation by the lung. Isolated lungs of 5 fed male Sprague-Dawley rats were perfused *in situ* via the right ventricle at 37 C in a recirculating circuit with oxygenated Krebs Hensleit buffer (pH 7.4) containing 5.5 mM glucose, 4% BSA and 2.8 ng/ml synthetic S-14, at a rate of 30 ml/min for 12 min. S-14-like immunoreactivity (S-14-LI) disappeared in a semi-logarithmic fashion with a $t_{1/2}$ of 23.8 ± 2.1 min. S-14 was also degraded, but to a lesser extent ($P < 0.01$), in perfusate which had previously recirculated through the lung for 15 min prior to the introduction of the peptide into the lung-free recirculating circuit (81 ± 6% of S-14 remained after 20 min of perfusion). By contrast, virtually 100% of S-14 was recovered after 20 min of lung-free perfusion with perfusate not previously passed through lungs. Non-recirculating perfusions (N=3) confirmed that arterio-venous ratios of S-14-LI remained constant over 12 min of the perfusion preparation. We conclude that S-14 is rapidly degraded in the lung and that the lung is capable of releasing into the circulation enzymes which may degrade S-14.

2373 LUTEINIZING-HORMONE (LH) RESPONSE TO PROSTAGLANDIN E2 (PGE2) AND NALOXONE (N) IS MODULATED BY TESTOSTERONE (T) FEEDBACK. U. Schweiger and K.M. Pirke* Max-Planck-Institut für Psychiatrie, Kraepelinstr. 10, D-800 München 40

Since LH response to PGE2 and N changes in situations that also show altered steroid feedback sensitivity (e.g. starvation), we studied the influence of different levels of T substitution on the PGE2 and N effect on LH secretion. Male Wistar rats (220g) were castrated, implanted with silastic tubes (0-2,6 cm) containing T and fitted with an indwelling jugular cannula. On day 4,6,8 post castration LHRH (25-400 ng/kg BW), PGE2 (0,05-1 mg/kg BW) and N (0,5-50 mg/kg BW) were injected i.v.. Blood samples (0,45ml) were drawn before and 10,20 and 30 minutes post injection. Stimulation by PGE2 and LHRH leads to comparable LH peak levels in non-substituted rats. In substituted rats peak levels attainable by PGE2 reach only a percentage of the values attainable by LHRH decreasing with the level of substitution. Ascending doses of N change the time structure of the LH response. Peak responses stay below the responses elicited by LHRH and PGE2. High levels of T substitution lead to a complete abolition of LH response even to very high doses of N. Our data show feedback inhibition of both the N effect and the PGE2 effect at the hypothalamic level, the N effect beeing more sensitive to inhibition. This fits well with the hypothesis that endorphinergic influences are situated at a higher leven than prostaglandin mediated processes in the cascade of regulation of LH secretion.

2374 ARCUATE NEURONS IN VITRO RESPOND TO MORE THAN ONE HYPOTHALAMIC HORMONE: AN ELECTROPHYSIOLOGICAL STUDY. Nancy E. Sirett*, A.E. Herbison and J.I. Hubbard, Department of Physiology, University of Otago School of Medicine, P.O. Box 913, Dunedin, New Zealand.

Extracellular recordings were made in vitro from spontaneously firing neurons (units) in the rat arcuate nucleus (ARC) and the effect of LHRH, TSH and somatostatin on frequency studied. Parasagittal slices (300 µm thick) containing the ARC were cut from the medial hypothalamus of rat brains using a Vibroslice. Neuronal activity was recorded for up to 12 hours from the slice which was held in an organ bath containing artificial CSF (37°C, flow rate 2 ml/min, 1/2 turnover time 3 min). Activity was located predominantly in the rostral arcuate, medial to the ventricular surface (mean frequency 2.5 s^{-1}; range 0.1-11.7 s^{-1}). When hypothalamic hormones were added to the perifusing solution over 50% of the units tested responded to one or the other and some units to all three hormones. At concentrations close to that in portal blood, LHRH was generally excitatory and somatostatin inhibitory. With LHRH at 10 pM to 100 nM (29 units), 15 were excited and 5 inhibited; with somatostatin at 1 nM to 100 nM (25 units), 2 were excited and 12 inhibited; with TRH at 100 pM to 100 nM (25 units), 6 were excited and 5 inhibited. Thirteen units were tested with 2 hormones, 6 responded to 2, 6 to one and one unit was unresponsive. This data provides further support for a neurotransmitter role for these hypothalamic hormones. This study was supported by the Medical Research Council of New Zealand.

2375 The Natriuretic Response To Acute Volume Expansion Is Mediated, In Part, By Renal Production of Dopamine From Its Precursor, Dopa. J.R. Sowers,* P.D. Crane, F.W.J. Beck, M. McClanahan, M.E. King, and P.K. Mohanty
V.A. Medical Center and Medical College of Virginia, Richmond, VA 23249

High concentrations of the enzyme dopa decarboxylase, which converts dopa to dopamine, are found in close proximitity to renal tubules. As dopamine is a putative intra-renal natriuretic factor, we have studied the effect of carbidopa (CD), a dopa decarboxylase inhibitor, on the renal excretion of sodium and catecholamines in 7 dogs which were infused iv with 0.9% saline (30cc/kg/hr over 2 hrs). Saline infusions were performed in the presence and absence of CD given by nasogastric tube (1mg/kg every 8 hrs beginning 24 hours prior to saline infusion). CD treatment did not alter the arterial blood pressure, left ventricular filling pressure, GFR or renal blood flow. Total sodium excretion (40 ± 8 mEq vs 72 ± 11 mEq), and the percent of the administered load excreted (26 ± 4% vs 47 ± 5%) were less ($P<0.01$) following carbidopa treatment than during the control period. Saline infusion was associated with a rise ($P<0.01$) in urinary excretion of dopamine, a decline ($P<0.001$) urinary excretion of norepinephrine and no effect on renal excretion of epinephrine. Carbidopa treatment abolished the increase in renal production of dopamine following saline infusion but had no effect on renal production of norepinephrine and epinephrine. Decreases in renal sympathetic nerve activity, as reflected by decreases in renal excretion of norepinephrine, probably account, in part, for the natriuresis associated with acute volume expansion. Since carbidopa blocks tissue conversion of dopa to dopamine, renal production of dopamine is probably an important mechanism mediating the natriuretic response to acute vascular volume expansion.

2376 DIFFERENCE IN MAGNITUDE OF THE STIMULATORY EFFECT OF ADRENALIN AND LH ON RAT LUTEAL PROGESTERONE PRODUCTION. G.Selstam*, E. Norjavaara and K. Ahrén, Depts of Physiology, Univ of Umeå and Univ of Göteborg, Sweden.

Both adrenalin and LH increase cAMP levels in 2 day old corpora lutea (CL) obtained from PMSG treated immature rats. In 8 day old CL adrenalin in contrast to LH only had a minimal effect(Acta endocr 1982,100:613). Also, 8 day old CL have fewer β-adrenergic receptors(Endocrinology 1984, in press). To test whether a difference in steroidogenesis also exists, isolated CL were incubated for 2 h in Krebs buffer with glucose and albumin. Progesterone (P_4) and 20αOH-P_4 were meassured with RIA in tissue and medium at end of incubation. Adrenalin (5μg/ml) and LH-B9 (5μg/ml) increased both tissue and medium content of P_4 in 2 and 8day old CL and 20αOH-P_4 in 2, but not in 8 day old CL. The increments, i.e. total content in tissue and medium in presence of adrenalin or LH minus control levels are shown in table (N=5-6):

	Progesterone			20αOH-prog.		(μg/mg protein)
	2	8		2	8	(days of CL age)
Adrenalin	1.2±0.3	2.2±0.3	$p<0.01$	1.2±0.2	-0.1±0.1	
LH	1.1±0.2	5.0±0.5		1.1±0.2	0.1±0.1	

The results show that the effects on P_4 production and conversion to 20αOH-P_4 is increased to the same degree by adrenalin and LH in 2 day old CL. In 8 day old CL a significant (paired t-test) lower production of P_4 was registered for adrenalin in comparison to LH. No increments on 20αOH-P_4 production was seen in 8 day old CL. The smaller effect of adrenalin on 8 day old CL is consonant with our findings on the cAMP system.

2377 CONTROL OF THE INITIATION OF FOLLICULAR AROMATASE ACTIVITY IN LACTATING SOWS. H.J. Shaw*, M.G. Hunter, C.A. Price and G.R. Foxcroft, ARC Research Group on Hormones and Farm Animal Reproduction, University of Nottingham Faculty of Agricultural Science, Sutton Bonington, Loughborough, Leics, LE12 5RD, UK.

Control of the initiation of follicular development was investigated in studies involving the manipulation of litter size during lactation in primiparous sows. Six control sows suckled entire litters until weaning/ slaughter at 4 weeks post-partum whilst litter size (LS) (8 to 12 piglets/ sow) were reduced to 5 piglets, 5 days prior to weaning in seven females. Ovaries were recovered at slaughter and the 10 largest follicles used to assess follicular fluid (FF) testosterone (T) and oestradiol (E_2) concentrations, granulosa cell aromatase activity (Ar.A) and the capacity of granulosa cells and thecal homogenates to bind hCG. FF concentrations of T exceeded those of E_2 in 67% of follicles studied but in all cases FF steroid levels were low, indicative of immaturity and a lack of endogenous steroidogenesis. Ar.A *in vitro* was however, significantly enhanced ($P<0.05$) in non-atretic follicles from reduced LS sows. The capacity of thecal homogenates to bind hCG was not affected by treatment. These data suggest that E_2 synthesis *in vivo* is not prevented by an inactive Ar. enzyme system but by a lack of available androgen precursor and that Ar.A may represent the first stage in the activation of follicular development. A significant correlation ($r = 0.794$; $P<0.05$) existed between Ar.A and the mean plasma FSH levels after LS reduction and implies that induction of Ar.A may be FSH dependent.

2378 PHORBOL ESTER INHIBITS GRANULOSA CELL DIFFERENTIATION IN VITRO. O. Shinohara*, M. Knecht, S. Hoffmann, and K.J. Catt, NICHD, NIH, Bethesda, MD, USA

FSH-induced differentiation of cultured granulosa cells is inhibited by GnRH and its agonist analogs. To investigate the role of protein kinase C as a mediator of GnRH action in the ovary, the effects of 12-0-tetradecanoylphorbol-13-acetate (TPA) were studied in granulosa cells obtained from immature, DES-primed rats. Added alone, TPA had no effect on LH receptor formation at concentrations up to 10 ng/ml during the 48 h culture period. However, FSH-induced LH receptor expression and progesterone production were inhibited by TPA with an ED_{50} of 0.05 ng/ml, and were suppressed to the control levels with 1 ng/ml TPA. Production of cAMP was markedly suppressed by TPA after 24 h of culture, consistent with the central role of cAMP in cellular differentiation. Addition of TPA (1 ng/ml) at times up to 30 h after initiation of culture completely suppressed LH receptor expression, while cAMP formation was reduced to 50% of the FSH-induced levels. Both [D-Ala^6]des-Gly^{10}-GnRH-ethylamide (GnRHa, 10^{-8}M) and TPA (1 ng/ml) suppressed formation of LH receptors induced by 8-bromo-cAMP (5 mM), cholera toxin (CT, 100 ng/ml) or forskolin (25 μg/ml) to the control levels. In contrast, cAMP levels induced by CT or forskolin were not altered by GnRHa or TPA. Also, addition of 8-bromo-cAMP, CT, or forskolin did not reverse the inhibitory effect of TPA when added 36 h after initiation of culture. An inactive phorbol derivative (4-α-phorbol) did not affect FSH-induced cell differentiation. These results indicate that both cAMP formation and post-cAMP action are sites of the inhibitory effects of GnRHa and TPA, and that protein kinase C is probably involved in the suppression of granulosa cell maturation by GnRH agonists.

2379 PREPARATION AND CHARACTERIZATION OF POLYCLONAL ANTIBODIES AGAINST AROMATASE CYTOCHROME P-450. Evan R. Simpson* and Carole R. Mendelson. Cecil H. and Ida Green Ctr. for Reprod. Biol. Sci., Univ. of Texas Health Science Center, Dallas, TX 75235, U.S.A.

The conversion of androgens to estrogens (aromatization) is catalyzed by an enzyme complex that is comprised of a flavoprotein, NADPH-cytochrome P-450 reductase, and a form of cytochrome P-450 known as aromatase cytochrome P-450. Aromatase cytochrome P-450 was partially purified from human placental microsomes by phenyl-Sepharose chromatography and DEAE-cellulose chromatography. The resulting preparation had a specific activity of 1-2 nmol x mg^{-1} protein with respect to cytochrome P-450 content and displayed a type I difference spectrum upon addition of the aromatase substrate, androstenedione, indicative that the P-450 was specific for aromatase. When the cytochrome P-450-enriched fractions were subjected to SDS-polyacrylamide gel electrophoresis and stained with Coomassie blue, two major bands, of 51 and 55 kDa, were observed. These bands were removed from unstained gels, suspended in Freund's adjuvant, and injected subcutaneously into rabbits. An IgG fraction from serum of the rabbit injected with the 55 kDa band, but not the 51 kDa band, inhibited aromatase activity of human placental microsomes by 80%. On the other hand, 17α-hydroxylase and 21-hydroxylase activities of human fetal adrenal microsomes were not inhibited by the IgG fraction. By immunoblot analysis, we found that this IgG fraction bound to the purified 55 kDa protein, as well as to a single protein of 55 kDa in human placental microsomes. This antibody appears to be a suitable tool to study the synthesis of aromatase cytochrome P-450 and its regulation by hormones in steroidogenic cells.

2380 ESSENTIAL ROLE OF LIPOPROTEIN IN HCG-INDUCED DECREASE OF CYTOCHROME P-450 IN PREOVULATORY RAT OVARIAN MICROSOMES. K. Suzuki* and B. Tamaoki, National Institute of Radiological Sciences, 9-1, Anagawa-4-chome, Chiba-shi 260, Japan.

Acute decrease in ovarian estradiol-17β secretion after ovulation was found due to drastic decrease in ovarian 17α-hydroxylase and C-17-C-20 lyase, but not in aromatase, as evidenced by our results of hCG effect upon PMSG-treated immature rats (Suzuki and Tamaoki, Endocrinology 104, 1317, 1979). Since the decrease in the two enzyme activities was proportional to the content of cytochrome P-450 in ovarian microsomes, the decrease in the activities was caused by decrease in enzymes themselves, but not by changes in activator or inhibitor. These decrease due to hCG (LH) could be partially prevented by administration of inhibitors to RNA and protein synthesis (*ibid.* 113, 1985, 1983). Recently we established a primary culture system of ovarian cells of the PMSG-treated rats, in which a small decrease in the lyase activity was demonstrated by addition of hCG into the medium. The lyase activity was measured with cell-free system using ^{14}C-17α-hydroxyprogesterone in the presence of NADPH. When a lipoprotein fraction obtained from rat sera was added together with hCG, the enzyme activity was decreased furthermore, even though the lipoprotein itself had no significant influence upon the enzyme. In this system, dibutyryl c-AMP also could decrease the lyase activity in the same manner as hCG. Finally, preovulatory LH surge or administration of hCG could be summarized to cause a drastic decrease in ovarian production of aromatizable androgens *via* synthesis of cAMP, new RNA and protein in the presence of lipoprotein.

2381 Evidence for prostaglandin F-2α stimulation of ovarian follicular growth & oestrogen synthesis in guinea-pigs. W.H. Tam* & Ellen L.P. Chan, Dept. of Zoology, University of Western Ontario, London, Ontario N6A 5B7, Canada.

The aim of this study is to demonstrate that a direct relationship exists between PGF-2α & follicular development. In Expt. 1, guinea-pigs were hysterectomized, allowed to recover & then the oestrous cycle was maintained by injection i.p. with PGF-2α (0.25 mg/day). When PGF-2α was administered on or before Day 11 of the cycle, the induced cycle length was normal (16.3±0.4 days), & the shortest duration of PGF-2α treatment for ovulation to occur was 6.2±0.4 days. In Expt. 2, not only did we confirm our previous finding that elimination of uterine PGF-2α synthesis by hysterectomy of indomethacin injection abolished the final growth phase of Graafian follicles but we also found that, if PGF-2α was injected simultaneously, the final growth phase resumed. In Expt. 3, granulosa cells were harvested from Day 15 guinea-pigs, previously injected from Days 9-14 with either sesame oil (carrier) or indomethacin to inhibit PGF-2α synthesis. The granulosa cells were cultured for 3 days in Medium 199 in the presence of exogenous testosterone. The amount of oestrogen synthesized by the indomethacin treated guinea-pigs was always lower than that of the carrier injected animals (1.74±0.2 vs 2.77±0.33 ng/10^6 cells, $p<0.0005$). Neither the addition of LH, FSH or PGF-2α in the cultures could reverse the situation. Evidence from these experiments suggested that for ovulation to occur PGF-2α was required during final follicular growth and that only in the presence of PGF-2α did granulosa cells achieve their full oestrogenic synthetic capacity.

2382 INHIBIN AND STEROID LEVELS IN PERIPHERAL AND OVARIAN VEIN BLOOD THROUGHOUT HUMAN MENSTRUAL CYCLE. K.Tanabe*, S.Shiraishi, K.Sugimura, Y.Kasuga, Y.Nakamura and R. Iizuka, Dept. of OB/GYN, School of Med. Keio University, 35 Shinanomachi, Shinjuku-ku, Tokyo, 160 Japan.

In order to determine the change of plasma inhibin levels throughout human menstrual cycle, peripheral and bilateral ovarian vein blood were sampled from 19 normal women at various stages of the menstrual cycle. Inhibin levels in vein blood were measured in rat anterior pituitary cell cultures after stripping of steroids with dextran-coated charcoal as reported previously (JCEM 57:24, 1983). Inhibin was expressed in terms of nanoliters of standard porcine follicular fluid. Steroids were determined by specific RIAs. Both follicular and luteal phases were divided into three stages (early, mid and late), respectively. Inhibin levels in ovarian vein blood increased from early follicular phase (24±5 units/100 µl, Mean±SE, n=4) toward late follicular phase (41±9, n=6). Inhibin level at early luteal phase (22±4, n=10) was significantly lower than that of late follicular phase and was lowest at mid luteal phase (4±2, n=6). Inhibin level at late luteal phase was again high (39±6, n=6). Inhibin levels were significantly different between in right and left ovarian vein blood at late follicular and late luteal phases. Inhibin levels in peripheral vein blood were essentially less than detectable levels. Estradiol and progesterone levels in both peripheral and ovarian vein blood showed typical pattern as reported previously. These data demostrate the first observation of inhibin in human vein blood throughout the menstrual cycle and suggest that inhibin might play an important role in human female reproduction. This study was supported by a Rockefeller Foundation grant RF 83002.

2383 INSULIN RECEPTORS AND STEROIDOGENIC RESPONSE IN RAT LUTEAL CELLS
M.Tesone*,R.G.Ladenheim,V.A.Chiauzzi and E.H.Charreau.Instituto de Biología y Medicina Experimental Obligado 2490,1428,Buenos Aires Argentina and School of Sciences,University of Buenos Aires

The binding and *in vitro* effect of insulin (Ins) on the steroidogenesis response were studied in collagenase dispersed luteal cell prepared from ovaries of PMSG/hCG-primed rats.Incubation with Ins during 4 hours at 34°C showed a dose dependent increase in progesterone production with a maximal stimulation at 10^{-8} M concentration.In comparison hCG produced the same effect at 10^{-11} M.An additive effect on progesterone synthesis was observed when both hormones were present in the incubation medium.However,Ins neither stimulated cAMP production nor enhanced the cAMP-hCG luteal response.Ins binding to luteal cells attained highest values after 30 min incubation at 20°C.A curvilinear Scatchard plot was obtained and it was analyzed using a two binding sites model.The affinity constant values were $2.1x10^{8}$ M^{-1} and $5.2x10^{6}$ M^{-1} and the number of binding sites 35,000 and 900,000/cell respectively.Bound Ins was not displaceable by hCG,hGH,hLH,EGF or oPrl and after trypsin digestion a marked loss of binding activity was observed.Subcellular fractionation was performed and the highest binding was obtained in the 105,000 xg pellet fraction.This study demonstrated that Ins binds specifically to rat luteal cells and stimulates steroidogenesis,adding support for the hypothesis that Ins acts directly upon the ovary.(Supported by CONICET and Roemmers Foundation)

2384 RECEPTORS FOR VASOPRESSIN ON THE RAT MESENTERIC ARTERY OF NORMAL AND SODIUM DEPLETED RATS. Jean St-Louis* and Ernesto L. Schiffrin, Clinical Research Institute of Montreal, Montreal, Quebec, H2W 1R7, Canada.

High affinity binding sites for ^{3}H-Arg-vasopressin (^{3}H-AVP) have been demonstrated on membrane preparations of rat mesenteric arteries. We have measured the biological activity of this peptide (AVP) and of analogues on the perfused rat mesenteric artery. There was a close relationship between the pD_2 of agonists or the pA_2 of agonists on the perfused tissue and the relative potency (EC_{50}) of analogues for displacing ^{3}H-AVP from the membrane preparation. The pD_2 were 7.69 ± 0.16 for AVP, 7.56 ± 0.06 for Lys-vasopressin and 5.68 ± 0.10 for oxytocin. Oxytocin produced 75% of the maximal response of AVP. In sodium depleted rats, we found an increase (27%) of the maximal response to AVP with no significant change in ED_{50} (from 2.8 ± 1.0 x 10^{-8} M to 1.3 ± 0.2 x 10^{-8} M). On the membrane preparation, the number of binding sites for ^{3}H-AVP was increased from 71 ± 17 fmole/mg protein (Kd 3.5 ± 0.5 nM) to 115 ± 10 fmole/mg protein (Kd 4.8 ± 0.3 nM) in sodium depleted rats in comparison to control animals. These results suggest that AVP and its analogues interact in a similar manner in the two preparations used in this study and that receptors for AVP and the biological response to this peptide are increased in this vascular bed by sodium depletion.

Supported by Quebec Heart Foundation and M.R.C. (Canada).

2385 EFFECTS OF WATER DEPRIVATION AND DESAMINO-D-ARGININE[8]-VASOPRESSIN ON [^{14}C] 2-DEOXYGLUCOSE UPTAKE BY THE HYPOTHALAMO-NEUROHYPOPHYSIAL SYSTEM IN MICE WITH HEREDITARY NEPHROGENIC DIABETES INSIPIDUS. R.C. Sutherland*, G. Fink and J.F. Morris†, MRC Brain Metabolism Unit, Edinburgh EH8 9JZ; †Department of Human Anatomy, Oxford OX1 3QX, U.K.

Quantitative autoradiography using [^{14}C] 2-deoxyglucose (2DG) showed that the relative metabolic activity (rma) of the pars nervosa (PN) was significantly greater in Brattleboro compared with normal Wistar rats (1). Injection of desamino-D-arginine[8] vasopressin (dDAVP) significantly reduced the rma of the PN in Brattleboro rats, and the aim of the present study was to determine whether this effect of dDAVP was due solely to its action on plasma osmolality or an action as well directly on the hypothalamo-neurohypophysial neurones. Water deprivation (4-5h) significantly increased the rma of the paraventricular nuclei (PVN) and PN in Di +/+ Severe diabetic mice (as was also the case in Brattleboro and Wistar rats, ref. 1) compared with either Di +/+ Non-severe or normal mice that had been similarly deprived of water. The increased rma of the PVN and PN produced by water deprivation in the Severe mice was not significantly reduced by administration of dDAVP. None of the treatments affected the rma of either the supraoptic nuclei (SON) or the other 19 areas of the brain examined. These data show (a) that the above changes in the rma of the PVN and PN are due mainly to changes in plasma osmolality, and (b) that, together with data from suckling and mammary nerve stimulation (2) and investigations with high resolution (^{3}H-2DG) autoradiography, the differences between the rma of the PVN and SON are likely to reflect differences in the activity of their afferent imputs.
(1) Brain Res. 271, 101, 1983. (2) Brain Res. 273, 291, 1983.

2386 OXYTOCIN IN PLASMA AND CEREBROSPINAL FLUID OF HUMAN. S. Takeda*, Y. Kuwabara, M. Mizuno and S. Sakamoto, Dept. of Ob-Gyn, Faculty of Medicine, Univ. of Tokyo, 7-3-1 Hongo, Bunkyo-ku, Tokyo, Japan

It is noticed that oxytocic neurosecretory fibers are located extensively in extrahypothalamic brains and some of these neurons terminate in close to the cerebral ventricle. In order to investigate the central action of oxytocin, oxytocin concentrations in cerebrospinal fluid (CSF) and plasma were determined. Plasma and CSF were taken simultaneously at spinal puncture for anesthesia of minor surgeries from 42 patients without endocrine and brain disease. Specific RIA of oxytocin was carried, following extraction procedure with Florisil. The sensitivity of method was 0.5μU/ml and the recovery of added hormone into plasma and CSF ranged from 75-85%. In 4 male patients mean plasma values($\pm$SE) were 3.8$\pm$1.1(μU/ml) and CSF values were 7.8$\pm$0.5. In 15 nonpregnant patients mean plasma and CSF values were 4.8$\pm$0.5 and 10.1$\pm$1.2, respectively. CSF levels were significantly higher than plasma levels in males and nonpregnants. In 11 pregnant patients without labor mean plasma and CSF values were 16.1$\pm$2.9 and 9.7$\pm$1.5, respectively. In 12 pregnant patients with labor mean plasma and CSF values were 19.7$\pm$3.3 and 18.6$\pm$2.3, respectively. CSF levels in pregnants with labor were significantly higher than in those without labor. No significant correlations were found between plasma and CSF levels. It is assumed that secretion mechanisms of oxytocin in CSF is defferent from those in peripheral circulation.

2387 PLASTICITY IN THE HYPOTHALAMIC SUPRAOPTIC NUCLEUS IN RESPONSE TO ENDOCRINE STIMULI. D.T. Theodosis*, D.A. Poulain, C. Montagnese, and J.D. Vincent. INSERM, U.176, Rue Camille St Saëns, 33077 BORDEAUX-Cedex, France.

Magnocellular neurons in the supraoptic nucleus (SON) are usually separated by glial fibers. Quantitative ultrastructural analyses indicate, however, that in lactating rats, close to 40% of all neurosecretory somata and dendrites are in direct apposition, without glial interposition. There is also a higher incidence of presynaptic terminals contacting two such cells simultaneously ("double" synapses). Immunocytochemistry shows that cells in apposition contain oxytocin. The SON appears unmodified during gestation but at parturition, the incidence of neuronal appositions is equivalent to that recorded at lactation. The anatomical modifications are reversible since 2 months after weaning, as in virgin rats, there are again few neuronal appositions. On the other hand, similar changes occur in the SON of virgin and primiparous rats induced to lactate without prior parturition, by continuous exposure to newborn litters ; in this case, an increase in neuronal appositions and "double" synapses is seen only with the onset of the milk ejection reflex. Our observations demonstrate a surprising plasticity in this neuronal center, that affects both neuron-glial and synaptic configurations. The anatomical rearrangement could facilitate the synchronisation of firing displayed by oxytocin neurons at milk ejection. Although its causes remain unknown, it does appear to be closely related to the endocrine events taking place at parturition and lactation.

2388 EXTRAHYPOTHALAMIC VASOPRESSIN IMMUNOREACTIVITY IN THE RAT CENTRAL NERVOUS SYSTEM. G.Valiquette*, G.Nilaver, G.M.Abrams, J.Haldar and E.A.Zimmerman. College of Physicians and Surgeons, Columbia University, New York, N.Y.

The neurohypophysial peptides, vasopressin (VP) and oxytocin (OT), are known to be present outside the hypothalamus and we as well as other laboratories have reported their presence in spinal cord as well as in a number of brain areas. By immunohistochemistry (IHC), the VP-associated neurophysin is present in spinal cord, although in lesser amounts than the OT-associated neurophysin. However, VP itself cannot be visualized in the cord, while OT is readily seen, mostly in periaqueductal grey and in intermediolateral grey. We therefore decided to look for VP in rat CNS by radioimmunoassay. Adult male rats were sacrificed by decapitation and the CNS, including spinal cord, dissected into various areas. Tissue from 5 animals were pooled and homogenized in 10 volumes of 2M acetic acid. The homogenates were clarified by centrifugation and the supernatants lyophilized and radioimmunoassayed with a sensitive and specific antiserum. Vasopressin levels are reported in the table below (ng/g wet weight):

Area:	Amygdala	L-S Cord	Medulla	Thor Cord	Cerv Cord	Mid-brain	Pons
Mean	25.45	5.244	4.785	2.350	1.760	1.198	0.8076
SEM	6.029	0.6077	2.288	0.4293	0.2725	0.2764	0.1737

Hippocampus, frontal cortex and cerebellum all contained less than 0.5 ng/g of VP. These results suggest that most antibodies used for VP IHC cannot recognize VP in cord, possible because of fixation artifacts due to formalin. They also confirm and extend previous reports by showing a non-homogeneous distribution in rat cord, as observed in the human cord.
Supported by NIH grant HL 13147

2389 ONTOGENY AND REGULATION OF THE RAT PINEAL α_1-ADRENOCEPTOR. D. Sugden* and D. C. Klein. Section on Neuroendocrinology, Laboratory of Developmental Neurobiology, NICHD, National Institutes of Health, Bethesda, MD 20205

The development of the rat pineal α_1-adrenoceptor and its regulation in the adult by the sympathetic nerves innervating the gland has been studied using ^{125}iodo-2-[β-(4-hydroxyphenyl)-ethylaminomethyl]tetralone (^{125}I-HEAT), a specific, high affinity α_1-adrenoceptor ligand. Binding studies were done in Tris HCl buffer (50 mM, pH 7.4) containing Mg^{2+} (10 mM) at 30 °C for 15 min, using HEAT (1 μM) to define non-specific binding. Rats housed in a diurnal lighting schedule (14:10 L:D) showed no statistically significant change in α_1-adrenoceptor density at any time of day although a large nocturnal elevation in pineal melatonin content was apparent. Computer analysis of saturation experiments on glands obtained at 1200 or 2400 h showed similar K_d values (30.9 vs. 32.6 pM) and no significant difference in B_{max}. Superior cervical ganglionectomy or exposure to constant light for 20 days gradually increased the number of α_1-adrenoceptors (LD, 331 ± 32; SCGX, 516 ± 29; LL, 686 ± 82 fmol/mg protein). Acute (4 h, i.p.) or chronic (9 day s.c. infusion) administration of α_1-agonists did not alter α_1-adrenoceptor density. Together these results indicate that the pineal α_1-adrenoceptor, like the pineal β_1-adrenoceptor, is under neural control. Pineal α_1-adrenoceptors are present 3 days before birth (100 fmol/mg protein), increase rapidly up to 10 days of age (336 fmol/mg protein), and then decrease with age. This pattern of development and the decline in density with age are strikingly similar to that seen previously for pineal β_1-adrenoceptors.

2390 RADIOIMMUNOASSAY OF MELATONIN AND IT'S APPLICATIONS. T.Taguchi*[1],H.Shimada[1] and W.Mori[2],1)Department of pathology,Tokyo Metropolitan Geriatric Hospital,Sakaecho,Tokyo 173,Japan. 2)Depaartment of pathology,Faculity of Medicine,University of Tokyo,Hongo,Tokyo 113,Japan.

Hormone assay is currently a rapidly expanding application of the radioimmunoassay(RIA). Recently,several practical RIA procedures for melatonin in serum or tissue have been reported and studied on melatonin content during various environmental and endocrinological studies initiated. We have developed a RIA suitable for melatonin in routine clinical practice. Rabbits immuninized with bovine serum albumin(BSA)conjugates of N-acetylserotonin(Grota et al),melatonin(Lemaitre & Hartmann) and 5-methoxytryptamine(Rollag & Niswender). Obtained antisera were examined binding of [H^3]melatonin. They were bound anti melatonin-BSA with approximately the same affinity as anti N-acetylserotonin-BSA. Good specificity was obtained by anti melatonin-BSA. Very low crossreactivities with N-acetylserotonin and 6-hydroxymelatonin were shown. Specimens intended for melatonin assay and melatonin standards were extracted by constant amount of chloroform. Separation of B and F was done using saturated ammonium sulfate after incubation for 48 hrs. at 4°C. Counting was done using liquid scintillation spectrometry with Bray's solution. Rat pineal melatonin was increased to large extent in dark environment. In the light environment was given no indication of an increase rate of melatonin. Melatonin content in various human organs obtained from autopsy were given only 100 pg/100 mg wet wt.,at most 300 pg/100 mg,except the pineal glands(2-10 ng/100 mg). Melatonin content in patient sera with various disease which obtained at the constant daytime for routine examination were shown various value(15-174 pg/ml).

2391 DIFFERENTIAL STEROID MODULATION OF PITUITARY GONADOTROPIN SECRETION.
M. Rush*, H. Jones, and M. Vernon, Anatomy and Obstetrics/Gynecology (M.V.), University of Kentucky Medical Center, Lexington, KY. 40536, USA.

We examined the effects of the differential administration of estrogen (E) and progesterone (P) on the pituitary secretion of follicle-stimulating hormone (FSH). Cycling rats (n=64) were ovariectomized (ovx) and after 5 days were implanted with Silastic capsules filled with crystalline E or P and grouped as follows: empty implant (control; C), E implant (E), E and P implants (E+P), E implants with P supplied intermittently (E→P) by implanting and withdrawing P capsules every 48 hours. On specific days postimplantation (2, 6, 10, and 14; which coincided with implanting the P into the E→P groups), rats were cannulated and serially bled every 4 hours for 24 hours to monitor gonadotropin levels in blood. The controls exhibited a consistent postcastration rise in plasma FSH levels, as expected, and this elevation was partially suppressed by all exogenous E treatments. Neither the control nor the E+P group had preovulatory-like surges of FSH throughout the experiment. However, on the day 6 sampling both the E and the E→P treatments significantly elevated plasma FSH levels at 1800h with the the E→P stimulation being greater than the E group. At the day 10 bleed only the E→P group had a significant elevation ($p < 0.02$) of FSH at 1800h. We conclude that (1) the "cyclic" presence of P is stimulatory to increased gonadotropin secretion, whereas its constant presence is inhibitory, (2) physiological levels of steroids alone are unable to return FSH to precastration levels, and (3) the hypothalamic-pituitary axis eventually becomes refractory to the E effects even in the presence of cyclic P stimulation.
Supported by NIH.

2392 DETECTION AND QUANTIFICATION OF 22K AND 20K FORMS OF HUMAN GROWTH HORMONE IN PITUITARY ADENOMAS.
J. Smal, J. Closset, A. Stevenaert and G. Hennen* Endocrinologie, Université de Liège, C.H.U. B23, B-4000 Liège, BELGIQUE Neurochirurgie, Hôpital de Bavière, bd de la Constitution, B-4020 LIEGE

The two main forms of hGH (20 and 22K) have been studied in normal pituitary tissues and in pituitary adenomas. Indeed, the 20K variant has been shown to lack the early insulin-like effect of the 22K form; moreover the synthetic and secretory process for these two forms could also differ in their regulation. Comparative quantification in both normal and pathological tissues was thus of biochemical and clinical interest. 12 pituitary adenomas obtained from patients with clinical acromegaly(6) prolactinoma(3) and non secreting adenoma(3) were obtained by transphenoïdal surgery. Part of the tissue was immediately frozen in liquid nitrogen. The lyophilized material from 0.3 M KCl adenoma extracts were analyzed by specific RIA, SDS polyacrylamide gel electrophoresis and high resolution isoelectricfocusing using an Immobiline gel, pH gradient 5-6.1. Internal standards were 22K and 20K hGH which had been highly purified by HPLC and preparative Immobiline gel. The gel were scanned using an LKB laser densitometer. In all adenomas a good correlation exists between the estimated content of growth hormone as measured by RIA and in scanned Immobiline gels. The ratio of 20K variant to 22K growth hormone in 7 pituitary adenoma was found to be 9 $\pm$3% even when the hGH content was considerabely elevated. These results suggest that the synthesis of both 22K and 20K forms of human GH appear not to be independantly regulated in pathological pituitary tissues.

2393 DUAL SECRETION OF ACTH AND LH FROM PITUITARY CELLS.

P.F. Smith*, J.L. Roberts and J.D. Neill. Dept. of Physiol. & Biophys., Univ. of Alabama in Birmingham, AL 35294 and Dept. of Biochem., Columbia Univ., N.Y. USA

A large proportion of corticotropes reportedly also contain LH during the neonatal period in the male rat (Childs et al., Endocrin. 110:1676, 1982). To assess whether or not such cells can secrete both ACTH and LH we have applied the reverse hemolytic plaque assay for measurement of hormone secretion from individual cells (Neill & Frawley, Endocrin. 112: 1135, 1983). Pituitary glands from male rats at 6, 9 or 15 days of age were monodispersed with trypsin. Plaque assays and PAP-ICC for ACTH and LH were performed and the percentage of hormone secreting and hormone containing cells calculated. The number of LH containing cells rose from ∿6% to ∿10% from day 6 to day 15; at each age approximately half of the LH containing cells secreted LH in response to GnRH (10^{-7}M). The number of ACTH containing cells remained constant over the three intervals (∿14%) while the number of ACTH-secreting cells dropped from 14% to 11%. Plaque assays for LH followed by PAP-ICC for ACTH demonstrated that a small percentage of the total pituitary population (0.5%) contained ACTH and secreted LH. Some pituitary cells from each age group were cultured for 24 h and used in a sequential plaque assay for both ACTH and LH. In each age group a small proportion (1 in 20) of the ACTH secreting cells also secreted LH. This data provides evidence for a small population of cells in the neonatal male rat pituitary that contain both ACTH and LH and secrete either hormone in response to the appropriate secretagogue. If a larger population of cells containing both ACTH and LH exists these cells are unresponsive to CRF and GnRH.

2394 RUDIMENTARY PITUITARY IS THE MOST COMMON CAUSE OF IDIOPATHIC PITUITARY DWARFISM.

S. Sobieszczyk*, J. Grądzki, J. Kosowicz, and M. Gembicki, Department of Endocrinology, Medical Academy, 60-355 Poznań, Poland. Al. Przybyszewskiego 49

Since the cause of idiopathic pituitary dwarfism is still not clarified we undertook intensive pituitary hormone assays and computerized tomography / CT / studies. In the group of 28 cases with pituitary dwarfism serum GH, prolactin, LH, FSH, TSH and cortisol were determined by radioimmunoassay. CT scans of the sella turcica were made by the use of fourth generation "Synerview" / Picker / scanner. The slice thickness was 2 milimetres. In all cases serum growth hormone concentrations was below 2 ng/ml and did not rise during insulin induced hypo glycemia. In 60% of cases hypoprolactinemia non responsive to TRH stimulation was found. In 50% cases there was no response in serum TSH to TRH stimulation. Serum LH and FSH were lowered in 80%, whereas serum cortisol was lowered in 70% of subjects. CT scans revealed pituitary abnormalities in 25 out of 28 patients: pituitary hypoplasia / rudimentary pituitary / in 15 cases and pituitary agenesia in 10 patients. The results of our studies demonstrated that the most common cause of idiopathic pituitary dwarfism is the rudimentary pituitary, a congenital developmental defect.

2395 PULSATILE GONADOTROPIN-RELEASING HORMONE (GnRH)-INDUCED OVULATION IN LACTATING RHESUS MONKEYS. H. G. Spies*, T. Oyama, D. L. Hess, R. L. Norman, M. Stobie and P. Gliessman, Reprod. Biol. and Behav., Oregon Reg. Primate Res. Center, 505 N.W. 185th Avenue, Beaverton, Oregon 97006.

The role of hyperprolactinemia in the anovulatory syndrome during primate lactation remains undefined despite intense investigation. To address this issue, we fitted jugular catheters to postpartum rhesus mothers suckling newborns. The catheters were exteriorized thereby permitting remote blood sampling and chronic GnRH infusion (1 μg/min for 6 min each h). Progesterone (P), E_2, FSH, LH and prolactin (PRL) were measured in maternal serum by specific RIAs. Episodic secretion of PRL occurred throughout 24 h in the presence of the infant and dramatic increments in serum PRL were observed within 60-90 min of suckling in 4 females when infants were returned after 12 h of isolation. Starting GnRH pulses by day 25 postpartum resulted in ovulation after 43 and 48 days of treatment in 2/3 suckling mothers as indicated by 2 or more days of > 200 pg E_2/ml serum, an attenuated LH surge, no FSH surge, and > 2 ng P/ml for 12 to 14 days. Ovulation occurred after only 13, 17, 23 and 35 days of GnRH treatment in 4/4 suckling females whose postpartum residual corpora lutea were removed. These data suggest that P suppresses pituitary responsiveness to exogenous GnRH during the postpartum period. More importantly, the data support the concept that lactational anovulation results from inadequate hypothalamic GnRH secretion consequent to suckling and hyperprolactinemia rather than PRL-induced inhibition of the pituitary-gonadal axis. Supported by NIH grants RR-00163, HD-07602 and HD-16631.

2396 INVASIVE PROLACTINOMAS: TREATMENTS' EFFICIENCY. T. Stoica*, M. Coculescu, Department of Endocrinology, Institute of Medicine, Bucharest - Romania.

The method of treatment of invasive pituitary adenomas is still in discussion. Twelve invasive prolactinomas were submitted to transfenoidal surgery (5 cases), transfrontal surgery (3 cases), both associated with conventional X-ray therapy, and 4 cases were exclusively treated by bromocriptine. The pituitary surgery moderately decreased serum PRL levels, and the tumoral volume. The association of X-ray therapy (10,000-20,000 r) did not allow the rapid reexpansion of the tumoral rests, but did not influence the serum PRL level. Bromocriptine, in high doses (20-40 mg/day, two years), as primary treatment, normalised serum PRL level and decreased the tumoral mass until the empty sella syndrome, in all cases. In one case the complete cure of the tumor was proved 10 months after withdrawal of bromocriptine. Bromocriptine seems to be the treatment of choice in invasive prolactinomas, if high doses are available for long term period.

2397 PITUITARY RESPONSE TO EXOGENOUSLY ADMINISTERED LUTEINIZING HORMONE RELEASING HORMONE (LHRH) IN THE MALE DOG. Ali H. Surve* and Paul Taistra. Sandoz, Inc., East Hanover, N.J. 07936

Quantitative studies of canine reproductive endocrinology are limited. In this investigation a total of 9 sexually mature (age: 1.5-3 yr) mongrels were used. Exploratory studies revealed: (1) LHRH (100 ng/kg iv) produced quantitatively consistent responses in all the dogs; (2) blood sampling at 0, 5, 10, 15, 30 and 60 min post injection adequately covered the stimulatory episode; and (3) this dose did not affect FSH levels. Using these conditions, the effect of anesthesia (pentobarbital, 35 mg/kg iv) on pituitary response to LHRH was studied. Mean ± SE basal levels of LH in conscious dogs were 1.8 ± .3 ng/ml, whereas levels in anesthetized animals were not detectable (ND) at the sensitivity of the assay (0.5 ng/ml). Responses to LHRH in conscious dogs were not significantly different from those in anesthetized - mean area under the curve (AUC) ± SE: 344 ± 54 vs 280 ± 27. All subsequent experiments were performed under the anesthesia. Solubilization of LHRH in normal or proteinacious saline (1% dog serum) yielded similar responses - AUC ± SE: 250 ± 50 vs 267 ± 61. When all the LH responses described above were combined, the mean ± SE LH concentration at 0, 5, 10, 15, 30 and 60 min post injection was, respectively, ND, 10.8 ± .7, 11.6 ± .9, 9.8 ± .7, 3.8 ± .5 and 0.8 ± .2. When samples were collected at 1 min intervals for the first 10 min, LH levels were elevated within 1 min post injection. There were more than one peak and nadir, however LH levels were highest in the 4 min sample. A dose effect relationship could not be shown when 4 dogs were given 25, 50, 100, 200 or 500 ng/kg LHRH iv randomly at 1 h intervals. Although quantitatively consistent responses were produced by 5 injections of 100 ng/kg iv at 1 h intervals, those produced by 500 ng/kg were initially higher and declined after the first two stimulations. These data indicate that pentobarbital anesthesia in dogs probably has an inhibitory effect on the hypothalamus while the pituitary remains responsive to LHRH; large and repeated doses of it, however, are less stimulatory.

2398 THE IMMUNOCYTOCHEMICAL PROFILE OF 135 PITUITARY ADENOMAS. G. Turpin*, H.M. Heshmati, M. Kujas, A. Carayon, R. Van Effenterre, J. Racadot and J.L. de Gennes, Departments of Endocrinology, Pathology, Biochemistry and Neurosurgery, CHU Pitié-Salpêtrière, 75013 Paris, France.

Pituitary tumor was obtained during surgery from 135 patients (70 males, 65 females) with clinical and biological presentation of prolactin (PRL) (60 cases), growth hormone (GH) (30 cases) and non-functioning (NF) (45 cases) adenomas. Tumor tissue was fixed in Bouin-Hollande sublimate solution. Immunocytochemical study was performed with the peroxidase method. Antisera were used against human PRL, GH, corticotropin (ACTH) (1-24), chorionic gonadotropin (hCG), β-subunits of thyrotropin (TSHβ), luteinizing hormone (LHβ), follicle-stimulating hormone (FSHβ), and α-subunit of glycoprotein hormones (for NF adenomas only). The immunostaining of the tumor was considered positive when more than 30 % of the cell population fixed the antisera. A positive correlation between biological and immunocytochemical findings was present in 63 % of PRL adenomas, 87 % of GH adenomas and 73 % of NF adenomas. A non-specific immunocytochemical response was observed in 2 % of PRL adenomas (for GH), 27 % of GH adenomas (for PRL and ACTH) and 27 % of NF adenomas (for PRL, GH, ACTH, TSHβ, LHβ and FSHβ). The immunostaining for the α-subunit was present in less than 30 % of the cell population in 23 % of NF adenomas. It is concluded that: 1° Immunocytochemical study is more reliable in the positive diagnosis of GH adenomas than in PRL adenomas, but may show some non-specific responses in the case of GH adenomas. 2° NF adenomas may show some secretory pattern of PRL, GH, ACTH, TSHβ, LHβ, FSHβ and α-subunit in a few cases.

2399 PROLACTIN-LIKE IMMUNOREACTIVE PROTEINS IN PLASMA PRECIPITATES. Y.N. Sinha*, T.A. Gilligan and D.W. Lee, The Whittier Institute for Diabetes and Endocrinology, La Jolla, California 92037

A form of prolactin (PRL) 2-3,000 M_r greater than the traditional PRL (referred to as 25K and 23K PRL, respectively) has been observed in the murine (Endocrinology 112(Suppl.):384, 1983, Abstr.#1214) and human (FEBS Letters 154:111, 1983) pituitary. Structural analysis of the 25K component in sheep has shown it to be a glycosylated form of PRL (PNAS, 81: Jan., 1984). The human and ovine 25K-PRL cross-react with antibodies to 23K-PRL, but the murine 25K-PRL does not. Our recent studies indicate that the 25K-PRL occurs in human plasma also (JCEM, submitted). During our search for 25K-PRL in human plasma, we observed that precipitates normally encountered in plasma contained several proteins (M_r 30K, 33K, 55K, 66K and 100K) that cross-reacted with hPRL antibodies. Further, the 30K protein co-migrated with 25K-PRL during electrophoresis. In one experiment, an immunoreactive component comigrating with 23K PRL was also found in the precipitates. We tested the material against 3 antibodies: VLS #1, AFP-777212, and an antibody raised against a synthetic peptide representing 13 N-terminus amino acids of hPRL (BBRC 115:346, 1983). The 30K and 55K proteins reacted with each antibody. We peptide mapped the 30K protein by iodinating the band in the gel, followed by tryptic digestion and 2-dimensional analysis. Its fingerprint resembled that of the 25K-PRL from human pituitary. If the various immunoreactive components seen here are different forms of PRL, these results suggest that a portion of these precipitates out from plasma during storage and thus does not participate in immunologic reaction. This would explain why RIA measurements of hPRL are often not correlated with physiologic manifestations of its secretion.

2400 THE NATURAL HISTORY OF UNTREATED MICROPROLACTINOMAS. D. Sisam*, G. Redmond, and L. Sheeler, Department of Endocrinology, The Cleveland Clinic, Cleveland, Ohio 44106.

Fifty patients with presumed microprolactinomas, based on chronically elevated plasma prolactin levels, CT evidence of microadenomas, and absence of other causes of hyperprolactinemia were followed in an attempt to determine the frequency of tumor progression. The mean duration of symptoms was 5.7 years, the mean duration of hyperprolactinemia was 4.3 years, and the mean duration of serial CT follow-up was 3.1 years. High resolution, coronal CT scans with IV contrast, was performed on all patients. No patient received radiation therapy, surgery or sustained medical therapy. The mean initial prolactin was 68 ng/ml. Seven women had ovulation induction with bromocriptine and had subsequent uneventful pregnancies. Plasma prolactin levels were measured annually, and CT scans were repeated every one to three years, with no patient showing any demonstrable evidence of tumor growth. The mean serum prolactin on follow-up was 47 ng/ml. The initial results of this ongoing study suggests that all patients with microprolactinomas can be safely followed with serial plasma prolactin levels and CT scans, with or without medical therapy.

2401 GLYCOSYLATION OF OVINE PROLACTIN DURING CELL-FREE BIOSYNTHESIS.

T.W. Strickland* and J.G. Pierce, Dept. of Biological Chemistry, UCLA School of Medicine, Los Angeles, CA 90024

Carbohydrate is not an usual component of prolactin. However, ovine prolactin which contains a carbohydrate unit at asparagine 31 has recently been isolated by Lewis et al. (PNAS 81, Jan. 1984). We have utilized cell free translation to study the biosynthesis of ovine prolactin. Translation of ovine pituitary mRNA followed by immunoprecipitation with antiprolactin results in a single ^{35}S-cysteine labeled protein, preprolactin, as shown by SDS gel electrophoresis. When microsomes were present during translation three forms, prolactin, preprolactin, and a putative glycosylated prolactin were detected. Three lines of evidence point to the formation of glycosylated ovine prolactin: (1) the presence of a low mobility species on SDS gels, (2) digestion with Endo H converts this species to prolactin, (3) no comparable form is seen upon translation of bovine pituitary mRNA as bovine prolactin lacks an asparagine residue at position 31. Runoff experiments were performed in which ovine and bovine pituitary microsomes were allowed to complete synthesis, *in vitro*, of prolactin which had been initiated *in vivo*. Bovine pituitary microsomes synthesized only prolactin and preprolactin. Ovine pituitary microsomes synthesized four forms, preprolactin, prolactin, and two high molecular weight forms. Both high MW forms are converted to prolactin by Endo H, again strongly suggesting that the increase in MW is due to glycosylation. Thus, these two forms may represent ovine prolactin containing one and two N-linked carbohydrate units. As the published sequence of ovine prolactin contains only one ASN-X-SER (THR) sequence, the signal for N-linked glycosylation, the presence of a second carbohydrate unit is unexpected. (Supported by USPHS AM 18005.)

2402 SYNTHESIS OF RADIOACTIVELY LABELED RAT PROLACTIN (PRL) cDNA PROBE UTILIZING BACTERIOPHAGE M13mp9 AND DEVELOPMENT OF SANDWICH HYBRIDIZATION METHOD.

N.Suganuma*, H. Seo, N. Matsui, D. Christophe, G. Vassart and S. Refetoff, The Research Institute of Environmental Medicine, Nagoya University, Nagoya, Japan and Free University of Brussels, Belgium.

A rat PRL cDNA clone, kindly provided by Dr. J.A. Martial, was digested with restriction enzyme Hae III and the resultant fragments were cloned in M13mp9 phage. Using ^{125}I-PRL mRNA, single stranded (S-S) recombinant phage DNAs containing coding strand of PRL cDNA were detected and purified. One of the S-S recombinant phage DNA was immobilized onto nitrocellulose filters and the other phage DNA having non-overlapping PRL cDNA sequence was labeled with radioactive iodine. When these two were incubated under annealing conditions, no radioactivity was associated with the filters. Only when the RNA from rat anterior pituitary was added in the reaction, the radioactive probe was attached to the filters.

This sandwich assay was quantitative and reproducible. Less than 15 ng of total pituitary RNA from normal male rats was needed to detect PRL mRNA sequence. Comparison of this method with RNA dot hybridization revealed that this method was approximately 50 times more sensitive.

Cloning of cDNA utilizing M13 phage provides a simple and rapid preparation of hybridization probe. Furthermore, the development of sandwich assay enables to detect specific mRNA sequence in a crude RNA extracts with high sensitivity. The method will be useful to elucidate the mechanism involved in the regulation of gene expression. Supported in part by Grant-in-Aid for Cancer Research from the Ministry of Education, Japan (No. 57010034).

2403 FIBROCYSTIC DISEASE OF BREAST, PROLACTIN AND VITAMIN E. G.S.Sundaram*, S.Manimekalai, R.London, M.Sundaram and P.J.Goldstein, Reproductive Endocrinology Research Division, Department of Obstetrics and Gynecology, Sinai Hospital of Baltimore, Inc., Baltimore, Maryland 21215, U.S.A

In this study we evaluated 1) the role of prolactin (P) in the pathophysiology of fibrocystic disease (FD) of breast in women and 2) the effect of different doses of dl-α-tocopherol (T) therapy on FD and P. Women with clinically confirmed FD were treated with placebo, 150, 300 or 600 I.U. of T by a double-blind and randomized protocol. After two months of therapy, the resulting four groups (I to IV) were further sub-divided into responders (R) and non-responders (NR) to T, using established criteria. FD women (n=124) had P (in ng/ml, by a radioimmunoassay technique) of 11.1 ± 0.4, higher ($p < 0.05$) than that (10.2 ± 0.3) in normal women (n=33). When treated with 150,300 or 600 I.U. of T, P further increased in II (n=34), III (n=31) and IV (n=30) to 12.8 ± 1.0, 11.6 ± 0.8 and 13.6 ± 1.1, respectively ($p < 0.05$ in only IV). About 50% of patients in II to IV showed clinical improvement in FD; however, there were no differences between P of R and NR in II to IV. Interestingly, 50% of those not treated with T (placebo group I, n=29), also had spontaneous clinical improvement in FD in two months; but, P decreased to 7.7 ± 1.1 ($p < 0.02$) in R and increased to 11.8 ± 1.2 in NR. The results show that 1) FD is associated with increased P or vice versa 2) spontaneous resolution of FD is associated with a lowering of P and 3) T therapy at 150 to 600 I.U. does not resolve FD but causes an increase in P. The results suggest that 1)agents capable of reducing P may be effective in treating FD and 2) T therapy for FD should be undertaken with caution since FD and higher P levels are associated with an increased incidence of breast cancer.

2404 IDENTIFICATION OF THE mRNA CODING FOR PROLACTIN IN THE DECIDUA. S. Taii, Y. Ihara and T. Mori, Dept. of Gynecol. & Obstet., Kyoto University, Fac. of Med., 54, Shogoin kawahara-cho, Sakyo-ku, Kyoto 606, Japan.

The presence of high concentrations of Prolactin(Prl) in the amniotic fluid atract special interest in the human reproduction. Although recent evidences suggest that the major source of this Prl is of peri-placental, most likely of decidual, origin, neither the origin nor the function of it is completely demonstrated. In order to prove conclusively the origin of this Prl, we used the cell-free translation system to detect the mRNA coding for Prl in the peri-placental tissues. Total RNAs extracted from the amnion, chorion and decidua of the human second trimester placentas were translated in the presence of [^{35}S[-methionine, followed by immunoprecipitation with antiserum to Prl and electrophoresis in the sodium dodecyl sulfate slab gel. Immunoreactive Prl-like peptides were formed with both decidual and chorionic RNA. The former had a molecular weight of approximately 25,000, about, 3,000 larger than authentic Prl, and competed completely with unlabeled Prl but not with unlabeled human placental lactogen(hPL)for binding to the antibody. In addition, the electrophoretic patterns of the fragments formed by partial enzymatic proteolysis of both the translation product and authentic Prl were similar. Therefore, this immunoreactive translation product formed with decidual RNA was identified as the Prl Precursor(PrePrl). The latter was, however, shown to be a minor crossreaction of the hPL precursor against the antibody to Prl by the same analyses as described above. These data demonstrate that only the decidua is the site of the de nove sysntesis of Prl in the peri-placental tissues and that the decidual Prl is derived from the large precursor(PrePrl) as in the case of other secretory proteins.

2405 ACUTE DECREASE IN DOPAMINE CONCENTRATION STMULATES RAT PROLACTIN RELEASE UNDER EXISTENCE OF TRH IN VITRO.

J. Takahara[1)*], M. Niimi[2)], K.Hashimoto[3)], J. Kageyama[3)] and S. Irino[1)]. 1st. Dept Med.[1)], Central Labs.[2)], Kagawa Medical School, Kagawa, and 3rd. Dept. Med.[3)], Okayama Univ. Medical School, Okayama, Japan.

We investigated an effect of acute decrease in dopamine(DA) concentration on prolactin(PRL) by cultured or non-cultured rat pituitary cells under an existence of TRH using an in vitro perifusion method. A continuous infusion of TRH at dose of 1-100 ng/ml elicited a marked PRL release at the initial period of infusion and then in spite of the continuous TRH infusion , PRL release gradually decreased and returned to a basal level. At the end of the TRH infusion, an additional short period TRH infusion at 10 fold high dose compared to the continuous TRH infusion had no effect of PRL release. A continuous infusion of DA at dose of 5 ng/ml partly suppressed the basal PRL level. Immediately after the end of the continuous DA infusion, a small but significant increase in PRL release was observed. In a perifusion system using non-cultured rat pituitary pieces, a concomitant infusion of TRH at dose of 50 ng/ml and DA at dose of 5 ng/ml caused a marked PRL release and gradually decreased PRL release in spite of the continuous TRH infusion. When PRL level was returned to the basal level, an interruption of DA infusion but not TRH enhanced a greater PRL release than that observed at the initial period of the infusion. These results indicate that an acute decrease in DA concentration stimulates PRL release by pituitary mammatrophs under an existence of TRH. Thus we suggest that under existence of TRH or another PRF at some concentration, acute decrease in DA concentration in the hypophysial portal vessels stimulate PRL release in vivo.

2406 EFFECTS OF BROMOCRIPTINE (BCT) ON HYPERPROLACTINEMIC-AMENORRHEA (H-A).

T. Tamura*, T. Satoh and T. Tamada, Dept. of OB/GYN, Jichi Medical School, Tochigi Prefecture, Japan, 329-04

The effects of BCT on pituitary responsiveness to LH-RH and on estradiol (E_2)-induced LH release were studied in patients with H-A with reference to the induction of ovulation. Among patients in this category, four with pituitary blunted response and also four with pituitary normal response were selected as study (s) and control (c) groups, recpectively. LH-RH tests (100 μg, iv) and serum E_2 determinations were carried out prior to and during (once a week) BCT treatment (7.5 mg daily for 8-12 weeks) in group s. Estrogen provocation tests (E_2 benzoate, 2.0 mg, im) were performed prior to and during (at 8-12 weeks for group s and 2-3 weeks for group c) BCT treatment. Before BCT both LH response to LH-RH and serum E_2 were lowered, whereas the responsiveness was improved and the serum LH increased gradually reaching normal LH response and serum E_2 level of 60-80 pg/ml respectively at 8th week of this therapy in group s. The E_2 injection prior to BCT treatment produced no feedback LH release either in group s or in group c. The same injection during BCT treatment elicited no or only a small amount of LH release in group s, although the same injection caused a marked positive feedback LH release in group c. While all in group c ovulated on BCT, none in group s ovulated on the same therapy. The present data demonstrate that BCT improves pituitary responsiveness to LH-RH probably through the increase of serum E_2, and suggest that there exists in group s an impairment in the hypothalamic feedback mechanism different from that of group c and this impairment is responsible for the failure in the induction of ovulation with BCT.

2407 STUDY ON ROLE OF OXYTOCIN AND PROLACTIN BY PASSIVE IMMUNIZATION IN LACTATING RATS. Satoshi Tanimoto*, Tsunehisa Makino, Takashi Nagai, Shigekazu Takayama, Zenjiro Kondo, and Rihachi Iizuka, Department of Obstetrics and Gynecology, School of Medicine, Keio University, Tokyo, Japan

Some of the physiological roles of Oxytocin (OT) and Prolactin (PRL) in lactating rats were studied by passive immunization. Antibody to synthetic OT (A/S OT) and antibody to rats PRL (A/S PRL) were produced in rabbits immunized with synthetic OT or rat PRL. Then the sera of the rabbits were tested for the potency and specificity of antibody by radioimmunoassay technique. One ml of antiserum was inferred to be capable of sufficiently neutralizing endogenous OT or PRL in lactating rats. From the 5th day of postpartum, rats were daily injected intraperitoneally with 1ml of A/S OT or A/S PRL. In the control group rats were daily injected with 1ml of normal rabbit serum. All pups in the A/S OT treated group were dead during 11th to 15th postpartum day, and great number of pups in the A/S PRL treated group were also dead during the 16th to 20th postpartum day. All pups in the control group grew normally. Serum PRL levels in both the control and the A/S OT treated group were virtually identical suggesting that OT might be independent of PRL release. Serum OT levels in the A/S PRL treated group were significantly increased suggesting that mechanical stimuli to nipples by pups might increase OT level presumably because of decreasing of milk production due to lacking of PRL. Furthermore the histology of the mammary glands suggested that the role of OT on lactation might not affect the phase of milk production while however affecting on milk ejection.

2408 DEPLETION-TRANSFORMATION (DT) STATUS OF THE DONOR PITUITARY ALTERS THE IN VITRO RESPONSE TO PROLACTIN RELEASING ACTIVITY. Jeri Taylor-ElHage*, Steven Eversley and Anna-Lisa Barofsky, Dept. of Physiology & Biophysics, Howard Univ. College of Medicine, Washington, D.C. 20059, USA.

To stabilize the responsiveness of hemi-pituitaries to prolactin (PRL) releasing activity (PRA) in an in vitro incubation system, the DT status of donor pituitaries (pits) from lactating rats was examined. Lactating mothers were separated from their litters (8 pups) for 5-6 h and either decapitated immediately (NS), after a 30-min suckling stimulus (S), or 1 h after a 30-min suckling stimulus (PS). Half the pits (N=29) were homogenized (0.1 ml/mg) in 0.05 M $NaHCO_3$ (pH 10) to extract total PRL, half (N=25) were homogenized in distilled water (pH 7) to extract only non-DT PRL. PRL content measured by RIA was pH 10: NS=5617±1052, S=1745±333, PS=1707±308; pH 7: NS=7296±1871, S=470±29, PS=378±59 ng rat PRL-RP2/mg pit; P (DT status) <0.025. Similarly treated glands (S or NS) were hemisected and incubated in 2 ml Medium-199 (pH 7.4; 37°C; 5% CO_2; 30 min control, test and post incubations) with or without continuous exposure to 50 ng/ml dopamine (DA). Hypothalamic extract (HE; 0 or 2 equivalents/0.4 ml 0.01N HCl) from lactating rats was neutralized and added to the test incubation. PRL released by 0 and 2 HE, expressed as the slope of the dose response, was +DA: NS = +31, S = +6.5: -DA: NS = -33, S = +13 ng increase in PRL (test-control)/mg pit /1HE; P(DTx DA) <0.025. The results suggest (1) that pituitary depletion-transformation can be measured by RIA, and (2) the DT status of the donor pit, which may be controllable by continuous DA exposure, markedly influences the in vitro response to PRA. Supported by NIH Grants HD-10676, RR-08016-11, 5-T32-GM-07800.

2409 INDOMETHACIN OR LOW SALT DIET PREVENT INCREASES IN RENAL FUNCTION ASSOCIATED WITH INTRAVENOUS (i.v.) AMINO ACID (AmAc) INFUSION.

L. Ruilope*, J. Rodicio, J. Sancho-Rof, R. Garcia-Robles, E. Minavalles, M.T. Ortuno, T.G. Hammond, F.G. Knox, and J.C. Romero. Dept. Nephrol. Endocrinol., Hospitals "1 de Octobre" and "Ramon y Cajal", Madrid, Spain, and Mayo Clinic, Rochester, MN 55905, USA.

Because of recent reports showing that protein diet influences glomerular dynamics, we investigated the renal haemodynamic and urine (U) excretory effects of i.v. infusion of a 10% amino acid solution frequently used for parenteral nutrition ("Vibram" 0.75 ml/kg/hr). Renal CIn and CPAH, plasma renin activity (PRA), plasma aldosterone (PA), UVol., U electrolytes(Na, K) were measured before and at 2, 4, and 6 hours during AmAc infusion in 5 human volunteers on 'normal' salt diet. Results are depicted in the table below: (mean±standard error).

	RPF ml/min	GFR ml/min	V ml/min	UNaV µEq/min
Control	554±42	111± 6	13.0±1.7	284±64
2 hours	562±53	111±17	10.0±2.3	259±65
4 hours	690±64*	161±13*	10.4±1.7	325±94
6 hours	849±87*	182±18*	11.4±2.6	267±87

(*$p<0.05$ by paired t-test)

Blood pressure and fractional Na excretion did not change. The increase in RPF and GFR were effectively prevented by indomethacin pretreatment (75 mg/day for 2 days) or dieting sodium restriction for 3 days. We conclude that AmAc infusion is associated with major renal haemodynamic changes which may be prostaglandin and volume dependent. Supported by NIH grants HL16414 and HL14133.

2410 EFFECTS OF OVARIAN STEROIDS ON PROSTAGANDIN $F_{2\alpha}$ OUTPUT BY HUMAN ENDOMETRIUM AND ENDOMETRIAL EPITHELIAL CELLS IN CULTURE.

F. Schatz*, L. Markiewicz, P. Barg, and E. Gurpide. Depts. of Obs, Gyn & Reprod. Sci., Mount Sinai School of Medicine, New York, NY 10029, USA

Levels of immunoreactive $PGF_{2\alpha}$ were measured in media changed daily during incubations of endometrium and during culture of epithelial cells derived from isolated endometrial glands. Basal output during the first day of incubation was 420 ng/(mg prot. x d) ± 79 (SE), n=10, for proliferative endometrium and 140 ± 28, n=14, for secretory tissue. Estradiol (10^{-8} M) stimulated $PGF_{2\alpha}$ output by endometrium under organ culture conditions, 1.5-fold ± 0.26, n=9, by proliferative and 3.5-fold ± 0.58, n=13, by more responsive secretory tissue. Similar increases in PGF_2 output were obtained in cultures of epithelial cells derived from proliferative (3.5-fold ± 0.52, n=7, day 1), and secretory (2.9-fold ± 0.77, n=6, day 1) tissue. Addition of progesterone (10^{-7} M) to the medium resulted in 55% ± 6, n=10, and 44% ± 9, n=8, decreases in the basal output of $PGF_{2\alpha}$ by proliferative and secretory endometrium, respectively. In contrast, P (10^{-6} M) increased $PGF_{2\alpha}$ output by epithelial cells in culture (1.7-fold ± 0.30, n=7, day 1). Progesterone (10^{-7}-10^{-6} M), when mixed with E_2 (10^{-8} M), reduced the estrogen effect on $PGF_{2\alpha}$ output completely in proliferative endometrium but only partially in secretory tissue and in cultures of epithelial cells. These results demonstrate that incubation of human endometrium, either as whole tissue fragments or as epithelial cell cultures, respond to ovarian hormones and provide convenient *in vitro* systems to study the physiologic regulation of prostaglandin synthesis and metabolism.

2411 THE JUVENILE-PERIPUBERTAL TRANSITION PERIOD IN THE FEMALE RAT: ESTABLISHMENT OF A DIURNAL PATTERN OF PULSATILE LH SECRETION. H.F. Urbanski* and S.R. Ojeda, Department of Physiology, University of Texas Health Science Center at Dallas, Dallas, TX 75235.

The mode of LH release in prepubertal female rats is pulsatile and the secretory pattern appears to change as puberty approaches. To establish such a change we examined in detail the plasma LH profiles of more than 40 rats during late juvenile - early peripubertal development (26-38 days of age, before first proestrus). Blood samples were obtained using an automated technique (in press) which permits continuous sampling for more than 5 hours while simultaneously replacing blood volume. At all ages, morning plasma LH levels were low and showed pulses of low amplitude. Similar LH profiles were observed during the afternoon in juvenile rats (26-29 days old) but were notably different in older animals. These showed an increase in mean LH levels and in most cases (16 out of 18) a concomitant appearance of large LH secretory pulses (6.8±0.7 pulses/rat/5h; mean amplitude = 34±4 ng LH-RP-1/ml). Interestingly, in 5 of the 16 peripubertal rats the pulses were accompanied by a midafternoon mini-surge of LH secretion lasting for ~ 2 hours and reaching peak levels of 174±19 ng/ml (LH surge at first proestrus is > 1,000 ng/ml). The results demonstrate the prepubertal development of an afternoon increase in LH pulse amplitude and the appearance of a more prolonged and larger secretory episode (mini-surge). Such changes in LH release may contribute to the enhancement of peripubertal steroidogenesis. (Supported by NIH Grant HD-09988-07).

2412 VOLUME AND NUMBER OF DELTOID AND TROCHANTER ADIPOCYTES. EFFECTS OF AGE,SEX, TESTOSTERONE,ESTROGENS AND CORTISOL. J.Vague*, J.Meignen, J.Negrin, M.Thomas, M.Tramoni, J.Jubelin, Endocrinologic Clinic. Med . Univ. 13005, Marseille, France.

In 181 control females, 180 males 5-90 years deltoid volume(DV) is steady, unsignificantly larger in males than in females. Trochanter volume(TV) identical in both sexes during childhood is later twice in females than in males. Deltoid number (DN) increases with growth, much less in males. After puberty trochanter number(TN) decreases in males, increases two-fold in females. After 70 it decreases in females. D and T adipocytes in 4 cases of testicular feminization are similar to female type. In 6 cases of Turner's syndrome DV a little larger and TV a little smaller than in normal females are respectively decreased and increased after 2 years treatment by ethinyl estradiol-chlormadinone. In 6 cases of male eunuchoidism D and T adipocytes similar to female type are virilized particularly TN decreased after 3 years treatment by testosterone (T). The same is observed in a female transsexualism (TS) after 45 months T Treatment. In a male TS given supraphysiologic doses of estrogens DV is strongly decreased and TV increased. In 10 female and 4 male Cushing's syndromes the main adipocytes feature is dramatic increase of DV in both sexes, decrease of TN in females only. 2 years after surgical recovery DV is normalized in both sexes; TN remains low in females, probable definitive result of concomitant androgen effect. Because of the different responses of D and T adipocytes to steroid hormones local adipocytometry is worth daily using in clinical practice.

2413 HEIGHT VELOCITY AND BONE MATURATION BEFORE AND DURING SPONTANEOUS AND TESTOSTERONE INDUCED PUBERTY IN hGH TREATED HYPOPITUITARY BOYS.

M.Vandeweghe*, Chr.Ernould and J.P.Bourguignon, Department of Endocrinology, University of Ghent and Pediatric Clinic, University of Liège, Belgium (Belgian Studygroup for Pediatric Endocrinology).

Height velocity (HV) and bone age (BA, TW_2 method) were longitudinally studied before and during puberty in 29 hypopituitary boys. All were treated using hGH (18 to 24 IU/week). In 20 gonadotropin deficient patients, testosterone enanthate 100 mg/month IM was given from a mean BA ± 1 SD of 13.8 ± 1.1 yr, height being 148.8 ± 7.2 cm; 9 patients started spontaneous puberty at a BA of 12.4 ± 1.0 yr, height being 136.3 ± 6.5 cm. In both groups pubic hair and genital score developed normally. During the last year before puberty, HV was similar in both groups : 3.6 ± 1.1 cm; a maximal increase up to 7.4 ± 1.1 cm/yr occured during the first year of testosterone therapy. During spontaneous puberty, HV was maximal during the 2nd yr of puberty : 6.8 ± 2.5 cm/yr. Variations in BA parallel those of HV. Therefore, mean ratio ΔHeight age/Δ BA did not significantly change (from 0.90 to 1.24) throughout the entire study. Differences in BA (11.4 to 15.4 yrs) at the onset of testosterone therapy did not result in marked changes in HV (10.5 to 14.4 cm/2 yr) during puberty. In contrast, increase in BA during the same period varied from 0.8 to 3.4 yr and was negatively correlated (r=0.92) with BA at the onset of testosterone treatment. In conclusion, during testosterone induced puberty, the ability to accelerate HV is not impaired in relation with advancement in BA. Accordingly, height after puberty depends on height attained at the onset of testosterone therapy, and not on bone age at that time.

2414 17α-SUBSTITUTED ESTRADIOL DERIVATIVES: CANDIDATES FOR DEVELOPMENT OF HIGH-AFFINITY FLUORESCEIN-ESTRADIOL CONJUGATES.

M. Salman, S. Ray, P. L. Stotter, and G. C. Chamness,* Department of Medicine, University of Texas Health Science Center, San Antonio, Texas 78284, U.S.A.

17α-allyl estradiol has almost as high affinity for estrogen receptor as estradiol itself, and its epoxide reacts with thiopropyl-Sepharose to yield an excellent affinity chromatography reagent (Greene et al.). In the course of developing a fluorescein conjugate based on this same epoxide, we found that the epoxide's affinity is at least ten-fold less than that of allyl estradiol. To identify the probable cause of this affinity loss and to define the optimum compound for preparation of a high affinity conjugate, we have synthesized six further 17α-(3'-hydroxypropyl) and 17α-(3'-hydroxyprop-1'-ynyl) estradiols, and have determined their receptor affinities. By comparison of these, we can exclude internal hydrogen bonding of the side-chain oxygen with the 17β-hydroxyl as the cause of the reduced affinity. Nor does the increased solvent affinity of the oxygen-containing side chains fully explain the receptor affinity results, though it is probably a factor. Steric interference close to the D-ring binding site of the receptor appears to be a major consideration, as shown in part by the fact that two constrained compounds, the hydroxyprop-1'-ynyl estradiol and the 17β-spirolactone resulting from oxidation of the 17α-hydroxypropyl estradiol, have much higher affinity than hydroxypropyl estradiol itself. Preliminary results using longer side chains also agree with our conclusion that 17α derivatives with 1'- or 2'-unsaturations will possess better estrogen receptor affinity than their saturated homologs, and will thus be good candidates for conjugate development.

2415 IMMUNOHISTOCHEMICAL LOCALIZATION OF ESTRADIOL RECEPTOR IN RAT BRAIN WITH MONOCLONAL ANTIBODIES TO CALF CYTOSOLIC RECEPTOR. M. Sar* and I. Parikh, Department of Anatomy, School of Medicine, University of North Carolina, Chapel Hill, NC 27514 and Molecular Biology Department, The Wellcome Research Laboratories, Research Triangle Park, NC 27709.

A monoclonal antibody (JS34/32) against calf uterine cytosolic estrogen receptor (Moncharmont, B., Su, J.-L. and Parikh, I., 1982, *Biochemistry* **21**, 6916-21) was used to define anatomical distribution of the receptor in rat brain. Female Sprague-Dawley rats, 24-day-old intact and 40-day-old ovariectomized (for 24 hrs), were each injected i.p. with 1 µg/100 g body wt. of 17-β estradiol. The rats were sacrificed after 1 hr. Brains including preoptic and hypothalamic region were dissected, and frozen in liquified propane. Four to 6 µm frozen sections were thaw-mounted on slides, fixed in 4% paraformaldehyde in PBS and stained immunohistochemically with monoclonal antibodies to estrogen receptor using avidin-biotin technique. Immunostaining in nuclei of cells was observed in certain specific hypothalamic and extrahypothalamic nuclear groups. When stained with a control monoclonal antibody, derived from spleen cells of an unimmunized mouse, neither nuclear nor cytoplasmic staining was observed. Glial and ependymal cells did not show any positive staining. In the forebrain nuclear immunostaining was found in certain nuclei of septum, preoptic region, anterior and central hypothalamus and amygdala. The topographical distribution of immunohistochemically identified estrogen receptor containing neurons in the rat brain concurs with previous autoradiographic studies on estrogen target neurons in the rat brain after 3H-estradiol. The results demonstrate the usefulness of the monoclonal antibody for the detection of estrogen receptor in target tissues. Supported by PHS grant #NS17479.

2416 CHARACTERIZATION OF A UNIQUE NUCLEAR ESTROGEN BINDER MEDIATING TUMOR GROWTH IN MOUSE LEYDIG CELL TUMOR. B. Sato*, Y. Maeda, K. Noma, S. Kishimoto and K. Matsumoto, The Third Dept of Internal Medicine and The Second Dept of Pathology, Osaka University Hospital, Fukushima-ku, Osaka 553, Japan.

An estrogen-responsive mouse Leydig cell tumor line (T-124958) has been found to contain only a low-affinity estrogen binder in the cytosol but an estrogen receptor (ER)-like component in the purified nuclei even without estrogenic stimuli. The binding specificity of this nuclear binder was similar to that of putative ER, but its affinity for estradiol (E_2) in Mg^{++} containing buffer was temperature dependent (Kd 3 nM at 30 C and 12 nM at 0 C) without significant alteration in the number of maximum binding sites. The addition of EDTA, however, abolished this temperature dependency, resulting in high-affinity even at 0 C. These Mg^{++} and temperature effects were reversible. Collagenase dispersed cells were also incubated with [^{3}H] E_2. The high-affinity binder was again identified only in nuclei at 0 C and 37 C. Further, an exposure of cell to 10 nM [^{3}H] E_2 at 37 C, but not at 0 C, markedly diminished the number of nuclear estrogen binding sites without an appearance of the high-affinity cytosol binder, similar to so-called processing of ER. The possibility of direct influences of estrogen on tumor cells was studied in culture system. The presence of 10^{-8} to 10^{-7}M E_2 in 10 % charcoal treated fetal calf serum in MEM resulted in a 3 fold increase in the number of Leydig cell as well as [^{3}H] thymidine incorporation into DNA on day 14 over those seen in nonestrogenized control. These results would suggest that estrogen directly exerts its effect on tumor cell via this unique nuclear binder. This study was supported by grants-in-aid from the Ministry of Education, Tokyo, Japan.

2417 CHARACTERISTICS OF ESTROGEN RECEPTORS IN MCF-7 BREAST CANCER CELLS.
Nahid A. Shahabi*, Yun-Ju He, Ronald D. Wiehle and James L. Wittliff, Hormone Receptor Laboratory, James Graham Brown Cancer Center, and Department of Biochemistry, University of Louisville, Louisville, KY 40292, USA.

Size, shape and surface charge properties of estrogen receptors (ER) in cytosol prepared from MCF-7 cells have been determined. MCF-7 cells were grown in Dulbecco's modified Eagle's medium supplemented with calf serum. Cytosol was prepared in 10mM potassium phosphate buffer containing 1.5mM EDTA, 1.0mM DTT and 10% glycerol and incubated with 2-3nM 16α-^{125}I-iodoestradiol-17β (^{125}IE). Non-specific binding was determined by incubating an identical cytosol with ^{125}IE and a 250-fold excess of DES. Sucrose density gradient centrifugation demonstrated ER with a sedimentation value of 8-9 S in low salt and 4-5 S in 400mM KCl. Parallel analysis by high performance size exclusion chromatography using a TSK 3000 SW column gave a single large species (~70 A) whereas conventional size exclusion chromatography using Sephacryl S-300 revealed two distinct species (Stokes radii = 85A and 65-70A). Using high performance ion exchange chromatography, two ER isoforms were eluted at <0.1M and at ~0.2M potassium phosphate. High performance chromatofocusing using AX-500 anion exchange columns also separated two species eluting at pH 6.2 and 4.2. The latter was the predominant receptor. Properties of these ER isoforms appear similar to those of human uterus and of rabbit endometrial carcinoma, as well as those from lactating mammary gland of the rat. Supported in part by the Marie Overbey Memorial Grant from the American Cancer Society, by Phi Beta Psi Sorority, and by the Graduate School, University of Louisville.

2418 IDENTIFICATION OF EOSINOPHIL PEROXIDASE AS THE UTERINE NUCLEAR TYPE II ESTROGEN BINDING SITE.
D.M. Sheehan*, K.L. Medlock and C.R. Lyttle, National Center for Toxicological Research, Jefferson, AR 72079 and the University of Pennsylvania Medical School, Philadelphia, PA 19104, USA.

We have reported that eosinophils contain the uterine nuclear type II estrogen binding site (II) (Lyttle et al., J. B. C., in press). Since estradiol (E_2) is a substrate for eosinophil peroxidase (P), we tested the hypothesis that P is II. When added to uterine homogenates lacking II, P conferred II characteristics to the nuclear fraction. Scatchard plots are "hook-shaped" at high P levels and curvilinear at lower levels. Uteri from E_2 implanted rats show "hook-shaped" plots which become curvilinear upon dilution with non-II containing homogenates. Thus, curve shapes for both II and P appear concentration dependent. P-containing samples, like II, bound E_2 at 0°C and 37°C, but not in the presence of reducing agent, while the steroid specificity was identical to that reported for II. Guaiacol, a substrate for P, competed with E_2 for binding to II, but not for binding to the estrogen receptor. $CaCl_2$ (0.5M) used to solubilize P for purification, extracted II from the nuclear fraction. A heat stable, acid extractable uterine fraction, reported to contain a competitive inhibitor of II also contains a competitive inhibitor of P enzyme activity. For all characteristics examined, P behaved identically to II, leading us to conclude that II is P. The postulated role of II in modulating gene expression appears untenable. Other low affinity steroid binding proteins have been described, and our results suggest that some may be enzymes which bind ligand with no product formation under the conditions of the binding assay.

2419 BINDING OF [^{3}H]ESTRADIOL- AND [^{3}H]H1285-RECEPTOR COMPLEXES TO RABBIT UTERINE CHROMATIN. Raj. K. Singh*, Mary F. Ruh and Thomas S. Ruh, Department of Physiology, St. Louis University School of Medicine, St. Louis, MO 63104, U.S.A.

We investigated the binding characteristics of estrogen and antiestrogen receptor complexes to rabbit uterine chromatin. Activated or non-activated estrogen receptors were partially purified by DEAE-cellulose chromatography using low (1mM) or high (10 mM) concentrations of sodium molybdate, respectively. Activated [^{3}H]estradiol-receptor complexes showed enhanced binding to chromatin acceptor sites unmasked by 1M, 4M and 6M GuHCl. We also examined the chromatin binding characteristics of the estrogen receptors when bound by the high affinity triphenylethylene antiestrogen, H1285 (4(N,N-diethylaminoethoxy)-4'-methoxy-α-(p-hydroxyphenyl)-α'-ethylstilbene). The acceptor site activity for the [^{3}H]H1285-receptor complexes was decreased 30% at sites unmasked by 4M GuHCl and was decreased 50% at sites unmasked by 6M GuHCl. For both [^{3}H]estradiol- and [^{3}H]H1285-receptor complexes, the non-activated receptor forms showed very low binding to deproteinized chromatin. The estrogen receptor chromatin acceptor sites were tissue-specific and saturable. These chromatin acceptor sites differed in their affinity and capacity (number of binding sites per cell) for the estrogen and antiestrogen-receptor complexes. Thus, we suggest that the differences in the physiological actions of estrogens and antiestrogens may be related to their differential interaction with uterine chromatin subfractions. (Supported by NIH HD 13425).

2420 ANDROGEN BINDING IN CULTURED HUMAN FIBROBLASTS FROM PATIENTS WITH IDIOPATHIC HYPOSPADIAS. H.U. Schweikert*, W. Knauf and G. Romalo, Dept. of Internal Medicine, University of Bonn, D 5300 Bonn, W.-Germany.

Androgens stimulate development and growth of the external male genitalia. Since hypospadias represents the most common congenital abnormality in the male newborn and systematic studies on the mechanism of androgen action are lacking in this disorder, androgen binding (utilizing ^{3}H-methyltrienolone) was assessed in cultured fibroblasts from biopsies from genital skin of 12 patients with idiopathic hypospadias (IH). Binding was also determined in corresponding samples from 8 patients with normal genital development and 9 patients with known androgen resistance syndromes (Testicular Feminization, Reifenstein-Syndrome, 5α-Reductase-Deficiency) which served as controls. Finally, binding was measured in 10 samples of nongenital skin. Results: 1. Maximum specific binding (Bmax) in IH varied from undetectable to 15.5 (medium 5.6) fmol/mg protein. 2. Bmax in patients with normal genital development was between 12.2 - 17.9 fmol/mg protein. 3. Bmax in samples of patients with known androgen resistance syndromes were exactly in the range reported in previous literature. It is evident that Bmax in samples of patients with IH differs significantly ($p = 0.00215$ Mann-Whitney U test) from those with normal genital development. Thus, it seems reasonable to conclude that in some patients with IH the genital defect is caused by receptor deficiency.

Supported By Deutsche Forschungsgemeinschaft Schw 168/5-6.

2421 EFFECT OF AFLATOXIN ON ANDROGEN RECEPTOR AND BIOGENIC AMINES IN RAT TESTICULAR CYTOSOL. A.K.Srivastava* and U.S.Singh, Division of Biochemistry and Food Science, Indian Veterinary Research Institute, Izatnagar-243122, INDIA

Recent studies on male reproductive tract have revealed a drop in testosterone level and disruption of spermatogenesis due to aflatoxin administration in animals but the effect of aflatoxin on androgen receptor in testis has not been elucidated. In the present study we report our results of aflatoxin administration on androgen receptor and biogenic amines on rat testis. In rats, intubated with aflatoxin B1 (3 mg/kg body wt), androgen receptors were determined in testicular cytosol (105,000xg supernatant) using 3H-dihydrotestosterone (DHT) as a radiolignad by charcoal adsorption technique. The presence of high affinity saturable binding protein was observed and its specificity was established by competition studies. The cytosol of animals administered with aflatoxin showed significantly low levels of androgen receptor as compared to normal rats. Dopamine norepinephrine contents were also decreased in testis due to aflatoxin treatment. These results suggest a depletion of androgen receptor as well as decline in biogenic amine levels in rat testis which may hamper fertility in aflatoxin administered rats.

2422 REGULATION OF ANDROGEN RECEPTOR SYNTHESIS AND DEGRADATION IN A DUCTUS DEFERENS TUMOR CELL LINE (DDT_1MF-2). A.J. Syms*, J.S. Norris and R.G. Smith; Depts. of Urology and Cell Biology, Baylor College of Med., Houston, TX and (JSN) Dept. Med., Univ. of Arkansas School of Med. Sci., Little Rock, AR.

The DDT_1MF-2 cell line is differentially sensitive to and contains receptors for androgens and glucocorticoids. Cells maintained in serum free media for 48h contain 6.0 fmoles androgen receptors/μg DNA. Following treatment with [^{3}H]-methyltrienolone (R1881), androgen receptor concentration increases to 12.1 fmoles in 5h. Simultaneous treatment with 10 nM triamcinolone acetonide (TA) however, completely inhibits this elevation without altering the binding affinity (Kd 0.5 nM) of R1881 for the androgen receptor. The mechanisms involved in this regulation were investigated by labeling cells with dense amino acids enriched in the isotopes ^{2}H, ^{13}C and ^{15}N. Newly synthesized dense receptor (5.2S) was resolved from pre-existing receptors of normal density (4.4S) in 5-20% sucrose gradients containing 0.4M KCl. The rate of disappearance of the normal density receptor during incubation with dense amino acids was used to determine the half life ($t\frac{1}{2}$) of the androgen receptor. In the absence of androgens, where receptor was quantitated by post-labeling, the rate of decay followed 1st order kinetics with $t\frac{1}{2}$=3.2h. In the presence of 1 nM [^{3}H]-R1881 however, receptor levels remained stable for 2h and then declined with $t\frac{1}{2}$=6.2h. Therefore the observed elevation in androgen receptors can be attributed to an increase in receptor half-life. The addition of 10 nM TA did not reduce $t\frac{1}{2}$ of the receptor in the presence of R1881; thus glucocorticoid mediated repression is associated with a decrease in the *de novo* synthesis of the androgen receptor. Supported by NIH Grant #CA36264.

2423 DIMERIC 17β CARBOXAMIDE STEROIDS AS A TOOL FOR GLUCOCORTICOID RECEPTOR SUBUNIT STUDY.

B.Sablonnière, P.Formstecher* and M.Dautrevaux, Laboratoire de Biochimie structurale, Faculté de Médecine, 59045 LILLE, France.

According to the experimental conditions (buffer, temperature) the glucocorticoid receptor can be resolved in two forms by sucrose gradient centrifugation. The 4S form is often considered as a monomer bearing a single steroid binding site and the 8S form as a tetramer of 4S subunits. In such a case incubation in presence of dimeric steroids should yield dimerization of the 4S form and polymerization of the 8S one:

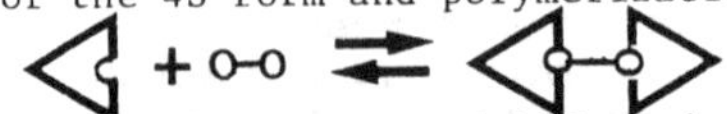

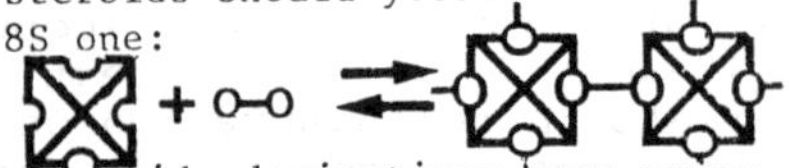

Thus various mono and bifonctional 17 βcarboxamide derivatives were prepared from [^{3}H] Dexamethasone, 40Ci/mM. Equilibrium and kinetic constants were determined in case of [^{3}H] DxB, a monomeric derivative: K_D = 0.7 10^{-7}M k_a =8.10^5 $M^{-1}.mn^{-1}$ and k_d =2.8 10^{-2} mn^{-1}. Owing to the short half life of the [^{3}H] DxB -receptor complex (25 mn), time consuming ultracentrifugation technique did not appear suitable for this complex characterization. Thus we resorted to high performance size-exclusion chromatography on TSK G3000 SW column, on which the 8S and 4S forms of the [^{3}H] Dexamethasone-receptor complexwere eluted in two peaks with retention times of 14mn and 19mn respectively (app.MW 390 KD and 98 KD); the [^{3}H] DxB-receptor complex giving a sharp 390 KD peak. In order to obtain the receptor concentration (2.10^{-7}M) needed to be in stoechiometric and saturating conditions with dimeric steroids, a partial purification of the unbound receptor was performed by protamine sulfate precipitation and hydroxyapatite adsorption. Work is now in progress with [^{3}H] dimeric 17 βcarboxamide derivatives.

2424 DECREASED HEPATIC GLUCOCORTICOID BINDING IN RATS DURING ACUTE INFECTION.

G.A. Saviolakis* and R.E. McCallum, U. S. Army Med. Res. Inst. Inf. Dis., Frederick, MD 21701 and Univ. of Oklahoma Health Sci. Ctr., Oklahoma City, OK 73190, USA

Acute infection is accompanied by complex changes in glucose (G) homeostasis. To determine the role of glucocorticoids (GC) in these changes we studied hepatic binding (B) of [^{3}H] dexamethasone (DEX) and GC induction of phosphoenolpyruvate carboxykinase (PEPCK), a key hepatic GC-induced gluconeogenic enzyme, activity in Fisher-Dunning rats infected (INF) with *Streptococcus pneumonieae* (1.8 x 10^3/100, i.p.). Control (C) rats were given heat-inactivated bacteria. Studies were performed at 48 hr, during the early phase of INF. Plasma insulin and GC values were 30% higher in INF than C animals, however, G levels were similar. High affinity specific B of DEX to hepatic cystosolic receptors was 59,540 ± 2,800 dpm/mg protein (P) in C but only 34,150 ± 2,000 dpm/mgP in INF rats. Scatchard analysis revealed that decreased binding was due to significant ($p <$ 0.05) reduction in the number of binding sites (596 ± 39 fmol/mgP in C vs 363 ± 24 fmol/mgP in INF) without a change in the DEX-receptor complex dissociation constant (K_D 10 nM). Parallel changes were observed in hepatic nuclear DEX binding. PEPCK activity was reduced in INF rats to 73% of C values (18.1 ± 1.6 U/mgP vs 24.8 ± 1.6 U/mgP). PEPCK activity could not be stimulated maximally in INF even with pharmacological doses of corticosterone (10 mg/100g), but it could be induced by dibutyryl cAMP. These data demonstrate that reduced GC binding sites are associated with impaired induction of PEPCK. Thus, glucocorticoid hormone resistance may partially explain altered glucoregulation during infection.

2425 HIGH AFFINITY BINDING OF THE PYRAZALOSTEROID, ^{3}H CORTIVAZOL, TO THE GLUCOCORTICOID RECEPTOR. J. Schlechte*, E. Thompson, S. Simons. Univ. of Iowa, Iowa City, Ia and Lab. Biochem/Chem, NIH, Bethesda, MD. USA

A ^{3}H ligand with greater potency than dexamethasone (DEX) would facilitate examination of glucocorticoid receptor regulation in cultured cells and human tissues. We compared the binding of ^{3}H cortivazol (CVZ), a pyrazalosteroid with potent glucocorticoid activity, and DEX to cytosol from the human leukemic cell line, CEM C7. As expected, ^{3}H DEX bound to a single class of receptors of uniform binding affinity (K_d 1x10^{-9}M; .46 pm/mg protein). In contrast, Scatchard analysis of ^{3}H CVZ binding revealed both high (6x10^{-10}M; .17 pm/mg protein) and low (9x10^{-9}M; .26 pm/mg protein) affinity binding sites. Two lines of evidence suggest that the CVZ binding sites are typical glucocorticoid receptors. In whole cells CVZ was 10 fold more potent than DEX in inducing glutamine synthetase, a marker of functional receptor activity. Cytosol receptor labeled with ^{3}H CVZ sedimented at ≃4S on 5-20% sucrose gradients with 0.4 M KCl. In addition, we covalently labeled receptor with ^{3}H dexamethasone mesylate and identified a single protein of MW≃90000 by polyacrylamide gel electrophoresis. We also studied a mutant CEM cell line (ICR-27) that has been previously characterized by ^{3}H DEX binding as lacking glucocorticoid receptor. Surprisingly, ^{3}H CVZ did bind to a single class of receptors in this cell line (K_d 1x10^{-9}M; .12 pm/mg protein). CVZ is a potent pyrazalosteroid that binds to 2 distinct binding sites that have characteristics of classical glucocorticoid receptors. This atypical steroid can be used to detect glucocorticoid binding sites in human leukemic cells that are not discernible by a more traditional ligand, and may be a superior ligand for examination of glucocorticoid hormone-receptor interaction.

2426 DECREASED INSULIN BINDING TO ERYTHROCYTES IN ACUTE HEPATITIS. Y.Nishimura*, I.Miyamoto, K.Ohsawa, A.Sanada, T.Yamamoto, H.Miyakoshi, Y.Noto and N.Hattori. First Department of Internal Medicine, Faculty of Medicine, Kanazawa University, Kanazawa, Ishikawa, Japan.

Decreased insulin binding to target tissues has been reported in liver diseases. This change is thought to be resulted from hyperinsulinemia often seen in the disorders and may lead to insulin resistance. However, the relationship between the change in insulin binding and the severity of hepatic damage has not been clarified. We studied, therefore, insulin binding to erythrocytes in 19 patients with acute hepatitis(AH) and 15 normal controls and related the changes in insulin binding to the severity of hepatic damage as represented by prothrombin time(PT). Insulin binding studies using erythrocytes were performed according to a modified method of Gambhir et al. Specific insulin binding to erythrocytes was significantly lower in patients with AH than in normal controls(4.78±0.17% vs. 6.14±0.35%; $p<0.001$). Scatchard analysis suggested that this difference was due to a decrease in the receptor number rather than the affinity. When patients with AH were divided into two groups according to their PT(Group A; PT≧13sec.: Group B; PT<13sec.), specific insulin binding was significantly lower in Group A than in Group B(4.34±0.17% vs. 5.17±0.24%; $p<0.02$). In addition, there was a significant inverse correlation between specific binding and PT. Fasting plasma glucose and insulin levels were comparable among Groups A, B and normal controls. Our results suggest that in acute hepatitis insulin binding to erythrocytes may be intimately related to the severity of hepatic damage itself rather than ambient insulin levels.

2427 GENETIC DEFECTS IN PROTEIN GLYCOSYLATION AND ABNORMAL INSULIN BINDING.
J.M. Podskalny*, A. McElduff, A. Robbins, and P. Gorden. Diabetes Branch, NIADDK, National Institutes of Health, Bethesda, Maryland 20205.

The insulin receptor is an integral membrane protein. Thus core glycosylation and complex carbohydrate processing can be important determinants of receptor function. We have studied insulin binding to parental Chinese hamster ovary (CHO) cells and to two mutants. B421 cells cannot synthesize mannosylphosphoryldolichol and are thus defective in core glycosylation while Lec 1.3c cells lack N-acetylglucosamine transferase I and are defective in complex carbohydrate processing. ^{125}I-Insulin bound to the wild type CHO cells and to both mutant cell lines. By the criteria of time and temperature dependence, competition for ^{125}I-insulin binding by anti-insulin receptor antibody, pH optimum, analogue specificity, curvilinear Scatchard analysis, and dissociability of bound hormone, the insulin was bound to a bona fide insulin receptor. The amount of insulin bound per mg protein in the cells were: wild type, 3.7 ± 1.5%; B421, 10.8 ± 2.3%; Lec 1.3c, 1.5 ± 0.4%. Likewise the 1/2 B_{max} for binding was different in the mutant cell lines. In parental CHO cells, 1/2 B_{max} was 2.6 ng/ml, in B421 0.75 ng/ml, and in Lec 1.3c 10 ng/ml. Thus, it appears that the binding of insulin to its receptor in B421 cells is of higher affinity than the wild type cells while the binding to Lec 1.3c cells is of lower affinity. These genetic studies indicate that insulin receptor carbohydrates are important determinants of receptor affinity.

2428 INSULIN RECEPTORS IN THE PREGNANT RAT'S MYOMETRIUM.
H. Sakamoto*, N. MacLusky, K. Den[1], S. Takagi[1] and F. Naftolin Dept. of Ob/Gyn, Yale University School of Medicine, New Haven, CT 06510 and (1) Dept. of Ob/Gyn, Nihon Univ., Tokyo, Japan

During pregnancy, uterine glycogen content rises until term, then decreases rapidly during labor (Chew and Renard, Biol. Reprod. 20:1111, 1979), suggesting its role as an energy source for uterine contractions. In nonpregnant animals, glycogen deposition is induced by estrogen (E). However, E treatment alone cannot achieve the high glycogen content found in pregnancy. Since muscle glucose uptake is stimulated by insulin (INS), we looked for INS binding in rat myometrium during pregnancy. Sprague-Dawley female rats were sacrificed on days 15, 20, 21 and 22 of pregnancy, and myometrium was processed to prepare cytosol, nuclear and plasma membrane fractions. E and progesterone receptors were determined in the cytosol and nuclei, and INS binding in the plasma membranes. The specificity of ^{125}I-INS binding was tested against porcine proinsulin, desalanine INS, desoctapeptide INS, rat prolactin, rat growth hormone and relaxin; the only effective inhibitor was desalanine INS. The Kd of INS binding was in the range of 6 x 10^{-11} to 10^{-10} M.

	Days Postconception				
	15	20	21	22	Postpartum
ERn[1]	1.07±0.05	1.58±0.09	1.71±0.06	3.25±0.20	0.89±0.20
PRn[1]	0.78±0.09	0.24±0.06	0.19±0.04	0.33±0.03	1.06±0.32
INS binding[1]	0.63±0.21	1.00±0.27	1.57±0.36	1.79±0.29	0.57±0.35
Glycogen[2]	0.41±0.09	0.81±0.13	0.66±0.32	1.38±0.17	0.50±0.21

(1) pmoles/mg DNA. ERn, PRn--nuclear E and P receptors. (2) g/100 g wet weight (Means±SEM)

The present data demonstrate INS specific binding sites in the pregnant rat's myometrium, which increase during the latter half of pregnancy in parallel with myometrial cell nuclear E receptor levels. Uterine glycogen content has been known to be influenced by sex steroids and blood sugar levels. Our demonstration of the presence of myometrial INS receptors and the concordance between ERn, INS binding and glycogen indicates a role for INS in the deposition of glycogen in preparation for labor.

2429 SOMATOSTATIN RECEPTORS IN RAT PITUITARY: LOCALIZATION BY AUTORADIOGRAPHY

D.C. Perry*, E.B. de Souza, D.C. Manning and S.H. Snyder, Department of Neuroscience, Johns Hopkins School of Medicine, 725 North Wolfe Street, Baltimore, MD 21205 U.S.A.

Somatostatin (SS) is widely distributed in mammalian tissues and potently inhibits the release of many peptide hormones. In the pituitary, SS inhibits release of growth hormone, TSH, ACTH and in certain circumstances, prolactin. Receptor binding sites for SS have been demonstrated in pituitary tumor cells and whole pituitary homogenates. In this study, we utilized iodinated analogs of SS ([^{125}I-Tyr^{11}]SS) and of SS28 ([Leu^{8}, DTrp^{22},^{125}I-Tyr^{25}]SS28) to label SS receptor sites in rat pituitary sections, according to the method of Young and Kuhar (Brain Res. 179: 255, 1979). Briefly, 10 micron frozen pituitary sections were incubated with ligand (15-25 pM) for 90 min at 22° in buffer containing bacitracin; blanks were defined as binding remaining in the presence of 100nM (DTrp^{22}) SS28. After rinsing twice for 30 min in buffer, sections were dried and apposed to LKB Ultrofilm or emulsion-coated coverslips. After suitable exposure and development, quantitation was performed by optical density measurement (film) or grain counting (coverslips). Specific binding of the SS and SS28 analogs was similar (O.D. 0.050±0.002 and 0.046±0.002, respectively). Labeling was uniform throughout the anterior pituitary. The binding potencies of several SS analogs in rat pituitary homogenates vs. both ligands correlated with the potency of the analogs in inhibiting growth hormone release. Thus, SS binding sites of appropriate pharmacology have been shown to be uniformly distributed throughout the rat anterior pituitary.

2430 [^{3}H]Dynorphin (1-8): A NEW USEFUL LIGAND TO CHARACTERIZE OPIOID RECEPTOR SUB-TYPES.

R. Quirion* and C. Pilapil, Douglas Hospital Research Centre, VERDUN, Québec, H4H 1R3, Canada.

The pro-dynorphin gene generates various opioid peptides such as Dynorphin A and B and the neo-endorphins. A dynorphin A fragment, dynorphin (1-8) appears to be the most abundant peptide derived from this precursor to be present in rat brain. Moreover, dynorphin A and its fragments probably act on their own opioid receptor sub-type (Corbett et al, Nature, 299, 79-81, 1982). Therefore, we decided to characterize the in vitro receptor binding profile of dynorphin (1-8) in brain. Under our incubation conditions (4°C plus 100 mM NaCl), [^{3}H]dynorphin (1-8) is stable for the duration of the incubation (60 min) with both rat and guinea pig membranes. [^{3}H]dynorphin (1-8) binds to a single class of sites in both species with K_d of 4.6 and 5.9 nM and B_{max} of 53 and 81 fmol/mg protein, respectively. Ligand selectivity pattern shows that under our incubation conditions, [^{3}H]dynorphin (1-8) binds almost exclusively to kappa opioid receptor sub-types (Dynorphins >>> enkephalins = β-endorphin; benzomorphans >>> morphine). The present data indicate that [^{3}H]dynorphin (1-8) is a suitable ligand to characterize opioid receptors and could be useful to precise the biochemical and pharmacological properties of the kappa sub-type.

2431 GROWTH HORMONE RESPONSES, BINDING AND RECEPTOR STRUCTURE IN RAT ADIPOCYTES
Jessica Schwartz* and C. Carter-Su, Dept Physiol, U Mich, Ann Arbor MI USA

Insulin-like responses to growth hormone (GH) can be demonstrated in a)adipose tissue from hypophysectomized (hypox) rats; b) adipose tissue from rats treated with antibodies to rat GH (ArGH) or c) preincubated adipose tissue or adipocytes from normal rats. The binding of ^{125}I-human GH (hGH*) to adipocytes did not correspond to the ability of tissue or cells to exhibit insulin-like responses to GH (stimulation of glucose oxidation). Cells from hypox rats bound less GH than cells from normal rats; ArGH treatment had no effect on the binding of hGH*, while in preincubated adipocytes GH binding was greater than that of freshly prepared cells. Since we have covalently labelled the GH receptor on adipocytes by cross-linking techniques, we further examined whether the properties of the GH receptor changed when either responses to or binding of GH changed. Bound hGH* was cross-linked to adipocytes with disuccinimidyl suberate, and membrane proteins labelled with hGH* were visualized using SDS polyacrylamide gels and autoradiography. Regardless of prior treatment, all adipocytes exhibited the prominent Mr=134,000 band and additional minor bands in the presence of reductant. Less Mr=134,000 protein was labelled in cells from hypox rats reflecting the decrease in GH binding. Otherwise, no significant differences in the overall banding pattern of membrane proteins were evident in reduced or non-reduced gels, using adipocytes from hypox or ArGH-treated rats, or in fresh vs preincubated cells. These findings suggest that changes in the ability of adipose tissue to show insulin-like responses to GH may not be associated with alterations in GH binding capability, or with large changes in the size or subunit structure of the GH receptor.

2432 TRANSLATION AND GLYCOSYLATION OF THE HUMAN EPIDERMAL GROWTH FACTOR RECEPTOR IN *XENOPUS LAEVIS* OOCYTES,
F. A. Simmen*, T. Z. Schulz, D. R. Headon, L. A. Gossett, and B. W. O'Malley, Dept. of Cell Biology, Baylor Coll. of Med., Houston, TX. 77030, USA; and G. Carpenter, Dept. of Biochemistry, Vanderbilt Univ., School of Med., Nashville, TN. 37232, USA.

The epidermal growth factor (EGF) receptor is a plasma membrane glycoprotein of MW 170K which mediates the multiple biological effects of EGF on target cells, including initiation of mitogenesis and cell differentiation. To initiate studies on the biosynthesis of this protein, we have undertaken translation of EGF receptor mRNA in *Xenopus* oocytes. Poly(A)$^+$-RNA from an epidermoid carcinoma cell line, A431, was microinjected into oocytes which were then incubated in Barth's medium containing [^{35}S]methionine. The oocytes were homogenized and the supernatant was incubated with a monospecific polyclonal antibody raised against purified A431 EGF receptor. The immunoprecipitate was collected and analyzed by SDS-PAGE. A [^{35}S]-labelled protein of MW 170K was synthesized and could be precipitated by several different antisera to EGF receptor. This protein comigrated with [^{35}S]-labelled EGF receptor from A431 cells. It was not synthesized by uninjected oocytes, nor did it precipitate with a control antiserum. Treatment with a deglycosylating agent, trifluoromethanesulfonic acid, caused a reduction in MW of the 170K protein. In conclusion, human EGF receptor mRNA can be translated in the *Xenopus* oocyte to yield a glycosylated protein of the correct MW. This now provides a suitable assay for EGF receptor mRNA and for the identification of cDNA clones. Supported by USPHS RR-05425 (TZS); NCl CA 24071, ACS BC-294 (G.C.)

2433 HIGH AFFINITY BINDING SITES (AEBS) FOR NON-STEROIDAL ANTIESTROGENS IN RAT LIVER MICROSOMES. C.K.W. Watts* and R.L. Sutherland, Ludwig Institute for Cancer Research, University of Sydney, Sydney, Australia.

The interactions of the non-steroidal antiestrogen Tamoxifen (TAM) with a specific binding site, which is distinct from the estrogen-receptor, were characterized in rat liver microsomal fraction. The subcellular distribution of the AEBS was determined following sub-cellular fractionation using differential centrifugation and discontinuous sucrose gradients. Conditions were defined which allowed solubilization of the microsomal AEBS with retention of binding activity. Scatchard analysis of equilibrium binding data obtained using [^{3}H] TAM showed that TAM binds to a single class of high affinity (K_D = 0.90±.05nM), non-interacting binding sites in rat liver microsomes (30.5 ± 4.9 pmol/mg microsomal protein). Competitive binding studies with triphenylethylene derivatives of the TAM and enclomiphene series established that the liver AEBS had a similar specificity to the AEBS present in other tissues. Structural changes in both the basic alkyl amino ether side chains and in the aromatic triphenylethylene portions of these compounds influenced binding affinity. The AEBS was concentrated in the rough microsomal fraction, most likely in the rough endoplasmic reticulum. Subsequent dissociation into ribosomal and membrane fractions showed that binding activity was associated only with the latter fraction. AEBS could not be solubilized from microsomes with 1M KCl, 0.5M acetic acid or by low concentrations of sodium cholate, but at higher detergent concentrations (>1%$^w/_v$) more than 20% of binding activity was solubilized. These results are consistent with the AEBS being an integral protein of rough endoplasmic reticulum in the rat liver.

2434 ALTERATIONS IN THE CONCENTRATIONS OF RETINOIC ACID BINDING PROTEINS (RABP) DURING CHEMICAL INDUCTION OF DYSPLASIA AND CANCER OF THE UTERINE CERVIX OF THE MOUSE. H. Zech*, W. M. Christopherson, J. L.Wittliff, Departments of Biochemistry and Pathology, University of Louisville, HSC, Louisville, Ky 4o 292, USA.

There is growing evidence, that the action of Vitamin A, an important nutrient for the maintenance of normal differentiation, is mediated by specific intracellular binding proteins in a manner similar to that of steroid hormones. Using topical application of the carcinogen methylcholanthrene to the mouse cervix three times a week for a total of 47 paintings, invasive cancer is preceeded by dysplasia, which is very similar to the human cervical carcinogenesis. 77% of the mice had developed invasive carcinomas and 16% dysplasia. Tissue samples were homogenized in phosphate buffer, centrifugated, an aliquot incubated with ^{3}H-Retinoic Acid (RA) alone or in the presence of a 1oo fold excess of RA, treated with charcoal, layered on a sucrose density gradient and centrifugated. RAPP sedimented in the 2 S region of the gradient. Normal cervices contained 465 fmol/mcp of the RAPP, as dysplasia developed, a significant rise to 1167 fmol /mcp of the RAPP was detectable. Cervices with squamous cell carcinomas contained 637 fmol/mcp of the RAPP. These data may indicate that the expression of the RAPP is altered during carcinogen induced tumor development, especially in its first phases, the development of dysplasias. Whether this simply reflects a change in the cellular composition of the cervix or in the state of differentiation of the cervical epithelium is presently unclear. This study was supported by the Marie Overbey Memorial Grant from the American Cancer Society.

2435 EFFECT OF DEXAMETHASONE ON THE ESTROGEN-LIKE STIMULATION OF UTERINE DNA SYNTHESIS BY DIMETHYLSULFOXIDE.

P.J. Stewart* and R.A. Webster. Department of Biological Sciences, University of Illinois at Chicago, Chicago, IL, 60680, USA.

Arachidonic acid metabolites (e.g. prostaglandins) have been suggested to play a key role in uterine hyperplasia. Previously we have shown that the intrauterine (i.u.) injection of cholera toxin in ovariectomized rats induces a uterine growth response similar in magnitude to that induced by the s.c. injection of estradiol. Dexamethasone (DEX), which interferes with arachidonic acid metabolism, inhibits the increase in DNA synthesis caused by either cholera toxin (i.u.) or estradiol (s.c.). In the present study we have examined the effect of dimethylsulfoxide (DMSO), which has various effects on cell membranes. The i.u. injection of DMSO in ovariectomized rats produced a 10.5-fold increase in uterine incorporation of ^{3}H-thymidine into DNA at 24 h after treatment (relative to uninjected control horns). Water (i.u.) increased incorporation 2-fold. Estradiol (s.c.) and cholera toxin (i.u.) increased incorporation 10.3-fold and 12-fold, respectively. The s.c. administration of DEX immediately prior to i.u. injection caused 89% inhibition of DMSO-increased thymidine incorporation. This degree of inhibition by DEX was comparable to that seen with estradiol (s.c.) and cholera toxin (i.u.). These results provide further evidence that arachidonic acid metabolites play an important role in uterine hyperplasia. Also, a common mechanism appears to be involved in the stimulation of uterine DNA synthesis by DMSO (i.u.), cholera toxin (i.u.) and estradiol (s.c.). (Supported by USPHS grant HD-14008).

2436 EFFECT OF HUMAN PLACENTAL AROMATASE INACTIVATORS ON RAT OVARIAN AROMATASE *IN VIVO*.

M. Tochigi*, C. Yarborough, Y. Osawa, †B. Tochigi, †T. Yoshida and †S. Takagi, Endo. Biochem. Dept., Medical Fndn. of Buffalo, NY 14203 USA; †Dept. of OB/GYN, Nihon Univ. Sch. of Med., Tokyo, Japan, 173.

An effective inactivator of aromatase may be useful in treatment of estrogen dependent disease and in the study of the mechanism of estrogen biosynthesis. 6β-Bromoandrostenedione (6β-BrA) and norethisterone (NET), known to be effective *in vitro*, were evaluated for *in vivo* activity in rats. In the first series, a suspension in sesame oil was injected subcutaneously to rats (BUF/N, 4 day cycling) at a dose of 50mg/Kg on the proestrous day, and the vaginal smear was checked every morning. For the second series, it was injected twice daily at 50mg/Kg/day for 4 days starting on the estrous day, and the pair of ovaries were homogenized in phosphate buffer and centrifuged at 105,000xg for 1 hr at 4°C. Aromatase activity of the precipitates was assayed by a ^{3}H-water method using [1β-^{3}H, 4-^{14}C]-androstenedione (6.16×10^5dpm^{3}H and 1.9×10^4dpm^{14}C, 48ng), NADPH (1mg), and BSA(5mg) in 1.5ml (0.1 M phosphate buffer, pH 7.5). NET stopped the estrus cycle at least for 16 days whereas the vehicle and 6β-BrA showed no effect. Aromatase activity of the rat ovary was 82±16.0 pmol/h/mg protein (mean ± SD) in the vehicle group, 37±16.1 with 6β-BrA and 60±17.6 with NET. The results indicate that both inactivators suppress rat ovarian aromatase activity *in vivo* but that the mechanism of action may be different. Supported by DHHS research grant HD04945 from NICHD and the J. H. Cummings Foundation.

2437 IDIOPATHIC HIRSUTISM:A POSSIBLE ROLE OF A PRIMITIVE ALTERATION IN PLASMA ANDROGEN BINDING. V. TOSCANO*, S. Caiola, M. Maroder, D. Casilli, R. Balducci°and F. Sciarra, Istituto di V Clinica Medica and °Istituto di Clinica Pediatrica,University of Rome,00100 Rome Italy.

Plasma 3α androstanediol(3αAd) is increased in all hirsute women and also in those with normal plasma levels of its precursors even if repeatedly evaluated during the menstrual cycle.The possible explanation of pathogenesis for this form of hirsutism may be:1)an increase in free testosterone fraction and MCR^{T},2)an increased utilization of normal plasma androgen at target tissue level.17 hirsute women (14-28 years)showing an isolated increase in plasma 3αAd (19.27±5.4SD ng/dl)were studied basally on day 6,7 of the menstrual cycle.An hirsute patient with CAH due to a 21OH deficiency (14 yrs)was also studied. Sex Hormone Binding Globulin (SHBG) was evaluated using a saturation method.Maximum binding number sites and Ka were calculated with Scatchard analysis. The results point out low plasma levels of SHBG in 13 cases and normal levels in 4 cases.The determination of Ka shows normal values in 7 cases and altered values in 10 cases.The patient with CAH presents low levels of SHBG and normal Ka value. On the basis of these results it may be concluded that some cases of peripheral hirsutism may be secondary to a primitive alteration of plasma androgen binding.

2438 PROGESTERONE STIMULATES THE AROMATASE ACTIVITY IN HUMAN ENDOMETRIAL STROMAL CELLS IN PRIMARY CELL CULTURE. L. Tseng, Dept. OB/GYN, HSC, SUNY @ Stony Brook, Stony Brook, New York 11794

Isolated human endometrial stromal cells were cultured in RPMI 1640 containing insulin, antibiotics and 10% fetal calf serum. After the stromal cells developed a confluent monolayer, estradiol (E2), progesterone (P) or both were separately added to the culture medium and cells were continuously incubated for various periods of time. Aromatase activities were measured in control and hormone treated cells by incubating the intact cells with [3H]testosterone (40 nM in medium = 200 nM in cells) and isolating the estrogens at the end of 3 hrs. E2 alone did not change the aromatase activity while P caused a 6->10 fold increase over the control values (1 to 5 fmol/mg protein-hour) and was further enhanced in the presence of E2 (20->100 fold). The stimulation of aromatase activity by P was found to be both time and dose dependent and blocked by actinomycin D. Maximal stimulation was reached after the stromal cells were treated with 300 nM P for 3 days. At 30 nM P, a concentration similar to the plasma level during the luteal phase of the menstrual cycle, 80% of maximal stimulation was noted. These results indicate that P stimulates the aromatase in endometrial stromal cells and E2 potentiates this stimulation. Much less effect of E2 and P on the aromatase activity was noted in endometrial epithelial glands. Supported by ACS.

2439 PLACENTAL AND LUTEAL STEROIDOGENESIS IN THE PREGNANT RAT. Meredith L. Warshaw*, Iqbal Khan, and Geula Gibori. Department of Physiology and Biophysics, College of Medicine, University of Illinois, Health Sciences Center, Chicago, Illinois 60612.

Recent investigations have suggested that both corpora lutea and placenta produce androgens in the pregnant rat and that high density lipoprotein serves as the major source of cholesterol for luteal steroidogenesis. The aim of this investigation was to compare the ability of luteal and placental tissues to produce androgens and to determine whether both tissues utilize cholesterol derived from high density lipoprotein for steroidogenesis. Corpora lutea or placental explants were incubated at 37°C for 3h in medium 199 containing 25mM Hepes under an atmosphere of 95% O_2- 5% CO_2. Corpora lutea produced 120 ± 20 pg/CL of testosterone and 252 ± 41 pg/CL of androstenedione, whereas placentas produced 651 ± 122 pg/placenta of testosterone versus $21{,}163 \pm 4423$ pg/placenta of androstenedione. Incubation with 500 ug of high density lipoprotein enhanced luteal production of progesterone and androgens by 69% and 70% respectively. In contrast, addition of high density lipoprotein to the media had no stimulatory effect on placental output of androgens. Results of this investigation indicate that placentas produce markedly more androgen than corpora lutea, and that placental steroidogenesis is less dependent on exogenous cholesterol than corpora lutea for maximal steroidogenesis. Supported by HD 11119.

2440 HYDROXYLATION OF [^{3}H]5α-ANDROSTANE-3β,17β-DIOL BY THE SAME HYPERPLASTIC HUMAN PROSTATE IN ORGAN AND CELL CULTURE. P. Ofner*, S.D. Spilman, R.L. Vena, P. Krinsky-Feibush and P.W. LeQuesne, Departments of Urology and Anatomy and Cellular Biology, Tufts University School of Medicine and Chemistry Department, Northeastern University, Boston, Massachusetts, USA.

Hydroxylation of 3β-hydroxy 5α-dihydro-C_{19}-steroids are terminal reactions by which male accessory sex organs dispose of intracellular androgens. Metabolic reactions facilitating cellular androgen egress are of particular interest in human benign prostatic hyperplasia where the elevated tissue contents of free total and bound nuclear 5α-dihydrotestosterone have been implicated in the etiology of the disease. Using TLC and HPLC for separation and subsequent crystallization to constant SA for identification of the radiometabolites, we here report substitution of hydroxyl groups at C-6α, C-7β and predominantly at C-7α of [^{3}H]5α-androstane-3β, 17β-diol on incubation of a physiological radiosubstrate concentration with the prostate adenoma in organ culture. Epithelial cells and fibroblasts were isolated from the same prostatectomy specimen by a collagenase-digestion differential-attachment procedure. Fibroblasts hydroxylated 5α-androstane-3β,17β-diol in primary monolayer culture mainly at C-6α, with extensive metabolism to 17-oxosteroids. Primary culture of epithelial cells substituted to the same extent at the three positions. Competing 3β-hydroxysteroid dehydrogenase exceeded hydroxylase activity only in epithelial-cell cultures. Our findings support previous evidence that both prostatic epithelial and stromal cells have the capacity to participate in androgen disposition by the 3β-hydroxysteroid pathway. (Supported by NSF grant PCM 7904073 and USPHS grant CA 29513).

2441 METABOLIC CLEARANCE RATE AND PRODUCTION RATE OF TESTOSTERONE IN A MALE WITH PROLACTINOMA. F. Oseko*, I. Umaki, M. Watanabe, S. Note, A. Taniguchi, T. Kono and H. Imura, Internal Medicine, Shimane Med. Univ. and Kyoto Univ., Shimane, Japan

In order to elucidate causes of hypogonadism seen in males with prolactin-secreting pituitary adenoma (PPA) rather often, metabolic clearance rate (MCR) and production rate (PR) of testosterone (T) and its plasma levels were measured in a man with PPA who had complained of sterility. The three parameters were determined before administration of bromocriptine (CB, 7.5 mg/day orally) and at two and half months after intitiation of CB when basal level of plasma prolactin had reduced to 12 ng/ml from 820 ng/ml. 1.5 μCi of tritiated T (^{3}H-T) in 10 ml saline was given intravenously to the patient and 12 ml of blood were drawn each time at 0, 5, 15, 25, 35, 45, 60, 90 and 120 min after the iv administration. ^{3}H-T in each sample was extracted and purified through two paper chromatographies and one thin layer chromatography. MCR was calculated from the two-hour long disappearance curve of ^{3}H-T. PR was obtained from a product of the MCR and concentration of plasma T assayed by RIA. The values of three parameters before and after CB treatment was 5.6 and 6.2 ng/ml for T, 752 and 1027 l/day for MCR and 4.3 and 6.4 mg/day for PR. The results suggested that low metabolism of T is partly responsible for hypogonadism in the male with PPA. After CB treatment his wife concieved.

2442 ISOLATION AND ANALYTICAL APPLICATIONS OF NOVEL BACTERIAL HYDROXYSTEROID DEHYDROGENASES (HSD). D. Payne* and P. Talalay, Dept. Pharmacology & Experimental Therapeutics, Johns Hopkins School of Medicine, Baltimore, MD 21205, U.S.A.

Many tissue steroids undergo reversible oxidoreductions of 3α-,3β-, and 17β-hydroxyl groups by positionally and sterically specific HSDs. We have isolated by enrichment culture several morphologically distinct soil bacteria which grow on estradiol-17β or testosterone as sole sources of carbon. These organisms contain various inducible, NAD-linked, highly active HSDs, that are suitable for steroid analyses (e.g. at subpicomol levels by enzymatic cycling; J. Biol. Chem. 257, 633, 1982). Significant quantities of 4 NAD-linked enzymes have been detected: 3α-, 3β-, 17β-, and (3 and 17)β-HSDs. Of most interest is an *Alcaligenes* sp. which contains 17β-HSD which (unlike the *P. testosteroni* enzyme) is chromatographically separable from a 3β-HSD. It has a specific activity 25-times that of the pure placental 17β-HSD and reacts at comparable rates with testosterone and estradiol-17β. We have purified this 17β-HSD from *Alcaligenes* sp. to homogeneity (specific activity > 200 I.U./mg) by ion exchange, affinity and adsorption chromatographies. The enzyme carries out highly selective oxidoreductions of 17β-hydroxyl groups of C_{18} and C_{19} steroids. The K_m for testosterone is 2.5 μM. No activity is observed with 3α-, 3β-, 6β-, 11α-, 11β-, 15α-, 20α-, or 20β-hydroxysteroids. This pure, and highly active 17β-HSD, is suitable for studies of androgen and estrogen metabolism in tissues and body fluids. (Supported by NIH Grant AM 07422).

2443 TESTOSTERONE SECRETION IS SEVERELY IMPAIRED AFTER HEPATECTOMY IN RATS AND DOGS. Ch. Sultan, B. St-Aubert, A. Bonardet, C. Astre, H. Joyeux and B. Descomps*, INSERM U.58 and C.R.L.C., C.H.U., 34060 Montpellier, France.

It is well established that the liver constitutes the principal site for androgen catabolism and inactivation. 90 % hepatectomy should therefore drastically alter the metabolic clearance of testosterone and increase its concentration in plasma. We studied the repercussion of 90 % hepatectomy on plasma testosterone in rats and dogs. In 90 % hepatectomized rats, plasma testosterone fell from 4.6 ± 0.5 (mean ± S.E.M.) ng/ml (controls) to 0.37 ± 0.07 and 0.39 ± 0.15 ng/ml at 24 h and 36 h respectively. These values are in the range of those obtained with castrated male rats : 0.10 ± 0.04 ng/ml. They are also significantly lower than those observed in sham operated male rats (1.7 ± 0.3 ng/ml, $p < 0.001$). By the same way, in 90 % hepatectomized dogs, the plasma testosterone level decreased from 3.22 ± 1.40 ng/ml (controls) to 0.15 ± 0.08 and 0.21 ± 0.1 ng/ml at 24 h and 48 h respectively. A general alteration of steroidogenic tissues by hepatectomy is unlikely since, at the same time, corticosterone secretion was not altered in hepatectomized animals. These results suggest that 90 % hepatectomy could sever a functional relationship between the liver and the testis in rats and dogs.

2444 SERUM STEROID RESPONSES TO A SINGLE INJECTION OF AN LHRH AGONIST IN DOG AND RAT. Y. Tremblay*, A. Bélanger and F. Labrie, MRC Group in Molecular Endocrinology, CHUL, Quebec G1V 4G2, Canada.

It has been recently demonstrated that there is species difference in the sensitivity of the hypophyso-gonadal response to chronic treatment with LHRH agonist in rat and dog. In the present study, we have investigated the effect of a single injection of [D-Tryp, des-Gly-NH_2^{10}] LHRH ethylamide on plasma progesterone (P), 17-hydroxyprogesterone (17-OH-P), dehydroepiandrosterone (DHEA), androstenedione (Δ^4-dione), androst-5-ene-3β,17β-diol (Δ^5-diol), androstane-3α,17β-diol (3α-diol), androstane-3β,17β-diol (3β-diol), testosterone (T) and dihydrotestosterone (DHT) levels in these two species. In the rat, the basal serum levels of P, 17-OH-P, DHEA, Δ^4, Δ^5, 3α-diol, 3β-diol, T and DHT were 3.5 ± 0.3, 0.5 ± 0.1, 0.09 ± 0.01, 3.0 ± 0.1, 0.2 ± 0.05, 1.3 ± 0.3, 0.4 ± 0.01, 2.7 ± 0.6, 0.3 ± 0.06 ng/ml, respectively. After injection of the agonist peptide in rat, a 1- to 3-fold increase of all steroids is observed while T levels is stimulated to 15 ± 1 ng/ml. In the dog, the basal steroid levels were 120 ± 35 (P), 105 ± 10 (17-OH-P), 300 ± 85 (DHEA), 455 ± 170 (Δ^4-dione), 165 ± 60 (Δ^5-diol), 190 ± 25 (3α-diol), 115 ± 20 (3β-diol), 2950 ± 1000 (T) and 130 ± 30 (DHT) pg/ml. In dog, LHRH agonist induces a marked stimulation of DHEA and Δ^5-diol (8-to 9-fold) while a small increase is observed for other steroid (1-2-fold). The present data indicate species difference in the testicular steroid response to LHRH analogue and show that plasma DHEA should be consider, in dog, as the marker of testicular steroid activity.

2445 PROOPIOMELANOCORTIN-DERIVED PEPTIDES ARE PRESENT IN TESTICULAR INTERSTITIAL FLUID (TIF) AND CHANGE IN RESPONSE TO ENDOCRINE MANIPULATIONS. M. Valenca* and A. Negro-Vilar, Reprod. Neuroendoc. Sect., Lab. Reprod. Devel. Tox., NIEHS, NIH, Research Triangle Park, NC 27709 USA.

Proopiomelanocortin (POMC)-derived peptides are present in the testis, but their role and the mechanism(s) regulating their production in the testis remain obscure. We searched for POMC-peptides in TIF, a functionally important compartment of the testis. Further, we evaluated the possible changes in POMC-peptide levels in TIF after administration of D-Ala^6, Gly^{10}, ethylamide LHRH (LHRH-A), a treatment that affects both the endocrine and gametogenic function of the testis. Using specific RIA's, we measured large amounts of β-Endorphin (β-End) and ACTH in TIF from adult rat testes. Serial dilutions of TIF showed parallelism with standards in both the β-End and ACTH RIA's. The levels of both peptides in TIF were many fold higher than those detected in peripheral plasma. At short intervals after intratesticular injection of the LHRH-A, TIF volume decreased and testosterone (T) levels increased. At longer time intervals and after systemic LHRH-A treatment, TIF vol. increased and T concentration decreased. Chronic treatment with the LHRH-A resulted in decreased testicular weight, and lower T levels and concentration in TIF. The effects of the LHRH-A on β-End levels in TIF were also biphasic, according to dose and length of treatment. Conclusions: 1) POMC-derived peptides are present in TIF; 2) treatments that affect androgen production and eventually germinal cell function concomitantly affect levels of those peptides in TIF. The data suggests important peptide-peptide interactions and paracrine-like functions for the above peptides in the testis.

2446 γ-GLUTAMYL TRANSPEPTIDASE (GTP) AND β-GLUCURONIDASE (GLR) IN NONGERMINAL CELL LINES OF TESTIS. T. Vanha-Perttula*, C.W. Bardin and J.P.Mather, The Population Council, New York, NY 10021, USA.

During early (0-30 d) testicular development in rat GTP rapidly increases and GLR decreases to adult levels. GTP has been proposed as a marker for Sertoli cells and GLR possibly for spermatogonia. In this study GTP and GLR were analysed in nongerminal cell lines originating from Sertoli (TM_4), Leydig (TM_3), myoid (TR-M) and endothelial (TR-1) cells of mouse and rat testes and propagated in serum-free F12/DME medium supplemented with 3F (Ins 10 μg/ml, TF 5 μg/ml, EGF 5 ng/ml), 3F+Cp (ibid + ceruloplasmin 10 IU/ml) or 8F (3F + FSH 100 ng/ml, HC 10^{-8}M, T 10^{-7}M, Prog 10^{-8}M, Vit E 200 ng/ml). GTP was measured with γ-GluNA and GlyGly as acceptor at pH 8.2 and GLR with p-NP-glucuronide at pH 4.0 in cell homogenates and chromatofocusing (pH-gradient 7-4 followed by NaCl-gradient 0-0.25 M) fractions. The highest specific activity (nmol/min.mg protein) of GTP in 3F medium was found in TR-M (2.51±0.28), while those in TM_4 (0.19±0.01), TM_3 (0.20±0.03) and TR-1 (0.26±0.01) were markedly lower. Neither 3F+Cp nor 8F caused any significant changes from these levels in any cell line. The highest GLR activity in 3F medium was found in TR-1 (8.64±1.02), while TM_4 (2.65±0.23), TM_3 (1.49±0.05) and TR-M (3.85±0.38) gave significantly lower activities with no obvious change in 3F+Cp and 8F medium. In chromatofocusing GTP was eluted close to pI 4.0 in all cell lines. In TR-M, however, another broad GLR peak was eluted at pI 6.2-5.2. These data suggest that GTP cannot unequivocally be ascribed as a marker for Sertoli cells or GLR for spermatogonia. Their activities in the nongerminal cell lines do not seem to be influenced by hormonal/growth factors.

2447 PITUITARY SECRETION OF LH AND FSH IN MALE HYPOGONADIC PATIENTS WITH SCHISTOSOMOSIS. I.T.N.Verreschi*, H.Vettorazzo Fº & J.G.H.Vieira. Div.of Endocrinology, Dept.of Medicine, Escola Paulista de Medicina,S.Paulo, Brazil.

Hypogonadism (Hg)is not uncommon among patients with Schistosomosis (Sch)-an endemic parasitic infection in Brazil-,mostly in forms involving the liver{hepato-intestinal(HI) and hepato-splenic(HS)},as opposed to its pure intestinal form(I).Also, the more severe the liver damage the more pronounced the degree of Hg. To characterize Hg we determined plasma testosterone(T) and gonadotropins responses to stimulation with LHRH in 33 adult males with different forms of Sch(I=15, HI=9, HS=9)and 10 age-matched healthy controls(C). Plasma T, LH and FSH were measured at hourly intervals during a continuous 4h IV infusion of 1 μg of LHRH in the recumbent and fasting subject. A 2h pre-infusion period was allowed to determine baseline and fluctuations of LH levels. Although clinical Hg was present in 10 patients(I=2, HI=4, HS=4),their basal T levels were not different from controls. No differences in LH fluctuations patterns were observed;also, averaged control values(I=18.6, HI=22.1, HS=23.7, C=17.5 mUI/ml) and its response to LHRH were not discriminative. FSH response to stimulation (mean± SEM) was significantly augmented in all Hg patients.

FSH(mUI/ml)	I	I Hg	HI	HI Hg	HS	HS Hg	C
control	4.3±0.2	10.8	5.5±0.9	9.5±2.2	7.6±1.1	10.8±3.1	4.4±0.6
peak (Δ%)	209	336	204	331	126	323	191

FSH but not T or LH responses to LHRH stimulation can discriminate Sch patients with Hg. Deficient LH or FSH reponses to LHRH were observed in none patient, excluding the pituitary as a cause of the Hg. The higher prevalence of Hg among patients with liver involvement suggests a possible defect in androgen metabolism. (This study was supported by CNPq, Brazil).

2448 IMMUNOREACTIVE CARCINOEMBRYONIC ANTIGEN-LIKE SUBSTANCE IN HUMAN SPERM. L.F. Wang, Y.C. Yan*, and S.S. Koide, The Population Council, New York, NY 10021

Membrane proteins extracted from human sperm with Triton X-100 interacted with monoclonal antibodies (MoAb) raised against carcinoembryonic antigen (CEA). The reaction was demonstrated by an ELISA method using second antibody conjugated with alkaline phosphatase. The amount of p-nitrophenylate released was determined by measuring the increase in absorbance at 405 nm. Absorbance values (corrected for background) were 0.940, 0.325, 0.171, and 0.095 with the anti-CEA MoAb diluted to 1:90, 1:270, 1:810, and 1:2430, respectively. The immunoreactive CEA-like substance was partially purified by gel filtration on Sephacryl S-100 column and was eluted in the void volume. Serum obtained from a mouse immunized with human sperm membrane proteins contained antibodies that interacted with CEA. The amount of ^{125}I-CEA bound by the antiserum diluted 1:128 was 10,497 cpm which decreased to 6,589 cpm on addition of authentic unlabeled CEA (20 ng) to the assay mixture. The absorbance (p-nitrophenylate hydrolyzed) obtained with the antiserum serially diluted to 1:50, 1:100, 1:500, and 1:2500 were 1.76, 1.51, 0.81, and 0.24, respectively. In conclusion, the human sperm contains immunoreactive CEA-like substance based on the findings that partially purified fraction of human sperm membrane proteins interacted with anti-CEA MoAb and that serum from mice immunized against human sperm membrane proteins possessed antibodies that reacted with authentic CEA. L.F. Wang and Y.C. Yan are fellows of the Rockefeller Foundation. Supported by Grant No. 8310 from the Rockefeller Foundation and from the Mellon Foundation. We thank Dr. Z. Liang, China and Dr. S. Leto for the semen.

2449 THE EFFECTS OF DIPHENYLHYDANTOIN (DPH) AND AMIODARONE ON THYROID HORMONE METABOLISM. M.C. Sheppard*, J.A. Franklyn, M. Gammage and D.B. Ramsden, Department of Medicine, University of Birmingham, Birmingham B15 2TH.

Several drugs may affect peripheral metabolism of thyroid hormones as well as their binding to transport proteins. We have measured free thyroxine and free triiodothyronine (fT4, fT3; Amerlex assays) in subjects receiving DPH and amiodarone to assess their effects on thyroid status. Euthyroid subjects on long-term DPH therapy (n=31) had lower free hormone levels compared to euthyroid controls (fT4 15.3±3.5* pmol/l, mean ± SD vs 17.2±3.9 in controls; fT3 5.9±1.6** pmol/l vs 7.4±1.8) with 6/31 subjects below normal for one or both values. Thyrotrophin (TSH) levels were unaltered. Addition of DPH at increasing concentrations to normal serum in vitro (therapeutic conc 7-17 μg/ml) increased fT4 and fT3 levels (fT4 21.7 ±0.7, fT3 6.2±0.3 untreated serum; fT4 23.1±1.7, fT3 6.4±0.1 at 12.5μg/ml DPH; fT4 26.2±1.2, fT3 6.9±0.4 at 25 μg/ml DPH, n=9). These changes are consistent with displacement of hormones from binding proteins and enhanced deiodination and clearance. Chronic amiodarone therapy in 21 clinically euthyroid subjects increased fT4 (22.3±6.6* vs 16.4±3.4 in controls) but decreased fT3 (3.9±0.8** vs 6.4±1.5) with 10/21 subjects below normal. TSH levels were significantly increased (3.8±2.2** mU/l vs 1.1±0.6). Addition of amiodarone to normal serum at therapeutic concentration (5 μg/ml) produced no change in measurements of fT4 or fT3. Free hormone changes in vivo were consistent with reduced conversion of T4 to T3. Conclusions: (a) low fT3 levels in euthyroid subjects on DPH suggest a change in cellular response to T3, or a T3 agonist action of DPH; (b) low fT3 and high TSH in patients on amiodarone may indicate mild hypothyroidism, a possible mechanism of therapeutic action of the drug. (*$p < 0.05$,** $p < 0.001$).

2450 RADIATION ASSOCIATED HYPERTHYROIDISM. K. Shimaoka*, S. Katayama, G. Osman and Y. Tsukada. Roswell Park Memorial Institute and SUNY at Buffalo, New York, U.S.A. and Saitama Medical School, Saitama, Japan.

Irradiation to the head and neck results in a higher incidence of both malignant and benign thyroid neoplasms as well as hypothyroidism. However, Graves' disease following thyroidal irradiation, manifested either by hyperthyroidism and/or exophthalmos is not a well-recognized entity. The present study, therefore, was designed to retrospectively find the therapeutic radiation exposure in 163 patients diagnosed to have hyperthyroidism at Roswell Park Memorial Institute from 1963 to 1983. Twenty-three patients (14%) had a previous irradiation history. Exophthalmos was observed in 5 cases. Eight patients had irradiation to the head and neck ranging up to 3,000 rads for benign diseases, mainly for acne. Another 6 cases received 3,000-7,700 rads to the head, neck and upper chest for malignant diseases. Their thyroid dose was calculated to be over 3,600 except two cases which had 260 and 300 rads. The other 9 patients received more than 2,800 rads to the abdomen and pelvis for gynecological malignancies. The thyroidal dose was estimated to be 30 to 200 rads, except one case which had 3,300 rads for concomitant supraclavicular irradiation. The mean latency between radiation exposure and onset of the disease was 14.2 ± 3.0 years, with a range of 3 months to 40 years. Anti-thyroglobulin and/or antimicrosomal antibodies were positive in 11 out of 16. LATS was also positive in 1 of 4. Positive TBII was observed in 3 of 4. The results suggest that irradiation to the head and neck as well as to the abdomen may precipitate the development of Grave's disease.

2451 THYROID FUNCTION IN NONTHYROIDAL ILLNESS: SPECIFIC CHANGES IN SERUM LEVELS OF THYROID HORMONES & CORRELATION OF THYROTROPIN(TSH) TO FREE THYROID HORMONES.

S.Shimoda,* H. Suzuki, M.Hiraiwa, Y. Suzuki and Y.Hashigami. Dept. of Endocrinology, Int. Med. Dokkyo Univ. Sch. Med., Tochigi, Japan.

In order to assess the thyroid function in patients with nonthyroidal illness, serum levels of thyroid hormones were examined in 292 sera from nonthyroidal illness(29 neoplastic patients, 22 patients with chronic hepatitis, 11 cirrhotic patients, 90 uremic patients under constant hemodialysis, 93 diabetics and 47 patients with cebrovascular accident) and 34 sera from healthy persons as a normal thyroid function. In these patients significant posirive correlations were found between age and total thyroxin(T4)(r=0.19, p<0.01), and age and reverse triiodothyronine(T3)(r=0.18, p<0.01). Significant negative correlation was also found between age and total T3(r=-o.23, p<0.01). As a whole the alterations in thyroid function in these patients were low total T3/free T3 and normal total T4/freeT4. Elevated serum level of reverse T3 was generally observed except for patients with uremia where significantly low level was observed. these characteristic changes were correlated with the severity of each original illness expressed as % motarity, serum levels of cholinesterase activity,blood urea hitrogen and diabetic control state. Performing multiple regression analysis in these patients, significant negative correlation coefficient was obtained between TSH and free T4. These findings suggest that decreased levels of serrum thyroid hormones in patients with nonthyroidal illness mean not only severity of suffered illness but also supposed presence of hypothyroid state, where free T4 would regulate strongly the secretion of TSH.

2452 A NEW TEST FOR ANTI-HUMAN THYROID TSH RECEPTOR ANTIBODIES USING PURIFIED TSH RECEPTOR.

T.Shinozawa*, Y.Ichikawa, T.Yoshida, K.Arikawa, S.Kawai, H.Oshima, H.Yamada, H.Tanaka, and M.Homma, Department of Internal Medicine, School of Medicine, Keio University, Shinjuku-ku, Tokyo, Japan.

We here describe a new method for directly detecting the anti-human thyroid TSH receptor antibodies (HTTRAb). (Method) Membrane fraction of Graves' thyroid was radioiodinated by a lactoperoxidase method, solubilized with Triton X-100 (^{125}I-soluble human thyroid membrane; SHTM*), and then purified for TSH receptor by affinity column (purified SHTM*). 1 μl of test serum is incubated with the anti-human IgG(Fc) antibody-Sepharose-4B bead complex at 4 C for 18 hrs, following which beads are incubated with SHTM*, or purified SHTM* at 22 C for 1 hr. The percent of SHTM* bound to the beads, minus the percent bound in serum-free blanks, is considered as specific. (Results) Specific binding using SHTM* (mean ± SD) were as follows: 10 Graves' disease, 1.7±1.0 %; 10 Hashimoto's disease, 1.0±0.8; 10 normals, 0.4±0.4, among which no significant differences were noticed. On the other hand, specific binding with purified SHTM*, considered as HTTRAb, of 10 Graves' patients including 3 with negative TDA (3.9±1.5%) were clearly separated from those in 10 Hashimoto's (-3.5±2.0)(P<0.001) and 9 normals (-3.3±2.0)(P<0.001). 2 TDA-positive nongoitrous hypothyroidism also showed positive HTTRAb. HTTRAb of Graves' serum, but not that of normal serum, increased dose-dependently, from 0.1 to 10 μl/tube, and displayed dose-dependent inhibition by b-TSH (up to 10 mU/tube). (Conclusion) We have developed a new sensitive and specific assay to detect directly the anti-human thyroid TSH receptor antibodies using the partially purified TSH receptors.

2453 EFFECT OF SEVERE IODINE DEFICIENCY ON KINETIC PARAMETERS FOR T_4 AND T_3 IN RATS. A. Shiroozu*, A. Taurog, and J.J. DiStefano III, UTHSCD, Dallas, TX 75235, and Biocybernetics Lab., UCLA, Los Angeles, CA 90024

Severe iodine deficiency was produced in rats fed a Remington low iodine diet (LID) and deionized drinking water for 2 months. Control rats received the same diet with KI-supplemented drinking water. Plasma disappearance curves for $^{125}I-T_4$ and $^{125}I-T_3$ were analyzed by a comprehensive kinetic procedure developed by DiStefano et al. (Endocrin. 110:198, 1982) Results for some of the kinetic parameters (expressed per 100g body wt) and for serum T_4 and T_3 levels are presented in the following table (m±SD).

Group		Serum Level T_4 (ng/ml)	Serum Level T_3 (ng/ml)	Plasma Clearance Rate (μl/min)	Production Rate (pg/min)	Mean Residence Time (min)	Total Body Pool (ng)
				T_4 kinetics			
LID	(6)	6±2	0.54±0.08	9.2±2.0	49±7.3	1229±269	60±17
LID+KI	(6)	52±8	0.76±0.13	12.1±1.2	626±108	898±38	564±114
p		<0.001	<0.01	<0.01	<<0.01	<0.01	<<0.01
				T_3 kinetics			
LID	(6)	8±2	0.66±0.23	235±58	170±14	675±50	100±14
LID+KI	(6)	52±2	0.69±0.09	264±45	205±26	757±126	135±24
p		<0.001	NS	NS	<0.05	NS	<0.01

Conclusions: T_4 production rate decreased more than 90% in severely iodine deficient rats, but T_3 production decreased only about 15%. Total body pools were similarly affected. Rats adapt to iodine deficiency by maintaining T_3 production at a nearly normal level.

2454 ACCUMULATION OF PROTEOGLYCAN IN PRETIBIAL MYXEDEMA TISSUE OF GRAVES' DISEASE. Y. Shishiba*, T. Tanaka, Y. Ozawa and T. Shimizu. Toranomon Hospital, Tokyo 105, Japan.

From the previous evidences indicating the accumulation of glycosaminoglycan (GAG) in pretibial myxedema (PM) tissue, we wondered if the GAG existed in a form of proteoglycan (PG). Biopsy specimens were obtained from the affected skin of two cases of PM and from the pretibial skin of two cases of non-thyroid disease and a case of hyperthyroid Graves' disease without PM. GAG was extracted with 4M guanidine-HCl and subjected to CsCl density gradient centrifugation. Bottom 1/4 fraction (D1) was examined for protein and GAG by measuring uronic acid. D1 from two cases of PM contained 143 and 333 μg of protein and 350 and 393 μg of uronic acid per g of tissue while those from other cases were less than detectable. With Sepharose 6B column chromatography, the uronic acid positive material was eluted at void volume. It was eluted at K_{av}=0.50 when digested with papain or treated with OH/BH_4 which extensively digested protein or released GAG from PG. The GAG was mainly composed of chondroitin sulfate or dermatan sulfate because the uronic acid positive material was destroyed by the digestion with chondroitinase ABC. To examine biosynthesis of PG, fibroblast culture obtained at skin biopsy was examined for the incorporation of $^{35}SO_4$. Radioactivity was incorporated into macromolecular moiety sensitive to papain digestion or OH/BH_4 treatment not only in fibroblast from cases of PM but also from non-thyroid disease or hyperthyroidism without PM. It is suggested that the accumulation of PG in PM is mainly due to the failure of tissue clearance of PG than to the enhanced biosynthesis.

2455 THYROTOXICOSIS IN ICELAND 1980-1982, AN EPIDEMIOLOGICAL SURVEY
G.SIGURDSSON *, A.HARALDSSON, S.Th.GUDMUNDSSON and G.LÁRUSSON
a working group on behalf of the Icelandic Endocrine Society, City Hospital, Reykjavík 108, Iceland.

Surveys of clinical thyrotoxicosis are rare and the incidence is still largely unknown. The Icelandic Endocrine Society instigated nationwide survey of clinical thyrotoxicosis in Iceland 1980-1982. Annual incidence was found to be 23.6/100 000 inhabitants with females outnumbering males by 4.2:1. 72% of all patients were aged 20-49. Grave´s disease was considered the cause in 83.3% of patients, uninodular goiter in 6,8% and multinodular goiter in 6.2%. Thyroiditis associated with transient thyrotoxicosis was found in 3.7% of cases. Silent thyroiditis seems thus to be comparatively rare cause of thyrotoxicosis in Iceland as in Europe. These Icelandic incidence figures are closely similiar to published figures from Denmark.

2456 TRIIODOTHYRONINE (T_3) TURNOVER IN NEONATAL RAT CEREBRAL CORTEX. RESPONSES TO HYPOTHYROIDISM.
J.E. Silva*, P. Matthews. Howard Hughes Medical Institute, Harvard Medical School, Boston, MA 02115 USA

Since 75% of the T_3 in rat cerebral cortex (Cx) is produced in situ from T_4, but only when serum T_4 is reduced by >80%, the Cx is biochemically hypothyroid, we examined the T_3 kinetics in this tissue and the responses to hypothyroidism. Congenitally hypothyroid (H) and euthyroid (Eu) 2 week old rats were injected with ^{125}I-T_4 and ^{131}I-T_3, the concentrations of which and those of the ^{125}I-T_3 were followed in Cx and serum. After injecting an excess of anti-T_3-antibody, Cx radioactive T_3 disappeared monoexponentially at a rate of 0.25 and $0.07h^{-1}$ in Eu and H rats respectively ($p < 0.001$). With this value and the equilibrium cortex/serum ratio of T_3, the rates of transfer of T_3 from plasma into the Cx and the local production rate of ^{125}I-T_3 from T_4 were derived. In spite of an 8-fold reduction in the Cx ^{125}I-T_4 in H rats, the production of ^{125}I-$T_3(T_4)$ was 4.8% of ^{125}I-T_4/g compared to 6.3 in Eu rats, representing a 6.3-fold greater efficiency in conversion. Because of the reduced removal rate of T_3 from Cx in H rats, the integrated local ^{125}I-$T_3(T_4)$ concentration was 70 (%/g).h vs only 26 in the Cx of Eu rats. In Eu rats, the calculated Cx T_4 and T_3 were 3.6 and 4.6 ng/g respectively. Total T_3 turnover was 1.17 ng/g/h; 82% of this was produced locally representing 14% of the total extrathyroidal T_3 production. Conclusions: Neonatal Cx has a high capacity to generate T_3. An increase of this capacity and, most importantly, a prolonged transit time of T_3 in the Cx, can protect this tissue from biochemical hypothyroidism in hypothyroxinemia during the neonatal period.

2457 ANGIOTENSIN-CONVERTING ENZYME ACTIVITY IS ALTERED IN THE HYPOTHYROID RAT.
R.C. Smallridge* and P.S. Verma, Walter Reed Army Institute of Research, Washington, D.C. 20307 USA

Serum angiotensin-converting enzyme (ACE) is affected by alterations in thyroid function in humans. To explore the effect of hypothyroidism on ACE, male Sprague-Dawley rats were thyroidectomized and, in selected studies groups received T_4 replacement (2.5 μg/100 g BW/day) for 14 days by osmotic minipump. ACE activity was measured in serum, and in lung and kidney homogenates, using a radiometric assay with ^{14}C-hippuryl-histidyl-leucine as substrate. Serum ACE rose by two weeks post-surgery and remained elevated at 5-8 weeks (59.6 ± 13.2 vs 47.2 ± 8.2 U/ml, $p < 0.0001$). Hypothyroid rats had an increase in both lung ACE activity (50.7 ± 9.8 vs 44.8 ± 5.8 U/mg protein in euthyroid rats; $p<0.05$) and kidney ACE (1.37 ± 0.37 vs 0.87 ± 0.15 U/mg protein; $p < 0.005$). T_4 therapy normalized enyzme activity in both tissues. Kinetic studies were performed on quadruplicate measurements from pooled group samples. In hypothyroid rats the Vmax was greater in both lung (65.58 vs. 54.26 U/mg protein; $p < 0.005$) and kidney (1.70 vs 1.29 U/mg protein; $p < 0.005$) and returned towards normal with T_4 treatment. The Kms were 1.36 and 2.15 mM in euthyroid lung and kidney, and were similar in the hypothyroid animals. Three enzyme inhibitors were tested: the IC_{50} was 7.5×10^{-9} M, 6×10^{-8} M, and 7×10^{-6} M for SQ 14,225, SQ 20,881, and angiotensin I, respectively, in both euthyroid and hypothyroid lung; similar results were obtained in kidney. These studies demonstrate that ACE activity increases in the hypothyroid rat. Hepatic angiotensinogen is known to be reduced and may be the proximate defect in the hypothyroid rat; ACE activity may increase as a compensatory response to low substrate levels.

2458 DEXAMETHASONE AND TRIIODOTHYRONINE INHIBIT GLYCOSAMINOGLYCAN SYNTHESIS THROUGH DIFFERENT PATHWAYS.
T.J. Smith*, Metabolic/Endocrine Disease Section, Medical College of Georgia and VA Medical Center, Augusta, Georgia.

Recent evidence suggests that Dexamethasone (Dex) and Triiodothyronine (T_3) can exert similar effects on specific cellular events. The present studies were designed to (1) characterize glucocorticoid inhibition of hyaluronate (HA) and glycosaminoglycan (GAG) accumulation in human skin fibroblasts, and (2) compare the effects of Dex with those recently described for T_3 (Smith et al, J Clin Invest 70:1066, 1982). Fibroblasts were grown to confluence in media containing 10% fetal calf serum. Dex (100nM) inhibited incorporation of either [^{3}H]acetate or [^{3}H]glucosamine into GAG and HA by 50-80% when added to culture medium 72 hrs prior to harvest. This inhibitory effect was half-maximal at 1 nM and maximal at 10nM. Inhibition occurred within 5 hrs and was near maximal by 25 hrs. To test stereospecificity, cultures were treated with testosterone (10nM) and progesterone (100nM). Neither inhibited GAG accumulation; however, progesterone (2μM) attenuated the response to Dex by ~57%. Analysis of Dex-treated cell layers which had been pulse-labeled and chased for 68 hrs failed to demonstrate any difference in the rate of [^{3}H]HA degradation. Both T_3 and Dex dose-dependently inhibited [^{3}H]GAG accumulation in cultures shifted to medium enriched with 10% thyroidectomized calf serum. Maximal effects of T_3 were achieved at 1 nM and those of Dex at 10 nM. Saturating concentrations of T_3 and Dex added alone inhibited [^{3}H]HA by 54% and 49% respectively. When both hormones were added, [^{3}H]HA accumulation was inhibited by 84%. These data suggest that different pathways were involved in the mediation of these effects on HA synthesis.

2459 REGULATIONS OF PHENOLIC AND NONPHENOLIC RING DEIODINASES BY SERUM COMPONENTS IN CULTURED CELLS. K. Sorimachi* and Y. Yasumura, Department of Microbiology, Dokkyo University School of Medicine, Mibu, Tochigi 321-02, Japan.

It was already reported that serum induced phenolic ring deiodinase, which contributes to the activation of T_4, in rat hepatoma cells. We have used monkey hepatocarcinoma cells (NCLP-6E), which retain much nonphenolic ring deiodinase contributing to the inactivation of T_4, for the investigation of the enzyme regulation by serum. Rat hepatoma cells (R-Y121B) were also used for the regulation of phenolic ring deiodinase. The cells, which had been cultured continuously at 0.5% serum, were treated with 10% serum (12 preparations) for 24 h at 37°C. Phenolic ring deiodinase activity was measured by the production of $^{125}I^-$ from [3',5'-^{125}I]T_3. A new method using [3',5'-^{125}I]T_4 was developed to measure nonphenolic ring deiodinase activity. When R-Y121B cells were treated with sera, 1-3 fold increases in phenolic ring deiodinase activity were observed. In NCLP-6E cells, 2-4 fold increases in nonphenolic ring deiodinase activity were observed. Dialysis of sera reduced the effect of serum on phenolic ring deiodinase activity (20-40%), but did not affect nonphenolic ring deiodinase activity in a few serum preparations and had a smaller effect on nonphenolic ring deiodinase in the others ($y = -0.142x + 95.37$, $r = -0.316$). These results indicate that at least two serum components, one dialyzable and the other undialyzable, regulate phenolic and nonphenolic ring deiodinase activities, and that the regulations of two enzyme activities are not identical in cell cultures.

2460 ROLE OF CORTISOL (C) IN THE PHYSIOLOGIC REGULATION OF TSH RELEASE IN MAN. C. Spencer*, M. Greenstadt, and J. Nicoloff, University of Southern California School of Medicine, Los Angeles, CA.

Although pharmacologic doses of cortisol (C) acutely inhibit TSH release in man, there is still controversy as to whether C exerts a regulatory influence on TSH under physiologic conditions. To address this issue, we obliterated C diurnal variation (DV), but maintained a physiologic C level by employing a 48-hour constant C infusion, (15-30 mg/d), together with metapyrone, (750 mg/p.o. q 4 hours) to block endogenous C, in 6 normals and 1 Addisonian subject. Blood was drawn every 4 hours for 2 days prior to, during and 2 days post infusion, for C and sensitive TSH measurement. C infusion (30 mg/d) produced similar mean C levels in the normal subjects as compared to the Addisonian (10.0±0.4 (S.E.) vs 11.0±0.9 ug/dl) indicating that all C was derived exogenously. The effect on TSH DV was assessed relative to the mean infusion C levels as percent of ambient mean C control. TSH DV was obliterated at high C levels, 173±5% of control, n=1; mostly suppressed in 2 studies at 128±4% and 155±6%, and blunted at 107±4%, n=5. In contrast, mean C below 70% produced an exaggerated, normally-timed TSH noctural surge in 3/4 subjects. Summary: 1) TSH DV is maintained when C DV is obliterated, provided that mean ambient C levels are not elevated. 2) Sustained C elevations within the physiologic range (>12 ug/dl), obliterate TSH DV. Since normal morning C values usually exceed 12 ug/dl and frequently persist above this value in non-thyroidal illness, we conclude that C levels do play a physiologic role in limiting the DV amplitude and possibly, the set-point of TSH release.

2461 EXTRANUCLEAR THYROID HORMONE ACTION.

Kenneth Sterling,* G. Tsuboyama and M.A. Brenner. VA Medical Center, Bronx, New York & Department of Medicine, Columbia University College of Physicians & Surgeons, New York, NY, USA.

The effect of triiodothyronine (T_3) on oxygen consumption (Q_{O_2}) at 37°C was measured polarographically in dispersed rat liver cells and cultured hepatocytes. The Q_{O_2} at 37°C was measured with the Clark oxygen electrode. In 22 preliminary experiments, enhancement (114% of control) was observed with T_3 in the medium for 2 hr at 3.3 nM ("physiological" level), and a greater effect (175%) with 300-1000 nM T_3 ("hyperthyroid" level). Thyroidectomized SD-NIH rats were kept on low I diet with $CaCl_2$ in drinking water over 4 wks to assure hypothyroidism (low serum T_4 and T_3). Liver cells were obtained by portal vein perfusion with oxygenated collagenase-enriched Krebs-Ringer bicarbonate buffer (Berry & Friend). Alternatively, cultured murine hepatocytes were grown by the MIT Cell Culture Center from seed cultures of the Naylor Dana Institute. Cells were grown to confluence in enriched (Williams) medium with serum depleted of thyroid hormones by treatment with Dowex AG 50W-X2 resin. Viability of cells from hypothyroid rats fasted 48 hr was shown by trypan blue exclusion and biochemical parameters prior to 2 hr incubations with or without added hormone. T_3 at 3.3 nM stimulated Q_{O_2} whether or not alanine (5-10 mM) was added as substrate. Cycloheximide (0.1 mM) was employed to inhibit new protein synthesis by incubated hepatocytes. In 6 experiments, T_3 at 3.3 nM enhanced Q_{O_2} by a mean of 137% ± 5.9% (SEM) of control despite the presence of the blocking agent. The results signify that liver cells show an early response to thyroid hormone by extranuclear pathways that do not require new protein synthesis.

2462 DIAGNOSIS OF PLASMA BINDING ABNORMALITIES IN EUTHYROID HYPERTHYROXINEMIA

J.R. Stockigt*, V. Stevens, S. Dyer, E.L. White, J.W. Barlow
Ewen Downie Metabolic Unit, Alfred Hospital, Melbourne 3181, Australia.

We have assessed the specificity of methods developed to identify familial dysalbuminemic hyperthyroxinemia (FDH), prealbumin-related hyperthyroxinemia (PRH) and autoantibody binding of T_4 (AAB). Subjects with hereditary TBG excess (>30 mg/l) and persistent hyperthyroxinemia without detectable binding abnormality (Unclass) were also studied. Euthyroidism was confirmed by TSH response to TRH.

Methods: 1. FDH: Charcoal uptake of ^{125}I T_4; Serum 1:100 + cold T_4 10^{-6}M; phosphate buffer; excess T_4 added to accentuate high-capacity binding.

2. PRH: ^{125}I T_4 immunopptn by anti-prealbumin; phosphate buffer.

3. AAB: Pptn of ^{125}I T_4 by 15% PEG 6000, barbitone buffer.

Results:

		Total T_4 nM	Percent ^{125}I T_4 Bound (mean±SD) Method 1	Method 2	Method 3
FDH	(≥10)	170-240	**85±3****	14±2	4±2
PRH	(5)	120-160	19±2	**44±6****	6±2
AAB	(5)	80-180	7±4	24±6	**16±6****
Unclass	(4)	175-220	14±5	24±5	5±2
TBG excess	(8)	120-290	12±5	11±3	5±1
Normal	(≥20)	60-150	14±6	24±4	4±1

**greater than normal, $p<.001$

Conclusion: As shown in the Table, each method is specific for one binding abnormality. Used together, these methods also identify euthyroid hyperthyroxinemia not due to known variations in plasma binding.

2463 PREVALENCE AND PATHOGENIC SIGNIFICANCE OF HYPOTHYROIDISM IN ESSENTIAL HYPERTENSION. D.H.P. Streeten*, G.H. Anderson, Jr., R. Chiang, H. Smulyan, SUNY Upstate Medical Center, Syracuse, NY 13210, USA.

Hypothyroidism sometimes causes reversible hypertension (Bing et al 1980, Streeten et al 1982). The prevalence of hypothyroidism, its relationship to hypertension, and the mechanism of its effect on BP, were studied in 433 untreated patients with essential hypertension. Twenty had primary hypothyroidism (serum T_4 <6 μg/dl, TSH >7 μIU/ml) while 3 had secondary hypothyroidism (serum T_4 <4.5 μg/dl, TSH <7 μIU/ml). All were treated with L-T_4 to restore normal serum T_4 and TSH levels. When BP was normal, antihypertensive medications were tapered. BP remained normal off all antihypertensive therapy (other than L-T_4) in 4 patients (1%) and fell strikingly or required reduced amounts of antihypertensive drugs to maintain normotension in 4 patients (1%). Among these 8 "L-T_4 responders", (1) plasma renin activity (after furosemide and standing 2 h) was normal (1.7-8.5 ng/ml/h) in 3, subnormal in 4 patients, (2) BP rose in 3 and was unchanged in 4 patients during saralasin infusion, and (3) plasma aldosterone was normally suppressed (below 8 ng/dl) by 0.9% NaCl, 2 Lit. I.V., in all 7 patients studied. Dye dilution studies revealed normal cardiac output and elevated systemic vascular resistance in 2 patients studied. L-T_4 replacement did not facilitate antihypertensive therapy in 7 patients, while the effects of L-T_4 therapy are not yet evident in 8 patients. Conclusion: Hypothyroidism was the cause of hypertension in at least 1% and an important pathogenic factor in another 1% of 433 essential hypertensive patients, acting by increasing peripheral vascular resistance, without mediation by the renin-angiotensin-aldosterone system.

2464 COUPLING OF IODOTYROSINE CATALYZED BY HUMAN THYROID PEROXIDASE IN VITRO. M. Sugawara* and C. Thayer, Endocrine Research Laboratory, Medical and Research Services, Wadsworth VA Medical Center, Department of Medicine, UCLA School of Medicine, Los Angeles, California, 90073, USA.

Coupling of iodotyrosine is the last step of thyroid hormone formation and is catalyzed by thyroid peroxidase (TPO). Because there has been no suitable method to demonstrate human TPO-catalyzed coupling reaction in vitro, we have developed a method. Human TPO was partially purified from 3 g of Graves' thyroid by Sephacryl S-300 filtration of trypsin-deoxycholate-treated TPO. Iodine-poor thyroglobulin (Tg) was obtained from a Graves' thyroid following propylthiouracil therapy by Bio-Gel filtration of the soluble fraction of the thyroid. Iodine-poor Tg (1 mg) was initially iodinated with 250 μM KI and 80 μM chloramine-T to provide hormonogenic iodotyrosines. Following dialysis, 0.3 mg of Tg was incubated with 10 μg Graves' TPO in the presence of an H_2O_2 source, coupling stimulator of 1 μM DIT, and 0.05 M phosphate buffer, pH 7.0 for 20 min at 37 C. The coupling activity was determined by the amount of newly formed T3 in Tg by radioimmunoassay following Pronase digestion of Tg. There was a linear increase in T3 formation up to 30 min. The optimal pH was 7.0 with T3 formation of 166 $\pm$ 14 ng/mg Tg (mean $\pm$ SD of triplicate samples). No coupling activity was seen at 0 or 70 C, or in the presence of 50 μM PTU. The coupling reaction was confirmed by the decrease of iodotyrosines and increase of iodothyronines when radiolabeled Tg in vitro was incubated under the identical conditions. This method should be useful for investigation of human TPO-catalyzed coupling reaction in vitro.

2465 IMPLICATIONS OF THE MATHEMATICAL MODELING OF TSH RESPONSE TO TRH. C.Swartz, Chicago Medical School, Chicago,IL.60064 and V.Wahby*, VA Medical Center and Yale Medical School, West Haven, CT.06516, U.S.A.

A simplified TRH test is suggested through a mathematical simulation for the TSH response on data from 57 TRH challenges. The equation representing the time course was derived to be: $C=P_1(e^{-P_3(T-P_4)}-e^{-P_2(T-P_4)})$, for T greater than P_4, where C is the elevation of TSH concentration over baseline, T is the time since TSH infusion, P_1 through P_4 are the coefficients for total TSH released, the rates of its release, elimination, and latency of release onset respectively and where C=0 for times less than or equal to P_4. Blood samples were collected at 15,30,45,60,90 and 120 minutes following 500 ug of IV TRH. A best fit of TSH response to time course equation was clearly defined in 45, whereas no realistic constraints had to be imposed on the coefficients in 25 of the 57 cases. Fit accuracy was within3.8% of peak elevation for the 45 cases and 4.5% for those with no clearly defined best fit.

For the 20 cases with best fit and no constraints, average release latency was 9.1 minutes, total TSH release was 13.7uU/ml and elimination half-life 49.5 minutes. These imply that the influence of release processes ends in 25 minutes. Peak blood levels correlated with total TSH release r=0.97 ($p < 0.001$). Only small variations were seen in the elimination rate, so a single blood level near the peak (average 35 minutes) along with the baseline are likely sufficient to determine the extent of TSH response. At least 2 blood levels are needed prior to the peak but after the latency period, to characterize the latency and rate of release. Best time for these may be when 1/3 and 2/3 of the release should have occurred, i.e. at 12.2 and 17.6 minutes after TRH.

2466 THE EFFECT OF MICROSOMAL ENZYME INDUCTION BY ZYXORIN /ALPHA-AETHYL-BENZHYDROL/ ON THE THYROXINE-TRIIODOTHYRONINE CONVERSION IN MAN. I.Szabolcs[+], G.Szilágyi, Zs.Kovács, G.Irsy and M.Góth, Postgraduate Medical School, 1389 Budapest, POB.112, Hungary

Zyxorin /alpha-aethyl-benzhydrol, Gedeon Richter ltd. Chemical Works, Hungary/ is a new compound with hepatic microsomal enzyme inducing activity and no other clinical effect. 3x900 mg/day was administered oral on 5 consecutive days and serum thyroxine /T-4/, triiodothyronine /T-3/, T-3-uptake and thyrotropin levels were measured before and on the 4th day of the treatment as well as 2 days after Zyxorin has been stopped. No significant change of hormone levels could be observed in 5 healthy adults and 4 patients with thyroxine treated hypothyroidism.In 8 euthyroid adults with vegetative complains this investigation was carried out on the basis of a prolonged Propranolol treatment /3x40 mg /day/.A significant T-4 decrease during Zyxorin treatment and a T-3 increase after Zyxorin withdrawal could be seen in this group. It is assumed, that Zyxorin induces the thyroxine metabolising microsomal enzymes inhibited by propranolol. Further investigations are necessary concerning a possible effect of Zyxorin in diseases with the "low T-3 syndrome".The work was supported by Gedeon Richter Pharmaceutical Works.

2467 REGULATION OF T_4 METABOLISM IN FASTED RAT LIVER. Y. Takabayashi*, M. Nishino, K. Kataoka, S. Matsuki and K. Itoh, Department of Internal Medicine, School of Medicine, Keio University and Itoh Hospital, Tokyo, Japan.

It is well known that the restriction of calorie intake, especially low carbohydrate diet, increases the conversion of T_4 to $_rT_3$. But the precise regulatory mechanism is still unclear. We studied how the intermediate metabolites of carbohydrate influence 5 or 5' -monodeiodination. SD rat livers fasted about 72 hrs, were homogenized in KRB buffer (Ph 7.4). And glucose, fructose, glucose 1-phosphate (G-1-P), glucose 6-phosphate (G-6-P), fructose 6-phosphate (F-6-P), fructose 1,6-bisphosphate (FBP), dehydroxyacetone phosphate (DHAP) or pyruvate, which was 50 to 100 times higher than physiological steady-state concentration except glucose and fructose, was added to the liver homogenate respectively. After 40 min preincubation with those chemicals, liver homogenate was incubated for further 10 min at 37°C with ℓ-T_4 (final concentration ; about 20 µg/dl) in triplicates. After these incubations liver homogenate was centrifuged at 3000 rpm (1630g), for 30 min. T_4, T_3 and $_rT_3$ in the supernatant were measured by RIA method. As the indicator of 5/5' monodeiodinase activity, $_rT_3/T_3$ ratio was calculated. In the pre-incubated groups with G-1-P, G-6-P, F-6-P, DHAP or pyruvate, $_rT_3/T_3$ ratios did not differ from the control group. But in the preincubated group with glucose, fructose or FBP, $_rT_3/T_3$ ratios decreased significantly ($P<0.05$). Especially FBP added group showed the lowest $_rT_3/T_3$ ratio. From these findings, we concluded that FBP has the potent regulatory role for the conversion of T_4 to T_3 or $_rT_3$.

2468 STUDIES ON T3 SUPPRESSION TEST: MECHANISM OF THE REBOUND PHASE OF POST T_3 UPTAKE FOLLOWING WITHDRAWAL OF ANTITHYROID DRUG THERAPY. M. Takahashi*, H. Shimizu, M. Murakami, K. Ohshima, M. Mori, Y. Shimomura, I. Kobayashi and S. Kobayashi, Division of Endocrinology, First Department of Internal Medicine, Gunma University School of Medicine, Maebashi 371, Japan.

The thyroid suppression test has been widely used to predict the outcome of medical treatment with antithyroid drug for Graves' disease. We have found that metylmercaptoimidazole(MMI) withdrawal resulted in a marked rebound of the post T_3 uptake in patients with sustained remission, while none of the patients showed the rebound after propylthiouracil(50 mg/day). An attempt was made to determine whether the rebound of the post T_3 uptake would relate to abnormal thyroid stimulator(s). Fifty patients with Graves' disease had been treated with MMI for 12 to 72 months . They were regarded as euthyroid in a maintenance of MMI(5 mg/day) at the time of investigation. Each patient was given 75 µg T_3 daily for 8 days and measured 24-h thyroid ^{131}I uptake(post T_3 uptake). Twenty patients had the post T_3 uptake less than 35 %(post T_3 uptake 20.7±2.2 %, Tg 47.8±7.1 ng/dl). Pronounced rebound of the post T_3 uptake occurred at one and 3 months after stopping MMI(one month 54.8±4.1 %, 3 months 41.9±4.3 %). On the other hand, circulating thyrotropin-receptor antibody(TRAb, Smith's kit) was not detected during the course of observation. Serum Tg did not change significantly. Serum T_4 and T_3 increased slightly, but were within normal ranges. Conclusion: The rebound phenomenon in the post T_3 uptake following goitrogen withdrawal was not associated with TRAb or TSH. Even in sustained remission, intrathyroidal mechanism may induce increased thyroid trapping which impedes their ability to relapse.

2469 COMPARISON OF SERUM T3/T4 RATIO BETWEEN PATIENTS WITH GRAVES' DISEASE AND THYROID HORMONE RESISTANCE.

J. Takamatsu*, K. Miki, H. Isaji, A. Kitazawa, K. Furukawa, T. Mozai, K. Kuma, Osaka Medical College, Takatsuki, Osaka 569, and Kuma Hospital, Kobe 652, Japan.

Chronic thyroid-stimulation by excessive thyrotropin(TSH) in man has not yet studied in vivo because of the methodological difficulties. Patients with thyroid hormone resistance(THR) have elevated serum T4 and T3 levels with inappropriately high serum TSH levels, so that the thyroid gland of THR was hyperactive secondary to chronic overstimulation by TSH. The present study aimed to compare the thyroid-stimulating effect of TSH and Graves' immunoglobulin. Forty patients who had been reported by some investigators to have THR (9 families and 10 sporadic patients including our two cases) were prospectively analyzed. At the time of diagnosis, 10 out of 40 patients had already undergone thyroidectomies or radioiodide therapy which may have caused a reduced thyroidal reserve, so that the group of treated patients were excluded in this study. Thyroid function of 30 untreated patients with THR was compared with that of 30 patients with untrated Graves' disease. Radioactive iodine uptake at 24 hours and serum T4 levels in THR were 43±13 % and 19.5 ± 4.8 μg/dl (mean ± SD), respectively, which were identical with those of Graves' patients (47 ± 20 % and 19.1 ± 5.2 μg/dl); while, serum T3 levels and serum T3/T4 ratios(ng/μg) in THR were significantly lower than those of Graves' patients (344 ± 82 vs 487 ± 205 ng/dl and 18.2 ± 5.7 vs 24.9 ± 6.5). The failure of T3-predominant production in patients with THR contrary to Graves' disease may merit further investigation.

2470 MODULATION BY ARACHIDONIC ACID CASCADE OF TSH-STIMULATED THYROID HORMONE RELEASE IN VITRO.

K. Takazawa*, Y. Kazama, T. Noguchi and T. Onaya, The Third Department of Internal Medicine, University of Yamanashi Medical School, Tamaho, Yamanashi-ken 409-38, Japan.

We previously reported that prostacyclin (PGI_2) markedly stimulated cyclic AMP formation and thyroid hormone release in vitro, and further that TSH-stimulated thyroid hormone release was significantly inhibited by PGI isomerase inhibitors, tranylcypromine and 15-HPETE. In the present study, various prostaglandins and their synthetic inhibitors in the arachidonic acid cascade were tested in vitro. Mouse thyroid lobes (one thyro-tracheal unit/tube) were incubated in Krebs-Ringer bicarbonate buffer at 37 C for 4 hours. Free thyroxine (fT_4) released in the incubation medium was measured by radioimmunoassay. PGD_2 significantly stimulated fT_4 release at 10^{-6}M. Thromboxane B_2, a known phagocytosis-stimulator, was not effective. Indomethacin, a well-known inhibitor of cyclo-oxygenase, did not inhibit TSH-stimulated fT_4 release at all at 3×10^{-5}M. In contrast, nordihydroguaiaretic acid, a lipoxygenase inhibitor, markedly depressed fT_4 release induced either by TSH or by dibutyryl cyclic AMP. Arachidonic acid itself significantly inhibited TSH stimulation and further bromophenacyl bromide, an inhibitor of phospholipase A_2, potentiated TSH stimulation. On the other hand, OKY-1580, an inhibitor of thyromboxane A_2 synthetase, significantly potentiated TSH stimulation at 10^{-7}M. Therefore, these results suggest that not only PGI_2 but other prostaglandins in the arachidonic acid cascade also play important roles in TSH stimulation of thyroid hormone release although more information is needed on the mechanisms of interactions among them.

2471 N^{α}-ACETYL-α- AND N^{α}-ACETYL-γ-ENDORPHIN: ENDOGENOUS,NON-OPIOID NEUROPEPTIDES WITH BIOLOGICAL ACTIVITY. V.M. Wiegant*, J.P.H. Burbach, J.E.C. Sykes, O. Gaffori, J. Verhoef and J.M.A. Sitsen, Rudolf Magnus Institute for Pharmacology, Univers. of Utrecht, Vondellaan 6, 3521 GD Utrecht, The Netherlands.

The β-endorphin (βE) fragments α-endorphin (αE; βE-(1-16)) and γ-endorphin (γE; βE-(1-17)), originally identified as opioid peptides, have been established as neuropeptides with distinct behavioural activities independent of their opioid properties. αE and γE occur in rat pituitary and brain. However, using combined HPLC- and RIA-techniques, we found that N^{α}-acetyl-α- and N^{α}-acetyl-γ-E represent the main forms of αE and γE in the neurointermediate lobe (NIL) of the pituitary and in brain structures remote from hypothalamus, whereas the anterior pituitary and the hypothalamus contained almost exclusively the non-acetylated forms. In addition, in vitro studies revealed that under basal, stimulatory and inhibitory conditions in addition to α-, β- and γ-E also the acetylated forms of these peptides were released from isolated NIL-cells. The peptides were purified from rat NILs and chemically characterized. N^{α}-acetyl-γE was further characterized with respect to its biological activities. In contrast to γE, the acetylated peptide appeared to be devoid of specific affinity for brain opiate binding sites. Yet, it retained the full γE-type behavioural activity. Similar observations were made with N^{α}-acetyl-αE. It is concluded that N^{α}-acetyl-α- and N^{α}-acetyl-γ-E are neuropeptides with non-opioid biological activities, produced and released by cells from the POMC system. It is suggested that N^{α}-acetylation represents not merely a mechanism for inactivation of opioid activities, but allows the organism to specifically select different sets of bioactivities enclosed in the endorphin sequence.

2472 IN SITU cDNA-mRNA HYBRIDIZATION HISTOCHEMISTRY OF POMC mRNA CONTAINING CELLS IN THE RAT BRAIN. J.N. Wilcox* and J.L. Roberts, Ctr. Repro. Sci., Colubia University College of Physicians and Surgeons, New York, N.Y. 10032 USA.

It has recently been shown that POMC peptides decrease in the hypothalamus after three weeks of estrogen exposure. We have done filter hybridizations on total RNA isolated from arcuate-median eminence microdissections to a POMC cDNA probe. Initial results from our laboratory suggest that POMC mRNA decreases in the rat hypothalamus after similar estrogen treatments. The POMC system in the brain is heterogeneous in that very few POMC cells concentrate radioactive estrogen. Therefore we have been developing the *in situ* cDNA-mRNA hybridization histochemistry technique to assess POMC gene expression at the level of the individual cell. We have thus demonstrated the presence of POMC mRNA and POMC peptides in a laminal layer of cells extending from the arcuate nucleus to the premammilary and mammilary nuclei. We have used the Bioquant II image analysis system to count silver grains and analyze data resulting from positive *in situ* hybridizations. Interestingly, we find that the density of silver grains (grains per sq mm) is consistent in different regions of positive cells, suggesting uniform distribution of the mRNA. The eventual goal of this research is to optimize the *in situ* technique to be able to use it to demonstrate regulatory changes in gene expression at the level of the individual neuron in the brain.

2473 PLASMA ACTH RESPONSES TO TRH IN PATIENTS WITH ACTH-SECRETING TUMORS. M.S. Zafar, R.C. Mellinger and M. Wisgerhof, Henry Ford Hospital, Detroit MI USA

Plasma ACTH concentrations have been reported to increase in response to TRH injection in some patients with Cushing's Syndrome. This observation suggests that the ACTH response to TRH might aid in distinguishing different classes of ACTH-secreting tumors. To assess the concept, we measured plasma ACTH, cortisol, TSH and prolactin levels before and after intravenous TRH administration in 10 patients with ACTH-secreting tumors.

Plasma ACTH, pg/ml before and after TRH

		CON	30 min.	60 min.
Cushing's Disease	1.	456	293	317
"	2.	56	-	83*
"	3.	272	289	291
"	4.	198	145	140
"	5.	99	91	-
Nelson's Syndrome	6.	103	66	45
"	7.	154	257*	165
"	8.	494	411	385
Ectopic ACTH se-	9.	765	747	775
creting tumor	10.	191	197	218*

Plasma ACTH concentration after TRH injection increased more than 10%* in three patients, one in each different class of ACTH-secreting tumor. Plasma cortisol did not change significantly after TRH injection but TSH and prolactin levels responded appropriately. A variable response of plasma ACTH to TRH in differing ACTH-secreting tumors - Cushing's Disease, Nelson's Syndrome and ectopic ACTH secreting tumors - suggests that this test is not useful to distinguish differing kinds of ACTH-secreting tumors.

2474 THE EFFECT OF OPIATE RECEPTORS BLOCKADE ON TSH RELEASE IN PATIENTS WITH HYPOTHYROIDISM. S.Zgliczyński*, B.Baranowska, M. Kaniewski, T.Górowski, A.Bednarski, Endocrinology Clinic, Cegłowska 80, 01-809 Warsaw, Poland

The aim of this study was to examine the effect of opiate receptors blockade with naloxone on the TSH release in patients with hypothyroidism. The material consisted of 10 women aged 26-78 years. The diagnosis of hypothyroidism was based on standard clinical and hormonal criteria. Serum triiodothyronine /T_3/, thyroxine /T_4/ and TSH concentrations were measured in all patients with RIA methods. Naloxone /Narcan/ was administered in bolus injection in a dose of 0.2 mg/kg of body weight. The blood samples were collected for TSH determination in basal conditions and 30,45 and 60 min after naloxone administration. The same procedure was applied after placebo. Serum TSH concentration significantly decreased 45 and 60 min after naloxone administration /$p < 0{,}01$, $p < 0{,}001$, respectively/. The decrease in serum TSH concentration was particularly pronounced in patients with severe hypothyroidism and with very high serum TSH concentrations. The opiate receptors blockade with naloxone had no effect on the TSH release in response to TRH. The results show the diminution of TSH release after opiate receptors blockade in patients with hypothyroidism and suggest that endogenous opiates may be important in the regulation of the hypothalamo- hypophyseal- thyroid system.

(Abstract 2770, p. 1645, also belongs to this section.)

2475 REGULATION OF THE CHOLESTEROL LYASE REACTION BY CYTOSOL IN THE RAT ADRENAL.

Y. Tamura*, T. Nishikawa, K. Mikami, Y. Saito and S. Yoshida, The 2nd Dept. of Internal Medicine, School of Medicine, Chiba Univ., Chiba 230, Japan.

The present experiments were carried out to clarify the mechanism of regulation of cholesterol lyase reaction which is the rate-limiting step in adrenal steroid biosynthesis by incubating adrenal mitochondria in the presence of emulsified cholesterol with cytosol protein prepared from control, hypox, and ACTH-treated rats. Pregnenolone formation was estimated by incubating isolated mitochondria with ^{14}C-cholesterol. The addition of native cytosols from control and ACTH-treated rats to an incubation mixture produced a dose-dependent decrease in the cholesterol lyase reaction, while delipidated cytosols did not show any inhibitory effect. A substrate mixture containing cholesterol and delipidated cytosol obtained from ACTH-treated animals produced a marked stimulation of the cholesterol lyase reaction. However, a substrate mixture containing cholesterol plus delipidated cytosols from control and hypophysectomized rats could not produce such an enhancement. The addition of both cAMP and protein kinase to the incubation mixture failed to increase pregnenolone formation. The present study has demonstrated that cAMP might not have a direct effect on the cholesterol lyase reaction, but some factor(s) in the delipidated cytosol induced by ACTH seems to regulate that reaction.

2476 A COMPARATIVE STUDY OF THE ACCELERATED METABOLISM OF VARIOUS GLUCOCORTICOIDS IN PATIENTS UNDER RIFAMPICIN THERAPY.

H. Tanaka*, S. Kawai, Y. Ichikawa, H. Oshima, H. Yamada, T. Yoshida, T. Shinozawa, K. Arikawa, and M. Homma, School of Medicine, Keio University, Tokyo 160, Japan.

A patient with active collagen disease who was treated with prednisolone and rifampicin (RFP) improved after discontinuance of RFP or after changing the kind of glucocorticoid (GC) from prednisolone to equivalent dose of cortisol under re-administered RFP. These phenomena prompted us to perform a comparative study of the metabolism of various GCs in patients under RFP. After 1 mg of betamethasone was administered on the previous night for suppression of endogenous cortisol, 1 mg each of cortisol, prednisolone and dexamethasone were given iv simultaneously. Plasma GC levels of periodically collected blood samples were assayed by respective RIA after separation by paper chromatography. The results of t1/2 and MCR of cortisol, prednisolone and dexamethasone in 11 patients under RFP were as follows: t1/2,1.6*± 0.4(M±SD), 1.4*±0.3 and 1.3*±0.3 h; MCR,150±60, 139*±57 and 775*±179 l/day/m^2, respectively (*P<0.01 vs. 16 normal controls: t1/2, 2.1±0.2,2.5±0.7 and 3.5±1.0 h; MCR, 114±20, 75±25 and 153±45 l/day/m^2). When these data were expressed as % of means of t1/2 and MCR in normals, the means of %-t1/2 were 75, 56, and 36 %, and those of %-MCR were 131, 186 and 506 %, in the same order. In addition, 5 patients examined also after discontinuance of RFP showed normalization of these parameters. In conclusion, marked differences in the degrees of accelerated metabolism, the order of which was dexamethasone, prednisolone and cortisol, in patients under RFP were observed. Although the reasons for the differences remain to be proved, these results are very important in concurrent clinical use of GC and RFP.

2477 **NORMATIVE VALUES OF 17-HYDROXYPROGESTERONE USING WHOLE BLOOD DISC FILTER PAPER SPECIMENS IN PREMATURE NEWBORNS.**
J.W. Temeck*, S. Pang, B. Burke, M.I. New, Division of Pediatric Endocrinology, The New York Hospital-Cornell Medical Center, 525 East 68th Street, New York, N.Y. 10021 U.S.A.

Due to the high incidence of false positive results in the premature newborn population in a newborn screening program for congenital adrenal hyperplasia (CAH), reference normative values of 17-hydroxyprogesterone (17-OHP) in premature newborns were established. The 17-OHP levels in 136 filter paper specimens impregnated with capillary whole blood from 80 premature newborns were compared to those of 4569 full-term newborns. Less than 1% of full-term infants had 17-OHP values greater than 20 pg/disc, compared to 16% of premature infants with values greater than 20 pg/disc. The data were analyzed according to the weight, equivalent gestational age (EGA = gestational age + post-natal age), age after birth, and degree of stress (the baby's medical condition) on the day the sample was obtained. There was a greater percentage of elevated 17-OHP levels in babies less than 2500 gms, under 37 wks EGA, and less than 10 days of life at the time of the specimen collection. In addition, stressed infants had significantly higher 17-OHP levels than well or non-stressed infants. There was a 1.25% (1/80) incidence of false positive 17-OHP levels in the group studied. This occurred in a ten-day old infant who was on a respirator, weighed 1,465 gms and was 32.4 wks EGA at the time of the specimen collection. This study emphasizes the importance of appropriate newborn reference data of 17-OHP when presented with an infant who has an elevated serum 17-OHP level.

2478 ATTEMPTS TO DEFINE A CORRELATION BETWEEN ADRENAL CONCENTRATIONS OF O,P'-DDD AND IN VITRO STEROID SYNTHESIS .
Y.Touitou*, A.J.Moolenar, A.Bogdan, A.Auzéby, J.P.Luton and C.Touitou, Laboratoire de Biochimie, Faculté de Médecine Pitié-Salpêtrière, 75013-Paris, France ; University Hospital, Leiden and Hopital Cochin Paris, France .

It is well known that plasma levels of o,p'-DDD are not related with the clinical and/or biological effects of the drug. In this study we looked for a possible correlation between concentrations of the drug in the adrenals of 7 patients (4 carcinomas, 3 hyperplasias) preoperatively treated with o,p'-DDD (total dose : 300-3400g) and *in vitro* steroid synthesis. o,p'-DDD was assayed by a GLC method previously published (Moolenar *et al*. Clin. Chim. Acta 1977, 76, 216) . *In vitro* incubations with tritiated precursors (progesterone, 17 OHP, 11-deoxycortisol) were performed as previously described (Touitou *et al*. J. Steroid Biochem. 1978, 9, 1217) . Due to the affinity of o,p'-DDD for lipids, the drug to lipid ratios (DLR) were also computed in each adrenal tissue . The following results were obtained : 1) o,p'-DDD concentrations were very different from one tissue to another, mean ± SEM : 61.5±28.9 μg per 400 mg tissue ; 2) using DLR these differences were obliterated (2.0 ± 0.2 μg per mg lipids) ; 3) cortisol and cortisone synthesis in adrenal carcinomas (3-17%) could not be correlated with drug concentration ; 4) In hyperplastic adrenals a strong inhibition of 11 β-hydroxylase activity (< 2% of steroids synthesized) occurred with DLR as low as 0.7 to 1.4. o,p'-DDD concentrations were strongly linked to the lipid content of adrenals and thus, only the drug to lipid ratio seems able to provide a reproductible index of the tissular impregnation .

2479 IMMUNOHISTOCHEMICAL DETECTION OF CHROMOGRANIN A-RELATED PROTEINS IN DIVERSE ENDOCRINE CELLS.

M. Tsukada*, T. Takano, M. Yoneda, K. Takatsuki and A. Tomita, 1st Department of Medicine, Nagoya University School of Medicine, Nagoya, Japan.

Chromogranin A (CGA) and parathyroid secretory protein (PSP) are glycoproteins contained in the secretory granules and released together with hormones, catecholamines and parathormone, respectively. Similarities between these proteins in their molecular weight, amino acid and carbohydrate compositions, N-terminal amino acid sequence and immunological properties have been reported recently. Moreover, we have demonstrated the presence of proteins immunologically indistinguishable from PSP in extracts of several endocrine tissues. The present studies were undertaken, therefore, to localize the cells containing CGA/PSP-related proteins in various bovine tissues. By an indirect immunoperoxydase method using antisera against highly purified bovine CGA, following cells were stained: most cells of the adrenal medulla, parathyroid parenchymal cells, a few cells scattering in the parafollicular space of the thyroid, some cells in the anterior pituitary and the cells in the periphery of the pancreatic islet. In addition to these classical endocrine cells, some gastric, duodenal and ileac epithelial cells, which showed a distribution similar to those producing gastrointestinal hormones, revealed positive reaction. Although function of CGA, PSP and related proteins is yet unknown, their presence in a certain endocrine cell types suggest that they are involved in the common secretory mechanism. Exact identification of the cells containing CGA/PSP-related proteins in respect to their specific hormone production appears to be important.

2480 RIA AND CLA ASSAYS OF PREGNENOLONE FORMATION IN RAT ADRENAL MITOCHONDRIAL INCUBATIONS WITH LIPOPROTEIN-CHOLESTEROL DEPLETED RAT PLASMA.

Frank Ungar* and Fortuna Kohen[1], Weizmann Institute of Science, Rehovot, Israel[1], and University of Minnesota, Minnesota, USA.

Rat adrenal preparations after *in vivo* treatment with 4-aminopyrazolopyrimidine (4-APP) were assayed for pregnenolone accumulated in the presence of cyanoketone blocking agent and with added normal or lipoprotein-cholesterol depleted plasma. Radioactive (RIA) and chemiluminescence (CLA) immunoassays used an antibody to pregnenolone-3-HS-alb obtained from P. Vecsei (Heidelberg). The ligand for CLA was a complex of N-hexylisoluminol linked by a C_{16}-thio group to Δ^{16}-pregnenolone starting material: assay range was 16 to 500 pg. Intact mitochondria were isolated in 0.25 M sucrose, or in 0.154 M KCL from controls and from rats pre-treated with 4-APP (20 mg/kg) for two days. The morning of the third day rats received saline, aminoglutethimide (AG), or cycloheximide (CHX), 10 mg/kg IP, one hour before, and all received 1 U ACTH ½-hr before decapitation. Low-Cholesterol plasma from 4-APP treated rat (A), or normal rat (D) plasma was added to mitochondria from (A) or (D). In all cases pregnenolone was increased (2 to 4 fold) by normal or cholesterol-depleted plasma; stimulation by A plasma $\geqq$ D plasma, both $\gg$ added adrenal cytosol. The greatest increase in pregnenolone formation was after 4-APP+AG+ACTH treatment and with added low cholesterol (A) plasma. Media also were assayed for corticosterone (RIA) or pregnenolone (RIA or CLA) with ACTH $\pm$ AG, using isolated intact adrenal cells and quartered adrenals obtained from 4-APP treated rats.

2481 ENKEPHALINS IN ADRENAL CORTEX: THE EFFECTS OF DENERVATION, SURGICAL STRESS, ACTH AND HYPOPHYSECTOMY. C.D. Unsworth and O.H. Viveros*, Dept. of Medicinal Biochemistry, The Wellcome Research Labs., Research Triangle Park, NC 27709, U.S.A.

Acid extracts of mammalian adrenal cortex (rat, ox, dog) displace ^{125}I-[D-ala^2,D-leu^5]-enkephalin from opioid receptors in rat brain membranes. Most of this native opioid peptide activity (NOP) co-eluted with met- and leu-enkephalin on HPLC. Total opioid activity (TOP) was measured after digesting the extracts with trypsin and carboxypeptidase B. Thus, cryptic opioid peptides (COP = TOP minus NOP) are a measure of precursor-contained enkephalin sequences. Rat adrenal glomerulosa (G), fasciculata-reticularis (FR) and medulla contain the following amounts of COP and NOP (pmole/gland of leu-enkephalin equivalents, mean ± S.E.), respectively: 6.07 ± 1.10/0.82 ± 0.14; 9.71 ± 1.42/1.52 ± 0.17; 8.26 ± 1.08/ 1.11 ± 0.21. Left adrenal denervation was performed to assess the contribution of enkephalinergic terminals to adrenocortical OP levels. This produced a bilateral decrease in NOP of the G and RF 24 hr later that recovered between 7 and 14 days postoperation and which was probably the result of surgical stress. Changes were larger and more prolonged in the right cortex. Reticularis-fasciculata COP showed an increase simultaneous with the recovery of NOP levels. The cortical OP changes differed in magnitude and time course from those observed in the adrenal medulla. Two weeks after hypophysectomy NOP and COP levels/gland in G and RF decreased to one-third and one-half, respectively, but OP/mg protein showed no change in G and doubled in the RF. ACTH (10 U/kg i.p.) resulted 24 hr later in a 70% increase in COP levels and no change of NOP in the FR; no changes were observed in G. In conclusion, OP of the adrenal cortex cannot be accounted for by nerve terminals of extraadrenal neurons nor by ectopic chromaffin tissue but are probably contained in adrenocortical cells. The control of adrenocortical OP seems to be a complex process involving neural and hormonal regulation of tissue levels, synthesis and processing.

2482 THE RELATIVE IMPORTANCE OF EPISODIC VERSUS CONTINUOUS CORTISOL SECRETION IN NORMAL MEN AND PATIENTS WITH CUSHING'S DISEASE OR BIPOLAR DEPRESSION. E. Van Cauter*, E. Honinckx, P. Linkowski and S. Refetoff, School of Medicine, Free University of Brussels, Belgium and Department of Medicine, The University of Chicago, Chicago, Illinois USA.

The normal 24-h profile of plasma cortisol (F) could result from either 1) a continuous circadian secretion with superimposed episodic bursts or 2) a circadian variation in the magnitude of episodic bursts without continuous secretion. To determine whether there exists a continuous secretion of F, we developed a computer program deducing the adrenal secretion from the plasma levels by fitting a 2-exponential model with a short (3.5-6 min) and a long (60-85 min) half-life for F distribution and metabolism. We computed the pattern of adrenal secretion from 24-h profiles of plasma F obtained by sampling every 15 min 8 normal subjects (mean level: 5.7 ± 0.7 μg/dl), 3 patients with Cushing's disease (CD; mean level: 15.9 ± 2.3 μg/dl) and 4 bipolar depressed patients (BPd) with hypercortisolism without clinical evidence of Cushing's (mean level: 18.4 ± 5.2 μg/dl). In normals, the best fit corresponded to a pattern of adrenal secretion consisting of pulses alternating with intervals without any secretion. The precision of the fit averaged 6.5 ± 1.7%. A similar result was obtained in BPd patients. In contrast, uninterrupted F release characterized patients with CD. These results indicate 1) that the normal secretion of F is entirely episodic without continuous component; 2) that hypercortisolism in CD is associated with continuous secretion and dampened pulsatile release; 3) that hypercortisolism in BPd is associated with enhanced pulsatility without continuous secretion.

2483 STIMULATION OF GONADAL STEROID SYNTHESIS BY CHRONIC ACTH EXCESS IN PATIENTS WITH ADRENOCORTICAL INSUFFICIENCY.

H.Vierhapper*, P.Nowotny, W.Waldhäusl and E.Nowotny, Division of Clinical Endocrinology and Diabetes mellitus, I.Medizinische Universitätsklinik, A-1090 Wien (Vienna) Austria.

Analysis of 24 hour urinary steroid excretion was performed by capillary gas-chromatography in 6 patients (5 men, one woman) with adrenocortical insufficiency. 10 healthy subjects (5 men, 5 women) served as controls. The excretion of cholesterol was similar in patients and in controls. A complete absence of all 21-hydroxylated steroid metabolites was seen in patients with adrenocortical insufficiency, whereas the excretion of several steroids lacking hydroxylation in the 21-position (pregnenolone, pregnenetriol, pregnanetriol, and 11-ketoandrosterone) was markedly increased. This pattern of steroid excretion was unchanged in patients with adrenocortical insufficiency both, following stimulation with 1-24 ACTH and after suppression with dexamethasone, whereas the healthy controls exhibited the expected changes in the excretion of steroids. These results indicate that pathologically elevated concentrations of ACTH in adrenocortical insufficiency stimulate early steps of gonadal steroid synthesis. In addition the presence of 11-ketoandrosterone in the urine of patients with adrenocortical insufficiency demonstrates that chronic ACTH excess in this disorder induces some activity of 11ß-hydroxylase, an enzyme not found in the gonads under physiological conditions.

2484 ADRENAL-VENOUS-BLOOD- AND PERIPHERAL-BLOOD-18-HYDROXYCORTICOSTERONE (18-OH-B) IN THE DIAGNOSTIC AND DIFFERENTIAL DIAGNOSTIC OF PRIMARY ALDOSTERONISM

G. von Mittelstaedt*, S. Abdelhamid+, P. Vecsei++, M. Strauch
Clinic of Nephrology, Klinikum Mannheim; +Deutsche Klinik für Diagnostik, Wiesbaden; ++Dept. of Pharmacology, University of Heidelberg; FRG

18-OH-B in adrenal-venous-blood- and peripheral-blood-plasma-extracts was determined by radioimmunoassay using a specific antibody and paperchromatography. The peripheral 18-OH-B-values of the patients with primary aldosteronism due to adrenal adenoma were significantly higher (pat.: n=14; det.: n=30; range: 56-470 ng/100ml) than the values of the patients with primary aldosteronism due to adrenal hyperplasia (pat.: n=5; det.: n=10, range: 18-75 ng/100ml). Plasma aldosterone values of the same groups of patients were: adenoma: range 8-150 ng/100ml (pat.: n=14; det.: n=30); hyperplasia: range 7,5-60 ng/100ml (pat.:n=5; det.: n=10; range: 18- 75 ng/100ml). However the 18-OH-B values have not allowed a clear cut distinction of adenoma and hyperplasia. 18-OH-B-determinations of the adrenal venous-blood were used for lateralisation diagnosis in 24 cases. The 18-OH-B-values were generally found to be parallel to the aldosterone concentrations. The fact, however, that the 18-OH-B-values are higher than the aldosterone values, provides methodological and diagnostical advantages. The 18-OH-B concentration is a valuable second parameter in the differential diagnosis of the primary aldosteronism.

2485 THE EFFECTS OF THE ANTIGLUCOCORTICOID AND ANTIPROGESTERONE RU38486, ON ADRENAL FUNCTION IN DOGS. C.E. Wade*, I.M. Spitz, D. Krieger and C.W. Bardin, Letterman Army Medical Center, San Francisco, Ca., Mount Sinai Medical Center and The Population Council, N.Y., N.Y.

To determine the effect of RU38486 on adrenal function, 5, 20 and 50 mg/kg of this agent was administered for 10 days to 7 female dogs at 10 week intervals. The drug was given twice daily after blood sampling. There was a 4% increase in body weight during the study. This was associated with a dilutional reduction in hemoglobin, hematocrit and plasma proteins. There were no alterations in plasma osmolality or electrolytes. No changes in cortisol or ACTH were apparent with 5 mg/kg RU38486. Cortisol levels rose significantly within two days of commencing the 50 mg/kg schedule and within three days following the 20 mg/kg dose; a 4-fold increase in cortisol levels was achieved with both doses. Plasma ACTH levels increased 3-fold with 20 mg/kg and even greater with 50 mg/kg. Plasma aldosterone concentrations increased significantly only with the highest dose schedule. To determine whether there was evidence for cortisol deficiency, 40 ml/kg of half normal saline was infused intravenously over 20 mins. on the last day of RU38486 treatment; water excretion was similar in the controls and treated dogs. Conclusion: 5 mg/kg RU38486 did not alter adrenal function; higher doses induced an increase in ACTH and cortisol; the rise in aldosterone suggested that RU38486 may have antimineralocorticoid action in the dog; despite the blockade of glucocorticoid receptors the ability to excrete a water load remained intact implying no objective evidence of cortisol deficiency at the renal tubule.

2486 STEROID EXCRETION IN CONGENITAL ADRENAL HYPERPLASIA: THE USE OF CAPILLARY GAS-CHROMATOGRAPHY, THIN LAYER CHROMATOGRAPHY AND MASS SPECTROMETRY. W.Waldhäusl*, H.Vierhapper, P.Nowotny, and H.Frisch, I.Med.Univ-Klinik, A-1090 Wien, Austria.

Urinary steroid excretion was studied by capillary gas-chromatography in 23 patients with congenital adrenal hyperplasia (CAH) due to 21-hydroxylase deficiency. Although excretion rates of pregnanetriol were in the normal range in 5 cases in whom substitution therapy had been discontinued for only 3 days the ratio of excreted pregnanetriol/tetrahydro-cortisone was increased in each case (range 5.9-466.0; healthy males: 1.0 ± 0.4; healthy females: 0.7 ± 0.3). In 4 patients an apparent preponderance of excreted pregnenetriol over pregnanetriol seemed to indicate impaired 3ß-steroiddehydrogenase activity; but additional analysis of the urine samples by gas-chromatography/mass-spectrometry following prepurification by TLC confirmed the data on pregnanetriol, but not on pregnenetriol indicating the interference of an as yet unidentified steroid metabolite with the initial analysis. In addition the steroid excretion in patients with CAH was characterized by a predominance of 5α- over 5ß-hydrogenated C19O3 steroids and an age-dependent rise in the excretion of C19O2 metabolites. It is concluded that capillary GC of urinary steroids is, within the limits of the method, a useful means to estimate the relative share of single metabolites in patients with CAH thus permitting a better characterization of individual enzyme defects.

2487 SITES OF ACTION OF ADRENAL MEDULLARY HORMONES IN FASTED EXERCISING RATS.
W.W. Winder*, V.M. Mitchell, and M.L. Terry, Division of Physiology and Anatomy, Zoology Department, Brigham Young University, Provo, Utah 84602.

We have investigated the physiological role of the marked increase in plasma epinephrine which occurs in fasted exercising rats. Fasted adrenal demedullated (ADM) rats show a marked reduction in endurance run times compared to sham operated (SO) controls (32 min for ADM vs 92 min for SO). After running for 30 min at 21 meters/min up a 10% grade, ADM rats' blood glucose concentration was 2.9 ± 0.1 mM compared to 4.3 ± 0.2 mM in SO rats. At the same time blood lactate was 3.0 ± 0.2 mM in SO rats compared to 1.0 ± 0.1 mM in ADM rats. Glycogen decreased in fast-twitch red muscle of the vastus lateralis (composed of Type IIA fibers) to the same extent in both ADM and SO rats during 30 min of exercise. In fast-twitch white muscle of the vastus lateralis (composed of Type IIB fibers) glycogen decreased 44% in SO rats but was not significantly decreased in ADM rats after 30 min of running. Soleus muscle (composed of Type I fibers) glycogen decreased 85% in SO rats vs 30% in ADM rats during the exercise. Hepatic cAMP was increased during exercise in both SO and ADM rats. Infusion of epinephrine into ADM rats during exercise corrected the hypoglycemia, restored lactate to normal, and stimulated glycogenolysis in the soleus and white vastus lateralis. We conclude that major sites of action of epinephrine during mild exercise in the fasted state include the Type IIB muscle fibers which are not likely to be recruited at these low work rates. Epinephrine-stimulated glycogenolysis in non-exercising muscle apparently provides essential quantities of lactate for hepatic gluconeogenesis in fasted exercising rats. (Supported by NIH AM32261).

2488 STUDIES ON CHOLESTEROL ESTER HYDROLASE IN THE HUMAN ADRENAL.
S. Yoshida*, T. Nishikawa, K. Mikami, Y. Saito and Y. Tamura, The 2nd Dept. of Internal Medicine, School of Medicine, Chiba University, Chiba 280, Japan.

We have investigated properties of cholesterol ester hydrolase (CEHase) in human adrenal cortex. Normal adrenal (N) tissue and specimens of diffuse hyperplasia (H) and adenoma (A) were surgically obtained from patients with Cushing's syndrome. A substrate mixture containing cholesteryl oleate and various concentrations of phosphatidylcholine (PC) was used for estimating CEHase activity. Optimum activity was observed at around pH 4.5 and 8.0, and each CEHase was associated with lysosome and microsome, respectively. The acid CEHase activity in the N tissue was increased by an increased concentration of PC in the substrate, while an increase in the acid CEHase activity was not observed in the A and H tissue when using a high concentration of PC. The alkaline CEHase activity in the N, H, and A tissues was not increased by PC. The cytosol from the H and A tissues enhanced the acid CEHase in the lysosomal fraction of the N tissue, while the cytosol fraction from the N tissue did not. This stimulating activity was inactivated by heat treatment. The dialyzed cytosol from the A tissue could not activate the activity but that from the H tissue could. The cytosol from the N tissue suppressed the acid CEHase activity in the lysosomal fraction of the H and A tissue. The present study clearly demonstrated two distinct types of CEHase in human adrenal glands and that the regulation of CEHase in the normal adrenal by PC and cytosol was different from that in the H and A tissues. It is also speculated that there may exist some activating factor(s) in the cytosol of the H and A for acid CEHase, resulting in a greater formation of free cholesterol for steroid biosynthesis in these tissues than in the N tissue.

2489 ROLE OF ADRENAL CATECHOLAMINE IN REGULATION OF BLOOD PRESSURE AND SODIUM HANDLING

M.Yoshimura*, H.Yamazaki, R.Takashina, K.Takeda, H.Takahashi, H.Ijichi. Department of Medicine II, Kyoto Prefectural University Of Medicine. Kawaramachi-hirokoji, Kamikyoku, Kyoto 602, Japan.

To evaluate a role of adrenal catecholamine(CA) in regulation of blood pressure and sodium handling, Wistar rats were treated adrenal medullectomy or sham-operation and were fed on regular(Na:0.24%) or high(Na:8%) salt diet for 4 weeks. Renal and urinary CA was measured by HPLC-ECD method and norepinephrine(NEp) turnover of kidney was estimated from % decrease after α-methyl-p-tyrosine iv. Salt loading induced to elevate blood pressure, augment urinary output of NEp and accelerate turnover of renal NEp. Adrenal medullectomy in rats fed on regular diet induced to maintain blood pressure and increase urinary output of NEp, augment renal content of NEp and accelarate turnover of renal NEp. Adrenal medullectomy in rats fed on high salt diet, on the other hand, showed to decrease blood pressure, increase urinary output of sodium but not change urinary output of NEp, renal content of NEp and turnover of renal NEp as compared with those of sham-rats. These results suggest that (1) salt loading accelerates renal NEp metabolism to result in elevation of blood pressure, (2) renal NEp metabolism is compensatively activated by adrenal medullectomy and works on maintaining blood pressure and sodium handling at regular diet and (3) salt loading with demedullation causes to enhance renal CA metabolism which is not enough to maintain blood pressure and sodium handling as compared with sham-rats. In conclusion, renal and adrenal CA may play an important role, working cooperatively, for regulation of blood pressure and sodium handling of kidney.

2490 RED BLOOD CELL (RBC) TRANSPORT OF 18-HYDROXYCORTICOSTERONE (18-OH-B),

P.G. Zager,* C.T. Spalding, H.J. Frey, M. Brittenham, Univ. of New Mexico School of Medicine, Albuquerque, New Mexico, USA.

Competition between 18-OH-B and cortisol for binding sites on nonalbumin plasma protein(s) (OP) may alter the distribution of 18-OH-B between plasma and RBC. Double equilibrium dialyses were performed in vitro at 37C to characterize the binding of 18-OH-B to OP. Plasma and 4.5% albumin were dialyzed in buffers containing ^{3}H-18-OH-B and increasing quantities of unlabeled cortisol. In a second series of experiments the buffers contained ^{3}H-cortisol and increasing amounts of unlabeled 18-OH-B. In both series of experiments increasing quantities of unlabeled steroid produced progressive decrements in the binding of ^{3}H-steroid to OP. The cortisol binding capacity of the OP binding 18-OH-B (23 μg cortisol/dl) was similar to that of transcortin. The affinity of 18-OH-B ($10^{6}M^{-1}$) for OP was lower than that of cortisol ($10^{7}M^{-1}$).

Heparinized whole blood was incubated with ^{3}H-18-OH-B in the presence of increasing quantities of unlabeled cortisol. Blood was separated at 4C or 37C and the ^{3}H-18-OH-B plasma: RBC ratio (ratio) was measured. Plasma cortisol correlated with the ratio when blood was separated at 4C ($r= 0.87$ $p < 0.01$) and 37C ($r= 0.62$ $p < 0.01$). The ratio ranged from 0.3 in low cortisol blood separated at 4C to 0.7 in high cortisol blood separated at 37C.

Conclusion: The OP binding 18-OH-B is transcortin. Plasma cortisol concentration and the temperature at which blood is separated alter the distribution of 18-OH-B between plasma and RBC.

2491 DECREASE OF VASOPRESSIN (VP) RELEASE WITH INCREASING AGE OF RATS STUDIED BY SUPERFUSION OF ISOLATED NEUROHYPOPHYSIS. V.Zbuzek*, V.K. Zbuzek and W.Wu. Dept. Anesthesiology, UMDNJ, New Jersey Medical School, Newark, NJ 07103, USA

Isolated neurohypophyses (NH) without pars intermedia of male Fisher 344 rats aged 2 months (n=17), 12 months (n=14) and 30 months (n=17) were individually superfused with Medium TC 199 for 3½ hours. Following the initial traumatic release (80 min), a steady basal VP release was established and the glands were stimulated electrically (trains of biphasic pulses, 0.2 ms, 8 mA, 30 Hz) for 10 min, followed by the resting period, and stimulated with 56 mM K^+ Locke's solution for 15 min. Age related VP release was analyzed in the following criteria: traumatic and basal release, response to the electrical and chemical stimulation, and the total release. VP content, expressed per mg NH, was significantly lower in all studied criteria in the old rats compared to the young ones. In the adult rats, the traumatic, basal and total release were all similar to those of young rats; while the response to the electrical and chemical stimulation was similar to that of the old rats. The percents of VP released during the entire superfusion, related to residual VP contents in the NHs, were 21 ± 2, 20 ± 3 and 13 ± 2% in the young, adult and old, respectively. The present data demonstrate a decreased VP release from NH of the old rats. They further suggest that during the aging process the impairment of VP release in response to chemical and electrical stimulation occurs at an earlier age than the impairment of spontaneous (traumatic and basal) VP release. Supported by NIA grant R01 AG02778.

2492 SEROTONIN STIMULATES ALDOSTERONE OUTPUT FROM RAT ADRENAL ZONA GLOMERULOSA CELLS BY ACTIVATION OF SPECIFIC 5HT RECEPTORS. B.C. Williams*, S. Shaikh and C.R.W. Edwards, Department of Medicine, Western General Hospital, Edinburgh EH4 2XU, U.K.

Serotonin (5HT) is a potent stimulant for aldosterone (aldo) secretion in vitro. To further investigate its mechanism of action in the zona glomerulosa (ZG) we employed the respective 5HT and $5HT_2$ receptor-antagonists methysergide (ME) and Ketanserin (KT) and the α_1-antagonist Prazosin (P). Rat ZG cells, prepared by collagenase digestion of adrenal capsules, were incubated in Krebs-Ringer bicarbonate buffer (0.2% BSA) for 30 min at 37°C with 5HT (10^{-9}-10^{-4} M), ACTH ($3x10^{-11}$-$3x10^{-9}$ M) or potassium (K^+)(8.4 mM) alone or with added ME, KT (10^{-8}-10^{-6} M) or P (10^{-6} M). Corticosterone (B), aldo and cyclic AMP (cAMP) outputs were measured in the cell supernatants by radioimmunoassay. 5HT produced correlative sigmoidal dose responses for cAMP, B and aldo which were competitively inhibited by ME at 10^{-7} and 10^{-6} M. KT at 10^{-6} M inhibited the cAMP, B and aldo responses to 5HT but had no significant effects at lower doses. Neither ME nor KT affected the cAMP, B or aldo responses to ACTH. Small inhibitions of the aldo response to K^+ were observed with ME (10^{-6} M) and KT (10^{-6} M) which were not significant. No effect of P was observed on the steroidogenic response to 5HT. These data indicate that the effects of 5HT on cAMP and steroidogenesis are correlated and specifically inhibited by 5HT receptor antagonists but not by an α_1-antagonist. We conclude that specific receptors for 5HT are present in ZG cells which are coupled to cAMP production which acts as second messenger for steroidogenesis.

2493 THE DOPAMINE AGONIST, BROMOCRIPTINE, DOES NOT DIMINISH THE ALDOSTERONE RESPONSE TO ANGIOTENSIN II OR TO ACTH IN IDIOPATHIC HYPERALDOSTERONISM

M.Wisgerhof* and R.C. Mellinger, Division of Endocrinology, Henry Ford Hospital, Detroit, Michigan 48202, USA.

The dopamine agonist, bromocriptine (Br), can diminish the plasma aldosterone (PA) response to angiotensin II (AII) in normal subjects. Insufficient dopamine effect thus might explain enchanced adrenal responsiveness in idiopathic hyperaldosteronism (IHA). To test this hypothesis, we measured the PA responses to AII and ACTH infusions before Br treatment (no Rx) and after Br treatment (2.5 mg TID for 5 days) (BrRx) in 3 white males (40, 55, 56 years old) with untreated IHA. We measured plasma AII (PAII) during the AII studies. The results are in mean±SE.

	pre-infusion		paired differences: noRx-BrRx	
	no Rx	BrRx	AII infusion	ACTH infusion
PA ng/dl	12±0.9	13±0.9*	1.1±0.68 inc*	no difference
PAII ng/ml	14±2.0	11±1.7*	3.5±3.46 dec*	not measured

*P > 0.05; inc=increased; dec= decreased

The slopes of the linear regression of PA and PAII were significant during the AII studies but not significantly different before (0.33;Sy.x =0.436;95%CI=0.300-0.360) and after (0.30;Sy.x=0.472;95%CI=0.275-0.331) BrRx, which significantly decreased plasma prolactin concentration to less than 2 ng/ml. BrRx did not significantly alter the increase in blood pressure during AII infusions or plasma corticosteroids during ACTH infusion. Plasma potassium did not change significantly during the studies. These results show that Br does not diminish PA responses to AII or ACTH in IHA. This suggests that insufficient dopamine effect does not account for enhanced adrenal responsiveness in IHA.

2494 ROLE OF SEROTONIN IN THE REGULATION OF ALDOSTERONE IN PATIENTS WITH CHRONIC RENAL FAILURE.

M. Yamakado*, H. Matsuoka, H. Tagawa and S. Tanaka, Mitsui Memorial Hospital, Tokyo and 2nd Department of Internal Medicine, University of Tokyo, Tokyo, Japan.

The regulation of aldosterone in patients with chronic renal failure (CRF) can not be completely explained by the known stimulators. Recently, it has been posturated that a serotonergic mechanism may be involved in the regulation of aldosterone in idiopathic hyperaldosteronism (IHA). In this study, in order to examine the role of serotonin in the regulation of aldosterone in patients with CRF, plasma aldosterone concentration (PAC, pg/ml), cortisol (F, ng/ml) and plasma renin activity (PRA) were measured by radioimmunoassay before and after the oral administration of 8 mg cyproheptadine (C), an antiserotonergic agent, at 30 minute intervals for 2 hours in 12 patients with CRF on maintenance hemodialysis (HD). Blood pressure (BP), heart rate (HR) and serum sodium (Na) and potassium (K) were also determined. After the administration of C, PAC decreased significantly from the basal level of 141 ± 32 to 118 ± 26 at 90 min ($p<0.05$). Also, F fell significantly from the basal of 86 ± 9 to 73 ± 9 at 60 min ($p<0.05$). Significant correlation existed between the basal level of PAC and the decrement in PAC ($r=-0.82$, $p<0.001$) and between the basal F and the change in F ($r=-0.94$, $p<0.001$). No changes occurred in PRA, Na, K, BP and HR. These results suggest that the serotonergic mechanism may play an important role in the regulation of aldosterone through its effect on hypothalamus or pituitary gland in patients with CRF on HD similar to that in IHA.

2495 SIMPLIFIED METHOD OF PURIFYING ANGIOTENSIN CONVERTING ENZYME (ACE).

T., YASUI*, T., SARUTA, F., ALHENC-GELAS°, P., CORVOL° and J., MENARD°. Dept. of Internal Medicine, School of Medicine, Keio Univ., Tokyo, JAPAN. ° INSERM U36, 17 rue du Fer-à-Moulin, 75005 Paris, FRANCE.

With the use of ACE-inhibitor in the treatment of hypertension and edematous states, the pathophysiological significance of ACE is coming to be clear and purified ACE is necessitated to study the role of ACE. We report here a simplified method of purifying ACE with greater efficiency and better reproducibility. Tryptic extract from human kidney microsomal fraction was applied onto ion-exchange cellulose column to attain appropriate volume and enzyme concentration. Several aliquots of the concentrate were applied, with 15 minutes intervals, onto ACE-inhibitor-coupled affinity column of n-α-[1-(S)-Carboxy-3-Phenylpropyl]-1-Lysyl-1-Proline (MK521) coupled epoxide-Sepharose CL4B (DORRY et al.). Elution was done by eliminating potassium chloride (0.33M) in 0.01M HEPES buffer (pH7.5). Specific activity of the eluate was 117 U(Cushman)/mGprotein and overall recovery rate was 34%. Polyacrylamide gel electrophoresis, with or without SDS-dimercaptoethanol treatment revealed one single band. Immunological identity with conventionally purified ACE (STEWART et al.) was verified by Ouchterlony method and radioimmunoassay (ALHENC-GELAS et al.). Dissociation constant of the affinity adsorbent for the protein was predicted to be less than 10^{-4}M. By taking advantage of feeble dissociation constant, we accomplished an affinity chromatography with great efficiency and high selectiity. It is noteworthy that two steps are sufficient to purify trypsin solubilized human kidney ACE as much as has been reported (WEARE et al.).

2496 OUTPATIENT DIAGNOSTIC PROCEDURE FOR MILD PRIMARY ALDOSTERONISM: THE 6 HOUR INTEGRATED ALDOSTERONE/RENIN RATIO.

Z. Zadik, P. Levin, B. Hamilton and A. Kowarski*, Departments of Pediatrics and Medicine, Universities of Maryland and Johns Hopkins Schools of Medicine, Baltimore, Maryland, USA.

Patients suspected of primary hyperaldosteronism, especially mild cases, are often hospitalized for complex multiple tests to achieve diagnosis. We have evaluated an outpatient diagnostic procedure based on measuring the 6 h integrated average plasma aldosterone (IC-ALDO) and plasma renin (IC-PRA). Blood was collected with a constant withdrawal pump while patients were on an unrestricted sodium diet. Primary hyperaldosteronism was found in 12 patients. This included 6 patients with low potassium but normal (<12 μg/24 h) urinary excretion of aldosterone levels.

The ratio of IC-ALDO/IC-PRA of the 12 patients (mean 339; range 116-700)(P <0.0001), did not overlap with the ratio of IC-ALDO/PRA measured in 105 normotensive controls (mean 28; range 5-97) or the ratio in 87 subjects with essential hypertension (mean 29; range 4-67).

Eight of the 12 patients had surgically proven adenomas. The remaining 4 patients had bilateral hyperplasia. The IC-PRA and blood pressure of all adenoma patients returned to normal following unilateral adrenalectomy. The blood pressure and potassium levels of the hyperplasia patients became normal on spironolactone.

Conclusion: The 6 h integrated aldosterone and renin ratio proved to be a sensitive and cost-effective outpatient diagnostic tool for hyperaldosteronism.

2497 THRESHOLD DOSES OF ANDROGENS REQUIRED FOR EJACULATION BY MALE RHESUS MONKEYS.

Richard P. Michael* and Doris Zumpe, Department of Psychiatry, Emory University School of Medicine and the Georgia Mental Health Institute, Atlanta, Georgia 30322, U.S.A.

To determine ejaculatory thresholds in castrated male rhesus monkeys, mating tests were conducted with 8 males during successive 4-week periods of treatment with testosterone propionate (TP) beginning at 25 µg and increasing in octaves to 12.8 mg s.c./day. All males were tested daily with the same 4 ovariectomized females. Because males are sensitive to the hormonal state of females, two were untreated while the other two received 5 µg and 15 µg estradiol benzoate s.c./day respectively (32 pairs, 1,408 1-hr mating tests). TP was given at 1600 h and plasma samples were obtained at 0800 h (352 samples). Ejaculatory thresholds ranged from 50 µg to 3.2 mg TP in different males. Males showed two types of responses; an all-or-none one and a graded response to increasing plasma levels of androgen. Male responses to TP were greatly influenced by the identity and hormonal status of the female partner (each male had 4 partners). Subsequently, retesting 4 of these males in identical fashion during treatment periods with dihydrotestosterone propionate (DHTP) beginning at 50 µg and increasing in octaves to 25.6 mg s.c./day (16 pairs, 704 1-hr tests) suggested that DHTP was considerably less effective than TP in stimulating ejaculatory performance. Small doses of estradiol benzoate (1 µg or 5 µg s.c./day) administered in conjunction with either TP or DHTP produced no further increases in male sexual activity.

Supported by USPHS Grant MH 19506.

2498 STUDIES ON INSULIN-INDUCED OBESITY: CHRONIC EFFECT OF INSULIN ADMINISTRATION ON FEEDING, DRINKING AND AMBULATION.

H. Shimizu*, Y. Shimomura, M. Takahashi, I. Kobayashi, S. Kobayashi and S. Tadokoro, First Department of Internal Medicine, Division of Endocrinology, Department of Medicine and Division for Behavior Analysis, Gunma University, Maebashi 371, Japan.

Hyperinsulinemia was reported to be an important role in the development of experimental obesity. We attempted to induce experimental obesity by insulin administration and determine the circadian rhythmicity of various behavior in insulin-induced obese animals.

Female Wistar rats were individually housed on a 12-12 light-dark cycles and maintained with Purina laboratory chow and tap water available ad lib. NPH-insulin(8 U/rat/day) was given just before light or dark cycles for 7 days. Their behaviors were analyzed using automatic apparatus for continuous and direct measurement of eating, drinking and ambulation. Insulin-induced obesity was proved in increased weight of brown adipose tissue and perimetrial adipose tissues. On insulin administration just before light cycle, both food intake and drinking during light cycle were significantly increased, in a sharp contrast to the dark cycle. Ambulation did not change throughout the both cycles. On insulin administration just before dark cycle, rhythm of food intake, drinking and ambulation did not change in the both cycles. Blood sugar levels decreased coincidentally in the two groups following insulin injection given just before light and dark cycles. In conclusion, insulin -induced obese rats was successfully made. Food intake and drinking, but not ambulation, were remarkably influenced by the time of insulin given.

2499 OVARIECTOMY-INDUCED OBESITY: THE IMPORTANT ROLE OF ADRENAL GLAND.

Y. Shimomura*, M. Takahashi, H. Shimizu, K. Ohshima, I. Kobayashi, S.Kobayashi and S. Tadokoro, Division of Endocrinology, First Department of Internal Medicine, and Division for Behavior Analysis, Gunma University School of Medicine, Maebashi 371, Japan.

Recent studies revealed that the adrenal gland of genetically obese(ob/ob) mice and VMH lesioned rats had an important role in the development of obesity. Little is known on the role of adrenal gland in the ovariectomized, obese animals. We investigated the role of the adrenal and circadian rhythmicity using automatic apparatus for continuous and direct measurement of eating, drinking and ambulation in ovariectomized(Ox) and adrenalectomized(Ax) rats. Female Wistar rats weighing 150-200 g were ovariectomized or ovariectomized-adrenalectomized(Ox + Ax). Studies were conducted with a special ambulo-drinkometer under 12 hr light/dark cycles. Six weeks after operation, the weight gain was 142.7±6.8 g in Ox and 119.6±11.7 g in Ox + Ax rats. Adrenalectomy resulted in reduction of weight gain in Ox rats. Ox + Ax rats were proved in decreased weight of brown adipose tissue, perimetrial fat and retroperitoneal fat. On the other hand, Ox + Ax animals showed an increased water intake, but not change of circadian rhythmicity. The circadian rhythm of eating and movement did not alter, while spontaneous movement and food intake decreased slightly in Ox + Ax animals. Conclusion: The adrenal gland has an important role in the development of ovariectomy-induced obese rats. Although we could not observe any change of circadian rhythmicity, a dissociation between drinking and food intake was demonstrated.

2500 HORMONES AND MOOD VARIABILITY AND BEHAVIOR PROBLEMS DURING EARLY ADOLESCENCE. E. J. Susman*, E. D. Nottelmann, J. H. Blue, L. D. Dorn, G. E. Inoff, NIMH, G. P. Chrousos, G. B. Cutler, D. L. Loriaux, NICHD, NIH, Bethesda, Maryland, 20205, U.S.A.

The purpose of this study was to examine relations between endocrine status and psychological development during puberty. We studied normal 9-14-year-old males (n=39) and females (n=25) enrolled in a longitudinal study. Pubertal staging according to Tanner was performed, and hormone status was assessed by measurement (X3) of plasma concentrations of luteinizing hormone, follicle stimulating hormone, testosterone, estradiol, dehydroepiandrosterone, dehydroepiandrosterone sulfate, and androstenedione. Adolescents' self-reports across five consecutive days were used to assess mood variability. Maternal ratings on the Child Behavior Checklist were used to assess the adolescents' behavior problems. Relationships reported are statistically significant ($p \leq .05$ and .01). For males, the correlations of hormone concentrations with mood variability were: a) negative for gonadotropins (nervous-calm and tired-energetic), b) positive for sex steroids (angry-friendly, happy-sad, and tired-energetic), and c) positive for adrenal androgens (happy-sad). A pattern of positive correlations emerged between hormones and behavior problems for males: between a) gonadotropins and hyperactive and somatic behavior problems, and between b) adrenal androgens and uncommunicative, obsessive, hostile, hyperactive, and somatic behavior problems. For females, there was no consistent pattern of relationships between hormones and moods or behavior problems. Thus, only for males, gonadal and adrenal changes during adolescence appear to increase mood variability as well as the incidence of behavior problems.

2501 MENTAL STATUS, T_4, AND SURVIVAL AFTER BURN INJURY. G.M. Vaughan*, A.D. Mason, Jr., and B.A. Pruitt, Jr., U.S. Army Institute of Surgical Research, Fort Sam Houston, Texas, 78234, U.S.A.

The relationships among T_4, level of obtundation (LO) and survival in nonthyroidal illness are not yet characterized. In 13 normal subjects and 16 burn patients including three nonsurvivors (NS), T_3 charcoal uptake-derived free indices (FT_4I and FT_3I) were correlated with respective dialysis-derived free concentrations (FT_4 and FT_3)(both $r \geq 0.95$). T_4, FT_4I, FT_4, T_3, FT_3I, and FT_3 were suppressed (all $p < 0.001$) in the patients. Therefore, FT_4I and FT_3I were used to represent free concentrations in 656 samples from 134 patients (burn size 6-96% skin area) including 45 NS, taken mainly from postburn day 1-30, all without steroid, dopamine, or iodine treatment. At each sampling, LO was determined on a six-point scale from normal to deep coma. Whereas mean FT_4I (initially 3.1) returned toward normal (> 5.0) in survivors (S), it remained low (2.3 - 3.1)from the earliest samples until death in the NS. In NS, mean LO worsened over the1st week and remained worse than in S even at 3-4 weeks before death. Multiple regression analysis showed that for a given age or burn size, nonsurvival was better correlated with lower T_4 or FT_4I than with T_3 or FT_3I but was even more closely correlated with worse LO ($p < 0.001$). Exclusion of data from within 24 h of narcotic or tranquilizer doses somewhat enhanced the relationship of nonsurvival with LO and FT_4I. Conclusion: Nonsurvival after burn injury is associated with reduced T_4, FT_4I, and mental status up to weeks before death, this association being independent of treatment with drugs acting on mental status or thyroid function.

2502 ANGIOTENSIN II INDUCED Na APPETITE IN SHEEP. R.S. Weisinger*, D.A. Denton, M.J. McKinley, J.B. Simpson and E. Tarjan. Howard Florey Institute, University of Melbourne, Australia.

The present experiments evaluated the effect of intracerebroventricular (IVT) or intravenous (IV) infusion of AII on Na intake and Na excretion of Na replete sheep. Sheep were trained to bar press for water and 0.5M NaCl. Water was available continuously while Na was available for 2h/day. At the end of a Na access period, a 48h IVT infusion of AII (3.8 μg/h) or IV infusion of AII (24 μg/h) was begun. Thus, the effect of AII on urinary Na loss as well as subsequent Na intake (i.e., after 22 and 46h of infusion) could be determined. IVT infusion of AII caused an increase in Na-excretion and a greater increase in Na intake. Without infusion of AII, the sheep (n=9) bar pressed for 9.5±2.4 deliveries or 119 mmol of Na. During IVT infusion of AII, Na intake was increased to 406 mmol of Na on day 1 and 502 mmol of Na on day 2. Daily Na deficit caused by urinary loss prior to the two Na access periods were 207 and 198 mmol. IV infusion of AII caused an increase in Na excretion and a greater increase in Na intake but not as much as with IVT AII. Without infusion of AII, the sheep (n=7) bar pressed for 5.0±1.4 deliveries or 62 mmol of Na. During IV infusion of AII, Na intake was increased to 261 mmol of Na on day 1 and 248 mmol of Na on day 2. Daily Na deficit caused by urinary loss prior to the two Na access periods were 84 and 33 mmol. This indicates that both IVT and IV AII increased Na intake in excess of previous loss. Thus, the increase in Na intake may be due to Na loss and to direct effects of AII on neural structures involved in salt appetite.

2503 HYPOPHOSPHATEMIC RICKETS WITH HYPERCALCIURIA AND ELEVATED SERUM LEVELS OF $1,25(OH)_2D$.

M. Tieder, R. Samuel, R. Arie, A. Halabe, D. Modai, D. Gabisõn and U.A. Liberman*. Pediatric Nephrology, Assaf Harofeh Hospital, Metabolic Unit, Beilinson Medical Center, Tel Aviv University, Israel.

A 14-year-old boy with short stature, severe deformities of the legs and active rickets, was investigated. The parents are unrelated and no one else in the family is affected. Kidney function was normal. Studies during hospitalization in a Metabolic Ward revealed: a) Hypercalciuria of 477±64 mg/24h (mean±SD), 10.8±1.4 mg/kg B.W./24h (upper normal 6 mg/kg/B.W./24h). Urinary Ca/Cr fell to 0.08 after 18h fast; b) Normocalcemia: 9.6±0.2mg/dl; c) Hypophosphatemia: 3.0±0.3mg/dl, in brackets, normal for age (4.4±0.5 mg/dl); d) low T_mP/GFR:2.6±0.4mg/dl GF (4.0±0.6mg/dl GF); e) Elevated serum, alkaline phosphatase; f) Urinary c-AMP: 1.25±0.27nmol/dl GF (2.9±0.7nmol/dl GF); g) Serum iPTH: 0.3,0.4ng/ml (0.9±0.3ng/ml); h) Serum vitamin D metabolites: $1,25(OH)_2D$-143pg/ml (30-70pg/ml), 25OHD and $24,25(OH)_2D$ normal; i) Oral calcium load (1.4g elemental Ca): a marked increase of urinary Ca/Cr: 0.76 mg/mg Cr (0.12±0.02 mg/mg Cr); j) Oral phosphate load (1.4g of elemental phosphorus): an increase in serum phosphorus of 2.4 mg/dl (1.2±0.2 mg/dl). The following sequence of events is proposed: primary renal phosphate leak, hypophosphatemia, stimulation of the renal 1-alpha-hydroxylase, elevated serum levels of $1,25(OH)_2D$, enhanced intestinal calcium and phosphorus absorption, increased renal filtered load of calcium and hypercalciuria. Treatment with oral neutral phosphate resulted in acceleration of linear growth rate, clinical radiological and biochemical cure of the rickets, and reduction of urinary calcium excretion to normal.

2504 EFFECT OF 1α-HYDROXYVITAMIN D_3 ON SERUM BGP LEVELS IN THE OSTEOPOROTIC AND NORMAL HUMAN AGED.

Y. Yamada*, K. Okano, C. Nawa, S. Kou, N. Sekita, K. Kida, K. Someya and S. Moriuchi, St. Marianna University School of Medicine, Kawasaki, Japan, Japan Women's University School of Home Economics, Tokyo, Japan.

Effect of 1α-hydroxyvitamin D_3 (1α-OHD_3) on serum bone γ-carboxyglutamic acid containing protein (BGP) levels was evaluated in 5 normal human aged subjects and 10 patients with senile osteoporosis. Serum BGP was determined by RIA using antiserum to bovine BGP, serum calcium by photon absorption method, serum inorganic phosphorus according to Chen et al. and serum Al-P'ase by Lowry's method using p-nitrophenyl phosphoric acid, before and after the oral administration of 1.5 μg/day 1α-OHD_3 for 16 weeks. Serum BGP in the normal aged group was 9.4 ± 1.9 ng/ml, and tended to increase after the administration of 1α-OHD_3. Serum BGP in the osteoporotic group were 6.1 ± 1.0 ng/ml (before), 11.2 ± 1.6 ng/ml (8 weeks) and 11.9 ± 1.9 ng/ml (16 weeks), and significantly increased after the administration of 1α-OHD_3. Serum calcium was significantly increased at 8 weeks of 1α-OHD_3 administration in the normal aged group, and at 8 and 16 weeks of 1α-OHD_3 administration in the osteoporotic group. Serum inorganic phosphorus was significantly increased at 8 weeks of 1α-OHD_3 administration in the normal aged group. Serum Al-P'ase level remained unaltered after 1α-OHD_3 administration in the both groups. There was a significant positive correlation between serum BGP and serum inorganic phosphorus or Al-P'ase in the osteoporotic group. These data suggest that serum BGP is decreased in senile osteoporosis and $1,25(OH)_2D_3$ converted from 1α-OHD_3 stimulates the production of BGP which will reflect an increase of bone turn over.

(Abstract 2771, p. 1646, also belongs to this section.)

2505 RAT VITAMIN-D-DEPENDENT CALCIUM BINDING PROTEIN : CELL-FREE SYNTHESIS AND WESTERN BLOTTING.

Roland Pochet* and Marc Parmentier, Lab. of Histology, School of Medicine, U.L.B., 2, rue Evers, B-1000 BRUSSELS. BELGIUM

Mammals are known to posses a 28,000 MW Vitamin D-dependent Calcium Binding Protein (D-CaBP) in their kidney and brain. We demonstrate here that two D-CaBP respectively of 27,000 and 23,000 daltons are present in the rat cerebellum and are directed by distinct mRNAs. Rat kidney contain only the 23,000 MW form. mRNAs were prepared using phenol extraction and poly-(U)-Sepharose chromatography. mRNAs were centrifuged through a linear sucrose gradient and fractions were translated in a rabbit reticulocyte lysate using (35S)-methionine as tracer. Two translations products with apparent MW of 23,000 and 27,000 on SDS-PAGE were immunoprecipitated with a rabbit anti-(chick intestinal D-CaBP)(gift from D.E.M. Lawson, Cambridge). The two D-CaBP forms were also detected in rat cerebellum homogenate using the Western Blotting method after SDS-PAGE. D-CaBP were revealed by ELISA method. Their MW were identical to the in vitro synthetised D-CaBP.

2506 SEX DIFFERENCES IN MOTILIN CONCENTRATION IN RAT BRAIN AND PITUITARY AND THE EFFECT OF CASTRATION. M. Poth* and D. Proia. Department of Pediatrics, Uniformed Services University, Bethesda, MD 20814, USA.

Motilin is a 22 amino acid peptide originally isolated from small intestine based on its ability to stimulate gastric motility. Although present in neuroendocrine tissue, its role has not yet been elucidated. We assayed brain and pituitary motilin concentrations by RIA, as previously described, in groups of 12 young adult Sprague-Dawley rats who 2 weeks previously were either castrated or had sham operations. Marked sex differences were found between male and female rats in cortex, cerebellum, midbrain and pituitary gland. Results in hypothalamus were quite variable as assayed in this particular experiment and were below the limits of the assay detection in many animals.

	Cortex(pg/gm)	Cerebellum(pg/gm)	Midbrain(pg/gm)	Pit.(pg/gland)
Male	12.8	66.0	56.0	0.6
" Castrate	10.0	51.9	95.0	0.6
Female	1.7	30.1	206.0	1.4
" Castrate	7.7	49.4	66.0	0.7

Cortex and cerebellum in male rats had higher concentrations than in females. Castration of the male rats had no effect. Castration of female rats resulted in an increase in the concentration in the cortex but no change in the cerebellum. Pituitary and midbrain concentrations were greater in female than male rats, and decreased to male levels after castration in females. Again, no change was seen after castration in males. These remarkable sex differences and changes with oophorectomy implicate interactions between sex hormones and this peptide in brain tissue. Understanding of these interactions await further experimentation.

2507 PROLACTIN-LIKE m RNA IN RAT BRAIN. B. Schachter*, S. Durgerian, R. Harlan, D. Pfaff, and B. Shivers, Mt. Sinai School of Medicine, and Rockefeller University, New York City, New York.

We have identified a polyadenylated RNA species in rat hypothalami which hybridized with a radiolabeled cloned DNA probe complementary to rat pituitary prolactin (PRL) mRNA (gift of J. Martial). Gel blot analysis showed that the reactive RNA in the hypothalamus was the same size as pituitary PRL mRNA. These results suggest that previously identified immunoreactive PRL-like material in hypothalamic neurons (Toubeau et al. (1979) J. Endocrinol. 83:261; Harlan et al. (1983) Science 219:1451) is synthesized locally in the brain. The amount of PRL-like mRNA in hypothalamic extracts varied considerably among animal preparations when compared to a single pituitary RNA standard. To determine whether this variablilty correlated with the efficiency of the extraction procedure, each gel blot was reprobed with radiolabeled DNA complementary to proopiomelanocortin (POMC) mRNA (gift of J. Eberwine and J. Roberts), for this mRNA is also made in the pituitary and hypothalamus, and is similar in size to the PRL mRNA. In contrast to the hypothalamic PRL-like mRNA, whose concentration varied by >100-fold among animal groups, the relative abundance of hypothalamic POMC mRNA varied by 4-fold or less among groups. Studies are underway to determine the factors regulating changes in PRL gene expression in the brain.

2508 VASOACTIVE INTESTINAL POLYPEPTIDE IN CEREBROSPINAL FLUID IN PATIENTS WITH HYPERPROLACTINEMIA AND ACROMEGALY. A. Shimatsu*, Y. Kato, Y. Tatsuoka, H. Ohta, Y. Kabayama, T. Inoue, K. Tojo and H. Imura, Second Medical Clinic, Department of Medicine, Kyoto University Faculty of Medicine, Kyoto, Japan.

Stimulation by vasoactive intestinal polypeptide (VIP) of the secretion of prolactin and growth hormone has been demonstrated in hyperprolactinemia and acromegaly both in vivo and in vitro. However, the role of endogenous VIP in these patients remains to be elucidated. In the present study, cerebrospinal fluid (CSF) levels of immunoreactive VIP were determined by a specific radioimmunoassay in control subjects and patients with hyperprolactinemia and acromegaly. In this assay the displacement curve obtained with serial dilution of pooled CSF was parallel to the displacement curve of synthetic VIP. Only one peak of VIP was eluted with authentic VIP by gel chromatography of CSF on Sephadex G-50. The mean(±SE) levels of CSF VIP were 98±6 pg/ml in controls without any endocrine and neurological disorders. CSF VIP levels in patients with hyperprolactinemia due to different etiologies were higher than those in controls (140±12 pg/ml, $p<0.01$). Among these patients, prolactinoma had the highest CSF VIP (149±15 pg/ml), which were remarkably decreased by bromocriptine treatment. CSF VIP levels were also increased in acromegalic cases associated with hyperprolactinemia, whereas those in acromegalics without hyperprolactinemia were within normal range (139±25 pg/ml and 108±12 pg/ml). CSF VIP levels were raised after successful transsphenoidal adenomectomy in 5 acromegalic cases from 103±8 pg/ml to 140 ±21 pg/ml ($p<0.05$). These findings suggest that CSF VIP is subject to change in connection with the pituitary function and that VIP plays a possible pathophysiological role in a part of hyperprolactinemia and acromegaly.

2509 VIP and PHI Stimulate Somatostatin Secretion from Fetal Cerebral Cortical and Diencephalic Cells in Dispersed Culture. L. Tapia-Arancibia* and S. Reichlin, Université de Montpellier II, Montpellier, and Endocrine Division, Tufts New England Medical Center, Boston, MA

VIP and somatostatin are among the most abundant peptides in cerebral cortex where they are individually localized to separate peptidergic systems. These studies were carried out to determine the effect of VIP on somatostatin secretion by cerebral cortical cells, and for comparison, diencephalic cells. Dispersed monolayer cultures of cerebral cortical and diencephalic cells were prepared by mechanoenzymatic dissociation of fetal day 17 rats (Robbins and Reichlin, Endocrinology 113:574, 1983) initially plated at 10^{-7} cells/dish (cortex) and $5x10^{-6}$ (diencephalon) and grown in MEM with Earle's salts, 10% Nu Serum and Penicillin-Streptomycin (5,000 U/ 5,000 ug/ml). Test incubations were carried out in Earle's balanced salt solution containing bacitracin, 30 ug/ml for a 60 min period after basal release had reached stable levels. VIP was found to stimulate immunoreactive somatostatin release from both cerebral cortex and diencephalic cells the lowest effective concentration being 10^{-9}M, with increasing effects up to 10^{-6}, the highest concentration tested. The specificity of this effect was examined by testing a series of VIP-related peptides. PHI-27 was approximately 0.06, as active as VIP, but secretin and hGRH 1-44-NH2 had no effect at concentration up to 10^{-6}M. These findings indicate that in fetal cells, VIP is a relatively specific excitatory neurotransmitter in both cortex and diencephalon. Because the effects of VIP and PHI were not additive at 10^{-7}M we also conclude that these peptides probably react with the same receptor. This study was supported by a grant from Fondation pour la Recherche Medicale & O.S.P.H.S. A16684

2510 SOMATOSTATIN (ST) IN THE HUMAN BRAIN AND SPINAL CORD. A. Weindl*, J. Unger, H. Lange and W. Lange, Department of Anatomy, University of Munich, Pettenkoferstr. 11, D-8000 Munich, FRG.

ST, a tetradecapeptide originally identified as a hypothalamic hormone which inhibits growth hormone release (GHRIH), is present in the central nervous system (CNS) of many vertebrates. Immunoperoxidase staining of BOUIN-fixed brain and spinal cord sections revealed ST in nerve cell bodies of the anterior hypothalamic nucleus, basal ganglia, amygdala, cerebral cortex and several brainstem nuclei, as well as in nerve fibers in the median eminence, several hypothalamic nuclei, stria terminalis, amygdala, hippocampus, basal ganglia, cerebral cortex, brainstem and spinal cord. RIA measurements of ST in extracts of dissected CNS areas showed good correlations with the immunohistochemical findings, revealing, e.g. high values in the anterior hypothalamus (177.2 ng/mg prot), moderate values in the hippocampus (68.8 ng/mg prot) and lower values in cerebral cortex (4.1 ng/mg prot). RIA determinations of ST in the cerebrospinal fluid of neurological patients revealed decreased levels in morbus Parkinson (41.6 ± 10.2 pg/ml), Chorea Huntington (66.5 ± 14.3 pg/ml), spasmodic torticollis (21.7 ± 4.1 pg/ml) and morbus Alzheimer (57.7 ± 25.1 pg/ml) as compared to controls (150.2 ± 9.3 pg/ml). The findings demonstrate that ST is a widely distributed peptide within the human CNS suggesting an involvement of ST in a variety of CNS functions, in addition to the regulation of growth hormone secretion. Furthermore, changes of ST levels in the cerebrospinal fluid of patients with movement disorders indicate that ST neurons are involved in the neural circuitry of central motor control. (Supported by DFG We 608/7).

2511 DEVELOPMENTAL CHANGES IN SOMATOSTATIN(SRIF)-14 AND SRIF-28 IN THE RAT CENTRAL NERVOUS SYSTEM (CNS). W.C.Wetsel*, P.A.Grubb, and J.D.Fernstrom, Department of Psychiatry, University of Pittsburgh School of Medicine, Pittsburgh, PA 15213.

The presence and distribution of immunoreactive SRIF is known in the adult rat CNS. Few data detail the changes in CNS during development. We have performed such studies, and have quantitated both SRIF-14 and SRIF-28 using reversed-phase, high-performance liquid chromatography (HPLC) followed by radioimmunoassay [see Van Itallie CM, Fernstrom JD, Brain Research 249: 177, 1982]. Sprague-Dawley rats, gestational ages 16, 18, and 20 days, birth, and postnatal ages 2 and 6 days, and adult were killed; brains and spinal cords were dissected and run on the HPLC. Fractions were subjected to RIA for SRIF-14 and SRIF-28. In all regions examined (brain stem, hypothalamus, cerebellum, cerebral cortex, midbrain, spinal cord), levels of both peptides were detectable by gestational day 16 or 18, and increased progressively to adult values. Of interest were the findings that: [1] the hypothalamus had a relatively high SRIF-28/SRIF-14 ratio throughout development (ca. 0.50); other brain regions were lower (e.g., cerebral cortex, 0.09-0.14); [2] SRIF-14 levels in spinal cord and brainstem were greater than in hypothalamus at gestational day 20, birth, and postnatal days 2 and 6, but not in adults; [3] in cortex, SRIF-14 level approximated that in hypothalamus from gestational day 18 to postnatal day 6. Adult values in cortex (47 ng/mg protein) were 50-60% those in hypothalamus. In contrast, SRIF-28 levels in cortex were always 10-20% those in hypothalamus (e.g., adult - 42 ng/mg protein). These and other data indicate that the maturation of SRIF synthesis may differ from region to region in the rat brain. These studies supported by the March of Dimes Birth Defects Foundation.

2512 HYDROCORTISONE INCREASES RECEPTORS FOR PARPTHYROID HORMONE IN CLONAL RAT OSTEOSARCOMA CELLS. I.Yamamoto*, J.T.Potts,Jr., and G.V.Segre,Kyoto University Hospital,Kyoto,Japan and Massachusetts General Hospital, Boston , MA, U.S.A.

We studied effects of hydrocortisone on receptors for PTH in clonal rat osteosarcoma cells (ROS 17/2), which possess properties of osteoblast. PTH-binding to ROS 17/2 cells was studied using ^{125}I-labeled[Nle^{8},Nel^{18},Tyr^{34}]bPTH-(1-34)amide,as radioligand. After exposure of cells to hydrocortisone (10^{-8} M), PTH-binding to the cells was gradually increased, reaching a plateau at 48 hours, and returned to the original value after 5 days by eliminating hydrocortisone from the medium. The increase of PTH-binding to ROS 17/2 cells is dependent on doses of hydrocortisone and occurs also by other glucocorticoids but not by other steroids such as sex steroids. Scatchard analysis showed that the increase in PTH-binding is attributable to an increase in numbers of receptor. PTH-stimulated adenylate cyclase on crude plasma membranes from ROS 17/2 cells was also potentiated after exposure to hydrocortisone and correlated well with the increase in PTH-binding. In conclusion, hydrocortisone increases receptors for PTH and, thus,the potentiation of cyclic AMP response to PTH by glucocorticoids(T.L.Chen,et al. 1978) can be explained, at least partly , by the increase in receptor number for PTH.

2513 TUBULAR REABSORPTION OF CALCIUM IN HYPOPARATHYROID PATIENTS AND ITS RELATION TO THE CALCEMIC RESPONSE TO THERAPY WITH ALPHACALCIDOL(1αOHD3).

M.Yamamoto*, Y.Kawanobe, Y.Takuwa and E.Ogata, The Fourth Department of Internal Medicine, Faculty of Medicine, University of Tokyo, 3-28-6 Mejirodai, Bunkyo-ku, Tokyo 112, Japan.

The possible relationship between renal handling of calcium(Ca) and rises in serum Ca during 1αOHD3 therapy for 2-8 years was evaluated in 11 hypoparathyroid patients (7 with idiopathic hypoparathyroidism(IHP) and 4 with pseudohypoparathyroidism(PHP)). In each patients, urine and serum samples were analyzed for Ca and creatinine every 1-2 month. The dose of 1αOHD3 was 1-4 μg/day. Since urinary Ca excretion (mg/dl GF) increased linearly with the elevation of serum Ca in all patients, renal handling of Ca was expressed as apparent renal Ca threshold defined as a serum Ca concentration at which Ca appeared in the urine. This value was determined using regression analysis of urine and serum Ca in each patient. The Ca threshold varied individually and directly correlated with the rises in serum Ca or inversely correlated with the doses of 1αOHD3 required to maintain a given serum Ca level. These results indicate that a patient who required a larger dose of 1αOHD3 have lower Ca threshold. The Ca threshold showed no correlation with age, sex, the degree of hypocalcemia prior to therapy, GFR, urinary sodium excretion, and serum level of 1,25(OH)2D. However, the Ca threshold was higher in patients with PHP than in those with IHP. Thus the present study demonstrates that the renal handling of Ca is an important determinant of calcemic response to 1αOHD3 in hypoparathyroid patients, and suggests that the higher Ca threshold may explain why patients with PHP respond better to 1αOHD3 than patients with IHP.

2514 HYPERCALCEMIA INHIBITS THE "RAPID" STIMULATORY EFFECT ON CALCIUM TRANSPORT IN PERFUSED DUODENA FROM NORMAL CHICKS MEDIATED *in vitro* BY $1,25(OH)_2$-VITAMIN D_3.

Y. Yoshimoto* and A. W. Norman, Department of Biochemistry, University of California, Riverside, CA 92521, U.S.A.

We have previously reported that vascular perfusion of normal vitamin D_3-replete chick duodena with physiological amounts of $1,25(OH)_2D_3$ increases the movement of ^{45}Ca from the lumen to the venous effluent within 14 min under conditions of normal Ca^{++} (10 mg/dl) concentration. Here we report the consequence of changing the Ca^{2+} concentrations in both the compartment bathing the brush border surface of the intestinal epithelial cells (IEC) and also the perfusate which bathes the basal lateral membrane of the IEC on (a) the basal level of ^{45}Ca transport and (b) the stimulatory effect of 650 pM $1,25(OH)_2D_3$ presented in the perfusate. Within the range from 6-14 mg/dl Ca^{++} in the intestinal lumen and in the perfusate, the basal ^{45}Ca transport ratios were not different from control preparations treated with 10 mg/dl of Ca^{++}. However, the effect of $1,25(OH)_2D_3$ on $^{45}Ca^{2+}$ transport was completely abolished in the group treated with 14 mg/dl of Ca^{++} concentration in the perfusate, but not in the groups treated with less than 12 mg/dl of Ca^{++}. In conclusion, we have shown in the perfused chick duodenum system that (i) rates of Ca transport (transfer) are relatively independent of the Ca^{++} concentration in the lumen and/or perfusate and (ii) hypercalcemia, but not hypocalcemia inhibits the $1,25(OH)_2D_3$ stimulatory effect. Thus the response to $1,25(OH)_2D_3$ may be modulated locally in part by the prevailing ionized Ca concentration. [Supported by USPHS AM-09012-020.]

2515 CALCITONIN-RESPONSIVE CYCLIC AMP-DEPENDENT PROTEIN KINASE IN A CALCITONIN SECRETING HUMAN LUNG CELL LINE. J.D. Zajac*, S.A. Livesey, S. Forrest, S. Omond, J. Moseley and T.J. Martin. University of Melbourne, Department of Medicine, Repatriation General Hospital, Heidelberg 3081, Australia.

A human lung cancer cell line (BEN cells) synthesises and secretes high molecular weight forms of immunoreactive human calcitonin (M.W. 10,000-40,000). These cells also have receptors for calcitonin, a calcitonin responsive adenylate cyclase, a rise in cAMP after calcitonin exposure and we have demonstrated that they contain cAMP-dependent protein kinase which is responsive to calcitonin. As is the case with most mammalian cells BEN cells contain two isoenzymes of cAMP-dependent protein kinase (types I and II), separable by ion exchange chromatography. The only known mechanism of action of cAMP in mammalian cells is via activation of this kinase, therefore calcitonin effects on this enzyme were investigated with a method which allows the assay of the state of activation of the two individual isoenzymes (Ng et al 1983). Calcitonin treatment resulted in dose-dependent activation of cAMP-dependent protein kinase in BEN cells, with a predominant effect on isoenzyme I. In this respect the calcitonin response in BEN cells is similar to that seen in a rat osteogenic sarcoma cell line but differs markedly from that in calcitonin-responsive human breast cancer cell lines (T 47D and MCF 7), in which selective activation of isoenzyme II occurs. The relationship between calcitonin production by BEN cells and the calcitonin response system is being investigated.

K.W. Ng, S.A. Livesey, R.G. Larkins and T.J. Martin. Cancer Research 43:794-800, 1983.

2516 IN VIVO BIOLOGICAL ACTIVITIES OF HUMAN 1-84 PARATHYROID HORMONE (PTH): DISCRIMINATION BETWEEN HUMAN (h) AND BOVINE (b) 1-84 PTH PEPTIDES AND THEIR 1-34 FRAGMENTS. Joan M. Zanelli*, E. Lane, T. Kimura+ and S. Sakakibara+. National Institute for Biological Standards and Control, London NW3 6RB, UK and +Peptide Institute, Osaka, Japan.

There are published reports on the biological activities of b1-84 PTH and synthetic b and h 1-34 fragments, but the scarcity of h 1-84 PTH has precluded study of its biological activities *in vivo*. We now report the results of *in vivo* bioassays of synthetic h 1-84 PTH in comparison with native b 1-84 PTH and synthetic b and h 1-34 PTH. The biological responses measured are those classically associated with the bioassay of PTH, ie. acute chick hypercalcaemia and mouse kidney and bone cAMP accumulation (a newly developed *in vivo* bioassay). Results show that all 4 peptides are approximately equipotent on a molar basis when given intravenously for the chick hypercalcaemia bioassay. In contrast, h 1-84 PTH had approx. 10-fold lower potency than b 1-84 and the b and h 1-34 peptides when given iv. for the mouse renal cAMP bioassay (confirming results obtained in *in vitro* rat renal cAMP assay). This discrimination against h 1-84 was not seen if chicks were used instead of mice for the *in vivo* renal cAMP response. Both 1-84 peptides were weakly active on mouse and chick calvaria cAMP accumulation whereas both the 1-34 peptides were markedly active in both species. These comparative studies demonstrate the difference between different peptides in different bioassay systems in different species. They also emphasize the need for clearly defined chemical and biological standardization procedures.

2517 GROWTH HORMONE RELEASING FACTOR STIMULATES RELEASE OF CALCITONIN IN A RAT C-CELL LINE. F Zeytin, S Ying*. Laboratories for Neuroendocrinology. The Salk Institute for Biological Studies, La Jolla, CA 92037.

The extrapituitary site(s) of action of GRF are not known. We reported previously that GRF stimulates release of neurotensin (NT) by a clonal line of rat C-cells (44-2C). We report here that GRF also stimulates calcitonin (CT) and cAMP release in these cells. The establishment of the cell line was described (Zeytin et al, Reg Pept 6:155, 1983). Cells are maintained in DMEM with 15% horse serum. For release experiments, replicate cultures are incubated for 5-180 min in a serum-free defined medium (BBM-T) at 37°C in a humidified atmosphere of 93% air and 7% CO_2. CT, NT and cAMP are measured by RIA. Human pancreas (1-44 NH_2) hGRF and rat GRF (rGRF) stimulate CT and NT release in a dose dependent manner. At a maximally effective concentration of GRF (1 μM) there is a 2-3 fold stimulation of CT release at 60-90 min with a peak release at 180 min. In contrast, GRF causes a rapid 4-6 fold increase of NT release within 5-15 min with a plateau at 60 min. There is a 6-10 fold stimulation of cAMP release by GRF. Incubation of MTC cells for 24-48 hr with DEX (10^{-8} M) enhances the stimulation of NT release by GRF 2-4 fold and markedly decreases (60%) the response of the same cells to GRF-stimulated CT release. In control and DEX-treated cells, norepinephrine (10^{-6} M) stimulates CT and NT release and has an additive effect on GRF-stimulated CT and NT release. GRF-stimulated cAMP efflux is potentiated by forskolin and inhibited by trifluoperazine and by somatostatin. We conclude that GRF stimulates release of NT and cAMP and show for the first time the effect of this peptide on release of CT. The 44-2 cells provide a stable, reproducible neurosecretory model to study the regulation of peptide release by GRF at extrapituitary sites.

2518 CALCIUM AND DEXAMETHASONE DIFFERENTIALLY MODULATE CALCITONIN, NEUROTENSIN AND SOMATOSTATIN RELEASE IN A RAT C-CELL LINE. F Zeytin* PE Brazeau, N. Ling. The Salk Institutefor Biological Studies, La Jolla, CA 92037.

The rat C-cell lines and clonal strains secreting calcitonin (CT) and neurotensin (NT) have been used extensively to show the modulation of Ca^{++}-dependent, short-term (5-180 min) release of NT and CT. We report here effects of 24 hr treatment of 44-2C cells with Ca^{++} on peptide release and the modulation of this effect by dexamethasone (DEX). Establishment of the 44-2C line was described (Zeytin et al, Reg Pept 6:155, 1983). Cultures are maintained in DMEM with 15% HS. Experiments are carried out in DMEM with 1.8 mM or 4.0 mM Ca^{++} which correspond to the ED_{50} and Emax respectively, for short-term peptide release. Replicate cultures are incubated for 24-48 hr in a humidified atmosphere of 93% air, 7% CO_2. CT, NT and somatostatin (SS) are quantitated by RIA. Incubation of cells with 4.0 mM Ca^{++} results in a marked stimulation of NT release and accumulation as compared to controls (1.8 mM Ca^{++}). Ca^{++} (4.0 mM) decreases CT release and intracellular CT accumulation. DEX at 10^{-8} M markedly stimulates NT release and accumulation and has an additive effect on NT secretion in the presence of 4.0 mM Ca^{++}. DEX also stimulates basal and Ca^{++}-dependent release of SS. In contrast, DEX alone or with 4.0 mM Ca^{++} markedly inhibits CT secretion. We conclude that Ca^{++} is required for short term release of CT and NT. Long term incubation with Ca^{++} stimulates NT and SS production and inhibits CT production. DEX is a potent inducer of NT and SS secretion and an equally potent inhibitor of CT secretion.

2519 PRODUCTION OF ACTIVE FRAGMENTS OF PARATHYROID HORMONE BY CATHEPSIN D AND BY ISOLATED KUPFER CELLS. J.E. Zull*, S. Pillai and Jacinta Chuang, Department of Biology, Case Western Reserve University, Cleveland, OH 44106.

Studies in several laboratories have shown that following secretion, 1-84 PTH is cleaved between residues 30 and 40 producing inactive C-terminal fragments. This cleavage occurs primarily in the Kupfer cells of the liver, although some PTH metabolism also occurs in the kidney. In our laboratory an enzyme producing very similar fragments of PTH was found and identified as cathepsin D. We have now studied further the cleavage of PTH by cathepsin D and have detected the production of two N-terminal fragments. The major one is 1-34 and the enzyme catalyzes virtually no further hydrolysis of this peptide. However, a second peptide is also generated which does not accumulate and appears to be an intermediate in the production of 1-34. Preliminary analysis showed that this peptide is either 1-37 or 1-40 PTH. Both peptides are of biological activity equal-to or greater-than the native hormone. Finally, we also found that cultured Kupfer cells produce 1-34, and secrete it into the medium. We propose that the metabolism of PTH by Kupfer cells is mediated through cathepsin D, and that its biological role is to generate and release active fragments of PTH which act on the target tissues for this hormone, i.e. kidney and bone. This study was supported by the NIH.

2520 GROWTH INHIBITION AND INDUCTION OF DIFFERENTIATION IN RAT MALIGNANT OSTEOBLASTS BY RETINOIC ACID. K.W. Ng*, S.A. Livesey, V.P. Michelangeli, T.J. Martin. University of Melbourne Department of Medicine, Repatriation General Hospital, Heidelberg, Victoria 3081, Australia.

A study was undertaken to determine the effects of retinoic acid on the growth and differentiation of UMR 106-06 cells, a subclone of rat malignant osteoblastic cells. The cells were grown as monolayer cultures in alpha modified MEM containing 2% FCS. Retinoic acid (RA) treatment resulted in morphological changes and significant growth inhibition in a reversible and dose-dependent manner. Maximal inhibition was observed at 10^{-6}M. Human PTH (1-34) had a biphasic effect on cell growth after 4 days. Growth was stimulated at $3x10^{-11}$M PTH and inhibited at $3x10^{-9}$M as well as $3x10^{-7}$M. When a submaximal dose of RA (10^{-8}M) was added simultaneously with PTH, a significant synergistic effect on growth inhibition was demonstrated. The interaction between RA and the cAMP dependent effects of PTH was investigated at 2 levels. Firstly, RA increased basal cAMP formation rates. Secondly, after pretreatment with RA, PTH activated both type I and type II cAMP dependent protein kinases isoenzymes. This pattern of activation resembles that demonstrated in rat calvarial cells (1) and contrasts with the selective activation of type I cAMP dependent protein kinase in the malignant cells by PTH alone. These results point to the therapeutic advantage of combining submaximal doses of RA with physiological doses of target hormones. They further demonstrate that RA treatment can change the response of malignant cells to a more differentiated pattern.

1. S.A. Livesey, B.E. Kemp, C.A. Re, N.C. Partridge, T.J. Martin. J.Biol.Chem. 257:14983-14987, 1982

2521 GLUCOCORTICOID RECEPTOR FORMS AND PEPTIDASE ACTIVITIES IN HUMAN LEUKEMIC CELL CYTOSOLS. M.R. Sherman,* F.B. Tuazon and Y.-W. Stevens, Endocrine Biochemistry Laboratory, Sloan-Kettering Institute, New York, NY 10021 USA.

Attempts to correlate the quantity and/or structure of glucocorticoid receptors (GR) in leukemic cell cytosols with the clinical course of patients are complicated by endogenous receptor-cleaving enzymes. Our objectives were 1) to evaluate the Stokes radii (R_S), sedimentation coefficients ($s_{20,w}$), molecular weights (M_r) and axial ratios (a/b) of the oligomeric and monomeric GR forms; 2) to quantitate and characterize the cytosolic peptidases, and 3) to determine the effects of rapidly freezing the cells on GR structure and peptidase activities. Enzymes were assayed fluorometrically with derivatives of 7-amino-4-methylcoumarin. GR, labeled with ^{3}H-triamcinolone acetonide, and enzymes were analyzed concomitantly by agarose filtration and glycerol gradient centrifugation in hypotonic buffer containing 20 mM Na_2MoO_4 (Buf-1) or molybdate-free buffer containing 0.4 M KCl (Buf-2). In Buf-1, parameters of GR from normal lymphocytes and specimens of acute lymphoblastic and non-lymphocytic leukemia and chronic lymphocytic and myelogenous leukemia were similar: $R_S = 8.1 \pm 0.5$ nm (mean ± SD, n = 48), $s_{20,w} = 9.5 \pm 0.3$ S (n = 37), $M_r = 325,000$, a/b = 12. In Buf-2, the latter complex was dissociated into subunits with R_S of 5.9 ± 0.3 nm (n = 10) and a/b of ~12. Fragmentation of GR, particularly in cytosols from frozen cells, was also detected in Buf-2. An aminopeptidase and three endopeptidases were detectable in 20 µl or less of leukemic cell cytosols. Their substrate specificities, R_S and effects of Na_2MoO_4 and $CaCl_2$ were evaluated. Removal or inhibition of such enzymes will be essential for definitive analyses of receptor structure and correlations with other leukemic cell properties or clinical data. (Supported by NCI grants CA28392, CA29564 and CA32178)

2522 PROLACTIN-INDUCIBLE PROTEINS IN HUMAN BREAST CANCER CELLS. R.P.C. Shiu*, G. Lima, and B. Iwasiow, Department of Physiology, Univ. of Manitoba, Winnipeg, Manitoba, R3E 0W3, Canada.

The role of prolactin(PRL) in human breast cancer(HBC) and the mechanism of action PRL in target cells are poorly understood phenomena. The present studies examined the effect of human(h) PRL on the synthesis of proteins by a HBC cancer cell line, T-47D, maintained in serum-free medium containing bovine serum albumin. [35S]methionine-labeled and [3H]glucosamine-labeled proteins secreted into the medium were analyzed by SDS slab polyacrylamide gel electrophoresis and fluorography. Treatment of cells with hPRL(1-1000 ng/ml) and hydrocortisone(F, 1 ug/ml) resulted in the induction of three proteins having molecular weights of 11K, 14K and 16K; the latter two were glycoproteins. Neither hPRL alone nor F alone induced these proteins. Of several other peptide hormones tested, only human growth hormone(hGH), being itself a lactogenic hormone, could replace hPRL in causing protein induction. About 36 hours of treatment with hPRL + F were required for new protein induction to occur. Protein induction was abolished by actinomycin D (1 ug/ml), an inhibitor of RNA synthesis, and was reduced by alpha-difluoromethylornithine(0.1 mM), a specific inhibitor of polyamine synthesis. Further, the PRL-inducible proteins were not immunoprecipitated by antisera to alpha-lactalbumin, casein and total milk proteins. Hence, the functional significance of the PRL-inducible proteins remains to be determined. Nevertheless, we have demonstrated that the two pituitary hormones, hPRL and hGH, are capable of inducing unique proteins, possibly via regulation of gene expression, in human breast cancer cells.(Supported by the Medical Research Council of Canada)

2523 ANTIESTROGENIC ACTIVITY OF LY 156758 IN RAT PITUITARY GONADOTROPHS IN PRIMARY CULTURE. J. Simard* and F. Labrie, MRC Group in Molecular Endocrinology, CHUL, Québec G1V 4G2, Canada.

Estrogens increase both basal and LHRH-induced LH release in rat anterior pituitary cells in culture, the main stimulatory effect being exerted on the sensitivity of LHRH action (ED_{50} value) (Endocrinology 99, 1477, 1976). Due to high degree of precision and sensitivity of measurements of changes of LH release, this parameter can be advantageously used as a bioassay of estrogenic compounds having potential agonistic and antagonistic activities. Following 48h of preincubation with 1 nM 17β-estradiol, the maximal LH response to LHRH is increased 3.2 fold ($p < 0.01$) while the ED_{50} value of LHRH action is decreased 3-fold from 210 to 70 pM ($p < 0.01$). The maximal 3-fold stimulation of 0.3 nM LHRH-induced LH release by 17β-estradiol is exerted at a K_D value of 14.4 PM LY 156756 (300 nM) completely blocks the potent stimulatory effect of 17β-estradiol up to 1 nM, the highest concentration of the estrogen used. As shown by the complete reversal of the stimulatory effect of 0.1 and 1.0 nM 17β-estradiol by LY 156 758 at IC_{50} values of 7.5 and 35 nM, respectively, the antiestrogen interacts competitively with 17β-estradiol at the estrogen binding site. The present data show that, under the experimental conditions described above, LY 156758 acts as a pure antiestrogen on the control of LHRH-induced LH release in rat pituitary gonadotrophs.

2524 METABOLIC PATHWAY OF ANDROGENS IN NON-CANCEROUS AND CANCEROUS HUMAN MAMMARY GLAND TISSUES. P. Singh*, K.R. Laumas and T.G. Muldoon, Dept. of Reproductive Biol. AIIMS, N.Delhi, India, and Dept. of Endocrinology, Med. Col. Georgia, Augusta, U.S.A.

Cancerous (CA) and histologically proven non-cancerous (NOR) breast tissues from women were removed on ice at the time of mastectomy. Unfractionated tissues and tissues fractionated in cytosol and nuclear fractions were then incubated in buffer containing co-factors at 37° C for 60 min with ten nM concentration of the radioactive androgenic steroid followed by extraction of the steroid from the incubates and separation and identification of the extracts by TLC and recrystalization to constant specific activity. The spectrum of metabolic transformation of androgens in both NOR and CA tissues was similar. The major metabolites of testosterone (T_4) were 5a-dihydrotestosterone (DHT) > 3β-diol > polar steroids > Δ 4-dione > 5α-diol > androsterone. The metabolites of DHT were 3α-diol > 3β-diol > polar steroids > T_4 > 5α-diol > 4α-diol > androsterone. Interestingly the oxidative and reductive pathways were distributed between the two sub-cellular fractions of cytosol and nuclei. In nuclear fractions the % metabolic conversion into the dihydroxylated and polar steroids was less compared to that in cytosol fractions, while the amount of 17-ketosteroids formed was higher in the nuclear fractions. The activity of 5 α-reductase, on the other hand, was similar in the two fractions. In the CA tissues the formation of DHT from T_4 was 1.6 times lower compared with that in NOR tissues. Thus a change in the metabolic potential of CA tissue, resulting in increased production of 17-ketosteroids from T_4 and deviation in the degree of formation of DHT from T_4 may be of an etiological importance in the tumorogenesis of hormone dependent tumors.

2525 ALTERED STEROIDOGENESIS IN HUMAN BREAST TUMOR CELLS. M. Smieja and J.P. Wiebe, Hormonal Regulatory Mechanisms Laboratory, Department of Zoology, University of Western Ontario, London N6A 5B7, Canada.

There is evidence linking cancer and altered steroidogenesis in certain tissues. However, no complete profile exists of the differences in steroid metabolism between normal and tumorous tissue. We studied the capacity of normal (NBT) and tumorous (TBT) human breast tissue to metabolize ^{14}C-labelled progesterone (P) and testosterone (T) in vitro. Metabolites were identified by TLC, GC, HPLC, GC/MS, derivatization and crystallization. On a per mg protein basis, NBT and TBT metabolized 1.87 and 3.5% per hour of P and 2.24 and 7.92% per hour of T, respectively. The main metabolites of P were T, 20α-hydroxy-4-pregnen-3-one (20P), and androstenedione (A); amounts of A and T produced showed no clear pattern but production of 20P was 2.8 to 3.5 fold greater by TBT than by NBT. The main metabolites of T were A, 5-androstane-3,17-diol and polar (unidentified) steroid(s). Amounts (ng/mg protein/h) of A produced from T were 13.5±1.1 by NBT and 171.4±29.1 by TBT; in the absence of added cofactor NBT and TBT produced the same amounts (13-16 ng/mg/h) of A. No estrogens were detected among the ^{14}C-labelled metabolites. We conclude that 20α-hydroxysteroid dehydrogenase (20α-HSD) and 17β-HSD activities are markedly (2.8 to 13 fold) greater in tumorous than in non-tumorous human breast tissue. (Supported by NSERC of Canada).

2526 COVALENT MODIFICATION OF AROMATASE BY A RADIOLABELED IRREVERSIBLE INHIBITOR. C.E. Snider* and R. W. Brueggemeier, College of Pharmacy and OSU Comprehensive Cancer Center, The Ohio State University, Columbus, Ohio 43210, USA.

7α-Substituted 4-androstene-3,17-diones are effective inhibitors of aromatase. The microsomal enzyme complex has a greater affinity for several of these inhibitors than for the substrate androstenedione, with 7α-(4'-amino)phenylthio-4-androstene-3,17-dione being the most potent competitive inhibitor of the series. Irreversible analogs have been prepared and are being utilized to examine the active site of aromatase. A bromoacetamide derivative of the amino compound has been synthesized in both unlabeled and ^{14}C-labeled forms via a condensation of bromoacetic acid with the amino compound using DCC. Inactivation studies with the unlabeled inhibitor showed a time-dependent, first-order inactivation of aromatase enzymatic activity. Androstenedione, when incubated in varying concentrations with the irreversible inhibitor, provided protection from inactivation. Binding studies with radiolabeled inhibitor and microsomal aromatase preparations showed that irreversible binding had occurred. SDS- and 2D-electrophoresis, followed by fluorography, identified four major microsomal proteins that were radiolabeled, with the protein band at 52,000 MW predominating. Similar studies with partially purified aromatase preparations decreased the amount of nonspecific binding. Thus, covalent bonds between the irreversible inhibitor and the aromatase cytochrome P450 molecule are formed. This study was supported by Grant HD 15014 from NIH.

2527 HUMAN BREAST CARCINOMAS PRODUCE SOMATOMEDIN-C. E.M. Spencer and J.L. Bennington, Children's Hospital, San Francisco, CA 94118, U.S.A.

Since somatomedins (SMs) are potent mitogens, they may have a role in malignant proliferation. SM production has been identified in human fibrosarcoma cells, cultured buffalo rat liver tumor cells, experimental mouse mammary tumors, and several lines of human mammary carcinoma cells. The objective of this study was to determine whether human, normal breast tissue and/or carcinomas produced SM-C. To detect cellular production a sensitive peroxidase-antiperoxidase (PAP) immunohistochemical (IHC) technique was developed. Tissues were fixed in neutral buffered formalin and embedded in paraffin prior to staining by a modification of the method of Sternberger. Positive staining was observed in normal hepatic tissue, the primary site of SM production, but not in staining controls or hepatomas. Using the GH-deficient lit/lit mouse plasma membrane binding of SM-C could also be detected in the chondrocytes of GH-treated, but not in untreated mice. Normal breast tissue and fibroadenomas did not stain for SM-C, but 6 of 6 mammary ductal carcinomas were positive. These studies demonstrate that: Immunohistochemical techniques can be used to detect SM-C cellular synthesis and plasma membrane binding. SM-C is synthesized by human breast ductal carcinomas and may be a factor in their development and course. SM-C production by mammary carcinoma cells may be very useful as an *in vitro* model to evaluate therapeutic agents if additional investigations establish a relationship between synthesis of this growth factor and the course and prognosis of mammary carcinomas.

2528 DISPARATE EFFECTS OF FETUIN ON ^{125}I-LUTEINIZING HORMONE BINDING TO MELANOMA AND LUTEAL TISSUE. R. Stouffer*, M. Grodin, D. Sander, and F. Meyskens, Jr. Departments of Physiology and Internal Medicine, College of Medicine, Univ. of Arizona, Tucson, Arizona, USA 85724.

We recently reported that murine and human melanoma contain binding sites for luteinizing hormone (LH) which appear qualitatively distinct from those in the gonads (J Steroid Biochem 19:128S). To compare the specificity of LH binding sites in melanoma and gonadal tissue, homogenates of murine (Cloudman S91) melanoma cells and ovaries of pseudopregnant rats were incubated with 10 ng ^{125}I-human (h) LH (NIH LH-I-1) for 20 h at 25C in the presence of various amounts of hormones and glycoproteins. Both chorionic gonadotropin (hCG) and hLH were effective inhibitors of ^{125}I-LH uptake by luteal tissue (ED_{50}=0.6 IU and 1.0 IU, respectively); however, hCG was 50-fold less potent than LH in displacing ^{125}I-LH uptake by melanoma. Other glycoproteins, including transferrin, interferon, and α_2-macroglobulin did not prevent ^{125}I-LH uptake by either tissue. In contrast, fetuin (Sigma Type III and IV, a glycoprotein in fetal calf serum) and asialofetuin inhibited ^{125}I-LH binding to melanoma, but not to luteal tissue, in a dose-dependent manner. Compared to control uptake (3.91 ± 0.52 ng LH bound/5×10^6 cells; $\bar{x}\pm$SE, n=4), optimal doses of fetuin ($\approx$serum levels) and LH (30 IU) suppressed ^{125}I-LH binding to a similar extent (1.89 ± 0.21 and 1.52 ± 0.18 ng, respectively, $p<0.05$). Addition of fetal calf serum also diminished LH binding to melanoma ($p<0.05$), but not to luteal tissue. We conclude that 1) melanoma contains binding sites with affinity for both fetuin-like and LH-like glycoproteins, or alternatively 2) pituitary LH preparations include a fetuin-like substance which binds to specific sites on melanoma, but not luteal, tissue. NIH CA 33336

2529 PLASMA LEVELS OF PROTEO- AND STEROID HORMONES AND OF MEDROXY-PROGESTERONE ACETATE (MPA) ESTIMATED IN HIGH DOSE MPA TREATED CANCER PATIENTS. G. Sturm*, P. Schmidt-Rhode, K.-D. Schulz and H. J. Künzig , Dept. Gynecol. Obstetrics, Philipps University D 3550 Marburg, FRG.

The mechanisms of the anti-tumor activity of 6α-methyl-17α-hydroxyprogesterone acetate in high dose MPA treated cancer patients are still under research and may partly correspond to the influence of MPA on endocrine control functions. We therefore correlated the plasma levels of MPA to hormones in patients with advanced breast cancer, treated with 1.000 mg MPA p.o. / day. MPA was determined by a mass fragmentographic controlled RIA , LH, FSH, hPRL, ACTH, cortisol, E_1, E_2, and E_1S by RIAs. MPA-metabolites were measured by HPLC, RIA and GC-MF. In the long term MPA treated patients (n=25) we observed increasing mean plasma MPA levels from 22 ng/ml on day 2 to 64 ng/ml on day 9 and 143 ng/ml on day 30 of treatment. Parallel to this increase of plasma MPA the plasma prolactin levels ascended to more than 200%, the LH and FSH values declined to 30% and the estrogens to 30-50% of their values before treatment. The interesting finding is that plasma cortisol levels decreased to 10% of the initial values, whereas plasma ACTH increased to about 150%. Furthermore tumor remission could be observed in such MPA treated patients, who´s plasma MPA levels exceeded 110 ng/ml. The study was supported by the P.E. Kempkes Stiftung.

2530 GROWTH INHIBITION OF GH_3 PITUITARY TUMOR IN RATS BY D-TRP^6-LH-RH. I. Torres-Aleman, T. W. Redding, B. F. Edwards and A. V. Schally*, VA Med. Center and Tulane Univ. Med. School, New Orleans, LA 70146, USA.
Previously we have shown that chronic administration of D-Trp^6-LH-RH and Somatostatin (SS) analogs inhibited the growth of the 7315a rat pituitary tumor (PNAS 80:3485,1983). We have now extended our observations to the prolactin(PRL)- and growth hormone(GH)-producing GH_3 pituitary tumor. Three days after transplantation of the tumor, female Wistar/Furth rats were injected s.c. with 25 μg/b.i.d. D-Trp^6-LH-RH or 5 μg/b.i.d. of SS analogs: cyclo(Pro-Phe-D-Trp-Lys-Thr-Phe) or D-Phe-Cys-Phe-D-Trp-Lys-Thr-Cys-Thr-NH_2 After seven weeks of treatment, rats were sacrificed and trunk blood collected. Tumor, body, pituitary and ovarian weights were recorded and tumor volume was measured. Serum and pituitary hormones were measured by RIA. In the D-Trp^6-LH-RH treated group, tumor volume was 34.5 ± 15 mm^3 vs. 538 ± 230 mm^3 for controls, a 93.6% decrease ($p<0.05$). D-Trp^6-LH-RH administration also diminished tumor weight from 0.52 ± 0.2 g (controls) to 0.04 ± 0.02 g, a 92.4% reduction ($p<0.05$). Body and pituitary weights were unaffected but ovarian weights were reduced. In contrast, tumor weight and volume increased by more than 40% after SS analogs administration vs. the controls, although these changes were not significant. Serum PRL, GH and insulin levels in D-Trp-6-LHRH treated animals were reduced by 94.7%, 83.7% and 29.7% respectively, as compared to controls. Pituitary PRL and LH, but not GH content were decreased after D-Trp^6-LH-RH administration. These results suggest that D-Trp^6-LH-RH should be considered for further research aimed at the development of a new therapy for certain human pituitary tumors. This work was supported by grants from NIH and VA.

2531 BETA-ENDORPHIN AND CANCER. K.Tsunashima, K.Ooya, K.Yoshitake, M.Soo, T.Yoshitake, N.Suzuki, H.Tokugawa and N. Iijima, 2nd Surgical Clinic, St. Marianna University, School of Medicine, 2095 Sugao, Kawasaki,Japan.

Beta-endorphin (0.2 to 2 mg/kg twice daily) was injected s.c. to C_3H male mice, 24 hours after transplantation of 5 x 10^6 MH_{134} cancer cells. The dose effect response of this peptide to promote cancers growth was observed with and the increase in fibrinonectin in P_2 of cancer cell. These effects were considerably reversed by twice daily injection of Naloxone (5 mg/kg). Naloxone increase antibody dependent cell mediated cytotoxity (ADCC) in spleen and thymus. In spontaneous mammary tumors (G_3H, GR) and transplantable lung cancer ($C_{57}BL$) bearing mice, the injection of Naloxone greatly increased the survival rate of the animals. And besides in about 50 human cancers including mammary, grastric and colono-rectal neoplasmas, Beta-endorphin remarkably increased in almost all cancers. According to the established fact that Beta-endorphin acts as stress-substance from brain, opioid antagonism may play an important role in cancer chemotherapy in relation to psycho-endocrino-immunological point of view.

2532 ESTRIOL AND CATECHOLESTROGEN BINDING SITES IN BREAST CANCER. B. Vandewalle, J. Bonneterre, JP. Peyrat, J. Lefebvre*, Laboratoire d'Endocrinologie Expérimentale, Centre de Lutte Contre le Cancer du Nord, BP 307, 59020 LILLE CEDEX (France)

The potential interaction between estradiol metabolites and estrogen receptors has been investigated in breast cancers. In these tumors, a significantly greater extent of 16-α-hydroxylation has been reported on one hand (Schneider et al., 1982 Proc. Nat. Acad. Sci. USA 79:3047) and the presence of the enzyme system catalyzing the synthesis of catecholestrogens has been described on the other hand (Hoffman et al. 1979 Cancer Res. 39:3584) ; therefore the selected E2 metabolites were estriol (E3) and catecholestrogens (CE) - 2-hydroxy and 4-hydroxyestrone - the end products of 2 and 4 hydroxylations. The mean levels of specific estrogen metabolite binding sites per mg protein, assayed in the cytosol of 53 breast tumors, were lower than those of E2 binding sites. A high correlation between E3 and E2 binding sites ($p<0.01$) and a weaker correlation between CE and E2 binding sites ($0.01<p<0.02$) were found. Contrary to E3 binding sites, essentially located in the cytosol, CE binding sites had subcellular distribution and ligand binding specificity different from those of E2 receptors ; no correlation between microsomal and cytosolic CE binding sites was found. E3 is now generally thought to be a potent estrogen agonist, the action of CE, however, is still bad-known ; they have been shown to be estrogenic, non estrogenic and even antiestrogenic. Our results show that CE action could be mediated through mechanisms other than E2 receptors and raise the question of the biological significance of estradiol metabolites in breast cancer.

2533 CHARACTERISTICS OF CLONED ANDROGEN-SENSITIVE (A+) AND ANDROGEN-INSENSITIVE (A^-) SC-115 CELLS IN CULTURE. R. Veilleux*, C. Kreis and F. Labrie, Dept of Molecular Endocrinology, CHUL, Québec G1V 4G2, Canada.

The mouse mammary tumor Shionogi cells (SC-115) grown in tissue culture show a 5-fold increase in cell density in the presence of maximal concentrations of DHT ($\geq$ 10 nM). When the cells are incubated in the absence of DHT for 5 months, the rate of cell growth is first decreased by approximately 60% while the response of cell growth to DHT measured during a 2-week exposure period is also decreased by 60%. At 9 months, the growth rate of cells incubated in the absence of DHT is similar to that measured in cells exposed to the androgen and the response to DHT is 90% lost. In addition, the prolonged absence (5 months) of DHT decreases the sensitivity of the response to the androgen by ~ 10-fold from 3 to 30 nM. Cells were then cloned on soft agar in order to examine the possibility of mixed populations of androgen-sensitive and androgen-insensitive cells in the original tumor. Following cloning, the androgen-sensitive cells showed an increased sensitivity of their response to DHT (K_D value of 0.3 nM). The stimulatory effect of DHT can be completely reversed by the pure antiandrogen Anandron. The A^+ cells show, in the presence of DHT, the typical fusiform morphology while the A^- cells show the cuboidal appearance. Analysis of proteins labelled with ^{35}S-methionine from A^+ and A^- cells by 2-D gel electrophoresis revealed the presence of androgen-sensitive proteins in A^+ cells, the level of incorporation of ^{35}S-methionine into these proteins being stimulated by DHT and reduced or inhibited in the presence of the antiandrogen. Proper analysis of A^+ and A^- tumor cells thus require repeated cloning of the cells in order to maintain homogeneity of the cell population.

2534 β-ENDORPHIN: CHARACTERISTICS OF BINDING SITES SPECIFIC FOR THE HUMAN HORMONE IN HUMAN GLIOBLASTOMA AND NEUROBLASTOMA CELLS. M. Westphal* and Choh Hao Li, Laboratory of Molecular Endocrinology, University of California, San Francisco, CA 94143.

Three established human neuroblastoma cell lines (IMR-32, Kelly, NMB) and one established human glioblastoma cell line (SF126) were investigated for binding sites for tritiated human beta-endorphin (^{3}H-β_h-EP) in whole cell binding assays. Binding of ^{3}H-β_h-EP to SF126 is saturable, maximal at 90 min at 22°C, instantaneously reversible and reduced by 80% in the presence of 150 mM NaCl. The ED_{50} is estimated to be 2.5 nM from competition binding experiments. Tritiated [D-Ala^2,D-Leu^5]-enkephalin and tritiated dihydromorphine did not bind to the cells.

All three human neuroblastoma cell lines bound ^{3}H-β_h-EP with affinities between 2.5 and 4 nM. In all cell lines the binding of ^{3}H-β_h-EP appears to be mediated through the COOH-terminus. The β_h-EP-(6-31) still retains high potency for displacing ^{3}H-β_h-EP (15%-75%) in all cell lines and the β_h-EP-(1-27) is without any detectable activity. The β_h-EP-(28-31) can still fully displace ^{3}H-β_h-EP. Camel β-EP has maximally only 1% of the displacing potency compared to the human hormone. β_h-EP may therefore be a molecule with two separate, opioid and non-opioid activities residing at the two ends of the peptide. This study was supported in part by NIH Grant GM-2907, NIDA Grant DA03434 and the Hormone Research Foundation. M.W. is a recipient of training grant from the Deutsche Forschungsgemeinschaft.

2535 THE EFFECT OF AROMATASE INHIBITOR, 4-HYDROXYANDROSTENEDIONE ON SEX STEROID TARGET TISSUES. L. Wing*, C. Tsai-Morris and A. Brodie, Dept. Pharm. & Exp. Therapeutics, U. of MD School of Medicine, Baltimore, MD 21201, USA.

4-Hydroxyandrostenedione (4-OHA) inhibits ovarian aromatase and causes marked regression of DMBA-induced, hormone-dependent mammary tumors in rats. Although estrogen secretion is also reduced, the level of LH does not increase during treatment nor does uterine weight decline as in ovariectomized (OVX) rats. Direct action of 4-OHA on the uterus and pituitary was therefore investigated. Although 2.5 μg/rat estradiol and E_2 + 4-OHA increased uterine weight 2-fold in immature rats after 48 hrs, 4-OHA (50 mg/kg/day) was without effect, suggesting no estrogenic or antiestrogenic action of the compound. However, treatment with 4-OHA for 2 weeks prevented uterine regression in OVX rats in a dose-response manner; 50 mg/kg/day was similar to intact diestrus controls and to 1.8 mg/kg/day dihydrotestosterone. The simultaneous injection of antiandrogen (flutamide) with 4-OHA completely blocked the effect of 4-OHA on the uterus. In rats OVX 2 weeks previously and primed with E_2 and progesterone on day 0, E_2 caused a 2-fold increase in the LH surge 20 mins after LHRH injection on day 2, whereas both DHT and 4-OHA treatment reduced LH by 30% of controls ($p < 0.05$). The results indicate that these actions of 4-OHA may be due to its weak androgenic activity. The effects may be beneficial for the proposed use of the aromatase inhibitor in breast cancer patients. 1) Inhibition of LH release by 4-OHA will prevent new aromatase synthesis under gonadotropin control. 2) The effect of 4-OHA on the uterus will prevent atrophy of the reproductive tract which otherwise occurs with reduced estrogen levels.

2536 ESTROGEN-INDUCED SECRETORY PROTEINS IN EXPERIMENTAL BREAST CANCER: BIOSYNTHETIC AND BIOLOGICAL STUDIES. C. Wright*, L. Baranao, P. Feil, and A. Manni, Dept. of Medicine, Div. of Endocrinology, The M.S. Hershey Medical Center, The Pennsylvania State University, Hershey, PA 17033

Prior studies indicate that estradiol (E_2) can stimulate breast cancer cells to synthesize specific secretory proteins. It is possible that these proteins might modulate the rate of tumor cell growth. We tested this hypothesis in the estrogen-responsive N-nitrosomethyl-urea (NMU)-induced rat mammary tumor grown in vitro in the soft agar clonogenic assay. The biosynthesis of secretory protein was confirmed by obtaining conditioned media (CM) from E_2 (10^{-8}M) treated tumors (incubated with ^{3}H-leucine) and from untreated tumors (incubated with ^{14}C-leucine). Pooled CM were subjected to SDS-PAGE and $^3H/^{14}C$ ratios calculated to follow the synthesis of specific E_2-induced proteins. This highly sensitive technique indicated that E_2 primarily stimulated the synthesis of 60,000 dalton protein(s). To evaluate the biologic significance of these secretory proteins, we tested the mitogenic potential of CM obtained from E_2 treated tumors. After charcoal stripping to remove E_2, serum-free CM was added to NMU-mammary tumors plated in soft agar. A consistent stimulation of colony formation to 136% of control was observed, a level more than double that of CM obtained from tumors not exposed to E_2 (114% of control). Such stimulatory activity was half of that produced by 10^{-8}M E_2 (174% of control). These data indicate that E_2 may stimulate NMU tumor growth through induction of specific secretory proteins by the cancer cells.

2537 IMMUNOHISTOCHEMICAL LOCALIZATION OF CYTOSKELETAL PROTEINS AND THYROGLOBULIN IN THYROID CANCERS.

Y. Yagi*, S. Yagi and T. Sakurami, Department of Biochemistry, Kagoshima Univ. School of Medicine, 1208-1 Usuki-cho, Kagoshima-city, Japan.

Using antibodies against three kinds of cytoskeletal proteins (actin, myosin and keratin) and thyroglobulin, the immunoperoxidase staining was performed in 18 cases of thyroid cancers (papillary carcinoma:14, follicular carcinoma:4). Both actin and myosin were distinctly found in almost all neoplastic cells of all patients with papillary and follicular carcinomas. Keratin was present in almost all or some neoplastic cells of 5 patients only with papillary carcinoma. Thyroglobulin was found in almost all tumor cells of 3 cases of papillary carcinoma and one of follicular carcinoma, and was also found in some tumor cells of 7 cases of papillary carcinoma and 2 of follicular carcinoma. However, stronger reaction for thyroglobulin seemed to be present in follicular carcinoma cells or keratin-negative tumor cells. These findings are suggested that actin and myosin may be one of the specific markers of neoplastic cells, and that keratin or thyroglobulin may be related to different degrees of cellular differentiation.

2538 VARIANTS OF HUMAN CHORIONIC GONADOTROPIN (hCG): BIOLOGICAL ACTIVITY OF CHORIOCARCINOMA-RELATED COMPONENTS

*K. Yazaki, M. Igarashi, K. Wakabayashi, S.S. Koide[1], Dept. of Obst. Gyn. Gunma Univ. Med School, Gunma, Japan, and [1]The Population Council, New York, New York

Microheterogeneity is a common property of glycoprotein hormones, e.g., hCG. We have previously analyzed sera of patients afflicted with choriocarcinoma (CCa) for variants of hCG by isoelectric focusing technique (IEF) and detected CCa-related components. In the present study CCa tissues were analyzed for variants of hCG and each separated component was tested for biological potencies. CCa tissues in uterine specimens removed by hysterectomy were immediately processed and the extracts subjected to IEF. In total 65 fractions were analyzed. hCG, $hCG\alpha$ and $hCG\beta$ in each component separated by IEF were determined by their respective homologous radioimmunoassay systems. The IEF pattern showed 12 peaks of immunoreactive hCG components with pIs ranging from 3.2 to 6.8. Components of pIs above 3.9 corresponded to the variants present in normal placenta and molar tissues; whereas components focusing at pI 3.2, 3.5 and 3.7 appeared to be unique to CCa. Biological potency was determined by measuring testosterone production by rat Leydig cells in vitro. The major component focused at pI 4.1 and possessed the highest biological potency. Components focusing at pI 3.5 and 3.7 also demonstrated comparatively high potency while components focusing in the alkaline range had low biological activity. In conclusion, CCa tissues contain unique variants of hCG (pI 3.2, 3.5 and 3.7) not found in placenta or molar tissues. The component focusing at pI 4.1 and the CCa-related variants (pI 3.5 and 3.7) possessed high biological potencies while those focusing further afield from pI 4.1 showed decreasing biological activities.

2539 DISPERSION OF FORMALIN-FIXED GLANDULAR TUMORS AND MEASUREMENT OF THE CELL CYCLE BY FLOW CYTOMETRY. M.A. Younes*, T.B. Nielsen, D. Dennison, P.K. Besch and M.O. Korhonen, Departments of Obstetrics/Gynecology, Medicine and Cell Biology, Baylor College of Medicine, Houston, Texas 77030.

Fixation of human endocrine gland tumors with formalin is a routine storage procedure. We reversed the fixation in hydatidiform moles, placentas and ovarian carcinomas by a 2 hour incubation with 0.2% collagenase, 0.5% trypsin and 0.15 M NH_4Cl. Isolated cells were then freed from tissue fragments and debris by gradient centrifugations using Ficoll and fetal calf serum. After staining with ethidium bromide for 10 minutes, the cells were analyzed by flow cytometry, which evaluates cells for DNA content. Control studies with placenta showed that fixed and normal tissue had a similar distribution of cells in the G_1 (a range of 60-81%), S (8-20%) and G_2-M (2-8%) parts of the cell cycle. Cells from ovarian tumor and molar tissue had a greater proportion of cells in S (17-45% and 30-42%, respectively) and in G_2-M (11-30% and 16-43%, respectively). Thus, fast-growing tumors had a greater proportion of cells in the S and G_2-M part of the cell cycle. Alternatively, the high proportion of cells in G_2-M could reflect a population of cells resting in G_2. In conclusion, fixed pathological specimens stored for months yielded dispersed cell preparations suitable for analysis of the cell cycle. (Supported in part by St. Luke's Episcopal Hospital, Reproductive Research Laboratory Special Projects #71002.)

2540 INCREASED IN VITRO PRODUCTION OF DHT-GLUCURONIDE(G) and 3αANDROSTANEDIOL(3αdiol) G FROM THE SKIN OF HIRSUTE WOMEN P. Serafini, F. Ablan and R. Lobo,* Univ. of So. Calif. Sch. of Med., L.A., Calif.

Steroid production in peripheral tissues is important in the manifistation of androgen excess. An androgen metabolite in serum (3αdiolG), which is extrasplanchnic in origin, has an excellent correlation with hirsutism (JCEM 57:393,1983). To further characterize peripheral tissue metabolism in hirsutism, genital skin biopsies were obtained from 22 patients and 23 age and weight-match premenopausal controls. Skin homogenates were incubated with ^{14}C-T in RPMI1640 media at 37°C with 95% C_{o2} and 5% C_{o2}. Serum from patients and controls was analysed for DHT, 3αdiol and 3αdiolG by RIA. In hirsute patients , $CR_{T\rightarrow DHT}$ (8.2±0.9%) $CR_{T\rightarrow 3\ diol}$ (4.8±0.5%), and PR DHT (1.6±0.3 pmol/mg/hr) were higher than values in controls (2.2±0.2, 1.6±0.2, 0.28±0.04 $p < .01$). While serum DHT and 3α diol were similar in patients and controls, serum 3αdiolG was significantly higher (268±68 vs 40±4 ng/dl. $p<.01$). In 10 skin homogenates, additional experiments verified in vitro production of DHT-G and 3αdiolG. $CR_{T\rightarrow DHTG}$and $_{T\rightarrow 3\ diolG}$ in hirsute patients (1.9±.7%, 0.53±.1%) was higher than in controls (0.34±0.2%, 0.25±.07%. $p<0.05$), as was the skin PR DHT→G and 3αdiol G (45.±12 and 218±38 vs 15±4 and 82±17 fmol/mg/hr. $p<.05$). There was a positive correlation between serum 3αdiolG and in vitro $CR_{T\rightarrow 3\ diolG}$, r=0.74, $p<.05$. These data confirm the importance of peripheral tissue enzymatic activity in hirsutism. Further, human skin has been shown to synthesize DHT-G and 3αdiolG. While serum DHT and 3αdiol may not correlate with hirsutism or tissue production of these steroids serum 3αdiolG, which is an excellent clinical marker, may arise from tissue 3αdiolG production.

2541 ACROMEGALY : LONG-TERM ASSESSMENT OF CURE BY TRANSSPHENOIDAL MICROSURGERY.
O. Serri*, R. Comtois, E. Rasio, J. Hardy and M. Somma, Notre-Dame Hospital, University of Montreal, Montreal, Canada.

We have reported that recurrence of hyperprolactinemia after successful surgical removal of prolactinomas is frequent and delayed (N Engl J Med 1983; 309: 280-3). To evaluate the long-term prognosis for acromegalic patients after selective transsphenoidal adenomectomy, we followed, for at least 5 years, 25 patients without any previous or simultaneous radiotherapy. Clinical, radiologic and biochemical assessments were made bofore and at various intervals after surgery. The patients, 14 men and 11 women, were classified in 2 groups. Group I (8 patients) presented microadenomas and a mean basal plasma GH value of 23.9 ± 2.4 ng/ml. Group II (17 patients) had macroadenomas and a mean basal GH value of 55.5 ± 14.3 ng/ml. After surgery, cure of acromegaly (basal GH values less than 5 ng/ml and normal GH response to hyperglycemia) was achieved in all 8 Group I patients and in 15 Group II patients. Relapse of acromegaly occurred in 3 Group II patients after a period of 6 months to 3 years of clinical and biochemical remission. Among the 20 cured patients five years after surgery, 3 showed paradoxical GH increase after TRH while maintaining normal GH suppression by oral hyperglycemia. All other cured patients had normal GH responses to hyperglycemia, insulin-induced hypoglycemia and TRH. The reported data emphasize that contrary to prolactinomas, GH-secreting pituitary adenomas rarely relapse after successful surgery.

2542 BIOACTIVE (BIO) LH AND THE BIO:IMMUNOREACTIVE (I) LH RATIO AFTER NALOXONE (NAL) AS A PROBE FOR ENDOGENOUS CENTRAL OPIOID ACTIVITY (COA) IN WOMEN. D. Shoupe*, R. Barnes, F.J. Montz, S.D. Brazal and R. Lobo. Univ. So. of California Sch. of Med., Los Angeles, Calif.

It has been demonstrated that BEP modulates GnRH neuronal activity. Responses of LH after Nal have been used, therefore, as a probe for COA. We studied the effect of Nal on bioLH, iLH and the bio:iLH ratio in 5 ovulatory women (OV) in the late follicular (LF) and midluteal (ML) phases as well as in 5 premenopausal women (PM) and 5 patients with polycystic ovary syndrome (PCO). BioLH was measured using the mouse interstitial cell assay and bio and iLH were measured using LER907. Blood samples were obtained at 15 min intervals before, during and after a 4-hr Nal infusion. In LF-OV, there was a significant increase in both iLH (43±6%), bioLH (55±8%) and a 20±5% increase in the bio:iLH ratio. Bio:iLH ratios were higher in MML of OV and iLH, bioLH and bio:iLH ratios increased significantly (48±7%, 61±10%, 30±5%, $p<.05$). PM had elevated baseline bio:iLH ratio and no responses of bioLH or iLH after Nal. Patients with PCO had minimal changes of iLH after Nal (17±2%) but significantly increased bioLH (49±5%) and bio:iLH ratios (51±4%). These data suggest that Nal results in the modulation of GnRH favoring LH secretion with greater biological activity. BioLH and bio:iLH ratios after Nal may be more sensitive markers than iLH as probes for COA. Decreased COA results in absent bio and iLH responses after Nal as in PM. When iLH responses are minimal or absent (PCO), bioLH and bio:iLH ratios suggest increased COA.

2543 ENDOGENOUS DOPAMINERGIC DYSFUNCTION: A NOVEL FORM OF HGH DEFICIENCY AND SHORT STATURE. M. Sibilia* and C.A. Huseman, Department of Pediatrics, University of Nebraska Medical Center, Omaha, NE 68105, USA.

The purpose of this study was to determine if combined therapy with dopaminergic drugs(DA) and exogenous hGH could increase growth velocity in hypopituitary children. Twelve prepubertal hypopituitary children(8 boys,4 girls,BA 3-11y) were studied. In a previous study 7 of these children had achieved normal growth for their BA by DA alone.The present study consisted of 2 groups.Grp 1(n=6) received L-dopa(L-D),15mg/kg po 6hrly for 6mo; then hGH,0.1IU/kg im 3x/wk for 6mo;and finally hGH & L-D at above dosages for a third 6mo period.Grp 2(n=6) received bromocriptine(BCT),1.25mg po every 12h for 6mo; hGH,0.1IU/kg 3x/wk for the next 6mo;and hGH & BCT at above dosages for a third 6mo period. Mean growth rates(cm/y±SE) in the 2 groups before, and during the 3 periods respectively,were: Grp 1: 3.5±0.2,6.6±0.7,6.8±0.3, 7.7±0.6, & 3 children showed a 12-21% growth increment on hGH & L-D as compared to hGH alone.Grp 2: 3±0.3,5±0.5,8±1.1 and 8±0.8, & 2 children showed a 22-32% growth increment on BCT & hGH as compared to hGH alone.Mean & peak hGH(ng/ml±SE) values measured every 30min for 6h at each study were significantly greater($p<0.05$) in the 5 patients with greater growth increments on hGH & L-D or BCT than hGH alone.Mean hGH values increased from 15±3 during hGH therapy to 30±5 during hGH & DA.Peak hGH values rose from 24±4 to 45±5.Somatomedin C,basal & GnRH induced LH & FSH,T_4,TSH,cortisol,estradiol and testosterone did not change significantly by combined DA & hGH therapy as compared with pre,DA or hGH. Conclusions: Addition of dopaminergic agents to hGH therapy potentiates hGH effects in some hypopituitary children. The increased hGH responses to L-D or BCT indicate impaired endogenous GH release. DA therapy may be uniquely efficacious in these children.

2544 Bioavailability of Rectally Administered Propylthiouracil (PTU). J.D.H. Silverberg*, W.R. Bartle, and S.E. Walker, Depts. of Medicine and Pharmacy, Sunnybrook Medical Centre, University of Toronto, Toronto, Ontario, Canada.

Thionamide drugs are useful in the management of thyrotoxicosis. Such drugs may be limited by their oral route of administration. Recently, methimazole was shown to exhibit sufficient circulating levels after rectal administration. This study examines the bioavailability of rectally administered propylthiouracil (PTU). Seven male subjects received 400 mg of PTU as an oral tablet and one week later as a rectal suppository prepared with Witepsol Wax H15 (suppository 1). Four of these subjects received a second PTU suppository formulated as a diethanolamine salt (suppository 2). Serum PTU was measured by reverse phase high pressure liquid chromatography serially after drug administration. Reverse triiodothyroxine (rT3) levels were also measured serially to assess the biological effect of PTU. The area under the curve (AUC) for the oral preparation (23.7 ± 3.2 ug.hr/ml) was significantly greater than either rectal preparation (6.2 ± 5.4 ug.hr/ml for suppository 1, 8.20 ± 3.9 ug.hr/ml for suppository 2). The AUCs for both rectal preparations were not significantly different. Both suppository preparations showed significantly lower peak serum concentrations (Cmax) and longer time to peak serum concentration (Tmax) relative to the oral preparation. Cmax and Tmax were not different with either suppository. The rT3 levels rose to the same extent with the oral and both rectal preparations. We conclude that rectally administered PTU gives lower circulating drug levels then the oral preparation; however the rise in the rT3 levels may imply a biological effect. Sunnybrook Trust for Medical Research supported.

2545 CUSHING'S DISEASE WITH NORMAL SIZE SELLA TURCICA: CURE BY TRANSSPHENOIDAL SURGERY. M. Somma*, E. Rasio, F. Robert and J. Hardy, Notre-Dame Hospital University of Montreal, Montreal, Quebec H2L 4K8, Canada.

Thirty-four patients (9 males, 25 females) out of a group of 42 with Cushing's disease, with normal size sella turcica and without previous radiotherapy, were cured by transsphenoidal microsurgery. Cure was achieved in 25 patients by adenomectomy. The tumors ranged in size from 2 to 9 mm in diameter. In the remaining 9 patients where no tumor was seen by the surgeon, 7 were cured by resection of the pituitary median region and 2 by total hypophysectomy: in these cases, 5 tumors were identified by the pathologist. Following surgery, clinical and biological cortisol deficiency was evident in all patients but one. Urinary excretion of free cortisol (UF) and plasma levels of cortisol (PF) fell respectively from 481 ± 51 mcg/24 h and 20.8 ± 1.3 mcg/dl (mean values ± S.E.M.) before surgery, to 8 ± 1 mcg/24 h and 2.2 ± 0.3 mcg/dl in the first week after surgery. In the patients who were not treated by total hypophysectomy, surgery induced partial deficits in 3. In 13 patients with a follow-up of at least one year, glucocorticoid therapy was withdrawn in all but one. In this group, UF averaged 36 ± 5 mcg/24 h and PF 13.9 ± 1.4 mcg/dl. In conclusion: i/ Over 80% of patients with normal size sella turcica are cured by transsphenoidal surgery. ii/ Removal of the pituitary median area is a successful treatment when there is no macroscopic evidence of tumor. iii/ Transient cortisol deficiency is a valuable index of cure.

2546 PITUITARY AND GONADAL RESPONSE TO PULSATILE LHRH THERAPY IN THE IDIOPATHIC HYPOGONADOTROPIC HYPOGONADAL (IHH) MALE. D. Spratt*, R. Katzin, J. Campbell, and W. Crowley. Depts Gyn and Med, Vincent Labs, Mass General Hospital, Boston, MA 02114.

Pulsatile LHRH was administered to 16 consecutive men with IHH by portable Ferring infusion pumps at 2° intervals sc for 3-30 mo. The dose was adjusted until normal adult testosterone levels (T) were achieved and varied from 25-300 ng/kg. T normalized in 15 men (mean pre-Rx T 55± 6 ng% SE vs 837 ± 97 ng% maximum during therapy); a marked increase in gonadal size occurred (mean pre-Rx 6 ± 1.5 ml vs 14 ± 1.5 ml peak); and mature spermatozoa appeared in the ejaculate of 66% in whom normal adult levels of serum T were maintained for>6 mo. Two men impregnanted their wives. Gonadotropin pulsations above the normal adult male range were required to initiate gonadal steroidogenesis whereas following gonadal maturation normal T levels could be maintained with normal LH and FSH levels thus documenting gonadal amplification. Identical doses of LHRH given prior to and following sexual maturation produced significantly greater serum levels of LH and FSH following sexual maturation suggesting the existence of pituitary amplification. Dose response testing to LHRH following pituitary priming revealed a linear-log relationship between the LH response and LHRH dose and documented that LHRH can alter the B/I ratio of these IHH men. Concl: 1) Pulsatile LHRH administered sc by portable infusion pumps is an effective therapy of IHH. 2) Pituitary and gonadal amplification occurs during sexual maturation. 3) LHRH is capable of altering both biologic and immunologic levels of gonadotropins in IHH males. (Supported by NIH Grant#1-R01-HD-15788.

2547 INLUENCE OF BROMOCRIPTINE ON TRIGLYCERIDE DYNAMICS IN PATIENTS WITH GENERALIZED LIPODYSTROPHY. N.T.Starkova*, E.K.Letova, Institute of Experimental Endocrinology and Hormone Chemistry, the USSR Academy of Medical Sciences, Moscow, USSR

Generalized lipodystrophy (GLD) is a rare poorly understood neuroendocrine disease. Taking into consideration its supposed hypothalamo-pituitary origin and favourable effect of bromocriptine on lipid metabolism in some other hypothalamo-pituitary diseases we tried to apply this drug in patients with TLD. In 3 such patients basal hyperlipidemia was revealed including highly elevated cholesterol, FFA and especially triglyceride levels as well as prominent pre-β -lipoprtein-aemia in plasma lipoprotein spectrum. Basal and stimulated IRI and glucagon levels were also markedly increased. Administration of bromocriptine (2,5-5,0 mg daily for 8-12 months) lead to quick normalization of mentioned above lipid metabolism indices except pre-β -lipoproteinaemia which had only a slight tendency to normalize after 3 months of treatment. The normalization was stable through the period of bromocriptine therapy. The drug did not influence high basal and stimulated IRI and glucagon levels. The results obtained suggest that in GLD bromocriptine might have extrapancreatic effects on lipid metabolism.

2548 TREATMENT OF HIRSUTE WOMEN WITH SPIRONOLACTONE: E. Stern, S. Leiba, Y. Rusecki*, I. Blum, H. Kaufman, B. Landau, S. Bruhis, B. Shindel, R. Weinstein, Dept. of Endocrinology, Beilinson Hospital, Petah Tikva, Israel 49 100

The antiandrogenic effect of spironolactone was investigated in 30 cases of hirsutism. In 6 cases with severe hirsutism, obesity and menstrual disorders treatment with doses from 100 to 300 mg/day for more than 5 months resulted in a total disappearance of the hirsutism and improvement in the menstrual cycles; in 5 of these ultrasound examination of the ovaries and hormonal tests, with the exception of free testosterone, were normal whereas in the sixth there was an ovarian cyst and increased levels of testosterone which showed no change during treatment. Twelve cases with the clinical and laboratory picture of polycystic ovary syndrome received only 50-100 mg/day because of side effects, including dizziness, hypotension and metrorrhagia; after more than 4 months of treatment there was a thinning of facial hair with less need for electrolysis of the hair follicles, the acne disappeared and there was an improvement in the menstrual cycles. In another 12 cases with the same syndrome the administration of the drug at these low doses for less than 4 months resulted only in the amelioration of the acne in 3 cases. It is concluded that spironolactone is an effective treatment for hirsutism when the patient can receive 100-300 mg/day for a period longer than 5 months.

2549 TRILOSTANE IN THE MANAGEMENT OF PRIMARY ALDOSTERONISM.
M. Stimpel*, H.Groth, W. Vetter, L. Neyses, H.-J. Winterberg, W. Siegenthaler and H. Vetter, Department of Internal Medicine, University Hospital Zurich, Switzerland and Medizinische Universitätspoliklinik Münster, Germany.

16 patients (5♀, 11♂) with primary aldosteronism (7 adrenal adenoma, APA; 9 idiopathic bilateral hyperplasia, IAH) were treated with trilostane, an inhibitor of the adrenal 3β-hydroxysteroid-dehydrogenase enzyme system. Starting with an initial oral dose of 120 mg/day, trilostane was increased up to 900 mg/day. After 12 weeks' treatment with trilostane (average dosage 400 mg/day) mean plasma aldosterone levels (PA) of the total group (n = 16) fell from 370 to 98 ng/ml. Normalisation of PA (< 120 ng/ml) was achieved in 10 (63%) of our patients. At the same time blood pressure (BP) dropped from 185/115 to 143/93 mmHg, which correlated well with the reduction of PA values. Patients with IAH had less severe hypertension (180/112 mmHg) and PA elevations (272 pg/ml) than those with APA (BP 193/119 mmHg, PA 510 ng/ml). Correspondingly, the IAH-group responded to lower doses of trilostane (mean 350 mg/day) than patients with APA (mean 470 mg/day). The observed inhibition of aldosterone biosynthesis was accompanied by an increase of mean serum potassium values from 3.6 to 4.0 mmol/l, a diminished urinary potassium and aldosterone-18-glucuronide excretion from 98 to 64 mmol/24h and 27 to 19 µg/24h, respectively. Mean plasma cortisol levels at 10 a.m. fell from 7.7 to 5.9 µg/100 ml. In none of our patients clinical or biochemical signs of an Addisonian crisis were observed.
Our results demonstrate that trilostane in dosages up to 900 mg/day is an effective therapeutic agent in the treatment of primary aldosteronism.

2550 EFFECT OF TRADITIONAL HERBAL MEDICINE, SHAKUYAKU-KANZO-TO (S-K-T), FOR LOWERING SERUM TESTOSTERONE LEVELS ON HYPERANDROGENIC WOMEN.
T.Takeuchi*, T.Okamura, T.Yaginuma and T.Kobayashi, Dept of Obstet and Gynecol, Faculty of Med, University of Tokyo at Mejirodai, Tokyo, Japan.

S-K-T contains equivalently Shakuyaku, extract of Paeonae Radix, and Kanzo, extract of Glycyrrhizae Radix. Hyperandrogenism was defined as the serum testosterone (T) levels of above 70ng/dl by the previous studies. Five gm of S-K-T was administered orally to 6 patients daily for 10 weeks, and 7.5g of only Kanzo was administered orally to 7 patients daily for 10 weeks. Blood samples were obtained every 2 weeks to measure serum FSH, LH and T levels. In 6 patients administered S-K-T, serum T levels began to decrease at 2 weeks, being reduced to 68%, 68% and 73% at 4, 6 and 8 weeks, respectively ($P<0.005$), and not significantly at 10 weeks. In 7 patients administered only Kanzo, serum T levels were reduced to 69%, 56% and 68% at 2, 4 and 10 weeks, respectively ($P<0.005$). Serum FSH levels decreased only at 2 weeks ($P<0.005$), and serum LH levels decreased at 4 and 6 weeks ($P<0.005$). In 4 of them there was a significant correlation ($r>0.7$) between serum T and LH levels. These results indicate that S-K-T, particularly Kanzo can lower serum T levels probably by suppressing ovarian secretions of T. No side effects were found during these administration.

2551 SERUM IMMUNOREACTIVE-BETAENDORPHIN (IR-β-EP) IN HUMAN OVULATORY CYCLE.
L.C.H. Tang*, S.Y.W. Chan and G.W.K. Tang, Department of Obstetrics and Gynaecology, University of Hong Kong, Queen Mary Hospital, Hong Kong.

Daily serum immunoreactive-beta endorphin (IR-β-EP) levels, in conjunction with luteinizing hormone, follicle-stimulating hormone, 17β-oestradiol, progesterone and prolactin were measured during the ovulatory cycle in five healthy Chinese women. IR-β-EP levels were determined by using ^{125}I-β-EP RIA kits from New England Nuclear, Boston, MA. The antibody cross-reacts with β-lipotropin (50%); but not with (< 0.01%) α-endorphin, leucine enkephalin, methionine enkephalin, or α melanocyte-stimulating hormone. The sensitivity is 50 picograms of IR-β-EP per milliliter of serum with an accuracy of within 5% in the 80 to 90 pg/ml range. Standardization of raw data by conversion to the statistical "Z scores" and composite plot of the 5 cycles showed that serum IR-β-EP levels fluctuated during the follicular, late luteal and menstrual phases. A preovulatory rise occurred 2-3 days prior to the luteinizing hormone surge followed by a post ovulatory dip for 2-3 days. The mean ± S.E.M. concentration of IR-β-EP were: 85.5 ± 10.5 pg/ml (n=36) in the follicular phase; 92.4 ± 36.5 pg/ml (n=5) in the ovulatory phase; 72.3 ± 16.6 pg/ml (n=7) in the early luteal phase; 100.02 ± 10.7 pg/ml (n=38) in the late luteal phase. The values in the luteal phase were highest in the ovulatory cycle. These findings suggest that the fluctuation of endogenous β-EP is under the influence of, among other factor, ovarian sex steroids. Whether the β-EP plays a significant role in the neurochemical mechanisms regulating gonadotropin release during normal menstrual cycle remains to be further investigated.

2552 THE ASSESSMENT OF SHORT TERM GROWTH USING NON-INVASIVE TECHNIQUES IN NORMAL GROWING CHILDREN AND IN CHILDREN WITH GROWTH DISORDERS.
I.M. Valk*[1], A.M.E. Langhout Chabloz[1], A.G.H. Smals[2] and W. van Gilst[3]. Dept. of Anatomy, Embryology and Physical Anthropology[1], Dept of Endocrinology[2], Univ. of Nijmegen the Netherlands, Erasmus Univ.[3] Rotterdam the Netherlands.

Shortterm growth (time intervals of one to three weeks) is an important tool for the research in human growth and the effects of medical treatment in growth disorders. Using non-invasive techniques (Valk, Growth 47,1983) the right lower leg length and the right ulnar length of 45 normal growing children (16 girls, 29 boys) and 5 children with growth disorders were measured over time intervals varying from one to three weeks during a study period of two years.

The one week lower leg growth rates were :

sex	age	millimeters	sex	age	millimeters
boys	6-12 yrs	0.31 P<0.05*	girls	6-10 yrs	0.30 P<0.05*
boys	12-15 yrs	0.60 P<0.05*	girls	10-14 yrs	0.45 P<0.05*

i Immediate growth acceleration was detected in a tall boy treated with sustanon (250 mg 1x2 weekly). ii Instant growth stop was seen in the same boy treated with bromocryptine (5 mg per day). iii Instant growth stop was seen in three tall girls treated with estrogens (100 mugr per day). iiii Immediate start of growth was seen in a boy with GH deficiency during treatment with HGH (8 i.u. weekly). In all cases the changes were significant. (P<0.05)*. From the results it is concluded that using non-invasive techniques growth can be scrutinized.

* Tukey's contrast method (Scheffé H. 1959 "The Analysis of Variance", J. Wiley, London).

2553 THE ENDOCRINE FEEDBACK OF PULSATILE ADMINISTRATION OF INTRAVENOUS HMG ON ENDOGENOUS GONADOTROPINS. J.F.H.M. van Uem M.D.*, Zev Rosenwaks M.D., Helen Liu Ph.D. and Georganna Seegar Jones M.D. The Howard and Georganna Jones Institute in the Department of Obstetrics and Gynaecology, Eastern Virginia Medical School, Norfolk Va 23507.

To elucidate the hormonal stimulatory and feedback mechanism of exogenous gonadotropins on pituitary and steroid hormones, pulsatile administration of intravenous human menopausal gonadotropins (HMG*) was utilized in seven male volunteers 23-38 years of age with proven fertility. HMG was administered on separate occasions at 30, 60 and 90 minute intervals for six hours in doses of 5, 10, 15 and 20 I.U. Blood was obtained every 20 minutes for 4 hours before, 6 hours during and for 2 hours after HMG administration. The serum was assayed for follicle stimulating hormone (FSH), luteinizing hormone (LH), testosterone and 17B estradiol by RIA. Whereas the FSH levels rose with increasing dose and/or frequency of HMG administered (at doses of15 and 20 I.U. and frequency of 30 and 60 minutes), LH pulses were significantly suppressed. With lower doses and frequency (5-10 I.U. administered every 90 minutes), there was no change in the LH pattern, though FSH continued to rise. Testosterone and 17B estradiol levels did not change during the 6 hours of HMG administration. The findings suggest that administered gonadotropins have a direct negative feedback on LH secretion and/or pulsatility.

* Pergonal 75 I.U. FSH and 75 I.U. LH/vial Serono Laboratories

2554 THE THYROGLOBULIN (Tg) AND THE ANTITHYROGLOBULIN ANTIBODIES (TgAb) IN THE DIFFUSE AND NODULAR GOITER. G. Vasilescu, M. Dimitriu, M. Hints, The Endocrinologycal Clinic Tg. Mures, Romania

212 patients were dosed with double antibody Tg (RIA) and with TgAb by the haemaglutination reaction of the tannated hematites. The determinations involved 198 women and 14 men between the age of 20 to 61. The cases were grouped by the thyroidian disfunction, and by the morphological and scintigraphic aspect, as follows:

	No. subjects	Tg (ng/ml) Mean ± SD	Ranges
EUTHYROIDISM			
Diffuse goiter	50	16.64 ± 1.00	7.03 - 38.50
Multinodular goiter (hot+cold)	50	136.47 ± 15.56	15.19 - 448.62
('cold') Thyroidian nodule	36	325.01 ± 31.87	28.70 - 673.0
HYPERTHYROIDISM			
Toxic multinodular goiter	22	64.62 ± 11.60	13.40 - 248.77
Toxic adenoma	16	72.65 ± 5.68	50.4 - 133.31
Graves disease	16	60.18 ± 10.19	21.32 - 167.38
HYPOTHYROIDISM	22	7.28 ± 1.21	1.82 - 20.25

The Tg increased level at the patients with euthyroidism is correlated to the larges volume of the goiter, the marked structural transformation and the presence of the 'cold' nodule. 44% of the cases (2/1280) were found TgAb, and in Graves disease it increased to 52%. The presence of TgAb coincided with significantly higher values of Tg in the 'cold' nodule as compared to the diffuse goiter.

2555 A CLINICAL SURVEY ON THE EPIDEMIOLOGY AND CAUSES OF SECONDARY AMENORRHOEA IN A HOSPITAL GYNAECOLOGICAL OUTPATIENT CLINIC. D. Vengadasalam*, T.K.Ong and Y.H. Chia, Dept of Obstetrics & Gynaecology, Alexandra Hospital, Singapore 0314.

Seventy-six cases of secondary amenorrhoea seen between January 1982 and December 1982 were analyzed. The incidence of secondary amenorrhoea was found to be 1.5% of new gynaecological outpatient attendance. The majority of the cases (84%) were between the 20 to 40 years age range. The racial ethnic composition in the study showed a slight preponderance in ethnic Indian as compared to the general population of Singapore. There was no significant correlation between secondary amenorrhoea and late menarche ($>$ 16 years old). Eighteen (23.7%) patients had previous history of irregular menstrual cycles. Of the 23 patients who had no previous pregnancies, 9 patients were investigated for primary subfertility. Of the remaining 53 patients who had one or more pregnancies, 7 patients were investigated for secondary subfertility. Pregnancy was excluded in all patients prior to any investigation or treatment. Two patients were found to have viable pregnancies. Three patients had missed abortion with histological confirmation. Four (5.3%) patients had associated galactorrhoea. Of these, one patient was diagnosed to have a pituitary microprolactinoma. There were 8 (10.5%) cases of post steroidal amenorrhoea. Five patients (6.6%) were diagnosed to have premature menopause ($>$ 35 years old). Asherman's syndrome was diagnosed in one patient. The commonest cause of secondary amenorrhoea in this study was infrequent ovulation of hypothalamic origin which constituted 64.5% of the cases.

2556 Adrenocortical Responsiveness to ACTH in Women Runners. A.L. Villanueva* and R.W. Rebar, Dept. Repro. Med., UCSD Sch. of Med., La Jolla, CA 92093

We have previously reported significantly higher basal cortisol levels among both amenorrheic (AR) and normal menstruating (i.e.,cycling) runners (NCR) compared to normal control women (NC) (Endo. Soc. Abst. #462, 1983). To assess adrenal responsiveness, the steroidogenic changes following exogenous ACTH 1-24 in 6 AR and 6 NCR were compared to those of 6 NC tested on days 3-7 of the menstrual cycle. AR and NCR ran at least 20 miles/wk, and the AR were amenorrheic for at least 1 year prior to study. Body weights did not differ among the groups. Each subject was suppressed with dexamethasone (0.5 mg po q 6h x4) prior to testing with 10 $\mu g/m^2$ ACTH given as an IV bolus. This dose of ACTH resulted in maximal steroid release. Blood samples for measurement of cortisol, progesterone, 17-hydroxyprogesterone (17Po), 17-hydroxypregnenolone (17Pe), androstenedione (A), dehydroepiandrosterone, testosterone, estrone and estradiol were obtained prior to and at frequent intervals following ACTH. NCR had higher cortisol ($p<0.005$), 17Po ($p<0.005$), 17Pe ($p<0.001$) and A ($p<0.01$) responses compared to NC, and higher 17Po ($p<0.001$), 17Pe ($p<0.005$) and A ($p<0.005$) responses compared to AR. No significant differences were noted between the steriodogenic responses of NC and AR to ACTH. These data suggest that adrenocortical responsiveness increases in women who exercise strenuously and continue to menstruate but decreases once more with the onset of amenorrhea. In view of the changes we have observed, further evaluation of the hypothalamic-pituitary-adrenal axis is clearly indicated in athletes. (Supported by HD-15162)

2557 DECREASED TESTOSTERONE AND PROLACTIN LEVELS IN HIGH MILEAGE MALE DISTANCE RUNNERS.

S.R. Wall*, G. Wheeler, A.N. Belcastro, D.C. Cumming. Depts of Phys Ed and Spts Sci, Ob/Gyn and Medicine (Div of Endocrinol), University of Alberta, Edmonton, Alberta, T6G 2G3.

Endurance training in women has been associated with decreased estradiol levels, decreased basal prolactin levels and impaired thyroid function. To evaluate whether chronic exercise has any similar effects on male distance runners we conducted a cross-sectional study of 18 sedentary controls (NC), 14 habitual runners averaging 20-40 miles per week (LMR), and 31 high mileage runners averaging >41 miles per week (HMR). A single resting, late afternoon blood sample was obtained from each subject for measurement of total (T), non-SHBG bound (Tu) and unbound (Tf) testosterone, LH, FSH, prolactin (PRL), cortisol, TSH, thyroxine, T3 uptake and free thyroxine index. Levels of T, Tu, Tf and PRL were significantly lower in HMR than NC (all $p<0.05$ on ANOVA) but no differences among the groups in the other hormones measured. These data suggest that reproductive hormones may be influenced by exercise in males as well as females. The lack of difference in LH, FSH and cortisol suggests that the underlying mechanism of lowered testosterone in runners does not involve these hormones. The normal free thyroid hormone levels even in HMR suggest that the previously reported change in thyroid function is a physiological adjustment to increased demand rather than occult hypothyroidism. Supported by UAH Special Services and U of A CRF.

2558 SKELETAL ABNORMALITIES IN YOUNG WOMEN WITH DELAYED MENARCHE AND SECONDARY AMENORRHEA.

M.P. Warren*, J. Brooks-Gunn, L.H. Homek, W.G. Hamilton and L.F. Warren. St. Luke's-Roosevelt Hospital, NY NY USA

A delay in menarche and a high incidence of secondary amenorrhea has been reported in young ballet dancers (Warren, JCEM 51:1150, 1980). To date, no permanent medical problems have been reported due to the delay in sexual maturity and intermittent hypoestrogenism although altered skeletal proportions have been noted. We surveyed 70 dancers in four professional ballet companies (mean age 24.8) and found an incidence of scoliosis of 23%. Dancers with scoliosis had a delay in menarche over non scoliotic dancers (15.5 years vs. 14.7 years) and had a higher incidence of secondary amenorrhea (65% vs. 30%). The scoliotic dancers with secondary amenorrhea had a menarche of 16.5 which was significantly delayed over normal dancers ($p < .025$). Scoliotic dancers also showed a higher incidence of anorectic behavior on the EAT 26 scale, a measure of anorectic behavior. In a subgroup of dancers studied, the amenorrheic intervals were marked by prolonged hypoestrogenism. In addition, a high incidence of fractures was noted in this group of professional dancers with the incidence of fractures directly related to the delay in menarche ($r = .87$). These data suggest that a delay in menarche and prolonged intervals of amenorrhea related to nutritional aberrations may predispose to skeletal abnormalities including scoliosis and stress fractures. This group should be followed for the development of skeletal abnormalities and the effects of prolonged hypoestrogenism and nutritional aberrations in adolescence warrant further investigation.

2559 HORMONAL HOMEOSTASIS IN FEMAL ANORECTICS DURING WEIGHT GAIN.
M.J. Wheeler*, J. Treasure+, and G.Russell+, Department of Chemical Pathology, St Thomas' Hospital, London, England and the Institute of Psychiatry+, Denmark Hill, London, England.

We have previously shown in male anorectics that during weight gain there is an exaggerated response of Lutenizing Hormone (LH) and Follicle Stimulating Hormone (FSH) to Luteinizing Hormone-Releasing Hormone (LHRH). This occurred between 45 kg and 50 kg. We have interpreted this as showing a loss of normal homeostatic control of LH and FSH due to rapid metabolic changes. We now report the responses of LH, FSH and Prolactin (PRL) to LHRH and Thyrotropin Releasing Hormone (TRH) in female anorectics. Fourteen anorectic women whose starting weights were below 42 kg were given LHRH and TRH stimulation tests at approximately 5 kg weight gains. An exaggerated response of LH and FSH and occasionally PRL was seen at about 47 kg. Basal levels of androgens, oestradiol and Sex Hormone Binding Globulin(SHBG) were not related to LH and FSH responses. In some patients the exaggerated response (loss of homeostatic control) occurred at a patient's calculated target weight. Return of menses occurred in those patients whose LH and FSH responses had returned to normal. We suggest that the LHRH stimulation test may be useful in predicting the return of menses in female anorectics. Some patients may require a weight gain above their calculated target weight before normal homeostatis is established.

2560 AN LH AND FSH SECRETING PITUITARY ADENOMA: LOSS OF GONADOTROPHIN PULSES, AND ABERRANT HORMONAL CONTROL.
M.C. White*, D. Mathias, P. Kendall-Taylor, and R. Perry. Royal Victoria Infirmary and General Hospital, Newcastle upon Tyne, UK.

A 68 year old male was incidentally found to have pituitary adrenal insufficiency and an enlarged pituitary fossa on x-ray. Examination revealed loss of secondary sexual hair, but testes were of normal size and consistency. Investigations showed elevated basal FSH levels, 24-32 u/l (NR 1-7), and elevated LH levels 6-8.5 u/l (NR 1-6). PRL, T4, TSH estimations were normal but testosterone was low at 5.9 nmol/l (NR 8.5-27). Measurement of serum LH and FSH every 20 min for 6h revealed a complete lack of LH pulsatility and only 4 FSH pulses in total, 2 at the start and 2 at the end of the study period. LH was consistently stimulated by i.v. TRH 200 μg (230-282% of basal), and i.v. LHRH 100 μg (333% of basal), but there was no significant change in FSH after either peptide. No acute change in either LH or FSH was observed over 24h, following either bromocriptine, 2.5 mg orally, or on a separate occasion, oestradiol benzoate 1 mg i.m. Following surgery immunocytochemistry of the tumor and in vitro culture studies confirmed an LH and FSH secreting adenoma. Testicular histology showed normally progressing spermatogenesis with some decrease in spermatogonia, and reduced Leydig cells, but no primary hypogonadism. The hormonal secretory pattern of LH and FSH in this case suggests autonomy from normal hypothalamic control; the dissociation of LH and FSH secretion both basally and following TRH and LHRH administration illustrates separate mechanisms exist for the control of tumorous LH and FSH secretion.

2561 THE INITIATION OF HUMAN PARTURITION: DISTRIBUTION OF PROGESTERONE, CORTISOL AND ESTRADIOL BETWEEN ACTIVE AND INACTIVE COMPONENTS IN PLASMA.

D.L.Willcox*, J.L. Yovich, J.M. Phillips and S.C. McColm, Speciality Laboratories Inc, Los Angeles, CA 90025 and Department of Obstetrics and Gynaecology, University of Western Australia, WA 6008.

We examined if "progesterone withdrawal" occurs in women prior to the onset of labor by a decrease in the free, physiologically-active fraction of the hormone in peripheral plasma. Blood samples were obtained from 26 women between 38 and 40 weeks of gestation, at the beginning of spontaneous (n=12) or induced (n=14) labor, after delivery, and 2-6 days post-partum. Total hormone concentrations were measured by specific radioimmunoassays and free hormone fractions were determined by a rate dialysis procedure. Total progesterone decreased gradually from 223±46 ng/ml (mean ± sem, spontaneous group) and 214±22 ng/ml (induced group) at 10 days pre-partum to 175±22 ng/ml and 185.5±24 ng/ml at the beginning of labor, and then fell rapidly to 38±7 ng/ml and 43±5 ng/ml after delivery of the placenta. Over this period, free progesterone remained at 2-3% of its total concentation. Total and free cortisol varied between 200-325 ng/ml and 4.5-5.5%, respectively, before labor but 12 h after the onset of labor increased to 451±30 ng/ml ($p<0.02$, spontaneous group) and 452±35 ng/ml ($p<0.001$ induced group) and increased to 7.7%±0.5% in both groups. Total estradiol- 17β varied between 28-38 ng/ml pre-partum in both groups and declined rapidly during labor to 5.2±0.9 ng/ml (spontaneous group) and 8.1± 1.4 ng/ml (induced group) by 12 h post-partum whilst its free fraction remained constant at 1.0-1.8%. We conclude that the relative amounts of free and bound progesterone do not redistribute in favor of the physiologically-inactive, bound form in women prior to labor.

2562 LOWER PREVALENCE OF BENIGN DISEASES OF THE BREAST AND BENIGN TUMORS OF THE REPRODUCTIVE SYSTEM AMONG FORMER COLLEGE ATHLETES COMPARED TO NON-ATHLETES.

G. Wyshak,* R.E. Frisch, N. Albright, T. Albright and I. Schiff, Harvard Center for Population Studies, 9 Bow Street, Cambridge, MA 02138, U.S.A.

The effect of strenuous physical activity on the long-term health of women is unknown. We collected self-reported lifetime menstrual, reproductive and medical histories from 5,400 women, 2,622 former college athletes and 2,778 non-athletes, ranging in age from 21 to 80 yr. We present data on the prevalence (lifetime occurrence) of benign diseases of the breast, reported as benign tumors and/or breast biopsies, and of benign tumors of the reproductive system. Cancers of the breast and reproductive system are reported elsewhere. Multiple logistic regression analyses were done to determine the relative risk (RR) of disease among non-athletes (controls) vs. athletes, adjusting for possible confounding factors including: age, leanness, age of menarche, family history of cancer, ever-pregnant, use of oral contraceptives, use of hormones for menopausal symptoms, smoking, coffee and decaffeinated coffee consumption. For women reporting benign breast disease, the unadjusted prevalence rates are: 11.3% for controls vs. 8.2% for athletes; the adjusted relative risk, RR is 1.30, P=0.006. For women reporting benign tumors of the reproductive system, unadjusted rates are 6.5% vs. 4.0%; the adjusted RR=1.42, P=0.006. We conclude that physical activity lowers the risk of benign diseases of the breast and benign tumors of the reproductive system. This work was supported by the Advanced Medical Research Foundation.

2563 IRREVERSIBLE INHIBITORY EFFECT OF TOBACCO EXTRACT ON PLACENTAL ESTROGEN BIOSYNTHESIS *IN VITRO*. C. Yarborough*, M. Tochigi and Y. Osawa, Endo. Biochem. Dept., Medical Fndn. of Buffalo, Buffalo, NY 14203.USA

Previously we found that cigarette smoke contains an inhibitor of human placental aromatase (Endocrinology, 112s, Abst. 458, 1983). In this study we observed that extract of cured tobacco leaf contains aromatase inhibitors, some of which are different from that of cigarette smoke in their chemical nature and mode of inhibition. Commercial cigarette leaf was extracted with 70% ethanol and the ingredients were separated by solvent partition and chromatography. Aromatase activity was assessed using a ^3H-water assay with [1β-^3H, 4-^{14}C]-androstenedione (1.5×10^5dpm^{3}H and 2.7×10^3 dpm^{14}C, 2μg) incubated with placental aromatase and NADPH. The ethanol extract showed a dose and time dependent inactivation of aromatase, and the concentration required for 50% inactivation was 0.025 cigarette equivalent (cig. eq.) at 30 min exposure at room temperature. No cofactor (NADPH) dependency was observed. The strongly acidic ether soluble fraction which possesses characteristic tobacco aroma showed the strongest aromatase inactivation among other weakly acidic, neutral, basic, and polar aqueous fractions. The 50% inactivation was achieved with 0.08 cig. eq. (400μg of extract). To our knowledge this is the first known case of the existence of a natural inactivator of aromatase in plants. Effective aromatase inactivators have a potential use in the study of the mechanism of estrogen biosynthesis and treatment of estrogen dependent diseases. Supported by DHHS research grant HD04945 from NICHD, grant no. RR05716 from the Division of Research Resources and grant no. 1643 from the Council for Tobacco Research - U.S.A., Inc.

2564 **CORTISOL, PROGESTERONE, ESTRONE AND CBG IN MYOCARDIAL INFARCTION : EVIDENCE FOR A PROGNOSTIC VALUE.*** H. Zouaghi*, L. Savu*, C. Guérot**, R. Gryman** A. Coulon* and E. Nunez*. - * ERA 881, CNRS - U. 224, INSERM - Faculté de Médecine Xavier Bichat - Laboratoire de Biochimie - 16, rue Henri Huchard 75018 PARIS - ** Service de Cardiologie - Hôpital Bichat - 75018 PARIS.

Day-of-admission (Day 0) sera from 34 myocardial infarction patients (MI) and 6 patients with non-MI cardiopathies were analyzed for total and unbound cortisol (F), progesterone (P_4) and estrone (E_1) and corticosteroid binding activities (CBG).
The MI who survived (n=28) showed with respect to healthy controls (n=24) important increases of total F, P_4 and E_1 ; the MI who died within 10 days of admission (n=6) had unchanged F, while their P_4 and E_1, though higher than normal, were significantly less increased than in survivors. The non-MI had higher F and E_1 than controls but normal P_4.
The unbound fractions of all steroids were highly increased in all cardiopathies, but the rises were much smaller in MI deceased than in MI survivors. Thus, means of ~ 220 nmol/l free F, ~ 350 pmol/l free P_4 or E_1, were associated with subsequent survival ; $<$ 100 nmol/l free F and $<$ 150 pmol/l free P_4 or E_1 have been followed by death.
The CBG activities of Day 0 sera were at least twice lower in MI (regardless of outcome) than in normals, but unchanged in non-MI.
These data suggest a prognostic value for responses of total and free F, P_4 and E_1 in early MI, the weaker increases predicting fatal outcome. Furthermore the rise of total P_4 and fall of CBG emerge as differential diagnostic parameters, discriminating MI from non-MI cardiopathies.

2565 ANTIBODY TITERS IN MARMOSET MONKEYS ACTIVELY IMMUNIZED WITH THE BETA SUBUNIT OF OVINE LUTEINIZING HORMONE(oLHBeta).

P. Spinola*, R. Thau, E. Coutinho and I. Barbosa. Maternidade Climerio de Oliveira, Rua do Limoeiro No. 1, Nazaré - 40.000 Salvador, Bahia, Brazil.

Immunization of marmoset monkeys (Callithrix Jacchus) with oLHβ provides a model for a new approach to human contraception. The animals were actively immunized against chorionic gonadotropin by injections of the Beta fraction of ovine luteinizing hormone(oLHBeta). The immunizing emulsion was prepared by dissolving 50μg of oLHBeta in 250μl of saline emulsified with equal volume of Freund's complete adjuvant. Multiple sites were injected subcutaneously in all animals on day 0 and 3 weeks later. Blood samples were drawn every week between 09:00 and 12:00 hours and plasma stored at -20°C until assayed. Antibody titers can be expressed as percent bindings of an iodinated hormone which shows partial or total cross-reactivity with the circulating antibodies to a known amount of serum at appropriate dilutions. All monkeys developed circulating antibodies which bound iodinated hCGβ. This study was supported by the Rockefeller Foundation.

2566 ANDROGEN INDUCED PROTEINS IN THE HUMAN EPIDIDYMIS. J.Tezon, M.Vazquez, M. Larminat, E. Ramella, L.Pineiro, J.Blaquier*. Instituto de Biologia y Medicina Experimental, Buenos Aires 1428, Argentina

We have previously shown that the human epididymis maintained in organ culture responds to androgenic stimulation with increased protein synthesis We now report the identification of the proteins synthesized, some of their physicochemical properties and their interaction with spermatozoa. Tissues obtained from patients undergoing orchidectomy for prostatic cancer were cultured for 3 days prior to the addition of 0.1 uM dihydrotestosterone (DHT) or vehicle alone. After 20 different cultures were analyzed, induction of a protein with Ra (relative mobility in PAGE) 1.01 was observed in 95% of the cases, a band Ra 0.68 was found in 75% and bands Ra 0.3 and 0.43 were observed in 55% of the experiments. The effect of DHT was suppresed by the simultaneous presence of cyproterone acetate. The caput and proximal corpus epididymis were found to be the most active sites of production of these proteins. Bands Ra 0.3; 0.43 and 1.01 were found in the luminal fluid and culture medium and also in the 0.5M NaCl extract of caudal sperm but not in caput sperm. Bands 0.43 and 1.01 had apparent Mr 24,000 when analyzed by SDS-PAGE, band 0.3: 38,000 and band 0.68: 82,000. All bands had acidic isoelectric points (pH range:5.2-6.8). The androgen-induced epididymal proteins associated with sperm were found localized over the acrosomal cap of sperm. These results suggest that the human epididymis in culture responds to androgens in a manner similar to that demonstrated *in vivo* for experimental animals.

(Supported by NICHD grant 1RO/HD15920)

2567 CLINICAL AND BLOOD CLOTTING RESPONSES IN ASIAN WOMEN ON THE TRIPHASIC PILL.
F. H. M. Tsakok*, S. Koh, S. E. Chua, B. L. Tan, R. Yuen and K. M. Kwok, University Department of Obstetrics and Gynaecology, Kandang Kerbau Hospital, Hampshire Road, Singapore 0821.

This paper examines the different responses to the triphasic pill in 3 ethnic groups viz Chinese, Malay and Indian. The parameters studied were (a) clinical i.e. blood pressure, weight change, bleeding patterns, skin changes, nausea, vomiting, breast changes, headaches and mood changes, (b) blood clotting i.e. coagulation factors and inhibitors, fibrinolytic activity and inhibition, platelet function. There were 127 women in the study group observed through 1300 pill cycles. There were 80 Chinese, 25 Malay and 22 Indian women in the study. The dropout rate was significantly higher in the Malays due to mainly subjective side effects. The coagulation changes were not significantly different between the 3 groups. However, all the study women had haemostatic changes after taking the pill.

2568 ANTIFERTILITY EFFECTS OF ANORDRIN.
Y.Y. Tsong* and C.C. Chang, Center for Biomedical Research, Population Council, New York, New York 10021

Anordrin (AN), 2α,17α-diethynyl-A-nor-5α-androstane-2β,17β-diol 2,17-dipropionate has been used as post-coital contraceptive but its sites of antifertility action have not been clearly established. In investigating the mechanism of action of AN, immature female rats treated with pregnant mare serum (PMS) were studied. To test the effect on ovulation, the drug was administered orally for 3 days beginning on the day of PMS treatment. All of the controls and 50% of the treated rats (7.5 mg/kg) ovulated. Among ovulating animals, the number of ova were 15.7 ± 1.5 and 8.0 ± 1.2 in the control and treated group, respectively. To test the effect of AN on ovum transport, the drug was given orally either as a single dose (5mg/kg) on the day of mating or on 3 days beginning at the day of mating. None of the treated rats had any implantation sites. To test the effect of AN on implantation, the drug (5mg/kg) was given orally as a single dose on the 5th day after mating, 20% of rats had normal implantation. No implantation sites were found when higher dose (7.5mg/kg) of AN was given. Administration of 5mg/kg per day orally to normal cycling female rats resulted in interrupting of normal cyclic pattern. We conclude that AN has multiple sites of action: (1) it inhibits the transport of ovum, although its direct cytoxic effects have not been ruled out; (2) it interferes with implantation more effectively at higher dose; and (3) it also can inhibit ovulation.

2569 INITIATION OF NORMAL OVARIAN CYCLE IN HYPOTHALAMIC AMENORRHEA WITH CHRONIC (PORTABLE PUMP) INTRAVENOUS, SUBCUTANEOUS PULSATILE OR "INTERMITTENT" PULSATILE LHRH ADMINISTRATION. Z. Voulgaris, A. Souvatzoglou*, R. Charitopoulou, and E. Rapti. Department of Clinical Therapeutics, 1st Department of Obst. and Gynecology, University of Athens, "Alexandra" Hospital, GR-115 28 Athens, Greece

In a patient with primary hypothalamic amenorrhea LHRH administration, pulsatile (15 μg every 90 min) intravenous (Iv-90P), subcutaneous (Sc-90P) and pulsatile "intermittent" (7.6 μg every 90 min, in this time period 2.3 μg every 22.5 min) intravenous (Iv-IP), subcutaneous (Sc-IP) were compared. Each regimen lasted 4 weeks. LHRH was administered by means of a portable pump devised by us. Serum LH, FSH, estradiol (E_2), progesterone (P) were estimated daily. Iv-IP resulted in increase of serum LH and E_2, a diminished FSH and P response and follicular maturation without ovulation and corpus luteum formation (sonogram). With Iv-90P a mormal cycle (adequate LH, FSH, E_2, P serum levels) with corpus luteum formation (sonogram) and subsequent bleeding occured. Sc-IP caused a flat curve response of serum LH, FSH, E_2, P. Sc-90P resulted in increase of serum LH, FSH, E_2, without P response, no subsequent bleeding occured. Frequent (every 5 min for 90 min) blood sampling showed in Iv-IP proper "episodic" secretion only for LH, in Sc-90P diminished LH fluctuation and flat FSH curve, in Sc-IP flat LH and FSH serum curve. In conclusion only Iv-90P resulted in a normal ovarian cycle. Iv-IP, Sc-90P, Sc-IP caused more and more a "desensitization" of the gonadotropic cell shown first by diminishing of serum FSH fluctuation and low serum P. This study was supported by the Greek Research Foundation.

2570 CONTROL OF MALE FERTILITY BY 1,2,3-TRIHYDROXYPROPANE: RAPID ARREST OF SPERMATOGENESIS WITHOUT ALTERING LIBIDO, ACCESSORY SEX ORGANS, GONADAL STEROIDOGENESIS, AND SERUM TESTOSTERONE, LH AND FSH. J.P. Wiebe* and K.J. Barr, Hormonal Regulatory Mechanisms Lab, Department of Zoology, University of Western Ontario, London N6A 5B7, Canada.

This study examines the effects of intratesticular injection of aqueous 1,2,3-trihydroxypropane (THP) solution on male reproductive biology. In a series of experiments, Sprague-Dawley rats of various ages (48-95d) were injected with 50-200 μl/testis and various parameters were studied for up to 21 weeks. An injection of THP resulted in testicular weight reduction of up to 45-60% within 2 weeks but the weights of prostate and seminal vesicles were not affected for the duration of the experiments. The number of sperm per epididimys in the THP treated rats declined rapidly and was reduced by 99.99% (of controls) after the 3rd mating. THP treated males mated with virgin females at the same frequency as control rats but were infertile after the 3rd mating and remained infertile for the duration of the tests. In vitro studies showed that metabolism of ^{14}C-progesterone by testicular homogenates was not altered quantitatively or qualitatively by THP treatment. Serum levels of androgens, LH and FSH of the THP treated rats did not differ significantly from the controls. Histologically and histochemically the Leydig cells appeared to be normal, but the seminiferous tubules of THP treated testes were devoid of spermatogenic cells within 2 weeks of a single treatment. We conclude that direct injection of THP acts as a potent inhibitor of spermatogenesis, resulting in long term infertility without affecting steroidogenesis, libido, secondary sex characteristics, mating behaviour, or serum hormone levels. (Supported by NSERC of Canada).

2571 INHIBITION OF FOLLICLE RECRUITMENT IN MONKEYS FOLLOWING EARLY FOLLICULAR PHASE ADMINISTRATION OF AN LHRH AGONIST. J.W. Wilks*, Fertility Research, The Upjohn Company, Kalamazoo, Michigan 49001 U.S.A.

Early follicular phase administration of an LHRH agonist to women has been reported to cause luteal phase defects. This study was undertaken to evaluate corpus luteum function in rhesus monkeys when [D-His(im-Bzl)^6, Pro^9]-LHRH N-ethylamide was administered on days 1-3 of the menstrual cycle at doses of 0.1, 1, 5 or 10 mg. Two responses were observed regardless of dose: a)anovulatory menstrual cycles of short duration (11.5 $\pm$ 0.5 days, n=4); or b)ovulatory menstrual cycles characterized by long follicular phases of 24.5 $\pm$ 3.2 days duration (n=8). Monkeys with shortened menstrual cycles had prominent increases in serum gonadotropin and estradiol concentrations during LHRH agonist treatment; early menses was attributed to uterine bleeding following estrogen withdrawal. Serum FSH concentrations were depressed immediately after LHRH agonist treatment in monkeys with ovulatory cycles; serum LH concentrations were not altered. Two of eight monkeys with ovulatory menstrual cycles had elevations in serum estradiol during LHRH treatment. Although follicular phases in ovulatory menstrual cycles were long, corpus luteum function was normal following treatment with the LHRH agonist. The results indicate that both the long and short menstrual cycles following administration of [D-His(im-Bzl)^6, Pro^9]-LHRH N-ethylamide to monkeys can be attributed to an inhibition in the recruitment of a cohort of follicles capable of yielding a dominant follicle. This effect of the LHRH agonist may be mediated at the level of the hypothalamus/pituitary gland by a down regulation of LHRH receptors or an alteration in the patterning of endogenous LHRH signals.

2572 Characterization of Leydig Cell Membrane Phosphorylation. C. Winters*, and M. Dufau, Mol. Endo. Section, ERRB, NIH, Bethesda, MD, USA, 20205

We have previously observed that the rapid plasma membrane events preceding LH activation of adenylate cyclase of rat Leydig cells include increased binding of guanyl nucleotides, and that guanyl nucleotides stimulate the cAMP-independent phosphorylation of a 44,500 Mr protein with characteristics similar to the adenylate cyclase nucleotide regulatory subunit, (Winters, et al, 1983). This phosphorylation is optimal at 10^{-4} M Gpp[NH]p and is Ca^{++}-dependent, being stimulated by 10^{-10} M and 10^{-9} M free [Ca^{++}] and inhibited by higher concentrations (10^{-8} M to 10^{-6} M). We have now analyzed the nature of this phosphorylation by partial acid hydrolysis and 2-D TLC electrophoresis at pH 3.5 and pH 1.9. Autoradiography and densitometry showed significant differences in phosphoaminoacid content between control and Gpp[NH]p-stimulated samples. The EGTA-washed membranes, in the absence of Ca^{++}, showed two labeled spots of equal intensity comigrating with the phosphoserine and phosphothreonine markers. In the membranes treated with 10^{-10} M free [Ca^{++}], the phosphoserine spot density was increased by 100% over control, and phosphothreonine was unchanged. In the presence of Gpp[NH]p plus 10^{-10} M [Ca^{++}], incorporation into phosphoserine was further increased by 55%, and labeled phosphothreonine was barely discernable. Phosphotyrosine was not found in control or stimulated membranes. These results demonstrate that not only an increase in the phosphorylation of the 44,500 Mr protein but also a GTP-induced change in phosphoaminoacid content may play a role in the rapid plasma membrane responses of the hormonally-activated Leydig cell.

2573 CARBOHYDRATE METABOLISM IN THE OFFSPRING OF ETHANOL-TREATED RATS: STUDIES IN RELATION TO FETAL ALCOHOL SYNDROME. A. Snyder*, S. Singh, G. Pullen and R. Sethi, Veterans Administration Medical Center and Chicago Medical School, North Chicago, Illinois 60064, USA.

We have reported hypoglycemia, hypoinsulinemia, and depletion of glycogen stores at term in rat fetuses exposed to ethanol. The present study examines the effects of fasting and reduced ethanol dose on hepatic glycogen metabolism in like animals. Pregnant rats were fed liquid diet containing ethanol (EF) as 20 or 36% of the caloric content. Controls received isocaloric diet without ethanol by pair-feeding (PF) or ad libitum (AF). Dams were sacrificed in the fed state or after a 24-hour fast and fetal liver glycogen (G), glycogen synthase (S), and phosphorylase (P) were determined. G was reduced in 36% EF fetuses from fed or fasted dams ($p<0.001$) and in 20% EF fetuses after maternal fast ($p<0.01$). S (I and I+D) activities were reduced by fasting in all groups. In addition, S I was reduced in 36% EF fetuses in the fed state (0.121 $\pm$ 0.020 U/g vs 0.195 $\pm$ 0.030 in PF and 0.169 $\pm$ 0.003 in AF) and after maternal fast (0.089 $\pm$ 0.011 U/g vs 0.140 $\pm$ 0.017 in PF and 0.124 $\pm$ 0.010 in AF). In the fed state, both active (a) and total (a+b) P activities were reduced ($p<0.01$) in 36% EF fetuses (a = 0.69 $\pm$ 0.30, 2.59 $\pm$ 0.09, and 2.63 $\pm$ 0.10 U/g and a+b = 1.79 $\pm$ 0.37, 4.30 $\pm$ 0.47 and 4.36 $\pm$ 0.44 U/g in EF, PF and AF respectively). Following a maternal fast, a+b was lower in 36% EF fetuses (2.74 $\pm$ 0.14 U/g) than in controls (3.54 $\pm$ 0.08 in PF and 4.97 $\pm$ 0.52 in AF). Exposure to high levels of ethanol in utero may thus interfere with glycogen metabolic pathways in the term fetus.

2574 THE PLASMA GROWTH HORMONE (GH) SECRETORY RESPONSE TO GROWTH HORMONE RELEASING FACTOR (GRF) IN THE ADULT AND NEONATAL RHESUS MONKEY. D. Styne*, Dept. of Pediatrics, University of California, Davis, California 95616, USA.

To determine whether the higher circulating plasma GH concentrations characteristic of the primate neonate and fetus are mediated by hypothalamic GRF secretion, synthetic GRF (generously provided by Drs. Ling and Guillemin) was administered by intravenous bolus to 2 male neonatal (less than 4 weeks of age) and 4 adult (3 male, 1 female) chair-trained rhesus monkeys. In the basal state plasma GH (measured by human GH radioimmunoassay) was higher in neonatal than adult animals, and spontaneous secretory episodes were noted in the neonates. A 1 µg/kg BW bolus of GRF elicited a greater than 100% rise in GH within 3-7 minutes in the 2 adult males tested, but had no effect on the 2 male neonates. A 10 µg/kg BW GRF bolus stimulated a greater than 100% rise in GH in 3 adults (2 male, 1 female) and the 2 male neonates; no rise occurred in 1 adult male. Peak GH values did not exceed 10 ng/ml in the responding adults. In summary, 1) a rise in plasma GH occurs after a 1 or 10 µg/kg BW bolus of GRF in adult male rhesus monkeys, 2) infant rhesus demonstrate spontaneous GH secretion, have higher baseline GH values and require a higher dose of GRF (10 µg/kg BW) than adults to respond with a rise in GH, 3) as previously noted in the adult female rhesus (Endo Soc, 1983, 290A), there is variability in GH response to GRF among adult males, 4) peak GRF stimulated GH values in the rhesus monkey are less than those reported in human beings given comparable doses of GRF. In conclusion, GRF can affect the secretion of GH in the infant and adult rhesus monkey and may mediate elevated plasma GH concentrations in the neonate.

2575 PARTICULARITIES OF URINARY STEROID EXCRETION IN INFANTS DURING THE FIRST FOUR WEEKS OF LIFE. W.M. Teller*, and J. Homoki, Center of Paediatrics, University of Ulm, FR Germany.

Newborn and young infants excrete steroids mainly as sulfoconjugates (1). However, quantitative data on their excretion are still lacking. We investigated the 24^h urinary steroid profiles (up to 23 metabolites) in 22 newborn infants (16 m; 6 f) during the first four weeks of life by capillary column gas chromatography. The method (2) used consisted of Sep-Pak extraction, column chromatography on Sephadex LH-20 for separation of glucuronides and sulfates, hydrolysis, derivative formation, capillary column gas chromatography and quantitation. The following results were obtained: During the first 4 weeks of life healthy neonates excrete more than ten times as much steroid monosulfates (0,8-9,3 mg/24^h) than glucuronides (0,06-1,4 mg/24^h). Steroids of the 3β-hydroxy-5-ene type, presumably originating in the fetal cortex, were excreted as sulfates, while cortisol and progesterone metabolites, which are produced in the adult cortex, were excreted in the urine in the free and glucuronic acid conjugated forms. The appearance in neonatal urine of 15β-hydroxy-pregnenetetrol (3β,15β,17α,20α-tetrahydroxy-5-pregnene), whose structure was confirmed by mass spectrometry, is reported for the first time. Supported by DFG Ho-471.

References: (1) SHACKLETON et al. J.steroid Biochem.11,523 (1979)
(2) HOMOKI et al. J.steroid Biochem.19,1061(1983)

2576 A COLORIMETRIC ENZYME IMMUNOASSAY (EIA) FOR THE DETERMINATION OF TSH IN DRIED BLOOD SPOTS: A VALID ALTERNATIVE TO RIA FOR NEONATAL THYROID SCREENING. T.Torresani*, E.Schuster and R.Illig, Department of Pediatrics, University of Zürich, CH 8032 Zürich, Switzerland.

Neonatal thyroid screening has been performed so far by RIA or fluorimetric EIA. Both methods depend on the availability of rather expensive equipment. We have adapted a colorimetric EIA, set up for TSH measurement in 200 µl serum, for the determination of TSH in filterpaper discs containing ca. 10 µl of dried blood. This EIA is based on a sandwich technique using a monoclonal anti-βTSH antibody coupled to the tube wall and a polyclonal anti-αTSH antibody coupled to horseradish peroxydase as the label. Substrate for the colorimetric reaction is the chromogen ABTS[R] and the endpoint is read with a photometer at 420 nm. The limit of detection is close to 10 mU/l. The intra- and interassay variation is 7.0% and 10.3% respectively, at the level of 25 mU/l which is the upper limit of normal for neonatal screening in our laboratory.
In order to compare the EIA with our routine RIA we have assayed so far 50 samples by both methods using the TSH MRC 68/38 as the reference preparation. The regression analysis showed a slope of 0.923 and a correlation of 0.98. The advantages of the TSH EIA are the long shelf life of reagents, the non radioactive label, and the possibility to read the endpoint with an ordinary photometer. However, interference of hemoglobin in the color reaction requires removal of filterpaper discs and, therefore, may complicate an automatisation of the assay system.
Supported by the Swiss National Science Foundation Grant no. 3.984.080
and by Boehringer Mannheim GmbH

2577 IMPAIRED LACTATION IN RATS WHICH HAD PREVIOUSLY RECEIVED PROPYLTHIOURACIL PERINATALLY. L. Van Middlesworth*, Dept. of Physiology & Biophysics, University of Tennessee Center for the Health Sciences, Memphis, TN 38163

Fifteen pregnant rats were given 0.03% propylthiouracil (PTU) in their drinking water 4 days before delivery and during the first 16 days of nursing, after which they were fed normal control diet and water. The pups were weaned at 23-24 days old. When 4 months old the females were bred with normal males. Thirteen became pregnant and delivered 96 pups. However, 50% of the pups died within 2 days, and 73% died within 10 days. After 2 months the dams were bred a second time. Again, 60% percent of the pups died within 2 days, and 70% died within 10 days. (Simultaneous normal controls weaned 93% of their pups.) Six healthy pups, 4-6 days old, from normal dams were substituted to each of 4 dams whose pups had died. In 3 of the 4 foster litters all pups gained weight poorly, and 12 died after 10 days; only one foster litter survived to weaning age. It is concluded that while perinatal exposure to PTU results in a syndrome involving damage to the auditory system (reported in Endocrinology 106:1686, 1980), it also results in systemic damage which impairs lactation and thereby threatens survival of future offspring. This study was supported by USPHS amnd USDOE.

2578 NEONATAL THYROID FUNCTIONS IN INFANTS OF THYROTOXIC MOTHERS. S. Varma*, M. Bourgeois, and S. Aiyar, Department of Pediatrics, Texas Tech University Health Sciences Center, Lubbock, Texas.

Twelve infants of thyrotoxic mothers (ITM) were closely monitored. Eight mothers were on thiocarbamides (Group I), 3 had radioactive iodine therapy and one had thyroidectomy prior to the pregnancy (Group II). In Group I, 6 patients were on Propylthiouracil (200-400 mg/day) and 2 were on Tapazole (20-30 mg/day). Mean serum T_4 level in this group was 17.0 ± 6.4 Ug/dl (n=7). The remaining patient in this group had high serum T_3 with normal T_4 levels. Group II patients were on replacement thyroid medication. Mean T_4 in this group was 10.8 ± 4.6 Ug/dl. Thyroid Function Tests were done on Days 1 (or cord blood), 3, 7 and 14 and onwards if indicated. There was no statistical correlation between maternal T_4 and neonatal T_4 levels of Day 3 or cord blood either in Group I or II. Three neonates were treated with Lugol's Solution in the first week of life for elevated T_4 levels and/or tachycardia. The treatment was discontinued between Days 14-21 on the basis of normal T_4 levels. One neonate was started on L-Thyroxine on Day 7 for low T_4 and elevated TSH levels and decreased thyroid activity on thyroid scan. In the remaining 8 neonates, serum T_4 was elevated up to Day 7 in 4 cases, whereas in other 4 it returned to normal levels by Day 14. Serum TSH was elevated (> 40 uIU/ml) along with normal serum T_4 levels in 2 cases, which returned to normal ranges by Day 14. Our study shows (1) there is no correlation between maternal T_4, mode of maternal treatment of Thyrotoxicosis and neonatal T_4 levels; (2) transient neonatal thyrotoxicosis is common in ITM (25%); (3) hypothyroidism in ITM has been reported for the first time and (4) Thyroid Function Tests should be monitored up to 2-3 weeks in ITM.

2579 PRIMARY TSH SCREENING BY EITHER CORD OR HEEL BLOOD IMPROVES DETECTION OF NEONATAL HYPOTHYROIDISM. P.G. Walfish*, E. Gera, F. Peter, G. Growcock, N. Duncan and R.M. Ehrlich, Mount Sinai Hospital, Central Laboratories, Ontario Ministry of Health, The Hospital for Sick Children, and Univ. of Toronto Medical School, Toronto, Ontario, M5G 1X5, Canada.

In order to determine the relative effectiveness of primary TSH as a screening program for detecting primary persistent neonatal hypothyroidism (PPH), we have studied primary dried blood TSH testing within the same population of 81,000 infants in Metro Toronto assessed from October 1980 to December 1982 using a commercial solid-phase (Sephadex) antibody radioimmunoassay method (Phadebas® Dry Spot TSH Test) simultaneously assayed from either neonatal 3-5 day old heel blood (H) or cord blood (C) in two different laboratories. Recall cut-off values for C and H screening programs for the dried blood TSH method were 35 and 25 uU/ml, respectively. 126 infants (0.16%) were recalled by C, resulting in 30 (24%) true PPH positives, 2 (2%) transient positives, and 94 (74%) false positives. By comparison, the H program recalled 74 (0.09%), of which 29 (39%) were true PPH positives, 0% transient positives, and 45 (61%) false positives. One infant with true PPH detected by the C program was missed by H, resulting in a detection incidence of 1:2700 for the C program and 1:2800 for H. Another PPH infant with hypoplasia was missed by H and undetected by C due to a missed sample. Time to diagnosis and institution of therapy for infants with PPH ranged from 7-18 days with the C program (mean = 8 days) compared to a range of 12-20 days (mean = 16 days) for H. Comparison of the recent primary TSH-H program to a previous H program of 63,000 infants tested by primary T4 and supplementary TSH on the lowest 10% indicated that: i) primary TSH improved ($p = < 0.05$) the detection incidence from 1:3900 to 1:2800 to result in a comparable H detection incidence to the primary TSH-C program; ii) was more cost-effective, and iii) reduced time to diagnosis and treatment by 7-10 days. These results indicate that, for an H screening program, primary TSH is better than primary T4 and supplementary TSH, and that primary TSH by a C program is the screening method of choice for instituting therapy before two weeks of age. This study was supported by Ontario Ministry of Health Grant #DM-467.

2580 HORMONAL REGULATION OF LH RECEPTORS AND TESTOSTERONE PRODUCTION IN THE RAT FETAL TESTIS IN VIVO. D. Warren*, I. Huhtaniemi, M. Dufau and K. Catt, Department of Physiology & Biophysics, University of Southern California, Los Angeles, California 90033 and ERRB, NICHHD, NIH, Bethesda, Maryland 20205.

We have previously shown that the neonatal testis, in vivo, and the fetal testis, in vitro, respond to high doses of LH or hCG with an increase in LH receptors and androgenic capacity. In contrast, the adult testis shows loss of LH receptors and induction of steroidogenic lesions to this stimulus. In this study, we have given high doses of hCG to the rat fetus in vivo and measured LH receptors and steroidogenic capacity to determine if the in vitro model reflects the in vivo response. Fetal rats were injected with 1.0 IU hCG on day 17.5 of gestation. One day after injection, LH receptors were 12% of control values (p 0.01), had returned to control levels by 3 days after injection and were 141% of control (p 0.05) by 4 days after injection, just before birth. The return to control values and the increase in LH receptors lag behind the neonatal response by 1 day. One possibility for this delay is that hCG clearance by the fetus may be slower because of intraamniotic circulation of the hormone. Three days after injection of 1 IU hCG, fetal testes were removed and incubated for 3 hr with or without 100 IU hCG. Basal testosterone (T) from injected fetuses was 780% (p 0.01) above saline injected controls and hCG stimulated T was 170% (p 0.01) above controls. These results show that the fetal testis is capable of increasing LH receptors and androgenic capacity when exposed to high levels of LH agonist, a phenomenon which would be beneficial in maintaining the high T levels needed for male genital tract organogenesis.

2581 EFFECT OF VASOACTIVE INTESTINAL POLYPEPTIDE (VIP) AND RELATED PEPTIDES ON ACTH AND GH SECRETION FROM RAT PITUITARY GLAND: DIFFERENTIAL RESPONSES OF NEONATAL AND ADULT TISSUE. S. M. Watts*, S. A. Nicholson, †R. A. Prysor-Jones, R. K. Coker, M. T. Jones and B. Gillham, Departments of Obstetrics and Gynaecology and Biochemistry, St. Thomas's Hospital Medical School, London SE1 7EH, and †Department of Medicine, St. George's Hospital Medical School, London SW17 ORE.

Whilst VIP has no effect on ACTH secretion in vitro from anterior pituitary segments removed from adult rats (>50 days old) it significantly stimulates ACTH secretion in a dose-dependent manner from hemipituitaries removed from neonatal (5-6 days old) rats. Neonatal and adult tissues respond similarly to various concentrations of ovine CRF (2.1 - 21.5 nM) and AVP (7.2 - 115.3 nM). The effects of four peptides structurally related to VIP, namely porcine histidine isoleucine amide-containing peptide (PHI), gastric inhibitory peptide (GIP), secretin and glucagon were also tested on ACTH release. PHI and GIP at a high concentration (100 nM) significantly increased release from neonatal tissue but had no effect on adult tissue. Glucagon significantly stimulated ACTH release, in a dose-dependent manner, from adult tissue. These results suggest that at an early stage in the ontogeny of the corticotroph, VIP (and to a lesser extent PHI and GIP) is capable of stimulating the release of ACTH but in the mature cell this facility is lost and replaced by a responsiveness to glucagon. GIP and PHI both markedly stimulated GH release from pituitary pieces removed from neonatal but not adult rats. It is concluded that VIP-related peptides show effects on both ACTH and GH secretion which are dependent on the maturity of the pituitary gland.

2582 EFFECT OF OVINE CORTICOTROPIN RELEASING FACTOR (CRF) & ANTIDIURETIC HORMONE (ADH) ON ACTH IN THE OVINE FETUS.

E.M. Wintour*, R.J. Bell, M. Congiu, D.T. Fei and X. Wang.
Howard Florey Institute of Experimental Physiology and Medicine, Dept. Physiology, University of Melbourne, Parkville, 3052, Australia.

Recently, it has been shown that a trend for increased ACTH can be seen in the ovine fetus over the last 3 weeks of gestation, if samples from stressed fetuses (urine osmolality > 200 msomol./kg H20) are excluded. (J. Dev. Physiol. 4, 339, 1982). In fetuses < 130 days of gestation there is a significant relationship between endogenous plasma ACTH and ADH concentrations. Plasma ACTH = 4.41 + 3.42 (ADH), n = 30, r = 0.7. On 15 occasions the injection I.V. of 0.1-1.0 μg CRF into fetuses 104-127 days failed to increase ACTH whereas the same dose caused significant increases in 22 cases, the fetuses being > 118 days. As gestational age increased the magnitude of the response increased. 10 μg CRF raised ACTH in 11/15 fetuses, 110-149 days of gestation. When ADH was infused for 2 hrs at a rate sufficient to produce negative Free Water Clearance, there was no elevation of ACTH values, nor was there any synergism with ACTH at any stage of gestation. Conclusions:- 1) Endogenous stress e.g. cord constriction, simultaneously releases ACTH and ADH. 2) The fetal pituitary becomes increasingly responsive to CRF as term approaches, but ADH is not a potent CRF in the fetus.

Supported by the N.H.M.R.C. of Australia.

2583 NEGATIVE FEEDBACK CONTROL OF OVINE FETAL ADRENOCORTICOTROPIN (ACTH) SECRETION: HIGH SENSITIVITY TO CORTISOL. Charles E. Wood*. Department of Physiology, University of Florida College of Medicine, Gainesville, Florida, USA.

ACTH secretion by the ovine fetal pituitary is partially controlled by corticosteroid negative feedback. In previous studies, Wood and Rudolph demonstrated that increases in fetal plasma cortisol concentration similar to maximal increases during fetal stress completely inhibited the fetal ACTH response to hypotension. The present study was designed to investigate the role of smaller increases in fetal plasma cortisol in modulating fetal ACTH secretion. Eleven experiments were performed on 5 fetal sheep (117-131 days) with chronically maintained vascular catheters. Vehicle or cortisol was infused into the fetus (IV) for 5h; one hour later, sodium nitroprusside (50 ug/min) was infused into the fetus (IV) for 10 min. Plasma cortisol concentrations during cortisol or vehicle infusions were measured by a cortisol-specific RIA. Plasma ACTH concentrations before and at the end of nitroprusside infusions were also measured by RIA. In vehicle-infused group, nitroprusside increased mean fetal plasma ACTH by 128 pg/ml. Infusion of cortisol at rates of 1 and 2 ug/min increased fetal plasma cortisol by 12.7 and 18.7 ng/ml and completely blocked the ACTH response to nitroprusside. These results demonstrate a high sensitivity of the late gestation ovine fetal hypothalamo-pituitary unit to cortisol negative feedback, such that apparently minor increases in fetal plasma cortisol markedly alter fetal ACTH responsiveness. (Supported by NIH and the American Heart Association).

2584 PLACENTAL UPTAKE AND TRANSPORT OF T4, T3 AND IODIDE IN EARLY AND LATE PREGNANCY IN RATS

R.J.Woods*, A.K.Sinha and R.P.Ekins, Department of Molecular Endocrinology, The Middlesex Hospital Medical School, London W1N 8AA, UK.

Neurological cretinism in children of mothers with low T4, high TSH and normal T3 serum levels in early pregnancy is well documented. However, the availability of thyroid hormone to the foetus in the critical stages of neuronal differentiation and proliferation has been a topic of controversy due to the apparent lack of placental transfer of T4 and T3 in early ontogeny. The role of TBG and its factorial increase in pregnancy also remain ambiguous, although its putative involvement in T4 delivery has been suggested[1]. To verify these assumptions, rats at different stages of pregnancy were injected with ^{125}I-T4, T3 and ^{131}Iodide; TCA soluble and insoluble radiolabel measured and ratios of soluble ^{125}I and ^{131}I in tissues compared with those in serum. On protein basis 9 $\pm$ 3, 3 $\pm$ 2, 2.4 $\pm$ 1.2 and 1 $\pm$ 1 % of serum T4 pool is transferred to the foetus at 9/10, 13/14, 15/16 and 18/19 days of gestation and 17 $\pm$ 7 and 46% of maternal serum T3 was also obtained in the 9/10 and 18/19 day foetuses respectively. Chromatography of acid insoluble fractions revealed that a high proportion of transported T4 was converted to T3 in early and to rT3 in late pregnancy. The soluble ^{125}I/^{131}I ratios were 1.23 $\pm$ 0.2 in 9/10 day foetuses with T4 and 2.42 $\pm$ 0.43 and 1.79 in 9/10 and 18/19 day foetuses with T3 tracers respectively. The placental uptake of T4 at 15/16 and 18/19 days of pregnancy were 21 $\pm$ 4% of maternal serum T4 value, and iodide ratio was 1.8. The placenta concentrated significantly more iodide than the maternal organs. Our results strongly indicate a placental control of the supply, metabolism and synthesis of T4 and T3 in the foetus.

1. Ekins, R.P. (1982) Recent Adv. Endoc. Metab. 2, 287.

2585 PREDICTION AND THERAPY OF INTRAUTERINE AND LATE-ONSET NEONATAL HYPERTHYROIDISM. M. Zakarija*, J.M. McKenzie, W. Hoffman**, Dept. of Med., Univ. Miami Sch. of Med., Miami, FL. and Children's Hospital, Detroit, MI**.

We have described (J Clin Invest 72:1352,1983) thyroid-stimulating antibody (TSAb) and TSAb-inhibiting antibody in serum of a woman (M) whose child was euthyroid at birth and hyperthyroid after 6 weeks. M's IgG stimulated human thyroid in vitro only when dilute (e.g. 5ug per ml) and not at 1-10mg per ml. Since an adult concentration of IgG occurs in fetal serum only after 26 weeks we hypothesized earlier low concentrations might stimulate the thyroid whereas later (equal to maternal) would not. With M's next child (C_3) tachycardia developed at about 12 weeks gestation so propylthiouracil, 200 mg per day, was prescribed for M until 28 weeks; fetal signs improved coincident with the therapy and remained normal through delivery (when Apgar score was 9). C_3 was euthyroid at birth but was started on PTU at 49 days for hyperthyroidism (T_4 27.3ug/100ml; T_3 452ng/100ml). Serum for TSAb and TSH-binding inhibition assays (latter data now shown) was obtained monthly. The characteristic negative dose response of M's IgG in an assay for TSAb (% increase in cAMP in human thyroid cells in culture) is: 5ug/ml, 791%; 50ug/ml, 476%; 500ug/ml, 177%; this pattern was duplicated by C's serum IgG in the first month and gradually changed to a low positive dose-response at 6 months; e.g., concentrations as above, IgG at 5 days, 589%, 415%, 152%; IgG at 186 days 111%, 185%, 377%. The data are compatible with the concept that a TSAb-inhibitor, when in high concentration, prevented third trimester and early neonatal hyperthyroidism, but at lower concentrations, in second trimester and after 6 weeks, did not, when TSAb effect predominated and hyperthyroidism developed.

2586 LACK OF LINKAGE BETWEEN HLA AND TYPE 2 MULTIPLE ENDOCRINE NEOPLASIA IN A FAMILY. Thomas J.L.*, Genton P., Gay G., Perrier F., Brunschwig A., Leclere J., Hartemann P. - Clinique Médicale E et Endocrinologique, CHU de Nancy Brabois, 54500 Vandoeuvre les Nancy, France.

The transmission of type 2 Multiple Endocrine Neoplasia (MEN 2) is autosomal dominant. In MEN 2 families, the systematic screening for affected or potential members requires calcitonin secretion tests and detection of carcinoembryonic antigen for medullary thyroid carcinoma and catecholamine assays for pheochromocytoma. When negative, these tests must be repeated. A genetic marker would be useful to identify potential cases once and for all. We studied a single caucasian family of 26 subjects spread over 3 successive generations. 8 had MEN 2 : 3 had died of pheochromocytoma and the 5 others had a pheochromocytoma or a medullary thyroid carcinoma confirmed by pathological examination. 4 had also parathyroid hyperplasia or adenoma. 12 members have been typed for HLA A, B and DR by microlymphocytotoxicity (NIH technique). 3 were affected and 1 had increased serum calcitonin levels after pentagastrin and will undergo thyroidectomy. Like the two previous family studies, our study found no linkage between MEN 2 and any particular HLA haplotype. These findings suggest that the locus of MEN 2 is not on chromosome 6.

2587 GLUCOCORTICOID STIMULATION OF HUMAN GROWTH HORMONE PRODUCTION IN TRANSGENIC MICE. T.E. Wagner, R. Portanova*, J. Yun and R. Seldon[+], Departments of Chemistry and Zoological-Biomedical Sciences and College of Osteopathic Medicine, Ohio University, Athens, OH, USA; [+]Department of Molecular Biology, Massachusetts General Hospital, Boston, MA, USA.

A gene construct, consisting of the promoter sequence of the mouse metallothionein gene fused to the structural gene which codes for human growth hormone (hGH), was introduced into mice by microinjection of one cell embryos, using procedures similar to those previously described (Wagner *et al.*, PNAS, 78,6376, 1981). At 7 weeks of age, the transgenic mice were approximately twice as large as control animals (37 g *vs* 17 g, BW). Using a highly sensitive and specific double monoclonal antibody RIA (Hybridtech, Inc.), plasma from transgenic animals was found to contain high concentrations of hGH (.007 μg/ml to 4.5 μg/ml); hGH was not detected in plasma from control animals (<.001 μg/ml). The metallothionein/human growth hormone fusion gene used in these studies contains a copy of the 21 base pair glucocorticoid regulation sequence in the first interon of the growth hormone portion of the gene. When the transgenic mice were given triamcinalone in their drinking water (50 μg/ml, 24 to 48 h) hGH levels were elevated approximately 3-fold; at about 1 week following removal of the steroid, hGH concentrations returned to pre-treatment levels. These findings are consistent with the view that; the metallothionein/human growth hormone fusion gene is incorporated into the genome of the mouse; the gene is functionally expressed, not only producing the specific growth hormone protein product, but also accelerating the growth rate of the transgenic animal; and, the gene is externally controllable by the administration of glucocorticoid.

2588 FAMILIAL DYSALBUMINEMIC HYPERTHYROXINEMIA (FDH): A FOUR GENERATION STUDY. Y. Yabu, J.R. Etzkorn, P.P.B. Yeo*, R. Rajatanavin, L.E. Braverman and S.H. Ingbar. Beth Israel Hospital, Boston, MA; St. Louis University School of Medicine, St. Louis, MO and University of Massachusetts Medical Center, Worcester, MA, U.S.A.

We present here evidence of the mode of inheritance of FDH in the largest family group yet reported, comprising 31 family members and 3 spouses across 4 generations. Diagnosis of FDH was established by demonstrating hyperthyroxinemia with normal free T_4, total T_3, TBG concentrations, and an increase in the binding of ^{125}I-T_4 by a serum albumin during paper electrophoresis. Results:

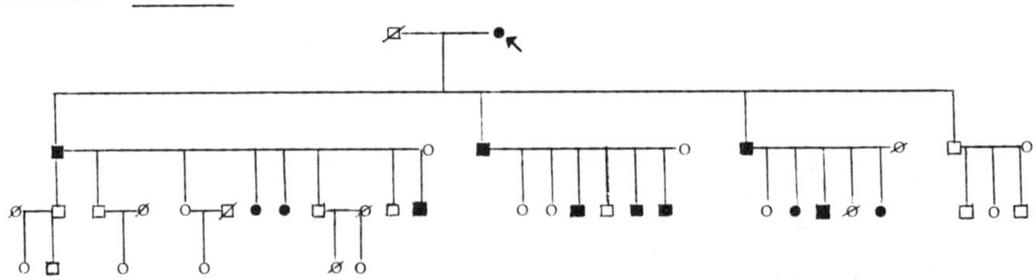

Key: ● or ■ - FDH; ø or ☐̸ - not studied; ↖ - proposita

Conclusion: These findings indicate that FDH is inherited by autosomal dominant transmission with strong penetrance.

2589 CHANGING PATTERNS OF PERIPHERAL HORMONES AND STEROLS DURING MATURATION IN THE FEMALE RABBIT. E.V. YoungLai*, Department of Obstetrics and Gynecology, McMaster University, Hamilton, Ontario, Canada L8N 3Z5.

Although female rabbits do not reproduce until at least 5 months old their hormonal patterns from birth to adulthood are not well defined. This study was therefore initiated to determine the peripheral levels of luteinizing hormone (LH), follicle stimulating hormone (FSH) and prolactin (PRL) at the following days - 1,3,5,7,9,15,22,30,35,40,50,80 and 100 with the day of birth being considered as day 1. These levels were correlated with total serum cholesterol determined by a colorimetric method. Hormones were determined by radioimmunoassay and expressed in ng/ml. Serum LH and FSH showed three distinct peaks occurring on day 3 (LH=3.34±1.97; FSH=1.92±0.86), day 9 (LH=4.05±0.76; FSH=3.62±0.67) and day 35 (LH=5.90±1.20) or day 40 (FSH=9.01±1.43). By day 100 levels of LH and FSH were in the adult range - (LH<1 ng/ml and FSH<0.6 ng/ml). Serum PRL showed a progressive increase from day 1 (1.04±0.07 ng/ml) to day 100 (16.30±2.50 ng/ml). Total serum cholesterol was high during the nursing period up to day 22 (291±25 mg%) and then progressively decreased to 75±8 mg% in adult. Since meiois does not begin until after birth in the rabbit and is completed within the first three weeks of life these results suggest that pituitary gonadotropins may have a role during meiosis and in the initiation of follicular development.

2590 BINDING-SITE SPECIFICITY OF MONOCLONAL ANTIBODIES TO HUMAN GROWTH HORMONE. M. Wallis* and M. Daniels, Biochemistry Laboratory, School of Biological Sciences, University of Sussex, Falmer, Brighton BN1 9QG, U.K.

Monoclonal antibodies (McAbs) to a complex protein antigen may bind to several different epitopes. In order to try to define the epitopes on the human growth hormone (hGH) molecule, the binding of a series of McAbs to variants and modified forms of the hormone has been investigated. The ability of 7 McAbs to bind to fragments produced by plasmin digestion of hGH was studied. Each of the antibodies bound well to plasmin-digested hormone (a two-chain form of hGH in which residues 135-140 are missing). Most of the antibodies bound poorly to peptides (hGH^{1-134} and $hGH^{141-191}$) produced after reduction, alkylation and fractionation of plasmin-digested hGH. However, 2 antibodies bound the plasmin fragment corresponding to residues 1-134 almost as well as they did the native hormone, suggesting that the epitope(s) to which they bind is largely located within the N-terminal two-thirds of hGH. Studies on binding to size variants of hGH showed that 3 of 4 McAbs tested were unable to distinguish between monomeric, dimeric and higher-molecular weight forms of the hormone, but that a fourth antibody bound more effectively to monomer than to dimer. Antibodies have also been raised against the dimeric form of hGH, and can distinguish between size variants. Such studies should help to define the epitopes on the hGH molecule. Supported by the MRC.

2591 ACUTE AND CHRONIC EFFECTS OF INSULIN AND GROWTH HORMONE ON PORCINE ADIPOSE TISSUE METABOLISM. P. E. Walton*, and T. D. Etherton. Pennsylvania State Univ., Univ. Park, PA 16802, USA.

The current study was undertaken to determine the effects of porcine growth hormone (pGH) and insulin (I) on lipogenesis (LPG), glucose oxidation (GO) and lipolysis (LP) in swine adipose tissue during acute (2 h) and chronic (24, 48 h) exposure to these hormones. Subcutaneous adipose tissue explants (~10 mg) were cultured for 0, 24 or 48 h in M-199 supplemented with I, pGH or I and pGH. Explants were removed and then incubated in KRB containing the hormone(s) in addition to [U-^{14}C]glucose. Insulin increased LPG and GO 2.1 and 1.8 fold respectively in short-term incubations. Rates of GO and LPG were maintained by I after 24 h whereas rates in tissue not exposed to I had significantly declined. After 48 h the decline in LPG was attenuated by I in a dose-dependent manner. LP was increased by I after 48 h. pGH was insulin-like with respect to LPG and GO in acute incubations. In long-term culture, pGH significantly inhibited these processes. pGH did not affect LP acutely. However, pGH increased LP after chronic exposure. Physiological concentrations of pGH significantly inhibited the effects of I on LPG and GO in both acute and chronic incubations. Results of the present study indicate that I is involved in maintaining lipogenic capacity of swine adipose tissue, but that other hormones are necessary for full maintenance of lipogenic capacity. Secondly, these data demonstrate a lipolytic effect of pGH on swine adipose tissue in the absence of theophylline or glucocorticoids. Furthermore, the observation that pGH antagonizes I action provides a model system to study the diabetogenic effects of pGH in domestic animals. This will be important in studies conducted to determine the efficacy with which pGH increases swine growth performance after long-term administration.

2592 CHARACTERIZATION OF BOVINE GROWTH HORMONE PRODUCED BY RECOMBINANT BACTERIA. Paul Wingfield, Gary Buell, Biogen S.A., Geneva 24, Switzerland, and B. Dan Burleigh*, International Minerals & Chemical Corporation, Terre Haute, Indiana 47808, U.S.A.

Recombinant bovine growth hormone (rbGH) has been purified from E. coli, strain MC-1061, transformed with a suitable expression vector, using a combination of conventional techniques. The purified rbGH has been characterized by amino acid analysis, N-terminal determination (Dansyl), gel electrophoresis (PAGE) under reducing and nonreducing conditions, molecular weight determination via gel filtration, isoelectric focusing (IEF), and tryptic peptide mapping using reversed-phase high performance liquid chromatography (HPLC). Parallel characterization using the same techniques was done on a natural bovine growth hormone preparation (bGH, AFP-671) purified from pituitaries. These studies confirm the identity of the rbGH preparation; the PAGE and IEF studies show it to be more homogeneous than natural bGH preparations, which have significant deamidation and proteolytic nicking. The biological activities of natural bGH and bacterial rbGH were measured using hypophysectomized rat tibia and rat growth assays; their comparative receptor binding properties were studied using a radioreceptor assay based on pregnant rabbit liver membrane. The biological activity and competitive receptor binding characteristics of the bGH and rbGH preparations were found to be nearly identical. The data demonstrate that purified bacterial rbGH does not differ significantly from natural pituitary bGH in its essential properties.

(Abstract 2772, p. 1646, also belongs to this section.)

2593 REGULATION OF PROTEIN PHOSPHORYLATION BY TRIIODOTHYRONINE (T3) IN PRIMARY ASTROCYTIC CULTURES. J. Ruel*, J.-M. Gavaret and J.H. Dussault, Thyroid Research Unit, Dept of Endocrinology and Metabolism, CHUL, Quebec, G1V 4G2, Canada.

In order to investigate the mechanism of action of thyroid hormone on the central nervous system, we examined the effects of T_3 on protein phosphorylation in cultured glial cells. Cerebral hemispheres from 2 day old rats were dissociated mechanically and cultured for 2 weeks in DME medium containing 10% of serum depleted of thyroid hormones. These cultures were incubated with T_3 (10^{-8} M) for 2.5, 24, 48 and 72 hours and then with ^{32}P-phosphate (100 μCi) for an additional 4 hours. Cell homogenates were centrifuged at 100,000 x g and phosphorylated proteins in both soluble and particulate fractions were analysed by one and/or two- dimensional polyacrylamide gel electrophoresis. The degree of phosphorylation was either increased or decreased by T_3 in a minimum of 12 soluble proteins. The major effects were 1) a rapid and transient increase in the phosphorylation of a 34 K dalton protein (pI = 5.0) and 2) a progressive decrease in the phosphorylation of two proteins (20 K and 21 K). The phosphorylation of the 34 K and 20 K proteins was increased by dbcAMP (10^{-3} M). The effects were less marked in the particulate fraction where an increased phosphorylation of two proteins (15 K and 21.5 K) was induced both by T_3 and dbcAMP. These results show that T_3 modulate the phosphorylation of specific proteins in cultured astrocytes, some of which are also under cAMP control. Hence thyroid hormones may influence metabolic pathways in this cell type through such modifications.

2594 CYCLIC VARIATION OF SUBSTANCE P IN THE NORMAL MENSTRUAL CYCLE. J. Sanfilippo*, R. Handy, and C. Osuampke, University of Louisville, Department of Obstetrics and Gynecology, Division of Reproductive Endocrinology and Infertility, Louisville, Kentucky, U.S.A.

Substance P is an 11 amino acid peptide found in both the central nervous system and the gastrointestinal tract. It is a neurotransmitter, active in the perception of pain, and located primarily in the dorsal horn gray matter of the spinal cord and dorsal root ganglia. Little is known about its role in the normal menstrual cycle. It was the purpose of this project to determine circulating levels of substance P throughout the menstrual cycle. Six females with regular menstrual cycles (on no medications) had peripheral blood samples drawn for determination of substance P. Seven samples were drawn throughout the cycle (one each in the early, mid, and late follicular phases; one at ovulation; and one each during the early, mid, and late luteal phases). The levels of substance P were determined by a radioimmunoassay using ^{125}I substance P. The assay has been previously evaluated for cross-reactivity with enkephalins, endorphins, eledoisin, and physalaemin. The antibody as tested had minimal cross-reactivity with these substances. In four patients there was a periovulatory peak in substance P. One patient had undetectable levels throughout the menstrual cycle. This study revealed variation in circulating levels of substance P throughout the menstrual cycle.

2595 ENDOGENOUS BRAIN STEROIDS: FAILURE TO RESPOND TO STRESS OR HYPOPHYSECTOMY. W. J. Shoemaker*, C. Corpéchot, F.E. Bloom and E. Baulieu. The Salk Institute, La Jolla, CA.

The steroids, dehydroepiandrosterone (DHA) and Δ-5 Pregnenolone (5P), have been measured using specific radioimmunoassays in brains of male rats. The regional distribution of these two steroids varies 10-fold for DHA and 4-fold for 5P in a study of eight brain regions. The ratio of DHA to 5P within a particular structure also varies considerably across brain regions. We have confirmed the earlier report of Corpechot, et al. (Brain Res 270:119) that neither adrenalectomy, orchiectomy nor both treatments alters the level of the steroids in most brain regions. We have extended those studies by determining the effect of a standardized stress on the steroid levels in eight brain regions; we have also studied the effect of hypophysectomy on the steroids in the brain. A 15 minute exposure to ether vapors was used as a stress to compare with barbiturate-anesthetized non-stressed "controls". All rats were decapitated 30 minutes later, brains removed, dissected and prepared for RIA. Comparisions of DHA or 5P in 8 regions revealed no significant effect of the stress. Surgically hypophysectomized male rats were given 1% saline for 14 days-post-op;shams and hypox were then sacrificed. Both steroids were virtually unchanged in any of the brain regions. In contrast to peripheral steroidogenic tissue, brain DHA and 5P fail to respond to stress and to hypophysectomy, strongly inferring a separate and independent brain steroid system. In other studies, rapid and specific changes in these brain steroids have been observed. (Soc. Neurosci. Abs. 9:1237, 1983). (Supported by NIAAA 03504).

2596 RAT HYPOTHALAMIC AROMATASE (HA) ACTIVITY IS RELATED TO ADULT ENDOCRINE STATUS Donald L. Wilke* and W. Emmett Braselton Jr. Dept. Pharmacology/Toxicology, Michigan State University, E. Lansing, MI 48824 U.S.A.

Aromatization of circulating androgens to estrogens in mammalian hypothalamus is critical to brain differentiation, regulation of gonadotropin secretion, and control of sexual behavior. Although male brain has higher HA activity than does female brain, we wished to determine whether this is due to perinatal differentiation of the hypothalamus, or to the hormonal status of adult animals. HA activity was measured in Sprague-Dawley rats by incubating ^{3}H-androst-4-ene-3,17-dione with pooled hypothalamic homogenate from 3 animals in the presence of an NADPH regenerating system. The ^{3}H-estrone produced by aromatization was isolated by two successive HPLC steps and quantified by liquid scintillation counting. Adult (60 days old) castration of male rats resulted in reduction of HA activity to female levels. Perinatal treatment of male pups (from day 15 of gestation to day 7 post-partum) with the aromatase inhibitor androsta-1,4,6-triene-3,17-dione failed to reduce HA activity of adults below that of control males. Castration of male pups on day 1 lowered HA activity to female levels. HA activity of day 1 castrates treated with testosterone (T) as adults was not different from that of normal males. Treatment of female pups with 100ug of T on day 3 failed to increase adult HA activity, but adult T treatment raised HA activity to male levels. These results indicate that in the rat, HA activity is related to adult T concentration. (Supported by BRSG #2S07RR05623-16)

2597 EFFECT OF GROWTH HORMONE ON SLEEP IN GROWTH HORMONE DEFICIENT CHILDREN.
R.H. Wu*. DEPARTMENT OF PEDIATRICS, ALBERT EINSTEIN COLLEGE OF MEDICINE, BRONX-LEBANON HOSPITAL CENTER, BRONX, N.Y., 10457.

Sleep related release of growth hormone, GH, has been associated with slow-wave sleep, SWS, stages 3-4. Any interruption of SWS will inhibit sleep entrained GH release. In order to assess the effect of GH administration on SWS in GH deficient children, total sleep time, sleep stages 1-4, REM, REM latency and sleep efficiency were studied in four children with growth hormone deficiency before and after GH therapy. Growth hormone therapy resulted in a significant change in the mean duration of stage 3 sleep, 58 ± 11 vs 39 ± 26 minutes, before and after GH respectively ($p < 0.05$). Individually, three of the four patients had decreases in stage 3 while the fourth had no change. The magnitude of the decrease in stage 3 was 19 minutes or a 33% change. When the sleep parameters were expressed as percentages of the total sleep period no significant changes were observed although three of four patients had increases in their percentages of stage 2 sleep and decreases in stage 3 sleep percentage. There was a 28% change in stage 3 percentage and a 7% change in stage 2 percentage. None of the other sleep parameters were significantly effected by GH therapy. No subjective changes in sleep were reported by the patients, despite the changes in sleep stages. These data indicate that GH therapy may effect sleep stages in GH deficient children without changing the duration of sleep or sleep efficiency. The significant changes observed in stage 3 sleep and the lack of any significant changes in REM sleep have not been described before in GH deficient children. They differ from animal studies which have shown that REM sleep increased with exogenous administration of growth hormone.

2598 THE RECURRENCE OF COMPLETE ESTROUS CYCLE IN SUPRACHIASMATIC NUCLEUS (SCN)-LESIONED RATS. Shinji Yoshioka and Michio Takahashi*, Laboratory of Vetrinary Physiology, Faculty of Agriculture, University of Tokyo, 1-1-1 Yayoi Bunkyo-ku, Tokyo 113, Japan.

Adult female rats with an isografted anterior pituitary (AP) recur the estrous cycle with a full expression of luteal activity for each cycle. Ovulation occurs spontaneously at 2 weeks intervals. We investigated the involvement of the neural mechanism governing the rhythmicity in the recurrence of this type of ovulation in the rat. Bilateral electrical lesions were placed at SCN. After confirming animals were rendered into constant estrus (CE), they were transplanted with AP and induced 1st ovulation by an injection of hCG. A group of rats with a relatively large lesion extending to the caudal portion of SCN (group-I) returned to CE after passing one luteal phase and were unable to ovulate spontaneously. The other group of rats with a small lesion restricted within the medio-rostal portion of SCN (group-II) recurred the complete estrous cycle as long as the AP explant existed. Blockade of prolactin secretion by bromocriptine in group-II rats lowered peripheral progesterone and resulted in ovulation. This induced ovulation was preceded by normal LH-surge. It is known that the neural circadian oscillatory device is a prerequisite for the occurrence of ovulation in the rat during 4-day estrous cycle. Introduction of the luteal phase between ovulations, however, nullifies the necessesity of the involvement of this neural mechanism. The ovulatory cycle in group-II rats will be proceeded to only by the steroidal feedback regulations as in primates and ungulates.

(Abstract 2773, p. 1647, also belongs to this section.)

2599 STRUCTURAL AND FUNCTIONAL INTERACTION OF PEPTIDE HORMONES.
Yu.A.Pankov, Institute of Experimental Endocrinology and Hormone Chemistry, the USSR Academy of Medical Sciences, Moscow, USSR.

Three approaches have been used for the study of peptide hormones structure and function interrelation: 1/research on amino acid sequence of hormones extracted from endocrine glands of different species; 2/computerizing for the comparative analysis of homologous hormones and for determination of their secondary structure and physico-chemical parameters; 3/ protein fragments of peptide hormones study for research of stuctural determinants of their various activities. The result of the research done is the established amino acid sequence of porcine, bovine and whale β-lipotropins, bovine and whale prolactins, whale corticotropin and whale somatotropin and spermwhale luteinizing hormone. By means of computer the study of homologous fragments of amino acid sequences has been carried out for superfamilies of a/opiate polyhormones' precursors; b/proinsulin; c/proglucagon; d/epidermal growth factor. Inside the precursors studied homologous parts of primary structures, unknown before, have been discovered. These parts might determine synthesis of new peptides. The study of somatotropin biologically active fragments has indicated the localization of structures which determined lipotropic, insulin-like, growth-stimulating and neurotropic activities of this hormone.

2600 MOTILIN (M) IS A PHYSIOLOGICAL PEPTIDE CONTROLLING VIA AN HORMONAL PATHWAY THE INTERDIGESTIVE MIGRATING COMPLEX (IDMC) OF THE SMALL INTESTINE IN DOG.
P. Poitras*, D. Tassé and L. Trudel. Clinical Research Center, Hôpital Saint-Luc, Montréal, Canada.

The IDMC is known to be regulated by hormonal mechanisms in dog. M cyclical increases in the peripheral circulation associated with the phase III's [or activity front (AF)] of the IDMC suggest that this peptide could be involved in the hormonal control of the IDMC. However, the simultaneous induction of AF and motilin release by morphine suggested that M rise could only be secondary to the intestinal contraction rather than being the cause of it. For this study, myoelectrical intestinal motility was recorded in 4 conscious dogs equipped with 7 chronically implanted monopolar electrodes on the small intestine, and M was measured by RIA. The following experiments were performed to elucidate the hormonal role of M in dog: 1) an IV infusion of pancreatic polypeptide (1 $\mu g\ Kg^{-1}hr^{-1}$ for 3 hrs) could abolish the regular occurrence of AF without influencing the cyclical variation of M blood levels. 2) Synthetic canine motilin was given IV (50, 100, 200 $\mu g\ Kg^{-1}$ 30 min^{-1}). The highest dose, reproducing physiological circulating increases, consistently elicitated duodenal migrating AF. 3) Immunoneutralisation of circulating M was performed by infusing a specific M antiserum (7921 antibody, 2.5 ml bolus IV, and then 1.5 ml hr^{-1}). During the 3 hr infusion, AF were undetectable in the proximal small intestine. Distally initiated AF (known to be independent of motilin control) were still documented. These experiments clearly suggest that M is a gastrointestinal hormone released from endocrine cells of the duodenojejunal mucosa in the peripheral circulation to control the induction of the phase III of the IDMC in the proximal intestine of the dog.

2601 AN ASSAY FOR METHIONINE IN PEPTIDES, WHICH IDENTIFIES (AFTER ELECTRO-FOCUSING) AND ESTIMATES BIOACTIVE FORMS OF CORTICOTROPIN AND OTHER HORMONES. P.L. Storring* and R.J. Tiplady, National Institute for Biological Standards and Control, London NW3 6RB, UK.

Many peptide hormones contain a single methionine residue per molecule, which is readily oxidized with a resultant loss of bioactivity. Estimates of non-oxidized methionine of such hormones are therefore useful for evaluating differences in the bioactivities between preparations and for monitoring their activity during isolation or synthesis, processing and storage. But the accurate estimation of non-oxidized methionine in peptides is a problem. A radioassay for methionine is described based on its specific reaction with iodo(2-^{14}C)acetic acid. The labelled peptide was isolated by carboxymethyl-cellulose chromatography or by isoelectric focusing (IEF) or electrophoresis in polyacrylamide gel, and its radioactivity measured. The assay was applied to corticotropins, α-melanotropin, bombesin, glucagon, substance P, parathormone and calcitonin. 24-30 samples were conveniently analyzed at a time with a lower detection limit of less than 1 nmole of methionine per sample. The accuracy of the assay, assessed also by reverse-phase high performance liquid chromatography, is due to its precision, the specificity of the reaction with iodoacetic acid and the use of an appropriate standard of the peptide being assayed. Methionine was identified, and could be estimated, in individual peptide components of a mixture by using IEF to separate simultaneously the labelled peptide from iodo(2-^{14}C)acetic acid and from other peptide and protein components. This was facilitated by a convenient method for detecting and quantifying these peptides after IEF.

2602 PURIFICATION AND IMMUNOLOGICAL CHARACTERIZATION OF INHIBIN FROM BOVINE FOLLICULAR FLUID (bFF). S. van Dijk*, J. Steenbergen, F.H. de Jong and H.J. van der Molen, Dept. of Biochemistry (Div. of Chemical Endocrinology), Erasmus University, P.O. Box 1738, 3000 DR Rotterdam, The Netherlands.

Inhibin was partially purified from bFF on immobilized Procion Red 3B, Sephadex G-25 and ion-exchange chromatography, using Fast Protein Liquid Chromatography (FPLC). Inhibin activity was determined measuring suppression of FSH release from cultured rat pituitary cells. Results of sodium dodecyl poly acrylamide gel electrophoresis (SDS-PAGE) analysis after FPLC on Mono Q at pH 7.9 suggested that inhibin was associated with a 65 kD band (relative specific activity ∼ 40). After rechromatography on Mono Q at pH 9.2, inhibin was found in a fraction with a single 65 kD band after SDS-PAGE. This fraction was radio-iodinated and immunoprecipitated with antisera against an inhibin fraction or a fraction of plasma from castrated cows (bPcas). The precipitated radioactivity was analyzed on SDS-PAGE. The difference in precipitated radioactivity was found as a 65 kD protein. In a radioimmunoassay system based on precipitation with Staphylococcus aureus bFF displaced this labelled inhibin preparation from the anti-inhibin antiserum. SDS-PAGE of the precipitated material showed that the displacement was caused by a 65 kD protein which was not displaced by bPcas. However, the purified inhibin preparations contain apart from the ovary-specific 65 kD protein some plasma-derived proteins with approximately the same molecular weight. It is concluded that inhibin has an apparent MW of 65 kD and an iso-electric point lower than 7.9.

2603 THE ROLE OF CARBOHYDRATE MOIETY IN THE GONADOTROPIN MOLECULE IN EVOKING CELLULAR RESPONSE TO THE HORMONE. U. Zor, M.R. Sairam†, P. Sentzer, A. Azrad and A. Amsterdam, Dept. Hormone Res., Weizmann Inst. of Science, Rehovot, Israel; and †Clinical. Res. Inst. of Montreal, Quebec, Canada.

We have examined whether various deglycosylated gonadotropins (DGLH, DGhCG and DGFSH), which serve as hormone antagonists, could affect desensitization of cyclic AMP response induced by continuous exposure to homologous agonists (LH, hCG, FSH), and whether they induce receptor "down regulation". Rat granulosa cells were cultured with antagonists and agonists concomitantly, for a period of 20 h, and subsequently washed in acidic medium to dissociate bound ligands from their receptors. The cells were then challenged with fresh agonists or with labelled ^{125}I-hormone. At 20 h of culture with LH, hCG and FSH, cyclic AMP response to challenge with reapplication of the same hormones was only 5-10% of maximal stimulation, while after 20 h of culture with DGLH, DGhCG and DGFSH alone, the response to the appropriate agonist was retained by 50-60%. DGLH as well as LH reduced the binding of ^{125}I-hCG to surface receptors by 90%. In contrast, DGhCG induced only 15% reduction in receptor density, while hCG induced 50% reduction. FSH induced a 35% reduction in receptor density, while DGFSH increased the receptor number by 25%. The fate of ^{125}I-hCG and ^{125}I-DGhCG was examined during the 20 h incubation. ^{125}I-hCG was internalized within lysosomes 5-fold greater than ^{125}I-DGhCG. The rate of degradation of the native internalized hormone was twice the degradation rate of the DGhCG. Thus ligand binding to receptor is essential but not sufficient to induce desensitization. The sugar moiety on the hormone protein core is therefore essential for expressing its biological activity.

2604 INHIBITION OF LACTATION WITH DEPOT-BROMOCRIPTINE. R. Rolland*, W. Nijdam, A. Weyer and I. Lancranjan[1], Department of Obstetrics and Gynaecology, St. Radboud University Hospital, Nijmegen, The Nederlands and [1]Clinical Research Department, Sandoz Ltd, Basel, Switserland.

Since the introduction of bromocriptine, this drug has been utilized widely for the inhibition or supression of post partum lactation. Concomitant with the normalization of prolactin, the menstrual cycle restores in women taking this drug. The only drawback is the need to take tablets for 14 to 21 days post partum to prevent rebound phenomena. Bromocriptine can however, be bound to polylactic acid and microcapsules of this substance show a sustained release of the drug. In 30 women 50 mg depot-bromocriptine (DB) was injected within three hours after delivery and the candidates were followed for 28 days. In all subjects the medication was well tolerated without any local or systemic side effect. Milk let down, engorgement or pain was absent in all women except in a few instances on days 2, 3 and 4 post partum when mild symptoms were present. Rebound phenomena did not occur. All women judged the treatment as extremely satisfactory and convenient. Within 48 hours post partum serum prolactin was within the normal nonpregnant range below 800 IU/l and remained so until day 28. 10 women started on oral contraceptives before day 28. Of the remaining 20, 12 had high progesterone values on day 28 indicating ovulation, whereas the remaining 8 showed LH, FSH and oestradiol levels in accordance with the periovulatory phase. It is concluded that DB has a high efficacy in the prevention of puerperal lactation with little or no side effects. It is more convenient for the client than the need to take tablets for 14 to 21 days and ovarian function is likely to restore within 28 days post partum.

2605 QUANTITATIVE DETERMINATION OF PLASMA CATECHOLESTROGENS DURING PREGNANCY WITH H.P.L.C.

Y. Sagara*, Y. Okatani, N. Morioka, and Y. Takeda, Dept. of OB/GYN, Kochi Medical School, Japan.

Present study was designed to develop a more convenient and rapid HPLC method for the simultaneous microdetermination of plasma 2 hydroxy estrogens. (2OHE1, 2OHE2) and their O-methylated derivatives (2mE1, 2mE2, 3mE1, 3mE2) using high sensitive electrochemical detector. In addtion, to clarify the metabolic pathway of catecholestrogens in normal pregnancy, gestational changes of plasma catecholestrogens levels or changes of their levels after volus injection of estrone sulfate (E1-S, 40mg) or DHAS (100mg) to normal pregnant women (36-40th week). The concentration of 2OHE1 increased toward term with wide variations. The pattern of 2mE1 and 2mE2 showed gradual increase from 24th week to 36th week and gradual decrease there after. The concentration of 3mE1 remained low level (less than 200pg/ml) throughout pregnancy. The injection of E1-S resulted in marked increase of 2mE1 (1205 $\pm$ 213%, M $\pm$ S.D. vs preinjection levels) and also significant increase of 2mE2 (268 $\pm$ 54%) at 60 min. The injection of DHAS resulted in more gradual increase of both 2mE1 and 2mE2 until 120 min accounted for 346 $\pm$ 140, 187 $\pm$ 89%, respectively. Significant correlations were demonstrated only between E1 and 2mE1, E1 and 2mE2, 2mE1 and 2mE2 in both DHAS and E1-S loaded groups. However significant correlation was not demonstrated between E2 and 2mE2. These indicated that the main metabolic pathway of catecholestrogens is E1$\rightarrow$2OHE1$\rightarrow$2mE1. Also it is suggested that estradiol participate in the synthesis of catecholestrogens mainly via its conversion to estrone.

2606 AN INCREASE OF PLASMINOGEN ACTIVATOR IN THE RAT INVOLUTING UTERUS.

H.Shimada*, H.Okamura and T.Mori, Department of Gynecology and Obstetrics, Kyoto University, Faculty of Medicine, Kyoto, 606, Japan.

Many reports have shown the correlation between plasminogen activator(PA) and a process of tissue remodeling. Significant increase of active collagenase at 3 day post partum was reported in rat involuting uterus with increasing attention to the possible role of plasmin in collagenase activation. But no study has been done to investigate PA activity in involuting uterus. PA activities were sequentially measured in rat uterine extract from parturition to 30 day post partum, using a chromogenic substrate S-2251 which we have recently developed for the determination of PA in rat ovary(Shimada et al, Thrombos Haemostas.1981). To investigate effects of 17β-estradiol(E_2) on PA synthesis and involution, various doses of E_2 were injected into rats for 3 days after parturition.
At 3 day post partum, uterine weight falled down to one quarter of those at parturition and reached a minimum level at 15 post partum. The PA activity at parturition was 0.033$\pm$0.018(m$\pm$S.D)μ moles/4mg uterine wet weight/30min and showed its peak value with an 4 fold-increase at 3 day post partum, then decreased sharply till 10 day post partum, though it was not until 25 day post partum that PA activity returned to the level at parturition. E_2 suppressed PA synthesis(50%) and involution(70%).
The results indicate that PA is involved in the process of tissue remodeling in involuting uterus and regulated by estrogen in this process. And it is assumed that PA acts on involution through enhancement of the activity of latent collagenase.

2607 ACTIVITIES OF GLYCOGEN SYNTHETASE AND GLYCOGEN PHOSPHORYLASE IN HUMAN ENDOMETRIUM: RELATIVE DISTRIBUTION IN ISOLATED GLANDS AND STROMA.

Y. Souda*, K. Fukuma, I. Matsuo, T. Souda and M. Maeyama, Department of Obstetrics and Gynecology, Kumamoto University Medical School, Kumamoto 860, Japan.

Human endometrial glycogen is improtant in nidation and in nutrition of the young fertilized ovum. In our previous study, we observed that ovarian steroids, estrogen and progesterone, regulate the endometrial glycogen synthetase (GS) and glycogen phosphorylase (GP) which are responsible for endometrial glycogen metabolism. But the roles of endometrial gland cells and stromal cells are unknown. In the present study, the relative distribution of GS and GP activities in isolated gland and stromal cells was determined following collagenase digestion of the endometrial specimens obtained from 22 premenopausal women undergoing hysterectomy. The GS activity in the glands was about three to eight times that in the stromal cells though the GS activities in both glands and stromal cells increased gradually from the proliferative phase to the secretory phase of the cycle and reached to peak during the mid secretory phase. There was no difference between GP activities of the glands and stromal cells while the GP reached its maximal activity on and after the mid secretory phase of the cycle. These data suggest that not only glands but also stromal cells play an important role in nutrition of the implanting blastocyst.

2608 DOES GnRH ADMINISTRATION TERMINATE PREGNANCY IN THE RAT BY SUPPRESSING OVARIAN TESTOSTERONE PRODUCTION?

R. Sridaran*, Department of Physiology, Morehouse School of Medicine, Atlanta, GA. 30310, U.S.A.

In the pregnant rat LH stimulates the ovarian production of testosterone (T) which is aromatized to estradiol (E_2) by the corpus luteum. In turn, E_2 promotes progesterone (P) synthesis by the ovary which maintains pregnancy. To determine if the administration of GnRH disrupts pregnancy by suppressing ovarian T production, pregnant rats were treated from day 7 to day 12 with 25, 50 or 100 ug/day of GnRH or 0.2, 1.0 or 5ug/day of a GnRH agonist (Wy-40972; Ag) using an osmotic minipump. Rats were bled daily from the jugular vein under light ether anesthesis and on days 10 or 12 of pregnancy both jugular and ovarian vein blood samples were obtained. The higher two doses of GnRH and Ag terminated pregnancy within 48h as indicated by vaginal bleeding. By day 12, peripheral levels of serum P in rats treated with 50 or 100 ug of GnRH or 1.0 or 5.0 ug of Ag were 17±2, 15±1, 12±1 and 8+1ng/ml respectively, compared to 71±6ng/ml in controls. In the same groups, levels in the ovarian vein were 732±438, 122±16, 48±4 and 43±13ng/ml compared to 1950±216ng/ml in controls. In contrast, the serum T levels in systemic blood on days 7-12 remained unchanged in all groups. Ovarian vein levels of T on days 10 or 12 of pregnancy were either not significantly different from controls at 2106±105 or 1357±256 pg/ml respectively or increased dramatically to 9547±1789 on day 10 and to 5243±2100 pg/ml on day 12 in rats treated with 0.2 ug of Ag. These results suggest that GnRH administration induces abortion in rats by suppressing ovarian production of P. We were unable to find any evidence that a GnRH-induced fall in ovarian secretion of T was involved in this process. (Supported by NIH, HD 17867-01).

2609 EFFECT OF CENTCHROMAN ON THE ACTIVITIES OF CERTAIN LYSOSOMAL ENZYMES DURING IMPLANTATION, A.D.Srivastava & S.K.Roy*, Central Drug Research Institute, LUCKNOW-226001, India

Three lysosomal enzymes viz., acid-DNase, acid-RNase and acid-cathepsin-D were observed in (i) ovariectomized rats (ii) differently treated hormonal regimes and (iii) in drug-administered groups. The compounds used are a post-coital anti-implantation agent viz., Centchroman (trans-2-2-dimethyl-3-phenyl-1-1-(p-(-pyrrolidinoethoxy) phenyl-7-methoxychroman) synthesized by CDRI. Both estrogen and progesterone when given separately, caused increase in the activities of the three enzymes but conjointly, they neutralised effect of each other. In progesterone-treated rats an elevation in activity was observed but in estrogen-treated and estrogen + progesterone-treated rats on inhibition in the activities was recorded. In contrast to the effects of estradiol on cathepsin-D synthesis, progesterone increases the role of synthesis of the enzyme without initiating increase in general protein synthesis or uterine growth. A decrease in activities of the three enzymes in rats is due to anti-estrogenicity of the drug. Presence of a chymotrypsin-like enzyme activity in uterine fluid has also been recorded in initiation of implantation whereas reports also exist about the dissolution of matrix present in intercellular spaces for displacing the cells leaving space for entry of trophoblast cells of embryo. Thus, a decrease in the activities of these lysosomal (essential for implantation) enzymes by the present drug Centchroman might be responsible for its anti-implantation activities.

2610 REGULATION OF THE UTERINE SECRETORY IMMUNE SYSTEM DURING PREGNANCY. J.E. Stern* and C.R. Wira, Department of Physiology, Dartmouth Medical School, Hanover, NH, U.S.A.

Sex steroid hormones play a central role in regulting the secretory immune system of the rat uterus by directly mediating the movement of IgA and its transport protein secretory component (SC) as well as uterine IgG (Wira et al. Ann NY Acad Sci 49:534, 1983). In the present study we investigated the secretory immune system in pregnant rats and in rats with induced decidual cell reactions (DCRs). SC and IgA were low in progesterone treated (2.5mg/day) ovariectomized animals with or without DCRs. The levels of IgG after induction of DCR were 10-fold greater (2545±636ng/flush) than in the absence of decidualization (275±53ng/flush). Timed pregnant rats were used to evaluate SC in later pregnancy. SC was found in low concentrations in amniotic fluid between days 14 and 20 of pregnancy. To measure uterine SC production, uteri were perfused with saline and incubated in RPMI 1640 for 24 hours at 37°C. Uteri from day 7 pregnant rats released 118±24ng/horn/24hrs whereas tissues from day 19 pregnancies released 3380±556ng. Uteri from rats at the diestrous stage of the estrous cycle released 1754±284ng. A 4-fold increase was also observed between days 7 and 19 when SC was expressed as ngSC/100mg tissue. SC accumulation was entirely inhibited when cycloheximide (100μg/ml) was added to the media, suggesting that SC synthesis was taking place. These results indicate that SC is present at low levels during early pregnancy and increases in later pregnancy. The studies also indicate that IgG is elevated at the time of decidualization and may play a part in blastocyst survival. This study was supported by AI-13541 from NIH.

2611 CRITICAL PERIOD FOR THE UTERUS TO INDUCE LUTEOLYSIS IN PREGNANT RATS.
K. Ueda*, H. Kato, H. Tamura and T. Torigoe, Dept. of Obstetrics and Gynecology, Yamaguchi University School of Medicine, 1144 Kogushi, Ube, 755, Japan.

We have reported the luteolytic effect of the non-gravid part of the uterus in the pregnant rat (Endocrinol., 111:2020, 1982). This paper shows when the uterus exerts the luteolytic effect during pregnancy. The possible role of the conceptus in the regulation of this effect is also demonstrated. Sprague-Dawley rats were used. On day 7 of pregnancy, all of the conceptuses except the one were removed by aspiration (Asp). In these rats, the uterine horns except the portion that containing a single conceptus were then removed by hysterectomy (Hyst) on day 8 (Asp plus Hyst-8) or day 9 (Asp plus Hyst-9). Other 3 groups of rats received only Hyst on day 7 (Hyst-7), day 8 (Hyst-8) or day 9 (Hyst-9). Serum progesterone levels were determined on days 12, 15 and 17 of pregnancy. In Hyst-7 and Hyst-8, but not in Hyst-9, serum progesterone levels increased on day 15 of pregnancy. In Asp, serum progesterone levels remained low on days 15 and 17. On the other hand, in Asp plus Hyst-8, serum progesterone levels did not rise on day 15, but did rise on day 17, while Asp plus Hyst-9 did not show any increase in serum progesterone levels either on day 15 or 17. These results indicated that the critical period for the non-gravid part of the uterus to exert the luteolytic effects would be between day 7 to 9 of pregnancy, which would, however, be controlled by the presence of large amounts of conceptus-derived substances.

2612 ARACHIDONIC ACID STIMULATES PHOSPHOLIPASE C ACTIVITY, CALCIUM EFFLUX AND HUMAN PLACENTAL LACTOGEN RELEASE FROM TROPHOBLAST CELLS.
P. Zeitler* and S. Handwerger, Dept. of Ped. and Phys.,Duke Med. Ctr., Durham, NC USA

Previous studies from this lab have demonstrated that arachidonic acid (AA) stimulates human placental lactogen (hPL) release *in vitro*. Since AA affects calcium flux and stimulates the activity of phosphatidylinositol (PI)-specific phospholipase C(PLC) in many tissue, we have examined the effects of AA on calcium efflux, phosphatidylinositol turnover and hPL release in an enriched fraction of hPL-secreting cells prepared by the isopycnic centrifugation of enzyme-dispersed trophoblast cells. The cells were incubated for 3 hrs with $^{45}CaCl_2$ or ^{3}H-myoinositol, layered on columns of acetylated Sephadex G-10 and were perfused with medium containing AA, palmitic acid or vehicle alone. Exposure of the cells to AA at conc of 10-100 uM caused dose-dependent increases in the rate of $^{45}Ca^{++}$ efflux (15.7-100.5%), ^{3}H-myoinositol release (20.6-75.1%) and hPL release (75.4-204.1%) within 10 min of exposure. The rates of release returned to baseline when AA was removed from the medium. In addition, when cells were prelabelled with $^{32}PO_4$ for 12 hrs and then exposed to 50 uM AA, the membrane content of ^{32}P-PI and ^{32}P-phosphatidylserine (as determined by 2D-TLC) decreased by 40.1% and 29.3% respectively within 2 mins, while there were no effects on other phospholipids. Palmitic acid, even at 100 uM, had no effects on calcium efflux, PI turnover or hPL release. Since changes in cellular calcium metabolism and PI turnover are associated with secretion in some endocrine tissues, these results suggest that changes in cellular calcium flux and PI cycle activity mediate the stimulation of hPL release by arachidonic acid. NIH grants HD07447 and GM07171.

2613 PEPTIDE PHI-27 STIMULATES ACTH SECRETION FROM THE RAT ANTERIOR PITUITARY GLAND IN VIVO AND IN VITRO. F.J.H. Tilders*, F. Berkenbosch and I. Vermes, Dept. Pharmacology, Free University, 1007 MC Amsterdam, The Netherlands.

PHI is a 27 aminoacid peptide isolated from porcine intestinal material (1). The presence of PHI immunoreactive nerve terminals in the median eminence and colocalization of PHI and CRF in neurones of the paraventricular nucleus prompted us to study the effect of synthetic PHI-27 on ACTH secretion. Freshly prepared anterior pituitary fragments of rats were superfused in vitro and ACTH was determined in effluent medium samples by radioimmunoassay. Rat Corticotropin Releasing Factor (r-CRF) causes a concentration dependent (0.2-10 nM) increase of basal ACTH secretion (maximum 7-9 fold). PHI-27 is without effect at 0.1-700 nM but stimulates ACTH secretion to 160% at 2000 nM. At concentrations that by itself are ineffective (100-300 nM), PHI-27 strongly potentiates the ACTH releasing effects of rat and ovine CRF. The structurally related peptide VIP shows similar effects. Administration of PHI-27 to chlorpromazine-morphine-nembutal treated rats causes a dose related increase of plasma ACTH level to 250% at 5 /ug/rat i.v. as measured 5 min later but in this in vivo model, the ACTH releasing effects of CRF and PHI-27 appear additive. The present results show that PHI-27 can fascilitate ACTH secretion by a direct action on the pituitary gland. We conclude that PHI-27 may be a factor of physiological significance for the control of pituitary-adrenal activity.

(1) Tatemoto, K. & Mutt, V. PNAS 78 (1981) 6603.

2614 LOCALIZATION CHARACTERIZATION AND BIOLOGICAL ACTION OF CRF IN THE FROG. M.C. Tonon*, A. Burlet[π], M. Lauber[§], P. Cuet, S. Jégou, L. Gouteux and H. Vaudry. Gr. Rech. Endocr. Mol., ERA 891, Lab. Endocrinol. Fac. Sci. Rouen, Mt-St-Aignan, France; [π]Lab. Histol. A, Fac. Méd., Vandoeuvre-les-Nancy, France. [§]Gr. Neurobioch. Cell. Mol., Univ. P. et M. Curie, Paris, France.

The distribution of corticotropin-releasing factor (CRF) in the frog brain was studied by means of a specific radioimmunoassay. High concentrations of CRF-like material were found in both chiasmatic and infundibular regions of the hypothalamus (1.2±0.03 and 1.7±0.1 ng/mg protein, respectively) and in the neurointermediate lobe (NIL) as well (12.5±2.9 ng/mg protein). Standard curves of synthetic CRF and the dilution curves for hypothalamic or NIL extracts were parallel. After Sephadex G-75 gel filtration, CRF-like immunoreactivity eluted in a single peak, in the same position as synthetic ovine CRF. Reversed-phase HPLC separated 5 components with CRF-like immunoreactivity, the major peak having a retention time of 21.8 min (25.4 min for ovine CRF and 36 min for rat CRF). The localization of CRF-containing perikarya was studied in colchicine treated frogs. The great majority of the CRF-positive cell bodies were observed in the ventral region of the preoptic nucleus and were distinct from vasotocin and mesotocin containing cell. A few scattered perikarya were also observed in the dorsal preoptic nucleus and in the retrochiasmatic region. Synthetic CRF stimulated ACTH release by frog distal lobe cells in a dose-dependent manner, but had no effect on α-MSH release by the NIL. The secretion of ACTH was also stimulated by vasopressin (10^{-9} to 10^{-6}M) whereas α-MSH release was not affected. These results indicate that CRF is located in the preoptic region of the frog hypothalamus and stimulates specifically ACTH secretion by the pars distalis.

2615 REDUCED BIOLOGICAL ACTIVITY PATTERN OF TSH IN PATIENTS WITH HYPOTHALAMIC OR PITUITARY TUMOR : INVOLVEMENT OF HYPOTHALAMIC COMPRESSION, DOPAMINE AND TRH DEFICIENCIES. P.Valensi*[1], A.Warnet, E.Lajeunie, M.Duet and J.Lubetzki. Hôpital Lariboisière, Paris and [1]Hôpital Avicenne, Bobigny - FRANCE.

8 patients with a pituitary adenoma extending above the fossa, and 6 patients with a hypothalamic tumor were thought to secrete TSH with reduced biological activity because of a subnormal free thyroxine index (FTI) and a normal TSH response to TRH (iv bolus of 200 µg) evaluated using a L index ($L = \log_{10} [(mTSH-bTSH)/bTSH]$, bTSH and mTSH being the basal and zenithal TSH levels). FTI and L were chosen because they were normally distributed in 30 normal subjects. None of the patients had goiter or antithyroid antibodies. 8 of these patients had functional hyperprolactinemia ; their bTSH was higher than normal (5.12 ± 2.64 - m $\pm$ sem - vs 2.30 ± 0.05, $p<0.01$) with a significant negative linear correlation with FTI ($r = -0.766$, $p<0.05$), as in primary hypothyroidism. A significant positive linear correlation was observed between basal prolactin and either bTSH ($r = 0.889$, $p<0.01$) or mTSH ($r = 0.826$, $p<0.02$). This suggests that dopamine reduction might be involved in sustaining the TSH secretion. Hypothalamic compression present in the 14 patients, was apparently necessary although no sufficient to produce a reduced biological activity pattern of TSH, because this pattern was not found in 28 patients with intrasellar adenoma. Such a hypothalamic involvement could act by reducing TRH secretion. It has been shown (1) that TRH stimulates thyroid secretion directly in vitro. TRH suppresion might reduce thyroid activity. Subsequent hypothyroidism as well as dopamine reduction could then induce a sustained TSH secretion.

(1) ATTALI J.R., VALENSI P., DARNIS D., SEBAOUN J., C.R.Acad.Sc.Paris 1983 III. 386.

2616 **Comparison of GnRH Concentrations in Third Ventricular CSF of Ovariectomized and Intact Monkeys.** **D.A. Van Vugt* and M. Ferin, Department of Obstetrics & Gynecology, Columbia University, New York, NY. 10032.**

We recently reported that gonadotropin releasing hormone (GnRH) is present in third ventricular CSF of ovariectomized monkeys and that it is released in a pulsatile manner. Here, we examine the effects of ovarian steroids on the GnRH oscillator by contrasting GnRH concentrations in third ventricular CSF of ovariectomized monkeys and monkeys in different phases of the menstrual cycle. A stainless steel cannula and inner silastic tubing were stereotactically implanted into the third ventricle of 12 ovariectomized and 8 intact rhesus monkeys. CSF was continuously withdrawn (6h) by an exfusion pump at a rate of 0.4 - 0.5ml/h while animals were seated in primate chairs. Samples were divided into 15 min fractions and assayed for GnRH (R-42). GnRH pulses were found in 24 of 33 CSF collections performed in ovariectomized animals and in 6 of 14 collections in the intact monkeys. Absence of detectable GnRH pulses is probably related to technical problems of collecting CSF, since there are several examples where GnRH pulses were detected in one collection but not in another from the same monkey. During the 24 collections totalling 120h in the ovariectomized group, 64 GnRH pulses occurred and had a mean amplitude of 87 ± 10pg/ml. In contrast, pulse amplitude was reduced in the intact animals, as mean amplitude was 30 ± 10pg/ml (n=11 pulses in 84h). The present results indicate that there is a marked difference in the amplitude of GnRH pulses in CSF of ovariectomized vs intact monkeys. We conclude that this difference is the result of an action of ovarian steroids at the hypothalamic level.

2617 COMPARISON OF LHRH AGONIST AND ANTAGONIST IN THE MALE RAT.

B. H. Vickery*, G.I. McRae, J. Goodpasture and J.J. Nestor Jr, Syntex Research, Palo Alto, California, USA.

Nafarelin acetate, an LHRH agonist 200x more potent than native LHRH, was administered to mature male rats (2µg per day, sc). After two weeks of treatment only marginal decreases in the weights of the testes and accessory organs were seen. After 4 weeks, although the weights were significantly lower than controls and the histology revealed focal inhibition of spermatogenesis and signs of testosterone deprivation, the weight decreases did not exceed 20%. Since studies in prostatic cancer patients, with high doses of LHRH agonists, document abolition of spermatogenesis and marked suppression of prostatic tissue, a higher dose of this agonist, 100µg/rat/day, was tested in the rat. A direct comparison was also made with the highly potent antagonist [N-Ac-D-Nal(2)^1,D-pCl-Phe^2,D-Trp^3, D-hArg(Et$_2$)^6,D-Ala^{10}]LHRH, at the same dose. By two weeks the antagonist reduced testicular weight, intratesticular sperm count and accessory organ weight by >65% in each case, while the agonist caused little change. By 6 weeks both analogs had achieved a high level of suppression of the reproductive tissues, but for each organ the antagonist caused greater suppression. These differences may be due in part to the initial stimulatory effects of LHRH agonists. If extrapolable to man, antagonists may be the agents of choice for both prostatic cancer and the inhibition of spermatogenesis.

2618 GROWTH HORMONE RELEASING FACTOR INFUSION DOES NOT SUSTAIN ELEVATED GH-LEVELS IN NORMAL SUBJECTS.

K. von Werder+, M.Losa, L. Bock, G.K.Stalla and O.A.Müller. Medizinische Klinik Innenstadt University of Munich, 8000 München 2, FRG

Human pancreatic growth hormone releasing factor (hpGRF$^{1-44}$) was infused over 2 respectively 5 hrs in a dosage of 100 µg GRF/hr into 11 healthy subjects. The infusion was started and terminated with a bolus injection of 50 µg GRF. In 5 subjects 200 µg TRH was given 4 hrs after starting the infusion. Four healthy subjects received three times 50 µg GRF (I, II, III) as a bolus every 2 hrs.

GH, PRL, TSH, and GRF immunoreactivity was measured, the latter by specifically developed radioimmunoassay.

50 µg GRF increased GH levels with a maximum at 30 min (24.1 ± 5.1 ng/ml ± SE). However, though GRF was continously infused and serum GRF levels remained elevated GH decreased to a minimum 270 min after start of the infusion (2.0 ± 0.7 ng/ml). The GH response to the second bolus at the end of the infusion was blunted compared to the first response (14.6 ± 3.4 ng/ml after 2 hrs and 7.6 ± 3.6 ng/ml after 5 hrs). TRH did not lead to a GH-increase during GRF infusion, though PRL and TSH rose normally. The intermittent bolus injection of 50 µg GRF leading to comparable endogenous GRF concentrations led to continously decreasing GH responses to the same GRF dosage (I: 16.5 ± 1.6 ng/ml; II: 4.2 ± 0.8 ng/ml; III: 3.4 ± 0.5 ng/ml). These findings show that GRF infusion or bolus injection in short intervals can not sustain elevated GH-levels. Pituitary GH is either not readily available for continous GRF stimulation or GH secretion may be antagonized by increasing somatostatin levels. (Supported by DFG)

2619 PLASMA CORTICOTROPIN (ACTH) AND CORTISOL RESPONSES TO CORTICOTROPIN-RELEASING FACTOR (CRF) IN THE MORNING AND EVENING IN MAN. T. Watabe*, K. Tanaka, M. Hasegawa, T. Horiuchi, K. Nakamura, S. Miyabe, H. Yoshida, T. Kinouchi and N. Shimizu, First Department of Medicine, Teikyo University School of Medicine, Tokyo, 173 Japan.

To evaluate the responsiveness of plasma ACTH and cortisol to CRF in the morning and evening, synthetic ovine CRF (1.0 µg/kg) was administered as an i.v. bolus injection to six normal males aged 25 to 43 yrs, weighing 50 to 80 kg. CRF was given at 900 h and 1700 h after overnight and 4-hour fasts, respectively. Blood samples were obtained before and 15, 30, 60, 90 and 120 min after each CRF injection for determination of plasma ACTH and cortisol levels by radioimmunoassay. The morning and evening experiments were performed at an interval of at least 7 days. Significant increases in ACTH and cortisol levels were observed in all subjects in both morning and evening experiments. The mean increment in the area under the ACTH concentration curve in the morning (74.9 ± 21.9 pg x min/ml) was not significantly different from that in the evening (83.4 ± 20.8 pg x min/ml). However, the increment in the area under the cortisol concentration curve in the evening (76.0 ± 11.1 µg x min/dl) was significantly ($p<0.05$) greater than that in the morning (36.1 ± 7.1 µg x min/dl). The results suggest that there is no significant difference in responsiveness of the pituitary to CRF in the morning and evening, although the response of the adrenal to ACTH in the evening is greater than in the morning.

2620 ANTIBODIES TO GROWTH HORMONE-RELEASING FACTOR (GRF) INHIBIT SOMATIC GROWTH. W.B. Wehrenberg* and B. Bloch. Laboratories for Neuroendocrinology, The Salk Institute, P.O. Box 85800, San Diego, CA 92138.

The primary role of GH in controlling postnatal somatic growth is well documented. Its secretion is in turn controlled by hypothalamic GRF. We have raised antibodies to rat GRF which when administered in vivo cause a complete inhibition of GH release. Using this passive immunization technique, we have evaluated the role of GRF in normal somatic growth. Twenty-two day old male Sprague-Dawley rats (61 ± 2 gm) were treated for 15 days (0.25 ml ip, qd) with either normal rabbit serum (nrs) (n=7) or rabbit antiserum raised against GRF (GRF-ab n=7). During this period the body weight of rats treated with nrs increased 8.3 ± 0.4 gm/day while rats treated with GRF-ab increased 4.3 ± 0.2 gm/day ($p<0.01$). These rats were then left untreated for an additional 22 days to determine whether the GRF-ab treated animals would have a period of catch-up growth. Rats treated with nrs continued to increase in body weight at 8.1 ± 0.4 gm/day. Remarkably, rats treated with GRF-ab continued to have a reduced growth rate, 5.4 ± 0.6 gm/day ($p<0.01$). This reduced growth rate was not due to long term suppression of GH since the patterns of pulsatile secretion and concentrations of plasma GH were not different between the two groups when measured three weeks after termination of the GRF-ab treatment. The inhibition of somatic growth by GRF-ab treatment was expected; however, upon cessation of this treatment we expected a period of accelerated growth. This absence of catch-up growth suggests that there is a critical period during postnatal development when GRF and GH are required for subsequent normal growth and development. Research supported by Andrew W. Mellon Foundation and grants from NIH (AM-18811 and HD-09690).

2621 MORPHOMETRIC AND CYTOCHEMICAL STUDIES OF CRF BINDING AND STIMULATION OF ANTERIOR PITUITARY CELLS.

K.N. Westlund*, G. Aguilera, P. Wynn, and G.V. Childs, Department of Anatomy, Univ. of Texas Med. Br., Galveston, Tx. ERBB, NICHD NIH, Bethesda, Md. USA

Morphological and physiological changes produced by CRF stimulation in vivo were studied in pituitary cell populations immunocytochemically stained for ACTH. Following 48 h ip minipump infusions of CRF, serum ACTH levels increased from control values of 60 ± 5 pg/ml or sham infused values of 74 ± 8.2 pg/ml to 127 ± 14 pg/ml and 145 ± 20 pg/ml with 10 and 50 ng/min CRF respectively. Serum ACTH was 320 ± 27 pg/ml in a separate group of rats adrenalectomized for 48 h. In the CRF infused rats, the percentage of stained ACTH cells detectable in tissue sections was decreased from control values of 8.5% to 5% due to degranulation. The average ACTH cell area was significantly increased in a dose dependent manner from control values of 69 ± 2.4 μm^2 and 60 ± 2.3 μm^2 in intact and sham infused rats to 116 ± 3.6 μm^2 and 132 ± 3.7 μm^2 with 10 and 50 ng/min respectively. The area or percentages after sham infusion of saline did not differ from control values (Duncan's Multiple Range test, $p < 0.01$ for all comparisons). In adrenalectomized rats, the percentage of corticotropes was 5.9%. The cell area was larger than in the CRF infused groups (269 ± 8 μm^2) correlating with the higher ACTH serum levels. The expansion in area probably reflects the lack of negative corticosterone feedback that is present in the CRF infused group and is known to block ACTH release. The present studies thus show dramatic changes in ACTH cell area and percentages following CRF treatment and an excellent correlation between morphological changes and ACTH serum levels. Supported by NIH post-doctoral fellowship to KNW. 1 F 32 NS 07309 01 BNS.

2622 DIMINISHED GROWTH HORMONE RELEASE IN RESPONSE TO HUMAN PANCREATIC GROWTH HORMONE RELEASING FACTOR (hpGRF-44) IN HYPERPROLACTINEMIC WOMEN.

N. Wiedlin, F. Culler*, A. Villanueva, J. Liu, R.W. Rebar and K.L. Jones, Departments of Pediatrics and Reproductive Medicine, University of California, San Diego, and The Whittier Institute, La Jolla, CA.

We have used synthetic hpGRF-44 to compare the growth hormone (GH) and prolactin (PRL) responses of hyperprolactinemic women to those of normal control women. The 6 hyperprolactinemic women had a mean (±SE) age of 30.8± 2.8 years, mean basal (PRL) of 113.1±30.9 ng/ml and bilateral galactorrhea. Three of the patients were amenorrheic and the others were studied between days 3-7 of the menstrual cycle. The control group included 6 regularly menstruating women with mean age 34.6±2.8 years and mean basal PRL of 14.2± 3.0 ng/ml studied between days 3-7. Blood was sampled basally and over a 120 min. span following bolus injection of 100 μg hpGRF-44. The mean maximal ΔGH after hpGRF-44 was 11.0±2.2 ng/ml in the hyperprolactinemic women compared to 33.0±6.8 in the controls ($p<0.05$). The hyperprolactinemic patients had a mean peak of 15.8 ng/ml (range 7.3-25.2) while the mean peak in the normals was 38.2 ng/ml (range 18.4-62.5 ng/ml). Mean PRL levels did not change following hpGRF-44 in either group. The mean basal estradiol levels in the 2 groups were not significantly different. Although the hyperprolactinemic women weighed somewhat more, the difference was not significant and there was no correlation of GH response with weight.

We conclude that women with hyperprolactinemia have a blunted GH response to hpGRF-44. This blunting does not appear to be due to differences in estrogen levels or body weight.

2623 DIFFERENTIAL PITUITARY BINDING AND INTERNALIZATION KINETICS OF [D-Lys^6]GnRH AGONIST AND ANTAGONIST ANALOGS IN VITRO AND IN VIVO. P. C. Wynn, G. V. Childs, C. Suárez-Quian, E. Loumaye, and K. J. Catt. NICHD, NIH, Bethesda, MD., U.S.A. Dept. Anatomy, University of Texas, Galveston, TX, U.S.A.

We have previously shown that the potent antagonist [N-Ac-D-p-Cl-Phe^{1,2},D-Trp^3,D-Lys^6,D-Ala^{10}]GnRH (GnRH antag) exhibits prolonged occupancy of GnRH surface receptors *in vitro*, whereas several studies have shown that the agonist [D-Ala^6] des-Gly^{10} GnRH-N-ethylamide is rapidly internalized (75% at 15 min) in dispersed pituitary cells. Since internalization of the [D-Ala^6] analog could be overestimated if surface-bound ligand is lost during glutaraldehyde fixation, we used [D-Lys^6]GnRH-N-ethylamide for agonist localization by EM-autoradiography and found that only 50% of the specifically bound ligand was internalized after 2 h *in vitro*. During *in vivo* studies, specific uptake of [D-Lys]^6 agonist was maximum at 30 min and had dissipated by 12 h, whereas the binding of [D-Lys^6] antag reached its maximum at 8 h and gradually decreased to 12% by 8 days. EM observation revealed that binding of agonist, but not antagonist, was associated with cell stimulation. The [D-Lys^6] analogs were internalized at different rates: 66% of specifically bound agonist was internalized 15 min after injection, but comparable internalization (60%) of GnRH antag was not observed until 4 h. Morphological analysis using ^{125}I-labelled and gold-conjugated analogs showed that each of the ligands became incorporated into multivesicular bodies or clustered in secondary lysosomes. The prolonged inhibitory effects of GnRH antag are accompanied by very slow cellular processing that is probably more associated with plasma membrane turnover than with hormone-stimulated receptor-mediated endocytosis.

2624 DIURNAL RHYTHM OF HYPOTHALAMO-PITUITARY-THYROID AXIS. J.Yamauchi*, K.Hashimoto, T.Ofuji and J.Takahara, Kobe Ekisaikai Hosp., Chuoku, Kobe, Okayama Univ. Medical School(K.H.,T.O.), Okayama and Kagawa Medical College (J.T.), Takamatsu, Japan.

Studies were performed to determine the specific hypothalamic area controlling the diurnal rhythm of pituitary TSH secretion. Adult male Wistar strain rats were used and divided into 6 groups of 4 to 5 rats. They were maintained under controlled illumination(light on 7:00-19:00) and temperature . The rats were sacrificed by decapitation every four hours from 0:00 and brains were dissected. Twenty-one brain regions including hypothalamin nuclei and areas were punched out and homogenized to determine thyrotropin releasing hormone(TRH) content by RIA. Serum TSH concentrations showed a significant 24-hr rhythm, with maximum level at 8:00(580±100ng/ml) and low concentration at 4:00(228±23). In contrast, pituitary TSH concentration had its peak at 4:00(1.13±0.06mg/mg prot.) and nadir at 0:00(0.85±0.11). The change of TSH in the serum level was paralleled those in this gland with 4 hr lag. Diurnal rhythm of TRH concentration in each portion of hypothalamic and extrahypothalamic areas were examined. In suprachiasmatic nucleus(SCN) and supraoptic nucleus(SON), peak values of TRH were found in 0:00(1.34±0.20 and 1.16±0.13ng/mg prot. respectively) and nadir at 16:00(0.77±0.11 and 0.62±0.05 respectively). These peak values were also 4 hr prior to the TSH value in the pituitary. The median eminence, arcuate nucleus and other brain regions did not show such significant synchronized fluctuations. These results suggest a physiolosical role of TRH in the SCN and SON for the regulation of daily pituitary and serum TSH rhythm.

2625 COMPARATIVE STUDIES ON THE DISTRIBUTION OF CRF (CORTICOTROPIN-RELEASING FACTOR) AND GRF (GROWTH HORMONE-RELEASING FACTOR) IN THE RAT CENTRAL NERVOUS SYSTEM (CNS). N. Yasuda*, G. Hostetter and Y. Yasuda, Division of Endocrinology and Anatomy, Oregon Health Sciences University, Portland, Oregon, 97201, U.S.A.

Structures of rat CRF and GRF have recently been elucidated. We have raised specific rabbit antisera against these peptides and studied their CNS distributions using radioimmunoassays and PAP immunocytochemistry. Various neural tissues were discretely dissected (approx. 0.1 mg wet weight [WW] for the median eminence and 6-20 mg WW for other neural tissues from each rat). Tissues pooled for each neural area from 10 male rats were extracted with 0.1 N-HCl and assayed for CRF and GRF. The CRF and GRF concentrations of the rat median eminence were 84.4 ng/mg WW and 63.0 ng/mg WW respectively. When CRF or GRF concentrations of the median eminence were taken as 100%, the relative concentrations of CRF (GRF) in other areas were; paraventricular nucleus (PVN) 0.42(2.71), medial basal hypothalamus (MBH, ventromedial + arcuate nucleus) 1.1 (0), preoptic area 0.65 (0), septum 0.2 (0.6), caudate nucleus 0.24 (0.67), thalamus 0.1 (0), amygdala 0.18 (0), hippocampus 0.11 (0), cerebral cortex 0.22 (0.21), cerebellum 0.12 (0.56), brain stem 0.15 (0.7), spinal cord 0.17 (1.1). The relative distribution pattern of CRF in this study is generally in good agreement with those previously reported. Despite numerous physiological evidence to indicate the MBH as the GRF center, GRF concentration in MBH was undetectable. Instead the highest concentration of GRF outside the median eminence was found in PVN. Immunocytochemical studies confirmed these findings. This work was supported by NIH grants AM-26896, AM-07331 and MRF 2-2-603-511.

2626 PRESENCE OF GROWTH HORMONE-RELEASING FACTOR (GRF) IN THE RAT EXTRAHYPOTHALAMIC TISSUES. Y. Yasuda* and N. Yasuda, Division of Endocrinology, Oregon Health Sciences University, Portland, Oregon 97201, U.S.A.

We have raised rabbit antisera against the 43-residue rat GRF and developed a specific radioimmunoassay (RIA). The antisera showed no cross-reactivity with hpGRF-44, rat CRF, AVP, TRH or LH-RH. A large hypothalamic block (30 mg wet weight [WW]), posterior pituitary (PP) and cerebral cortex (CC) dissected from each rat were extracted (0.1N-HCl) and the extracts were pooled from 10-20 male rats. Extracts of the hypothalamus (H) and PP both contained high concentrations of GRF which showed RIA displacement curves parallel to that for rat GRF standard. The average GRF concentration in H and PP were 4.1±0.3 ng/mg WW and 3.8±0.4 ng/mg WW respectively. The RIA displacement curves for CC showed two components, one parallel to the rat GRF standard and the other nonparallel. When calculated using the parallel portion, the average GRF concentration of CC was 0.3±0.02 ng/mg WW. Extracts of H and CC were fractionated on Sephadex G-100. H showed a single GRF peak at the elution position of synthetic rat GRF. In contrast approximately 50% of the total GRF of CC was found in the void volume with the remainder coeluting with synthetic rat GRF. In some batches of CC extracts, GRF immunoreactivity was detected also in more retarded fractions which might represent GRF fragment(s). Conclusions: 1) Average concentrations of GRF in the hypothalamus and posterior pituitary are comparable in rats. 2) The 43-residue GRF is the only GRF form in the rat hypothalamus whereas about 50% of the total GRF in the rat cerebral cortex is associated with high molecular weight substance(s). This work was supported by NIH grants AM-26896 and AM-07331.

2627 AN "ULTRASHORT-LOOP" FEEDBACK IN THE CONTROL OF HYPOTHALAMIC LHRH.

M. Zanisi*, E. Messi, L. Martini and M. Motta, Department of Endocrinology, Via A. del Sarto, 21, 20129 Milano, Italy.

An "ultrashort-loop" feedback mechanism has been supposed to be involved in the control of two hypothalamic hormones: 1) the still hypothetical FSH-RF (Hyyppa et al., Neuroendocrinology 7: 221, 1971) and 2) SRIF (Lumpkin et al. Sciences 211: 1072, 1981). In order to test the possible involvement of such a mechanism in the regulation of LHRH, adult male rats, submitted to hypophysectomy and castration have been treated chronically (7 days) with a superactive analogue of LHRH (D-Ser-(tBU)^{6} desGly^{10} -LHRH N-ethylamide, Buserelin). This analogue has been shown in a series of assays performed in our laboratory not to cross-react with the antiserum against LHRH used for RIA-LHRH. At autopsy the brains of experimental and control animals were dissected, the medio-basal region of the hypothalamus homogenized in HCl and the extracts were assayed for their content in LHRH. The results obtained indicate: 1) hypophysectomy performed in addition to castration markedly reduces the hypothalamic LHRH stores; 2) chronic treatment with Buserelin further decreases the content of the hormone when compared to saline-treated controls. Since in the experimental animals both the pituitary and the gonads had been removed, these results point to a direct effect of exogenous LHRH at hypothalamic level. (Supported by the CNR through the Project "Preventive and Rehabilitative Medicine").

2628 GROWTH HORMONE RELEASING FACTOR STIMULATES RELEASE OF STORED POOLS OF GROWTH HORMONE IN NORMAL RAT PITUITARY CELLS IN MONOLAYER CULTURE.

F Zeytin, N Ling, FS Esch, WB Wehrenberg, A Baird, R Guillemin*. The Salk Institute for Biological Studies, La Jolla, CA 92037.

We report here results of studies carried out to ascertain whether GRF stimulates release of newly synthesized or stored pools of GH from rat pituitary cells in monolayer culture. Pituitary monolayer cultures were as described (Brazeau et al, Proc. Natl Acad Sci 79:7909, 1982). Single or double labeling of cells with [^{3}H] or [^{14}C] leucine was carried out in culture medium containing 1/20 of the normal leucine concentration. Effect of GRF on GH release was studied by incubation of cells for 15 min to 24 hr in medium containing excess leucine. GH was measured by RIA using Sinha's anti-murine GH antiserum. The [^{3}H]- or [^{14}C]-labeled GH was quantitated by immunoprecipitation. Identity of the immune precipitate with cold or [^{125}I]-labeled rat GH standards was demonstrated by SDS PAGE. Incorporation of label into cytoplasmic GH is quantitated within 20 min, increases linearly up to 60 min and is maximal at 8-12 hr. In cells labeled continuously for 60 min or in cells in which a 30 or 60 min [^{3}H]-leu pulse is followed by a chase with excess leucine, release of immunoreactive and [^{3}H]-labeled (new pool) occurs within 10-15 min. Following a 30-60 min labeling, incubation of cells with GRF (10^{-12} to 10^{-9} M) for 3-8 hr causes a 4-6 fold stimulation of GH release. There is no difference in the amount of [^{3}H]-labeled new pool of GH release in control vs GRF-treated cells. When double-labeled cells [^{14}C]-leu for 12-18h; [^{3}H]-leu for 30-60 min, are incubated with GRF (10^{-9} M) for 1-4 hr, the GH released into the medium by GRF is the [^{14}C]-leucine labeled old pool. Release of the [^{3}H]-labeled GH in response to GRF is observed 12-24 hr after the pulse. We show for the first time that GRF preferentially stimulates release of stored GH and does not affect the basal, tonic release of newly synthesized GH by pituitary cells. Thus the mechanism of action of GRF is analogous to that of TRF which stimulates release of stored pools of pituitary prolactin.

2629 DEVELOPMENTAL EXPRESSION OF THE RAT SOMATOSTATIN GENE. H.H. Zingg*, R.H. Goodman and Joel F. Habener, Laboratory of Molecular Endocrinology, Massachusetts General Hospital and Howard Hughes Medical Institute, Harvard Medical School, Boston, MA 02114, USA.

Prosomatostatin-derived peptides, including the tetradecapeptide somatostatin, are produced by neural cells as well as endocrine-like cells present in pancreas, stomach and intestine. To investigate the developmental expression of the somatostatin gene, the levels of mRNA encoding somatostatin were determined in rat brain and stomach during fetal and early postnatal development. Tissue levels of somatostatin mRNA were measured using a quantitative radiodensitometric hybridization assay and a cloned rat pre-prosomatostatin cDNA (J Biol Chem 257:1156; 1982). Throughout ontogenesis, a single band of mRNA which hybridized specifically to the rat somatostatin cDNA was detected in both tissues examined. This suggests that the same somatostatin gene is expressed in both tissues, in the developing as well as in the adult rat. In gastric tissues, somatostatin mRNA was undetectable in the fetus, rose gradually after birth and reached, at day 28, a level which corresponded to only ∿50% of the concentration present in the adult. By contrast, brain somatostatin mRNA was already detectable at day 7 of embryonic life and reached concentrations corresponding to the adult brain at embryonic day 20. These marked differences may reflect basic differences in the developmental regulation of somatostatin gene expression in neural vs. non-neural tissues and/or may be related to the onset of functional activity in the organs studied.

2630 PULSATILE SUBCUTANEOUS LHRH TREATMENT OF ANOVULATORY INFERTILITY. G. Skarin*, S. J. Nillius and L. Wide, Departments of Obstetrics and Gynecology and Clinical Chemistry, University Hospital, Uppsala, Sweden.

Long-term pulsatile subcutaneous administration of low doses of LHRH was given to 19 normo-hypogonadotropic, clomiphene-nonresponding women with 2-18 years of amenorrhea. Two of them had hyperprolactinemia (PRL 150 and 270 µg/l, respectively) one of whom had not responded to bromocriptine therapy. The LHRH therapy was given by means of a small, computerized infusion pump (Zyklomat, Ferring GmbH, Kiel, FRG) which was connected to an indwelling subcutaneous catheter in the lower abdominal wall. The catheter was changed approximately once every month. The women were mostly treated with 20 µg LHRH once every 90 min. Some received 1 or 5 µg/90 min. The treatment was given until menstruation or pregnancy occurred.

Fourtysix ovulatory menstrual cycles were induced in 15 out of the 17 normoprolactinemic women. The two hyperprolactinemic women responded with follicular maturation and ovulation during the LHRH therapy and nine ovulatory menstrual cycles were induced, one of which was conceptual. In all twelve pregnancies occurred. Five term pregnancies resulted in six healthy children (4 single, 1 duplex). Four pregnancies are developing normally. Three women had early spontaneous abortions. The subcutaneous pulsatile LHRH therapy was safe and well accepted. The only side-effect was a subcutaneous infection.

Thus, pulsatile subcutaneous low dose LHRH therapy is a very promising alternative to human gonadotropin therapy of anovulatory infertility.

2631 AN ATTEMPT AT ESTABLISHING INDICATIONS FOR BROMOCRIPTINE TREATMENT IN INFERTILITY. U.Stopińska, B.Baranowska* and G.Rozbicka, Endocrinology Clinic, Cegłowska 80, 01-809 Warsaw, Poland

The aim of the study was to evaluate the indications and the results of bromocriptine treatment in some forms of infertility in women and men. The material consisted of 48 women /21- with "functional" amenorrhoea-galactorrhoea syndrome, 17 women with PCO syndrome and 13 men with idiopathic oligozoospermia/. Serum prolactin /Prl/ was estimated before and after metoclopramide /MCP/. Serum LH and FSH was measured before and after LH-RH /Relisorm-Serono/ stimulation. Basic serum Prl concentrations increased only in 10 out of 21 patients with "functional" amenorrhoea-galactorrhoea syndrome, in 2 out of 17 with PCO syndrome and in no patient with oligozoospermia. However, an enhanced response of Prl to MCP in the majority of patients was observed. Bromocriptine /Parlodel-Sandoz/ was administered in a dose of 5.0-7.0 mg daily from 6 months to 2 years. After treatment galactorrhoea disappeared and normal menstruations were restored in all women. Ten out of 19 infertile women and 6 out of 13 wives of sterile men became pregnant. The normalization of Prl release and the increase in frequency and amplitude of LH pulsatility was observed. In conclusion: the estimation of Prl release in response to dopaminoergic receptors blockade is important in determining indications to bromocriptine treatment in patients with infertility.

2632 INDUCTION OF OVULATION - RISK FACTORS. Z M van der Spuy*, P J Steer, M McCusker, S J Steele and H S Jacobs, Middlesex Hospital Medical School and St Mary's Hospital Medical School, London, United Kingdom

Since the commonest cause of amenorrhoea with infertility is subnormal body weight, and many underweight women have induction of ovulation, we have studied pregnancy outcome in 2 groups of women. The first group consisted of 1212 women with spontaneous singleton pregnancies who booked for antenatal care before 16 weeks gestation and who had a booking ponderal index (PI = $\frac{wt(kg)}{ht^2(m)}$) of 25.1 or less. Women were classified "underweight" if their PI was < 19.1 and "normal weight" with a PI 19.1 -25.1. Women with a low PI had more low birthweight infants ($p < 0.005$) and more preterm deliveries ($p < 0.01$) than women with normal PI. The differences could not be explained by differences in social class or pregnancy weight gain. The second group comprised 25 women having induction of ovulation with human menopausal gonadotrophin. - 40% of them had PI < 19.1 compared with 15.3% in the general population ($p < 0.001$) and they had more low birthweight infants ($p < 0.001$). In the induction group there was a trend for underweight women to have more low birthweight babies than the normal weight women. We conclude that preconception nutritional status is related to pregnancy outcome in women with spontaneous and induced ovulation. It is therefore preferable that underweight women with amenorrhoea should be treated nutritionally rather than with hormonal therapy.

2633 "SLOW PULSING OLIGOSPERMIA" - HYPOTHALAMIC MALFUNCTION AS A POSSIBLE CAUSE OF MALE INFERTILITY. T.O.F. Wagner*, G. Brabant, F. Warsch, G. Daehne, C. Dette, and A. von zur Mühlen. Dept. Clinical Endocrinology, Medizinische Hochschule Hannover, D-3000 Hannover, West Germany.

A decreased LHRH pulse frequency was shown to result in normal LH but elevated FSH levels in hypothalamic lesioned animals. We, therefore, studied the 24-hour secretory pattern of gonadotropins in five patients with severe oligospermia having normal LH and testosterone but elevated FSH levels (group I) under basal conditions and during six months of pulsatile LHRH therapy (Zyklomat, Ferring, West Germany). As control three patients with normogonadotropic oligospermia (group II) and 12 normal male volunteers (group III, basal conditions only) were included in the study. Three different methods of pulse frequency analysis were employed: visual examination, "Cycle Detector" (Clifton and Steiner), and "Pulsar" (Merriam and Waechter). In group I the basal LH pulse frequency was significantly reduced as compared to the other groups. During LHRH therapy LH pulses were synchronized (12 pulses/24 hours) in all patients. A dramatic decrease in FSH levels was observed in group I as early as four weeks after the start of treatment while improved sperm counts (+80 to +300%) were only reached after four months. Even after six months, though, normal FSH values were not reached. No changes in FSH levels were observed in the other patients. In conclusion it is tempting to speculate that "slow pulsing oligospermia" is a pathophysiologic entity due to a hypothalamic defect easily overcome by pulsatile LHRH treatment, once dosage and time interval have been optimized. Supported by Ferring, West Germany

2634 LEYDIG CELL DENSITY AND ITS RELATION TO GONADOTROPINS AND TESTOSTERONE IN INFERTILE MEN. D. B. Weiss*, Shaare Zedek Medical Center, Jerusalem 91002, Israel.

Testicular Leydig cell density, circulating levels of gonadotropins (FSH and LH) and testosterone (T) were correlated in 35 infertile azoospermic or severely oligospermic (sperm count below 4.2 million per ml) patients in whom neither varicocele nor epididymal or vas deferens pathology could be detected. Leydig cell density was evaluated quantitatively in bilateral testicular biopsies of each patient and expressed as Leydig cell clusters per seminiferous tubule. In this group of patients, no significant correlations were found between Leydig cell density and T, LH, T to LH ratio or FSH. However, when these patients were subdivided, Leydig cell density was negatively correlated, in the azoospermic group of patients, with T, T to LH ratio, positively to FSH and unrelated to LH levels. In the oligospermic patients, Leydig cell density was positively correlated with T, T to LH ratio and negatively to LH and FSH. Sperm motility, but not count, correlated with Leydig cell density. These findings suggest that two mechanisms involving Leydig cell function are responsible for the infertility in these patients.

2635 INDUCTION OF TYPE 1 DIABETES BY GLUCOSE LOAD IN THE NONOBESE DIABETIC (NOD) MOUSE ACCOMPANIED WITH SPONTANEOUS INSULITIS. K. Yamada*, A. Miyazaki, T. Hanafusa, J. Miyagawa, H. Nakajima, K. Nonaka, and S. Tarui, The Second Department of Internal Medicine, Osaka University Medical School, Japan.

Strict blood glucose regulation by insulin proved to be required at the early stage of type 1 diabetes to promote a remission and to protect islet cells from further degeneration. But unlike type 2 diabetes, it is still obscure whether type 1 diabetes can be induced by excess uptake of carbohydrates. We studied the effect of intraperitoneal glucose load on the onset of type 1 diabetes using the NOD mouse, an animal model for type 1 diabetes. In female NOD mice insulitis can generally be observed from the age of 5 weeks; overt diabetes occurs abruptly from around the age of 15 weeks. We injected glucose intraperitoneally into 70 aglycosuric 14-week old female NOD mice at a dose of 1 mg/g wt in 10% aqueous solution. Persistent glycosuria began to occur in 10 (14%) of the mice on the next day. Plasma glucose patterns just after the loading were not so markedly different between the diabetes-induced group and the non diabetes-induced group except a significantly high level at 60 min in the former (249 ± 163 vs 183 ± 50 mg/dl, mean ± SD). The same tests were repeated three times in aglycosuric mice at the age of 27, 34, and 44 weeks. Incidence of persistent glycosuria on the next day of the load was 11%, 22%, and 21%, respectively. These rates were markedly high comparing with the mean incidence of diabetes per day (0.7%) throughout the period of 34 weeks during which 56 mice became diabetic and 3 mice died without glycosuria. This result suggests excess uptake or load of carbohydrate could induce type 1 diabetes in the presence of insulitis.

2636 THE ENHANCING EFFECT OF CLOFIBRATE ON INSULIN SENSITIVITY IN THE PERIPHERAL TISSUES. H. YASHIRO*, T. IRIE, K. TAKEBE, THE THIRD DEPARTMENT OF INTERNAL MEDICINE, HIROSKI UNIVERSITY SCHOOL OF MEDICINE, HIROSAKI, JAPAN.

In addition to the hypolipidemic action of clofibrate,there are many reports that the drug improves glucose intolerance in diabetic patients. But the mechanism of lowering blood glucose concentration is unclear. The purpose of this study is to investigate whether clofibrate mediates the enhanced sensitivity to insulin in the peripheral tissues. Male rats of the Wisar strain,weighing 260-280g,were given an intraperitoneal injection of 300 mg clofibrate per Kg body weight daily for 8 days. The right hindquarters of rats were perfused by the procedure described by Ruderman et al with minor modifications. After equilibration with KRB buffer containing 0.5% BSA and 10 mM glucose, the perfusate was replaced by the buffer containing 20 ng/ml porcine insulin for 20 min,followed by the buffer without insulin for 20 min. Immediately after insulin infusion,the glucose concentration of the outflow perfusate in the clofibrate-treated and the control groups gradually lowered,and 14 min after insulin infusion,its decline was steeper in the clofibrate than in the control. Glucose concentration of the outflow perfusate after interuption of insulin infusion remained lower in the clofibrate than in the control. The following results,glucose uptake(pmol/min/g muscle),were obtained:

	preperfusion	insulin infusion 0 - 9 min	insulin infusion 10 - 19 min	postperfusion
Clofibrate	62.6 ± 10.6	104.4 ± 6.9	190.5 ± 6.6*	252.7 ± 11.6**
Control	68.8 ± 14.7	100.0 ± 8.2	161.8 ± 11.0	220.8 ± 9.3

Values are mean ± s.e.. *; $p<0.05$, **; $p<0.10$

These results suggest that clofibrate enhances the glucose uptake action of insulin in the peripheral tissues.

2637 EFFECT OF 2-DEOXYGLUCOSE AND ITS ANALOGUES ON MAINTENANCE IN CULTURE OF NEONATAL B CELLS OF RAT.

K. Yoshida,* S. Kagawa, K. Nakao, S. Wakabayashi, N. Tanaka, K. Murakoso and A. Matsuoka, Clinical Laboratory, Hyogo College of Medicine, 1-1 Mukogawa, Nishinomiya, 663 Japan.

The effect of 2-deoxyglucose, 2-deoxy-2-fluoroglucose and 3-amino-3-deoxyglucose on maintenance in culture of B cells of the neonatal rat was examined. Culturing of monolayer islet cells in basal medium with 5.5mM glucose alone for 7 days underwent a remarkable drop of insulin in cells and medium. By contrast, the medium supplemented with 1mM 2-deoxyglucose or its analogues maintained insulin content in cells and medium and the capacity of 16.7mM glucose-induced insulin release and biosynthesis in B cells at levels several times higher than at culture day 0. Also, insulin release evoked by 10mM leucine and 2-ketoisocaprorate was enhanced 3-4 fold over the initial levels. Moreover, the addition of the sugars allowed a selective survival of endocrine cells, and prevented the deterioration of islet cells in basal medium. In these cells, glucose showed a significant increase in cAMP response. In conclusion, these results suggest an increased oxidative catabolism of medium nutrients in B cells grown in the media containing glycolytic inhibitors, and the present culture systems provide a useful tool for the functional and morphological studies of B cells in culture.

2638 INSULIN SENSITIVITY AS ASSESSED BY THE GLUCOSE CLAMP TECHNIQUE IN ANOREXIA NERVOSA.

S. Zuniga-Guajardo*, P. Garfinkel and B. Zinman, Dept. of Medicine and Psychiatry, University of Toronto, Toronto, Ontario, M5G 1L7, Canada.

Anorexia nervosa (AN) is a state of self-induced malnutrition resulting in altered insulin binding to erythrocytes and monocytes. To measure insulin sensitivity in AN we performed euglycemic insulin clamp studies (1mU/kg/min) in 7 females with clinical anorexia nervosa (age 26.1±2.3 yr and 74.7±4.2% ideal body wt (IBW) as compared to 7 normal control (NC) females (age 23.6±1.0 yr and 92.7±2.6% IBW). Fasting plasma glucose and immunoreactive insulin (IRI) were significantly lower in AN as compared to NC (82.8±2.6 vs 91.4±1.6 mg/dl and 8.8±1.5 vs 13.5±1.4 uU/ml, $p<0.05$). Plasma glucose concentration was kept constant during the 2h insulin infusion and glucose uptake (M), metabolic clearance of glucose (MCR_G), IRI, and the metabolic clearance of insulin (MCR_I) were measured during the last h. M and MCR_G were increased in AN as compared to NC (9.47±1.5 vs 6.93±0.6 mg/kg/min and 11.0±1.8 vs 7.4±0.6 ml/kg/minx100) but these differences were not statistically significant because of large individual variations. Interestingly IRI concentrations were lower in AN (92.4±9.6 vs 137.3±5.8 uU/ml, $p<0.005$) despite similar infusion rates. This appears to be related to increased MCR_I in AN (15.6±1.9 vs 9.04±0.5 ml/kg/min, $p<0.01$). Insulin sensitivity as assessed by the M/IRI ratio (glucose metabolized per unit insulin) was significantly elevated in AN (11.5±2.9 vs 5.0±0.3, $p<0.05$). In summary anorexia nervosa is associated with both increased insulin sensitivity and metabolic clearance of insulin. This later effect may be important in protecting against severe hypoglycemia with malnutrition.

2639 SPECIFIC BINDING OF GH_3 CELL NON-HISTONE CHROMATIN PROTEINS TO CLONED PROLACTIN (PRL) GENOMIC DNA. Bruce A. White*[1], Thomas Lufkin[2] and F. Carter Bancroft[2], Dept. of Anatomy, U. Conn. Health Center, Farmington, CT[1] 06032 and Molecular Biology and Virology Dept., Sloan-kettering Inst., New York, NY[2] 10021, U.S.A.

Since non-histone chromatin proteins are likely to be important components of mechanisms by which the expression of the PRL gene is regulated, we have begun searching for nuclear proteins which bind preferentially to or near the PRL gene. We have adapted procedures for probing protein (Western) blots of chromatin proteins with ^{32}P-labeled cloned PRL genomic DNA. Using the clone pl.21, which contains 3 kilobase pairs (kbp) of the 5' end of the PRL gene and 8 kbp of 5' flanking DNA in the vector pUC9, we have detected two major binding proteins with M_r 44 kDal and 48 kDal that reside in the 0.2M - 0.4M NaCl chromatin extract fraction. These two nuclear proteins (termed NP44 and NP48) preferentially bind pl.21 over wild type pUC9 or a prolactin cDNA in pBR322. No binding activity is detected in chromatin proteins from rat liver or rat osteosarcoma cells. Binding activity is similar in fractions obtained from hormonally-induced and hormonally-withdrawn GH_3 cells, and from GC cells, a subclone of GH_3 cells which produce little or no PRL. Western blots from 2-dimensional gels indicate multiple isoelectric variants of both NP44 and NP48, with isoelectric points in the range of 6.2 - 7.2. Thus, we have detected two proteins that bind to or near the PRL gene preferentially and are cell type-specific. Binding activity is not related to the level of PRL gene expression in cells that have a potentially-active PRL gene, but presence of isoelectric variants suggest covalent modifications of NP44 and NP48 which may be related to changes in PRL gene expression.

2640 RAPID INHIBITION OF ACTH SECRETION *IN VITRO*. E. P. Widmaier* and M. F. Dallman. Dept. Physiology, University of California, San Francisco, CA 94143 USA.

We have shown that glucocorticoids inhibit within 20 min CRF-stimulatedACTH release from rat anterior pituitaries perifused *in vitro*. The inhibition was not blocked by pretreatment with cycloheximide. To further elucidate the mechanism of this inhibition, rat pituitaries were perifused with a modified KREBS buffer for a 30 min baseline period followed by a 30 min period with added test substances. Co-addition of 2nM CRF and 10^{-7}M corticosterone, cortisol, or dexamethasone, but not cortisone, produced significantly less secretion over 30 min than that caused by CRF alone. The 2-3 fold increase in ACTH secretion induced by 2nM CRF was also significantly blunted within 20 min when Ca^{++} was removed from the medium. We considered interference of Ca^{++} entry as a possible mechanism of steroid action. Recent evidence suggests that vasopressin (VP) does not increase cAMP levels in corticotrophs, but may require Ca^{++} as a second messenger. In our experiments, VP stimulated ACTH release with an $ED_{50} \approx 10nM$. Co-perifusion with 10^{-7}M corticosterone, however, did not inhibit the effect of VP at any dose tested. Of all ACTH-releasing substances examined, only CRF is known to increase cellular levels of cAMP. We found that corticosterone did not inhibit stimulation of ACTH induced by 5mM 8-Br-cAMP. Further, there was no effect of corticosterone on pituitary content of ACTH either when given alone or with CRF. Thus, the independence of protein synthesis, lack of effect on ACTH synthesis, selectivity for CRF and not VP, and failure to block 8-Br-cAMP-induced release suggests that rapid steroid inhibition of stimulated ACTH release *in vitro* may occur by directly interfering with the generation of cAMP induced by CRF. Supported by AM28172.

2641 ESTROGEN CONTROL OF SECRETORY COMPONENT IN THE RAT UTERUS: EVIDENCE FOR THE INVOLVEMENT OF RNA SYNTHESIS. C.R. Wira*and J.E. Stern, Department of Physiology, Dartmouth Medical School, Hanover, NH, USA.

Secretory component (SC) plays a central role in immune protection by regulating the movement of IgA into external secretions. Previous studies from our laboratory have shown that SC is under hormonal control (Wira et al. Ann. N.Y. Acad. Sci. 49:534, 1983). Following estradiol (E_2) administration to ovariectomized rats, SC increases in uterine luminal secretions. Enhanced SC production is also observed when uterine segments from E_2-treated rats are incubated in vitro. The purpose of the present study was to determine whether RNA synthesis is involved in the increase in SC production in response to E_2. Uterine segments from E_2-treated rats (1 μg/day for 3 days) were perfused with saline and incubated at 37° in RPMI-1640. SC in media was measured by an RIA which recognizes primarily free SC. Uteri from E_2-treated rats released 2.3±0.22 μg SC/ml/24 hrs whereas saline controls released 0.04±0.01 μg. In the presence of actinomycin D (20 μg/ml), an inhibitor of RNA synthesis, SC release by uteri from E_2-treated animals was reduced to 0.75±0.06 μg. Accumulation of SC in media of uteri from E_2-treated rats was also blocked by α-amanitin (0.02 μg/ml), which is known to inhibit Type II polymerase from catalyzing the synthesis of mRNA. These results indicate that E_2-stimulated SC production in the presence of RNA inhibitors is markedly reduced and suggests that E_2 regulation of uterine SC is mediated through the stimulation of uterine mRNA synthesis. This study was supported by AI-13541 from NIH.

2642 STIMULATION OF PYRUVATE DEHYDROGENASE ACTIVITY IN INTACT RAT ADIPOCYTES BY INSULIN MEDIATOR FROM RAT SKELETAL MUSCLE. E. H. A. Wong*, L. Jarett, S. L. Macaulay and J. Smith, University of Pennsylvania School of Medicine, Philadelphia, PA USA

This study investigates the effects on adipocyte pyruvate dehydrogenase (PDH) of insulin mediator partially purified from skeletal muscle of control (CM) and insulin-treated (IM) rats. CM and IM stimulated PDH activity of isolated mitochondria by three-fold and five-fold, respectively, at a 1/20 dilution. CM or IM stimulated mitochondrial PDH activity of intact adipocytes in a linear manner up to a 1/10 final dilution, with IM having a four-fold effect, twice that of CM. These findings indicate that the mediator preparations contained PDH stimulating mediator which can penetrate the plasma membrane of the adipocyte and the outer membrane of the intact mitochondria. CM and IM at a 1/20 dilution caused peak stimulation of adipocyte PDH activity after 10 minutes of incubation with adipocytes. A rapid decline in PDH activity occurred thereafter, with the stimulation by CM falling faster than the stimulation by IM, suggesting degradation of mediator by the adipocytes. On the other hand, a two-fold peak stimulation of PDH reached after 10 minutes of insulin treatment of adipocytes was sustained for at least 40 minutes, indicating that insulin caused a limited but continual production of mediator. The stimulatory effect of CM or IM on adipocyte PDH was additive to that of insulin. This study further substantiates the physiological relevance of this putative insulin second messenger. Supported by NIH, Reynolds Foundation, J.D.F. and Am. Assoc. Univ. Women.

2643 THE TERNARY COMPLEX MODEL: PROPERTIES AND APPLICATION TO THE PITUITARY DOPAMINE RECEPTOR.

K.A. Wreggett* and A. De Léan, Institut de Recherches Cliniques de Montréal, Montréal, Québec, H2W 1R7, Canada.

Common properties of receptor systems involved in the regulation of adenylate cyclase activity appear to be complex agonist/radiolabeled antagonist competition data and an allosteric effect of guanine nucleotides on agonist binding. The majority of ligand binding data can be adequately accounted for by proposing that the receptor(R) interacts reversibly with another membrane component which binds guanine nucleotides(N). This ternary complex model, which we originally applied to the stimulatory β-adrenergic receptor, has only been presumed by analogy with this system, in studies of another receptor systems. Interestingly, there are distinct differences in the binding properties of the β-adrenergic receptor and those of the inhibitory D_2-dopamine receptor. By extensive simulations of the properties of the ternary complex model, several experimentally testable properties of this model were recognized; the relevance of this model was also strengthened by its successful application to the D_2-dopamine receptor. However, some predictions of the model are contradicted by experimental data, namely the existence of residual high-affinity agonist binding in the presence of excess guanine nucleotide and the apparent insensitivity of R-N interaction to receptor alkylation by specific dopamine receptor alkylators. An extension of the model to explicity incorporate the characteristics of N might provide a more definitive description of receptor systems regulated by guanine nucleotides.

2644 THERMIC EFFECT OF ORAL GLUCOSE AND FRUCTOSE IN LEAN HUMAN SUBJECTS.

L. Tappy*, JP. Randin, RA. DeFronzo, E. Jéquier, JP. Felber. Divisions d'Endocrinologie et Biochimie Clinique et de Physiologie Clinique, CHUV, 1011 Lausanne, Switzerland.

Since it has been suggested that insulin is required for diet-induced thermogenesis, we have studied the effect of the non-insulin releasing sugar fructose on energy expenditure. The rates of carbohydrate and lipid oxidation and the total energy expenditure were measured in the fasting state and during the 4 hours following the ingestion of 75 g of either glucose or fructose in 9 lean subjects (age 28 $\pm$ 3 yr, body weight 61 $\pm$ 3 kg) by means of indirect calorimetry. The mean increase in plasma insulin concentration over 4 hr was markedly inferior after fructose than after glucose ingestion (8.3 $\pm$ 1.7 vs 32.9 $\pm$ 4.0 µU/ml, $p < 0.001$). The thermic effect of the load, expressed as the mean percent increase in resting metabolic rate over 4 hr, was more important after fructose than after glucose ingestion (11.2 $\pm$ 0.9 vs 7.4 $\pm$ 1.3 %, $p < 0.05$) ; the increase in carbohydrate oxidation and the decrease in lipid oxidation over 4 hr occurred faster and were greater after fructose than after glucose ingestion (396 $\pm$ 30 vs 307 $\pm$ 1.3 and 144 $\pm$ 12 vs 106 $\pm$ 19 mg/kg body weight respectively, $p < 0.05$ in both cases). Net de novo lipogenesis, as shown by respiratory quotients > 1.0 occurred in 6 out of the 9 subjects at some time following the fructose ingestion. These results show that carbohydrate-induced thermogenesis is not dependent on insulin. They suggest that it might be related to stimulation of carbohydrate metabolism or, in the case of fructose, to the energetic cost of conversion to fat.

2645 LONG TERM REVERSAL OF LIPID RISK FACTORS BY SURGICAL INTERVENTION IN OBESITY. K. Tassie, M. Hooper*, and D. Thomas. Royal Adelaide Hospital and Institute of Medical and Veterinary Science, Adelaide, Australia.

Since the increased mortality from vascular disease in the morbidly obese is presumably reversed by correction of lipid risk factors we have studied patients in long term follow up of Roux-en-Y gastric bypass surgery to establish that the improvement in lipid abnormalities shown earlier, is maintained. Fasting blood levels of total triglyceride (TG), total cholesterol (C), high density lipoprotein cholesterol (HDL-C) and low density lipoprotein cholesterol (LDL-C) were measured in 32 patients, 3-5 years after surgery and in 29 control obese patients similar in age, sex and pre-operative weight [mean preoperative weight, index population 110 ± 16 (SD)kg, control population 115 ± 19 (SD)kg].

GROUP:	WEIGHT kg M±SD	TG mmol/l M±SD	C mmol/l M±SD	HDL-C mmol/l M±SD	LDL-C mmol/l M±SD
CONTROL:	115±19	1.94±0.89	5.30±0.78	1.12±0.23	3.37±0.86
SURGICAL:	88±18	1.42±0.86	5.05±0.82	1.60±0.45	2.83±0.72
SIGNIFICANCE:	$p < 0.01$	$p < 0.05$	NS	$p < 0.01$	$p < 0.01$

This study shows significant differences in lipid risk factors and presumed decreased atherogenicity and lends support to the justification of surgical intervention in obesity. These results must be validated by further long term studies showing a reduced incidence of coronary heart and cerebrovascular disease.

2646 MICROSCOPIC STUDY OF EMBRYONARY AND EARLY POSTNATAL DEVELOPMENT OF BROWN ADIPOSE TISSUE AND ONSET OF ITS THERMOGENIC CAPACITY. M. Tolszczuk*, M. Cadrin, and L. Bukowiecki. Laval University, Med. Sch., Dept. Physiol., and Laboratory of Physical Activity Sciences, Québec, G1K 7P4, Canada.

It is well established that the uncoupling protein (thermogenin) is responsible for the high capacity of brown adipose tissue mitochondria for thermogenesis. The presence of this protein was sought in the embryo and newborn rat. Using the peroxidase-antiperoxidase immunohistochemical method, the protein was localized in the embryo's brown adipose mitochondria as early as the 18th day of gestation. Up to now, no biochemical method has allowed the detection of such small quantity of protein. At this stage of differentiation, the labelled cells did not seem to contain lipid droplets. At birth, most cells were labelled and many of them, while still very small, started to be filled with lipids. Three days after birth, both cell size and lipid content had increased significantly. Concurrently, the labelling appeared to be less uniform than at birth and unilocular fat cells were observed. In conclusion, the transition from homogenous to heterogenous labelling between the first and the third day after birth suggests that brown adipocytes gradually lose their thermogenic activity by differentiating into white adipocytes. This study was supported by the MRC and the LABSAP.

2647 HIGH DENSITY LIPOPROTEINS (HDL)2 AND HDL3 METABOLISM IN HYPERTHYROIDISM.

C. Valentin*, L. Richard, L. Perrot, F. Berthezène. Hôpital Antiquaille, INSERM U 197; Lab. Biochimie Médicale, Faculté A. Carrel, Lyon, France.

Hepatic triglyceride lipase has been directly implicated in HDL2 to HDL3 transformation. Since thyroid hormones modulate this enzyme activity, hyperthyroidism is a good model to study HDL metabolism. Six women and five men have been studied in hyperthyroid (period I) and euthyroid(period II) states. Apoplipoprotein AI and AII (apo AI, apo AII) were measured by RIA, HDL2 and HDL3 were separated by polyacrylamide gel electrophoresis with continuous gradient. Post heparin lipasic activity (PHLA) was determined using a highly sensitive radioenzymatic assay (hepatic triglyceride lipase + lipoprotein lipase).

	apo AI (mg/dl)	apo AII (mg/dl)	HDL2/HDL3	PHLA (pm/s/ml)
Period I	93.2 ± 4.2	21.1 ± 1	0.36 ± 0.1	46.2 ± 1.7
Period II	107.9 ± 5.9	19.3 ± 1	0.76 ± 0.2	42.6 ± 2.8
mean ± SEM	$p < 0.05$	NS	$p < 0.01$	$p < 0.05$

Thus, hyperthyroidism induces a decrease in apo AI and HDL2/HDL3 and an increase in PHLA. PHLA values were negatively correlated with apo AI ($r = -0.53$; $p < 0.02$) and HDL2/HDL3 values ($r = -0.63$; $p < 0.01$). In addition, an inverse correlation was found between PHLA variations and HDL2/HDL3 variations ($r = -0.69$; $p < 0.05$). Therefore the present data support the hypothesis of an hepatic triglyceride lipase action on HDL2 to HDL3 transformation.

2648 TRANSPORT ASSOCIATED PHOSPHORYLATION OF GLUCOSE IN RAT ADIPOCYTES.

Tj. Wieringa, M.P. Bos and H.M.J. Krans*, Laboratory for Diabetes Research, University Hospital, 2333 AA Leiden, The Netherlands.

Adipocytes of epididymal fat pads of the rat possess an insulin-sensitive glucose transport system. It is generally accepted that the uptake process of glucose occurs through facilitated diffusion. However, when glucose is incubated with pure membrane vesicles (established by electronmicroscope and biochemical methods) and ATP we found that the glucose was phosphorylated at the level of the plasma membrane. Transport and phosphorylation are inhibited by specific transport inhibitors like cytochalasin B and phlorizin. Phosphorylation of glucose is stimulated by Mg^{2+} (maximum at 6 mM) and is inhibited by Ca^{2+} (upto 30%). The phosphorylation is pH-dependent, with an optimum at pH 8.2. The glucose analogue 2-deoxyglucose inhibits transport and phosphorylation competatively in contrast to 3-O-methylglucose, which has no effect. Phosphorylation is markedly inhibited by glucose-6-phosphate but not by 2-deoxyglucose-6-phosphate, suggesting the involvement of a hexokinase. Treatment of the membranes with NaOH or NaI was without effect, implicating that the phosphorylation occurs by an integral membrane protein. The present data demonstrate that besides facilitated diffusion processes, transport-associated-phosphorylation mechanism plays a role in glucose uptake.

(Abstract 2774, p. 1647, also belongs to this section.)

2649 DOPA AND DOPAMINE METABOLISM BY ISOLATED PERFUSED RAT KIDNEY. H.Suzuki*, H. Nakane, M.Kawamura, M.Yoshizawa, E.Takeshita, T.Uchida, and T. Saruta. Dpt of Internal Med. and Dpt of Laboratory Med., Keio University Hospital, Tokyo, and Dpt of Internal Med., Urawa City Hospital, Urawa, Japan.

The renal metabolism and handling of DOPA and dopamine (DA) were studied using isolated perfused rat kidney to elucidate the source of urinary DA. The right kidney of male Wistar rats was isolated and perfused in vitro. DOPA added to the synthetic perfusate was rapidly metabolized, and a significant amount of urinary DA excretion was observed, whereas DOPA was hardly detected in the urine. When the perfusate DOPA concentration was comparable with the plasma DOPA concentration in normal rats(0.5-1.5 ng/ml), urinary DA excretion was comparable with physiological values(50-100 ng/ml). Carbidopa, a DOPA decarboxylase inhibitor, added to the perfusate markedly reduced the urinary DA excretion. When the physiological concentration of plasma DA (50-100 pg/ml) was added to the medium, the perfusate DA rapidly decreased and urinary DA excretion was much less than that seen in normal rats. In studies using nonfiltering kidneys, a marked decrease of DOPA and slight increase of DA in the perfusate were observed. It is suggested that the process of glomerular filtration and tubular reuptake of DOPA is not essential for the renal DA formation. In the experiments of DOPA metabolism by perfused kidney of sodium restricted and sodium loaded rats, there was no difference in urinary DA excretion and metabolic clearance rate of DOPA between two groups. It is suggested that the changes in the activity of DOPA decarboxylase may not contribute ot the difference of urinary DA excretion observed between sodium restricted and sodium loaded rats in vivo. These data indicate that urinary free DA is derived mainly from DOPA, which is converted by DOPA decarboxylase in the kidney.

2650 IMPAIRMENT OF THE ADRENOCORTICOTROPIC FUNCTION BY A SELECTIVE NORADRENERGIC INNERVATION OF THE HYPOTHALAMUS IN THE RAT. A. Szafarczyk*, G. Alonso, G. Ixart, F. Malaval and I. Assenmacher, Lab. Neuroendocrinology,ERA 85 CNRS, University of Montpellier II, France.

The effects of various suppressive procedures of the noradrenergic (NA) innervation of the hypothalamus on the diurnal fluctuations of plasma ACTH and corticosterone (C) was explored in individual chronically cannulated female rats. After a single injection of 300 µg/kg 6-OHDA into the 3rd ventricle, or three successive injections of 150 µg/kg 6-OHDA into the lateral ventricle, or bilateral electrolytical lesions of the locus coeruleus (LC), which all led to a dramatic decrease -checked by histofluorescence- of the NA innervation of the arcuate nucleus, the anterior hypothalamic area and of the sole periventricular area of the paraventricular nuclei (PVN), the adrenocorticotropic function (AC) was unaffected. On the other hand,bilateral injections of 6-OHDA (3,5 µg) into the lateral part of the medial forebrain bundle, which suppressed all the NA fibers from the LC but also from the central medullary A1 group and from the dorsal vagal complex (A2),and led to a total NA denervation of the PVN and the supraoptic nuclei,plus a 85 % drop in the hypothalamic NA content, as measured by HPLC, split the circadian rhythms of both ACTH and C into an ultradian pattern, associated with a 40 % to 55 % downfall of the oscillations' amplitudes and mean levels. Considering both, the prominent role of the PVN in the control of ACTH secretion and the specific origin of the NA axons distributed to the PVN areas were selectively impaired by the latter procedure, the data point to the NA innervation of the PVN originating in the A1 group as to a significant component of the central control of AC.

2651 HEMORRHAGE(H) INDUCED CHANGES IN ELECTROCHEMICAL(EC) ACTIVITY IN THE LOCUS CERULEUS OF THE CAT:CORRELATION WITH CHANGES IN ACTH.

K.V.Thrivikraman*, D.E. Carlson, D.S. Gann, Brown Univ/RI Hospital, Providence, RI 02902 USA.

Release of ACTH after H depends upon the input from arterial and atrial baroreceptor afferents. Signals pass from the terminations of these afferents in the medulla through ACTH-active areas in the dorsal rostral pons that include the locus ceruleus(LC). This area contains both norepinephrine (NE) and serotonin(5HT). The roles and possible interrelations of these transmitters in the control of ACTH have not been defined. These studies in chloralose-urethane anesthetized cats were designed to examine the activity of this region during H using an in vivo EC technique that is sensitive to NE,5HT and their metabolites. Blood was sampled for the measurement of plasma ACTH by RIA. Differential pulse voltammetric scans were obtained every other min during an H(20%/3min) of 30min and subsequent reinfusion. H was repeated at 90min. ACTH increased during both H's, with a potentiation of the response seen after the second H. EC signals during H were related to the anatomical distribution of the recording sites. Two sites in the anteroventral LC yielded immediate and transient increases in the oxidative current(I)in response to the first H that preceded increases in plasma ACTH. Three sites in the dorsal LC and one site in the parabrachial LC yielded sustained decreases in I in response to the first H that also preceded increases in plasma ACTH. However, the magnitude of the changes in I obtained from both of these groups decreased during the second H. Three sites on the ventral and dorsal borders of the LC yielded no change or an increase in I at 10min following the first H, but all of these sites yielded an increase in I at 10min following the second H. Two sites in the posteromedial LC yielded no change in I in response to either H. These results indicate that H mediates specific changes in the concentration of aminergic transmitters in various regions of the LC that may be involved in the control of ACTH release. Supported by NIH AM26831.

2652 CARBAMYLCHOLINE STIMULATION OF HUMAN THYROID CELL FUNCTION.

R. Toccafondi*, M.L. Brandi, C.M. Rotella and A. Tanini, Clinica Medica III, Università di Firenze, I-50134 Firenze, Italy

Cholinergic fibers between and around thyroid follicles have been found in man and other mammals. To assess the possible influence of cholinergic agents on human thyroid function and its control exerted by TSH, the effect of carbamylcholine (Cch), a cholinesterase resistant analog of acetylcholine, on cAMP and cGMP cellular content has been studied in human thyroid cells, prepared by enzymatic digestion and mechanical dispersion, and kept in culture for 7 days. Cch (10 μM) produced a significant cAMP increase after 15 min incubation, returning to baseline after 30 min; at this time Cch exerted a dose dependent (0.1-10 pM) cAMP activation. Cch produced also a dose--dependent (1 nM-10 μM) increase of cGMP levels. High Cch amounts (10 μM) significantly inhibited TSH effect on cAMP content. The simultaneous stimulation with low doses of Cch (0.1 nM) and TSH (10 pM) resulted in an additive effect on cAMP levels. Finally, atropine, a muscarinic receptor antagonist, blocked Cch effects on both adenylate and guanylate cyclase systems, leaving unchanged the effect of TSH on cAMP. In conclusion, present data demonstrate that Cch is able to regulate cyclic nucleotide metabolism of human thyroid cell through muscarinic receptors. Besides we can argue that a cholinergic stimulation may exert either potentiating or inhibitory effects on TSH action as function of the release of the neurotransmitter.

2653 RELATIONSHIP OF URINARY NOREPINEPHRINE (NE) TO HYPOTHALAMIC-PITUITARY-ADRENOCORTICAL (HPA) ACTIVITY IN MALES. V.Wahby*and J.Mason,Psychoendocrine Lab, VA Medical Center and Yale University, West Haven, CT 06516, U.S.A.
RATIONALE: (1)Central NE is thought to inhibit the HPA axis. (2)Plasma NE is variably considered to correlate positively, negatively, or not at all with central NE. (3)Plasma NE was again reported by some investigators to correlate positively and by others negatively, with HPA activity. (4)Recently, 24 hour urinary excretion rates of NE were reported to reflect its total production in the body. (5)We examined the relationship between 24-hour urinary content of NE and HPA activity as measured by 8am plasma cortisol, 24-hour urinary free cortisol levels and the response to dexamethasone suppression(DST).
METHODS: This study was done in the course of a protocol on HPA activity in 24 male psychiatric patients representing a cross-sectional diagnostic sample. None had medical illnesses. Eleven patients were on no medication, 13 on medications known not to interfere with HPA activity. Cortisol was measured by RIA and catecholamines by radio-enzymatic assay. All tests were done under basal unstimulated physical or emotional activity. A 1 mg overnight DST was performed. Non-suppression was defined as post-DST plasma cortisol level of 5.0 ug/dl at either 8am, 4 or 11 p.m.
RESULTS: Urinary NE correlated positively with basal (8am pre-DST), 4 and 11 pm post-DST plasma cortisol levels, $p < 0.001$, < 0.05 and < 0.01 respectively. DST non-suppressors had significantly higher NE levels than suppressors($t = 2.5$, $p < 0.05$). No significant correlation was found between urinary NE and free cortisol.
CONCLUSIONS: In this population, urinary NE correlated positively with indices of HPA axis overactivity. Larger patient and control populations of both sexes need to be stuided in order to evaluate this finding.

2654 FURTHER EVIDENCE FOR THE EXISTENCE OF ESTROGEN (E) RECEPTIVE PREOPTIC NEURONS WHICH UTILIZE GABA TO MEDIATE NEGATIVE AND POSITIVE E-FEEDBACK SIGNALS. W. Wuttke*, J. Demling and E. Fuchs, Dept. of Reproductive Biology, German Primate Center, 3400 Göttingen, FRG.

Recently we proposed the existence of estrogen (E) receptive neurons in the preoptic-anterior hypothalamic area (MPAH) which utilize GABA as neurotransmitter. These neurons are believed to interact with noradrenergic axon terminals which innervate LHRH neurons. Thereby the E-receptive neurons influence circulating blood LH levels. Focal perfusion of the MPAH using the push-pull cannula technique revealed high NE release rates ($\bar{X} = 103 \pm 9$ fmol / 15 min fraction) in ovariectomized (ovx) and low ($\bar{X} = 45 \pm 8$ fmol / 15 min fraction) in animals under the negative E-feedback action. NE release into the MPAH increased in E-treated animals in the afternoon, i.e. at the time of the positive feedback action of E. GABA release rates measured in the same samples were low in ovx (37 ± 7 pmol/ 15 min), high in ovx-E treated animals in the morning (71 ± 9 pmol /15 min) and low in the afternoon (39 ± 4 pmol / 15 min). Hence mean preoptic NE release parallels blood LH levels whereas GABA release exibits an inverse relation. Preoptic epinephrine release was also higher in animals with high blood LH levels than in those under negative E-feedback action. Conspicuous high NE and dopamine release episodes into the MPAH were measured in E-primed animals at noon, i.e. at the time of the "critical period". This and the morphological demonstration of E-receptive neurons (by autoradiography) and simultaneous staining with glutamic acid decarboxylase antibodies (the marker enzyme for GABAergic neurons) corroborate and extend the above outlined working hypothesis.

(Abstract 2775, p. 1648, also belongs to this section.)

2655 HORMONE-INDUCED MEIOTIC NON-DISJUNCTION. E.Theuring* and I.Hansmann,Dpt. of Human Genetics,Univ. of Göttingen,FRG

With the use of gonadotropins and gonadotropin-releasing hormone(GnRH) it is possible to generate hormone-induced chromosomal aneuploidy by meiotic non-disjunction (ND) in oocytes from Djungarian hamsters.The aneuploid oocytes are neither generated by non-ovulated follicles of the preceding cycle nor by immature oocytes,which didn't have reached the acquisition for resumption of meiosis.Stimulatory and inhibitory effects were obtained after GnRH-treatment with respect to follicular maturation,resumption of meiosis and ovulation.The involvement of preferentially large metacentric chromosomes in ND implicates,that chromosomal properties,e.g. length and position of the spindle predispose to non-disjunction.The Djungarian hamster is a suitable model for studying the molecular mechanisms involved in the neuroendocrine control of mammalian meiosis (hypothalamus-pituitary-ovary)and that of ND.Explanations for the process of ND have to consider the interactions of the germ cell with the adjacent somatic cells in the follicle itself and the communication between the follicles of the ovary might be as important as processes involved in the cytoplasmic and nuclear differentiation of the oocyte.

2656 CHARACTERIZATION OF THE ADENYLYL CYCLASE OF CORPUS LUTEUM IN CONNECTION WITH $PGF_{2\alpha}$ INDUCED LUTEOLYSIS. P.A. Torjesen* and A. Aakvaag, University of Oslo Hospitals, Hormone Laboratory, Aker Hospital, Oslo 5*, and University of Bergen, Hormone Laboratory, Bergen, Norway.

Prostaglandin $F_{2\alpha}$ ($PGF_{2\alpha}$) administration to the superluteinized rat leads to a sharp decline in the serum level of progesterone. This reduction is accompanied by decreased adenylyl cyclase (AC) response to hCG and isoproterenol while the response to forskolin remains unchanged. In addition to activation by hormone binding to its receptor, cAMP production can be activated through direct stimulation of the N-component of the AC complex by Mg^{2+} and the non-hydrolyzable GTP analogue GMP-P(NH)P. Furthermore, activation of AC seems to be modified by phosphorylation/dephosporylation reactions, which in the present case were studied by the addition of alkaline phosphatase and the phosphatase inhibitor Na_2MoO_4. Wistar rats, 25 days of age, were treated with pmSG and hCG to achieve superluteinization. Seven days after hCG each animal received 5 μg of the $PGF_{2\alpha}$ analogue cloprostenol (ICI, UK) to induce luteolysis. Ninety min later the animals were decapitated, and the ovaries homogenized and assayed for AC activity. AC activity was stimulated maximally - 4 to 30 times above basal - with 1000 IU hCG/ml, 0.1 mM isoproterenol, 0.1 mM forskolin, 40 mM Mg^{2+}, 0.5 mM GMP-P(NH)P, 2.3 U/ml alkaline phosphatase, and 20 mM Na_2MoO_4, but only the response to hCG and isoproterenol was reduced following cloprostenol treatment. It is suggested that $PGF_{2\alpha}$ induced attenuation of ovarian AC response to activation is caused by a modification in the coupling of hormone receptor to the N-component of the AC while the rest of the AC complex remains unchanged.

2657 MULTIPLE CYSTIC OVARIAN DISEASE - A NEW CLASSIFICATION M. Tucker, J. Adams, W.P. Mason, D.V.Morris, S.Franks, and H.S.Jacobs*. Middlesex Hospital, London, W.1, U.K.

Based on ultrasound scans of ovaries and response to treatment with pulsatile LHRH therapy we now distinguish two distinct groups of patients with multiple cystic ovarian disease. Those with Stein-Leventhal polycystic ovaries (PCOS) are fatter than normal (mean body mass index±SD= 31.0±5.1), have hirsutism with raised plasma testosterone and low SHBG concentrations. Their ovaries are enlarged with numerous small cysts, of diameter 2-4 mm. Patients with megalocystic ovaries are often thinner than normal (mean BMI±SD=20.8±2.7), and 60% have a history of weight loss. Testosterone and SHBG concentrations are normal. On ultrasound the enlarged ovaries contain 10-12 cysts, 6-10 mm in diameter. In both groups the ratio of LH to FSH is raised. 42 clomiphene resistant, progestogen negative amenorrhoeic patients were studied. In PCOS cases 2 of 17 cycles in 8 women treated with sc LHRH were ovulatory and there was 1 conception. 3 of 7 cycles in 4 women treated with the same dose of LHRH given iv were ovulatory. In contrast 16 of 34 cycles in 15 women with megalocystic ovaries treated with sc LHRH were ovulatory and there were 6 pregnancies. All 13 cycles of iv therapy in 9 patients were ovulatory and there were 8 conceptions. These results suggest megalocystic ovaries are caused by an LHRH responsive disorder of gonadotrophin secretion, while PCOS is resistant to this treatment and is perhaps caused by a primary ovarian disturbance.

2658 PREMATURE MENOPAUSE-DELETION IN THE LONG ARM OF X CHROMOSOME. R.N. TURKSOY*, A. Luciano, L. Atkins, T. Beatty, I. Irwin, Div. of Reproductive Endocrinology, Dept. of Obs. & Gyn. Tufts-N.E. Med. Ctr. Hospital, Boston, MA. U.S.A.

We report a family in which the patient (pt.), her mother, maternal aunt and maternal grandmother developed premature menopause between 24-37 years. Pt., age 27, gravida 0, female, was the 2nd of 3 offspring of age 32 father and age 30 mother. Mother and maternal aunt had irregular menses, developing menopause at ages 37 and 32. They were the only offspring of the grandmother who experienced menopause at age 34. The pt's sister (age 31) has irregular menses. A brother (age 24) has two children. Pt. experienced menarche at age 13, then irregular menses (6-12 wks) x 3 days. She developed hypergonadotropic amenorrhea and vasomotor symptoms at age 24. Pt. is phenotypically well developed female, height 155cm, with arm span of 154cm, weight 74kgm. Serum prolactin, testosterone, thyroxin and thyroid stimulating hormone values were normal. Antiovarian, antiadrenal, antithyroid antibodies were negative. Laporotomy revealed normal uterus and Fallopian tubes. Both ovaries were small, each measuring 2 x 0.8 x 0.5cm and 1.8 x 0.8 x 0.5cm. Histologic examination of ovarian biopsies showed 2 primordial follicles, a corpora albicantia, and normal stroma. Karyotype and banding studies by Giemsa staining revealed 46X del(X)pter-q24, (having a break at 24). Chromosomal studies of the other family members are in progress, results will be presented. Comment: Genetic studies of this pt. are consistent with the theory that genes essential for normal ovarian development are located on both arms of the X chromosome and at least one of the gene(s) is located between q24 and the end of the long arm. Family history of this pt. suggests X linked dominant and sex limited inheritance. Inheritance of premature menopause requires early reproductive counseling in affected families.

2659 INHIBITION OF FSH AUGMENTED ADENYLATE CYCLASE ACTIVITY (AC) IN PORCINE GRANULOSA CELLS BY OVARIAN PROTEIN (OP).

E. L. Ujita, J. D. Campeau and G. S. diZerega*, Department of Obstetrics and Gynecology, USC; L. A., CA.

Previously, we identified a fraction of porcine follicular fluid (pFF) which inhibited granulosa cell aromatase, FSH induction of LH receptor, and hMG induced rat ovarian weight gain. Since these FSH actions are mediated by AC, we evaluated the effects of partially purified [$(NH_4)_2SO_4$, dialysis, Orange A chromatography, lyophilization] pFF on FSH induced AC in broken granulosa cell preparations. Maximum AC activity was present 20 min (10x basal) after incubation with FSH (3.3 μM) which fell to a constant level (2x basal) at 45 min. OP (500 μg/ml) induced a parallel reduction in AC throughout a 5-20 min incubation. After a 20 min incubation, a decrease in AC was found (OP, 100 μg/ml) with maximal inhibition at 1 mg/ml. AC in OP (350 μg/ml) treated cells was less than in cells incubated with both FSH and OP ($p < .05$). AC in OP treated cells was unchanged in the presence or absence of methyl-isobutyl-xanthine (.4 mM). Further, when OP was heated (56 C, 45 min) or precipitated with 10% TCA, inhibition of AC was lost. OP induced a reduction in Gpp(NH)p (25 μM) stimulated AC with an OP ID_{50} of 350 μg/ml with FSH and 80 μg/ml without FSH preincubation (3.3 μM, 20 min). The ID_{50} for OP inhibition of forskolin (10 μM) stimulated AC was 350 μg/ml. Gpp(NH)p stimulated AC was more sensitive to inhibition by OP than forskolin stimulated AC throughout a 5-20 min incubation interval ($p < .05$). In conclusion, OP specifically inhibited FSH responsive AC activity in porcine granulosa cells. The differential degree of AC inhibition with OP suggests that the G/F regulatory subunit of AC may be an important site for intracellular control.

2660 DIRECT EFFECTS OF LH-RH AND ITS ANALOGUES ON THE OVARY IN PSEUDOPREGNANT RATS.

B.Varga+, E.Horváth and R.Tarnai, Inst Exptl Med Hung Acad Sci. Budapest, P.O.Box 67, 1450-Hungary

Rats on day 5 of pseudopregnancy were anesthetized with pentobarbital and hypophysectomized. Polyethylene cannulas were inserted into one of the femoral arteries and utero-ovarian veins. A polyethylene catheter was fixed in the ovarian bursa and the uterine branch of utero-ovarian vein was ligated. Five minute blood samples were collected from the ovarian vein for 40 minutes. Following the first five minute blood fractions LH-RH, an agonist (D-Phe^6, des Gly-$NH_2{}^{10}$-LH-RH-ethylamide) and an antagonist analogue (Formyl-D-$Trp^{1,3}$,D-pCl-Phe^2,D-Phe^6-LH-RH) were injected to the surface of ovary. Blood pressure, ovarian venous outflow and hematocrit were continuously recorded. From the blood samples progesterone(P) and 17β-estradiol(E_2) were determined by RIA and the secretion rate was calculated. Luteal cells from pseudopregnant rats on day 5 were incubated with HCG, LH-RH and its analogues. In pseudopregnant rats LH-RH(100 ng) and LH-RH antagonist(100 ng) were ineffective. LH-RH agonist(10 ng) increased ovarian blood flow. No change in P and E_2 secretion was observed. LH-RH agonist(50 ng) given to intact pseudopregnant rats increased also ovarian blood flow and E_2 secretion. In isolated luteal cells HCG and LH-RH agonist stimulated P synthesis.

2661 ESTROGEN REGULATES CHOLESTEROL METABOLISM IN CULTURED SWINE OVARIAN CELLS.
JD Veldhuis*, JT Gwynne, JF Strauss, University of Virginia, Charlottesville, VA, University of North Carolina, Chapel Hill, NC, University of Pennsylvania, Philadelphia, PA, USA.
Peptide hormones are recognized to control one or more steps associated with the utilization of cholesterol in ovarian steroidogenesis. In contrast, the actions of steroid hormones on ovarian cholesterol metabolism are poorly defined. We utilized serum-free cultures of swine granulosa cells to examine estrogen's regulation of lipoprotein binding and degradation, cholesterol esterification, and de novo biosynthesis of cholesterol. Under these conditions, pig granulosa cells exhibited high-affinity receptors for ^{125}I-swine LDL with an estimated Kd of 2.4 µg/ml (range 1.3-5.1 µg/ml), and a binding capacity of 370 ng swine LDL/mg DNA (range 320-440 ng LDL/mg DNA). Treatment with estradiol did not alter the Kd for LDL binding, but increased specific LDL binding capacity two-fold, and enhanced time-dependent LDL degradation. To assess the importance of partitioning cholesterol into cholesteryl ester storage pools, granulosa cells were treated with an inhibitor of the acetyltransferase reaction (Sandoz 58-035). This fatty acyl amide effectively blocked ^{3}H-oleic acid incorporation into cholesteryl esters in microsomes and intact granulosa cells, and significantly augmented the stimulatory effects of long-term (48-96 hours) estrogen treatment on progesterone biosynthesis. Conversely, the stimulatory effect of estrogen in serum-free cultures could be partially inhibited by compactin, a competitive antagonist of de novo cholesterol biosynthesis. We conclude that actions of estradiol impinge upon key steps in the metabolism of both extracellularly and intracellularly derived cholesterol in the ovary. (Support: HD16393,HD12314,HD06274)

2662 INSULIN ACTION IN THE OVARY: EVIDENCE THAT THE INSULIN RECEPTOR ON SWINE GRANULOSA CELLS IS SPECIFICALLY PHOSPHORYLATED BY INSULIN. JD Veldhuis, L Kolp,* S Tamura, D Juchter, RW Furlanetto, J Larner, Univ. Virginia, Charlottesville, VA, Univ. Pennsylvania, Philadelphia, PA, USA.
Insulin augments progesterone biosynthesis by cultured swine granulosa cells. We now demonstrate that multiplication stimulating activity (MSA) and insulin-like growth factor type I (IGF-I) also do so, but at 20 to 50-fold lower concentrations than insulin. Thus, insulin might act via receptors for IGF-I or MSA, or via a classical insulin receptor pathway (or both). To further dissect the mechanism(s) of insulin action in ovarian cells, we tested: (1) the ability of anti-insulin receptor antibody to inhibit the trophic actions of insulin; and (2) the capacity of insulin, MSA, and IGF-I to induce specific phosphorylation of the beta subunit of the immunoprecipitated insulin receptor. Insulin receptor antibody (B-9 of C.R. Kahn) produced dose-dependent inhibition of insulin's stimulation of progesterone biosynthesis, with 70-85% inhibition expressed at dilutions of 1/150-1/50, without significantly affecting basal progesterone production. Moreover, when partially purified soluble receptor preparations from swine granulosa cells were incubated with or without hormones for 30 minutes at 4°C, insulin (but not IGF-I, MSA, or desoctapeptide insulin) specifically induced phosphorylation of a 95,000-dalton polypeptide that was immunoprecipitated with anti-insulin receptor antibody, and resolved by SDS-gel electrophoresis. In summary, while we do not exclude the operation of more than one receptor mechanism in the ovary, our results provide direct evidence that insulin can act via a classical insulin-receptor pathway in the gonad. (Support HD16393, & ADA.)

2663 EFFECT OF CYCLOHEXIMIDE (CYCLO) ON OVARIAN PROTEIN SYNTHESIS, SERUM LEVELS OF PEPTIDE AND STEROID HORMONES AND OVULATION IN THE PROESTROUS HAMSTER. S.-C. Wang* and G.S. Greenwald, Dept. of Physiology, Univ. of Kansas Med. Ctr., Kansas City, KS 66103, U.S.A.

Hamsters (6 per group) were injected s.c. at 1400 h proestrus (onset of LH surge) with either saline (SAL) or 2,4 & 8 mg CYCLO. CYCLO prevents ovulation by 0900h of estrus, which normally occurs at 0200h. Ovaries collected 2,8,16 & 24h after treatment were incubated for 1h with ^{3}H-leucine. CYCLO inhibited protein synthesis at 1600h (for 2,4 & 8mg CYCLO = 75,36 & 34% of control values) and at 2200h (68,64 & 43% respectively). During this time span, serum FSH & LH did not differ between the 2 groups, whereas serum P_4 was decreased in a dose dependent manner in the CYCLO groups (e.g. at 2200h-in SAL group-18.3±0.8ng/ml vs. 6.6±0.8ng/ml in 4mg CYCLO groups). In contrast, at 2200h when serum E_2 declined to 15pg/ml in the SAL group, it was 50 & 100pg/ml respectively in the 4 & 8mg CYCLO groups & even at 0600h estrus, E_2 was still detectable. Compared to 2200h, ovarian protein synthesis declined in the control groups at 0600 & 1400h estrus (when ovulation had occurred) but it increased in the CYCLO groups (e.g. at 0400h-an increase of 57% in 4mg group). At 0900h estrus, in the CYCLO groups antral follicles were not atretic but showed histologic signs of arrested preovulatory changes but none had ovulated. By 1400h all hamsters treated with 2mg CYCLO ovulated 10.5±1 ova & after 4mg CYCLO 4/6 animals ovulated 8.5±1.2 ova. By 0900h of the next day only 2/6 hamsters ovulated (3 ova) ater 4mg CYCLO & instead the ovaries contained huge cystic follicles and corpora hemorrhagica. Thus, by inhibiting protein synthesis, ovarian steroidogenesis was temporarily altered and serum E_2 did not abruptly collapse as normally occurs after the LH surge.

2664 CHARACTERIZATION OF THE EFFECT OF A GnRH ANALOG ON THE RAT OVARY IN VIVO M. Zilberstein*[1,2], H. Zakut[2], D.M. Phillips[3], I. Sherizly[1], and N. Dekel[1], [1]Department of Hormone Research, The Weizmann Institute of Science, Rehovot 76100, Israel; [2]Department of Obstetrics and Gynecology, Sackler Faculty of Medicine, Tel Aviv University, The Edith Wolfson Hospital, Holon, Israel, and [3]The Population Council, New York, U.S.A.

The present study was undertaken to characterize the effect of a GnRH analog (D-Ala^6 des-gly^{10}-GnRH N ethylamide, GnRHa) on the rat ovary *in vivo*. GnRHa (2 g/rat) was administered to either PMSG-primed or non-primed hypophysectomized immature female rats. At different time intervals after administration of the hormone cumulus-oocyte complexes were recovered. Interference contrast microscopy was used to assess maturation in the oocytes. Cumulus cell masses were analyzed by scanning electronmicroscopy. Ovulation was indicated by the presence of ova in the oviduct. Analysis of the timing of GnRHa action revealed that oocyte maturation and ovulation are induced by 4 and 10 h after administration of the hormone, respectively. This timing is very similar to that of LH action in the ovary Expansion of the cumulus mass and secretion of the hyaluronidase sensitive mucoid material, which are characteristic responses of the cumulus cells to LH, were also observed following GnRHa administration. However, while LH action on the ovary is mediated by cAMP, no accumulation of the nucleotide could be detected in the follicular cells exposed to GnRHa. Moreover, unlike LH, GnRHa action on the follicular oocyte of hypophysectomized immature rat did not require PMSG priming. We conclude that even though GnRHa and LH can elicit similar responses in the rat ovary they do not share the same mechanistic pathways.

2665 RESETTING OF THE OSMOTIC THRESHOLD FOR VASOPRESSIN SECRETION IN PATIENTS WITH CONGESTIVE HEART FAILURE.

J.G. Verbalis*, B.F. Uretsky, T. Generalovich, A. Valdes and P.S. Reddy, Department of Medicine, University of Pittsburgh, Pittsburgh, PA, USA.

Many patients with congestive heart failure (CHF) have elevated levels of plasma vasopressin (AVP) which are inappropriate for their osmolality and possibly contribute to the hyponatremia often seen in this syndrome. To study osmotic regulation of AVP secretion in CHF, plasma AVP levels were measured by RIA in 10 normal patients and 10 patients with severe heart failure (NYHA Class III-IV) before and after injection of contrast media (Renografin-76) during diagnostic cardiac catheterization. Patients with CHF had both significantly elevated basal AVP levels and an exaggerated AVP response to osmotic stimulation:

	pOsm (mOsm/kg)		pAVP (μU/ml)	
	BASAL	POST-DYE	BASAL	POST-DYE
NORMAL (10)	283 ± 1	290 ± 2**	2.0 ± 0.3	3.6 ± 0.4***
CHF (10)	275 ± 4	288 ± 5**	7.2 ± 2.0#	32.6 ± 7.7#***

(#p<.05, NL vs CHF; **p<.01, ***p<.001, basal vs post-dye)

Three CHF patients remained hypo-osmolar even after contrast media (260, 273 and 280 mOsm/kg) but still had similar AVP responses (+36, +15 and +70 μU/ml, respectively). Thus, patients with CHF have a lower osmotic threshold for AVP secretion and a greater slope of plasma AVP rise with changes in osmolality. This is similar to alterations of AVP secretion seen following volume depletion, suggesting that decreased effective blood volume and/or pressure accompanying CHF resets the response of vasopressinergic neurons to osmotic stimuli.

2666 CHANGES IN THE OSMOREGULATION OF THIRST AND VASOPRESSIN (VP) DURING THE NORMAL MENSTRUAL CYCLE (MC).

T. Vokes*, M. Gaskill and G. Robertson, Department of Medicine, University of Chicago, Chicago, Illinois, USA.

To evaluate the influence of the MC on the osmoregulation of thirst and VP, we studied 5 healthy women during the early follicular(F), midcycle (O) and late luteal(L) phases of the MC. Plasma osmolality(pOS), sodium (pNa), VP(pVP), urine osmolality(uOS), body weight(BW) and mean arterial pressure(MAP) were measured under basal conditions and every 30 min. during an acute oral water load followed by infusion of 3% saline. During the latter, thirst threshold(T_t) was also assessed on a visual rating scale. The linear regression of pVP and pOS defined the precision (correlation=r), sensitivity (slope=b) and threshold (x-intercept=T_v) of osmoregulation.

	BASAL VALUES (mean±SEM)					
MC Phase	BW(kg)	pOS	pNa	pVP(pg/ml)	uOS	MAP
F	66±6	290±1	140±1	1.9±.6	808±142	79±5
O	66±6	288±1	139±1	2.6±.9	810±132	81±5
L	66±6	285±1*	138±1	1.4±.2	920±28	78±4

	WATER LOAD				SALINE INFUSION			
	pOS	pVP	uOS	% out/2°	r	b	T_v	T_t
F	285±1	.7±.1	62±5	102±10	.93±.03	.8±.1	285±1	292±1
O	281±2	.7±.2	60±5	96±14	.97±.01	.9±.1	284±2	287±2
L	278±1*	.5±.1	57±4	99±10	.95±.01	.8±.2	280±1*	282±1*#

*p<.05 - L vs F, #p<.05 - L vs O by paired t-test

The results show that the precision and sensitivity of osmoregulation are not altered during the normal MC. However, basal pOS as well as the osmotic thresholds for thirst and VP secretion are reduced during the luteal phase. These changes may facilitate premenstrual water retention.

2667 CHARACTERIZATION OF NEUROPHYSIN FROM THE SHEEP ANTERIOR PITUITARY GLAND

W.B. Watkins* and L.G.Moore, J.E.Rivier and J.Spiess, Postgraduate School of Obstetrics and Gynaecology,University of Auckland,Auckland,New Zealand and Peptide Biology Laboratory,Salk Institute,San Diego,CA 92138, U.S.A.

Formalin-fixed sheep anterior pituitary gland tissue was prepared for histology and treated in the immunoperoxidase procedure with an antiserum raised against neurophysin. A positive staining for neurophysin-like immunoreactivity was observed in the cells identified as corticotrophs. The anterior pituitary tissues was extracted with hydrochloric acid and assayed by RIA for the ovine neurophysins, oN-I/II and oN-III. In all specimens of the pituitary tissue examined oN-I/II and oN-III immunoreactivities were detected. The neurophysins of the anterior pituitary behaved identical to that of oN-I/II and oN-III on polyacrylamide gel electrophoresis and isoelectric focussing on polyacrylamide gel. N-III from the anterior pituitary was purified by affinity chromatography by passage through a column of vasopressin bound to Sepharose and finally by HPLC. The neurophysin was shown to possess an amino acid composition similar to that of oN-III and an N-terminal amino acid sequence identical to that of oN-III up to at least residue No 35. The findings support the conclusions of others that oxytocin and/or vasopressin may be present in the anterior pituitary gland and thus may be involved in the modulation of hormone release from this tissue.

This work was financed by the Medical Research Council of New Zealand.

2668 VASOPRESSIN AND THE CONTROL OF URINARY KININS. N. Weiss*, M. Conder and G. Robertson, University of Chicago, Dept. of Medicine, Chicago, IL, USA.

Urinary kinins are known to arise in the distal nephron where vasopressin (VP) dependent urinary concentration also occurs. We showed previously that water loading suppresses the rate of urinary kinin excretion ($\dot{u}$k) in healthy adults. To determine if this suppression was mediated by the associated fall in plasma VP (pVP) we measured the effect of graded, 90 minute IV infusions of low doses of synthetic VP on pVP and $\dot{u}$K, as well as on plasma and urine osmolality (pOS and uOS) in 5 water loaded normal subjects and 3 patients with severe neurogenic diabetes insipidus (DI). In the water loaded normal subjects, infusion of VP at 2.1 μU/kg/min raised (mean±SE) pVP from 1.4±0.1 to 2.8±0.7 pg/ml (p<.02). At the same time, there was a rise in uOS from 80±11 to 130±13 mosmol/kg (p<.001) and in $\dot{u}$K from 12.5±3.3 to 27.7±4.1 ng/mg creatinine (p<.05). Increasing the rate of VP infusion to 7.0 μU/kg/min and then to 12.6 μU/kg/min, further increased pVP to 4.8±.3 and 6.2±.8 pg/ml (p<.05) and uOS to 418±91 and 655±158 mosmol/kg (p<.05) respectively. However, the higher VP infusion rates did not further increase $\dot{u}$K, which plateaued at 31±8.4 and 26.5±7.0 ng/mg creatinine. pOS remained constant at 280±0.85 mosmol/kg throughout the infusions. In the DI patients, basal pVP, uOS and $\dot{u}$K were also low (<0.5 pg/ml, 48±6 mosmol/kg and 9.8±1.2 ng/mg respectively) and responded similarly to the same graded infusions of VP (pVP to 0.7±0.05, 1.4±0.4 and 2.2±0.9 pg/ml, uOS to 137±32, 273±33 and 394±15 mosmol/kg and $\dot{u}$K to 25.1±13.6, 32.4 ±14.1 and 22.5±6.1 ng/mg creatinine). These results confirm that $\dot{u}$K is sensitive to small physiologic changes in pVP. We conclude that urinary kinins are regulated at least in part by VP and may modulate the antidiuretic effects of this hormone.

2669 EFFECTS OF PROSTAGLANDIN INHIBITION ON THE ANTIDIURETIC ACTION OF VASOPRESSIN R.L. Woods* and W.P. Anderson, Baker Medical Research Institute, Prahran, Victoria, Australia.

Renal prostaglandins (PGs) have been suggested to modulate the antidiuretic action of arginine vasopressin (AVP) via a negative feedback system. Much of the evidence for this concept is from *in vitro* studies. Only a few *in vivo* studies have been performed and interpretation of these is confounded by the use of anesthetized animals, unphysiological amounts of AVP, and administration of AVP systemically, which causes significant hemodynamic effects. In the present study low doses of AVP were infused directly into the renal artery of chronically-instrumented, conscious dogs (n=5) with and without pre-treatment by the PG synthesis inhibitor, ibuprofen (1.2-2.0 g, orally). Control experiments were performed by vehicle infusion into the renal artery with and without ibuprofen. During all experiments a mild diuresis was induced in the dogs by continuous 5% dextrose infusion i.v. (1.5 $ml.min^{-1}$). PG inhibition in control experiments attenuated the dextrose diuresis. AVP infusions either with or without ibuprofen increased aortic AVP levels by less than 1 $pg.min^{-1}$, even at the highest dose, and were without significant changes in cardiovascular hemodynamics or changes in renal blood flow. AVP infusions (0.2, 0.7, 2.0 $ng.min^{-1}$) decreased urine flow by 39±14%, 58±12%, 76±7%, respectively. Ibuprofen pre-treatment did not significantly alter these antidiuretic responses to AVP. It is concluded that in conscious dogs with levels of AVP within the physiological range, renal prostaglandins are not important modulators of the antidiuretic action of AVP but they may have effects on water excretion independent of AVP.

(Abstract 2776, p. 1648, also belongs to this section.)

2670 **TROPHIC RESPONSE OF HAMSTER BROWN ADIPOSE TISSUE (BAT) TO COLD OR TO DIET: NO ROLE FOR NORADRENALINE (NA) OR THE PINEAL AND A DEFECT IN THE HAMSTER WITH MUSCULAR DYSTROPHY.** Joan Triandafillou, Jean Himms-Hagen*, Wiebke Hellenbrand. Department of Biochemistry, University of Ottawa, Ottawa, K1H 8M5, Canada.

The objective was to identify the mediator of the cold- or diet-induced hypertrophy of BAT in hamsters. Such hypertrophy in rats is mediated by NA. Chronic treatment with NA failed to produce BAT hypertrophy (increase in protein content) in hamsters, as it does in rats. NA treatment also failed to cause BAT hypertrophy in pinealectomized (Px) hamsters, indicating that NA-induced suppression of pineal secretion of melatonin (MT), known to have a trophic effect on BAT during short photoperiod, could not explain the lack of effect of NA. In Px hamsters, BAT hypertrophy in response to cold-acclimation or to a high-fat diet occurred normally. Regression of testes induced by cold-acclimation also occurred normally in Px hamsters. In hamsters with muscular dystrophy (BIO 14.6) diet- or short photoperiod-induced trophic response of BAT was absent. Regression of testes did occur in myopathic hamsters in short photoperiod. Cold-induced BAT hypertrophy does occur in the myopathic hamster (Himms-Hagen, Gwilliam, Am.J.Physiol. 239:C18,1980). It is concluded that (1) neither NA nor pineal-derived MT mediates the trophic response of hamster BAT to cold or to diet; (2) cold-induced regression of testes is not mediated by pineal-derived MT; (3) the defect in the myopathic hamster that prevents the BAT trophic response to both short photoperiod and diet but not to cold is unlikely to involve defective pineal function but is most probably a central one, perhaps in the hypothalamus. (Supported by the Muscular Dystrophy Association of Canada and the Medical Research Council of Canada).

2671 INJECTIONS AND/OR IMPLANTS OF 5-METHOXYTRYPTAMINE AND MELATONIN: EFFECTS ON PLASMA THYROXINE IN MALE AND FEMALE SYRIAN HAMSTERS. M.K. Vaughan,* B.A. Richardson, L.J. Petterborg, A.P. Holtorf, G.M. Vaughan, R.J. Reiter and T.H. Champney. Dept. of Cellular & Structural Biology, The University of Texas Health Science Center at San Antonio, San Antonio, TX 78284.

Daily injections of 25 µg melatonin (MEL) but not 5-methoxytryptamine (5MT) inhibited plasma thyroxine (T_4) titers in male (Exp. 1) and female (Exp. 2) Syrian hamsters; this effect was prevented in both sexes by a sc 1 mg MEL or 5MT pellet. In Exp. 3, various doses of MEL or 5MT were injected each afternoon to compare the effectiveness of these 2 indoles in reducing T_4 in hamsters kept in 14:10 LD. Only the 200 µg dose of 5MT significantly suppressed T_4 whereas all doses of MEL ($\geq$ 5 µg) were effective. MEL or 5MT were implanted as pellets in male hamsters exposed to short photoperiod (SP; 10:14 LD) to determine if either indole could prevent the SP-induced suppression of T_4 (Exps. 4 & 5). Regression analysis showed a significant log-dose related degree of prevention of SP-induced suppression of T_4 by using either MEL or 5MT in doses up to 1000 µg/pellet. Analysis of covariance and multiple regression analysis detected no differences between MEL and 5MT in their effectiveness in raising T_4. In conclusion, MEL appears considerably more effective than 5MT in inhibiting T_4 concentration when administered as a daily afternoon injection. On the other hand, sc 5MT implants appear to be as effective as MEL in preventing the suppression of T_4 that otherwise occurs as a result of either repeated afternoon injections of MEL or exposure to SP. (Supported by NSF grant PCM 8304706).

2672 DAY-NIGHT SYNTHESIS OF 5-METHOXYINDOLES IN THE PINEAL GLAND OF THE TORTOISE (TESTUDO HERMANNI GMELIN),DURING THE ANNUAL REPRODUCTIVE CYCLE. B.Vivien-Roels*[1],P.Pévet[1,2],J.Van Benthem[3],M.Sommer[3],A.Steinen[3],M.G.M. Balemans[3] 1,Lab.Zool.exp.Embryol.,Strasbourg,France,2, The Netherlands Inst.Brain Res. Amsterdam, The Netherlands,3, Zool.Lab.,Utrecht, The Netherlands.

Since it is now evident that, not only melatonin (aMT), but also other 5-methoxyindoles (MI) are effector compounds mediating the effects of environmental factors on seasonal reproduction, we have investigated the day and night capacity of the pineal gland of a reptile to synthetize the different MI during the annual reproductive cycle(technique of Balemans et al.,Experientia,34,1334,1978). Male tortoises, kept in a natural environment, were killed every 3hrs during 24hrs, at different times of the seasonal reproductive cycle (January, April, July, October). 5-methoxytryptophol (ML) appears by far, the most abundantly MI synthetized in this species; it represents 55 to 70% of all MI, independently of the period of the year,while aMT represents, depending on the season, 4 to 8%. Day-night studies show significant diurnal variations of synthesis of MI. For example, in July, during the period of reproduction, ML and 5-methoxyindole acetic acid (MA) show two peaks of synthesis, one during day-time (12h) and another during night-time (24h), while aMT synthesis is the highest during the night and that of 5-methoxytryptamine (MT) during the day.Except a night peak of synthesis for aMT in October,all these rhythms disappear from October until April, which corresponds to the period of hibernation and sexual quiescence.

If seasonal variations in the synthesis of MI are present, it is clear nevertheless, that MI are synthetized both during day and night and that ML is probably an important physiological compound in this species.

2673 PINEAL ARYLAMINE N-ACETYLTRANSFERASE AND ARYLALKYLAMINE N-ACETYLTRANSFERASE. P. Voisin*, M. A. A. Namboodiri and D. C. Klein, Section on Neuroendocrinology, Laboratory of Developmental Neurobiology, NICHD, National Institutes of Health, Bethesda, MD 20205

Acetylation of serotonin in the pineal gland is a key step in the synthesis of melatonin. The enzyme responsible for this reaction has been thought to be an arylamine N-acetyltransferase (NAT). We have investigated this issue and have found that the rat and ovine pineal glands contain two distinct enzymes which acetylate aromatic amines. One has narrow specificity for arylamines, including aniline and phenetidine. The second enzyme acts on arylalkylamines, including serotonin, tryptamine, 5-methoxytryptamine, 6-fluorotryptamine and phenylethylamine. It has little or no detectable activity towards phenetidine or aniline. These enzymes are separated using high performance size exclusion chromatography: the arylamine N-acetyltransferase has an apparent molecular weight of 35,000 daltons and the arylalkylamine N-acetyltransferase has two peaks of activity; one (75-90%) at about 100,000 MW and the second (10-25% total activity) at about 20,000 MW. The two enzymes are further differentiated by marked differences in their rate of inactivation at 4 °C. Finally, in the rat and sheep large changes in pineal arylalkylamine NAT activity can be caused by either adrenergic stimulation or protein synthesis inhibition without changing the arylamine NAT activity. The presence of two N-acetyltransferases in the pineal gland probably reflects the need to independently regulate serotonin N-acetylation for the generation of the melatonin rhythm, without affecting detoxification of arylamines by N-acetylation.

2674 COMPARISON OF THE PINEAL SENSITIVITY TO LIGHT IRRADIANCE IN A NOCTURNALLY AND A DIURNALLY ACTIVE RODENT. S. Webb*, A. Lewiński, T.H. Champney and R.J. Reiter, Dept. of Anatomy, The University of Texas Health Science Center, 7703 Floyd Curl Drive, San Antonio, Texas 78284, U.S.A.

The inhibitory effect of light on pineal metabolism is well known; however, the sensitivity of this gland to light may vary in different species. We compared the sensitivity of the pineal to different light irradiances in a diurnally (Richardson's ground squirrel) and a nocturnally (Sprague-Dawley albino rats) active rodent; we also evaluated the effect of photoreceptor atrophy on this sensitivity. Fifty-nine rats were in constant light for 6 weeks to induce photoreceptor atrophy; they were then returned to a 14:10 light:dark cycle for 2 weeks. Fifty-six rats and 64 squirrels were kept in a 14:10 cycle. Animals (6-8/group) were killed in the dark period between 0130 and 0300h (lights out 2000h), either before, or 15 or 30 min after exposure to cool white fluorescent light. Pineals were analyzed for NAT activity and melatonin levels. Squirrels: an irradiance of 1850 $\mu W/cm^2$ was required to depress pineal NAT and melatonin levels at night ($p<0.02$). Rats: 0.0005 $\mu W/cm^2$ significantly inhibited nocturnal NAT and melatonin levels in intact animals ($p<0.01$). In rats with photoreceptor atrophy, nighttime pineal NAT activity was significantly greater than in intact animals ($p<0.02$); 0.0005 $\mu W/cm^2$ was ineffective in lowering NAT and melatonin, while 0.175 $\mu W/cm^2$ partially, and 3.33 $\mu W/cm^2$ totally decreased these levels. Conclusions: 1) The pineal of the rat is 3.7×10^6 times more sensitive to light than that of the squirrel. 2) Photoreceptor atrophy reduces the sensitivity of the rat pineal to light. (Supported by NSF grant no. PCM 8003441).

2675 THE EFFECT OF MELATONIN ON LH-STIMULATED STEROIDOGENESIS FROM TESTIS INTERSTITIAL CELLS OF ADULT RATS. J. Y.-L. Yu* and T.-P. Lin, Endocrinology Laboratory, Institute of Zoology, Academia Sinica, Nankang, Taipei, Taiwan 115, R. O. C.

The purpose of this study was to demonstrate the direct effect of melatonin on androgen synthesis and release from rat testis interstitial cells, and to elucidate the mode of action of melatonin in this system. Testis interstitial cells from 10-12-wk old rats were isolated by collagenase dispersion and incubated with varying doses of ovine LH or dibutyryl cyclic AMP with/without melatonin, for 4 h at 34 C in Medium 199 under continuous aeration of 95% O_2-5% CO_2. Androgen (A) and progesterone (P) in the cells and in the incubation medium were determined by radioimmunoassays prior to and post incubation. Melatonin inhibited LH-evoked androgen synthesis in a dose related manner; on the other hand, it markedly enhanced progesterone formation. Both A and P contents in the cells were low and similar between LH and LH+Melatonin groups. Melatonin also affected steroidogenesis as evoked by cyclic AMP; the patterns being similar to that observed with LH+Melatonin. These findings indicate: 1) melatonin exhibits a direct inhibition on androgen synthesis; 2) its site of action is not at membrane receptors, but at intracellular steps of conversion from P to A without affecting the release of A from Leydig cells; and 3) it does not interfere the de novo synthesis of progesterone. This study was supported by NSC, R.O.C..

2676 **Peptide Alpha-Amidation Activity in Human Plasma and Tissues.** **G. Wand*, S. Baylin, R. Ney, and E. Eipper. Departments of Internal Medicine and Neuroscience, The Johns Hopkins University, Baltimore, Maryland.**

Many biologically active peptides contain carboxy terminal α-amide moieties which are essential for full potency (e.g. TRH, CRF, calcitonin). Recently an α-amidation activity was identified in rat and beef pituitary secretory granules (Eipper et al, PNAS, USA, 80:5144-[1983]). Full activity was dependent on copper, ascorbate and molecular oxygen. We have now identified similar α-amidation activity in several human tissues and plasma, measuring conversion of ^{125}I-D-Tyr-Val-Gly to ^{125}I-D-Tyr-Val-NH_2. Extracts of an ACTH-secreting pituitary adenoma contained α-amidation activity (0.7 pmole/mg tissue/hr). The level of activity in adult plasma (n=17) was 106 ± 3 pmole/ml/hr (mean ± SEM), with no difference between male (n=7) and female (n=10) subjects. In subjects under 15 years old (n=8), mean plasma activity was 128 ± 10 pmole/ml/hr, higher than the adult control plasma($p < .025$). Plasma from hyperthyroid (n=8) and hypothyroid (n=5) adults contained 155 ± 10 and 140 ± 10 pmole/ml/hr respectively, values higher than euthyroid controls ($p < .0005$ for both). However the most striking elevations occurred in patients with medullary thyroid carcinoma (n=8, 175 ± 90 pmole/ml/hr, range 98-480), with a positive correlation between plasma calcitonin and α-amidation activity (R = 0.928). Extracts of medullary thyroid tumor which stained for calcitonin contained 4.2 pmole/mg tissue/hr α-amidation activity. Conclusion: α-amidation activity has been identified in human plasma, medullary thyroid carcinoma, and an ACTH secreting pituitary adenoma. This activity may be co-secreted along with amidated peptide hormones and be altered in states of abnormal hormone secretion.

2677 A PROSPECTIVE TRIAL OF BROMOCRIPTINE IN THE TREATMENT OF GROWTH HORMONE SECRETING TUMOURS. J.A.H. Wass*, M. Charlesworth, D.P.E. Kingsley, Lesley H. Rees and G.M. Besser, Depts. of Endocrinology, Radiology and Chemical Endocrinology, St. Bartholomew's Hospital, London, UK.

Bromocriptine can decrease the size of prolactin and growth hormone (GH) secreting pituitary tumours in rats and prolactinomas in man. There are only anecdotal reports of GH secreting tumours changing in size and it has been suggested that this may be related to coexistent hyperprolactinaemia. We have therefore carried out a prospective trial to assess the frequency of tumour shrinkage in a consecutive series of 12 newly diagnosed acromegalic patients without significant hyperprolactinaemia. The patients (3F, aged 19-70y) had clinical and biochemical acromegaly (pretreatment GH 22-642mU/l, mean 144; prolactin 137-468mU/l, mean 299). After assessment of pituitary function and radiology using a GE8800 scanner making coronal and sagittal reformats in 1.5mm contiguous slices, they were treated with bromocriptine alone for 1 to 10 months (mean 3.8) (dose 10 to 60mg/day) and then reassessed. CT scans were assessed by two radiologists independantly. GH levels fell in all but three patients by more than 50% (range 6-320mU/l, mean 67). Follow up CT scans are available so far in 9 patients and in 4 there was clear evidence of a decrease in pituitary tumour size, which was associated with a growth hormone fall (mean GH fall in 4 responders 81%, 5 non responders 41%). No tumour enlarged during treatment. We have shown that a significant proportion of pure growth hormone secreting pituitary tumours can decrease in size (44%) on treatment with dopamine agonist therapy alone. This is important when considering permanent ablative therapy with surgery or external pituitary irradiation.

2678 **Dibutyryl Adenosine 3',5'-Cyclic Monophosphate (dbcAMP) Preincubation Potentiates the Gonadotropin-Releasing Hormone (GnRH)-Induced Biphasic Release of Luteinizing Hormone (LH) in Cultured Rat Pituitary Cells.** **W.W. Wilfinger* and T. Downs, Dept. of Physiology, College of Medicine, Univ. of Cincinnati, OH, USA.**

The cyclic nucleotides have been implicated in the physiologic regulation of LH release. In this study, we have examined the effects of dbcAMP preincubation on the temporal pattern of GnRH-induced LH release. Dispersed pituitary cells (♀) were cultured in α-modified Eagle's medium + 10% charcoal-stripped horse serum + 0.18 nM estradiol (Control medium, CM). On the third day of culture, the medium was discarded and the cells were treated for 6h with either CM, CM + 1 mM dbcAMP + 1 mM theophylline (cAMP), or cAMP + 2.5 μM cycloheximide (cAMP + CH). After the preincubation period, the cells were washed and incubated with CM for an additional 3h period before GnRH stimulation (5h, $\pm$ 10 nM GnRH). Preincubation with cAMP significantly enhanced ($p < .05$) GnRH-induced LH release in comparison to CM (34%↑); however, this increase was completely blocked in cAMP + CH-treated cultures. The rate of LH release during the initial (0-60 min) and late (180-300 min) phase of GnRH stimulation was significantly enhanced by cAMP treatment in comparison to CM; however, compared to CM, cAMP + CH only significantly altered (↓) the initial phase of the LH response. The total quantity of immunoreactive LH recovered from the cells and medium was unaffected by treatment. In an additional experiment, dbcAMP concentrations ranging from .1 to 10 mM also produced a dose-dependent increase in LH release (21 to 114% ↑ LH release). When the interval between cAMP preincubation and GnRH stimulation was extended from 0 to 12h (1.5h intervals), the cAMP-mediated increase in LH release decayed at a linear rate ($T_{1/2}$ = 6.4h). In conclusion, cAMP preincubation, prior to GnRH stimulation, appears to alter the synthesis of a labile protein(s) which is involved in GnRH-mediated LH release. Supported by NIH HD-13739.

2679 OCCURRENCE AND DISTRIBUTION OF CALMODULIN AND CALMODULIN-BINDING PROTEINS IN BOVINE PITUITARY.

T. Yap Nelson, M. Y. Lorenson, L. S. Jacobs and A. E. Boyd III*, Dept. of Medicine, Baylor College of Medicine, Houston, TX and University of Rochester, NY, USA.

Ca^{2+} is necessary for secretion of pituitary hormones. Many of the biological effects of Ca^{2+} are mediated by the Ca^{2+}-binding protein calmodulin (CaM) which interacts with proteins regulated by the Ca^{2+}-CaM complex. We determined the quantity and distribution of CaM and CaM-binding proteins in bovine pituitary homogenates, subcellular fractions, secretory granules isolated by discontinuous sucrose gradient centrifugation, and secretory granule membranes. CaM, measured by radioimmunoassay, was found in each fraction and was not enriched in the secretory granule. CaM-binding proteins were identified by an ^{125}I-CaM gel overlay technique and quantitated by densitometric analysis of the autoradiograms. Pituitary homogenates contain 8 major CaM-binding proteins of M_r = 142, 126, 91, 64, 58, 56, 31, and 22.5 kDa. Binding to all the bands was specific, Ca^{2+}-sensitive, and displaceable with a 100-fold excess of unlabeled CaM. Heat treatment (100°C, 15 min) which results in a 75% reduction in phosphodiesterase activation by CaM markedly decreased ^{125}I-CaM binding to all protein bands. In contrast to the CaM distribution, the secretory granule membranes showed 3-8 fold enhancement for CaM-binding proteins 142, 126, 91, and 56 kDa. The enrichment of CaM-binding proteins in the secretory granule membranes suggests a role for CaM in the Ca^{2+}-dependent movement of the secretory granules to the plasma membrane prior to exocytosis.

2680 STUDY ON HUMAN PITUITARY GONADOTROPIN SYNTHESIS AND RELEASE BY LH-RH TWO STEP TEST AND LAPAROSCOPY IN OVARIAN DYSFUNCTION.

Tsuneo Yokokura*, Tsunehisa Makino+, Hiroshi Ochiai and Rihachi Iizuka+. Department of Obstetrics and Gynecology, Tokyo Saiseikai Central Hospital and Keio University+, Tokyo, Japan.

Pituitary gonadotropin response of synthesis and release to two-step stimulation by 100μg of LH-RH at 60 minutes interval was studied by radioimmunoassay for hLH and hFSH in normal menstrual cycle (n=15) and ovarian dysfunction (n=17). The definitions of Δ_1 and Δ_2 were; Δ_1=30(or 60) min. value - 0 min. value. Δ_2=90(or 120, 180) min. value - 60 min. value. Δ_1, Δ_2 ratio=Δ_2/Δ_1. Ovarian morphology was confirmed by laparoscopy in all cases after LH-RH two-step test. In normal follicular phase, the second LH-RH administration increased serum hLH levels further than the first peak induced by the first LH-RH, indicating that "priming effect" by the first LH-RH on the second peak. The first peak is presumed as the pituitary gonadotropin release by the first injection of LH-RH, and second peak can be composed in part by newly synthesized LH by the first LH-RH stimulation. The response of hLH in ovarian anovulation increased after the first LH-RH stimulation, but showed no significant peak after the second administration. In contrast, LH-RH two-step test in PCO type amenorrhea demonstrated two peaks. The Δ_1, Δ_2 ratio of hLH and hFSH in follicular phase were more than 1.0, indicating dominant pattern of synthesis of pituitary gonadotropin. The Δ_1, Δ_2 ratio of gonadotropin in ovarian anovulation and PCO type amenorrhea were smaller than 1.0, suggesting dominant pattern of release of pituitary gonadotropin. Thus LH-RH two step test was useful to clarify anterior pituitary function in both synthesis and release of gonadotropin.

2681 LEUMORPHIN STIMULATES PROLACTIN SECRETION IN THE RAT. K. Tojo*, Y. Kato, H. Ohta, A. Shimatsu, Y. Kabayama, T. Inoue, N. Yanaihara and H. Imura, Second Medical Clinic, Department of Medicine, Kyoto University Faculty of Medicine, Kyoto 606, and Laboratory of Bioorganic Chemistry, Shizuoka College of Pharmacy, Shizuoka 422, Japan.

Leumorphin (LM) is one of "big" leu-enkephalins derived from prepro-enkephalin B and contains leu-enkephalin (LEK) and rimorphin (RM) sequence at the N-terminus. LM has a potent opioid activity but the effect of LM on the pituitary function remains to be elucidated. We studied the effect of LM and related peptides on prolactin (PRL) secretion in the rat. Intraventricular injection of synthetic porcine LM (0.06, 0.6 and 6 nmol/rat) caused a dose-related increase in plasma PRL levels in urethane-anesthetized male rats. Peak values of plasma PRL were obtained 10-20 min after the injection and mean±SE values were 33.5±6.3 ng/ml, 286.5±29.5 ng/ml and 626.1 ±44.1 ng/ml, respectively. Saline injection icv as a control did not change plasma PRL levels (14.0±1.6 ng/ml). Intraventricular injection of LEK and RM (6 nmol/rat) resulted in an increase of plasma PRL with mean±SE peak values of 87.8±8.5 ng/ml and 102.1±8.0 ng/ml, but LM was the most potent to stimulate PRL release among these peptides. Plasma PRL response to LM (0.6 nmol/rat) was blunted by naloxone (125 µg/100 g BW, iv) (peak values: 92.0± 8.4 ng/ml vs control, $p<0.05$). Intraventricular injection of LM (0.6 and 6 nmol/rat) also raised plasma PRL levels in conscious freely moving rats. In in vitro studies, PRL release from perfused pituitary cells was stimulated by LM (10^{-7}M) and the effect was blunted by naloxone (10^{-5}M). These results suggest that LM has a potent stimulating effect on PRL secretion from the pituitary lactotroph in the rat through an opiate receptor.

2682 HYPERPROLACTINEMIA ASSOCIATED WITH CHRONIC RENAL FAILUE (CRF) IN THE RAT J. Torres-Noriega* and L. A. Frohman, Division of Endocrinology and Metabolism, Univ. of Cincinnati College of Medicine, Cincinnati, Ohio.

Patients with CRF exhibit hyperprolactinemia and resistance to the prolactin-suppressive effects of dopamine. In order to explore the pathogenetic mechanisms involved, an animal model of CRF was developed in the adult male rat bearing an indwelling right atrial catheter by performing a two stage 5/6 nephrectomy (NX). Following NX, serum creatinine levels rose to a value of 1.3±0.2 mg/dl at 8 weeks as compared to sham-operated controls (0.3±0.1, $p<0.001$). There was a parallel increase in plasma prolactin levels in NX animals with values significantly greater than in controls by 8 weeks (49±11 vs 17±2 ng/ml, $p<0.02$). At 8 weeks, the plasma prolactin responses to metoclopramide (500 µg/kg, iv) were similar in unanesthetized NX and sham-operated control animals (incremental rise: 180±8 vs 150±13 ng/ml). The prolactin-suppressive effects of an iv dopamine infusion (6 ug/kg/min x 30 min) was also similar in the two groups (46±8% vs 40±10% suppression). The responses of lactotrophs in vitro were compared in NX and control animals at 8 weeks in dispersed adenohypophyseal monolayer cultures grown for 3 days in autologous serum-containing medium. Basal prolactin release during 4 h was similar in the two groups as were the suppressive responses to dopamine and bromocriptine. The results indicate that the rat with CRF, like the human, develops hyperprolactinemia. In contrast to the human, however, responses to dopaminergic agonists and antagonists in vivo and in vitro are unimpaired, indicating that hyperprolactinemia in rats with CRF occurs on a non-dopaminergic basis.

2683 PROLACTIN SUPPRESSES PROSTAGLANDIN E_2 PRODUCTION BY HUMAN FETAL MEMBRANE.
J.E. Tyson*, J.A. McCoshen and N. Dubin, Dept. of Obstet., Gynecol., and Reprod. Sci., Univ. of Manitoba, Winnipeg, MB, and Dept. of Gynecol. and Obstet., The Johns Hopkins University, Baltimore, MD.

Prolactin elaborated by human decidua and transported across reflected fetal membrane may affect prostaglandin synthesis by those membranes. Since prostaglandins synthesized by fetal membrane may be involved in the initiation of parturition our study evaluated the effect of ovine prolactin (oPRL) and prostaglandin synthesis by sections of reflected human amnion, choriodecidua and amniochorion with adherent decidua all of which were obtained from elective Caesarean sections. Membranes were secured in two-sided perfusion chambers and exposed to oPRL in concentrations of 0, 1,000 and 10,000 ng/ml of incubation medium. Aliquots of medium were obtained at 0, 30, 60, 120 and 240 minutes from each chamber, quickly frozen and later assayed for prostaglandin E_2 (PGE_2). Multifactorial analysis of variance revealed that PGE_2 production was significantly suppressed in those membranes exposed to 10,000 ng/ml oPRL ($F=13.42$, $P<0.001$). Most obvious was the effect on amnion [3581.0 ± 596.0 SEM versus 1818.8 ± 451.5 pg/ml/mg (n=20)]. PGE_2 production by other membrane combinations was only 9-15% that of amnion. However, production was similarly suppressed by 34-59% when compared to control membranes in the same set. oPRL did not affect PGE_2 production when used in a concentration of 1,000 ng/ml. However, in all instances PGE_2 production was specific to incubation time and type of membrane. Thus, the production of PRL by human decidua and its accumulation in reflected human membrane may affect the elaboration of PGE_2 by such membranes. Supported by the MRC of Canada.

2684 ECTOPIC PITUITARY GRAFTS REDUCE HYPERPROLACTINAEMIA IN ESTROGENIZED FEMALE RATS.
M.D. Vaticón*, C. Fernández Galaz, E. Aguilar and A. Tejero, Depto. Fisiología, Fac. Medicina, Univ. Complutense, Madrid-3, SPAIN.

It is a well known feature that neonatally estrogenized female rats show an elevation of plasma prolactin (PRL) levels in the adult age. In order to assess the effects induced by pituitary grafts from both control and neonatally treated animals on the PRL secretion pattern in control and treated hosts, the following experimental groups (no less than 9 rats each) were utilized: 90 days old female Wistar rats treated on day 5 of life with 100 ug of estradiol benzoate (E) and their age-matched controls (C) received a pituitary transplant from (C) or (E) donors under the right kidney capsule. Additional (C) and (E) animals were sham operated to serve as controls (SC and SE, respectively). Bleeding was performed from jugular vein under light ether anaesthesia 5, 10 and 16 days after the operation. All estimates of PRL are given in terms of the reference preparation NIAMDD Rat-PRL-RP-1. Values are expressed as means ± S.E.M. from the whole studied days. Significance was determined by Student's t-test. In (C) animals an ectopic graft from another control rats significantly increased prolactinaemia (CC 120.8 ± 10.8 vs 13.2 ± 1.5; $P<0.01$) whereas a transplant from (E) resulted in a less marked elevation (CE 46 ± 6.1 vs SC 13.2 ± 1.5; $P<0.001$). In (E) hosts both types of grafts depressed PRL concentrations (EC 54.6 ± 7.7. vs SE 254.5 ± 31.5; $P<0.01$) (EE 53.2 ± 4.8 vs SE 264.5 ± 31.5; $P<0.01$). Nearly identical results were obtained when the pituitary grafting was performed in gonadectomized rats. It is concluded that 1/ ectopic pituitary grafts from (E) rats showed less ability to increase PRL levels, 2/ the transplantation of (C) or (E) pituitaries resulted in a marked modification of PRL control mechanisms in (E) hosts, and 3/ these effects were probably not mediated by gonadal function. This work has been possible trough of the CAICYT nº 4290. Prolactin kit was supplied by the NIAMDD.

2685 A METHOD FOR THE PURIFICATION OF PITUITARY PROLACTIN (PRL) CELLS BY AUTO-FLUORESCENCE-ACTIVATED CELL SORTING (FACS). B. Velkeniers*, G. Smets[1], S. De Boel, M. Van de Winkel[2], D. Pipeleers[2], W. Gepts[1] and L. Vanhaelst. *Dept. of Pharmacology, [1]Dept. of Experimental Pathology and [2]Dept. of Metabolism and Endocrinology, Vrije Universiteit Brussel, Brussels, Belgium.*

The cellular heterogeneity of the pituitary hinders a complete understanding of the physiological and pharmacological regulation of pituitary hormone release. The availability of pituitary cell lines or of purified cell preparations from normal tissue might provide suitable models for the study of these interactions. In the present report, a method is described for the purification of single PRL cells from rat pituitary.

The anterior pituitary was isolated from adult female rats and dissociated until 60 % single cells were obtained. Approximately 2.10^6 cells were prepared per gland; cell viability exceeded 90 %. The pituitary cell suspension was submitted to isopycnic gradient centrifugation employing linear Percoll density gradients (from d 1.045 to 1.090 g/ml). The fractions with density 1.051 to 1.065 g/ml were collected and rinced with Earle's Hepes medium (EH, pH 7.35). This cell fraction was then further purified by FACS according to the cells' light scatter activity and their NAD(P)H-related autofluorescence. The enrichment in PRL cells was assessed by electronmicroscopical and immunocytochemical analysis of the various cell fractions. The present procedure was then found to yield single pituitary cells consisting of 85 % PRL cells. Dopamine (10^{-7} M) prevented degranulation of the PRL cells and was therefore included in the cell medium. The purified cell preparation contained more than 90 % viable cells as measured by neutral red uptake and by cell survival after 48 hrs culture. It is concluded that PRL cells can be purified by a combination of isopycnic gradient centrifugation and FACS.

2686 SEX-RELATED DIFFERENCE OF THE RAT PROLACTIN RESERVE BY TRH ENSUES THROUGH THE INHIBITORY EFFECT OF POSTNATAL TESTOSTERONE OVER THE ANTERIOR PITUITARY TRH RECEPTOR ONTOGENESIS

H.WATANOBE,M.KITAOKA,K.ENDO and K.TAKEBE,Third Department of Internal Medicine,Hirosaki University School of Medicine, 5 Zaifu-cho,Hirosaki-shi,Aomori-ken,Japan.

Upon in vivo thyrotropin releasing hormone(TRH) stimulation following estradiol priming,adult-castrated(AC) female rats and neonatally castrated(NC) males exhibited 4-fold greater plasma PRL responses than that of AC-males. Inhibitory effect of testosterone propionate(TP) substitution(200μg/rat) following NC was apparent at 4 weeks(w),2w and 0w,in descending order of potency. The AP PRL concentration was almost identical among AC-,NC-,and NC+TP(4w)-males with exception of AC-females harboring a 3-fold greater concentration than those of these groups. On the other hand,the AP TRH receptor density of AC-females or NC-males was 2-fold or 3-fold greater than that of AC-males,respectively. These results indicate that(1) the sexual dimorphism of AP PRL reserve by TRH is determined by testosterone less of early postnatal than of later developmental period with marked contrast to its time of action in determining the cyclic secretability of PRL and that(2) this inhibitory effect of testosterone seems to be exerted at least partially by way of its detrimental influence over the AP TRH receptor ontogenesis in male rats.

2687 LACTATION AND BIRTH-SPACING IN HIGHLAND NEW GUINEA. J. Wood*, I. Maslar, P. Johnson and K. Campbell, Reproductive Endocrinology Program and Department of Anthropology, U. of Michigan, Ann Arbor, MI 48109, and Department of Biology, U. of Massachusetts, Boston, MA 02125.

The Gainj are a noncontracepting tribal people of highland New Guinea with low reproductive output (total fertility rate = 4.3), prolonged breastfeeding (median age of children at weaning = 38.6 mos) and long inter-livebirth intervals (mean = 45.4 mos). Endocrinological and behavioral data were used to gauge the impact of breastfeeding on birth intervals in this population. Serum samples were collected from 30 lactating women and analyzed by RIA for P_4, LH/hCG, E_2 and PRL in order to classify the subjects by ovarian function (i.e., luteal, follicular, pregnant or acyclic). Probit analysis of the results indicates that the median duration of puerperal infecundability in lactating mothers is 20.4 ± 4.7 mos, one of the longest ever recorded. Serum PRL levels are consistent with this finding: PRL remains significantly elevated in nursing mothers until about 26 mos postpartum. Nursing bouts were timed in 21 mother-offspring pairs during a standardized 8 hr period (8 am-4 pm). These observations reveal a pattern of frequent bouts of short duration, changing very slowly as the nursing child grows older. The mean interval between nursing bouts is ~30 min among children aged <1 mo and rises to ~70 min in children >36 mos. Path analysis suggests that the frequency of nursing is the principal determinant of maternal PRL levels, with nursing child's age influencing PRL only insofar as it affects the pattern of nursing. We conclude that breastfeeding is the single most important birth-spacing mechanism in this population, primarily because its frequency is high and declines slowly with time.

2688 EFFECTS OF REDUCTION AND ALKYLATION ON HORMONE BINDING TO THE PROLACTIN RECEPTOR ON HEPATOCYTES FROM PREGNANT RATS.
K. Yamada*, K.E. Lipson and D.B. Donner, Memorial Sloan-Kettering Cancer Center, New York, NY 10021

^{125}I-human growth hormone was covalently incorporated into lactogenic complexes of M_r 65,000 and 50,000 on hepatocytes from pregnant rats. The apparent molecular size of these complexes increased slightly after reduction suggesting that intrachain disulfide bonds compact the structure of the prolactin receptor. Digestion of hepatocytes with dithiothreitol diminished the affinity of lactogenic sites for prolactin without altering cellular binding capacity. This was not due to a non-specific effect of dithiothreitol on the cell membrane as reduction augmented the release of ^{125}I-prolactin from solubilized, partially purified receptor. N-ethylmaleimide inhibited the specific binding of ^{125}I-prolactin to lactogenic sites. This resulted from a loss of receptor binding capacity without any substantial effect on the affinity of the prolactin receptor for hormone. These observations suggest that thio and sulfhydryl groups are present in the prolactin receptor and that these functional moieties regulate the formation and properties of prolactin receptor complexes. This study was supported by grants from NIH.

(Abstracts 2777 and 2778, p. 1649, also belong to this section.)

2689 DETECTION OF PROSTAGLANDIN E_2-9-OXOREDUCTASE IN HUMAN DECIDUAL TISSUES.

W. Schlegel[x], S. Krüger and K. Korte, Universitäts-Frauenklinik, Domagkstraße 11, 44oo Münster, Germany

Prostaglandin E_2-9-oxoreductase (PGE_2-9-OR), the enzyme, which converts prostaglandin E_2 (PGE_2) to prostaglandin $F_{2\alpha}$ ($PGF_{2\alpha}$) has been detected in the human decidual vera. The cytoplasmatic fractions of these tissues were used for purification. The enzymatic reaction was monitored by measuring the conversion of PGE_2 to $PGF_{2\alpha}$ in the presence of NADPH. $PGF_{2\alpha}$ was isolated and identified by thin-layer chromatography, radioimmunoassay, autoradiography and HPLC-technique. 22-fold purification was achieved by DEAE-Trisacryl Ultrogel ACA 44 and Hydroxyapatite-Agarosegel chromatographies The final specific activity was 93.3 pmol/min/mg protein. The pH-profile of the enzymatic reaction showed a steep maximum at pH 8.o. A linear regression analysis yielded limiting Michaelis constants (Km(PGE_2) = 64.1 μM, Km(NADPH) = o.72 μM).
Enzyme activities have also been found in the human chorion. The occurence of PGE_2-9-OR in decidua and chorion suggests that this enzyme may be responsible for the transformation of PGE_2 to $PGF_{2\alpha}$ in these tissues. This may be an important mechanism for the initiation and maintainance of uterine contractions. The control mechanism of this enzyme has to be studied in more detail, therefore.

2690 PROSTACYCLIN PRODUCTION AND STEROIDOGENESIS IN GOAT OVARIAN CELLS.

Vimla Sharma*, S.M. Kharbanda, R. Kumar, A.H. Band, K. Murugesan and A. Farooq, Departments of Reproductive Biology, Pathology (Haematology Unit) and Pharmacology, All India Institute of Medical Sciences, NEW DELHI-110029, India.

Prostacyclin (PGI_2) production by granulosa (G), theca (TH) and corpus luteum (CL) cells of the goat ovary was studied in vitro. PGI_2 like activity was measured by the inhibition of adenosine diphosphate induced aggregation of human platelets. CL cells showed the highest spontaneous production of PGI_2 (27.54$\pm$2.61 ng/10^6 cells) followed by G cells (2.32$\pm$0.27 ng/10^6 cells). Addition of arachidonic acid (AA, 2 mM) enhanced PGI_2 production in both CL and G cells. TH cells did not show any detectable PGI_2 like activity even when provided with AA. The production of PGI_2 was further enhanced in both the cell types when trapidil, 100 μg/ml was added alongwith AA, whereas it was completely blocked with U-51605, 10 μg/ml. PGI_2 as well as its stable analog 6β PGI_1 did not affect progesterone (P_4) and estradiol 17B (E_2) production in small doses; with higher doses (1 μg & 10 μg) an increase in P_4 and E_2 production by all the three cell types was observed. AA produced increase in steroid production by all the three cell types which was blocked by aspirin and indomethacin but not by U-51605. AA induced increase in steroids was not enhanced by trapidil. This study revealed that PGI_2 is produced in the goat ovary. Although ovarian steroid production can be modulated by exogenous PGI_2, it is most likely a pharmacologic effect.

2691 RAPID HISTAMINE- AND STEROID-MEDIATED EFFECTS ON PGF PRODUCTION BY HUMAN ENDOMETRIAL CELLS.
S.J.M.Skinner*, G.C.Liggins and T.Wilson, Postgraduate School of Obstetrics and Gynaecology, University of Auckland, Auckland, New Zealand.

The effects of cortisol, progesterone, estradiol and histamine on PGF production by cultured human endometrial cells were studied in perifusion and static incubation systems. Endometrial tissue obtained at hysterectomy was dispersed with collagenase, filtered, washed and the cells cultured overnight. The cells were then washed, aliquots (10^5 cells) placed in filtration chambers and perifused (0.1 ml/min). Fractions (30 min) were collected for RIA of PGF. A stable base-line production of PGF (<0.1 pmol/10^5 cells/h) was achieved after 90 min of perifusion. When histamine (10^{-5}M) was introduced after 120 min, either continuously or as a "pulse" (2.4 min duration), a single peak of PGF (1.1 - 3.8 pmol/10^5 cells/h) was rapidly released into the culture medium. When mepacrine (10^{-5}M), progesterone (10^{-6}M) or cortisol (5 x 10^{-6}M) was introduced into the perifusion medium for 180 min before histamine, the response was inhibited (87 - 95%). When cells in incubation cultures were exposed to estradiol (10^{-7} - 10^{-5}M) for 180 min there was significant stimulation of PGF production (0.8 - 3.9 pmol/10^5 cells/h). The induction of the inhibitory response to progesterone and cortisol, and of the stimulatory response to estradiol, is rapid (<180 min) in comparison with the time necessary for the induction of protein synthesis (e.g. lipomodulin) via steroid receptor-mediated events.

2692 EFFECT OF INHIBITION OF CYCLOOXYGENASE (CO) AND LIPOXYGENASE (LO) PATHWAYS ON ACTH-STIMULATED CORTICOSTEROID AND c-AMP PRODUCTION IN RAT ADRENOCORTICAL CELLS.
K. Tahara*, A. Hirai, H. Saito, Y. Tamura and S. Yoshida, The 2nd Department of Internal Medicine, Chiba University Medical School, Inohana 1-8-1, Chiba 280, Japan.

As an enhancement of PGs synthesis in adrenal glands by ACTH has been reported, the in vitro effect of CO and LO inhibition on corticosteroid and c-AMP production was studied in rat adrenocortical cells when stimulated by ACTH. Indomethacin (CO inhibitor, final conc 12.5∿50 μM) had no effect on both corticosteroid and c-AMP production in ACTH-stimulated adrenocortical cells. Nordihydroguaiaretic acid (NDGA, LO inhibitor 12.5∿50 μM), AA-861 (5LO inhibitor, 13.7∿54.8 μM) and Bromophenacyl bromide (BPB, phospholipase A_2 inhibitor 2.5∿10 μM) markedly decreased corticosteroid production, but had no effect on c-AMP generation. BW755c (CO and LO inhibitor 62.5∿250 μM) showed a significant decrease in both corticosteroid and c-AMP production. No effect on corticosteroid production by indomethacin may suggest that metabolites of CO pathway may not play a role as mediator in steroidogenesis. Uniform suppression of corticosteroid production by inhibition of LO pathway without any change of c-AMP production (except BW755c) indicate that LO metabolites may play an important role in adrenal steroidogenesis, though its mechanism is still unknown.

2693 ROLE OF PROSTAGLANDINS FOR NOREPINEPHRINE(NE) CLEARANCE IN BORDERLINE ESSENTIAL HYPERTENSION.
R.Takeda*, I.Miyamori and H.Koshida, The Second Department of Internal Medicine, School of Medicine, Kanazawa University, Kanazawa 920, Japan.

Studies were done to determine the role of endogenous prostaglandins(PGs) for NE clearance in 10 male borderline hypertensives(age 23 ± 3) and age matched six male controls. 100 ng/Kg/min of ℓ-NE was infused for 60 min at supine. Blood was withdrawn from indwelling catheter at every minute for 10 min. Plasma NE was measured by THI method using HPLC. Disappearance curve of plasma NE was analyzed following the two compartment open model after stopping the infusion. The same protocol was repeated after all the subjects were given 150 mg/day of indomethacin for three days. Basal plasma NE concentration in normotensive controls was 180.8 ± 28.0 pg/ml and in hypertensives 196.9 ± 37.7 pg/ml. These values were not significantly different. Initial half life ($T_{1/2\alpha}$) was 1.50 ± 0.07 min at baseline which decreased to 0.98 ± 0.08min ($P < 0.01$) after indomethacin. In borderline hypertensives $T_{1/2\alpha}$ was 1.03 ± 0.08 ($P < 0.01$ vs normotensive controls) at baseline which was not significantly changed after indomethacin pretreatment. These results may suggest that endogenous PGs have some role for NE clearance in normotensives, possibly exerts inhibitory action at neuronal uptake, whereas in hypertension this effect of PGs will be diminished.

2694 A ROLE OF PHOSPHOLIPASE (A_2&C) AND PROSTAGLANDIN BIOSYNTHESIS FROM THE AMNION IN THE INITIATION OF LABOR.
T. Tsukamoto*, N. Masaoka, K. Akamine, M. Matsuura, B. Tochigi, H. Sakata, T. Yoshida and S. Takagi, Dept. of OB/GYN. Nihon Unive. Sch. of Med. Tokyo, Japan, 173.

The biosynthesis of prostaglandin (PG) which induces a myometrial contractile activity in human is thought to play an important role during the mechanism of labor. Arachidonic acid (AA), which is a precursor of PG, is released from phospholipids by the action of phospholipase A_2 (PLA_2) and C (PLC). In order to study the relationship between PG biosynthesis and labor, PLA_2 and PLC activities and PG biosynthetic activity (PG-BA) in the amnion during spontaneous vaginal deliveries and elective cesarean sections (ECS) in the absence of labor were assayed in vitro. PLA_2 a derivative of AA-^{14}C (PC-SA) and PLC a derivative of inositol-^{14}C (PI) were assayed. PG-BA was estimated for PGE_2 and $F_2\alpha$ and 6keto-$PGF_1\alpha$ synthesized from AA-^{14}C. PLA_2 (60.1pmole/hr/mg pro.) and PLC (1.8nmole/hr/mg pro.) activities in amnions obtained from spontaneous labor are similar to amnions obtained at ECS, and PLC activity is thirty times that of PLA_2. While, PG-BA in amnions with spontaneous labor is higher than that without, and the major PG among the three PGs measured was PGE_2. Thus, PLA_2 and PLC in the amnion are not thought to be the initiating step of human labor.

2695 **ENDOGENOUS PROSTAGLANDINS AND CARDIOSELECTIVE BETA-ADRENOCEPTOR-BLOCKERS IN HYPERTENSION.** S. Vajpeyee*, U. H. Shah, M. P. Patel, G. M. Panchal and S. M. Mansuri, Department of Pharmacology, B. J. Medical College, Ahmedabad 380 016 Gujarat, India.

Renal prostaglandins (PGs) are considered to be the hypotensive substances which maintain a physiological balance with the renin - angiotensin - aldosterone system for regulation of blood pressure. Alterations in the activity of any of these may lead to hypertension. We have studied the effect of PG synthesis inhibition by indomethacin treatment on the hypotensive action of a cardioselective beta-blocker metoprolol vis a vis propranolol, in anaesthetized cats. Mean arterial pressure (MAP) was recorded by cannulating one of the carotid arteries. Propranolol (2 mg/kg i.v.) and metoprolol (0.5 mg/kg i.v.) caused a mean fall of 73.75 ± 14.05 and 78.25 ± 10.73 mm of Hg respectively in the MAP. The fall was steep but recovery was gradual. Indomethacin (20 mg/kg i.p.) caused a slight fall in MAP lasting for not more than 10 min. However, the mean reduction in MAP produced by propranolol and metoprolol in indomethacin treated animals was 53.75 ± 14.19 and 63.7 ± 12.48 mm of Hg respectively. Moreover the recovery was much quicker in the latter. These findings indicate that indomethacin treatment attenuates the hypotensive effect of both the cardioselective as well as non-selective beta-blockers suggesting that the endogenous PGs are possibly involved in this effect at least in this experimental model and probably in other clinical situations as well. (This work was supported by a financial grant from the Medical Research Centre, Bombay Hospital Trust, Bombay).

2696 Prostaglandins: a first investigation of their actions on blood pressure, renal function and steroid production in a lower vertebrate.
N. A. M. Wales* and T. Gaunt. Department of Zoology, The University of Sheffield, Sheffield, S10 2TN and Department of Biological Sciences, Sheffield City Polytechnic, Sheffield, S1 1WB, England.
Seawater adapted eels were implanted with both venous and arterial cannulae and catheterised. Prostaglandins (PGs) in 0.9% saline was given either by 10 μl injection or by infusion (40 ng/min.) whilst blood pressure and blood samples were taken from the dorsal aorta. Glomerular filtration rates were calculated from the clearance of 3H inulin, renal plasma flow from the clearance of PAH and functional tubular mass from measurements of glucose reabsorption maxima (TmG). Cortisol levels were measured by radioimmunoassay. Injections of PGs E_1, E_2 and A_2 (0.01-1.0ng/k) induced transient reductions in dorsal aortic blood pressure whilst concentrations of between 10-100 ng/k caused both prolonged vasodepression and glomerular antidiuresis, with decreased TmG and decreased CPAH. Relative electrolyte excretion rates remained unchanged. Doses of 10-50 µg/k caused an initial glomerular diuresis, increased TmG and CPAH but were without effect on relative electrolyte excretion rates. This diuretic action was followed by a longer period of antidiuresis. Similar doses of PGs $F_{2\alpha}$ were slightly vasopressor but with no obvious effect on kidney function. The vasodepression during 24h PG infusion became less severe after an initial 2h period, indicating a degree of tachyphylaxis. All PGs so far used, given either by infusion or injection caused a significant increase in cortisol production. These results suggest that prostaglandins may play similar roles throughout a range of vertebrates.

2697 COMPARISON OF STORAGE TEMPERATURES ON LEVELS OF PROSTANOIDS IN UTERINE AND PLACENTAL TISSUE OF THE RAT. L. Wilson,Jr.* and L. S. Huang, Dept. of Obstet. Gynecol., Univ. of IL. Med. Sch., Chicago, IL 60612 USA.

Although several studies have reported on the stability of plasma prostanoids at different temperatures, similar reports on tissue levels are mostly anecdotal. The purpose of the present study was to compare the levels of Prostaglandin (PG)E, PGF, Thromboxane B_2 (TxB_2) and 6-Keto-PGF_1 (6KF) in uterine and placental tissue stored frozen at -20°C, -70°C and -196°C (liquid nitrogen) for 6 months. These tissues were collected from rats sacrificed on day 21 of pregnancy. The prostanoids were analyzed by radioimmunoassay after extraction and column chromatography. Results:

PG (ng/g)	Uterus -20°	Uterus -70°	Uterus -196°	Placenta -20°	Placenta -70°	Placenta -196°
PGF	510*($p<.05$)	79	105	20*	3	3
PGE	224*	24	26	26*	2	2
TxB_2	299	310	320	4	3	3
6KF	216	194	153	7*	2	2

Tissues stored at -20°C had levels of PGF and PGE 6 to 9 x greater than at -70 or -196. Similarly, 6KF was higher in the placenta. In distinct contrast, TxB_2 in uterine and placental tissue and 6KF in uterine tissue showed no statistical differences ($p>.05$). In conclusion, these results indicate that: 1) -20°C is not an adequate temperature to prevent PGF and PGE production in uterine and placental tissue and 6KF synthesis in the placenta, but can prevent TxB_2 production in the uterus and placenta and 6KF synthesis in the uterus; 2) the pathways for production of these prostanoids show a differential sensitivity to temperature within the same tissue and between different tissues.

2698 PARTIAL PURIFICATION AND CHARACTERISATION OF TWO PHOSPHOLIPASE INHIBITORS IN HUMAN AMNIOTIC FLUID. T.Wilson*, and G.C.Liggins, Postgraduate School of Obstetrics and Gynaecology, National Women's Hospital, Claude Road, Auckland, 3, New Zealand.

A current hypothesis proposes that parturition is prevented during pregnancy by a factor that inhibits prostaglandin synthesis within the uterus. To test the hypothesis we sought such a factor in amniotic fluid of term patients who had not started labor. As an assay system we used human endometrial cells in which prostaglandin synthesis was stimulated by histamine (10^{-5}M) or bradykinin (10^{-6}M). We determined the presence of inhibitors of prostaglandin synthesis by a decrease in prostaglandin F (PGF) production or [^{3}H]-arachidonate ([^{3}H]-aa) release. Two inhibitors having respective molecular weights of 160,000 - 180,000 (Inhibitor I) and 75,000 - 80,000 (Inhibitor II) as estimated by gel filtration in 2 systems were found. Both caused a decrease in prostaglandin production. Inhibitor I (10^{-7}M) reduced histamine stimulated PGF production by 52 ± 22% and Inhibitor II (5 x 10^{-6}M) reduced production of PGF by 39% ± 9.2%. Neither inhibitor reduced arachidonic acid - stimulated production of PGF. Inhibitor I at a concentration below 10^{-8}M caused a reduction in [^{3}H]-aa release stimulated by histamine (70 ± 14% reduction) or bradykinin (51 ± 22% reduction). Inhibitor II at a concentration below 5 x 10^{-7}M caused a reduction in the same system stimulated by histamine (67 ± 9%) or bradykinin (82%). Activity of both inhibitors was lost on digestion with trypsin or on heating. These highly potent compounds could act to regulate prostaglandin synthesis during pregnancy.

2699 ANTI-MULLERIAN HORMONE IN BOVINE FREEMARTINS. B. Vigier*, D. Tran, J.Y. Picard, J. Bézard, L. Legeai, and N. Josso, Unité de Recherches de Génétique Médicale INSERM, Hôpital des Enfants-Malades, 75743 Paris Cedex 15, France.

Freemartin heifers, bovine females united by chorionic anastomoses to a male twin, are characterized by extensive regression of their Müllerian ducts, which occurs simultaneously in both twins early in fetal life. Virilization may also affect the gonads of the freemartins, in which seminiferous tubules may develop in late pregnancy. To determine whether anti-Müllerian hormone (AMH) in the freemartin is of exogenous or endogenous origin, we studied 28 freemartin fetuses and 3 newborns. At the time their Müllerian ducts regress, serum AMH, measured by a 2-site RIA using 2 distinct monoclonal antibodies, is high and identical in both twins. In contrast, in vitro production of AMH by the freemartin gonad is seen in only 2 out of 13 fetuses, and is negligible compared to the testicular output of AMH. After 80 days of gestation, serum AMH levels decrease, as they do in the normal male fetus, and AMH production can be detected in 6 out of 15 freemartin gonads, those which happen to have developed seminiferous tubules. The amount of endogenous AMH produced by the freemartin is, however, negligible compared to that contributed by the male twin, as shown by comparison of in vitro production of AMH by freemartin and male gonads and by the fact that serum AMH is not significantly higher in those freemartins whose gonads do produce AMH. At birth, AMH disappears from the serum of freemartin heifers within 10 days, its half-life being similar to that measured in males after castration. In conclusion, our results show that regression of Müllerian ducts in the freemartin fetus is induced by exogenous AMH of testicular origin. Production of AMH by the freemartin gonad itself occurs too late to affect Müllerian development, and represents both an acceleration and an increase of the capacity of normal bovine granulosa cells to produce AMH (Vigier et al. 1984).

2700 EFFECTIVE LONG-TERM SUPPRESSION OF CENTRAL PRECOCIOUS PUBERTY (CPP) IN A 3 YEAR OLD MALE WITH LHRH ANALOGUE D-SER (TBU)^{6} - LHRH 1-9E^{10} (HOE 766). G. Wielgosz*, A. Fazekas, M.R. Jenner. Dept. of Paediatrics, University of Western Ontario, London, Canada and Hoechst-Canada, Montreal, Canada.

A boy with central precocious puberty (CPP) resistant to depo Provera and cyproterone acetate was treated with HOE 766. Treatment for 2 months with 120 ug/kg t.i.d. intranasally followed by 12 months with 30 ug/kg b.i.d. subcutaneously resulted in clinical improvement as demonstrated by a reduction in sebaceous activity, decreased height velocity [1.4 cm/mo (pre Rx) vs. 0.2 cm/mo (post Rx)] and rate of bone maturation. Serum androgen levels fell from 1641 ng/dl (pre Rx) to 46 ng/dl (post Rx). However, the HOE 766 treatment resulted in an increase in both basal and peak serum LH levels following LHRH stimulation test suggesting an incomplete 'down regulation' effect on the pituitary in the presence of clinical improvement. In summary, our data indicate that HOE 766 is effective in the treatment of a male with CPP resistent to other forms of therapy.

2701 USE OF AN LHRH ANALOGUE ($LHRH_a$) IN THE TREATMENT OF CENTRAL PRECOCIOUS PUBERTY (CPP). M. Wierman*, D. Beardsworth, J. Mansfield, D. Kushner, J. Crawford, J. Crigler, H. Bode and W. Crowley. Depts Gyn, Med and Ped, Vincent Labs, Massachusetts General Hospital, Children's Hospital, Boston, MA 02114.

$LHRH_a$ (4-8 ug/kg sc qd) was administered to 42 children (38♀, 4♂), with central precocious puberty (CPP) for 3-42 months. Prior to therapy, all patients demonstrated a pulsatile pattern of gonadotropin release and a mature response to LHRH. $LHRH_a$ administration uniformly resulted in an arrest or regression of the clinical signs of puberty, suppression of sex steroid levels, ablation of the pulsatile pattern of gonadotropin secretion, and a return to a prepubertal response to exogenous LHRH. Growth velocities fell to prepubertal levels and the rate of skeletal advancement for chronological advancement ($\Delta BA/\Delta CA$) was also slowed significantly (≤ 1) so that predicted height increased in the majority of patients. Dehydroepiandrosterone sulfate levels (DS), as an index of adrenal maturation, were constant or increased in an age expected fashion. In 18 girls evaluated, DS values pre- and post-$LHRH_a$ therapy were positively correlated with rate of skeletal advancement ($r = .72$, $p < .001$) and negatively correlated ($r = -.62$, $p = .006$) with increase in predicted height suggesting a direct role of adrenal androgens upon bone maturation during puberty. Summary: 1) $LHRH_a$ therapy is uniformly effective in the treatment of central precocious puberty. 2) Removal of gonadal sex steroids with $LHRH_a$ reveals an effect of adrenal androgens upon skeletal maturation. 3) $LHRH_a$ is a selective probe with which to investigate the complex processes involved in pubertal development. Supported by HD18169.

2702 PUBERTY WITHOUT GONADOTROPINS - A NOVEL MECHANISM OF SEXUAL DEVELOPMENT. M. Wierman*, D. Beardsworth, T. Badger, J. Mansfield, J. Crawford, J. Crigler, H. Bode, R. Scully, W. Hoffman and W. Crowley. Depts Gyn, Med and Ped, Vincent Labs, Mass. General Hospital, Children's Hospital, Boston, MA.

Precocious sexual development may be classified into pseudoprecocity, central precocious puberty (CPP) and a new subset of sexual maturation - gonadotropin independent precocity (GIP). To define GIP more precisely, 4♂ and 5♀ with CPP were contrasted with 6♂ and 1♀ with GIP. The two subsets (CPP vs GIP) were similar in terms of age of onset of precocity (5.87±.91 vs 3.2±.98 yrs), degree of sexual maturation (Tanner stage 3.5±.29 vs 3.4±.34), growth velocity (13.45±2.73 vs 10.58±1.42 cm/yr) and skeletal development (12.94±.36 vs 12.04±.62 yrs). In ♂ with GIP, a family history of precocity was noted in 3/5 families. Children with CPP demonstrated pulsatile release of gonadotropins, mature responses to LHRH and uniform suppression of gonadarche on an LHRH analogue ($LHRH_a$). By contrast, children with GIP demonstrated absence of gonadotropin pulsations, variable responses to LHRH and uniform progression of gonadarche despite $LHRH_a$. A cyclic pattern of sex steroid secretion was noted in GIP on or off $LHRH_a$. Bioassayable LH ranged from undetectable to prepubertal in GIP. Testicular biopsies in 5/6 boys with GIP ranged from normal to Leydig cell hyperplasia. Conclusions: 1) A subset of children exists in which sexual development is mediated independent of gonadotropin secretion. 2) Cyclicity of sex hormone release and a familial occurrence are common features of this disorder. 3) Prepubertal bio- and immunoassayable LH levels, a variable response to LHRH, and resistance to $LHRH_a$ are consistent features which document the gonadotropin independent pathophysiology of this syndrome. Supported by HD18169.

2703 REPRODUCTIVE HORMONE SECRETION AND TESTICULAR GONADOTROPIN RECEPTORS IN THE RAM LAMB. T.A. Yarney*[1], L.M. Sanford[1,2] and M.R. Sairam[3]. McGill Centre for the Study of Reproduction, Departments of Animal Science[1] and Obstetrics and Gynecology[2], Macdonald College of McGill University, Ste Anne de Bellevue, Clinical Research Institute of Montreal[3], H9X 1C0, Canada.

Testicular gonadotropin receptors and testis weight, and serum levels of LH, FSH, prolactin (PRL) and testosterone (T) were examined for March-born ram lambs. Serial blood samples were obtained from groups of four lambs at 30, 60, 90, 120, 150 and 200 days of age. Lambs were then sacrificed and their testes removed, weighed and stored at -75°C until receptor analysis. Testis weight and serum T level increased progressively from 60 through 200 days of age; increases in testis weight and T level became prominent between 90 and 120 days, and between 150 and 200 days, respectively. FSH receptors per g testis increased from 30 days to peak concentrations at 60 and 90 days and then declined. The total number of FSH receptors per testis increased with advancing age. Mean FSH levels increased from 30 days to a maximum between 60 and 90 days of age and decreased thereafter. Basal LH levels and LH-pulse frequency increased between 30 and 90 days, declined slightly by 150 days, and increased again to their highest values at 200 days of age. The magnitude of LH pulses was relatively high between 30 and 90 days and then decreased steadily. Increases in total number of LH receptors paralleled testis growth. Marked increases in LH-receptor concentration occurred concurrently with elevations in T secretion. Mean PRL levels were relatively high between 120 and 150 days of age. Data indicate that increases in gonadotropin receptor numbers enhance the stimulatory effects of gonadotropic hormones on testicular development of ram lambs. (Supported by MRC of Canada).

2704 CONTROL OF PROGESTERONE RECEPTOR SYNTHESIS IN THE FETAL GUINEA PIG UTERUS IN CULTURE. C. Sumida*, C. Gelly and J.R. Pasqualini, CNRS Steroid Hormone Research Unit, Foundation for Hormone Res., 26 Bd Brune, 75014 Paris, France

Recent studies from this laboratory have demonstrated synthesis of progesterone receptor (PR) in explants of fetal guinea pig uterus in organ culture, but PR increased even in hormone-free medium. The present series of studies was undertaken to see whether PR synthesis effectively escapes estrogen (E) control. Explants of fetal uterus (50-65 days of gestation) were cultured in Medium 199. In the absence of any estrogens, PR rises between 1 and 2 days of culture from 3.20 ± 1.26 (SD) pmol/mg DNA to 11.00 ± 4.14. This increase is inhibited by Actinomycin D and Cycloheximide (10 μg/ml) indicating new synthesis of PR protein. Simultaneously, ER (cytosol + nuclear) decreases from 12.81 ± 1.96 before culture to values between non-detectable and 2.14 after only 1 day in culture with no further significant variation. The synthesis of PR in culture is inhibited by progesterone (P) but can be restored by removal of P from the medium. Even when fetuses are first E-primed (1 mg E/kg b.w. to the mother 1 day prior to sacrifice) so that PR is 18.24 ± 5.8 before culture, PR synthesizing capacity is not exhausted since after a transitory drop in PR to 3.63 ± 0.91 new synthesis of PR reappears on day 2. Adding 5×10^{-8}M P to the medium rapidly decreases PR but the explants retain their PR synthesizing capability since subsequent removal of P leads to a second rise in PR, the entire process occurring in the presence of less than 1 pmol/mg DNA of ER and with no response to 5×10^{-8}M E. The present data show that fetal uterine explants retain their ability to synthesize PR in organ culture even after prior inhibition by progesterone and in the apparent absence of estrogens and with very low levels of ER.

2705 IMMUNOLOGICAL STUDIES OF THE SUBUNIT STRUCTURE OF THE 8.5S RABBIT UTERINE PROGESTIN RECEPTOR. P.-K., K. Tai*, and L. Faber, Medical College of Ohio, C.S. #10008, Toledo, Ohio 43699, USA.

Employing our monoclonal antiprogestin receptor antibody, we found that nonactivated 8.5S rabbit progestin receptor contains Mr ≅ 92,000 and Mr ≅ 60,000 peptides. Sucrose gradient analyses revealed that the two subunits dissociate during a 16-17 hr ultracentrifugation in the absence of Na_2MoO_4. SDS PAGE analysis of receptor, affinity purified with monoclonal antibody coupled to Affigel-10, suggested that the Mr ≅ 92,000 peptide may be a steroid binding component and that the Mr ≅ 60,000 peptide is a non-steroid binding peptide containing the epitopic site. Further work with the immuno adsorbant suggests that the Mr ≅ 92,000 and Mr ≅ 60,000 components associate with a greater affinity than previously suspected. In the absence of Na_2MoO_4 neither incubation at 20°C for 2 hr, 300 mM KCl (30 min 20°C, +3 hr 4°C), nor $(NH_4)_2SO_4$ precipitation completely dissociate the subunits. Surprisingly the 300 mM KCl treatment resulted in release of bound steroid prior to immunoadsorption. Both subunits were isolated from the immunosupport indicating that the above treatments did not result in complete dissociation. The two subunits apparently could be separated only by a 16-17 hr ultracentrifugation in sucrose gradients lacking Na_2MoO_4. Under these conditions the Mr ≅ 60,000 peptide (free of Mr ≅ 92,000 peptide) could be immunoadsorbed from the low molecular weight region of the gradient. From these and additional studies we have concluded that KCl causes release of the progestin prior to separation of the subunits, that sucrose gradient analysis may result in dissociation of components, and that the dissociation of the subunits and the steroid is a highly complex process. Supported by HD-09367 and AG-02776.

2706 BIOLOGICAL IMPLICATION OF STEROID RECEPTOR LEVELS IN HUMAN UTERINE STROMA AND DECIDUA FOR THE PROCESS OF DECIDUALIZATION. T. Tamaya*, N. Ide and H. Okada, Dept. of OB/GYN, Kyoto Pref. Univ. of Med., Kyoto 602, Japan.

This study was designed to understand steroid action for decidualization of stromal cells from the steroid receptor interaction in the human uterine endometrium. Dispersed endometrial stroma cells contained receptors for estrogen (ER), progesterone (PR) and androgen (AR). Dissected uterine and ovarian arteries contained cytosol ER, and AR, but not PR. Human pregnant uterine decidua contained ER, PR and AR, which increased at the level as the advance of the gestation, at least during the first trimester. In cultured endometrial fibroblasts, these three receptors were detected and estrogen stimulated such receptor syntheses, but progesterone decreased these stimulations. These findings suggested that estrogen stimulates steroid receptor synthesis in mesenchymal fibroblasts around the uterine spiral arteries and that progesterone together with estrogen via these receptors differentiates fibroblasts to decidual cells, where steroid receptor levels increase as decidua for steroid action during the early pregnancy.

2707 INTERPRETATION OF ESTROGEN RECEPTOR-NEGATIVE, PROGESTERONE RECEPTOR-POSITIVE HUMAN BREAST TUMOR ASSAYS. H. D. Tildesley and W. A. McBlain*, Department of Medicine, University of Alberta, Edmonton, Alberta, Canada T6G 2G3

Progesterone receptor (PgR) of human breast tumors is probably synthesized as an end-product of estrogen action; thus tumors containing PgR should have a functional estrogen-response pathway including estrogen receptor (ER) and ER-negative, PgR-positive (ER-ve, PgR+ve) tumors should be rare. Of 1197 tumors assayed over 17 mos we found 104 (8.7%) to be ER-ve, PgR+ve and we have investigated this finding. Tumors homogenized in buffer (10 mM Tris, 1.5 mM EDTA, 12 mM thioglycerol, 10% (v/v glycerol, pH 7.4 at 22°C, ±10 mM Na_2MoO_4) were centrifuged 30 min at 200,000 × g. The cytosol was incubated 18h with 0.1-5 nM [^{3}H]estradiol or [^{3}H]R5020 plus 10-fold excesses of dexamethasone and dihydrotestosterone with or without 100-fold excesses of unlabeled DES or R5020, respectively. Binding data from dextran-coated charcoal (DCC) assays were analyzed by the method of Scatchard. Preliminary data analyses indicate 3 variables which preferentially stabilize PgR: 1. Molybdate buffer prevents a 78.1±4.6% loss of PgR and a 46.9±8.2% loss of ER (means±SEM, $p<0.05$, analysis of covariance, n=20). 2. Excess homogenization (30 sec Polytron) of powdered tumors results in more loss of ER than PgR (65.8±4.5 and 33.4±1.1% losses, respectively, n=3). Shaking of plastic assay tubes during the DCC assay causes a 54.2±3.2% loss of ER but a PgR loss of only 20.5±5.6% ($p<0.05$, n=11). In addition, ER could be occupied by endogenous estrogen and a 30°C steroid exchange revealed ER in 5 of 42 (11.9%) ER-ve, PgR+ve tumors. Benign tissues can also be ER-ve, PgR+ve. To interpret ER-ve, PgR+ve results correctly, stabilization of ER, tissue pathology and repeat or exchange assays should be considered.

2708 CELLULAR STEROID RECEPTORS IN HUMAN ENDOMETRIA. Urmila Verma*, K. Murugesan, V.L. Bhargava, K.R. Laumas and A. Farooq, Department of Reproductive Biology and Obstetrics & Gynecology, All India Institute of Medical Sciences, NEW DELHI-110029, India.

Estrogen and progesterone receptors in human endometrial tissue from normal and pathological tissues were determined. Throughout the normal menstrual cycle, the receptor levels showed changes in relation with the circulating endogenous hormone concentration. Characterization of receptors revealed similarity between the biochemical properties of estrogen and progesterone receptors of normal endometrium and those of endometrial carcinoma. After radiotherapy, both estrogen and progesterone receptor levels decreased in endometrial carcinoma. Using a large number of progestins and antiprogestins the specificity of progesterone receptor was comparable in normal proliferative and secretory endometrium, endometrial hyperplasia and endometrial carcinoma. This study revealed that the presence of progesterone receptor system is a critical factor in the effectiveness of hormone therapy in endometrial carcinoma.

2709 INDUCTION OF RAT PITUITARY PROGESTERONE RECEPTORS BY A NON-AROMATIZABLE A-RING REDUCED METABOLITE OF NORETHISTERONE (NET). F. Vilchis*, B. Chávez, A. E. Pérez, G.A. García, S. Poucell and G. Pérez-Palacios, Department of Reproductive Biology, National Institute of Nutrition S.Z., 14000 México, D. F., México.

Previous studies from this laboratory have demonstrated that 17α-ethynyl-5α-estran-3β,17β-diol (3β,5α-NET), a metabolite of NET, specifically interacts with cytosol estradiol receptors. To assess the biological expression of such interaction, the effect of varying doses of 3β,5α-NET upon the induction of pituitary progesterone receptors (PR) was studied in castrated rats. 3β,5α-NET was s.c. administered (300,600, or 1000 μg) to castrated female rats. Pituitary PR were labeled *in vitro* by a post-gradient technique using [^{3}H]-ORG 2058 as radioligand. Receptor binding specificity was assessed by the addition of an excess of radioinert natural and synthetic steroids. The results indicated that 3β,5α-NET induced the synthesis of the pituitary cytosol specific 7S PR in an identical manner to that observed in the estradiol (E_2)-treated control rats. The pituitary PR induction by 3β,5α-NET exhibited a dose-response parallelism. In addition 3β,5α-NET also induced uterine growth and vaginal keratinization. The morphological uterine changes were identical to those obtained with E_2. The overall data demonstrated that a non-aromatizable NET metabolite induced typical biochemical and morphological estrogenic responses, thus providing support to the understanding of the *in vivo* estrogen-like effects of NET.

(Supported by the W.H.O. (HRP), The Rockefeller Foundation, and CONACYT).

2710 **ISOLATION OF PROTEIN KINASES FROM CHICKEN OVIDUCT WHICH PHOSPHORYLATE THE PROGESTERONE RECEPTOR *IN VITRO*,** **N. L. Weigel*, Department of Cell Biology, Baylor College of Medicine, Houston, Tx. 77030 U.S.A.**

The chicken progesterone receptor contains two hormone binding subunits, A(M_r=79,000) and B(M_r=108,000). We have previously reported that the B subunit, and to a lesser extent, the A subunit can be phosphorylated by the catalytic subunit of cAMP dependent protein kinase from bovine heart (Weigel *et al.*, (1981) Biochem. Biophys. Res. Commun. 102, 513). We have now found a protein kinase which co-purifies with the A subunit and which phosphorylates the A protein more effectively than the cAMP dependent protein kinase. This kinase is partially resolved by chromatography on heparin sepharose and can be completely separated from the A by passing the preparation through an anti-A IgM affinity column. The eluted A, which has no kinase activity, can be phosphorylated by the kinase present in the flow through fraction. This endogenous kinase will be useful in studies of the effects of phosphorylation on receptor function and regulation. A second kinase which phosphorylates the B subunit has been found in partially purified B preparations. This kinase is partially separated from B by chromatography on DEAE Sephadex and has been further purified by chromatography using immobilized cibacron blue F3GA. The receptor is not retained by the column and the enzyme can be eluted with ATP and NaCl. These results suggest that the B subunit is not itself a kinase as reported by other workers. **This study was supported by the Chicago Community Trust/Searle Scholars Program.**

2711 NUCLEAR AND CYTOSOLIC ESTROGEN RECEPTORS IN THE MACAQUE CERVIX, ENDOMETRIUM AND OVIDUCT DURING SEQUENTIAL ESTRADIOL-PROGESTERONE TREATMENT.
N. B. West* and R. M. Brenner, Reproductive Biology and Behavior, Oregon Regional Primate Research Center, Beaverton, OR 97006

We compared nuclear and cytosolic estrogen receptor levels in reproductive tracts of spayed cynomolgus macaques that were either untreated, treated for 14 days with implants of estradiol (E_2), or treated first for 14 days with E_2 and then for various periods with combinations of E_2 and either one or two progesterone (P) implants (sequential treatment). In the endometrium, nuclear receptors (fmol/mg DNA) increased significantly from 86 $\pm$ 20 (n=4) in untreated animals to 1582 $\pm$ 233 (n=5) after 14 days E_2; cytosolic receptors (fmol/mg DNA) in the endometrium increased significantly from 4387 $\pm$ 1116 (n=4) to 7634 $\pm$ 657 (n=5) in the same groups. In the cervix, nuclear receptors increased significantly from 472 $\pm$ 212 (n=4) to 1201 $\pm$ 167 (n=12) after 14 days E_2. Sequential treatment with one P implant for 14 days reduced endometrial nuclear receptors to 352 $\pm$ 184 (n=6) and also reduced cytosolic receptors similarly to 924 $\pm$ 112 (n=6). Cervical nuclear receptor levels were not reduced by sequential treatment with one P implant for either 14 or 21 days, but were significantly reduced to 510 $\pm$ 99 (n=7) when two P implants were used for 14 days. In both the oviduct and the endometrium, nuclear and cytosolic receptor levels were significantly decreased by 6 days of sequential treatment and in some animals substantial decreases were apparent by 1 or 2 days. Thus, higher serum P levels appear to be required to suppress estrogen receptors in the cervix than in the oviduct or endometrium of cynomolgus macaques. Supported by NIH grants HD-05969 and RR-00163.

2712 ISOFORMS OF ESTROGEN RECEPTORS DETECTED BY HIGH PERFORMANCE LIQUID CHROMATOGRAPHY (HPLC) METHODOLOGIES. Ronald D. Wiehle*, Nahid A. Shahabi, and James L. Wittliff, Hormone Receptor Laboratory, James Graham Brown Cancer Center and Department of Biochemistry, University of Louisville, Louisville, KY 40292, USA

Characterization of isoforms of the estrogen receptor from hormone responsive organs, such as human uterus and breast cancer and mammary gland of the lactating rat, has been accomplished using HPLC in size exclusion, chromatofocusing and ion-exchange modes. Previously we reported our use of high performance size exclusion chromatography (HPSEC) with TSK 3000 SW columns and high performance chromatofocusing (HPCF) using the AX-500 column. We have recently developed high performance ion exchange chromatography (HPIEC) using the AX-300, AX-500, and AX-1000 columns with linear gradients of potassium phosphate for receptor elution. HPSEC separated as many as 3 isoforms of the receptor on the basis of size. HPCF distinguished up to 5 isoforms on the basis of surface change in a fashion somewhat unlike isoelectric focusing or open column chromatofocusing. Two isoforms were identified by HPIEC similar to profiles obtained with conventional DE-52 chromatography. In each case, the apparent hydrophobic nature of the high performance column complicated the interpretation of the results although unambiguous data can now be obtained with appropriate controls. The effect of various modifiers of receptor structure (molybdate, leupeptin, TLCK) are being explored with regard to isoform profile. Supported in part by the Marie Overbey Memorial Grant from the American Cancer Society, by Phi Beta Psi Sorority and by the Graduate School, University of Louisville.

2713 MOLECULAR SPECIES DIFFERENCE OF CYTOPLASMIC PROGESTERONE RECEPTORS IN OVIDUCT OF REPRODUCTIVE ACTIVE AND QUIESCENT TURKEYS (MELEAGRIS GALLAPAVA).
Winston C. Y. Yu*, Benjamin S. Leung, M. El Halawani, Larry S. Stout, Dept. of OB/GYN and Dept. of Animal Science, University of Minnesota, Minneapolis MN 55455

Cytoplasmic progesterone receptors (PRc) from the reproductive tract of female turkeys at different stages of their reproductive cycle were analyzed by HPLC using a DEAE ion-exchange column. Four groups of turkeys were used: 1) laying birds that have laid eggs regularly up to the date of experiment; 2) broody birds that were on the nest 6 or 7 times each day for at least 2 weeks without producing eggs, and showed aggressive nest-protective behavior when disturbed; 3) photorefractory birds that had neither laid nor nested for at least 2 weeks despite the 15L :9D long-day photoperiod; 4) dark birds that were under the 9L : 15D short-day photoperiod and ready to be photostimulated into egg production. Laying bird uterus contained only one species of PRc which was eluted around 0.260M of salt concentration from DEAE column whereas two molecular species of PRc with elution salt concentrations of 0.226M and 0.260, respectively, were identified in the reproductive tract of broody, photorefractory and dark birds. When analyzed by ultracentrifugation on a 10-30% sucrose gradient, both species of the PRc showed sedimentation coefficient around 4S suggesting that they were about equal in molecular weight. However, with the presence of molybdate in buffer system, only one type of PRc was detected at about 0.224M. Quantitatively, laying bird uterus contained the most PRc than any of the other three reproductive quiescent tissues. PRc binding to DNA-cellulose were observed with all the reproductive stages.
(Supported in part by PHS grant number RO1 CA25998 awarded by NCI, DHHS).

2714 PUTATIVE PHYSIOLOGIC HIGH AFFINITY BINDING SITES FOR ESTRADIOL 17-β (E_2) IN THE ANTERIOR PITUITARY.
J. Zolman* and T. Theodoropoulos. The University of Texas Medical Branch, Galveston, Texas, U.S.A.

$^{125}I-E_2$ specific binding to subcellular fractions of the bovine anterior pituitary is dependent on the amount of protein, hormone concentration and time of hormone exposure. To characterize the putative binding sites in such fractions, we employed physiologic concentrations of $^{125}I-E_2$ of high specific activity (1500 Ci/mmol). The subcellular fractions were obtained by differential centrifugation on discontinuous sucrose gradients. The binding was measured after incubation in Tris-HCl buffer (pH 7.4, 37°C) for 15, 30, 60, 90, 120 min and 24 hrs in the 10^{-11} to 10^{-10}M concentration range. The binding capacities were 0.20 ± 0.02, 0.36 ± 0.03, 0.02 ± 0.004 and 0.06 ± 0.009 (mean ± SE, fmol/μg protein) at 10^{-10}M E_2 for isolated plasma membranes, nuclei, microsomes and secretory granules respectively. The association kinetics suggested the presence of more than one binding sites of high affinity. Scatchard plots were curvilinear and Hill coefficients were >1, suggesting positively cooperative interaction. The binding to membranes and nuclei was highest at 24 hrs of incubation, while the binding to microsomes and granules culminated at 90 min. We conclude that E_2 in physiologic concentrations binds to specific binding sites in the subcellular fractions of the bovine anterior pituitary with high affinity and the binding exhibits complex kinetics compatible with positive cooperativity. E_2 bound with high affinity to plasma membranes probably modulates GnRH receptor.

2715 ISOLATION OF CHEMICALLY DEMONSTRABLE QUANTITIES OF NUCLEAR ANDROGEN RECEPTOR. M. To*, N. Bruchovsky, P.S. Rennie and Y. Lefebvre, Department of Cancer Endocrinology, Cancer Control Agency of British Columbia, Vancouver, British Columbia, V5Z 3J3, Canada.

Owing to the high concentration of nuclear androgen receptor (NAR) in rat ventral prostate, it is theoretically possible to recover enough receptor from this source to enable its direct visualization by silver nitrate staining (threshold sensitivity, 5-10 ng). Since we have shown that the prostatic nucleus contains about 20,000 molecules of NAR with a MW of 33,000, each gram of tissue containing an average of 1.5×10^8 nuclei and 3 mg of nuclear protein would yield 165 ng of NAR; thus, purification to homogeneity would require an 18,000-fold enrichment. We are developing methods suitable for processing 2000 ng of NAR through a series of purification steps. Micrococcal nuclease digestion (1) of chromatin leads to precipitation of 95% of NAR which is then incubated with Matrex Gel Green A (2) and eluted with a 0-2M NaCl gradient. After (2) 35% of NAR is recovered and can be identified using polyacrylamide gel electrophoresis and silver staining as a 34,000 MW band which is greatly reduced by castration. NAR can be further processed through gel-exclusion chromatography on Sephadex G-75 (3), lyophilization (4) and affinity chromatography with dihydrotestosterone (DHT)-17β-succinyl agarose (5). The yield after (5) is about 400 ng NAR which can be eluted with 75 μM DHT and recovered using (2) with on column labelling in the presence of ^{3}H-DHT. Using these techniques the purification of chemically detectable quantities of NAR may be possible. (Supported by MRC).

2716 EFFECTS OF MOLYBDATE AND KCl ON DISAGGREGATION OF CYTOSOLIC ANDROGEN RECEPTORS OF RAT VENTRAL PROSTATE, A.M. Traish*, R.E. Müller and H.H. Wotiz. Boston University School of Medicine, 80 E. Concord Street Boston, MA 02118 USA

Cytosolic androgen receptor complexes (AR) formed *in vitro* at 0°C sediment as 8-10S entities on low salt sucrose density gradients (SDG) and 4-5S on SDG containing 0.4M KCl. Similar sedimentation profiles were obtained with cytosols prepared and analyzed in the presence of 10mM molybdate. Increasing the molybdate concentration in the homogenization and gradient buffers to 50mM resulted in sedimentation values of 10S on low salt and 7-8S on 0.4M KCl SDG. Thus, higher concentrations of molybdate reduced the ability of KCl (0.4M) to induce disaggregation of the AR into subunits. This effect is observed only with unactivated untransformed AR, suggesting that once dissociated into the 4-5S subunits, the androgen receptor can no longer reassociate into 7-8S on 0.4M KCl gradients even in the presence of 50mM molybdate. The ability of $MoO_4^{=}$ to maintain 7-8S AR state in presence of 0.4M KCl is no longer observed at pH $>$ 7.4. Higher KCl concentrations (0.8-1.2M) induced dissociation of the 7-8S AR into 4-5S entities even in the presence of 50mM $MoO_4^{=}$, suggesting that the aggregating effect of molybdate is reversible. Urea (2M), NaSCN (0.1-0.2M) and SH directed reagents (5-10mM) reduced the effectiveness of molybdate (50mM) to maintain AR in the 7-8S state in high salt. Chromatography of AR on Sephacryl-S200 with 0.4M KCl buffer showed that in the presence of molybdate (50mM) AR eluted as a single macromolecule with stokes radius of 69A°. In absence of molybdate however, AR with 54A° and 27A° were detected.

2717 THERMAL ACTIVATION OF PURIFIED RAT HEPATIC GLUCOCORTICOID-RECEPTOR COMPLEXES - POSSIBLY A TWO-STEP MECHANISM. T.J. Schmidt*, A. Miller, M.L. Webb, P. Grandics and G. Litwack. Dept. of Physiology and Biophysics, The University of Iowa, Iowa City, IA 52242 and Fels Research Institute, Temple University School of Medicine, Philadelphia, PA 19140 USA.

The thermal activation of rat hepatic glucocorticoid-receptor complexes (GRC) has been analyzed using reconstitution experiments. The unactivated GRC have been purified to near homogeneity by a three step procedure which includes affinity chromatography. Subsequent activation has been quantitated by the DNA-cellulose binding assay and by chromatography (salt elution) of the GRC on DEAE-cellulose. Thermal activation (25°C for 30 min) has consistently resulted in a shift from the high (unactivated) to the low salt eluting (activated) form of the purified GRC but only in a minimal increase in DNA-cellulose binding when compared to the unactivated control (2-fold versus 8-10 fold in crude cytosol). However, after addition of Na_2MoO_4 to the thermally activated GRC, an additional incubation with an aliquot of crude cytosol at 0°C for 30 min results in maximal binding to DNA-cellulose. The cytoplasmic factor(s) which facilitates DNA-cellulose binding in a dose dependent manner is stable at 90°C and sensitive to trypsin. These data suggest that thermal activation may involve two steps. The first step, which is inhibited by Na_2MoO_4 and is temperature dependent, results in the elution of activated complexes from DEAE-cellulose which bind minimally to DNA-cellulose. The second step, which is not inhibited by Na_2MoO_4 and may not be temperature dependent, appears to require the presence of a cytoplasmic factor(s) which confers full DNA-cellulose binding capability on the GRC.

Supported by AM-32870 and AM-13531 (NIH).

2718 CHARACTERISTICS OF THE GLUCOCORTICOID RECEPTOR IN MEN WITH PRIMARY CORTISOL RESISTANCE. M. Tomita*, D. Brandon, G.P. Chrousos, S. Taylor, C. Foster, A.C.M. Vingerhoeds, D.L. Loriaux, M.B. Lipsett. NICHD, National Institutes of Health, Bethesda, Md. U.S.A.

We examined the biochemical properties of the glucocorticoid receptor (GR) in two members of a family with primary cortisol resistance. Epstein-Barr virus-transformed lymphocytes from these patients (severely affected patient, SP, and mildly affected patient, MP) were used as sources of GR. These cells were resistant to the actions of dexamethasone (DEX) as assessed by the decreased ability of DEX to suppress 2-deoxyglucose uptake (SP<MP<Control). Compared to the controls, both patients had decreased concentration of GR, and the SP had a GR with decreased affinity for DEX. GR from both patients, covalently labelled with [^{3}H]-Dex-21-mesylate, was identified by SDS polyacrylamide gel electrophoresis, as a protein moiety with $M_r \cong 92{,}000$, similar to that obtained from controls. We studied the thermolability of the DEX-bound GR complexes (D-GR) in these cells in the presence of excess labelled DEX and found that loss of D-GR with time of incubation at 28°C occurred more rapidly in the patients (SP>MP>control). We analyzed the process of thermal activation, in isotonic buffer, of D-GR in these cells using phosphocellulose chromatography. Approximately 25% of the D-GR was activated to a form (GR*) that bound to phosphocellulose under these conditions in both the patients and controls. GR* from control and patients bound to nuclei equally. We conclude that the GR in these two patients had 1) increased thermolability, 2) a normal molecular weight, and 3) a normal pattern of thermal activation and ability to bind to nuclei.

2719 ALKALINE PHOSPHATASE PROMOTION OF THE 9.1S TO 5.2S TRANSFORMATION OF THE MOUSE GLUCOCORTICOID RECEPTOR.

Wayne V. Vedeckis* and Cheryl E. Reker, Dept. of Biochemistry, LSU Medical Center, New Orleans, LA. 70112, USA.

Addition of calf intestinal alkaline phosphatase (AP) promotes conversion of the mouse AtT-20 cell glucocorticoid receptor (GC-R) from the untransformed, 9.1S species to the transformed, 5.2S receptor. The reaction is dependent on added enzyme concentration and is linear for up to 2 h at 10°C. The most potent phosphatase inhibitors which blocked AP-promoted transformation were 20 mM molybdate, 2 mM tungstate and 2 mM arsenate. Levamisole (10 mM) and NaF (50 mM) were partially inhibitory, whereas 100 mM glucose-1-phosphate had no effect. Although the effects of these inhibitors on AP-promoted receptor transformation did not correlate well with paranitrophenyl phosphate hydrolysis by AP, a much better correlation was obtained when endogenous (cytosolic) phosphatase activity was assayed. For example, NaF was a potent inhibitor of both G-25 promoted GC-R transformation as well as cytosolic phosphatase activity. Protease inhibitors such as phenylmethylsulfonyl fluoride and antipain had no effect on the 9.1S to 5.2S GC-R transformation, while leupeptin was inhibitory. Thus, a contaminating protease in the AP could be responsible for the 9.1S to 5.2S conversion. Nevertheless, the involvement of dephosphorylation in GC-R transformation seems likely because 1) identical receptor transformation is obtained with two different commercial sources of AP and 2) NaF (a poor protease inhibitor) blocks endogenous GC-R transformation. The possibility that leupeptin inhibits AP-promoted transformation by a mechanism other than protease inhibition is being explored. Supported by American Cancer Society Grant BC-436.

2720 QUANTITATION AND CHARACTERIZATION OF GLUCOCORTICOID RECEPTOR (GR)IN LYMPHOID CELLS: THEIR RELATIONSHIP TO THE STAGE OF CELLULAR DIFFERENTIATION.

W. Voigt,* R.E. Garola, G.E. Byrne Jr., and C.C. Whitcomb, Department of Pathology, University of Miami School of Medicine, Miami, FL. U.S.A.

Non-B, Non-T lymphoid cells have been reported to have high levels of GR (Lipman, M. Am. J. Physiol. 243: E103,1982). It has also been reported that abnormal forms of GR's are found in the leukemic cells of some patients (McCaffrey et al. Blood: 59, 2, 393, 1982). We have evaluated these two aspects of the GR concomitantly in 17 patients with lymphoproliferative diseases (12 peripheral blood and 5 lymph nodes), and 7 patients with non lymphoid proliferation. Cells were analyzed by the dextran charcoal technique and 16-41% glycerol gradient centrifugation in tris buffer containing EDTA, monothioglycerol and sodium molybdate. Binding sites and dissociation constant (Kd) of the receptor were estimated by Scatchard plot. The stage of cellular differentiation was defined by immunological, cytochemical, and morphological studies. Significant amounts of GR's were found in all 15 lymphoid-type cells as well as in 3/3 acute myeloid leukemias. In contrast, cells from plasmocytoma (1/1), angioimmunoblastic lymphadenopathy (1/1), chronic myeloid (3/3), and acute monomyelocytic leukemia (1/1) did not show any binding activity. Highest GR values were observed in "null" (immature) acute lymphoblastic leukemia. No significant variations in the Kd (9.85×10^{-9} M ± 4.02) or in the sedimentation coefficient (9.29 ± 0.19) of the receptor were observed. Our data suggest a) that higher concentrations of GR are related to the immaturity of lymphoid cells and b) that in all cell types studied, only one molecular species of GR exists. This last observation is in disagreement with McCaffrey reported results.

2721 PURIFICATION, CHARACTERIZATION, AND ACTIVATION OF RAT KIDNEY CORTEX GLUCOCORTICOID RECEPTOR. M.L. Webb*, A.S. Miller, P. Grandics, and G. Litwack, Fels Research Institute, Temple University School of Medicine, Philadelphia, PA 19140.

Glucocorticoid receptor (GcR) was purified from rat kidney cortex (K_c) using a modification of the procedure previously described for rat hepatic GcR. This procedure includes affinity, BioGel A1.5m, and ion-exchange chromatography in the presence of sodium molybdate. Preliminary physicochemical results indicate that the purified, unactivated, molybdate-stabilized GcR has a Stokes radius of 6.1 nm (rechromatography on BioGel A1.5m), a sedimentation coefficient of 9S (glycerol gradient centrifugation), and a Mr=90,000 (SDS-PAGE). Following removal of sodium molybdate by gel filtration and thermal activation (25°/30 min) DNA-cellulose binding increased 1.5-2 fold over the unheated control. Thermal activation in the presence of kidney or hepatic cytosol (endogenous receptors heat inactivated) increased DNA-cellulose binding 4-6 fold over the unheated control. Activation was also observed on DEAE-cellulose as a shift in elution pattern from 0.25M to 0.09M salt concentration. Addition of sodium molybdate during both thermal and thermal plus cytosol activation treatments blocked the increase in DNA-cellulose binding. These results suggest that purified, unactivated, molybdate-stabilized GcR from Kc had physicochemical properties similar to those previously described for hepatic GcR, and following removal of sodium molybdate, can be thermally and thermal plus cytosol activated. Further investigation using this purification scheme is underway to determine the presence of other forms of GcR in Kc in order to study the concept of receptor polymorphism. Supported by grants AM-32870 and AM-13531.

2722 INTERACTION OF RAT LIVER CYTOSOLIC GLUCOCORTICOID RECEPTOR WITH HEPARIN. A. Weisz*, G.A. Puca, R. Pagnotta, C. Masi, A. Petrillo, M.T. Masucci and V. Sica, Istituto di Patologia Generale e Oncologia, I Facoltà di Medicina e Chirurgia, Università di Napoli, Naples, 80138 Italy. Sponsor: F. Bresciani.

When rat liver cytosol containing ^{3}H-Dexamethasone-receptor complex is incubated with Sepharose-heparin (S-hep) the steroid-receptor complex binds to the substituted Sepharose avidly (K_d 3.5±1.7 x 10^{-10}M). Under appropriate conditions up to 85% of the receptor present is adsorbed to the solid phase after 40 min at 0°C. The binding is enhanced by cations, with Mn^{++} being more efficient than Mg^{++}; Ca^{++} and Sr^{++} are ineffective. Sodium molybdate, a salt very effective in receptor stabilization, does not influence the reaction. The binding is dependent on the ionic strength of the medium and is totally reversed by 300 mM KCl. Both native and temperature transformed glucocorticoid receptors interact with S-hep. Furthermore, while the ^{3}H-Dexamethasone-receptor complex can be eluted from S-hep by washing the column with a solution of heparin, no elution is achieved by a solution of sheared calf thymus DNA. These results strongly suggest that the receptor site that binds heparin is distinct from that binding DNA. Among the applications of the glucocorticoid receptor interaction with heparin are:a) purification of the receptor; b) utilization for the study of nucleic acid-receptor interactions.
Supported by: Progetto Finalizzato "Oncologia" of the Consiglio Nazionale delle Ricerche, Italy.

2723 ULTRASTRUCTURAL OBSERVATION OF MICROAGGREGATION AND REDISTRIBUTION OF OCCUPIED INSULIN RECEPTORS ON 3T3-L1 ADIPOCYTES. R.M. Smith*, M. Cobb, O.M. Rosen and L. Jarett, University of Pennsylvania School of Medicine, Philadelphia, PA and Albert Einstein College of Medicine, Bronx, NY.

Biologically active monomeric ferritin-insulin (Fm-I) was used to study insulin receptors (IR) on the 3T3-L1 adipocyte (3T3-L1 adip). The initial distribution of IR was determined by prefixation 3T3-L1 adip prior to incubation with Fm-I to binding equilibrium. Fresh 3T3-L1 adip were incubated with Fm-I for 1 to 60 min at 37°. Electron micrographs of prefixed cells revealed that IR were primarily on the cell microvilli with few molecules on the intervillous cell surface. IR were organized into a few small groups of 2 or 3 receptors or single receptors (31, 5 and 61% of the total IR, respectively). Microaggregation of occupied IR occurred rapidly on fresh 3T3-L1 adip. Within 1 min at 37° the single IR decreased to 30% of the total; by 15 min 60% of the IR were found in groups of 4-6 and 16% were in clusters of 7 to >18 molecules. Redistribution of IR occurred, with virtually all of the groups being on the intervillous cell surface within 15 min. Groups of IR also were observed in both pinocytotic invaginations and coated pits with no significant difference in the concentration of Fm-I in either structure. Morphometric analysis of 3T3-L1 adip stained for coated pits revealed a 10:1 ratio in the number of invaginations to coated pits. This study demonstrated that on 3T3-L1 adip dispersed IR on the microvilli bound insulin and rapidly microaggregated and relocated to the intervillous cell surface and as well were associated with the numerous invaginations and the less numerous coated pits. Supported by NIH grant and the Reynolds Foundation.

2724 AN INVESTIGATION OF THE Ca^{2+} REGULATION OF INSULIN RECEPTOR AFFINITY. P.F.Williams* & J.R. Turtle, Dept. of Endocrinology, Royal Prince Alfred Hospital & Dept. of Medicine, University of Sydney, NSW, Australia.

The specificity and nature of the binding site through which Ca^{2+},Ba^{2+}, Mg^{2+} and Sr^{2+} increased human placental insulin receptor (HPIR) affinity was investigated using as probes, ions from the Lanthanide series and ethyl dimethylaminopropyl carbodiimide (EDAC) an agent that reacts with carboxylate groups. The trivalent lanthanide ions share many properties of Ca^{2+} including co-ordination number and ionic radius, they substitute for Ca^{2+} in a number of proteins and because of an increased ratio of charge to ionic radius they are effective at lower concentrations. Thus ½-maximal stimulation of insulin binding occurred at 0.1 mM for lanthanides vs 2.5 mM for Ca^{2+}. Lanthanides with an ionic radius smaller than Ca^{2+} (Dy^{3+},Ho^{3+} Er^{3+},Tm^{3+},Yb^{3+},Lu^{3+})did not stimulate insulin binding to the same degree as the other lanthanides (100-125% vs 150% stimulation of binding). Na^{+} with a similar ionic radius to Ca^{2+} is not effective. Like Ca^{2+},Tb^{3+} ions were displaced by insulin from their binding site (determined by Tb^{3+} fluorescence at 545 nm after excitation at 292 nm). The decrease in Tb^{3+} emission was proportional to the amount of hormone bound and was consistent with a conformational change in the HPIR caused by insulin binding. EDAC 1-2 mM was reacted with the HPIR (10-30 mg/ml, 50 mM Hepes pH 7.8) for 1.5h at 22° and did not alter HPIR binding but it did block the ability of Ca^{2+} to stimulate HPIR affinity. Pre-incubation with Ca^{2+} prevented the effect of EDAC. These results are consistent with a carboxylic acid binding site on or near the receptor that requires a cation with a similar ionic structure to Ca^{2+} in order to increase HPIR affinity.

2725 REDOX REGULATION OF INSULIN RECEPTOR KINASE. K.-T. Yu* and M. P. Czech, University of Massachusetts Medical Center, Worcester, MA 01605

Partially purified insulin receptor immobilized on insulin-agarose exhibits tyrosine kinase activity towards its own β subunit and exogenous substrates. The kinase activity of the receptor was increased more than five-fold when dithiothreitol (DTT) was included in the phosphorylation buffer. The effect of DTT was concentration dependent and was maximal betwee 2-5mM. Other reductants such as reduced glutathione and mercapto-ethanol were also effective in activating the receptor kinase. The time course of activation of the receptor kinase with maximal concentrations of DTT was very rapid and was maximal after 3 min of incubation with the reductant. The elevated activity of the receptor kinase was dependent on the continuous presence of DTT and was rapidly reversed upon the removal of the reductant by washing. These results suggest that the insulin receptor kinase is activated when it is in the reduced state. In order to investigate whether the activation of the receptor kinase towards exogenous substrates by DTT is mediated through increased autophosphorylation of the receptor which causes its kinase activation, the insulin receptor preparation was incubated with increasing concentrations of ATP in the presence and absence of DTT, followed by extensive washing to remove the unreacted ATP and DTT. The receptor mediated histone phosphorylation was increased progressively when the concentrations of ATP used in the preincubation were raised. Significantly, the ATP-activated histone kinase activity was further enhanced by more than 10 fold when DTT was present in the first incubation and persisted after extensive washing. These results suggest that the activation of the receptor histone kinase activity by DTT is mediated through the autophosphorylation of the insulin receptor.

(Abstract 2779, p. 1650, also belongs to this section.)

2726 CHARACTERIZATION OF FUNCTIONAL RECEPTORS FOR SOMATOSTATIN (SRIF) IN A RAT INSULINOMA CELL LINE. Susan J. Sullivan* and Agnes Schonbrunn, Lab of Toxicology, Harvard School of Public Health, Boston, MA 02115, U.S.A.

Direct analysis of the interaction of SRIF with receptors on pancreatic beta cells has been complicated in islet preparations by cell population heterogeneity and low levels of saturable binding. We have used the RIN5F cell line cloned from a rat islet cell tumor (PNAS 77:3519, 1980) and [^{125}I-Tyr^{11}]SRIF to characterize pancreatic SRIF receptors. At 37C, equilibrium binding of trace concentrations (5×10^{-11}M) of [^{125}I-Tyr^{11}]SRIF was reached in 4 hrs and greater than 80% of the cell associated radioactivity was bound to saturable, high affinity sites. The radiolabelled ligand was not rapidly degraded by RIN5F cells: after incubation at 37C for 6 hr, 95% remained intact. The half-time for dissociation of saturably bound ligand was 7 hrs and was not affected by the presence of 100nM unlabelled SRIF. Saturable binding of trace amounts of [^{125}I-Tyr^{11}]SRIF diluted with known amounts of unlabelled SRIF gave a linear Scatchard plot characteristic of a single class of binding sites. The Kd for SRIF was 0.5 ± 0.1 nM and there were 10^4 sites per cell. [^{125}I-Tyr^{11}]SRIF binding was not inhibited by unrelated peptides such as TRH, insulin, met-enkephalin, substance P or ACTH. The affinities for SRIF and unlabelled [Tyr^{11}]SRIF (Kd = 0.7 nM) were essentially the same. SRIF 25 and SRIF 28 bound with slightly lower affinities (Kd = 0.9 nM). Thus, we have demonstrated the existence of specific, high affinity binding sites for SRIF on RIN5F cells. Since addition of 100 nM SRIF inhibits both basal and glucagon-stimulated insulin secretion by about 40% in these cells, the characterized binding sites are functional receptors. Supported by a JDF postdoctoral fellowship and NIADDK (AM 32234).

2727 CHARACTERIZATION OF BOMBESIN (BBS) RECEPTORS IN A PANCREATIC β CELL LINE.
S. L. Swope* and A. Schonbrunn, Harvard Medical School and Harvard School of Public Health, Boston, MA, U.S.A.

BBS rapidly and potently stimulates insulin release by HIT cells, a clonal line of hamster pancreatic β cells (PNAS, in press). To characterize the receptors which mediate the effect of BBS, we have examined the binding of [^{125}I-Tyr^4]BBS (I-BBS) to HIT cells. Saturable binding of I-BBS at 4C reached a plateau by 10 h and remained constant for up to 24 h. Binding studies at 4C with increasing concentrations of I-BBS resulted in a linear Scatchard plot with a Kd of 0.87±.11 nM and R_T of 85,000±35,000 sites/cell. Peptides structurally unrelated to BBS did not compete for receptor binding. However, BBS inhibited I-BBS binding with an ID_{50} of 1.12±.35 nM which agrees with the ED_{50} (0.5 nM) observed for stimulation of insulin release. In addition, the potencies of 5 BBS analogs to compete for receptor binding and to stimulate insulin secretion correlated well. After binding for 90 min at 4C, over 85% of the I-BBS was dissociated by an acid/salt wash, indicating that it was on the cell surface. Increasing the temperature to 37C, resulted in internalization of 75% of receptor bound peptide within 3 min. After binding of I-BBS at 4C and shifting to 37C, radioactivity dissociated from the cell with a $t_{1/2}$ of 20±1 min. Only 12±1% of the radioactivity released during 30 min was intact I-BBS. The lysosomotropic agent, chloroquine increased the amount of cell associated radioactivity at 37C and slowed the rate of release of radioactivity. These results demonstrate that HIT cells possess saturable, high affinity receptors for BBS. Furthermore, at 37C, initial binding of peptide at the cell surface is rapidly followed by internalization, degradation via a lysosomal pathway and release of the degradative byproducts from the cell.

2728 Nb2 LYMPHOMA CELL RADIORECEPTOR AND RECEPTOR MODULATION ASSAYS FOR PROLACTIN.
T. Tanaka* and Y. Shishiba. Department of Pediatrics and Endocrinology, Toranomon Hospital and Okinaka Memorial Institute for Medical Research, Akasaka, Tokyo 105, Japan.

We have previously demonstrated that serum from a patient with giant prolactinoma have contained big-big, medium-big, big and little forms of hPRL with different bioactivity/immunoactivity ratio (BA/RIA ratio). Big-big hPRL had higher BA/RIA ratio and big hPRL had lower BA/RIA ratio than little hPRL determined by Nb2 cell bioassay and RIA. To determine whether this difference in BA/RIA ratio of heterogeneous hPRLs attributes to the difference in receptor binding activity, we have established the Nb2 lymphoma cell radioreceptor (RRA) and receptor modulation assays (RMA) for prolactin. In the RRA, 0.5 ml of stationary phase Nb2 lymphoma cells were distributed to culture tubes in Fischer medium containing 10% horse serum at a concentration of 2 - 5 x 10^6 cells/ml. Cell plus [^{125}I] hPRL (2 - 8 x 10^6 cpm) were incubated with standard hPRL or sample at 37°C for 90 min. Cell suspension, 0.5 ml, was withdrawn and layered onto 3 ml cold PBS in a fresh tube. These tubes were then centrifuged for 5 min at 1000xg at 4°C. After decanting and draining, the radioactivity in the cell pellet was counted. In the RMA, 0.5 ml of cells from suspension culture (5 - 10 x 10^6 cells/ml) in the stationary phase were aliquoted into culture tubes containing hPRL standards or samples. After 4 h incubation at 37°C in CO_2 incubator, cells were spun, washed and resuspended in fresh medium containing [^{125}I] hPRL. After 90 min incubation, cells were treated as described in RRA method. Big hPRL showed lower activity in both assays than RIA.

2729 HPL AND INSULIN BINDING SITES IN RAT LIVER AND FAT TISSUES DURING ONTOGENESIS AND PREGNANCY. Y. Ueda*, H. Morikawa, Y. Tokiwa, M. Deguchi, and M. Mochizuki, Department of Obstetrics and Gynecology, School of Medicine, Kobe University, Kobe, Hyogo, Japan.

Human placental lactogen(HPL) and insulin have very important roles on the regulation of carbohydrate-lipid metabolism in pregnancy. The dynamics of hPL and insulin binding sites were investigated in livers and fat tissues in rats during ontogenesis and pregnancy. HPL binding sites were very few in liver cell membranes in fetal and immature rats. They were increased strikingly after mid-pregnancy(L12), reaching more than 300-400% of control level (nonpregnant adult female, fed state) in late pregnancy. And they were reduced soon after parturition. On the other hand, insulin binding were almost constant at all stages examined except in late pregnancy in liver. They were decreased in late pregnancy(L20) in contrast with hPL ($p<0.05$). Such reduction of insulin binding sites observed in late pregnancy was more dominant in fed state than in fasted state. Similar results were observed in rat and human fat tissues (both isolated fat cells and fat cell membranes - 10^5g pellets). Scatchard analyses indicated that the changes of both hPL and insulin binding sites were due to the changes of binding capacities rather than binding affinities. In conclusion, insulin binding sites were supressed in the maternal liver and fat tissues, which means the "insulin resistance" in periphery. Conversely, hPL binding sites were much dominant in maternal liver. In fetal liver and placenta only insulin binding was observed. This phenomenon seems to be a metabolic adaptation for the fetal growth in feto-maternal systems.

2730 INCREASES OF GONADOTROPIN-RELEASING HORMONE RECEPTORS BY GONADOTROPIN-RELEASING HORMONE IN THE GRANULOSA CELLS. T. Uemura*, K. Shirasu, A. Kimura, T. Namiki and H. Minaguchi, Department of Obstetrics and Gynecology, Yokohama City University, School of Medicine, Yokohama, 232, Japan.

In vivo and *in vitro* studies were undertaken to examine the regulatory mechanism of gonadotropin-releasing hormone(GnRH) binding capacity in the granulosa cells(G-cells). ^{125}I-[D-Ser(TBu)^6 des-Gly-NH_2^{10}] LHRH ethylamide(GnRHa) was used as a ligand.

1).Autoradiographic studies demonstrated GnRH receptors(GnRH-R) in all components of granulosa, theca, and interstitial cells of the ovary. 2). *In vitro* assay of GnRH binding has shown that PMSG(10-200iu/rat) injections to diethylstilbestrol primed hypophysectomized 28-day-old immature decreased GnRH-R binding in residual tissue($p<0.01$) as well as in the whole ovary, but not in G-cells. 3).*In vivo* administrations of GnRH(0.1-100ug$\times$3$\times$2days) caused significant increases in GnRH-R of the whole ovary in PMSG treated rats($p<0.01$), but not in saline treated rats. 4).G-cells exhibited increases of GnRH-R binding(from 17.9 ± 0.8 to 53.2 ± 2.4fmol/mg protein, $p<0.01$) more than residual tissue did and exhibited decreases of HCG receptor binding($p<0.01$) by GnRH administrations. 5).*in vitro* experiment, rat FSH(1ug) stimulated cAMP accumulation, progesterone production and HCG receptor in G-cells cultured with 3-isobutyl-1-methylxanthine, but not GnRH-R induction in G-cells. GnRHa(10^{-6}M) inhibited these FSH-induced rises and stimulated GnRH-R induction.

These results suggested that GnRH in combination with FSH has stimulatory effects on GnRH-R binding of G-cells.

2731 COVALENT CROSSLINKING OF ^{125}I-VASOACTIVE INTESTINAL POLYPEPTIDE TO A HUMAN LYMPHOBLASTIC CELL LINE.
C.L. Wood* and M.S. O'Dorisio (Spon: S. Cataland), Department of Medicine, The Ohio State University, Columbus, Ohio 43210, USA.

Cultured Molt 4b lymphoblasts possess a high affinity receptor for vasoactive intestinal polypeptide (VIP) which is pharmacologically specific and which is functionally linked to the plasma membrane adenylate cyclase complex (Beed, et al., Reg Peptides 6,1, 1983). In order to characterize the VIP receptor further, viable Molt cells were pre-incubated with ^{125}I-VIP, exposed to the bifunctional reagent disuccinimidyl suberate, solubilized, and subjected to sodium dodecyl sulfate-polyacrylamide gel electrophoresis and autoradiography. A band with an apparent molecular weight of 51,000 was labelled. The light-sensitive crosslinker N-succinimidyl 6-(4'-azido-2'-nitrophenylamino) hexanoate (SANAH) gave similar results, whereas N-hydroxysuccinimidyl 4-azidobenzoate (HSAB), with a shorter chain length, was much less effective. The crosslinking of ^{125}I-VIP to the binding site required the presence of a bifunctional reagent, and was blocked by excess unlabelled VIP in the pre-incubation. The apparent molecular weight of the labelled protein was unchanged by treatment with dithiothreitol. These observations are consistent with the VIP receptor containing a protein subunit of 48,000 molecular weight which lacks disulfide bonds to other peptides. To our knowledge this is the first demonstration of crosslinking of ^{125}I-VIP to intact cells or human cells.

2732 BINDING OF A SUBSTANCE P-DIPHTHERIA TOXIN CONJUGATE TO A RAT PANCREATIC CELL LINE.
P. Wu*, T.M. Jessell, P. Bacha and S. Reichlin. Endocrinology Division, Tuft's-New England Medical Center, Boston, MA 02111 and Dept. Neurobiology, Harvard Medical School, Boston, MA 02115, USA.
Substitution of TRH for the eukaryotic cell receptor domain of diphtheria toxin forms a TRH-toxin hybrid (TRH-CRM45) that includes both the toxic, enzymically active and hydrophobic domains of the toxin and will bind specifically to cells with TRH receptors (Bacha et al, J. Biol. Chem. 258, 1565-1570, 1983). We have now synthesized an analogous substance P-CRM45 hybrid (SP-CRM45) and studied its specific binding to a rat pancreatic cell line AR4-2J (Hanley and Jessell, J. Physiol. 1984 in press) which is rich in SP receptors. SP was thiolated with 2-imidothiolane at α and ε amino groups (SP-SH). CRM45 was modified with SPDP (N-Succinimidyl 3-(2-pyridothio) propionate) to give a 1:1 PDP:CRM45 molar ratio. Desalted PDP-CRM and SP-SH were reacted at equimolar concentrations to form a disulfide-linked SP-CRM45 hybrid molecule which, after desalting, displaced ^{125}I-Tyr^{8} SP in an RIA and which actively adenylated elongation factor 2. SP binding sites on AR4-2J cells in dissociated cell culture were determined with ^{125}I-labelled Bolton Hunter SP (^{125}I-BHSP, 220Ci/mmole; 80pM; gift of Dr. C. Pazoles). Binding was inhibited by SP(IC-10^{10}M) fragments of SP and other tachykinins indicating the presence of SP-P type receptors on these cells and by both SP-SH (IC_{50}-5×10^{-10}M) and SP-CRM45 (IC_{50}-5×10^{-9}M. These results suggest that SP-CRM45 binds to the same sites on these cells as ^{125}I-BHSP and may demonstrate SP receptor-mediated binding of a 45000 dalton protein to these cells. Supported by grants from Seragen Inc., Pfizer, Inc. and NIH grant NS 17369.

(Abstract 2780, p. 1650, also belongs to this section.)

2733 DISPARATE EFFECTS OF "ANTI-ESTROGENS" ON ESTROGEN AND PROGESTIN BIOSYNTHESIS BY CULTURED RAT GRANULOSA CELLS. T.H. Welsh, Jr.*, P.B.C. Jones, L.Z. Zhuang, X.C. Jia and Aaron J.W. Hsueh. Dept. of Reproductive Medicine, Univ. of California, San Diego, La Jolla, CA 92093 U.S.A.

The influence of "anti-estrogens" on FSH-stimulated estrogen, progesterone and 20α-hydroxy-4-pregnen-3-one (20α-OH-P) production was examined in primary cultures of rat granulosa cells. Cells were cultured with FSH, with or without DES or various "anti-estrogens". After 3 days, medium progesterone and 20α-OH-P content was determined by RIA. Cells were then reincubated for an additional 8h with androstenedione and estrogen formation was measured by RIA. Estrogen and progestin production was negligible for control cultures and cultures treated with DES or "anti-estrogens" alone. FSH treatment increased estrogen and progestin production in a dose-dependent manner. Concomitant treatment with DES (10^{-7} M) enhanced FSH-stimulated estrogen and progestin production. Similarly, treatment with 10^{-6} M of "anti-estrogens", tamoxifen (Tam), nafoxidine (Naf) or clomiphene citrate (CC), also enhanced FSH-stimulated aromatase activity. In contrast, each "anti-estrogen" inhibited FSH-stimulated progestin production (85% inhibition at 300 ng/ml of FSH). Increasing concentrations (3×10^{-8} -10^{-6} M) of the "anti-estrogens" augmented FSH-stimulated estrogen production in a dose-related manner (CC>Tam >Naf). Similar doses of the "anti-estrogens" inhibited the stimulatory effect of FSH on progestin production (Tam>CC>Naf). These studies demonstrate that "anti-estrogens" exert disparate actions upon granulosa cell estrogen and progestin biosynthesis and suggest the mediation of these functions by ovarian estrogen and "anti-estrogen" receptors.

2734 MICROBIOLOGICAL HYDROXYLATION OF ESTRADIOL: FORMATION OF 4- AND 2-HYDROXY-CATECHOL ESTROGENS. J. Williamson, D. Van Orden and J.P. Rosazza*, Division of Medicinal Chemistry and Natural Products, and Department of Obstetrics and Gynecology, University of Iowa, Iowa City, IA 52242, USA.

Microorganisms and their enzymes have been widely exploited for their highly selective abilities to achieve chemical changes in the structures of numerous steroids. These biocatalysts have the properties of selectively introducing molecular oxygen into substrate molecules under mild reaction conditions which prevail in fermentation media. Experiments designed to provide catechol estrogens in quantity by the microbial transformation route have been conducted. Twenty microorganisms known to introduce oxygen into the aromatic rings of several alkaloidal and amino acid substrates were examined for their abilities to hydroxylate estradiol (E_2), and estrone. A variety of reactions were observed by thin-layer chromatographic examination of culture extracts supplemented with these estrogenic steroid substrates. Of cultures examined, *Aspergillus alliaceus* smoothly converted E_2 to mixtures of catechol products, but estrone was not metabolized. Analytical experiments (HPLC, Lichrosorb-Diol, $CHCl_3$:MeOH 99:1) revealed that within 48 hours, *A. alliaceus* formed 4-hydroxy-E_2 in 63% yield while 2-hydroxy-E_2 was formed in 10% yield. Preparative scale incubations were conducted using 2 gm of E_2 as substrate in a 3 liter fermentation. Ascorbic acid was added in doses to incubations containing E_2 and catechol products at time intervals to prevent oxidative decomposition of catechols. The catechol metabolites were isolated and characterized by ^{1}H-NMR and mass spectroscopy. The microbial transformation of E_2 provides an efficient and rapid method for the preparation of catechol estrogens.

2735 AROMATASE ACTIVITY OF ANDROSTENEDIONE IN LEIOMYOMA AND MYOMETRIUM OF THE SAME UTERUS.

T. Yamamoto*, K. Takamori and H. Okada, Dept. of OB/GYN, Kyoto Pref. Univ. Med., Kyoto 602, Japan

The growth of uterine leiomyoma is closely associated with estrogen, but there is no report, to our knowledge, whether or not estrogen synthesis (aromatase activity of androgen) proceeds in myoma tissue or in normal myometrial tissue obtained from the same uterus, involving in the mechanism of the growth of this tumor. We have investigated the conversion of androstenedione to estrogens in leiomyoma tissue and in myometrial tissue obtained from the same uterus, and moreover demonstrated the distribution of the enzyme activity in the tumor. The homogenate (500 mg W.W in 3 ml of 0.1M-PBS, pH7.4) of leiomyoma and myometrial tissue obtained from the coincident uterus was incubated with (1,2,6,7-^{3}H)-androstenedione (100 pmol) and NADPH (1.5 mg) at 37° C for 1 h in air, respectively. After incubation, E_1 and E_2 were purified by Bio-Rad AG1-X2 column chromatography, T.L.C. and co-crystallization. It was demonstrated that estrogen formed from androstenedione by leiomyoma (E_1: 36~466 fmol/h/g, E_2: ~78 fmol/h/g) was significantly higher than that by myometrium (E_1: ~32 fmol/h/g, E_2: ~10 fmol/h/g) from the same uterus. Moreover, the amount of estrogen biosynthesized in leiomyoma was high in the order of edge > middle > center. This finding indicates that the aromatization of androstenedione in uterine leiomyoma may contribute to the growth of this tumor. This study was supported in part by grant (No.58771082, 1983) from the Ministry of Education, Science and Culture, Japan.

2736 EFFECTS OF IPRIFLAVONE ON THE RESPONSE OF UTERUS AND THYROID TO ESTROGEN

I. Yamazaki*, Biology Laboratories, Central Research Division, Takeda Chemical Industries, Ltd., 17-85, Jusohonmachi 2-Chome, Yodogawaku, Osaka 532, Japan.

An isoflavone derivative, 7-isopropoxy-isoflavone (ipriflavone), showed a uterotropic activity on immature normal rats but not on ovariectomized rats, suggesting its activity requires the presence of estrogen. When administered with estrogen to ovariectomized rats, ipriflavone exaggerated the response of uterus to estrogen. Plasma calcitonin response to calcium-load was decreased in ovariectomized rats. Three week-administration of ipriflavone and/or estrogen was carried out in ovariectomized rats. Estrogen restored calcitonin response to calcium dose dependently but ipriflavone did not. However, the combination administration of ipriflavone with estrogen increased the basal calcitonin level and the response to calcium more markedly than estrogen alone. Ipriflavone had neither of gonadotropin-releasing, gonadotropic nor inhibiting action on estrogen metabolism. From these results, ipriflavone appears to increase the actions of estrogen on the uterus and thyroid.

2737 A SIMPLE METHOD FOR THE DETERMINATION OF SEX HORMONE BINDING GLOBULIN (SHBG) IN HUMAN SERUM. N. Y. Zachariah, Z. H. Chakmakjian,* R. Thornblom and G. Sumner, Division of Endocrinology and Metabolism, Baylor University Medical Center, Dallas, Texas, U. S. A.

A simple and rapid method for serum sex hormone binding globulin (SHBG) was developed. Serum from pregnant women was pooled and the SHBG concentration was measured (6.8 ug/dl) by previously established method (Rosner, et al). This pool was diluted with charcoal treated and heated serum to give standards ranging in concentrations from 2.68 - 0.08 ug/dl. Two sets of dihydrotestosterone (DHT) coated tubes were prepared; assay tubes with 1 ng per tube and control tubes with 100 ng per tube. Standards and unknown samples were diluted 8-fold and 400 ul added to assay and control tubes followed by the addition of 100 ul of tritiated DHT (20,000 cpm, with counting efficiency of 34.6%). Following incubation at room temperature for 10 minutes, cold saturated ammonium sulfate (500 ul) was added to each tube, mixed, centrifuged and the supernatant counted. With an Apple II computer, a program was developed for data reduction. Mean SHBG concentration (ug/dl ± SEM) in nonobese normal men (n=14) was 0.36 ± 0.04, nonobese normal women (n=10) 1.14 ± 0.22, pregnant women (n=14) 5.8 ± 0.26, hirsute women (n=25) 0.72 ± 0.08, hypothyroid women (n=11) 0.77 ± 0.16, and hyperthyroid women (n=13) 2.62 ± 0.22. These results correlate well with previous reports. This fast and convenient method can easily be set up in a laboratory and up to forty samples can be analyzed in one assay.

2738 CHARACTERIZATION OF THE SUBUNIT MOLECULAR STRUCTURE OF THE SEX STEROID-BINDING PROTEIN (SBP) OF PLASMA. Philip H. Petra*, Kenneth A. Walsh, and Koiti Titani. Depts. of OB/GYN and Biochemistry, Univ. of Washington, Seattle, WA 98195, U.S.A

The sex steroid-binding protein (SBP) isolated from human or rabbit serum is a glycoprotein composed of two 44K polypeptide chains which associate noncovalently (Petra, J. Steroid Biochem. 11, 245, 1979). The native molecular weights of human and rabbit SBPs are 85,440 ± 3,360 and 85,750 ± 5,290, respectively. These are refined values calculated from recently reported ultracentrifuge data (Petra *et al*., J. Steroid Biochem. 19, 699, 1983). The purpose of these studies is to establish whether or not the subunits are similar in primary structure. Both SBPs were reduced and alkylated with ^{3}H-iodoacetate and digested with trypsin. Each digest was separated on an LKB UltroPac TSK-G2000SW column (7.5 x 600 mm) in 6M Gu·HCl - 0.1M PO_4, pH 6.0 at flow rate 0.5 ml/min. Fractions were pooled and each was rechromatographed by reverse phase HPLC on a SynchroPak RP-P (4.1 x 250 mm) column using gradients of 0.1% trifluoroacetic acid and acetonitrile at a flow rate of 2 ml/min. The amino acid composition of each pure peptide was determined. The results are as follow: For human SBP, a total of about 23 tryptic peptides were isolated, of which only four contained carboxymethyl cysteine, and four contained methionine. Since human SBP is composed of 24 lysine, 29 arginine, 8 cysteine, and 8 methionine residues per 85,440 MW, the results strongly suggest that the SBP molecule is made up of two identical polypeptide chains. Similar results were obtained for rabbit SBP. Supported by HD 13956 and GM 15731.

2739 SKIN & ENDOCRINE CHANGES DURING TREATMENT WITH THE ANTIANDROGEN CYPROTERONE ACETATE (CPA), & OESTROGEN. Valerie A. Randall, F.J.G. Ebling, and R.S. Sawers, Depts. of Zoology & Obstetrics and Gynecology, The University of Sheffield, U.K.

To throw light on the causes of androgen-potentiated skin disorders and the mechanism of therapy we have monitored both skin and endocrine parameters in hirsute women. They were examined at 28-day intervals before and during oral administration of CPA (10 days, generally 100 mg) and/or ethinyl estradiol (EE_2) (21 days, 30 or 50 µg). Combined therapy decreased sebum excretion by about 60% within 1-2 cycles, but reduced thigh hair growth rate and diameter much more slowly. CPA by itself lowered sebum excretion in 1 cycle, but EE_2 alone had only slight effects even after 3-4 months. Before treatment, levels of plasma testosterone were within, and those of andostenedione slightly above, the normal range. However, sex hormone binding globulin (SHBG) levels were low, suggesting that "free" testosterone, ie. that not bound to plasma binding proteins, was high. The combined treatment decreased plasma androgens and raised SHBG. CPA by itself decreased SHBG, androgens and oestradiol; EE_2 alone dramatically increased SHBG. It was concluded that the antiandrogen was the major agent in the cutaneous effects. The reduction in free testosterone induced by EE_2 had little effect on sebum, suggesting a less important role for SHBG than previously believed. CPA seems to act via suppression of androgen production and also, probably, by interference with hormone binding to the intracellular androgen receptors in skin tissues.

2740 PRENATAL SEX DIAGNOSIS OF MALE FOETUS BY BLOOD SMEARS. S. Sharma* Dept. of Anatomoy, K.G's Medical College, Lucknow, 226 003, U.P. India.

The diagnosis of X-Chromatin in amniotic cells is the most common occasion of prenatal diagnosis. Therefore, the present study was conducted to diagnose the sex of male foetus, prenatally, by blood smears of pregnant women between 14th-16th weeks of gestation, which is considered to be the most favourable time for sex diagnosis as well as for amniocentesis. The blood smears from pregnant women were made, stained with 0.2 per cent quinacrine dihydrochloride (sigma) and examined under the fluorescence microscope. The percentage of Y-chromatin in blood cells of women carrying male foetus was found to be from 9 to 24 per cent. This study was also confirmed by the fluorescent study of amniotic cells.

2741 MULTIPLE SITES OF ANDROGEN HYDROXYLATION BY THE LIVER MICROSOMAL P-450 SYSTEM: PRIMARY AND SECONDARY METABOLISM.

J.J. Sheets*, J.I. Mason, and R. Estabrook, Dept. Biochem., U. Texas Hlth. Sci. Ctr., Dallas, TX 75235.

Liver microsomal cytochromes P-450 metabolize a variety of steroids to more polar metabolites. To investigate the interaction of the various pathways of androgen hydroxylation we have conducted studies to identify the profile of products formed during the time-course of metabolism of androst-4-ene-3,17-dione (AD). Incubates containing 10 to 100 μM [^{14}C]-AD, NADPH, and microsomes (from rats pretreated with phenobarbital) were sampled at times between 30 sec. and 20 min. and extracted with dichloromethane. Both metabolized and nonmetabolized steroids were resolved by reverse phase (C_{18}) hplc using a linear gradient of 20-45% CH_3CN over 40 min. Elution of metabolites was monitored at 254 nm and by measuring radioactivity. By this method the pattern of formation (and utilization) of at least 21 primary and secondary metabolites of AD was determined. Identification of metabolites was made by co-retention with known standards on hplc and by gas chromatography-mass spectrometry. We report here the formation of a previously unidentified major metabolite of AD; 6β, 16α-dihydroxyandrost-4-ene-3,17-dione. We propose that liver microsomal P-450's can sequentially hydroxylate AD at multiple sites. The multiple hydroxylase activities result in a transient time course for the appearance of primary metabolites which may lead to erroneous conclusions when determining enzyme activities. These results provide the opportunity to determine the presence of a unique transport mechanism and/or regiospecific positioning of different P-450 isozymes in the microsomal membrane.

2742 CELLULAR LOCALIZATION OF TESTICULAR AROMATASE (AASE) ACTIVITY DURING RAT DEVELOPMENT.

C.H. Tsai-Morris*, D.R. Aquilano and M.L. Dufau. ERRB, NICHD, NIH, Bethesda, MD. 20205, USA

Estrogen plays a significant role in regulating testicular steroidogenesis through modulation of microsomal enzymes (17α-hydroxylase/ 17,20 desmolase) in the adult rat. To determine the contributions of Leydig (LC) and Sertoli cells (SC) to aromatization of androgen during maturation, both cell types were isolated, purified and assayed for Aase activity with a tritiated water release method using 1β-[^{3}H]-testosterone as substrate. Electron microscopic analysis indicated that LC underwent ultrastructual changes during development (appearance of thicker nuclear heterochromatin and plate-like mitochondria) that support the existence of fetal and mature LC populations. The number of LH/hCG receptors increased with age in the LC preparation whereas the highest number of FSH receptors in SC was observed at 15 days of age. cAMP increased significantly in LC after hCG, and in SC after FSH stimulation. This morphological and biochemical evidence indicated that LC were separated from SC. Aase activity increased in the LC (810 ± 35, 1351 ± 228, 2346 ± 220 pg/mg protein, mean ± S.D.), but decreased in the SC (901 ± 82, 550 ± 25, 458 ± 26 pg/mg protein) during development (5, 15 and 60 days of age). In LC the change in E_2 levels measured by RIA after hCG stimulation was not significant from basal in 5-day old rats but increased from 2.3 ± 0.4 to 8.8 ± 1.0 pg/10^6 cells following Aase stimulation at 30 min in 60-day old rats. These findings indicated that: 1) LC is a major cellular source for the estrogen synthesis in adult rats; 2) The age-dependent change in the Aase activity of LC could contribute to the differential response of LC to hCG in neonatal and adult rats.

2743 VIBUNAZOLE, AN ORALE TRIAZOLE ANTIMYCOTICUM DOES NOT INFLUENCE SIGNIFICANTLY THE STEROID HORMONE LEVELS. P. Vecsei+(*), K. Lichtwald+,K.-H. Graefe, W. Ritter, G. Gruenwaldt, H. Schmitz, U. Lietz, R. Ziegler.+Dept. of Pharmacology, University Heidelberg, FRG, BAYER AG, Dept.of Clin. Pharmacology, Wuppertal, FRG.

Vibunazole (V) (BAY n 7133, 1-(4-chlorophenoxy)-3,3dimethyl-2-, (1,2,4-triazol-1-yl)methyl-butan-2-ol), an effective antimycoticum with similar pharmakokinetic to ketoconazole (K), another azole derivative, was studied on the plasma testosterone (T), dihydrotestosteron (DHT), cortisol (F) and dehydroepiandrosterone (DHEA) and comparison was made with ketoconazole in a double blind cross-over study in 8 healthy volunteers. Blood samples for drug- and hormone levels in plasma were taken at regular intervals up to 24 hours after dosing. K was determined by HPTLC, V by GC. The steroids were analyzed by RIA. T-concentration fell to a minimum of 64% of the pre-value following V. After K 200 mg and 400 mg the lowest T-concentrations were found 8 hours after drug administration: 40% and 16% of prevalues. The decrease of T in percentage correlated with the log C_{max} after K (r=0.969) but not with that of V. The lowest DHT value following V was 72.8% and 51.8% after K 200 mg and 38.2% after K 400 mg. ACTH stimulation (0.25 mg Synacthen i.m.) provoked an increase in F and DHEA plasma levels with peak values after 2 hours, F (mcg/100ml: 21.7 (K 200 mg), 17.3 (K 400 mg) and 27.4 (V), DHEA (ng/100ml) 484 (K 200 mg), 315 (K 400 mg), 734 (V). The reduction of T and DHT after V was in accordance with diurnal variation. The effect of another oral antimycoticum: BAY I 9139 which will not be further developed was also studied. This has also no significant endocrinological side effects.

2744 ANDROGEN-DEPENDENT PEPTIDES ASSOCIATED WITH THE NUCLEAR ENVELOPE OF THE RAT VENTRAL PROSTATE. J.T. Venkatraman, G.M. Howell* and Y.A. Lefebvre, Department of Medical Biochemistry, The University of Calgary, Calgary, Alberta, T2N 4N1, Canada.

Relatively little is known about the dynamics of nuclear envelope (NE) components which accompany morphological changes of the nucleus during cellular metabolic processes. Ventral prostate nuclear volumes and nuclear pore densities decrease following castration. We have quantitated NE peptides of the rat ventral prostate in different hormonal environments. NE's isolated after treatment of purified nuclei with DNAse at pH 8.5 contained inner and outer nuclear membranes, as well as nuclear pore complexes. The polypeptide profile obtained after SDS-Page of NE preparations from ventral prostates of intact animals was similar to that obtained from rat liver. Peptides corresponding to the lamins were observed in the molecular weight range 60,000 to 68,000. SDS-Page analysis of NE's from ventral prostates of 7-day castrates did not show a diminution of the peptides in this molecular weight range. Therefore, these peptides remain as components of the NE during loss of the nuclear pores following castration. Castration did, however, result in the disappearance of peptides in the molecular weight range 18,000 to 21,000. Moreover, the administration of testosterone for 2 weeks to 7-day castrates restored these peptides. These changes were not seen in liver nuclei or NE's from the same animals. Sham castration and subsequent oil injection did not alter the peptide profiles. The identification and role of these androgen-regulated peptides in the NE is being further investigated. (Supported by MRC and AHFMR).

2745 METABOLISM OF GONADAL STEROIDS BY NORMAL AND NEOPLASTIC GLIAL CELLS.
J. Weidenfeld, O. Abramsky and H. Ovadia, Labs of Exp. Endocrinology and Neuroimmunology, Dept.of Neurology, Hadassah Hebrew Univ. Hosp. and Dept. of Internal Medicine, Bikur Cholim Hospital, Jerusalem, Israel.

It is well established that gonadal steroids can be metabolized by specific brain tissues and that these intracerebral transformations of steroids are essential for some of their CNS effects. The relative importance of the various CNS cell types i.e., neurons and glia for brain steroid metabolism is not yet clear. In the present study we investigated whether oligodendrocytes and cultured glioma cells are capable of metabolizing testosterone(T) and estradiol(E_2). Oligodendrocytes isolated from male rat brains and monolayers of rat glioma (10^6 cells) were incubated with either tritiated T or E_2. Both cell types could aromatize T to E_2 (approx. 1.5 pmol/h) as measured by loss of tritium to water during the incubation. Only oligodendrocytes could convert T to dihydrotestosterone (5 pmol/h). Oligodendrocytes and glioma cells could metabolize E_2 to catechol-E_2 (5 pmol/h). Catechol-E_2 was identified by formation of specific phenazine derative and by radioenzymatic methylation with ^{3}H-S-adenosylmethionine in the presence of catechol-o-methyltransferase. These results suggest that (1) Oligodendrocytes are involved in brain metabolism of gonadal steroids and that both oligodendrocytes and glioma cells are capable of transforming these hormones to metabolites with altered biologic activity. (2) The presence of steroid metabolizing enzymes in these cell types may be useful as a biochemical parameter for characterization of normal and neoplastic glial cells.

2746 EFFECT OF THREE AROMATASE INHIBITING STEROIDS ON THE 5α-REDUCTION OF ANDROGENS IN THE PROSTATE. S. Zoppi, L. Martini and M. Motta* - Dept. of Endocrinology, University of Milano, 21 Via A. del Sarto - 20129 Milano, Italy.

The steroids 1,4,6-androstantriene-3,17-dione (ATD), 4-hydroxy-4-androstene-3,17-dione (4-OH-A) and 4-acetoxy-4-androstene-3,17-dione (4-Ac-A), previously shown to inhibit aromatization, have been studied as possible blockers of the 5α-reduction of testosterone (T) and Δ_4-androstenedione (Δ_4-A). ATD, 4-OH-A and 4-Ac-A, when added at the concentrations of $6x10^{-7}$, $3x10^{-6}$, $6x10^{-6}$, $3x10^{-5}$, and $6x10^{-5}$M to incubation media containing rat prostatic tissue and labelled T, prevent the transformation of T into dihydrotestosterone (DHT) (maximal inhibition 61%) and into the 5α-androstandiols (3α- and 3β-diols). On the contrary the formation of Δ_4-A is enhanced up to 4 fold; also the formation of 5α-androstanedione (5α-A), the 5α-reduced metabolite of Δ_4-A, is increased up to 2 fold. When Δ_4-A is used as labelled substrate, the conversion of Δ_4-A into 5α-A is not modified by the presence of ATD, 4-OH-A and 4-Ac-A; Δ_4-A is converted back into T and the reduction of T into DHT is decreased. When DHT is used as labelled substrate, the formation of the diols is not influenced by the added steroids. These data suggest that the enzymes responsible for the 5α-reduction of T to DHT and of Δ_4-A to 5α-A are probably different. Only that which directly reduces in position 5α- the molecule of T is sensitive to the addition of the three steroids. Preliminary experiments indicate that these steroids are able to interfere with the 5α reduction of T in human prostatic tissue (BPH). (Supported by the C.N.R. through the Projects "Medicina Preventiva e Riabilitativa", and "Controllo della Crescita Neoplastica").

2747 POTASSIUM DEPLETION DECREASED TESTICULAR FUNCTIONS IN RATS. C Wang*[1], JP Qiu[2], WM Lee[2], A Tsang[2], CL Au[3], A Leung[1], WO Fu[2], & PYD Wong[2], Departments of Medicine[1] & Physiology[2], University of Hong Kong & Department of Physiology[3], Chinese University of Hong Kong, Hong Kong.

Reproductive and endocrine functions were studied in 40 and 60 days old Sprague Dawley male rats fed with a normal or low potassium (K) diet (K<0.01%) for up to 9 weeks. Plasma K fell from 4.5 to around 2 mmol/l after one week feeding with low K diet and then stabilized at this level. After 9 weeks of K depletion, although the testicular weights were slightly decreased (10-20%), the rate of testicular fluid secretion measured by efferent duct ligation was markedly reduced by 82% and 78% in 40 and 60 days old rats respectively. At this time, spermatozoa flushed out from the cauda epididymidis of the low K rats could initiate forward motility and these animals were fertile. After one week of treatment with low K diet, serum testosterone (T) fell from 5.6 ± 2.2 in control rats to 2.6 ± 1.5 nmol/l in 40 days old rats ($P<0.01$). This was associated with a reduction in seminal vesicle weight. Despite the persistently low serum T, serum FSH and LH were not elevated above control values throughout the treatment period. The fall in T was due to an impairment in Leydig cell function, since isolated testes from the K depleted rats produced 50% less T *in vitro* compared to that of control rats. The testicular LH receptor content measured by ^{125}I-hCG binding to testes decreased by 20% with K depletion. The endocrine effects of low K were less marked in 60 days old rats. Refeeding the low K rats for 5 days with normal diet restored plasma K, serum T, seminal vesicle weight, testicular fluid secretion, T production and LH receptor content to normal. It is concluded that K plays an important role in testicular functions.

2748 IMMATURE MOUSE LEYDIG CELLS BEAR Fc RECEPTORS - STUDIES WITH MONOCLONAL ANTIBODIES. S.D. Wolpe* and J.P. Mather, Population Council New York, USA

Immature (15-17 d) $CB6F_1$ mouse interstitial cells were prepared by mechanical dissociation and cultured in serum-free medium with Ins, Trans and EGF. Cells were trypsinized off the plate after two days in culture and tested for reactivity with monoclonal antibodies. Trypsin-purified interstitial cells (macrophages cannot be removed from tissue culture plates with trypsin) were positive for 2.4G2, a monoclonal antibody directed towards the macrophage Fc receptor. They were negative for B21-2, an antibody directed against Ia antigens (which are present on macrophages). Further, cells purified on Percoll gradients showed a single, coincident peak of hCG binding and 2.4G2 reactivity. The fact that these cells are removed with trypsin, bind hCG and are Ia negative, yet have 2.4G2 reactivity equivalent to an equal number of peritoneal macrophages, suggests that immature Leydig cells bear receptors for the Fc portion of immunoglobulin.

2749 EFFECT OF PHORBOL ESTERS ON LEYDIG TUMOR CELL PROGESTERONE PRODUCTION.
S. Zimniski*, M.R. Clark, D. Puett, REPSCEND Laboratories, Univ of Miami School of Med, Miami, Florida 33101, USA

Phorbol esters are thought to act by stimulating a calcium-and phospholipid-dependent protein kinase (protein kinase-C). Since phospholipid metabolism is altered by many steroidogenic agents, these studies were undertaken to examine the effects of 12-0-tetradecanoyl-phorbol-13-acetate (TPA) on steroid production by the Leydig cell tumor (M5480A). Dispersed Leydig tumor cells were maintained in primary culture for various periods of time under basal or gonadotropin-stimulated conditions. TPA (25 ng/ml) was added to Leydig cell cultures in the presence or absence of 50 ng/ml human chorionic gonadotropin (hCG). In addition, an equimolar amount of an inactive phorbol ester, 4β-phorbol-13α-monoacetate (PMA) was added to parallel cell cultures. Since progesterone is the primary steroid produced by this tumor line, effects on steroidogenesis were monitored by specific progesterone radioimmunoassay. TPA was found to significantly stimulate basal progesterone levels at 3 and 6h of culture. At 6h TPA-stimulated progesterone levels were increased nearly 3-fold (13.3±0.7 vs. 33.0±1.5 ng/ml). In contrast, PMA did not alter media progesterone levels. Furthermore, neither TPA nor PMA changed hCG-stimulated progesterone levels regardless of incubation time. These results demonstrate a specific stimulatory effect of active phorbol esters on Leydig tumor cell progesterone production, presumably through activation of protein kinase-C. Further experiments may elucidate the role of this enzyme in Leydig tumor cell steroidogenesis. (Supported by NIH:AM 33973, HD 07129 and HD 17942.

(Abstract 2781, p. 1651, also belongs to this section.)

2750 TRH REGULATION OF TSH SUBUNIT BIOSYNTHESIS AND GLYCOSYLATION.
T. Taylor* and B. D. Weintraub, NIADDK, NIH, Bethesda, Md., USA.

We have recently shown that TSH from thyroidectomized (TX) rats is more glycosylated that normal TSH. To determine the kinetics, subunit specificity and regulation of this response, 21d post-TX rat pituitary minces (PIT) were incubated in quadruplicate with both ^{3}H-glucosamine (GLN) and ^{14}C-alanine (ALA) for 1-6h with various doses of TRH. Total proteins (TP) were acid precipitated and TSH was immunoprecipitated with β then α subunit anti-sera and analyzed by gel electrophoresis. TP incorporation of GLN and ALA was not changed by TRH. In secreted TSH at 6h, TRH (10^{-7}M) stimulated incorporation of both GLN (TSH-GLN, 4095±736 dpm/pit vs 1171±78, $p<.02$) and ALA (TSH-ALA, 414±62 vs 148±7, $p<.02$) with a half maximal response at 8×10^{-10}M. Stimulation of TSH-GLN and TSH-ALA was first noted at 4h with continuous TRH but was more rapid (GLN at 2h, ALA at 3h) with TRH pulses (10 min/h). TRH stimulation of TSH synthesis reflected increases in both combined α and β subunits. In the control at both 4 and 6h, the GLN/ALA ratio, reflecting relative glycosylation, was similar in secreted combined α and β. GLN/ALA ratio with 10^{-8}M TRH was increased in secreted combined β at 4h (12±0.9 vs 6±2.3, $p<.05$) and 6h (14±1.8 vs 9±0.6, $p<.05$) but was not changed in secreted combined α. This selective 1.5-2 fold stimulation of the GLN/ALA ratio by TRH was noted in secreted but not PIT combined β. TRH did not change synthesis or glycosylation of free α. We conclude, 1)TRH stimulates both TSH combined α and β apoprotein and carbohydrate biosynthesis, more rapidly with pulsatile than continuous exposure. 2)TRH stimulates the glycosylation of the β subunit of secreted TSH. Such specific regulation of TSH β subunit glycosylation may be important for hormone release, bioactivity or clearance.

2751 BIOSYNTHESIS OF THYROTROPIN RELEASING HORMONE (TRH) IN THE NEONATAL RAT PANCREAS: EVIDENCE FOR TWO DISTINCT TRH-LIKE ACTIVITIES.

T. Theodoropoulos*, W. Banks, and J. Zolman. The University of Texas Medical Branch, Galveston, Texas, U.S.A.

The presence of high TRH levels in the neonatal rat pancreas suggests that this organ may actively synthesize TRH. To verify this hypothesis, we studied the in vitro synthesis of TRH by pancreatic cells, using ^{14}C-histidine incorporation and RIA. Neonatal pancreases were incubated in Krebs-Ringer-Bicarbonate (KRB) buffer, pH 7.4, at 37°C, under 95% O_2-5% CO_2. ^{14}C-histidine was added and its incorporation into the tissue proteins was followed up to 4 hours. The methanolic pancreatic extracts obtained were subjected to sephadex G-10 chromatography. Two peaks of ^{14}C radioactivity were eluted, one small (20% of total radioactivity) with the void volume and one large in a position identical to synthetic TRH. Both radioactive peaks corresponded to immunoreactive TRH peaks present in the same samples. Mean recoveries were 95%. Similar data were obtained with high performance liquid chromatography (HPLC). In pulse-chase experiments, excess cold histidine (40 µg/ml) was used and samples were taken at 15, 30, 60, 90, 120 and 150 min from the beginning of the tissue incubation with labeled histidine. Methanolic extracts of these samples showed again similar radioactive peaks to the ones described earlier with an initial increase and a later decrease in the size of the small peak. We conclude that the neonatal rat pancreas actively synthesizes TRH and/or a higher molecular weight TRH-like protein, which may represent a TRH precursor.

2752 METABOLIC EVALUATION (SHBG, STI, ART) AND SPONTANEOUS EVOLUTION OF "PRE-CLINICAL HYPERTHYROIDISM". F. Tortosa*, J.J. Staub, R. Oetiker, D. Burckhardt, P. Huber, K. Scheidegger. Div. of Endocrinology, Dept. Medicine, University Hospital, CH - 4031 Basle

TRH testing is the most sensitive parameter in assessment of thyroid dysfunction. The lack of a TSH response to TRH, in the presence of euthyroid T3 and T4 serum levels, has been previously described by our group as "preclinical hyperthyroidism" (JCEM 42: 810, 1976). In order to further elucidate the clinical relevance of this syndrome, we conducted a prospective study on 22 clinically euthyroid women with a previously absent TSH response to TRH (Δ TSH < 1 mU/l) and compared them to a control group of 20 euthyroid women with normal TRH tests. They were examined 3 to 36 months (mean 20 months) later. A Crooks-Wayne index was calculated for each subject and baseline TSH, T4, T3, free T4, free T4 index, free T3 index, sex hormone binding globuline (SHBG), systolic time intervals (STI, PEPc) and ankle reflex time (ART) were determined. Intravenous (200 mg) and oral (40 mg) TRH tests were performed. Our methods have been described previously (J. Mol. Med. 4: 49, 1980). In 9/22 women TSH response was normalised, in 13 TSH suppression persisted. In the latter, all metabolic parameters and baseline hormone levels did not differ significantly when compared to the controls (SHBG, nmol/l, 31.8 ± 2.5 v.s. 30.5 ± 2.4; PEPc, msec, 129 ± 2 v.s. 128 ± 3; ART, msec, 341 ± 8 v.s. 333 ± 8). Such patients must be considered clinically euthyroid and therapeutic measures are most often unnecessary and should be evaluated carefully.

2753 PREOPERATIVE DIAGNOSIS OF THE THYROID CARCINOMA WITH SPECIAL EMPHASIS ON ASPIRATION CYTOLOGY OF THE TUMOR. H. Uchida*, G. Nakayama, K. Yokota, N. Akiyama, H. Nemoto, M. Oba, K. Aso and T. Imai, Departments of Surgery and Pathology, Kitasato University, Sagamihara, Japan.

Clinical diagnosis for carcinoma of the thyroid gland is occasionally difficult even with taking into considerations for intraoperative findings of the tumor. A preoperative precise diagnosis for the malignant and/or benign lesion, however, is imperative for making a plan for the radical treatment. Before December 1980, preoperative diagnostic procedures for the tumor of the thyroid in our institution were based on a combination of the physical findings, plain neck X-ray films, echographies, scintigraphies, and CT scannings. As a result, 53 out of 58 malignant thyroid lesions (confirmed after surgery) were diagnosed as malignant (true positive rate: 91.4 %) and 104 out of 108 benign thyroid tumors (confirmed after surgery) were diagnosed as benign (true negative rate: 96.3%) before surgery. Since January 1981, a technique of aspiration cytology was introduced to the conventional procedures. Briefly, the aspirate of the thyroid nodule obtained by using a 21 gauge needle attatched to a 10 ml of disporsable plastic syringe was sprayed on a slide glass, which was immediately immersed into 95% ethanol for 30 minutes for fixation. The sample was stained by Papanicolaou and examined under a light microscope. As a result, in 16 malignant and 114 benign tumors (both were confirmed after surgery), 15 out of 16 were diagnosed as malignant (true positive rate: 93.8%) and 114 out of 114 were diagnosed as benign (true negative rate: 100%) before surgery. Therefore, we conclude that the aspiration cytology of the thyroid tumor is an excellent adjunct to the conventional diagnostic procedures.

2754 EXPERIMENTAL EVIDENCES THAT AMIODARONE (AM) DOES NOT INHIBIT T4 TO T3 INTRAPITUITARY CONVERSION. MA. Valenzuela and G.Pineda*FACP, IEMA Endocrine Laboratory and Universidad de Chile (Div.Oriente), Santiago, Chile.

Previous works from our group had suggested that AM did not interfere with the feed-back mechanisms of pituitary-thyroid axis as evidenced by the findings of a significant negative correlation between T4/TSH and T4/TSH-induced rise by TRH in patients on chronic AM therapy (Rev Med Chile in press). In order to demonstrate lack of intrapituitary inhibition of T4 to T3 conversion by AM, 12 Sprague-Dawley males rats were studied 44 d after ip administration of 0.43 mCi 131-I. Hypothyroidism was certified by elevation of TSH levels as compared to 7 normal controls (258.9 ± 8.1 vs 185.6 ± 6.6 mU/ml, $\bar{x} \pm$ SE, $p < 0.001$). Vehicle(N=4) AM (N=4) 8.9 mg/100 g bw were given ip 24,16 and 1.5 h prior to T4 administration (800 ng/100 g bw) and new blood samples were obtained 3 h later; the remaining 4 rats received only T4 and were considered as controls.

		Control	Vehicle	AM
	N =	4	4	4
rTSH $\bar{x} \pm$ SE	Basal	241.6 ± 8.4	285.5 ± 5.8	250.0 ± 14.7 mU/ml
	post T4	168.1 ± 11.2	190.2 ± 19.1	182.0 ± 13.5 mU/ml
paired t test		< 0.01	< 0.0125	< 0.025

Since acute T4 administration produced similar TSH diminution in the 3 groups under study it is concluded that AM does not interfere with pituitary 5' deiodinase as other iodine-containg drugs do.

2755 INCOMPLETE GLYCOSYLATION OF THYROGLOBULIN IMPAIRES IODOTHYRONINES FORMATION.
M.F. van den Hove , M. Couvreur and I. Dehart, Hormones and Metabolic Research Unit, ICP, University of Louvain, B-1200 Brussels, Belgium.

It has been proposed that T_3 and T_4 may originate from membrane-bound incompletely glycosylated thyroglobulin (Tg) through a short-loop mechanism. To test this hypothesis, we have analyzed iodine incorporation and iodothyronine formation in asialo- and asialoagalacto-Tg using "in vitro" conditions. Rat 19S Tg was fractionated by RbCl centrifugation and the fraction containing 33 iodine atoms, 4 T_4 residues and 0.7 T_3 residues per molecule was selected. Asialo-Tg was prepared by incubating native Tg with neuraminidase. Asialoagalacto-Tg was prepared by subsequent incubation with β-galactosidase. "In vitro" iodination and coupling were performed using a lactoperoxidase-glucose oxidase system. Iodinated residues were analyzed by chromatography. The release of terminal sialic acid and galactose residues from the B-oligosaccharidic chain of Tg did not affect the incorporation of iodine in the molecule. However, iodothyronine synthesis was impaired. After iodination of asialo-Tg with increasing amounts of iodide, T_4 formation reached a lower value. T_3 residues were formed but at iodine levels higher than in control Tg. With asialoagalacto-Tg, T_4 synthesis was dramatically reduced at all iodine levels and T_3 formation required even more iodine to reach control values. In contrast, rT_3 was synthesized. In conclusion, the number of tyrosine residues exposed to iodination in Tg with incomplete B-carbohydrate chains is not affected but the spacial alignment is modified reducing the reactivity for coupling. These results indicate that a short-loop route of incompletely glycosylated Tg would be able to provide T_3 and T_4 but with a lower efficiency than the normal pathway.

2756 VITAMIN D_3 METABOLISM IN THYROTOXICOSIS. C. Velentzas Military Hospital of Athens, Messogion 140, Greece - Toronto Western Hospital, Toronto 399, Bathurst Street, Canada.

Since thyroid hormones are potent stimulators of microsomal liver enzymes activity, we studied the hepatic conversion of vitamin D_3 to 25 OH D_3 in thyrotoxicosis estimating 25 OH D_3 plasma levels before and after (six hourly intervals for 48 hrs) the i.v. injection of 1 mg vitamin D_3 in five thyrotoxic patients and in four healthy euthyroid subjects matched for age and body weight. In the euthyroid subjects no changes were observed during 48 hours post injection intervals. In thyrotoxic patients the transformation of the intravenously injected vitamin D_3 into 25 OHD_3 had already begun in the sixth hour, reached the maximum in the thirthy-sixth hr ($8,6 \pm 4,5$ ng/ml) and subsided before the forty eighth hr. The maximum increase was noted between the twelth and thirty sixth hr. The mean increase of 25 OHD_3 plasma level in the group of thyrotoxic subjects at 42 hrs ($5,41 \pm 3,75$ ng/ml) and at 48 hrs ($5,46 \pm 3,73$ ng/ml) was higher than the corresponding increases in the euthyroid healthy subjects at the same intervals ($-0,05 \pm 2,18$ ng/ml and $+0,16 \pm 2,3$ ng/ml). The difference is statistically significant ($p < 0,001$). If we consider the fact that euthyroid healthy subjects show maximum increase in 25 OHD_3 plasma levels at the ninety-sixth hr onwards following injection of 1 mg of vitamin D_3, it is concluded that hepatic hydroxylation of vitamin D_3 in thyrotoxicosis is 2,5 to 8 times faster than in euthyroid healthy subjects.

2757 SERUM THYROGLOBULIN IN THE ASSESSMENT OF AUTONOMOUSLY FUNCTIONING THYROID TISSUE. C. von Westarp*, Department of Medicine, University of Alberta, Edmonton, Alta., T6G 2G3, Canada.

To determine whether serum thyroglobulin (Tg) levels were suppressible or not with thyroxine in patients with and without autonomously functioning thyroid tissue, serial Tg measurements were made in a group of 19 patients (2 males, 17 females) with benign thyroid nodules. All had initial serum T4, T3, Tg levels measured and a technetium thyroid scan done. Tg was determined by radioimmunoassay, with a lower limit of detectability of 1 ng/ml and a normal range up to 15.5 ng/ml. All patients were given thyroxine (T4Rx) to bring the serum T4 level up to or above the upper limits of normal. Tg levels were elevated in 17/19 patients (Tg range 16.2-400.0 ng/ml). With T4Rx 5/17 patients had Tg fall from high levels to within the normal range. Scans showed "hot" nodules (HN) in 10 and "cold" nodules (CN) in 9 patients. Tg fell by >50% in 6/10 patients in the HN group and 3/7 of the CN patients with initially high Tg levels. Pre-treatment Tg levels were not significantly different between the two groups. TRH stimulation tests done in 4 of the CN non-responding patients had a normal release of TSH. This preliminary study suggests that the response of serum Tg levels to T4Rx does not allow one to predict the presence or absence of autonomously functioning thyroid tissue. Tg could not be suppressed even in patients with a normal TRH test and a cold nodule on thyroid scanning. These data do not support the hypothesis that autonomously functioning thyroid tissue can be distinguished from "cold" thyroid nodules by the response of Tg to thyroxine treatment. This study was supported by The M.S.I. Foundation.

2758 ABNORMAL PITUITARY T_4-5'DEIODINASE (5'DI) ACTIVITY IN ADULT RATS FOLLOWING NEONATAL HYPERTHYROIDISM (NH). P. Walker* and F. Courtin. Unité de recherche en biologie du développement, CHUL, Québec, G1V 4G2, Canada.

NH leads to change in the adult rat suggestive of hypothyroidism. Although pituitary 5'DI activity is increased and pituitary GH concentration is decreased, serum TSH concentration is decreased. We therefore examined acute (4 hr) pituitary responses to graded T_4 doses of hypothyroid adult control and NH male rats (methimozole 0.02% in water for 30 days). Linearization of the relationships between 5'DI and TSH vs T_4 was obtained by log-log transformation of the data. The regression curve of TSH vs T_4 ($r=-0.69$; $n=48$) in NH rats was parallel and significantly displaced to the left of that of control rats ($r=-0.86$; $n=40$; $p < 0.001$). The slope of the regression line defining 5'DI vs T_4 in NH rats (-1.12; $r=-0.93$) was significantly decreased compared to that in control rats (-0.94; $r=-.93$; $p < 0.05$). Pituitary GH was measured after 4 days T_4 administration to hypothyroid control and NH rats. The log-log regression curve of the NH rats ($r=0.90$; $n=29$) was parallel to that of control rats but significantly shifted to the right ($r=0.88$; $n=19$; $p < 0.005$). Administration of increasing doses of T_3 resulted in similar increases in pituitary GH concentration thus eliminating abnormal receptor and post-receptor responses to T_3. Conclusions: Pituitary 5'DI activity is abnormally regulated in adult NH rats. Decreased pituitary GH content suggests insufficient intracellular T_3 generation and inappropriately low somatotrope 5'DI activity. The increased pituitary 5'DI activity also suggests that increased intrathyrotrope T_3 production may be responsible for decreased TSH secretion in adult NH rats.

2759 Abstract withdrawn.

2760 METHIMAZOLE (MMI) UPTAKE BY MONOCYTES.

AP. Weetman*, C. Gunn, AM. McGregor, R. Hall. Department of Medicine, Welsh National School of Medicine, Cardiff, Wales, UK

We have recently shown that the immunosuppressive action of the antithyroid drug methimazole (MMI) is exerted at a cellular level on antigen-presenting cells such as the monocyte in which it inhibits oxygen radical formation. To determine whether this effect is related to drug concentration by the monocytes, we have measured {^{35}S}-MMI uptake by these and other cells. The radiolabelled drug (1 μCi/ml) was added to cells (1×10^6/ml). Adherent cells were released after 1 hour with trypsin-EDTA and the cells collected with an automatic harvester. Uptake was assessed as counts per minute (CPM) by scintillation counting and compared with background CPM, that is, {^{35}S}-MMI in wells with no cells. Significant differences indicating uptake were seen with monocytes, neutrophils and thyroid cells (all $P < 0.01$) but not with lymphocytes, myeloma cells or the L929 and K562 tumour cell lines ($P > 0.1$). Typical mean CPM/2×10^5 cells (six replicates) were thyroid 7351, neutrophils 6740, monocytes 5013, lymphocytes 3384, background 1791. Uptake of {^{35}S}-MMI was temperature dependent, being negligible at 4°C. Basal uptake values at 37°C were increased by 30% (monocytes) or 100% (neutrophils) with the phagocytic stimulus, opsonised Candida. Thus, immunosuppression by MMI is probably due to an action on monocytes since the drug is taken up by these cells but not by lymphocytes, and uptake in enhanced during phagocytosis.

2761 HYPOTHYROIDISM : A NEW MODEL TO STUDY THE CELLULAR LOCATION AND THE FUNCTION OF PANCREATIC TRH (P.TRH). B.Wolf, P.Leduque, P.M.Dubois, P.Czernichow* and S. Aratan-Spire. INSERM U.30, 149, rue de Sèvres, 75743 PARIS 15 FRANCE.

Though TRH has been detected in the pancreas for 6 years, its role is still unknown. This study was undertaken to test the role of hypothyroidism on P.TRH content using RIA measurement and immunocytochemistry. Adult rats were rendered hypothyroid (HyT) by PTU-low iodine treatment for 6 wks. Two groups served as control : control I, adult rats fed a normal diet ; control II, previously HyT rats made euthyroid with 5 wks normal diet. Intensity of hypothyroidism was attested by undetectable T_3 and increased TSH levels. P.TRH was measured by RIA and P.TRH-degrading activity (P.TRH-DA) was quantified following incubation of pancreatic homogenates with tritiated TRH and chromatography, by measurement of TRH degraded by min. In a parallel experiment, pancreatic fragments fixed in glutaraldehyde, embedded in araldite were prepared for immunocytochemical detection of P.TRH and P.insulin, by light and electron microscopy, using a well-characterized TRH antibody at 1:1000 dilution and an insulin antibody at 1:5000 dilution with appropriate controls. Compared to controls I and II, hypothyroid rats have increased TRH content: 0.55 ± 0.39, 0.65 ± 0.08 vs 6.95 ± 2.09 pg/mg/100g BW$\pm$SEM, respectively, while P.TRH-DA was abolished compared to controls. Intense staining for TRH in insulin containing cells were visualized in HyT rats but not in controls. Immunoreactive TRH was found over the secretory granules of insulin-containing cells at ultrastructural level. In conclusion :1) In hypothyroid rats, increased P.TRH may be related to decreased P.TRH-DA. 2)PTU-induced hypothyroidism provides a suitable model to study the role of P.TRH. 3) A regulatory role of TRH on insulin secretion is postulated.

2762 CATECHOLAMINERGIC AND SERTONINERGIC INFLUENCE ON THYROXINE METABOLISM IN VIVO. C.C.Wong*, K.-D.Doehler & A. von zur Muehlen , Dept. of Physiology Chinese University, Hong Kong & Dept. of Clinical Endocrinology ,Med. Ho. Hannover,F.R.G.

Adult male rats were pre-treated with repeated doses of 1-DOPA, methyl-DOPA, tyramine, 5- hydroxytryptophan (5-HTP) and p-chlorophenylalanine (PCPA) to alter their catecholaminergic and serotoninergic activity. Following a subcutaneous injection of 100 μg/kg T_4 in the morning of the 5th day, serial blood samplings were taken 3, 7, 24 and in some 48 hours afterward. Repeated loading with 1.97 mg/kg 1-DOPA, 2.11 mg/kg methyl-DOPA and 200 mg/kg tyramine to rats showed a tendency of catecholaminergic involvement in increasing the clearance of serum T_4 . Pre-treatment with 4 doses of 100 mg/kg 1-DOPA significantly decreased serum T_4 & T_3 levels ($P < 0.01$), while same doses of methyl-DOPA increased their levels ($P < 0.01$, 2-way analysis of variance followed by Tukey's test). Repeated injections with 300 mg/kg 5-HTP to rats increased the clearance of both T_4 & T_3 ($P < 0.01$), while in rats treated at 1st and 3rd day with 300 mg/kg PCPA showed no significant differences of thyroid hormone levels 3, 7 & 24 hours after T_4 injection. At 48-hour , serum T_3 levels were significantly higher in the PCPA treated than in the normal rats. This indicated a slow down of thyroid hormone clearance in serotonin depleted rats. In this study, an enhancement of T_4 turnover under increased activity of both catechoaminergic and serotoninergic systems was found.

2763 THYROTROPIN CONCENTRATIONS IN NORMAL AND HYPERTHYROID SUBJECTS.

J.S. Woodhead*, I. Weeks, M.K. Jones, M. Sturgess and K. Siddle+, Dept. of Medical Biochemistry, Welsh National School of Medicine, Cardiff and +Dept. of Clinical Biochemistry, University of Cambridge, Addenbrookes Hospital, Cambridge, U.K.

Lack of sensitivity of conventional immunoassays for thyrotropin (TSH) using radioisotopic labels precludes their use in distinguishing between euthyroid and hyperthyroid states. We have developed an immunochemiluminometric assay (ICMA) for TSH utilizing a monoclonal antibody labelled with a chemiluminescent acridinium ester. The assay has a sensitivity of 0.003 mU/l with a reaction time of only 3h and shows no cross reactivity with other glycoprotein hormones. Serum samples were obtained at around 11.00h from 104 healthy volunteers who were clinically euthyroid as well as from 16 overtly hyperthyroid patients. Hourly samples were obtained throughout 24h from 5 euthyroid and 5 hyperthyroid subjects in whom TRH tests were also carried out. Of the healthy volunteers, 20 were excluded as a result of raised free T3 levels or circulating thyroid antibodies. In the remainder, the mean TSH was 1.4 mU/l with a range from 0.4 to 4.0 mU/l. All hyperthyroid patients had TSH levels < 0.03 mU/l. The normal subjects showed circadian rhythms with a nadir around midday and peak values during the night. No rhythm was observed in the hyperthyroid group though night values were slightly higher. Following TRH, there was no rise in TSH in these latter patients. This distinction in TSH levels between normal and hyperthyroid subjects suggests this assay may provide a useful first line test of thyroid function.

2764 INCREASED ACTIVITIES OF CYCLIC NUCLEOTIDE PHOSPHODIESTERASE (PDE) AND CALMODULIN (CaM) IN THYROID OF GRAVES' DISEASE.

T. Yagura*, I. Nagata and H. Uchino, Tenri Hospital, Tenri, Kansai Denryoku Hospital, Osaka and Kyoto University, Kyoto, Japan.

Activities of cyclic nucleotide phosphodiesterase (PDE) and calmodulin (CaM) were measured in soluble fractions of normal and Graves' thyroid. PDE activities were assayed by method of Thompson and Appleman with a slight modification. 0.4 μM cAMP or cGMP was used as substrate usually in the presence of 0.1 mM Ca^{2+}. CaM activity was measured as ability of boiled sample to enhance bovine CaM-dependent PDE. When a sample increased cGMP PDE activity 100%, its CaM activity was defined 10 units.

Thyroid	cAMP PDE activity* pmol/min/μg DNA equivalent soluble fraction	cGMP PDE activity* pmol/min/μg DNA equivalent soluble fraction	CaM activity* unit /μg DNA equivalent soluble fraction
Normal	0.561 ± 0.065 (7)	0.845 ± 0.087 (7)	14.2 ± 2.2 (5)
Graves'	0.846 ± 0.094 (8)[a]	1.839 ± 0.287 (8)[b]	22.4 ± 3.0 (5)[c]

* Mean ± S.E. (Number of subjects).
[a] $p<0.025$, [b] $p<0.005$ and [c] $p<0.05$ vs. normal.

Enhancement of PDE activities by Ca^{2+} was greater in Graves' thyroid than in normal ($p<0.025$). Addition of CaM to soluble fraction of normal thyroid did not increase Ca^{2+}-dependency to an extent comparable to that of Graves' thyroid. Conclusions: 1) PDE and CaM activities of Graves' thyroid were increased compared to normal thyroid. 2) Graves' thyroid had greater Ca^{2+}-dependency of PDE activities than normal thyroid and further study is necessary for elucidation of its mechanism.

2765 DISTRIBUTION OF THYROID HORMONE RECEPTORS IN THE CHROMATIN.

J. Yamakawa*†, N. Hamada†, H. Morii†, R. Ogawa, K. Enomoto, M. Yukioka, S. Morisawa and A. Inoue, Dept. of the 2nd Div. of Internal Medicine+ and Biochemistry, Osaka City University Medical School, Osaka, Japan.

Thyroid hormone is known to regulate transcription, most probably through nuclear receptor proteins. Localization of the receptors in the chromatin was studied with respect to the transcriptionally active region. Rat liver nuclei were mildly digested with micrococcal nuclease in a 3 mM $MgCl_2$-containing medium, and resulting chromatin fragments in the 1st and the 2nd supernatants (the latter was isolated with EDTA from the residual nuclei) were fractionated and assayed for the receptor and RNA polymerase II activities. In contrast to RNA polymerase, the receptor was easily liberated into S1 as 6.5S fragments with high specific activities. On the other hand, in S2 both receptor and polymerase activities were recovered bound to larger chromatin fragments. Redigestion of S2 revealed that the receptor-containing chromatin paused at 10.5S, which was further degraded to 6.5S. The polymerase in S2 behaved, in various fractionations, coincidently with the nascent RNA labelled in vivo, and could be measured for its activity at 250 mM $(NH_4)_2SO_4$ in the absence of exogenous template (it is hence thought to be in the transcriptional complexes engaged in elongation of RNA chains). Upon fractionations in Bio-Gel A-15m filtration, electrophoresis on a column of Sephadex G-10 and sucrose density gradient centrifugation, the receptor and polymerase activities in S2 were resolved from each other and from bulk chromatin. These results suggest that the receptor may exist at specific loci of the nuclease sensitive chromatin differing from bulk chromatin and from that containing elongating RNA polymerases.

2766 THE COMPARISON OF VARIOUS METHODS FOR MEASUREMENT OF THYROID ADENYLATE CYCLASE STIMULATING EFFECTS OF GRAVES' IgG

S. Yamashita*, M. Izumi, N. Yokoyama, S. Morita, S. Ohtakara, T. Tanabe, S. Okamoto and S. Nagataki. The First Department of Internal Medicine, Nagasaki University, Nagasaki 852, Japan.

Although various methods for measurement of thyroid stimulating antibody (TSAb) have been employed, there have few reports on the study of the comparison of these methods. In the present study, the following five systems to detect TSAb were chosen using 1) human thyroid membrane (HTACS) 2) porcine thyroid membrane (PTACS), 3) human thyroid slice (HTS), 4) human thyroid organ culture (HTOC) and 5) FRTL5 cell line supplied by Dr. Kohn. The minimum concentration of TSH to increase cAMP production was 0.1-1.0mIU/ml in HTACS, 1.0mIU/ml in PTACS, 0.01-0.1mIU/ml in HTS and HTOC, and 0.01mIU/ml in FRTL5. The increment of cAMP production in response to 10mIU/ml TSH was 300-450% in HTACS, 200% in PTACS, 400-600% in HTS, 300-650% in HTOC. and 25000% in FRTL5. When one of our strong TSAb was used, the lowest concentration of Graves' IgG to stimulate adenylate cyclase was 0.1-1.0mg/ml in HTACS, 1mg/ml PTACS, HTS and HTOC, and 0.1mg/ml in FRTL5. TSAb was detected in 50-65% of untreated patients with Graves' disease by HTACS, 40% by PTACS, 60-80% by HTS, 55-70% by HTOC and 80% by FRTL5. The broad ranges of % observed in HTACS, HTS and HTOC were due to variable results obtained among individual human thyroids employed. In summary, the methods for detection of TSAb using human thyroids were sensitive but not so good reproducible. On the contrary, PTACS was reproducible but not sensitive. On the other hand, both the sensitivity and reproducibility were excellent in FRTL5 cell line system.

2767 EFFECT OF THYROID HORMONE ON THE INTERNALIZATION OF β-ADRENERGIC RECEPTORS IN RAT HEPATOCYTES. K. Yamauchi*, K. Hashizume, M. Kobayashi and K. Ichikawa, Department of Gerontology, Endocrinology and Metabolism, Shinshu University School of Medicine, Matsumoto 390, JAPAN

Although it is well known that thyroid hormone decreases the number of plasma membrane-associated β-adrenergic receptors in liver, the mechanism of this modification is not known. We have studied the effect of thyroid hormone on the internalization of β-receptor using isolated rat hepatocytes.

Young male rats were thyroidectomized, and 14 days after operation, saline(T_x+saline) or T_4(20 μg)(T_x+T_4) was administered. The total uptake(membrane bound + internalized) of [^{3}H]-dihydroalprenolol(DHA) by the cells was not significantly different between T_x+saline and T_x+T_4 animals. However, the rate of disappearance of cell surface bound-[^{3}H]-DHA was greater in T_x+T_4 rats compared to that in T_x+saline rats. The number of membrane-associated β-receptor, after preincubation of the cells in the presence of 10^{-5}M of d,l-isoproterenol, was significantly lower in T_x+T_4 animals. The amount of internalized-[^{3}H]-DHA-receptor complex was significantly higher in T_x+T_4 rats than that in T_x+saline rats. The internalization of DHA-receptor complex was inhibited by methylamine or monodasylcadaverine. The results suggest that thyroid hormone induces an acceleration of β-adrenergic receptor internalization in hepatocytes.

2768 SPECTRUM OF THYROID DISEASE IN SINGAPORE. P.P.B.Yeo, K.W.Wang *, L.Chan, K.C.Lun, K.Hughes, A.C.Thai, K.F.Lui, J.Sng, S.P.Sothy, J.S.Cheah, P.Lim, W.O.Phoon. National University of Singapore; Dept. of Medicine, Alexandra Hospital; Singapore.

A national study of the population was conducted to ascertain the prevalence and spectrum of thyroid disease in Singapore. 1210 subjects 18 years and above were recruited. They were interviewed and examined for evidence of thyroid disorders. Blood was taken for estimation of total serum thyroxine and tiiodothyronine, thyrotrophin (TSH), thyroid antibodies, resin-uptake study and serum iodine level. 2.7% of sample had history of thyroid disease but no new clinically overt cases of hyper or hypothyroidism were found. Goitres were detected in 4.3% of females and 0.9% of males ($p<0.01$), 87.5% were under 45 years. Thyroid antibodies were found in 10.9% of females and 4.7% of males, ($p<0.01$). Raised TSH level was found in 2.1% of males and 4.7% of females ($p>0.05$). No significant difference found in the lipid profile and incidence of ischaemic heart disease between those with and without positive antibody and/or raised TSH. Frequency of antibodies did not increase with age in males but showed an increasing trend in females.

2769 EFFECT OF ALTERATION IN THYROID STATUS ON RAT AND HUMAN PLACENTAL T_4 INNER RING DEIODINASE.

K. Yoshida*, M. Suzuki, T. Sakurada, N. Kaise, K. Kaise, H. Fukazawa, T. Nomura, Y. Itagaki, K. Yonemitsu, M. Yamamoto, S. Saito and K. Yoshinaga, Dept. of Internal Med., Tohoku Univ. Sch. of Med., Sendai, Japan

We have recently shown (XIIIth ETA, 1983) that the activity of human placental T_4 inner ring deiodinase (PT_4ase) decreased with advancing gestational age, and rT_3 concentration in amniotic fluid ($AFrT_3$) was correlated with the PT_4ase. In the present paper the effect of alteration of thyroid status on the metabolism of T_4 was studied in the homogenates of placenta and liver obtained from the same rat, and human placenta incubated in vitro with stable T_4 in the presence of 5～50mM dithiothreitol. Administration of 10 μg/100g B.W./day T_4 (hyperthyroid) or 0.05% methylmercaptoimidazole in drinking water (hypothyroid) to pregnant Sprague-Dawley rats from 10th to 17th day of gestation resulted in significant increase or decrease in serum T_4 and $AFrT_3$ concentrations, respectively. The conversion of T_4 to T_3 in liver homogenates was significantly increased in hyperthyroid and decreased in hypothyroid rat. The net placental rT_3 production from T_4 in control, hyperthyroid and hypothyroid was 20.3 ± 3.0 (mean ± SD, n=6), 17.2 ± 2.8 (n=8) and 17.9 ± 4.1 (n=7) ng/mg prot/μg T_4/h, respectively, and there was no significant difference between them. In four patients with hyperthyroidism who had elevated maternal serum T_4 and $AFrT_3$ concentrations at delivery (38～41 weeks), the mean net placental rT_3 production from T_4 was 9.0 ± 0.8 ng/mg prot/μg T_4/h, which was not significantly differnt from that (8.5 ± 2.4, n=18) in normal pregnancy at equivalent gestational age. These results indicate that PT_4ase is not affected by thyroid status, and elevated $AFrT_3$ in hyperthyroidism might be due to elevated maternal serum T_4 level.

2770 OPIOID PEPTIDES IN HUMAN PERITONEAL FLUID.

Petraglia F., Segre A., Facchinetti F., D'Ambrogio G., Genazzani A.R.°

Dept. Obstet.Ginecol. University of Modena, ITALY

Considering the peritoneal fluid (PF)as delivered from peritoneal/ovarian secretion we evaluated its possible contents of β-EP, ACTH, β-LPH and M-E on the basis of β-EP and ACTH presence in ovarian homogenates. Twenty-five women (18-51 yrs.) partecipated to the study; PF or follicular (FF)(2 cases) fluids, collected throughout laparoscopy for pelvic pain (18 cases) or for tubal ligation (4 cases) and in 3 cases ovarian cyst fluid (CF) collected at laparotomy, were immediatly freeze-dried . Single specific assayes, performed on pool of redissolved samples, demonstrated the presence of different peptides in PF, FF and CF. The similarity of the immunoreacting materials to the standard peptides was assessed by the parallelism between dilution curves of PF and the single standard hormones assayed. Immunoreactive profile of redissolved fluids submitted to Sephadex G-75 columns (45 x1.5 cm) showed the presence of β-LPH (Kav=0.54) ACTH (Kav=0.75) and β-EP (Kav=0.82)-like coeluting materials while the elution on Sephadex G-25 columns (30x1 cm) showed the presence of M-E-like (Kav=0.86) coeluting materials. β-EP and β-LPH PF contents (after chrom.)(range 30-322 and 9-116 fmol/ml respec.) were higher($P<0.01$) than circulating levels. M-E peritoneal concentrations were in the highest range, varying between 1.17 and 18.8 pmol /ml. In the menopausal women the PF concentrations of the different peptides were undetectable ovarian cyst contents of M-E, β-EP, β-LPH and ACTH were almost in the same range than in PF while higher concentrations were found in FF. These results suggest the ovarian origin of peritoneal M-E and POMC -related peptides, confirming a different processing of POMC in the extrapituitary sources.

2771 THE EFFECT OF EXERCISE-INDUCED AMENORRHEA ON BONE DENSITY. J. Lindberg*, W. Fears, M. Hunt, M. Powell, D. Boll and C. Wade, Letterman Army Medical Center, Presidio of San Francisco, California, 94129, U.S.A.

To assess the effect of exercise-induced amenorrhea on bone density, we measured bone density using single photon absorptiometry in 11 amenorrheic runners, 5 oligomenorrheic runners, 15 eumenorrheic runners, 14 age-matched non-running controls and 10 postmenopausual women. There was no difference in height or serum levels of calcium, phosphate, prolactin and parathyroid hormone between groups. Weight was lower and ponderal index higher in the amenorrheic runners ($p<0.05$). Luteinizing hormone and follicle-stimulating hormone were increased in the postmenopausal women. Estradiol levels were consistently low in the dysfunction groups, whereas both progesterone and estradiol levels reflected random cyclic function in the other groups. There was a reduction in bone density in amenorrheic runners when compared with non-running controls, both in cortical and trabecular bone (0.71 ± 0.04 gm/cm^2 vs 0.77 ± 0.07 gm/cm^2 and 0.46 ± 0.07 gm/cm^2 vs 0.56 ± 0.05 gm/cm^2 respectively, $p<0.05$). There was also a difference between amenorrheic runners and normal runners in both cortical and trabecular bone density (0.71 ± 0.04 vs 0.79 ± 0.08 and 0.46 ± 0.07 vs 0.56 ± 0.07 respectively, $p<0.05$). Amenorrheic runners and postmenopausal controls had lower bone density than the other groups but not different from each other. In addition, spinal bone density assessed with dual photon absorptiometry in 9 subjects from the amenorrheic running group was found to be reduced. Our results show that women with exercise-induced amenorrhea have reduced bone density and consequently are at risk for developing stress fractures and premature osteoporosis.

2772 LATE REMOVAL OF THE LEADER SEQUENCE IN THE FORMATION OF THE GH IN THE PITUITARY. N.H. Scherberg* and K. Barokas, Thyroid Unit, Billings Hospital, The University of Chicago, Chicago, Illinois 60637, USA.

The segregation and processing of nascent growth hormone (GH) has been investigated by the addition of ^{125}I-tyrosyl tRNA to homogenates of rat pituitary. Maximal transfer into peptide linkage, of up to half the iodotyrosines, occurred by 5 min at 37°. 10% of protein-bound isotope was in GH. The nascent GH was associated with a particulate fraction and was resistant to proteolysis in the absence of detergents. If synthesis was interrupted by the addition of EDTA, five proteins, between 5 and 20K, were prominent in acrylamide gel electrophoresis patterns. These early proteins, which were bound in the pellet fraction, diminished in amount with time. They were shown to be intermediates in the elongation of GH on the basis of immunoreactivity and by conversion into full-sized GH. The pauses in GH formation did not occur during translation of GH messenger in initiation synchronized reticulocyte lysates. The pauses in elongation of GH in the pituitary were not due to a tRNA deficiency and were not specific to a pituitary co-factor since they also occurred during the elongation of GH in the livers of GH-transgenic mice. The same intermediates occurred during the elongation of GH in pituitary disrupted in the presence of triton, in which condition pre-GH was the principal end product. This contrasted to the lack of full length pre-GH formation in the absence of triton. Since the highest weight GH-intermediate (approx. 20,000 daltons) was common to both the ultimate formation of GH and pre-GH, we conclude that the leader sequence of GH must be present when GH is 90% completed.

2773 AROMATASE ACTIVITY AND LUTEINIZING HORMONE-RELEASING HORMONE CONTENT IN DISCRETE REGIONS OF THE MONKEY BRAIN. C. E. Roselli* and J. A. Resko, Physiol. Dept., Oregon Health Sciences University, Portland, OR and Reprod. Biol., Oregon Regional Primate Research Center, Beaverton, OR, USA.

Aromatization of androgens appears to be an important step whereby androgens regulate neuroendocrine processes at the cellular level. We determined aromatase activity (AA) in 12 nuclei and brain regions from five intact adult female cynomolgus monkeys. Microdissections (punches) were performed on 300 μm frozen brain sections and AA was measured in these tissues by an in vitro assay based on the release of ^3H_2O from [1β-^3H] androstenedione. The luteinizing hormone-releasing hormone (LHRH) contents of these same areas were measured by RIA. AA was distributed heterogeneously throughout the monkey brain. The highest activity (1.4 pmol/h/mg protein) was found in the n. medialis amygdalae. AA was intermediate (0.4 pmol/h/mg protein) in the medial preoptic-anterior hypothalamic area (APM/AMH) and the n. ventromedialis hypothalami (VMH), and low but detectable (0.01 pmol/h/mg protein) in the n. infundibularis-median eminence (IH/EM). The n. caudatus and putamen were devoid of detectable activity. High concentrations of LHRH were found in the IH/EM and were 25 times greater than the amounts measured in the AMP/AMH and VMH. The contents of the medial diencephalic regions were eight times greater than the adjacent lateral regions. Other regions contained little or no LHRH. Our results indicate that AA is discretely localized in the monkey brain. Although the highest concentrations of LHRH are found in the IH/EM, an area low in AA, there is overlap between AA and the content of LHRH within the AMP/AMH and VMH, thus suggesting that aromatization of androgen may be involved in neuropeptide regulation. Supported by NIH grants 1-P50-HD-1190 & RR-00163.

2774 EFFECTS OF DIAZEPAM ON LIPID METABOLISM AND PLASMA AND ADRENAL CATECHOLAMINES DURING REGRESSION OF ATHEROMATOSIS IN ROOSTERS. H.Y.C. Wong*, N.B. Thoa, K.S. Cheng and D.T. Ng. Department of Physiology, College of Medicine, Howard University, Washington, D. C. 20059 and Dept. of Anesthesiol., Uniformed Service University of Health Sciences, Bethesda, Maryland 20814.

We have studied the effects of diazepam (D) on plasma cholesterol (TPC) and triglycerides (TG) levels and changes in plasma and adrenal gland catecholamines during regression of induced atherogenesis in atherogenic-fed roosters. After atherosclerosis was induced in birds by an atherogenic diet (AD), consisting of 2% cholesterol plus 5% cotton-seed oil added to plain mash (PM), 40-week-old Hyline roosters were divided into the following groups: I. Controls on PM; II. PM + 0.4 mg/kg of D; III. AD; IV. AD + 0.4 mg/kg of D. After 12 weeks the following data were obtained: 1) TPC and TG levels of groups I and II were not significantly different when compared to the initial data before D was administered; TPC and TG concentrations of group IV were lower than group III; 2) norepinephrine (NE) levels of groups II and IV were significantly reduced compared to group I ($P<0.005$); epinephrine (E) levels of groups II, III and IV were significantly less than group I ($P<0.001$); dopamine values of group IV were statistically lower than groups I, II and III ($P<0.05$); and 3) no significant differences in catecholamine levels were noted in the adrenal glands. Conclusions: Administration of D resulted in lower TPC and TG levels in AD group and NE and E values in both PM and AD groups. This study was supported by grants from US PHS 2S06RR0816, 1-TO-2 GM-05010-01 (MARC), GM-07800, Hoffman-La Roche Inc., and Hunt Food Industries.

2775 PROLACTIN AND LH SECRETION FOLLOWING MICROINFUSION OF AMINO ACIDS INTO THE PREOPTIC-ANTERIOR HYPOTHALAMUS. J.G. Ondo* and R. Dom, Depts. of Physiology and Anatomy, Medical Univ. of S.Carolina, Charleston, S.C.

Studies from this laboratory suggested that neurally active amino acids (AA) act as mediators in the neuroendocrine system regulating gonadotrophic functions. Inorder to localize their site of action and because of our interest in the nature of the transmitters acting in the rostral hypothalamus we examined the sensitivity of the preoptic-AH neurons to the microinfusion of AA. The receptor agonists N-methyl aspartate (NMA) and muscimol, for glutamate and GABA respectively, were used in unanesthetized male rats. Blood samples were removed at -15,0,5,15,30 min. and analyzed for LH and PRL, followed by an ANOVA-RM over time. Microinfusion of A-CSF (.25ul), used as a control, did not alter baseline LH or PRL. Muscimol (500 pmoles) increased PRL levels slightly (4.5 ng/ml at 0 min. to 13.5 at 15 min. p<.05), but did not alter LH. NMA (500 pmole) was highly stimulatory to LH, increasing plasma levels 3-fold by 15 min. (p<.001). NMA (50 pmoles) also increased LH levels significantly (p<.001). Both doses of NMA elevated plasma PRL when infused into the preoptic area. The study supports a role for the excitatory amino acids in the rostral hypothalamus in the control of PRL and LH. Although inhibitory amino acid receptors are found in the preoptic area, the actions of muscimol were not definitive. (Supported by NICHHD HD10132).

2776 DISTRIBUTION OF VASOPRESSIN (AVP) BETWEEN PLATELETS AND PLASMA IN HUMANS, DOGS, AND RATS. L. Share*, J.T. Crofton, and D.P. Brooks, Dept. of Physiology & Biophysics, UTCHS, Memphis, TN 38163, U.S.A.

It has recently been reported (Preibisz et al., Hypertension 5: I-129, 1983) that, in normal humans, 90% of the circulating immunoreactive AVP is in the platelets. In confirmation of this, we have found that, in normal humans (n = 4), the concentrations of immunoreactive AVP in platelet-rich (PRP) and platelet-poor (PPP) plasma were 3.74 ± 1.34 (SE) μU/ml and 0.33 ± 0.06 μU/ml, respectively ($p<0.05$). On the other hand, only 40% of circulating immunoreactive AVP was found in platelets in conscious dogs (n = 7; PRP = 1.67 ± 0.34 μU/ml; PPP = 0.94 ± 0.29 μU/ml; $p<0.01$) and anesthetized dogs (n = 6; PRP = 6.46 ± 1.85 μU/ml; PPP = 3.69 ± 1.14 μU/ml; $p<0.01$). When these anesthetized dogs were hydrated by infusing 5% dextrose i.v. for 2 h (0.2ml/kg•min) the platelets failed to release a significant quantity of AVP, even though the concentration of AVP in PPP was reduced 75%. When AVP levels in PPP were then increased to approximately 35 μU/ml by the infusion of arginine vasopressin i.v. for 2 h (800 μU/kg•min), there was no increase in the platelet AVP content after one h. After 2 h of infusion, it appeared that AVP was taken up by platelets. Thus, in dogs, platelet immunoreactive AVP does not appear to exchange readily with plasma AVP. In conscious Long-Evans rats (n = 16), concentrations of AVP in PRP (1.09 ± 0.12 μU/ml) and PPP (0.94 ± 0.15 μU/ml) were not statistically different. In conclusion, although platelet immunoreactive AVP may be important in humans, it may be of limited physiological significance in dogs and rats. (Supported by USPHS grants HL-12990 and HL-19209).

2777 ENDOCRINE EFFECTS OF THE ERGOLINE DERIVATIVE FCE 21336, A NEW LONG-LASTING PROLACTIN LOWERING DRUG. E. di Salle*, D. Giudici, G. Briatico, G. Ornati and P. Ragazzi, Farmitalia Carlo Erba, Biological Research and Development, Nerviano (Milan), Italy.

The effects of FCE 21336 (1-ethyl-3-(3'-dimethylamino-propyl)-3-(6'-allylergoline-8'β-carbonyl)-urea diphosphate) on prolactin (PRL) secretion, on PRL-dependent processes (egg nidation and lactation) and on luteinizing hormone (LH) secretion were studied after oral administration in different laboratory animals. FCE 21336 caused a lasting reduction of the hyperprolactinemia induced in the male rat by reserpine (2 mg/kg i.p.,7 h before killing); at the dose of 30 mcg/kg the effect reached its maximum 4-8 hours after treatment and persisted for at least 2 days, the ED_{50} at 48 hours being 17 mcg/kg. The compound administered to rats on day 5 of pregnancy inhibited egg nidation, the ED_{50} being 25 mcg/kg. FCE 21336, administered to rats, rabbits and bitches for 4 days during established lactation inhibited the pups' growth rate, the ED_{50} being 29, 15 and 1.3 mcg/kg/day, respectively. The compound was well tolerated by lactating bitches; no emesis was induced up to 15 mcg/kg. FCE 21336, 1 mg/kg given at 2 p.m. during proestrus in the rat, did not influence the preovulatory LH surge and ovulation, but completely suppressed the PRL surge. The compound thus appears to be a potent and extremely long-lasting PRL-lowering drug.

2778 EFFECTS OF PROTEIN MALNUTRITION ON PROLACTIN RELEASE AND HYPOTHALAMIC DOPAMINE ACTIVITY DURING SUCKLING. H.H. Huang*, J.Q. Kissane and E.J. Hawrylewicz. Department of Research, Mercy Hospital and Medical Center, Chicago, Illinois 60616, U.S.A.

Female rats were fed, ad libitum, isocaloric diets consisting of 8% (LP) or 19.5% (NP) casein for a period of 3 weeks before mating. The diets were maintained throughout the mating, gestation and lactation periods. The litters were reduced to eight pups on the second day of birth. On the fifth day postpartum, the mother rats were separated from their pups for 4 hours. Some of the mother rats were returned to their pups and were suckled for 30 minutes, then were decapitated for measuring prolactin and dopamine. The remaining mothers were sacrificed without suckling. Non-suckled LP and NP mother rats showed no difference in levels of serum prolactin (165.0 ± 16.3 vs. 165.6 ± 17.2 ng/ml, N=12). However, 30 minutes after initiation of suckling, LP animals release significantly less prolactin as compared to NP animals (296.0 ± 51.8 vs. 852.0 ± 76.3 ng/ml, N=14, $p < 0.001$). Also the dopamine turnover rate in the median eminence of LP mother rats was significantly higher than NP animals (62% vs. 27% decreased 60 minutes after α-methyl-para-tyrosine injection, $p < 0.01$). These results suggest that the reduced milk secretion in LP rats can partly be attributed to the high dopamine activity which, in turn, inhibits the release of prolactin. This study was supported by grant #AG02626 from the National Institutes of Health and grant #83-36 from the American Cancer Society, Illinois Division.

2779 INSULIN BINDING AND INSULIN SECRETION INDUCED BY HIGH FRUCTOSE FEEDING. A. Claro, National Institute of Endocrinology, Havana 4, Cuba.

We have studied whether fructose induced decrease of cellular insulin binding or change in the insulin secretion in rats. Rats (150-170 gs weight) were fed high fructose diet (67%) for 10 days. There were no statiscally significant differences between body weight of control and diets. High fructose feeding caused significant changes in plasma concentrations of glucose, insulin, colesterol ($p < 0,05$) and a significant reduction of insulin binding in adipocites ($p < 0,01$). However in isolated islet of rats feeding with high fructose diet, the glucose has no stimulatory effect on insulin secretion. We concluoed that fructose decreased the insulin binding without affecting directly the beta cells, the observed effect could adscrite may be a reduction in the number of receptor to insulin in perifery.

2780 IDENTIFICATION OF GONADOTROPIN-RELEASING HORMONE BINDING SITES IN THE CENTRAL NERVOUS SYSTEM USING A BIOLUMINESCENT LIGAND RECEPTOR ASSAY. J.M. Schaeffer* and A.J.W. Hsueh, Dept. Reproductive Medicine, Univ. of California, San Diego, La Jolla, CA 92093 U.S.A.

Firefly luciferin has been covalently linked to a gonadotropin-releasing hormone (GnRH) analog and is being used as a nonradioactive probe to study GnRH receptors. GnRH-luciferin has approximately the same bioactivity as the non-derivatized GnRH analog and competes with ^{125}I-Buserelin (a GnRH agonist) for specific binding to the anterior pituitary. The amount of GnRH-luciferin was quantitated by adding excess ATP and luciferase to each sample and measuring light production with a liquid scintillation spectrophotometer. Under these conditions, the amount of light emission is proportional to the GnRH-luciferin present. The sensitivity of the present bioluminescent ligand assay is approximately 50-fold greater than the radioreceptor assay using ^{125}I-Buserelin. Washed membranes were incubated with varying concentrations of GnRH-luciferin in the presence or absence of excess unlabeled GnRH. After a 90 minute incubation at 4°C, the membranes were washed and resuspended in 100 mM sodium phosphate buffer. The amount of GnRH-luciferin bound to the tissue was then determined. The highest concentrations of GnRH-luciferin binding sites were observed in the anterior pituitary, interpeduncular nucleus, habenula, and periaquaductal grey (120-300 fmol/mg protein), with significantly lower concentrations in the ovary, testes and posterior pituitary. These results provide the basis for using nonradioactive bioluminescent probes in the quantitation of GnRH receptors. The high sensitivity of the bioluminescent ligand assay permits the quantitation of GnRH receptors in brain regions and suggests a central action for this peptide.

2781 DECREASED SEMINIFEROUS TUBULE ANDROGEN RECEPTORS IN EXPERIMENTAL CRYPTORCHIDISM. Stephen J. Winters.* Department of Medicine, Montefiore Hospital, University of Pittsburgh, Pittsburgh, PA 15213.

The spermatogenic effect of testosterone is well established. Some of the effects of androgens on germ cell development are likely to be mediated by androgen receptors (AR) located in the seminiferous tubule. We therefore chose to examine the seminiferous tubule AR in rats with experimental hypospermatogenesis. Unilateral cryptorchidism was produced in six wk old rats. Two wks later the animals were hypophysectomized and one wk later they were sacrificed to study cytosol receptor binding. Tubules were prepared by microscopic dissection. Saturation plots revealed high affinity, saturable, androgen-specific binding of ^{3}H-methyltrienolone to rat tubule cytosol when excess dexamethasone was added to occupy putative glucocorticoid binding sites. Sodium molybdate stabilized binding at 0°C, 15°C and 25°C similarly in cryptorchid and control cytosol. The content of AR was markedly ($p<0.05$) reduced in cryptorchid tubule cytosol (88 ± 56 (m$\pm$SD) vs 210 ± 240 fmol/testis); equilibrium binding constants were similar (0.70 ± 0.15 vs 0.82 ± 0.34 nM). Nuclear androgen receptors, studied by 0.6 M KCl extraction, were also markedly reduced ($p<0.05$) in the cryptorchid (219 ± 125 fmol/testis) vs the scrotal testis (440 ± 45 fmol/testis) of nonhypophysectomized rats. Testis weights were 0.63 ± 0.16 gm and 1.55 ± 0.09 gm, respectively ($p<0.01$). These experiments indicate that the AR content of the seminiferous tubules of cryptorchid rat testis is marked reduced. The cause and effect relationship between the hypospermatogenesis and the receptor decrease remains to be clarified.

Index of authors

Figures refer to abstract nos.